Dermatopathology

A Volume in the Series Foundations in Diagnostic Pathology

Other books in this series

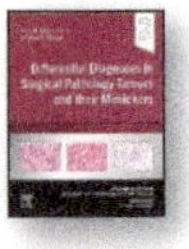

Abdul Karim: *Differential Diagnoses in Surgical Pathology Tumors and their Mimickers*
978-0-323-75611-2

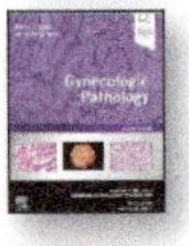

Nucci and Parra-Herran: *Gynecologic Pathology*, 2e
978-0-323-35909-2

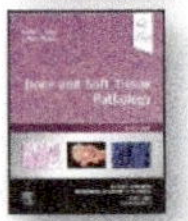

Folpe and Nielsen: *Bone and Soft Tissue Pathology,* 2e
978-0-323-75871-0

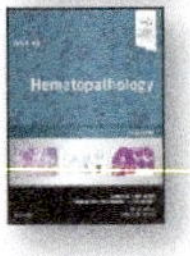

Hsi: *Hematopathology,* 3e
978-0-323-47913-4

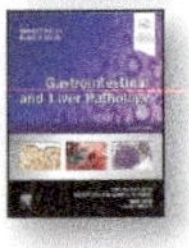

Srivastava and Allende: *Gastrointestinal and Liver Pathology,* 3e
978-0-323-52794-1

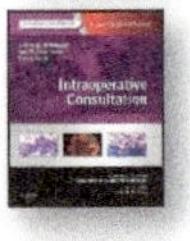

Marchesvsky, Abdul-Karim, and Balzer: *Intraoperative Consultation*
978-1-455-74823-5

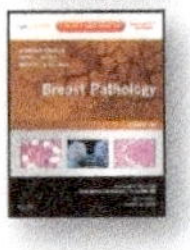

O' Malley, Pinder, and Mulligan: *Breast Pathology*, 2e
978-1-437-71757-0

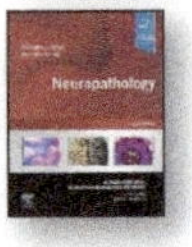

Prayson: *Neuropathology*, 3e
978-0-3237-1344-3

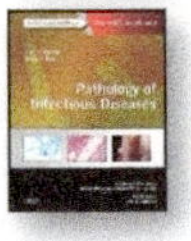

Procop and Pritt: *Pathology of Infectious Diseases*
978-1-437-70762-5

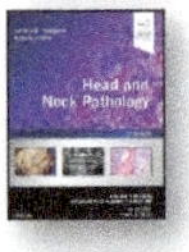

Thompson: *Head and Neck*, 3e
978-0-323-47916-5

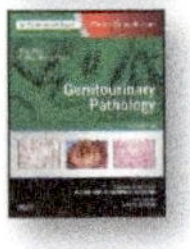

Zhou and Magi-Galluzzi: *Genitourinary Pathology*, 2e
978-0-323-18827-2

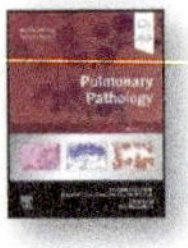

Zander: *Pulmonary Pathology*, 3e
978-0-323-93548-7

Dermatopathology

A Volume in the Series Foundations in Diagnostic Pathology

Third Edition

Klaus J. Busam, MD
Director of Dermatopathology
Department of Pathology
Memorial Sloan Kettering Cancer Center
Professor
Department of Pathology and Laboratory Medicine
Cornell University
New York, New York

Pedram Gerami, MD
Professor of Dermatology
Department of Dermatology
Pediatrics and Pathology
Northwestern University Feinberg School of Medicine
Chicago, Illinois

ELSEVIER

Elsevier
1600 John F. Kennedy Blvd.
Ste 1800
Philadelphia, PA 19103-2899

DERMATOPATHOLOGY, THIRD EDITION ISBN: 978-0-323-83071-3

Content Strategist: Belinda Kuhn
Senior Content Development Specialist: Suddha Sen
Publishing Services Manager: Deepthi Unni
Project Manager: Haritha Dharmarajan
Design Direction: Margaret Reid

Printed in the United States of America

Last digit is the print number: 9 8 7 6 5 4 3 2

This book is dedicated to my wife and children.
To Vinita—for your tireless love and support.
You put up with a lot!
To Jonathan and Sophia—for the joy of your company.
Dr. Klaus J. Busam

"To my dear wife Rana, thank you for all your love and support. To my daughters, Lily, Ella and Gigi, you are the light of my life. I love you all dearly."
Dr. Gerami's

Contributors

Rami Al-Rohil, MBBS
Associate Professor
Department of Pathology and Dermatology
Duke University
Durham, North Carolina

Bijal Amin, MD
Assistant Professor
Department of Pathology
Montefiore Medical Center-Albert Einstein College of Medicine
Bronx, New York

Sepideh Nikki Asadbeigi, MD
Assistant Professor
Department of Pathology
University of Oklahoma Health Sciences Center
Oklahoma City, Oklahoma;

Scott C. Bresler, MD, PhD
Assistant Professor
Department of Pathology and Dermatology
Michigan Medicine, University of Michigan
Ann Arbor, Michigan

Darya Buehler, MD
Associate Professor
Pathology and Laboratory Medicine
School of Medicine and Public Health, University of Wisconsin
Madison, Wisconsin

Klaus J. Busam, MD
Director of Dermatopathology
Department of Pathology
Memorial Sloan Kettering Cancer Center
Professor
Department of Pathology and Laboratory Medicine
Cornell University
New York, New York

Helen M. Chen, MD
Pathology
Palos Community Hospital
Palos Heights
Illinois

Loren E. Clarke, MD
Dermatopathologist
Vice President of Medical Affairs
Dermatology Unit
Myriad Genetic Laboratories, Inc.
Salt Lake City, Utah

Shawn E. Cowper, MD
Professor of Dermatology and Pathology
Department of Dermatology
Yale University
New Haven, Connecticut

Jasmine H. Francis, MD, FACS
Attending
Ophthalmic Oncology Service
Department of Surgery
Memorial Sloan Kettering Cancer Center
New York, New York

Douglas R. Fullen, MD
Professor of Pathology and Dermatology
Department of Pathology
University of Michigan
Ann Arbor, Michigan

Maxwell Alexander Fung, MD
Professor
Department of Dermatology
University of California
Sacramento, California

Pedram Gerami, MD
Professor of Dermatology
Department of Dermatology
Pediatrics and Pathology
Northwestern University Feinberg School of Medicine
Chicago, Illinois

Jacqueline M. Junkins-Hopkins, MD
Dermatopathologist
Department of Pathology
Geisinger Medical Center
Danville, Pennsylvania

Hideko Kamino, MD
Clinical Associate Professor of Dermatology and Pathology
New York University School of Medicine
New York, New York

Jennifer S. Ko, MD, PhD
Associate Professor of Pathology
Department of Anatomic Pathology
Cleveland Clinic
Cleveland, Ohio

Julia Lehman, MD
Professor
Department of Dermatology
Laboratory Medicine and Pathology
Laboratory Director
Immunodermatology Laboratory
Mayo Clinic
Rochester, Minnesota

Brian P. Marr, MD
Ophthalmologist
Columbia University Medical Center
New York, NY

Michael E. Ming, MD, MSCE
Director
Pigmented Lesion Clinic
Associate Professor of Dermatology
Hospital of the University of Pennsylvania
University of Pennsylvania School of Medicine
Philadelphia, Pennsylvania

Cuong Nguyen, MD
Assistant Professor
Department of Dermatology
Northwestern University
Chicago, Illinois

Victor G. Prieto, MD, PhD
Professor
Department of Pathology
University of Texas MD Anderson Cancer Center
Houston, Texas

Melissa Pia Pulitzer, MD
Assistant Attending
Department of Pathology
Memorial Hospital for Cancer and Allied Diseases
Assistant Professor
Department of Pathology and Laboratory Medicine
Weill Medical College of Cornell University
New York, New York

Marcia Ramos-e-Silva, MD, PhD
Associate Professor of Dermatology
Head of the Sector of Dermatology
University Hospital of the Federal University of Rio de Janeiro
Rio de Janeiro, Brazil

Luis Requena, MD
Department of Dermatology
University Hospital Fundacion Jimemez Diaz
Autonomous University Madrid
Spain

Franco Rongioletti, MD
Professor of Dermatology
DISSAL, Department of Health Science
University of Genoa
Genoa, Italy

Beth Ruben, MD
Director of Dermatopathology
Department of Dermatology
Palo Alto Medical Foundation
Palo Alto, California
Professor
Department of Dermatology/Dermatopathology
University of California
San Francisco, California

Richard A. Scolyer, BMedSci, MBBS, MD, FRCPA, FRCPath, FAHMS
Senior Staff Specialist
Department of Tissue Pathology and Diagnostic Oncology
Royal Prince Alfred Hospital and NSW Health Pathology
Conjoint Professor
Faculty of Medicine and Health
The University of Sydney
Co-Medical Director
Melanoma Institute Australia
Sydney, New South Wales, Australia

Sharlene See, MD
Anatomic & Clinical Pathologist
Northwestern Memorial Hospital
Chicago, Illinois

Christopher Richard Shea, MD
Eugene J. Van Scott Professor in Dermatology
Department of Medicine
University of Chicago
Chicago, Illinois

Nathaniel Smith, BS, MD, ABP Board Certification in Anatomic and Clinical Pathology and Dermatopathology
Staff Dermatopathologist
Department of Pathology and Laboratory Services
Brooke Army Medical Center
San Antonio, Texas
Assistant Professor
Department of Pathology
Uniformed Services University
Bethesda, Maryland

Kerith Spicknall, MD
Associate Professor
Dermatology
University of Cincinnati
Cincinnati, Ohio

Brian Swick, MD
Clinical Professor
Department of Dermatology and Pathology
University of Iowa—Iowa City VAMC
Iowa City, Iowa

Ravi R. Ubriani, MD, FAAD
Assistant Professor of Clinical Dermatology
Department of Dermatology Education
Columbia University
New York, New York

Angela J. Wyatt, MD
Clinical Assistant Professor
Department of Dermatology
Baylor College of Medicine
Physician
Dermatology
Flagstaff Medical Center
Flagstaff, Arizona

Preface

The goal of the third edition of this textbook remains the same as before: an introductory to midlevel no-nonsense practical guide to the histopathologic diagnosis of skin disorders. We want to provide a book for residents in pathology or dermatology and fellows in dermatopathology that they can manage to read and use to deal with most daily encountered diagnostic challenges. In an effort to keep the book compact, compromises were necessary, which meant leaving out entities or mentioning some only briefly. As before, we minimized references to save space for text and illustrations with the same rationale—that we do not aim to provide an encyclopedic book, and readers can easily query online libraries on the Internet for primary references. We decided to put together a third edition of the book because significant updates were necessary. The field has advanced, especially in the area of molecular diagnostics. Most importantly, however, the third edition provides an opportunity to bring in a coeditor (Dr. Gerami) and new authors for major revisions of prior chapters and to add yet another new chapter (Pediatric Dermatopathology). The editors would like to thank all the contributing prior and new authors who made this book possible. The book is the result of teamwork. We also want to express our appreciation for the great support I received for this book from the publisher.

Contents

Section 1

Non-Neoplastic Disorders

1 Inflammatory Diseases of the Dermis and Epidermis

Maxwell A. Fung

Inflammatory disorders of the skin may be classified by etiology (suspected or confirmed), clinical features, histopathologic features (e.g., reaction patterns), site(s) of involvement, or all of the above, as remains the tradition in *Foundations in Diagnostic Pathology*. As our collective understanding of inflammatory skin disorders continues to evolve, no single uniform classification of disease has proved perfect for all uses. Instead, disorders tend to be classified by etiology when possible, with the large remainder based on tradition or "most distinctive" features. The subject headings in this chapter represent *clinically relevant* topics that are biopsied with reasonable frequency and embody a traditional and fairly comprehensive presentation of the material in this field in a way that is designed to be useful as a reference as well as from the standpoint of evaluating new cases.

In terms of a routine and systematic approach to interpretation, the pathologist should ideally avoid bias by first examining the slide without any clinical data whatsoever. In some cases, the diagnosis will be apparent within a split second, and the clinical data will merely confirm the diagnosis. At the other extreme, the histology alone may be nonspecific and require clinical correlation to produce a clinically relevant interpretation, directing the pathologist to additional findings initially "missed" or additional stains or deeper sections. Advanced learners appreciate that many diseases have more than one clinical or histopathologic expression and that some unrelated diseases may have identical clinical or histopathologic appearances. Ultimately, nearly all inflammatory skin disorders require clinical confirmation.

Successful dermatopathologists thrive on the perpetual challenge of rendering diagnostic interpretations based primarily on microscopic features, sometimes with very limited clinical information. For an increasing subset of submitted specimens, the advent of integrated electronic health records has significantly obviated clinical data gaps to improve patient care via diagnostic precision and relevance, albeit often at the expense of pathologist efficiency. With the exception of identifying distinctive pathogens, the instant pattern recognition that is often possible for tumors is much less frequently encountered when examining a biopsy of a rash. The likelihood of a correct diagnosis is maximized via a composite assessment of everything known about the patient: both clinical data and histologic features, with a case-by-case recognition and judgment of the relative importance of the most decisive clinical and histopathologic features.

While the dermatopathologist is responsible for providing the best possible pathologic interpretation, final responsibility falls on the patient's direct provider (submitting physician). The aim of the dermatopathologist should be to provide the submitting physician with a clinically relevant differential diagnosis (using the standard language of clinical dermatology) based primarily on the microscopic features and, whenever justified, a specific diagnosis. If the pathologist obtains a diagnosis *by histology alone* that turns out, upon review of the requisition form, to be the clinician's suspected diagnosis, or at least within their clinical differential diagnosis, this generally represents strong diagnostic support if not outright confirmation. Caveat: Specific diagnoses issued in pathology reports that are clinically disproved (read: wrong per the submitting dermatologist) carry little weight and tend to be ignored. (Having such reports consistently associated with one pathologist may represent a quality improvement opportunity for the pathologist.) Maintaining an open mind and maintaining communication with submitting physicians are essential to refining one's diagnostic skills (and reputation) in the area of inflammatory skin disease. At the other extreme, wholly noncommittal pathology reports do not advance patient care; as a rule, the pathologist should strive to mention at least one clinical disorder, and any histologic differential should indicate an order of likelihood and degree of confidence. Even if no single diagnosis can be favored, addressing the clinical differential diagnosis can be helpful.

SPONGIOTIC DERMATITIS

Clinical Findings

It is essential to recognize that although spongiotic dermatitis is perhaps the most frequently biopsied inflammatory skin disease, it is not a clinical disorder (Table 1.1). Rather, spongiotic dermatitis is a descriptive diagnosis that corresponds to a variety of clinical

TABLE 1.1

Basic Differential Diagnosis of Spongiotic Dermatitis

	Atopic Dermatitis	Nummular Dermatitis	Dyshidrosis	Seborrheic Dermatitis	Allergic Contact Dermatitis	Irritant Contact Dermatitis	Papular Dermatitis	Urticarial Dermatitis	Pityriasis Rosacea
Superficial perivascular lymphocytes	++	++	++	++	++	++	++	++	++
Deep perivascular lymphocytes	o	o	o	o	o	o	o	±	o
Epidermal necrosis	o	o	o	o	o	++	±	o	o
Follicular spongiosis	±	o	o	++	o	o	±	o	o
Dermal eosinophils	±	±	±	±	±	±	++	++	±
Lymphocyte exocytosis	±	±	±	±	±	±	o	o	++
Erythrocyte extravasation	o	o	o	o	o	o	o	o	++

++, characteristic; ±, variable; o, unusual or not classic.

disorders, some of which are completely unrelated from the clinical point of view. The fact that the most common group of disorders manifesting as spongiotic dermatitis is designated variably and imprecisely by submitting physicians, including dermatologists, is a source of confusion for both students and practitioners. These designations include eczema, dermatitis, and eczematous dermatitis. Unless further specified, these terms are considered synonymous and are referred to herein as eczematous dermatitis. The term *eczematous dermatitis* still does not correspond to a single clinical disorder, but it does correspond to a more limited number of specific, common clinical disorders, including atopic dermatitis (designated by some as atopic eczema, or simply eczema), allergic contact dermatitis, photoallergic contact dermatitis, nummular dermatitis (or nummular eczema), dyshidrotic dermatitis (or dyshidrotic eczema), and the Id reaction. Stasis dermatitis, xerotic dermatitis (Fig. 1.1), and pityriasis alba may also be added to this list. A subgroup of these disorders clinically exhibits superimposed urticarial features and may be designated urticarial dermatitis, either provisionally or as an idiopathic diagnosis of exclusion.

To confuse matters further, submitting physicians sometimes refer to any one of these specific disorders simply as eczema or dermatitis. The most common example is *eczema* as a synonym for atopic dermatitis or atopic eczema. However, many clinicians seem satisfied with a pathologic diagnosis of "spongiotic dermatitis" in the pathology report and do expect additional diagnostic precision from the pathologist.

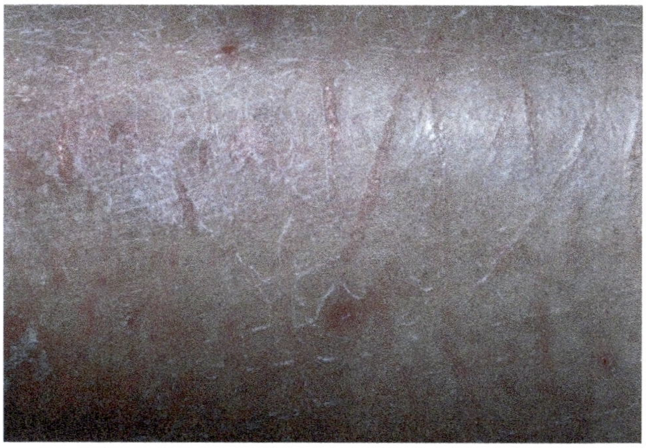

FIG. 1.1

Xerotic (asteatotic) dermatitis, also known as eczema craquelé and winter itch, is very common and is sometimes associated with nummular dermatitis. Exceptionally, it may be associated with systemic lymphoma.

The clinical common denominators of eczematous dermatitis are acutely pruritic, erythematous, and variably edematous papules and papulovesicles that quickly rupture, leaving discrete or coalescent foci of crusts and scale. Often, the vesicles are fragile and pruritic enough that intact vesicles are not observed because they are promptly excoriated. With chronicity, papules and vesicles may coalesce into poorly demarcated (e.g., compared with psoriasis) erythematous plaques containing crust and scale. As the dermatitis persists further, lesions become lichenified and may evolve into lichen simplex

ECZEMATOUS DERMATITIS—DISEASE FACT SHEET

Eczema does not represent one disease but rather a spectrum of clinical disorders that share the histologic appearance of spongiotic dermatitis.

Patient Group

- Children and adults
- May be associated with a personal or family history of asthma (atopic dermatitis)

Site of Involvement (Varies From Disease to Disease)

- Atopic dermatitis:
  - Children in acute phase: extensor surfaces and face
  - Chronic form: flexural sites
- Seborrheic dermatitis: scalp, ear, face, and central chest
- Allergic or contact dermatitis: site of exposure

Clinical Findings (Vary From Phase to Phase)

- Acute phase
  - Erythematous or edematous papules and plaques
  - Vesicles may develop with oozing, serous crusts
- Subacute phase
  - Erythematous papules and plaques
  - Scales and excoriations common
- Chronic phase
  - Thickened hyperkeratotic (lichenified) plaques (lichen simplex chronicus)
  - Nodule formation (prurigo nodularis)
  - Postinflammatory pigment changes
- Pruritus
- Xerosis (dry skin)

Prognosis and Treatment

- Atopic dermatitis tends to be chronic
  - Contact dermatitis may be acute or chronic
  - Topical steroids for atopic dermatitis
- Topical azoles and zinc pyrithione shampoos for seborrheic dermatitis
- Moisturizers
- Avoidance of exposure to triggers or stimulants

chronicus (LSC), becoming less erythematous but more thickened, hyperpigmented or hypopigmented, and lichenified, with more prominent skin lines.

Histologic Features

The essential finding in spongiotic dermatitis is spongiosis. Spongiosis is defined as intercellular edema between epidermal and/or adnexal epithelial keratinocytes, appearing on light microscopy as widened intercellular spaces that allow the intercellular bridges between keratinocytes to be observed more easily. Prominent spongiosis eventuates in the formation of intraepithelial spongiotic vesicles that correspond to clinically observed papulovesicles when large enough to be appreciated grossly. Spongiotic vesicles exhibit a round or inverted flask shape, usually contain lymphocytes or Langerhans cells, and exhibit spongiosis at their periphery. The underlying dermis usually exhibits a superficial perivascular and variably interstitial, predominantly lymphocytic infiltrate. Histiocytes, eosinophils, or neutrophils are variably present. Spongiotic vesicles must be distinguished from Pautrier microabscesses of mycosis fungoides (MF), i.e., intraepidermal collections of atypical lymphocytes without significant associated spongiosis and not containing Langerhans cells.

In acute spongiotic dermatitis, the stratum corneum exhibits undisturbed basket-weave orthokeratosis (Fig. 1.2A). The presence of parakeratosis signifies subacute spongiotic dermatitis. In chronic spongiotic dermatitis, there is epidermal hyperplasia characterized by a thickened (acanthotic) epidermis with elongated rete ridges and hypergranulosis, although hypogranulosis may be present in areas exhibiting spongiosis. In chronic spongiotic dermatitis, spongiosis is often minimal (e.g., often lacking spongiotic microvesiculation).

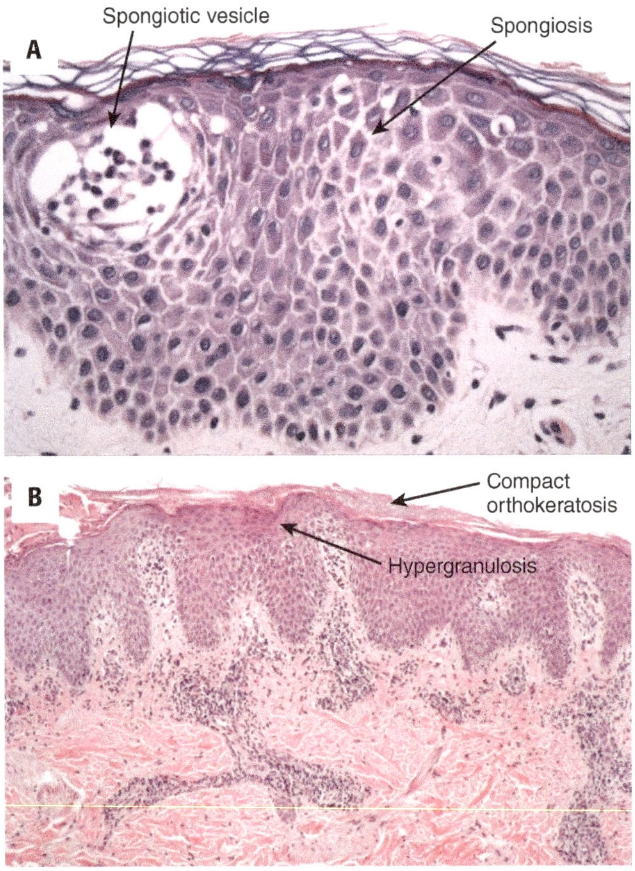

FIG. 1.2

A, Acute spongiotic dermatitis. Spongiotic vesiculation is the full expression of intercellular edema (spongiosis), which is the hallmark of all forms of spongiotic dermatitis, including allergic contact, nummular, dyshidrotic, and atopic dermatitis. In most cases, the diagnosis is established without biopsy. **B,** Chronic spongiotic dermatitis is characterized by compact orthokeratosis and irregular psoriasiform epidermal hyperplasia. Compared with psoriasis, the granular layer tends to be retained or thickened in many areas; spongiosis may be less prominent.

ECZEMATOUS DERMATITIS—PATHOLOGIC FEATURES

Histologic Features

- Spongiotic dermatitis
  - Acute: spongiosis with or without intraepidermal vesicle
  - Subacute: spongiosis and parakeratosis
  - Chronic: psoriasiform epidermal hyperplasia
- Superficial dermal lymphocytic infiltrate with or without eosinophils and/or neutrophils

Ancillary Studies

- PAS, PAS-D, or GMS stain to exclude fungal infection

Differential Diagnosis

- Spongiotic drug reaction
- Mycosis fungoides
- Tinea (dermatophytosis)

GMS, Gomori methenamine; *PAS*, periodic acid-Schiff; *PAS-D*, periodic acid-Schiff with diastase digestion.

With sufficient chronicity, the histopathologic picture evolves to LSC, with compact orthokeratosis and papillary dermal fibrosis (Fig. 1.2B). Superimposed excoriation is frequent, with variable erosion or ulceration, junctional fibrin, extravasated erythrocytes, and superficial fibrovascular granulation tissue.

Ancillary Studies

Histochemical stains (periodic acid-Schiff [PAS], PAS with diastase digestion [PAS-D], or Gomori methenamine silver [GMS]) are routinely used in spongiotic dermatitis to exclude dermatophytosis. Direct immunofluorescence (DIF) may be required if immunobullous disorders such as pemphigoid or pemphigus are clinical concerns.

Differential Diagnosis

The pathologist may narrow the differential diagnosis based on the biopsy site and clinical information but should not attempt to unequivocally distinguish different forms of spongiotic dermatitis based on histopathologic features alone. The clinician determines the final clinical-pathologic diagnosis based on clinical-pathologic correlation. Histopathologic features that may suggest a specific disorder are discussed in the sections below.

Failure to identify dermatophytosis is a diagnostic pitfall. This should be most strongly suspected when there is clinical suspicion for tinea or when central clearing or annular lesions (e.g., granuloma annulare [GA]) are described. Histologically, a parakeratotic neutrophilic crust or prominent dermal eosinophils are typical of dermatophytosis.

Drug reactions may be suspected when eosinophils are prominent or when a mixed pattern is present (e.g., combined spongiotic and interface). Ultimately, drug reactions require clinical correlation and cannot be confirmed or excluded by histology alone.

The early prebullous phase of pemphigus and pemphigoid requires DIF testing. Early pemphigus and pemphigoid usually exhibit eosinophilic spongiosis or neutrophilic spongiosis and may exhibit subtle acantholysis (pemphigus) or focal subepidermal clefting (pemphigoid).

Distinction between spongiotic dermatitis, parapsoriasis, and patch or plaque (stages Ia–Ib) mycosis fungoid can be difficult because of overlapping clinical, histologic, and immunophenotypic features. This differential diagnosis is discussed in detail in Chapter 15. Briefly, classic lesions of MF are characterized by increased numbers of atypical lymphocytes in the basilar epidermis and minimal or absent spongiosis compared to conventional spongiotic dermatitis.

Spongiosis (usually mild) may also occur as a nonspecific, secondary feature in other inflammatory processes, including interface dermatitis, vasculitis, diffuse dermal infiltrates (e.g., Sweet's syndrome), or cases with marked papillary dermal edema.

In chronic spongiotic dermatitis exhibiting psoriasiform hyperplasia but only minimal spongiosis, it is sometimes impossible to exclude psoriasis. Moreover, contact dermatitis may be superimposed upon psoriasis. Typically, psoriasis exhibits more prominent or consistent loss or diminution of the granular layer (hypogranulosis), chronic spongiotic dermatitis exhibits hypergranulosis (except in areas of active spongiosis, where hypogranulosis may be present). The presence of nonneutrophilic spongiotic microvesiculation is not typical of psoriasis. Other typical features of psoriasis are described in the following section.

Prognosis and Treatment

Because spongiotic dermatitis is not a disease *sui generis*, the prognosis, natural history, and management of spongiotic dermatitis depend on the specific clinical-pathologic diagnosis, the major forms of which are discussed in the sections that immediately follow. Nevertheless, most cases of spongiotic dermatitis respond to topical corticosteroids. Mid- to super-high (class 1) potency may be required on the hands and feet. Occlusion of topical steroids, intralesional injection of corticosteroids, and short courses of systemic corticosteroids (intramuscular or oral) may be helpful in refractory areas. Nonsteroidal topical agents include tacrolimus ointment and pimecrolimus cream. Oral antihistamines help to suppress pruritus, and their sedative effects may be beneficial. Phototherapy may be helpful in severe or refractory cases. Dupilumab is approved for moderate to severe atopic dermis in children and adults and has anecdotally reported efficacy in other forms of spongiotic dermatitis such as allergic contact dermatitis and refractory pruritus with dermal hypersensitivity reaction (DHR) on biopsy.

ALLERGIC CONTACT DERMATITIS

Clinical Findings

Acute allergic contact dermatitis frequently manifests as papules, vesicles, or plaques in linear array at the sites where the offending agent (commonly poison ivy and poison oak) brushed the skin (Fig. 1.3A). In these cases, the diagnosis is usually obvious, and patients are only rarely biopsied. Subacute or chronic allergic contact dermatitis may be clinically indistinguishable from atopic, nummular, or dyshidrotic dermatitis or LSC. In some cases, the diagnosis may be established based on the suggestive shape or distribution of lesions, the clinical history, or patch testing. Common allergen sources include plants, metals (Fig. 1.3B), and skin care products (fragrances, antibiotics, preservatives). Allergic contact dermatitis on the face or groin may present as diffuse edema resembling cellulitis.

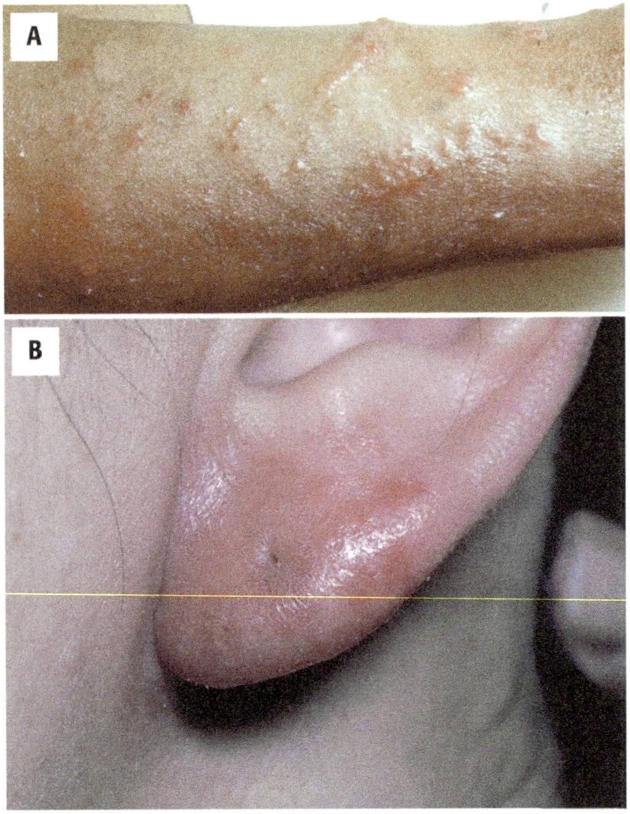

FIG. 1.3

Allergic contact dermatitis. **A,** Vesicles in linear array secondary to poison oak exposure. **B,** Secondary to nickel in jewelry.

Histologic Features

For general features, see "Spongiotic Dermatitis." Allergic contact dermatitis cannot be reliably or consistently distinguished from other forms of eczematous dermatitis based on assessment of histopathologic features alone. The presence of eosinophils has traditionally been regarded as characteristic, although there is recent evidence that intraepidermal Langerhans cell collections (spongiotic vesicles) are more specific. Dermal eosinophils, eosinophilic spongiosis, dermal dendritic multinucleated cells, and papillary dermal edema may be present, but their absence does not preclude the diagnosis. Likewise, the presence of dermal neutrophils is variable and not required. Chronic photoallergic contact dermatitis may exhibit deep perivascular extension of the dermal infiltrates. Rare variants of allergic contact dermatitis include urticarial (e.g., latex), systemic, pustular (e.g., cement), purpuric (e.g., textile dyes), granulomatous (e.g., gold), lymphomatoid (e.g., nickel), and contact dermatitis with prominent postinflammatory hypopigmentation (leukodermic variant).

Ancillary Studies

If the culprit is not revealed by a detailed exposure history, diagnostic patch testing may reveal the etiology. However, not all patch test results are clinically relevant, and interpretation of test results may be confounded by false-negative or false-positive (irritant) reactions.

Differential Diagnosis

Photocontact dermatitis, particularly chronic cases, may exhibit deep perivascular extension of the dermal inflammatory cells (see "Spongiotic Dermatitis").

Prognosis and Treatment

Allergic contact dermatitis subsides if the allergen is withdrawn. The challenges in most cases are the identification and effective removal of the allergen from the patient's environment (see "Spongiotic Dermatitis").

IRRITANT CONTACT DERMATITIS

Clinical Findings

Irritant contact dermatitis is often clinically obvious, as suggested by the pattern of inflammation corresponding to the site of contact with the irritant. The severity of the reaction is proportional to the severity of the exposure or the nature of the irritant in dose-dependent fashion. In contrast to allergic contact dermatitis, prior sensitization is not required. Compared with allergic contact dermatitis, atopic dermatitis, nummular dermatitis, and dyshidrotic dermatitis, pruritus is less characteristic. Mild reactions resemble allergic contact dermatitis. Severe irritants (e.g., chemical burn) may cause large blisters (bullae), erosion or ulceration, and may leave scars. Dermatitis associated with dry skin (xerotic dermatitis, asteatotic dermatitis, eczema craquelé) may be regarded as a variant of irritant dermatitis.

Histologic Features

For general features, see "Spongiotic Dermatitis." The histopathologic features of irritant contact dermatitis depend on the severity of the irritant and extent of exposure. Severe irritants cause confluent epidermal necrosis with "ghost" nuclei manifesting as loss of nuclear basophilia, either confluently within the superficial epidermis or full thickness. Mild irritants or lesser exposure may result in single necrotic keratinocytes within the suprabasal epidermis associated with spongiosis. Dermal neutrophils are characteristic of acute irritant contact reactions, but eosinophils and neutrophils may be variable.

Differential Diagnosis

Single necrotic keratinocytes are usually located above the basal layer in irritant dermatitis, but in interface dermatitis, they are found mostly along the dermal-epidermal junction. Single necrotic keratinocytes at the junction may also reflect wound healing from secondary excoriation by the patient (see "Spongiotic Dermatitis").

Prognosis and Treatment

Removal of the offending agent is curative. Otherwise, the condition persists depending on the frequency and severity of exposure (see "Spongiotic Dermatitis").

NUMMULAR DERMATITIS

Clinical Findings

Round erythematous plaques that typically manifest in the shape and approximate size of coins characterize nummular dermatitis. There is a predilection for the extremities. Plaques may be crusted (wet) or dry and scaly and may appear annular with a hint of central clearing. Outbreaks are often seasonal, associated with the onset of hot and humid, or more often, cold and dry winter weather. Emotional stress may also play a role in some cases.

Histologic Features

For general features, see "Spongiotic Dermatitis." Nummular dermatitis cannot be distinguished from other forms of eczematous dermatitis based on histopathologic features alone, although the anatomic site might be more or less typical (see "Differential Diagnosis").

Ancillary Studies

Nummular dermatitis is usually diagnosed based on clinical features alone, without biopsy. It is essential for the pathologist to exclude dermatophytosis.

Differential Diagnosis

Clinically, nummular dermatitis may resemble other forms of spongiotic dermatitis, as well as dermatophytosis, psoriasis, parapsoriasis, patches or plaques MF, as well as Bowen's disease or superficial basal cell carcinoma. If lesions are located on the legs, the differential diagnosis may include xerotic dermatitis and stasis dermatitis. Xerotic dermatitis is primarily a clinical diagnosis. Stasis dermatitis should exhibit concomitant changes of venous stasis, including clusters of small, thick-walled vessels in the upper dermis or full thickness of the dermis, associated with extravasated erythrocytes and hemosiderin. If venous stasis change is minimal or inactive (e.g., vascular changes but no hemorrhage), the possibility of nummular or other spongiotic dermatitis superimposed on a background of venous insufficiency cannot be excluded. A biopsy from acral skin would suggest that lesions are limited to or most prominent on acral skin, generally favoring dyshidrosis or contact dermatitis over nummular dermatitis. A biopsy from the head and neck region would also be unusual for nummular dermatitis with the possible exception of Sulzberger-Garbe disease, also known as exudative discoid and lichenoid chronic dermatosis or "oid-oid" disease, and historically regarded as an unusually extensive and recalcitrant expression of nummular dermatitis.

Prognosis and Treatment

There is a chronic waxing and waning course (see "Spongiotic Dermatitis").

ATOPIC DERMATITIS

Clinical Findings

Atopic dermatitis (commonly designated eczema) is associated with a personal or family history of atopy, including asthma, allergic rhinitis, and allergic conjunctivitis. Atopic dermatitis is most common in infancy and childhood. Atopic dermatitis is known as the "itch that scratches" because pruritus often appears before a significant visible skin lesion. The earliest lesions are believed to be papulovesicles, akin to those that may be observed in acute spongiotic dermatitis. However, in atopic dermatitis, intact vesicles are rarely observed because papulovesicles are promptly excoriated, resulting in crusted papules that coalesce into ill-defined plaques. Atopic dermatitis is most common in childhood, and plaques involve the antecubital and popliteal fossae. Chronically manipulated lesions become scaly, lichenified, and dyspigmented (Fig. 1.4A). Secondary impetiginization with *Staphylococcus aureus* or secondary herpes simplex virus (HSV) infection (eczema herpeticum) may occur. Papular or follicular atopic dermatitis is most common in dark-complected children (Fig. 1.4B).

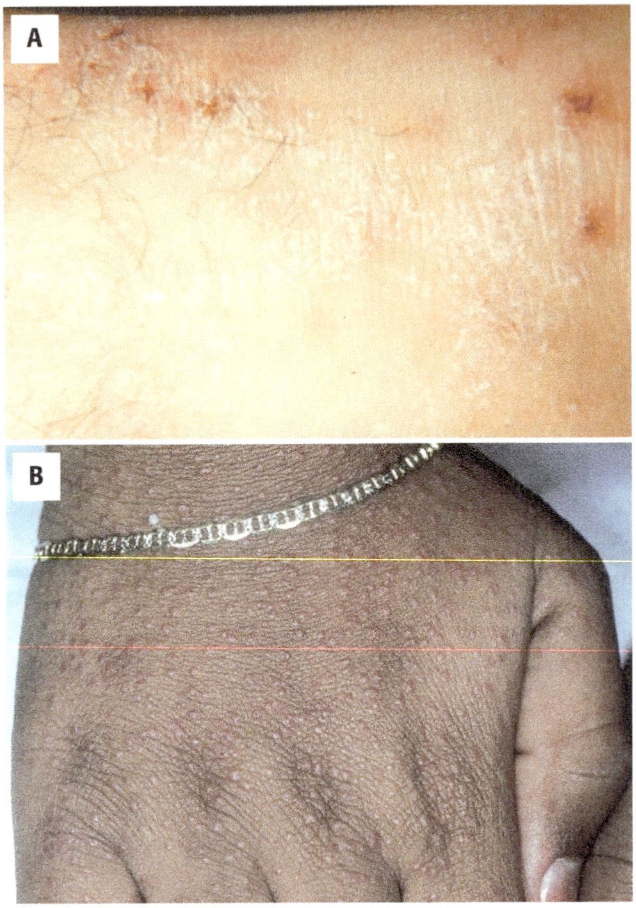

FIG. 1.4

Atopic dermatitis. **A,** Ill-defined plaques composed of pruritic focally crusted papules (in many instances ruptured papulovesicles) that become lichenified secondary to chronic rubbing. **B,** Papular or follicular atopic dermatitis is more common in dark-skinned children and clinically resembles lichen nitidus.

Histologic Features

For general features, see "Spongiotic Dermatitis." Atopic dermatitis cannot be reliably or consistently distinguished from other forms of eczematous dermatitis based on the assessment of histopathologic features alone, but a biopsy is rarely required for diagnosis. Biopsies of atopic dermatitis are usually taken from subacute or chronic lesions, so parakeratosis, epidermal hyperplasia with hypergranulosis, and superimposed LSC (see following section) are typical, and spongiosis itself is often mild. Papular or follicular atopic dermatitis is characterized by spongiosis involving the infundibula of hair follicles. Lesions of atopic dermatitis are particularly susceptible to secondary bacterial impetiginization by *S. aureus* or HSV superinfection. Impetiginized lesions are characterized by clusters of gram-positive cocci within a crusted stratum corneum often with some neutrophils. HSV infections are characterized by intraepidermal vesiculation, variable acantholysis, and epithelial necrosis, with viral cytopathic changes of ballooning and reticular degeneration, multinucleation with nuclear molding of keratinocytes, and steel gray nuclei with peripheral margination of nuclear chromatin.

Differential Diagnosis

The diagnosis of atopy is determined by the patient's personal and family history and clinical findings. Atopic dermatitis is invariably pruritic and characteristically involves the antecubital and popliteal fossae. Atopic dermatitis may exhibit prominent lichenification and postinflammatory hyperpigmentation or hypopigmentation. Most cases do not require biopsy for diagnosis.

However, atypical cases may be biopsied to evaluate for MF, psoriasis, pityriasis rubra pilaris (PRP), or other disorders. Follicular atopic dermatitis is clinically and histologically indistinguishable from a rare disorder, recurrent and disseminate infundibulofolliculitis, which has been reported in individuals without history of atopy. Miliaria rubra and Fox-Fordyce disease (apocrine miliaria) are clinically distinctive disorders characterized by spongiosis of acrosyringium and apocrine duct, respectively. However, depending on the plane of section, it may be difficult to determine whether focal spongiosis is associated with follicular, eccrine ductal, or apocrine ductal epithelium. Pityriasis alba is characterized by hypopigmented patches with a fine pityriasiform scale, most commonly on the face of dark-complected children, on whom it is generally not biopsied. The process may be generalized and involve the trunk and extremities. It is widely believed to represent postinflammatory hypopigmentation secondary to atopic dermatitis.

Prognosis and Treatment

See "Spongiotic Dermatitis." Atopic dermatitis is common in infancy and childhood and tends to resolve or diminish in severity with advancing age (so-called extrinsic or allergic eczema). Atopic individuals are particularly susceptible to *S. aureus* superinfection, and a 2-week course of dicloxacillin or cephalexin will often improve refractory cases, especially if there is significant crusting of lesions. New-onset, unexplained, generalized eczema or atopic dermatitis in older adults may be classified as intrinsic or nonallergic eczema, has been attributed to immunosenescence, and should evoke consideration of a drug reaction or, rarely, occult malignancy.

DYSHIDROTIC DERMATITIS

Clinical Findings

Dyshidrotic dermatitis (also designated *pompholyx*) is characterized by small tapioca pearl-like vesicles bilaterally on the fingers or toes. There is a tendency to involve the lateral aspects of the digits (Fig. 1.5). Vesicles may coalesce or extend onto the palms or soles but generally not beyond the wrist or ankle. Milder cases may present with erythematous papules rather than visible vesicles. In severe acute cases, there may be extension to the distal extremities.

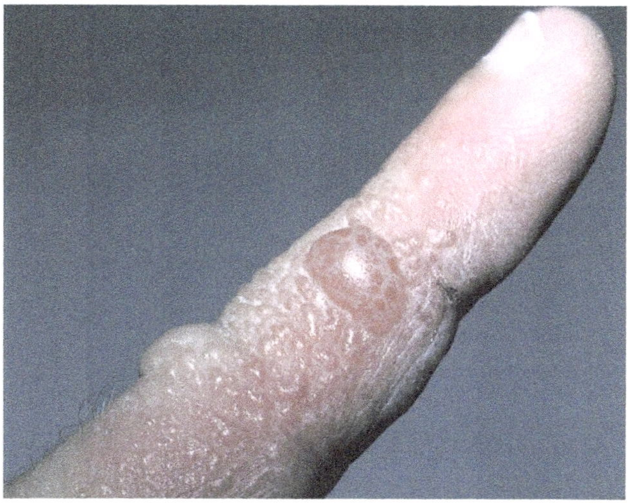

FIG. 1.5

Dyshidrotic dermatitis consists of pruritic vesicles that tend to arise on the lateral fingers and hands. In contrast to spongiotic vesicles at other sites, they often remain intact in dyshidrosis.

Histologic Features

For general histologic features, see "Spongiotic Dermatitis." Except for the requirement of acral involvement, dyshidrotic dermatitis cannot be distinguished from other forms of eczematous dermatitis by histology alone. However, the diagnosis may only be considered when the hands or feet are involved, usually symmetrically.

Differential Diagnosis

Dyshidrotic dermatitis is usually diagnosed based on clinical features alone, without biopsy. The pathologist should exclude vesiculobullous lesions caused by dermatophytes or allergic contact dermatitis, since these may clinically resemble dyshidrotic dermatitis. Patients with tinea pedis may develop an Id reaction with dyshidrotic dermatitis on the hands and sometimes a generalized eczematous dermatitis. Id reactions may occur during initiation of systemic antifungal therapy for tinea pedis or onychomycosis.

Prognosis and Treatment

See "Spongiotic Dermatitis." Unless a cause can be identified and removed (see Id reaction), dyshidrotic dermatitis usually exhibits a chronic, waxing and waning course. Emotional stress has been implicated as a cause.

SEBORRHEIC DERMATITIS

Clinical Findings

Seborrheic dermatitis is common in adulthood, exhibiting a soft, greasy scale and erythema, with a predilection for the scalp, eyebrows, nasolabial and retroauricular skin folds (Fig. 1.6), and upper trunk. Inguinal skin folds are less commonly involved. Seborrheic dermatitis is also common in newborns.

Histologic Features

Seborrheic dermatitis cannot be reliably or consistently distinguished from other forms of eczematous dermatitis based on assessment of histopathologic features alone. However, classic examples of seborrheic dermatitis exhibit spongiosis localized to the ostia or upper infundibula of hair follicles. A neutrophilic crust or some neutrophilic exocytosis is commonly present. Colonizing *Pityrosporum* (*Malassezia*) yeast spores may be present in the stratum corneum or superficial follicular orifice.

See "Spongiotic Dermatitis." Seborrheic dermatitis is usually clinically sufficiently diagnostic. Occasionally, chronic seborrheic dermatitis is clinically or histologically indistinguishable from psoriasis.

Prognosis and Treatment

See "Spongiotic Dermatitis." Seborrheic dermatitis usually exhibits a chronic, waxing and waning course. In addition to topical corticosteroids, topical ketoconazole, medicated (e.g., coal tar, selenium sulfide, zinc sulfate) shampoos, and topical tacrolimus are also often helpful.

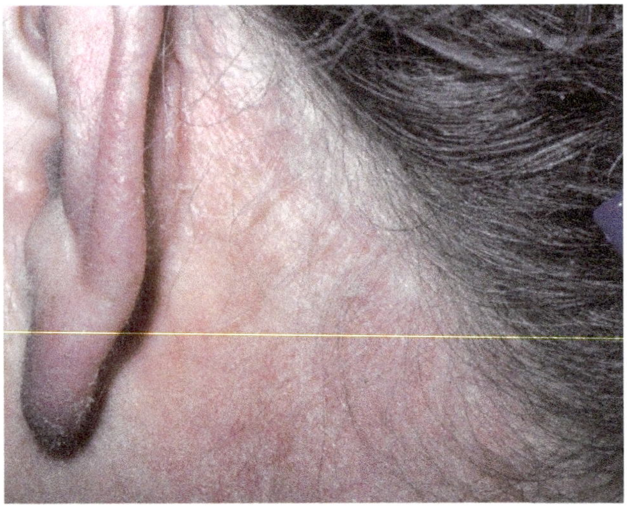

FIG. 1.6
Seborrheic dermatitis is rarely biopsied. There is usually ill-defined, greasy, soft scale involving the scalp, and nasolabial and retroauricular skin folds.

PAPULAR DERMATITIS

Clinical Findings

Papular dermatitis describes adults with refractory pruritic papules of unknown etiology with a predilection for the trunk, pelvis, and proximal extremities (Fig. 1.7A). Papular dermatitis has been equated to what other observers have previously designated subacute prurigo and itchy red bump disease. Individuals with papular dermatitis may have some atopic features but not enough to warrant a diagnosis of atopic dermatitis. The incidence of papular dermatitis is unknown but is believed to be underrecognized, with cases likely being "lumped" into established diagnostic categories (e.g., atopic dermatitis, arthropod bite reactions).

Histologic Features

Papular dermatitis is characterized by minimal spongiosis and dermal perivascular lymphocytes with eosinophils (Fig. 1.7B–D). These nonspecific changes have historically been reported descriptively or classified under various headings, particularly DHR pattern, by many pathologists and, subsequently, some clinicians. In contrast to urticaria, lesions may exhibit limited epidermal spongiotic and/or interface changes and may be excoriated. In subacute prurigo, the spongiosis has been reported to be localized to the follicular infundibula.

Differential Diagnosis

As with most forms of spongiotic dermatitis, the diagnosis of papular dermatitis is primarily based on clinical features. Cases entirely devoid of spongiosis exhibiting otherwise identical dermal changes may represent nondiagnostic samplings of papular dermatitis. Papular presentations of other forms of spongiotic dermatitis, most commonly follicular atopic dermatitis, cannot be reliably distinguished from papular dermatitis without clinical correlation. Likewise, the diagnosis of pruritic urticarial papules and plaques of pregnancy (PUPPP) requires clinical correlation. Arthropod bite reactions typically exhibit denser and deeper dermal perivascular involvement and more prominent eosinophils but sparse, so-called "timid" arthropod bite reactions may

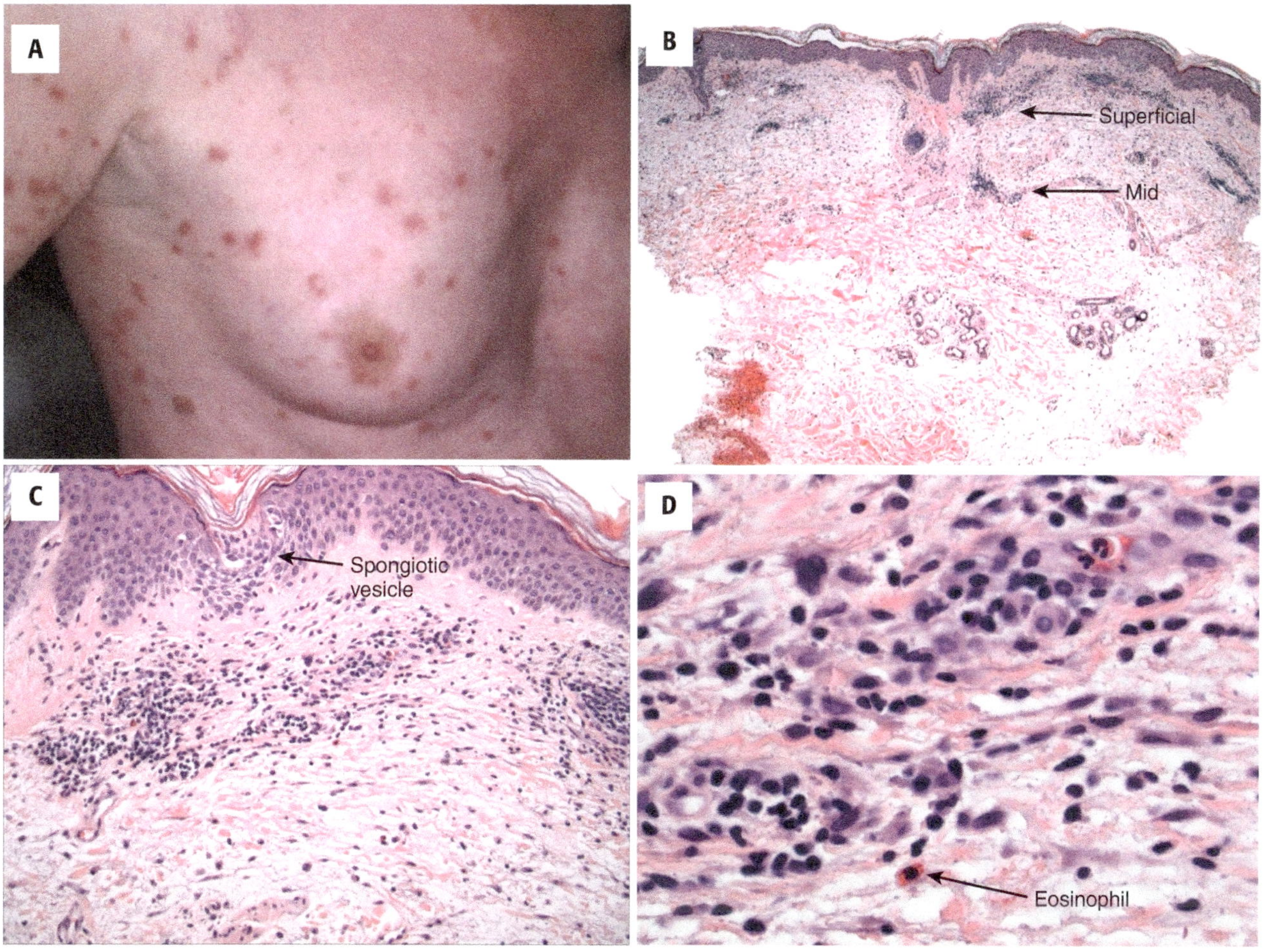

FIG. 1.7

Papular dermatitis (subacute prurigo, itchy red bump disease). **A,** Numerous edematous red pruritic papules with variable crusting (from excoriation) on the trunk and proximal extremities. **B,** Scanning magnification reveals superficial, mid perivascular, and interstitial lymphocytes. **C** and **D,** Scattered eosinophils are present, and limited or focal spongiosis may be present. Urticarial dermatitis may be histologically identical to papular dermatitis, although spongiotic vesicles would not be typical.

still be considered. Scabies typically exhibits very prominent eosinophils and crust. Drug reactions can never be confirmed or excluded by histology alone; clinical correlation is always required. The urticarial stage of bullous pemphigoid can be confirmed by DIF analysis. Papular acrodermatitis (Gianotti-Crosti disease) exhibits variable histopathologic features that may include spongiotic or lichenoid features.

Prognosis and Treatment

Papular dermatitis typically exhibits a chronic, waxing and waning course. Topical corticosteroids, oral antihistamines, and phototherapy may be beneficial. Systemic immunosuppressive therapy (mycophenolate mofetil) has been reported.

URTICARIAL DERMATITIS

Clinical Findings

The term *urticarial dermatitis* includes many patients with DHR who present clinically with pruritic urticarial eczematous plaques with or without papules. The incidence of urticarial dermatitis is unknown, but, akin to papular dermatitis, may be underrecognized; case series from the United States and Australia have been reported.

Histologic Features

Urticarial dermatitis designates a subset of the DHR histologic reaction pattern. Urticarial dermatitis is characterized by minimal spongiosis with normal stratum corneum (e.g., no parakeratosis) and upper dermal perivascular lymphocytes with eosinophils (i.e., identical to papular dermatitis) (Fig. 1.7B–D).

Differential Diagnosis

As with most forms of spongiotic or eczematous dermatitis, the diagnosis of urticarial dermatitis is primarily based on clinical features and does not designate a specific disease entity. With clinical correlation, some cases can be classified more specifically, including drug reactions, urticarial pemphigoid, atopic dermatitis, or contact dermatitis. In contrast to papular dermatitis, the differential diagnosis for urticarial dermatitis does not usually include arthropod bite reactions, but scabies, PUPPP, dermatitis herpetiformis, viral exanthems, and cutaneous T-cell lymphoma have rarely been documented.

Prognosis and Treatment

Urticarial dermatitis may be managed with topical corticosteroids and oral antihistamines. Phototherapy, dapsone, and systemic immunosuppressive or targeted biologic agents may be beneficial based on limited data.

PITYRIASIS ROSEA

Clinical Findings

Pityriasis rosea (PR) is a common, seasonal (spring, fall), self-limited eruption usually affecting children and young adults, manifesting as multiple round or oval erythematous papules, patches, or plaques with a collarette of pityriasiform (branlike) scale (Fig. 1.8A) distributed in a "Christmas tree" pattern on the trunk (following relaxed skin tension lines on either side of the midline). The inguinal and axillary skin folds may be involved in inverse PR. A single lesion preceding by 1 to 2 weeks the onset of the generalized eruption is often identified (herald patch or mother patch) and is often larger than all subsequent lesions. Many individuals experience flu-like symptoms before the onset of the herald patch or during the early stages of the eruption. PR is widely suspected of being virus-induced (e.g., HHV-7), but no specific etiology has been consistently identified to date. COVID-19 vaccination has been reported to trigger PR or PR-like reactions.

Histologic Features

PR cannot always be reliably or consistently distinguished from other forms of spongiotic dermatitis based on histopathologic features alone. Classic biopsies of PR exhibit periodic foci ("caps") of spongiosis with overlying focal parakeratosis (Fig. 1.8B and C), relatively prominent exocytosis of small lymphocytes, and extravasated erythrocytes in the papillary dermis or epidermis (Fig. 1.8D). Scattered single dyskeratotic keratinocytes may be identified and may be more prominent in the herald patch. However, the pattern of inflammation is predominantly spongiotic rather than interface. Inflammation within the dermis is usually confined to the upper dermis and is predominantly lymphocytic. Eosinophils are variable. Although PR is clinically classified by dermatologists as a papulosquamous disorder, psoriasiform hyperplasia is not required.

Differential Diagnosis

See "Spongiotic Dermatitis." PR is usually diagnosed based on clinical features alone, without biopsy.

If epidermal changes are focal, the appearances may be indistinguishable from the superficial variant of erythema annulare centrifugum (EAC). Because biopsies from acute lesions of EAC may sometimes exhibit multiple foci of parakeratosis with spongiosis, including spongiotic vesiculation, clinical correlation is required to distinguish EAC from PR. Lymphocyte exocytosis, scattered single necrotic keratinocytes, and extravasation of erythrocytes are also shared features with pityriasis lichenoides and morbilliform viral exanthems. Pityriasis lichenoides is primarily an interface dermatitis with more keratinocyte necrosis and junctional vacuolar alteration than spongiosis. Morbilliform viral exanthems are characterized by sparse lymphocytes with extravasated erythrocytes, mild vacuolar alteration, minimal spongiosis with lymphocyte exocytosis, or no epidermal alteration at all. PR-like drug reactions have been associated with captopril, COVID-19 vaccination, gold, barbiturates, clonidine, isotretinoin, metronidazole, and penicillamine and require clinical correlation to establish.

Prognosis and Treatment

PR invariably resolves within 2 weeks to 3 months. Recurrence is unusual. Most patients are managed symptomatically with such agents as low- to midpotency topical corticosteroids or oral antihistamines. Ultraviolet B phototherapy may shorten the disease course, especially if initiated early.

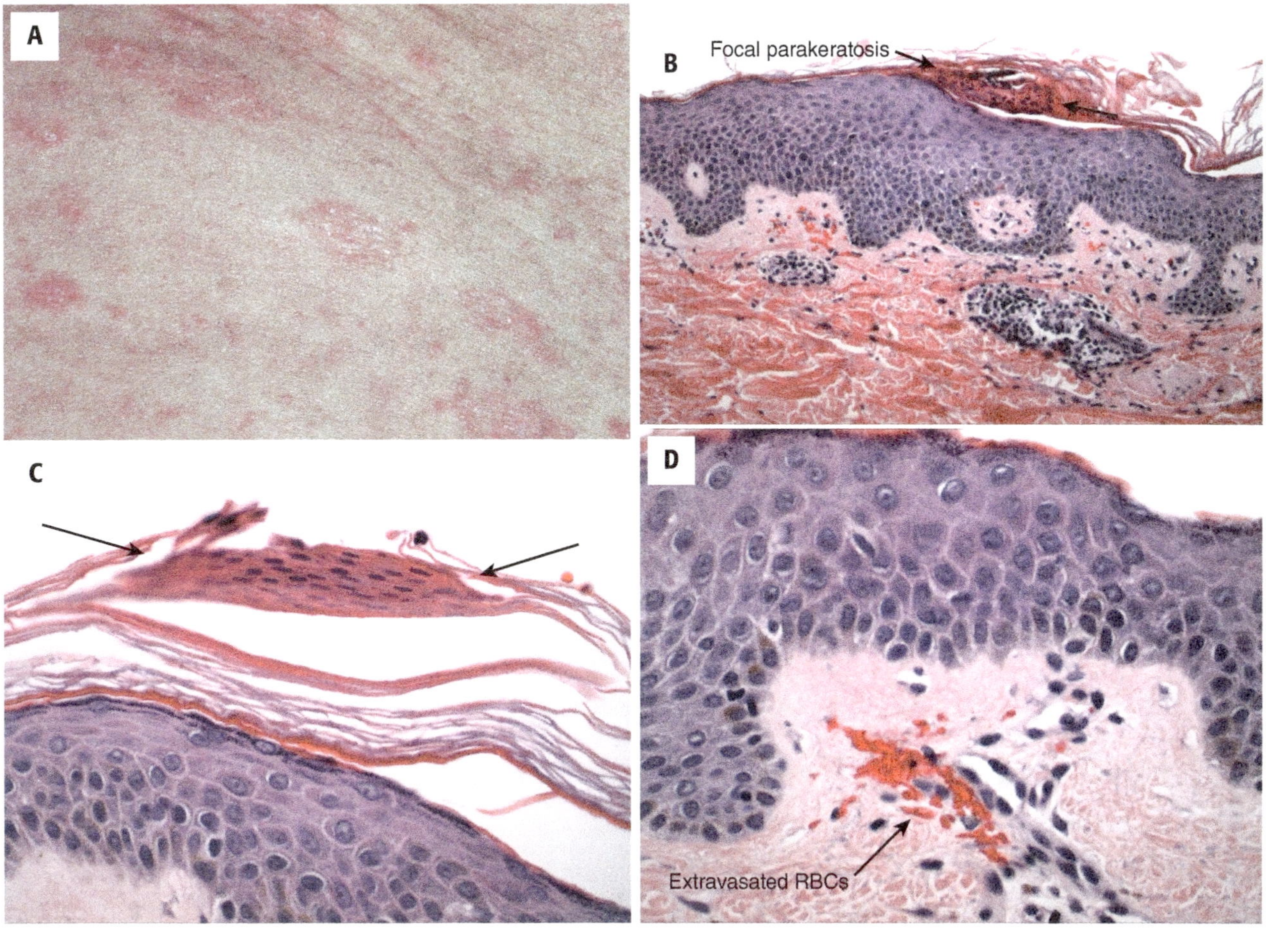

FIG. 1.8

Pityriasis rosea. **A,** Characteristic oval plaque with collarette of pityriasiform (branlike) scale oriented along relaxed skin tension lines. **B** and **C,** Focal "caps" of parakeratosis and spongiosis. **D,** Extravasated erythrocytes in the papillary dermis.

PSORIASIFORM DERMATITIS

Similar to spongiotic dermatitis, psoriasiform dermatitis is a descriptive "diagnosis" used by pathologists in dermatopathology reports that does not correspond to a single clinical disorder. Rather, it describes a specific feature, psoriasiform epidermal hyperplasia, that is characteristic of a variety of inflammatory disorders, the prototype being psoriasis (Table 1.2).

PSORIASIS

Clinical Findings

Classic plaque-type psoriasis (psoriasis vulgaris) is characterized by well-circumscribed erythematous plaques with a thick, silvery scale with a predilection for the elbows, knees, scalp, and gluteal fold (Fig. 1.9A and B). Fingernail plate involvement includes pitting and distal onycholysis. Lesions often arise at sites of superficial trauma (Koebner phenomenon). Involvement of the face is uncommon. Flexural skin fold involvement characterizes inverse psoriasis. Guttate psoriasis is characterized by the acute onset of innumerate papules or small plaques, classically in association with streptococcal pharyngitis. Pustular psoriasis may be generalized or localized to the distal extremities (Fig. 1.9C). Psoriasis is one of the more common etiologies underlying diffuse erythroderma, or exfoliative dermatitis (Fig. 1.9D). Individuals with psoriasis often have concomitant psoriatic arthritis and/or metabolic syndrome. Approximately one-third of patients have a family history of psoriasis.

Histologic Features

Psoriatic plaques exhibit a distinctive profile of parakeratosis containing horizontally flattened layers of neutrophils, psoriasiform epidermal hyperplasia characterized by hypogranulosis and regular elongation of slender rete ridges often with club-shaped profiles and fusion of adjacent rete ridges, thinned suprapapillary

TABLE 1.2
Basic Differential Diagnosis of Psoriasiform Dermatitis

	Psoriasis	Chronic Spongiotic Dermatitis	Lichen Simplex Chronicus or Prurigo Nodularis	Pityriasis Rubra Pilaris
Superficial perivascular lymphocytes	++	++	±	++
Deep perivascular lymphocytes	o	o	o	o
Hypogranulosis	++	±	o	o
Hypergranulosis	o	±	++	±
Dermal eosinophils	o	±	±	o
"Checkerboard" parakeratosis pattern	±	±	±	++
Parakeratosis with neutrophils	++	±	±	o
Papillary dermal fibrosis	±	±	++	±

++, characteristic; ±, variable; o, unusual or not classic.

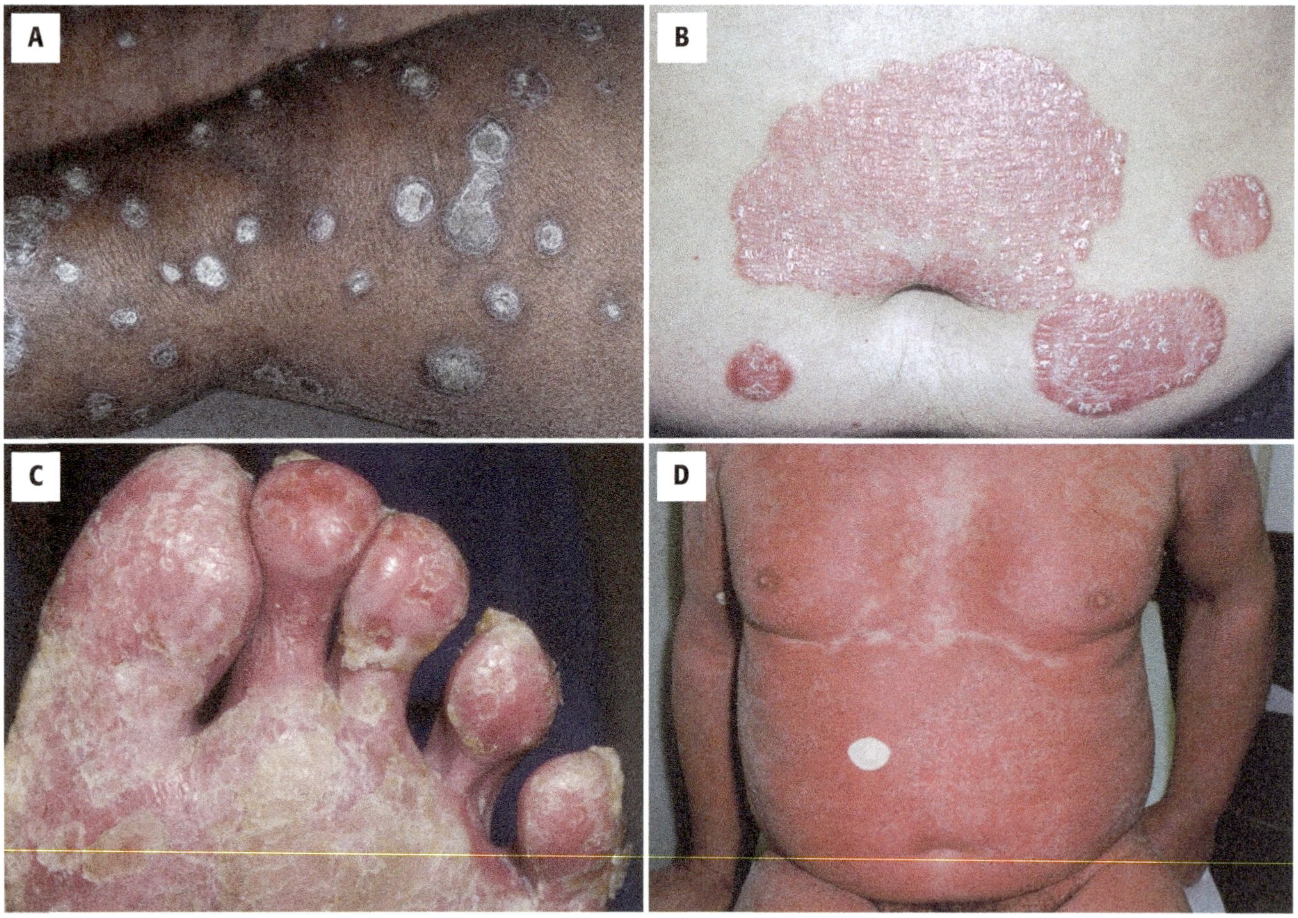

FIG. 1.9
Psoriasis. **A** and **B,** Classic well-demarcated plaques with a thick scale. **C,** Pustular psoriasis. A few intact pustules are present at the base of the great toe. **D,** Erythrodermic psoriasis.

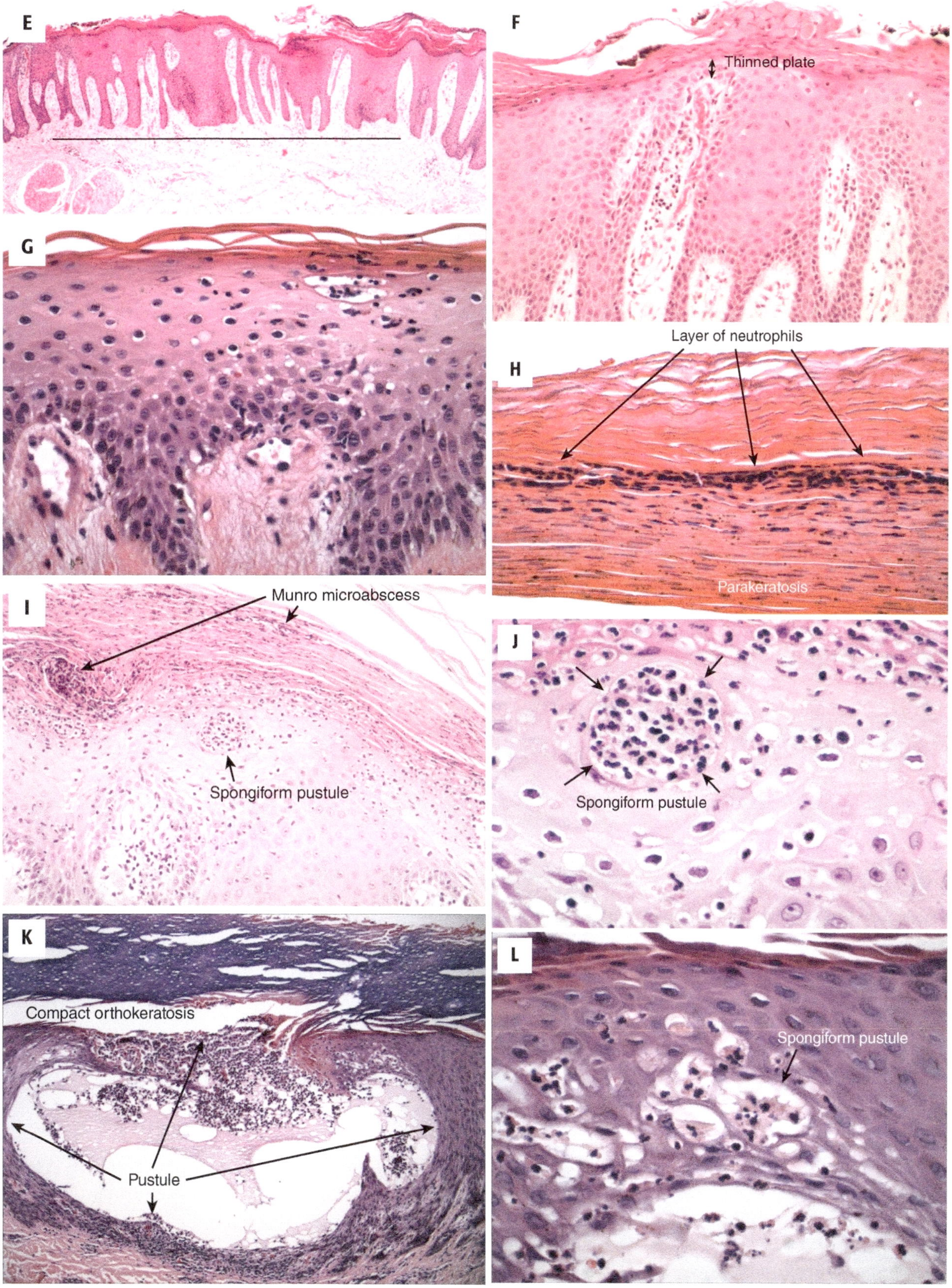

FIG. 1.9, cont'd

E, At scanning magnification, there is regular elongation of the rete ridges. An imaginary line connecting the rete tips would be fairly straight. **F,** Parakeratotic crust, hypogranulosis, and a thinned suprapapillary plate. **G,** Neutrophilic spongiosis (intraepidermal neutrophils) includes single neutrophils or clusters (spongiform pustule of Kogoj). **H,** Layered neutrophils within parakeratosis. **I,** Collections of neutrophils in the stratum corneum (Munro microabscess) and in the stratum malpighii (spongiform pustule of Kogoj). **J,** Spongiform pustule at higher magnification. **K** and **L,** Pustular psoriasis may be generalized or localized to acral skin (whereupon the clinician has no choice but to biopsy an acral site, as evidenced by the presence of compact orthokeratosis in **K**).

PSORIASIS—DISEASE FACT SHEET

Patient Group

- May occur at any age (bimodal onset between 20 to 30 and 50 to 60 years)
- Familial predisposition; eruption often triggered by events (e.g., trauma, infection, medication)

Site of Involvement

- Scalp, elbow, knees—most common
- Nails, hands, feet, and trunk may also be affected

Clinical Findings (Variable)

Chronic Plaque Disease (Most Common):

- Erythematous plaques with a silvery scale; sharply demarcated

Guttate (Eruptive) Psoriasis (Rare):

- Discrete papules and plaques

Pustular Psoriasis (Rare):

- Pustules

Erythrodermic Psoriasis (Rare):

- Generalized erythroderma and scaling: associated arthritis found in a subset of patients (5%–30%)

Prognosis

- Chronic disorder

Treatment

- Topical vitamin D analogs
- Topical corticosteroids
- Topical calcineurin inhibitors, tar, tazarotene, or anthralin
- Phototherapy (ultraviolet light)
- Systemic immunosuppressive therapy (acitretin, apremilast, methotrexate, cyclosporine)
- Systemic biological therapies against tumor necrosis factor-α, interleukin-17 (IL17) pathway, IL23, and related cytokines

plates, prominent blood vessels within edematous papillary dermal tips, and superficial perivascular predominantly lymphocytic dermal infiltrates (Fig. 1.9E–H). Acute, guttate, or pustular lesions most frequently exhibit neutrophilic spongiosis often with intraepidermal neutrophil collections (spongiform pustules of Kogoj) and intracorneal neutrophil collections (Munro microabscesses) (Fig. 1.9I–L). Despite the prominence of neutrophils within the epidermis, they are not prominent within the dermis. Eosinophils are usually not prominent in psoriasis. Early lesions of guttate psoriasis may not have well-developed epidermal changes, and the granular layer may still be somewhat intact, making them difficult to distinguish from other forms of subacute spongiotic dermatitis. Neutrophils in the stratum corneum may be helpful in these cases.

PSORIASIS—PATHOLOGIC FEATURES

Histologic Features

- Chronic plaque lesions
  - Psoriasiform epidermal hyperplasia
  - Multilayered mounds of parakeratosis and orthohyperkeratosis
  - Neutrophils cluster in a parakeratotic stratum corneum (microabscess of Munro)
  - Neutrophil cluster in stratum malpighii (spongiform pustule of Kogoj)
  - Diminished or absent granular cell layer (hypogranulosis)
  - Thinning of suprapapillary plate
  - Hypervascular edematous dermal papillae
- Guttate psoriasis
  - Less hyperplasia, more inflammation, and spongiosis
- Pustular psoriasis
  - Dense accumulations of intraepidermal neutrophils

Ancillary Studies

- Consider PAS stain to exclude fungal infection

Differential Diagnosis

- Chronic spongiotic dermatitis
- Lichen simplex chronicus
- Drug reaction
- Mycosis fungoides
- Dermatophytosis
- Pustular psoriasis: immunobullous disorders, pustular drug reactions, infection

PAS, periodic acid-Schiff.

Ancillary Studies

A PAS or GMS stain may help exclude a fungal infection associated with a psoriasiform histologic reaction pattern. However, while onychomycosis is common in patients with psoriasis, in classic cases of psoriasis, superimposed tinea corporis is uncommon and may be reasonably excluded by H&E alone.

Differential Diagnosis

Most cases are diagnosed clinically, without biopsy. Biopsy is more likely to be performed when the clinical features or response to therapy is unusual. For classic plaques, dermatophytosis, chronic spongiotic dermatitis, psoriasiform drug reactions, necrolytic migratory erythema (NME), and patch or plaque stage MF may enter the differential diagnosis. Reiter syndrome is histopathologically indistinguishable from pustular psoriasis. In chronic spongiotic dermatitis, the elongated rete ridges are usually less uniform in length, the granular layer tends to be preserved or even thickened at least variably, and spongiosis is more prominent. For pustular eruptions, vesiculopustular dermatophytosis needs to be excluded; clinical correlation is often sufficient (rather than a PAS stain). Psoriasis may represent a common underlying etiology of exfoliative erythroderma. However, erythroderma is a final common pathway of several disorders, including MF, Sézary syndrome, atopic dermatitis, PRP, drug reactions, and others. Diagnosis of erythroderma depends on identification of specific histopathologic attributes of the underlying disorder. In many examples of erythroderma, specific histopathologic features may be subtle. Spongiotic dermatitis is more likely to become impetiginized than psoriasis, so clusters of coccobacteria may be present within the neutrophilic crusts of spongiotic dermatitis. NME may present as psoriasiform dermatitis and neutrophilic spongiosis, without the prominent necrolysis that would most easily identify it. NME usually exhibits pronounced pallor in the upper epidermis. Patch-stage MF often displays psoriasiform hyperplasia with a denser lichenoid infiltrate and disproportionate exocytosis of atypical lymphocytes (epidermotropism). Plasma cells may represent a clue to syphilis.

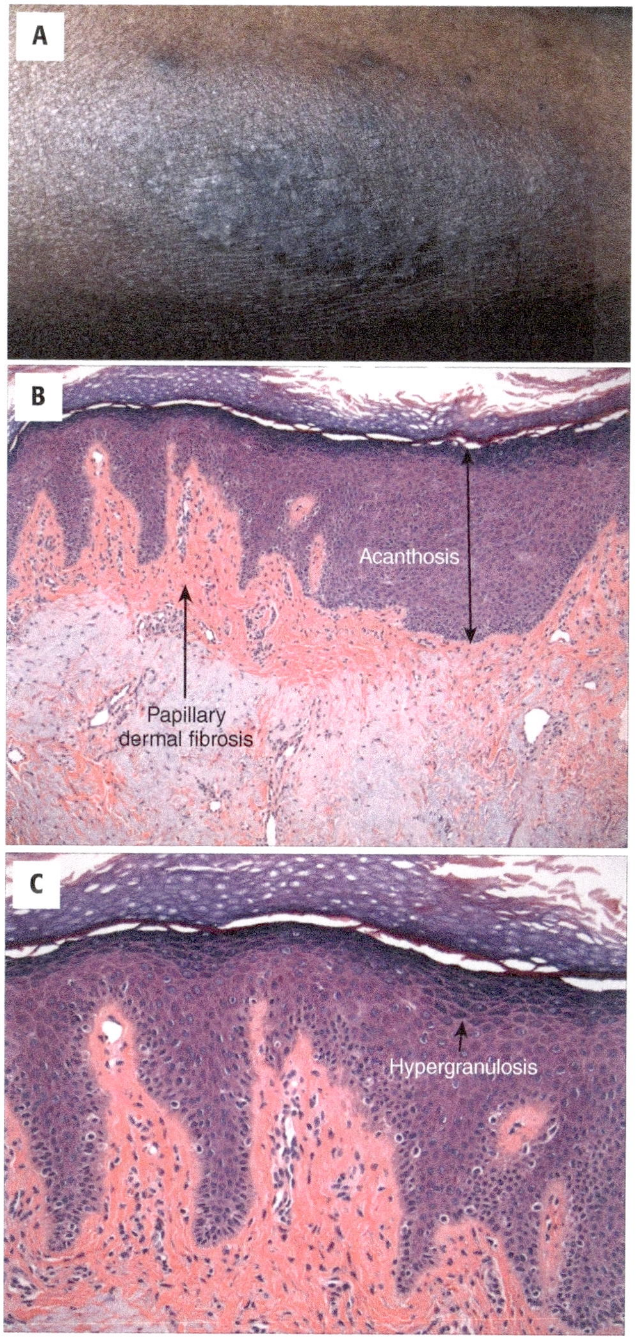

FIG. 1.10

Lichen simplex chronicus. **A,** Thickened, hyperpigmented plaque with decreased numbers of more prominent skin lines. **B, C,** Compact orthokeratosis, hypergranulosis, papillary dermal fibrosis, and vertically oriented blood vessels within papillary dermal tips. In this case, the dermal fibrosis is more obvious because it displaces solar elastosis.

Prognosis and Treatment

Psoriasis exhibits a variable, unpredictable course that is frequently chronic or waxing and waning. Guttate eruptions in children and young adults may have the highest chance of complete remission. Therapy is individualized, largely based on disease severity, and includes topical and intralesional steroids; topical retinoids; topical calcipotriene; topical coal tar or anthralin; broad- or narrowband ultraviolet B phototherapy; photochemotherapy (psoralen plus ultraviolet A [PUVA]); or systemic agents such as methotrexate, cyclosporine, and acitretin. Biologic agents include etanercept, infliximab, adalimumab, and ustekinumab.

LICHEN SIMPLEX CHRONICUS AND PRURIGO NODULARIS

Clinical Findings

LSC is a localized thickening, hyperpigmentation, and lichenification secondary to chronic rubbing (Fig. 1.10A). The cause of the rubbing is usually pruritus, which produces a habitual, intractable, itch-scratch cycle. Lesions may appear to arise de novo, but more often lichenification occurs in the setting of chronic spongiotic dermatitis, particularly atopic dermatitis. Prurigo nodularis (picker's nodule, chronic prurigo) can be regarded as the papulonodular counterpart of LSC. Prurigo nodularis may arise at focal sites of inflammation, such as insect bites or folliculitis, regressed warts, or in patients with generalized pruritus associated with systemic disease such as chronic renal failure. Prurigo nodules are firm, smooth, or slightly rough dome-shaped papules or nodules that are often hyperpigmented or crusted. Patients generally admit to manipulating the lesions.

Histologic Features

Lichen simplex chronicus and prurigo nodularis are characterized by compact orthokeratosis with marked hypergranulosis and epidermal and follicular epithelial hyperplasia with follicular plugging resembling acral skin (except for the presence of hair follicles: hairy palm sign) and papillary dermal fibrosis with vertically oriented blood vessels within fibrotic dermal papillae (Fig. 1.10B and C). Residual mild spongiosis is often present. In prurigo nodularis, a dome-shaped configuration is evident, and follicular epithelial hyperplasia and hypergranulosis can be quite prominent.

Differential Diagnosis

Any chronic spongiotic dermatitis may eventuate in LSC. Dermatophytosis should still be excluded. Psoriasis may resemble LSC, but LSC typically exhibits a thickened stratum corneum containing predominantly orthokeratosis rather than parakeratosis, hypergranulosis, and more irregular elongation of rete ridges. If hypogranulosis is present, it is confined to areas of visible spongiosis or evidence of excoriation. In LSC, there is no tendency to thinned suprapapillary plates, and papillary dermal fibrosis, often with a scarlike configuration of collagen fibers oriented parallel to the epidermal surface, is characteristic. To the extent that papillomatosis is present, an antecedent or regressing verruca vulgaris may be suspected.

Prognosis and Treatment

Lichen simplex chronicus is often refractory to treatment. The itch-scratch cycle may be broken by treatment with potent topical or intralesional corticosteroids or sedating oral antihistamines such as hydroxyzine, diphenhydramine, or doxepin. Occlusive therapy, with or without corticosteroids, may be helpful. Refractory prurigo nodularis has been reported to improve with phototherapy or thalidomide.

PITYRIASIS RUBRA PILARIS

Clinical Findings

PRP is a chronic, idiopathic disorder characterized by red-orange follicular papules that coalesce into well-demarcated confluent plaques, leaving characteristic islands of sparing (Fig. 1.11A). Lesions typically progress from rostral to caudal, with many patients presenting with initial involvement of the face and scalp (hair and teeth are normal), followed by palmoplantar keratoderma and generalized involvement. Erythroderma may ensue. Many patients are photosensitive. Erythroderma may result in severe cases. Localized, familial (e.g., CARD14-associated), and juvenile variants have been described, as well as drug-induced PRP (e.g., tyrosine kinase inhibitors). Acquired cases often exhibit an abrupt onset, but familial cases may have a more gradual onset. Nail changes include splinter hemorrhages, yellow-brown discoloration, and nail plate thickening.

Histologic Features

PRP is characterized by alternating orthokeratosis and parakeratosis, both vertically and horizontally, producing a distinctive checkerboard pattern in the stratum corneum in histologic sections (Fig. 1.11B). There is usually psoriasiform hyperplasia, preservation of the granular layer, follicular plugging, and sparse superficial perivascular lymphocytes. Spongiosis, if present at all, is minimal. Focal acantholytic dyskeratosis may be present.

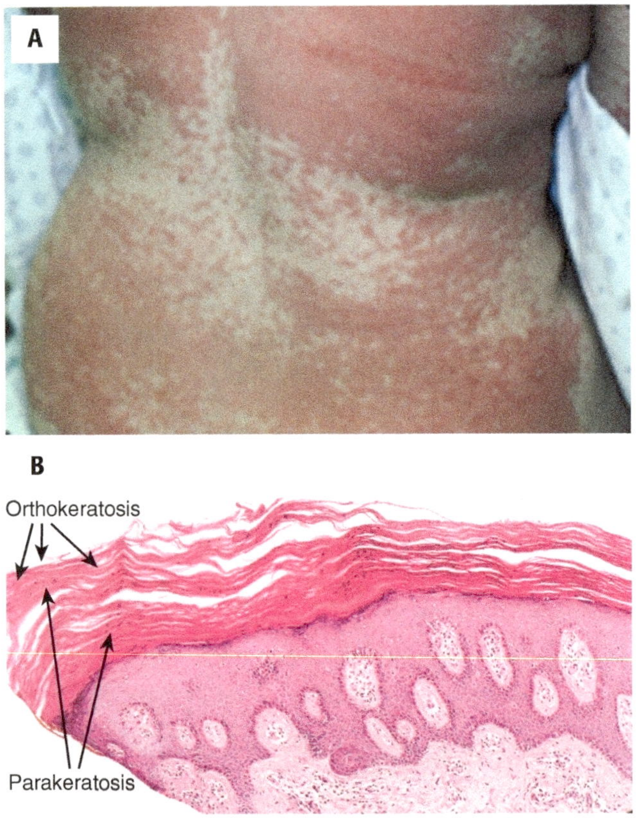

FIG. 1.11

Pityriasis rubra pilaris. **A,** Coalescent orange-red papules with islands of sparing. **B,** Alternating orthokeratosis and parakeratosis (checkerboard pattern), psoriasiform epidermal hyperplasia with preserved granular layer, and sparse superficial perivascular lymphocytes.

Differential Diagnosis

Compared with psoriasis, the epidermal hyperplasia in PRP is usually more irregular (rete ridges are more variable in length), the granular layer is preserved, and neutrophils in the stratum corneum are not typical of PRP. Follicular plugging is not characteristic of psoriasis. Focal acantholytic dyskeratosis may represent a somewhat characteristic finding in this histologic context but is not present in most examples of PRP.

The superficial dermal perivascular lymphocytes in PRP are typically sparse compared with psoriasis and chronic spongiotic dermatitis. If regressing chronic spongiotic dermatitis is sampled, the findings may be indistinguishable from PRP unless additional features, such as follicular plugging or a classic checkerboard pattern in the stratum corneum, are identified. When the histopathologic features are not diagnostic, clinical correlation is essential to establish the diagnosis.

Prognosis and Treatment

Classic, acquired, generalized PRP runs a chronic, waxing and waning course. Familial PRP persists throughout life. Therapy includes topical emollients and keratolytics; topical corticosteroids; IL17 or IL23 inhibitors, retinoids (including isotretinoin and acitretin); and for refractory cases, cyclosporine, low-dose methotrexate, or other systemic agents.

NECROLYTIC MIGRATORY ERYTHEMA

Clinical Findings

NME is a paraneoplastic reaction usually associated with an islet cell glucagon-secreting neuroendocrine pancreatic carcinoma (glucagonoma). Patients present with diabetes mellitus, weight loss, anemia, glossitis, and erythematous erosive desquamating plaques that tend to develop in flexural skin folds such as the groin and axilla (Fig. 1.12A).

Histologic Features

The histologic features are variable, but the most distinctive finding is pronounced pallor of the upper epidermis associated with necrolysis, which is characterized by vacuoles within the cytoplasm of superficial epidermal keratinocytes, resulting in confluent necrosis in the upper epidermis (Fig. 1.12B). Confluent/diffuse parakeratosis is usually present. Plaques in NME often exhibit psoriasiform hyperplasia. Other findings may include neutrophilic crust, neutrophilic spongiosis, subcorneal pustule formation (Fig. 1.12C), sparse eosinophils, or single necrotic keratinocytes.

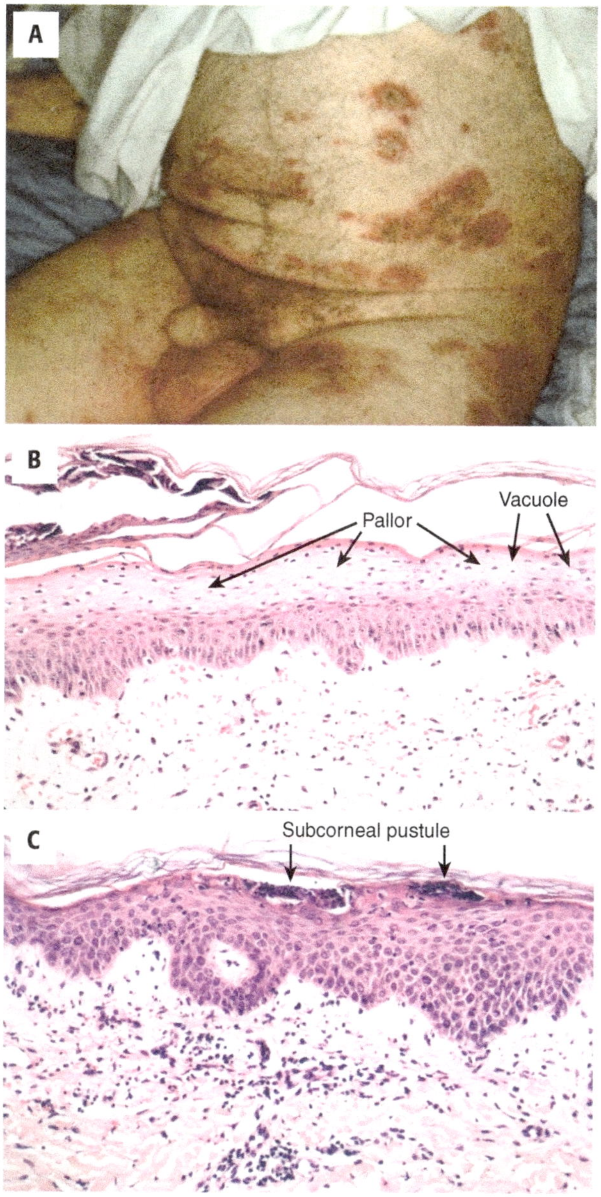

FIG. 1.12
Necrolytic migratory erythema (glucagonoma syndrome) in a 74-year-old man with markedly elevated serum glucagon level and pancreatic mass. **A,** Erythematous, erosive desquamating plaques in a flexural distribution. **B,** Initial biopsy revealed vacuolization and pronounced pallor in the superficial epidermis. Necrolysis is not yet evident. **C,** Subsequent biopsy revealed only focal subcorneal pustule formation. Thus, prominent necrolysis is not always a feature, and the findings may resemble psoriasis or other inflammatory disorders. Confluent/diffuse parakeratosis is characteristic but not shown.

Ancillary Studies

Serum glucagon levels are typically elevated. Imaging studies usually reveal a pancreatic mass lesion.

Differential Diagnosis

Psoriasis, particularly early lesions, and PRP may exhibit pallor in the upper epidermis but not to the degree that is achieved in the fullest expression of NME, wherein the accompanying necrolytic changes are quite distinctive. Necrolysis is not a feature of psoriasis or PRP. Other forms of deficiency dermatitis, such as zinc deficiency (acrodermatitis enteropathica), riboflavin, and niacin (vitamin B_3) deficiency (pellagra), may also exhibit necrolysis and keratinocyte pallor and are best distinguished based on clinical and laboratory features. Plasma cells may reflect chronicity or represent a clue to syphilis.

Prognosis and Treatment

Patients with NME often respond dramatically (within hours to days) to surgical removal of the glucagonoma. Patients are typically amino acid deficient, and intravenous amino acid infusion has also been associated with rapid resolution of the skin lesions.

INTERFACE DERMATITIS

Similar to spongiotic dermatitis and psoriasiform dermatitis, interface dermatitis is a descriptive phrase used by pathologists in dermatopathology reports that is not a specific disease entity (Table 1.3). Interface dermatitis describes a pattern of inflammation in which lymphocytes aggregate around and obscure the interface of the dermal-epidermal junction. T lymphocytes mediate damage to the basement membrane zone and the keratinocytes above them, the microscopic hallmarks being junctional vacuolar alteration and single keratinocyte necrosis. Vacuolar alteration is characterized by small, empty, round spaces of variable diameter along the dermal-epidermal junction. Necrotic keratinocytes exhibit homogeneous (nongranular) eosinophilic cytoplasm and a shrunken, pyknotic, intensely basophilic nucleus. Depending on the plane of the section, the nucleus may not be visible. In some examples of interface dermatitis, such as lichen planus (LP), the necrotic keratinocytes have been shown to be undergoing apoptosis. In other examples, such as acantholytic dyskeratosis (see Grover's disease or Darier's disease), similar-appearing cells are attributable to abnormal differentiation ("dyskeratosis"). Thus, from the standpoint of routine practice, necrotic, dyskeratotic, and apoptotic keratinocytes ("dead reds") are interchangeable when evaluating routine stained sections of a specimen without presumption of diagnosis. Secondary spongiosis is invariably present in interface dermatitis, but interface changes generally prevail over spongiosis for the purposes of differential diagnosis. Overlapping or combined patterns suggest a drug reaction. In addition to mild "secondary" spongiosis, limited exocytosis of lymphocytes into the epidermis is expected. Exocytosis is characteristically more prominent in pityriasis lichenoides (see Table 1.3) or viral exanthems.

Interface dermatitis is typically subdivided based on the pattern of inflammation (Ackerman), but

TABLE 1.3

Basic Differential Diagnosis of Interface Dermatitis

	Erythema Multiforme	Stevens-Johnson/Toxic Epidermal Necrolysis	Lichen Planus	Pityriasis Lichenoides	Lupus Erythematosus	Lichen Striatus	Graft versus Host Disease	Fixed Drug Reaction
Vacuolar interface	++	++	o	±	±	±	±	±
Lichenoid interface	±	o	++	±	±	±	±	±
Basilar squamatization	o	o	++	o	±	o	±	±
Deep perivascular inflammation	o	o	o	±	++	±	o	++
Follicular involvement	o	o	±	o	++	±	++	o
Eccrine involvement	o	o	o	o	++	++	±	o
Dermal eosinophils	o	±	±	o	o	±	o	++
Dermal neutrophils	o	±	o	o	±	o	o	±
Lymphocyte exocytosis	±	±	±	++	±	±	±	±
Erythrocyte extravasation	±	±	o	++	o	o	o	o
Epidermal necrosis	±	++	o	±	o	o	±	±

++, characteristic; ±, variable; o, unusual or not classic.

alternatively, it may be subdivided based on associated epidermal changes (LeBoit) as well as the predominant types of inflammatory cells. Classification based on associated epidermal changes is beyond the scope of this text but is recommended for those striving to master this subject. Based on the pattern of inflammation, vacuolar interface dermatitis is characterized by sparse lymphocytes along the dermal-epidermal junction with junctional vacuolar alteration and single and/or clustered necrotic keratinocytes. Erythema multiforme (EM) is considered a prototype for this pattern. Lichenoid interface reactions have a bandlike predominantly lymphocytic infiltrate along the dermal-epidermal junction, sometimes filling the entire papillary dermis. LP is the prototype for lichenoid dermatitis. Thus, the term *lichenoid* has both a clinical meaning (lesions resembling lichen, typified by LP) and a histologic one (lesions with a bandlike lymphocytic infiltrate below the dermal-epidermal junction). Less commonly, lymphocytes forming a bandlike pattern in the papillary dermis with minimal or absent vacuolar alteration or necrotic keratinocytes may still be classified as lichenoid dermatitis, e.g., the lichenoid variant of pigmented purpura (lichenoid purpura of Gougerot and Blum).

ERYTHEMA MULTIFORME, STEVENS-JOHNSON SYNDROME, AND TOXIC EPIDERMAL NECROLYSIS

Clinical Findings

EM encompasses a wide clinical spectrum of severity. The three disorders included under this heading are clinically distinct. Classic EM ("EM minor" if no mucosal involvement; "EM major" if mucosa is involved) is also considered pathogenetically distinct from Stevens-Johnson syndrome (SJS) and toxic epidermal necrolysis (TEN), but all three are united here because they cannot be distinguished based on histology alone. EM is an acute, self-limited, benign disorder characterized by targetoid papules, papulovesicles, or plaques on the extremities and trunk, often with involvement of the palms. Classic targetoid lesions have a dusky or violaceous center surrounded by two concentric rings or zones of pallor and erythema (Fig. 1.13A). As the name suggests, multiple morphologies are possible, including bullous lesions (Fig. 1.13B). EM is most commonly associated with the HSV carrier state, and outbreaks may be accompanied by cold sores

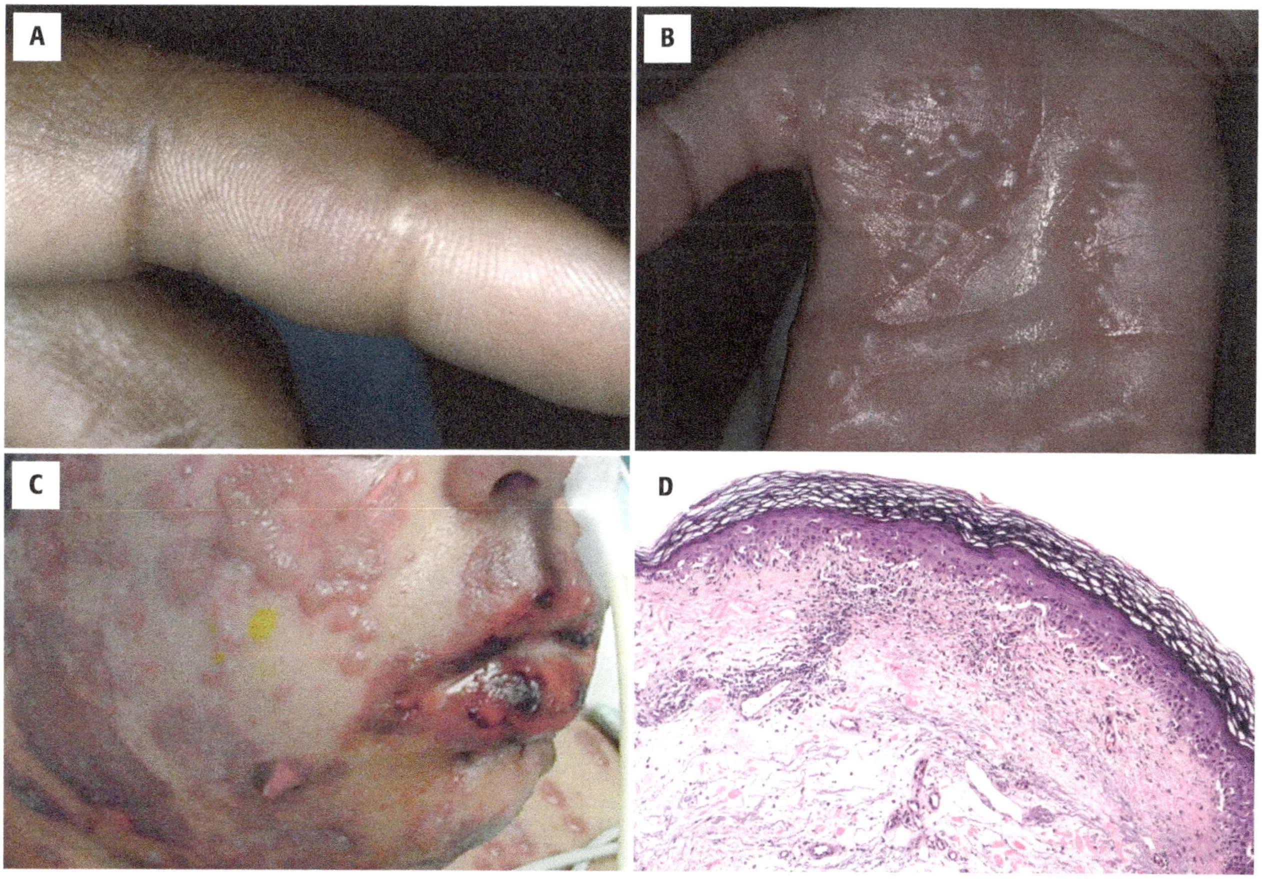

FIG. 1.13

Erythema multiforme (EM) and Stevens-Johnson syndrome (SJS). **A,** Targetoid papule on the lateral finger that resolved with acyclovir therapy. **B,** Bullous eruption on the palms associated with a cold sore. **C,** Hemorrhagic crusted lesion with lip involvement in SJS. **D,** Basket-weave orthokeratosis, vacuolar interface dermatitis, and superficial lymphocytes in the dermis.

Continued

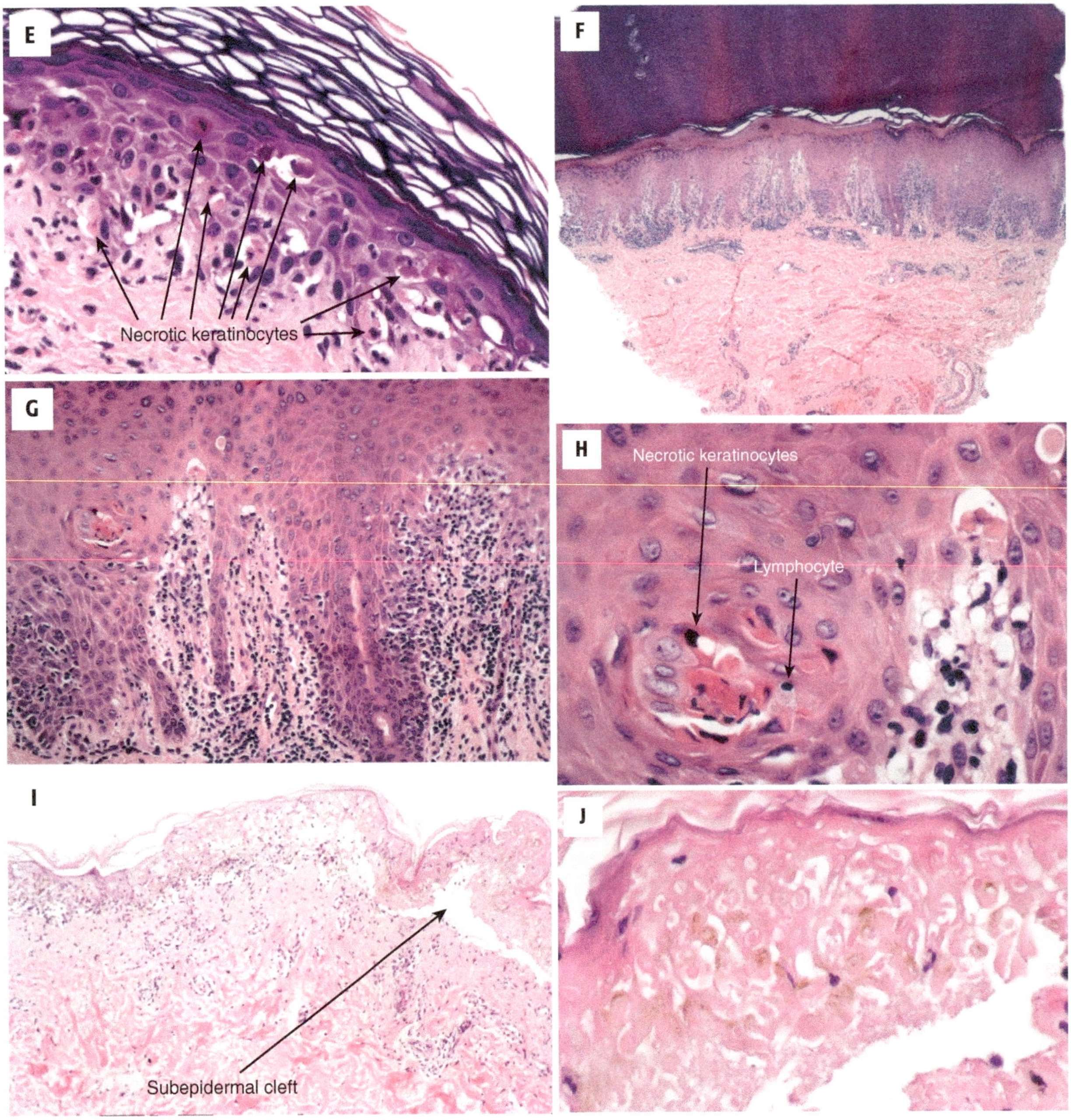

FIG. 1.13, cont'd

E, Prominent single necrotic keratinocytes at all levels of the epidermis. **F,** Biopsy from the patient in part A reveals a sparse lichenoid infiltrate. **G,** Prominent keratinocyte necrosis. **H,** Satellite cell necrosis. **I** and **J,** SJS is characterized by confluent epidermal necrosis and subepidermal clefting. These changes are indistinguishable from some cases of bullous EM. In toxic epidermal necrolysis, inflammation tends to be minimal, but biopsy of perilesional skin may reveal changes indistinguishable from SJS or bullous EM.

or reactivation of latent HSV by ultraviolet light exposure. SJS is a severe acute generalized reaction characterized by involvement of multiple mucosal sites (oral, ocular, genital) in which the disease manifests with prominent hemorrhagic crusting (Fig. 1.13C). Associated discrete or coalescent variably purpuric atypical targetoid lesions (two zones, rather than three) may coexist on the trunk and extremities. SJS is usually associated with recent drug exposure but may also be triggered by infection, including *Mycoplasma pneumoniae*. TEN is the most severe reaction, defined as widespread sloughing of the epidermal surface on greater than 30% of the total body surface area. Between 10% and 30% surface area involvement has been classified as SJS/TEN overlap. TEN is characterized by disproportionate sloughing with minimal erythema compared with EM minor or SJS; a recently introduced medication is the typical trigger, and several are highly associated (e.g., allopurinol, phenobarbital, sulfamethoxazole). Assessment of

ERYTHEMA MULTIFORME—DISEASE FACT SHEET

Erythema multiforme shows similar histologic features but is clinically distinct from Stevens-Johnson syndrome and toxic epidermal necrolysis.

Patient Group

- ▸▸ Most often young adults but may occur at any age
- ▸▸ Eruption triggered by infection (herpes simplex virus most common) or medication

Site of Involvement

- ▸▸ Extremities (usually upper, especially the dorsum of hands and forearms)
- ▸▸ Face

Clinical Findings

- ▸▸ Abrupt onset of classic target lesions (acrofacial sites)
- ▸▸ Erythematous urticarial papules and plaques
- ▸▸ Coalescence of lesions produces a polycyclic appearance

Prognosis and Treatment

- ▸▸ Acute self-limited disease
- ▸▸ Acyclovir or valacyclovir if associated with herpes simplex

prognosis may be facilitated by the SCORTEN clinical/laboratory score.

Histologic Features

Because EM is acute, there is usually basket-weave orthokeratosis and vacuolar interface dermatitis with prominent necrosis of single and clustered necrotic keratinocytes both along and above the basal layer (Fig. 1.13D and E). Prominent reactions may display a denser lichenoid infiltrate from scanning magnification (Fig. 1.13F–H), but junctional vacuolar alteration and keratinocyte necrosis remain prominent, and sparse superficial perivascular lymphocytes in the upper dermis are usual. When lymphocytes are juxtaposed against necrotic keratinocytes, the term *satellite cell necrosis* has been used (Fig. 1.13H). (Satellite cell necrosis is also seen in other acute interface reactions and is not specific for EM.) Dermal eosinophils are typically rare or absent. In bullous variants, confluent keratinocyte necrosis and junctional vacuolar alteration result in full-thickness epidermal necrosis and subepidermal blistering (Fig. 1.13I and J). Marked papillary dermal edema is less commonly a second means by which subepidermal blistering may occur. In TEN, perilesional skin may reveal changes indistinguishable from EM or SJS. However, in TEN, there is rapid progression to full-thickness epidermal necrosis and widespread subepidermal blistering and sloughing typically associated with sparse lymphocytes relative to typical EM or SJS.

ERYTHEMA MULTIFORME—PATHOLOGIC FEATURES

Histologic Features

- ▸▸ Acute vacuolar interface dermatitis
- ▸▸ Epidermal necrosis, variable
- ▸▸ May be associated with a secondary subepidermal blister

Differential Diagnosis

- ▸▸ Stevens-Johnson syndrome/toxic epidermal necrolysis (distinction requires clinical context: prodrome of upper respiratory tract syndrome, mucous membrane involvement, extensive exfoliation, association with medication use)
- ▸▸ Erythema multiforme-like graft versus host disease
- ▸▸ Rowell syndrome (erythema multiforme-like lesions in patients with lupus erythematosus)

Ancillary Studies

Frozen section analysis of a freshly formed blister roof can facilitate rapid distinction between TEN and staphylococcal scalded skin syndrome.

Differential Diagnosis

Although their clinical contexts tend to be mutually exclusive, acute graft versus host disease (GVHD) may be histologically indistinguishable from EM/SJS/TEN. GVHD is more likely to exhibit extension of the vacuolar interface reaction within the adnexal epithelium. A frequent clinical differential diagnosis is TEN versus staphylococcal scalded skin syndrome. The latter exhibits a superficial intraepidermal cleavage plane, as per pemphigus foliaceus (see "Ancillary Studies"). Fixed drug reactions may exhibit similar epidermal changes to EM but usually exhibit neutrophils and/or eosinophils, may exhibit greater spongiosis, and the inflammation typically involves the deep vascular plexus in the reticular dermis. After repeated episodes, fixed drug reactions also typically contain increased melanophages in the papillary dermis. Pityriasis lichenoides usually exhibit neutrophilic crust, greater lymphocyte exocytosis, and erythrocyte extravasation in the papillary dermis with deep perivascular extension of lymphocytes. However, early lesions of pityriasis lichenoides et varioliformis acuta (PLEVA) may resemble EM. Acute cutaneous lupus erythematosus (LE) may also resemble EM. Acute lupus usually exhibits compact orthokeratosis, epidermal atrophy, relatively sparse single necrotic keratinocytes, and increased interstitial mucin in the reticular dermis. Chemotherapy-induced interface dermatitis may contain cytologically atypical keratinocytes. Finally, consistent with its etiologic role in EM, HSV and varicella zoster virus infections usually exhibit vacuolar interface dermatitis extending along the dermal-epidermal junction peripheral to viral cytopathologic changes within the epidermis and/or follicular epithelium.

Prognosis and Treatment

EM is self-limited, but episodes may recur chronically. Sun protection and avoidance may minimize HSV outbreaks. Episodic or suppressive systemic antiviral therapy is usually helpful. SJS and TEN are debilitating and potentially life-threatening conditions that warrant hospitalization. Because of the significant morbidity and mortality and special management challenges associated with TEN, these patients are optimally managed in a surgical intensive care burn unit to use frequent dressing changes, management of fluid and electrolyte status, and monitoring for and treatment of sepsis (the most frequent cause of death). The mortality rate may approach 10% to 25%. The role of systemic corticosteroids in the acute management of SJS and TEN is controversial though historically frequently administered. Cyclosporine, intravenous immune globulin plus systemic corticosteroids, and the tumor necrosis factor inhibitor, etanercept, represent additional therapeutic options.

FIXED DRUG REACTION

Clinical Findings

Fixed drug reactions are round, erythematous or violaceous macules or patches that occur on one or a few fixed sites repetitively after repeat exposure to the offending agent. Atypical variants include generalized or bullous fixed drug reactions. Tetracycline, penicillin, acetaminophen, aspirin, nonsteroidal antiinflammatory agents, dapsone, benzodiazepines, and barbiturates are commonly implicated culprits. The face, extremities, and genitalia are common sites, but any site may be involved. The lesions may vesiculate (Fig. 1.14A). Postinflammatory hyperpigmentation persists for several weeks to months after a single exposure to the offending agent. With repeat exposure, persistent pigmentation intensifies, and additional sites may manifest. The pigmentation is said to have a mercurochrome hue owing to the combination of erythema superimposed on post inflammatory hyperpigmentation.

Histologic Features

Fixed drug reactions display junctional vacuolar alteration, single or clustered necrotic keratinocytes within the basal and often upper levels of the epidermis (Fig. 1.14B). Spongiosis is variable but may predominate. Confluent epidermal necrosis is associated with subepidermal cleavage in bullous fixed drug reactions. The dermis contains superficial or superficial and deep perivascular lymphocytes, usually with eosinophils, neutrophils, or both. After repeated flares, melanophages are prominent in the papillary dermis. Vasculitis may be present.

Differential Diagnosis

The epidermal changes in EM may be indistinguishable from those of fixed drug reactions. Clues that may favor fixed drug reaction include melanophages, psoriasiform epidermal hyperplasia, a retained polygonal configuration of the necrotic keratinocytes in the stratum spinosum, and greater spongiosis. Fixed drug reactions are more likely than EM to involve the deep dermal perivascular plexus and contain eosinophils, neutrophils, or both. In the context of vacuolar interface dermatitis,

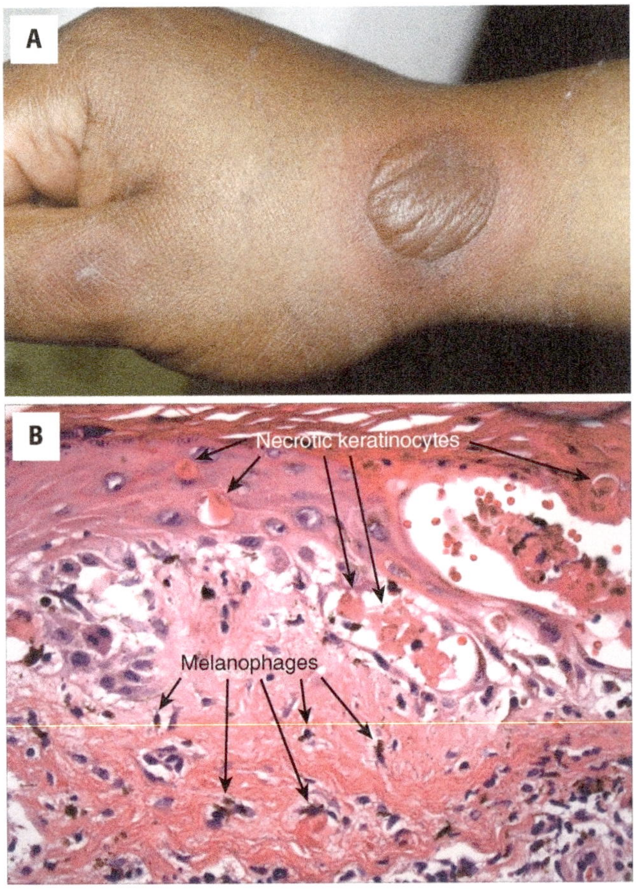

FIG. 1.14

Fixed drug reaction. **A,** Dusky red, hemorrhagic, bullous, round plaque on the wrist. Smaller lesion on the thumb. **B,** Vacuolar and lichenoid interface dermatitis with prominent necrotic keratinocytes. Dermal eosinophils are expected (but not required). Melanophages are often prominent.

prominent melanophages are generally a clue to the diagnosis of a fixed drug reaction.

Prognosis and Treatment

Fixed drug reactions usually resolve within several days. However, with repeat exposure to the offending agent, progressive hyperpigmentation persists. Generalized lesions may develop rarely. Avoidance of the offending drug is curative.

LICHEN PLANUS

Clinical Findings

LP is a relatively common disorder characterized by flat-topped erythematous or violaceous, pruritic papules most commonly involving the wrists or ankles in a symmetric fashion. The papules classically have an angulated or polygonal shape (Fig. 1.15A). Reticulated white lines may be appreciated on the surface of the papules, known as Wickham striae. Oral and genital skin are also

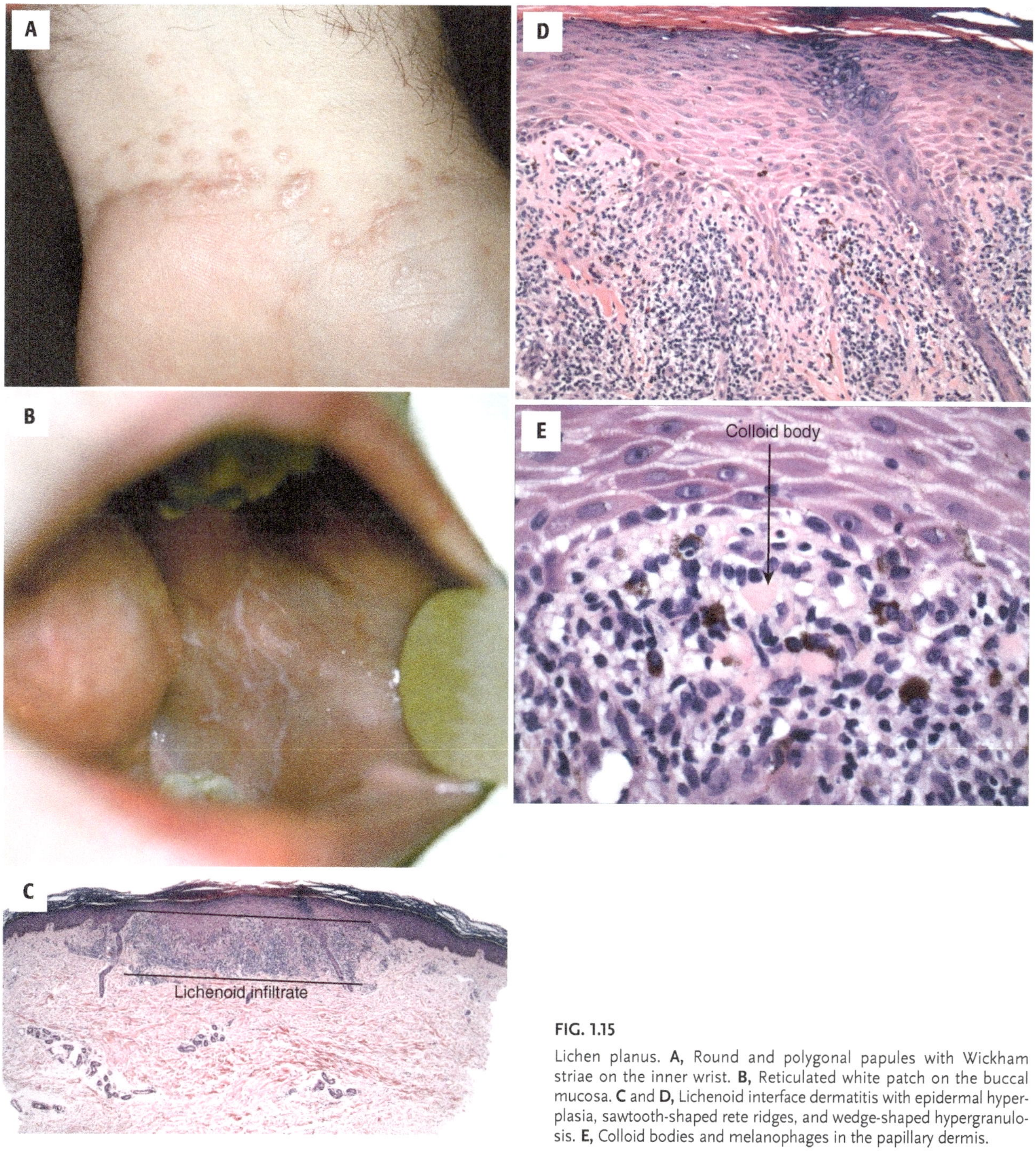

FIG. 1.15

Lichen planus. **A,** Round and polygonal papules with Wickham striae on the inner wrist. **B,** Reticulated white patch on the buccal mucosa. **C** and **D,** Lichenoid interface dermatitis with epidermal hyperplasia, sawtooth-shaped rete ridges, and wedge-shaped hypergranulosis. **E,** Colloid bodies and melanophages in the papillary dermis.

LICHEN PLANUS—DISEASE FACT SHEET

Patient Group

- Usually middle-aged adults (onset usually between ages 30 and 60 years)

Site of Involvement

- Oral mucosa (up to 75% of patients)
- Skin of the wrist, forearm, genitalia, distal lower extremity

Clinical Findings

- Classic skin lesions: flat-topped violaceous papules and plaques
- Variants: linear, bullous, hypertrophic, atrophic, annular skin lesions
- Wickham striae (network of fine white lines on the surface of lesions)
- Mucosa: reticular pattern (most common) of whitish linear streaks; atrophic, erosive, papular, or plaque lesions
- Nail: lateral thinning, longitudinal ridging, fissuring pterygium

Prognosis

- Clinical course variable (self-limited to chronic persistent)
- Ulcerative oral, hypertrophic, and nail lichen planus tend to persist

Treatment

- Corticosteroids
- Retinoids
- Phototherapy

commonly involved. In oral LP, the Wickham striae may be the most prominent finding (Fig. 1.15B). Involvement of the nail unit may result in pterygium formation. Hypertrophic LP is common on the shins. In dark-complected individuals, the erythema may be subtle, with hyperpigmentation as the predominant feature. In lichen planopilaris (follicular LP), the disorder is centered on the lower infundibulum and isthmus of hair follicles, where scarring alopecia may result. Annular, atrophic, vesiculobullous, actinic, erosive, and hyperpigmented LP are other clinical variants. An association with hepatitis C virus (HCV) infection has been documented. Two rare overlap syndromes are the LP-LE overlap and LP pemphigoides.

Histologic Features

Fully developed LP is the prototype of lichenoid interface dermatitis, typified by a dense lichenoid (bandlike) infiltrate obscuring the dermal-epidermal junction (Fig. 1.15C–E). The epidermal changes are most characteristic. Classic LP exhibits compact orthokeratosis, wedge-shaped hypergranulosis overlying jagged, sawtooth-shaped rete ridges, and squamatization of the basal layer (basilar squamatization). Squamatization of the basal layer refers to the flattening of basilar keratinocytes, resembling the physiologic flattening of keratinocytes in the stratum granulosum just prior to terminal differentiation into the stratum corneum. Basilar squamatization is often best appreciated in areas where the rete ridges exhibit a jagged or sawtooth shape and overlying hypergranulosis provides optimal contrast. The areas of hypergranulosis represent an exaggeration of the physiologic hypergranulosis associated with the adnexal (follicular, sweat duct) epithelium. In hypertrophic LP, there is even greater epidermal hyperplasia with acanthosis, variable papillomatosis, and elongated rete ridges. In atrophic LP, there may be attenuation of the rete ridges and a thinned, atrophic epidermis resembling lupus. In hypertrophic LP, which is typically very pruritic, there is epidermal hyperplasia with papillomatosis and often papillary dermal fibrosis secondary to chronic rubbing. In mucosal LP, the epidermal changes may be less specific, with rounded rather than pointed rete ridges and parakeratosis. In all variants, the lichenoid infiltrate is composed predominantly of lymphocytes. Melanophages are usually present. Pertinent negative findings include the absence of prominent dermal eosinophils and the absence of deep perivascular extension of the dermal infiltrate. Hypertrophic LP may exhibit greater numbers of eosinophils. Mucosal LP usually contains some plasma cells that may be attributable to the mucosal site. The apoptotic keratinocytes exhibit homogeneous eosinophilic cytoplasm and sometimes a pyknotic basophilic nucleus (the nucleus may not be observed depending on the plane of the section). They are mostly present along the dermal-epidermal junction but may also be found in the upper levels of the epidermis or in the papillary dermal lichenoid infiltrate. In the context of LP, the anucleate remnants of these apoptotic keratinocytes have been named Civatte bodies (colloid bodies, cytoid bodies) when present in the papillary dermis. Focal subepidermal clefts formed by confluent vacuoles have been termed Max-Joseph spaces.

LICHEN PLANUS—PATHOLOGIC FEATURES

Histologic Features

- Epidermal hyperplasia with compact orthokeratosis, hypergranulosis, and lichenoid (bandlike) lymphocytic infiltrate
- Sawtoothing of rete ridges
- Civatte bodies

Ancillary Studies

- If crust or eosinophils are present, consider PAS stain to exclude dermatophyte
- Direct immunofluorescence: basement membrane zone linear/shaggy fibrinogen

Differential Diagnosis

- Lichen planus-like keratosis
- Lichenoid drug reaction (distinction best done clinically: nonclassic sites involved, mucous membranes often spared; history of medication use)

Ancillary Studies

Although biopsy is typically performed to confirm the diagnosis of LP, DIF studies are not routinely required to establish the diagnosis. However, immunofluorescence studies routinely show linear "shaggy" fibrinogen along the junction and globular deposition of IgM at the dermal-epidermal junction (Civatte bodies). LP may be associated with HCV infection in fewer than 30% of cases.

Differential Diagnosis

LP may be histologically indistinguishable from an LP-like keratosis (lichenoid keratosis, benign lichenoid keratosis), but the clinical setting is usually sufficient to distinguish these two disorders. Whereas LP is characterized by multiple lesions and is usually sampled by punch (trephine) biopsy, LP-like keratoses are solitary lesions, most commonly on the trunk of an adult, and are sampled by shave biopsy to rule out carcinoma. Compared with LP, LP-like keratosis usually exhibits some parakeratosis and does not invariably contain the distinctive epidermal changes (basilar squamatization, jagged rete, wedge-shaped hypergranulosis) requisite for LP. Lichenoid drug reactions (e.g., thiazide diuretics, beta-blockers, antimalarials, furosemide, spironolactone) also tend to exhibit parakeratosis, dermal eosinophils, and deep dermal perivascular extension. Lichenoid drug reactions also do not invariably contain the epidermal changes of LP, and single necrotic keratinocytes may be present in the upper epidermis, including the stratum corneum. Lichenoid variants of the pigmented purpuric dermatoses, including lichenoid purpura (Gougerot-Blum) and lichen aureus, contain extravasated erythrocytes or hemosiderin-containing histiocytes (siderophages), whose pigment can be highlighted by hemosiderin stain if needed. The lichenoid variant of chronic GVHD may resemble LP clinically and histopathologically; clinical correlation is required. In lichenoid GVHD, the lichenoid infiltrate is typically sparse, and dermal eosinophils or plasma cells may be present. Discoid LE may exhibit basilar squamatization but, additionally, epithelial atrophy, basement membrane thickening, deeper and denser perivascular and perifollicular lymphocytes (usually devoid of eosinophils), and increased interstitial mucin deposition in the reticular dermis. Some instances in which features of both LP and lupus were present have been termed *lupus erythematosus-LP overlap*. Lichen striatus may resemble LP but typically exhibits lymphocytes with admixed histiocytes and, most distinctively, perieccrine lymphocytes. Lichen nitidus exhibits a ball-in-claw configuration of rete ridges surrounding the lichenoid lymphohistiocytic infiltrate that may exhibit granulomatous features with prominent histiocytes, some multinucleated. Lichenoid mucositis secondary to candida exhibits spongiosis, neutrophilic pustules, eosinophils, and pseudohyphae within the superficial epithelium.

Prognosis and Treatment

LP typically runs a chronic but self-limited course, often resolving after 3 to 5 years. Therapeutic options include potent topical and/or intralesional corticosteroids; short courses of systemic corticosteroids; photochemotherapy; systemic retinoids; and, for refractory cases, other systemic immune suppressive agents. Chronic erosive lesions should be examined regularly to rule out secondary squamous cell carcinoma.

PITYRIASIS LICHENOIDES

Clinical Findings

Pityriasis lichenoides is an idiopathic disorder that can be viewed as a clinical and histopathologic spectrum with the clinical disorders PLEVA (Mucha-Habermann disease) and pityriasis lichenoides chronica (PLC). PLEVA usually affects children and young adults, with widespread vesicles and hemorrhagic, erythematous, minimally symptomatic papules that ulcerate and leave focal varioliform (smallpox-like) scars (Fig. 1.16A and B). Plaques or patches are not a feature. A rare but severe hyperacute ulceronecrotic variant of PLEVA is characterized by fever, constitutional symptoms, and larger ulcerations and has been associated with Epstein-Barr virus or cytomegalovirus infections. PLC runs a mild chronic course with randomly scattered, minimally symptomatic erythematous papules in children or adults. PLC typically does not ulcerate or scar. Cases with intermediate or overlapping features of PLEVA and PLC may occur.

Histologic Features

Pityriasis lichenoides et varioliformis acuta is characterized by parakeratotic neutrophilic crust, vacuolar interface dermatitis with lymphocyte exocytosis, papillary dermal hemorrhage, and superficial and deep wedge-shaped lymphocytic infiltrates (Fig. 1.16C and D). Despite the characteristic neutrophilic crust in PLEVA, neutrophilic spongiosis or dermal neutrophilia are not prominent. Eosinophils are usually absent. Fully developed lesions have a lichenoid and perivascular/periadnexal infiltrate of lymphocytes, sometimes with evidence of lymphocytic vasculitis. In PLC, the lymphocytes tend to be sparser and

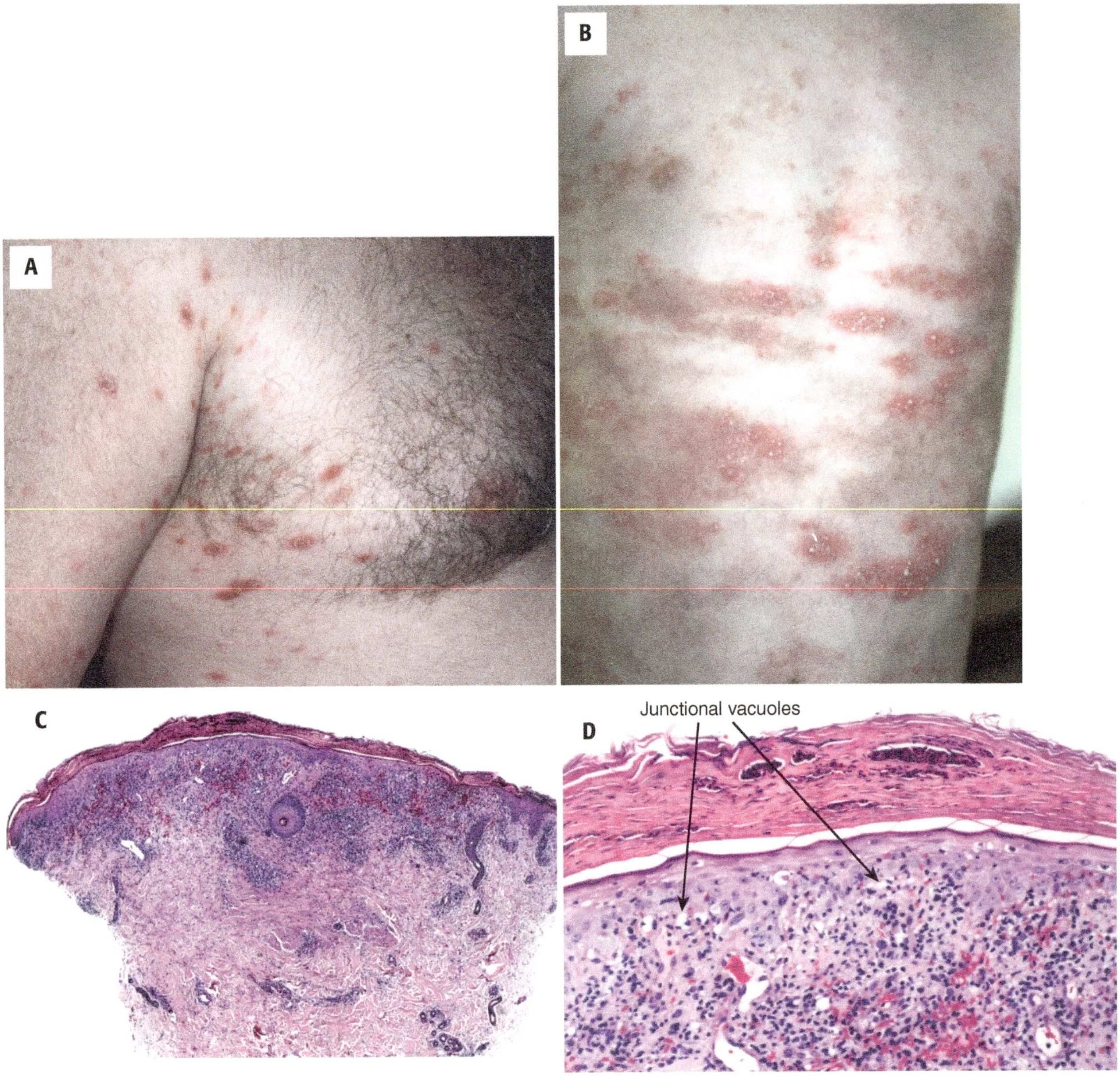

FIG. 1.16

Pityriasis lichenoides. **A,** Erythematous papules on the trunk and extremities. **B,** Papulovesicles in pityriasis lichenoides et varioliformis acuta (Mucha Habermann disease). **C,** Scanning magnification reveals lichenoid interface dermatitis associated with a dense wedge-shaped lymphocytic infiltrate with deep perivascular and periadnexal extension and erythrocyte extravasation in the upper dermis. **D,** Higher magnification reveals neutrophilic crust, lymphocyte exocytosis, junctional vacuolar alteration, necrotic keratinocytes, and erythrocyte extravasation. Eosinophils are rare/absent.

confined to the upper dermis. Parakeratosis, interface dermatitis, and lymphocyte exocytosis are usually present, but a neutrophilic crust and erythrocyte extravasation may be minimal or absent.

Differential Diagnosis

PR may resemble pityriasis lichenoides. Both conditions may exhibit overlapping spongiotic and interface features with lymphocyte exocytosis and erythrocyte extravasation. However, epidermal changes in PR are predominantly spongiotic, whereas, in pityriasis lichenoides, they are predominantly interface. The presence of a neutrophilic crust—dense, deep dermal perivascular involvement—or lymphocytic vasculitis favors PLEVA over PR. The neutrophilic crust is also typical of psoriasis, spongiotic dermatitis, and dermatophytosis, but interface dermatitis is not typical of any of these, and histochemical staining for fungi will identify rare cases of dermatophytosis manifesting an interface reaction.

Pityriasis lichenoides should not contain atypical lymphocytes. In the past, the designation *lymphomatoid pityriasis lichenoides* was proposed. However, if atypical lymphocytes with convoluted or cerebriform nuclear contours are present, lymphomatoid papulosis or MF should be suspected. If scattered large atypical CD30-positive lymphocytes with prominent nucleoli are present in the dermis, lymphomatoid papulosis (type A pattern) should be suspected. If small to medium convoluted or cerebriform lymphocytes are present within the epidermis, then lymphomatoid papulosis (type B pattern) is a consideration. Lymphocyte exocytosis without overt atypia may be observed in both pityriasis lichenoides and patches of MF. In MF, lymphocytes tend to aggregate in the basilar epidermis, and necrotic keratinocytes, vacuolar alteration, and spongiosis are usually not prominent. Prominent eosinophils are not typical of pityriasis lichenoides or early patch-stage MF. In pityriasis lichenoides, intraepidermal lymphocytes are scattered throughout all levels of the epidermis with greater spongiosis or interface changes, and deep perivascular lymphocytes are typical.

Prognosis and Treatment

Pityriasis lichenoides et varioliformis acuta is usually self-limited. Therapeutic options include topical corticosteroids, phototherapy, and oral erythromycin or tetracyclines. Longitudinal observation is advisable because refractory "pityriasis lichenoides" may represent lymphomatoid papulosis or MF.

LUPUS ERYTHEMATOSUS

Clinical Findings

LE is a systemic autoimmune disorder that exhibits both specific and nonspecific cutaneous manifestations (e.g., leukocytoclastic vasculitis, livedo reticularis). The specific lesions can be classified into acute, subacute, and chronic cutaneous LE. Whereas acute cutaneous lesions are usually associated with systemic lupus, systemic involvement in subacute or chronic cutaneous lupus lesions may be milder or, in the case of chronic lesions, usually absent. Acute cutaneous lupus lesions include the localized malar (butterfly) rash or more generalized morbilliform (measles-like) eruptions that may extend to involve the dorsal fingers, characteristically sparing the skin overlying the interphalangeal joints. Subacute lesions have a predilection for the trunk and upper extremities and are typically scaly, erythematous, circumscribed plaques with an annular or psoriasiform appearance. Neonatal LE morphologically, histopathologically, and serologically resembles subacute LE lesions but has a tendency to involve the scalp (Fig. 1.17A). The most common chronic cutaneous manifestation is discoid lupus, characterized by circumscribed scaly atrophic plaques on the head, neck, or upper trunk that frequently produce atrophy, dyspigmented scars, and follicular plugging (Fig. 1.17B). Systemic LE (SLE) and subacute LE may rarely produce nonscarring alopecia, but discoid LE usually produces scarring alopecia when it involves the scalp. Variants of chronic cutaneous LE include LE profundus (lupus panniculitis), which involves the subcutaneous fat and manifests as indurated, variably ulcerated deep-seated plaques usually above the waist, and tumid lupus erythematosus, characterized by smooth, infiltrated erythematous plaques with minimal to absent epidermal involvement. Bullous LE represents a rare manifestation of acute LE and is discussed elsewhere.

CUTANEOUS LUPUS ERYTHEMATOSUS—DISEASE FACT SHEET

Patient Group

- Adults; female predominance
- More common in the Black population than White

Site of Involvement

- Often face, scalp, ears (discoid LE)
- May occur anywhere (variable)

Clinical Findings

- Acute cutaneous LE
  - Malar erythema (butterfly rash)
- Subacute cutaneous LE
  - Annular or psoriasiform lesions
  - Papulosquamous lesions
- Chronic cutaneous LE
  - Discoid LE (most common form of chronic cutaneous LE)
    - Erythematous scaly plaques
    - Atrophy and hyperpigmentation common
    - May result in scarring
    - Hypertrophic/verrucous variant exists
  - Tumid LE
    - Indurated erythematous plaques without scale
  - Panniculitis (lupus profundus)
    - Subcutaneous nodules
  - Chilblain lupus
    - Red or purple papules/plaques on the nose or acral sites
- Other variants
  - Bullous LE
  - Erythema multiforme-like (Rowell syndrome)
  - Neonatal LE (infants from mothers with anti-Ro antibodies manifest subacute cutaneous LE-like lesions)

Prognosis

- Acute cutaneous LE is usually associated with systemic LE
- Most patients with subacute and chronic forms of cutaneous LE do not have significant systemic disease

Treatment

- Corticosteroids
- Antimalarials
- Sun protection

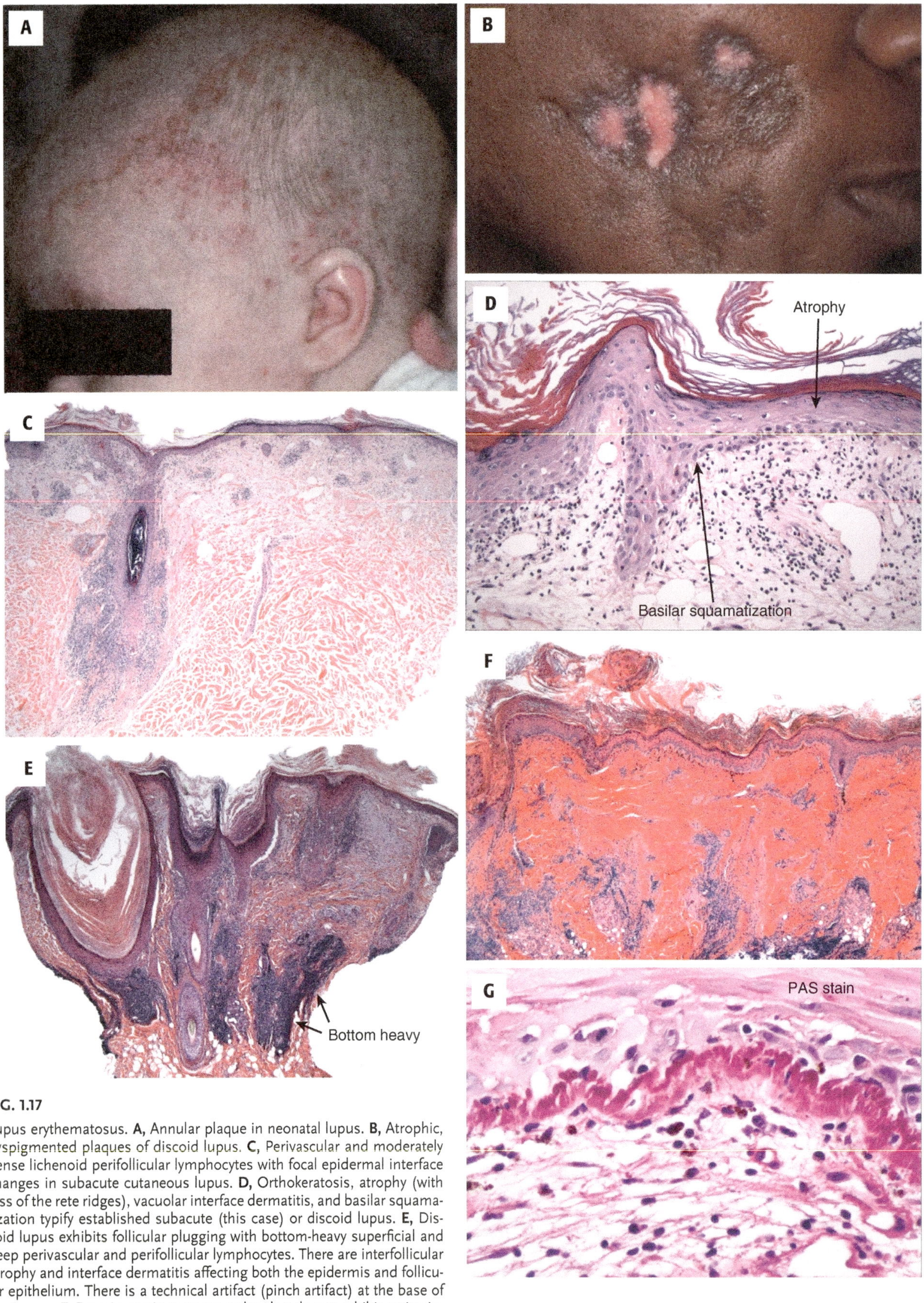

FIG. 1.17

Lupus erythematosus. **A,** Annular plaque in neonatal lupus. **B,** Atrophic, dyspigmented plaques of discoid lupus. **C,** Perivascular and moderately dense lichenoid perifollicular lymphocytes with focal epidermal interface changes in subacute cutaneous lupus. **D,** Orthokeratosis, atrophy (with loss of the rete ridges), vacuolar interface dermatitis, and basilar squamatization typify established subacute (this case) or discoid lupus. **E,** Discoid lupus exhibits follicular plugging with bottom-heavy superficial and deep perivascular and perifollicular lymphocytes. There are interfollicular atrophy and interface dermatitis affecting both the epidermis and follicular epithelium. There is a technical artifact (pinch artifact) at the base of the image. **F,** Even in sections or examples that do not exhibit active interface dermatitis, the balance of the dermal inflammation is centered in the deep dermis and surrounds adnexal structures. **G,** Basement membrane thickening may be highlighted by periodic acid-Schiff stain.

Histologic Features

All forms of LE, with the exception of many cases of tumid LE and LE profundus, are characterized by interface dermatitis, with single necrotic keratinocytes and vacuolar alteration at the dermal-epidermal junction. There is compact or lamellar ortho(hyper)keratosis, yet the stratum malpighi is often atrophic. In acute LE, subacute LE, neonatal LE, and early discoid LE, dermal lymphocytes may be sparse enough that a vacuolar, rather than lichenoid pattern, and a superficial, rather than superficial and deep pattern, are observed (Fig. 1.17C and D). Fully developed lesions exhibit moderately dense superficial and deep perivascular and periadnexal (perifollicular and perieccrine) lymphocytes, generally devoid of eosinophils. Plasma cells are typically present. Interstitial acid mucopolysaccharide (mucin) is typically increased. More variable findings include fibrin thrombi or lymphocytic leukocytoclastic debris (nuclear dust) within and around vessels (lymphocytic vasculitis) or in the subepidermal or subcutaneous zones. Discoid lesions exhibit follicular plugging and basilar squamatization (see "Lichen Planus") (Fig. 1.17D–G). Discoid lesions may also exhibit papillated or verrucous epithelial hyperplasia. In acute, subacute, and especially chronic discoid LE, the PAS-positive basement membrane may be thickened. In tumid LE, moderately dense perivascular and periadnexal lymphocytes are associated with increased interstitial mucin deposition in the reticular dermis, but overlying interface changes are minimal or absent. LE profundus is characterized by lymphocytes in the lobules of the subcutaneous fat and a hyaline-type homogeneous eosinophilic necrosis of the fat lobules. As in tumid LE, overlying interface dermatitis may be limited or absent. Unlike other forms of LE, in lupus profundus, eosinophils are often present. Bullous LE is characterized by subepidermal vesiculation with neutrophils. These latter two variants are discussed in detail elsewhere.

Ancillary Studies

Serum antinuclear antibody titers are positive in most cases of SLE but are usually negative when LE is confined to the skin. Subacute LE is associated with anti-Ro or anti-La antibodies. Continuous granular or linear deposition of IgG, IgM, IgA, or C3 along the dermal-epidermal junction by DIF represents the lupus band test. Lesional lupus bands are observed in most cases of acute, subacute, and chronic LE. Nonlesional lupus bands from sun-protected sites are specific for SLE.

CUTANEOUS LUPUS ERYTHEMATOSUS—PATHOLOGIC FEATURES

Histologic Features

- Interface dermatitis
- Variable epidermal thickness, often atrophy
- Hyperkeratosis (discoid LE)[1]
- Follicular plugging (discoid LE)[1]
- Basement membrane thickening (discoid LE)[1]
- Moderately dense superficial and deep perivascular lymphocytic infiltrate
- Periadnexal lymphocytic infiltrate (discoid LE)[1]
- Melanophages in superficial dermis
- Increased interstitial mucin deposition in reticular dermis
- Mild vascular damage may be seen

Ancillary Studies

- Special stains are not usually required but may assist
  - PAS or PAS-D stain to highlight thickened basement membrane zone
  - Alcian blue or colloidal iron stain to highlight interstitial mucin
- Lupus band test: direct immunofluorescence[1]
  - Granular or linear IgG, IgA, IgM, or C3 at the dermal-epidermal junction (lesional in all forms of LE; nonlesional in systemic LE)

Differential Diagnosis

- Drug reaction
- Lichen planus
- Lichenoid keratosis
- Polymorphous light eruption
- Tumid LE: erythema migrans (Lyme disease)
- Hypertrophic discoid LE: squamous cell carcinoma
- Lupus profundus: primary cutaneous subcutaneous panniculitis-like T-cell lymphoma

Ig, Immunoglobulin; *LE*, lupus erythematosus; *PAS*, periodic acid-Schiff; *PAS-D*, periodic acid-Schiff with diastase digestion.
[1]The histologic features are for classic discoid LE. Acute cutaneous LE often shows less well-developed features and may manifest with a "nonspecific" interface dermatitis. Subacute LE tends to lack basement membrane thickening, follicular plugging, or a marked periadnexal infiltrate.

Differential Diagnosis

Clinical-pathologic correlation is the most effective means of distinguishing acute, subacute, and chronic LE lesions. Likewise, other connective tissue disorders such as dermatomyositis and mixed connective tissue disease may exhibit changes indistinguishable from acute, subacute, or early discoid LE and must be distinguished by correlation of clinical and laboratory features. If scarring alopecia, prominent follicular plugging, or marked basement membrane thickening is present, discoid lesions may be specifically identified based on histology alone.

The presence of eosinophils favors a drug reaction over LE.

LP may resemble LE both histologically and clinically by its propensity to cause scarring alopecia (lichen planopilaris). Compared with LP, LE usually exhibits relatively dense and deep dermal inflammation with perieccrine involvement, increased interstitial mucin, in the reticular dermis, basement membrane thickening, and epidermal atrophy (often juxtaposed with focally hyperplastic areas). The presence of plasma cells and CD123-positive dendritic cells may favor a diagnosis of cutaneous lupus. The clinical context of a solitary lesion is generally sufficient to favor lichenoid keratosis over LP or LE.

Marked papillary dermal edema is a hallmark of polymorphous light eruption (PMLE) that may rarely be seen in LE. Most cases of PMLE do not exhibit significant interface or other epidermal changes. Clinical correlation is required.

Superficial and deep dermal perivascular and periadnexal lymphocytes with plasma cells are shared features of tumid LE and erythema migrans (Lyme disease). The infiltrates in tumid LE tend to be denser and accompanied by increased interstitial mucin. Clinical correlation is required.

Prognosis and Treatment

LE, whether associated with systemic involvement or not, runs a chronic course. Morbidity and mortality correlate with the severity of systemic disease. Approximately 10% of patients with chronic lesions only at the time of diagnosis subsequently develop evidence of SLE. Subacute LE patients are more likely than discoid patients to develop systemic disease (≈50%), but this subset typically exhibits milder systemic disease than those with acute LE lesions. Neonatal LE is self-limited but may result in heart block if not recognized and managed promptly. Prednisone is generally reserved for SLE. Cutaneous LE may respond to sun avoidance, topical or intralesional corticosteroids, antimalarials, thalidomide, dapsone, retinoids, methotrexate, azathioprine, cyclosporine, or sulfasalazine.

DERMATOMYOSITIS

Clinical Findings

Gottren's papules, violaceous papules over the knuckles, are considered pathognomonic for dermatomyositis. In contrast, when the dorsal hands are involved in acute cutaneous LE, the knuckles are characteristically spared. Other manifestations include Gottren's sign (scaly papules over the elbows or knees); periocular or facial erythema and edema with a pink/violet (heliotrope) hue; urticarial, erythematous, or poikilodermatous patches or plaques on the trunk or extremities or in a V or shawl (upper trunk, neck, and shoulder) pattern; periungual telangiectasia; and calcinosis cutis. Pruritus may be significant. Dermatomyositis *sine myositis* (clinically amyopathic dermatomyositis [CADM]) describes patients with typical skin lesions in the absence of muscle involvement. Subclinical evidence of muscle involvement may be present, and a subset of these patients eventually develop dermatomyositis. There is bimodal incidence, with distinct juvenile and adult subsets, the latter associated with systemic malignancy. Myositis-specific antibody profiling may further stratify clinical subsets, e.g., anti-MDA-5 associated with more aggressive interstitial lung disease in CADM patients. Atherosclerosis is a potential comorbidity.

Histologic Features

Biopsies from Gottren's papules, Gottren's sign, heliotrope rash, and poikilodermatous lesions usually

DERMATOMYOSITIS—DISEASE FACT SHEET

Patient Group

- Children (juvenile DM): most 10 to 15 years old at diagnosis
- Adults: peak onset between ages 45 and 60 years
- Women are more likely to be affected than men

Site of Involvement

- Face, especially periocular region
- Extensor surfaces of extremities, especially knuckles

Clinical Findings

- Violaceous poikiloderma (hyper- or hypopigmentation, telangiectasia, atrophy)
- Heliotrope sign (periocular pink-purple discoloration)
- Gottron's papules (violaceous discoloration over the knuckles)
- Ragged cuticles (cuticular dystrophy)
- Nailfold telangiectasia
- Pruritus
- Calcinosis cutis (juvenile DM)

Prognosis

- Depends on extent of systemic disease (myopathy, interstitial lung disease, cardiac disease)
- Depends on associated malignancy (adult DM; incidence of associated malignancy increases with older age at presentation)

Treatment

- Systemic corticosteroids
- Antimalarials

DM, Dermatomyositis.

exhibit findings similar or indistinguishable from the vacuolar interface dermatitis of acute cutaneous LE. The appearances may be subtle with only sparse superficial perivascular lymphocytes or only dermal edema and interstitial mucin. Compared with lupus, the histopathologic abnormalities are generally less pronounced and more variably present. As in acute lupus, eosinophils are usually absent. DIF is not routinely required to establish the diagnosis and is typically negative. Vascular deposits of C5b-9 (membrane attack complex) have been documented in dermatomyositis. Dermatomyositis may be associated with a lobular lymphocytic panniculitis that is indistinguishable from LE profundus.

Ancillary Studies

Characteristic dermatologic features comprise one diagnostic criterion for dermatomyositis. Other criteria include the presence of myositis as determined by the results of one or more of the following: neurologic examination, serum muscle enzymes (creatine phosphokinase, aldolase, lactate dehydrogenase) and myositis-specific antibodies, electromyogram, skeletal muscle biopsy, barium swallow, and magnetic resonance imaging.

Differential Diagnosis

The histopathologic features overlap significantly with cutaneous LE as well as other forms of connective tissue disease, including mixed connective tissue disease. Correlation with clinical and laboratory features is required. The histopathologic features of dermatomyositis tend to be milder and more variable than those of LE.

DERMATOMYOSITIS—PATHOLOGIC FEATURES

Histologic Features

- Vacuolar interface dermatitis: often subtle
- Epidermal atrophy (except for Gottron's papules)
- Sparse lymphocytic infiltrate
- Evidence of mild vascular damage

Ancillary Studies

- Direct immunofluorescence studies: nonspecific or negative using routine test panels

Differential Diagnosis

- Lupus erythematosus
- Drug reaction
- Poikilodermatous graft versus host disease

Prognosis and Treatment

Dermatomyositis is a chronic illness but is generally associated with a fairly good prognosis if appropriately managed with systemic immunosuppressive therapy (usually including corticosteroids), although adult dermatomyositis has been associated with an increased risk of systemic malignancy. In addition to topical therapy, hydroxychloroquine may be useful for nondisabling cases, whereas methotrexate may be favored for severe, disabling disease. Juvenile dermatomyositis usually exhibits a slow, progressive course but may rarely evolve rapidly with potentially fatal outcome.

GRAFT VERSUS HOST DISEASE

Clinical Findings

GVHD encompasses a spectrum of disease with characteristic cutaneous and systemic manifestations, arising in the setting of bone marrow or other hematopoietic cell transplantation and, rarely, solid organ transplantation or blood product transfusion, wherein donor or autologous lymphocytes react against various targets within the host recipient, most commonly the skin, liver, and gastrointestinal (GI) tract. GVHD is classified as acute or chronic. Acute GVHD typically presents as numerous erythematous macules on the face or palms and soles. Generalized eruptions are often morbilliform (Fig. 1.18A). Acute GVHD usually arises within 100 days of bone marrow transplantation. Chronic GVHD evolves from acute GVHD and occurs weeks to months (>100 days) after transplantation and may appear lichenoid (LP-like) and eventually sclerodermoid (scleroderma-like) in appearance (Fig. 1.18B). Similar to acute GVHD, chronic GVHD typically starts on the distal extremities. Chronic GVHD is often associated with pigmentary alterations, typically manifesting as poikiloderma or diffuse hyperpigmentation. Histopathologic features of acute GVHD may be present in patients more than 60 days after transplantation. GI involvement results in nausea, vomiting, and diarrhea.

Histologic Features

Acute GVHD is vacuolar interface dermatitis (Fig. 1.18C), including the pattern of satellite cell necrosis, which refers to intraepidermal lymphocytes associated with single or clustered apoptotic (dyskeratotic, necrotic) keratinocytes. The interface dermatitis characteristically involves both the epidermis and follicular epithelium (Fig. 1.18D).

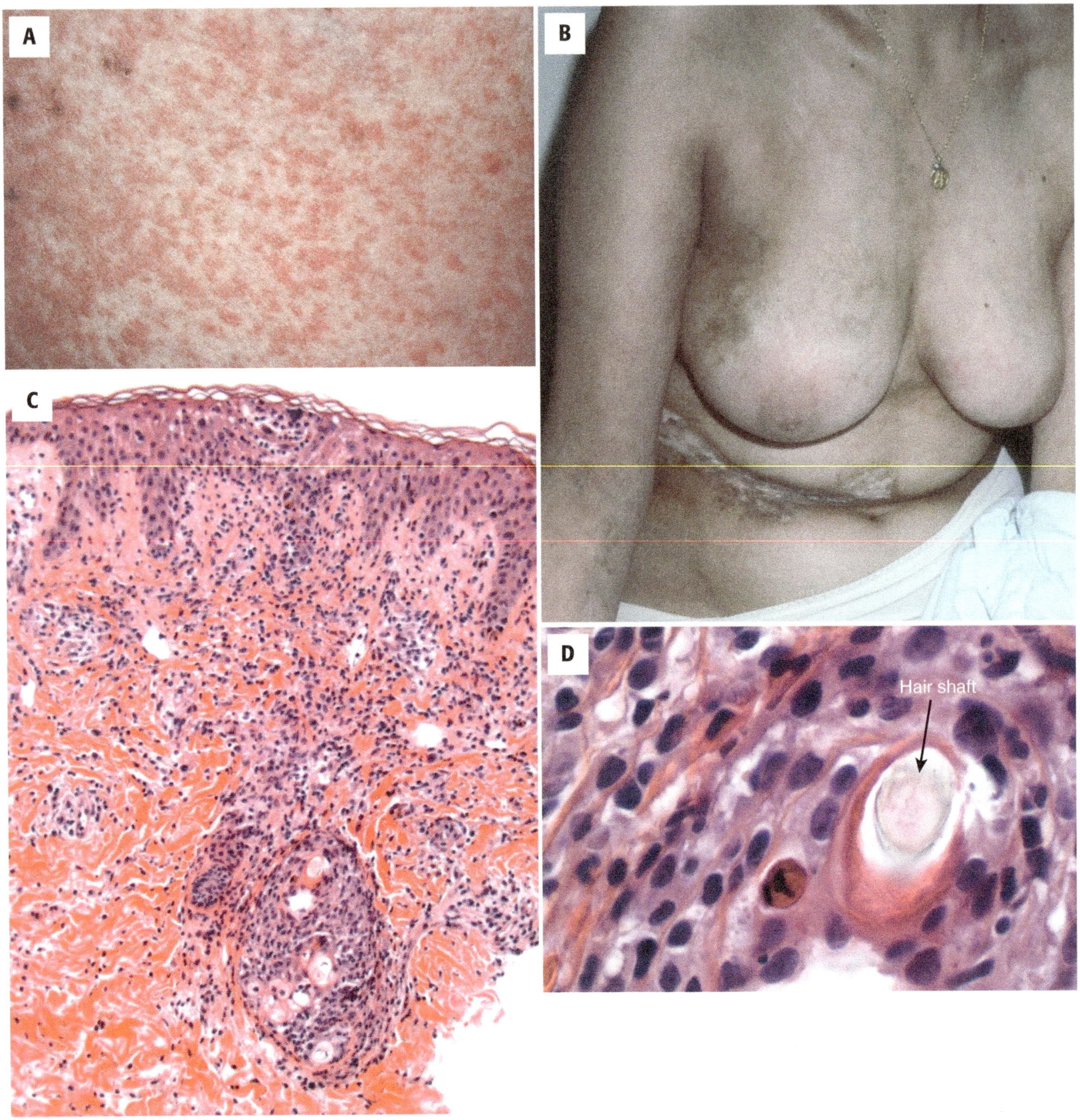

FIG. 1.18

Graft versus host disease (GVHD). **A,** Acute GVHD may be localized, usually to the distal extremities, or generalized, as exemplified by this morbilliform eruption in a recent bone marrow transplant recipient. **B,** Chronic GVHD may consist of sclerotic plaques and dyspigmentation. **C,** Acute GVHD is characterized by a vacuolar interface dermatitis with relatively sparse dermal inflammation. **D,** Interface dermatitis involving adnexal epithelium (hair follicle, sweat duct) is characteristic.

The superficial dermis usually contains a lymphocytic infiltrate, which may be sparse in neutropenic patients. Eosinophils are usually rare or absent, but their presence does not exclude GVHD. A grading scale has been applied to the continuum of interface changes in acute GVHD as follows: vacuolar alteration (grade 1), necrotic keratinocytes (grade 2), subepidermal microvesicles (grade 3), and epidermal separation (grade 4). Chronic GVHD may simulate LP with a dense bandlike lymphocytic infiltrate and associated epidermal hyperplasia, jagged rete ridges, and squamatization of the basal cell layer. In late lesions, melanophages may be prominent in the papillary dermis with only rare lymphocytes and scattered Civatte bodies (i.e., postinflammatory hyperpigmentation secondary

GRAFT VERSUS HOST DISEASE—DISEASE FACT SHEET

Patient Group

- Status post-hematopoietic cell transplantation, allogeneic > autologous

Site of Involvement

- Eruption tends to begin at acral sites, distal extremities, ears, sides of the neck
- May become generalized

Clinical Findings

- Acute cutaneous eruption (within 3 months of engraftment)
  - Erythematous macules and papules (maculopapular)
  - Blisters
  - Erythroderma
- Chronic cutaneous disease (usually ≤100 days after engraftment)
  - Lichenoid papules
  - Sclerodermoid lesions
  - Dyschromia, poikiloderma

Prognosis

- Variable, depending on extent of graft versus host disease and susceptibility to infection

Treatment

- Systemic immunosuppression with corticosteroids, tacrolimus, cyclosporine

interface dermatitis). Chronic GVHD may have a sclerodermatous (morphea-like) or poikilodermatous appearance. Features of acute and chronic GVHD may coexist (chronic active GVHD). An uncommon manifestation of chronic GVHD may be panniculitis or fasciitis.

GRAFT VERSUS HOST DISEASE—PATHOLOGIC FEATURES

Histologic Features

- Acute graft versus host disease (GVHD)
  - Interface dermatitis with follicular or sweat ductal involvement
  - Necrotic or apoptotic keratinocytes with satellitosis
  - Lymphocytic infiltrate
  - Eosinophils are usually rare or absent but may be present
- Chronic GVHD
  - Features of morphea
  - Features of lichen planus
  - Features of poikiloderma (atrophy, telangiectasia, melanophages)

Ancillary Studies

- If eosinophils, consider periodic acid-Schiff stain to exclude dermatophytosis
- Biopsies of other organ sites (gastrointestinal tract)

Differential Diagnosis

- Drug reaction
- Viral exanthema

Ancillary Studies

GVHD frequently involves the GI tract (including the oral mucosa) and hepatobiliary tract. Elevated bilirubin and alkaline phosphatase levels are present.

Differential Diagnosis

Clinical correlation is paramount. Acute GVHD may be indistinguishable from EM, the eruption of lymphocyte recovery (which may, in fact, represent a transient, mild acute cutaneous GVHD reaction associated with engraftment), drug eruptions, and some viral exanthema if only basket-weave orthokeratosis is present. However, in acute GVHD, vacuolar interface dermatitis typically involves the adnexal epithelium. Acute GVHD may also be indistinguishable from lupus or dermatomyositis if interstitial mucin deposition is not evident. The sclerosis present in some cases of chronic GVHD is not a feature of LP. Drug reactions typically have eosinophils, but drug reactions with few or absent eosinophils may be impossible to differentiate from GVHD without clinical correlation.

Prognosis and Treatment

Histologic grading of acute GVHD does not correlate highly with the clinical severity of GVHD. Management of GVHD may require intensification of the patient's systemic immunosuppression with systemic agents such as prednisone, cyclosporine, ruxolitinib, belumosudil, and/or others. Topical corticosteroids, topical tacrolimus ointment, systemic photochemotherapy (PUVA), and extracorporeal photochemotherapy (photopheresis) may be helpful in chronic GVHD.

LICHEN SCLEROSUS

Clinical Findings

Lichen sclerosus (LS), formerly known as lichen sclerosus et atrophicus, is characterized by atrophic, porcelain white papules and plaques. Lesions most commonly arise on genital skin but may arise anywhere on the body, sometimes at sites of trauma (Fig. 1.19A). Chronic genital lesions may be associated with ulceration, secondary squamous cell carcinoma, and phimosis. Historically, male genital involvement has been termed balanitis xerotica obliterans, and its occurrence is

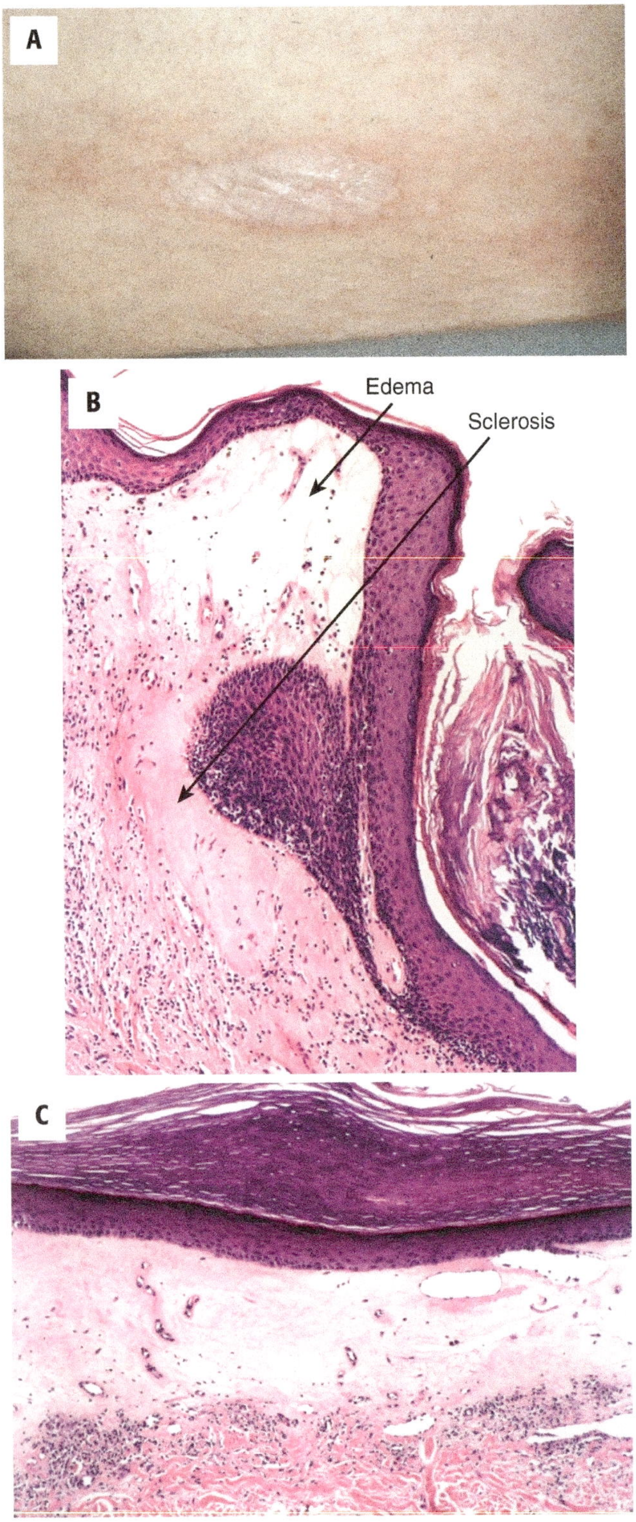

FIG. 1.19

Lichen sclerosus. **A,** Porcelain white plaque with peripheral erythema. **B,** Atrophy, follicular plugging, papillary dermal edema, and sclerosis. **C,** A lichenoid lymphocytic infiltrate is typically present beneath the zone of altered connective tissue in the subepidermal zone. Analysis of early lesions or the peripheral area of fully developed lesions exhibit vacuolar interface dermatitis before the advent of identifiable edema or sclerosis.

LICHEN SCLEROSUS—DISEASE FACT SHEET

Patient Group

- May occur in children or adults
- Women are more commonly affected

Site of Involvement

- Most commonly affects genitalia
- May occur elsewhere (trunk, proximal extremities)

Clinical Findings

- Sclerotic white plaques with epidermal atrophy
- May cause scarring (e.g., phimosis in men)
- Pruritus

Prognosis

- No association with systemic disease, but secondary squamous cell carcinoma may develop
- Chronic disease

Treatment

- Patient education
- Potent or ultrapotent topical steroids
- Topical calcineurin inhibitors
- Other topical or systemic agents

Ceftriaxone or penicillin (if *Borrelia* sp. is suspected)

generally restricted to uncircumcised men, commonly causing phimosis. Female genital involvement has been termed kraurosis vulvae. Vulvar LS is typically pruritic, painful, and disabling. Extragenital LS is often asymptomatic.

Histologic Features

LS is characterized by lichenoid dermatitis, which is often accompanied by compact orthokeratosis, epidermal atrophy, and (at extramucosal sites) follicular plugging (Fig. 1.19B) in combination with superficial stromal edema and eventually sclerosis. The sclerotic collagen assumes a distinctive homogeneous or hyaline appearance with complete or nearly complete loss of the normal fibrillary pattern of collagen fibers (Fig. 1.19C). The loss of the normal collagenous support for the superficial papillary vessels may lead to ectatic and hemorrhagic vessels in the papillary dermis. Lymphocytes are usually present in a patchy or lichenoid pattern beneath the altered connective tissue or at the junction of fibrosed stroma and normal stroma. Eosinophils are variable. The earliest changes in LS are not specifically diagnostic but include psoriasiform hyperplasia and lichenoid infiltrates of lymphocytes

LICHEN SCLEROSUS—PATHOLOGIC FEATURES

Histologic Features

- Interface dermatitis
- Layer of hyalinized stroma
- Band of lymphocytes

Differential Diagnosis

- Chronic graft versus host disease
- Radiation dermatitis

with lymphocyte exocytosis into the basilar epidermis to an extent that may resemble patch-stage MF. In diagnostically difficult cases, an elastic stain may be helpful as it should confirm the disintegration of the elastic fibers in the papillary dermis.

Differential Diagnosis

Features similar (or identical) to LS can be seen in chronic radiation dermatitis. Chronic radiation dermatitis tends to contain ectatic vessels and atypical radiation fibroblasts. The differential diagnosis of LS also includes chronic LS-like GVHD and superficial morphea, including guttate morphea (which some authorities regard as indistinguishable from LS). If sclerosis extends into the reticular dermis or subcutis, then LS-morphea overlap is most likely.

Prognosis and Treatment

LS is usually chronic and persistent or progressive, although some cases may remit. Ultrapotent (class 1) topical corticosteroids represent the first-line treatment. Topical calcineurin inhibitors or topical or systemic retinoids may be used. Phimosis or scarring that impairs function must be managed surgically. Chronically eroded or ulcerated lesions should be monitored for secondary squamous cell carcinoma.

LICHEN NITIDUS

Clinical Findings

Lichen nitidus is an idiopathic benign disorder that usually occurs in children and young adults, mostly males. It is characterized by innumerate discrete pinhead-sized 1- to 2-mm flesh-colored, erythematous, or hypopigmented papules in localized or generalized distribution. The papules usually have a glistening, smooth, or minimally scaly surface. The Koebner phenomenon may be present. Wickham striae are absent. The papules are usually asymptomatic but may be pruritic. Papules may be clustered or grouped, with a predilection for the flexural skin folds on the trunk and extremities, including the genitalia.

Histologic Features

Lichen nitidus characteristically exhibits a "ball-in-claw" pattern at scanning magnification, in which a very focal lichenoid infiltrate (ball) composed of lymphocytes and histiocytes spans only one or a few rete ridges and is surrounded by inward-bending rete ridges (claw) (Fig. 1.20A and B). There is often epidermal hyperplasia surrounding a central zone of atrophy, hypogranulosis, and parakeratosis overlying the lichenoid infiltrate. The infiltrate tends to exhibit a prominent histiocytic component that could be characterized as granulomatous, that is, discrete granulomas are not present, although multinucleated histiocytes may be present (Fig. 1.20C).

Differential Diagnosis

Clinically, lichen striatus may resemble lichen nitidus or follicular/papular atopic dermatitis in dark-complected children. Like lichen nitidus, lichen striatus may also exhibit a granulomatous (i.e., histiocyte predominant) infiltrate, but the lichenoid interface reaction typically affects the epidermis more broadly, and underlying perieccrine lymphocytes are relatively specific for lichen striatus. Small papules of superficial sarcoid may resemble lichen nitidus, but sarcoid is characterized by sarcoidal granulomas. LP may occasionally resemble lichen nitidus, but DIF studies are negative in lichen nitidus (colloid bodies absent), and junctional fibrinogen is present in LP.

Prognosis and Treatment

Most cases of lichen nitidus resolve within the first year, and, if not, within a few years of onset. Because the lesions are usually asymptomatic, reassurance is sometimes all that is necessary. Therapy includes topical corticosteroids or retinoids, and ultraviolet B and PUVA phototherapy.

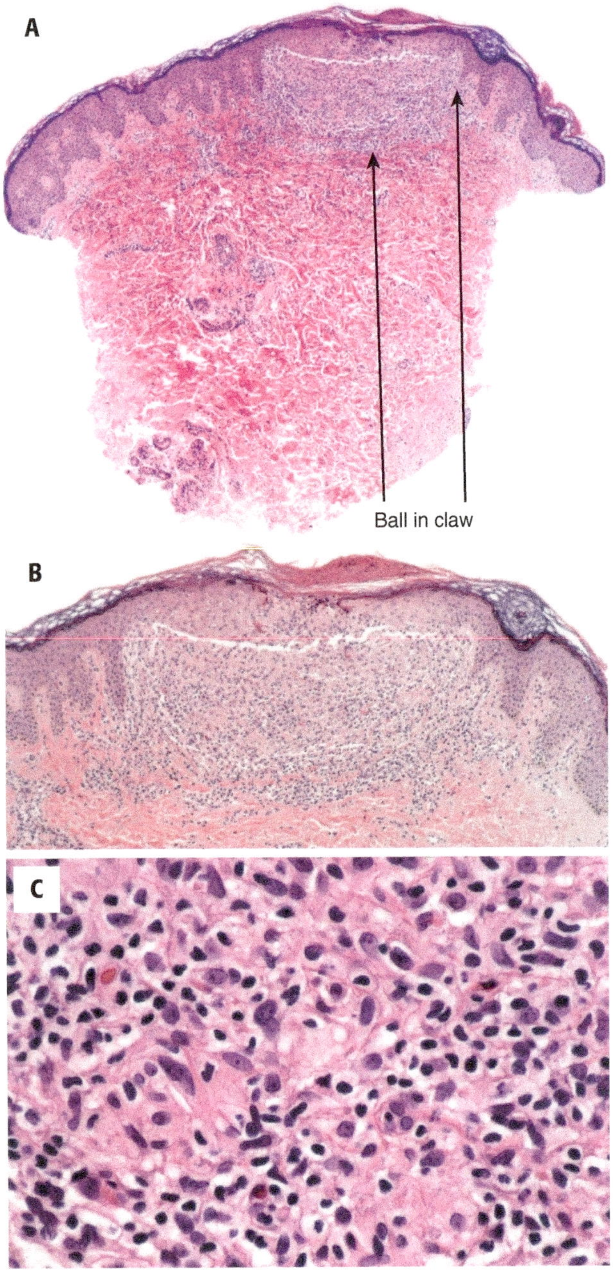

FIG. 1.20
Lichen nitidus. **A,** Scanning magnification best depicts the "ball-in-claw" configuration of the focal lichenoid interface dermatitis. **B,** The overlying epidermis is typically parakeratotic, thinned, and hypogranulotic. **C,** Histiocytes often predominate in the lichenoid infiltrate.

LICHEN STRIATUS

Clinical Findings

Lichen striatus is an idiopathic, self-limited, linear dermatosis that usually occurs in children or young adults. It is characterized by 1- to 3-mm smooth or scaly papules that coalesce in linear array usually on one extremity, occasionally extending to the trunk or nails. Pruritus is mild or absent. Genital involvement may occur. Lesions often follow Blaschko's lines (embryonic migration lines) and may have a somewhat linear appearance.

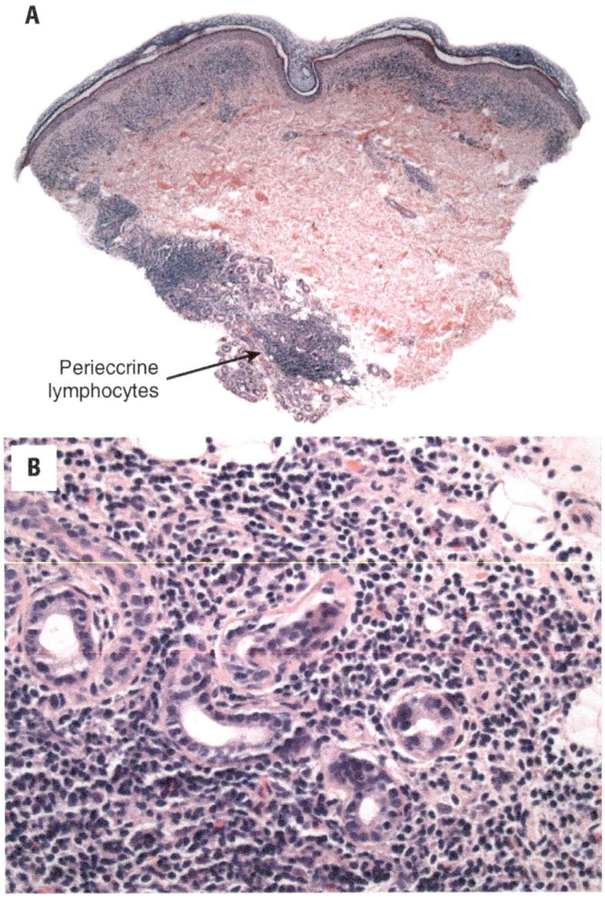

FIG. 1.21
Lichen striatus. **A,** Lichenoid lymphocytic infiltrates with deep perivascular and periadnexal involvement. **B,** Perieccrine lymphocytes are relatively specific for lichen striatus but are not always present.

Histologic Features

Lichen striatus usually exhibits a patchy or bandlike lichenoid lymphocytic interface reaction associated with superficial and deep perivascular and periadnexal involvement (Fig. 1.21A). Perieccrine lymphocytes are believed to be a relatively characteristic finding (Fig. 1.21B). Psoriasiform epidermal hyperplasia may be present. A relatively prominent histiocyte population may be present, rendering a focally granulomatous appearance to the upper dermis.

Differential Diagnosis

Lichen nitidus may also exhibit focal lichenoid dermatitis with a relatively prominent histiocytic component, but the "ball-in-claw" configuration with overlying parakeratosis and epidermal atrophy is distinctive. LE may resemble lichen striatus but typically exhibits denser perifollicular lymphocytes and increased interstitial mucin deposition. The epidermal and interface changes of lichen striatus may closely resemble those of LP, but LP typically lacks deep perivascular or periadnexal involvement.

Prognosis and Treatment

Lichen striatus usually resolves after several months or years. Therapy includes topical corticosteroids.

GRANULOMATOUS DERMATITIS

Granulomatous dermatitis is a phrase that broadly encompasses reactive skin disorders that are characterized by a relative predominance of histiocytes, rather than lymphocytes, in the dermis. (Nonspecific perivascular and interstitial inflammation in the dermis is sometimes termed *lymphohistiocytic*, but this term refers to lymphocyte-predominant infiltrates.) A broad spectrum of disorders can manifest with a granulomatous tissue reaction (Table 1.4). Not all granulomatous dermatitides contain granulomas per se, although granulomas are the discrete nodular aggregates of epithelioid histiocytes that are the most specific hallmark of granulomatous dermatitis. Different types of granulomas typify sarcoid (sarcoidal-type granuloma), infection (tuberculoid granulomas), and others; different types of granulomas may coexist and are not completely specific. For example, some foreign body reactions may appear sarcoidal. Also, not all disorders characterized by tuberculoid granulomas are infectious (e.g., granulomatous rosacea). Other forms of granulomatous dermatitis are characterized by palisaded and/or diffuse/interstitial patterns of histiocytes in the dermis, even if discrete granulomas are lacking. Examples include the interstitial variant of GA and lichen nitidus. When evaluating granulomatous dermatitis, general rules of practice are to exclude the presence of birefringent foreign material (using polarized light) and infection.

SARCOID

Clinical Findings

Sarcoid (sarcoidosis) is a chronic systemic granulomatous disorder of unknown etiology with frequent pulmonary and cutaneous involvement that may arise in adults and children. Cutaneous lesions occur in at least 20% to 25% of cases and may have a wide variety of appearances, most typically smooth, variably flesh-colored to red, purple, or yellow-brown papules or plaques (Fig. 1.22A), often preferentially arising at sites of prior injection or trauma. Other manifestations include macular, lupus pernio (pernio-like lesions on the face and fingers), subcutaneous, annular (Fig. 1.22B), follicular, ulcerative, and ichthyosiform lesions. In the United States, sarcoid is more common among Black Americans. Erythema nodosum may represent a nonspecific manifestation of sarcoid. Acute sarcoid presenting with erythema nodosum, hilar adenopathy, fever, and arthritis is historically known as Löfgren syndrome.

Histologic Features

Despite the varied clinical appearances, the histopathologic least common denominator is the presence of sarcoidal granulomas in the dermis or subcutis. The classic sarcoidal granuloma is a circumscribed collection of epithelioid histiocytes that, compared with other types of granulomas, is relatively devoid of lymphocytes (*naked granulomas*) or central necrosis (Fig. 1.22C–E). In practice, many exceptions to the classic profile may

TABLE 1.4

Basic Differential Diagnosis of Granulomatous Dermatitis

	Sarcoid	Granuloma Annulare	Rheumatoid Nodule	Necrobiosis Lipoidica	Necrobiotic Xanthogranuloma	Foreign Body Reaction	Infection
Sarcoidal granuloma	++	o	o	o	o	±	o
Palisaded granuloma	o	++	++	++	++	±	±
Tuberculoid granuloma	±	o	o	o	o	±	++
Interstitial granulomatous pattern	±	++	o	±	±	±	±
Foreign body identified	±	o	o	o	o	++	o
Plasma cells	o	o	o	++	±	±	±

++, characteristic; ±, variable; o, unusual or not classic.

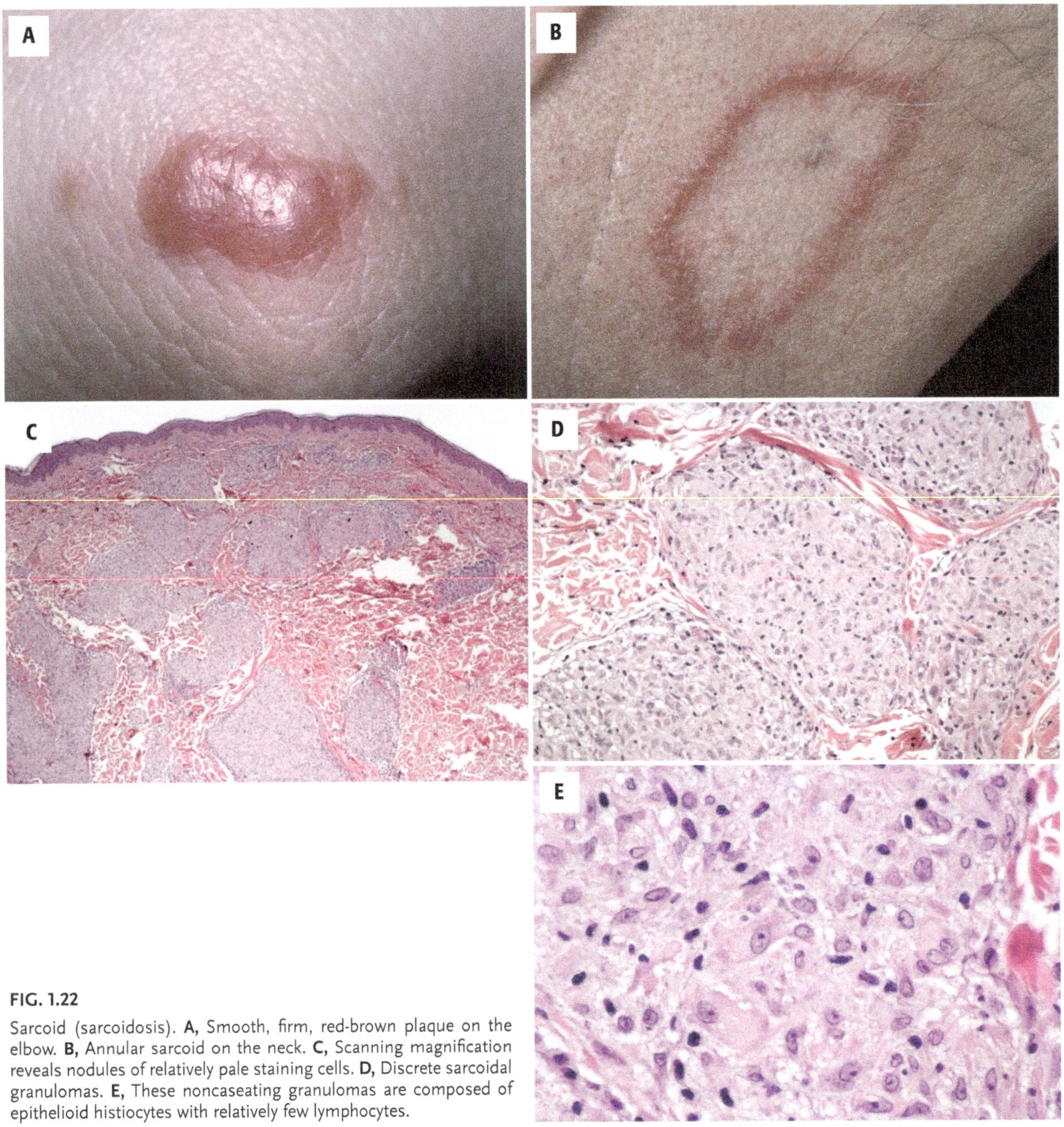

FIG. 1.22

Sarcoid (sarcoidosis). **A,** Smooth, firm, red-brown plaque on the elbow. **B,** Annular sarcoid on the neck. **C,** Scanning magnification reveals nodules of relatively pale staining cells. **D,** Discrete sarcoidal granulomas. **E,** These noncaseating granulomas are composed of epithelioid histiocytes with relatively few lymphocytes.

occur, including tuberculoid granulomas, suppurative granulomas, lichenoid inflammation, and interstitial histiocytic infiltrates. Likewise, the presence of a foreign body does not exclude the diagnosis because sarcoid has a tendency to develop at sites of trauma.

Ancillary Studies

Systemic evaluation may reveal evidence of systemic involvement, most often on chest radiographs (lymphadenopathy or parenchymal involvement). Serum angiotensin-converting enzyme (ACE) levels are typically elevated, although an elevated ACE level is not specific for sarcoid. Infection should be reasonably excluded clinically and with special stains or cultures if needed.

Differential Diagnosis

Foreign body granulomas may sometimes exhibit sarcoidal features. Polarized microscopy will reveal birefringent foreign bodies, but sarcoid may be more likely to develop at sites of foreign body implantation (so-called "scar sarcoid"), so clinical correlation is ultimately required to establish a diagnosis of sarcoid.

Prognosis and Treatment

Sarcoid is a chronic, incurable disorder. The number of skin lesions does not correlate with the severity of systemic disease. However, the type of cutaneous lesion may be relevant. Patients with macular and papular lesions (with the exception of eyelid papules) tend to have the lowest risk of systemic disease, but those with annular lesions, plaques, scalp involvement, and ichthyosiform lesions have been reported to have a higher risk of chronic, systemic disease. Lupus pernio is associated with upper airway and bone involvement. While localized lesions may be treated with topical or intralesional corticosteroids, systemic corticosteroids are the mainstay of treatment for rapidly progressive or disfiguring diseases. Patients with extensive or refractory sarcoid may be candidates for antimalarials, methotrexate, tetracyclines, or TNF-alpha inhibition.

GRANULOMA ANNULARE

Clinical Findings

GA is an idiopathic, self-limited disorder characterized by smooth annular papules and plaques that may be asymptomatic or pruritic. Lesions may be localized, generalized, perforating (transepidermal elimination of collagen), and subcutaneous. Localized lesions usually appear on the distal extremities of children and young adults as smooth, flesh-colored to erythematous, firm papules that may coalesce, with central clearing, into an annular papule or plaque (Fig. 1.23A). Subcutaneous lesions, also known as pseudorheumatoid nodules, occur in children and may also involve the scalp or forehead. Perforating GA is associated with overlying hyperkeratosis (Fig. 1.23B). In the arcuate dermal erythema variant, lesions appear as round or arcuate erythematous patches that may clinically resemble erythema migrans (Lyme disease) (Fig. 1.23C).

Histologic Features

GA is characterized by palisaded granulomas consisting of palisades of histiocytes with central alteration of collagen fibers and increased interstitial mucin deposition (Fig. 1.23D and E). Subtle palisading is often easiest to appreciate at scanning magnification. The altered (degenerating, necrobiotic) collagen fibers are smudgy and indistinct and may be more intensely eosinophilic or basophilic. Associated with these palisaded granulomas are perivascular and interstitial lymphocytes and occasionally neutrophils and nuclear dust (leukocytoclastic or karyorrhectic nuclear debris). In the incomplete or interstitial variant, there is only an interstitial histiocytic infiltrate with minimal or absent palisading or increased mucin (Fig. 1.23F). In the perforating variant GA, there is overlying epidermal hyperplasia and transepidermal elimination of abnormal collagen fibers. In subcutaneous GA, palisaded granulomas are centered in the subcutis.

GRANULOMA ANNULARE—DISEASE FACT SHEET

Patient Group
- Children and young adults
- Affects women more often than men

Site of Involvement
- Extremities (majority of lesions are on hands and arms)
- May occur at sites of trauma (e.g., insect bite reaction, zoster)
- May occur anywhere, especially in generalized GA

Clinical Findings
- Papules coalescing into an arciform/annular plaque
- Solitary papules may be umbilicated
- Clinical variants: generalized, perforating (crusted), subcutaneous GA

Prognosis
- Benign self-limited disease
- May be associated with systemic disease (e.g., diabetes mellitus)

Treatment
- Watch and wait
- Topical steroids
- Local destructive therapy (e.g., cryotherapy, laser)

GA, Granuloma annulare

Ancillary Studies

An Alcian blue stain can assist in identifying interstitial mucin deposition.

GRANULOMA ANNULARE—PATHOLOGIC FEATURES

Histologic Features
- Palisading granuloma surrounding areas of dermis with mucin deposition
- Often multiple small foci separated by normal dermis
- Granulomas and eosinophils are common
- May also show interstitial pattern of histiocytes

Ancillary Studies
- Alcian blue to highlight mucin

Differential Diagnosis
- Necrobiosis lipoidica (little or no normal dermis between granulomatous foci, minimal or no mucin)
- Deep granulomata annulare: rheumatoid nodule, epithelioid sarcoma
- Infection
- Interstitial mycosis fungoides
- Interstitial granulomatous drug reaction

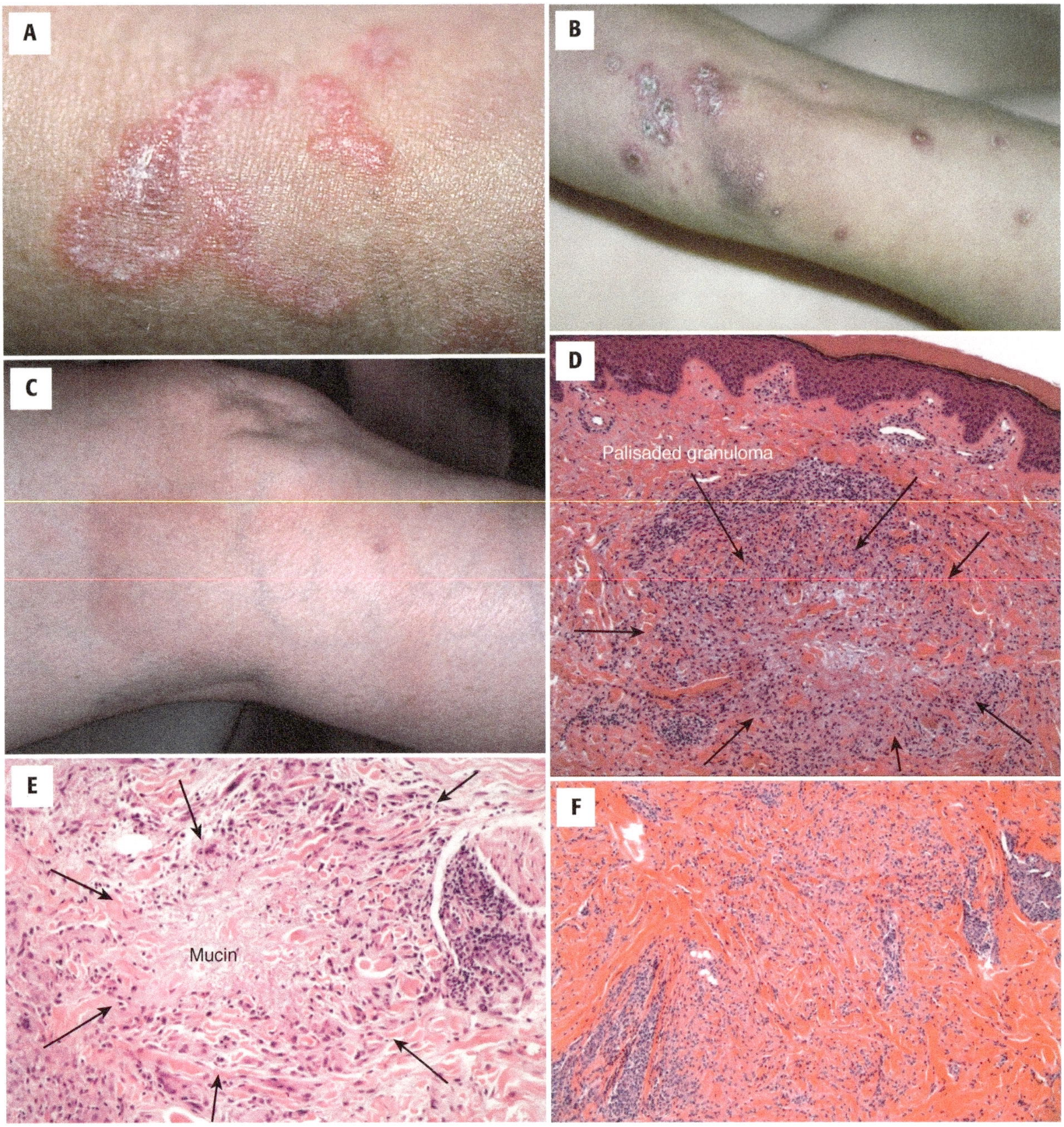

FIG. 1.23

Granuloma annulare (GA). **A,** Typical annular red plaques. **B,** Perforating GA. **C,** Arcuate dermal erythema variant. **D** and **E,** Palisaded granuloma *(arrows)* containing central interstitial mucin. **F,** Interstitial or incomplete variant.

Differential Diagnosis

Rheumatoid nodules contain fibrin rather than mucin in the center of the palisaded granulomas that are large, irregular, and confluent with well-defined palisades centered in the subcutis, where they may resemble subcutaneous GA. Whereas the presence of multinucleated histiocytes within the palisaded granulomas favors the diagnosis of rheumatoid nodule, the presence of mucin within the center of the palisaded granulomas favors subcutaneous GA. Necrobiosis lipoidica (NL) is characterized by diffuse, rather than focal, involvement of the dermis or subcutis; plasma cells are usually present, and there is minimal, if any, increase in mucin. Dermatofibroma may mimic the interstitial pattern of granulomas annulare, but the factor 13a-positive spindle cells in dermatofibroma are surrounded by thickened collagen fibers cut in cross section and often overlying epidermal hyperplasia and hyperpigmentation. Patch-stage Kaposi sarcoma may also resemble the interstitial variant of GA but is characterized by slitlike vascular channels surrounding preexisting vessels (promontory sign), plasma cells, erythrocyte extravasation with degenerated erythrocytes, and hemosiderin, as well as immunopositivity for HHV-8 latent nuclear antigen. Moreover, each of these disorders in the histologic differential diagnosis is clinically distinct. Palisaded neutrophilic and granulomatous dermatitis usually presents as symmetric nonannular erythematous, variably crusted papules, usually on the extremities, in patients with connective tissue disorders such as lupus or rheumatoid arthritis. In early lesions, there is leukocytoclastic vasculitis with broad collars of fibrin surrounding affected vessels. In fully developed lesions, palisaded granulomas are present. In older lesions, palisaded granulomas are associated with fibrosis, and neutrophils or vasculitis are absent.

Prognosis and Treatment

Localized GA is usually self-limited within months to a few years. Generalized GA may be self-limited or chronic. Topical and intralesional corticosteroids, topical calcineurin inhibitors, cryotherapy, and diagnostic biopsy have been used. Generalized and adult-onset lesions tend to persist. Various therapeutic modalities include hydroxychloroquine, isotretinoin, dapsone, niacinamide, and narrowband ultraviolet B photochemotherapy.

RHEUMATOID NODULE

Rheumatoid nodules are subcutaneous nodules that typically arise on the extensor surfaces of the extremities of patients with rheumatoid arthritis (Fig. 1.24A). They are also described in Chapter 2 but are mentioned here to complete the differential diagnosis.

Histologically, the nodules are characterized by palisaded granulomas in the subcutis containing increased fibrin within their centers (Fig. 1.24B–D). Leukocytoclasis and strands of basophilic nuclear debris may also be present, but mucin is typically minimal/absent.

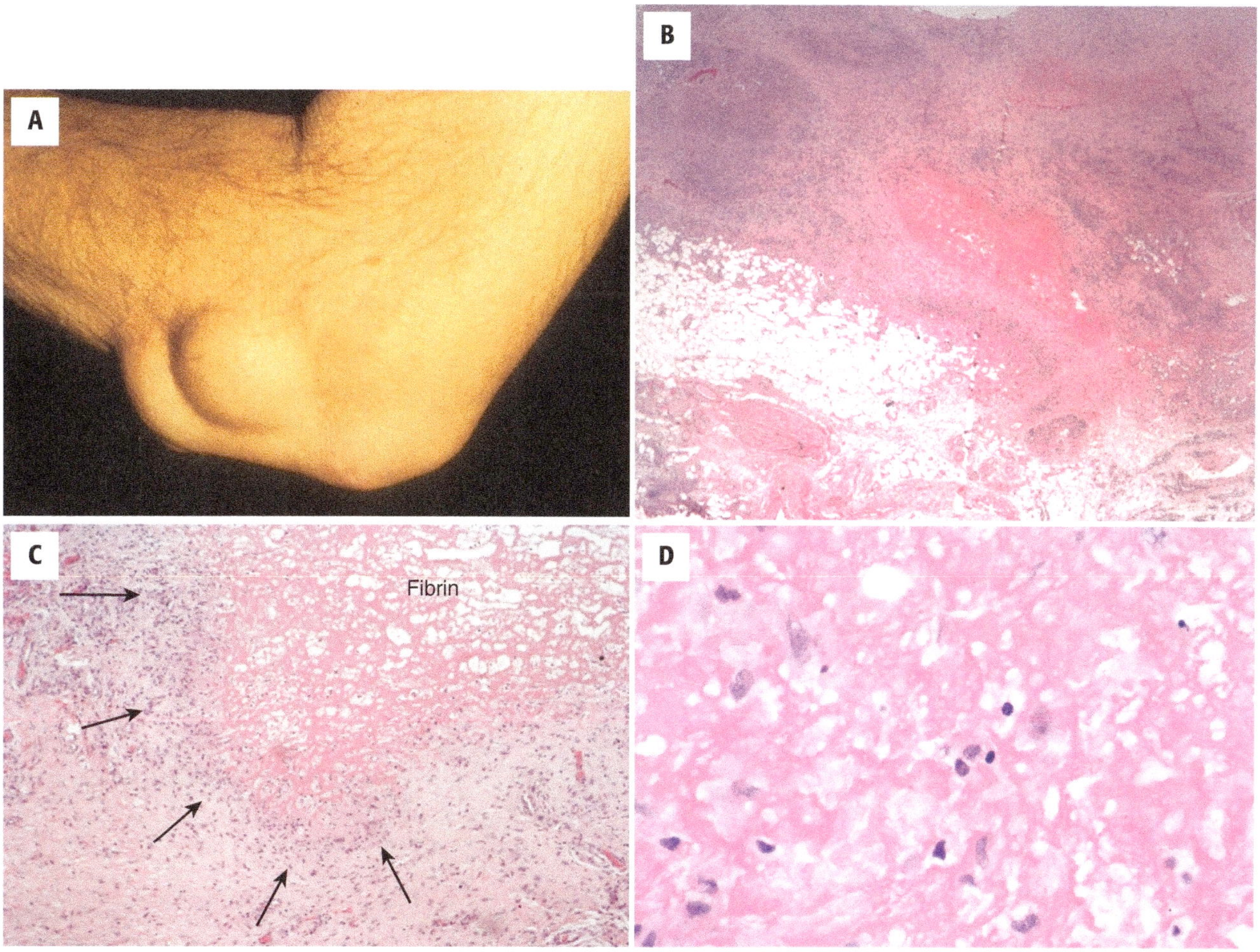

FIG. 1.24

Rheumatoid nodule. **A,** Subcutaneous nodule on the elbow. **B,** Palisaded granulomas are typically situated in the subcutis. **C** and **D,** The palisade of histiocytes *(arrows)* surrounds a more intensely eosinophilic, homogeneous, smudgy-appearing substance, fibrin.

NECROBIOSIS LIPOIDICA

Clinical Findings

Formerly known as NL diabeticorum, up to two-thirds of individuals with NL have been said to have diabetes mellitus, although some studies have suggested a lower incidence (as low as 11%) or at least a wider range of associated diabetes. Few (<1%) of individuals with diabetes mellitus develop NL.

NL may occur at any site but usually occurs on one (usually eventually both) pretibial surfaces in individuals with diabetes mellitus (Fig. 1.25A). The lesions appear as well-demarcated red-brown papules that coalesce into flat yellow-brown atrophic plaques with telangiectasia and peripheral erythema. Some lesions ulcerate. The severity of disease does not correlate highly with the severity or control of diabetes. Other sites of involvement include the ankles, calves, thighs, and feet, and less commonly above the waist. The lesions are usually asymptomatic but may be pruritic or painful.

Histologic Features

The palisaded granulomas in NL involve the dermis diffusely (and sometimes subcutis), so the histologic features typically extend broadly to peripheral and deep edges of a punch or incisional biopsy. From scanning magnification, a distinctive pattern is appreciated that has been compared with a layer cake (Fig. 1.25B). The centers of palisaded granulomas contain eosinophilic, smudgy (degenerating or necrobiotic) collagen fibers similar to those of GA. However, in NL the palisades of histiocytes tend to be flattened and incomplete (not annular), and thus histiocytes do not completely encircle the degenerating collagen. As incompletely palisaded granulomas merge together, confluent zones of abnormal collagen fibers form broad zones of necrobiosis oriented parallel to the epidermal surface (Fig. 1.25C). Fully developed lesions of NL usually contain predominantly lymphocytes and

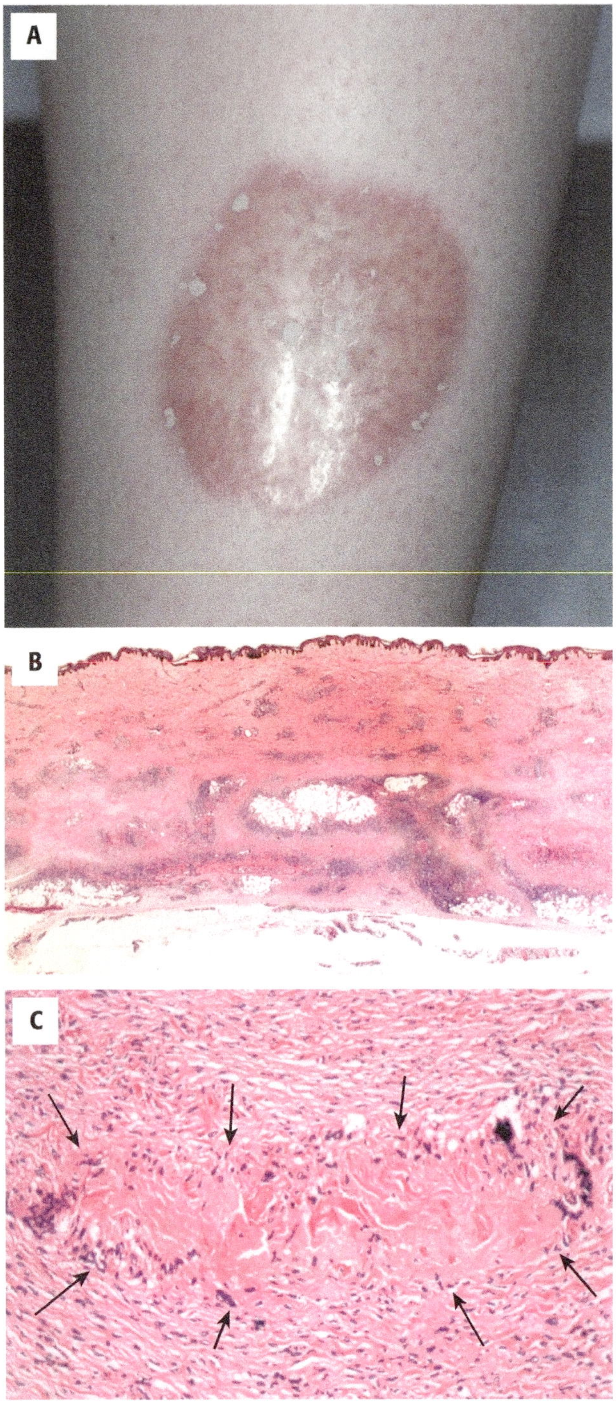

FIG. 1.25

Necrobiosis lipoidica. **A,** Red and yellow, atrophic, telangiectatic plaques most commonly arise on the shins of patients with diabetes. **B,** Scanning magnification best depicts the layer cake pattern of horizontally oriented tiers of degenerating, necrobiotic collagen extending to the deep and lateral biopsy margins. **C,** Palisaded granulomas *(arrows)* are often incomplete and flattened; that is, oriented parallel to the epidermal surface. Plasma cells and scattered multinucleated histiocytes are usually present.

NECROBIOSIS LIPOIDICA—DISEASE FACT SHEET

Patient Group
- Adults
- A subset of patients (15%–65%) have diabetes mellitus

Site of Involvement
- Shin

Clinical Findings
- Plaques (violaceous to red-brown rim with yellow-brown center)
- Atrophy and telangiectasia

Prognosis and Treatment
- Benign condition; may persist or resolve spontaneously
- Topical steroids may be effective

histiocytes, with occasional multinucleated cells, including Touton giant cells. Plasma cells are characteristic. Early lesions may contain neutrophils. Vasculitis is not a typical feature but has been described in early lesions.

Differential Diagnosis

Compared with GA, the granulomas in NL involve the dermis more extensively, but the individual granulomas are less discrete. The presence of plasma cells supports NL. Necrobiotic xanthogranuloma (NXG) may also exhibit a similar "layer cake" appearance at scanning magnification, but NXG exhibits more prominent necrobiosis of collagen, more prominent Touton giant cells, and is much more likely to exhibit cholesterol cleft formation. As with all inflammatory skin diseases, clinical correlation is often essential in attaining the best clinical-pathologic diagnosis.

Prognosis and Treatment

NL is usually chronic and does not necessarily resolve if the diabetes is more tightly controlled. Spontaneous remission may occur but is unpredictable. Therapy is symptomatic and includes topical and intralesional corticosteroids and local wound care for ulcerated lesions. Anecdotally effective modalities include oral niacinamide, aspirin, and cyclosporine, but no treatment is consistently highly effective.

NECROBIOTIC XANTHOGRANULOMA

Clinical Findings

Necrobiotic xanthogranuloma is a rare disorder that usually presents as smooth yellow papules or plaques on the head, neck, or upper trunk with predilection for the periorbital region. The vast majority of cases are associated with paraproteinemia, although the onset of skin involvement may precede detectable serum paraproteins. Paraproteinemia may evolve into multiple myeloma. Many cases are also associated with cryoglobulinemia. Less commonly, cases conforming to established histopathologic criteria have been reported without periorbital lesions or paraproteinemia.

NECROBIOSIS LIPOIDICA—PATHOLOGIC FEATURES

Histologic Features

- Palisading granulomatous dermatitis
- Involvement of most of the dermis (little or no intervening normal dermis)
- Necrobiotic granulomas without increased mucin
- Plasma cells

Ancillary Studies

- Alcian blue can assess for mucin, if needed

Differential Diagnosis

- Granuloma annulare (necrobiotic granulomas with mucin)
- Necrobiotic xanthogranuloma (necrobiotic granulomas, cholesterol clefts)

Histologic Features

Necrobiotic xanthogranuloma is characterized by broad zones of degenerating or necrobiotic collagen surrounded by palisades of histiocytes, including foamy histiocytes and Touton giant cells, throughout the dermis, often extending into the subcutis. Multinucleated histiocytes may be large or bizarre-appearing. Cholesterol clefts are characteristically present (Fig. 1.26A–C). Plasma cells and reactive lymphoid follicles may also be present.

Ancillary Studies

Serum or urine protein electrophoresis study results are usually positive. Histochemical stains to exclude acid-fast or fungal infection may be indicated. As with any granulomatous disorder, polarized microscopy to screen for birefringent foreign material is prudent.

Differential Diagnosis

Histologically, NL may overlap significantly with NXG, including the "layer cake" pattern of necrobiosis that is associated with NL. NXG atypically exhibits more prominent necrobiosis, more prominent Touton giant cells, and cholesterol clefts. The multinucleated histiocytes in NXG are often larger, more prominent, and more atypical appearing compared with NL. Infection should be reasonably excluded.

Prognosis and Treatment

Necrobiotic xanthogranuloma exhibits a chronic, progressive course. It may precede the development of hematologic malignancies. Chlorambucil, alone or in combination with corticosteroids, has been recommended for treatment of malignancy-associated cases. Partial or temporary remission has been associated with prednisone, radiation therapy, and plasmapheresis.

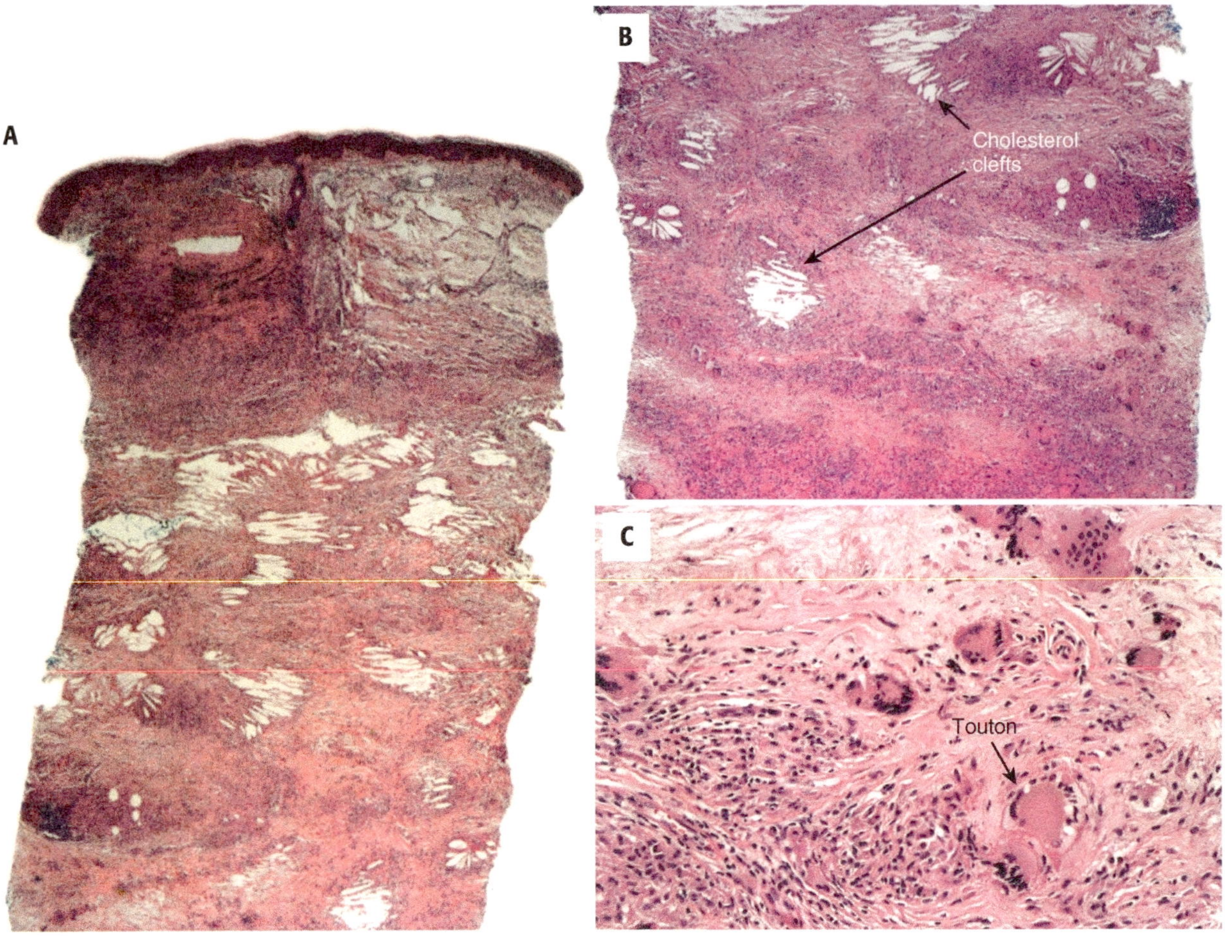

FIG. 1.26
Necrobiotic xanthogranuloma (NXG). **A,** Scanning magnification may be similar to necrobiosis lipoidica (see Fig. 1.25B), with broad zones of necrobiotic collagen extending to the biopsy margins. **B,** Cholesterol clefts are relatively specific for NXG but are not always present. **C,** Touton giant cells are required for the diagnosis.

FOREIGN BODY GRANULOMAS

Clinical Findings

There is no single clinical presentation for foreign body granulomatous reactions. Similar to contact dermatitis, the distribution of lesions depends on the distribution of exposure (unilesional, localized, generalized) and may be obvious from the clinical history. Thus, some of the specimens submitted for microscopic analysis escaped clinical detection, whereas others represent therapeutic procedures.

Histologic Features

Foreign body granulomas may assume a variety of microscopic appearances, including sarcoidal, tuberculoid, or palisaded patterns. One classic example is the "Swiss cheese" pattern caused by paraffin or silicone that is removed during tissue processing and leaves innumerate empty circular spaces associated with histiocytes (Fig. 1.27A and B). Solitary or sparse round, empty lipid vacuoles characterize chalazion of the eyelid. Nonpolarizable (nonbirefringent) foreign materials include tattoo pigments (all colors), injectable collagen, zirconium, gut suture, and injected triamcinolone. Commonly encountered birefringent foreign materials include retained synthetic suture material, silica (glass), and cotton gauze fibers.

Ancillary Studies

Polarized microscopy should be performed on any granulomatous dermatitis of unconfirmed etiology, particularly if granulomas are present.

Differential Diagnosis

The presence of a foreign body in association with sarcoidal granulomas does not exclude the diagnosis of sarcoid because sarcoid has a tendency to develop at sites of trauma. Zirconium may produce a sarcoidal

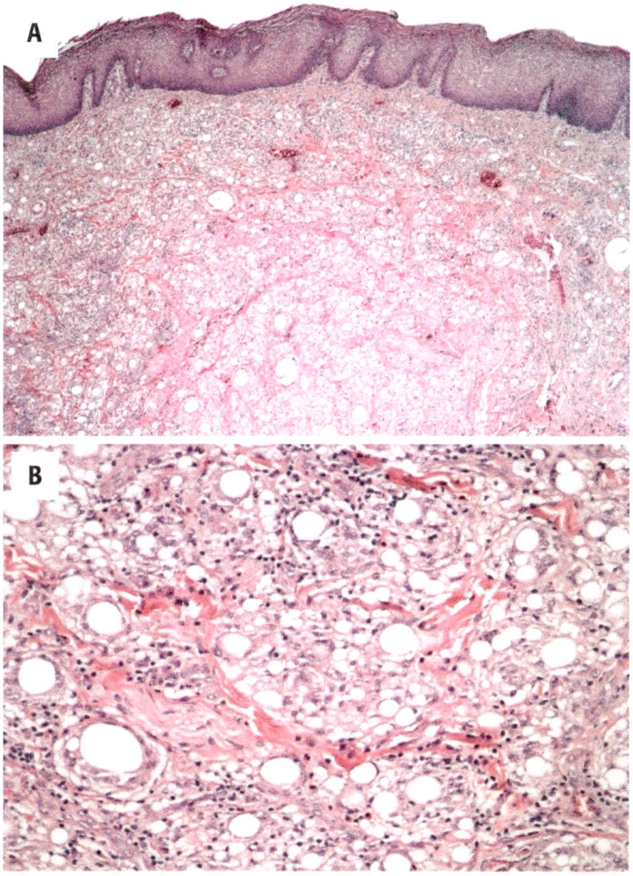

FIG. 1.27

Foreign body granuloma (paraffinoma). **A,** Histiocyte predominant dermal infiltrate. **B,** Numerous round, empty spaces correspond to the foreign body that was removed during tissue processing. Mineral oil and silicone may also impart this Swiss cheese appearance.

foreign body reaction pattern. Histochemical stains for microorganisms, particularly mycobacteria and fungi, should be at least considered in every instance.

Prognosis and Treatment

Surgical removal is the only effective method of therapy for disfiguring or disabling persistent foreign body reactions. Implanted foreign bodies usually persist, although some may undergo transepidermal elimination or be broken down by macrophages and gradually cleared. Many foreign body reactions are clinically stable and do not impart significant morbidity.

CUTANEOUS CROHN'S DISEASE

Clinical Findings

The most common cutaneous manifestations of Crohn's disease (also ulcerative colitis) are the reaction patterns of erythema nodosum and pyoderma gangrenosum (covered elsewhere in this chapter). Some patients with Crohn's disease develop specific cutaneous lesions that are histopathologically analogous to those involving the GI tract. Perianal skin tags; fistulas; abscesses; and oral lip swelling, ulceration or fissuring, and mucosal "cobblestoning" are characteristic. Metastatic Crohn's disease describes such lesions occurring at sites other than the mouth or anus, often presenting around a stoma, or as nodules or plaques with a predilection for flexural skin folds.

Histologic Features

Cutaneous Crohn's disease is characterized by lymphocytes, plasma cells, and noncaseating granulomas in the dermis, in some cases extending into the subcutis. Palisaded granulomas and neutrophils may be present. Granulomatous vasculitis is a variable feature.

Ancillary Studies

Ancillary studies include cultures or special stains to exclude infection.

Differential Diagnosis

Granulomatous rosacea, granulomatous perioral dermatitis, cheilitis granulomatosa (Miescher-Melkersson-Rosenthal syndrome), superficial sarcoid, and granulomatous reactions to infection may enter the differential diagnosis for perioral lesions. Clinical correlation is generally required to distinguish among these entities. The granulomas in granulomatous rosacea and granulomatous perioral dermatitis are typically perifollicular. In Miescher-Melkersson-Rosenthal syndrome, lip swelling (cheilitis granulomatosa) is accompanied by unilateral facial paralysis and geographic tongue. Sarcoidal granulomas are composed of a more homogenous population of epithelioid histiocytes, with relatively few admixed lymphocytes and plasma cells. Caseating granulomas are most associated with infectious etiologies.

Prognosis and Treatment

Cutaneous Crohn's disease may arise before or after GI manifestations. Cutaneous lesions may or may not respond to therapy directed against Crohn's disease.

SWEET'S SYNDROME

Sweet's syndrome (acute febrile neutrophilic dermatosis) may be regarded as a prototype of neutrophilic dermatoses. Vasculitis is typically associated with neutrophils (e.g., leukocytoclastic vasculitis) and is discussed elsewhere.

SWEET'S SYNDROME AND SWEET'S-LIKE REACTIONS

Clinical Findings

Cutaneous lesions of Sweet's syndrome are typically accompanied by acute fever and peripheral neutrophilia and consist of tender, intensely erythematous or violaceous, firm, sharply bordered, elevated papules, plaques, or nodules on the face, neck, trunk, and extremities (Fig. 1.28A). Pseudovesicular, pseudopustular, or pseudobullous lesions are common. Pustular, bullous, and subcutaneous nodules may occur. Periocular edema is a rare but distinctive presentation. Patients may experience arthralgias, myalgias, headache, and malaise. Oropharyngeal, ocular, and internal organ involvement occurs less commonly. Sweet's syndrome is often associated with systemic disease, including various malignancies, including acute myeloid leukemia, and other conditions, including inflammatory bowel disease, upper respiratory tract infection, or pregnancy. Medications such as minocycline, trimethoprim–sulfamethoxazole, all-*trans* retinoic acid, and granulocyte colony-stimulating factor have been reported to induce Sweet's syndrome.

SWEET'S SYNDROME—DISEASE FACT SHEET

Patient Group

- Usually middle-aged adults
- May be associated with infection (e.g., *Streptococcus, Yersinia*), chronic disease (e.g., Crohn's disease, rheumatoid arthritis), malignancy (e.g., leukemia, lymphoma), or drug-induced (e.g., G-CSF)

Site of Involvement

- Head and neck regions and upper extremities are most often affected
- May occur anywhere
- Neutrophilic dermatosis of the dorsal hands is a localized variant

Clinical Findings

- Smooth erythematous plaques, may be hyperkeratotic or annular
- Tender, usually not pruritic
- Associated fever and malaise

Prognosis and Treatment

- Benign condition, which may resolve on its own, but usually rapidly responds to oral steroids

G-CSF, Granulocyte colony-stimulating factor.

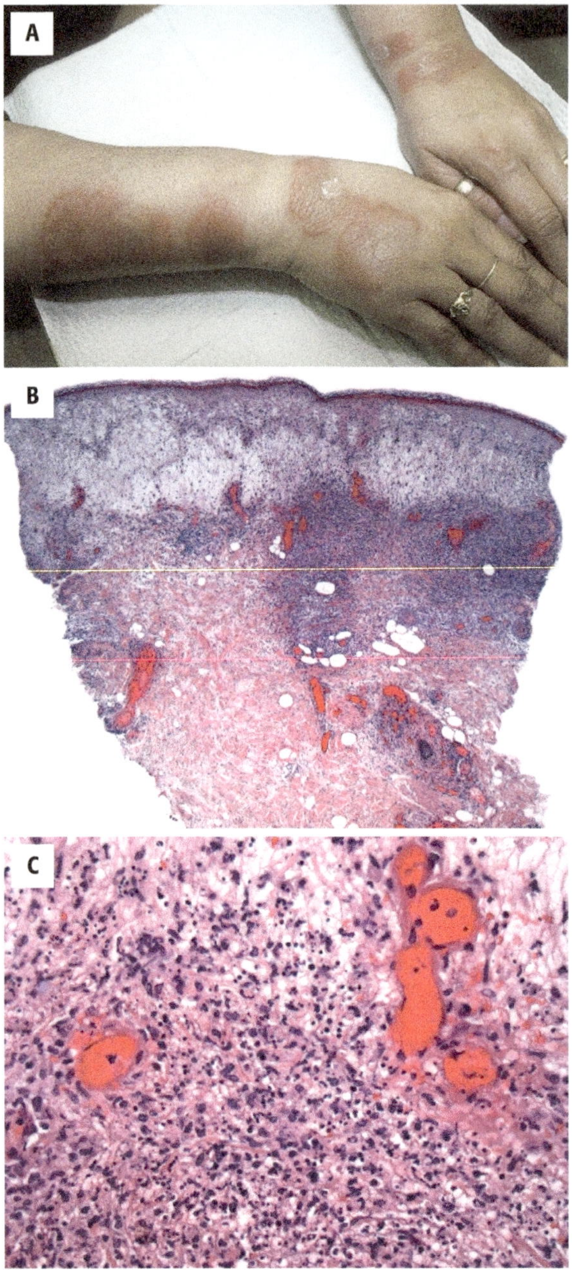

FIG. 1.28
Acute febrile neutrophilic dermatosis (Sweet's syndrome). **A,** Acute onset of tender, edematous plaques on the arms and hands. **B,** Scanning magnification reveals marked papillary dermal edema and dense inflammation in the upper dermis. **C,** Most of the cells are neutrophils, and nuclear dust (leukocytoclasis), but not vasculitis, is prominent.

Histologic Features

Sweet's syndrome is characterized microscopically by a diffuse, variably dense infiltrate of neutrophils with marked papillary dermal edema that may involve the entire dermis but typically only the upper dermis (Fig. 1.28B and C). Leukocytoclastic nuclear debris (nuclear dust) is typically prominent, but as a rule, there is no primary vasculitis. Vasculitis has been observed in a minority of cases, wherein it has been regarded as a minor or secondary feature. If

NEUTROPHILIC DERMATOSIS—PATHOLOGIC FEATURES

Histologic Features

- Dense infiltrate of neutrophils with nuclear dust in the upper dermis
- Marked papillary dermal edema
- Vasculitis typically absent

Ancillary Studies

- Special stains for bacterial, mycobacterial, or fungal organisms (negative)
- Cultures (negative)

Differential Diagnosis

- Infection (cellulitis)
- Pyoderma gangrenosum
- Behçet's disease
- Bullous lesions
  - Pustular drug reactions
  - Bullous lupus erythematosus
  - Dermatitis herpetiformis
  - Linear bullous IgA dermatosis

present, the vasculitic changes are not the focal point or the epicenter of the inflammatory reaction. The histopathologic correlate of the pseudobullous lesions that are often observed clinically is the marked papillary dermal edema with impending or actual subepidermal blister formation. Similar to leukocytoclastic vasculitis, the overlying epidermis may exhibit a variety of nonspecific secondary changes, including neutrophilic spongiosis, neutrophilic spongiotic vesicles, or subcorneal pustules.

Ancillary Studies

An elevated neutrophil cell count and an elevated erythrocyte sedimentation rate are typically present. A Gram stain may help exclude bacterial infection. In the absence of concomitant granulomatous inflammation, fungal or mycobacterial infection is less likely but must still be reasonably excluded with histochemical stains or lesional tissue culture.

Distinction from other rare forms of neutrophilic dermatitis such as bowel bypass syndrome and rheumatoid neutrophilic dermatitis requires clinical correlation to distinguish them from Sweet's syndrome. Infection should be excluded. In cellulitis, interstitial neutrophils within an edematous dermis are usually relatively sparse. The histopathology of pyoderma gangrenosum is variable but may include in its superficial expression features that are indistinguishable from Sweet's syndrome. The evanescent macular eruption associated with juvenile rheumatoid arthritis (Still's disease) is most prominent when the patient is febrile and, microscopically, is characterized by superficial perivascular neutrophils and papillary dermal edema. Subcutaneous Sweet's syndrome may resemble other forms of lobular neutrophilic panniculitis, including alpha-1-antitrypsin deficiency panniculitis, factitial panniculitis, infection, pancreatic panniculitis, and drug-induced neutrophilic panniculitis, e.g., BRAF inhibitor.

Prognosis and Treatment

Sweet's syndrome is self-limited within weeks to months, especially if an underlying cause can be identified and managed. Lesions usually resolve without scarring. Even in cases associated with chronic disease or malignancy, systemic corticosteroids are the first-line treatment. Other options include topical or intralesional corticosteroids, potassium iodide, colchicine, indomethacin, and clofazimine.

NEUTROPHILIC ECCRINE HIDRADENITIS

Clinical Findings

Neutrophilic eccrine hidradenitis (NEH) is a reaction pattern originally described in association with systemic administration of certain chemotherapeutic agents such as cytarabine and subsequently other chemotherapeutic agents. NEH may manifest clinically as tender erythematous papules, plaques, or nodules most often on the trunk. A second clinical subset occurs on the palms or soles of children (idiopathic plantar hidradenitis, palmoplantar eccrine hidradenitis, PlayStation palmar hidradenitis) and is not associated with chemotherapy or systemic disease.

Histologic Features

NEH is characterized by predominantly neutrophilic infiltrates surrounding and infiltrating eccrine glands. Associated vacuolar alteration and necrosis of the eccrine gland and squamous metaplasia (squamous syringometaplasia) may be present.

Ancillary Studies

Special stains should be performed to evaluate for infectious eccrine hidradenitis (e.g., *Staphylococcus* sp., *Nocardia* spp.).

Differential Diagnosis

The differential diagnosis of NEH includes other neutrophilic dermatitides, including Sweet's syndrome, pyoderma gangrenosum, neutrophilic urticarial dermatosis (NUD), and infectious eccrine hidradenitis. Preferential involvement of the eccrine glands by neutrophils is the distinguishing feature of NEH. Most cases of palmoplantar eccrine hidradenitis are indistinguishable from chemotherapy-associated NEH, but in addition to the differing clinical presentation and anatomic site, squamous metaplasia is typically absent in palmoplantar eccrine hidradenitis. NUD is associated with autoimmune or autoinflammatory disorders.

Prognosis and Treatment

The lesions of NEH typically resolve within several days to weeks after exposure to the causative agent and usually resolves but may episodically recur.

CELLULITIS

Clinical Findings

Cellulitis refers to the clinical presence of dermal inflammation secondary to a skin infection, usually bacteria. A single extremity is typically affected. *S. aureus* is the most common etiology, but a variety of bacteria and occasionally fungi may cause clinical cellulitis. Cellulitis is characterized clinically by a diffuse, variably circumscribed zone of erythema, swelling, heat, pain, and tenderness that may extend several centimeters, sometimes involving the majority of the affected extremity. Disproportionate pain may signify subcutaneous or fascial involvement, i.e., necrotizing fasciitis, a medical emergency often requiring surgical intervention. Erysipelas is a clinically distinct form of cellulitis that typically occurs on the face, characterized by an erythematous plaque with a well-demarcated, rapidly advancing edge. Ecthyma is characterized by punched-out crusted ulcers and is usually associated with *Streptococcus pyogenes* or *S. aureus* and regarded as a deep variant of impetigo rather than cellulitis. The term *pyoderma* is a more general term sometimes used to describe localized cellulitis.

Histologic Features

The diagnosis of cellulitis is usually established clinically without biopsy. Histopathologic features include sparse perivascular and interstitial neutrophils and usually some lymphocytes. Dermal edema and dermal necrosis are variable findings.

Ancillary Studies

Blood culture is the most sensitive and specific diagnostic test. Demonstration of microorganisms in tissue sections or from culture of lesional skin biopsy is helpful if positive but insensitive enough that negative study results do not exclude the diagnosis of cellulitis.

Differential Diagnosis

The diagnosis may be confirmed by culturing a pathogen from lesional tissue or blood, or it may be presumed based on an expected response to antibiotics. Other disorders characterized histopathologically by dermal neutrophils can usually be distinguished from cellulitis through clinical-pathologic correlation. Infectious or noninfectious vasculitis usually presents as purpuric papules and microscopically with perivascular leukocytoclasis, erythrocyte extravasation, vascular thrombosis, and fibrin obscuring vessel walls. Because the diagnostic features of vasculitis may be focal, deeper sections may be required. Acute febrile neutrophilic dermatosis (Sweet's syndrome), bowel bypass syndrome, rheumatoid neutrophilic dermatosis, and pyoderma gangrenosum (see the following) may all exhibit dermal neutrophils, but typically the neutrophil infiltrates are substantially denser than those in cellulitis. Erythema marginatum, the transient erythema associated with acute rheumatic fever, is clinically quite distinct from cellulitis and typically exhibits perivascular neutrophils usually confined to the upper dermis.

Prognosis and Treatment

Cellulitis typically responds to oral or intravenous antistaphylococcal antibiotic therapy. Uncommonly, cellulitis secondary to infection by *S. aureus* or other organisms may progress to potentially fatal septic shock.

PYODERMA GANGRENOSUM

Clinical Findings

Pyoderma gangrenosum is an idiopathic ulcerative disorder characterized by one or more painful ulcers with elevated, ragged borders, usually on the extremities (Fig. 1.29A). Lesions characteristically exhibit pathergy, meaning they flare or progress in response to trauma such as surgical debridement. Clinical variants include the classic ulcer, superficial pustules, bullous, and superficial granulomatous. Analogous to Sweet's syndrome, pyoderma gangrenosum may be associated with a variety of systemic disorders, including myeloid leukemia, inflammatory bowel disease, and arthritis. In contrast to Sweet's syndrome, there are no associated constitutional symptoms.

Histologic Features

The histologic features of pyoderma gangrenosum can be somewhat characteristic but are variable and not diagnostic on histology alone (Fig. 1.29B and C). In all

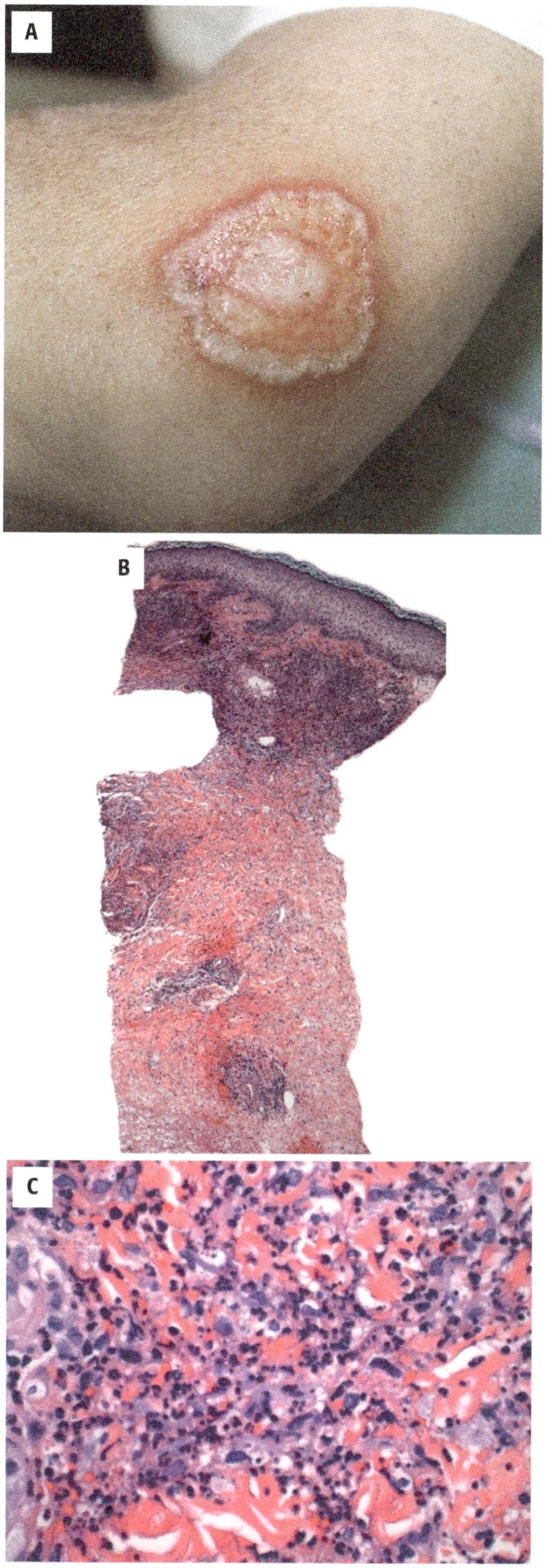

FIG. 1.29

Pyoderma gangrenosum. **A,** Ulcer with an elevated, ragged border. **B,** In this example, there is a nodular infiltrate of mostly neutrophils, although there is no single characteristic pattern. **C,** Although pyoderma gangrenosum is never diagnosed by histology alone, some degree of tissue neutrophilia is expected, and a biopsy is generally recommended to exclude infection or other causes such as vasculitis.

forms, there are typically neutrophils in the dermis or subcutis. Suppurative folliculitis has been posited to be the earliest manifestation, but more nodular or diffuse neutrophilic infiltrates are typical. The clinically characteristic undermining inflammation at the ulcer edge may be appreciated, as well as dermal edema, microabscess formation, vascular thrombosis, and dermal necrosis. Vasculitis, if present, is typically a secondary finding limited to the ulcer base. Superimposed granulomatous inflammation characterizes the superficial granulomatous variant.

Ancillary Studies

Ancillary studies include cultures and special stains to exclude infection.

Differential Diagnosis

Infection must be ruled out. The neutrophilic infiltrates in cellulitis are typically sparse. Clinical correlation is required to distinguish pyoderma gangrenosum from other neutrophilic dermatoses such as Sweet's syndrome or bowel bypass syndrome, but the presence of folliculitis or perifollicular neutrophilic abscess formation favors early pyoderma gangrenosum. While a characteristic undermining edge may be perceived microscopically, ultimately, the diagnosis of pyoderma gangrenosum is primarily made clinically. Usually, the pathologist's contribution is to exclude other diagnoses such as infection or malignancy and to confirm the presence of findings compatible with pyoderma gangrenosum.

Prognosis and Treatment

Pyoderma gangrenosum exhibits a variable, but often chronic, waxing and waning course; however, complete remission is possible. Mild cases may be managed with topical or intralesional corticosteroids. Appropriate wound care and avoidance of trauma are essential. In addition to topical or intralesional corticosteroids, systemic corticosteroids, cyclosporine, and biologic therapies may be used.

PERIVASCULAR DERMATITIS WITHOUT EPIDERMAL CHANGES

Considering the frequency that perivascular dermatitis is encountered in routine practice, relatively little attention has been devoted to the subject. The somewhat disarming (or boring) simplicity of this pattern belies the inherent challenges in managing these cases because they are only rarely diagnostic on histology alone. Diagnostic considerations unique to perivascular dermatitis include the following: (1) *Perivascular dermatitis is the least common denominator for virtually all inflammatory skin disorders.* Thus, deeper sections should be considered to avoid missing other diagnostic features, such as parakeratosis, spongiosis, interface dermatitis, or folliculitis. (2) *Because inflammatory skin lesions evolve and exhibit recognizable differences in their early versus late stages, a biopsy of perivascular dermatitis may represent an early or waning stage or a partially treated expression of a disorder that exhibits more specific diagnostic features in its fullest expression.* One example is the urticarial stage of bullous pemphigoid, which may be histologically indistinguishable from a drug reaction, urticaria, or a mild arthropod bite reaction. (3) *Perivascular dermatitis also represents the fullest expression or primary pattern of some disorders.* Examples include urticaria, some urticarial drug reactions, some examples of PUPPP, some paraneoplastic reactions, and a variety of poorly documented pruritic eruptions designated variably by dermatologists (e.g., itchy red bump disease, urticarial dermatitis) and dermatopathologists (e.g., DHRs, urticarial hypersensitivity reactions). After multiple sections have established that no additional diagnostic features are present, attention may turn to the pattern (superficial, superficial and mid, or superficial and deep) and the presence of cell types, usually eosinophils or neutrophils. Superficial perivascular dermatitis involves the papillary dermis. Superficial and deep perivascular dermatitis involve both the papillary and reticular dermis. *Superficial and mid perivascular dermatitis* describes perivascular infiltrates that fall in between (i.e., perivascular lymphocytes extend into the upper reticular dermis but not the deep reticular dermis). On most of the trunk and extremities, the reticular dermis is many times thicker than the papillary dermis, so the superficial and mid pattern is commonly encountered.

URTICARIA—DISEASE FACT SHEET

Patient Group

- May occur at any age
- Associated allergies

Site of Involvement

- May occur anywhere

Clinical Findings

- Wheals: pruritic pink or pale transient superficial dermal plaques (individual lesions disappear within 24–48 hours)
- Angioedema: deep dermal, subcutaneous, or submucosal swellings
- May occur spontaneously or be induced (physical or mechanical urticaria, cold/heat urticaria, contact urticaria)

Prognosis

- Benign condition, may become chronic with frequent recurrences

Treatment

- Avoidance of triggers
- H1 antihistamines
- Systemic corticosteroids
- Leukotriene modifiers, e.g., montelukast

URTICARIA

Clinical Findings

Urticaria is a common disorder characterized by pruritic, erythematous edematous papules or plaques (wheals) that occur transiently on any part of the body (Fig. 1.30A). The lesions are smooth-surfaced and often surrounded by a peripheral rim of pallor secondary to dermal edema. As a rule, excoriation does not occur because individual lesions generally resolve within hours or 1 to 2 days at most. Urticaria can be classified as acute (<6 weeks) or chronic (>6 weeks) depending on overall disease duration, but in all instances, individual lesions come and go within hours to days. Many cases are idiopathic. A wide variety of drugs (aspirin, opiates, radiocontrast media), infections (parasites), and food allergies (shellfish, nuts, chocolate) have been implicated. Physical urticaria may be induced by cold, heat, pressure, or sun exposure. Cholinergic urticaria is a common, self-limited variant arising in young adults as numerous small red macules and papules in association with heat, exercise, or emotional stress. Urticaria may represent a sign of systemic malignancy, although this is generally not the case in otherwise healthy individuals with chronic urticaria.

Histologic Features

The vast majority of urticaria is diagnosed clinically, without biopsy. However, lesions of urticaria may be biopsied to rule out urticarial vasculitis, urticarial pemphigoid, urticarial eczematous dermatitis, urticarial drug reactions, urticarial dermatitis herpetiformis, urticarial arthropod bite reactions (papular urticaria), and others. Although the histopathologic features alone in urticaria are not pathognomonic, the clinical history will facilitate specific diagnosis. Urticaria is characterized by sparse superficial and mid or deep perivascular and interstitial lymphocytes with variable numbers of

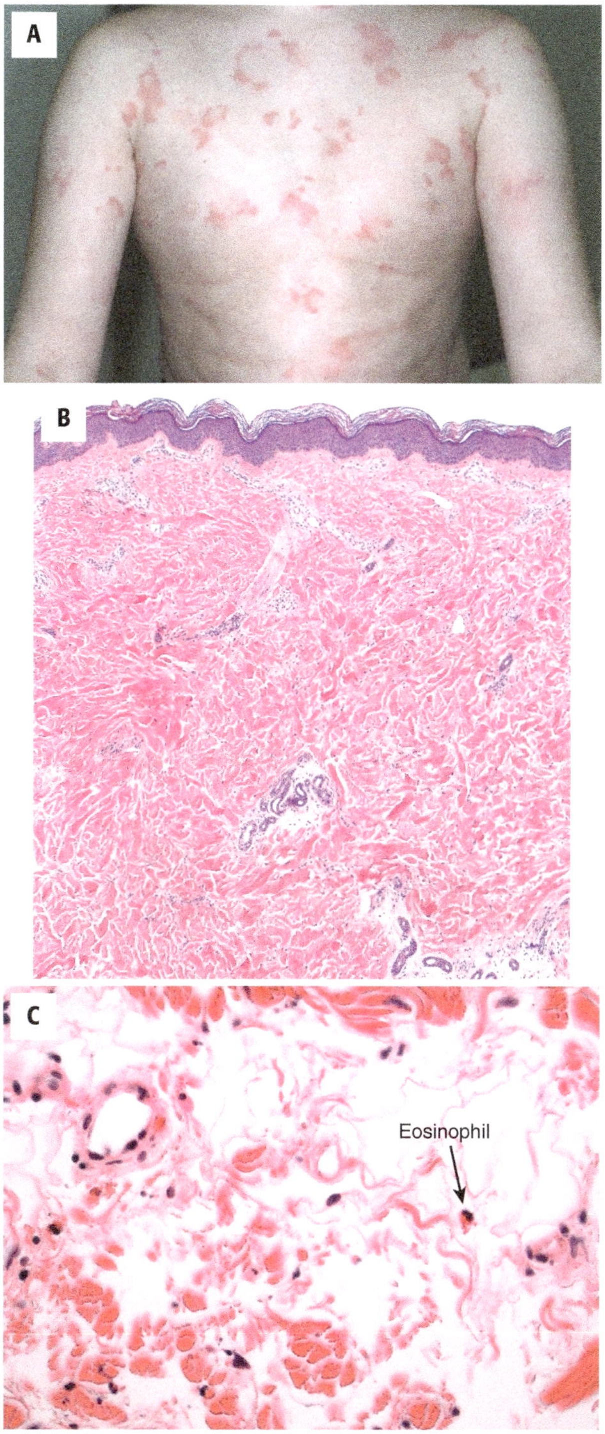

FIG. 1.30
Urticaria. **A,** Transient, edematous, red, often annular plaques that resolve within 24 hours. **B,** Scanning magnification reveals sparse perivascular and interstitial lymphocytes without overlying epidermal alteration. Dermal edema may not be obvious. **C,** Collagen fibers are relatively widely spaced (evidence of dermal edema), and a few eosinophils are noted at high magnification.

neutrophils or eosinophils. Diffuse dermal edema may be appreciated, manifesting as diffusely exaggerated "empty" spaces between dermal collagen fibers. The overlying epidermis should be uninvolved (Fig. 1.30B and C).

URTICARIA—PATHOLOGIC FEATURES

Histologic Features

- Dermal edema
- Variably dense (minimal to moderate) perivascular inflammatory cell infiltrate
- Lymphocytes with neutrophils and/or eosinophils
  - No epidermal changes

Differential Diagnosis

- Urticarial vasculitis (evidence of vascular damage)
- Drug reaction
  - Urticarial dermatitis

Ancillary Studies

Urticaria can be associated with a wide variety of possible systemic food or medication allergies or infections. A much smaller proportion of individuals, mostly adults, who present with urticaria, have an associated systemic malignancy. Thus, a detailed review of systems, routine laboratory screening, imaging studies, and allergy testing may be performed on patients with unexplained chronic urticaria. Contact allergens may rarely cause urticaria and may be diagnosed by patch, prick, or serum radioallergosorbent testing (RAST) (e.g., latex rubber).

Differential Diagnosis

Multiple sections should be obtained to rule out more specific findings. Fully developed lesions of urticarial vasculitis are essentially identical to those of small-vessel leukocytoclastic vasculitis, but not infrequently, biopsies from patients fulfilling other criteria for the diagnosis of urticarial vasculitis exhibit only minimal evidence of vasculitis, such as perivascular neutrophils and leukocytoclasis but no significant fibrin deposition around vessel walls. Thus, the histopathologic findings of urticarial vasculitis may fall on a spectrum ranging from an appearance that is only minimally beyond, if not indistinguishable from, classic urticaria to those of fully developed vasculitis. Other disorders presenting with urticarial lesions should exhibit histologic evidence of those disorders. One exception is urticarial pemphigoid, wherein eosinophils tend to aggregate in the papillary dermis near the dermal-epidermal junction. This may be associated with exocytosis of eosinophils into the epidermis (eosinophilic spongiosis), but subepidermal vesiculation may not be present. DIF studies should reveal linear deposition of C3 and often IgG in the urticarial pemphigoid; in some instances, an n-serrated staining pattern may be evident. PUPPP, usually arising during the third trimester, often exhibit mild spongiosis but may be histologically indistinguishable from urticaria, but clinical correlation is generally sufficient to establish this diagnosis. Similarly, a condition that often frustrates patients and their physicians is urticarial dermatitis, characterized by edematous pruritic papules and/or plaques that can be histologically identical to urticaria. If exclusively papular, lesions may resemble those of papular urticaria (arthropod bite reactions) or idiopathic itchy bump disease, but there is no history of pets or arthropod exposure. Histologically, biopsies of urticarial dermatitis or itchy red bump disease may show minimal epidermal alteration, in contrast to urticaria itself.

Prognosis and Treatment

Urticaria, especially acute urticaria, is usually self-limited. If an underlying cause can be identified and removed, the disease abates. However, many cases go unsolved despite extensive inquiry and testing. Symptomatic therapy includes daily administration of sedating (e.g., hydroxyzine, diphenhydramine, doxepin) and minimally sedating (e.g., cetirizine), levocetirizine, or nonsedating (e.g., fexofenadine) oral H1 antihistamines, either alone or in combination, and sometimes with up-dosing. In contrast to most inflammatory skin disorders, topical agents, including corticosteroids, are ineffective.

ERYTHEMA ANNULARE CENTRIFUGUM

Clinical Findings

EAC is a cutaneous reaction pattern with multiple possible underlying causes. EAC has been divided into two clinical-pathologic variants, superficial and deep. The superficial variant is characterized by erythematous macules or edematous papules that rapidly clear centrally, leaving only thin annular, serpiginous, or polycyclic rings of erythema and a ridge of scale on the trailing edge of the advancing border (Fig. 1.31A). The buttocks

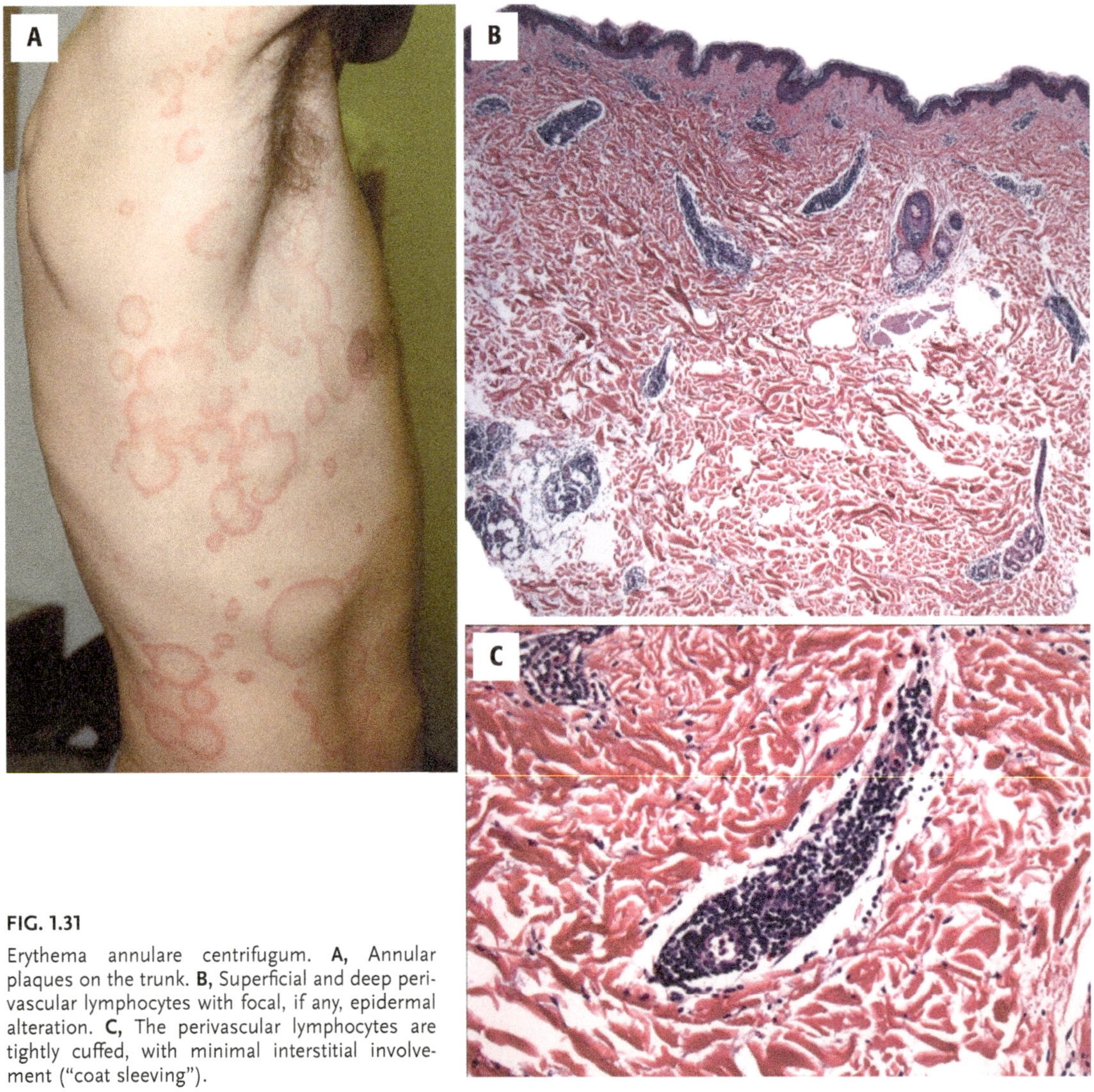

FIG. 1.31

Erythema annulare centrifugum. **A,** Annular plaques on the trunk. **B,** Superficial and deep perivascular lymphocytes with focal, if any, epidermal alteration. **C,** The perivascular lymphocytes are tightly cuffed, with minimal interstitial involvement ("coat sleeving").

and trunk are most commonly affected. Some cases are associated with dermatophytosis, but most are idiopathic despite extensive inquiry. In the deep variant, the plaques do not exhibit an overlying scale.

Histologic Features

EAC is characterized by perivascular lymphocytes that are "tightly cuffed" around blood vessels (also known as coat sleeving), meaning that there is minimal interstitial extension of inflammatory cells. Coat sleeving is most consistently observed in the deep variant of EAC. In the deep variant of EAC, epidermal changes are usually absent. The dermis contains superficial and deep, tightly cuffed perivascular lymphocytes (Fig. 1.31B and C). In superficial EAC, sections through the ring of scale at the lesion edge reveal focal spongiosis and parakeratosis. Spongiotic microvesiculation may be present. Rarely, multiple areas of spongiosis may be present. A minority component of dermal eosinophils, and less commonly, neutrophils, are variably present within the predominantly lymphocytic infiltrate. Plasma cells are not prominent.

Differential Diagnosis

A fungal stain may be considered to exclude dermatophytosis in the superficial variant. Some authors consider the histopathologic features of the superficial variant of EAC to be often indistinguishable from those of PR (see preceding section), although lymphocyte exocytosis and papillary dermal extravasation of erythrocytes are more characteristic of PR. Both disorders are usually diagnosed clinically by dermatologists and not routinely biopsied unless the clinical features are atypical. The deep variant of EAC is more likely to present a diagnostic challenge as it may closely resemble tumid LE; Jessner's lymphocytic infiltrate; and, if the infiltrates are dense enough, pseudolymphoma (cutaneous lymphoid hyperplasia) or cutaneous marginal zone (B-cell) lymphoma may enter the differential diagnosis. Dermal lymphocytes in lupus, with its prominent perifollicular infiltrates, are usually situated in the deep dermis, imparting a slightly bottom-heavy profile, in concert with increased interstitial mucopolysaccharide (mucin). However, increased interstitial mucin has been reported in EAC, so it may not be possible to distinguish the deep variant of EAC from tumid LE in patients who do not have additional evidence of LE. Erythema migrans (see following section) is characterized by plasma cells accompanying superficial and deep perivascular lymphocytes. PMLE (see following section) and erythema gyratum repens, a rare paraneoplastic disorder, may also exhibit similar features, and such cases require confirmation via clinical correlation. Clinically, erythema gyratum repens is characterized by greater induration and a dense (zebralike) concentric banding pattern. Erythema marginatum, the eruption of rheumatic fever, is a transient eruption that typically exhibits neutrophils accompanying superficial perivascular lymphocytes.

Prognosis and Treatment

EAC is a benign disorder. Superficial EAC is usually self-limited. Deep EAC may run a chronic waxing and waning course. Symptomatic therapy includes topical corticosteroids and antihistamines. Refractory cases may require intermittent systemic corticosteroid therapy.

ERYTHEMA MIGRANS

Clinical Findings

Erythema migrans (formerly erythema chronicum migrans) is the most common cutaneous manifestation of Lyme disease (*Borrelia burgdorferi*) in the United States, consisting of one or a few round or oval, minimally symptomatic, erythematous, smooth patches up to several centimeters in diameter (Fig. 1.32A). Central clearing routinely produces an annular configuration. The primary lesion starts at the site where the individual was bitten by an infected tick (ticks generally must be attached for more than 48 hours to transmit Lyme disease), but if untreated, secondary lesions may subsequently develop elsewhere. Fever, arthralgia, myalgia, and headache may accompany the initial infection. In oral pathology, the term *erythema migrans* is synonymous with geographic tongue, an unrelated disorder.

Histologic Features

The annular border of lesions of erythema migrans is characterized by superficial or superficial and deep perivascular lymphocytes and plasma cells (Fig. 1.32B and C). Eosinophils and neutrophils are variable. There is usually no overlying epidermal alteration. Biopsy of the central portion of a lesion reveals nonspecific changes compatible with an arthropod bite reaction.

Ancillary Studies

Warthin-Starry stain may reveal small numbers of spirochetal forms in the upper dermis; however, a negative or

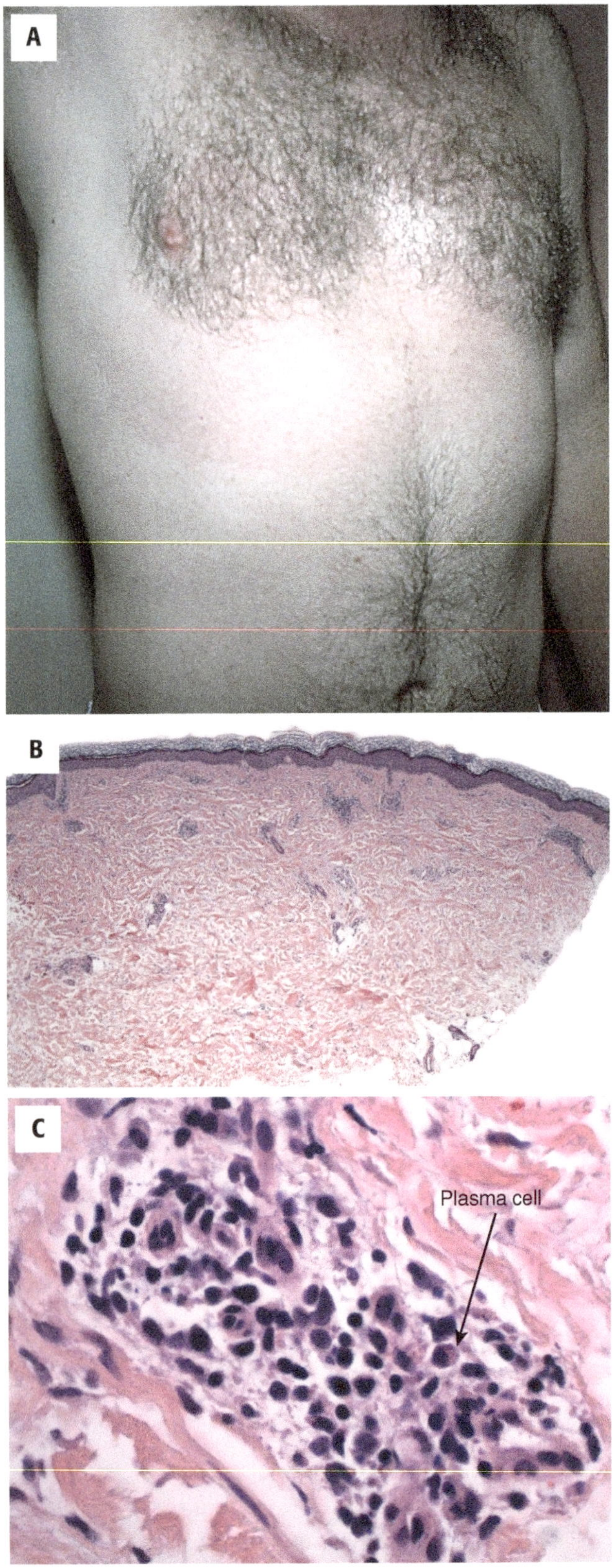

FIG. 1.32
Erythema migrans. **A,** A hiker from upstate New York with a large erythematous patch expanding centrifugally from the site of an infected tick's bite. **B,** Superficial and deep perivascular lymphocytes without epidermal alteration. **C,** Plasma cells are typically present.

equivocal study result does not exclude the diagnosis. Serum titers for *B. burgdorferi* usually confirm the diagnosis of Lyme disease in clinically ambiguous cases. The testing methods and pathogenic strains of *B. burgdorferi* differ among the United States, Europe, and elsewhere. Thus, intercontinental travelers whose exposure and testing occur in different locations may have a higher chance of false-negative test results.

Differential Diagnosis

The deep variant of EAC may exhibit nearly identical features. Typically, the perivascular lymphocytes are relatively sparse, so tumid LE and pseudolymphoma bear less resemblance than some cases of deep EAC might. The presence of plasma cells is the best available histopathologic clue to the diagnosis of erythema migrans. Early lesions of secondary syphilis may exhibit perivascular lymphocytes and plasma cells, but fully developed lesions typically display epidermal hyperplasia with variable spongiosis, slight interface dermatitis, and a neutrophilic crust.

Prognosis and Treatment

Erythema migrans is effectively treated by appropriate antibiotic regimens. Untreated cases may potentially progress to disabling systemic involvement.

TELANGIECTASIA MACULARIS ERUPTIVA PERSTANS

Clinical Findings

Telangiectasia macularis eruptiva perstans (TMEP) is a variant of cutaneous mastocytosis that typically arises in adults and is characterized by numerous telangiectatic macules, usually on the trunk. In contrast to urticaria pigmentosa, Darier's sign (urtication on scratching) is only variably elicited.

Histologic Features

In contrast to other forms of mastocytosis, the mast cell infiltrates in TMEP are typically subtle, with slightly increased numbers of perivascular and interstitial mast cells in the upper dermis, in concert with slightly dilated thin-walled dermal blood vessels. The changes may be subtle enough that a definite histopathologic diagnosis cannot be established without clinical correlation. Comparison with nonlesional skin may be helpful to establish the presence of increased mast cells in lesional skin. Roughly three to seven perivascular mast cells can usually be identified, on average, in normal skin. Hyperpigmentation of the overlying epidermis may be present.

Ancillary Studies

Ancillary studies include histochemical (e.g., Giemsa, toluidine blue, Von Leder) or immunohistochemical studies for tryptase or c-kit (CD117) to identify mast cells.

Differential Diagnosis

TMEP may resemble nonspecific, sparse perivascular dermatitis because the increase in mast cells relative to nonlesional skin may be subtle without mast cell-specific stains or comparison with nonlesional skin. In some examples of the urticaria pigmentosa variant of mastocytosis, the increase in mast cells may be mild, but mast cells are usually more than twice normal in number. In mastocytosis, the mast cells tend to be larger and acquire a fusiform shape.

Prognosis and Treatment

TMEP is usually chronic and progressive. Topical corticosteroids and systemic antihistamines may be used. It is prudent to equip patients with injectable epinephrine (EpiPen).

PLASMACYTOSIS MUCOSAE

Clinical Findings

Plasmacytosis mucosae encompasses a group of idiopathic, noninfectious inflammatory disorders affecting mucosal surfaces, typically genital skin (Zoon's balanitis or balanitis circumscripta plasmacellularis in men; Zoon's vulvitis, vulvitis circumscripta plasmacellularis in women) or lips (plasma cell cheilitis). Other terms include circumorificial plasmacytosis, plasmacytosis circumorificialis, and mucous membrane plasmacytosis. Lesions are usually solitary, erythematous, smooth, variably eroded, and often disproportionately minimally symptomatic patches.

Histologic Features

Plasmacytosis mucosae is characterized by a lichenoid or nodular accumulation of mature plasma cells (plasmacytes) in the upper dermis or lamina propria. Plasma cells are readily identified on H&E by their medium size, with relatively abundant cytoplasm, eccentrically situated nucleus, pale paranuclear halo or clearing (paranuclear or perinuclear Hof), and clumped peripheral chromatin (clock-face nucleus). The paranuclear Halo results from a prominent Golgi apparatus that reflects increased immunoglobulin secretion. Vascularity and dermal edema may be prominent. Extravasated erythrocytes, other lymphocytes, mast cells, eosinophils, or neutrophils may be present. There is no significant cytologic atypia. Russell bodies (intracytoplasmic eosinophilic accumulations of immunoglobulins and glycoproteins) may be present.

Ancillary Studies

Immunohistochemistry or in situ hybridization of kappa (κ) and lambda (λ) light chain expression, if performed, reveal a $\kappa:\lambda$ ratio within physiologic limits ($\approx$2:1).

Differential Diagnosis

Several other disorders are also characterized by plasma cell-rich infiltrates, most notably primary or secondary syphilis. In addition to distinct clinical and serologic features, the inflammatory infiltrates in syphilitic chancre (primary) and syphilids (secondary) usually contain lymphocytes and neutrophils, as well as plasmacytes, and secondary lesions typically exhibit psoriasiform epidermal hyperplasia. Primary syphilis (chancre) is typically ulcerated. In contrast, the epithelium is often crusted and eroded, but ulceration is uncommon. Spirochetes may be visualized in primary and secondary lesions with a Steiner stain. Plasma cells may be prominent at any chronically inflamed site and are often a prominent component of the host response directed against squamous cell carcinoma or basal cell carcinoma. If the infiltrate is unusually homogenous and dense, serum protein electrophoresis studies may be worthwhile to search for an occult plasma cell dyscrasia. Sinus histiocytosis with massive lymphadenopathy (Destombes-Rosai-Dorfman disease) may also show numerous plasma cells but is associated with a florid xanthogranulomatous infiltrate containing S100 protein-positive histiocytes. Cutaneous plasmacytoma may rarely represent a slowly growing primary cutaneous disorder but most commonly represents a cutaneous manifestation of multiple myeloma, plasma cell leukemia, or extramedullary plasmacytomas. The presence of high-grade atypia and large atypical cells with plasmacytic features (plasmablasts) correlates with a poor prognosis even in cases that appear to be primarily cutaneous at presentation.

Prognosis and Treatment

Plasmacytosis mucosae is a benign but chronic disorder. There is no association with increased risk of plasma cell malignancy. Anecdotally, lesions may respond to topical corticosteroid therapy.

MISCELLANEOUS INFLAMMATORY DISORDERS

A few selected inflammatory dermatoses are discussed here that show variable features that do not neatly fit into any of the other categories used to broadly classify inflammatory diseases in this chapter.

POLYMORPHOUS LIGHT ERUPTION

Clinical Findings

True to its name, the clinical appearance of PMLE is polymorphous and may take the form of papules, plaques, papulovesicles, vesicles, targetoid lesions, or other. Lesional morphology varies more among individuals, with individual patients tending to manifest the same morphologic pattern from season to season. PMLE usually arises acutely on newly sun-exposed areas such as the V of the neck and upper extremities (rather than the face or dorsal hands) within days of the individual's first significant exposure to ultraviolet light, generally in the spring (Fig. 1.33A). The eruption is usually less severe with subsequent exposure (hardening), but the ultraviolet sensitivity is reset during the winter, so the process repeats itself the following spring. Patients may have mild, transient eruptions and not need medical attention.

Histologic Features

PMLE usually exhibits a superficial and deep, moderately dense, predominantly lymphocytic perivascular dermatitis (Fig. 1.33B and C). Additional findings generally correlate with the clinical morphology. Marked papillary dermal edema with impending or actual

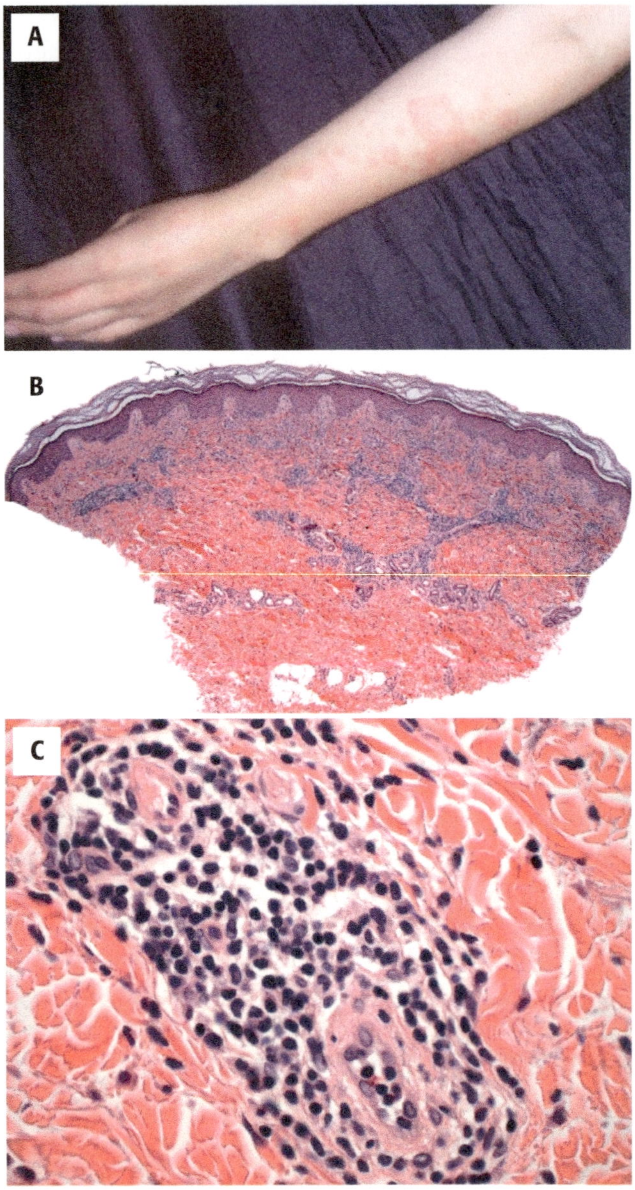

FIG. 1.33

Polymorphous light eruption. **A,** Erythematous papules and plaques on the extensor surface of the forearm and dorsal hand. **B,** Moderately dense dermal infiltrate with deep perivascular involvement. Papillary dermal edema is typical but is minimal in this case. **C,** Lymphocytes predominate. Variable histopathologic findings, as the name suggests, include papillary dermal edema, spongiosis, and some eosinophils or neutrophils in the infiltrate.

subepidermal blister formation may be present (clinical correlate: urticarial lesions, blisters). Spongiosis is variable (clinical correlate: eczematous or papulovesicular lesions). Erythrocyte extravasation is variable (clinical correlate: purpuric lesions).

Ancillary Studies

Phototesting usually reveals increased sensitivity to ultraviolet A, or less commonly, ultraviolet B light, or both.

Differential Diagnosis

Actinic prurigo is a genetically inherited eruption that clinically and histologically may be identical to PMLE. However, actinic prurigo is most common in Mestizos (individuals of mixed European and Amerindian ancestry) and usually presents with distinctive conjunctivitis and cheilitis. The inflammatory infiltrate in actinic prurigo may be deeper and denser, often containing eosinophils and reactive lymphoid follicles, and there are usually psoriasiform spongiotic epidermal changes. If spongiosis and eosinophils are present, photoallergic contact dermatitis should also be considered. Acute radiation dermatitis and phototoxic dermatitis are characterized by scattered single necrotic keratinocytes in the mid epidermis (sunburn cells) and junctional vacuolar alteration.

Prognosis and Treatment

PMLE often improves in adulthood. Sun protection and avoidance are usually sufficient to manage PMLE. Incremental ultraviolet light exposure under medical supervision can induce "hardening" before significant environmental exposure, minimizing the initial eruption.

ARTHROPOD BITE REACTIONS

Clinical Findings

Typical arthropod bite reactions in the United States are presumably caused by bites of mosquitoes, fleas, animal mites, bedbugs, chiggers, ticks, and others. Bite reactions are typically pruritic erythematous papules. Papular urticaria is a descriptive synonym for a common presentation of arthropod bite reactions, most common in children. Lesions are usually distributed on the distal extremities or other exposed sites. The lesions are often clustered or grouped, suggesting multiple bites from the same assailant (breakfast, lunch, dinner). Family members and close contacts are often not affected because the reaction depends mostly on the host immune response.

Histologic Features

Typical arthropod bite reactions are focal, wedge-shaped reactions (corresponding to a papule) that extend into the reticular dermis or even subcutis (Fig. 1.34A). Optimal sections will reveal a centrally situated focus of epidermal disruption (spongiosis, necrosis, erosion, ulcer) and sometimes retained arthropod parts within the overlying epidermis, most commonly tick mouthparts (Fig. 1.34B). Eosinophils are characteristically present and typically numerous (Fig. 1.34C). Flame figures may be seen. Neutrophils are variable and may be more prominent in bites from fleas, mosquitoes, and fire ants.

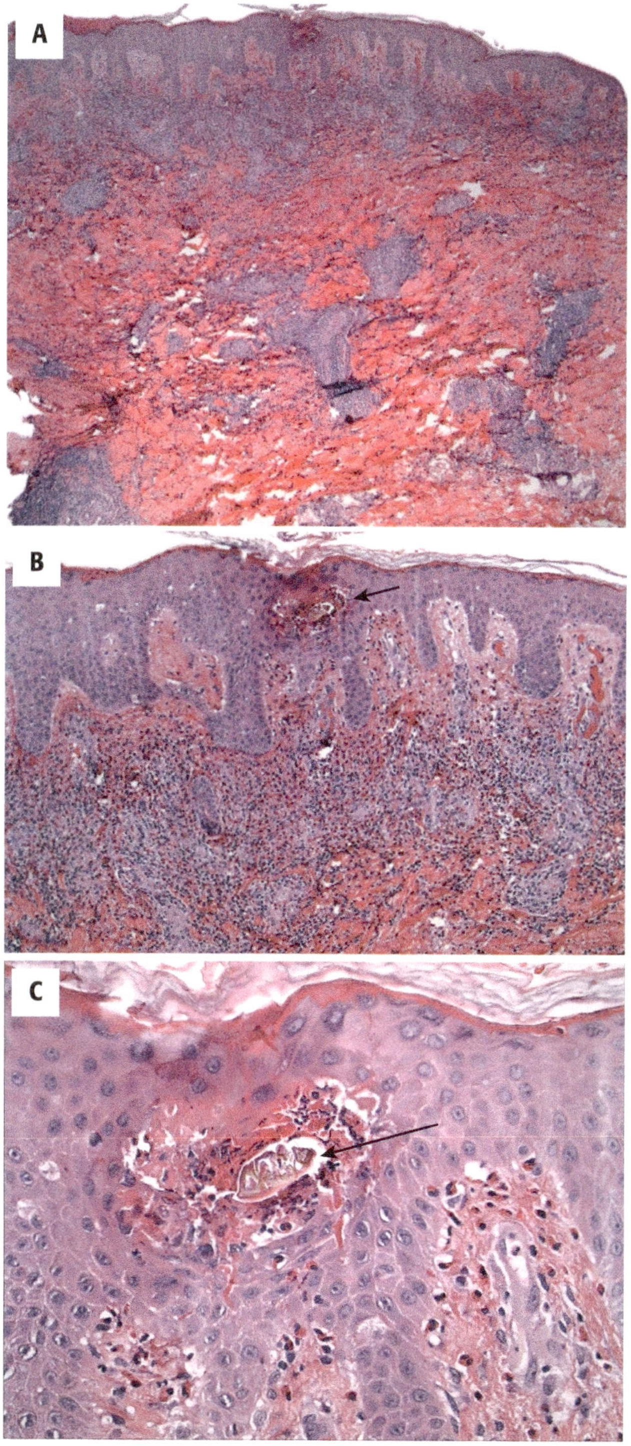

FIG. 1.34

Arthropod bite reaction. **A,** Scanning magnification reveals superficial and deep, often wedge-shaped, perivascular dermatitis. Depending on the plane of the section, central epidermal disruption may be present *(arrow)*. **B** and **C,** Eosinophils are typically prominent. A portion of the arthropod is retained in the tissue specimen *(arrow)*.

Differential Diagnosis

Excoriated lesions of papular dermatitis, folliculitis, some drug/medication reactions, or the urticarial stage of bullous pemphigoid may be histologically indistinguishable from an arthropod bite reaction. The differential diagnosis for crusted lesions also includes scabies. Multiple sections will typically reveal folliculitis, if present. However, arthropod bites may be centered on hair follicles. Papular dermatitis, PUPPP, and drug reactions should be distinguished primarily by clinical correlation but often exhibit more superficial and sparse dermal inflammation compared with arthropod bite reactions. Pemphigoid may be diagnosed by direct immunofluorescent analysis of perilesional skin. Lymphomatoid papulosis (type A) exhibits wedge-shaped mixed cell infiltrates with eosinophils but contains large atypical CD30+ T cells with prominent nucleoli. CD30 may be present in reactive infiltrates, including arthropod bite reactions, usually in smaller numbers and with solid clusters of cells compared to lymphomatoid papulosis.

Prognosis and Treatment

Arthropod bite reactions are self-limited. Insect repellents are effective. Symptomatic therapy consists of topical corticosteroids and oral antihistamines.

TRANSIENT ACANTHOLYTIC DERMATOSIS (GROVER'S DISEASE)

Clinical Findings

Transient acantholytic dermatosis (Grover's disease) is characterized by multiple small variably pruritic erythematous or skin-colored papules and crusted papulovesicles usually involving the trunk of adults (Fig. 1.35A). Men and women are approximately equally affected, although men older than 40 years of age are most commonly affected. Grover's disease may be precipitated by excessive sweating or fever.

Histologic Features

As per the exclusively papular lesions that characterize Grover's disease clinically, the microscopic findings in Grover's disease are focal. The five histologic variants include Darier's pattern (acantholytic dyskeratosis) (Fig. 1.35B), Hailey-Hailey pattern (full-thickness acantholysis), pemphigus vulgaris pattern (suprabasilar acantholysis) (Fig. 1.35C), pemphigus foliaceus pattern

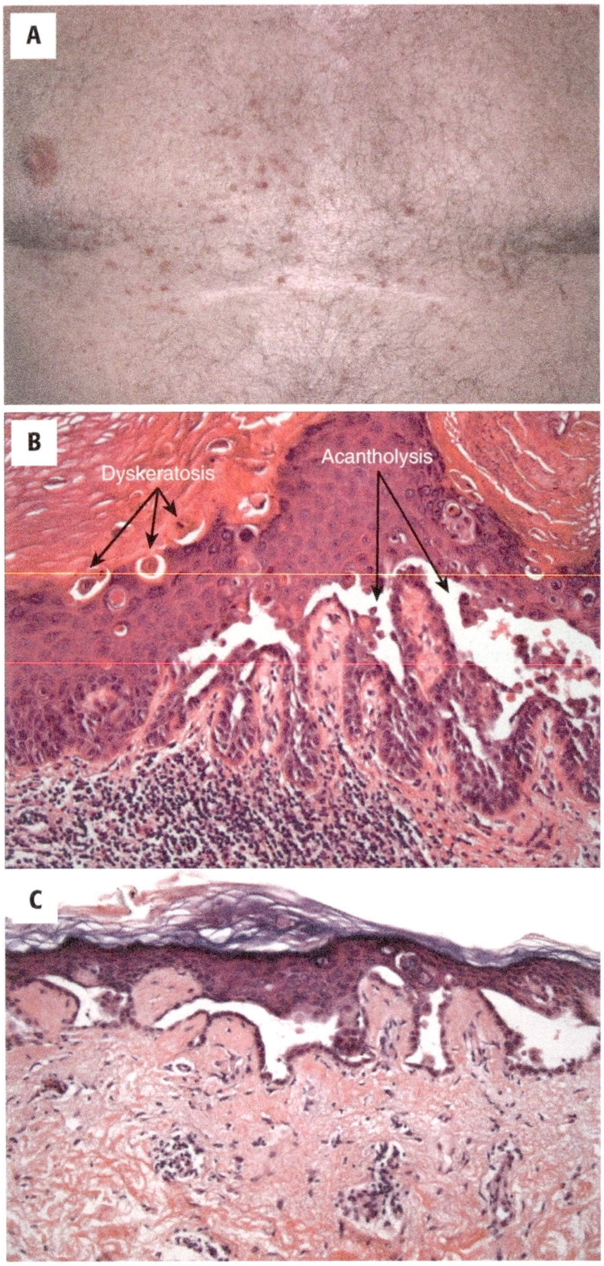

FIG. 1.35
Transient acantholytic dermatosis (Grover's disease). **A,** Numerous red, variably crusted papules on the trunk. **B,** Focal acantholytic dyskeratosis (Darier's disease pattern). **C,** Focal suprabasilar clefting (pemphigus vulgaris pattern).

(intragranular acantholysis), and spongiotic pattern. Combined patterns may be observed in single biopsy specimens or different specimens from the same patient. The findings are variably associated with sweat ducts or glands.

Differential Diagnosis

Compared with other disorders whose patterns it may resemble, the changes in Grover's disease are, as a rule, focal, usually extending no more than a few millimeters along the surface of the biopsy. If the changes affect the epidermis more broadly, clinical correlation may be required to distinguish Grover's disease from the diseases it mimics. Other disorders exhibiting acantholytic dyskeratosis include Darier's disease (keratosis follicularis) and acantholytic acanthoma. In Darier's disease, acantholytic dyskeratosis affects the epidermis more broadly and is associated with epidermal hyperplasia, follicular plugging, and relatively prominent dyskeratosis. In acantholytic acanthoma, the changes affect one circumscribed zone of acanthotic epidermis, and the clinical context is a single or multiple lesions, not an inflammatory disorder. Focal acantholytic dyskeratosis is a frequent incidental finding in excision specimens.

Prognosis and Treatment

Grover's disease may run a transient or chronic course. Symptomatic therapy includes topical corticosteroids or oral antihistamines.

FIBROSING DERMATITIS

Fibrosing disorders are characterized by increased dermal collagen deposition and usually increased numbers of cytologically bland spindled mononuclear cells (fibrocytes and dermal dendritic cells). Sclerosis is a subset of fibrosis characterized by thickened collagen fibers with disproportionately decreased density of spindle cells compared to typical fibrosis, e.g., scar.

SCAR

Clinical Findings

Scars represent a stereotypical wound healing response secondary to compromise of dermal integrity. Scarring may result from external trauma or other inflammatory processes that are significant enough to cause permanent loss or alteration of the collagen fiber architecture, such as folliculitis. Scars are smooth and firm and may appear erythematous, telangiectatic, hyperpigmented, hypopigmented, or depigmented. Hypertrophic scars are elevated but do not extend clinically beyond the confines of the initial trauma. Acne scars often result in focal depressions in the skin surface (termed *ice pick* scars when the scars are very well-demarcated). In contrast, keloids extend beyond the site of the initial trauma and may be very large and disfiguring. Keloids tend to occur along the jawline, earlobe (secondary to ear piercing), sternum, and shoulder girdle, more often in dark-complected individuals.

Histologic Features

Initially, the wound healing reaction is characterized by fibromyxoid stroma with increased vascularity (i.e., granulation tissue). Fully developed conventional scars exhibit increased collagen fiber deposition in which the fibers and spindled fibrocyte nuclei are oriented parallel to one another as well as to the overlying atrophic epidermal surface ("East-West"). Blood vessels are oriented perpendicular ("North-South") to the collagen fibers and epidermal surface. The atrophic epidermis is thinned, with attenuation or loss of the rete ridge pattern. Conventional scars are generally flat and do not significantly displace the underlying subcutis or adjacent adnexal structures. Hypertrophic scars are characterized by a nodular proliferation of haphazardly oriented fascicles whose collagen fibers maintain a parallel array within one another within a given fascicle. The fascicles are demarcated by small, thin-walled blood vessels. Keloids invariably contain a background of hypertrophic scar but additionally exhibit zones containing markedly broad or thickened collagen fibers (keloidal collagen, so-called "red crayons") that are typically situated in the centers of the fibrotic nodules. Keloids may be quite large. The diagnosis of keloid is usually clinically apparent.

Differential Diagnosis

Hypertrophic scars and keloids represent points along a histopathologic continuum. Dermal or subcutaneous neoplasms may resemble hypertrophic scars or keloids. Examples include desmoplastic melanoma, dermatofibroma, dermatofibrosarcoma protuberans, and the fibrotic stroma of cutaneous endometriosis. Immunohistochemical studies or analysis of incisional or excisional biopsy specimens may be required to arrive at a specific diagnosis. Keloidal collagen fibers may develop within a variety of disorders, including dermatofibroma, desmoid fibromatosis, and basal cell carcinoma.

Prognosis and Treatment

Scars are usually a cosmetic concern, and the erythema and dyspigmentation of scars may continue to slowly improve for at least a year, after which the appearance usually stabilizes. Pitted scars may be temporarily improved using injectable fillers (e.g., collagen, hyaluronic acid). Laser or intense pulsed light, dermabrasion, or chemical peels offer a variable degree of partial improvement in contour and dyspigmentation. Intralesional corticosteroids, administered monthly, usually flatten and soften hypertrophic scars and keloids. Silicone gel sheeting has been used. Surgical excision of keloids is effective in the short term, but there is a significant risk of keloid recurrence. Occasionally, small keloids spontaneously regress.

MORPHEA

Clinical Findings

Morphea (localized scleroderma) is a disorder of unknown etiology characterized by indurated, hard plaques with variable surface erythema or dyspigmentation. Lesions may be few in number, generalized, linear (*coup de sabre* on the forehead), or quite deep (morphea profunda).

MORPHEA—DISEASE FACT SHEET

Patient Group

- Usually adults but may also occur in children (especially the linear variant)
- Women are more commonly affected than men

Site of Involvement

- Scalp, trunk, or extremities

Clinical Findings

- Indurated plaque
- May be erythematous with a lilac border
- May show pigmentary alteration
- Clinical variants: linear (e.g., *en coup de sabre* is a manifestation of linear morphea of the forehead), generalized, guttate, deep, nodular or keloidal, or bullous

Prognosis and Treatment

- In contrast to systemic sclerosis, no associated extracutaneous disease
- Difficult to treat; may spontaneously regress or progress
- Generalized progressive morphea can lead to disabling constrictions

MORPHEA—PATHOLOGIC FEATURES

Histologic Features

- "Square punch biopsy"
- Reticular dermal fibrosis extending into subcutis
- Inflammation at dermal/subcutaneous junction
- Lymphocytes and plasma cells

Differential Diagnosis

- Postradiation dermatitis or panniculitis
- Chronic graft versus host disease
- Sclerosing injection site reaction

Histologic Features

In early lesions, there are perivascular lymphocytes and plasma cells, sometimes accompanied by increased interstitial mucin deposition without obvious sclerosis. Fully developed lesions become progressively less inflamed, with a predominance of thickened (sclerotic) collagen fibers and narrowing or virtual elimination of the empty spaces between adjacent fibers. At scanning magnification, tissue sections from a punch biopsy exhibit notably straight, parallel edges or squared-off edges (cookie cutter sign, square biopsy). If the dermal-subcutaneous junction is present, it may be prominent and straight (line sign). (Fig. 1.36). The deep dermal sclerosis causes eccrine glands to appear displaced superficially into the mid dermis. Sparse perivascular lymphocytes with plasma cells and often eosinophils characteristically surround vessels, especially at the junction of the reticular dermis and subcutis. Although the sclerosis is typically centered in the deep dermis, it may extend within the subcutaneous septa (morphea profunda) or more superficially into the papillary dermis. Rarely, the histopathologic features may be limited to the upper dermis (superficial morphea), where superimposed features of LS may be present.

Differential Diagnosis

Cutaneous lesions of systemic scleroderma, including limited (CREST [calcinosis, Raynaud's phenomenon, esophageal dysmotility, sclerodactyly, and telangiectasia

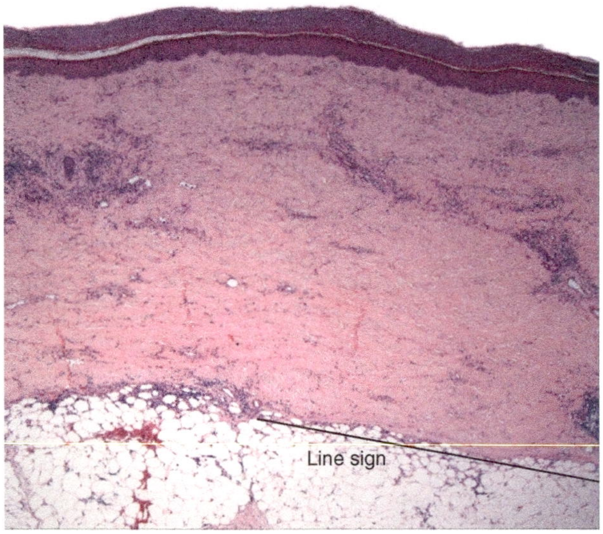

FIG. 1.36

Morphea. Sclerosis of collagen fibers is centered in the deep reticular dermis. At scanning magnification, the junction between the reticular dermis and subcutaneous fat is often smoother and more prominent (line sign). Perivascular lymphocytes, including plasma cells, encircle blood vessels in the reticular dermis; subcutis; and characteristically, the juncture between these two compartments.

in limited systemic scleroderma] syndrome) and generalized (progressive systemic sclerosis) forms, are typically less inflammatory than morphea but cannot be reliably distinguished from morphea based on histology alone. Sclerodermoid porphyria cutanea tarda and sclerodermoid GVHD are best distinguished from morphea by clinical correlation. Chronic radiation dermatitis may exhibit sclerosis at all levels of the dermis and is typically associated with scattered, large, bizarre mononuclear cells (radiation fibroblasts). Eosinophilic fasciitis (Schulman's syndrome) is clinically very distinct but microscopically overlaps significantly with morphea profunda; the changes in eosinophilic fasciitis are centered in the fascia rather than overlying deep dermis or subcutis, and eosinophils are usually, although not always, present in concert with peripheral eosinophilia.

Prognosis and Treatment

The prognosis in patients with morphea is good with most patients achieving complete remission within several months to years. There are no proven, consistently highly effective treatments, but topical corticosteroids, oral calcitriol, phototherapy, and systemic agents such as methotrexate have been used depending on the extent of the disease. In contrast, management of systemic sclerosis is typically dictated by the nature of extracutaneous organ involvement.

NEPHROGENIC SYSTEMIC FIBROSIS

Clinical Findings

Nephrogenic systemic fibrosis (NSF, aka nephrogenic fibrosing dermopathy) is highly associated with renal insufficiency in a variety of clinical settings that include acute or chronic renal failure and renal transplantation. The majority of patients were also previously exposed to gadolinium-containing radiocontrast media; incidence has dramatically reduced since 2007. NSF usually affects adults and is characterized by one or a few indurated papules that coalesce into plaques most commonly arising on the extremities in a symmetric fashion. The advancing edge of plaques may have an irregular amoeboid shape. Lesions often arise between the ankle and mid-thigh or between the wrist and mid-upper arm.

Histologic Features

Early lesions are characterized by a diffuse dermal proliferation of epithelioid, spindled, and dendritic fibrocytes, increased thick and thin collagen fibers, and variably increased interstitial mucin broadly affecting the dermis often with prominent involvement of the subcutaneous septa. Multinucleated giant cells are occasionally present in small numbers. The dermal fibrocytes appear to be derived from circulating fibrocytes coexpressing CD34 and procollagen-1 that are recruited to the dermis in NSF. In older lesions, interstitial mucin is decreased or absent. Regressed lesions resemble scars.

Differential Diagnosis

NSF was originally reported as a scleromyxedema-like disorder associated with renal disease. Scleromyxedema (papular mucinosis, lichen myxedematosus) typically exhibits more prominent interstitial mucin deposition and an accompanying inflammatory infiltrate of lymphocytes, including plasma cells. The plasma cells in scleromyxedema may be clonally restricted. In clinical practice, the presence or absence of CD34 or procollagen-1 immunohistochemical staining is insufficient to confirm or exclude NSF. Clinically, scleromyxedema typically involves the face and trunk rather than the extremities. Marked involvement of the subcutaneous septae is also more characteristic of NSF.

Prognosis and Treatment

The course to date has been variable, with some cases persisting or progressing but others exhibiting regression. The clinical subset associated with chronic renal failure appears to have the lowest chance of spontaneous remission. There are no established effective therapies for NSF, but physical therapy is important. Extracorporeal phototherapy has been used.

FOLLICULITIS

ACNE VULGARIS

Clinical Findings

Acne vulgaris (pimples) is a very common disorder affecting, to some extent, the majority of adolescents. Typical adolescent acne begins at the onset of puberty and usually subsides by the end of the second or third decade of life. However, acne may occasionally persist throughout the third decade or even beyond. The individual lesions may be noninflammatory; for example, they may be open comedones (blackheads) and closed comedones (whiteheads), erythematous papules or pustules, or larger nodules and cysts. Typically, the face is primarily involved, with additional involvement of the neck, upper trunk, and shoulders in moderate-to-severe cases. Acne lesions frequently leave postinflammatory hyperpigmentation and scars. Keloids may rarely form. The lesions are usually minimally symptomatic or tender (when inflamed). Acne may be pruritic. Some patients habitually pick their lesions, leaving only crusted papules or scars rather than primary lesions. Distinct clinical subsets of acne include neonatal acne, steroid acne (Fig. 1.37A), chloracne, and acne fulminans.

Histologic Features

The diagnosis of acne is usually made clinically; biopsy confirmation is exceptional. The histopathologic features correlate with the clinical lesions. Comedones resemble milia, essentially representing small follicular cysts. However, comedones differ from milia in that their content includes not just orthokeratin and hair shafts but also secretory lipid products of the sebaceous gland (sebum) and bacteria, usually *Propionibacterium acnes*. Comedones arise from the lower infundibulum or upper isthmic portion of the follicle (i.e., at the entrance of the sebaceous duct). Open comedones (blackheads) extend to the epidermal surface with a wide opening, but closed comedones (whiteheads) do not. Although lymphocytes have been reported to be the earliest inflammatory cells affecting the hair follicle, inflamed papules and pustules promptly attract neutrophils, leading to suppurative folliculitis with variable follicular rupture (Fig. 1.37B and C). The precursor lesion to inflammatory acne lesions is usually the closed comedone or a microcomedone (subclinical comedone). Granulomatous inflammation may follow follicular rupture, but discrete granuloma formation is often lacking.

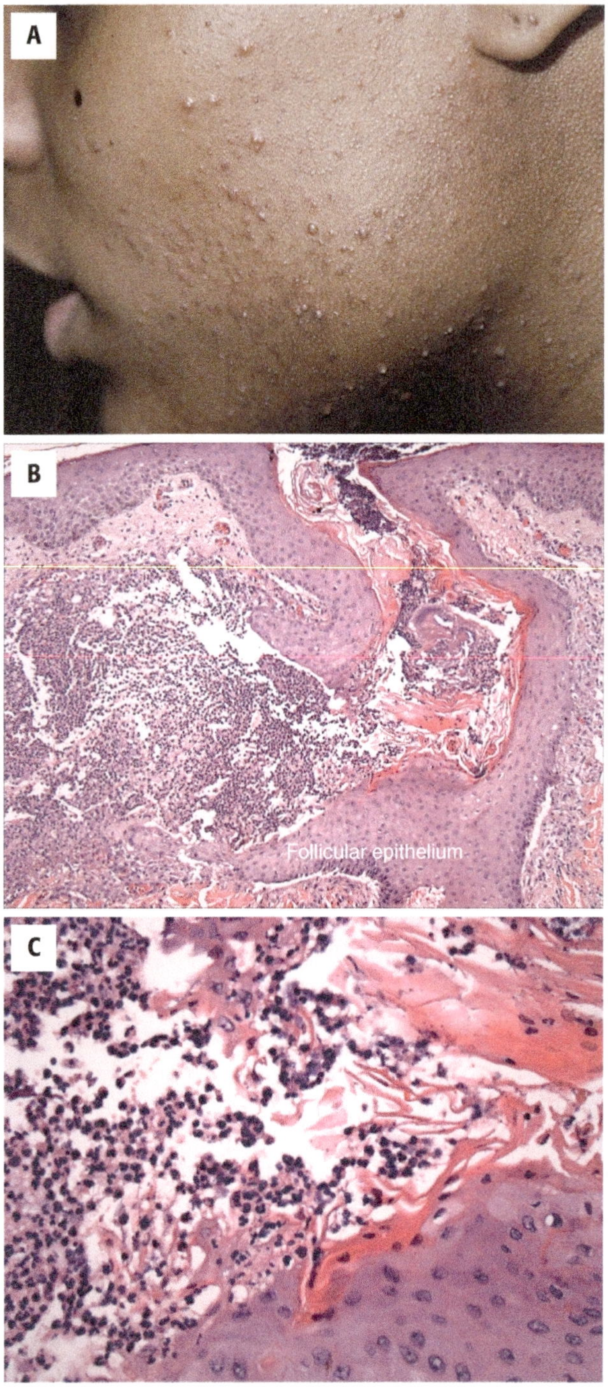

FIG. 1.37

Steroid-induced acne. **A,** Acneiform papules (i.e., comedones and pustules) on the cheek of a 16-year-old girl hospitalized for an acute asthma attack. The skin lesions arose within a few days of the initiation of systemic corticosteroid therapy. **B, C,** Suppurative folliculitis. Neutrophils surround and infiltrate the follicular epithelium, typically present in large numbers within the follicular canal. This pattern of inflammation may be observed in any acneiform disorder, including acne vulgaris, rosacea, perioral dermatitis, and infectious folliculitis.

Differential Diagnosis

The differential diagnosis for acne vulgaris includes all variants of acne and rosacea, including steroid acne, perioral dermatitis, and steroid rosacea. Clinical correlation is required to distinguish among these acneiform disorders. Suppurative folliculitis (Fig. 1.38) secondary to infection (usually *S. aureus*) is also indistinguishable from acutely inflamed papules of acne or rosacea unless microorganisms can be identified. The comedones in chloracne have been reported to possess a bottle or column shape in histologic sections. Other halogenoderma may exhibit nodular and diffuse suppurative and granulomatous inflammation with prominent pseudocarcinomatous epithelial hyperplasia. An acneiform drug reaction can be seen in association with novel cancer treatments aimed at inhibiting the epidermal growth factor receptor pathway.

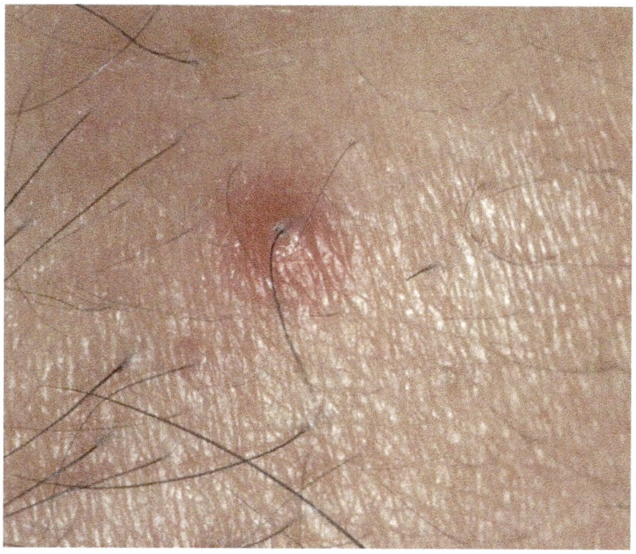

FIG. 1.38
Suppurative folliculitis. An erythematous pustule, most commonly associated with *Staphylococcus aureus* infection.

Prognosis and Treatment

Although acne often persists into the third decade, it usually slowly improves and eventually resolves. Topical therapy options include benzoyl peroxide, tretinoin, clindamycin or other antibiotics, or dapsone gel. Systemic therapy includes oral tetracyclines and isotretinoin. Women may occasionally benefit from certain oral contraceptives and spironolactone.

EOSINOPHILIC FOLLICULITIS

Clinical Findings

As a clinical term, *eosinophilic folliculitis* corresponds to a trio of uncommon but distinctive disorders characterized by folliculitis with numerous eosinophils. The classic variant, eosinophilic pustular folliculitis (Ofuji), is more common in Japan and rare in the United States, usually manifesting as pustules, sometimes forming circinate plaques on the face, proximal extremities, and trunk, and sometimes the palms and soles. Before the advent of improved antiretroviral therapy directed against HIV infection, the most commonly encountered variant was HIV-associated eosinophilic folliculitis, typified by numerous pruritic urticarial papules on the upper trunk, head, and neck in patients with AIDS with a helper T-cell count below 300/μL. Pustules may not be present. Pediatric eosinophilic folliculitis is a self-limited disorder characterized by multiple papules and pustules on the scalp.

Histologic Features

In all of the clinical variants of eosinophilic folliculitis, there is folliculitis with lymphocytes and prominent eosinophils centered in the infundibulum with inflammation often extending superficially to the epidermis, where pustules may be observed, and inferiorly to the follicular isthmus (Fig. 1.39). Follicular rupture is variable. Granuloma formation is not typical.

Ancillary Studies

Ancillary studies include PAS-D or GMS stain to rule out *Pityrosporum* folliculitis or a follicular dermatophyte infection. Patients with eosinophilic folliculitis may have circulating or bone marrow eosinophilia.

Differential Diagnosis

Fungal folliculitis, including tinea capitis and Majocchi's granuloma, and scabies often contain numerous eosinophils. Multiple tissue sections may be required to identify the etiologic agent in both cases.

Prognosis and Treatment

HIV-associated eosinophilic folliculitis is usually extremely pruritic and may be managed with topical and

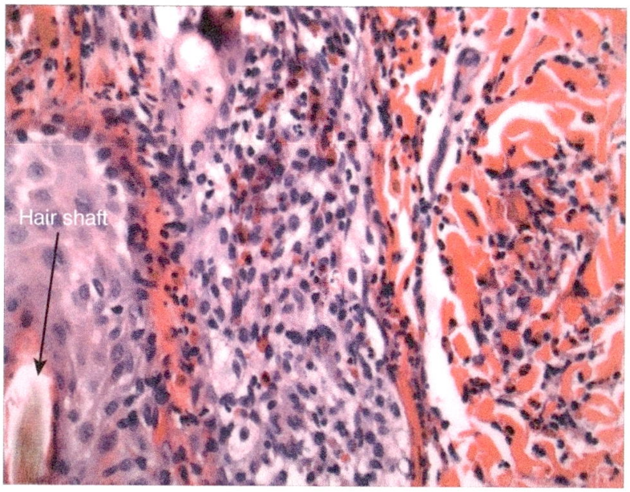

FIG. 1.39
Eosinophilic folliculitis. Eosinophils surround and infiltrate the follicular epithelium at the level of the infundibulum and isthmus. Clinical correlation is required to distinguish the classic, HIV-associated, and pediatric variants. The differential diagnosis includes an infectious etiology.

systemic corticosteroids, oral antihistamines, or other antiinflammatory agents. Many other agents, including phototherapy, have been reported to be effective. Ofuji's eosinophilic pustular folliculitis is usually less pruritic.

INFECTIOUS FOLLICULITIS

Clinical Findings

In clinical practice, the most common cause of infectious folliculitis is *S. aureus*, which presents as tender erythematous pustules, often on the buttock or trunk. However, a wide variety of organisms may infect the hair follicle, including other bacteria, e.g., *Pseudomonas aeruginosa* (hot tub folliculitis) or fungal folliculitis including dermatophytes (Majocchi's granuloma, tinea capitis, tinea barbae), *Malassezia (Pityrosporum)* sp., or *Candida* sp. Varicella zoster virus and molluscum contagiosum virus also affect the follicular unit. *Demodex* mites colonize the follicular canal in many individuals and occasionally mediate clinical folliculitis in predisposed individuals.

Histologic Features

Similar to the inflammatory lesions of acne vulgaris, *S. aureus* folliculitis is a suppurative (neutrophilic) folliculitis with variable follicular rupture. Clusters of gram-positive coccobacteria may be observed within the follicle. A neutrophilic abscess may surround the follicular unit, resulting in furunculosis or carbunculosis (multiple affected follicles). Other forms of folliculitis may exhibit suppurative, eosinophilic, granulomatous, or mixed patterns of inflammation centered on the follicular unit. Syphilitic folliculitis is usually associated with plasma cells. Fungal folliculitis usually has eosinophils in the inflammatory infiltrate.

Ancillary Studies

Culture or microbial genomic analysis of pustule content or lesional skin is a sensitive and specific means of identifying most forms of infection when histologic analysis is insufficient. As a rule, negative histochemical stains do not exclude infection.

Differential Diagnosis

Because the diagnostic findings are focal, deeper sections are recommended whenever the clinical description or clinical differential diagnosis includes folliculitis, but initial sections are nonspecific. Likewise, if folliculitis is identified but no organisms are seen, additional histochemical stains should be considered. If pathogenic organisms cannot be visualized or cultured, the differential diagnosis includes the acneiform disorders, acne, and, to a lesser extent, rosacea are rarely biopsied in clinical practice. Clinical correlation is essential to establish the diagnosis of acneiform disorders. Spongiosis, particularly atopic dermatitis and seborrheic dermatitis, occasionally is localized to the follicular infundibula (*infundibulofolliculitis*) and may resemble true folliculitis. In follicular spongiosis, there is infundibular follicular epithelial intercellular edema; if there is exocytosis of inflammatory cells into the follicular epithelium, the cells are mostly lymphocytes or Langerhans cells (or both), not neutrophils. Recurrent and disseminate infundibulofolliculitis is a rare disorder characterized by widespread follicular papules resembling papular atopic dermatitis but occurring in individuals without atopy. Follicular mucinosis may affect deeper portions of the follicular epithelium and may appear similar to follicular spongiosis with the additional presence of mucin between follicular keratinocytes that is readily appreciated on H&E. Follicular mucinosis may represent an idiopathic condition, be associated with alopecia (alopecia mucinosa) and may represent a manifestation of the folliculotropic variant of MF (Fig. 1.40).

Prognosis and Treatment

If the pathogens can be identified or at least suspected, appropriate antibiotic therapy is generally curative. Systemic therapy is often required because topical antibiotics do not always penetrate the follicular canal effectively. Hot tub folliculitis is self-limited but may recur unless the hot tub water is adequately treated.

ROSACEA

Clinical Findings

Rosacea (acne rosacea) is very common but rarely biopsied, usually to rule out skin cancer. The earliest manifestation is central facial erythema, typically exacerbated by exposure to heat (e.g., sunlight, exercise, hot drinks, spicy foods). Over time, repeated episodes of erythema and flushing eventuate in persistent erythema and telangiectasia. Acneiform lesions (comedones, inflamed papules, pustules) may be superimposed on the erythema. Chronic involvement of the nose in men may lead to

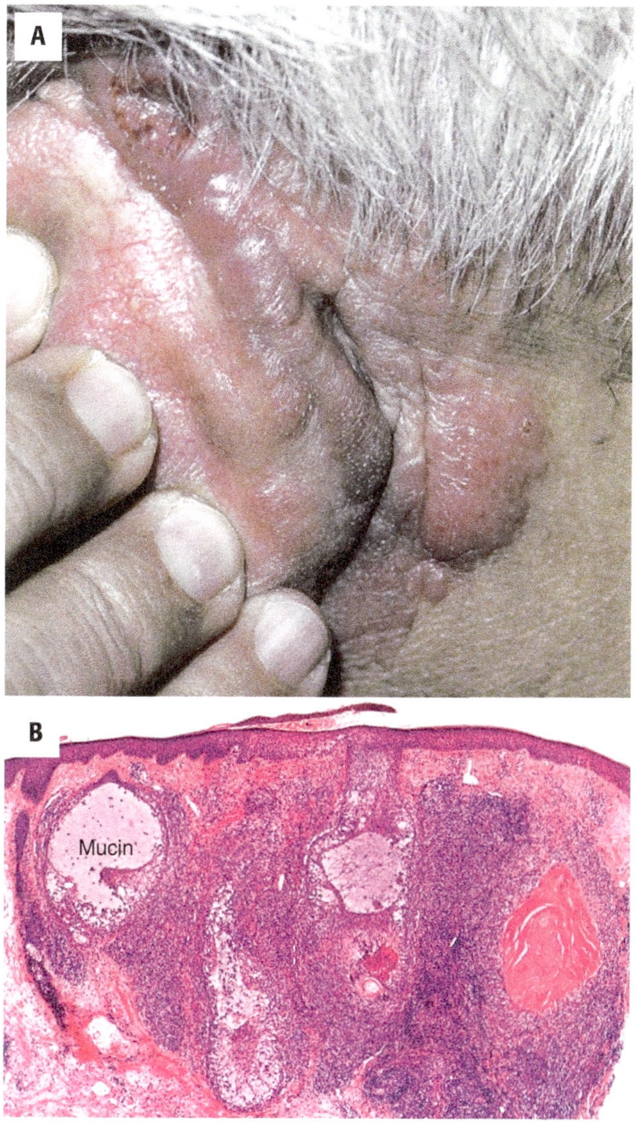

FIG. 1.40
Follicular mucinosis. **A,** Smooth, infiltrated plaques behind the ears in a man with biopsy-proven generalized patch or plaque stage mycosis fungoides (cutaneous T-cell lymphoma). **B,** Dense infiltrates of atypical lymphocytes surround and infiltrate follicular the epithelium, whose keratinocytes are separated by basophilic mucin (acid mucopolysaccharide).

rhinophyma. More persistent, firm papules in rosacea may represent granulomatous rosacea.

Histologic Features

Perivascular and perifollicular lymphocytes are typically associated with vascular dilation (telangiectasia). Acneiform papules usually represent folliculitis that may be suppurative, lymphocytic, or granulomatous. Plasma cells, neutrophils, or eosinophils may be present but not predominant. Rhinophyma specimens contain features consistent with localized chronic lymphedema with increased fibrosis, vascularity, nodular solar elastosis, and sebaceous gland hyperplasia. The histopathologic features of rhinophyma are not specifically diagnostic, but tissue is often submitted from a cosmetic procedure in which the diagnosis is not in question.

Ancillary Studies

Infection and foreign body granuloma should be excluded with special stains. Granulomatous lesions should be examined under polarized light.

Differential Diagnosis

Perioral or periorificial dermatitis is an acneiform disorder with acneiform papules localized around the mouth (sparing the vermilion border of the lips) and sometimes the nose and eyes. There is variable photosensitivity and superimposed seborrheic dermatitis, but the follicular inflammation in perioral dermatitis is histologically indistinguishable from rosacea, including variable secondary granulomatous inflammation. Both perioral dermatitis and a more generalized facial eruption, steroid rosacea, are associated with the use of halogenated topical steroids on the face. If a patient has been using halogenated topical steroids (usually mid to high potency), the condition often flares temporarily on withdrawal of the steroid.

Granulomatous rosacea must be distinguished from granulomatous infection, sarcoid, and foreign body granulomas. Severe presentations of granulomatous rosacea may be classified as rosacea fulminans, pyoderma faciale, or lupus miliaris disseminatus faciei. To the extent that a perifollicular distribution of granulomas can be discerned, the diagnosis favors the granulomatous rosacea group of disorders. Occasionally, a prominent papule within the rhinophyma may be sampled to rule out basal cell carcinoma.

Prognosis and Treatment

Rosacea is a chronic, slowly progressive disorder. The rate of progression may be stalled by preventive measures (e.g., avoidance of sun, ethanol ingestion), topical metronidazole, sulfacetamide, tretinoin, or azelaic acid, or oral administration of tetracycline antibiotics. Rhinophyma is largely irreversible and requires surgical ablation or resurfacing.

DRUG REACTIONS

Clinical Findings

The most common drug reaction is a morbilliform (measles-like) maculopapular rash concentrated on the trunk and spreading peripherally toward the distal extremities in a symmetric fashion. Pruritus is variable. Other distinctive reactions include fixed drug reactions, pustular drug reactions (e.g., acute generalized exanthematous pustulosis), urticaria, and drug reactions with eosinophilia and systemic symptoms (DRESS syndrome). However, drug reactions may mimic or mediate any inflammatory skin disorder (e.g., pseudoporphyria, drug-induced pemphigoid, lymphomatoid drug reactions, acneiform drug reactions, psoriasiform drug reactions, spongiotic drug reactions, interstitial granulomatous drug reactions, erythema nodosum, telogen effluvium, to name a few), and a comprehensive review is beyond the scope of this chapter. Likewise, virtually any drug may elicit skin changes. The diagnosis is usually based primarily on the temporal relationship between initiation of the offending agent and the onset of the eruption, combined with the reputation of the suspected drug. Some of the most common offending agents include trimethoprim-sulfamethoxazole and other sulfa-containing agents such as hydrochlorothiazide, penicillin and its derivatives, other antibiotics, and antiseizure medications. Drug reactions typically arise within 1 or 2 weeks of initiation of the medication. Severe reactions may occur within hours, and delayed reactions may arise several months after a medication has been introduced. The advent of targeted biologic anticancer therapies has introduced a new spectrum of reactions (e.g., eruptions associated with epidermal growth factor receptor inhibitors). Drug reactions are not restricted to inflammatory changes ("rashes") but also include tumor induction (e.g., verrucous keratoses, keratoacanthomas, or squamous cell carcinoma secondary to treatment with BRAF inhibitors).

In summary, a drug reaction is never confirmed or excluded by histology alone; clinical correlation is always required.

DRUG REACTIONS—DISEASE FACT SHEET

Patient Group

- Individuals taking medication (especially antibiotics, nonsteroidal antiinflammatory agents, psychotropic drugs, and beta-blockers)

Site of Involvement

- Lesions tend to appear first on the trunk and spread peripherally to extremities

Clinical Findings

- Erythematous macules and papules (most common)
- May simulate any pattern of inflammatory dermatosis
- May induce pigmentary alterations

Prognosis and Treatment

- Resolution with cessation of drug
- Prognosis depends on severity of eruption (e.g., significant morbidity and mortality associated with Stevens-Johnson syndrome and toxic epidermal necrolysis)

DRUG REACTIONS—PATHOLOGIC FEATURES

Histologic Features

- Any inflammatory reaction pattern may be seen
- Clues to drug reaction
  - Mixed histologic pattern (e.g., spongiosis + interface)
  - Eosinophils (but their absence does not exclude a drug etiology)
  - Maturational disturbance of keratinocytes (cytotoxic drug reaction)

Ancillary Studies

- Special stains to exclude infection (depending on the reaction pattern, e.g., granulomatous, pustular, or neutrophilic)

Differential Diagnosis

- Miscellaneous inflammatory dermatoses
- Infection
- Paraneoplastic process
- Nonmedication-related hypersensitivity reaction (e.g., food allergy)

Histologic Features

The classic morbilliform drug reaction exhibits a spongiotic and/or interface reaction pattern with single necrotic keratinocytes and vacuolar alteration along the dermal-epidermal junction and/or spongiosis, with superficial and deep perivascular lymphocytes and, often, eosinophils. However, the absence of eosinophils does not exclude a drug reaction. Often there is also mild, patchy spongiosis. However, drug reactions can mimic virtually any pattern of inflammatory skin disease; combined patterns (e.g., spongiotic and interface) may represent a clue to the diagnosis of drug reaction. Pleomorphic, dyskeratotic epidermal keratinocytes may reflect chemotherapy-induced dysmaturation.

Ancillary Studies

The diagnosis of a drug reaction is established by correlation of the clinical history with the estimated likelihood of candidates from the patient's medication list. Allergy testing (prick, intradermal, provocation) can provide more specific confirmation but is not widely available in dermatology practices and should only be conducted in a supervised setting. Rechallenge or desensitization is usually not attempted unless medically mandated.

Differential Diagnosis

Drug reactions may mimic any pattern of inflammatory skin disease. In disorders usually characterized by superficial perivascular inflammation such as spongiotic, interface, or psoriasiform dermatitis or perivascular dermatitis without epidermal alteration, the presence of deep perivascular inflammation with eosinophils is often invoked as evidence to include the differential diagnosis of a drug reaction.

Prognosis and Treatment

By definition, drug reactions resolve after discontinuation of the drug, but in some cases, the reaction may persist for days, weeks, or months and may worsen for a few days after the drug has been discontinued. Symptomatic therapy with topical corticosteroids and oral antihistamines is usually sufficient to manage a morbilliform drug reaction. In rare circumstances, patients may be allergic to the very topical or systemic corticosteroids or oral antihistamines used to manage drug reactions.

SUGGESTED FURTHER READING

Ackerman, A. B. (1978). *Histologic diagnosis of inflammatory skin diseases.* Philadelphia: Lea & Febiger.

Fung, M. A. (2002) The clinical and histopathologic spectrum of "dermal hypersensitivity reactions," a nonspecific histologic diagnosis that is not very useful in clinical practice, and the concept of a "dermal hypersensitivity reaction pattern". *Journal of the American Academy of Dermatology*, *47*, 898–907.

Hannon, G. R., Wetter, D. A., & Gibson, L. E. (2014). Urticarial dermatitis: Clinical features, diagnostic evaluation, and etiologic associations in a series of 146 patients at Mayo Clinic (2006-2012). *Journal of the American Academy of Dermatology*, *70*(2), 263–268.

LeBoit, P. E. (1993). Interface dermatitis. How specific are its histopathologic features? *Archives of Dermatology*, *129*, 1324–1328.

Patterson, J. W., Gregory, A. H., & Karyn L. P. (2021). Section 2: Tissue Reaction Patterns. In *Weedon's skin pathology* (5th ed., pp 49-240). Elsevier.

Phelps, R. G., Miller, M. K., & Singh, F. (2003). The varieties of "eczema": clinicopathologic correlation. *Clinics in Dermatology*, *21*, 95–100.

Rabinowitz, L. O., & Zaim, M. T. (1996). A clinicopathologic approach to granulomatous dermatoses. *Journal of the American Academy of Dermatology*, *35*, 588–600.

2 Panniculitis

Maxwell A. Fung

This chapter reviews inflammatory diseases involving the subcutaneous fat tissue (panniculitis). Although panniculitis is definitionally centered within the subcutis, some forms of panniculitis are associated with internal organ involvement or represent a manifestation of a systemic disease. The focus here will be on the most distinctive and commonly encountered histopathologic features of the major forms of panniculitis. Panniculitis is classically divided into mostly septal (i.e., those affecting predominantly the subcutaneous fibrous septa) versus mostly lobular (i.e., those predominantly affecting the fat lobules). An important consideration is that a 4-mm punch biopsy may not capture both the fat lobules and the septae. Hence, for panniculitic disease, a minimum of a 6- or 8-mm punch and, in some cases, a wedge biopsy may be necessary.

VASCULITIS INVOLVING THE SUBCUTIS

In addition to assessing for a mostly septal versus mostly lobular pattern at scanning magnification, another initial step in the evaluation of panniculitis is to determine if vasculitis is present and, if present, whether the vasculitis is a primary or predominant feature of the case, and which type of vessel is involved. Small arteries, arterioles, veins, and venules may be involved. Vasculitis involving subcutaneous vessels may be regarded as a distinct subset of panniculitis and of vasculitis. Examples include cutaneous polyarteritis nodosa, erythema induratum (nodular vasculitis), granulomatosis with polyangiitis (Wegener's), eosinophilic granulomatosis with polyangiitis (Churg-Strauss), and Behçet's disease. With the exception of erythema induratum (nodular vasculitis), vasculitis is further discussed in Chapter 4.

PANNICULITIS WITHOUT VASCULITIS

The following classification is based on an initial assessment at scanning magnification for a mostly septal versus mostly lobular pattern (in the absence of significant vasculitis) followed by assessment of cell types, the type(s) of adipocyte necrosis, and other distinctive features. In some cases, a specific diagnosis may be favored. However, it is commonly the case that only a differential diagnosis can be derived, and correlation with clinical features will be required for a specific diagnosis or to provide the differential diagnosis, ideally listed in order of likelihood.

Classification of Panniculitis

Mostly Septal Inflammation

1. Erythema nodosum
2. Subcutaneous involvement by granulomatous dermatitis
3. Subcutaneous involvement by sclerosing disorders

Mostly Lobular Inflammation

1. Neutrophilic and/or granulomatous
   a. Reaction secondary to ruptured follicular cyst
   b. Infectious panniculitis
   c. Pancreatic panniculitis
   d. α-1-Antitrypsin deficiency panniculitis
2. Lymphocytic
   a. Lupus panniculitis (lupus profundus)
   b. Dermatomyositis
   c. Subcutaneous panniculitis-like T-cell lymphoma
3. Granulomatous or histiocytic
   a. Erythema induratum (nodular vasculitis)
   b. Lipodermatosclerosis (sclerosing panniculitis)
   c. Traumatic panniculitis
   d. Factitial panniculitis
   e. Sclerosing postradiation panniculitis
   f. Subcutaneous fat necrosis of the newborn
   g. Sclerema neonatorum
   h. Gout
   i. Oxalosis
   j. Calciphylaxis
   k. Cold panniculitis
   l. Poststeroid panniculitis
   m. Cytophagic histiocytic panniculitis
4. Eosinophilic panniculitis
5. Neutrophilic panniculitis
6. Drug-induced panniculitis
7. Loss of fat
   a. Lipoatrophy and lipodystrophy
   b. Lipedema

MOSTLY SEPTAL PANNICULITIS

ERYTHEMA NODOSUM

Clinical Features

Erythema nodosum (EN) is a distinctive acute reaction pattern that is considered to be the most common form of panniculitis. EN typically affects adolescents and young adults, and women are more often affected than men. Localization is symmetrical and usually involves the anterior shins (Fig. 2.1). Less commonly, the thighs, hands, forearms, and face may be involved. Usually, there are multiple smooth, erythematous, tender nodules. The nodules may resemble a bruise (erythema contusiformis). The lesions do not ulcerate and generally involute within a few weeks without leaving a depressed scar.

Affected individuals may experience an acute disease phase characterized by fever, headache, malaise, or arthropathy.

Systemic disorders associated with EN include infections (bacterial, fungal, protozoal, viral), malignancies, reactions to medications, and other miscellaneous conditions. Associated bacterial infections include streptococcal infection, tuberculosis, *Yersinia enterocolitica* infection, brucellosis, leptospirosis, tularemia, *Chlamydia* infection, and *Mycoplasma pneumoniae* infection. Associated fungal infections include coccidioidomycosis, histoplasmosis, dermatophytosis, aspergillosis, and blastomycosis, depending on the geographic location and immune status of the patient. Protozoal infections, such as toxoplasmosis, amebiasis, and *Giardia* infections, can cause EN. Associated infections include rickettsial, viral (herpes simplex, infectious mononucleosis resulting from Epstein-Barr virus infection), lymphogranuloma venereum, and psittacosis.

EN may occur in the setting of leukemia, Hodgkin's disease, and non-Hodgkin's lymphomas, as well as with some other cancers, particularly after irradiation or other treatment releases antigens into the circulation by tumor necrosis.

Among the miscellaneous associations is sarcoid, which can have EN as part of a symptom complex, including fever, hilar adenopathy, and arthralgias (Lofgren's syndrome) or fever, uveitis, and parotitis (uveoparotid fever or Heerford's syndrome).

Medications implicated in EN include sulfonamides, estrogens, and oral contraceptives.

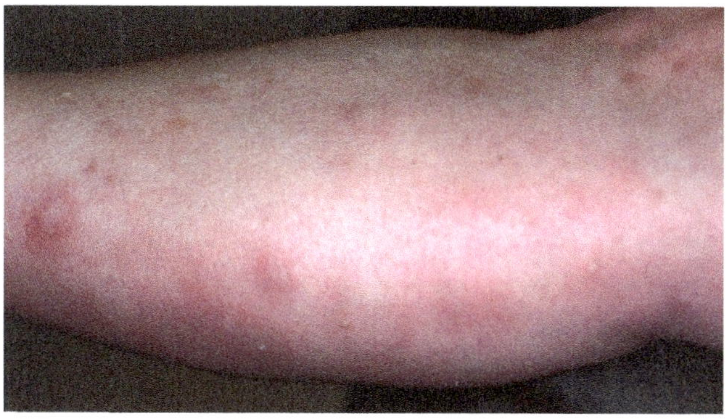

FIG. 2.1
Erythema nodosum. Discrete, nonulcerated, erythematous subcutaneous nodules on the legs.

ERYTHEMA NODOSUM—DISEASE FACT SHEET

Patient Group
- Most often young adults (20 to 40 years of age)
- Women are more often affected than men

Site of Involvement
- Lower extremities (shins), usually bilateral

Clinical Features
- Skin: erythematous nonulcerated nodules, often tender; may arise in crops
- Commonly associated with other diseases (e.g., poststreptococcal infection, sarcoidosis, paraneoplastic), drugs (e.g., sulfonamides), or pregnancy but may be idiopathic
- Systemic symptoms: fever, aches, possible arthralgias

Pathophysiology
- Delayed hypersensitivity reaction (e.g., to bacterial antigens, medication)

Prognosis
- Lesions tend to resolve spontaneously without a scar

Treatment
- Directed at associated symptoms (e.g., nonsteroidal antiinflammatory drugs, bedrest)
- Directed at underlying disease or causes: antibiotics for associated infection
- Cessation of possible causative medication
- Colchicine, if associated with Behçet's disease
- Steroids or potassium iodide if necessary

Histologic Features

The histologic changes in EN are centered on the subcutaneous septa (Fig. 2.2A). Epidermal and dermal involvement is typically minimal to absent, with sparse superficial and deep perivascular lymphocytes at most. In early EN, there is septal edema with a mixed lymphohistiocytic infiltrate with neutrophils (sometimes prominent) and, often, eosinophils. Focal fibrin deposition and extravasation of erythrocytes may be seen. Often the inflammation is most intense at the periphery of the edematous septa and extends into the periphery of the fat lobules, creating a "paraseptal" or mixed septal and lobular pattern involving those regions of the fat lobules directly adjacent to the septa.

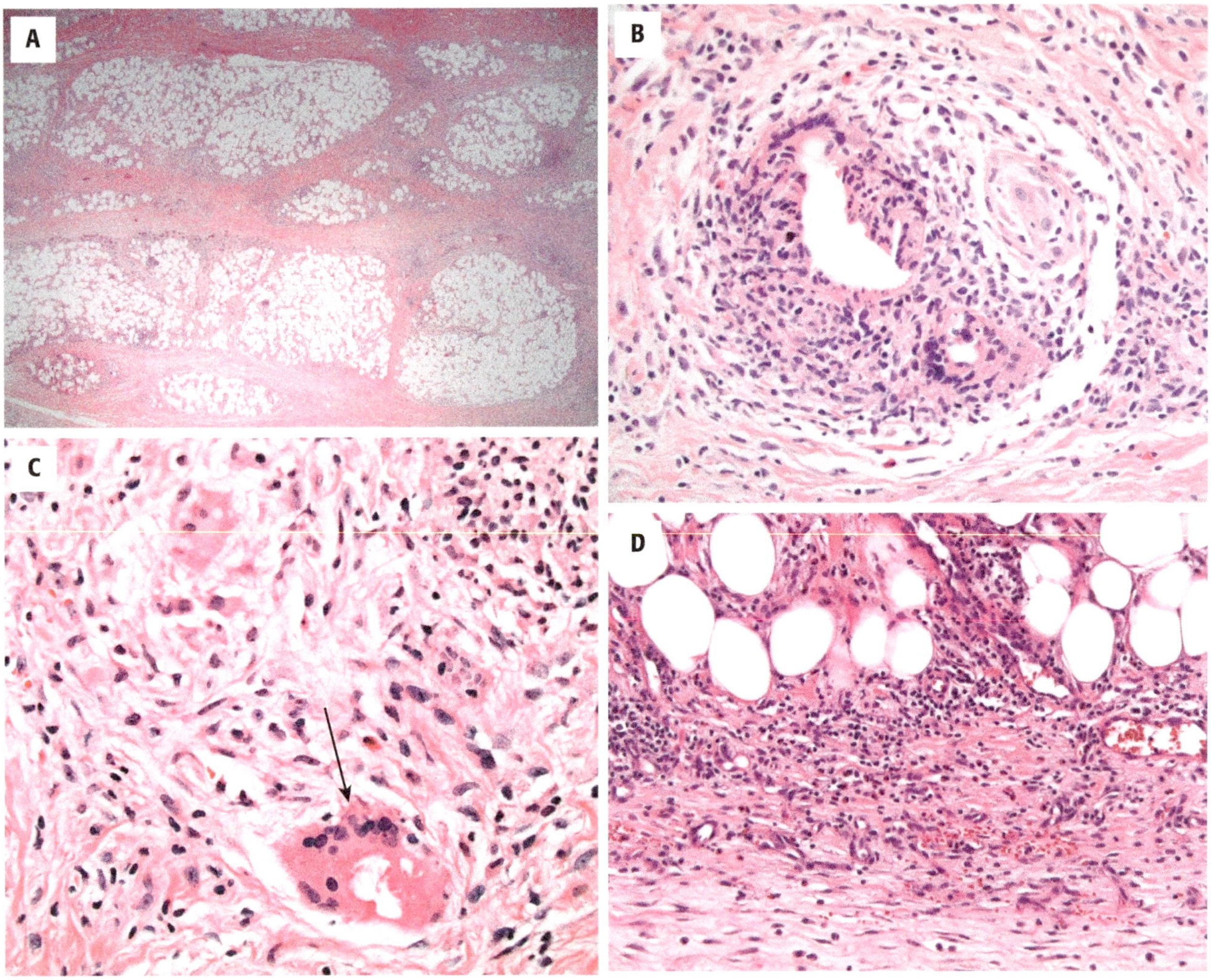

FIG. 2.2

Erythema nodosum. **A,** Inflammation is concentrated within the subcutaneous septa, especially at the junction between septa and lobules. **B,** Miescher's radial granuloma is a collection of nonenlarged macrophages and often also neutrophils surrounding an empty cleft-shaped space. **C,** Multinucleated giant cells in the septa may contain intracytoplasmic clefts *(arrow)*. **D,** Eosinophils are commonly present within widened, edematous septa. Extravasated erythrocytes may be present, but vasculitis is not typical.

A fairly sensitive and specific feature of EN, including early lesions, is Miescher's radial granuloma, a cluster of nonenlarged macrophages, often with neutrophils, surrounding an empty cleft-shaped space (Fig. 2.2B). Multinucleated histiocytes are typically most prominent in the late stages of EN, sometimes in loosely formed granulomas. Multinucleated histiocytes with central clefts likely reflect the disintegration or late stage of Miescher's radial granuloma (Fig. 2.2C). The typical infiltrate is mixed, with mostly small lymphocytes in concert with histiocytes, neutrophils, and eosinophils. Eosinophils within widened edematous septa are common (Fig. 2.2D). Adipocyte necrosis is not prominent. Vasculitis is not characteristic but has rarely been documented in patients with acute EN secondary to infections, in Behçet's syndrome, and secondary to medications, including estrogenic oral contraceptives.

ERYTHEMA NODOSUM—PATHOLOGIC FEATURES

Histologic Features

- Mostly septal panniculitis (fibrosis and inflammation)
- Miescher's radial granulomas (small aggregates of histiocytes associated with cleftlike spaces; neutrophils variable)
- Mixed infiltrate. Neutrophils prominent in early lesions. Multinucleated histiocytes prominent in late or chronic lesions

Ancillary Studies

- Special stains, cultures, or antistreptolysin titers to exclude infection
- Chest radiography to assess for sarcoid or pneumonia

Differential Diagnosis

- Infection
- Subcutaneous involvement by granulomatous dermatitis

Ancillary Studies

Special stains and cultures for microorganisms are needed to exclude an infectious etiology. Differential studies reveal only nonspecific findings.

Differential Diagnosis

EN must be distinguished from erythema induratum (nodular vasculitis). Vasculitis and prominent fat necrosis are usually absent in EN and are typical of erythema induratum. Also, erythema induratum typically involves the posterior lower legs as opposed to the anterior lower legs seen in EN. In exceptionally rare patients suspected of having EN but with arteritis, rather than venulitis, cutaneous polyarteritis nodosa must be considered. In polyarteritis, arteries rather than veins or venules are affected. Mycobacterial and fungal infections typically evoke a granulomatous host response. Subcutaneous tuberculosis can mimic EN in lesions that extend into the subcutis from underlying organs, soft tissues, or bone. Whereas subcutaneous tuberculosis can spare the upper portion of the panniculus, EN usually does not. Syphilitic gummas are ulcerative, irregular granulomatous lesions that produce depressed scars. EN does not have discrete granulomas or dermal sclerosis and thus can be distinguished from most cases of sarcoidosis, scleroderma, ruptured follicular cysts, and factitial traumatic panniculitis.

Crohn's disease can be associated with EN, and the two diseases can be difficult to distinguish from each other histologically in the skin unless there is ulceration, which does not occur in EN. Other associated conditions are ulcerative colitis and Behçet's disease. The panniculitis in Behçet's disease may resemble EN clinically.

Prognosis and Treatment

Most cases of EN are self-limited and resolve spontaneously. Drug-induced EN must be clinically excluded. Beyond symptomatic care, prognosis and specific treatment are dictated by the underlying systemic condition. Symptomatic treatments for uncomplicated EN include nonsteroidal antiinflammatory agents and bed rest.

CHRONIC ERYTHEMA NODOSUM

Clinical Features

The rare chronic form of EN is also known as EN migrans or subacute nodular migratory panniculitis. Chronic EN is predominantly found in women. In contrast to classic acute EN, the presentation is more often unilateral or even a solitary lesion, and constitutional symptoms are usually absent. The lesions may migrate. Individual nodules tend to enlarge by peripheral extension into plaques, often with central clearing. The duration may range from several months to several years.

Histologic Features

In chronic EN, the microscopic appearances are essentially those of late-stage classic EN with widened, fibrotic septa and more chronic inflammation (Fig. 2.3). Multinucleated histiocytes and lipophages may be sparse or prominent. There is vascular proliferation and thickening of the endothelium with the extravasation of erythrocytes. In some lesions, numerous discrete granulomas can be found and consist of epithelioid and multinucleated histiocytes without caseous necrosis. Although vasculitis has been observed by some authors, others have found vascular changes to be slight or absent.

Ancillary Studies

As for classic EN, mycobacterial or fungal infections in particular should be ruled out.

Differential Diagnosis

The distinction from classic acute EN is primarily clinical. As per classic EN, infection, and subcutaneous involvement by granulomatous dermatitis must be excluded.

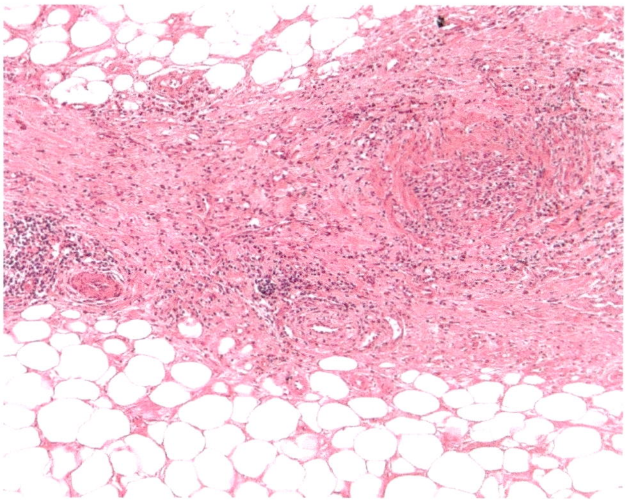

FIG. 2.3
Erythema nodosum (EN), late stage. The septa are widened and fibrotic in the late stage of classic or acute EN as well as chronic EN.

Prognosis and Treatment

The evaluation and management for classic acute EN applies. However, chronic EN is usually idiopathic and follows a chronic course spanning several months or years. Tetracycline and minocycline have been reported to be effective in refractory cases of chronic EN.

SUBCUTANEOUS INVOLVEMENT BY GRANULOMATOUS DERMATITIS

Granulomatous dermatitis is characterized by prominent histiocytes within a dermal inflammatory infiltrate and is reviewed in detail in Chapter 1. Discrete nodular collections of histiocytes are termed *granulomas* and may exhibit sarcoidal (lymphocyte-poor), tuberculoid (lymphocyte-rich), or palisaded appearances. Palisaded granulomas have an organized peripheral palisade of enlarged histiocytes around a central zone of altered stroma, including necrobiotic degenerated collagen, fibrin, and/or interstitial mucin; granuloma annulare (GA) is the prototype (Fig. 2.4A). Subcutaneous GA is characterized by palisaded granulomas that contain mucin (Fig. 2.4B) and sometimes also fibrin (Fig. 2.4C). Fibrin is most characteristic of rheumatoid nodules, which typically involve the subcutis but occur in patients with pre-existing rheumatoid arthritis. Other forms of granulomatous dermatitis that may occasionally involve the subcutis include necrobiosis lipoidica and necrobiotic xanthogranuloma; in these cases, there is direct extension into the septa from the overlying reticular dermis. A significant differential diagnosis is epithelioid sarcoma, a rare sarcoma that is notorious for its resemblance to palisaded granulomatous dermatitis. In addition, both epithelioid sarcoma and GA frequently involve the deep dermis or subcutis of the distal upper extremities in young persons. The tumor cells in epithelioid sarcoma exhibit cytologic atypia and eosinophilic cytoplasm. The immunophenotypic profile of epithelioid sarcoma is also distinctive, with immunopositivity for vimentin, cytokeratin, EMA, often CD34, and loss of staining for INI-1.

Subcutaneous sarcoid tends to exhibit a lobular or mixed septal and lobular pattern (Fig. 2.5A). Although lymphocytes are typically sparse, fibrosis can be prominent around subcutaneous sarcoidal granulomas (Fig. 2.5B).

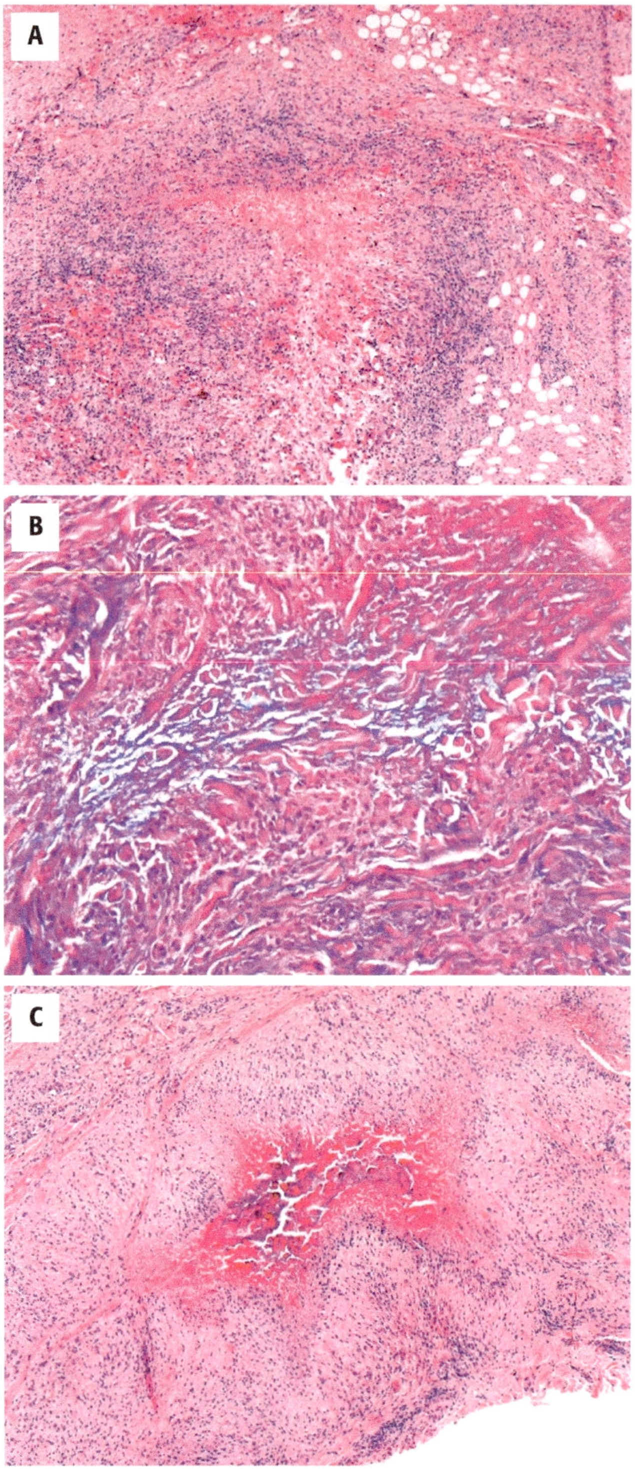

FIG. 2.4

Subcutaneous granuloma annulare (GA). **A,** The fat lobule is largely obscured by a palisaded granulomatous infiltrate. **B,** Alcian blue stain highlights mucin *(blue)* in the center of the palisaded granuloma. **C,** Deep GA may also contain fibrin *(pink)* (hence the term *pseudorheumatoid nodule*).

SUBCUTANEOUS INVOLVEMENT BY SCLEROSING DISORDERS

Fibrosis and sclerosis are characterized by excess collagen. In fibrosis (e.g., scar), reactive fibroblasts and

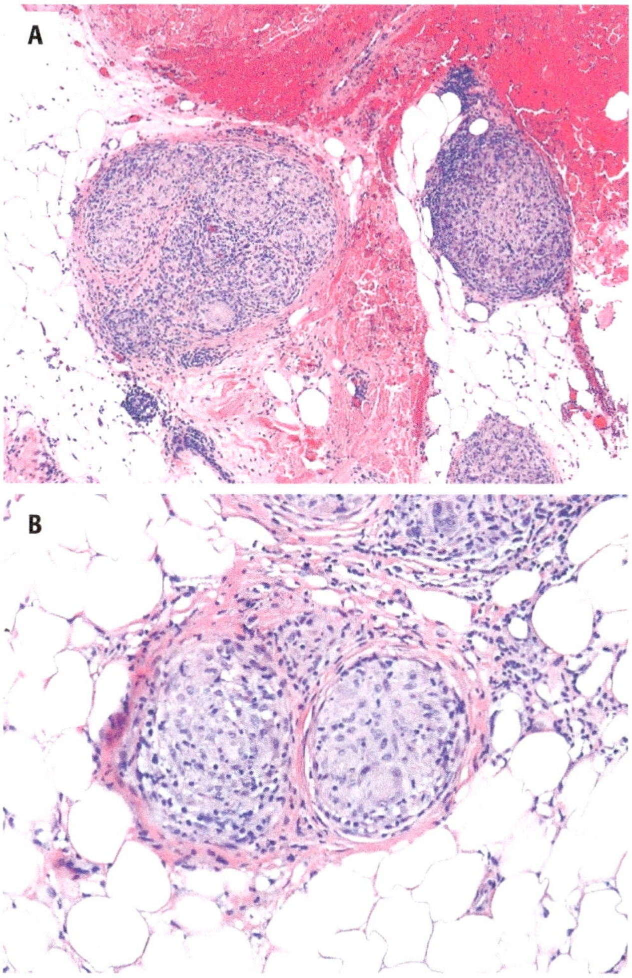

FIG. 2.5

Subcutaneous sarcoidosis. **A,** Discrete noncaseating granulomas involve the septa and the lobules of the subcutis. **B,** Fibrosis surrounding subcutaneous granulomas is characteristic.

fibrocytes are proportionally increased, but in sclerosis, they are relatively decreased in number. Thus sclerosing disorders may be classified as a subset of fibrosing disorders or fibrosing dermatitis, in some cases representing the end stage of a fibrotic process. Sclerotic disorders may begin in the superficial dermis (e.g., lichen sclerosus), deep dermis (e.g., morphea), subcutaneous septa (e.g., morphea profunda), or underlying connective tissue fascia (e.g., eosinophilic fasciitis). Sclerosing disorders enter the differential diagnosis of septal panniculitis when septa are widened secondary to sclerosis of collagen. With the exception of eosinophilic fasciitis, most sclerosing disorders typically involve the dermis with only variable involvement of the subcutis and are discussed in detail in Chapter 1. Lipodermatosclerosis (sclerosing panniculitis) and sclerosing postradiation panniculitis also exhibit septal sclerosis and are each addressed later in this chapter.

Involvement of the subcutaneous septa may occur in the deep variant of morphea (*localized scleroderma*), also known as morphea profunda, as well as in systemic scleroderma (including limited and diffuse variants). Morphea profunda typically involves the deep dermis in continuity with significant involvement of subcutaneous septa (Fig. 2.6A), with associated inflammatory infiltrates centered at the junction between the reticular dermis and subcutis and containing plasma cells (Fig. 2.6B). The distinction between morphea and systemic scleroderma is made clinically (one or more discrete plaques in morphea; calcinosis, Raynaud's phenomenon, esophageal dysmotility, sclerodactyly, and telangiectasia in limited systemic scleroderma [CREST syndrome]) and more diffuse sclerosis and systemic involvement in diffuse systemic scleroderma (progressive systemic sclerosis).

Eosinophilic fasciitis (Shulman syndrome) exhibits histologic overlap with morphea profunda. Clinically, eosinophilic fasciitis is distinctive, presenting as an acute, bilateral, symmetrical fasciitis often occurring after an episode of exceptionally strenuous physical exertion. Biopsies deep enough to sample fascia show sclerosis and edema of the collagenous fascia associated with lymphocytes, plasma cells, and eosinophils (Fig. 2.6C and D). Fibrin may be present. Eosinophilic fasciitis responds promptly to systemic steroids, but scleroderma usually does not. In some cases where only the more superficial aspect of the fascia is sampled, the eosinophils may not be as immediately obvious; hence, if the clinical presentation still suggests eosinophilic fasciitis, then it should still be considered in the differential diagnosis.

Injections of substances (e.g., Talwin) or foreign material such as silica can induce sclerosis that histologically resembles scleroderma. Examination of tissue sections under polarized light may detect silica or other birefringent foreign material. Of historical note, in 1981, the ingestion of contaminated cooking oil was implicated in the toxic oil syndrome in Spain, with vasculitis and systemic manifestations resembling scleroderma as well as neurotoxicity and several hundred fatalities.

MOSTLY LOBULAR PANNICULITIS

Lobular panniculitis reflects inflammation that is localized *predominantly* (almost never exclusively) to the subcutaneous fat lobule. In other words, the inflammatory infiltrate secondarily involves the septa, resulting in a mixed septal and lobular pattern, so the predominant pattern may be used to generate the differential diagnosis, at least initially. Because the

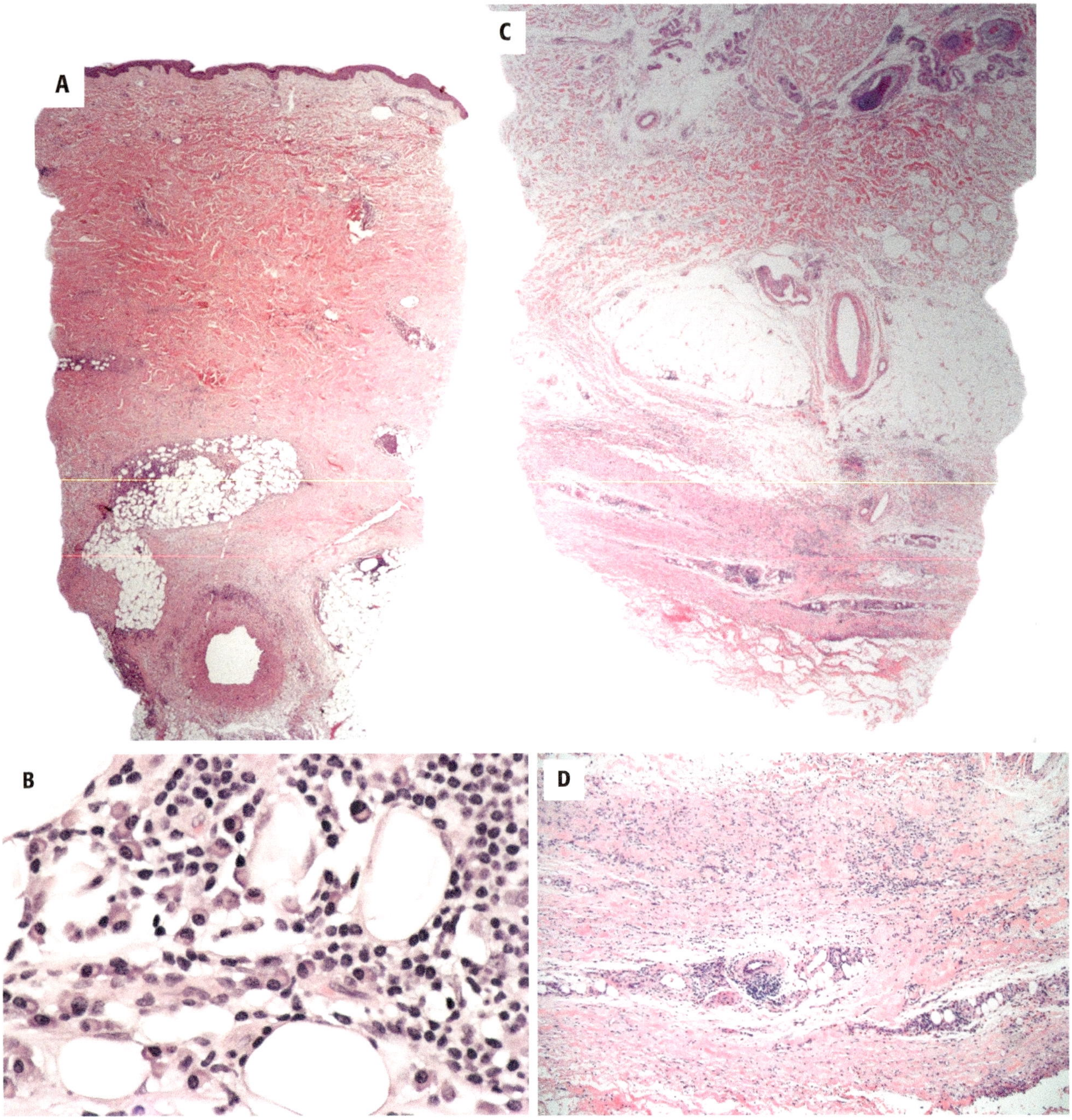

FIG. 2.6

Morphea. **A,** Sclerosis of the deep dermis is associated with widened, sclerotic septa in morphea profunda. There is a perivascular and periadnexal lymphocytic host response with aggregates along the dermal subcutaneous junction. **B,** Plasma cells are usually present in morphea. **C,** In eosinophilic fasciitis, the sclerosis usually involves subcutis but is centered on the underlying fascia. **D,** Variable sclerosis and edema are associated with a mixed inflammatory infiltrate that usually contains eosinophils.

differential diagnosis for lobular panniculitis is lengthy, key attributes also include the predominant cells of the inflammatory infiltrate (neutrophilic, lymphocytic, granulomatous, eosinophilic) and the type(s) of adipocyte necrosis present. Subclassification based on the composition of the inflammatory infiltrate may be limited, as neutrophils or histiocytes may stereotypically predominate at early or late stages, respectively, of many forms of lobular panniculitis (e.g., infectious, traumatic).

INFECTIOUS PANNICULITIS—DISEASE FACT SHEET

Patient Group
- Any age or gender
- Immunocompromised at greater risk

Site of Involvement
- Any site. Direct inoculation results in localized lesions. Systemic infection (septicemia) is associated with multiple or generalized lesions

Clinical Features
- Erythematous tender nodules
- May be ulcerated and drain pus

Prognosis and Treatment
- Depends on immune status, comorbidities, virulence of the pathogen
- Antibiotics

INFECTIOUS PANNICULITIS—PATHOLOGIC FEATURES

Histologic Features
- Any pattern (septal, lobular or mixed) (Fig. 2.7)
- Typically a mixed neutrophilic (suppurative) or granulomatous infiltrate

Ancillary Studies
- Lesional cultures
- Histochemical stains for bacterial, mycobacterial, or fungal pathogens
- Specific serologic, immunohistochemical, or molecular studies

Differential Diagnosis
- Ruptured follicular cyst
- Noninfectious neutrophilic or granulomatous panniculitis

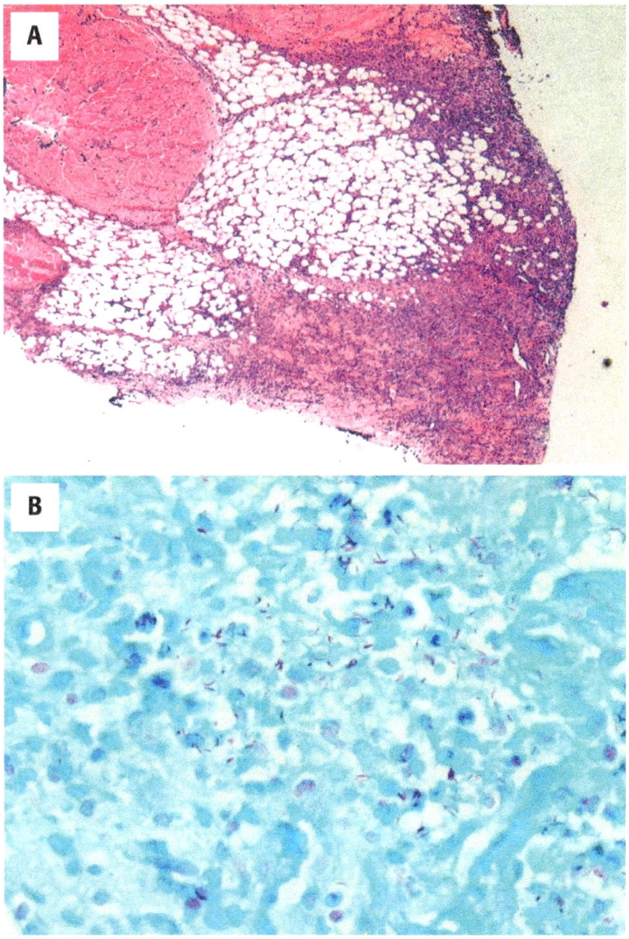

FIG. 2.7

Infectious panniculitis secondary to *Mycobacterium tuberculosis*, direct infection of the subcutis. **A,** Septa are widened and the inflammation is around the periphery of the fat lobules. **B,** Numerous mycobacteria are detected on acid-fast staining.

PANCREATIC PANNICULITIS

Clinical Features

Pancreatic panniculitis usually arises in the setting of pancreatic insufficiency, most commonly acute or

PANCREATIC PANNICULITIS—DISEASE FACT SHEET

Patient Group
- Patients with pancreatic disease (pancreatitis, cancer, cyst, or fistula)

Site of Involvement
- Most often on legs but may occur elsewhere

Clinical Features
- Erythematous nodules
- May be painful, ulcerate, and discharge oily material

Prognosis
- Variable; depends on underlying disease

Treatment
- Lesions may resolve weeks after acute pancreatitis
- Lesions may resolve after surgical resection of tumor
- Octreotide

PANCREATIC PANNICULITIS—PATHOLOGIC FEATURES

Histologic Features
- Mostly lobular panniculitis with neutrophils
- "Ghost cells" are the outlines of necrotic lipocytes with loss of nuclear staining (enzymatic fat necrosis)
- Calcification

Ancillary Studies
- Infection must be ruled out

Differential Diagnosis
- Infectious panniculitis (ghost cells may be seen in mucormycosis and aspergillosis)
- α-1-Antitrypsin deficiency panniculitis

chronic pancreatitis. Rare associations include pancreatic cancer; vaccine therapy for pancreatic cancer; hepatic cancer; pancreas divisum; or other rare causes of pancreatitis, including viral hepatitis, lupus pancreatitis, medication-induced pancreatitis (sulindac), or allograft pancreatitis. Lesions typically arise on the legs, often the ankles and knees, but may also arise on the proximal upper and lower extremities, buttocks, trunk, or scalp. Ulcerated lesions emit an oily brown exudate.

Histologic Features

In the early stage of pancreatic panniculitis, there is neutrophilic lobular panniculitis (Fig. 2.8A). Established lesions exhibit enzymatic fat necrosis, with "ghost" adipocytes characterized by the faintly stained outlines of adipocyte membranes with loss of nuclear staining and associated calcification (Fig. 2.8B and C). Enzymatic fat necrosis, in the absence of overt fungal pathogens, is nearly pathognomonic for pancreatic panniculitis.

Ancillary Studies

Serologic or imaging studies may be required to determine the nature of the pancreatic or other underlying disease. Fungal stains may be considered to definitively rule out infections that may rarely produce ghost adipocytes.

Differential Diagnosis

In an early lesion, infection and α-1-antitrypsin (AAT) deficiency panniculitis may be considered. Neutrophilic panniculitis may also be seen in early factitial panniculitis, myelodysplasia, and as a medication reaction (e.g., vemurafenib). In fully developed lesions, the histologic appearances are distinctive. However, ghost-type adipocytes have rarely been documented in mucormycosis and aspergillosis.

Prognosis and Treatment

The prognosis is favorable to the extent that the underlying cause can be successfully managed. In addition to supportive care and the identification and management of complications, there is limited evidence supporting the use of somatostatin analogues such as octreotide. Surgical excision of a pancreatic tumor may induce remission of the panniculitis.

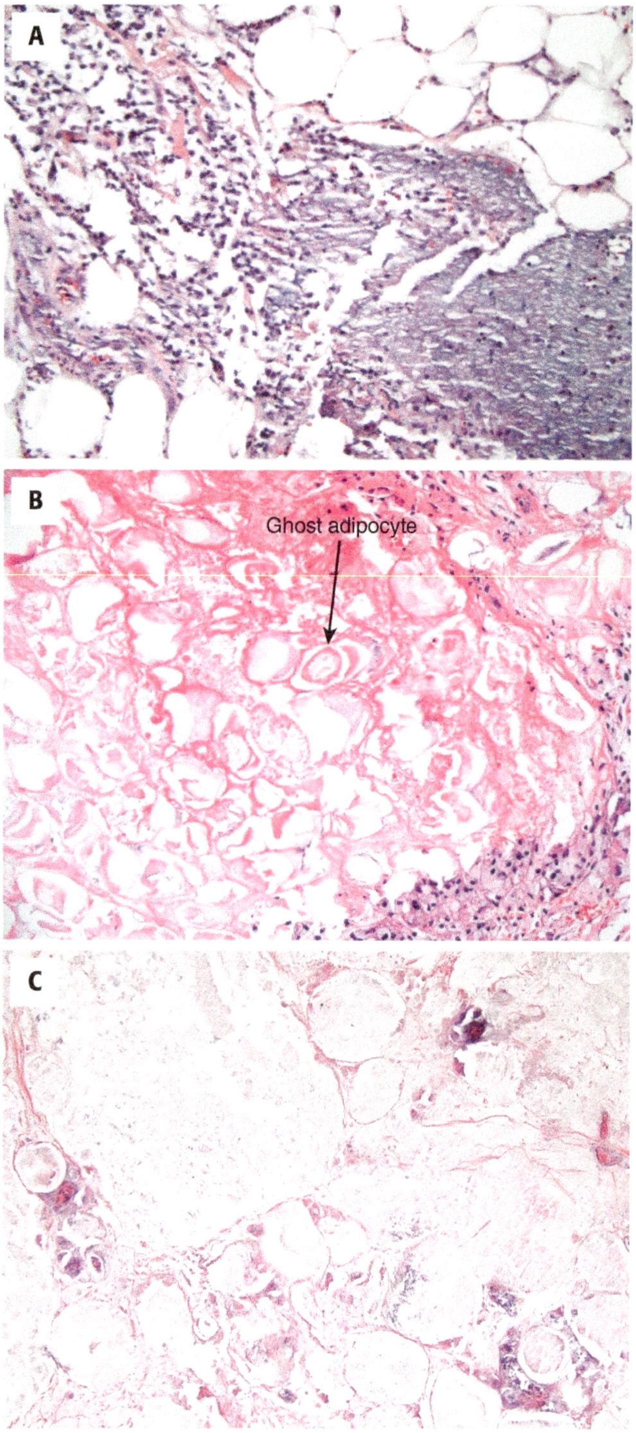

FIG. 2.8

Pancreatic panniculitis. **A,** Neutrophils and granular basophilic material reflecting mostly nuclear debris characterize early lesions. Fully developed (**B**) and late-stage (**C**) lesions contain ghost adipocytes and calcification.

α-1-ANTITRYPSIN DEFICIENCY PANNICULITIS

Clinical Features

ATT deficiency panniculitis is associated with mutations in the *SERPINA1* gene that encodes the serine protease,

AAT. *SERPINA1* has more than 120 alleles; these alleles are classified into four major variants—F (fast), M (medium), S (slow), or Z (very slow)—based on their motility on an acid starch gel. Most people have an MM phenotype. AAT panniculitis and AAT-related disease are most typical of patients with a ZZ phenotype but have been reported in patients with normal clinical values of AAT but with abnormal phenotypes including patients with MS, SS, or MZ. Hepatic cirrhosis and panlobular emphysema of the lungs are other possible complications, mostly seen in patients with the ZZ phenotype. The clinical onset may be in childhood or adulthood. Similar to pancreatic panniculitis, the skin nodules almost always ulcerate at some point in the disease course and discharge oily fluid. Lesions typically arise on the thighs but may also arise on the trunk, upper extremities, or face. Trauma has been cited as an inciting factor.

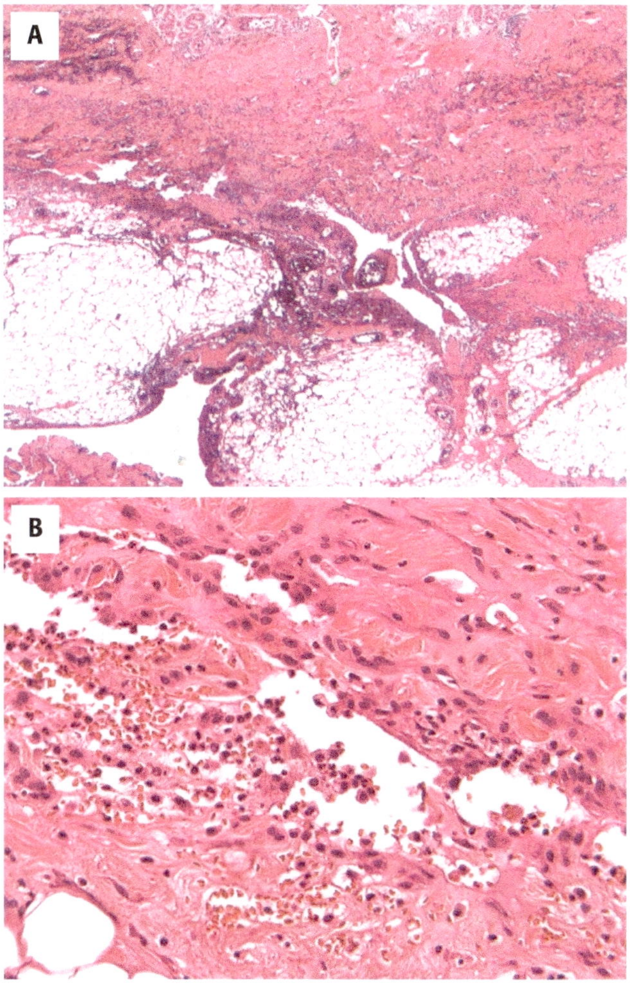

FIG. 2.9

α-1-Antitrypsin deficiency panniculitis. **A,** Panniculitis associated with separation of lobules from surrounding septa. **B,** Neutrophils dissect through the collagen of the septa and the deep dermis.

Histologic Features

The overall pattern in AAT deficiency panniculitis may be mostly lobular, mixed septal and lobular, or occasionally mostly septal. Separation or lysis of the septa from the lobules may result in "floating" lobules (Fig. 2.9A). Neutrophils can be found in the septa of the subcutis and interstitium of the deep reticular dermis (Fig. 2.9B) most typically in an earlier-stage lesion. A granular or amphophilic liquefactive-type necrosis may be present. Secondary vasculitis may be present. Later-stage lesions may be predominantly granulomatous.

Ancillary Studies

Decreased serum AAT levels (usually <20 μmol/L) and abnormal serum electrophoresis (isoelectric focusing) can establish the diagnosis.

Differential Diagnosis

The differential diagnosis for neutrophilic panniculitis applies, including infection, early pancreatic panniculitis, early factitial panniculitis, myelodysplasia, and as a medication reaction (e.g., vemurafenib).

Prognosis and Treatment

The prognosis depends on the degree of severity of the genetic abnormality. Treatment is symptomatic and often difficult and may include antiinflammatory agents such as corticosteroids, colchicine, cyclophosphamide, dapsone, or doxycycline; intravenous augmentation therapy with AAT; plasma exchange; and liver transplantation.

LUPUS ERYTHEMATOSUS PROFUNDUS

Clinical Features

Lupus erythematosus (LE) profundus (lupus panniculitis) represents one subset of chronic cutaneous LE and may or may not be associated with systemic LE. Young to middle-aged adults, mostly women, are most commonly affected, but children also develop LE profundus (often on the face). In contrast to most forms of panniculitis that involve the legs, LE profundus tends to involve the trunk and proximal extremities as well as sites exposed to trauma; the lateral upper arms, thighs, buttocks, or chest may be involved. The lesions are painful and can ulcerate.

LUPUS PROFUNDUS—DISEASE FACT SHEET

Patient Group

- Young to middle-aged adults (typical onset in the third to fourth decades of life) and children
- A subset of chronic cutaneous lupus erythematosus (LE). Many patients also have discoid LE
- A minority of patients have associated systemic LE

Site of Involvement

- Face, upper arms, trunk, and hips
- Sites of trauma

Clinical Features

- Erythematous tender subcutaneous nodules or plaques; ulceration variable

Prognosis

- Chronic relapsing course
- May precede onset of other manifestations of LE

Treatment

- Antimalarials

LUPUS PROFUNDUS—PATHOLOGIC FEATURES

Histologic Features

- Lobular lymphocytic panniculitis
- Hyaline fat necrosis
- Lymphoid follicles with reactive germinal centers
- Plasma cells typically present
- Eosinophils may be present

Ancillary Studies

- No detectable clonal T-cell receptor gene rearrangement by polymerase chain reaction

Differential Diagnosis

- Dermatomyositis
- Primary cutaneous subcutaneous panniculitis-like T-cell lymphoma
- Sclerodermoid panniculitis

Histologic Features

LE profundus is the prototype for lobular lymphocytic panniculitis. The associated epidermal interface changes and dermal perivascular or periadnexal lymphocytes with interstitial mucin expected in most other forms of cutaneous LE are variably present (Fig. 2.10A). Hyaline fat necrosis is the characteristic form of fat necrosis in LE profundus, characterized by eosinophilic hyalinized proteinaceous material between adipocytes and variably replacing them (Fig. 2.10B). Lymphocytic vasculitis and leukocytoclastic nuclear debris (nuclear "dust") are variable features (Fig. 2.10C). Reactive lymphoid follicles with germinal centers may be present (Fig. 2.10D). As in most forms of cutaneous LE, plasma cells are present. In contrast to most forms of cutaneous LE, eosinophils are often present.

Ancillary Studies

In addition to clinical correlation, serologic studies may facilitate screening for evidence of systemic LE.

Differential Diagnosis

Rare cases of panniculitis due to dermatomyositis require clinical correlation. More commonly, the differential diagnosis is between LE profundus and primary subcutaneous panniculitis-like T-cell lymphoma (SPTCL) or other lymphomas involving the subcutis, a distinction that can be difficult or, in rare cases, impossible at a single point in time. Features favoring LE profundus include changes of LE in the epidermis and dermis, the presence of plasma cells and lymphocyte follicles with reactive germinal centers, and the absence of a detectable T-cell clone by polymerase chain reaction. SPTCL typically involves the lower extremities and histologically exhibits a dense population of atypical lymphocytes with rimming of neoplastic lymphocytes around adipocyte lobules (Fig. 2.11). The neoplastic lymphocytes in SPTCL are immunopositive for CD8, cytotoxic markers (TIA-1, granzyme), and βF1 (β chain of T-cell receptor) and exhibit clonal T-cell receptor gene rearrangements. However, cases of SPTCL either evolving from or indistinguishable from LE profundus have been documented, and a fatal case of subcutaneous T-cell lymphoma lacking atypia has also been documented. The terms *indeterminate lymphocytic lobular panniculitis* and *atypical lymphocytic lobular panniculitis* have been used to provisionally classify disorders with indeterminate or overlapping features. Whether patients with such diagnostically problematic lesions have lymphoma can sometimes only be determined by the clinical course and follow-up biopsies of persistent or recurrent lesions. The presence of clusters of CD123-positive plasmacytoid dendritic cells or significant immunopositivity for human myxovirus resistance protein 1 (MxA) in the lesional histiocytes favors LE profundus over SPTCL.

Cytophagic histiocytic panniculitis (CHP) is another form of panniculitis that may overlap significantly with SPTCL or other forms of subcutaneous lymphoma. Some authorities regard CHP as an indolent stage or granulomatous cytophagic variant of lymphoma because a subset of cases of CHP has been fatal, either evolving from CHP to lymphoma or originally misclassified as CHP. However, there also seems to be a subset of cases of CHP that display long-term indolent behavior. Furthermore,

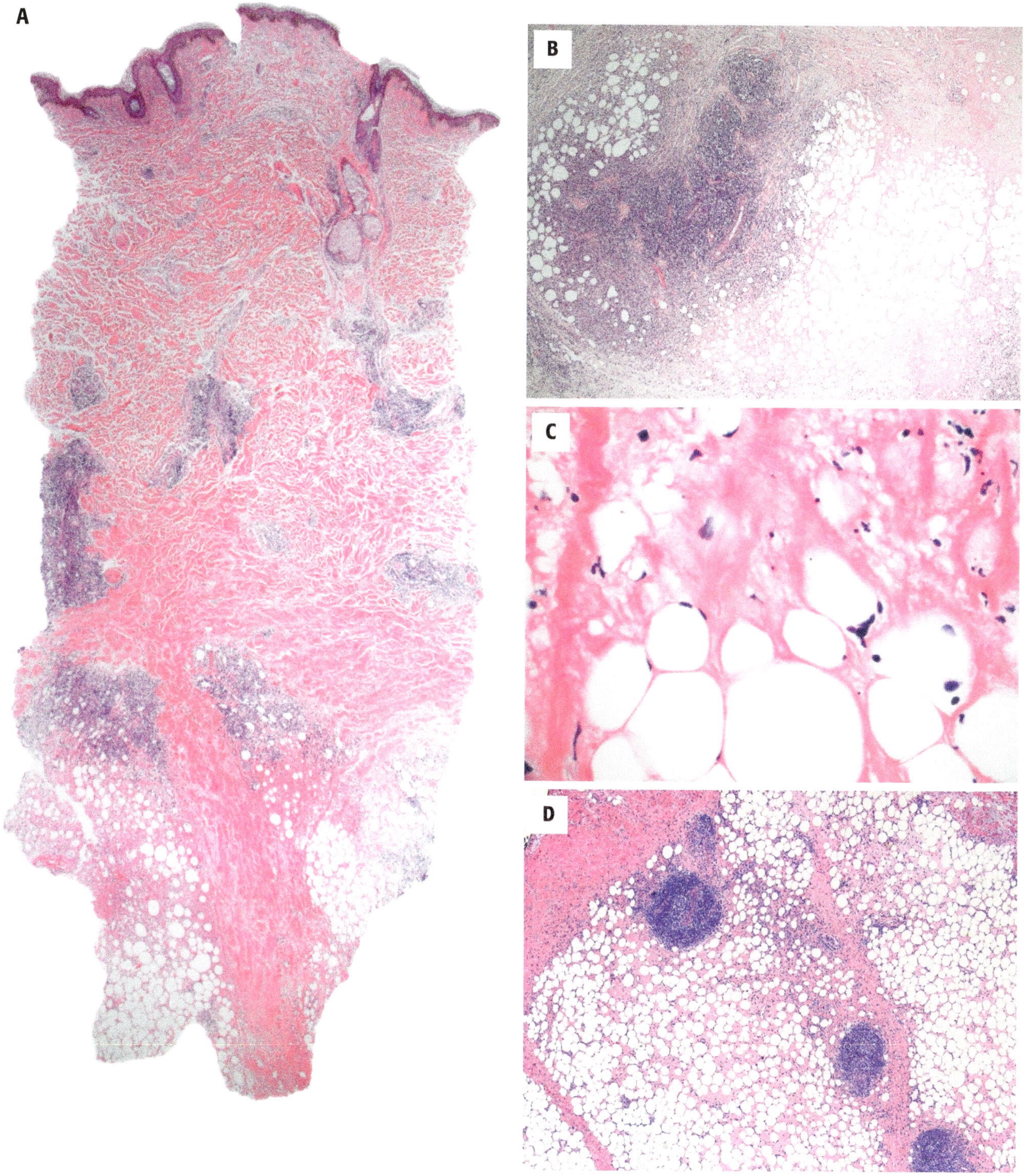

FIG. 2.10

Lupus erythematosus profundus (lupus panniculitis). **A,** Lobular lymphocytic panniculitis with overlying dermal changes of lupus (i.e., superficial and deep perivascular and periadnexal lymphocytes). **B,** Infiltration mostly within the lobules by lymphocytes with associated hyaline fat necrosis. **C,** Nuclear "dust" may also be present in lupus profundus. **D,** Reactive lymphoid follicles are present in the lobules and along the septa.

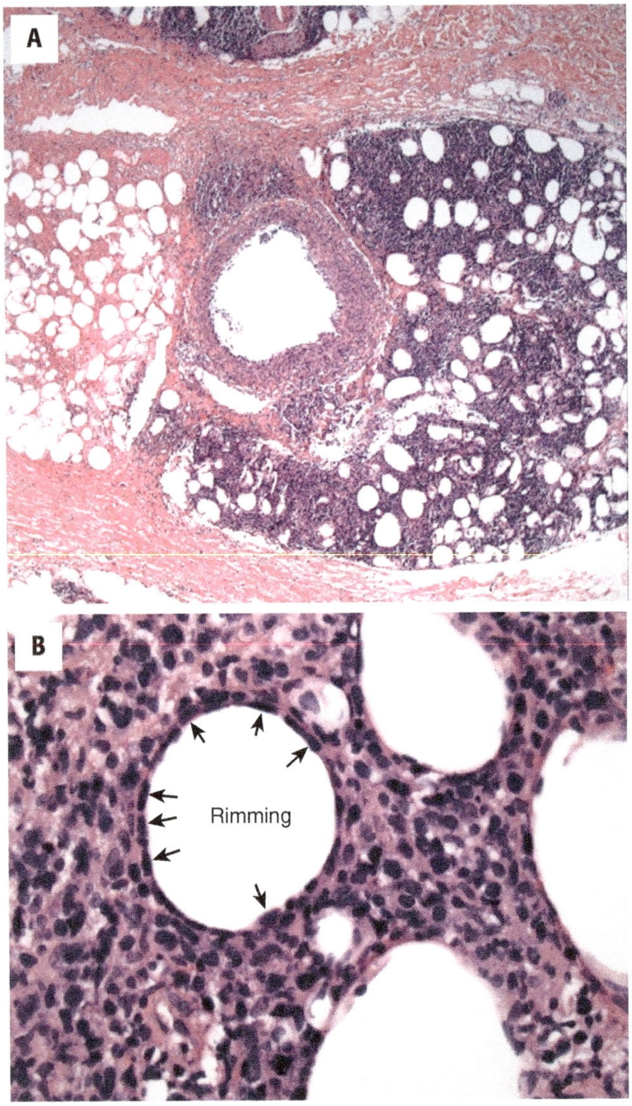

FIG. 2.11

Primary cutaneous subcutaneous panniculitis-like T-cell lymphoma (SPTCL). **A,** Lobular lymphocytic infiltrate resembling lupus profundus. **B,** In SPTCL, lesional CD8-positive lymphocytes are atypical and aggregate around individual adipocytes (rimming) *(arrows)*.

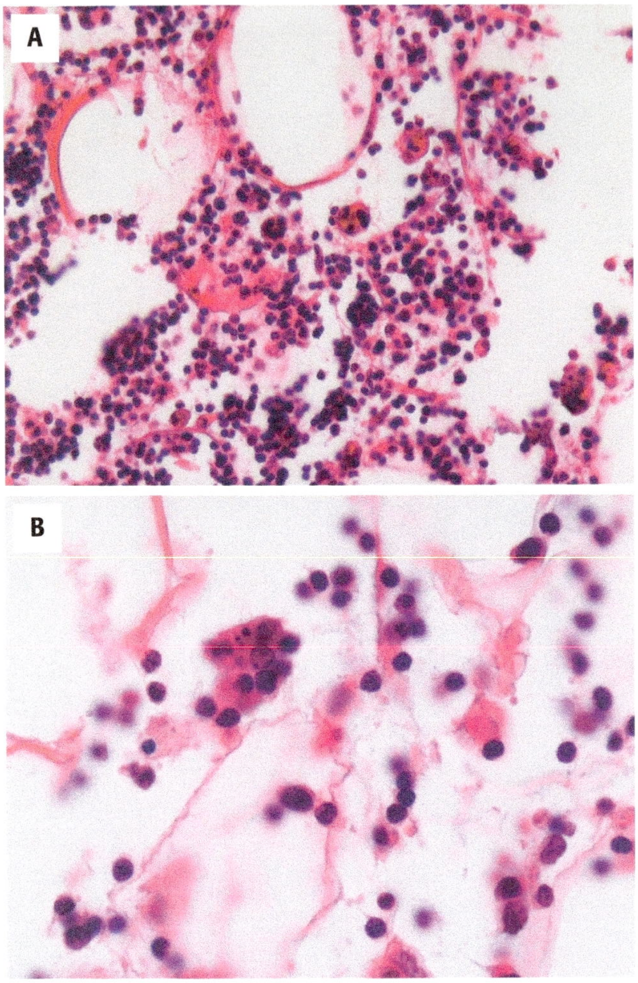

FIG. 2.12

Cytophagic histiocytic panniculitis. **A,** Lobular lymphocytic panniculitis associated with "beanbag" histiocytes displaying lymphophagocytosis and erythrophagocytosis within an edematous subcutis. **B,** Degradation of the lymphocyte nuclei (nuclear "dust," lymphocytoclasis) within the cytoplasm in *beanbag* histiocytes parallels the hemophagocytosis that may be seen in other organ systems but differs from emperiopolesis in which entire cells are phagocytosed.

some cases of CHP are virus associated, and a case associated with H1N1 vaccination was recently reported. Thus CHP may also be viewed as a manifestation of macrophage activation. Typically, there is lymphogranulomatous lobular panniculitis with fragmented nuclei (nuclear "dust") of inflammatory cells within macrophages, termed *beanbag* histiocytes (Fig. 2.12). The cytophagic histiocytes are immunopositive for CD68 and negative for S100 and CD1a.

Prognosis and Treatment

LE profundus is chronic, and the disease course depends in part on the immune status of the patient. Treatment has been with antimalarial drugs for long-term management or systemic corticosteroids for short-term initial treatment or very inflammatory flares. Resistant cases may be treated with cyclophosphamide or low-dose methotrexate. As noted earlier, SPTCL must be reasonably excluded, and long-term follow-up is mandated for possible evolution to SPTCL.

ERYTHEMA INDURATUM (NODULAR VASCULITIS)

Clinical Features

In locations and times of prevalent tuberculosis, the persons affected by erythema induratum were those most likely to contract tuberculosis. Thin, young to

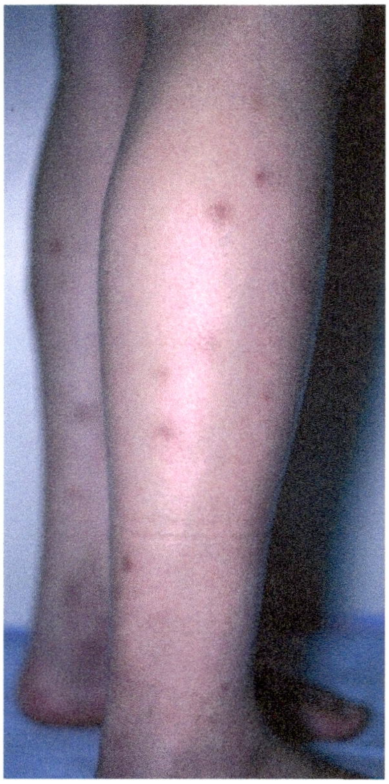

FIG. 2.13
Erythema induratum (nodular vasculitis). The posterior leg is a favored site. Nodules may ulcerate.

middle-aged women were the classic stereotype for "consumption" caused by *Mycobacterium tuberculosis*. Erythema induratum is one form of cutaneous tuberculid in which pathogens cannot be identified by staining or culture from lesional skin; however, when the distant infection is successfully treated, erythema induratum also resolves. Cases not associated with tuberculosis have been classified as nodular vasculitis, although some authorities use these two terms synonymously; they are regarded as synonymous herein.

Erythema induratum classically affects the lower legs, with a predilection for the calves and with a tendency to show symmetric involvement (Fig. 2.13). Individual lesions present as deep, often recurrent erythematous nodules that may ulcerate. Healing leaves depressed scars.

Histologic Features

Erythema induratum displays a mostly lobular pattern with granulomatous inflammation, including discrete granulomas, in the subcutaneous lobules in conjunction with vasculitis (Fig. 2.14A). Vessel involvement by vasculitis in erythema induratum is variable and may involve centrilobular venules, septal veins, or septal arteries. Moreover, in some biopsies or tissue sections, vasculitis may be absent, although the diagnosis of erythema induratum may still be suspected based on the presence of distinctive extravascular changes, including a mixed infiltrate obscuring the subcutaneous lobules with extensive granulomatous inflammation with lipophages, plasma cells, eosinophils, neutrophils, and zones of extravascular caseous (eosinophilic) necrosis (Fig. 2.14B). Nuclear "dust" is present within the zones of necrosis (Fig. 2.14C). Adipocyte pallor additionally identifies areas of ischemic necrosis. The vasculitis in erythema induratum is fundamentally a neutrophilic leukocytoclastic vasculitis; however, sampling of chronic lesions often produces an appearance of lymphocytic vasculitis. In very long-standing lesions, the histologic appearance can be that of granulomatous vasculitis (Fig. 2.15). In ulcerated lesions, there is associated necrosis of the overlying epidermis and dermis, but the epidermis itself is not infiltrated by granulomas, as can be the case in ulcerative sarcoidosis.

Ancillary Studies

In erythema induratum, by definition, special stains and lesional tissue cultures are negative for mycobacteria or any other lesional pathogen. However, polymerase chain reaction studies have detected evidence of *Mycobacterium tuberculosis* DNA in a subset of tuberculosis-associated cases.

Differential Diagnosis

The differential diagnosis for erythema induratum includes other causes of subcutaneous vasculitis, including cutaneous polyarteritis nodosa, eosinophilic granulomatosis with polyangiitis (EGP; Churg-Strauss), granulomatosis with polyangiitis (GP; Wegener), and thrombophlebitis. Although clinical correlation remains paramount, only EGP exhibits strikingly prominent eosinophils. A distinctive palisaded granuloma (Churg-Strauss granuloma) typifies both EGP and GP. Whereas in polyarteritis, the inflammatory infiltrates are typically confined to the immediate vicinity of the affected artery, in erythema induratum, other veins may be affected, and there is significant extravascular extension into the fat lobules with granulomatous features and zonal necrosis. Because of the granulomatous inflammation and necrosis, infection must be excluded. Factitial injection of foreign material can mimic individual lesions of erythema induratum, so screening for birefringent foreign material by polarized microscopy is

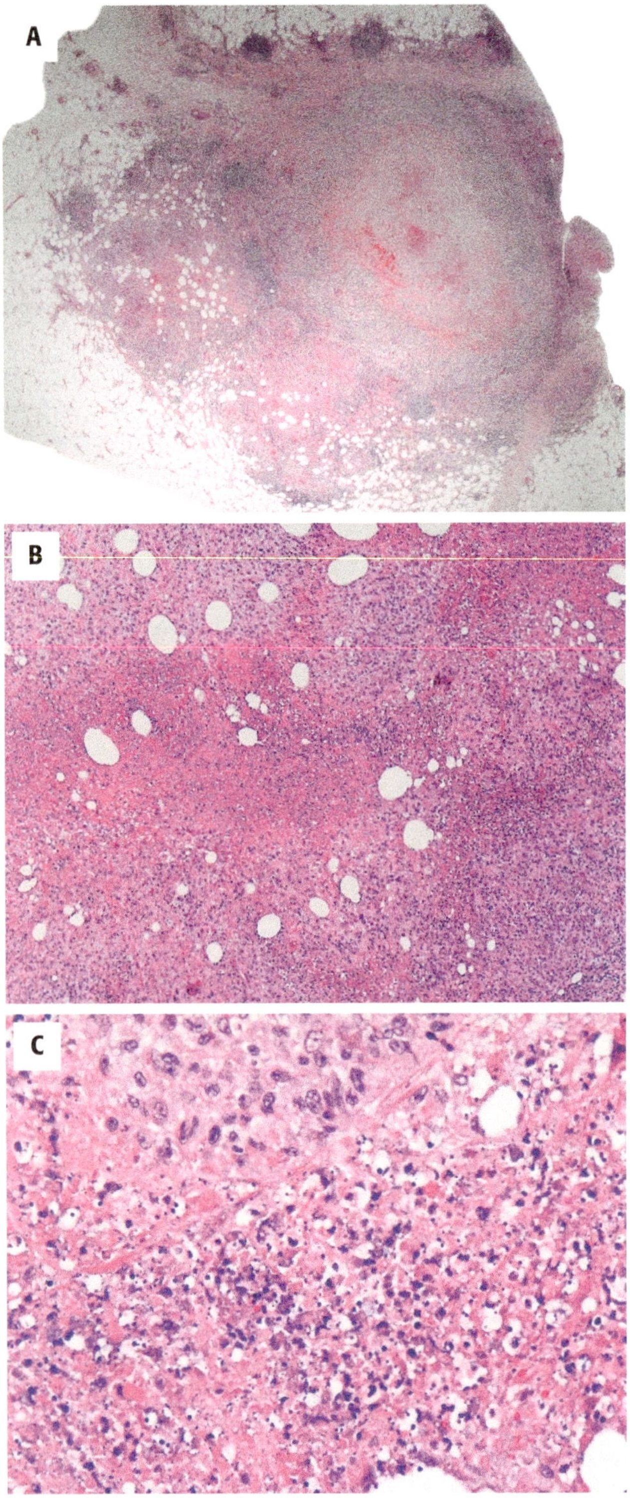

FIG. 2.14

Erythema induratum (nodular vasculitis). **A,** Mostly lobular panniculitis with vasculitis. The vessel type involved by vasculitis is variable and may include centrilobular venules, septal veins, or septal arteries; vasculitis may not be demonstrated in every biopsy or every tissue section. **B,** There is a mixed granulomatous infiltrate replacing the lobules with zones of extravascular necrosis. **C,** The zones of necrosis are associated with cellular debris.

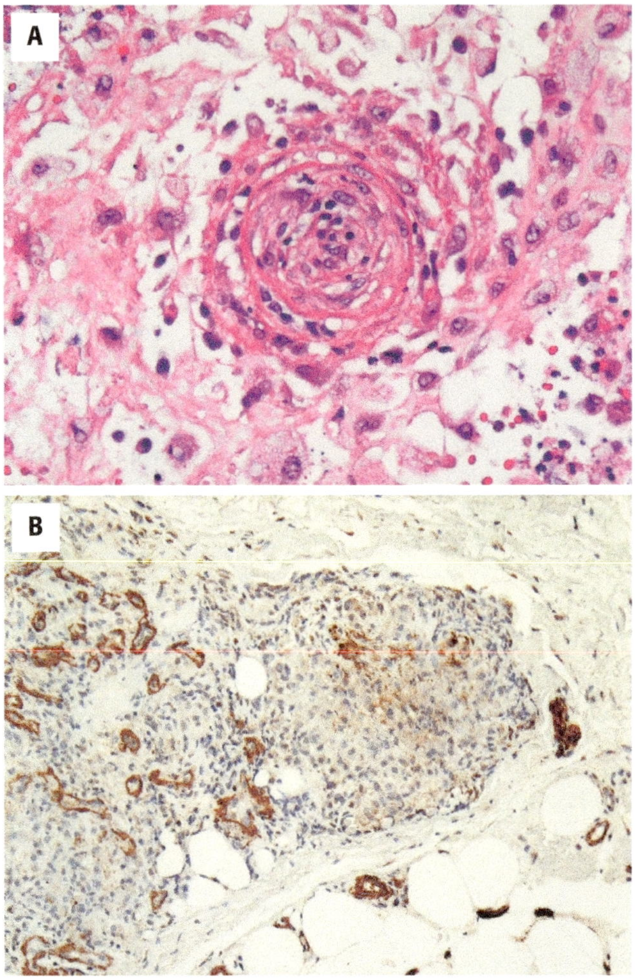

FIG. 2.15

Erythema induratum (nodular vasculitis). **A,** In this example of granulomatous vasculitis, a small artery is surrounded by macrophages and edema, and the lumen is occluded. **B,** Immunopositivity for smooth muscle actin reveals the destruction of a blood vessel wall by lymphogranulomatous inflammation.

prudent (as for any granulomatous condition). Clinical correlation is required to distinguish Crohn's disease, which usually involves orificial sites, although "metastatic" Crohn's disease may also rarely occur.

Prognosis and Treatment

The prognosis in tuberculosis-associated cases of erythema induratum is favorable in patients with treatable mycobacterial infection because antituberculous multidrug treatment usually results in a good response. If an underlying cause is not identified, the prognosis is variable. In addition to conservative and supportive measures, systemic immunosuppressive therapy may be considered in select cases.

ERYTHEMA INDURATUM (NODULAR VASCULITIS)—DISEASE FACT SHEET

Patient Group
- Women

Site of Involvement
- Legs, especially calves
- Usually bilateral and symmetrical

Clinical Features
- Erythematous tender subcutaneous nodules or plaques; ulceration variable

Prognosis
- Favorable if underlying tuberculosis can be successfully identified and treated

Treatment
- Treatment of underlying tuberculosis or other cause
- Conservative, symptomatic care
- Consider immunosuppressive therapy in refractory idiopathic cases

ERYTHEMA INDURATUM (NODULAR VASCULITIS)—PATHOLOGIC FEATURES

Histologic Features
- Lobular panniculitis with vasculitis and granulomatous inflammation
- Zones of extravascular necrosis
- Mixed infiltrate with granulomas, lipophages, eosinophils, neutrophils, plasma cells

Ancillary Studies
- Negative cultures and histochemical stains for infection
- Evidence of *Mycobacterium tuberculosis* sometimes detectable by polymerase chain reaction

Differential Diagnosis
- Other forms of subcutaneous vasculitis
- Other forms of granulomatous panniculitis
- Infectious panniculitis
- Factitial panniculitis

LIPODERMATOSCLEROSIS

Clinical Features

Lipodermatosclerosis (sclerosing panniculitis, hypodermitis sclerodermiformis) usually affects older women in the setting of pre-existing venous stasis. Lesions are confined to one or both lower extremities, characteristically arising on the medial lower leg. Acute lipodermatosclerosis can be exquisitely painful and clinically resembles bacterial cellulitis with ill-defined erythema. Established lesions are hyperpigmented, with "bound down" ill-defined sclerosis of the lower legs, which creates an appearance that has been compared to an inverted champagne glass (Fig. 2.16A).

LIPODERMATOSCLEROSIS—DISEASE FACT SHEET

Patient Group
- Women with venous stasis

Site of Involvement
- One or both lower medial legs

Clinical Features
- Sclerotic hyperpigmented plaques
- Acute lesions resemble bacterial cellulitis

Prognosis and Treatment
- Generally progressive
- Leg elevation, compressive therapy

LIPODERMATOSCLEROSIS—PATHOLOGIC FEATURES

Histologic Features
- Mixed septal and lobular pattern
- Septal sclerosis
- Lipomembranous fat necrosis
- Microcystic fat necrosis
- Lipophages
- Venous stasis changes

Differential Diagnosis
- Late stage of other forms of lobular panniculitis

Histologic Features

Although often classified as mostly lobular panniculitis, biopsies from established lesions of lipodermatosclerosis exhibit a mixed septal and lobular pattern with septal sclerosis in concert with distortion and variable obscuration of the fat lobules with prominent adipocyte necrosis (Fig. 2.16B). Usually, a few forms of adipocyte necrosis are present concomitantly, the most distinctive being lipomembranous (membranocystic) fat necrosis. The lipomembranous change gets its name from the fine, feathery projections of material extending from the periphery toward the center of the distorted fat cells (Fig. 2.16C). Importantly, this characteristic feature may not be seen in more acute forms of lipodermatosclerosis which may have relatively sparse histologic findings. *Microcystic fat necrosis* refers to marked pleomorphism of the size of the adipocyte vacuoles, forming microcysts and macrocysts, and is typically present concomitantly with lipomembranous fat necrosis. Lipophages (lipophagic fat necrosis, "lipophagic granuloma"), foamy histiocytes within the subcutaneous lobules, are also usually present. Calcification and elastosis may be seen, sometimes resembling the calcified, fragmented elastic fibers that typify pseudoxanthoma elasticum.

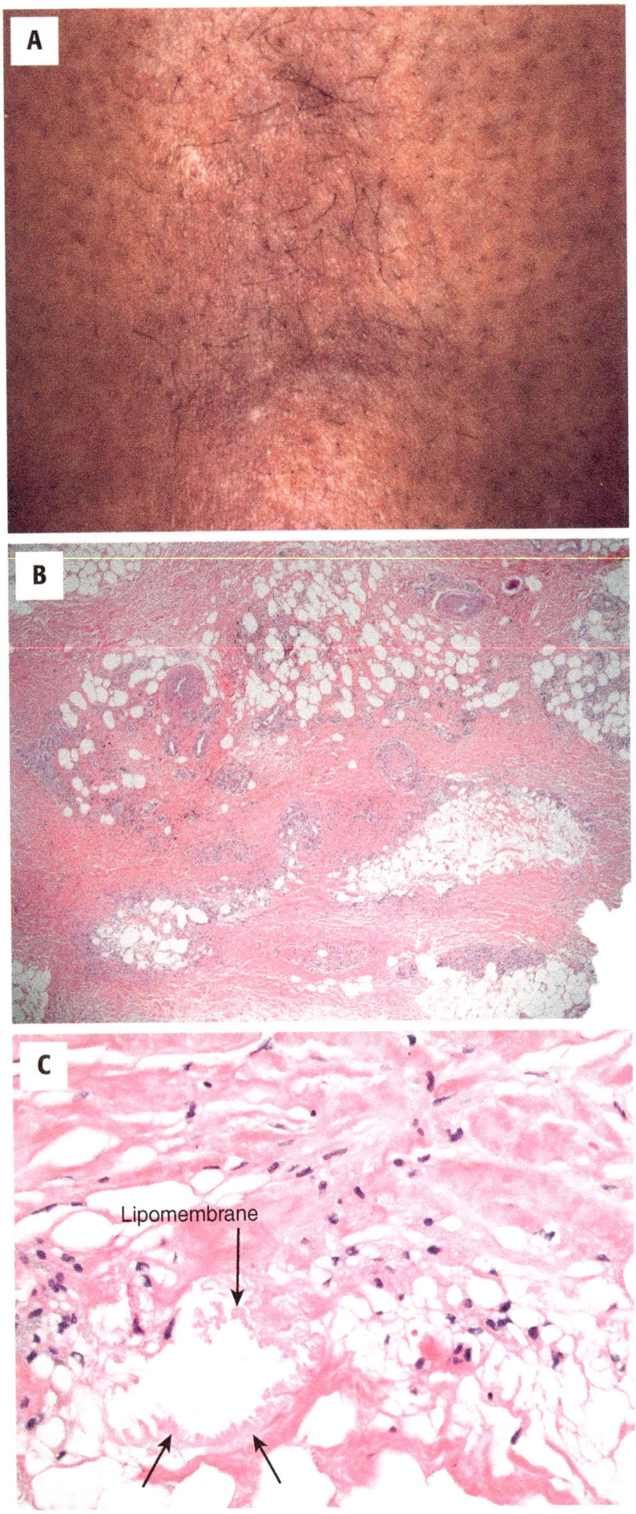

FIG. 2.16

Lipodermatosclerosis (sclerosing panniculitis). **A,** Clinically a firm depressed region of the lower leg is a common presentation. (Case courtesy of John T. Headington, MD.) **B,** Mixed septal and lobular pattern with widened sclerotic septa and fat lobules altered by fat necrosis (lipomembranous, microcystic, lipophagic). **C,** Lipomembranous fat necrosis *(arrows)* is most characteristic of but not specific for lipodermatosclerosis.

Superimposed venous stasis changes are typically present and include increased vascularity, extravasated erythrocytes, and hemosiderin in the papillary and sometimes also the reticular dermis.

Ancillary Studies

Lipomembranes are periodic acid-Schiff positive; however, this is not required for diagnosis.

Differential Diagnosis

Lipodermatosclerosis is usually diagnosed clinically without biopsy. Involvement is confined to the legs of adults, the vast majority of whom are women, most with elevated body mass indexes. In this clinical context, the combined presence of venous stasis changes, septal sclerosis, and lipomembranous and microcystic fat necrosis is specific. However, lipomembranous fat necrosis and microcystic fat necrosis may be seen in many other disorders, including traumatic panniculitis (i.e., the late stage of essentially any lobular panniculitis), LE and EN.

Prognosis and Treatment

Management of lipodermatosclerosis is symptomatic and directed at management of venous stasis. Leg elevation and compressive therapy are usually advised. Systemic therapy may include pentoxifylline or fibrinolytic agents.

TRAUMATIC PANNICULITIS

Clinical Features

Traumatic panniculitis most commonly presents as a solitary lesion at a site of recent trauma. The trauma may be confirmed by the clinical history or occult. The extremities, especially the lower extremities, are typically affected. In the broader sense of trauma encompassing any external force or agent, either externally applied or injected, traumatic panniculitis may include the more specific entities of nodular cystic fat necrosis (mobile encapsulated lipoma), factitial panniculitis, and cold panniculitis.

Factitial panniculitis may be regarded as a distinct subset of traumatic panniculitis with a varied presentation. In factitial panniculitis, a deliberate human action results in panniculitis secondary to the injection of foreign material into the subcutis. The injection could be performed by the affected individual themself, by their proxy (Munchausen syndrome by proxy), or by a medical provider as a cosmetic procedure or unintended side effect of medical therapy. Similar to other forms of traumatic panniculitis, the number of lesions is usually limited; in addition, the distribution of lesions is restricted to anatomic sites that are accessible to injection or where cosmetic enhancement has been requested (e.g., face, penis).

Cold panniculitis arises in the distinctive clinical settings of cold exposure, including popsicle panniculitis (cheeks of children), equestrian panniculitis (lateral thighs of equestrians and cyclists), and on the scrotum.

Histologic Features

Traumatic panniculitis is a mostly lobular or mixed septal and lobular panniculitis (Fig. 2.17A), typically with prominent lipophages (Fig. 2.17B). Lipomembranous fat necrosis, hemorrhage, hemosiderin, and calcification are also commonly present. In the early stages of traumatic panniculitis, particularly factitial panniculitis, neutrophils may predominate.

In nodular cystic fat necrosis, the affected fat lobules appear encapsulated by a sclerotic fibrous capsule with a loss of nuclear adipocyte staining and variable superimposed lipophages, lipomembranous fat necrosis, or calcification.

In cold panniculitis, lymphocytes and histiocytes aggregate at the junction of the dermis and subcutis and variably within the subcutaneous lobules. Neutrophils may be present in early lesions. Eosinophils are variable. "Fluffy edema" of vessel walls has been described.

The effects of foreign materials are commonly identified in reactions secondary to cosmetic fillers. Historically, injection of paraffin and silicone resulted in a granulomatous reaction with numerous empty vacuoles, creating a "Swiss cheese" appearance at scanning magnification. Liquid silicone may be associated with similar changes when an associated granulomatous reaction becomes clinically evident (Fig. 2.18). The appearances of a wide variety of injected substances have been reviewed in detail by Requena and colleagues (Dadzie et al., 2008; Requena, Cerroni, & Kutzner, 2012) and also by Dadzie and colleagues (Dadzie et al., 2008).

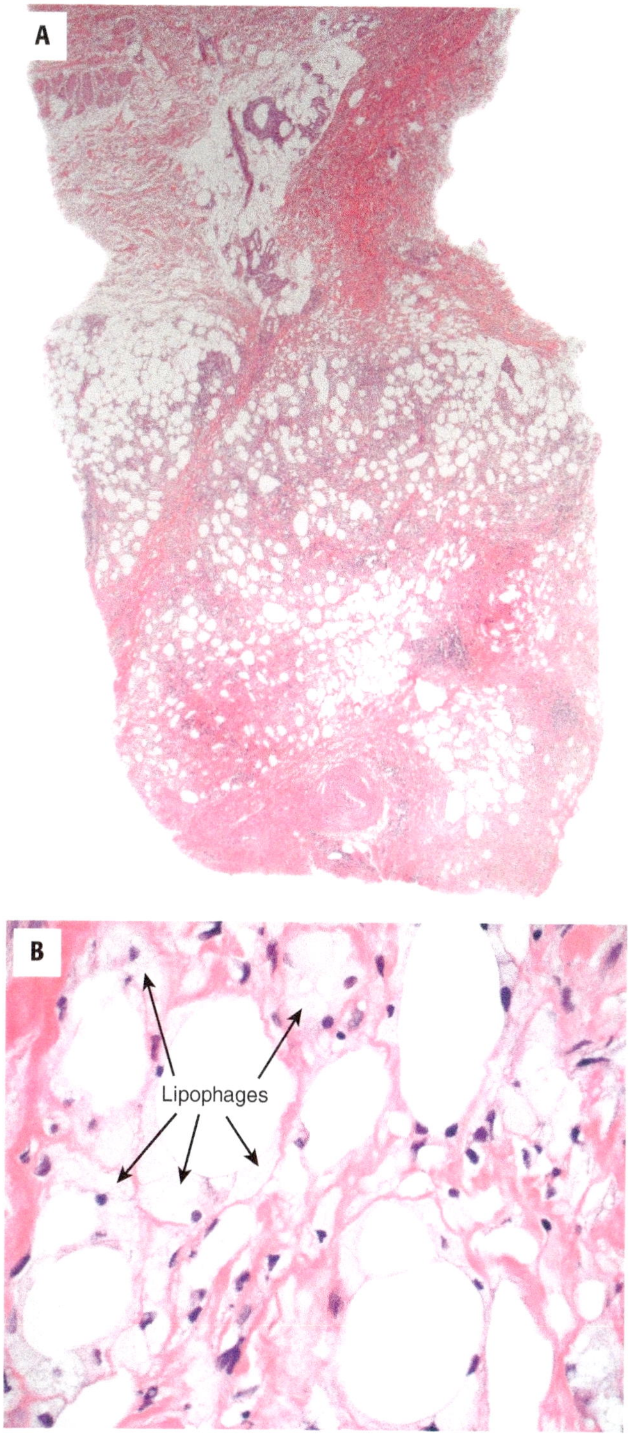

FIG. 2.17
Traumatic panniculitis. **A,** Mostly lobular panniculitis. **B,** Lipophages are prominent *(arrows)*.

Ancillary Studies

Although some cases of traumatic panniculitis are obvious, other cases may require a detailed clinical history and negative medical workup to establish the diagnosis. Special stains for infection and polarized microscopy are generally advised if neutrophils or granulomatous inflammation is present.

Prognosis and Treatment

The prognosis is variable and depends on whether a causative agent can be identified and removed. Discontinuation of the causative agent is generally curative. For reactions to cosmetic fillers, intralesional corticosteroid may be attempted.

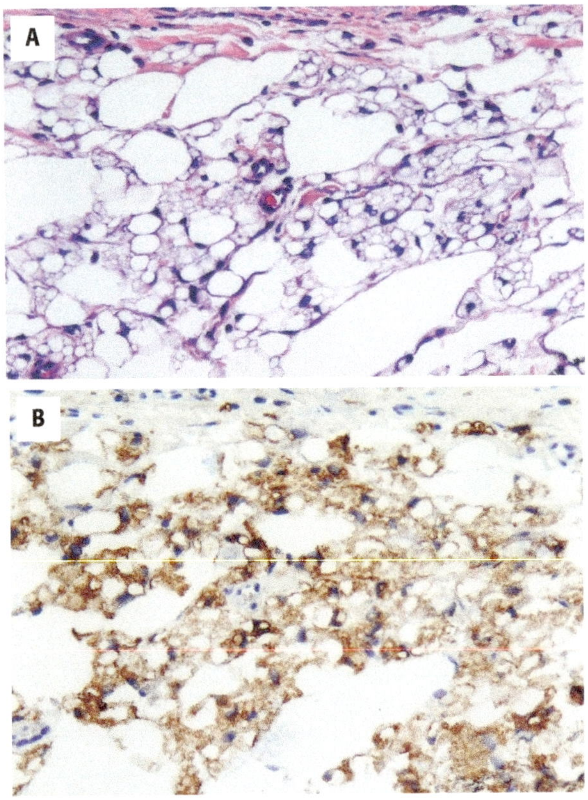

FIG. 2.18
Factitial panniculitis secondary to liquid silicone injection. **A,** Vacuolated cells are numerous. Liquid silicone produces multiple cavities or cystlike spaces that are irregular in outline. **B,** Cytoplasmic immunopositivity for CD68, a lysosomal marker, confirms that these cells are macrophages rather than lipoblasts.

SCLEROSING POSTIRRADIATION PANNICULITIS

Clinical Features

Sclerosing postirradiation panniculitis (postirradiation sclerodermoid panniculitis, postirradiation pseudosclerodermatous panniculitis) occurs secondary to megavoltage radiation therapy, usually for treatment of breast cancer. Nodular lesions appear on the chest within several months (but sometimes several years or even longer than a decade) of megavoltage radiation therapy within the field of treatment.

Histologic Features

Sclerosing postirradiation panniculitis exhibits a mostly lobular or mixed septal and lobular pattern with the combined presence of lobular lymphohistiocytic infiltrates with lipophages, plasma cells, and eosinophils, and septal sclerosis (Fig. 2.19). Ischemic fat necrosis is also expected. Enlarged fibroblasts (radiation fibroblasts) and endothelial cells (radiation vasculopathy) with hyperchromatic atypical nuclei are also expected.

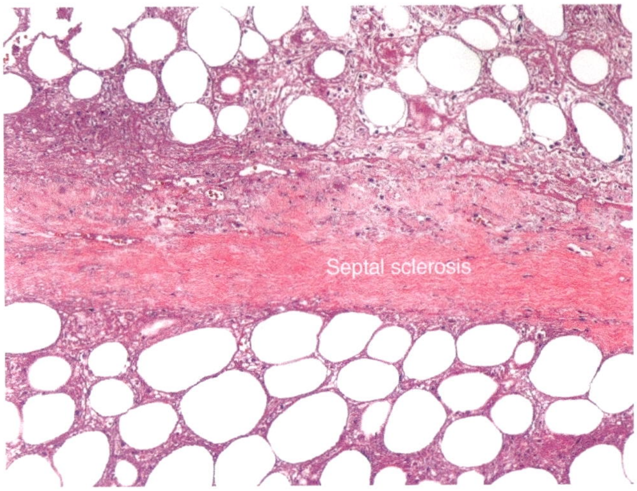

FIG. 2.19
Postirradiation sclerosing panniculitis. There is septal sclerosis and lipophages within the lobules. (Image courtesy Luis Requena, MD, Madrid, Spain.)

Ancillary Studies

A history of megavoltage radiation to the affected area is requisite and sufficient for diagnosis if the histopathologic features are compatible.

Differential Diagnosis

Lesions can be difficult to distinguish from inflammatory morphea. Clinical correlation (cutaneous manifestations limited to radiation field) is essential. Histologic clues to a probable radiation-related process include the presence of radiation fibroblasts, vasculopathy, and a usually more florid mixed inflammatory cell infiltrate than typically seen in morphea.

Prognosis and Treatment

Biopsy is typically performed to rule out recurrent carcinoma, infection, or angiosarcoma. Reassurance may be provided.

SUBCUTANEOUS FAT NECROSIS OF THE NEWBORN

Clinical Features

Subcutaneous fat necrosis of the newborn usually affects term newborns, with erythematous nodules or plaques with variable ulceration and caseous discharge. Risk factors include scenarios involving hypothermia or

DIFFERENTIAL DIAGNOSIS OF PANNICULITIS WITH NEEDLE-SHAPED CLEFTS

Disease	Patients	Onset	Histology
Subcutaneous fat necrosis of the newborn	Full-term neonates	First 2 weeks of life	Panniculitis with needle-shaped clefts in adipocytes and giant cells
Sclerema neonatorum	Premature neonates	First week of life; rare in developed countries	Panniculitis with needle-shaped clefts in adipocytes and minimal inflammation
Poststeroid panniculitis	Children	Follows cessation of systemic steroids	Panniculitis with needle-shaped clefts in adipocytes and giant cells

hypoxia, including whole-body cooling or a complicated forceps delivery. The trunk and proximal extremities are the most frequently involved, although the head and neck regions may also be involved. Systemic complications include hypercalcemia (sometimes associated with nephrocalcinosis), thrombocytopenia, and hypertriglyceridemia.

Histologic Features

Subcutaneous fat necrosis of the newborn is a lobular panniculitis with macrophages containing distinctive cleft-shaped spaces in stellate or radial array within the cytoplasm of the macrophages and lipocytes that represent the artifact of crystallized saturated fat (Fig. 2.20). Neutrophils may be present in early lesions.

Differential Diagnosis

Crystalline triglyceride arrays in adipocytes and macrophages can occur in subcutaneous fat necrosis in newborns, sclerema neonatorum, and poststeroid panniculitis. Withdrawal of systemic steroid treatment is the risk factor for poststeroid panniculitis and is distinguishable from subcutaneous fat necrosis of the newborn only by clinical correlation. Sclerema neonatorum is a devastating and rapid condition that can be fatal. It is a vanishing disorder in developed countries, attributable to adequate postnatal care. Before the advent of heated incubators, sclerema neonatorum was manifested by a rapid hardening of the subcutaneous fat in plaques and confluent areas. The child was usually premature, hypothermic, and often septic. In sclerema neonatorum, there is no inflammatory infiltration, and the crystals tend to be smaller (microsized) and present only within adipocytes because there is no host response (Fig. 2.21). In oxalosis, the crystals are birefringent in formalin-fixed sections. In gout, crystals are not birefringent in formalin-fixed tissue. Mucormycosis, aspergillosis, etanercept, and gemcitabine-associated microangiopathy have rarely been associated with crystal formation.

Prognosis and Treatment

Subcutaneous fat necrosis of the newborn usually resolves in weeks to months, but associated sequelae such as nephrocalcinosis may persist. Beyond supportive care, pamidronate may be used to manage significant hypercalcemia or to reduce the risk of nephrocalcinosis.

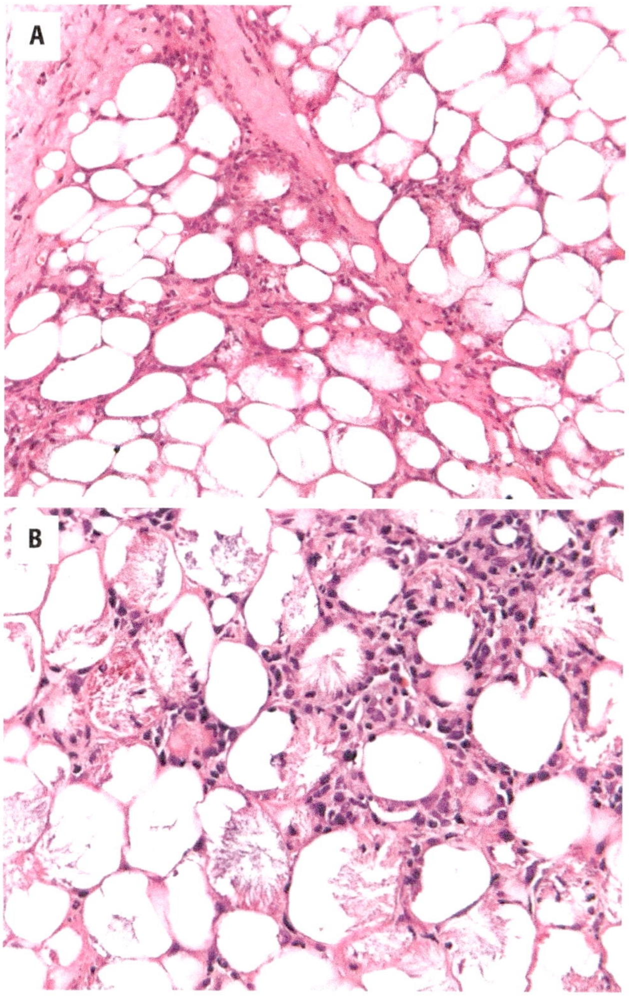

FIG. 2.20

Subcutaneous fat necrosis of the newborn. **A,** The periphery of the fat lobules is most affected, with macrophage infiltration. **B,** The fat cells have undergone crystallization of the triglycerides in their cytoplasm. Stellate protein precipitates remain to outline the clefts where the triglyceride crystals were present.

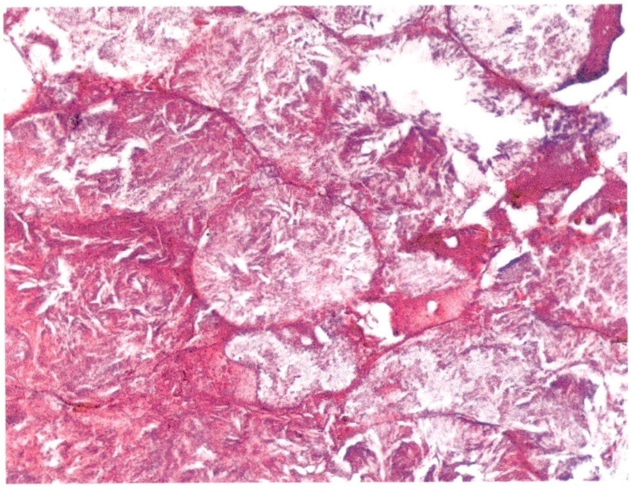

FIG. 2.21
Sclerema neonatorum. Adipocytes are filled with crystals. The associated host response is minimal. (Image courtesy Luis Requena, MD, Madrid, Spain.)

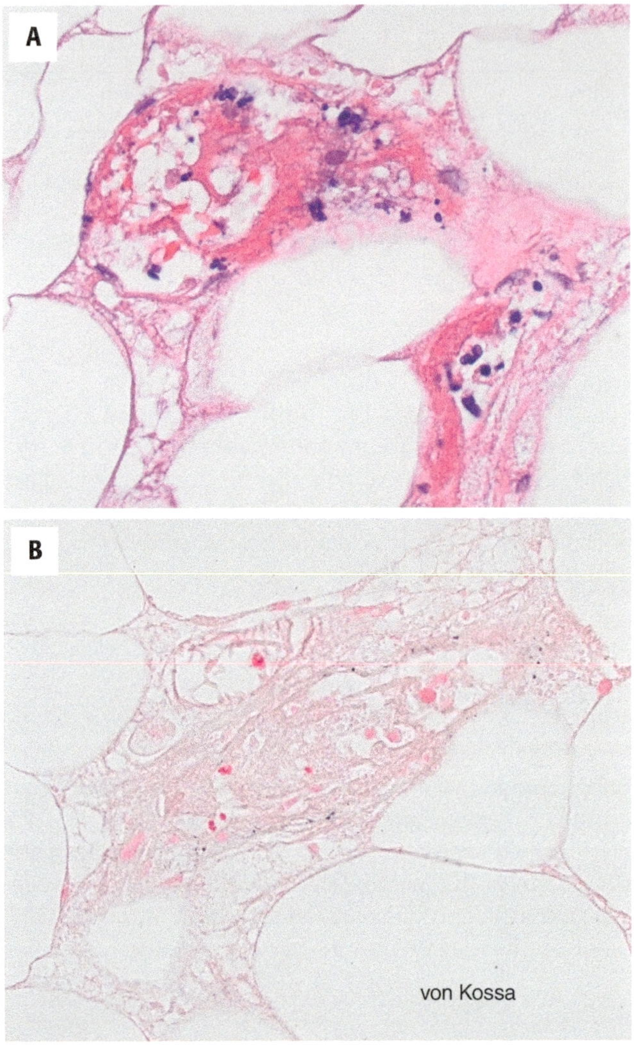

FIG. 2.22
Calciphylaxis. The combination of subcutaneous small vessel thrombosis and vascular calcification supports the diagnosis. **A,** Thrombosis with lipophages (hematoxylin and eosin [H&E]). **B,** The *von Kossa* stain highlights subtle vascular calcification not evident on H&E.

CALCIPHYLAXIS

Clinical Features

Calciphylaxis (calcific uremic arteriolopathy) is a life-threatening disorder that usually occurs in the setting of end-stage renal insufficiency, with hard, tender, erythematous but cold necrotic plaques with subsequent eschar formation, usually on the lower extremities or abdomen. Most cases progress acutely, although a more protracted, subacute presentation may also occur.

Histologic Features

The hallmark of calciphylaxis is the calcification of the subcutaneous vessel walls. However, nondiagnostic biopsies are not uncommon, especially in smaller biopsy specimens. An important finding also includes vasocclusive changes, which are a critical component of the diagnosis. This may include ischemic necrosis with secondary subepidermal clefting, sparse neutrophils, calcification of capillaries, or eccrine gland basement membrane. As even patients without calciphlaxis but with renal disease and abnormalities in their calcium phosphate metabolism may show evidence of calcifications, it is the combination of changes within the appropriate clinical context that establishes the diagnosis. Subtle calcification of capillaries or the eccrine gland basement membrane zone may not be evident on hematoxylin and eosin (H&E) but can be identified using von Kossa stain (Fig. 2.22).

Ancillary Studies

Serum calcium and phosphate levels may be elevated. Elevated parathyroid hormone levels are also expected. Exceptional cases in patients without renal insufficiency have been associated with metastatic breast cancer or Crohn's disease.

Prognosis and Treatment

Calciphylaxis may be fatal. Management is directed at control of calcium and phosphate levels and may include sodium thiosulfate, bisphosphonates, or vitamin K supplementation. Trigger factor cessation may entail discontinuation of warfarin or calcium-containing phosphate binders or parathyroidectomy.

EOSINOPHILIC PANNICULITIS

Lobular panniculitis with prominent eosinophils is a distinctive histologic picture, but a number of conditions can produce it (Fig. 2.23) from infancy to old age. By this designation is implied only the histologic picture and a differential diagnosis, usually a hypersensitivity reaction from a drug or arthropod bite. Reported drugs are diverse, including subcutaneous heparin, intramuscular penicillin, and apomorphine. Eosinophilic panniculitis may also be seen in the clinical setting of human immunodeficiency virus (HIV) infection, atopy, and hypereosinophilic syndrome (as a diagnosis of exclusion) and has even been documented in EN. Depending on the etiology, eosinophilic panniculitis may be accompanied by fever, pruritus, and malaise, particularly in association with hypersensitivity reactions to medications. The fat lobules contain mostly eosinophils, usually with a few lymphocytes and sometimes neutrophils, with variable septal involvement. Depending on the clinical context, a complete blood count with differential may be worthwhile to screen for eosinophilia. A stool sample to screen for ova and parasites may be worthwhile. The prognosis of eosinophilic panniculitis is variable but generally favorable, with a very favorable prognosis if the cause can be identified and removed.

NEUTROPHILIC PANNICULITIS

Similar to eosinophilic panniculitis, neutrophilic panniculitis is a histologic reaction pattern, not a specific clinical entity. The differential diagnosis includes infection, myelodysplasia, early pancreatic panniculitis, or AAT deficiency panniculitis. Subcutaneous Sweet's syndrome or a nondiagnostic sampling of vasculitis should be considered if nuclear dust is prominent. Neutrophilic panniculitis has also been associated with a variety of medications, including granulocyte colony-stimulating factor, filgrastim, pegfilgrastim, interleukin-2, all-*trans*-retinoic acid (ATRA), azacitidine, and vemurafenib. The histologic appearance is mostly lobular panniculitis of predominantly neutrophils. Special stains or cultures may be needed to reasonably exclude pathogens.

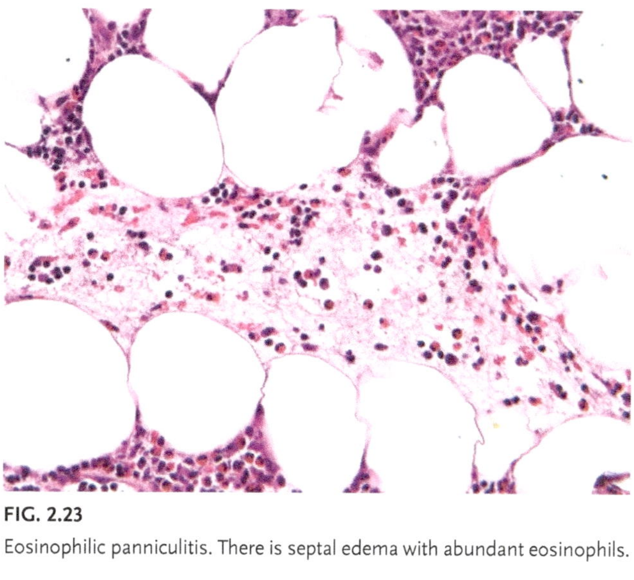

FIG. 2.23
Eosinophilic panniculitis. There is septal edema with abundant eosinophils.

DRUG-INDUCED PANNICULITIS

Drugs can recapitulate virtually any pattern of inflammatory skin disease, including mostly lobular or mostly septal panniculitis. Eosinophils are traditionally associated with medication reactions, although many drugs have been associated with neutrophilic panniculitis (see earlier discussion). Most recently targeted therapy drugs such as BRAF inhibitors have been associated with neutrophilic panniculitis. Lymphohistiocytic lobular panniculitis may also occur (e.g., the late stage of reactions secondary to granulocyte-monocyte-colony-stimulating factor [GMCSF]). EN, the prototype of mostly septal panniculitis, may be triggered by numerous medications, including oral contraceptives, sulfa drugs, and dozens of others. Drug-induced polyarteritis nodosa has been associated with minocycline.

LIPOATROPHY AND LIPODYSTROPHY

Clinical Features

The loss of subcutaneous fat lobules may be ascribed to noninflammatory or inflammatory conditions that may be focal, partial, or total and inherited or acquired. The terms *lipoatrophy* and *lipodystrophy* have been used variably and sometimes interchangeably in the medical literature. Some authorities define *lipoatrophy* as having an inflammatory component (*lipodystrophy*, having no evidence of inflammation); others use *lipoatrophy* to describe localized fat loss and *lipodystrophy* for more generalized involvement. Given the prevalence of HIV infection, HIV-positive patients on antiretroviral therapy represent the most common acquired lipodystrophy syndrome; in this context, the term *lipodystrophy* has been defined as fat redistribution rather than loss of fat tissue. Over a dozen rare genetic lipodystrophies, partial or generalized, have been documented. Lipoatrophic panniculitis of the ankles represents a distinctive inflammatory lipoatrophy that typically affects the ankle region of children.

The clinical appearance can be dramatic when generalized, with total loss of all fat, loss from the face and upper body in partial lipodystrophy, or loss of fat from the cheeks, arms, and legs in HIV-associated lipodystrophy. Otherwise, the localized loss of fat produces a localized, nonulcerated depression of the skin surface. The concomitant presence of erythema suggests an inflammatory component.

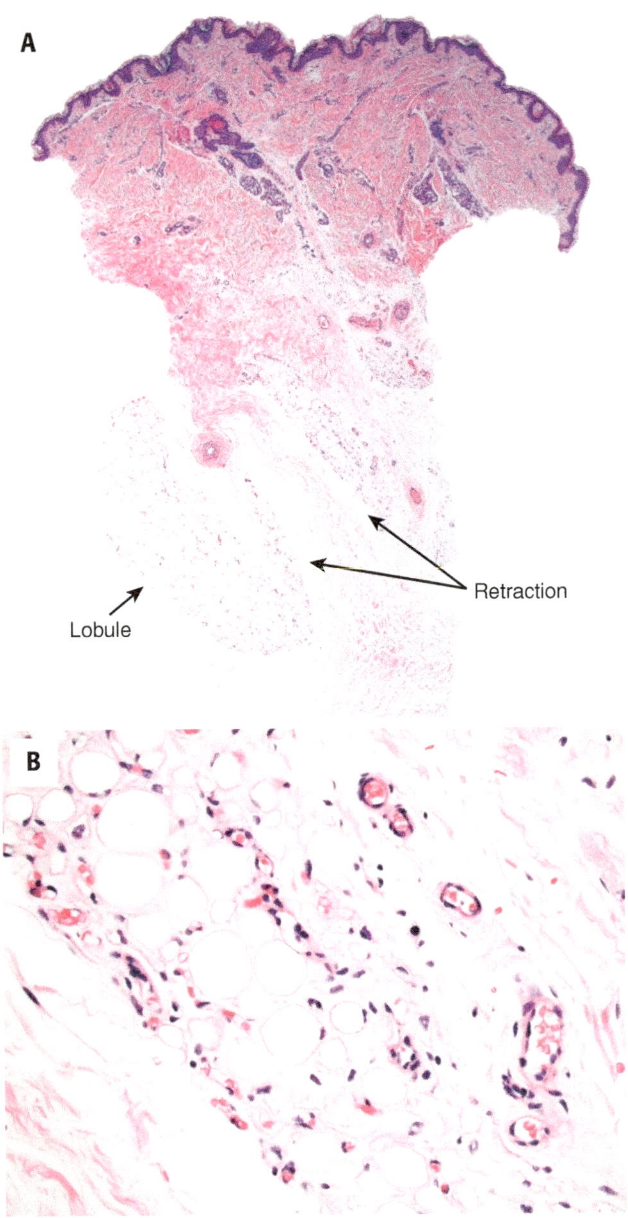

FIG. 2.24

Localized lipoatrophy or lipodystrophy, noninflammatory. **A,** Fat lobules are shrunken and retracted from their surrounding septa. **B,** Small vessels and myxoid stroma are evident within affected fat lobules.

Histologic Features

In lipoatrophy and lipodystrophy, the least common histologic denominator is a loss of fat, with a reduction in the size of the individual fat lobules and retraction of the shrunken lobules from the surrounding septa (Fig. 2.24A). The individual adipocytes are also smaller and retracted from each other, resembling embryonic fat tissue with myxoid stroma and increased vascularity (Fig. 2.24B). In inflammatory variants, lymphocytes are also present. Multiple biopsies may be required to document the progression of the disease and whether an inflammatory component is present. However, HIV-associated lipodystrophy is usually an easy clinical diagnosis.

Differential Diagnosis

Although the histologic appearances are distinctive, clinical correlation is required because the clinical appearance and the patient history are most important in determining the correct diagnostic category from among numerous inherited and acquired possibilities.

Prognosis and Treatment

Tesamorelin, a growth hormone-releasing factor analog, is approved by the Food and Drug Administration for HIV-associated lipodystrophy. Cosmetic fillers, such as poly-l-lactic acid and calcium hydroxyapatite, or lipotransfer may achieve semidurable results in HIV-associated lipodystrophy.

ACKNOWLEDGMENT

The late N. Scott McNutt, MD, is gratefully acknowledged for providing the foundation of the previous edition's chapter.

SUGGESTED FURTHER READING

Dadzie, O. E., Mahalingam, M., Parada, M., El Helou, T., Philips, T., & Bhawan, J. (2008). Adverse cutaneous reactions to soft tissue fillers—a review of the histological features. *Journal of Cutaneous Pathology*, *35*, 536–548.

Diaz-Cascajo, C., Borghi, S., & Weyers, W. (2000). Panniculitis: Definition of terms and diagnostic strategy. *American Journal of Dermatopathology*, *22*, 530–549.

Gilchrest, H., & Patterson, J. W. (2010). Erythema nodosum and erythema induratum (nodular vasculitis): Diagnosis and management. *Dermatologic Therapy*, *23*, 320–327.

Pincus, L.B., LeBoit, P.E., McCalmont, T.H., Ricci, R., Buzio, C., Fox, L.P., et al. (2009). Subcutaneous panniculitis-like T-cell lymphoma with overlapping clinicopathologic features of lupus erythematosus: Coexistence of 2 entities? *American Journal of Dermatopathology*, *31*, 520–526.

Requena, L., Cerroni, L., & Kutzner, H. (2012). Histopathologic patterns associated with external agents. *Dermatologic Clinics*, *30*, 731–748.

Requena, L., & Sanchez Yus, E. (2001). Panniculitis. Part I. Mostly septal panniculitis. *Journal of the American Academy of Dermatology*, *45*, 163–183.

Requena, L., & Sanchez Yus, E. (2001). Panniculitis. Part II. Mostly lobular panniculitis. *Journal of the American Academy of Dermatology*, *45*, 325–361.

Infectious Diseases of the Skin

3

Brian L. Swick • Helen M. Chen • Marcia Ramos-e-Silva
Hideko Kamino • Klaus J. Busam

VIRAL INFECTIONS

HUMAN PAPILLOMA VIRUS

WARTS (VERRUCAE)

The human papilloma virus (HPV) is the most prominent member of the papovaviruses group. There are more than 100 distinct HPV genotypes, some of which have oncogenic potential.

Clinical Findings

Different HPV strains have different clinical manifestations. Verruca vulgaris (common wart) may present as solitary or multiple, rough-surfaced (verrucous) papules on exposed surfaces, frequently affecting fingers (Fig. 3.1). Palmoplantar warts are often painful and covered by a thick callus (Fig. 3.2). The deep variant that resembles an anthill histologically is called myrmecia (inclusion wart). Plane warts (verrucae planae) are flat-topped smooth papules; some appear pigmented (Fig. 3.3). The clinical lesions of epidermodysplasia verruciformis (EDV) may present as persistent, widely distributed flat warts that may coalesce and form plaques. Squamous cell carcinoma may arise in association with EDV (highest risk for HPV-5 and -8). Susceptibility to EV is inherited, but EDV may also occur in immunosuppressed individuals.

HUMAN PAPILLOMA VIRUS INFECTION—DISEASE FACT SHEET

Patient Group

- Cutaneous warts
  - Children (up to 10% of 2- to 12-year-old children have warts)
  - Adults at any age
- Condylomas: genital human papillomavirus (HPV) is the most common sexually transmitted disease among adolescents and adults; it is uncommon in prepubertal children, in whom it may be caused by sexual abuse

Site of Involvement

- Hands and feet
- Genital region
- Oral mucosa

Clinical Findings

Common Warts (HPV-1, -2, -4)

- Hyperkeratotic exophytic papules or plaques with digitated surface

Flat Warts (HPV-3, -10)

- Skin-colored, smooth-surfaced, flat-topped papules

Myrmecial (Deep Palmoplantar) Warts (HPV-1, -60)

- Endophytic growth on palms and soles

Epidermodysplasia Verruciformis (HPV-3, -5, -8)

- Scaly guttate, red macules, and thin plaques

Condyloma Acuminata (HPV-6, -11)

- Skin-colored, discrete, sessile, smooth-surfaced papules

Bowenoid Papulosis (HPV-16)

- Multiple red-brown verrucous papules or confluent plaques

Prognosis

- Common warts tend to persist but may regress spontaneously
- Squamous cell carcinoma may arise in association with warts, especially in immunocompromised individuals (HPV types with oncogenic potential include HPV-16, -18, -31, and -33)

Treatment

- Surgical: shave removal or excision
- Nonsurgical destruction: chemical, liquid nitrogen, electrodesiccation, laser
- Immunologic (imiquimod)
- Vaccine against HPV types 6, 11, 16, and 18 to minimize the risk of cervical cancer

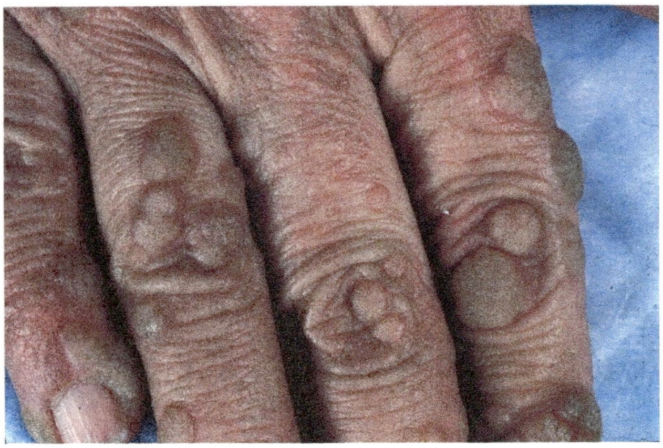

FIG. 3.1
Verruca vulgaris. Multiple papules with a rough surface are present on the dorsal aspect of the fingers.

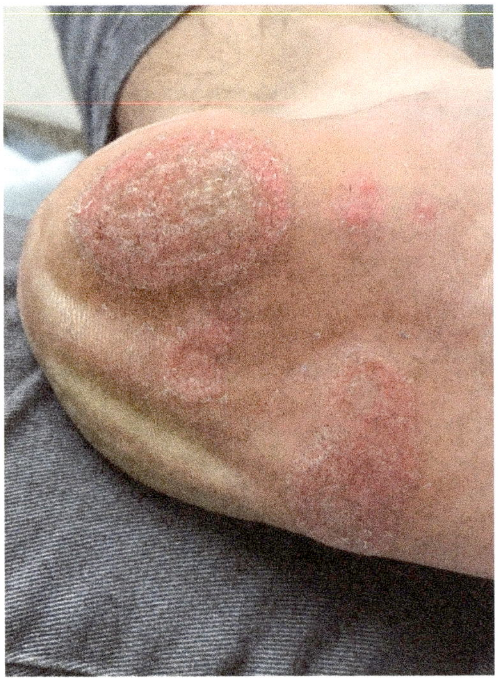

FIG. 3.2
Verruca plantaris. Thickened keratotic plaques with interruption of skin lines and thrombosed capillaries.

Focal epithelial hyperplasia (Heck's disease), a chronic disease with a higher incidence among Inuit peoples and Native Americans, is characterized by the presence of multiple soft, pink papules and plaques on the mucosa of lips (most commonly the lower lip) and cheeks.

Histologic Features

There are prominent hyperkeratosis and acanthosis with elongation of the rete ridges, which at the periphery tend to curve inward and point toward the center

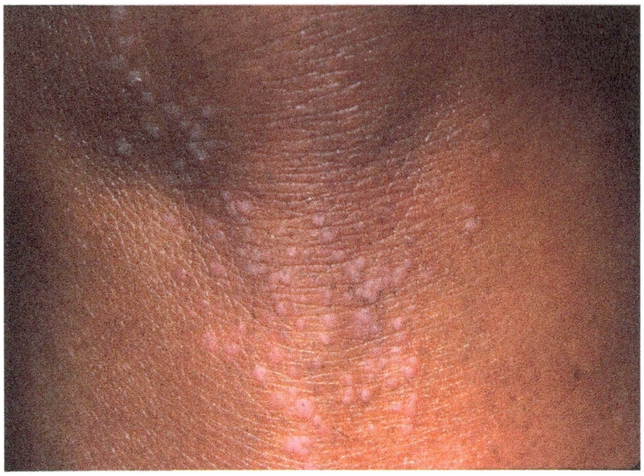

FIG. 3.3
Verruca plana. Multiple small flat topped hypopigmented papules.

(Fig. 3.4). Columns of parakeratosis overlie the tips of the papillomatous peaks. Hypergranulosis with coarse keratohyalin clumps (Fig. 3.4B) is present in the valleys between these peaks. Large, characteristically vacuolated cells are seen in the upper epidermis. These cells have a small, dark, hyperchromatic nucleus, which may have irregular contours, giving rise to a "raisinoid" appearance, surrounded by clear cytoplasm (koilocytes). Filiform warts are characterized by papillomatous epidermal hyperplasia over a narrow base with long, thin columns of hyperkeratosis and parakeratosis (Fig. 3.5). Commonly, warts are inflamed. There may be a prominent lichenoid inflammatory reaction at the junction of the base of the lesion and the surrounding dermis.

HUMAN PAPILLOMA VIRUS—PATHOLOGIC FEATURES

Histologic Features

Common Wart

- Hyperkeratosis and acanthosis
- Papillomatosis with columns of parakeratosis at the peaks
- Hypergranulosis with coarse keratohyaline granules
- Large vacuolated keratinocytes with deeply basophilic "raisinoid" nuclei in the upper levels of epidermis and/or binucleated keratinocytes
- Serum or hemorrhage in the stratum corneum

Flat Wart

- Only slight epidermal hyperplasia with a prominent granular cell layer
- Keratinocytes with haloed nuclei (bird's eyes) in upper spinous and granular cell layer

Myrmecial Wart (Deep Palmoplantar Warts)

- Papillomatous surface, but significant endophytic growth
- Bright, large eosinophilic keratohyaline granules

Condyloma Acuminatum

- Papillomatous mammillated epithelial hyperplasia
- Koilocytes (keratinocytes with hyperchromatic raisinoid nuclei surrounded by a clear halo) and binucleated cells

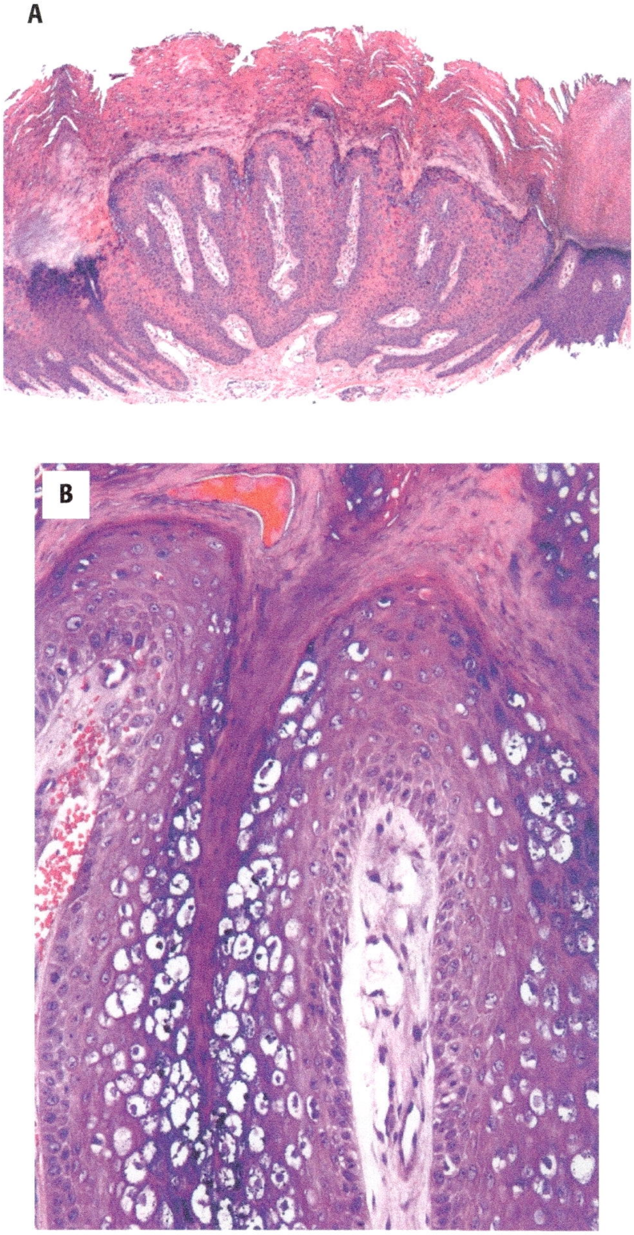

FIG. 3.4

Verruca vulgaris. **A,** Silhouette: there is papillomatous epidermal hyperplasia with hyperparakeratosis. **B,** Viral cytopathic changes (keratinocytes with hyperchromatic small nuclei surrounded by a clear halo) are present. There is associated hypergranulosis. Serum is present in the stratum corneum, and the dermal papillae show ectatic capillaries.

Ancillary Studies

- Molecular studies (polymerase chain reaction or in situ hybridization) to test for high-risk HPV types
- Condyloma: MIB1 labeling of keratinocytes in the upper epithelial layer

Differential Diagnosis

- Squamous cell carcinoma
- Digitated (verrucoid) keratoses
- Prurigo nodularis
- Epidermal nevus

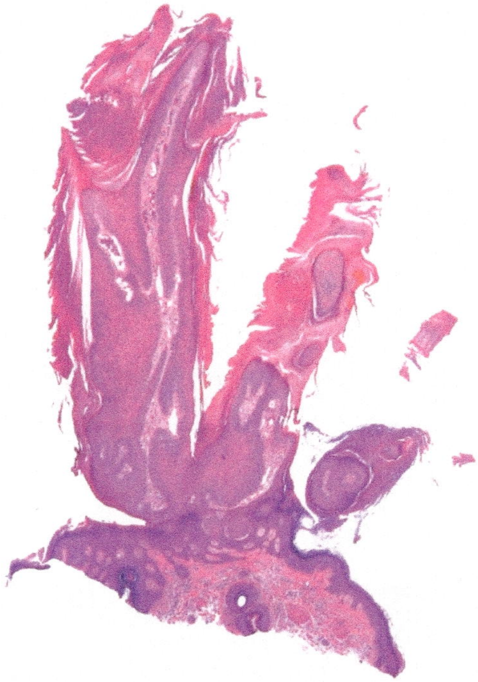

FIG. 3.5

Filiform wart. Note the long, pointed papillomatous projections.

A flat wart (verruca plana) lacks papillomatosis and has a basket-weaved stratum corneum. Layers of keratinocytes with "bird's eye" nuclei in the upper spinous and granular cell layers are commonly seen in flat warts (Fig. 3.6). Myrmecial warts are characterized by marked acanthosis and abundant eosinophilic keratohyaline granules that coalesce and form large homogeneous intracytoplasmic inclusion bodies reminiscent of molluscum bodies (Fig. 3.7). The nucleus, which is not displaced by the inclusions, persists in the cornified layer, where it appears deeply basophilic and surrounded by a clear halo.

EDV lesions show similar but more pronounced epidermal changes than planar warts. A distinct cytopathic effect is seen: large keratinocytes present mostly in the upper epidermis with pale blue-gray cytoplasm and perinuclear clear halo (Fig. 3.8). In focal epithelial hyperplasia, there are acanthosis, blunt and thick elongated rete ridges, pale upper epidermal cells, and occasional binucleated keratinocytes.

Ancillary Studies

Immunohistochemical stains with polyclonal antibodies directed against the viral capsid can be used to detect HPV in paraffin-embedded tissue (Fig. 3.9), but this

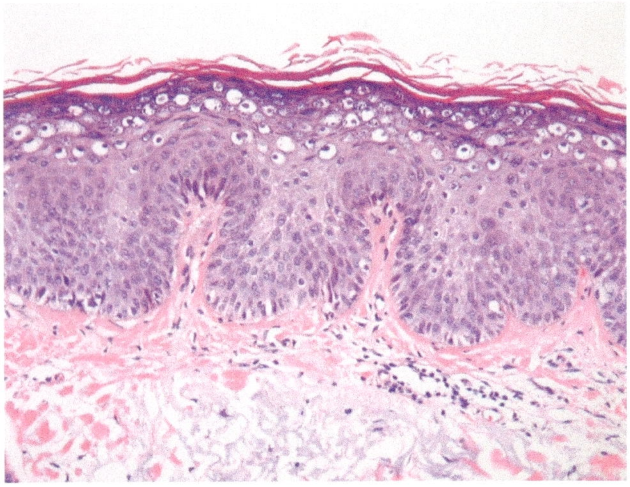

FIG. 3.6

Verruca plana. Multiple "bird's eye" nuclei are present in the granular cell layer.

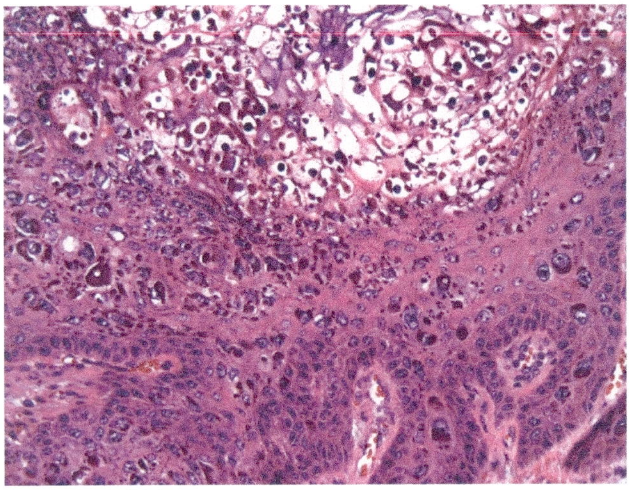

FIG. 3.7

Myrmecia wart. Multiple eosinophilic keratohyaline granules are characteristic.

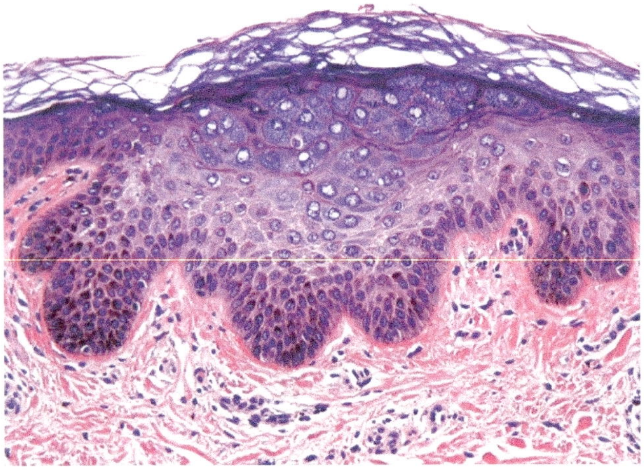

FIG. 3.8

Epidermodysplasia verruciformis. Note the enlarged keratinocytes with abundant slate gray bluish cytoplasm.

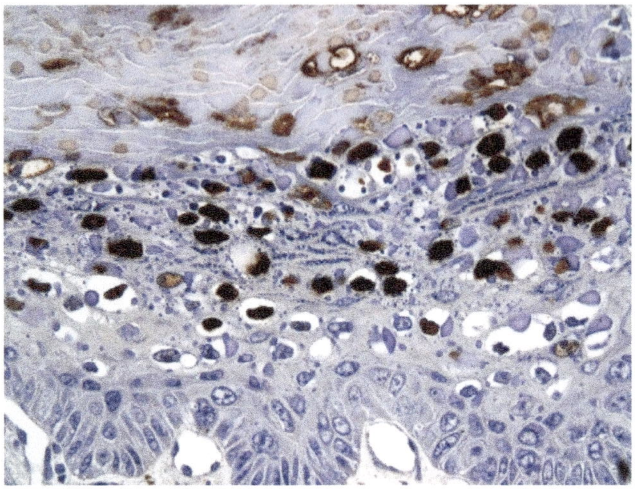

FIG. 3.9

Immunohistochemistry for human papilloma virus. Staining of keratinocytic nuclei indicates a positive result (immunoperoxidase reaction).

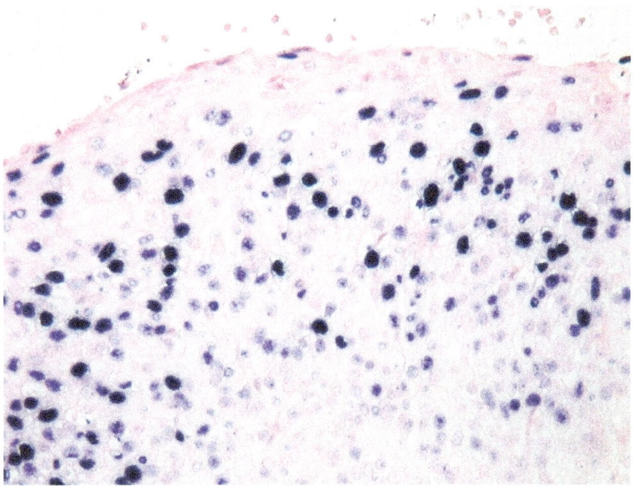

FIG. 3.10

In situ hybridization for human papilloma virus. Grainy deposits are found over infected keratinocytic nuclei.

method is not very sensitive. In situ hybridization (Fig. 3.10) and polymerase chain reaction (PCR) studies are more sensitive and specific assays, which may be helpful if, in a particular case, the relationship of the lesion to HPV is uncertain or if subtyping of HPV into high- or low-risk viruses is clinically desired.

Differential Diagnosis

The most important distinction is from squamous cell carcinoma, which may arise in association with a wart or simulate the growth pattern of a wart. Mild atypia of keratinocytes is common in warts, but they lack the full-thickness atypia and loss of polarity associated with in situ squamous cell carcinoma.

Because diagnostic viral pathologic changes may not always be detectable in warts, they may be confused with other benign papillomatous squamous proliferations, such as verrucoid or digitated variants of seborrheic or actinic keratosis.

The presence of a wart may be falsely assumed by incidental, often tissue-processing-related changes of keratinocytes associated with "halo" phenomena around nuclei.

Prognosis and Treatment

Warts may resolve spontaneously but often persist and require treatment, which includes topical application of salicylic acid, cryotherapy, and surgery. In immunocompromised patients, the lesions may be widespread and resistant to treatment, and there is an increased risk of the development of squamous cell carcinoma.

CONDYLOMA ACUMINATUM

Condylomas are associated mostly with HPV-6 and -11 but also with other types, some of which have oncogenic potential, such as HPV-16, -18, -31, -33, -51, and others. They are sexually transmitted and can be extensive in immunosuppressed patients.

Clinical Findings

Condyloma acuminatum is characterized by small, soft, pink to brown, round-topped papules (Fig. 3.11) distributed in the anogenital region, which sometimes coalesce into a large cauliflower-like mass (Fig. 3.12).

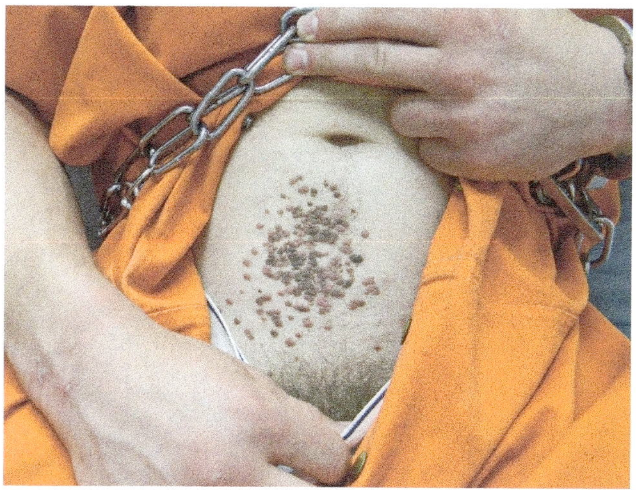

FIG. 3.11

Condyloma acuminatum. Multiple small, soft, hyperpigmented, round-topped papules.

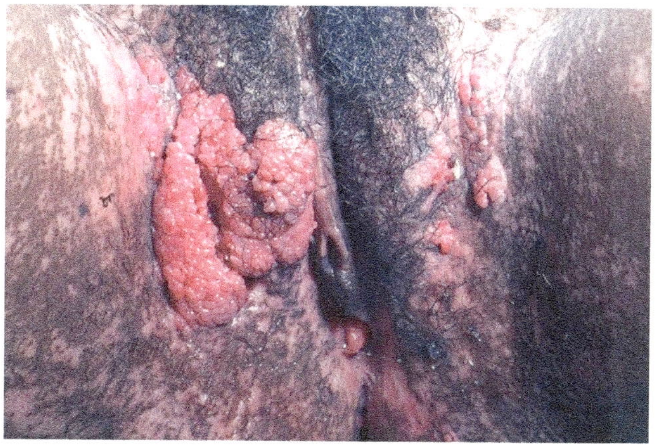

FIG. 3.12

Condyloma acuminatum. Flesh-colored exophytic lesions are present in the genital region.

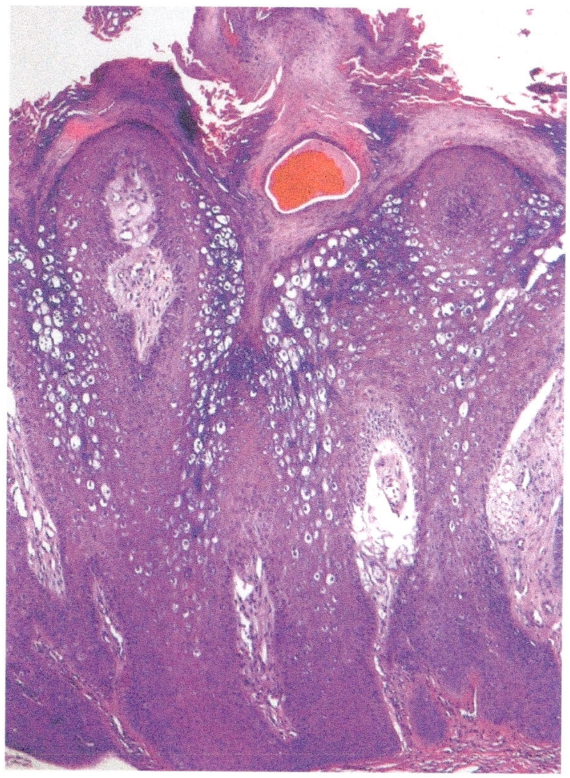

FIG. 3.13

Condyloma acuminatum. There is papillomatous mamillated epithelial hyperplasia with hyperkeratosis and koilocytic changes (hyperchromatic nuclei surrounded by a clear halo).

Histologic Features

The epidermis is acanthotic, with expansion of the stratum spinulosum, and shows mammillated papillomatosis (Fig. 3.13), mild hyperkeratosis or parakeratosis, and vacuolated keratinocytes with round hyperchromatic nuclei in the upper stratum spinosum. Koilocytes with "raisin-like" hyperchromatic nuclei and an irregular perinuclear halo, or binucleated cells, may be seen, especially within the papillomatous pits.

Ancillary Studies

Molecular studies (in situ hybridization or PCR studies) may be used to identify the subtype of the virus. Immunostains for Ki-67 (labeling limited to the basilar or lower part of the stratified squamous epithelium) and p16 (overexpression in high-risk HPV lesions) can help in the distinction of condylomas from high-grade squamous intraepithelial lesions or squamous cell carcinoma in situ.

Differential Diagnosis

Squamous cell carcinoma may arise in association with or simulate the pattern of a condyloma (papillary or digitated squamous cell carcinoma). Carcinoma is primarily distinguished from condyloma by the lack of maturation and presence of full-thickness keratinocytic atypia.

Prognosis and Treatment

In up to 30% of patients, the lesions regress spontaneously, but subclinical infection can persist for life. The recurrence rate is high and depends on the virus type. HPV types 16 and 18 (and others) are associated with the development of intraepithelial neoplasia (dysplasia) and invasive squamous carcinoma of the cervix, vulva, perineum, and penis. Treatment is aimed at removal of the lesions and includes surgery, cryotherapy, laser ablation, and topical reagents. More recently, a vaccine has become available for protection against infection by high-risk HPV types.

BOWENOID PAPULOSIS

Bowenoid papulosis has been associated with HPV-16 and in a smaller percentage of cases with HPV-18, -35, -39, or other types.

Clinical Findings

Bowenoid papulosis is characterized by the presence of multiple red-brown, small verrucous papules on the genitalia (Fig. 3.14). It has a predilection for young adults and can regress spontaneously.

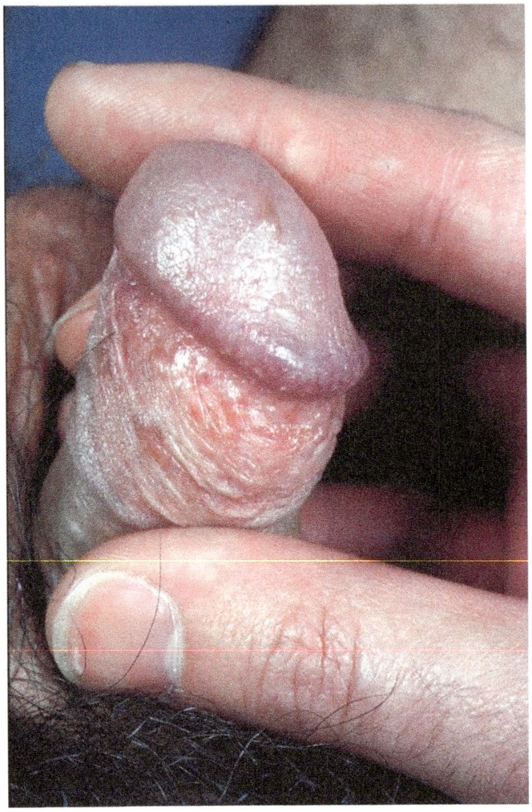

FIG. 3.14
Bowenoid papulosis. Multiple small, red-brown papules are seen.

Histologic Features

Histologic findings include epidermal thickening and abnormal maturation (Fig. 3.15) with a "wind-blown" appearance. Atypia is present, involving the full thickness of the epithelium. Mitotic figures in suprabasilar keratinocytes are commonly seen. Hyperchromatic, dyskeratotic, or multinucleated cells may be seen.

Differential Diagnosis

Clinical features (multiplicity, small size of the lesions, young age) help in differentiating bowenoid papulosis from conventional Bowen's disease. However, this can be difficult at times.

Prognosis and Treatment

Treatment is directed toward eradication of intraepithelial disease and includes cryotherapy, laser treatment, or topical treatment (e.g., imiquimod).

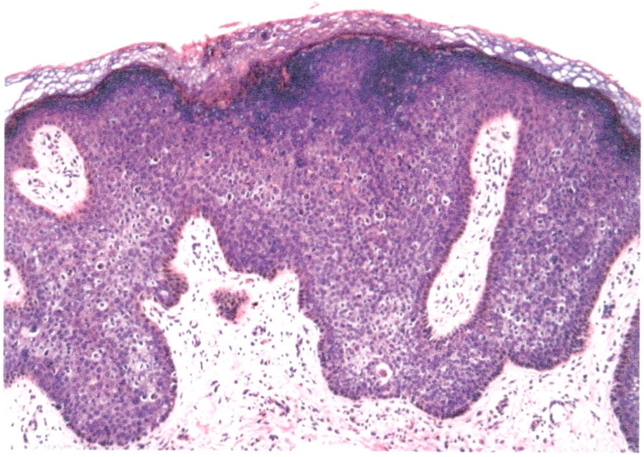

FIG. 3.15

Bowenoid papulosis. There is acanthosis and full-thickness epithelial atypia with loss of polarity in keratinocytes. Mitoses are frequent.

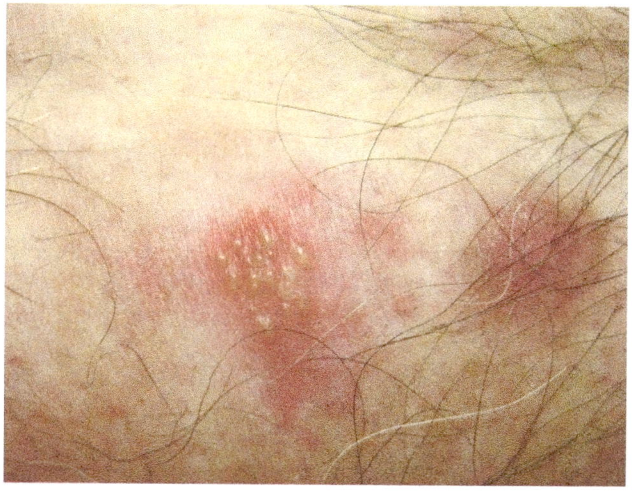

FIG. 3.17

Herpes simplex. Multiple grouped vesicles and pustules on an erythematous base.

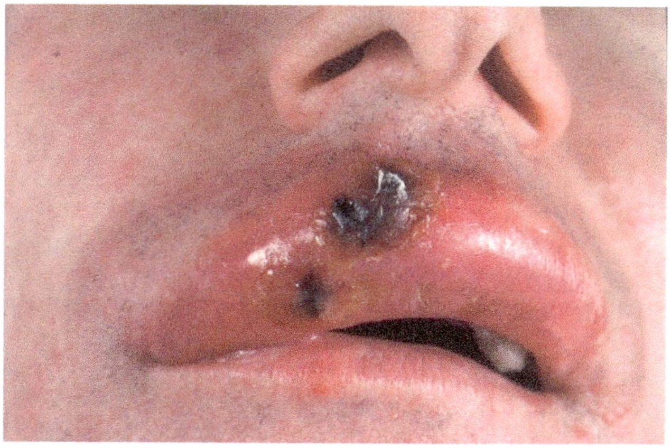

FIG. 3.16

Herpes simplex. Crusted labial vesicles.

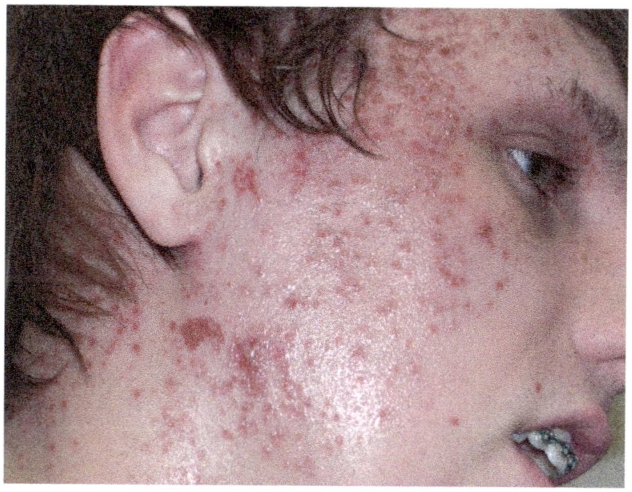

FIG. 3.18

Herpes simplex. Eczema herpeticum with multiple punched out, often grouped, ulcers in atopic patients.

HERPESVIRUS FAMILY

The family of *Herpesviridae* includes three major subgroups. The a-subgroup includes herpes simplex virus (HSV) and varicella-zoster virus (VZV). Both are neurotropic. Cytomegalovirus (CMV) and herpesviruses 6 and 7 belong to the b-subgroup. The g-subgroup includes the lymphotropic viruses Epstein-Barr virus (EBV) and human herpesvirus (HHV) type 8.

HERPES SIMPLEX

HSV types 1 and 2 are similar to *Herpesviridae*, which contain double-stranded linear DNA, produce primary and recurrent infections, and are transmitted by direct skin-to-skin or mucous membrane contact. Infection with HSV-1 is usually subclinical and occurs in childhood. Recurrences are very common, most frequently around the lips ("cold sores") (Fig. 3.16). Infection with type 2 (HSV-2) is the result of sexual transmission during symptomatic or asymptomatic viral shedding, occurs within 2 weeks of exposure, and has increased in incidence in past decades.

Clinical Findings

Lesions of HSV consist of clusters of small vesicles filled with clear fluid on an erythematous base (Fig. 3.17), which may become pustules before crusting, and if present on mucosal surfaces, erode quickly. They heal without scarring. There are several distinct clinical variants: herpetic whitlow (painful vesicles usually on the distal fingers of medical personnel after direct contact with affected patients), eczema herpeticum (generalized infection in atopic patients) (Fig. 3.18), and herpes gladiatorum (in wrestlers).

HERPES SIMPLEX VIRUS—DISEASE FACT SHEET

Primary and recurrent infection caused by human herpes simplex virus (HSV) type 1 (orolabial) and type 2 (genital)

Worldwide Incidence

- HSV-1 antibodies in serum of 90% of individuals by the age of 20 to 40 years
- HSV-2 seroprevalence in the United States increased in the last two decades by more than 30%

Patient Group

- HSV-1 primary infection occurs in childhood and persists through adult life
- HSV-2 primary infection occurs after initiation of sexual activity

Site of Involvement

- HSV-1—typically face (lips, perioral, perinasal)
- HSV-2—genital region

Clinical Findings

- HSV-1
  - Clusters of vesicles on an erythematous base that ulcerate and become covered by crust
- HSV-2
  - Erosive vulvitis and vaginitis in women
  - Erosive papules on glans penis and shaft in males
- Recurrent eruptions are often related to triggers such as stress, trauma, fever, or immunosuppression

Prognosis

- Lifelong infection with variable frequency of recurrences
- Neonatal herpes has significant morbidity and mortality

Treatment

- Oral and topical antiviral therapy instituted early results in decreased duration of lesions, viral shedding, and pain

Histologic Features

Intraepidermal and subepidermal vesicles form because of ballooning, acantholysis, necrosis, and spongiosis (Fig. 3.19A). The keratinocytic nuclei show peripheral condensation of chromatin (margination) with a central gray ground-glass appearance or eosinophilic inclusion bodies surrounded by a clear halo (Fig. 3.19B). Multinucleate cells (Tzanck cells) with "molding" nuclei are present. The dermis shows marked perivascular, periadnexal, and perineural lymphocytic inflammatory infiltrate. Adnexal structures may be primarily involved (herpetic folliculitis or syringitis). Sometimes there is localized necrotizing small vessel vasculitis. In late stages, the vesicles rupture and form ulcers covered by crust.

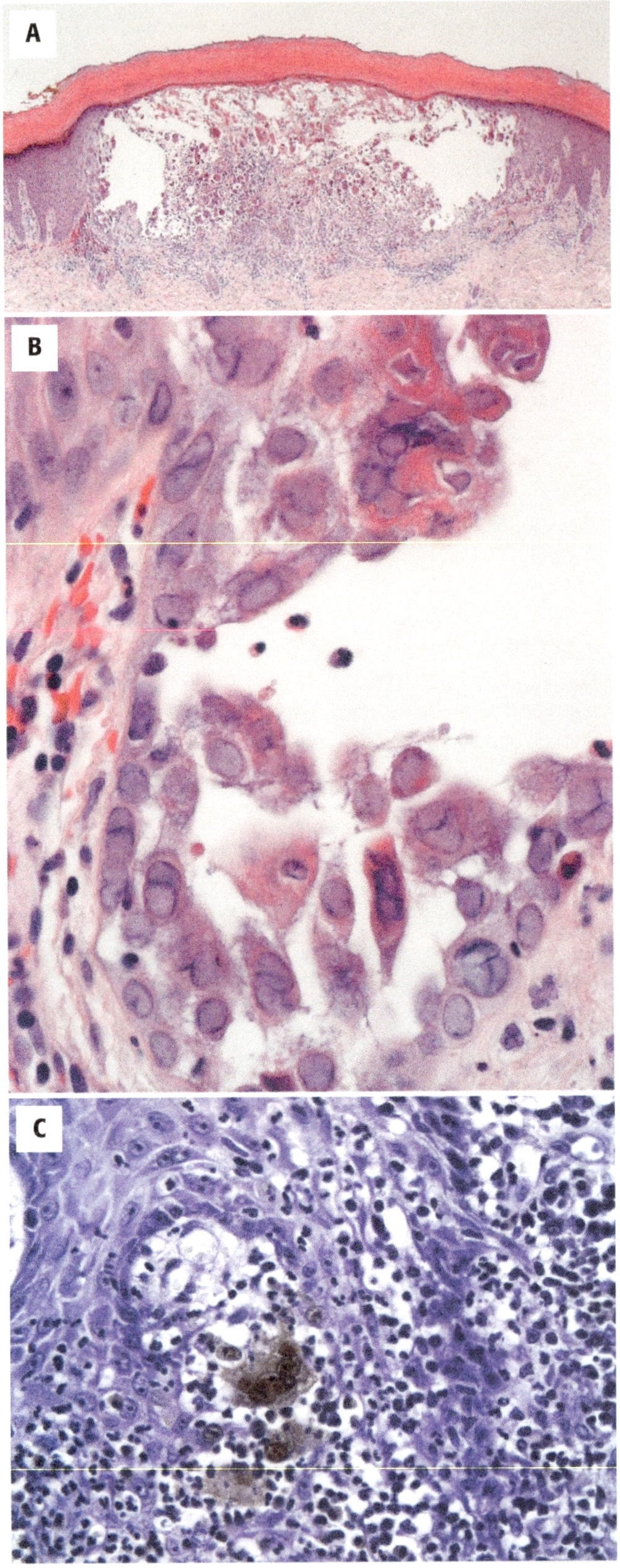

FIG. 3.19

Herpes simplex. **A,** There is an intraepidermal acantholytic vesicular dermatitis. **B,** Viral cytopathic changes are present characterized by multinucleated keratinocytes and pale nuclei with peripheral condensation of chromatin. **C,** Multinucleated cells are common.

Ancillary Studies

Rapid diagnosis can be made by staining a smear from the base of a freshly unroofed vesicle with Giemsa stain and

HERPES SIMPLEX VIRUS—PATHOLOGIC FEATURES

Histologic Features

- Keratinocytes with slate-gray, ground-glass nuclei
- Multinucleated giant cells (Tzanck cells)
- Intraepidermal and subepidermal vesiculation
- Ulcers
- Dermal lymphocytic inflammatory infiltrate

Ancillary Studies

- Immunohistochemistry or immunofluorescence studies for virus detection and subtyping (HSV-1, -2, distinction from varicella-zoster virus)
- Tzanck smear

Differential Diagnosis

- Varicella zoster infection (distinction clinically and by immunostains)
- Nonviral acantholytic disorders (e.g., pemphigus)

identifying multinucleated giant cells with typical intranuclear inclusions (Tzanck smear). Monoclonal antibodies against HSV-1 and HSV-2 may be used on smears and paraffin sections for rapid detection and differentiation.

Differential Diagnosis

Herpetic dermatitis caused by HSV-1 or -2 can be histologically indistinguishable from VZV. Immunostains should allow a definitive distinction (Fig. 3.19C). On occasion, herpetic dermatitis may be associated with a dense lymphoid infiltrate simulating lymphoma (pseudolymphoma).

Prognosis and Treatment

Primary infection is followed by lifelong latent infection. Reactivation can be triggered by factors such as stress, trauma, surgery, fever, immunosuppression, or pregnancy. If HSV infection is transmitted at birth from a mother to her infant, the fatality rate is high. In immunocompromised patients, the disease is more severe and extensive and may become disseminated. Herpes labialis may be treated with topical acyclovir. First-episode genital lesions are treated with oral antiviral agents (acyclovir, famciclovir, or valacyclovir). If recurrent episodes are treated with oral antiviral agents within the first 2 days after onset, they may have a shorter duration and reduced severity. Immunocompromised patients require continuous, daily therapy.

VARICELLA AND HERPES ZOSTER

VZV is also a member of the *Herpesviridae* family. It has a double-stranded linear DNA genome and an icosahedral capsid. Primary infection results in varicella (chickenpox), a highly contagious childhood disease. Reactivation of latent infection results in herpes zoster (shingles), with incidence increasing with advancing age. Transmission is through inhalation of airborne droplets and direct contact. The incubation period is approximately 2 weeks.

Clinical Findings

The rash appears on the head and spreads to the trunk. Lesions develop in successive crops and are found at clinical examination in different stages of development: papules, vesicles on an erythematous base resembling "dew drops on rose petals," pustules, crusts, and pink depressions left after crusts fall (Fig. 3.20). Scarring occurs if there is bacterial superinfection. After primary infection, VZV establishes latency in the dorsal root ganglia. Reactivation results in herpes zoster (Fig. 3.21). This illness affects adults and begins with a prodrome of pain in the area, most frequently the lumbar and thoracic regions (Fig. 3.22), innervated by the sensory ganglia harboring the virus. The rash is unilateral, does not cross the midline, and typically has a dermatomal distribution. It consists of closely grouped vesicles on an erythematous base.

Histologic Features

Varicella and herpes zoster share similar histopathological changes and cannot reliably be distinguished from each other without special studies. VZV is more likely to present with prominent follicular (Fig. 3.23) involvement (herpetic folliculitis) than HSV-1 or -2. Similar to HSV,

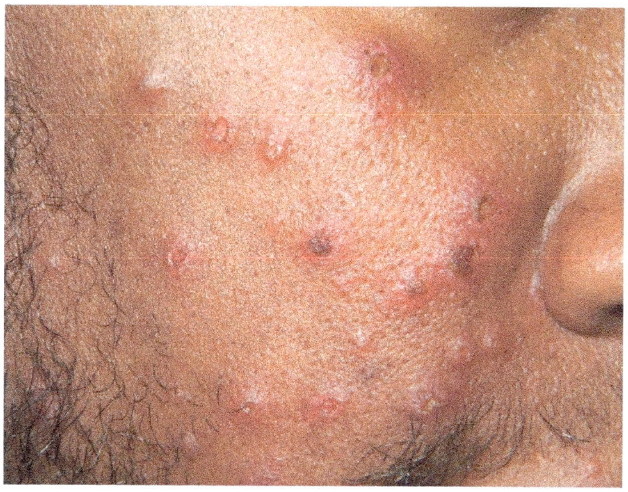

FIG. 3.20

Varicella. Inflammatory papules and vesicles on an erythematous base resembling "dew drops on rose petals." Crusted papules and pink depressions with resolution of individual lesions.

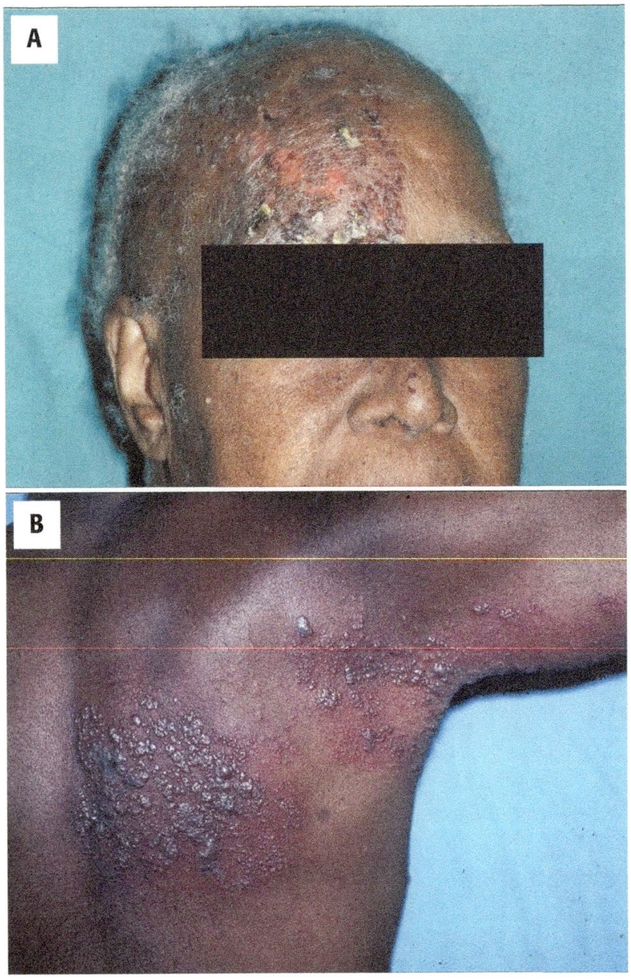

FIG. 3.21
Herpes zoster (shingles). **A,** Crusted lesions in the region of the ophthalmic nerve. **B,** Unilateral grouped vesicles.

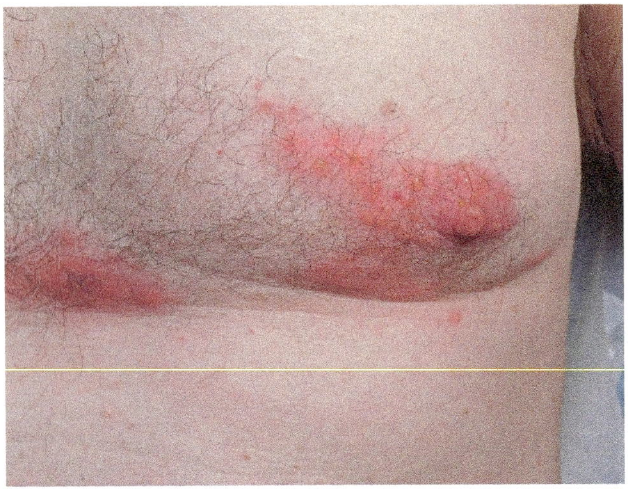

FIG. 3.22
Herpes zoster (shingles). Grouped vesicles on an erythematous base in a unilateral thoracic dermatomal distribution.

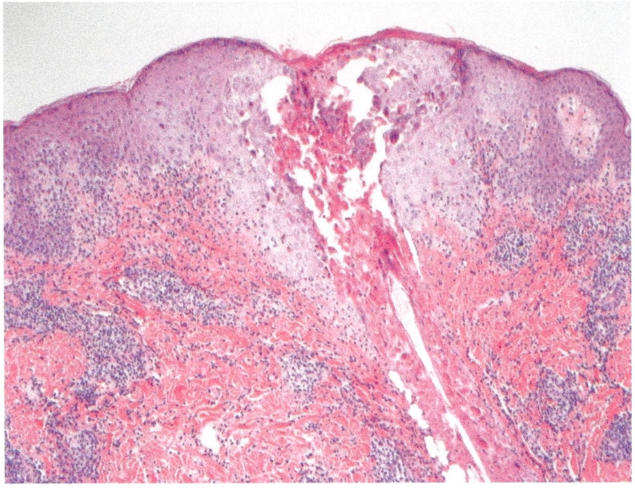

FIG. 3.23
Herpes zoster (shingles). Herpetic folliculitis with folliculocentric viral cytopathic change consisting of balloon cell degeneration of the outer root sheath with multinucleated keratinocytes and acantholysis.

VZV may induce a secondary localized necrotizing vasculitis at the site of the clinical lesion. Recent reports have described a granulomatous pattern in the biopsies of patients with herpes zoster in the setting of concurrent chronic lymphocytic B-cell lymphoma or drug-induced hypersensitivity syndrome.

Ancillary Studies

Tzanck smear helps to identify the presence of multinucleated giant cells and intranuclear inclusions, but it does not differentiate VZV from other herpesviruses. Direct immunofluorescence and immunoperoxidase methods allow rapid, sensitive, and specific diagnosis.

Differential Diagnosis

The distinction from herpes simplex infection can often readily be accomplished clinically. Immunostains for HSV versus VZV can confirm the diagnosis. On occasion, a nonviral vesicular dermatitis, such as from a drug reaction or pemphigus, may show acantholysis and multinucleation of keratinocytes that may simulate a herpesvirus infection. Similar to HSV, VZV infection of the skin may result in a deep, pseudolymphomatous inflammatory reaction.

Prognosis and Treatment

Live attenuated vaccine from the Oka strain is now administered for protection against varicella. Antiviral agents such as acyclovir, famciclovir, and valacyclovir can be used in high-risk patients to decrease morbidity and mortality. They are most effective if therapy is initiated in the first 24 to 48 hours after the onset of the rash. The most common complication is bacterial superinfection. Serious complications in immunocompetent children infected with varicella are rare but may include Reye's syndrome and varicella pneumonia. In adults, varicella is more severe, and primary varicella pneumonia is more frequent. Complications of herpes zoster include postherpetic neuralgia and ocular damage. The incidence and severity of herpes zoster are greater in immunocompromised hosts, who may develop disseminated skin lesions and fatal systemic disease.

CYTOMEGALOVIRUS

Infection with CMV is common and usually asymptomatic.

Clinical Findings

A small percentage of newborns who acquire CMV infection in utero develop mobile blue-gray cutaneous nodules ("blueberry muffin" baby). In healthy adults, CMV produces a morbilliform eruption, especially with prior administration of ampicillin. Ulcers and petechial macules and papules may develop in immunocompromised patients. Vasculitis may be a complication of CMV.

Histologic Features

The characteristic findings are enlarged, irregularly shaped endothelial and interstitial cells that contain large intracytoplasmic and nuclear viral inclusions (Fig. 3.24). The intranuclear inclusions are large, single, eosinophilic, round to oval, and surrounded by a clear halo. The intracytoplasmic viral inclusions tend to be multiple, granular, irregular, and basophilic. The blue-gray nodules of congenital CMV infection correspond histologically to foci of dermal extramedullary hematopoiesis.

Ancillary Studies

The CMV virus can be rapidly identified in paraffin-embedded tissue sections using monoclonal antibodies (Fig. 3.24C). PCR or in situ hybridization methods can also be helpful in more difficult cases.

Prognosis and Treatment

It is important to promptly identify skin infection with CMV, especially in immunocompromised patients in whom early treatment with antiviral agents such as ganciclovir may prevent a potentially fatal systemic spread.

INFECTIONS BY OTHER MEMBERS OF THE HERPESVIRUS FAMILY

New HHV types have been identified since 1980. HHV6 is a widespread T-lymphotropic virus that causes primary infection in early childhood. It has been identified as the cause of roseola infantum, an exanthem similar to measles or rubella (exanthem subitum), the most common cause of fever-induced seizures in children. It is believed to possibly play a role in pityriasis rosea in adults. The diagnosis of roseola infantum is clinical. HHV7 is also a T-lymphotropic virus possibly associated with roseola and pityriasis rosea. HHV8 is related to EBV and causes primary effusion lymphoma and Kaposi sarcoma. HHV8 infects CD19-positive B cells and endothelial-derived spindle cells in Kaposi sarcoma.

POX VIRUS FAMILY

Pox viruses contain DNA surrounded by a capsid. Infections by members of the poxvirus family include molluscum contagiosum, milker's nodule and orf, variola (smallpox), vaccinia, cowpox, and monkeypox.

MOLLUSCUM CONTAGIOSUM

Molluscum contagiosum is a poxvirus distributed worldwide that tends to infect the pediatric population and is transmitted by direct skin-to-skin contact. It causes the most common poxvirus infection seen after smallpox eradication. There are four genomic subtypes described, of which type 1 affects predominantly children. Types 2 and 3 are prevalent in HIV-positive patients.

Clinical Findings

The lesions consist of dome-shaped, discrete, skin-colored papules with central umbilication (Fig. 3.25) that can be solitary or multiple and often involute spontaneously. Sexually transmitted lesions in adults are usually seen on the lower abdomen and genitalia. In immunocompromised patients, the lesions tend to be larger, widely disseminated, and more persistent.

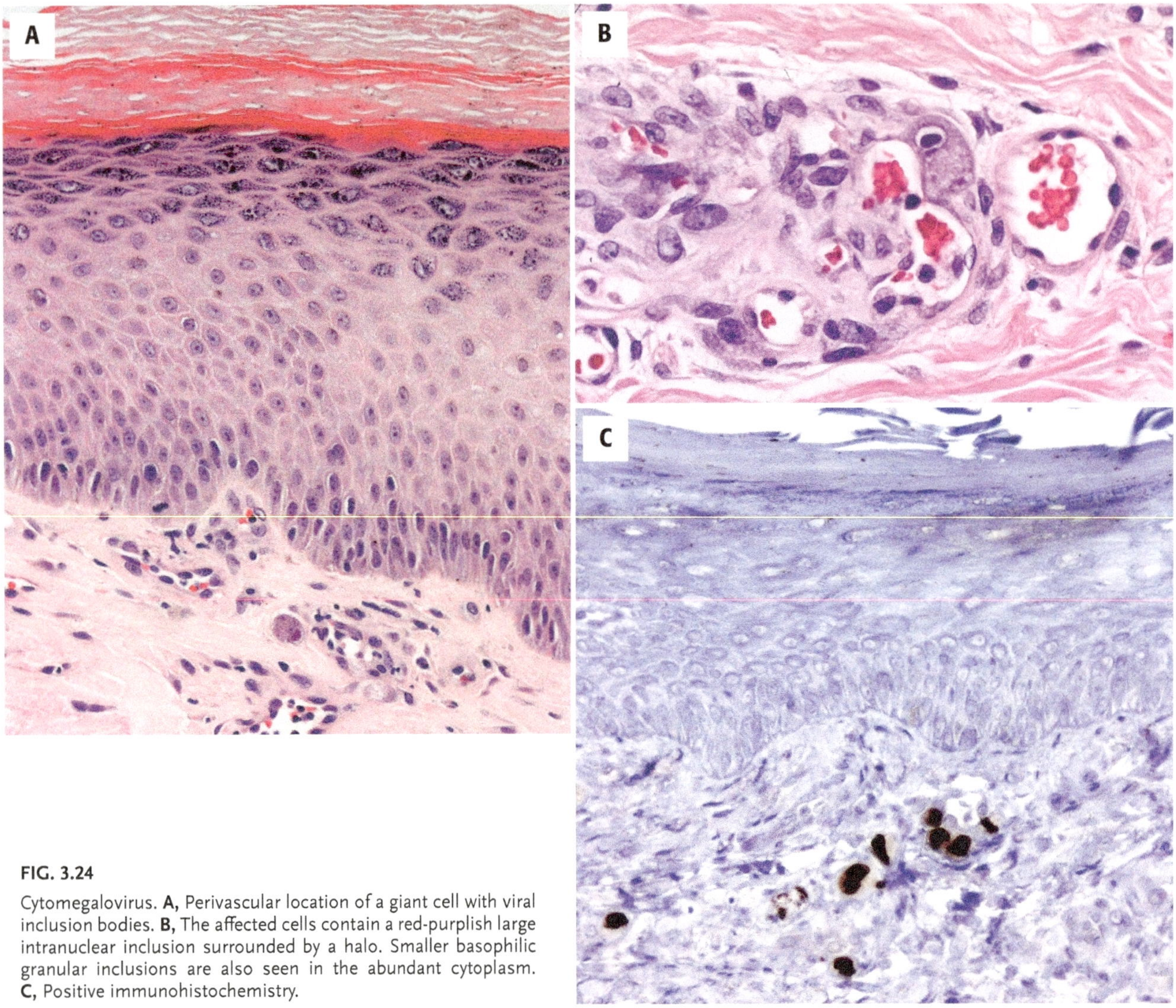

FIG. 3.24

Cytomegalovirus. **A,** Perivascular location of a giant cell with viral inclusion bodies. **B,** The affected cells contain a red-purplish large intranuclear inclusion surrounded by a halo. Smaller basophilic granular inclusions are also seen in the abundant cytoplasm. **C,** Positive immunohistochemistry.

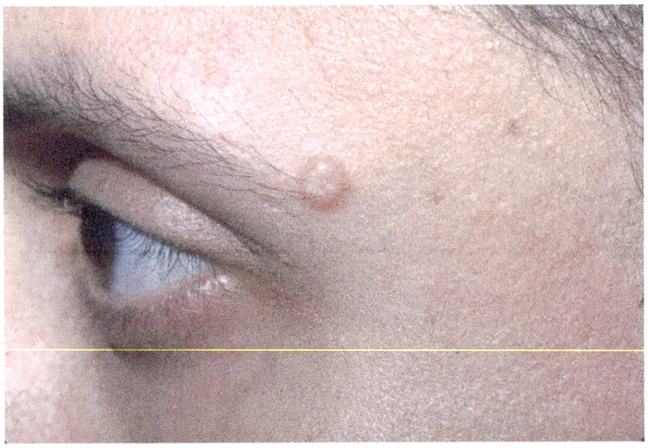

FIG. 3.25

Molluscum contagiosum. Papules with central umbilication are typical.

MOLLUSCUM CONTAGIOSUM—DISEASE FACT SHEET

Benign, self-limited infection caused by molluscum contagiosum virus of the *Molluscipox* genus of the Poxviridae viruses with worldwide distribution.

Patient Group

- Highest incidence in children
- Increased frequency in immunocompromised individuals
- May be sexually transmitted in adults

Site of Involvement

- Face and trunk

Clinical Findings

- Firm, centrally umbilicated, pearly papules

Prognosis and Treatment

- Resolves spontaneously in immunocompetent individuals
- Long-lasting, disfiguring lesions in patients with advanced immunosuppression with immune dysregulation (HIV)
- Therapeutic modalities include cantharidin application, cryotherapy, or surgical excision

MOLLUSCUM CONTAGIOSUM—PATHOLOGIC FEATURES

Histologic Features

- Inverted, cup-shaped lobules of acanthotic squamous epithelium
- Eosinophilic inclusion bodies (Henderson-Patterson bodies)
- Central crater-like ostium

Differential Diagnosis

- Henderson-Patterson bodies are pathognomonic
- Primary inflammatory dermatoses or atypical lymphoid proliferations if the molluscum lesions are traumatized, inflamed, and Henderson-Patterson bodies are difficult to visualize

Histologic Features

Molluscum contagiosum shows characteristic endophytic, cup-shaped lobules of acanthotic squamous epithelium (Fig. 3.26). Eosinophilic intracytoplasmic inclusions (Henderson-Patterson bodies) accumulate and progressively enlarge until they replace the entire cell (Fig. 3.26). They are ultimately extruded at the surface through the central craterlike ostium. Many lesions are not inflamed, but some show a florid, dense lymphocytic infiltrate.

Differential Diagnosis

The presence of molluscum bodies is pathognomonic.

Prognosis and Treatment

In immunocompetent patients, spontaneous involution occurs within 6 to 12 months, and recurrence is rare. Lesions that fail to involute can be treated with a variety of destructive methods, including liquid nitrogen, cantharidin, cryotherapy, laser, electrodesiccation, trichloroacetic acid, curettage, or by topical application of immune modulators (imiquimod). Patients with acquired immunodeficiency syndrome (AIDS) develop extensive molluscum lesions that are recalcitrant to treatment; topical cidofovir has been successfully used in these patients.

MILKER'S NODULE AND ORF

Milker's nodule and orf are poxvirus infections caused by parapoxviruses. Infection can be accidentally transmitted to humans by direct contact with infected animals (milker's nodule in cattle; orf in sheep and goats) through minor breaks in the skin.

Clinical Findings

Infection usually manifests as a solitary papule on a finger (Fig. 3.27). An individual lesion classically evolves through six stages, each about a week long: papular, targetoid, weeping, regenerative, papillomatous, and regressive.

Histologic Features

In the early stage, there are spongiosis, vacuolization, and ballooning of the cells in the upper third of the epidermis, which can result in multilocular vesicle

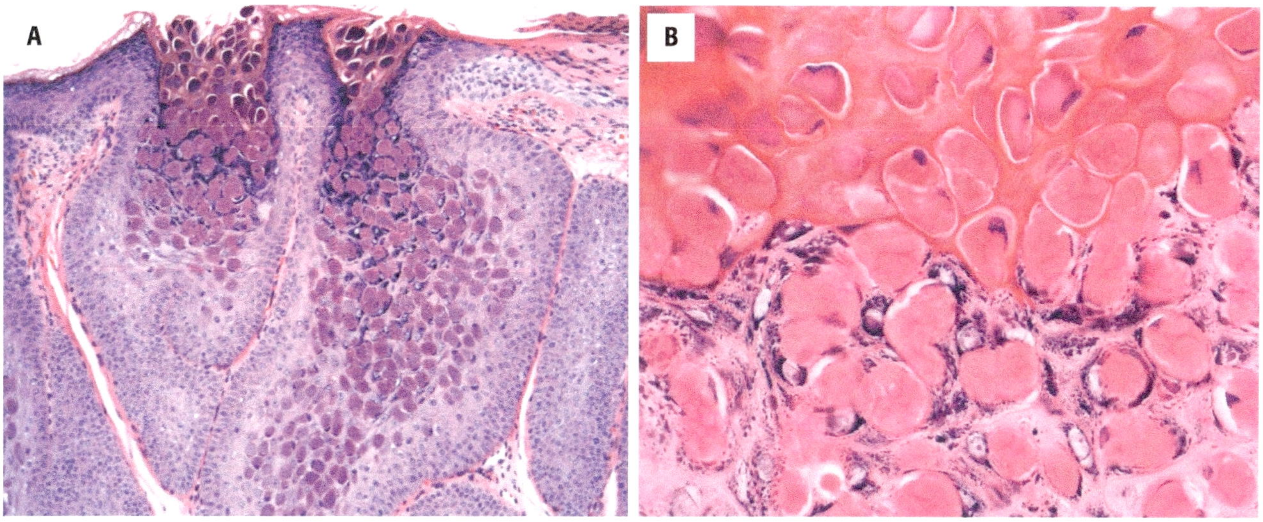

FIG. 3.26

Molluscum contagiosum. **A,** Cup-shaped, endophytic epithelial lobules. **B,** Characteristic intracytoplasmic eosinophilic inclusions (Henderson-Patterson bodies) are present.

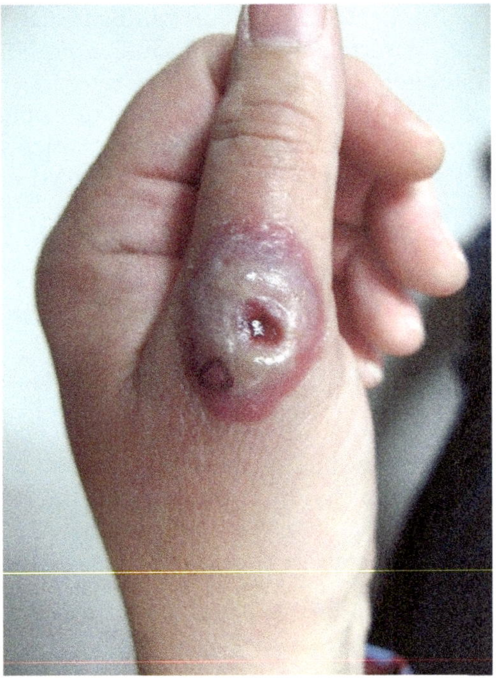

FIG. 3.27
Orf. Solitary edematous inflammatory nodule on a finger.

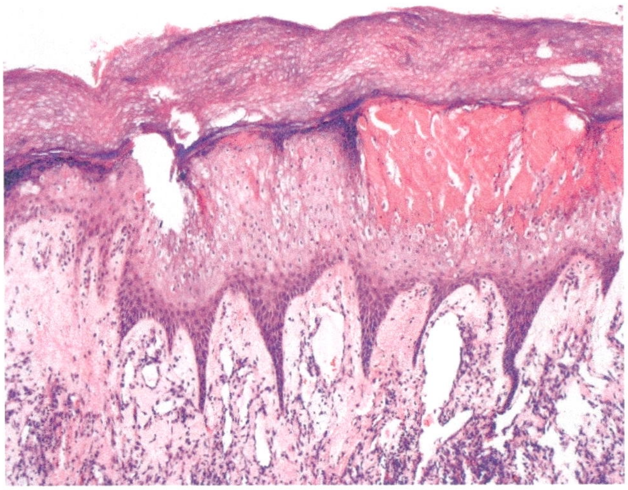

FIG. 3.28
Orf. Crusted spongiotic epidermis with characteristic elongated "dagger-like" rete ridges.

formation (Fig. 3.28). In addition, the epidermis often demonstrates characteristic "dagger-like" elongated rete ridges (Fig. 3.28). Intracytoplasmic eosinophilic inclusions (Fig. 3.29) (Guarnieri bodies) may be seen. In the acute weeping stage, there is focal epidermal necrosis with neutrophils in the epidermis and papillary dermis followed by ulceration and scale crust formation. The black dots seen clinically in the regenerative stage consist of extruded, degenerated hair follicle cells. Mature lesions show acanthosis with thin, elongated rete ridges; prominent edema of papillary dermis with an inflammatory infiltrate composed of lymphocytes, histiocytes,

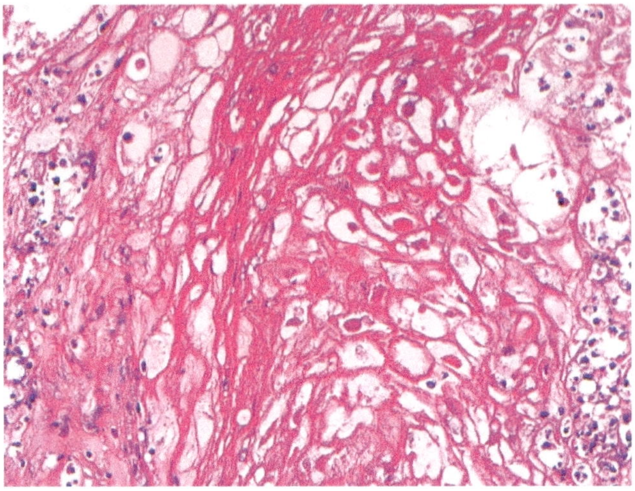

FIG. 3.29
Orf. Small, round eosinophilic intracytoplasmic inclusions are characteristic.

plasma cells, and occasional eosinophils; and numerous dilated small blood vessels. In the regressive stage, acanthosis and inflammation progressively diminish.

Ancillary Studies

Electron microscopy can reveal the oval viral particles in the crust of an early lesion.

Differential Diagnosis

The clinical differential diagnosis is broad and includes anthrax, fungal infections, atypical mycobacterial infections, and spider bites. The history of contact with an infected animal plays a crucial role.

Prognosis and Treatment

The disease is usually self-limited. Most lesions resolve spontaneously. Bacterial superinfection is a potential complication. Some have suggested cryotherapy or shave removal of a lesion.

SMALLPOX, COWPOX, AND MPOX

Smallpox, cowpox, and mpox (aka monkeypox) viruses are members of the *Orthopox* virus genus. Although smallpox, the most aggressive and notorious orthopoxvirus, has been completely eradicated, it is still of concern as a potential weapon of bioterrorism. Transmission is by aerosols, and patients are infectious from the time the rash appears until all lesions are completely healed. Vaccination against smallpox is accomplished by inoculation with vaccinia virus, which results in localized, attenuated disease limited by the host response. Complications of vaccination include bacterial superinfection, autoinoculation, generalized vaccinia, progressive vaccinia, and encephalitis.

Cowpox was first described by Edward Jenner in 1798; it is rarely seen today and consists of lesions similar to smallpox but less extensive. Monkeypox lesions are also similar to smallpox but are much less severe and are self-limited. In 2003, an outbreak of monkeypox occurred in the Midwestern United States because of direct contact of individuals with infected prairie dogs sold as pets.

Recent outbreaks of mpox were predominantly related to contact with mpox lesions on the skin or mucosal surfaces during sexual activity. Transmission may also result from close nonsexual contact or direct injury, such as piercing. Affected individuals may develop fever, lymphadenopathy, and a skin rash. The rash often involves the perioral or anogenital region and is characterized by a vesiculopapular eruption.

Clinical Findings

Firm papules rapidly transform into characteristic clouded, pustule-like vesicles with central umbilication. A crust then forms and, after it falls off, leaves a scar.

Histologic Features

In the early stages, the epidermis shows marked spongiosis, reticular degeneration and ballooning of keratinocytes, and eosinophilic intracytoplasmic inclusions (Guarnieri bodies). Vesicle formation and focal epidermal necrosis with neutrophils may occur, followed by ulceration, scale crust formation, and re-epithelialization. In the dermis, there is a dense inflammatory infiltrate with neutrophils, occasional eosinophils, and marked edema. Cowpox lesions show larger intracytoplasmic inclusions, less necrosis, and more hemorrhage.

Biopsies of mpox lesions are typically associated with a lichenoid dermatitis and/or folliculitis. Lesions may be ulcerated and densely inflamed. If the surface is ulcerated, characteristic features are best seen in the follicles (Fig. 3.30). Epidermal or follicular epithelial cells may show ballooning degeneration with swollen cytoplasm and/or epithelial apoptosis and necrosis. Nuclei may be enlarged and hyperchromatic. Multinucleation may be seen. Some epithelial cells may have a syncytial appearance. Immunohistochemically, viral antigen can be detected in epithelial cells.

Differential Diagnosis

If the diagnosis of smallpox is suspected, the patient should be immediately isolated and the Centers for Disease Control and Prevention (CDC) in Atlanta notified.

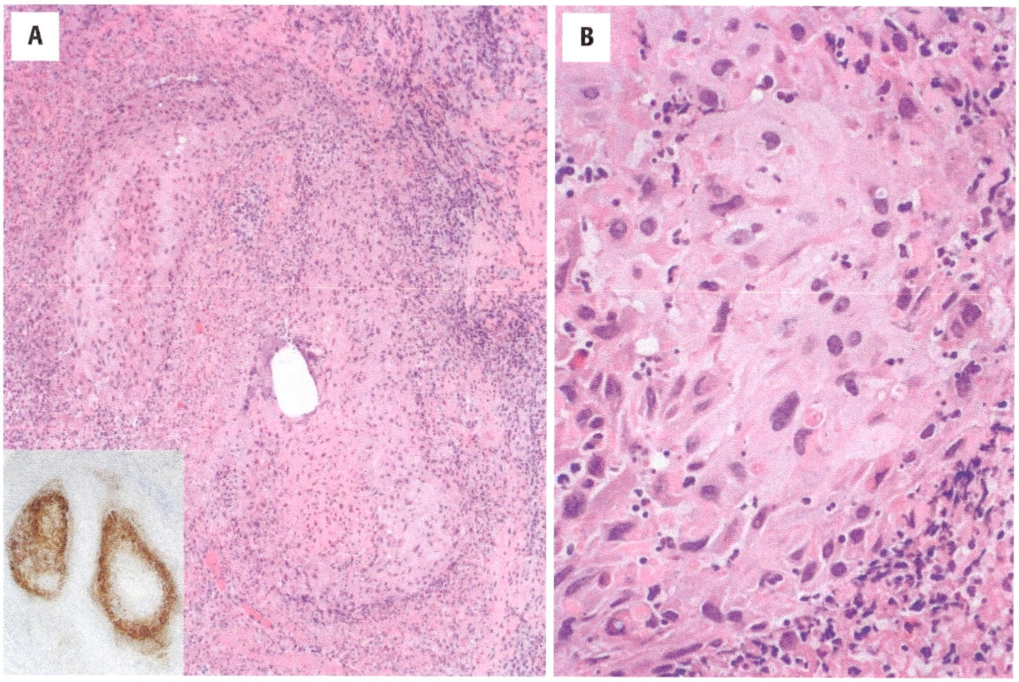

FIG. 3.30

Monkeypox. **A**, Inflamed follicles with epithelial cells being immunoreactive for the Poxvirus. **B**, The cytoplasm of epithelial cells is swollen, some of the nuclei are hyperchromatic, a few multinucleated cells are present. There is associated inflammation and apoptosis.

(The procedure is detailed at www.bt.cdc.gov/agent/smallpox/index.asp.) The differential diagnosis for cowpox and mpox include parapoxvirus infection, herpesvirus infection, and anthrax.

Prognosis and Treatment

Vaccination has eliminated smallpox. Cowpox and mpox may require supportive care but are usually self-limited.

MISCELLANEOUS VIRAL EXANTHEMS

HAND-FOOT-AND-MOUTH DISEASE

Hand-foot-and-mouth disease (HFMD) is a mild viral exanthem caused by a variety of enteroviruses, most commonly coxsackievirus serotype A16.

Clinical Findings

The HFMD exanthem is nonpruritic and is characterized by oval vesicles with an erythematous rim, localized on the hands and distal lower extremities, associated with concomitant erosive stomatitis (Fig. 3.31). The diagnosis is primarily clinical.

Histologic Features

The histologic features include intraepidermal spongiosis, ballooning and reticular degeneration with intraepidermal vesicle formation, papillary dermal edema, and a scant superficial perivascular dermal lymphocytic infiltrate (Fig. 3.32).

Differential Diagnosis

The differential diagnosis includes herpesvirus infections, in which there are characteristic viral cytopathic effects, and erythema multiforme, in which there is vacuolar alteration at the dermoepidermal junction and necrotic keratinocytes in the lower levels of the epidermis.

Prognosis and Treatment

The treatment is supportive, the disease is self-limited, and the prognosis is excellent in the majority of cases. Several recent outbreaks in East Asia, caused by enterovirus 71, were associated with neurologic complications and even fatalities.

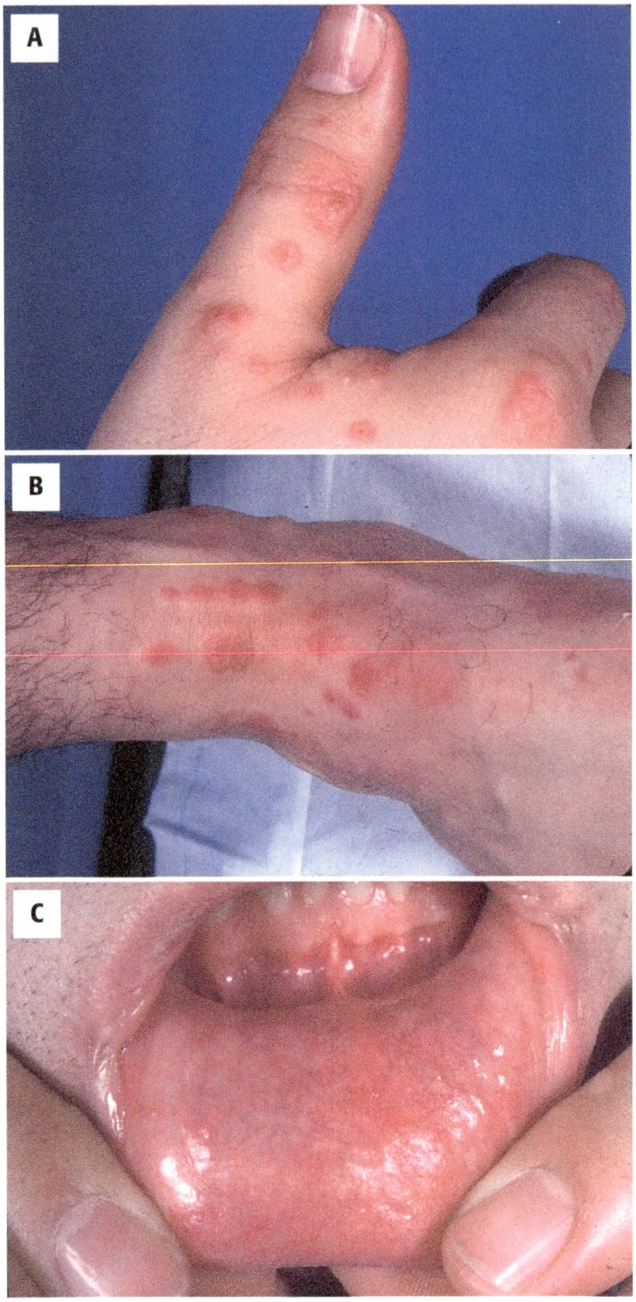

FIG. 3.31
Hand-foot-and-mouth disease. Oval vesicles on an erythematous base on the hand (**A**) and distal lower extremity (**B**). Erosive stomatitis with multiple small oral ulcers (**C**).

VIRUS-ASSOCIATED TRICHODYSPLASIA SPINULOSA

Clinical Findings

Virus-associated trichodysplasia spinulosa (VATS) is a rare condition that was historically first seen in patients

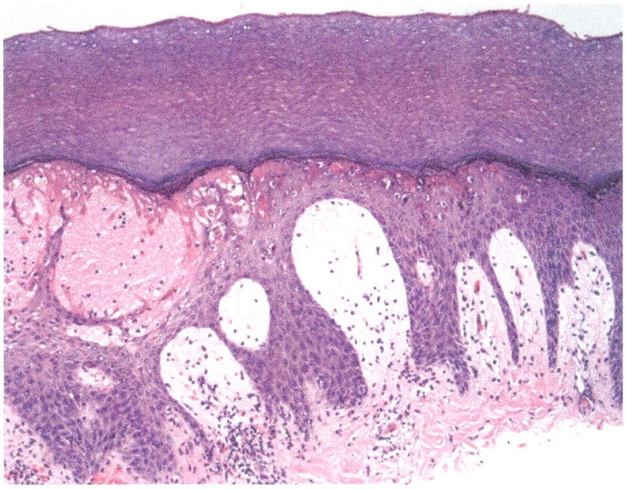

FIG. 3.32

Hand-foot-and-mouth disease. There is an intraepidermal vesicular dermatitis associated with marked papillary dermal edema. There is partial necrosis of keratinocytes in the upper epidermis.

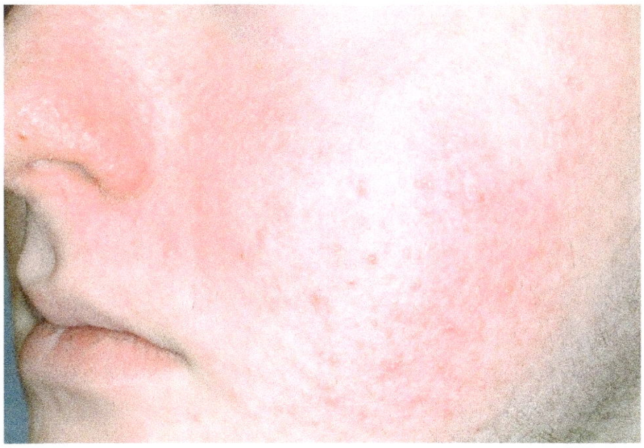

FIG. 3.33

Virus-associated trichodysplasia spinulosa. Multiple small follicular papules are present on the face.

after solid organ transplantation. However, it has subsequently been found to occur also in bone marrow transplant patients and lymphoma patients who did not have a transplant. Clinically, cutaneous disease is characterized by multiple small, spiky papules, primarily affecting the face (Fig. 3.33).

Histologic Features

The essential finding is the presence of abnormal hair follicles with excessive inner root sheath production (Fig. 3.34). The hair bulb may lack a papilla. Above the cells of the hair matrix, a column of nucleated eosinophilic cells with trichohyalin granules is typically present. Eventually, this column turns superficially into compact keratinous material without ever maturing into a fully cornified hair shaft. The follicles are typically distended with an ectatic infundibulum.

Differential Diagnosis

Similar histologic features can be seen in drug-induced (e.g., cyclosporine) follicular dystrophy. It is possible that follicular dystrophy and VATS are the same entity.

Ancillary Studies

A diagnosis of VATS requires the ultrastructural demonstration of (polyoma-like) viral particles in keratinocytes of affected hair follicles (Fig. 3.35). The identity of the virus has not been determined yet at the molecular level.

Prognosis and Treatment

The VATS-related skin eruption raises mainly cosmetic concerns. Anecdotal evidence suggests that topical cidofovir may be beneficial.

COVID-19 INFECTION

Clinical Findings

Skin manifestations are common in patients with COVID-19 (SARS-CoV2) infections. The spectrum of clinical presentations includes a morbilliform rash, vesicular and urticarial eruptions, and purpuric and vasculitic lesions (Fig. 3.36). Chilblain-like changes may affect the fingers or toes.

Histopathologic Features

The histopathologic findings mirror the spectrum of clinical findings. Morbilliform and urticarial lesions may be associated with a perivascular dermatitis. Other lesions may show a lichenoid and/or purpuric dermatitis (Fig. 3.37). Vascular damage and other findings may also be seen.

BACTERIAL INFECTIONS

IMPETIGO—IMPETIGO CONTAGIOSA, BULLOUS IMPETIGO, AND ECTHYMA

Impetigo represents a group of contagious, superficial, pyogenic infections of the skin that heal without scarring. It is typically subdivided into bullous impetigo and nonbullous impetigo (impetigo contagiosa). Impetigo contagiosa has been related to both *Staphylococcus aureus* and

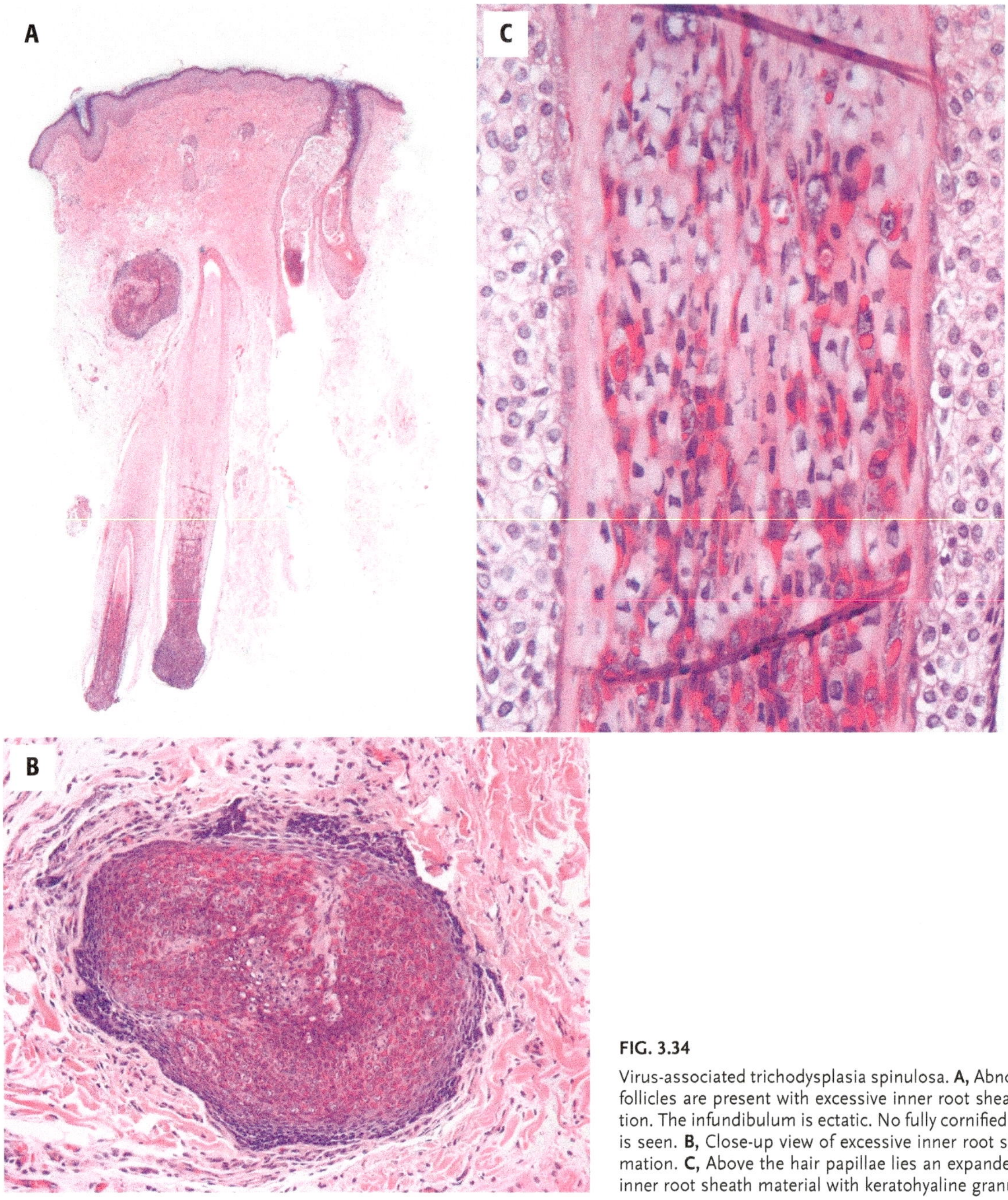

FIG. 3.34

Virus-associated trichodysplasia spinulosa. **A,** Abnormal hair follicles are present with excessive inner root sheath formation. The infundibulum is ectatic. No fully cornified hair shaft is seen. **B,** Close-up view of excessive inner root sheath formation. **C,** Above the hair papillae lies an expanded layer of inner root sheath material with keratohyaline granules.

group A β-hemolytic streptococci. Ecthyma is essentially an ulcerated impetigo caused by group A streptococcal infection. Bullous impetigo, including staphylococcal scalded skin syndrome (SSSS), is caused by *S. aureus*, phage group II. The latter syndrome will be discussed separately.

Clinical Findings

IMPETIGO CONTAGIOSA

Impetigo contagiosa typically affects preschool-age children (Fig. 3.38). After minor trauma, impetigo contagiosa usually begins on the face and extremities. Predisposing factors may include chickenpox, arthropod bites, abrasions, and burns, or systemic diseases such as diabetes mellitus and AIDS or other diseases that disrupt the integrity of the skin barrier. Impetigo contagiosa starts as small superficial vesicles or pustules that rapidly burst, progressing into honey-colored crusted plaques, usually less than 2 cm in diameter. The infection may spread rapidly by direct contact, especially in crowded or warm, humid conditions with poor hygiene. If left untreated, the lesions tend to slowly enlarge, involving new sites over several weeks. The lesions may either spontaneously resolve without scarring, or ulcerate, a condition known as ecthyma.

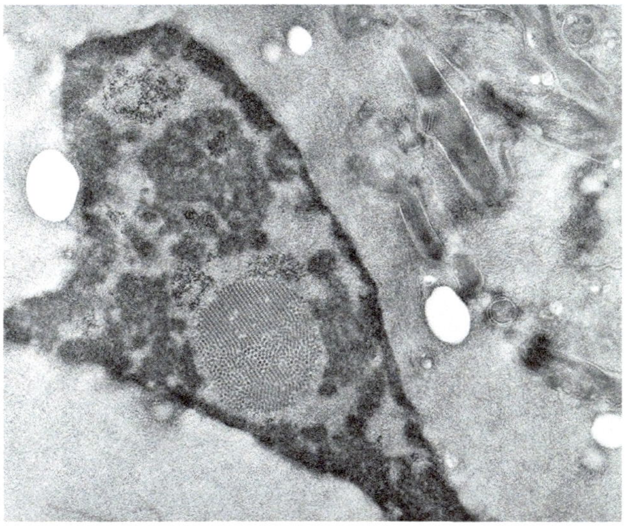

FIG. 3.35
Virus-associated trichodysplasia spinulosa. Viral inclusions are seen by electron microscopy.

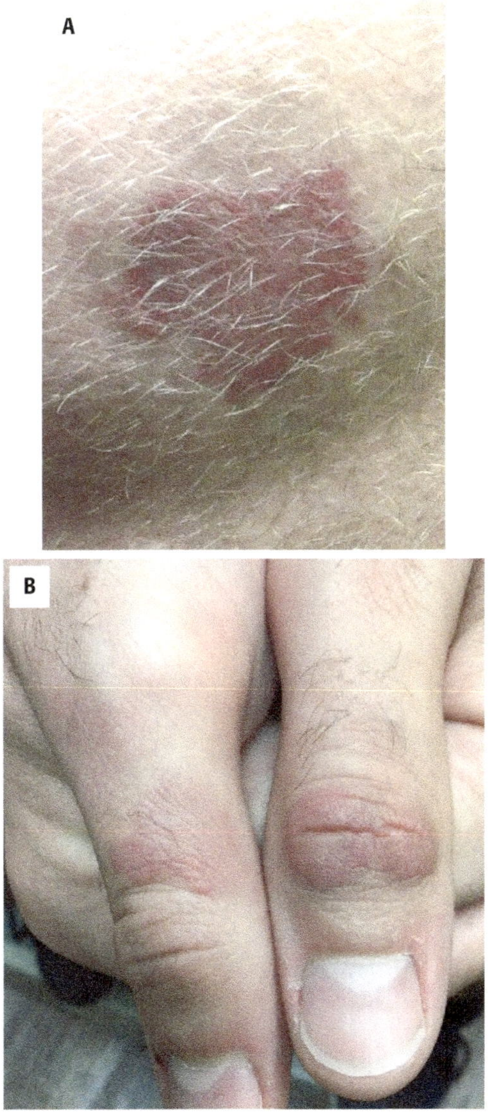

FIG. 3.36
COVID-19. **A**, Erythematous purpuric patch. **B**, Erythema and swelling of the fingers.

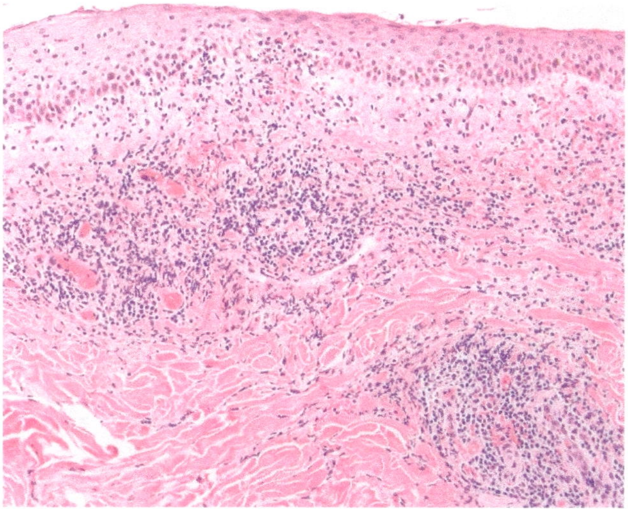

FIG. 3.37
COVID-19. Spongiotic interface and purpuric dermatitis with lymphocytes and extravasated red blood cells.

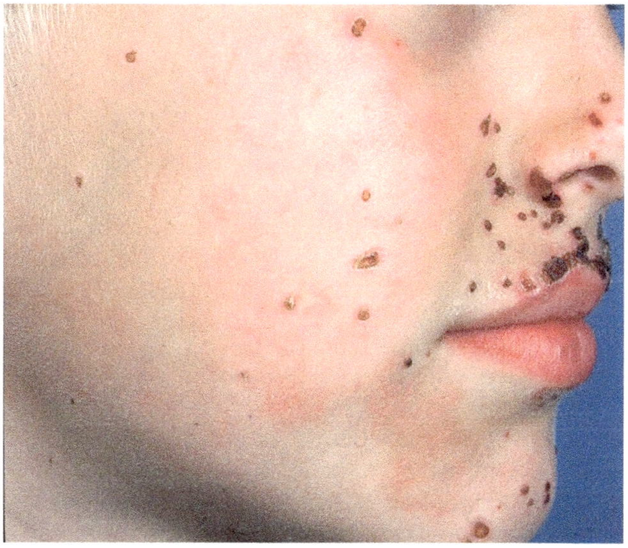

FIG. 3.38
Impetigo contagiosa. Multiple crusted papulovesicular lesions are present on the face.

BULLOUS IMPETIGO

Bullous impetigo occurs mainly in newborns, infants, and young children and only occasionally in adults. In nontraumatized skin, it is characterized by flaccid blisters up to 2 cm across or moist erosions with surrounding erythema. Initially, the bullae contain clear yellow fluid that turns dark yellow and turbid. The lesions, which are distributed mainly on the face, buttocks, trunk, and perineum, spontaneously resolve in 2 to 3 weeks.

Histologic Features

Bullous impetigo and impetigo contagiosa share similar histologic findings. They are characterized by formation

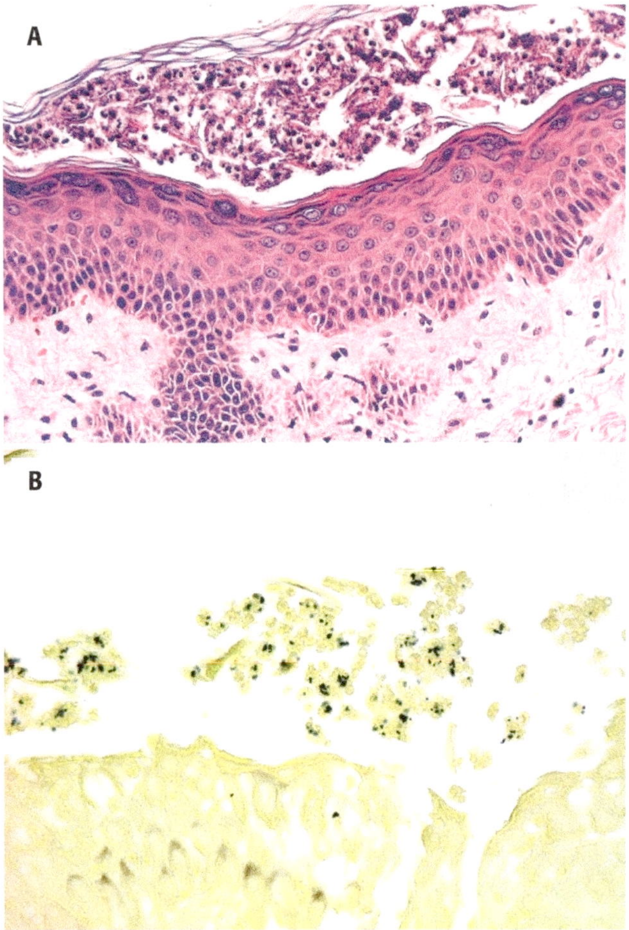

FIG. 3.39

Bullous impetigo. **A,** Intracorneal aggregates of neutrophils are present (pustule). **B,** Gram-positive cocci are identified.

of a subcorneal pustule beneath the granular layer (Fig. 3.39A), with an associated superficial perivascular infiltrate of lymphocytes and interstitial infiltrate of neutrophils. Within the pustule, gram-positive cocci can be found both within the neutrophils and extracellularly (Fig. 3.39B). Occasionally, acantholytic keratinocytes are also present. Ecthyma shows ulceration and inflamed granulation tissue with neutrophils and gram-positive cocci.

Differential Diagnosis

Impetigo is usually a clinical diagnosis, but it can be supported by positive microbiologic cultures. Histologically, impetigo should be distinguished from subcorneal pustular dermatosis and pustular psoriasis, which are devoid of gram-positive cocci in the pustules. The distinction from pemphigus foliaceus may be difficult because the latter can be secondarily infected. In contrast to superficial pemphigus, impetigo generally contains numerous neutrophils and gram-positive cocci but only mild acantholysis.

Prognosis and Treatment

Topical treatment with mupirocin ointment with removal of crusts and maintenance of cleanliness are sufficient to cure mild cases. In more extensive diseases, systemic antibiotic therapy may be needed.

STAPHYLOCOCCAL SCALDED SKIN SYNDROME

Staphylococcal scalded skin syndrome, a blistering skin disease induced by the exfoliative (epidermolytic) toxins A and B of *S. aureus*, phage groups 71 and 55, clinically resembles a scald. It is only briefly described here. Its histology is illustrated in the chapter on bullous disorders of the skin.

Infants and young children younger than 5 years of age are primarily affected. The syndrome begins abruptly with fever, macular scarlatiniform erythema, and tenderness of the skin followed by formation of flaccid, fluid-filled bullae in the axillae, groin, and around the body orifices (Fig. 3.40). The bullae quickly rupture on slight pressure, leaving extensively desquamated areas. In the absence of secondary infection, children rapidly recover from SSSS, re-epithelializing their skin within 1 to 2 weeks.

Histologically, one finds an intraepidermal cleavage at the granular layer, containing few acantholytic cells and sparse neutrophils (Fig. 3.41). The underlying dermis is either free of inflammation or contains a sparse, superficial perivascular and interstitial mixed infiltrate of lymphocytes and neutrophils. Gram-positive cocci are absent because the lesions are induced by diffusible toxins rather than the bacterium itself.

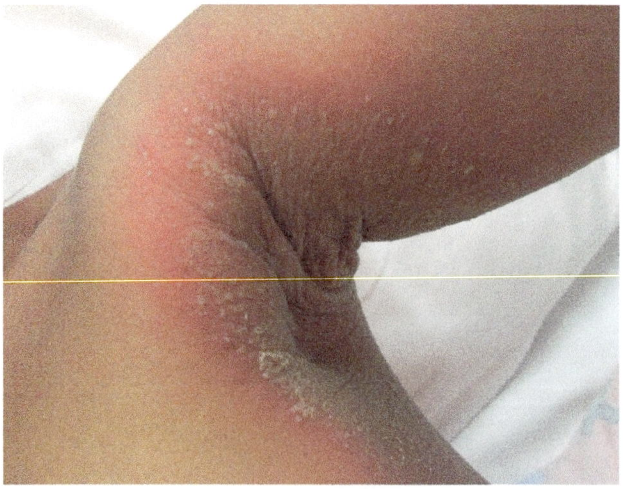

FIG. 3.40

Staphylococcal scalded skin syndrome. Flaccid, fluid-filled bullae in the axilla.

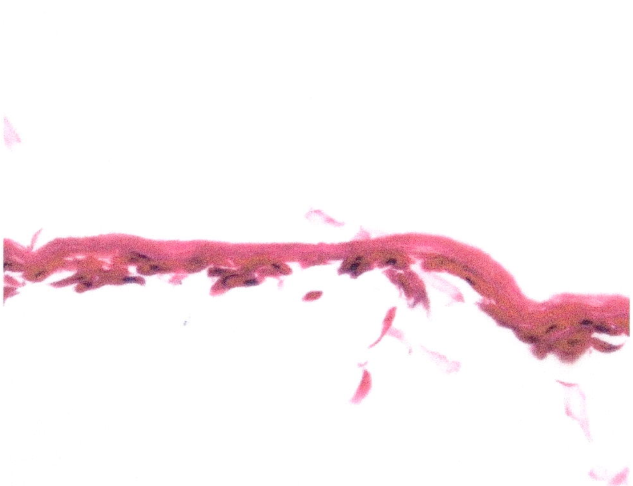

FIG. 3.41
Staphylococcal scalded skin syndrome. Superficial intraepidermal cleavage at the granular layer.

When SSSS is treated with intravenous penicillinase-resistant antistaphylococcal antibiotics followed by oral antibiotics along with appropriate topical skin care, most patients rapidly recover within 5 to 7 days. Adults with SSSS have a higher rate of sepsis because of higher rates of renal failure and underlying illness.

CELLULITIS AND ERYSIPELAS

Cellulitis is an infection-related acute suppurative inflammation (pyogenic infection) of the dermis, subcutis, or both. It may be caused by any bacteria but is most often the result of an infection by streptococci and staphylococci. Erysipelas is a clinical variant of superficial cellulitis characterized by elevated borders and common involvement of lymphatics.

Clinical Findings

Cellulitis is often preceded by a wound and usually manifests as a tender erythematous patch or plaque. Vesicles may form, and pus may be discharged (Fig. 3.42). It may be complicated by lymphangitis, abscess formation, or sepsis. Historically, erysipelas has often affected the face and was caused by *Streptococcus pyogenes* infection. However, more recently, infections seem more common on the legs.

Histologic Features

Depending on the stage of the evolution of the infection, there is usually a mixed inflammatory cell infiltrate

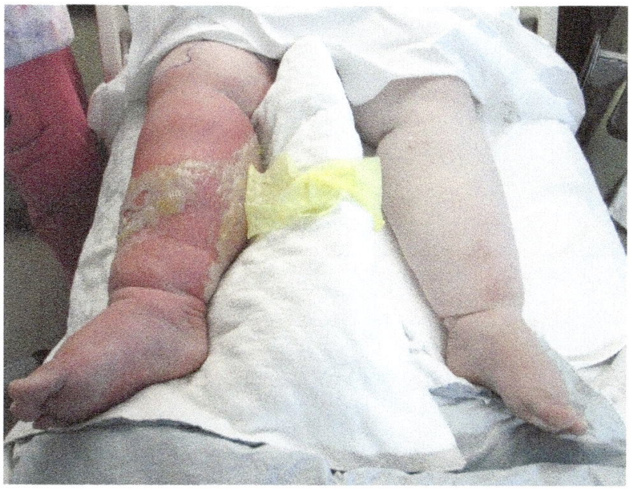

FIG. 3.42
Cellulitis. Unilateral erythematous edematous extremity with purulent bullae.

(Fig. 3.43). Neutrophils may be numerous and predominate in the early stages. There is usually a background of vascular ectasia, edema, or later fibrosis. In the later stages of cellulitis, the proportion of lymphocytes and histiocytes increases.

NECROTIZING FASCIITIS

Necrotizing fasciitis is an acute necrotizing infectious process of the skin and deep soft tissue. It tends to be rapidly progressive and can be fatal. Immunosuppressed patients and individuals with diabetes mellitus are particularly susceptible. Many different forms of bacteria have been cultured, including streptococci and staphylococci, enterococci, *Pseudomonas* sp., and others. It is indeed often a polymicrobial condition.

Clinical Findings

Within a day or two after trauma (often a surgical procedure), there is erythema and edema, simulating cellulitis, which is then followed by bluish or purplish discoloration (cyanosis), pain, and skin or soft tissue necrosis. Necrotizing fasciitis usually occurs on the extremities or trunk but may occur anywhere. Fournier's gangrene is essentially a variant of necrotizing fasciitis involving the genital, perineal, and abdominal region(s).

Histologic Features

The histology shows nonspecific edema, inflammation, and necrosis involving the skin and deep soft tissues. Histology and, in particular, intraoperative frozen sections may be

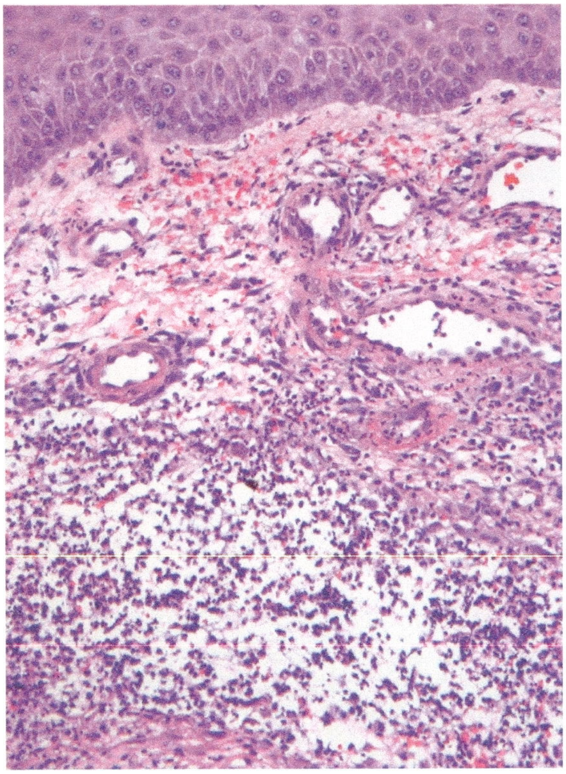

FIG. 3.43
Cellulitis. Many neutrophils are present (suppurative dermatitis) associated with edema and ectatic vessels.

useful to confirm the presence of deep tissue necrosis and assess the viability of the residual tissue after debridement.

Ancillary Studies

A Gram stain readily identifies the presence of microorganisms. Cultures are usually positive.

Differential Diagnosis

Cellulitis differs from necrotizing fasciitis by its limitation to the dermis and superficial subcutis. However, necrotizing cellulitis may develop into fasciitis. Pyoderma gangrenosum and neutrophilic dermatoses (Sweet's-like dermatoses) differ from necrotizing fasciitis by the lack of necrosis and the fact that the inflammatory reaction is usually centered in the dermis. Autolytic tissue with bacterial overgrowth may also simulate fasciitis.

Prognosis and Treatment

Early surgical debridement and intravenous antibiotics are critical. The process can be fatal.

ERYTHRASMA

Erythrasma is a chronic infection of intertriginous skin caused by the lipophilic gram-positive bacterium *Corynebacterium minutissimum*.

Clinical Findings

Erythrasma can occur at any age. It is found worldwide but most often in the tropics and subtropics. The incidence increases with age. Predisposing factors include a humid environment, obesity, diabetes, and immunosuppression. Patients present with asymptomatic or pruritic reddish-brown patches. The usually well-defined but irregular lesions may show a fine scale resembling dermatophytosis (Fig. 3.44). Erythrasma commonly involves the groin, the feet between toe web spaces, and other intertriginous areas such as the axillae and submammary regions.

Histologic Features

Although the hematoxylin and eosin (H&E)–stained skin sections usually appear normal, filamentous branching bacilli may be seen in the superficial cornified layer (Fig. 3.45). They are gram positive. Mild hyperkeratosis, parakeratosis, or acanthosis may be identified.

Ancillary Studies

Clinically, Wood's lamp examination is helpful. Under the Wood's lamp, the lesions characteristically fluoresce

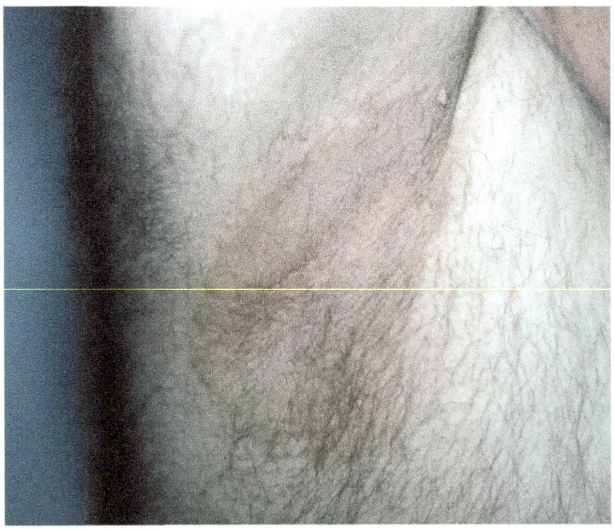

FIG. 3.44
Erythrasma. Well-demarcated red patch in the axilla.

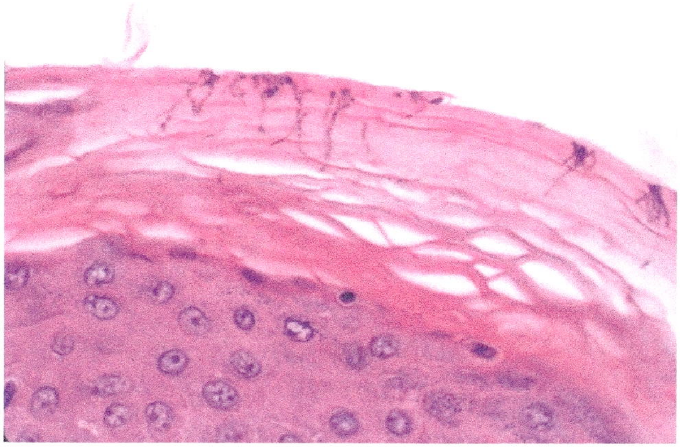

FIG. 3.45
Erythrasma. Bacilli (*Corynebacterium minutissimum*) are present in the stratum corneum.

coral-red because of coproporphyrin III produced by the bacterium. Histologically, a Gram stain highlights the gram-positive organisms.

Differential Diagnosis

Candidiasis and dermatophytosis can be differentiated from erythrasma by the presence of epidermal and dermal inflammatory changes (usually absent in erythrasma), the detection of fungal elements on Gomori methenamine silver (GMS) stain, and lack of reaction for a Gram stain.

Prognosis and Treatment

The disease can remain asymptomatic for years, or it can undergo periodic exacerbations even after antibiotic treatment. Benzoyl peroxide wash or topical clindamycin solution is effective for treating localized symptomatic erythrasma.

BACTERIAL FOLLICULITIS

A number of different bacterial organisms can affect hair follicles, such as staphylococci (impetigo of Bockhart) and *Pseudomonas* sp.

Clinical Findings

Folliculitis typically manifests as an erythematous papule (Fig. 3.46) that may become vesicular and pustular. A hair shaft may or may not be clinically apparent. Some inflammatory reactions result in nodules, plaques, or abscesses.

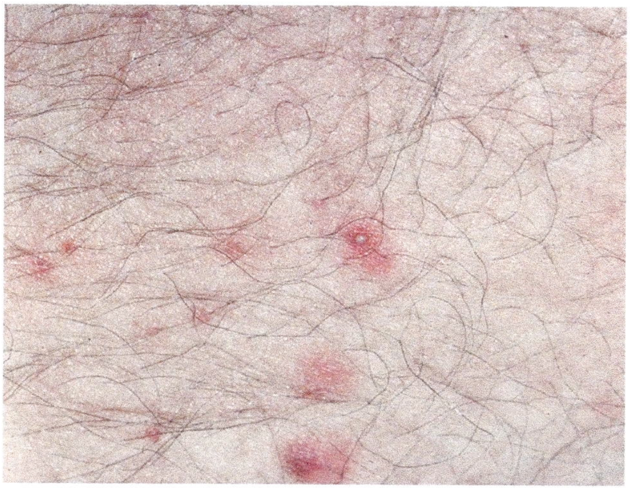

FIG. 3.46
Bacterial folliculitis. Erythematous papules and pustules are present.

Histologic Features

Early lesions typically show an inflammatory cell infiltrate predominantly composed of neutrophils (Fig. 3.47). The inflammation may affect the superficial portion of the hair (superficial folliculitis), often involving the infundibulum, or be centered in the deep dermis and subcutis (deep folliculitis). If there is rupture of the epithelium and keratin or hair shaft material leaks into the dermis, a granulomatous foreign body-type giant cell reaction is usually found.

Ancillary Studies

The bacterial origin of the inflammatory process is confirmed by the detection of microorganisms on Gram stains or by cultures.

Differential Diagnosis

A bacterial suppurative superficial folliculitis needs to be distinguished from a fungal or viral infection of the hair, acne, and acneiform drug reactions, such as from inhibitors of the epidermal growth factor receptor (EGFR)–mediated signaling pathway. Special stains for microorganisms and clinical review of the potential causative medication are important for the correct diagnosis. The differential diagnosis of deep folliculitides includes the "follicular occlusion triad" of hidradenitis

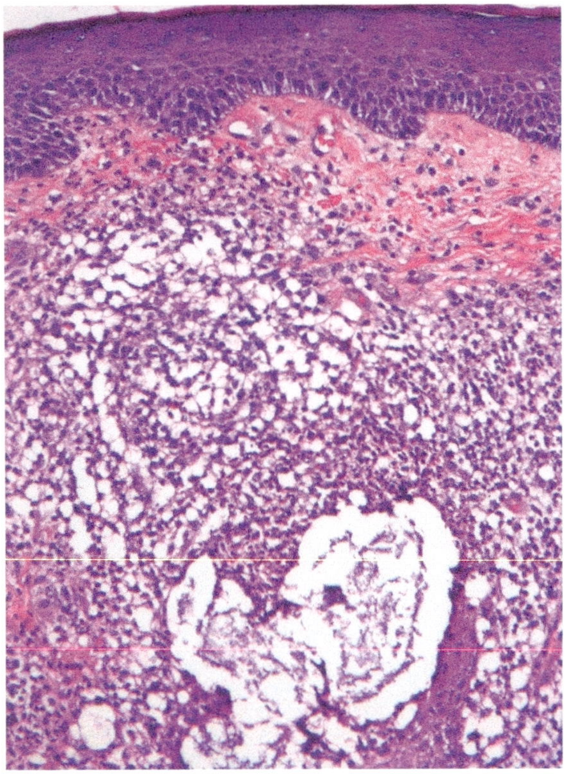

FIG. 3.47
Bacterial folliculitis. A superficial suppurative dermatitis is present with rupture of the follicular infundibulum.

suppurative, acne conglobata, and perifolliculitis capitis abscedens et suffodiens. The histologic picture of those conditions reveals mixed suppurative and chronic inflammation with ruptured follicular cyst(s) and foreign body–type giant cell reactions. The differential diagnosis also includes eosinophilic folliculitis, a superficial folliculitis rich in eosinophils, which is often associated with immunosuppression (related to HIV, lymphoma, or treatment).

Prognosis and Treatment

An isolated folliculitis is often self-limited. Treatment consists of cleansing the affected area with an antibacterial soap solution and/or topical application of an antibiotic ointment or cream.

PITTED KERATOLYSIS

Pitted keratolysis, a superficial infection of the cornified layer of the web spaces and plantar surface, forms multiple pits and superficial erosions. The pits result from the catalyzing activity of mixed organisms, including *Corynebacterium*, *Dermatophilus congolensis*, and *Micrococcus sedentarius*.

Clinical Findings

Although pitted keratolysis can occur in adults and children of either gender, it affects men with sweaty feet most often. The lesions consist of numerous superficial crateriform pits in the horny layer of the soles and ventral surfaces of the toes (Fig. 3.48). Discrete, shallow, punched-out lesions then tend to coalesce, forming a large defect with serpiginous outlines. This causes brownish discoloration, hyperhidrosis, maceration, a foul odor, and mild pruritus.

Histologic Features

The early lesions consist of multiple, sharply circumscribed invaginations with pallor in the cornified layer. Eosinophilic debris containing clumps of cocci, bacilli, and filamentous organisms can be found at the base and margins of the pits (Fig. 3.49).

Ancillary Studies

The microorganisms are gram positive. They also stain positive for GMS.

Differential Diagnosis

Pitted keratolysis is distinguished from erythrasma by differences in clinical distribution and appearance, as well as pits in the compact cornified layer.

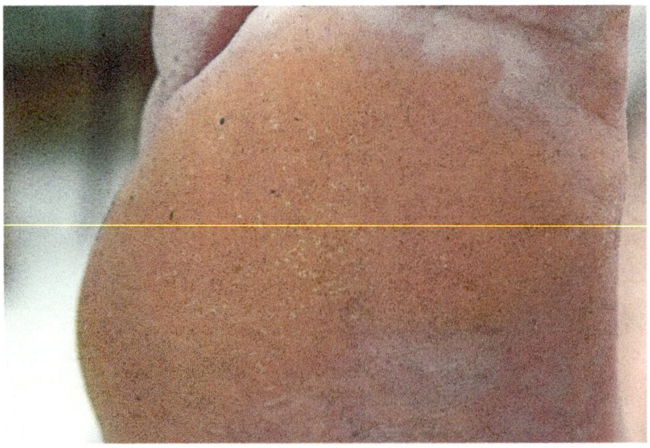

FIG. 3.48
Pitted keratolysis. Numerous superficial crateriform pits in the horny layer of the soles.

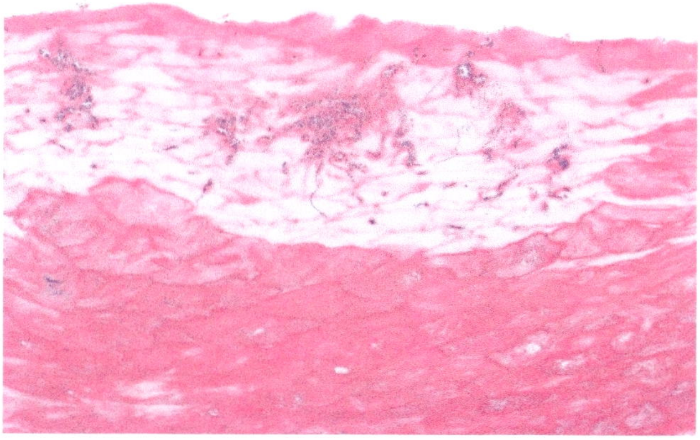

FIG. 3.49
Pitted keratolysis. Multiple invaginations, with pallor, in the cornified layer containing filamentous bacteria.

Prognosis and Treatment

Benzoyl peroxide wash and topical antibiotics are effective treatments.

SEPTIC VASCULITIS

Septic vasculitis, a variant of acute vasculitis, may develop from any infection but is most commonly associated with disseminated *Neisseria meningitidis, Neisseria gonorrhoeae, S. aureus, Pseudomonas aeruginosa,* or *Streptococcus* sp.

Clinical Findings

Cutaneous lesions can be observed in more than 80% of patients with acute meningococcemia along with other symptoms such as fever, chills, myalgia, nausea, or vomiting. Petechiae begin on the ankles, wrists, or axillae. In the fulminant condition known as purpura fulminans, purpuric or ecchymotic lesions are associated with septic shock and disseminated intravascular coagulopathy (DIC). In chronic meningococcal infection, the cutaneous lesions are variable, manifesting as erythematous macules, papules, petechiae, pustules, vesicles, or hemorrhagic tender plaques or nodules (Fig. 3.50). The symptoms of disseminated gonococcal infections resemble those of acute meningococcemia, except that skin lesions are fewer in number and usually involve distal extremities near joints.

Pseudomonas septicemia (ecthyma gangrenosum), which usually occurs in immunocompromised patients, is often caused by trauma or indwelling venous and urinary catheters. The typical cutaneous lesion consists of a sharply demarcated, painless, indurated, necrotic ulcer or an eschar with surrounding erythema. Hemorrhagic bullae may be present.

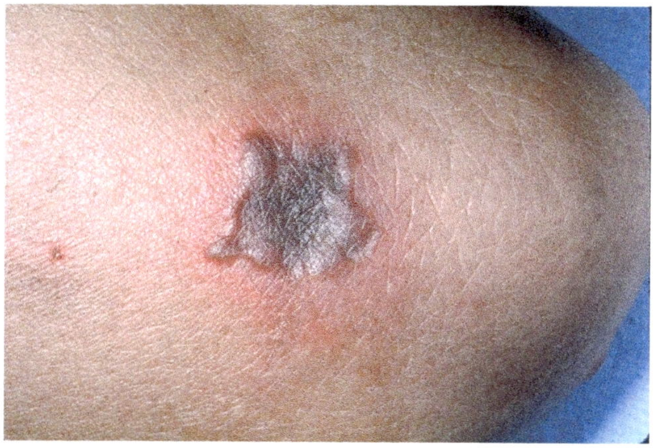

FIG. 3.50
Gonococcal sepsis. A hemorrhagic plaque is present.

Histologic Features

Septic bacterial infections with cutaneous dissemination share common histopathologic findings characterized by a necrotizing vasculitis and variable degree of inflammatory and secondary reactive changes, such as edema or infarct-type necrosis or ulceration (Fig. 3.51). Gram stains often reveal the presence of microorganisms (gram-negative cocci in the case of meningococci, gram-positive organisms in the case of staphylococcal sepsis) (Fig. 3.51). In ecthyma gangrenosum, the epidermis and upper dermis necrose and red blood cells extravasate (Fig. 3.52). Numerous gram-negative bacilli (Fig. 3.53) can be identified in the blood vessels or between the collagen bundles.

Differential Diagnosis

Meningococcemia, gonococcemia, and ecthyma gangrenosum are best distinguished from each other and from other causes of infectious septicemia by the constellation of clinical findings and identification of the microorganisms through culture of blood and skin lesions.

Prognosis and Treatment

Septic infections may be fatal. Therapy is focused on antibiotic treatment, replenishing the coagulating factors, controlling hemorrhage, and stabilizing the cardiovascular system (hypotension from septic shock).

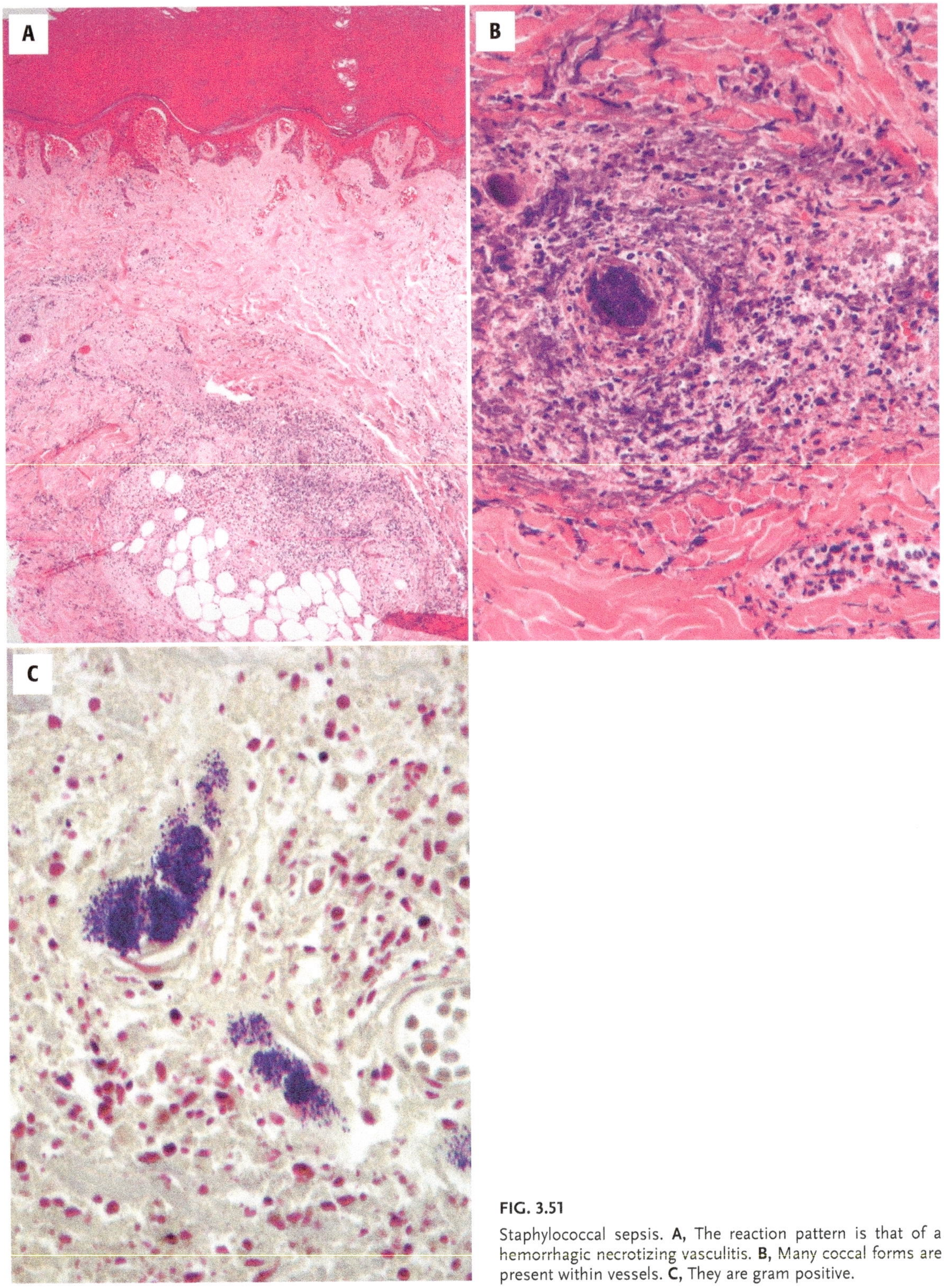

FIG. 3.51

Staphylococcal sepsis. **A,** The reaction pattern is that of a hemorrhagic necrotizing vasculitis. **B,** Many coccal forms are present within vessels. **C,** They are gram positive.

CAT-SCRATCH DISEASE AND BACILLARY ANGIOMATOSIS

In an immunocompetent host, *Bartonella henselae* causes cat-scratch disease, a self-limited, zoonotic lymphadenitis. Bacillary angiomatosis (BA) is caused by either *B. henselae* or *Bartonella quintana*.

Clinical Findings

Cat-scratch disease is distributed worldwide, often affecting normal children and adolescents. Most patients report a history of animal contact. The cutaneous manifestations occur in 4% to 5% of patients. They may be

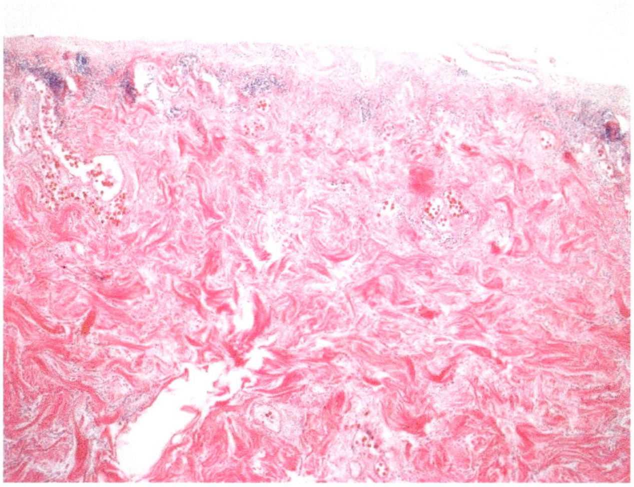

FIG. 3.52
Ecthyma gangrenosum. Epidermal and dermal ischemic necrosis with vascular occlusion by fibrin.

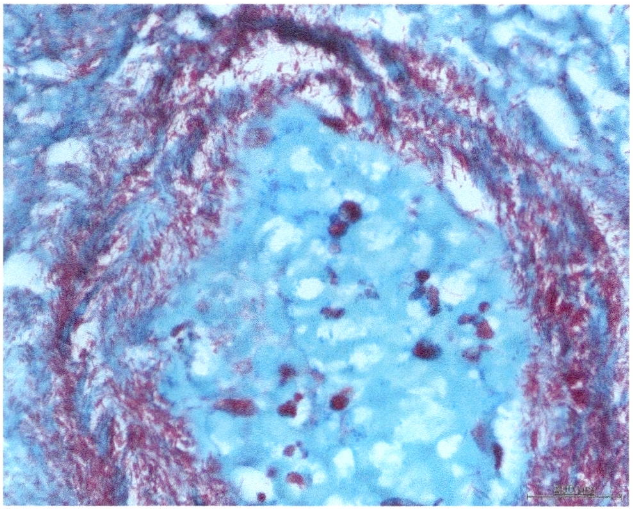

FIG. 3.53
Ecthyma gangrenosum. Numerous gram-negative bacilli in blood vessel walls.

maculopapular, pustular, morbilliform, or purpuric. The skin lesions often resolve within 2 weeks as regional lymphadenitis develops.

BA usually occurs in immunocompromised hosts, especially in HIV-infected individuals. It usually manifests as angiomatoid red to violaceous papules or nodules on the trunk or extremities, resembling pyogenic granuloma or Kaposi sarcoma, but may also form lichenoid plaques or subcutaneous nodules.

Histologic Features

In cat-scratch disease, there is a zone of stellate necrosis surrounded by a rim of histiocytes, neutrophils, and occasional giant cells. The epidermal changes are variable and may include acanthosis and ulceration. Silver stains confirm the presence of small, pleomorphic coccobacilli in the area of necrosis.

In BA, there is a proliferation of blood vessels with prominent endothelial cells (Fig. 3.54). Among the vascular proliferation are dispersed neutrophils with leukocytoclasis and purplish material that represent clumps of bacilli.

Ancillary Studies

The bacilli can be visualized with the Warthin-Starry stain. Cultures are definitive, but PCR tests are highly sensitive and much faster than cultures.

Differential Diagnosis

Cat-scratch disease is distinguished from other necrotizing granulomatous diseases, such as mycobacterial infections, fungal infections, or lymphogranuloma venereum (LGV), by the demonstration of the causative pleomorphic bacilli using a silver stain. BA should be differentiated from other vascular neoplasms, particularly pyogenic granuloma and Kaposi sarcoma. In Kaposi sarcoma, there is often a plasmacytic infiltrate, and the blood vessels are more often slitlike with a pronounced dissecting growth pattern. In pyogenic granuloma, there is a distinctive lobular architecture, which is absent in BA.

Prognosis and Treatment

Cat-scratch disease is self-limited. The currently recommended therapy for BA is oral antibiotics (e.g., erythromycin).

RICKETTSIAL INFECTIONS

Rickettsia is an obligate intracellular bacterium. Various species cause a group of heterogeneous infectious diseases: Rocky Mountain spotted fever, Boutonneuse fever, rickettsialpox, murine typhus, scrub typhus, regional variants of (e.g., Queensland or Siberian) tick typhus, and Q-fever (Table 3.1). In the United States, Rocky Mountain spotted fever, which is caused by *Rickettsia rickettsii*, is the most frequent and severe rickettsial infection. Most rickettsial infections, except for Q fever, are associated with skin lesions.

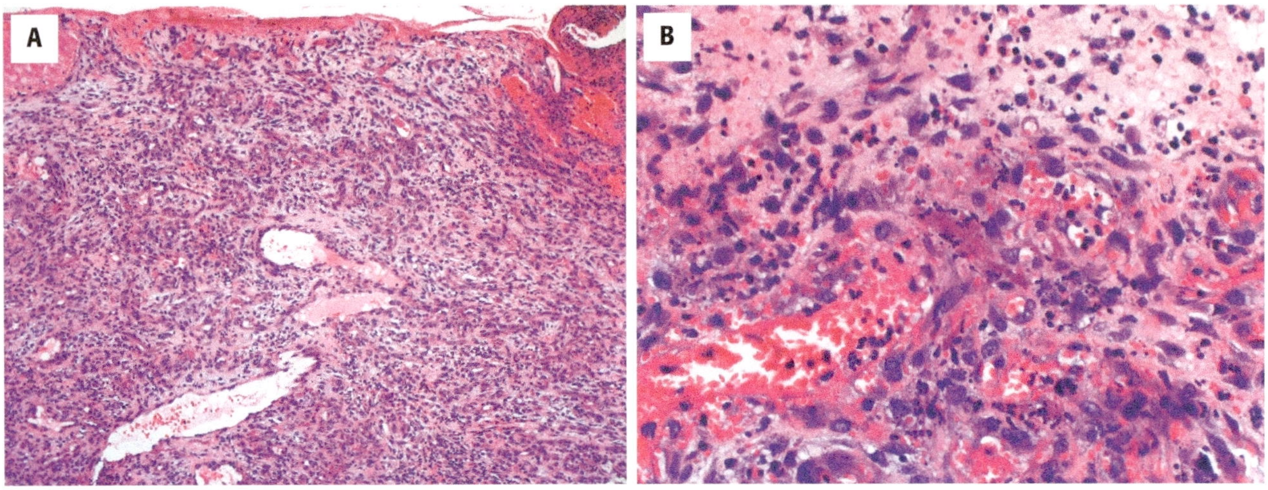

FIG. 3.54

Bacillary angiomatosis. **A**, Vascular proliferation with prominent endothelial cells and neutrophilic inflammation. **B,** Blood vessel with neutrophils, leukocystoclastic nuclear debris, and purplish material that represent clumps of bacilli.

TABLE 3.1

Rickettsial Infections With Skin Lesions

Disease	Organisms	Transmission or Vector
Rocky mountain spotted fever	*Rickettsia rickettsii*	Tick
Boutonneuse fever	*Rickettsia conorii*	Tick
Rickettsialpox	*Rickettsia akari*	Mite
Epidemic typhus	*Rickettsia prowazekii*	Human body louse

Clinical Findings

Rickettsiae are endemic in different geographic areas; they can be transmitted by various arthropod bites. Rickettsial infections usually induce an acute febrile illness with headache, malaise, and characteristic skin lesions, except in Q-fever. The rash usually begins as erythematous macules that may spread centripetally to the trunk with relative sparing of the face. The lesions may become maculopapular, petechial, or purpuric. Although eschar formation at a tick bite site is frequent in rickettsialpox infection, it is rare in Rocky Mountain spotted fever.

Histologic Features

The histologic hallmark of rickettsial infection is lymphocytic vasculitis with fibrin thrombi, endothelial swelling, and extravasation of erythrocytes (Fig. 3.55). Basal layer vacuolar changes with mild to moderate exocytosis are common in Rocky Mountain spotted fever, and marked subepidermal edema with lymphocytic exocytosis is frequent in rickettsialpox. Coagulative necrosis of the epidermis and underlying dermis occurs in the area of eschar formation. There is often a superficial and deep perivascular and interstitial infiltrate of lymphocytes, histiocytes, neutrophils, and plasma cells.

Ancillary Studies

The presence of rickettsial microorganisms can be demonstrated in the endothelium by immunofluorescence or immunohistochemistry using antirickettsial antibodies.

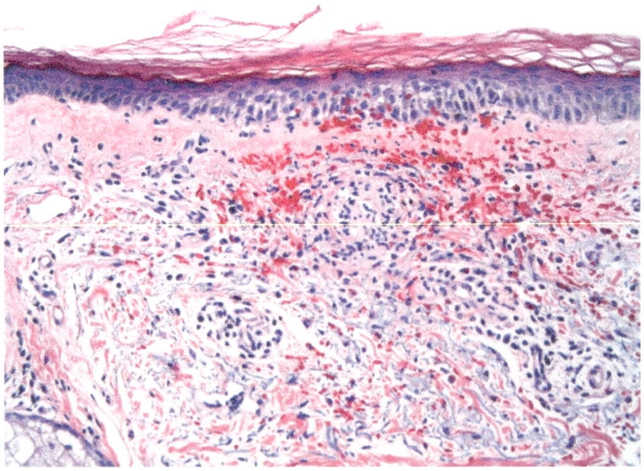

FIG. 3.55

Rocky Mountain spotted fever. Hemorrhagic lymphocytic dermatitis.

Differential Diagnosis

Insect bite reaction is characterized by a wedge-shaped, superficial and deep, mixed infiltrate with eosinophils. In contrast, the vasculitic changes with rickettsial infections are not as prominently seen in an insect bite. Other causes of lymphocytic or leukocytoclastic vasculitis must be differentiated from rickettsial infection by clinical, immunohistochemical, and serologic studies.

Prognosis and Treatment

Prompt initiation of antibiotic therapy usually leads to rapid recovery.

CHANCROID

Chancroid is a sexually transmitted ulcerative disease caused by *Haemophilus ducreyi* infection.

Clinical Findings

Chancroid is most prevalent among adult men in the tropical countries of Africa and Central and South America. After an incubation period of 4 to 7 days, the lesions develop in the genital area as one or more painful papules surrounded by erythema. The papules rapidly ulcerate with ragged, undermined edges, and the granulated bases become covered by a yellowish-gray exudate. Unilateral or bilateral inguinal lymphadenopathy is common.

Histologic Features

Classically, a triple-zone underneath the ulcerated epidermis is found: a narrow surface zone at the floor of the ulcer consists of degenerated neutrophils, fibrin, necrotic tissue, and erythrocytes; the broader middle zone is composed of granulation tissue rich in newly formed blood vessels with prominent endothelial swelling and occasional thrombi; and the deep zone contains a dense infiltrate of plasma cells and lymphocytes.

Ancillary Studies

Tissue sections stained with Gram or Giemsa may reveal short, gram-negative coccobacilli. The *H. ducreyi* microorganisms are arranged in parallel chains, resembling a school of fish. The diagnosis is confirmed by culture.

Differential Diagnosis

Chancroid may be confused with the chancre of primary syphilis or granuloma inguinale. Gram-negative coccobacilli in smears and isolation of *H. ducreyi* bacilli in culture help establish a definitive diagnosis.

Prognosis and Treatment

Appropriate oral antibiotics are effective, usually clearing lesions completely within 1 to 2 weeks.

GRANULOMA INGUINALE

Granuloma inguinale (Donovanosis) is a chronic, sexually transmitted ulcerative disease that causes ulcerations in the genital area. It is caused by infections by *Calymmatobacterium granulomatis*.

Clinical Findings

Granuloma inguinale is endemic in the tropical and subtropical regions of Southeast Asia, New Guinea, Australia, South America, and Africa. After an incubation period of 3 weeks, the initial lesion appears as a firm papule or nodule in the genital, perianal, or inguinal areas. The lesion may disappear or rapidly break, forming an ulcer of variable morphology. The classic ulcer in the granulomatous variant is painless, friable, and beefy-red with an elevated, serpiginous border and a granulated base that bleeds easily. Less common clinical variants include hypertrophic, necrotic, and sclerotic types. Lymphadenopathy is usually absent, in contrast to LGV. Spontaneous healing is extremely slow, often occurring with fibrosis, scarring, and lymphatic obstruction.

Histologic Features

Granuloma inguinale is characterized by a collection of vacuolated histiocytes with intracellular inclusion bodies (Donovan bodies). The epidermal changes are variable and may include partial or complete ulceration, acanthosis, pseudoepitheliomatous hyperplasia, parakeratosis, spongiosis, and exocytosis of neutrophils. A dense dermal infiltrate with numerous neutrophils, histiocytes, plasma cells, and scant lymphocytes is often present. The lesion may extend into the subcutaneous tissue. Dermal fibrosis is common in chronic disease.

Special Studies

The coccobacilli (*C. granulomatis*) are gram negative. They are best seen using a Giemsa stain, which highlights the "safety pin" morphology.

Differential Diagnosis

Granuloma inguinale may be confused with other infectious ulcers. Chancroid is distinguished from granuloma inguinale by the detection of gram-negative bacilli in parallel chains.

Prognosis and Treatment

Oral antibiotic therapy is recommended. The lesions clear from the majority of patients within a few weeks. However, relapse and recurrence have been reported.

LYMPHOGRANULOMA VENEREUM

LGV is a sexually transmitted disease caused by serotypes L1, L2, and L3 of *Chlamydia trachomatis*.

Clinical Findings

Endemic in parts of Africa, India, Southeast Asia, and South America, LGV is characterized by three clinical stages: the initial lesion, a painless papule, vesicle, or ulcer, resolves within a few days; several weeks later, painful regional lymphadenopathy appears along with constitutional symptoms; finally, the tertiary stage is characterized by the genitoanorectal syndrome, which is more common in untreated women, in which the patient develops ulcers, fistulae, strictures, and lymphedema.

Histologic Features

The primary lesions are often not biopsied because the histologic changes of the skin appear nonspecific: an ulcerated epidermis with granulation tissue and a mixed inflammatory cell infiltrate. In the second stage, the regional lymph node demonstrates characteristic stellate necrosis surrounded by a rim of palisading histiocytes, plasma cells, and neutrophils; large lymphoid follicles and germinal centers are prominent.

Differential Diagnosis

LGV should be differentiated from cat-scratch disease, deep fungal infection, and tularemia by identifying the causative microorganisms and noting the characteristic clinical presentations.

Prognosis and Treatment

Oral antibiotic treatment usually leads to cure within a few weeks.

RHINOSCLEROMA

Rhinoscleroma is a chronic infectious granulomatous disease of the nasal and oral mucosa caused by *Klebsiella rhinoscleromatis*, a gram-negative bacillus.

Clinical Findings

Rhinoscleroma is endemic in isolated tropical areas of Latin America, Africa, and Asia, where crowding and poor hygiene are prevalent. It is spread by direct or indirect contact with nasal secretion. Adult patients of either gender are affected equally. Granulomas originate in the nose and in the advanced cases can spread to the nasopharynx, larynx, pharynx, trachea, and bronchi. The early stage of rhinoscleroma begins as nonspecific rhinorrhea with a purulent discharge and mucous membrane hypertrophy. Later granulomatous nodules and friable masses infiltrate the nasal cavity, the skin of the nose, and the upper lip, eventually obstructing the nose and deforming and destroying the surrounding tissues.

Histologic Features

Microscopically, the fully developed lesion is characterized by a mixed granulomatous infiltrate consisting of numerous plasma cells, large histiocytes with vacuolated cytoplasm (Mikulicz cells), lymphocytes, and neutrophils. Russell bodies are a frequent finding in the plasma cells.

Ancillary Studies

Clumps of encapsulated gram-negative bacilli in the cytoplasm of Mikulicz cells stain positively with periodic acid-Schiff (PAS) or Giemsa. However, the organisms are best revealed by the Warthin-Starry stain.

Differential Diagnosis

Foamy vacuolated macrophages may be seen in other chronic inflammatory or infectious diseases such as leprosy, leishmaniasis, granuloma inguinale, and histoplasmosis. Clinical presentation, gram-negative bacilli within Mikulicz cells, and culture of the microorganisms can help differentiate rhinoscleroma from these other conditions that appear histologically similar.

Prognosis and Treatment

Antibiotic therapy, especially streptomycin, is effective in most patients. Surgery may be indicated in recalcitrant cases.

MYCOBACTERIAL INFECTIONS

TUBERCULOSIS

Cutaneous mycobacterial infections include tuberculosis, infections by nontuberculous (previously called "atypical") mycobacteria, and leprosy. Infection by *Mycobacterium tuberculosis* may result from exogenous inoculation, direct extension from an underlying source, autoinoculation, or hematogenous spread. Cutaneous tuberculosis is traditionally classified into primary tuberculosis (tuberculous chancre or tuberculous primary complex) and secondary tuberculosis, which is caused by reinfection. Based on clinical presentation, secondary tuberculosis can be further divided into tuberculosis verrucosa cutis, lupus vulgaris, scrofuloderma, orificial tuberculosis, and disseminated cutaneous tuberculosis. The variable clinical manifestations of cutaneous tuberculosis are determined by the number and virulence of the infecting strain, route of infection, presence or absence of an internal source, and status of host cellular immunity. In the past two decades, tuberculosis has resurged, and new strains have emerged, which are resistant to conventional treatment regimens.

CUTANEOUS MYCOBACTERIAL INFECTIONS (EXCLUDING LEPROSY)—DISEASE FACT SHEET

Tuberculosis

Infection by *Mycobacterium tuberculosis*

Clinical Variants

- Primary-inoculation TB (tuberculous chancre): direct inoculation at a site of trauma (usually in children) resulting in an ulcerative nodule typically associated with lymphadenopathy
- TB verrucosa cutis: warty plaques typically occurring on the hands after direct inoculation of individuals previously infected with *M. tuberculosis* or *M. bovis.* May resolve spontaneously with scarring
- Miliary TB to the skin: rare event; occurs in the setting of fulminant miliary TB, usually in severely immunocompromised individuals
- Scrofuloderma: subcutaneous nodules with ulceration and sinus tract formation
- TB cutis orificialis: typically peri- or intraoral (especially tongue) and perianal involvement; results from autoinoculation into periorificial skin
- Lupus vulgaris
  - Most common type of cutaneous TB; chronic progressive disease
  - Usually solitary nodules or plaques, typically affecting the head and neck region
  - May result from lymphatic or hematogenous spread or primary inoculation
- Tuberculids
  - Erythema induratum (Bazin disease)
  - Papulonecrotic tuberculid
  - Lichen scrofulosorum

Treatment

- Multidrug regimen

Nontuberculous Mycobacteria

Infection by mycobacteria other than *M. tuberculosis*

Mycobacterium Subtypes and Related Clinical Findings

M. marinum

- Most common nontuberculous mycobacterium to cause skin infections
- Results from exposure of traumatized skin to infected aqueous environment (fish tank, lake)
- Nodule(s) form at inoculation site (swimming pool or fish tank granuloma)

M. ulcerans (Buruli Ulcer)

- Firm papules or nodules, which become necrotizing and ulcerative
- Ulceration and underlying necrosis may be extensive
- Underlying bone involvement is common

M. haemophilum

- Papules or nodules typically occurring in immunocompromised patients

Prognosis

- Depends on the patient's immune status
- Depends on whether or not strain is sensitive to common drugs

Treatment

- *M. marinum:* Medical treatment; surgical debridement may be necessary
- *M. ulcerans:* Excision is the treatment of choice
- *M. haemophilum:* Medical treatment

Clinical Findings

In an individual who has not been previously exposed to *M. tuberculosis,* primary tuberculosis is caused by exogenous inoculation. The chancre of the skin together with the affected regional lymph nodes constitutes the tuberculous primary complex. Primary tuberculosis of the skin is most commonly seen in healthcare workers and children in endemic areas. Primary tuberculosis usually presents 2 to 4 weeks after inoculation as a small papule, indurated plaque, or nonhealing ulcer. Fever, pain, and swelling of the surrounding tissues sometimes simulate bacterial infection. In patients with acquired immunity, the process remains localized regionally and usually heals with scarring. Rarely, lupus vulgaris can develop at the site of a healed tuberculous chancre.

Lupus vulgaris is the most common form of secondary tuberculosis; it usually develops in a host with moderate immunity and high sensitivity to tuberculin. It is less common in the United States than in Europe. Women are affected about two to three times more often than men, and all age groups are affected equally. The usually solitary lesions most commonly involve the head and neck area, followed by the extremities. The lesion starts as an ill-defined, smooth, soft macule or papule that may progress to form a plaque or nodule (Fig. 3.56). In the absence of treatment, lupus vulgaris runs a chronic course: prominent atrophic scarring, lymphatic obstruction, and recurrent erysipelas can lead to gross deformity or disfiguration. Squamous cell carcinomas develop in up to 10% of longstanding cases.

Tuberculosis verrucosa cutis is an uncommon form of secondary tuberculosis caused by exogenous inoculation in previously sensitized patients. It is more frequently seen in men in the tropical climate, accounting for more than 40% of cutaneous tuberculosis in Hong Kong. The lesion presents in an otherwise asymptomatic patient as an expanding papule or pustule on an indurated base, which becomes a verrucous plaque with an irregular outline and fissures. The lesion may clinically resemble a common wart. Lymphadenopathy is absent. Without treatment, the lesion can persist for many years or spontaneously involute with an atrophic scar.

Scrofuloderma, a rare form of secondary tuberculosis, results from contiguous spreading of tuberculous infection from an underlying lymph node or joint. It is often seen in the head and neck region. Scrofuloderma generally starts as a fixed, well-defined, subcutaneous swelling that eventuates into linear sinus tracts, with watery discharge, and purulent or caseous material (Fig. 3.57). The clinical course is protracted, and healing with residual scars usually occurs over many years.

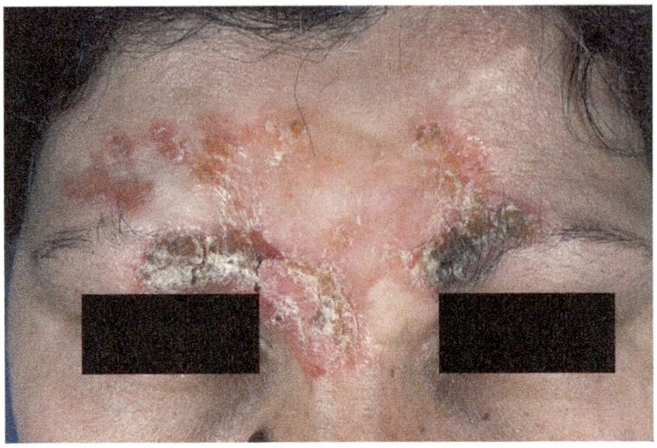

FIG. 3.56
Lupus vulgaris. Chronic infiltrative process in the face with crusts.

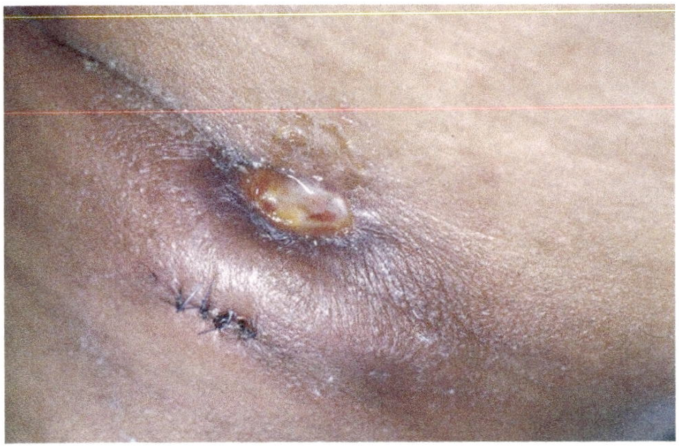

FIG. 3.57
Scrofuloderma. Subcutaneous nodule with pus.

Orificial tuberculosis, another rare form, is caused by autoinoculation of the mucous membrane and surrounding skin. It often occurs in infants and immunocompromised patients. The lesions, which begin as yellow-to-red nodules, develop into shallow, tender ulcers.

Histologic Features

The early lesions of primary tuberculosis contain a mixed dermal infiltrate of neutrophils, lymphocytes, and plasma cells. After the lesions ulcerate, tuberculoid granulomas with epithelioid histiocytes form, which are surrounded by a cuff of lymphocytes. Diffuse granulomatous reactions may be seen in more developed lesions. In the center of the tubercle, one can occasionally see central caseating necrosis with pink, granular material lacking cell outlines. In early lesions, the Fite or Ziehl-Neelsen stains can identify microorganisms within the center of the tubercle.

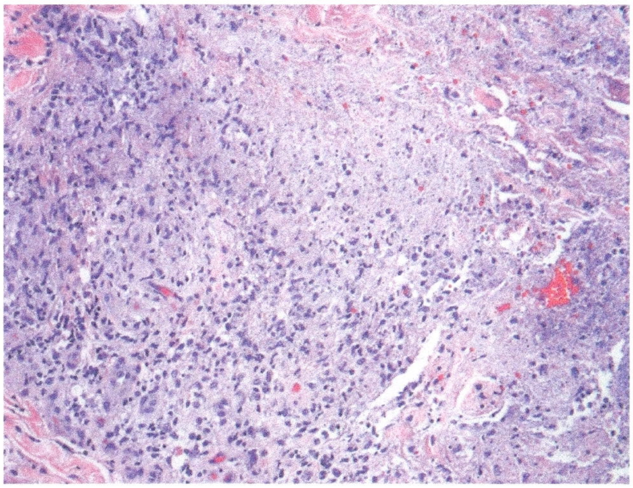

FIG. 3.58
Cutaneous tuberculosis. A suppurative and necrotizing granulomatous dermatitis is present.

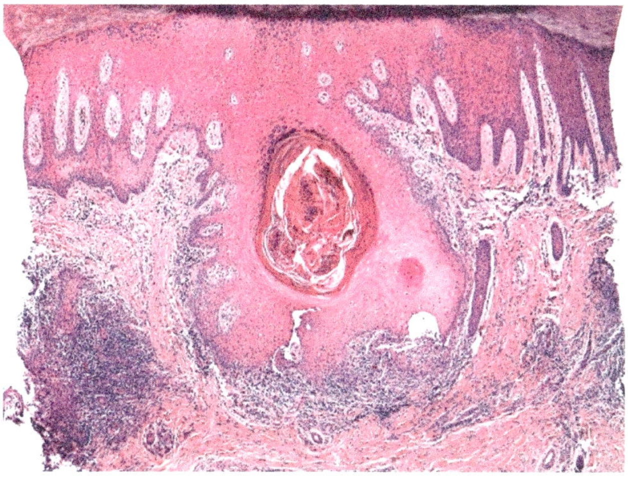

FIG. 3.59
Cutaneous tuberculosis. The epidermis is acanthotic and hyperkeratotic. There is a lymphocytic and neutrophilic infiltrate. Such lesions are often seen in association with verrucous tuberculosis.

The histologic findings in lupus vulgaris are variable but typically show a combination of suppurative and granulomatous dermatitis with necrosis (Fig. 3.58). Tuberculoid granulomas in the upper half of the dermis, which are composed of epithelioid cells with lymphocytic cuffing, may impinge on an atrophic, acanthotic, or ulcerated epidermis. Although necrosis is common, acid-fast bacilli (AFB) are usually sparse and difficult to find. The histologic features may simulate sarcoidosis.

Tuberculosis verrucosa cutis is characterized by verrucous hyperkeratosis with focal parakeratosis, hypergranulosis, and prominent epidermal hyperplasia, which may be pseudoepitheliomatous (Fig. 3.59). The dermal infiltrate is mainly neutrophilic; abscesses can form in the superficial dermis or within the pseudoepitheliomatous rete pegs. Although epithelioid granuloma is often present, central caseation is rare. AFB are rarely identified.

In scrofuloderma, massive necrotic tissue forms a sinus tract that extends to the ulcerated or atrophic epidermis. Epithelioid granulomas are present at the periphery. Although AFB usually can be found in smears from the affected area, they cannot always be demonstrated in tissue sections.

In orificial tuberculosis, there are ulcers with extensive necrosis and deep caseating granulomas containing numerous AFB.

CUTANEOUS MYCOBACTERIAL INFECTIONS (EXCLUDING LEPROSY)—PATHOLOGIC FEATURES

Histologic Features

- Suppurative and granulomatous dermatitis
- Necrosis or caseation is often, but not always, present
- Associated epidermal hyperplasia, especially in verrucous tuberculosis
- Ulceration and granulation tissue
- Other histologic reaction patterns include panniculitis, interstitial granulomatous dermatitis, vasculitis, abscess

Ancillary Studies

- Acid-fast (Ziehl-Neelsen) stain
- Immunohistochemistry
- Cultures
- Polymerase chain reaction studies

Differential Diagnosis

- Leprosy
- Other infections with granulomatous reactions, such as deep fungal infections
- Noninfectious granulomatous disease (e.g., foreign body reactions, drug reactions, Crohn's disease, sarcoidosis, and others)

Ancillary Studies

Fite stain or Ziehl-Neelsen (AFB stain) highlight AFB. Cultures allow a definitive diagnosis. PCR-based tests have proved useful in detecting and subclassifying AFB. Immunohistochemical detection systems for mycobacteria have also been developed, which are more sensitive than conventional histochemical stains.

Differential Diagnosis

The differential diagnosis includes other infections with suppurative and granulomatous reaction, in particular nontuberculous mycobacteria, leprosy, fungal infections, leishmaniasis, and syphilis.

Clinical correlation, special stains, or cultures are needed for the distinction of tuberculosis from noninfectious granulomatous reactions, such as sarcoidosis, cutaneous Crohn's disease, granulomatous drug reactions, granulomatous rosacea, and many other processes. Foreign body granulomas may contain polarizable material under the light microscope.

Prognosis and Treatment

Antituberculous chemotherapy remains the treatment of choice.

NONTUBERCULOUS MYCOBACTERIAL INFECTIONS (EXCLUDING LEPROSY)

Nontuberculous ("atypical") mycobacterial infections are caused by a heterogeneous group that excludes *M. tuberculosis.* They are AFB that are present in many different environments worldwide. There has been an increase in the incidence of infections caused by these organisms over the past decades. Although they often lead to systemic disease in immunocompromised patients, they may affect the skin in many ways. The microorganisms are often introduced at a site of trauma. They are generally classified according to colony pigmentation, optimal temperature, and growth rate. A few of them merit brief discussion here.

Clinical Findings

MYCOBACTERIUM MARINUM

Mycobacterium marinum is found worldwide in salt or fresh water. Lesions are usually limited to the skin because the organisms require a temperature of 30 to 32°C for optimal growth. Systemic dissemination is rare except for immunocompromised hosts. Cutaneous infections are often referred to as *swimming pool granuloma* or *fish tank granuloma*. Because of widespread use of chlorination, *M. marinum* infections today are rarely acquired in swimming pools and are more likely obtained in lakes. After an incubation period of 2 to 3 weeks, solitary erythematous to violaceous, hyperkeratotic papules form on the elbows, hands, feet, or knees (Fig. 3.60). These lesions subsequently develop into psoriasiform or verrucous nodules or plaques, with or without ulceration. Multiple lesions may be present and extend proximally along sites of lymphatic drainage (so-called sporotrichoid distribution). The lesions either spontaneously resolve in months or persist for years to heal with scarring. Most experts recommend antibiotic therapy for faster clearance of the infection. Superimposed bacterial infection can occur, which should be confirmed by culture or Gram stain.

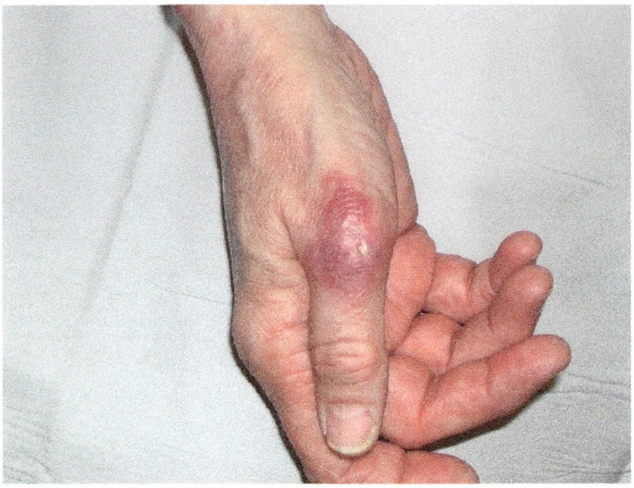

FIG. 3.60
Nontuberculous mycobacterial infection. Solitary erythematous nodule on a finger.

MYCOBACTERIUM ULCERANS (BURULI ULCER)

Infections caused by *M. ulcerans* generally occur in Central and West Africa, New Guinea, Australia, Southeast Asia, and Mexico. The disease, usually limited to extremities, is more frequent among children and young adults with a female preponderance. Because *M. ulcerans* preferentially proliferates at 32 to 33°C, the disease involves skin and subcutaneous tissue. Transmission requires contact through abraded, cut, or pricked skin with contaminated water, soil, or vegetation. After incubating for about 3 months, papules or pustules begin to appear, typically on the lower extremities; these soon evolve into a painless swelling that eventually ulcerates. The ulcer is deeply undermined with a characteristic edge. The ulceration and tissue necrosis result from an exotoxin, mycolactone, which the microorganism produces. The ulcer may persist for months to years, leading to significant scarring or lymphedema. Wide surgical excision and debridement are the best treatment.

MYCOBACTERIUM AVIUM COMPLEX (*M. AVIUM, M. INTRACELLULARE*, AND OTHERS)

Infections by this organism are common in individuals with HIV infection. *Mycobacterium avium* is primarily a pulmonary pathogen. Cutaneous involvement most often occurs through dissemination from a systemic infection in immunocompromised patients. However, cutaneous infections may occur via direct inoculation by a contaminated object. Skin lesions usually present as panniculitis, including subcutaneous nodules, which may ulcerate.

MYCOBACTERIUM HAEMOPHILUM

This organism was first identified in 1978 in a skin ulcer from a woman with Hodgkin's disease. It causes cutaneous, joint, bone, muscle, and pulmonary infections in immunocompromised patients and lymphadenitis in immunocompetent children. The spectrum of cutaneous lesions ranges from isolated, indistinct papules and nodules to panniculitis and vasculitis. *Mycobacterium haemophilum* is a slowly growing organism that grows best at 30 to 32°C and requires iron-supplement or ferric iron–containing compounds for growth. This bacillus is not usually isolated using standard culture techniques for mycobacteria.

OTHER NONTUBERCULOUS MYCOBACTERIAL INFECTIONS

Other nontuberculous mycobacteria rarely involve the skin. Infections are transmitted by abrasion or direct implantation through surgical procedures in immunocompromised individuals. The clinical features, which are highly variable, can include solitary verrucous nodules, abscesses, ulcerations, pseudotumors, and rosacea-like lesions.

Histologic Features

MYCOBACTERIUM MARINUM INFECTION

The histologic findings in *M. marinum* infection vary. They range from suppurative dermatitis with ulceration and necrosis in early lesions to tuberculoid granulomas at the late stage (Fig. 3.61). The epidermis often shows hyperkeratosis and papillomatosis and is occasionally ulcerated. The early lesions may have AFB evident with Fite stain.

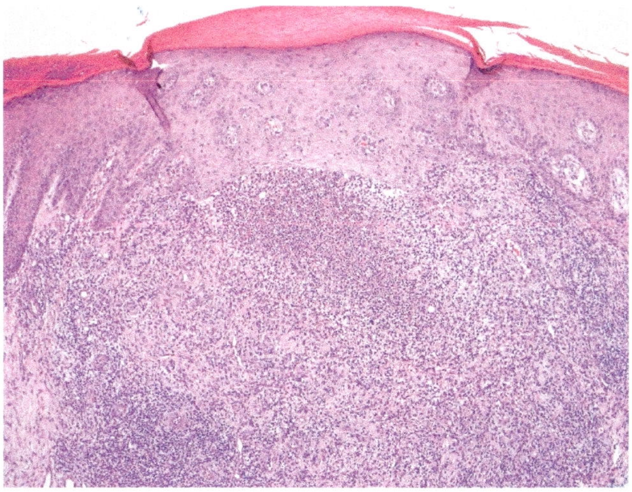

FIG. 3.61
Nontuberculous mycobacterial infection. Suppurative nodular dermatitis.

MYCOBACTERIUM ULCERANS INFECTION

In *M. ulcerans* infection, there is strikingly extensive coagulative necrosis that involves the dermis and the subcutaneous fat. A relatively sparse mixed inflammatory cell infiltrate can be found at the peripheral viable areas. Pseudoepitheliomatous hyperplasia or subcutaneous small vessel vasculitis may be present. Clumps of extracellular AFB are usually identified in the necrotic tissue.

MYCOBACTERIUM AVIUM COMPLEX

The histology is nonspecific but usually associated with granuloma formation. Staining for AFB usually shows many organisms within histiocytes.

MYCOBACTERIUM HAEMOPHILUM

The histologic spectrum includes a diffuse suppurative and granulomatous dermatitis, necrotizing or nonnecrotizing dermal granulomas, leukocytoclastic vasculitis, erythema nodosum–like reaction, lobular panniculitis (Fig. 3.62), or a mixed pattern of lichenoid and interstitial granulomatous dermatitis. Multiple Fite or AFB stains may be necessary to visualize rare bacilli. Occasionally, many organisms are found (Fig. 3.62).

OTHER NONTUBERCULOUS MYCOBACTERIAL INFECTIONS

The histopathologic changes are variable and rather nonspecific. Most often there is granulomatous dermatitis with poorly formed granulomas or a diffuse histiocytic infiltrate. Suppuration, folliculitis, or panniculitis may also be present. Microorganisms are generally difficult to find except in certain cases of *M. avium-intracellulare* infection.

Differential Diagnosis

The differential diagnosis is similar to that of cutaneous tuberculosis and includes other infectious as well as miscellaneous noninfectious granulomatous inflammatory reactions (sarcoidosis, Crohn's disease, drug reactions, reactions to foreign material).

Prognosis and Treatment

Infections by different types of nontuberculous mycobacteria require different treatment considerations. *M. marinum* infection usually spontaneously heals. However, most experts recommend antibiotic therapy to speed up clearance of the infection. For *M. ulcerans*, the

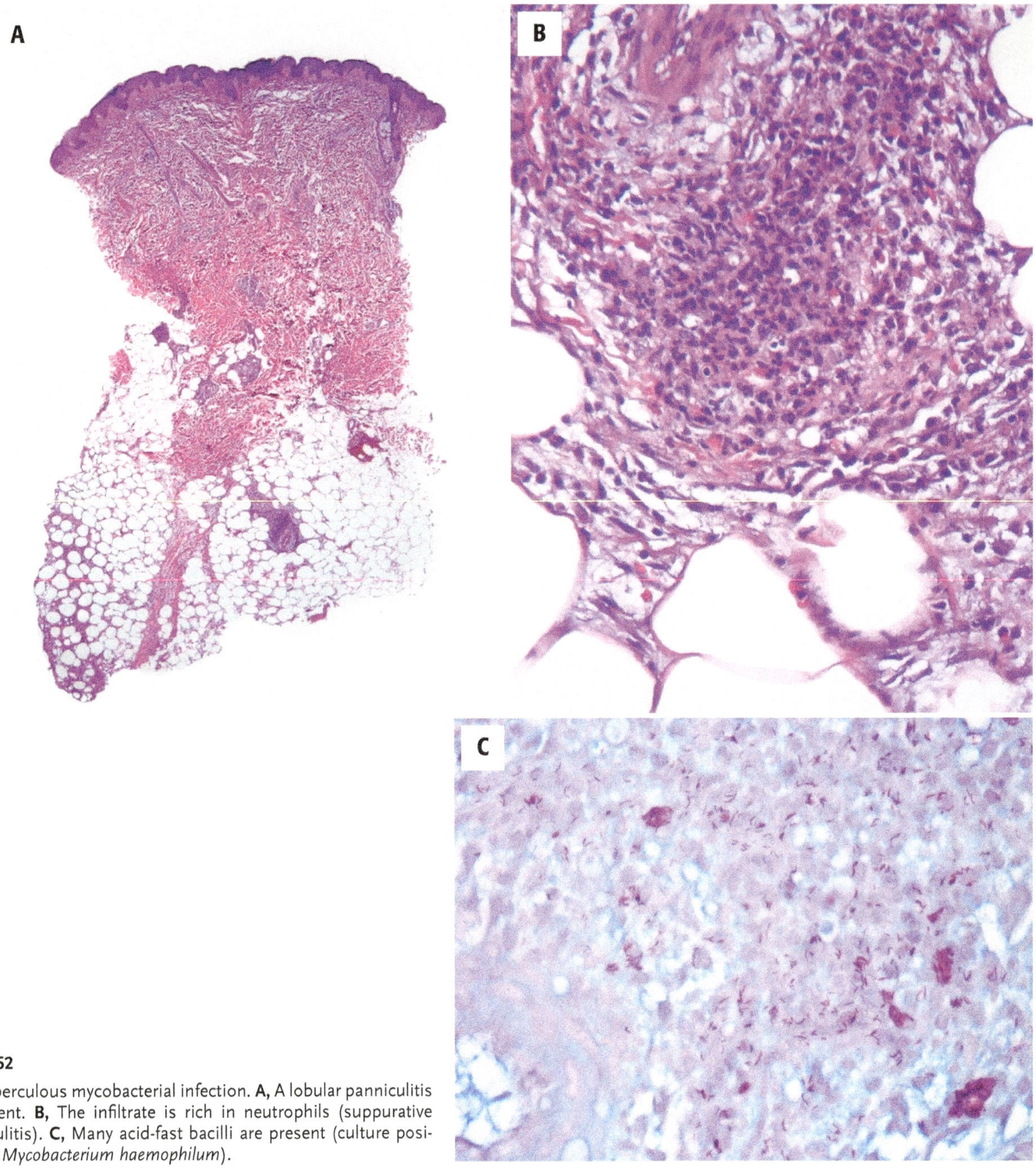

FIG. 3.62

Nontuberculous mycobacterial infection. **A,** A lobular panniculitis is present. **B,** The infiltrate is rich in neutrophils (suppurative panniculitis). **C,** Many acid-fast bacilli are present (culture positive for *Mycobacterium haemophilum*).

treatment of choice is surgical excision and debridement. Infections by *M. avium* complex should be treated aggressively with multidrug regimens.

LEPROSY

Leprosy is a chronic infection caused by *Mycobacterium leprae*, an obligate, intracellular, gram-positive, acid-fast microorganism. The disease mainly affects skin, nasal mucosa, and peripheral nerves.

Clinical Findings

Leprosy is primarily a disease of developing countries, especially in the tropical areas. India has two-thirds of the global leprosy burden. In the United States, new indigenous cases are reported mainly in Louisiana and Texas. The prevalence of leprosy has been decreasing in the past decade because of the effectiveness of multidrug therapy.

M. leprae is an intracellular organism most commonly transmitted from human to human. The course and presentation of an individual infected with *M. leprae* depend on the host response to the bacillus. The incubation period for leprosy is variable, on average 5 years. The organism is of low infectivity, and transmission requires prolonged or close contact. The portals of entries are thought to be skin and upper respiratory tract, particularly the nasal mucosa. The spectrum of clinical presentation and histopathologic findings of leprosy are currently classified according to the Ridley-Jopling classification. At one end of the spectrum is tuberculoid leprosy, which is a paucibacillary form with few lesions. On the other end is lepromatous leprosy, in which there are numerous lesions with myriad bacilli. In between are the clinical forms classified as borderline-tuberculoid, borderline, and borderline-lepromatous leprosy. This clinical-histologic classification has been shown to correlate closely with the level of cell-mediated immunity to the pathogen.

Indeterminate leprosy is a form better recognized in the endemic regions, seen before the appearance of well-developed lesions of leprosy. It usually manifests as single or multiple ill-defined hypopigmented or slightly erythematous macules, usually on the limbs. Slight impairment of sensation may be present. Most indeterminate leprosy lesions heal spontaneously, but approximately 25% of cases progress.

Tuberculoid leprosy is a relatively stable form seen in patients with strong immunologic host resistance and a markedly positive lepromin test result. Very well-demarcated annular patches or plaques with raised erythematous borders and central clearing are distributed asymmetrically on the trunk or extremities. Sensory impairment is an essential feature, and enlarging regional nerves often leads to palsy. The lesion is characteristically anesthetic and anhidrotic.

Borderline-tuberculoid leprosy is usually associated with more numerous, smaller lesions than classic tuberculoid leprosy. Hair impairment and hypoesthesia are more prevalent.

Borderline leprosy represents the middle of the spectrum, but it is unstable, with patients quickly upgrading or downgrading to a more stable stage. Cutaneous lesions are larger, usually ill-defined, erythematous or copper-colored, annular patches (Fig. 3.63) or ill-defined plaques (Fig. 3.64). Borderline-lepromatous leprosy has more numerous and poorly defined lesions than borderline-tuberculoid leprosy. These lesions are shinier and less anesthetic than the tuberculoid type. Nodular lesions may be present.

Lepromatous leprosy occurs in patients with minimal or absent host response (Fig. 3.65). The cutaneous lesions are usually symmetric, poorly demarcated, erythematous and hypopigmented macules, patches, and nodules, frequently involving the earlobes and nasal mucosa. Multiple facial nodules, which spare the eyebrows, give a classical leonine appearance. When local nerves are involved, lepromatous leprosy causes hypoesthesia of the affected areas. Multiple autoantibodies are frequently detected in lepromatous leprosy, and there is an increased incidence of vitiligo.

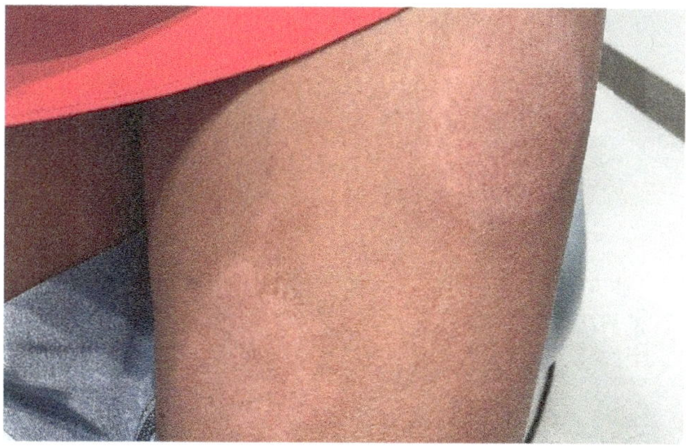

FIG. 3.63

Leprosy. Borderline-lepromatous leprosy with more numerous and poorly defined lesions than borderline-tuberculoid leprosy.

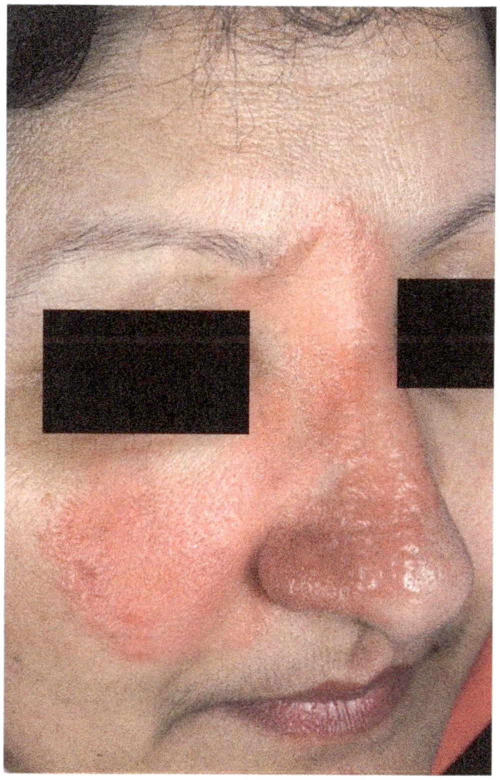

FIG. 3.64

Leprosy. Ill-defined erythematous patches and plaques are present on the face (borderline leprosy).

Histoid leprosy—a rare, nodular variant of lepromatous leprosy—usually develops in longstanding cases, possibly associated with drug resistance. It is characterized by cutaneous, or dermal, or subcutaneous nodules and plaques (Fig. 3.66).

Erythema nodosum leprosum is an immune complex–mediated reaction associated with multidrug therapy (Fig. 3.67). It occurs in 25% to 70% of lepromatous leprosy cases and occasionally in borderline-lepromatous

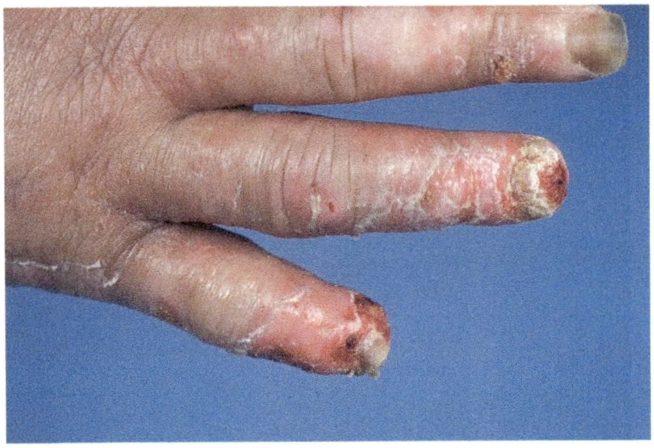

FIG. 3.65
Leprosy. Digits with neurosensory loss undergo tissue destruction (lepromatous leprosy).

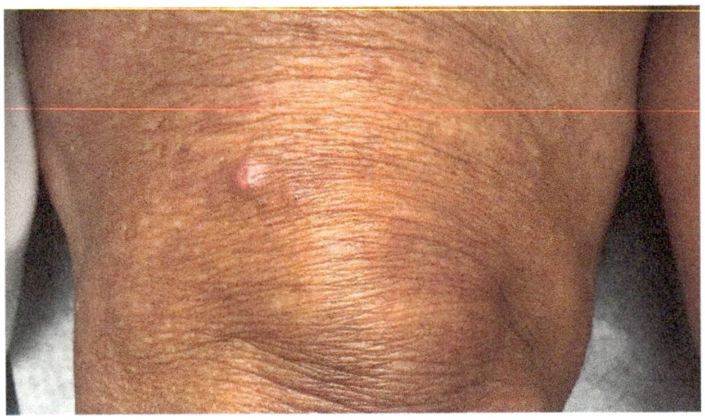

FIG. 3.66
Histoid leprosy. Dome-shaped erythematous cutaneous or subcutaneous nodules and plaques.

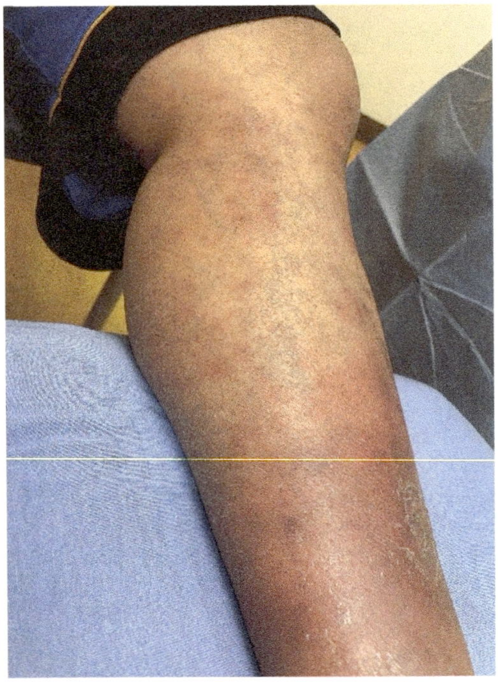

FIG. 3.67
Erythema nodosum leprosum. Painful, erythematous, and violaceous nodules, often involving the extremities.

cases during therapy. The clinical features include widespread eruptions of painful, erythematous, and violaceous nodules, often involving the extremities, and associated with systemic symptoms. Individual lesions last for 1 to 3 weeks. Lucio's phenomenon, a diffuse nonnodular form of lepromatous leprosy, is primarily observed in Mexican patients and is associated with irregularly shaped, jagged purpuric lesions and hemorrhagic ulcers as a result of the underlying vasculitic changes.

Histologic Features

Indeterminate leprosy is characterized by a superficial and deep perivascular and periadnexal lymphohistiocytic infiltrate that involves less than 5% of the dermis. A mild proliferation of Schwann cells may be observed, but marked neural thickening is usually absent. Bacilli are only occasionally seen with Fite stain. Skin biopsies of tuberculoid leprosy resemble those of cutaneous tuberculosis, especially lupus vulgaris (Fig. 3.68). Well-formed granulomas without caseation can be seen throughout the dermis without a Grenz zone; they are composed of epithelioid cells, giant cells, and lymphocytes, and they frequently surround neurovascular bundles and erector pili muscle and may destroy the eccrine glands. They can erode the overlying epidermis or extend into peripheral nerves or pilar muscles. AFB are rarely identified with the Fite stain.

In borderline-tuberculoid leprosy, the noncaseating granulomas are less evident, and nerve destruction is less prominent. The lymphocytic mantles about tubercles may be incomplete or poorly developed. A subepidermal grenz zone may or may not be present. AFB are often absent.

Borderline leprosy shows collections of epithelioid histiocytes with no giant cells and very few lymphocytes. AFB are easy to find in this condition.

Borderline-lepromatous granulomas consist of aggregates of lymphocytes and macrophages containing abundant granular to foamy cytoplasm (Fig. 3.69). Numerous AFB are seen with Fite stain. Lymphocytes and histiocytes infiltrate the nerve, producing laminated perineurium. Sheets of macrophages with a granular to foamy cytoplasm arranged in a perineural, perivascular, and periappendiceal fashion characterize lepromatous leprosy. The foamy histiocytes of leprosy resemble those seen in xanthoma; they are called lepra or Virchow cells. AFB load the cytoplasm of macrophages, endothelial cells, sweat glands, nerves, and Schwann cells. Effacement of the epidermal rete ridges with a distinct Grenz zone is often present along with scattered lymphocytes and plasma cells.

The histology of histoid leprosy (Fig. 3.70) is characterized by relatively circumscribed nodules that are composed of predominantly spindle cells intermixed with small collections of foamy macrophages and arranged in a storiform pattern. Because the spindle-shaped cells are

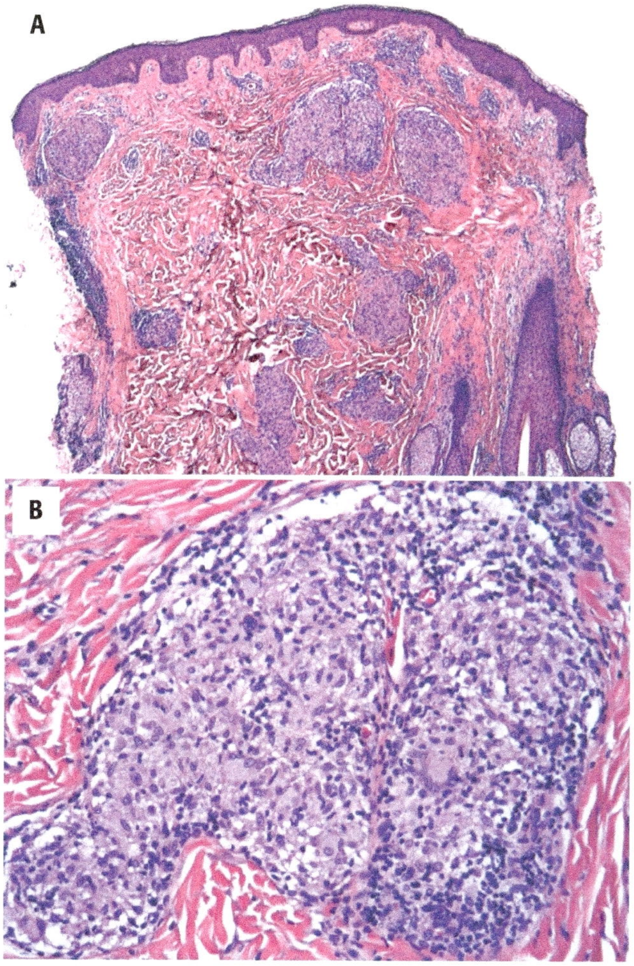

FIG. 3.68

Tuberculoid leprosy. **A,** A nonnecrotizing granulomatous reaction is present. **B,** Well-formed epithelioid granulomas are noted with a rim of lymphocytes.

of dermal dendritic origin (expressing factor XIIIa), the histologic findings may closely resemble a fibrous histiocytoma. Lesions of histoid leprosy are usually heavily infected with numerous AFB.

At the sites of preexisting lepromatous leprosy, erythema nodosum leprosum shows a mixed dermal infiltrate of lymphocytes and a variable number of neutrophils (Fig. 3.71). The cytoplasm of dermal macrophages contains fragmented AFB. Leukocytoclastic vasculitis or panniculitis may also be present.

In Lucio's phenomenon, necrotizing vasculitis of the small dermal vessels is found, often associated with epidermal infarction. Less commonly, vascular occlusion occurs when the superficial vessels are thrombosed or endothelial cells swell.

Ancillary Studies

Fite stain helps to identify microorganisms. PCR tests are more sensitive.

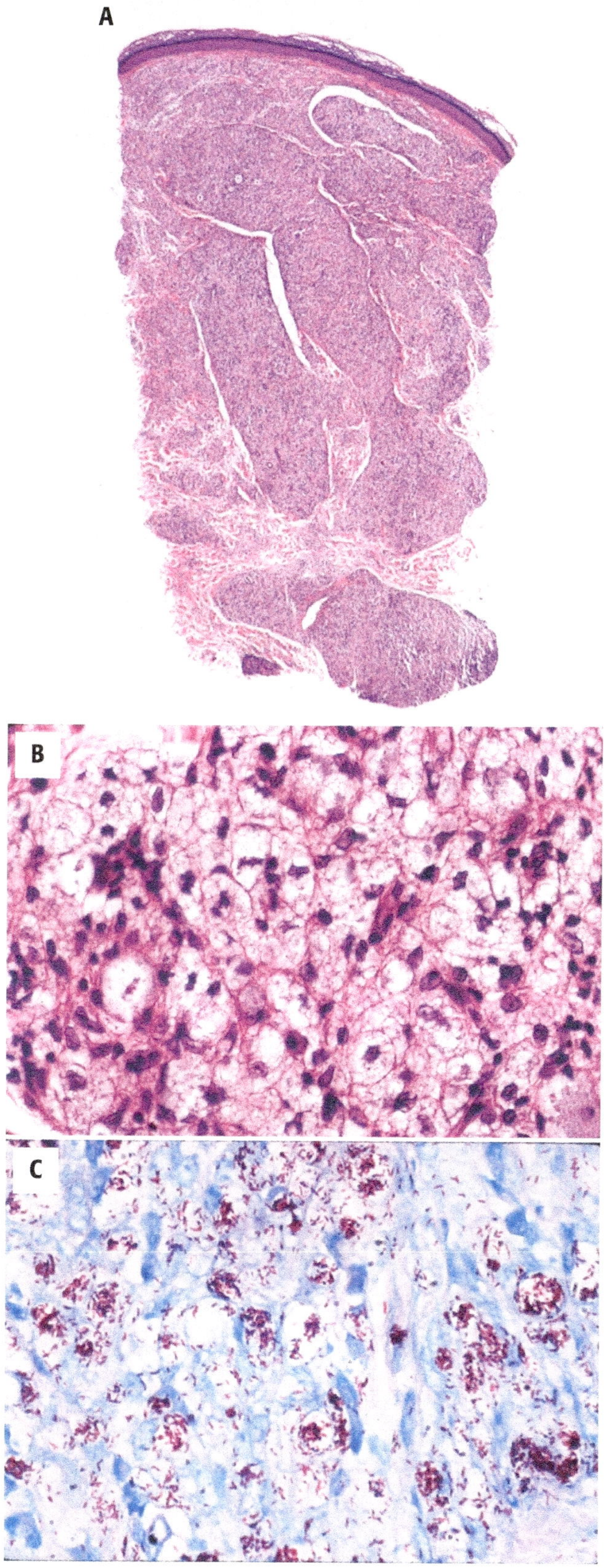

FIG. 3.69

Lepromatous leprosy. **A,** Dense diffuse sheets of histiocytes are present. **B,** The infiltrate includes many foamy histiocytes. **C,** Acid-fast bacilli are numerous.

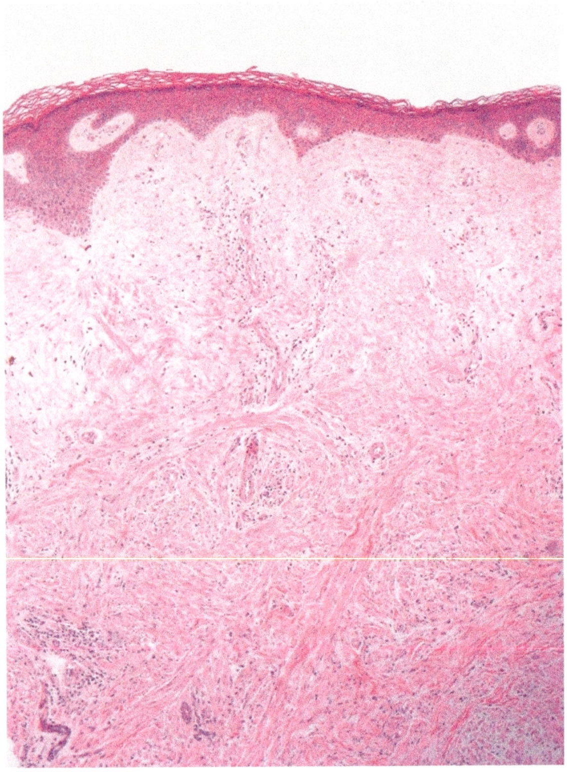

FIG. 3.70
Histiocytoid leprosy. A dermal fibroma–like lesion is identified.

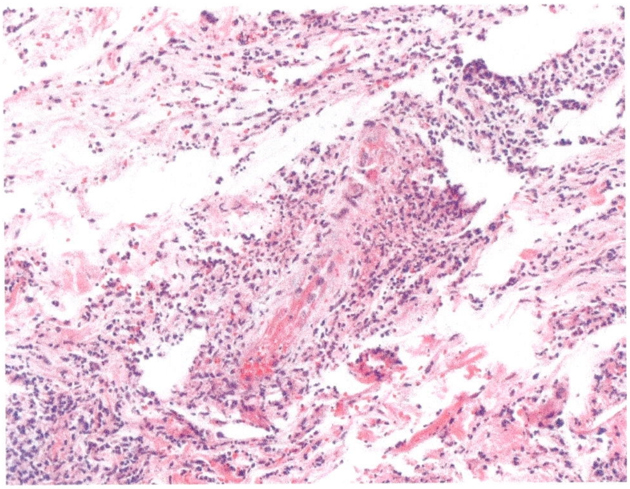

FIG. 3.71
Erythema nodosum leprosum. Mixed neutrophil-rich infiltrate with features of leukocytoclastic vasculitis.

Differential Diagnosis

Sarcoidosis may be difficult to differentiate from tuberculoid leprosy if the Fite stain findings are negative. Finding the elongated tuberculoid leprosy lesions that follow neurovascular bundles and the remnants of nerves (via silver stain) within granulomas are helpful clues. Cutaneous tuberculosis and tuberculoid leprosy are histologically similar. Culture and clinical findings are important in differentiating these two diseases. Any tendency to involve the nerves points toward a diagnosis of leprosy. Similar to lepromatous leprosy, sheets of foamy histiocytes occur in xanthoma. However, Fite stain results are negative in the latter. The round intracytoplasmic inclusions within the histiocytes of rhinoscleroma and histoplasmosis distinguish these from lepromatous leprosy. Granular cell tumor may mimic lepromatous leprosy because the neoplastic cells have a perineural distribution and granular cytoplasm. However, a granular cell tumor is usually overlaid by pseudoepitheliomatous hyperplasia, and the cytoplasm appears more eosinophilic than the macrophages in leprosy.

Prognosis and Treatment

Multidrug chemotherapy is directed at the infection itself or at a reactional state. Multiple different regimens are currently available; the cure rate is greater than 80%.

ACTINOMYCOSIS, NOCARDIOSIS, AND BOTRYOMYCOSIS

Cutaneous actinomycosis, nocardiosis, and botryomycosis are uncommon, chronic, localized infections with characteristic small, yellow, or white granules composed of bacteria. Gram-positive filamentous bacteria, predominantly *Actinomyces israelii* and *Nocardia brasiliensis*, cause actinomycosis and nocardiosis, respectively. The pathogenic organisms in botryomycosis are either gram-positive or gram-negative bacteria.

Clinical Findings

Although cutaneous actinomycosis and nocardiosis are rare, they are distributed throughout the world. In the United States, actinomycosis typically infects young farm workers. Botryomycosis affects rural patients in developing countries worldwide. It has been reported in immunocompromised individuals and patients with diabetes. In all three diseases, trauma or surgery can implant the microorganisms. Actinomycosis predominantly manifests as cervicofacial involvement associated with poor oral hygiene or dental extraction; whereas nocardiosis primarily affects the extremities, botryomycosis usually afflicts hands, feet, head, and inguinal and gluteal areas. The lesions present as fluctuant swellings, subcutaneous abscesses, and formations of draining sinuses (Fig. 3.72). Pus extruding through the sinus tracts eliminates the bacteria as yellow grains (sulfur granules in actinomycosis) or as white grains (in nocardiosis and botryomycosis).

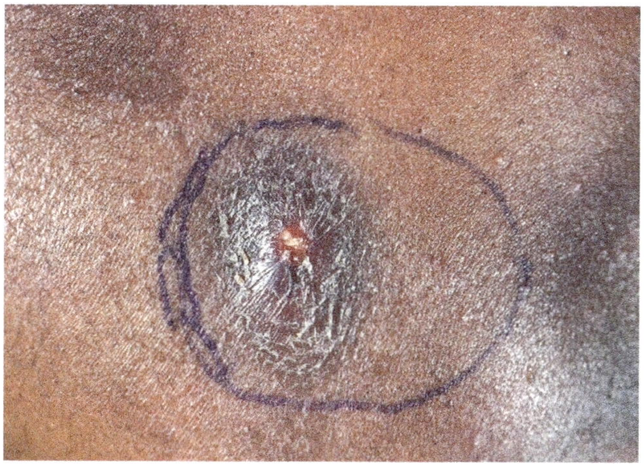

FIG. 3.72
Actinomycetoma. A dermal and subcutaneous nodule is present with focal drainage of pus.

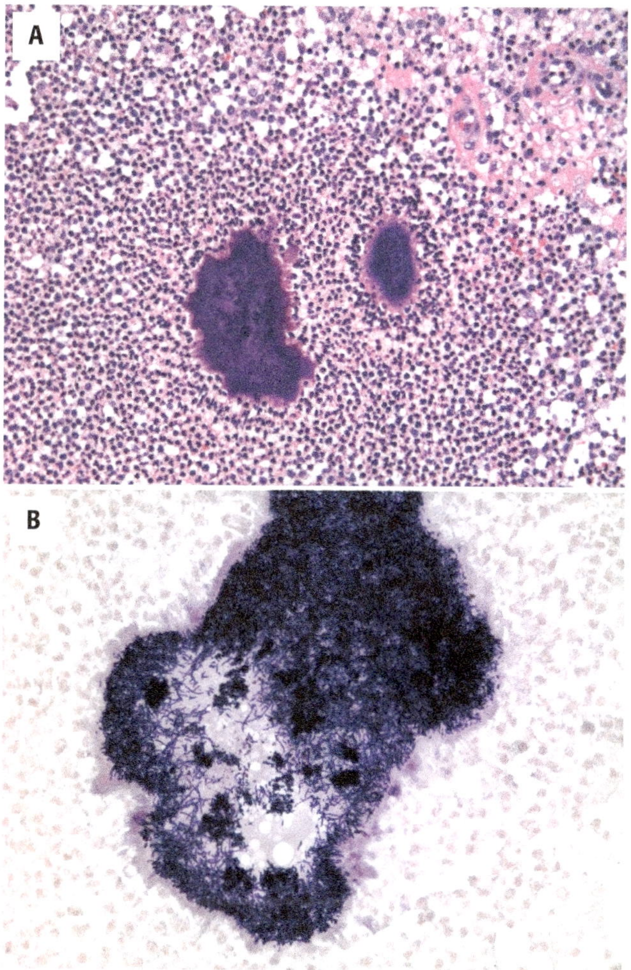

FIG. 3.73
Actinomyces. **A,** Colonies of filamentous bacteria are associated with suppurative inflammatory cell infiltrate. **B,** The bacilli are gram positive.

Histologic Features

There is usually a subcutaneous neutrophilic abscess surrounded by granulation tissue and fibrosis. In actinomycosis, one or more sulfur granules, 20 μm to 4 mm in diameter, are present in a microabscess (Fig. 3.73). The granules are composed of thin filamentous, branching, bacteria, 1 μm in diameter, with a beaded appearance. The microorganisms tend to be crowded, radiating in parallel at the periphery, and associated with deposits of eosinophilic material or Hoeppli-Splendore reaction. Nocardia is another gram-positive bacillus that may form grains similar to actinomyces (Fig. 3.74). Actinomyces is usually easier to find on routine H&E-stained sections than Nocardia. The granules of botryomycosis are composed of clusters of cocci with a peripheral, radial deposition of intensely eosinophilic material; the granules may range from 2 μm to 2 mm in size (Fig. 3.75).

Ancillary Studies

Actinomyces organisms are gram positive but acid-fast negative. They also stain positively with the PAS and GMS stains. Nocardia is also gram and PAS positive. In contrast to actinomyces, the acid-fast stain is often weakly positive. Botryomycosis may stain either gram positive or negative.

Differential Diagnosis

Actinomycosis, nocardiosis, and botryomycosis are distinguished from each other and from other causes of deep abscesses by their characteristic morphology and by Gram and acid-fast staining reactions.

Prognosis and Treatment

To penetrate fibrosis and suppuration with antibiotics, it is often necessary to treat patients for prolonged periods with high doses to reach adequate serum drug concentrations. Although the prognosis of patients with localized infection is generally favorable, the mortality rate can be high in patients with disseminated infection.

TREPONEMAL INFECTIONS

SYPHILIS

Syphilis—a generalized infectious disease caused by the spirochete *Treponema pallidum*—is usually transmitted via sexual contact. Congenital infection and nonsexual

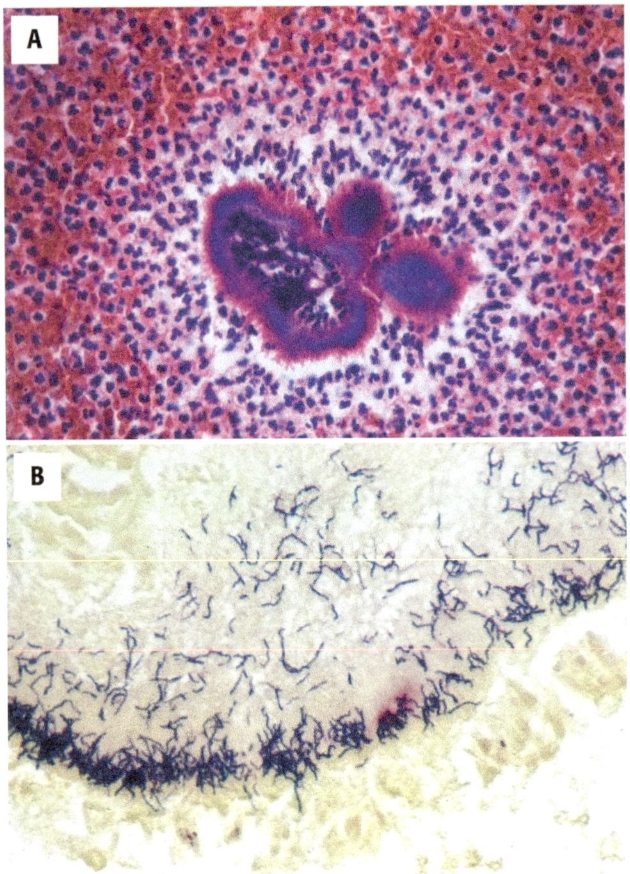

FIG. 3.74

Nocardia. **A,** Colonies of filamentous bacteria are present in association with a suppurative infiltrate. **B,** The bacilli are gram positive.

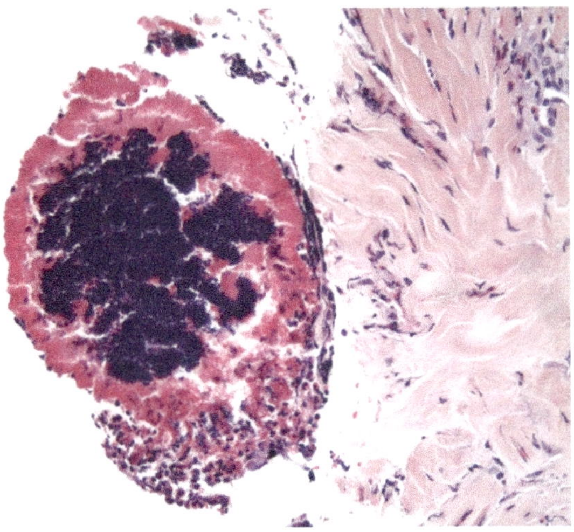

FIG. 3.75

Botryomycosis. A peripheral eosinophilic layer surrounds central blue-staining bacteria (Splendore-Hoeppli phenomenon).

transmission to children from affected parents rarely occur. Acquired syphilis is classified into four stages: primary, secondary, latent, and tertiary. Latent syphilis refers to a period after the cessation of manifestation of secondary syphilis with no apparent disease but positive serology. The spirochetes are easily identified from specimens obtained during the early stages, primary and secondary syphilis. The spirochetes usually cannot be found in late stages.

SYPHILIS—DISEASE FACT SHEET

Chronic venereal disease caused by infection by *Treponema pallidum*

Patient Group

- Sexually active adults
- Increased incidence among HIV-infected men

Site of Involvement

- Primary syphilis: anogenital region
- Secondary syphilis: generalized, trunk, and extremities
- Tertiary syphilis: CNS, lung, bone, skin

Clinical Findings

- Primary syphilis
  - Chancre ulcer
- Secondary syphilis
  - Maculopapular or papulosquamous eruption (may simulate miscellaneous inflammatory dermatoses)
  - Alopecia
  - Condyloma lata
- Tertiary syphilis
  - Gummas–Neurosyphilis
  - Cardiovascular complications

Prognosis and Treatment

- Favorable, if treated (penicillin)

Clinical Findings

PRIMARY SYPHILIS

The initial lesion of syphilis that arises at the site of treponemal penetration involving genital or perianal skin is called the primary chancre (Fig. 3.76). After an incubation period that ranges from 10 to 90 days, the primary chancre begins as a solitary, dusty red papule. Later it becomes a well-demarcated, firm, painless ulcer with indurated borders. Regional lymphadenopathy is often present. Untreated, the chancre may persist for 1 to 6 weeks. It usually resolves within 2 weeks after treatment.

SECONDARY SYPHILIS

In untreated patients, multiplying treponemes leads to secondary syphilis approximately 3 to 12 weeks after the appearance of primary chancre. In 80% to 95% of secondary syphilis cases, skin eruptions develop. The rash may be accompanied by constitutional flu-like symptoms, including fever, hepatitis, and lymphadenopathy. Secondary syphilis is clinically variable: it may mimic a wide variety of skin diseases. Most commonly, there is a generalized eruption of erythematous to copper-colored macules or papules with a guttate psoriatic appearance

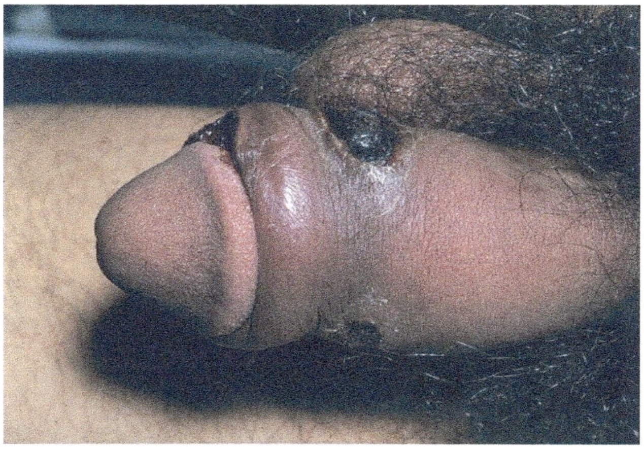

FIG. 3.76
Syphilis. Primary lesion (chancre).

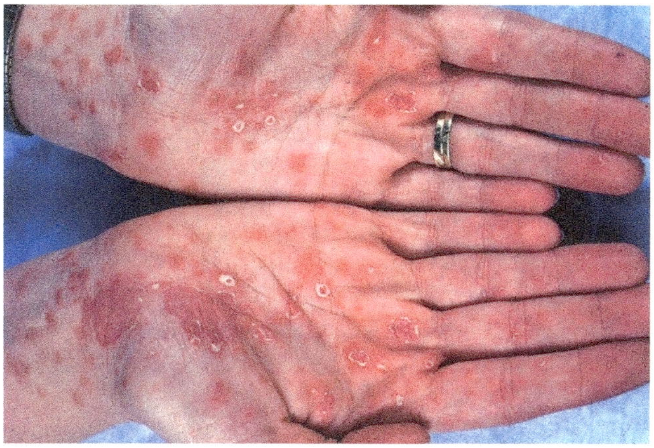

FIG. 3.77
Secondary syphilis. Maculopapular erythematous eruption on palms.

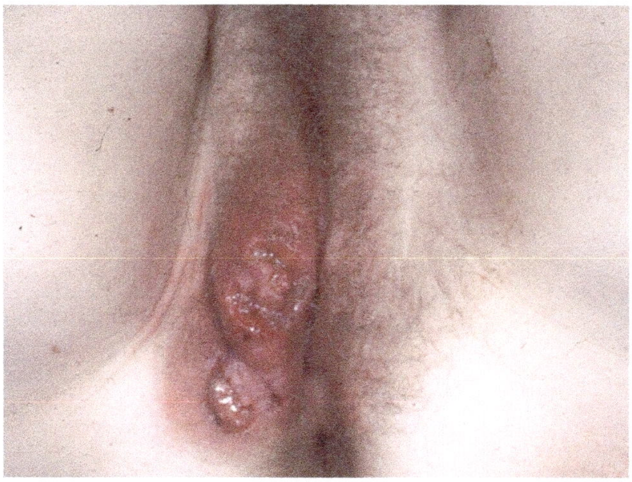

FIG. 3.78
Syphilis. Condyloma latum.

(Fig. 3.77). However, the lesions may be lichenoid, annular, follicular, pustular, nodular, or ulcerated. Palmoplantar involvement is often prominent, and a "moth-eaten" alopecia is characteristic. The lesions termed condylomata lata (Fig. 3.78) are the moist plaques in the anogenital area that may resemble condyloma acuminata. In patients with concurrent HIV infection, there may be an atypical presentation with more accelerated progression with ulceration, and necrosis, "lues maligna," may occur. If untreated, the symptoms of secondary syphilis may resolve and relapse over several years.

LATENT SYPHILIS

The symptoms of secondary syphilis subside spontaneously over time even in the absence of treatment. In this latent phase of syphilis without clinical symptoms, only serologic testing results remain positive.

TERTIARY SYPHILIS

In approximately one-third of patients with latent syphilis, tertiary syphilis appears 6 months to many years after the primary infection. Multiple organ systems can be affected; cardiovascular disease and neurologic disease are especially life threatening. Cutaneous manifestation may be either nodular or gummatous. The nodular form manifests as superficial, firm, painless nodules, often in a group. Mild necrosis may be present. The gummas are characterized by deep-pink to dusky-red nodules or plaques with extensive necrosis and various geometric configurations.

Histologic Features

PRIMARY SYPHILIS

The epidermis is acanthotic at the margins of the ulcer or erosion, becoming thinner and more edematous toward the eroded center (Fig. 3.79). The perivascular and diffuse dermal infiltrate is composed of lymphocytes, plasma cells, histiocytes, and a few neutrophils. Endothelial proliferation and swelling are characteristic (Fig. 3.79B). Spirochetes may be seen with silver (Warthin-Starry or Levaditi) or immunohistochemical stains in a perivascular distribution or in the epidermis (Fig. 3.80).

SYPHILIS—PATHOLOGIC FEATURES

Histologic Features

- Primary syphilis
  - Ulcer with lymphoplasmacellular and neutrophilic infiltrate
  - Positive for spirochetes on special stains
- Secondary syphilis
  - Psoriasiform, lichenoid, spongiotic or perivascular patterns
  - Mixed patterns (especially lichenoid and psoriasiform) are common
  - Lymphocytes are often accompanied by plasma cells and neutrophils
  - Granulomas may be present

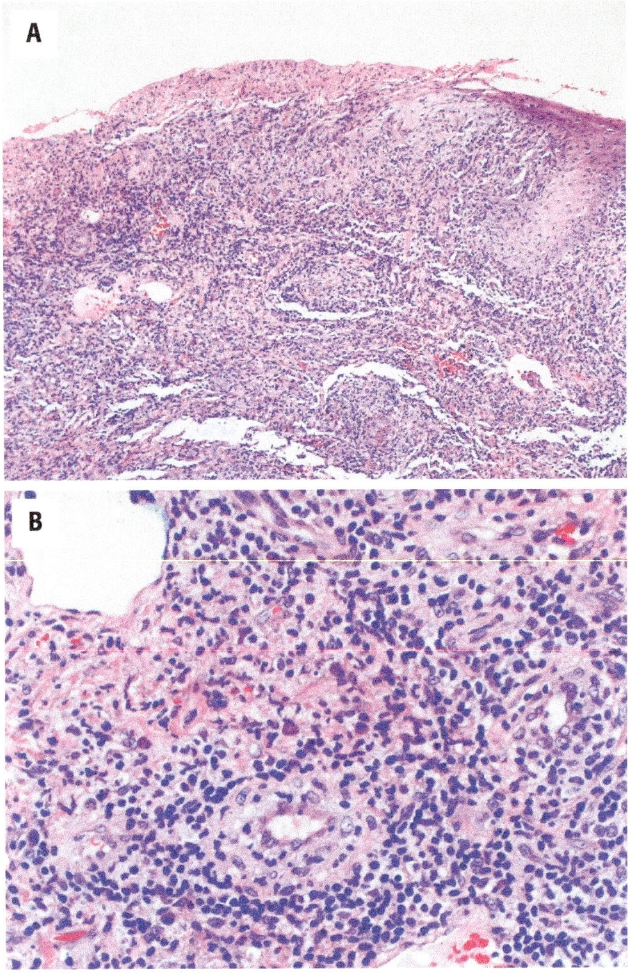

FIG. 3.79

Primary syphilis. **A,** The epidermis is acanthotic at the margins of the ulcer, becoming thinner and more edematous toward the ulcerated center. **B,** Prominent endothelial proliferation and swelling.

- ▸▸ Tertiary syphilis
  - Necrotizing granulomas

Ancillary Studies

- ▸▸ Immunohistochemistry for *T. pallidum*
- ▸▸ Dark field examination
- ▸▸ Warthin-Starry or Levaditi stain
- ▸▸ Serologic studies

Differential Diagnosis

- ▸▸ Miscellaneous inflammatory dermatoses
- ▸▸ Other spirochetal infections (Lyme disease, *Borrelia*, endemic syphilis)

SECONDARY SYPHILIS

Lesions of secondary syphilis demonstrate considerable histologic variability. A superficial and deep, perivascular or periadnexal plasma cell infiltrate is present in 70% to 80% of cases. Plasma cells are less pronounced in the macular lesions. The dermal infiltrate may also become lichenoid, obscuring the dermal-epidermal interface. Epidermal involvement is common, especially in the papulosquamous lesions (Fig. 3.81). Psoriasiform epidermal hyperplasia, parakeratosis, spongiosis, basal vacuolar changes, and microabscesses with neutrophils or other less common reactions such as granulomatous, vesicular, ulcerative, neutrophilic, and vascular patterns have been reported. A combined psoriasiform and lichenoid dermatitis with plasma cells is a common pattern. Tuberculoid granulomas may be identified, particularly in lesions that have been present for months. Spirochetes can be seen with the silver stain in about 30% of cases (Fig. 3.80C). In syphilitic alopecia, perifollicular lymphoid infiltrate, with follicular plugging is a constant finding.

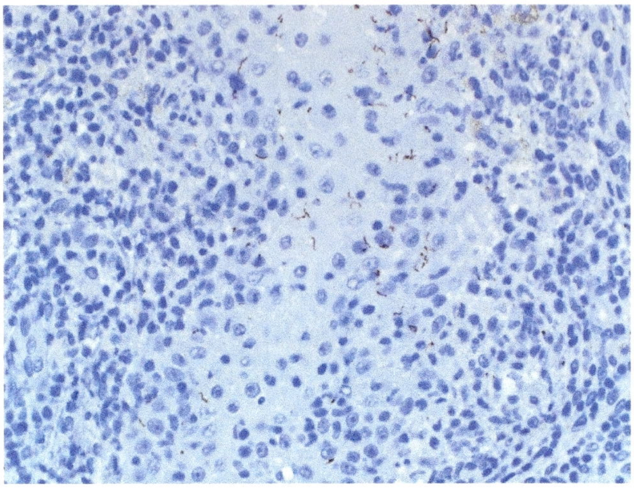

FIG. 3.80

Primary syphilis. Immunohistochemical staining for *T. pallidum* in the epidermis.

TERTIARY SYPHILIS

The nodular form is characterized by dermal tuberculoid granulomas with surrounding plasma cells and lymphocytes. The deeper and more destructive gummatous form produces extensive central caseation necrosis, which is surrounded by a peripheral mixed-cell infiltrate. Spirochetes are absent in tertiary syphilis.

Ancillary Studies

TISSUE TESTS

Treponemes may be visualized in exudates from genital ulcers using darkfield examination. The Warthin-Starry silver stain can help identify the organisms with a "corkscrew" shape in primary or secondary lesions. Reagents for immunohistochemical detection and specific primers for sensitive rapid PCR tests have also been developed.

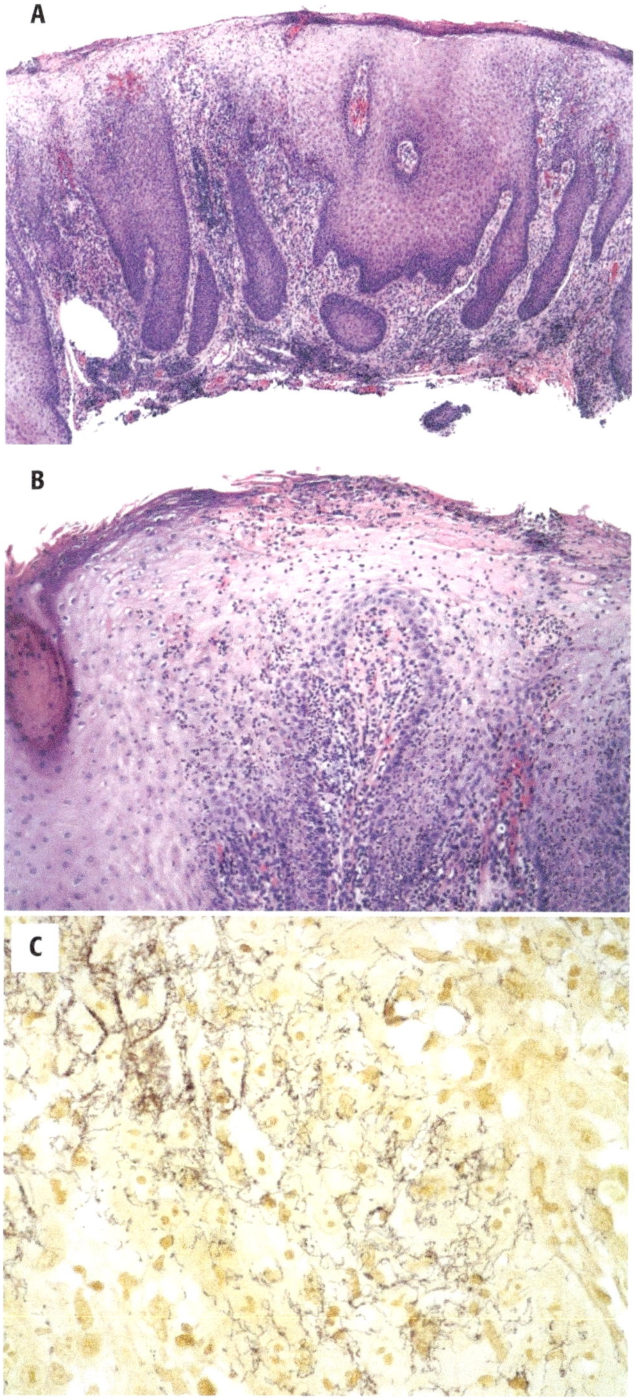

FIG. 3.81

Secondary syphilis. **A,** Psoriasiform dermatitis. **B,** There is a mixed inflammatory cell infiltrate. **C,** Spirochetes are identified on a silver stain (modified Steiner).

SEROLOGIC TESTS

The nontreponemal serologic tests, including rapid plasma regain (RPR) and Venereal Disease Research Laboratory (VDRL) tests, are 78% to 100% sensitive in various stages of syphilis. Positive results are verified by treponemal-specific testing, such as fluorescent treponemal antibody absorption (FTA-abs). Despite adequate treatment, the FTA-abs remains reactive for life in most patients.

Differential Diagnosis

Primary syphilis is histologically differentiated from chancroid by the absence of the three distinctive zones and by the Gram-negative coccobacilli characteristic of chancroid. The differential diagnosis is broad. In lichen planus, lichen striatus, or lichenoid drug reaction, the lichenoid infiltrate may resemble secondary syphilis. However, plasma cells and endothelial swelling are not prominent features of these conditions. Although swollen endothelial cells and a lichenoid infiltrate could be seen in both pityriasis lichenoides varioliformis acuta and secondary syphilis, pityriasis lichenoides et varioliformis acuta (PLEVA) has characteristic erythrocyte extravasation and basal layer vacuolization. PLEVA usually lacks plasma cells. Granulomatous secondary syphilis may closely resemble sarcoidosis and tuberculoid leprosy except for the presence of prominent plasma cells in the former. A positive silver stain result helps establish the diagnosis of treponemal infection.

Compared with tertiary syphilis, lupus vulgaris lacks the prominent plasmacytic infiltrate.

Prognosis and Treatment

Parenteral penicillin remains the treatment of choice for all stages of syphilis. The vast majority of patients are cured, improved, or stabilized if the correct dosage is administered.

NONVENEREAL TREPONEMAL INFECTIONS—YAWS, BEJEL, AND PINTA

Brief mention is made of yaws, endemic syphilis (bejel), and pinta, all nonvenereal treponematoses. Yaws is caused by *Treponema pertenue* infection through direct contact among children in tropical countries. The primary and secondary lesions are usually ulcerated, and the tertiary lesions are gummatous. Histologically, the ulcerated lesions resemble syphilis. Endemic syphilis is a chronic childhood disease involving skin, bone, and cartilage. It is transmitted through close contact and is more prevalent in dry, arid climates, particularly in the Middle East. The clinical and histologic findings overlap with venereally acquired syphilis and yaws. The disease has been essentially eradicated, and the primary lesion is rarely encountered. Pinta is a contagious tropical disease in the Caribbean area and Central and South

America caused by *Treponema carateum* infection. There is significant clinical and histologic overlap among its three stages.

LYME DISEASE

Lyme disease—a multisystemic disease caused by the spirochete *Borrelia burgdorferi*—produces characteristic cutaneous manifestations such as erythema chronicum migrans (ECM) in early stages and acrodermatitis chronica atrophicans in late stages.

Clinical Findings

Lyme disease is the most prevalent arthropod-borne infection in the United States. It is more commonly seen among children and adolescents. It is transmitted via a bite of an infected deer tick in the summer months in endemic areas of Connecticut, New York, New Jersey, Rhode Island, Delaware, Pennsylvania, Wisconsin, and Maryland (*Ixodes scapularis*) or Pacific Coast (*Ixodex pacificus*). The primary clinical manifestations include dermatologic, rheumatologic, neurologic, and cardiac abnormalities. The disease is loosely divided into three overlapping clinical stages: early localized infection, early disseminated infection, and late infection.

Early localized infection occurs 3 to 30 days after the tick bite. It is characterized by ECM, typically at the site of the tick bite, in 60% to 83% of patients. The lesion of ECM typically begins as a centrifugally expanding warm, erythematous, smooth macule or patch that forms a large, round lesion 20 cm or larger in diameter, often with central clearing (Fig. 3.82). ECM is frequently associated with constitutional flu-like symptoms and lymphadenopathy. These lesions usually fade within 3 to 4 weeks. Early disseminated infection is presumably caused by hematogenous spread of *B. burgdorferi*. Multiple ECM lesions are reported in more than 50% of patients along with malaise, severe fatigue, headache, and transient neck stiffness. A significant proportion of patients develop neurologic, cardiac, or musculoskeletal manifestations. Late infection is characterized by arthritis and neurologic complications. Cutaneous manifestations include acrodermatitis chronica atrophicans and the sclerodermoid lesions. The acrodermatitis chronica atrophicans lesions begin as erythematous nodules or plaques having a doughy consistency, often involving bilateral distal extremities. As the lesions expand, the central areas may show atrophic changes with loss of hair and poikiloderma. In the late atrophic stage, the skin has a glistening appearance with prominent blood vessels.

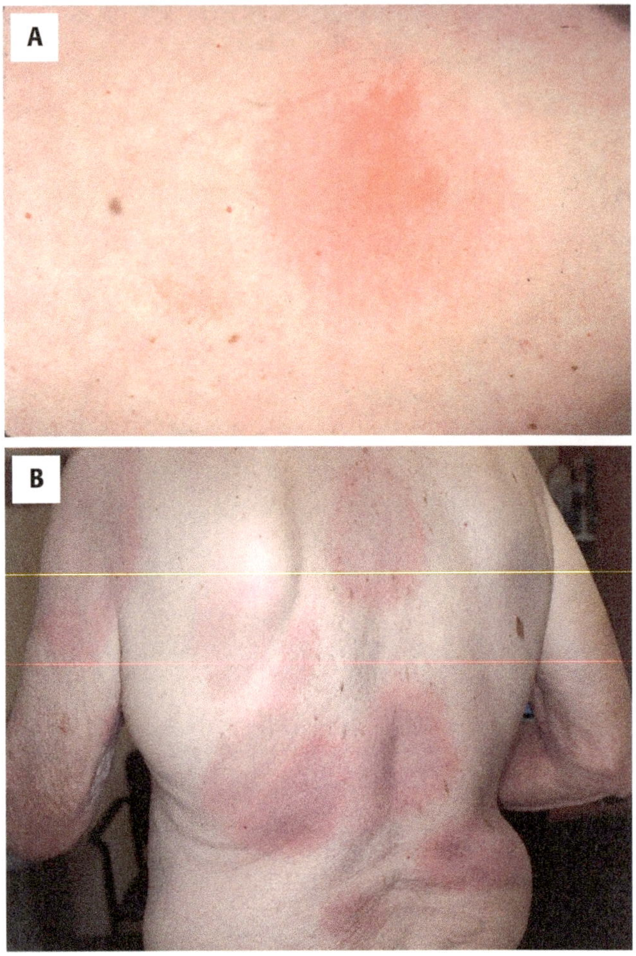

FIG. 3.82

Cutaneous Lyme disease. Erythema chronicum migrans. **A**, Single annular erythematous lesion. **B**, Multiple annular lesions.

Histologic Features

Histologically, ECM typically demonstrates a moderately dense superficial and deep perivascular and interstitial infiltrate of lymphocytes, histiocytes, and plasma cells, extending into the subcutaneous tissue in some cases (Fig. 3.83). Eosinophils may be present in the center of the lesion. At the center, the epidermis is unremarkable, but at the advancing border, variable epidermal changes, including acanthosis and spongiosis, are often observed. In the upper dermis, vascular dilatation with fibrin deposition, nuclear debris, and extravasated erythrocytes may be prominent features. Significant dermal edema or perineural inflammation also may be present in some cases.

Ancillary Studies

Spirochetes can be detected in the dermis with Warthin-Starry or Steiner stains in some cases (Fig. 3.83C).

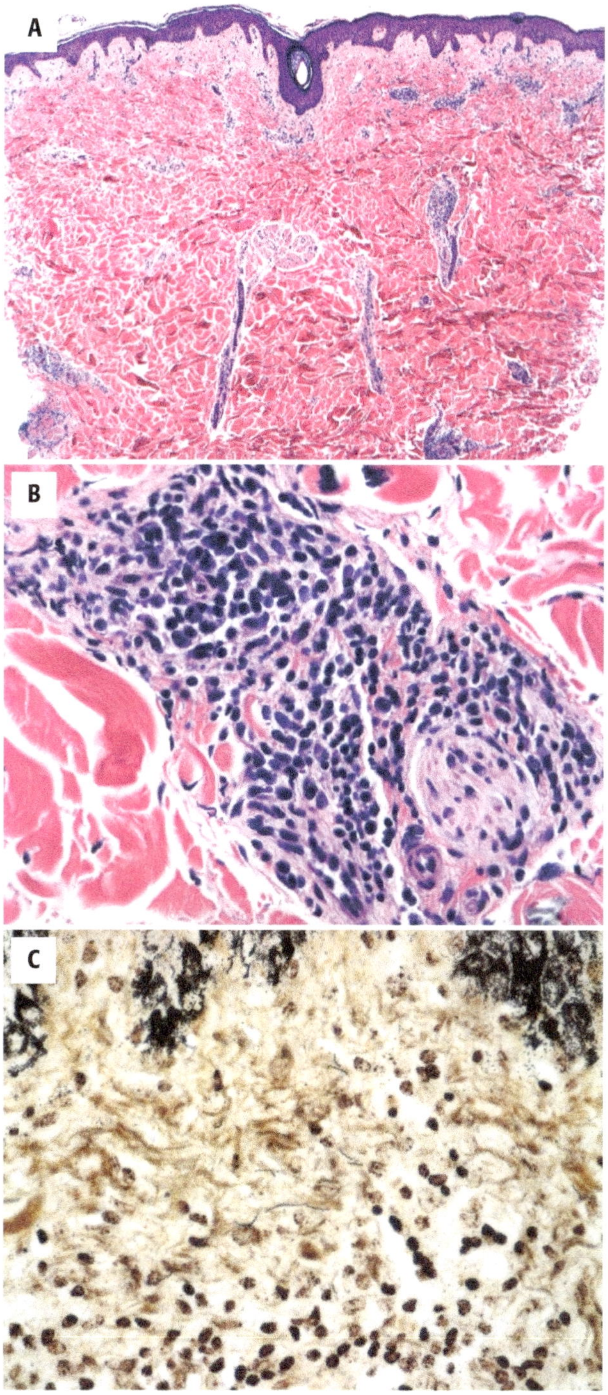

FIG. 3.83

Cutaneous Lyme disease. **A,** A common histologic feature is a perivascular mononuclear infiltrate. **B,** The infiltrate is composed of lymphocytes and plasma cells. **C,** A silver stain (modified Steiner) reveals the presence of spirochetes (*Borrelia* sp.).

Correlation of clinical and histologic findings with serologic studies is important to establish the diagnosis. For serologic testing, it is recommended to first perform a (more sensitive) enzyme-linked immunosorbent assay (ELISA). If it is positive, it should be followed by a (more specific) Western blot analysis.

Differential Diagnosis

Gyrate erythema is distinguished from ECM by the absence of plasma cells and eosinophils and the presence of a usually denser cuff of perivascular lymphocytic infiltrate. In contrast with ECM, insect bite reaction usually demonstrates a dense, wedge-shaped lymphohistiocytic infiltrate containing numerous eosinophils and only rare plasma cells.

Prognosis and Treatment

Prompt oral antibiotic therapy with tetracycline or doxycycline in the early stages leads to rapid recovery and prevents long-term sequelae. Intravenous regimens may be required for the meningitic and cardiac manifestations of late-stage Lyme disease.

FUNGAL INFECTIONS

SUPERFICIAL FUNGAL INFECTIONS

DERMATOPHYTOSES

Dermatophytes are fungi of the genera *Trichophyton*, *Microsporum*, and *Epidermophyton* that obtain nutrients from keratinized material present in the stratum corneum, nails, and hair but do not invade the host living tissues. The fungus and its metabolic products usually induce an allergic and inflammatory eczematous response in the host. Dermatophytes are found worldwide. The source of infection can be human (anthropophilic), animal (zoophilic), or the soil (geophilic).

Clinical Findings

Superficial skin infection with dermatophytes presents as an erythematous annular lesion that extends centrifugally, clearing centrally and showing fine peripheral scaling. Involvement of a specific site results in different clinical subtypes: tinea corporis (Fig. 3.84), tinea cruris (Fig. 3.85), tinea capitis (Fig. 3.86), tinea barbae (Fig. 3.87), and tinea pedis (Fig. 3.88). The classic clinical presentation can be modified after topical treatment with steroids (tinea incognito). Favus is a crusted scalp infection with *Trichophyton schoenleinii*, with secondary hair loss. Tinea imbricata, caused by *Trichophyton concentricum*, consists of concentric rings of scales over large areas of the body. Nail infection presents clinically as dystrophic nails

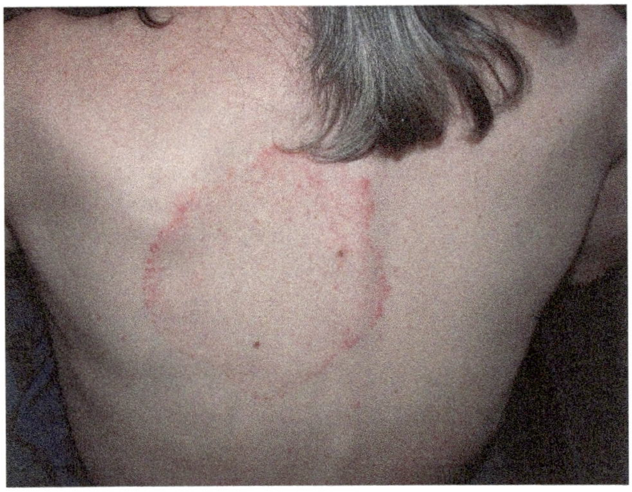

FIG. 3.84
Tinea corporis. Annular scaly erythematous patch with central clearing.

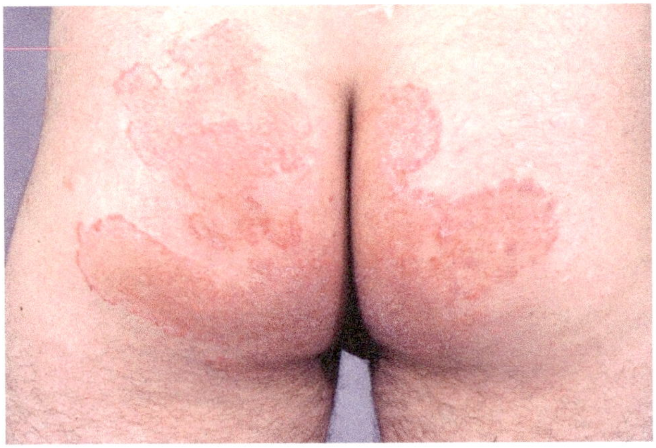

FIG. 3.85
Tinea cruris. Arciform erythematous patch.

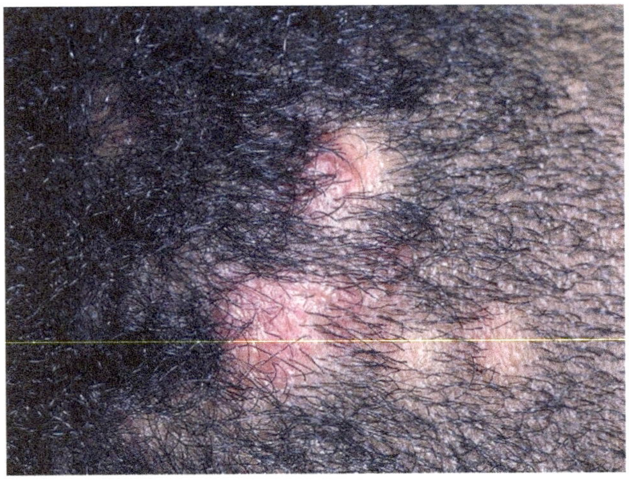

FIG. 3.86
Tinea capitis. Hair breakage and loss, scale, and erythema.

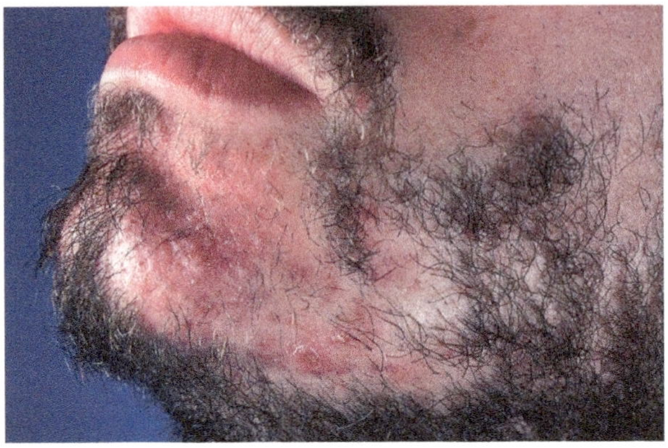

FIG. 3.87
Tinea barbae. Hair loss and crusted erythematous papules.

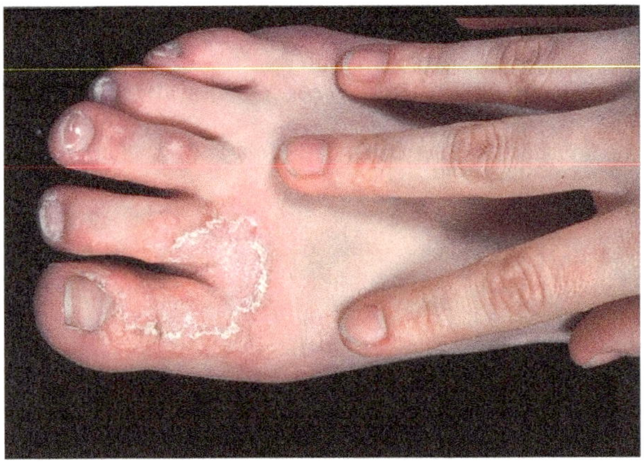

FIG. 3.88
Tinea pedis. Arcuate erythematous lesions with a peripheral scale.

DERMATOPHYTOSIS—DISEASE FACT SHEET

Definition

- Superficial fungal infection caused by three genera of fungi (*Microsporum*, *Trichophyton*, and *Epidermophyton*) that invade and multiply within keratinized tissue.
- Transmitted from human to human (anthropophilic: *T. rubrum. T. tonsurans, E. floccosum, T. concentricum, T. mentagrophytes* var. *interdigitale*), animals to humans (zoophilic: *T. mentagrophytes var. mentagrophytes, M. canis, T. verrucosum*), and from soil to humans (geophilic: *M. gypseum*)

Patient Group

- Children and adults, more common in males
- Tinea capitis seen more frequently in children

Site of Involvement

- Variable; may be anywhere

Clinical Findings

- Different clinical presentations arise from the various causative organisms at different body sites.
- *T. corporis:* Pruritic, annular, erythematous lesions with scale and central clearing (*T. rubrum, T. mentagrophytes*)
- *T. capitis:* Endothrix (*T. tonsurans*) with hair breakage near scalp ("black dot"), ectothrix (*M. audouinii*) with dry, scaly patches

of alopecia ("gray patch"); or favus with thick, yellow crusts (scutula), fluorescent with Wood's light (*T. schoenleinii*)
- T. pedis: Moccasin (*E. floccosum*), interdigital (*T. mentagrophytes* var. *interdigitale*), inflammatory (*T. mentagrophytes*), and ulcerative (*T. rubrum*) types
- T. unguium: Thick yellow nails with distal onycholysis (*T. rubrum, T. mentagrophytes, E. floccosum*)
- *T. cruris:* Arciform erythematous borders (*T. rubrum*); well-demarcated borders with many small vesicles (*E. floccosum*)

Prognosis and Treatment
- Topical and systemic antifungals are beneficial in treating most cases
- High incidence of recurrence is a significant problem, especially with *T. unguium*

that are thick and yellow. Hair shafts can be colonized on the surface (ectothrix) or within (endothrix); as a result, they are weakened and break easily.

Histologic Features

There is epidermal spongiosis, papillary dermal edema, and a superficial perivascular and/or bandlike inflammatory infiltrate composed of lymphocytes, histiocytes, neutrophils, and eosinophils (Fig. 3.89). The spongiosis can progress to intraepidermal vesiculation, especially on the palms and soles. While the hyphae and small spores can often be seen on H&E sections (Fig. 3.90), sometimes it is difficult to recognize them. They can be better identified by fungal stains (PAS-D or GMS stains). The PAS stain is best combined with diastase digestion (PAS-D), which removes background glycogen, thereby highlighting diastase-resistant fungal polysaccharides (Fig. 3.89C).

DERMATOPHYTOSIS—PATHOLOGIC FEATURES

Histologic Features
- Hyphae seen between an upper basket-weave layer and a lower compact orthokeratotic or parakeratotic layer ("sandwich" sign) in the cornified layer
- The hyphae are regular, septate, and best identified with PAS or GMS stains
- Superficial dermal perivascular inflammatory infiltrate

Ancillary Studies
- Special stains: PAS-D, GMS

Cultures
- *T. rubrum:* suede cream color front, pink to dark red reverse
- *T. mentagrophytes* var. *mentagrophytes*: cream front, brown reverse
- *T. mentagrophytes* var. *interdigitale:* granular front, buff reverse
- *T. tonsurans:* granular front, mahogany reverse
- *T. schoenleinii:* folded front, antler hyphae (favic chandeliers)
- *M. canis:* cream cottony front, bright yellow reverse
- *M. audouinii:* flat tan front, salmon reverse
- *E. floccosum:* khaki green, suede to granular front

A

B

C

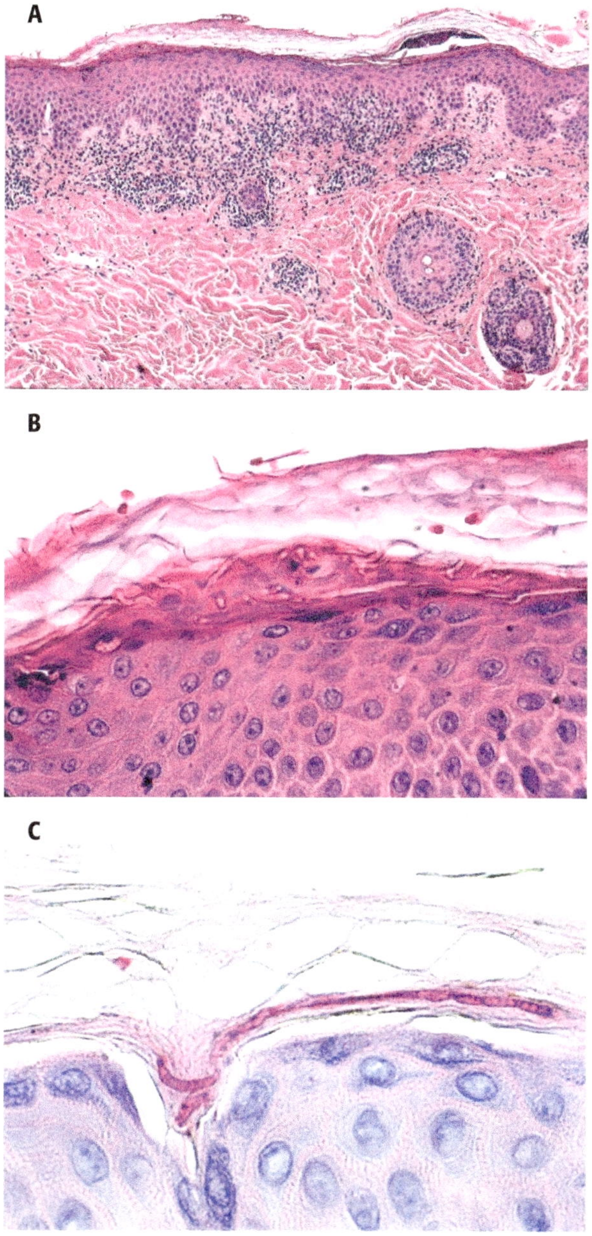

FIG. 3.89

Dermatophytosis. **A,** There is hyperkeratosis, mild spongiosis, and a superficial dermal inflammatory reaction. **B,** Fungal elements are often not seen on hematoxylin and eosin–stained sections but can be visualized when the microscope condenser is lowered. **C,** Dermatophytes are best seen on periodic acid-Schiff with diastase digestion stain.

Differential Diagnosis
- *T. corporis:* dermatitis (nummular, atopic, stasis, contact, seborrheic), annular psoriasis, erythema annulare centrifugum, pityriasis rosea, pityriasis versicolor, parapsoriasis, impetigo
- *T. cruris:* candidiasis, dermatitis (seborrheic, contact), psoriasis, erythrasma, lichen simplex chronicus, parapsoriasis
- *T. capitis:* seborrheic dermatitis, folliculitis, trichotillomania, alopecia areata, psoriasis, lichen planus, discoid lupus erythematosus
- *T. pedis:* dermatitis (dyshidrotic, contact), psoriasis, syphilis, erythrasma

GMS, Gomori methenamine silver; *PAS-D,* periodic acid-Schiff with diastase digestion.

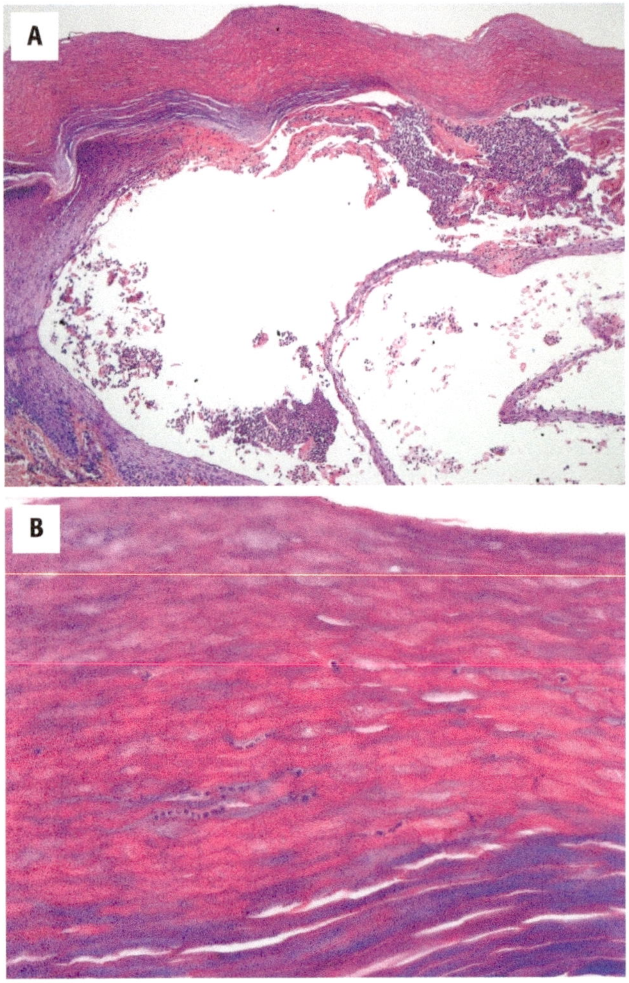

FIG. 3.90

Dermatophytosis. **A,** Spongiotic vesicle with purulent inflammation in tinea pedis. **B,** Septate hyphae in stratum corneum.

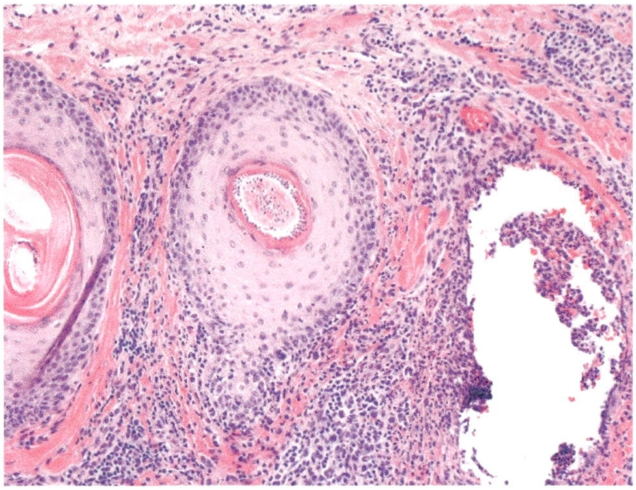

FIG. 3.91

Majocchi's granuloma. Suppurative and chronic perifolliculitis with intrafollicular arthrospores.

The fungi can be seen in a compact orthokeratotic stratum corneum, sometimes between an upper basket-weaved layer and a lower compact orthokeratotic or parakeratotic layer ("sandwich" sign), and may be accompanied by collections of neutrophils. The hyphae are regular and septate, have parallel walls, and tend to break into arthrospores. Majocchi's granuloma is characterized by chronic dermal inflammation and perifollicular suppurative granulomas (Fig. 3.91). In dermatophytoses affecting the hair, hyphae can be identified within hair shafts (endothrix) or around them (ectothrix) (Fig. 3.92). In onychomycosis, the hyperkeratotic subungual debris has a higher yield of hyphae than the nail plates on microscopic examination.

Ancillary Studies

Potassium hydroxide preparation of skin scraping shows septated, branched fungal hyphae. Nail clippings and subungual keratinous debris can be examined histopathologically to diagnose onychomycosis. Special stains (PAS-D or GMS) are helpful on histologic sections. Fungal culture identifies the pathogen in skin scrapings, hair, and nails. Bacterial culture can rule out superinfection.

Differential Diagnosis

For tinea pedis, the differential diagnosis includes interdigital erythrasma, candidiasis, impetigo, moccasin-type psoriasis, and eczematous dermatitis (allergic contact, dyshidrotic, or atopic dermatitis). Tinea cruris has to be differentiated from candidiasis, intertrigo, and inverse psoriasis. Tinea corporis can resemble allergic contact dermatitis, annular erythemas, psoriasis, and Lyme disease. Tinea capitis simulates seborrheic dermatitis and scalp involvement by psoriasis.

Prognosis and Treatment

Topical and systemic antifungal medications are used for treatment; avoidance of hot, humid, and occlusive conditions helps healing and prevents infections. In immunocompromised individuals, atypical deeper infections can develop. Patients with diabetes may have chronic or recurrent infections.

CANDIDIASIS

Candida albicans, the species most frequently involved in human infections, is a normal constituent of the

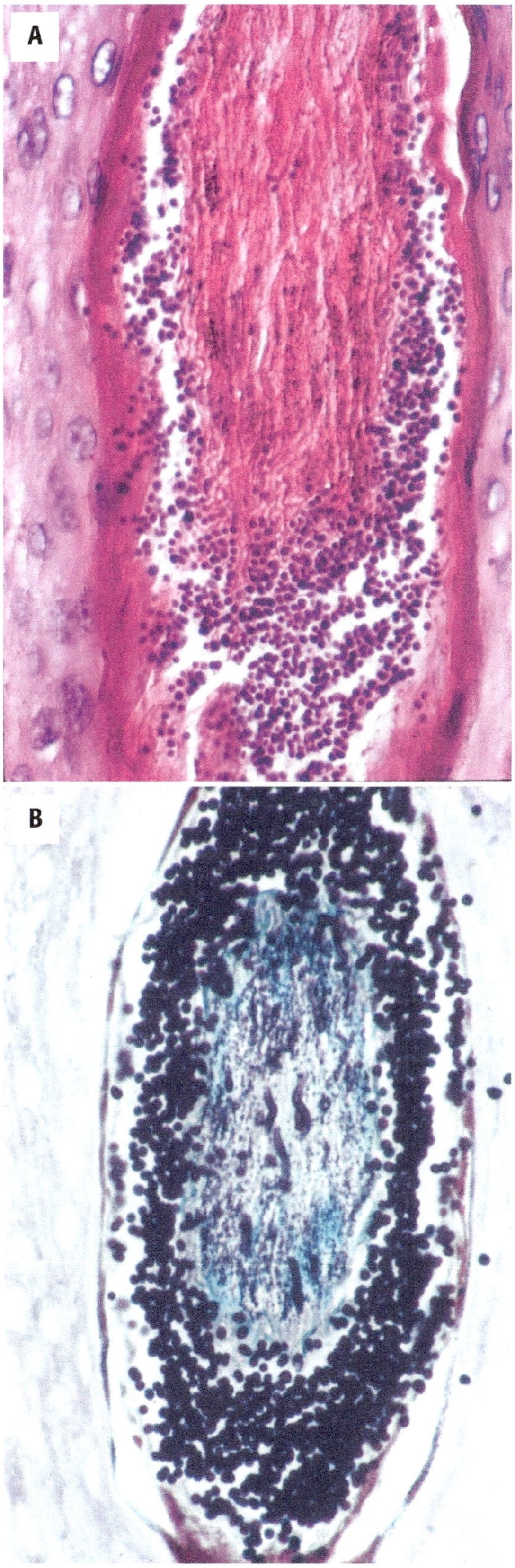

FIG. 3.92
Dermatophytes in hair. **A,** Fungal forms surround and involve a hair shaft. **B,** They are highlighted by a Gomori methenamine silver stain.

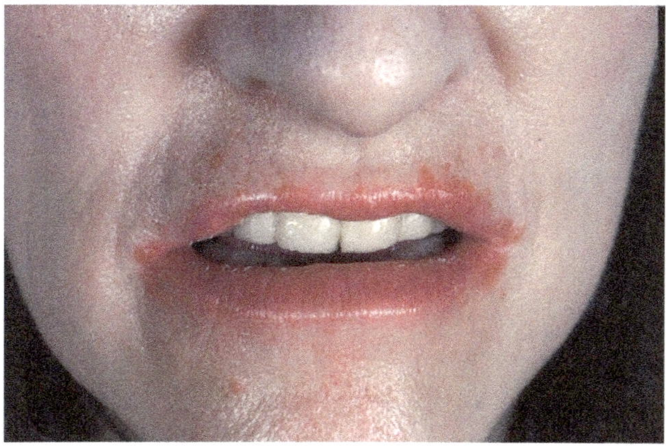

FIG. 3.93
Candidiasis. Perioral erythematous macules and papules are present.

gastrointestinal flora. Predisposing factors for infection include immunosuppression, neutropenia, diabetes and other endocrinopathies, corticosteroid use, prolonged antibiotic use, obesity, and persistent moisture.

Clinical Findings

Acute superficial infection involves the skin folds and manifests as small erythematous papules and pustules that become confluent. At the center, there are erythema and superficial erosion, and at the periphery, satellite papules and fine white scaling (Fig. 3.93). Mucosal lesions show characteristic white, curdlike plaques that can be easily removed to reveal an erythematous or bleeding surface.

Histologic Features

Lesions are characterized by compact orthokeratosis, scale crust, and scattered neutrophils within the epidermis, permeating and accumulating in the cornified layer. There are also focal spongiosis, mild epidermal acanthosis, and a superficial perivascular mixed inflammatory infiltrate. Oval budding yeast forms that elongate and form pseudohyphae can be seen. On H&E-stained sections, they have a lilac color (Fig. 3.94A) but can be better visualized with PAS (Fig. 3.94B) and GMS stains. The oval yeast (blastospores) measure 3 to 6 μm in diameter; the pseudohyphae are 3 to 5 μm wide. Epithelial hyperplasia is seen in mucosal lesions.

Ancillary Studies

Potassium hydroxide preparation of lesion scrapings shows oval budding yeast and pseudohyphae with

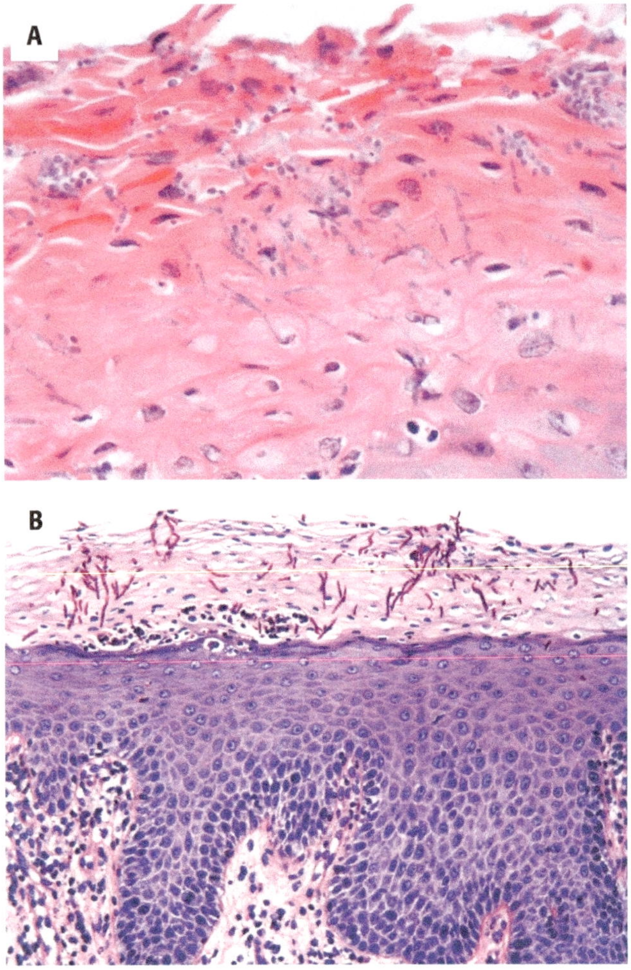

FIG. 3.94

Candida. **A,** Fungal spores and pseudohyphal structures are seen in the epidermis and stratum corneum. **B,** Oval budding yeasts and pseudohyphae oriented perpendicular to the surface of epidermis are highlighted by a periodic acid-Schiff with diastase digestion stain; they are usually oriented perpendicular to the surface.

periodic constrictions at the points at which the budding yeast cells are joined end to end ("sausage-like"). PAS-D and GMS stains are useful to highlight the organisms in tissue sections.

Differential Diagnosis

Cutaneous candidiasis has to be differentiated from intertrigo, inverse psoriasis, seborrheic dermatitis, scabies, and dermatophytosis. The differential diagnosis of oral candidiasis includes hairy leukoplakia and oral lichen planus.

Prognosis and Treatment

Topical antifungal medications are effective in the majority of cases; oral antifungals are reserved for resistant infections or immunocompromised patients, in whom disseminated disease may occur. Chronic mucocutaneous candidiasis may be associated with immunodeficiency, endocrinopathy, or thymoma.

TINEA VERSICOLOR AND PITYROSPORUM FOLLICULITIS

Malassezia furfur (*Pityrosporum ovale*) is a lipophilic yeastlike fungus that causes tinea versicolor (pityriasis versicolor), a common superficial fungal infection, and folliculitis (*Pityrosporum* folliculitis). It can be cultured by adding olive oil to the isolation medium.

Clinical Findings

Tinea versicolor involves mostly the upper trunk or arms of young adults (Fig. 3.95). The lesions are well-demarcated macules and patches with variable color ranging from tan-brown to white, sometimes confluent, and covered by fine scales. High humidity and sebum production predispose to infection.

Histologic Features

The organisms can be seen on H&E stain in the cornified layer (Fig. 3.96) as budding yeasts and short,

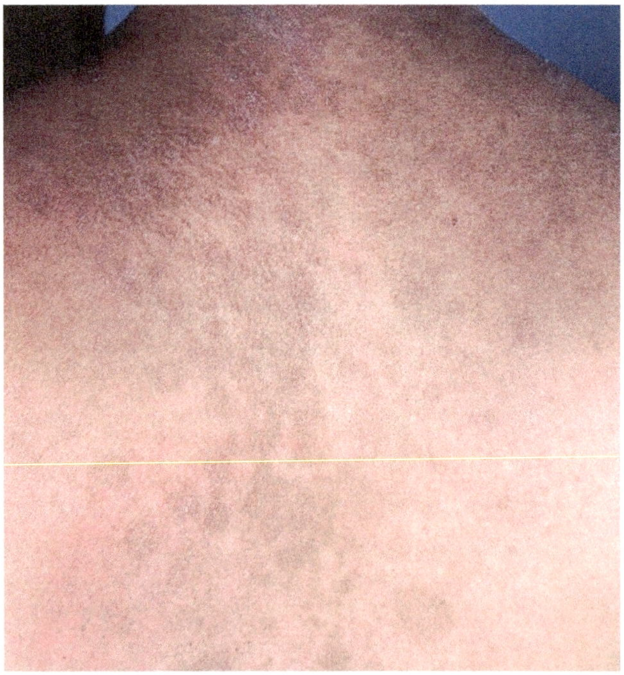

FIG. 3.95

Tinea versicolor. Upper trunk with irregular confluent tan-brown macules with fine scale.

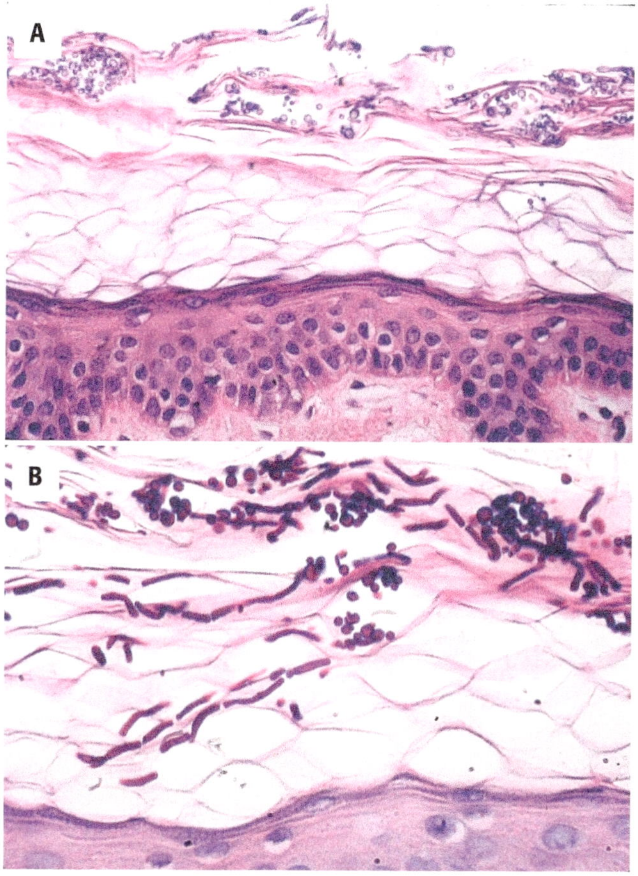

FIG. 3.96

Tinea versicolor. **A,** Spores and short, stubby pseudohyphae are present in the hyperkeratotic stratum corneum. **B,** Many fungal organisms are seen on the periodic acid-Schiff with diastase digestion stain ("spaghetti and meatballs").

stubby, infrequently branched, slightly curved pseudohyphae reminiscent of spaghetti and meatballs. The epidermis shows hyperkeratosis and slight acanthosis, and in the dermis, there is a mild superficial perivascular lymphocytic infiltrate. Pityrosporum folliculitis is characterized by dilated hair follicles filled with keratinous material with a rim of basophilic granular debris and numerous oval or round yeasts (Fig. 3.97).

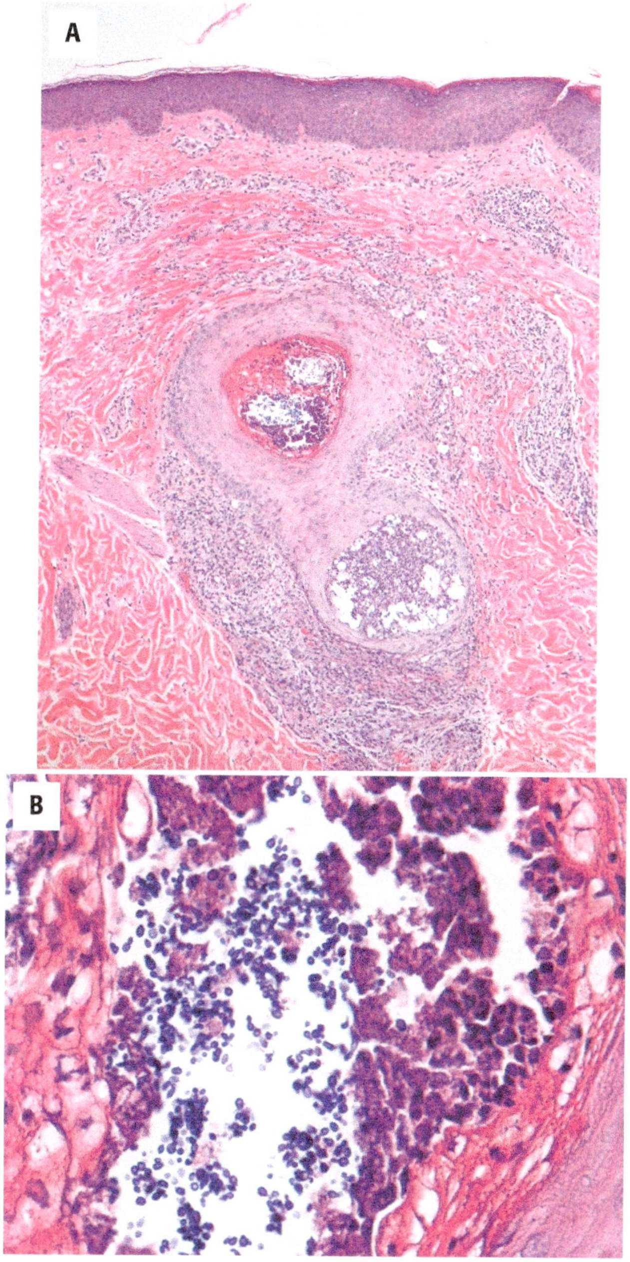

FIG. 3.97

Pityrosporum folliculitis. **A,** Superficial suppurative folliculitis. **B,** Fungal spores and basophilic debris are identified in the dilated hair follicle.

Ancillary Studies

Wood's lamp examination of the clinical lesions shows yellow fluorescence. PAS-D and GMS stains can highlight the organisms.

Differential Diagnosis

The clinical differential diagnosis includes pityriasis alba, seborrheic dermatitis, and postinflammatory pigmentary changes.

Prognosis and Treatment

The treatment consists of topical antifungal agents and selenium sulfide shampoo.

SUPERFICIAL AND DEEP FUNGAL INFECTIONS

PHAEOHYPHOMYCOSIS

Many different genera of dematiaceous fungi (Exophiala, Phialophora, Wangiella, Bipolaris, Exserohilum,

Cladophialophora, Phaeoannellomyces, Aureobasidium, Cladosporium, Curvularia, and Alternaria) can produce cutaneous or subcutaneous infection characterized by the presence of pigmented hyphae. Superficial infection of the hair shaft by *Piedraia hortae* causes the disease known as "black piedra."

Clinical Findings

Clinical forms of phaeohyphomycosis range from superficial colonization of the stratum corneum (tinea nigra) or hair shafts (black piedra) to subcutaneous cystic or nodular lesions. The latter are found most commonly on distal extremities, where the organism is inoculated as a result of trauma, such as a splinter implantation (Fig. 3.98). In black piedra, infected scalp hairs have several hard, adherent, gritty black nodules on the shaft. Tinea nigra is caused by *Phaeoannellomyces werneckii*, and the lesions consist of brown-black macules, usually located on the palms, that enlarge slowly and can be confused clinically with a melanocytic proliferation (Fig. 3.99).

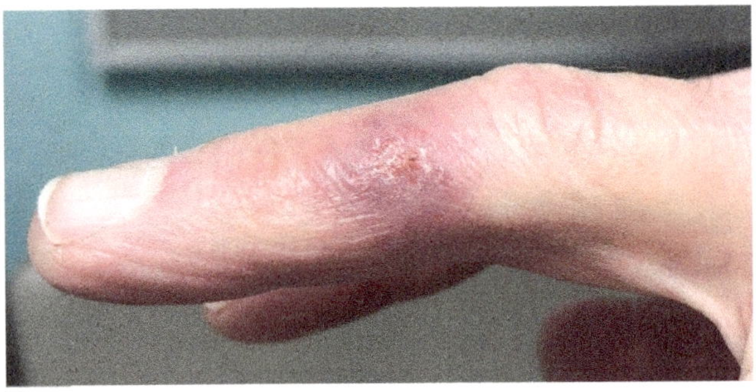

FIG. 3.98
Phaeohyphomycosis. Inflammatory nodule at the site of traumatic implantation on a finger.

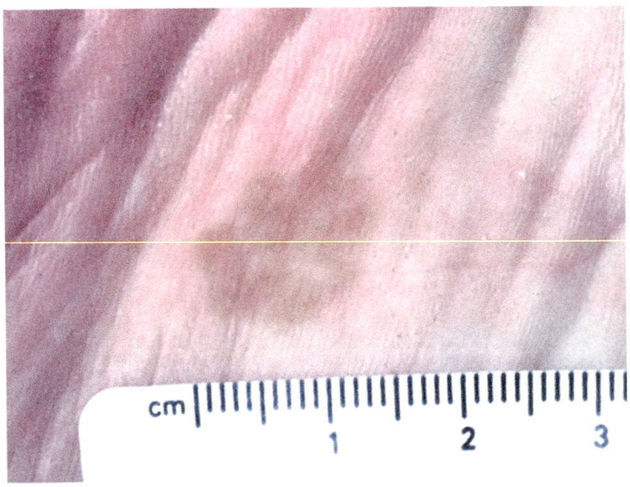

FIG. 3.99
Phaeohyphomycosis. Hyperpigmented macule with arcuate borders.

Histologic Features

In black piedra, the black nodules are composed of thick-walled fungal cells (ascostroma) in the center and hyphae at the periphery. Tinea nigra is characterized by black-brown, septate hyphae present in a compact stratum corneum (Fig. 3.100). Deeper forms of infection show an abscess contained by a fibrous wall with a chronic granulomatous inflammatory response and located in the dermis or subcutaneous tissue (Fig. 3.101). Hyphae and, occasionally, a wood splinter can be found in the necrotic debris in the center. The hyphae are brown, irregular, septate, and 4 to 6 μm in width (Fig. 3.101).

Ancillary Studies

The hyphae stain positive with Fontana-Masson stain.

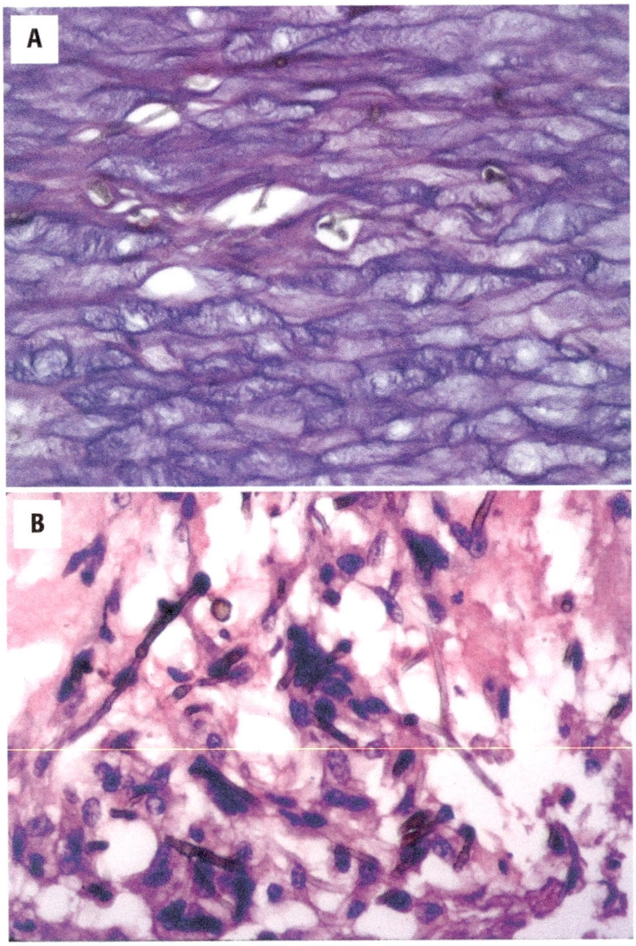

FIG. 3.100
Phaeohyphomycosis. **A,** Pigmented fungi are present in the stratum corneum. **B,** An inflammatory tissue reaction is seen surrounding pigmented septate hyphae.

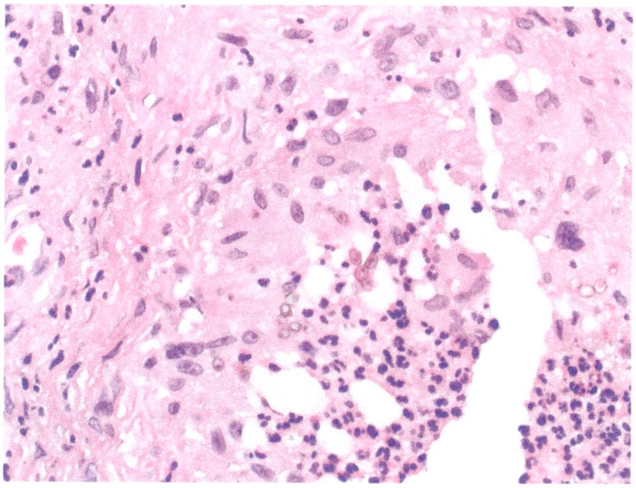

FIG. 3.101
Phaeohyphomycosis. Pigmented hyphal forms surrounding by suppurative and granulomatous inflammation.

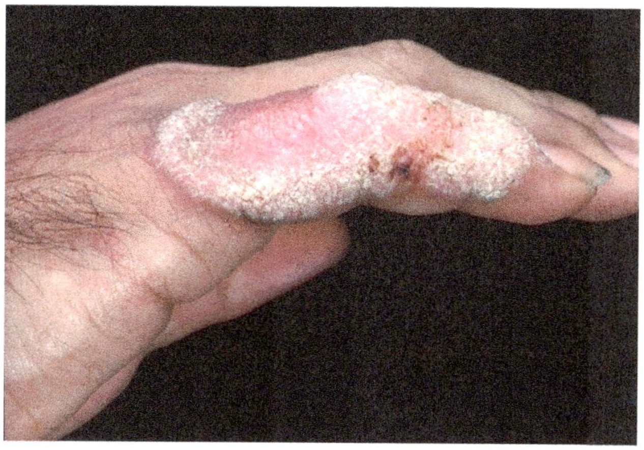

FIG. 3.102
Chromomycosis. A verrucous scaly erythematous plaque is present on finger.

Differential Diagnosis

The differential diagnosis includes chromomycosis, characterized by sclerotic bodies (not hyphae) and overlying florid pseudoepitheliomatous hyperplasia, and eumycotic mycetomas caused by *Madurella mycetomatis,* in which the interwoven mycelial aggregates form distinct grains. Black piedra may be confused with trichorrhexis nodosa or pediculosis. It can be easily differentiated from white piedra, caused by *Trichosporon beigelii*, characterized by softer, white nodules present on scalp or genital hair that can be detached without difficulty and are microscopically composed of hyphae oriented perpendicular to the hair shaft.

Prognosis and Treatment

The treatment consists of surgical excision and amphotericin B in disseminated infections. Black or white piedra can be treated by shaving the hair.

CHROMOMYCOSIS

Six fungal species may cause chromomycosis, a chronic superficial infection. The most frequently involved are *Fonsecaea pedrosoi* (*Phialophora pedrosoi*) and, in Australia, *Cladosporium carrionii.*

Clinical Findings

The lesions typically appear at the site of trauma, during which the pathologic agent is implanted. They consist of slowly expanding verrucous nodules or plaques, sometimes ulcerated and crusted (Fig. 3.102).

Histologic Features

The overlying epidermis shows hyperkeratosis and pseudoepitheliomatous hyperplasia (Fig. 3.103). The upper and mid dermis contain a chronic granulomatous inflammatory infiltrate. Less frequently, suppurative granulomas or intradermal microabscesses may be seen. The fungi are easily identified and are seen free or within giant cells (Fig. 3.103). They consist of round to polyhedral, golden brown to chestnut brown fungal cells that measure 5 to 12 μm in diameter; divide by septation; are considered vegetative forms intermediate between yeast and hyphae; and have been named Medlar bodies, sclerotic bodies, or muriform cells. The center is paler than the periphery.

Differential Diagnosis

The differential diagnosis includes sporotrichosis, characterized by very rare fungal forms accompanied by a more prominent suppurative inflammation, phaeohyphomycosis, leishmaniasis, tuberculosis, and sarcoidosis. Monoclonal antibodies can identify *F. pedrosoi.* Culture can be used to isolate the causal fungi.

Prognosis and Treatment

The treatment includes oral antifungal agents and local application of heat. Rare cases of hematogenous

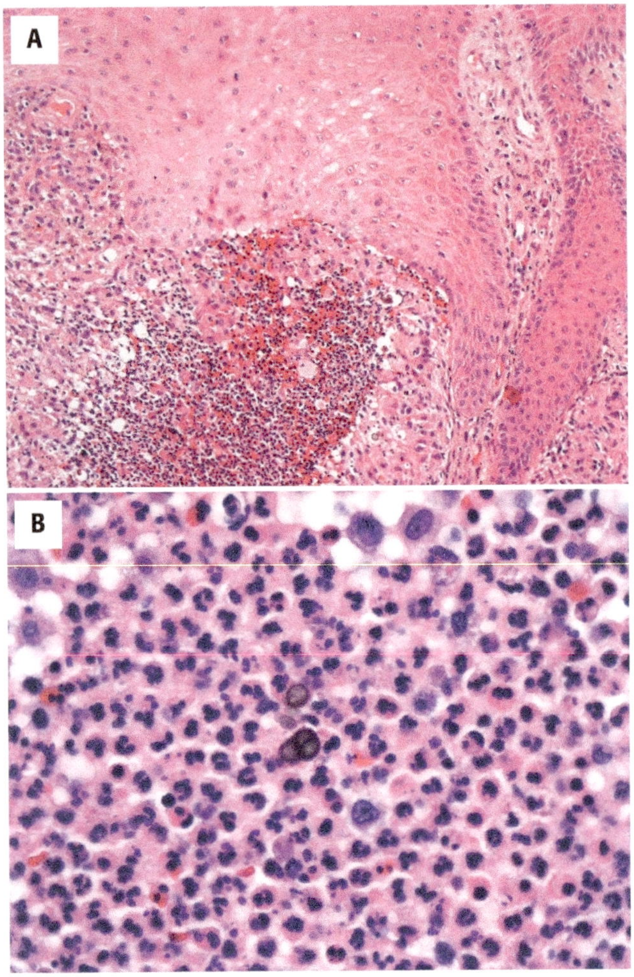

FIG. 3.103
Chromomycosis. **A,** Epidermal hyperplasia is associated with a suppurative dermal inflammatory process. **B,** Polyhedral, golden brown fungal forms with septation are characteristic.

dissemination of *F. pedrosoi* in immunosuppressed patients have been reported and have a grave prognosis.

SPOROTRICHOSIS

Sporothrix schenckii is a dimorphic fungus found worldwide that may produce lymphangitic or localized infection after inoculation as a result of trauma such as a wood splinter implantation or a rose thorn injury. The first case of sporotrichosis was described at Johns Hopkins Hospital in 1898 by Benjamin Schenck. In the United States, the largest epidemic occurred among forestry workers after exposure to sphagnum moss.

Clinical Findings

In the lymphangitic form, the most common form, a single erythematous plaque or nodule appears at the site of trauma and later becomes ulcerated, sometimes discharging purulent material (Fig. 3.104). Inflammation of the draining lymphatics follows, and clusters of similar nodules form along them. Deep extension of the infection may occur, especially in immunosuppressed patients. The localized form is seen more frequently in children on the face and consists of an ulcerated nodule, with or without satellite lesions developing at the periphery. Unlike the lymphangitic form, which results from primary exposure to *S. schenckii*, the solitary, fixed lesions are usually due to repeated infection.

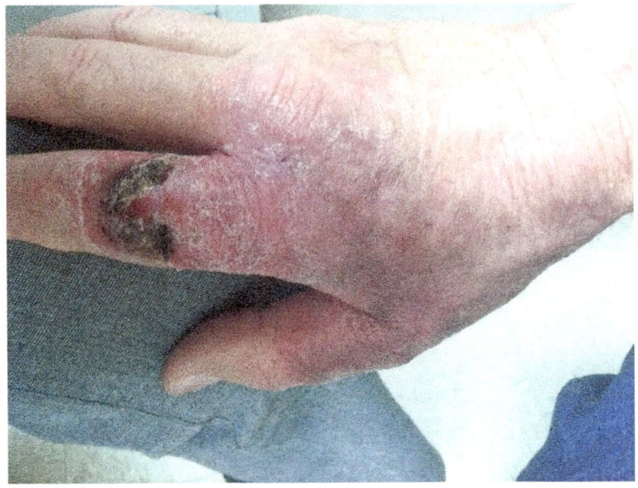

FIG. 3.104
Sporotrichosis. Crusted erythematous plaque at the site of inoculation.

Histologic Features

The primary lesions are characterized by pseudoepitheliomatous epidermal hyperplasia overlying a superficial and deep localized mixed granulomatous inflammatory infiltrate with central microabscesses. Ulceration can occur. The fungal forms are rare; multiple serial sections may be required to identify them. They consist of oval or elongated forms ("cigar bodies") measuring 2 to 8 μm in diameter, scarce hyphae, or asteroid forms (Fig. 3.105). The characteristic sporothrix asteroid (Fig. 3.106) consists of a yeast form surrounded at the periphery by eosinophilic, finely granular material arranged radially. In cutaneous lesions caused by *S. schenckii* var *luriei*, large, thick-walled yeast cells can be seen, with optically clear centers and transverse septa.

Ancillary Studies

Stains for PAS-D and GMS aid in the detection of the fungi.

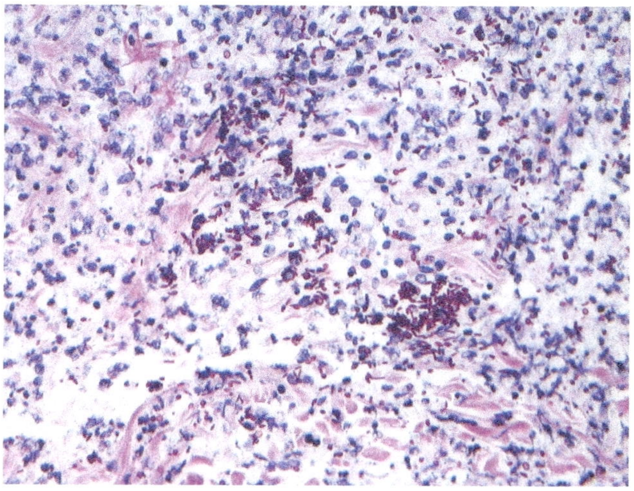

FIG. 3.105
Sporotrichosis. Elongated ("cigar bodies") budding yeast.

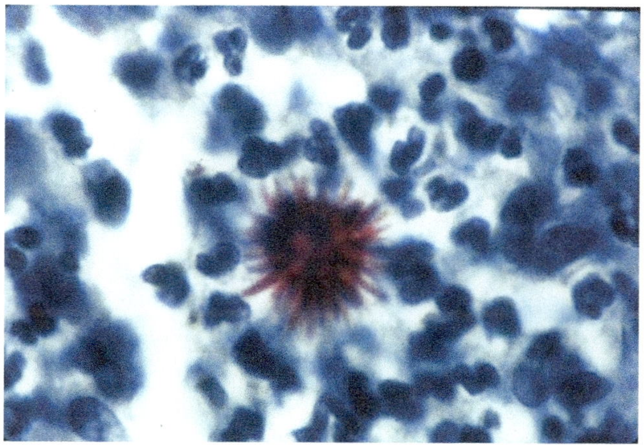

FIG. 3.106
Sporotrichosis. Yeast organisms with radiating spikes (asteroid body).

Differential Diagnosis

The differential diagnosis includes sarcoidosis, coccidioidomycosis, and blastomycosis. Fungal cultures can render a definitive diagnosis.

Prognosis and Treatment

Treatment consists of oral antifungal agents (itraconazole, fluconazole, ketoconazole) and local hyperthermia.

ALTERNARIOSIS

Human infection with fungi belonging to the *Alternaria* genus is rare and occurs mostly in patients with immunologic impairment, diabetes, or hypercorticism or those receiving systemic steroids.

Clinical Findings

Chronic crusted nodules, pustules, or ulcers are seen on exposed surfaces in infections caused by *Alternaria alternata*, the most frequently involved species.

Histologic Features

Septate brown hyphae of variable width and large, oval, thick, sometimes double-walled yeast cells may be identified both in the epidermis and dermis accompanied by suppurative granulomatous inflammation, intraepidermal microabscesses, and a thick scale crust with neutrophils.

Ancillary Studies

PAS-D or GMS stains highlight the fungal elements. Fungal culture and demonstration of macroconidia with longitudinal and transverse septae confirm the diagnosis.

Prognosis and Treatment

The prognosis depends on the immune status of the patient. There is no consensus on the best treatment. Surgical debridement may be part of the therapy. Intravenous antifungal drugs, such as amphotericin B or voriconazole, may be used.

BLASTOMYCOSIS

Blastomycosis (Gilchrist's disease) is endemic along the Mississippi and Ohio rivers, the Great Lakes, and the Southeast United States.

Clinical Findings

Cutaneous disease may be a manifestation of systemic involvement or, less frequently, a result of direct inoculation with the dimorphic fungus *Blastomyces dermatitidis*. The lesions show predilection for exposed skin and consist of slowly enlarging verrucous crusted nodules, which may have central ulceration or scarring (Fig. 3.107). They have a characteristic raised, violaceous, verrucous, arciform border with tiny crusted pustules.

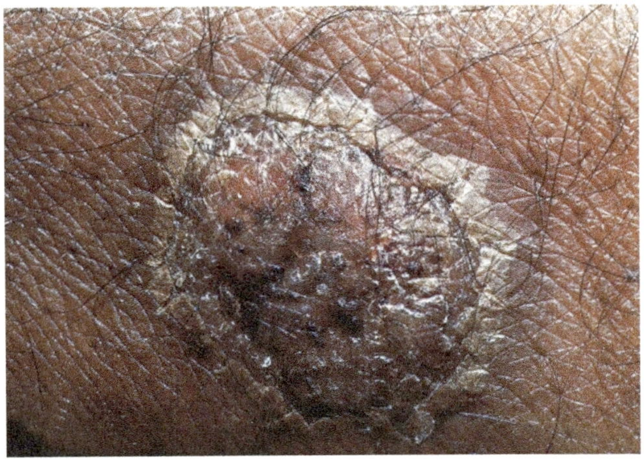

FIG. 3.107
Blastomycosis. Note the verrucous, crusted nodule.

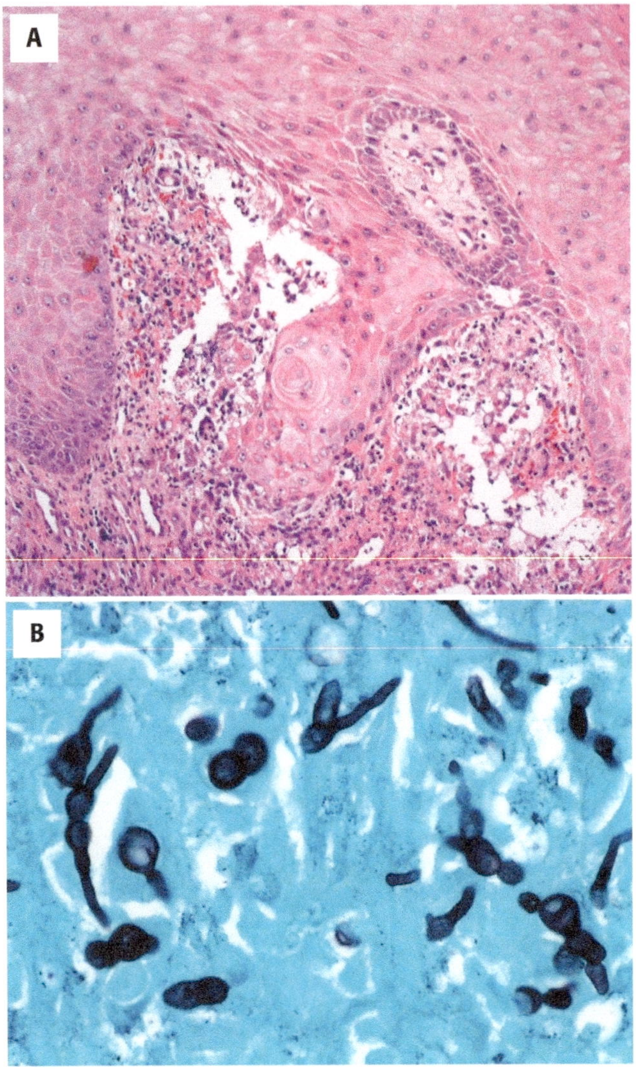

FIG. 3.108
Blastomycosis. **A,** Epidermal hyperplasia is associated with a suppurative dermatitis. **B,** Budding yeast forms (single bud with a broad base) are seen on Gomori methenamine silver stain.

BLASTOMYCOSIS—DISEASE FACT SHEET

Pulmonary disease with secondary cutaneous involvement or (infrequently) primary cutaneous disease caused by the dimorphic fungus *Blastomyces dermatitidis.* Blastomyces is endemic in the southeastern United States.

Patient Group

- Adult men are more likely to develop systemic infection; children are more likely to develop acute pulmonary infection

Site of Involvement

- Exposed skin

Clinical Findings

- Various clinical manifestations: papulopustules and well-demarcated verrucous plaques with scale crust and pustules seen more frequently
- Healing begins centrally

Prognosis and Treatment

- Most lesions resolve with systemic treatment with amphotericin B; occasionally, surgical treatment is also required
- Primary cutaneous infections progressively enlarge but remain localized
- Systemic infections are often severe and have high mortality rate if not treated

Histologic Features

The histologic findings consist of florid pseudoepitheliomatous epidermal hyperplasia overlying dermal suppurative granulomatous inflammation with giant cells (Fig. 3.108). Microabscesses are found both in the dermis and in the epidermis. The fungi can be identified within giant cells and in the center of the microabscesses. They consist of round, hyaline, multinucleated yeast cells with thick double contour walls that measure 8 to 15 μm in diameter and have a single bud with a broad base (Fig. 3.108).

BLASTOMYCOSIS—PATHOLOGIC FEATURES

Histologic Features

- Florid pseudoepitheliomatous hyperplasia
- Microabscesses
- 7- to 15-μm hyaline yeast cells with thick double contour walls and single, broad-based buds

Ancillary Studies

- GMS stain
- Culture: at 37°C, the broad-based budding yeast cells can be seen; at 25°C the colonies have characteristic white spikes

Differential Diagnosis

- *Histoplasma capsulatum* var. *duboisii*
- Squamous cell carcinoma

GMS, Gomori methenamine silver.

Ancillary Studies

Direct immunofluorescence with a specific conjugate directed against the cell wall antigens can be used in difficult cases. PAS-D and GMS stains can help identify rare organisms.

Differential Diagnosis

Blastomycosis needs to be distinguished from other yeast infections, particularly *Cryptococcus neoformans*. The yeast buds of the latter have a narrower base, and the capsule of *Cryptococcus* stains positive with mucicarmine, which is not the case for blastomycosis. The pseudoepitheliomatous epidermal hyperplasia associated with blastomycosis may be confused with squamous cell carcinoma if the organisms are not recognized.

Prognosis and Treatment

Without treatment, the cutaneous lesions tend to grow and ulcerate. The lesions heal with central scarring. Itraconazole is often given for 6 months. Systemic involvement carries a very high mortality rate if not treated with amphotericin B.

PARACOCCIDIOIDOMYCOSIS

The disease is caused by the dimorphic fungus *Paracoccidioides brasiliensis*, which is endemic in South America. It primarily affects men (estradiol inhibits the mycelium-to-yeast conversion) and represents the most important deep mycosis of Latin America.

Clinical Findings

The head and neck region, in particular the oral mucosa, is the most frequently affected site (Figs. 3.109 and 3.110). Nodules and painful ulcerations develop and slowly progress, and if left untreated, they can lead to extensive disfigurement. The majority of cutaneous lesions occur after hematogenous spread from a respiratory tract infection.

Histologic Features

Dermal granulomatous inflammation, including giant cell formation, focal suppuration, and overlying pseudoepitheliomatous hyperplasia, is typically seen. Large, thick-walled yeast forms are present both intracellularly and extracellularly, measure up to 60 μm in diameter, and have a characteristic multiple budding pattern (Fig. 3.111) with daughter cells attached by a narrow-necked bud resembling a mariner's wheel or steering wheel. They are best visualized with a GMS stain because they are difficult to identify on H&E stain. They appear globose, with refractive walls, and have a clear halo between cytoplasm and cell walls.

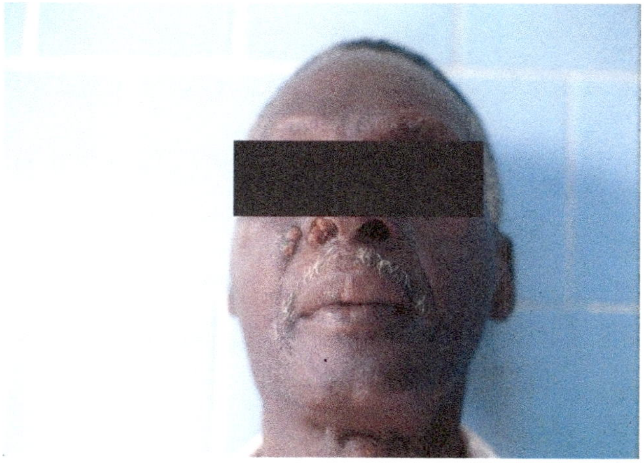

FIG. 3.109
Paracoccidioidomycosis. Note the intranasal and paranasal nodules.

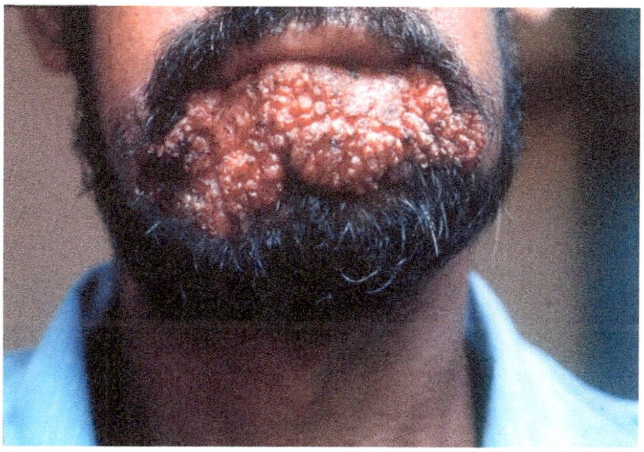

FIG. 3.110
Paracoccidioidomycosis. Perioral nodules.

Prognosis and Treatment

Detection of *Paracoccidioides brasiliensis*-gp43 circulating antigen is a practical approach for obtaining a fast, specific diagnosis in cases with pulmonary involvement. Long-term treatment with sulfa drugs may be required because the relapse rate is high. In patients with depressed immune systems, the prognosis is poor. Itraconazole or voriconazole have been used for treatment.

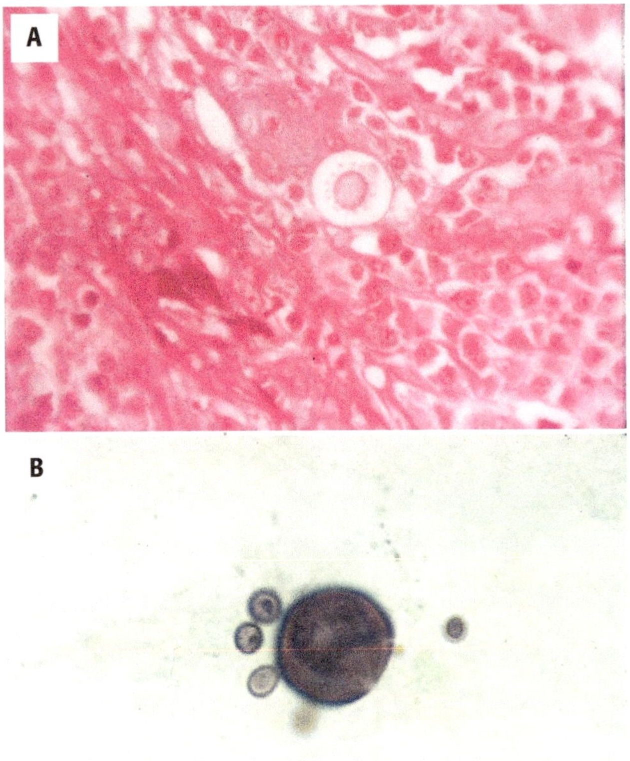

FIG. 3.111

Paracoccidioidomycosis. The "mariner's wheel" type of budding is characteristic (**A** and **B**).

COCCIDIOIDOMYCOSIS

Coccidioides immitis is a dimorphic fungus endemic in the southwestern United States. Pulmonary infection is the result of inhalation of arthroconidia aerosolized from dry soil in late summer. Primary skin disease is extremely rare and generally occurs after local trauma.

Clinical Findings

In 5% of cases, patients develop valley fever complex, manifested by erythema nodosum and erythema multiforme. Approximately 1% of patients with primary coccidioidomycosis develop disseminated disease; in these cases, lesions in the skin may present as verrucous plaques, ulcerated nodules, or verrucous ulcers.

Histologic Features

Granulomatous inflammation with central suppuration and overlying pseudoepitheliomatous hyperplasia are

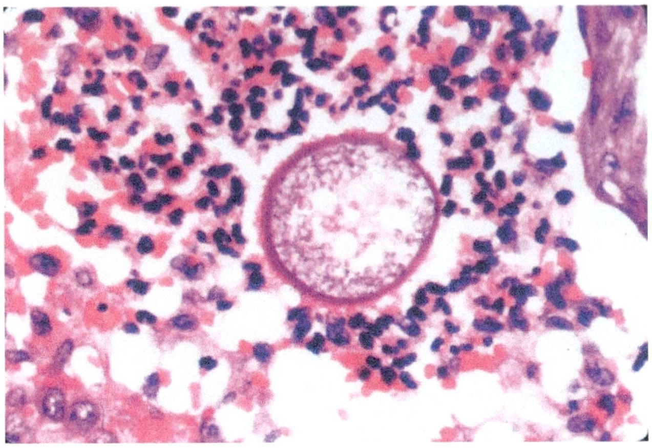

FIG. 3.112

Coccidioidomycosis. Note the thick-walled spherule with numerous endospores.

the usual findings. The fungal forms consist of large, thick-walled spherules measuring up to 80 μm in diameter, containing small endospores (2 to 4 μm in diameter), easy to identify in regular H&E sections (Fig. 3.112).

Ancillary Studies

GMS stain highlights the organisms. With PAS stain, only the endospores stain positively, and the walls of the spherules are negative because of high phospholipid content. The same pattern is observed with direct immunofluorescence using monoclonal or polyclonal-specific antibodies.

Differential Diagnosis

Sometimes the immature spherules may have to be distinguished from the yeast forms of *Blastomyces dermatitidis*, which show broad-based buds.

Prognosis and Treatment

The usually self-limited primary lesions affect the lungs in young people. In cases with dissemination, treatment with fluconazole and itraconazole is required; voriconazole and amphotericin B are reserved for severe or recalcitrant cases.

CRYPTOCOCCOSIS

In humans, *Cryptococcus neoformans* var. *neoformans* and var. *gattii* are the major pathogens. *C. neoformans* var. *neoformans* is found worldwide in dried bat and pigeon droppings, and in immunocompetent hosts causes

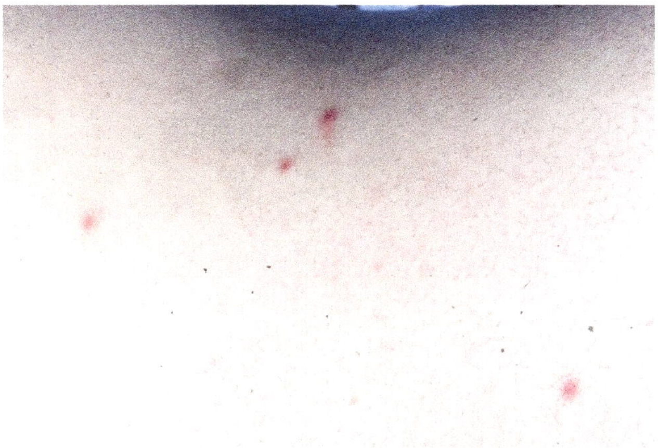

FIG. 3.113

Cryptococcosis. Multiple small erythematous papules are seen.

subclinical disease. Disseminated cryptococcosis occurs in immunocompromised patients and is the most common cause of fungal meningitis. Secondary cutaneous infection occurs in 10% to 20% of patients with disseminated cryptococcosis, usually as small papules that subsequently ulcerate. Primary skin infection after direct cutaneous inoculation is rare.

C. neoformans var. *gattii* is present in tropical and subtropical areas in decaying wood found in the hollow of trees (e.g., eucalyptus trees), affects immunocompetent hosts, and forms large masses in the lungs or brain (cryptococcomas).

Clinical Findings

In immunocompetent patients, the lesions involve mostly the face and fingers and are solitary or confined to a limited area. In disseminated disease and immunocompromised patients, the skin lesions are multiple, scattered, and seen more frequently on the lower extremities and trunk (Fig. 3.113). Various cutaneous presentations have been described and include papules, nodules, plaques, pustules, ulcers, and cellulitis.

CRYPTOCOCCOSIS—DISEASE FACT SHEET

Systemic mycotic infection with secondary cutaneous involvement or, rarely, primary cutaneous disease caused by *Cryptococcus neoformans*

Patient Group

- Rarely seen in immunocompetent hosts
- Incidence in HIV patients has decreased following the use of fluconazole and HAART therapy

Site of Involvement

- Immunocompetent host: localized—face, fingers
- Immunocompromised host: multiple lesions, may be disseminated, often involving lower extremities and trunk

Clinical Findings

- Varied: papules, nodules, ulcers, or abscesses

Prognosis and Treatment

- Poor prognosis in disseminated disease

HAART, Highly active antiretroviral therapy.

CRYPTOCOCCOSIS—PATHOLOGIC FEATURES

Histologic Features

- Gelatinous or granulomatous reaction patterns
- Thick, clear capsule better seen with mucicarmine or Alcian blue stains
- 4 to 12 μm diameter, refractile walls (positive with PAS or GMS stain)
- Narrow-based budding

Ancillary Studies

- GMS or PAS-D stain
- Mucin stain may highlight capsule

Differential Diagnosis

- *Histoplasma capsulatum* var. *capsulatum*
- *Blastomyces dermatitidis* with small tissue forms
- *Sporothrix schenckii*

GMS, Gomori methenamine silver; *PAS*, periodic acid-Schiff; *PAS-D*, periodic acid-Schiff with diastase digestion.

Histologic Features

The dermis shows gelatinous or granulomatous tissue reaction patterns. In the gelatinous type of cutaneous cryptococcosis, numerous organisms are scattered in a "shotgun" manner with little inflammatory response (Fig. 3.114). On low magnification, clustering of spores with very thick, clear capsules gives the appearance of soap bubbles. They measure 4 to 12 μm and have refractile walls. A thick mucinous capsule usually appears clear on H&E-stained sections. Spores may be found free or within the cytoplasm of multinucleated giant cells. Occasional budding spores, attached by a narrow base, may be seen.

Ancillary Studies

Rapid diagnosis may be made by examining Tzanck smears or aspirates from lesions stained with India ink. The organisms stain positive with PAS or GMS stain. The presence of a mucinous capsule can be demonstrated with mucicarmine or Alcian blue stains. Although a positive mucin stain is characteristic of encapsulated strains of *C. neoformans*, mucin positivity is not specific to this particular fungus. *Blastomyces dermatitidis* and

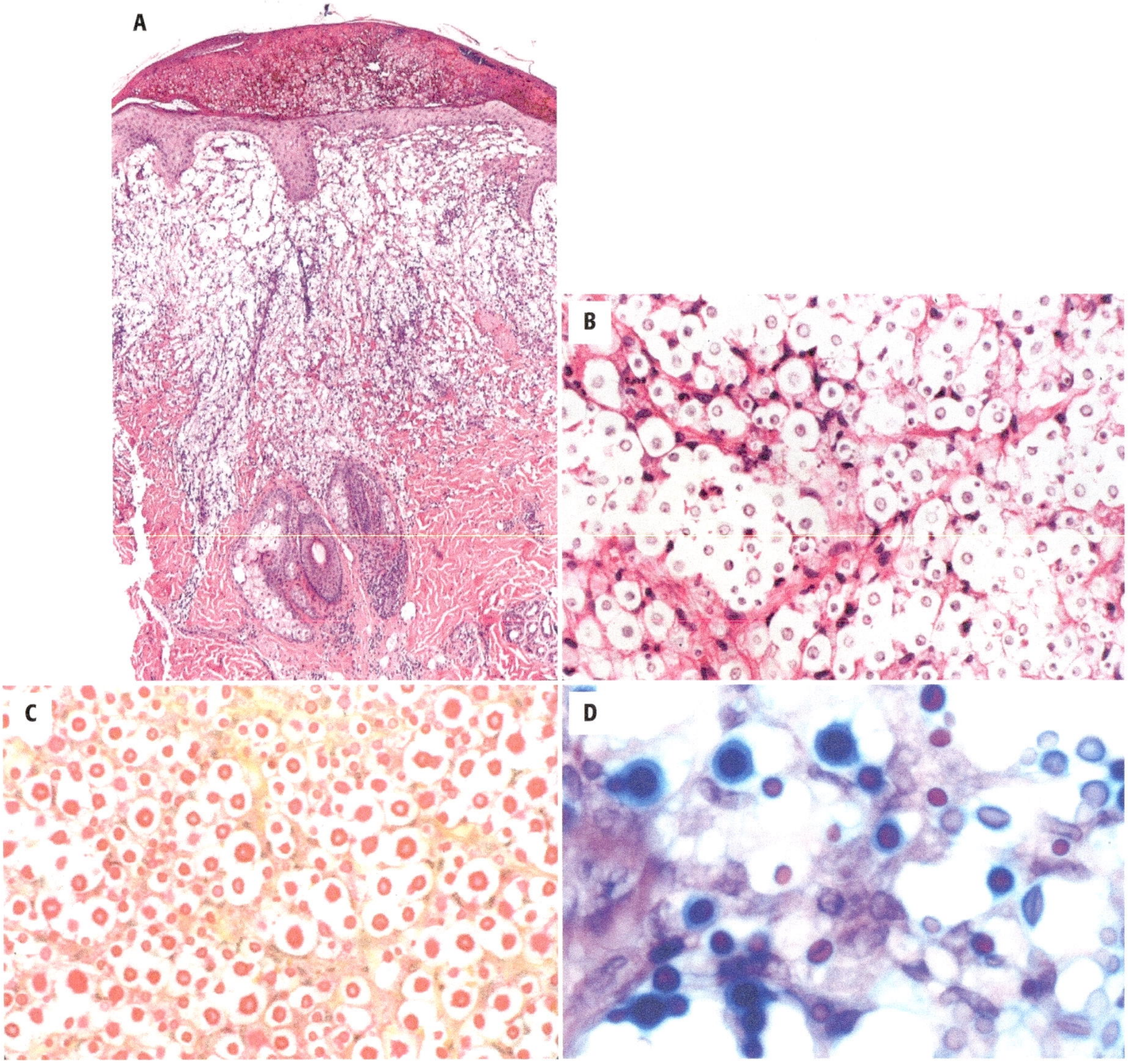

FIG. 3.114

Cryptococcosis. **A,** Gelatinous form with numerous fungi but little inflammation. **B,** Multiple encapsulated spores are present giving a "soap bubble" appearance. **C,** The spores are mucicarmine-positive. **D,** The capsule can also be stained with periodic acid-Schiff and Alcian blue.

Rhinosporidium seeberi may also stain for mucin. Immunoperoxidase methods can be used to identify the organisms on routine paraffin sections. Commercially available latex-agglutination tests that detect cryptococcal polysaccharide capsular antigen in serum or spinal fluid with very high sensitivity and specificity can also be used. In situ hybridization probes have also become available.

Differential Diagnosis

The gelatinous form is diagnostic. In the granulomatous variant, because of the pleomorphism of the spores, the differential diagnosis includes virtually any yeast-form fungal infection. The spherical shape, irregular size, and presence of a capsule strongly positive with mucicarmine are helpful clues to identification.

Prognosis and Treatment

Primary cutaneous lesions have a good prognosis, but patients have to be monitored for possible dissemination to the central nervous system. Disseminated cryptococcosis has a high morbidity and mortality. Amphotericin B and fluorocytosine are used for initial treatment followed by lifelong maintenance antifungal regimen with fluconazole in immunocompromised patients.

HISTOPLASMOSIS

Histoplasma capsulatum is a dimorphic fungus endemic to the Ohio and Mississippi river valleys, Mexico, Peru, Guatemala, Africa, and Asia. Two varieties of *H. capsulatum* are recognized: var. *capsulatum* or North American histoplasmosis, which causes pulmonary or disseminated disease, and var. *duboisii* or African histoplasmosis, which causes skin or bone disease.

Clinical Findings

Cutaneous disease is rare and usually secondary to systemic involvement in patients with deficient immune systems. It may present as papules, ulcerated nodules, or cellulite-like areas (Fig. 3.115).

Histologic Features

The dermis shows a chronic granulomatous inflammatory infiltrate with numerous macrophages containing the clustered round to oval hyaline yeast forms (Fig. 3.116) with a diameter of up to 5 μm, thin-walled, with basophilic cytoplasm separated by a clear halo from the fungal cell wall (Fig. 3.116). *H. capsulatum* var. *duboisii* is characterized by larger organisms, measuring up to 15 μm in diameter, present within the cytoplasm of multinucleated giant cells. The lesions heal with fibrosis.

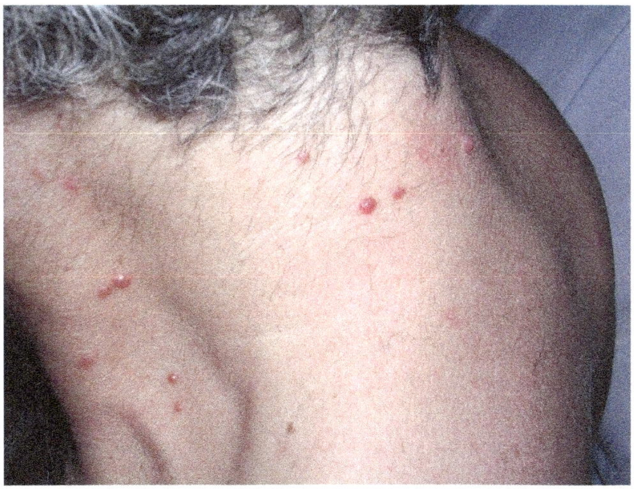

FIG. 3.115

Histoplasmosis. Multiple nonspecific inflammatory papules in disseminated histoplasmosis in an immunocompromised patient.

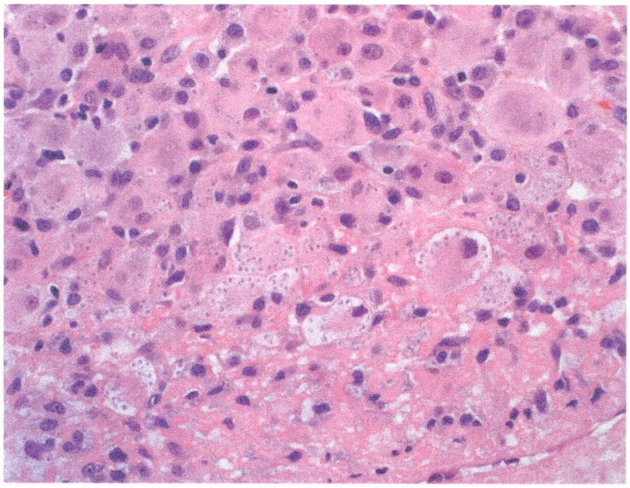

FIG. 3.116

Histoplasmosis. Yeast forms, with a surrounding clear halo, within the cytoplasm of multinucleated giant cells ("parasitized histiocytes").

Ancillary Studies

Fungal stains are typically needed to adequately visualize the organisms. GMS and PAS-D stains color the walls intensely, but there is no halo artifact.

Differential Diagnosis

The differential diagnosis includes *Torulopsis glabrata*, in which the fungal cells resemble *Histoplasma* but are amphophilic and do not have a halo, and *Penicillium marneffei*, in which the fungal cells also resemble *Histoplasma* but do not bud, do not have a halo, and divide by transverse septation. Amastigotes of *Leishmania* mimic *Histoplasma*, but the characteristic bar-shaped kinetoplast can be seen under oil immersion.

Prognosis and Treatment

The severity and duration of pulmonary disease depend on the host immune system and the load of conidia inhaled. Disseminated histoplasmosis is treated with amphotericin B; less severe forms may be treated with ketoconazole, itraconazole, or fluconazole.

MYCETOMA (EUMYCETOMA)

Mycetomas may be caused by bacteria (actinomycetic) or fungi (eumycetic or maduromycotic).

Clinical Findings

Eumycetic mycetomas are found predominantly in the tropics, affect the feet (Madura foot) in the majority of cases, and consist of a slowly enlarging subcutaneous nodule. Draining sinuses develop later in the disease, and deeper structures may become infected by contiguous spread.

Histologic Features

There is a dermal and subcutaneous central area of suppuration surrounded by palisading histiocytes, chronic inflammatory infiltrate, and fibrosis. Characteristic grains are present in the area of suppuration and later may be extruded through draining sinuses. Actinomycotic grains are white, red, or yellow and measure 0.5 mm. They have a homogeneous center and eosinophilic material around the edges (Splendore-Hoeppli phenomenon) and contain delicate branching bacterial filaments less than 1 μm thick (Fig. 3.117). Eumycetic mycetomas usually have larger grains, up to 5 mm in diameter, either black (dematiaceous) or white (hyaline), depending on the causal agent. The fungal hyphae comprising them are septate, 2 to 6 μm thick, often with distorted shapes, and spherical, thick-walled, terminal chlamydoconidium. *Madurella mycetomatis* has hard, brown-black grains, with thick hyphae embedded in a cementlike substance and arranged radially at the periphery. *Pseudallescheria boydii* grains are white and soft, and on routine H&E-stained sections have a pale center, abundant vesicles, or swollen hyphae and an eosinophilic fringe at the periphery.

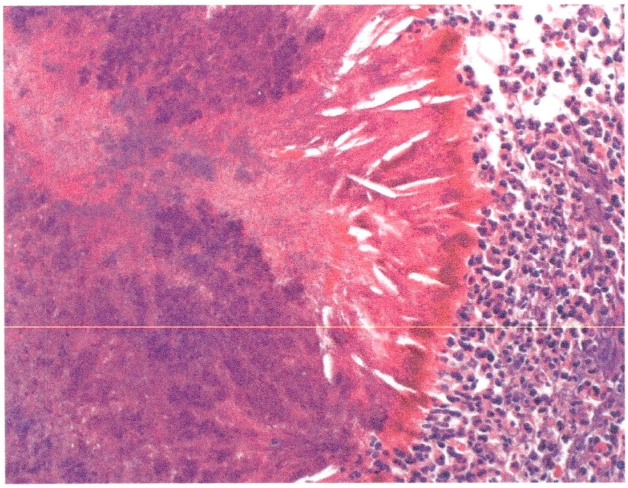

FIG. 3.117
Mycetoma. Actinomycotic grain consisting of a large mass of delicate branching bacterial filaments with eosinophilic immunoglobulin material around the edges (Splendore-Hoeppli phenomenon) and surrounding suppurative inflammation.

Ancillary Studies

The organisms stain positive with both the Gram and PAS-D stains.

Differential Diagnosis

The differential diagnosis includes botryomycosis, in which bacteria form compact aggregates.

Prognosis and Treatment

Mycetomas are usually an insidious localized infection. Treatment is limited to surgical debridement.

ZYGOMYCOSIS

Zygomycosis may be caused by fungi of the order Mucorales, genera *Rhizopus*, *Mucor*, or *Absidia* (mucormycosis), or by fungi of the order Entomophthorales, genera *Basidiobolus* and *Conidiobolus* (subcutaneous phycomycosis). The fungi that cause mucormycosis are found worldwide and are present in soil and decaying matter. They infect mainly patients who are immunocompromised, have diabetes, or have an underlying hematologic malignancy, and they have a fulminant clinical course. Zygomycosis resulting from entomophthoraceous fungi is chronic, slowly progressive, and restricted to the subcutaneous tissue in otherwise healthy individuals.

Clinical Findings

Primary skin mucormycosis is rare and seen in patients with burns or after local trauma. Skin disease tends to develop secondary to hematogenous spread. Lesions are characterized by necrosis, either as indurated tender plaques with a dusky center or as necrotizing cellulitis (Fig. 3.118). Subcutaneous phycomycosis caused by *Basidiobolus* sp. manifests as subcutaneous nodules, primarily occurring in boys. Subcutaneous phycomycosis caused by *Conidiobolus* sp. is typically restricted to the nasal submucosa and characterized by nasal polyps, nasal obstruction, drainage, and sinus pain. It has a male predominance.

Histologic Features

Fungi of the order Mucorales characteristically have a propensity to invade vessel walls, causing thrombosis

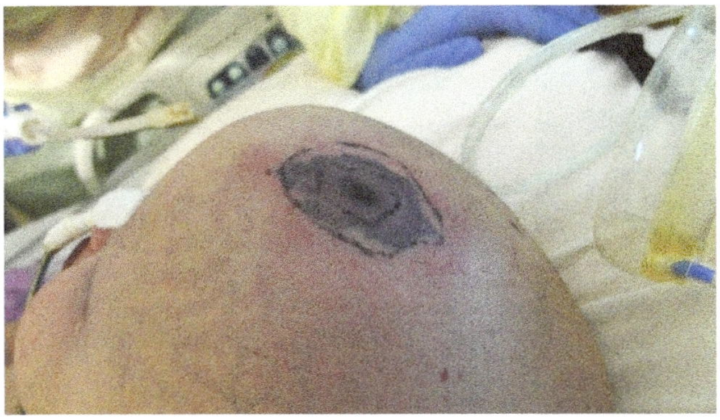

FIG. 3.118
Zygomycosis (mucormycosis). Necrotic patch with a dusky center.

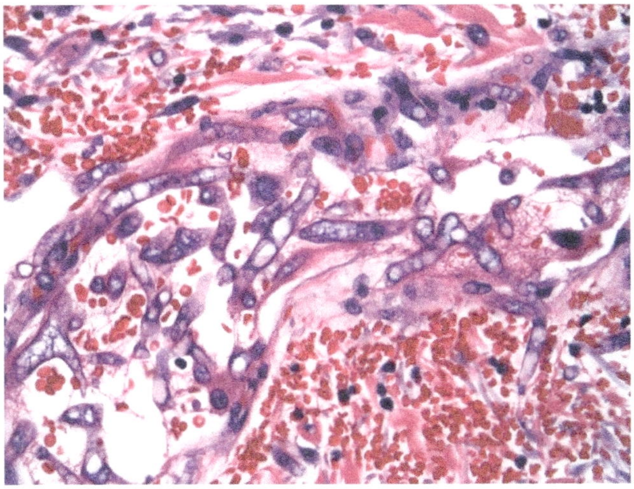

FIG. 3.119
Zygomycosis (mucormycosis). The hyphae are broad and nonseptate.

and infarction. Areas of necrosis with or without suppuration may be seen, accompanied by a variable inflammatory host response. The hyphae are broad, ribbon-like, irregularly contoured, non-septate or infrequently septate, and branch at 90-degree angles (Figs. 3.119 and 3.120). They are visible in H&E-stained sections, where the thin walls are basophilic or amphophilic and nonparallel and the center is optically clear (Figs. 3.119 and 3.120). They grow to form spongiophores and sporangia (Fig. 3.121). Subcutaneous phycomycosis is characterized by dermal and subcutaneous granulomatous inflammation containing eosinophils, scattered abscesses, and sometimes focal necrosis. The hyphae are sparse, short, and surrounded by a homogeneous eosinophilic material (Splendore-Hoeppli phenomenon). Angioinvasion is usually not present.

Ancillary Studies

GMS and PAS-D stains can be used to highlight the fungal hyphae. Culture can give a definitive identification.

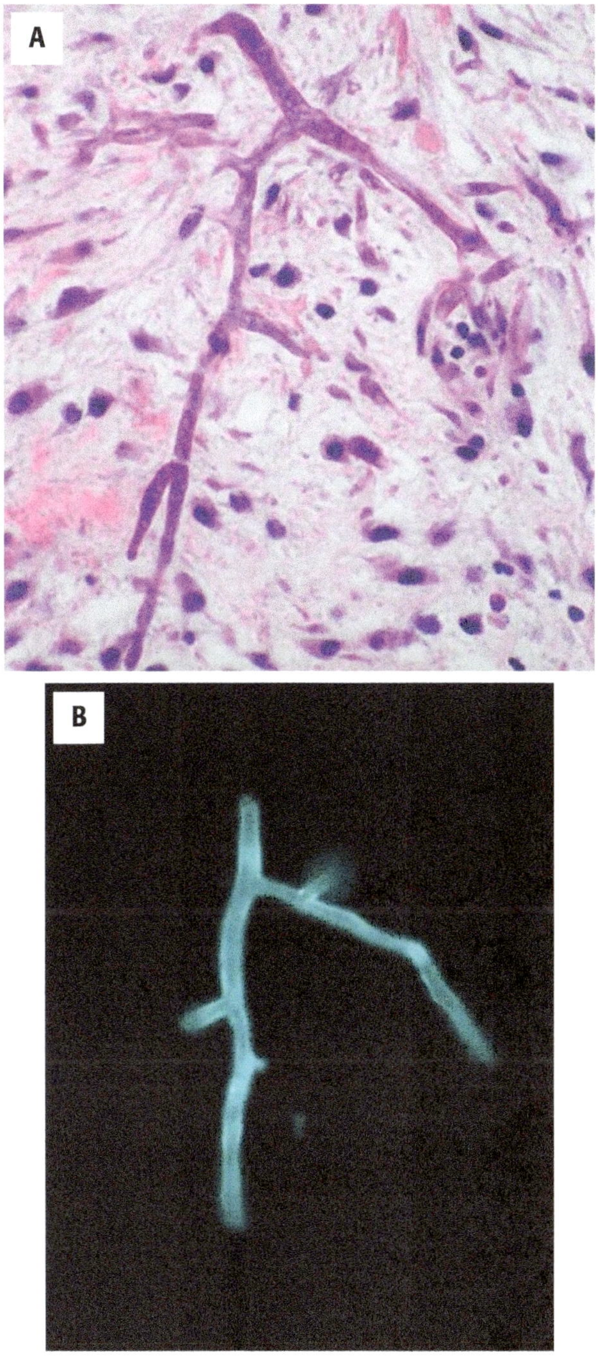

FIG. 3.120
Mucormycosis. **A,** Aseptate branching hyphae (H&E). **B,** Calcofluor white stain showing broad hyphae branching at 90-degree angles.

Differential Diagnosis

The main differential diagnosis is aspergillosis, in which the hyphae are septate and characteristically branch at 45 degrees. *Fusarium* hyphae may resemble Zygomycetes, branch at right angles, produce terminal or intercalated chlamydoconidium, and are constricted at their site of origin.

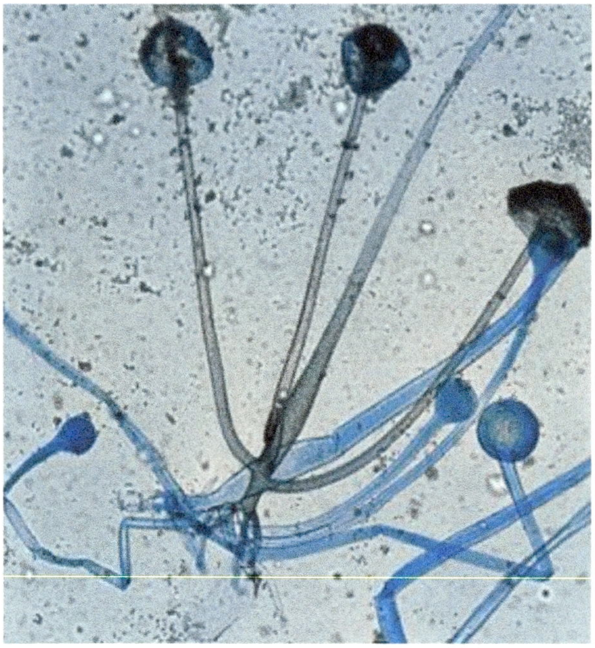

FIG. 3. 121

Lactophenol cotton blue stain showing rhizoid with unbranched sporangiophores and burst sporangia.

Prognosis and Treatment

Zygomycosis is highly aggressive and has a high fatality rate. Treatment consists of surgical debridement and amphotericin B. Subcutaneous phycomycosis is treated with potassium iodide and azoles; surgery can cause the infection to spread.

ASPERGILLOSIS

Cutaneous aspergillosis is uncommon and occurs mainly in patients with compromised immune status, hematologic disorders, diabetes, burns; in premature neonates; or at the site of intravenous catheters or occlusive dressings.

Clinical Findings

The lesions consist of erythematous tender macules, papules, or plaques with scattered pustules that evolve into violaceous nodules with central necrosis and ulceration.

ASPERGILLOSIS—DISEASE FACT SHEET

Opportunistic mycotic infection caused by fungi of the genus Aspergillus, more commonly *A. fumigatus* and *A. flavus*

Patient Group

- ▸▸ Immunosuppressed individuals

Site of Involvement

- ▸▸ Primary: Site of trauma, burns, wounds, intravenous catheters
- ▸▸ Secondary: Anywhere (hematogenous dissemination)

Clinical Findings

- ▸▸ Variable: Papules, nodules, and/or necrotic ulcers

Prognosis and Treatment

- ▸▸ Primary lesions have a better prognosis; the treatment consists of surgical excision and oral antifungals
- ▸▸ Secondary cutaneous aspergillosis carries a very poor prognosis and is frequently fatal

Histologic Features

Histologic findings are variable. Granulomatous inflammation with abscess formation is usually seen. The hyphae have characteristic 45-degree dichotomous branching, are septate and regular in outline, and have parallel walls (Fig. 3.122). Aspergillus may invade the vessel walls and cause thrombosis. Characteristic fruiting bodies are rarely seen in tissues (Fig. 3.123). *Aspergillus niger* is pigmented (Fig. 3.123).

Ancillary Studies

The hyphae are best highlighted by PAS-D or GMS stains but can often already be seen on routine H&E-stained sections.

ASPERGILLOSIS—PATHOLOGIC FEATURES

Histologic Features

- ▸▸ Granuloma or abscess formation
- ▸▸ Septate, hyaline, dichotomous hyphae with 45-degree branching, highlighted by GMS or PAS stain
- ▸▸ Vascular invasion and occlusion

Ancillary Studies

- ▸▸ Fungal stains (GMS, PAS-D)
- ▸▸ Cultures
- ▸▸ *A. flavus* colonies have khaki-green center, *A. fumigatus* colonies have blue-gray center
- ▸▸ Colonies with white to yellow rim ("South Sea islands")

Differential Diagnosis

- ▸▸ Mucormycosis
- ▸▸ *Fusarium* infections

GMS, Gomori methenamine silver; *PAS*, periodic acid-Schiff; *PAS-D*, periodic Wacid-Schiff with diastase digestion.

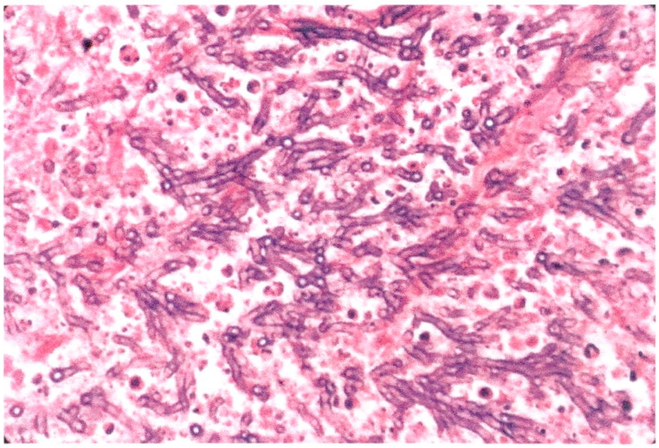

FIG. 3.122
Aspergillosis. Numerous hyphae are present. They are septate and branch at 45 degrees.

Differential Diagnosis

The differential diagnosis includes mucormycosis, usually easily distinguished by hyphal morphology, and *Fusarium* infection, in which the similar hyphae branch at right angles but also show constrictions at the site of branching, terminal, or intercalated chlamydoconidia, and intrahyphal vesicles. Definitive diagnosis may require culture on standard mycologic media.

Prognosis and Treatment

Prompt treatment with systemic amphotericin B is required to prevent widespread infection and thrombosis, which may be fatal.

LOBOMYCOSIS

Lobomycosis is an infection caused by the fungus *Lacazia loboi*, previously called *Loboa loboi*, found in Central and South America. Natural disease has been described only in humans and dolphins. The disease is also known as keloidal blastomycosis or Lobo's disease.

Clinical Findings

The disease manifests as keloid-like lesions, slowly growing, firm, verrucous nodules or plaques developing on exposed skin (Fig. 3.124), usually at a site of trauma. Older lesions may ulcerate. Satellite lesions may develop from autoinoculation.

Histologic Features

The dermis contains a dense granulomatous histiocytic inflammatory infiltrate with multinucleated giant cells. The fungi measure 7 to 14 μm in diameter and have a lemon shape and a slightly refractile double-contoured wall. They form single chains of budding cells united by narrow tube-like bridges. They may be present within the cytoplasm of multinucleated giant cells but often occur extracellularly (Fig. 3.125). Because they do not stain with H&E stain, they impart a sieve-like appearance at low power.

Ancillary Studies

The fungal cell walls and cytoplasm are strongly positive with PAS-D and GMS stains.

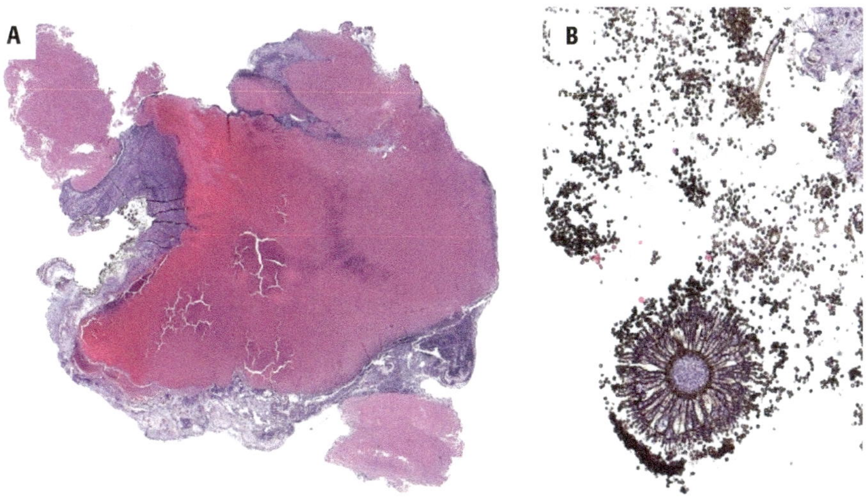

FIG. 3.123
Aspergillus niger. **A,** purulent exudate with fungus. **B,** Fruiting body.

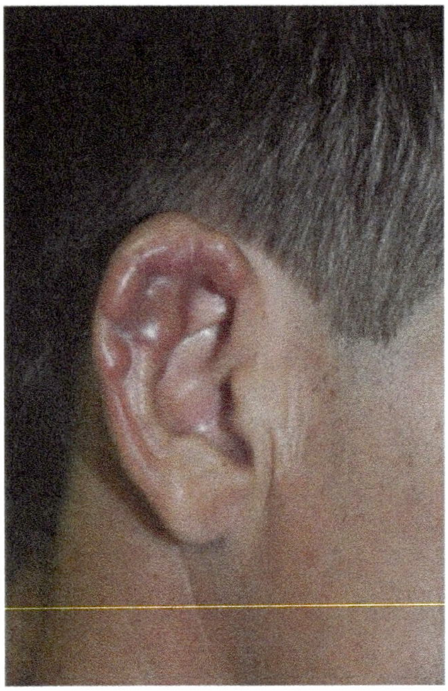

FIG. 3.124
Lobomycosis: indurated nodules. The ear is commonly involved. (From Talhari, S., & Talhari, C. (2012). Lobomycosis. *Clinics in Dermatology*, 30(4), 420–424.)

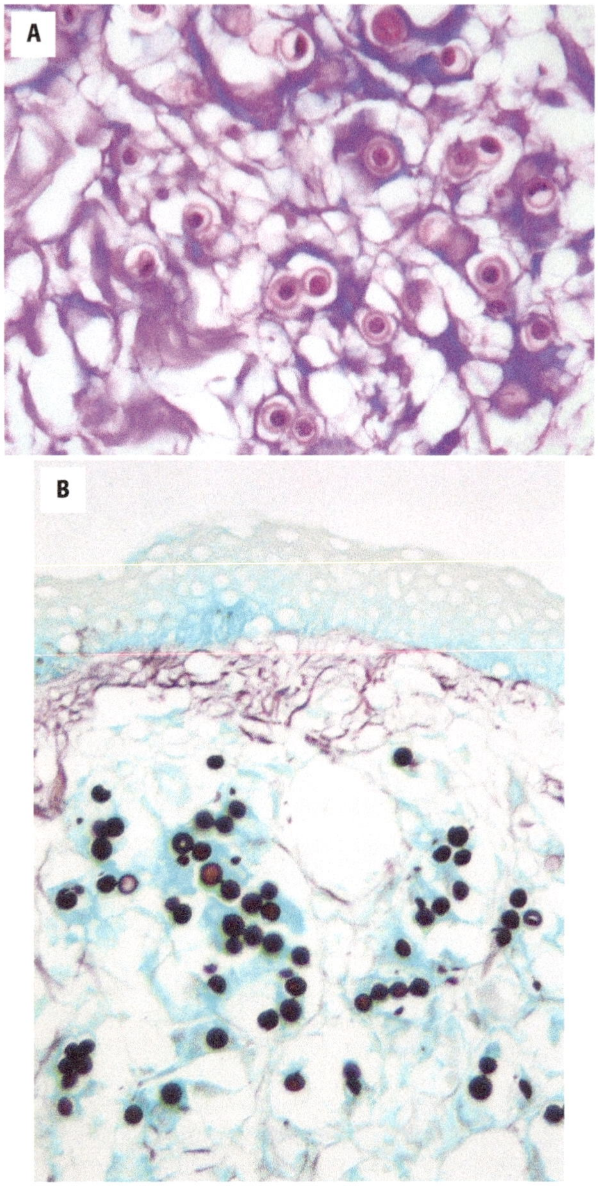

FIG. 3.125
Lobomycosis. **A,** The fungi have thick walls and tend to be arranged in chains. **B,** Positive staining by Gomori methenamine silver.

Differential Diagnosis

Mucicarmine stain is negative, helping to differentiate lobomycosis from cryptococcosis.

Prognosis and Treatment

The disease has a slow but progressive course. Treatment is surgical removal with wide margins.

RHINOSPORIDIOSIS

Rhinosporidium seeberi, the causative agent of rhinosporidiosis, is endemic in India and Sri Lanka. It has been recently demonstrated to be a protist belonging to a novel group of fish parasites, phylogenetically situated at the divergence between fungi and animals.

Clinical Findings

The clinical picture consists of pink, friable polypoid lesions on the nasal or ocular mucosa. In very rare cases, solitary nodules may occur in other areas of the body.

Histologic Features

Spherical sporangia measuring up to 400 μm in diameter and containing numerous tiny endospores are seen (Fig. 3.126), often accompanied by a mixed granulomatous inflammatory infiltrate. Sometimes transepidermal elimination can be seen.

Ancillary Studies

The thick, trilaminate walls of sporangia are positive with PAS and GMS stains. Sporangiospores and the

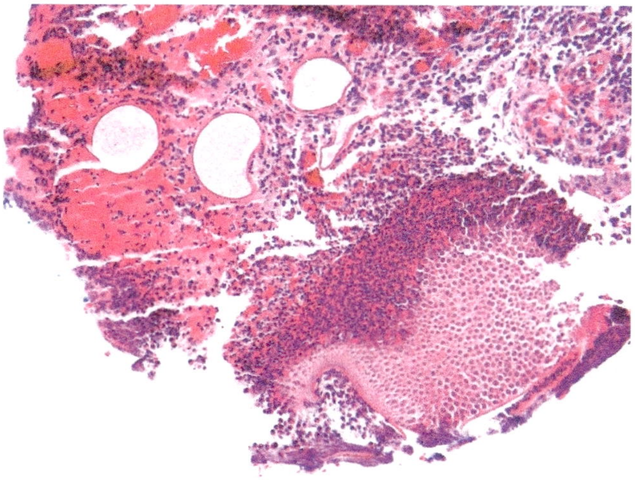

FIG. 3.126
Rhinosporidiosis. Sporangium with numerous endospores associated with inflammation.

inner surface of sporangial walls are also positive when stained with Mayer's mucicarmine.

Differential Diagnosis

The constellation of clinical and histologic findings is pathognomonic.

Prognosis and Treatment

Treatment consists of surgical excision and topical amphotericin B.

PROTOZOAN DISEASE, PARASITIC INFESTATIONS, ALGAL INFECTIONS, AND BITES

AMEBIASIS

Cutaneous infection with amoeba can be caused by *Acanthamoeba* sp. free living in water and soil or *Entamoeba histolytica* in patients with amoebic colitis. Cutaneous involvement can be a presenting sign of disseminated disease in immunocompromised patients, a very rare and, in most cases, fatal occurrence.

Clinical Findings

Cutaneous lesions are polymorphic but tend to evolve into ulcerated suppurative lesions, forming necrotic eschars.

Histologic Features

The ulcerated lesions of cutaneous amebiasis show extensive necrotic debris in which the trophozoites can be found singly or in clusters. *Entamoeba histolytica* trophozoites have a sharply defined cell membrane, ameboid shape, finely granular amphophilic vacuolated cytoplasm, and a single eccentric nucleus, 2 to 4 μm in diameter with a small karyosome. Phagocytized red blood cells may be seen in the cytoplasm. *Acanthamoeba* trophozoites have a central nucleus with large karyosome and abundant granular vacuolated cytoplasm (Fig. 3.127). Cyst forms have wrinkled, star-shaped double walls and are often found around vessels.

Ancillary Studies

Rapid identification may be done by examining wet drop preparation of the pus from the ulcer and observing trophozoites exhibiting motility. Identification of trophozoites on histologic examination is diagnostic. Immunocytochemistry, chemofluorescent dye staining, and PCR have also been used for laboratory diagnosis. Specimens can be transported on Page's amoeba saline for culture on nonnutrient agar overlaid with *Escherichia coli*.

Differential Diagnosis

The amoebas need to be differentiated from histiocytes or macrophages, ganglion cells, and CMV-infected cells.

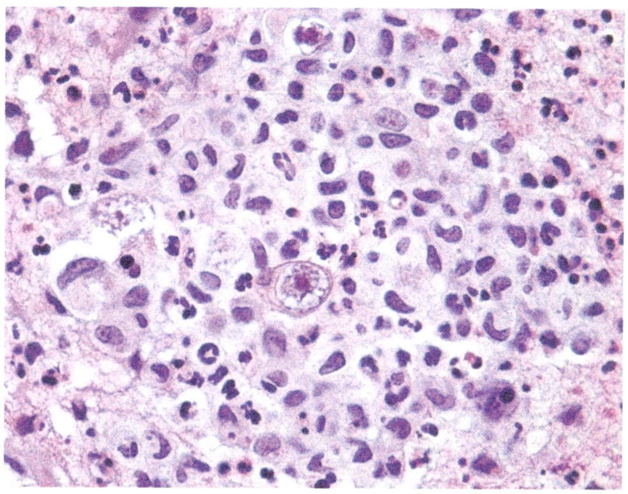

FIG. 3.127
Amebiasis. A trophozoite is present in a background of suppurative and granulomatous dermatitis.

Prognosis and Treatment

Medications used include oral or intravenous metronidazole (Flagyl) followed by luminal amebicides (paromomycin, iodoquinol, or diloxanide furoate) to eradicate the source of organisms in patients with amoebic colitis. In disseminated disease, prompt and aggressive multidrug therapy may offer a chance of survival.

LEISHMANIASIS

Leishmaniasis is an infection caused by a hemoflagellate parasite of the genus *Leishmania* (L.), which may affect the skin, the mucous membranes (espundia), and the internal organs. Leishmaniasis was classified into two major types: cutaneous (Old World and New World leishmaniasis) and visceral (kala-azar). Approximately 21 species may affect humans. The form of disease is determined by factors such as leishmanial species, geographic location, and immune response of the host.

Cutaneous lesions have been known by many names, such as chiclero ulcer, Uta, Delhi boil, Baghdad boil, Aleppo boil, button de Crete, and Biskra button. The vector sandfly may belong to the genus *Phlebotomus* in the "Old World" and *Lutzomyia* in the "New World." They breed in dark, moist environments and are nocturnal. The reservoir may be humans or animals (rodents and canines). Infection occurs when the promastigotes are injected from the proboscis of the female sandfly at the time of feeding. They invade the cells of the reticuloendothelial system, where they transform into amastigotes and multiply.

Clinical Findings

Cutaneous leishmaniasis can present as acute, chronic, mucocutaneous, and disseminated forms. Acute lesions are single pruritic papules that develop at the site of inoculation. In 2 to 8 weeks, they become nodules and then ulcerate (Fig. 3.128). The ulcers have erythematous raised margins and a shallow bed, resembling a volcano.

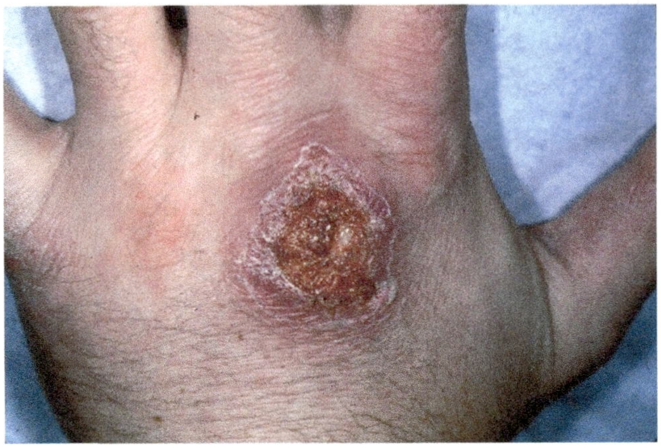

FIG. 3.128

Cutaneous leishmaniasis. An ulcerated papule with erythematous raised margins is present.

The best areas to be sampled to find the organisms are beneath the ulcer margins. The ulcers heal, leaving a residual scar. Mucocutaneous leishmaniasis consists of similar lesions developing initially at the site of inoculation and later spreading to the mucous membranes, more frequently first to the nasal mucosa. Destructive ulcerating lesions may develop, causing major disfigurement, a complication known as espundia. Chronic lesions are rare; they consist of raised single or occasionally multiple erythematous plaques that persist for 1 to 2 years and sometimes have a verrucous surface. The disseminated form may develop in immunocompromised patients as multiple nodules and macules that do not ulcerate.

CUTANEOUS LEISHMANIASIS—DISEASE FACT SHEET

Chronic disease is caused by protozoan parasites of the genus Leishmania. They spend part of their life cycle in the gut of the sandfly, but complete it in a vertebrate host.

Patient Group

- Both genders and all ages may be infected
- In the United States, infection is seen in individuals who traveled to endemic areas

Site of Involvement

- Usually located on exposed areas

Clinical Findings

- Cutaneous disease: Ulcerated pruritic papules, sometimes verrucous
- Mucocutaneous disease: Edema, ulceration, destruction of local structures (nasal cartilage)

Prognosis and Treatment

- Cutaneous leishmaniasis is self-limited in many cases; mucocutaneous disease can lead to massive tissue loss and disfigurement
- Treatment is local (surgical excision, heat therapy) and systemic (pentavalent antimonials)

LEISHMANIASIS—PATHOLOGIC FEATURES

Histologic Features

- Marked dermal inflammatory infiltrate, granulomatous in late stages
- Oval amastigotes, 3 μm in diameter, with darkly basophilic nucleus, distinct cell membrane, and kinetoplasts located in the anterior half ("safety pin")

- Highlighted by Giemsa stain
- Localized at the periphery of macrophage cytoplasm ("marquee" sign)
- Pseudoepitheliomatous hyperplasia

Ancillary Studies

- Giemsa stain can highlight organisms
- Cultures
- Montenegro skin test
- Polymerase chain reaction studies

Differential Diagnosis

- *Toxoplasma gondii*
- *Histoplasma capsulatum*
- Sarcoidosis
- Tuberculosis
- Squamous cell carcinoma

In approximately 6% of the cases of treated visceral leishmaniasis, there is also cutaneous involvement, usually several years after the onset of systemic disease. Erythema may occur on the face, with hypopigmented or hyperpigmented macules on the trunk, and later develop into firm nodules. The nodules are reminiscent of leprosy, but sensory loss is not observed.

Histologic Features

In acute cutaneous leishmaniasis, there is a marked dermal inflammatory infiltrate composed of macrophages, lymphocytes, plasma cells, neutrophils, and eosinophils. The parasites can be identified in the cytoplasm of macrophages (Fig. 3.129), localized mostly at the periphery (the "marquee" sign). As the host responds, there is dermal necrosis followed by ulceration. The amastigotes are oval, 3 μm in diameter, have a darkly basophilic nucleus; a distinct cell membrane; and a kinetoplast located in the anterior half, resembling a safety pin. In tissue sections, Giemsa stain highlights the details of the parasite better than H&E stain. Epidermal changes are nonspecific and include hyperplasia, sometimes pseudoepitheliomatous, and atrophy. Disseminated lesions of cutaneous leishmaniasis are similar, except that the inflammatory infiltrate consists mostly of macrophages containing parasites. Tuberculoid granulomas develop in chronic forms, there is rarely central necrosis, and the number of parasitized macrophages is lower. Mucocutaneous leishmaniasis is characterized by tuberculoid granulomas, areas of necrosis, numerous parasites, and epidermal hyperplasia. The cutaneous lesions occurring years after successful treatment of visceral leishmaniasis show a sparse inflammatory infiltrate separated by a Grenz zone from an atrophic epidermis. Parasites are rare. Weigert iron H&E stain or Wilder's reticulum stain is used for detection of *L. donovani*.

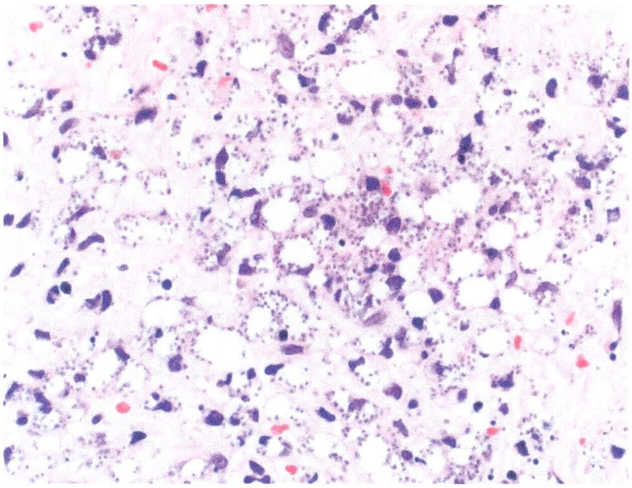

FIG. 3.129

Cutaneous leishmaniasis. Parasites within the cytoplasm of histiocytes ("parasitized histiocytes"), mostly localized to the periphery of the cells ("marquee" sign).

Ancillary Studies

The amastigotes can be rapidly identified in touch preparation of biopsy specimens using alcohol fixation and Giemsa stain. The Giemsa stain is also very helpful to better visualize the organisms on histologic sections. Immunohistochemistry or PCR can be used to identify the organism in tissues. Promastigotes can be identified in cultures on modified Novy-McNeal-Nicolle medium. The Montenegro skin test has been used in the past; a positive reaction consists of erythema and induration measuring more than 5 mm in diameter appearing 48 to 72 hours after intradermal injection of leishmanial antigen. The test has low sensitivity and does not distinguish between active disease and prior exposure, and the test result is negative in immunosuppressed patients.

Differential Diagnosis

History of travel to an endemic area is extremely important, especially because different species from different geographic areas can produce different clinical manifestations. Similar in size and shape are *Toxoplasma gondii* and *H. capsulatum*. The presence of the kinetoplast is an essential feature in identifying leishmania amastigotes. PAS-D or GMS stains help exclude histoplasmosis.

Prognosis and Treatment

Cutaneous leishmaniasis presents in a clinical spectrum of disease. At one end, there is acute disease with spontaneous healing (the vast majority of cases), and at the other end, chronic disease with relapsing and disseminated forms. Old World cutaneous leishmaniasis tends to resolve spontaneously, and the indications for treatment include lesions that are disfiguring or slow to heal. Thermosurgery is approved by the Food and Drug Administration (FDA) for the treatment of cutaneous leishmaniasis. The classic treatment of visceral leishmaniasis consists of pentavalent antimonials (sodium stibogluconate and meglumine antimoniate), available only from the CDC. Newer options include liposomal amphotericin B.

CUTANEOUS LARVA MIGRANS

Cutaneous larva migrans is the result of the migration of the larvae of several nematode species through the skin toward blood vessels. Most cases are caused by *Ancylostoma braziliensis* or *Strongyloides stercoralis*. After contact with contaminated soil or sand, infectious larvae penetrate the skin in exposed areas (most commonly the hands, feet, knees, and buttocks) with the help of potent digestive enzymes.

Clinical Findings

Lesions consist of pruritic papules that form linear or serpiginous tunnels (Fig. 3.130), first erythematous, later elevated and vesicular, and crusted in the end. The lesions advance at a rate of several millimeters per day. *Strongyloides stercoralis* may cause tunnels that advance as fast as 5 to 15 cm per hour, provoking an intensely itchy wheal along the tortuous tract (linear urticaria). These cases are known as larva currens, or racing larva. Chronic cases related to an autoinfective cycle were described in former World War II British prisoners of war imprisoned in Thailand and Burma.

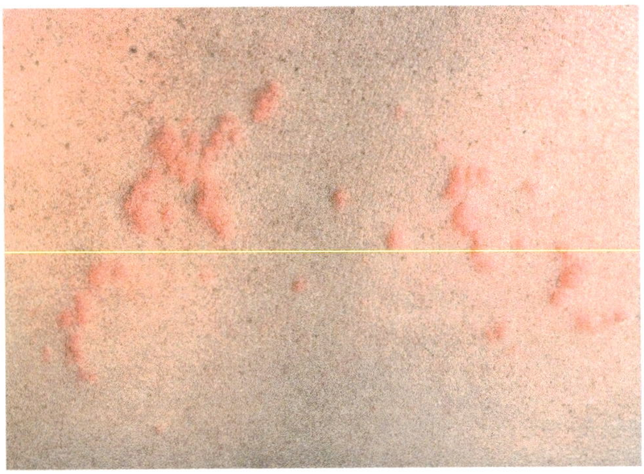

FIG. 3.130
Cutaneous larva migrans. Irregular serpiginous erythematous lesions reflect tracts formed by the larvae.

Histologic Features

The migrating larvae are seen burrowed above the dermal-epidermal junction, a few centimeters ahead of the visible track (Fig. 3.131). In most cases, only the tunnel of the larvae is seen, sometimes surrounded by spongiosis and intraepidermal vesicles containing eosinophils. The dermis contains a superficial mixed-inflammatory infiltrate with abundant eosinophils. *Gnathostoma spinigerum* may cause deeper tracks. *Ancylostoma* filariform larvae measure 500 to 700 μm in length and 20 to 24 μm in diameter and have pointed tails. *Strongyloides* filariform larvae are shorter (500 to 550 μm in length) and have notched tails.

Differential Diagnosis

The differential diagnosis includes, in rare cases, a migratory myasis caused by the horse botfly or cattle crab fly.

Prognosis and Treatment

Treatment consists of oral and topical thiabendazole.

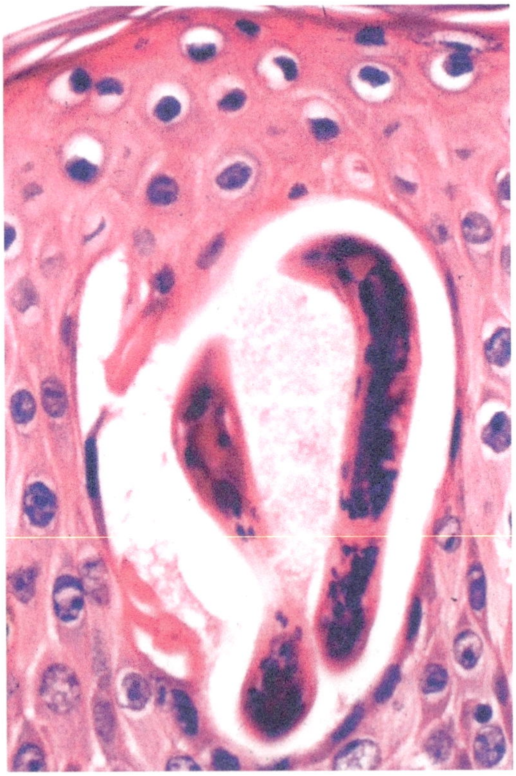

FIG. 3.131
Cutaneous larva migrans. Larvae are present in tunnels within the epidermis.

DEMODICOSIS

Demodex folliculorum and *Demodex brevis* are the most common permanent ectoparasites of humans. *Demodex folliculorum* was first described by Jakob Henle in 1841. *Demodex folliculorum* mites are long and thin, and they aggregate in the infundibular region of the hair follicles. *Demodex brevis* mites are usually solitary and smaller and target the deeper sebaceous glands. The mites are seen in normal skin with increased frequency as age increases and prefer the forehead, nose, and malar areas, where there is more abundant sebum production.

Clinical Findings

Three forms of *Demodex* infestation are described: a rosacea-like eruption (rosacea-like demodicosis), facial erythema with follicular plugging (pityriasis folliculorum), and granulomatous rosacea-like demodicidosis gravis. Because of the initial papers by Ayres, *Demodex* mites have been incriminated as putative pathogens in a wide variety of skin conditions, but these associations are still controversial.

Histologic Features

Follicular dilatation and plugging by keratinous material, folliculitis, and perifolliculitis are the most frequent histologic findings. *Demodex folliculorum* can be identified in the follicular ostia, buried with the head toward the dermis (Fig. 3.132). The mites have adapted to life in a hair follicle by assuming a thin, elongated shape (wormlike) and rudimentary legs. The finding of an occasional mite in a skin biopsy is of no significance, but increased numbers (more than 5 per 1 low-power field was the number proposed by Ayres) may be causative of skin pathology.

Differential Diagnosis

Demodex can readily be found on routine sections or by examining expressed contents of a sebaceous gland under the microscope. It is distinctive.

Prognosis and Treatment

Eruptions in which demodices are thought to be involved may be treated by topical application of benzyl benzoate emulsion, permethrin, or ivermectin. Oral ivermectin can also be used.

SCABIES

Scabies is a common infestation of the skin with the mite *Sarcoptes scabiei*, found worldwide and affecting all races and social classes since antiquity. The disease is highly contagious, and it is transmitted by prolonged direct contact or in overcrowded communities.

Clinical Findings

Patients complain of intense pruritus, mostly nocturnal. The most characteristic lesion is the burrow made by the female mite on her way to lay eggs. The burrows appear as fine, wavy, brown, or dirty appearing lines in the interdigital skin folds (Fig. 3.133). Other manifestations include papules, nodules (Fig. 3.134), vesicles, or eczematous changes with a predilection for the palms and wrists, soles, nipples, inframammary folds, waist (belt line), and male genitalia. Dermoscopy is helpful for mite and excreta detection and for guiding the skin scraping because the parasite is found at a small distance from the clinically visible burrow and not in its axis. Nodular persistent lesions, located mainly in the lower trunk, thighs, and scrotum, are seen mainly in younger age groups and are considered a form of delayed hypersensitivity reaction. Norwegian or crusted scabies is characterized by widespread crusted hyperkeratotic lesions with a heavy load of mites and occurs in debilitated and immunocompromised patients (Fig. 3.135).

SCABIES—DISEASE FACT SHEET

Infestation by *Sarcoptes scabiei* var. *hominis* mite

Patient Group

- Prevalence higher in children and sexually active adults
- Norwegian scabies seen usually in immunodeficient patients or patients with Down syndrome

Site of Involvement

- Predilection for interdigital and flexural areas, waist, ankles, and intergluteal fold

Clinical Findings

- Intensely pruritic, symmetrical, small erythematous papules with wavy, threadlike, elevated gray-white burrows are pathognomonic

Prognosis and Treatment

- Several courses of topical treatment with antiscabietic agents for the patient and all close contacts are effective in the majority of cases; oral ivermectin has also been successfully used recently
- The disease is highly contagious

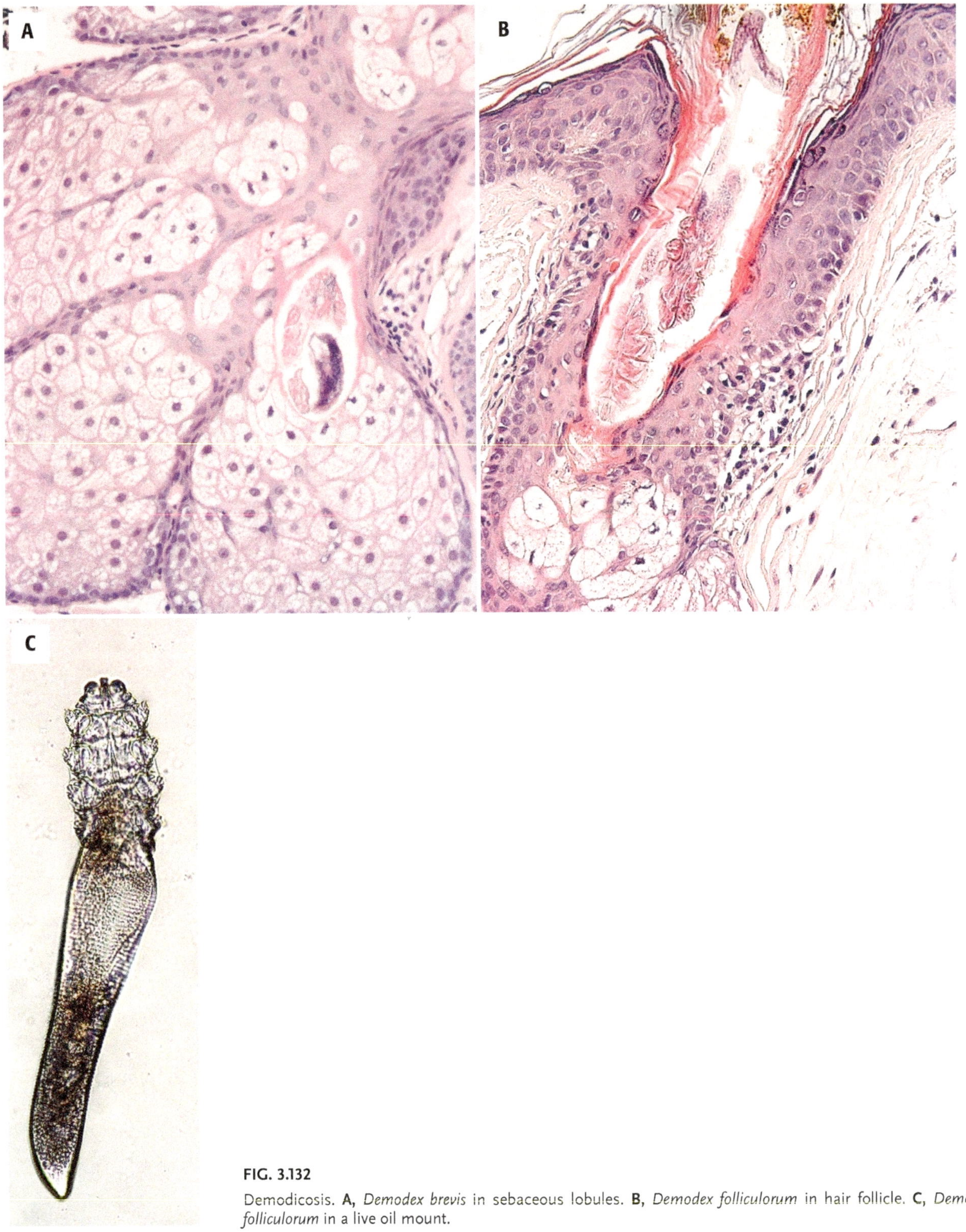

FIG. 3.132
Demodicosis. **A,** *Demodex brevis* in sebaceous lobules. **B,** *Demodex folliculorum* in hair follicle. **C,** *Demodex folliculorum* in a live oil mount.

Histologic Features

Mites, eggs, larvae, and excreta may be found in stratum corneum (Fig. 3.136). The female mite measures 0.3 to 0.4 mm in length and can be found at the blind end of the burrow. It has an ovoid shape with four pairs of legs. The first two are located at the anterior end; the other two are located laterally on the ventral surface and have long hairs that point posteriorly. The male mite is approximately half the size and dies after copulation. Spongiotic epidermal vesicles containing eosinophils can be seen. In the dermis, there is a perivascular superficial and deep inflammatory infiltrate containing

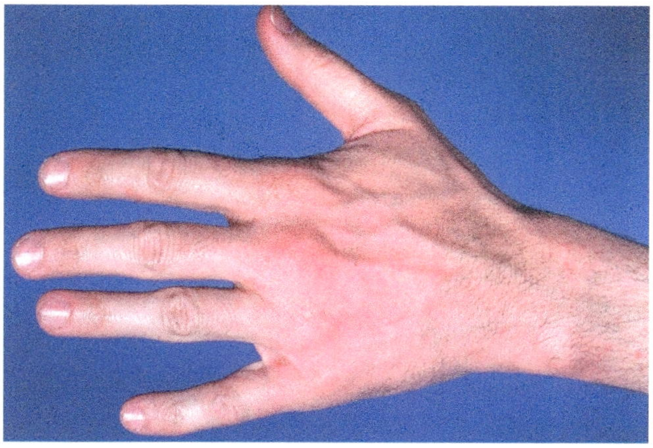

FIG. 3.133

Scabies. Papulovesicular pruritic lesions are present in the hand. Burrows are seen between the web spaces.

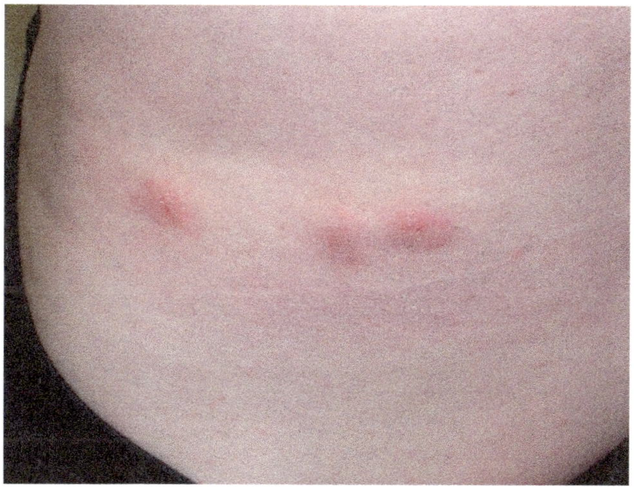

FIG. 3.134

Scabies. Scabetic nodules at the waist-line.

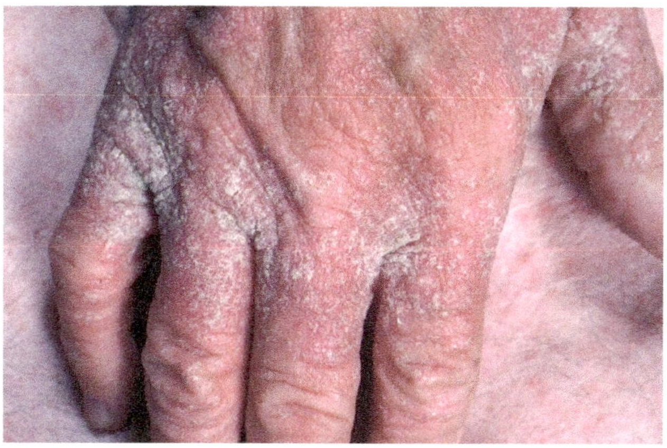

FIG. 3.135

Norwegian scabies. Scaling and crusting are typical of this hyperkeratotic variant.

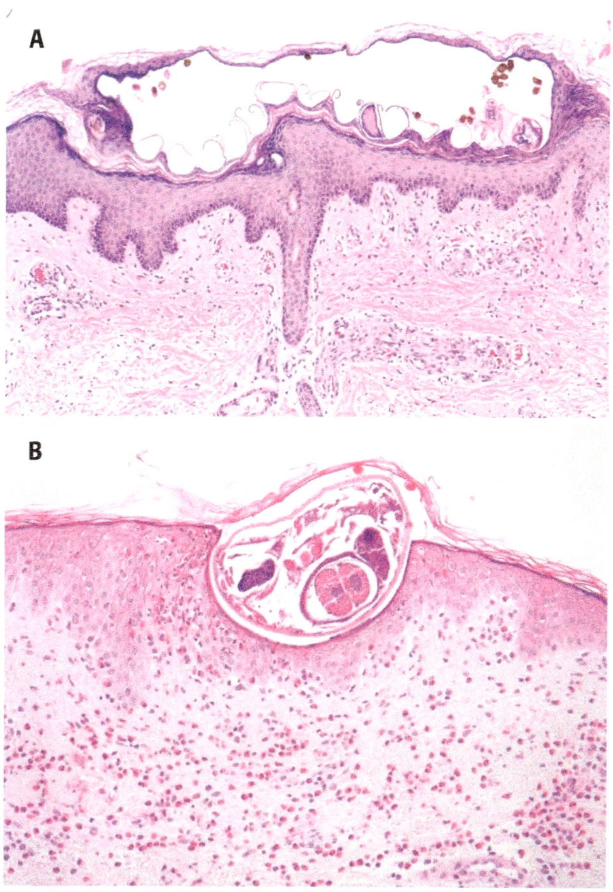

FIG. 3.136

Scabies. **A,** Mites, eggs, larvae, and excreta in the cornified layer. **B,** There is an eosinophilic inflammatory reaction to a mite.

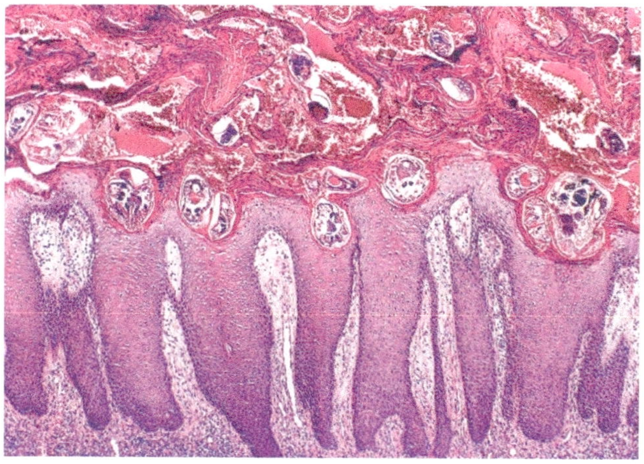

FIG. 3.137

Norwegian scabies. Numerous mites and eggs are present in multilayered burrows. There is massive hyperkeratosis.

eosinophils, which can also be identified scattered between the collagen bundles. In persistent nodular forms, mites are rarely found, and the inflammatory infiltrate is denser and deeper. In Norwegian scabies, there are epidermal psoriasiform hyperplasia and overlying massive ortho- and parakeratosis containing multilayered burrows, abundant mites, eggs, and excreta (Fig. 3.137).

SCABIES—PATHOLOGIC FEATURES

Histologic Features

- Mites, eggs, larvae, and excreta in stratum corneum burrows
- Mites located at the blind end of the burrow, which may extend into stratum spinosum
- Female mite is ovoid, up to 0.4 mm in length, and has four pairs of legs
- Perivascular superficial and deep inflammatory infiltrate with eosinophils

Differential Diagnosis

- Arthropod bite
- Cutaneous larva migrans
- Cercarial dermatitis
- Urticarial allergic reactions
- Drug reactions

Lesions of nodular scabies show a dense nodular dermal infiltrate of lymphocytes, histiocytes, and usually many eosinophils (Fig. 3.137).

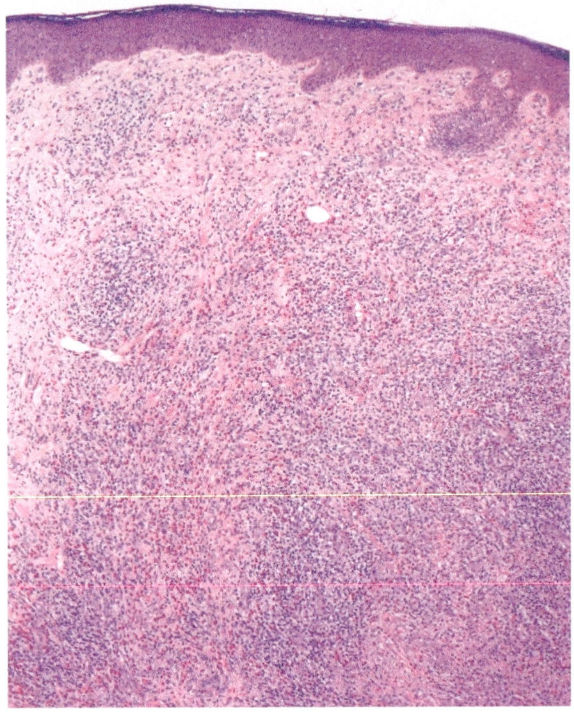

FIG. 3.138
Nodular scabies. A dense nodular infiltrate of lymphocytes, histiocytes, and eosinophils is present.

Differential Diagnosis

The diagnosis requires identification of mites, eggs, or excreta in burrows. If these are not found, the differential diagnosis is broad and includes arthropod bite, cutaneous larva migrans, cercarial dermatitis, urticarial allergic reactions, and drug reactions.

Prognosis and Treatment

Most cases resolve after treatment. Pruritus may persist for several weeks after eradication of the mites. The treatment consists of topical permethrin and has to be applied not only to the patient but also to all the persons who are close physical contacts.

PEDICULOSIS

Pediculosis has affected humans since prehistoric times. There are three types of lice that infest humans, generally site specific.

Clinical Findings

Pediculus humanus capitis (the head louse) usually infests children aged 3 to 12 years. Transmission occurs through close contact or contact with fomites. Nits (Fig. 3.138) are found more often in the occipital and retroauricular areas, and combing makes identification easier. Body louse (*Pediculus humanus humanus*) affects mainly homeless individuals in urban areas. It acts as a vector for *Bartonella quintana*, producing fever and endocarditis. Worldwide, body lice are important, especially among poor individuals and refugees, and may act as vectors for relapsing fever, trench fever, and epidemic typhus. Crab louse (*Pthirus pubis*) infestation is commonly sexually transmitted. Up to one-third of patients may have another concomitant sexually transmitted disease. The crab louse attaches to hair on pubis, trunk, legs, and buttocks and infrequently to scalp hair. Secondary to bites, characteristic blue-gray macules (maculae caeruleae) appear on the lower abdomen and thighs.

Histologic Features

The head louse is the size of a sesame seed, has three pairs of clawed legs, crawls rapidly, and lays nits (ova within a chitinous case) firmly cemented to hairs within 1 to 2 mm of the scalp (Fig. 3.139). The body louse is larger, measuring 2 to 4 mm in length. Females lay in their lifetime up to 300 nits; live in the seams of clothing, especially in areas of higher temperature (e.g., waistbands); and can survive up to 3 days without a blood meal. The crab louse is 0.8 to 1.2 mm long and almost as wide, in contrast to the oval, elongated shape of body and head lice.

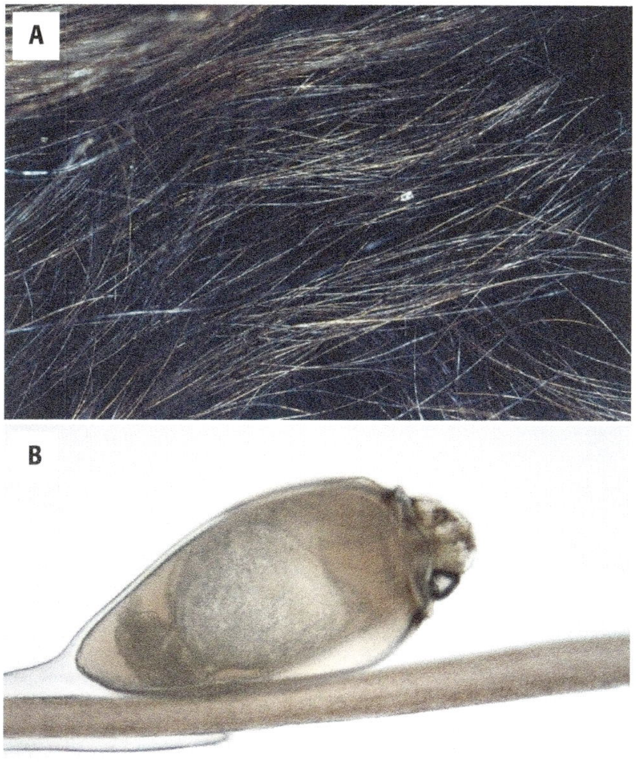

FIG. 3.139
Pediculosis. **A,** Note the white nit on the hair shaft. **B,** Nit in a close-up view.

Differential Diagnosis

Definitive diagnosis of head lice infestation requires lice identification. Hair casts, black and white piedra, flakes of seborrheic dermatitis, debris from hair spray, monilethrix, and trichorrhexis nodosa can be mistaken for nits. Psocid infestation can be confused with lice, but the insect has a larger head and larger antennae. For body lice, the diagnosis requires finding nits or lice in clothing. The crab lice are easy to identify; nits may be mistaken for white piedra.

Prognosis and Treatment

Head lice are a community-wide problem, and frequent screening in schools reduces the spread of infestation. Mechanical removal combined with chemical agents (permethrin, lindane) is successful in most cases. For body and pubic lice, proper hygiene and topical chemical agents are recommended. In cases of resistance to permethrin or lindane, oral ivermectin can be used.

CIMICOSIS (BEDBUGS)

Clinical Findings

Cimex lectularius, the common bedbug, is found hiding in cracks and crevices in walls, mattresses, or furniture or under carpeting. Bedbugs are usually only active during the night, and infestation can be suspected when an unpleasant odor or rusty excreta is detected. Adult bed bugs are reddish-brown, oval, flat, and approximately one-fifth of an inch long. They greatly engorge after feeding. The bite is painless but may induce formation of a firm, small papule (Fig. 3.140). Rows of several lesions are characteristic.

Histologic Features

Histologically, the findings typically reveal a nonspecific hypersensitivity reaction pattern with upper dermal edema and a perivascular inflammatory infiltrate containing eosinophils and mast cells, with eosinophils also infiltrating the interstitium.

Differential Diagnosis

The lesions need to be distinguished primarily by clinical history from other infestations and bite reactions.

Prognosis and Treatment

Treatment is primarily directed toward relief from itching using menthol, phenol, or steroids.

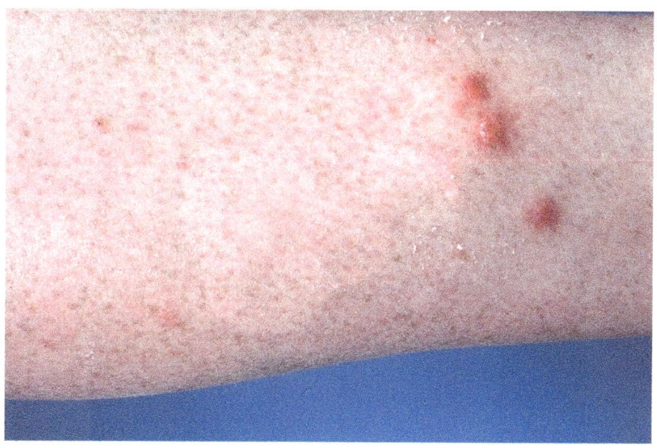

FIG. 3.140
Cimicosis. Several erythematous papules are arranged in a row.

MYIASIS

Infestation of living tissues with larvae of flies (maggots) is called myiasis. The flies belong to the order *Diptera*, and the species varies depending on geographic distribution. In the United States, human botfly (*Dermatobia hominis*) eggs are transmitted by mosquitoes; in Africa, the tumbu fly (*Cordylobia anthropophaga*) larvae penetrate the skin after hatching on the soil or clothing. Because the maggots feed on necrotic tissue, a few species have been used medicinally for wound care, the most widely used species being the green bottle blowfly, *Lucilia sericata*.

Clinical Findings

The lesions are similar to furuncles, may be very painful as they enlarge, and culminate in ulceration as the larva migrates outside the skin (Fig. 3.141).

Histologic Features

The larva is usually contained in a dermal or subcutaneous cavity with a surrounding heavy inflammatory infiltrate containing eosinophils and fibrosis. The larva has a thick chitinous cuticle with spines on the surface (Fig. 3.142). On cut sections, respiratory tubes and striated muscle can be seen.

Differential Diagnosis

The presence of striated muscle distinguishes the fly larva from helminths. The differential diagnosis also includes tungiasis and pentastomiasis (arthropods resembling worms but have sclerotized dark brown openings in the cuticle).

Prognosis and Treatment

Treatment consists of surgical removal of the larva.

TUNGIASIS

Tungiasis is the result of skin infestation by the sand flea *Tunga penetrans*, found in Central and South America, India, Pakistan, and tropical Africa. The pregnant flea burrows into the skin of the host near the plantar surfaces of the foot and between toes after a person has been walking in contaminated sand without shoes.

Clinical Findings

The first manifestation is the presence of a black dot at the penetration site followed by the formation of white papules that enlarge to form pea-sized nodules with a central black dot and erythematous halo. The nodules ulcerate after the tunga sheds the eggs and dies.

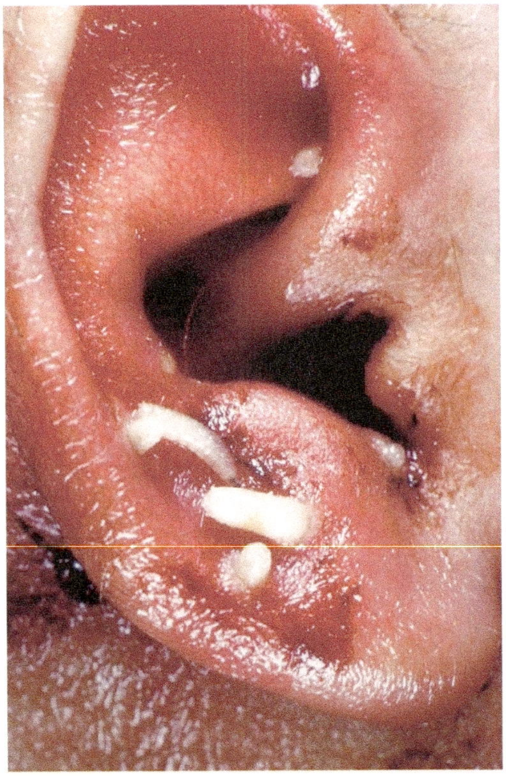

FIG. 3.141
Myiasis. Larvae are seen on the skin surface feeding on necrotic tissue.

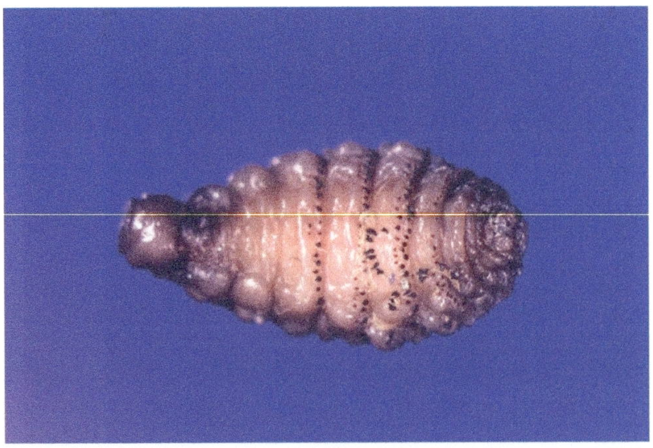

FIG. 3.142
Myiasis. Larval *Dermatobia hominis* with characteristic rows of spines.

Histologic Features

The pregnant tunga has a characteristic exoskeleton, eggs, and internal organs. It burrows with the head down in the epidermis and the terminal segment opening to the surface of the skin (Fig. 3.143). The eggs are white, smooth, and oval; measure approximately 0.6 cm in length; and have a thin shell. The flea has a thick tegument with hypertrophied hypodermal cells. Mature fleas become swollen with eggs and enfolded by elongated rete ridges. Their heads are small and have an elongated stylus that penetrates into the dermis, through which the tunga draws blood, and a prominent striated muscle band attached to the tegument behind them. Surrounding the tunga is a mixed inflammatory infiltrate containing neutrophils and eosinophils.

Prognosis and Treatment

Treatment consists of removal of the intact parasite. Complications include secondary infection.

TICK BITES

Ticks can cause disease through several mechanisms. They can function as vectors for infectious agents, indirectly causing diseases such as ECM (Lyme disease), Rocky Mountain spotted fever, ehrlichiosis, or babesiosis. Their embedded mouthparts can produce local reactions in the form of an acute response or a chronic one with a hypersensitivity component. Finally, the saliva injected at the time of the bite has antihemostatic, anti-inflammatory, and immunosuppressive local effects or can induce systemic toxemia. The two major families of ticks are soft ticks (*Argasidae*) and hard ticks (*Ixodidae*).

Clinical Findings

The hard ticks of the *Iodex* genera, named for their sclerotized dorsal plate or scutum (smaller in females), are important because of their role as a vector for Lyme disease or babesiosis. They attach to the skin (Fig. 3.144) and engorge with blood slowly in 7 to 9 days. Soft ticks, named for their flexible, leathery cuticle, detach from skin in minutes and may not be noticed by the victim. Within 1 to 3 days of both a soft and a hard tick bite, an erythematous macule, papule, or thin plaque may form, slightly indurated, with an erythematous halo that can measure up to several centimeters. Soft ticks are more often implicated in serious reactions, such as local necrosis progressing to necrotic ulcers several centimeters in size that heal with scarring. Fortunately, these are rare. In the majority of cases, only mild edema, vesiculation, or bullae formation has been reported. Tick bites can become secondarily infected or may exacerbate preexisting dermatoses. Chronic lesions with retained tick mouth parts in the dermis may persist for months or years as papules, nodules, or plaques.

Histologic Features

The histologic diagnosis may be difficult in the absence of tick body parts. Mouth parts of the tick can be identified

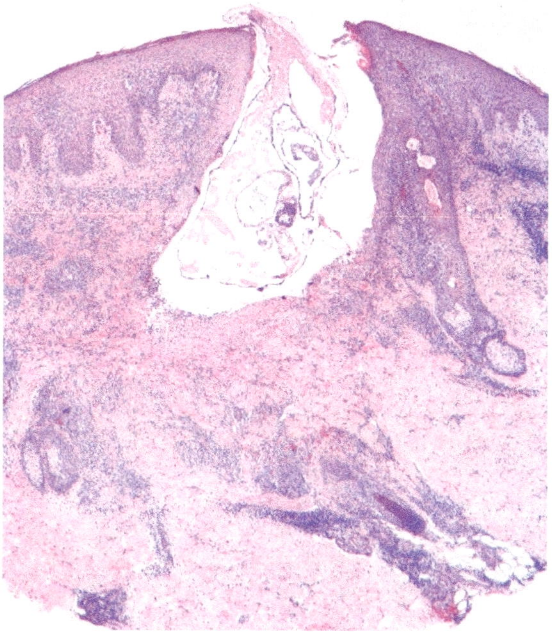

FIG. 3.143
Tungiasis. The tunga is embedded vertically in an epidermal cavity.

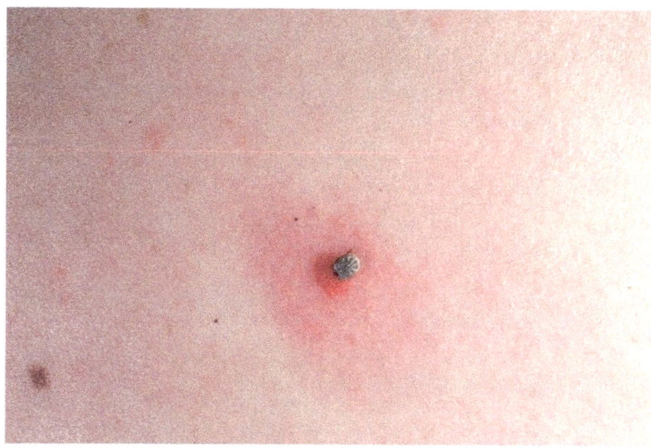

FIG. 3.144
Tick bite. A feeding tick is attached to the skin. The bite site is erythematous.

in the dermis (Fig. 3.145) accompanied by a moderately dense superficial perivascular and interstitial inflammatory infiltrate composed of lymphocytes, histiocytes, plasma cells, eosinophils, and neutrophils. In some cases, the infiltrate may be deep, extending to subcutis, resulting in panniculitis. A clue to the diagnosis is the presence of fibrin thrombi in the superficial dermal small vessels. In persistent lesions, the inflammatory infiltrate contains far fewer neutrophils, and there may be granulomatous inflammatory response and dermal fibrosis. If the inflammatory infiltrate is very dense, it may mimic a lymphoproliferative disease (pseudolymphoma).

Differential Diagnosis

Tick examination is required for taxonomic identification. The capitulum is visible from above, the four pairs of legs are seen laterally, and the females can be differentiated from males by the presence of a short scutum. *Ixodes* ticks have the anal groove located in front of the anal pore (Fig. 3.146). *Amblyomma americanum* (lone star ticks) have long mouthparts, and the females have a white spot on the tip of the scutum. *Dermacentor* ticks (wood tick, dog tick) have ornate scutums with white markings. In the soft ticks, the capitulum cannot be seen from above, and the scutum is absent. Persistent reaction to a tick bite can be accompanied by a prominent lymphocytic infiltrate that may mimic a lymphoproliferative disorder.

Prognosis and Treatment

Removal of the tick within 18 to 24 hours after attachment may prevent transmission of disease. Unfortunately, many bites are asymptomatic. For Lyme disease, doxycycline is the drug of choice.

SPIDER BITES

Spider bites can cause a wide spectrum of clinical effects, ranging from minor local pain (most of the cases) to necrotic ulcers and envenomation, depending on the species involved.

Clinical Findings

The brown recluse spider (*Loxosceles reclusa*) has a fiddle-shaped marking on the back of the thorax. If the bite causes a serious reaction, local necrosis can develop in 1 to 3 days, accompanied by fever, weakness, nausea, and

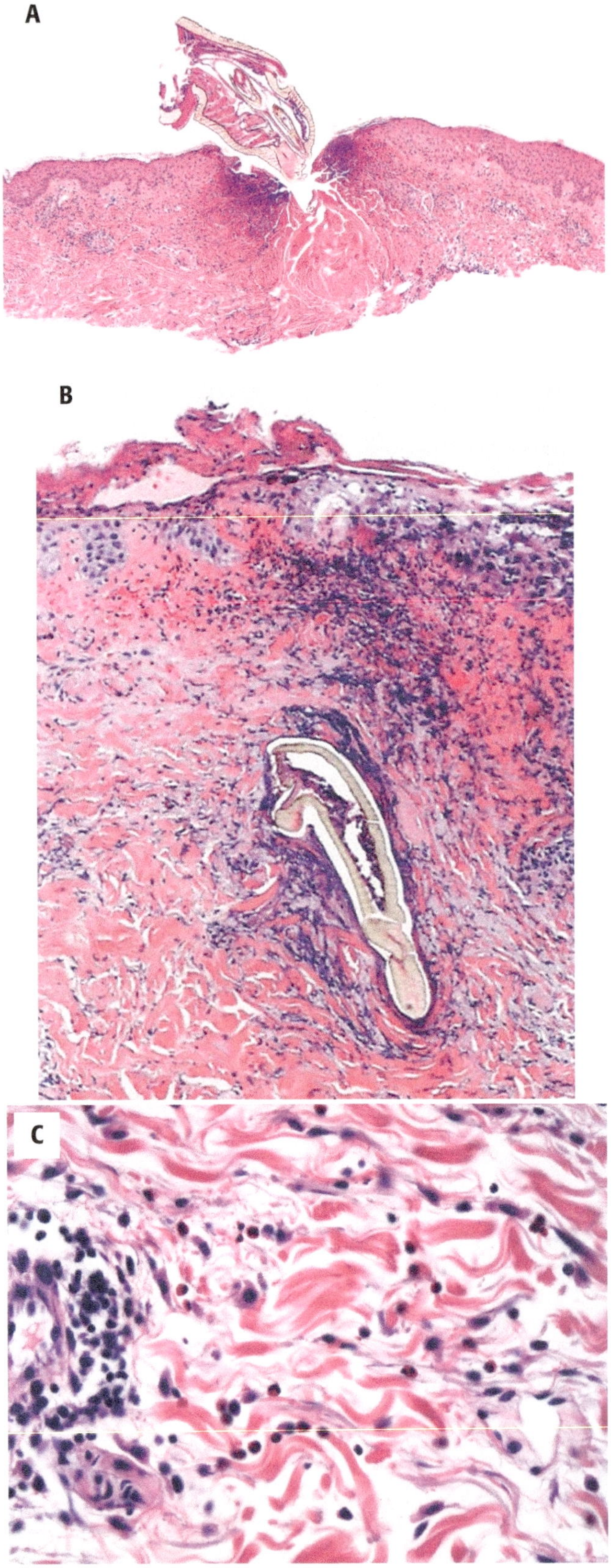

FIG. 3.145

Tick bite. **A,** The thick chitinous body is attached to the skin. **B,** The mouthpart is embedded within the dermis and surrounded by inflammation. **C,** Lymphoeosinophilic inflammatory reaction at a tick bite site.

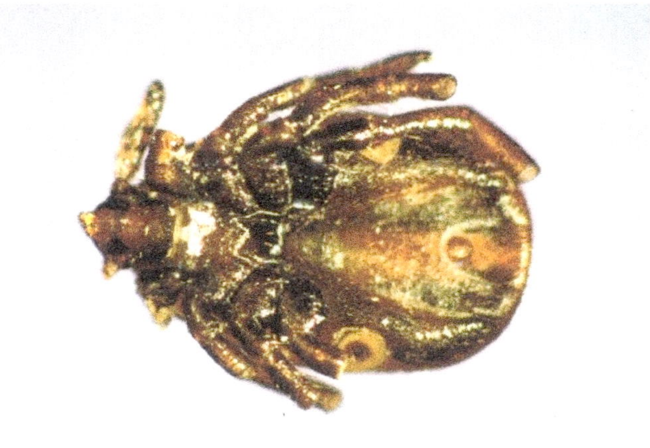

FIG. 3.146
Tick. *Ixodes* tick with a characteristic anal grove located anterior to the anal pore.

pain. Early necrosis at the center manifests as a deep blue discoloration at the site of the bite. It is surrounded by a pale halo (vasoconstriction) with a red rim (reactive erythema). This "red, white, and blue" sign is characteristic. The widow spiders are members of the genus *Latrodectus* and have a worldwide distribution. Most bites are on the extremities and may be followed by envenomation in addition to local necrosis. The black widow spider (*Latrodectus mactans*) has a globose black abdomen with a red hourglass marking. The red-back spider (*Latrodectus hasselti*) is ubiquitous in Australia. The larger and more dangerous female spiders are black and have an abdomen the size of a pea with an orange-red or gray stripe. Their venom is a neurotoxin called latrotoxin, which depletes neurotransmitters from nerve terminal vesicles and causes presynaptic blockade. The venoms of all *Latrodectus* sp. are thought to contain similar toxic components. Latrodectism, the clinical syndrome of envenomation resulting from a bite, may vary in severity depending on the species and size of the widow spider, the season, and the amount of venom injected.

Histologic Features

Early lesions may show a superficial and deep perivascular inflammatory infiltrate containing eosinophils and neutrophils, hemorrhage, thrombosis, and vasculitis. Eosinophils found in the edematous dermis between collagen fibers are characteristic. Later vessel wall necrosis, liquefactive or coagulative necrosis, and ulceration may be seen.

Prognosis and Treatment

For most cases, only supportive treatment is needed (rest, ice, compresses, elevation). If necrosis and systemic reactions occur, oral dapsone is recommended. Antivenom use is not approved by the FDA.

PROTOTHECOSIS

A rare infection caused by algae of the genus *Prototheca*, protothecosis is usually the result of traumatic direct inoculation.

Clinical Findings

There may be a variety of clinical appearances, including eczematous, herpetiform, or coalescing papules with plaque formation.

Histologic Features

The dermis shows a chronic granulomatous inflammatory infiltrate that contains histiocytes, lymphocytes, giant cells, and occasional eosinophils. Areas of necrosis may be seen. The organisms stain positively with Gram, PAS, and GMS stains and can be found free or in the cytoplasm of multinucleated giant cells and macrophages. They have a thick wall and internal septations, measure 3 to 11 μm in diameter (*Prototheca wickerhamii* is the species most commonly affecting humans), and have very small wedge-shaped endospores arranged radially and molded (morula-like form) (Fig. 3.147).

Ancillary Studies

Immunohistochemistry using monoclonal antibodies allows specific identification of the organisms.

Differential Diagnosis

Protothecal sporangia may be confused with those of *Coccidioides immitis*, which are much larger.

Prognosis and Treatment

Protothecosis is difficult to treat. Surgical removal and antifungal therapy have been shown to be effective for immunocompetent individuals. Immunocompromised patients with systemic infections are treated with amphotericin B.

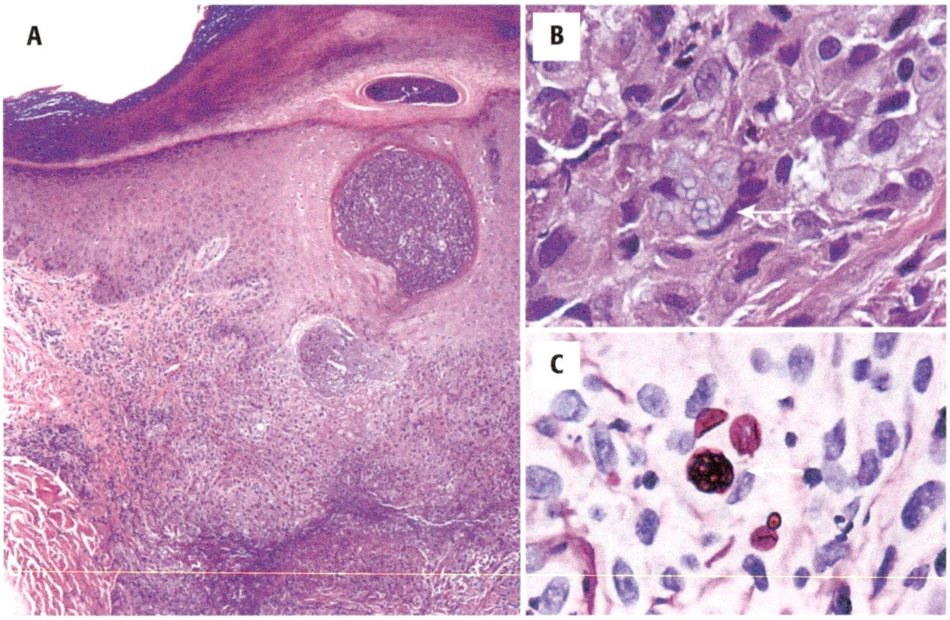

FIG. 3.147

Protothecosis. **A,** Suppurative folliculitis **B,** The organisms have a morula-like appearance septations for internal spores *(arrow)*. **C,** Morula *(arrow)* with septations seen on periodic acid-Schiff with diastase digestion stain.

NEMATODES

CYSTICERCOSIS

Humans may become accidental intermediate hosts for the larval form of *Taenia solium* (pork tapeworm). *Taenia solium* has worldwide distribution. Cysticercosis occurs in countries with poor sanitation or immigrants from these countries. The disease is the result of ingestion of viable eggs from water or food contaminated with human feces. After hatching and penetrating the intestinal wall, larvae enter the circulation and lodge in various sites.

Clinical Findings

Solitary or multiple asymptomatic cystic nodules may form, distributed with predilection on the chest and proximal extremities.

Histologic Features

Milky white oval to round cysts, filled with clear fluid, up to 1 to 2 cm in diameter, each containing a single larva with a single invaginated scolex, may be identified in the dermis and subcutaneous tissue (Fig. 3.148). Fibrous tissue encases the cysts. The cysticercus wall has an outer mammillated tegumental layer with surface microvilli, smooth muscle fibers, and stroma containing characteristic calcareous bodies (Fig. 3.148). These are laminated mineralized oval structures present in the stroma of many cestodes. The scolex has four suckers and up to 30 birefringent and acid-fast hooklets arranged in a double circular row. In early lesions, there is no surrounding inflammation. Later in the disease, there is degeneration of the parasite, and acute inflammation with eosinophils can be found followed by chronic granulomatous inflammation and finally fibrosis. The burnt-out lesions may still be identified by residual hooklets or calcareous bodies.

Differential Diagnosis

Sparganosis, occurring mainly in China, Japan, and Southeast Asia, is caused by larvae of the genus *Spirometra* tapeworm. Subcutaneous tender, sometimes migratory nodules may form, which contain a white worm varying abruptly in width between different segments, and measuring between a few centimeters and half a meter. The sparganum has a longitudinal excretory canal and muscle bundles arranged in longitudinal and horizontal fascicles ("checkerboard" pattern) and lacks a scolex or internal organoid structures. When it migrates, it leaves behind a tract of necrosis surrounded by chronic inflammation with abundant eosinophils. With degeneration, a necrotic and granulomatous reaction follows.

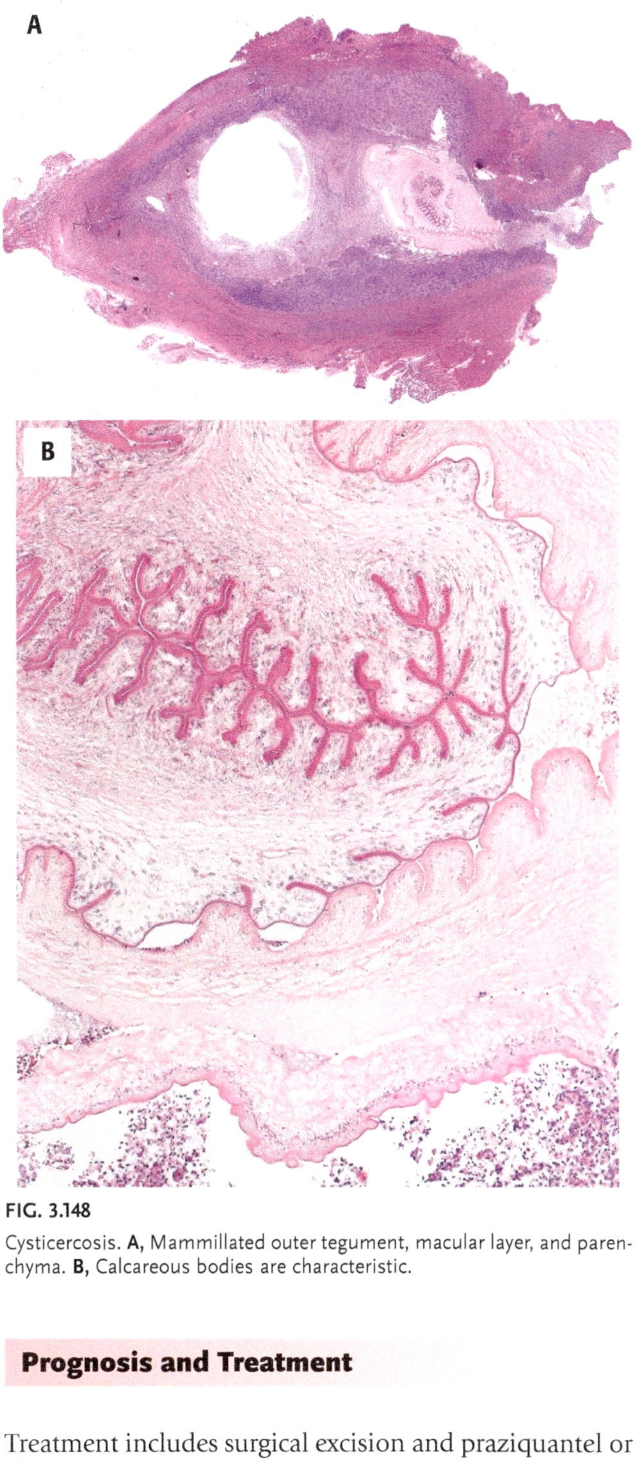

FIG. 3.148

Cysticercosis. **A,** Mammillated outer tegument, macular layer, and parenchyma. **B,** Calcareous bodies are characteristic.

Prognosis and Treatment

Treatment includes surgical excision and praziquantel or albendazole combined with corticosteroids. Cysticerci in the skin and subcutaneous tissue have a benign course, but if they are localized in the eye may cause blindness and if in the brain or heart may kill the patient.

ONCHOCERCIASIS

Onchocerciasis is caused by larvae of *Onchocerca volvulus* transmitted through blackflies of the genus *Simulium*, present on river banks. It is common in tropical Africa and Central and South America.

Clinical Findings

After inoculation in the subcutaneous tissue, the larvae mature into adult worms, and subcutaneous nodules 2 to 10 cm in diameter are formed. These nodules may contain one or several tightly coiled worms. The worms produce microfilariae, which migrate through the lymphatics. A pruritic papular rash (onchocercal dermatitis) with lichenification and pigmentary changes ("leopard skin") can result because of an inflammatory reaction to antigens from degenerating microfilariae.

Histologic Features

In the subcutaneous nodules, the tightly coiled worms are encased in a wall of fibrous tissue, in which at early stages a mixed inflammatory infiltrate with eosinophils and granulation tissue may be found (Fig. 3.149). In later stages, the dense fibrous tissue contains only scanty chronic inflammatory infiltrate, foreign body giant cells, eosinophils, and focal calcifications. *O. volvulus* is a threadlike white worm, measuring 0.25 to 0.45 mm in diameter and 20 to 50 cm in length. Microfilariae can be identified in lymphatic vessels or dermis, concentrating in the dermal papillae. They have a cephalic and a caudal clear space and are 200 to 360 μm long and 5 to 9 μm wide.

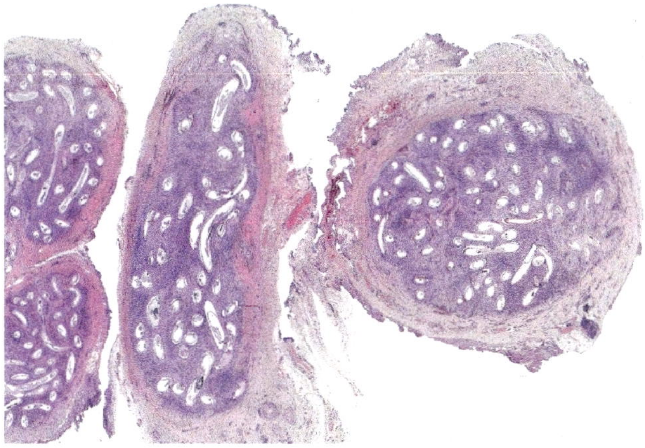

FIG. 3.149

Onchocerciasis. Worms are within a wall of fibrous tissue, with chronic inflammation.

Differential Diagnosis

Onchocercal microfilaria have the first two to three anterior nuclei arranged side by side. This is a feature that distinguishes them from *Mansonella streptocerca*, the other microfilaria that can be seen in the dermis.

Prognosis and Treatment

Adult worms may survive in the subcutaneous tissues for 15 years or more. If the microfilariae reach the eyes, they can cause blindness (river blindness). Obstruction of lymphatics by microfilaria can result in lymphadenitis or adenolymphocele (hanging groin). Treatment consists of excision of nodules, diethylcarbamazine, and suramin.

DIROFILARIA

Infection with *Dirofilaria* sp. is endemic in the Mediterranean region but rare in other parts of the world. The most common species causing subcutaneous dirofilariasis in humans are *Dirofilaria tenuis* (endemic in south Florida), *Dirofilaria ursi* and *Dirofilaria subserrate* (North America), and *Dirofilaria repens* (Europe). Mosquitoes are the vector.

Clinical Findings

Skin lesions consist of solitary erythematous subcutaneous nodules that may be tender or give a sensation of movement under the skin.

Histologic Features

The nodules contain a degenerating filaria and suppurative inflammation in the center, and surrounding it a marked chronic inflammatory infiltrate containing abundant eosinophils. The filaria has a thick, multilaminated cuticle with external longitudinal cuticular ridges. Underneath the cuticle, the thick muscular layer is arranged radially. If the parasite has been dead for a long time, degenerative changes might make identification difficult.

Differential Diagnosis

D. tenuis worms measure 40 to 130 mm in length and 260 mm in diameter. *D. repens* worms are larger, measuring 70 to 170 mm in length and 370 to 450 mm in diameter. Females are larger than males.

Prognosis and Treatment

Surgical excision is curative.

SCHISTOSOMIASIS

Schistosomiasis, human disease caused by trematodes of the genus *Schistosoma*, may manifest as cercarial dermatitis (swimmer's itch) or late cutaneous bilharziasis. Cercarial dermatitis is caused by "nonhuman" species of schistosomes, which cannot complete their life cycle in humans and are destroyed shortly after skin penetration. Late cutaneous bilharziasis is rare and is caused by deposition of ova in the dermis in patients with severe systemic invasion by the major species of schistosome fluke (*S. japonicum*, *S. haematobium*, and *S. mansoni*).

Clinical Findings

Cercarial dermatitis is a hypersensitivity reaction characterized by a pruritic erythematous urticarial papular rash developing on exposed skin areas after bathing in infested waters. Late cutaneous bilharziasis consists of papular or verrucous lesions that can develop in the genital and perigenital skin after the deposition of ova in the dermis.

Histologic Features

Cercarial dermatitis is characterized by spongiosis and permeation of the epidermis by eosinophils and neutrophils. Cercaria may be identified in the epidermis only if the biopsy is taken soon after penetration. Late cutaneous bilharziasis is characterized by the presence of calcified or degenerating ova in the dermis associated with a surrounding palisading necrotizing granulomatous reaction with numerous eosinophils. The epidermis is hyperkeratotic, sometimes pseudoepitheliomatous, and may show draining sinuses (transepithelial elimination). The causative parasite can be identified by examining the characteristic ova, which have a PAS-positive chitinous shell. Ova of *S. mansoni* measure 150 by 80 μm and have lateral spines; those of *S. haematobium* are smaller and have apical spines. The ova of *S. japonicum* have no spines and are smaller than those of *S. mansoni*. If modified acid-fast Ziehl-Neelsen stain is used, the spines of *S. haematobium* are positive, but for

S. japonicum and *S. mansoni,* both the egg shells and spines are positive. The mature miracidia inside the ova have a ring-shaped nerve center and intensely basophilic gonadal cells.

Differential Diagnosis

The diagnosis of cercarial dermatitis is made clinically and is linked to a history of swimming in potentially infested waters. Seabather's eruption is caused by larval forms of the thimble jellyfish (Florida, the Caribbean) or the sea anemone *Edwardsiella lineata* (Long Island, NY). It consists of a papular pruritic rash that develops on areas covered by swimming suits, but cercarial dermatitis occurs on exposed areas.

Prognosis and Treatment

Cercarial dermatitis requires only symptomatic treatment and resolves spontaneously in 1 to 2 weeks. Bilharziasis is treated with praziquantel.

ACKNOWLEDGMENTS

The authors also want to acknowledge and express their gratitude to contributions to this chapter in prior editions by Drs. Anca G. Prundeanu Croitoru and Stefanie Hu.

SUGGESTED FURTHER READING

General

Brown, T. J., Yen-Moore, A., & Tyring, S. K. (1999). An overview of sexually transmitted disease. Part I. *Journal of the American Academy of Dermatology*, *41*, 511–532.

Connor, D.H., Chandler, F.W., Schwartz, D.A., Manz, H.J., Lack, E.E. (1997). *Pathology of infectious diseases* (Vols. 1–2). New York: Appleton & Lange.

Diven, D. G. (2001). Color atlas and textbook of diagnostic microbiology. An overview of poxviruses. *Journal of the American Academy of Dermatology*, *44*, 1–14.

Clebak, K. T., & Malone, M. A. (2018). Skin infections. *Primary Care*, *45*, 433–454.

Lipozencić, J., Skerlev, M., Pasić, A. (2002). An overview: The changing face of cutaneous infections and infestations. *Clinics in Dermatology*, *20*, 104–108.

Viral Infections

Ahmed, A. M., Madkan, V., & Tyring, S. K. (2006). Human papilloma viruses and genital disease. *Dermatologic Clinics*, *24*, 157–165.

Genovese, G., Moltrasio, C., Berti, E., & Marzano, A. V. (2021). Skin Manifestations associated with COVID-19: Current knowledge and future perspectives. *Dermatology*, *237*, 1–12.

Ramdass, P., Mullick, S., & Farber, H. F. (2015). Viral skin diseases. *Primary Care*, *42*, 517–567.

Bacterial Infections

Barbagallo, J., Tager, P., Ingleton, R., Hirsch, R. J., & Weinberg, J. M. (2002). Cutaneous tuberculosis: Diagnosis and treatment. *American Journal of Clinical Dermatology*, *3*, 319–328.

Britton, W. J., & Lockwood, D. N. (2004). Leprosy. *Lancet*, *363*, 1209–1219.

Ghosn, S. H., & Kibbi, A. G. (2004). Cutaneous gonococcal infections. *Clinics in Dermatology*, *22*, 476–480.

Lupi, O., Madkan, V., & Tyring, S. K. (2006). Tropical dermatology: Bacterial tropical diseases. *Journal of the American Academy of Dermatology*, *54*, 559–578.

Weitzul, S., Eichhorn, P. J., & Pandya, A. G. (2000). Nontuberculous mycobacterial infections of the skin. *Dermatologic Clinics*, *18*, 5.

Zeltser, R., & Kurban, A. K. (2004). Syphilis. *Clinics in Dermatology*, *22*, 461–468.

Fungal Infections

Borgers, M., Degreef, H., & Cauwenbergh, G. (2005). Fungal infections of the skin: Infection process and antimycotic therapy. *Current Drug Targets*, *6*, 849–862.

Dixon, D. M., & Polak-Wyss, A. (1991). The medically important dematiaceous fungi and their identification. *Mycoses*, *34*, 1–18.

Lupi, O., Tyring, S. K., & McGinnis, M. R. (2005). Tropical dermatology: Fungal tropical diseases. *Journal of the American Academy of Dermatology*, *53*, 931–951.

Schwarz, J. (1982). The diagnosis of deep mycoses by morphologic methods. *Human Pathology*, *13*, 519–533.

Arthropod Bites, Infestation, Other

Goddard, J. (2002). *Physician's guide to arthropods of medical importance* (4th ed.). Boca Raton, CRC Press.

Heukelbach, J., & Feldmeier, H. (2006). Scabies. *Lancet*, *27*, 1767–1774.

Ko, C. J., & Elston, D. M. (2004). Pediculosis. *Journal of the American Academy of Dermatology*, *50*, 1–12.

Mehregan, D. R., Mehregan, A. H., & Mehregan, D. A. (1999). Histologic diagnosis of cutaneous leishmaniasis. *Clinics in Dermatology*, *17*, 297–304.

Prickett, K. A., & Ferringer, T. C. (2014). Helminths: A clinical review and update. *Seminars in Cutaneous Medicine and Surgery*, *33*(3), 128–132.

4 Cutaneous Vasculitis

Cuong V. Nguyen • Rami N. Al-Rohil

Vasculitis is a histopathologic diagnosis defined as inflammatory cell infiltration and destruction of blood vessels. Vasculitis can be classified as primary vasculitis (idiopathic, e.g., cutaneous leukocytoclastic angiitis [CLA], granulomatosis with polyangiitis [GPA]); secondary vasculitis (a manifestation of connective tissue diseases [CTDs], infections, adverse drug eruptions, or a paraneoplastic phenomenon); or incidental vasculitis, a histologic finding that is the consequence of another pathologic process such as traumatic ulceration or diffuse neutrophilic infiltrates. Clinically, cutaneous vasculitis can present in a panoply of morphologies that include urticarial papules and plaques, purpura, hemorrhagic vesicles, ulcers, nodules, livedo, infarcts, and digital gangrene. These findings may represent the cutaneous manifestation of systemic disease, or, as is the case in most instances, represent a benign, self-limited, single-episode phenomenon.

The diagnosis of vasculitic syndromes is problematic. Specific clinical vasculitic entities do not always correlate exactly with mechanisms, and any patient with vasculitis may have a constellation of morphologic signs that overlap with another clinical entity that prevents confident clinical diagnosis. Currently, the most widely adopted vasculitis classification system is that of 2012 Revised International Chapel Hill Consensus Conference (CHCC) with a 2018 dermatologic addendum to better standardize cutaneous disease. The other widely used system is that of the American College of Rheumatology (ACR), which is based predominantly on clinical findings. More recently, the ACR/EULAR (European Alliance of Associations for Rheumatology) released a 2022 updated classification criteria, focusing on giant cell arteritis (GCA), Takayasu arteritis, and the antineutrophil cytoplasmic antibody (ANCA)–associated vasculitides. All of these classification proposals have merits, but also significant limitations for skin-predominant disease.

A definitive diagnosis of vasculitis often requires histopathologic confirmation because few vasculitic syndromes have pathognomonic clinical, radiographic, and/or laboratory findings. Nonetheless, a biopsy diagnosis of vasculitis cannot stand by itself, as it must be correlated with clinical history, physical and laboratory findings, and/or angiographic features. For example, a diagnosis of vasculitis restricted to the skin (also known as hypersensitivity vasculitis, CLA, or leukocytoclastic vasculitis [LCV]) requires that the systemic manifestations of vasculitis be sought and found absent. If systemic vasculitis is present, imaging studies (e.g., renal angiogram in PAN) can provide a useful means to determine disease extent and activity. Furthermore, serology, such as C-reactive protein (CRP), can be used to monitor disease activity and may predict mortality risk. The classification of cutaneous vasculitis into specific syndromes is usually approached morphologically by determining vessel size and principal inflammatory response. The histopathologic features in context with clinical findings, direct immunofluorescence (DIF) examination, ANCA status, and findings from workup for systemic disease often allow for specific diagnoses and provide guidance for the most effective therapy (Fig. 4.1 and Table 4.1).

Clinical Findings

Cutaneous vasculitis affects all ages, with slight female predominance, and adults more often than children. The onset of vasculitis after exposure to a trigger such as a drug or infection is typically 7 to 10 days. A mean interval of 6 months (range, weeks to years) exists between the onset of symptoms and signs of systemic disease and the onset of secondary cutaneous vasculitis. Three patterns of disease evolution occur in cutaneous vasculitis: (1) single acute, self-limited episode (resolves in ≤6 months) of vasculitis which can be associated with a drug or infectious trigger; (2) relapsing disease with symptom-free periods usually found in patients with IgAV and CTD-associated vasculitis (~20%); and (3) a chronic, unremitting disease often associated with cryoglobulinemia and malignancy (~20%). The duration may be highly variable, with some studies documenting mean and median durations of 28 and 3.7 months, respectively. Up to 30% of patients with cutaneous vasculitis will have extracutaneous (visceral) involvement. Fatal disease occurs in a minority of patients (<7%).

In the majority of patients, vasculitic lesions affect the lower extremities. Upper extremity, trunk, and head and neck involvement are infrequent and often signal the presence of more severe disease or coexisting systemic vasculitis.

TABLE 4.1
Classification of Cutaneous Vasculitis by Histologic Findings and Laboratory Studies

SMALL VESSEL VASCULITIS	**SMALL VESSEL VASCULITIS**
Neutrophilic	ANCA-associated or pauci-immune (DIF−)
Immune complex mediated (DIF+)	Granulomatosis with polyangiitis
CLA (also known as hypersensitivity vasculitis and LCV)	Microscopic polyangiitis (microscopic polyarteritis nodosa)
IgA vasculitis	EGPA
Acute infantile hemorrhagic edema	Drug-induced ANCA vasculitis
Urticarial vasculitis	Miscellaneous or other
Chronic localized fibrosing vasculitis: EED, granuloma faciale, inflammatory pseudotumors	Behçet's disease
Incidental vasculitis (DIF−)	Septic vasculitis
Sweet's syndrome and pustular vasculitis of the dorsa of the hands	***Lymphocytic***
Eosinophilic	Degos' disease
Eosinophilic vasculitis, primary or secondary to connective tissue disease, or parasites	Rickettsial and viral infections
Some cases of EGPA	Collagen tissue disease vasculitis (e.g., Sjögren's syndrome, lupus vasculitis)
Granulomatous	Behçet's disease
Postherpetic eruptions	**MEDIUM (TO LARGE) MUSCULAR VESSEL VASCULITIS**
Necrobiosis lipoidica (some lesions)	***Neutrophilic***
Lymphocytic	Polyarteritis nodosa, classic and cutaneous
Rickettsial and viral infections	Nodular vasculitis (erythema induratum)
Lichenoid dermatitides, some cases (e.g., pityriasis lichenoides, GVHD, perniosis)	***Eosinophilic***
T-cell lymphomas: angiocentric T-cell lymphoma, lymphomatoid papulosis, mycosis fungoides	Juvenile temporal arteritis
Rare drug reactions and arthropod assaults	***Granulomatous***
MIXED, PREDOMINANTLY SMALL AND MEDIUM VESSEL VASCULITIS	Giant cell (temporal) arteritis
Neutrophilic	Takayasu's arteritis
Immune complex mediated (DIF+)	Postherpetic eruptions
Cryoglobulinemic vasculitis	***Lymphocytic***
Hypocomplemententemic urticarial vasculitis syndrome	Sneddon's syndrome
CTD vasculitis (e.g., lupus, rheumatoid arthritis, Sjögren's syndrome)	Degos' disease
	Buerger's disease (thromboangiitis obliterans)
	Superficial thrombophlebitis (Mondor's disease, sclerosing lymphangitis)
	Kawasaki's disease

ANCA, Antineutrophil cytoplasmic antibody; *CLA,* cutaneous leukocytoclastic angiitis; *CTD,* connective tissue disease; *DIF +*, direct immunofluorescence examination of skin lesions shows vessel wall immune complexes or complement deposition; *EED,* erythema elevatum diutinum; *EGPA,* eosinophilic granulomatosis with polyangiitis; *GVHD,* graft versus host disease.
Data from Carlson, J. A., & Chen, K. R. (2006). Cutaneous vasculitis update: neutrophilic small vessel vasculitic syndromes. *The American Journal of Dermatopathology,* 28(6), 486–506.

An understanding of the skin's vascular anatomy helps in characterizing the cutaneous manifestation of vasculitis. In terms of the Chapel Hill Criteria and from the perspective of internists or rheumatologists, all skin vessels are considered small to medium in size. The skin receives its blood supply from penetrating vessels within the underlying subcutaneous fat, which would be considered medium-sized vessels. These medium-sized skin vessels branch out to give rise to two intercommunicating vascular plexuses: the deep vascular plexus lying at the interface between the dermis and subcutaneous fat, and the superficial plexus located in the superficial aspects of the reticular dermis. This supplies the papillary dermis by forming capillary loops composed of terminal arterioles, capillaries (arterial and venous), and postcapillary venules.

The type of cutaneous lesion closely correlates with the size of the vessel affected by vasculitis (Table 4.2). The predominant small vessel affected in cutaneous LCV is the postcapillary venule, but arterioles and capillaries may also be involved. Targeting of the small vessels results in palpable purpura with lesions typically 2 to 4 mm in size but potentially fusing together to form larger plaques with rounded edges. An exception to this may be with IgA vasculitis (IgAV) which may also have a retiform clinical appearance. When medium to larger vessels are involved, because they supply multiple papillae, large purpuric lesions with retiform configuration,

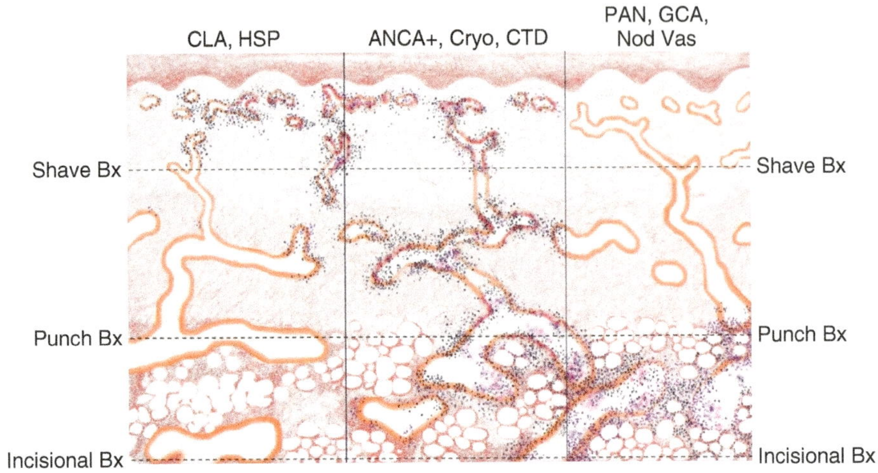

FIG. 4.1
Cutaneous vasculitis classification. Classification of cutaneous vasculitis can be initially based on vessel size(s) affected and extent of skin and subcutaneous involvement. In general, whereas IgA vasculitis (previously known as Henoch-Schönlein purpura [HSP]) and cutaneous leukocytoclastic angiitis (CLA) affect the superficial vessels of the skin, polyarteritis nodosa (PAN), nodular vasculitis (Nod Vas), and giant cell arteritis (GCA) affect deep muscular vessels found at the dermal-subcutis interface and within the subcutis. Most other forms of vasculitis such as cryoglobulinemic vasculitis, connective tissue disease (CTD) vasculitis, and antineutrophilic antibody-associated vasculitides (ANCA-positive vasculitis) can affect both small and muscular vessels (although not necessarily in the same biopsy [Bx]). The diagnostic yield of a skin biopsy is greatly influenced by the depth of the biopsy. In general, punch biopsy or excision biopsy extending into the subcutis is the preferred means to sample a vasculitic lesion in order to sample vessels of all sizes. (Reproduced with permission from Carlson, J. A., Ng, B. T., & Chen, K. R. (2005). Cutaneous vasculitis update: diagnostic criteria, classification, epidemiology, etiology, pathogenesis, evaluation and prognosis. *The American Journal of Dermatopathology*, 27, 504–528.)

TABLE 4.2

Clinical Manifestations of Vasculitis Based on Vessel Size Affected

Large	Medium	Small
Limb claudication	Subcutaneous nodules	Purpura
Asymmetric blood pressure	Ulcers	Urticarial lesions
Absence of pulses	Livedo reticularis	Vesiculobullous lesions
Aortic dilation	Pitted palmar or digital scars	Splinter hemorrhages
Bruits	Digital gangrene	Scleritis, episcleritis, uveitis
	Mononeuritis	Palisaded neutrophilic granulomatous dermatitis[1]
	Aneurysms	Glomerulonephritis
	Infarct	Gastric colic
	Hypertension (renal artery)	Pulmonary hemorrhage

Constitutional symptoms: fever, weight loss, malaise, arthralgias, and arthritis are common to vasculitic syndromes of all vessel sizes

[1]Also called extravascular necrotizing granuloma. Small vessel neutrophilic vasculitis is frequently seen in the vicinity of granulomas and necrosis.
Adapted from Saleh, A., & Stone, J. H. 2005. Classification and diagnostic criteria in systemic vasculitis. *Best Practice & Research. Clinical Rheumatology*, 19(2), 209–221.

livedo reticularis, ulcers, nodules, and pitted scars may form. These medium to large vessels are located at the dermal-subcutis interface or within the subcutis.

Biopsy: Timing and Choice of Lesions

The choice of clinical lesions and type of pathologic assessment have great impact on the diagnostic yield of cutaneous biopsies. First, the optimal time for skin biopsy is 24 to 48 hours after the appearance of a vasculitic lesion. If the biopsy is poorly timed, the pathologic features of vasculitis may be absent, a fact that clinicians must bear in mind when interpreting a negative biopsy finding from a patient whose clinical findings suggest vasculitis. A punch biopsy of a lesion at the appropriate stage will enable histopathologic confirmation of most small vessel vasculitic syndromes. The earliest findings often involve the presence of neutrophils with karyorrhectic debris and red cell extravasation. This is followed by fibrin deposition. Newly developed lesions may not show good fibrin deposition. More developed lesions but less than 24 hours old are characterized by fibrin deposits within the vessel wall accompanied by neutrophilic infiltration of the wall and surrounding hemorrhage and nuclear debris. In older lesions, neutrophils are replaced by lymphocytes and macrophages. Biopsy of lesions more than 48 hours old, regardless of the underlying form of vasculitis, may show lymphocyte-rich infiltrates. Second, the choice of a shave biopsy, punch biopsy, or excisional biopsy affects which vessels are examined because the type of vessel depends on the location within the skin and subcutis (i.e., the deeper the location, the larger the vessel). Thus, if a medium vessel vasculitis such as PAN is suspected, the biopsy must include the subcutaneous fat where medium-sized vessels of the skin are situated. Incisional biopsy is required for some conditions such as nodular vasculitis and GCA (Fig. 4.1). In the case of livedo reticularis, a deep biopsy extending to the subcutis should be taken from the center of the circular livedo segment (the white center, not the red periphery) because this is where the stenosed vessel responsible for the cyanotic periphery is located. Third, biopsies should be obtained from nonulcerated sites or, if not possible, from the edge of an ulcer. Last, omission of a biopsy for DIF studies wastes an opportunity to collect potentially valuable information and often leads to misdiagnosis. It is best to take two biopsies, one for light microscopy and one for DIF examination, rather than split one specimen. The specimen taken for DIF should be taken from lesional skin, usually fewer than 48 hours old. In fact, multiple biopsies and extending the biopsy depth to the subcutis and fascia can significantly increase the diagnostic yield for vasculitis.

TABLE 4.3

Histologic Diagnostic Criteria for Cutaneous Vasculitis

Criteria
HISTOLOGIC SIGNS OF ACUTE (ACTIVE) VASCULITIS
Dermal Small Vessels (Venules and Arterioles) (Two of Three[1] Criteria Needed)
Angiocentric[2] or angioinvasive inflammatory infiltrates[1]
Disruption or destruction of vessel wall by inflammatory infiltrate[1]
Intramural or intraluminal fibrin deposition ("fibrinoid necrosis")[1]
Dermal-Subcutaneous Muscular Vessels (Small Arteries and Veins)
Infiltration of muscular vessel wall by inflammatory cells[1]
Intramural and/or intraluminal fibrin deposition ("fibrinoid necrosis")[1,3]
Secondary Changes of Active Vasculitis (Suggestive, but Not Diagnostic, of Vasculitis)[2]
RBC extravasation (petechiae, purpura, hematoma)
Nuclear dust, perivascular (leukocytoclasia)
Endothelial swelling, sloughing, or necrosis
Eccrine gland necrosis (or regeneration with basal cell hyperplasia)
Ulceration
Necrosis or infarction
HISTOLOGIC SEQUELAE OF VASCULITIS (CHRONIC SIGNS AND HEALED LESIONS OF VASCULITIS)
Lamination (onion skinning) of vessel wall constituents[2] (concentric proliferation of pericytes and smooth muscle cells)
Luminal obliteration (endarteritis obliterans)[2]
Intimal or medial proliferation of cellular elements leading to luminal occlusion with preservation of the internal elastic lamina
Segmental or complete loss of elastic lamina in medium and large vessels associated with acellular scar tissue[1]
Reactive angioendotheliomatosis
Neovascularization of vessel adventitia

RBC, Red blood cell.
[1]Required for diagnosis of vasculitis.
[2]Other types of vessel injury can cause same pattern.
[3]Intraluminal fibrin deposition can be found in nonvasculitic arterial lesions such as malignant hypertension and antiphospholipid antibody syndrome.
Adapted from Carlson, J. A., Ng, B. T., & Chen, K. R. 2005. Cutaneous vasculitis update: diagnostic criteria, classification, epidemiology, etiology, pathogenesis, evaluation and prognosis. *The American Journal of Dermatopathology*, 27(6), 504–528.

Histopathologic Findings

HISTOPATHOLOGIC DIAGNOSIS OF VASCULITIS

The diagnosis of cutaneous vasculitis is made primarily by examination of hematoxylin and eosin (H&E)–stained sections. Table 4.3 lists criteria for diagnosis of cutaneous vasculitis. Fibrinoid necrosis (fibrin deposition within and around the vessel wall) is caused by the accumulation of plasma proteins, including coagulation factors that are converted to fibrin, at sites of vessel wall destruction (Figs. 4.2 and 4.3). The diagnosis of vasculitis can be made unequivocally, if there are inflammatory infiltrates within and around the walls of vessels accompanied by fibrin deposition. This typically consists of neutrophils with karyorrhectic debris. These changes coexist with signs of endothelial damage in the form of endothelial swelling, shrinkage (apoptosis), or sloughing. Secondary changes in which vascular damage can be inferred are the histopathologic findings of extravasation of RBCs (purpura), epidermal necrosis (infarct), and ulceration secondary to the ischemia from vessel obstruction or destruction by the inflammatory insult. The type of inflammatory cell mediating vessel damage and vessel sizes affected roughly correlate with pathogenic mechanisms, which are listed in Table 4.4.

Circumstantial evidence of vessel wall damage, thus vasculitis, includes lamination of the adventitia, media, or intima of vessels (so-called onion skinning); perivascular nuclear dust (leukocytoclasia) without

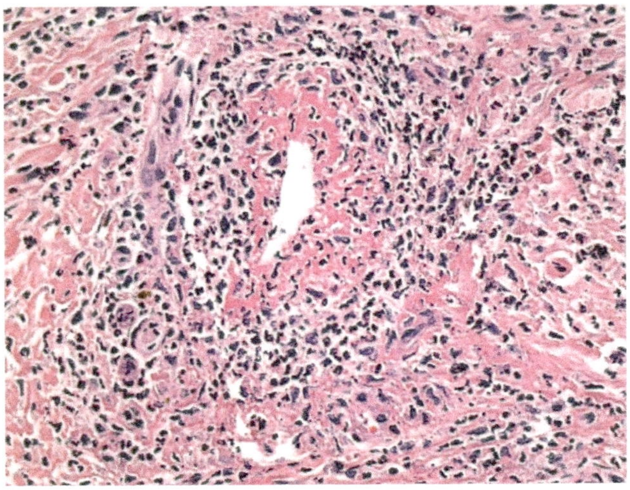

FIG. 4.2

Small vessel neutrophilic vasculitis (leukocytoclastic vasculitis) is identified by the presence of fibrin deposits, nuclear debris, and neutrophils disrupting a postcapillary venule.

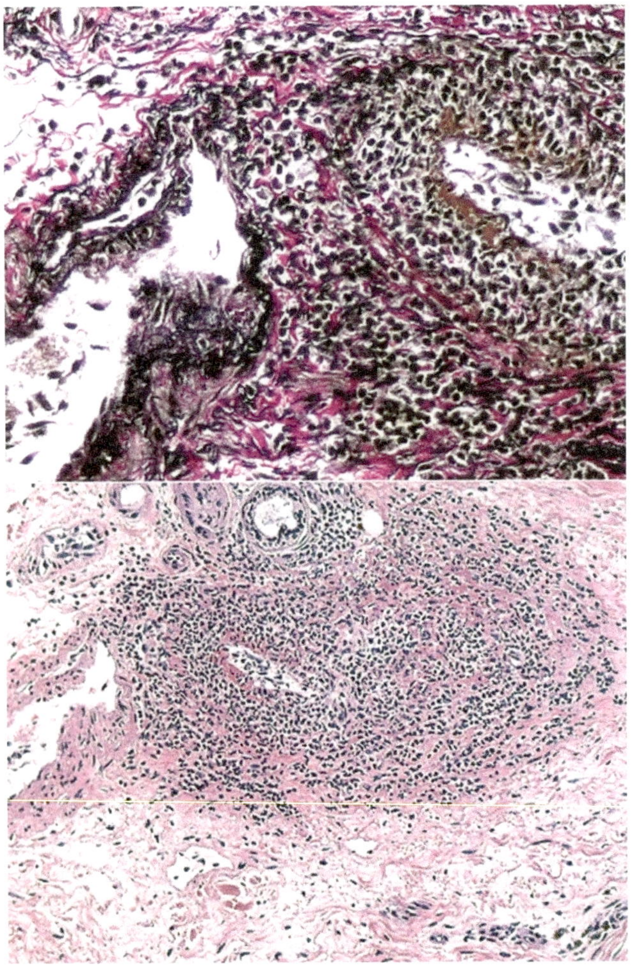

FIG. 4.3

Neutrophilic muscular vessel vasculitis associated with loss of the elastic lamina (elastic tissue stain, *top*).

fibrin deposits (early, evolving LCV); sharply defined loss of the elastic lamina associated with acellular scar tissue (the healed stage of muscular vessel vasculitis); or in the case of muscular (large) vessels, subendothelial, intramuscular, or adventitial inflammatory cells. In addition, neovascularization of the adventitia, the formation of small capillaries, is a prominent feature of mature and older lesions of medium vessel vasculitis, such as PAN, or mixed vessel vasculitis, such as GC, and a component of chronic localized small vessel vasculitis (SVV) such as erythema elevatum diutinum (EED). Last, luminal obliteration (endarteritis obliterans) is an irreversible, ischemic consequence of some forms of vasculitis such as lymphocytic and granulomatous arteritis. Endarteritis obliterans typically affects small- to medium-sized arteries. Healed lesions of muscular vessel vasculitis, the acellular scar stage, do not progress to endarteritis obliterans and can be associated with either luminal stenosis or aneurysm formation; however, persistence of vessel wall inflammation, either medial or intimal, can eventually lead to luminal obliteration or aneurysm rupture. Endarteritis obliterans can be broken down into stages. Initially, a lymphocytic endothelialitis (endarteritis) is evident, followed by the formation of a sponge-like plug composed of mononuclear cells, fibrin, and RBCs that results in partial to complete obstruction. A perivascular lymphohistiocytic (nonneutrophilic) inflammatory infiltrate develops around affected arteries, which is then followed by formation of dilated capillaries in obstructed vessels' adventitia. Smooth muscle cells immigrate and proliferate in the subendothelial zone, organizing the occluding plug during the intermediate stage. The final stage is characterized by fibrosis, shrinkage, and atrophy of the occluded artery.

INCIDENTAL VASCULITIS

It is common to find changes in neutrophilic SVV underlying an ulcer formed by another process (trauma or surgery). This is incidental vascular injury and can usually be differentiated from primary vasculitis by correlation with history and the focal nature of the vessel damage that is restricted to the area of trauma or ulceration; the vessels in the surrounding skin will be unaffected. (The term *secondary vasculitis* is not used because it refers to vasculitis developing *secondarily* in systemic disease, e.g., rheumatoid or lupus vasculitis.) Neutrophilic dermatoses (e.g., Sweet's syndrome) can also exhibit neutrophil-mediated vessel damage that can resemble small vessel neutrophilic vasculitis in approximately one-third of cases, typically affecting vessels within the diffuse dermal neutrophilic infiltrate compared with the angiocentric neutrophilic infiltrate of LCV. In addition, vasoocclusion can also be seen as an incidental finding at sites of ulceration.

TABLE 4.4

Pathogenic Mechanisms of Vasculitis and Their Clinical Diagnostic and Histologic Correlates

Pathogenic Mechanism	Vasculitic Syndrome	Vasculitis Pattern
Direct infection	Rickettsial infections	Lymphocytic small vessel vasculitis
Type I anaphylactic	Eosinophilic vasculitis	Eosinophilic small vessel vasculitis
	Eosinophilic granulomatosis with polyangiitis	Eosinophilic small and medium vessel vasculitis[1]
Type II cytotoxic–cytolytic antibody	Granulomatosis with polyangiitis	Neutrophilic mostly small and medium vessel vasculitis
	Microscopic polyangiitis	Neutrophilic mostly small and medium vessel vasculitis
Type III immune complex	IgA vasculitis	Neutrophilic small vessel vasculitis
	Cutaneous leukocytoclastic angiitis	Neutrophilic small vessel vasculitis
	Cryoglobulinemic vasculitis	Neutrophilic mostly small and medium vessel vasculitis
	Polyarteritis nodosa	Neutrophilic medium vessel vasculitis
Type IV delayed hypersensitivity	Giant cell arteritis	Granulomatous medium vessel vasculitis
	Chronic graft versus host disease	Lymphocytic small vessel vasculitis
	Sneddon's syndrome; Degos' disease	Lymphocytic medium vessel vasculitis followed by endarteritis obliterans

[1]Eosinophils are as or more numerous than neutrophils.

Adapted from Carlson, J. A., Ng, B. T., & Chen, K. R. (2005). Cutaneous vasculitis update: diagnostic criteria, classification, epidemiology, etiology, pathogenesis, evaluation and prognosis. *The American Journal of Dermatopathology*, 27, 504–528.

Other Histopathologic Findings Associated With Vasculitis

Some cutaneous vasculitis patients with systemic disease exhibit histopathologic findings concomitant to the vasculitis that will point to etiology and/or diagnosis, such as granulomatous dermatitis, dermal eosinophilia, or dermal neutrophilia (Table 4.5). Angiocentric fibrosis associated with foci of leukocytoclasis can be seen in some cases of cutaneous inflammatory pseudotumor and mature lesions of EED and granuloma faciale (Fig. 4.4). Eosinophilic or "red" extravascular granulomas (palisaded neutrophilic granulomatous dermatitis with eosinophils) are found in the papular and nodular extremity lesions of eosinophilic granulomatosis with polyangiitis (EGPA). "Blue" extravascular granulomas (palisaded neutrophilic granulomatous dermatitis) are found in some papular and nodular lesions in rheumatoid vasculitis (RV) and GPA. The term "palisaded and neutrophilic granulomatous dermatitis" was previously distinguished from "interstitial granulomatous dermatitis" by the presence of vasculitis. More recently, reactive granulomatous dermatitis has been proposed as an umbrella term for these overlapping diagnoses. Sub- and intraepidermal pustules may be seen in the setting of cutaneous vasculitis triggered by bacterial pharyngitis as well as in septic vasculitis and IgAV. Cases of septic vasculitis, mixed cryoglobulinemic vasculitis (CV), and levamisole-associated vasculitis can present with concurrent intraluminal thrombosis (vasculopathy) along with typical changes of LCV. In some instances, robust neutrophilic infiltrates may result in haloed areas that resemble yeast forms, or cryptococcus. Fungal stains and culture are negative, ruling out a true infectious process.

Ancillary Studies

DIRECT IMMUNOFLUORESCENT STUDIES

The absence of immune complexes, so-called pauci-immune vasculitis, is the expected finding in GPA, EGPA, and microscopic polyangiitis (MPA) with or without medium-sized vessel involvement. Deposition of IgG, IgM, IgA, or C3 in or around the vessels characterizes immune complex–mediated vasculitis such as CV and most cases of CLA. The most common immunoreactant found in vessels by DIF is C3 followed by IgM, IgA, and IgG (Fig. 4.5). Fibrinogen vascular deposits are also commonly found. Similar to H&E evaluation, the presence of diagnostic immunofluorescence patterns is inversely related to the age of the lesion biopsied. One hundred percent of biopsies will harbor immunoglobulins within the first 48 hours; 30% will be negative at 48 to 72 hours; and after 72 hours, only C3 is detected in positive DIF samples. In addition, the type of immunoglobulin and pattern of deposits in DIF exams can add diagnostic value. Predominant IgA vascular deposits are found in IgAV, increasing the need for renal monitoring. However, IgA deposits have also been reported in the setting of malignancy, Sweet's syndrome, infection, and even GPA. Immunoreactants at the basement membrane zone, mostly IgG, can be found in CTD vasculitis such as lupus vasculitis. In the evaluation of urticarial vasculitis (UV), the finding of basement membrane zone fluorescence

TABLE 4.5

Histologic Patterns Associated With Systemic Vasculitis or Indicative of Etiology

Lamellar or Storiform Fibrosis
Erythema elevatum diutinum, granuloma faciale, IgG4-related disease, or inflammatory pseudotumor
Diffuse (Sparse) Dermal Granulocytic Infiltrates
Tissue neutrophilia: urticarial vasculitis associated with systemic lupus erythematosus
Tissue eosinophilia: eosinophilic granulomatosis with polyangiitis, hypereosinophilic syndrome with vasculitis
Palisaded and Neutrophilic Granulomatous Dermatitis[1]
"Red" extravascular granuloma (eosinophils, flame figures): eosinophilic granulomatosis with polyangiitis, granulomatosis with polyangiitis (rare)
"Blue" extravascular granuloma (neutrophils, nuclear dust): granulomatosis with polyangiitis, rheumatoid vasculitis
Eosinophilic granulomatosis with polyangiitis (rarely)
Vacuolar Interface Dermatitis (Sometimes Dermal Mucin Deposition)
Connective tissue diseases: lupus erythematosus, dermatomyositis
"Pustular" Dermatosis With Intraepidermal or Subepidermal Neutrophilic Abscesses
Infectious trigger, septic vasculitis

[1]Also known as Winkelmann's granuloma, Churg-Strauss granuloma, extravascular necrotizing granuloma, and rheumatoid papules.
Adapted from Carlson, J. A., Ng, B. T., & Chen, K. R. (2005). Cutaneous vasculitis update: diagnostic criteria, classification, epidemiology, etiology, pathogenesis, evaluation and prognosis. *The American Journal of Dermatopathology*, 27, 504–528.

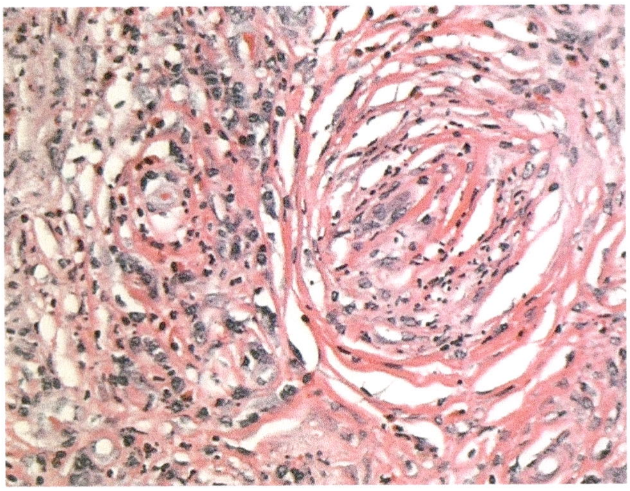

FIG. 4.4

Angiocentric fibrosis and focal small vessel vasculitis found in a cutaneous inflammatory pseudotumor.

may be seen in patients with hypocomplemententemic states and who have CTD. In addition, IgM deposition in blood vessels may be readily seen in cases of vasculitis with a circulating rheumatoid factor (RF) or with monoclonal production of IgM as found in CV.

Laboratory Studies

Active vasculitis is typically associated with an acute phase response with an increase in CRP and erythrocyte sedimentation rate (ESR). Other serologic tests useful in the workup of vasculitis include RF, antinuclear antibody (ANA) with reflex panel, C3 and C4 levels,

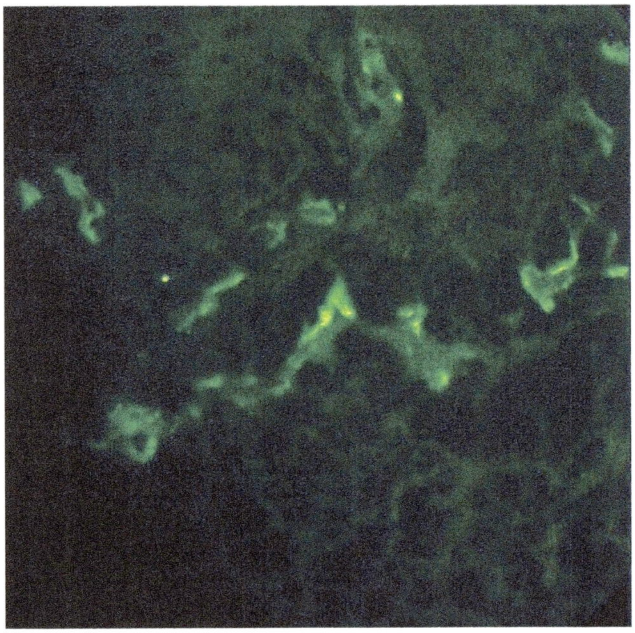

FIG. 4.5

Vascular C3 deposition is the most frequent immunofluorescent finding in patients with cutaneous vasculitis.

cryoglobulins, and ANCAs, as well as performing a chest radiography and serum and urine electrophoresis. In addition, monitoring levels of acute phase reactants (e.g., CRP, ESR) can potentially measure disease activity and response to therapy.

ANTINEUTROPHIL CYTOPLASMIC ANTIBODIES

ANCA-associated vasculitides include GPA, MPA, EGPA, and some drug-related vasculitis, but ANCA can also be found in patients with inflammatory bowel disease, CTD, and other chronic inflammatory diseases. Positive ANCA patterns should be separated into pANCA and cANCA. The perinuclear pattern of ANCA, pANCA, may be seen with myeloperoxidase (MPO) antibodies as well as others (e.g., lactoferrin, cathepsin) and is found in MPA and EGPA. The cytoplasmic pattern of ANCA, cANCA, is mostly antiproteinase 3 (anti-PR3), which is strongly associated with GPA. However, the presence of ANCA is not diagnostic of systemic vasculitis because up to 60% of patients with cutaneous LCV can have a positive ANCA result, and ANCA is found at low levels in many systemic inflammatory and pulmonary disorders that mimic vasculitis. In this latter group, atypical indirect immunofluorescent patterns are present, and antibodies to PR-3 and MPO are rare by antigen-specific enzyme-linked immunosorbent assay (ELISA) testing. The presence of pANCA in addition to dsDNA and antihistone antibodies may point to a drug-associated etiology (particularly hydralazine).

Evaluation of Patients With Cutaneous Vasculitis

If cutaneous vasculitis is documented histopathologically, then the clinician must seek an explanation for it by evaluating the presence and extent of systemic disease, identifying any treatable etiology such as drug, infection, malignancy, or coexisting systemic disease, and treating this condition. These steps will include a careful clinical history determining whether this is an acute or chronic condition and searching for triggers such as drugs or infections or symptoms indicative of pre-existing or concomitant disease, physical examination, chest radiography, and routine laboratory tests (blood and urine). If specific symptoms or signs of systemic disease, such as mononeuritis or microhematuria, are evident, further studies should be considered to arrive at specific diagnosis of a primary systemic vasculitis (PSV) or secondary systemic vasculitis. Symptoms indicating systemic involvement include arthralgias, myalgias, fever, hemoptysis, shortness of breath, cough, wheezing, eye or ear symptoms, sinusitis, hoarseness, numbness or paresthesias, abdominal pain, melena, hematuria, and testicular pain. Questioning for the presence of night sweats and weight loss or complaints of dry eyes or mouth, photosensitivity or facial cutaneous eruption, oral lesions, or muscle weakness will help determine if the vasculitis is associated with malignancy or CTD. Clinical examination helps to determine the size of vessel involvement, which can narrow the differential diagnosis (Table 4.2). For patients suspected of having chronic or systemic vasculitis, the following laboratory studies are recommended: complete blood cell count with differential, blood urea nitrogen or creatinine, liver function panel, urinalysis, hepatitis B and C virus serologies, cryoglobulins, complement levels (CH50, C3, C4), ANCA, ANA, and RF. Additional tests to consider are SPEP/UPEP with reflex immunofixation, blood cultures, and echocardiography if the patient has a high fever or a heart murmur, and antistreptolysin O titers in children. Although most cases of cutaneous vasculitis are benign and self-limited, a significant minority of cutaneous vasculitis patients will have extracutaneous disease, frequently renal involvement; contrarily, cutaneous disease occurs in up to 50% of PSV patients, and it can be the first presenting sign of disease in up to a quarter of patients with EGPA. Table 4.6 lists the clinical, pathologic, and laboratory findings that signal a high probability of systemic vasculitis or coexisting systemic disease. Table 4.7 lists the mean frequencies of cutaneous, laboratory, and systemic findings for the major vasculitic syndromes affecting the skin. After cutaneous vasculitis is documented pathologically, the clinician must correlate clinical and laboratory data to arrive at a specific diagnosis.

Differential Diagnosis

The differential diagnosis of cutaneous vasculitis is broad and involves many different clinical settings. The correct diagnosis often depends on correlating clinical findings with a number of laboratory parameters, of which a skin biopsy is only one part. When a skin biopsy confirms the presence of vasculitis, certain histologic features or additional ancillary studies may help narrow the differential diagnosis. Most important, however, is the clinical context. For example, information on whether or not a patient has received a new medication before the onset of the vasculitis, is septic, or has a history and associated other symptoms of CTD is critical for the correct interpretation of a cutaneous vasculitis.

Prognosis

The distinction between localized (cutaneous) and systemic vasculitis is thought to be the most crucial point in determining patient outcome. Patients with strictly cutaneous disease have an excellent prognosis, but those with evidence of systemic disease are at risk for permanent organ damage and death. Pooled data from retrospective studies have shown that fewer than 20% (up to 43% in one study) of patients have evidence of visceral vasculitis, most commonly kidney involvement (so-called renal-dermal vasculitis). Certain clinical and histologic findings correlate with prognosis and signal a higher probability of systemic vasculitis (Table 4.6).

TABLE 4.6

Clinical, Pathologic, and Laboratory Findings Indicating a High Probability of Systemic Disease

Findings	Suspected Systemic Vasculitis Syndrome
Clinical Signs or Symptoms	
High fever	Infection, systemic inflammatory disorders
Paresthesias, foot drop	EGPA, PAN
Abdominal pain	IgAV, EGPA
Frank arthritis	RV, infection, PAN, systemic inflammatory disorder
Hypertension	PAN
Purpura above waist, upper extremities	IgAV, MPA, GPA, EGPA
>One type of vasculitic lesion[1]	IgAV, MPA, GPA, EGPA
Punctuate palmar lesions	LV
Laboratory Evaluation	
ESR >40 mm/h	Infection, hematologic malignancies, systemic inflammatory disorders
Elevated RF and cryoglobulins and low complement	CV (Types II and III)
Chest radiograph: infiltrates or cavities	GPA, EGPA, MPA, malignancy
Hematuria or proteinuria or abnormal creatinine	Dermal-renal vasculitis syndrome: GPA, MPA, PAN, IgAV, SLE
Hypocomplemententemia	UV associated with SLE
Abnormal blood count	Infection, hematologic malignancy, systemic inflammatory disorders
cANCA (PR3)	GPA
pANCA (MPO)	MPA, EGPA
Histologic Examination	
Deep dermal and/or subcutaneous small and/or muscular vessel vasculitis	Systemic vasculitis syndrome (GPA, EGPA, MPA, CV, RV, LV, septic vasculitis)
Palisaded neutrophilic and granulomatous dermatitis	GPA, EGPA, LV, RV
Tissue neutrophilia or tissue eosinophilia	SLE or EGPA, respectively
Direct Immunofluorescence	
Isolated or predominant IgA vascular deposits	IgAV
Lupus band (IgG, IgM, and/or C3 at the BMZ)	LV, UV associated with SLE

CV, Cryoglobulinemic vasculitis; *EGPA*, eosinophilic granulomatosis with polyangiitis; *GPA*, granulomatosis with polyangiitis; *IgAV*, IgA vasculitis; *LV*, lupus vasculitis; *MPA*, microscopic polyangiitis; *MPO*, myeloperoxidase; *PAN*, polyarteritis nodosa; *PR3*, proteinase 3; *RF*, rheumatoid factor; *RV*, rheumatoid vasculitis; *SLE*, systemic lupus erythematosus; *UV*, urticarial vasculitis.

[1]Purpura plus ulcers, nodules, bullae, livedo reticularis, and so on.

Adapted from Russell, J. P., & Gibson, L. E. (2006). Primary cutaneous small vessel vasculitis: approach to diagnosis and treatment. *International Journal of Dermatology*, 45(1), 3–13.

Disease prognosis is highly correlated with the specific diagnosis. For example, patients with IgAV have higher propensity to develop renal disease. Coexistence of deep dermal and subcutaneous vasculitis is often seen in mixed vessel or medium vessel vasculitis and is associated with malignancy, systemic vasculitis such as ANCA-positive vasculitis or PAN, CTD vasculitis, and Behçet's disease. Systemic disease, most often systemic lupus erythematosus (SLE), can also be found in patients who have coexisting tissue (dermal) neutrophilia. Palisaded neutrophilic or extravascular granulomas exhibiting eosinophilic or basophilic debris around degenerated collagen bundles can be found in EGPA, GPA, and RV. Tissue eosinophilia can be a sign of drug-induced vasculitis or EGPA.

Treatment

Therapy depends on the nature and severity of the vasculitis. Here, we discuss general guidelines that are followed for cutaneous vasculitis. For mild hypersensitivity vasculitis caused by a drug reaction, discontinuing the offending drug may be sufficient enough; antihistamines might be used for pruritus. While topical steroids may be adequate for many cases of cutaneous small vessel vasculitis (CSVV), a short course of corticosteroids may be necessary for more severe cases or in those with systemic organ involvement. In addition, simple observation may be adequate for transitory vasculitis confined to the skin, as with mild cases of IgAV.

TABLE 4.7

Broad Overlap Exists in the Range of Clinicopathologic Findings Found in Cutaneous and Systemic Vasculitic Syndromes

Affected Organs	CLA	IgAV	UV[1]	CV	PAN	EGPA	MPA	GPA	GCA	LV	RV
Skin disease	100%	100%	100%	90%	28%–60%	50%–78%	50%–65%	40%–50%	<50%[5]	90%	80%–90%
DIF + (C_3 or Ig), vessels	82%–100%	87%–93% (IgA)	50%, 30%–100%[1]	83%, 67%–100%	≤60%[2]	0%	0%	54%, 25%–75%	—	~53%	~79% (IgM)
BMZ	—	—	34%, 1%–96%[1]		20%			Rare		~60%	
ANCA (any type, IIF)	Rare	IgA ANCA	NR	10%	10%–27%	40%–75%	~75%	90%, 65%–100%	Rare	11%–31%	32%, 16%–43%
PR3/cANCA	—			1%	8%	3%–35%	10%–50%	75%–90%		0%	0%
MPO/pANCA	—			2%	11%	38%–59%	50%–80%	5%–20%		31%	<2%
Systemic symptoms[3]	6%–23%	<10%	7%	100%	31%–76%	72%–100%	41%–79%	27%–51%	40%–50%	50%–100%	45%–72%
Upper respiratory tract	—	<5%	<5%	<5%	<5%	50%–75%	None	95%	9%	Rare	—
Lung disease	—	<5%	10%	<5%	<5%	≤100%	≤70%	≤85%	—	12% (1.4 OR)	9%–34%
Asthma		Rare	7%			90%–100%	None	None		Rare	
Radiographic findings			3%			40%–50%	15%–70%	70%–85%			
Alveolar hemorrhage			—			7%	10%–50%	5%–15%			
Genitourinary	3%–7%	40%–50%	<5%	30%–55%	60%–80%[4]	≤40%	≤90%	≤80%	—	16%–38%	6%–25%
Glomerulonephritis		12%	3%		None	10%–40%	75%–90%	70%–80%			
Lower tract disease		Rare	—		5%–10%	<2%	<5%	<2%			
Gastrointestinal	3%–5%	35%–65%	15%	<40%	14%–53%	30%–40%	30%	<5%	—	18%	4%–10%
Nervous system	—	10%	<5%	40%–80%	≤72%	≤80%	≤70%	≤50%	≤15%	12%–21%	36%–45%
Central			Rare	Rare	3%–28%	5%–30%	10%–15%	5%–10%	3%–15%	(2.1 OR)	
Peripheral			<5%	≤80%	38%–72%	70%–80%	60%–70%	40%–50%	—	5%	
Cardiac disease	—	Rare	Rare	<40%	5%–30%	10%–40%	10%–15%	10%–25%	—	15% (3.1 OR)	6%–34%
Ocular disease	—	Rare	4%	40%	<5%	<5%	<5%	50%–60%	14%–16%	—	4%–25%
Arthralgias or arthritis	14%–65%	75%	33%	70%	50%–75%	40%–50%	40%–60%	60%–70%	15%–39%	62%–7%	100%

ANCA, Antineutrophil cytoplasmic antibody; *BMZ*, basement membrane zone; *CLA*, cutaneous leukocytoclastic angiitis; *DIF*, direct immunofluorescence; *EGPA*, eosinophilic granulomatosis with polyangiitis; *GCA*, giant cell (temporal) arteritis; *GPA*, granulomatosis with polyangiitis; *IgAV*, IgA vasculitis; *IIF*, indirect immunofluorescence; *LV*, lupus vasculitis; *MPA*, microscopic polyangiitis; *NR*, not reported; *OR*, odds ratio of likelihood that patient with lupus vasculitis will have disease affecting that organ compared with an SLE patient with vasculitis; *PAN*, polyarteritis nodosa; *RV*, rheumatoid vasculitis; *UV*, urticarial vasculitis.

[1]For patients with hypocomplementemic UV, the frequency of positive DIF results and extracutaneous symptoms is significantly elevated.

[2]DIF evaluation on cases of cutaneous PAN.

[3]Symptoms of weight loss, anorexia, malaise, fever, fatigue, or weakness.

[4]Renal involvement in PAN affects arteries and results in nephrogenic hypertension.

[5]Scalp or artery tenderness, scalp necrosis, scalp cords or artery swelling, or decreased or absent temporal artery pulses.

Adapted from Carlson, J. A., & Chen, K. R. (2006). Cutaneous vasculitis update: neutrophilic small vessel vasculitic syndromes. *The American Journal of Dermatopathology*, 28(6), 486–506.

Nonsteroidal antiinflammatory agents may help with skin or joint pain. Colchicine and dapsone may be helpful in selected cases and may be used before the administration of a more potent regimen of glucocorticoids or cytotoxic drugs. Prior to starting colchicine, the patient's renal function should be evaluated. Evaluation for glucose-6-phosphate dehydrogenase (G6PD) deficiency is necessary prior to initiating dapsone.

Patients with rapidly progressive vasculitic diseases, such as GPA or PAN, are likely to require combination therapy consisting of a cytotoxic drug and steroids; after 1 or 2 months of combined therapy, the steroid dose may be reduced; therapy is usually continued for 6 to 12 months to diminish the risk of relapse. Azathioprine and methotrexate have been used in less severe forms of vasculitis and as maintenance therapy after remission has been induced by cyclophosphamide. Other drugs such as mycophenolate mofetil and biologic agents appear to be useful in some instances. For both refractory systemic and cutaneous vasculitis, intravenous immunoglobulin and plasmapheresis have been shown to be effective in case reports and case series.

Targeted therapy is playing a major and advancing role in the treatment of systemic vasculitis; with further understanding of the underlying pathophysiology of each systemic vasculitis, more targeted therapy can be used for more successful treatments with fewer side effects. The two most tested and trialed agents to this date are infliximab (antitumor necrosis factor α [TNF-α]) and rituximab (monoclonal antibody against CD20 [B lymphocytes]).

Rituximab is a promising agent for the treatment of systemic vasculitis (mostly for ANCA-positive vasculitis and CV), yet larger studies with guidelines are needed. Rituximab has equivalent remission-induction efficacy as cyclophosphamide in ANCA-associated vasculitides in conjunction with corticosteroids. However, rituximab demonstrates a less severe side effect profile compared to cyclophosphamide.

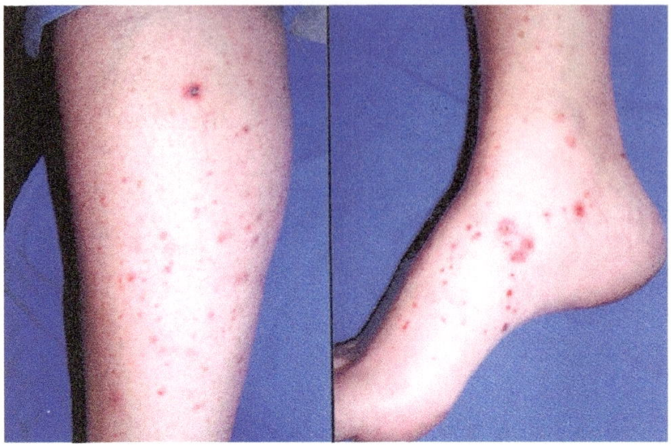

FIG. 4.6

Petechial and purpuric macules in a patient with cutaneous leukocytoclastic vasculitis secondary to an adverse drug reaction.

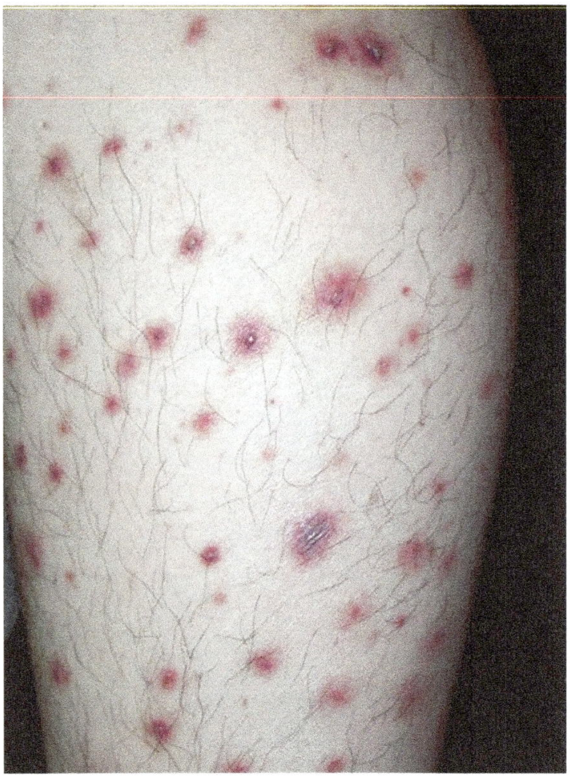

FIG. 4.7

Purpuric papules in cutaneous vasculitis. (Courtesy of Henry Foong, MBBS, Ipoh, Malaysia.)

VASCULITIDES AFFECTING PREDOMINANTLY SMALL VESSELS

CUTANEOUS SMALL VESSEL VASCULITIS

Other names for CSVV include CLA, LCV, hypersensitivity vasculitis, allergic vasculitis, and necrotizing vasculitis.

Clinical Findings

Patients with CSVV may first present with erythematous macules in the early stages but soon develop into palpable purpura (Figs. 4.6 and 4.7) over the lower extremities that develop and evolve relatively synchronously. The lower extremity involvement is typical of immune complex vasculitis since the immune complexes deposit in a dependent distribution. For bedridden patients, the dependent distribution may be different and involve the buttocks and upper thighs. These lesions may demonstrate symptoms of pruritus, stinging, tenderness, or burning. The diagnosis of CSVV is based on the exclusion of visceral disease. Most patients are middle-aged adults who have history of recent drug ingestion, infection, exposure to an environmental agent, or prolonged exercise in hot weather (e.g., a summer day at the golf course). Lesions resolve over 3 to 4 weeks, leaving residual ecchymoses and hyperpigmentation.

Histopathologic Findings

The histopathologic findings include small vessel neutrophilic vasculitis affecting the superficial dermal plexus, mostly of postcapillary venules and sometimes arterioles. Fragmented nuclei (karyorrhectic debris) around small vessels are characteristic. Focal fibrinoid necrosis may be seen (see Figs. 4.2 and 4.3).

Ancillary Studies

DIF examination shows both complement and immunoglobulins (most often IgM and IgG) in vessel walls (Fig. 4.5).

IGA VASCULITIS

Clinical Findings

IgAV was previously known as Henoch-Schönlein purpura (HSP). It is the most common vasculitis in children but also occurs in adults. A preceding upper respiratory tract infection occurs in up to 50%, and a history of recent drug or food ingestion triggers is reported in a minority. The classical clinical presentation includes the tetrad of skin involvement, arthritis, gastrointestinal (GI) involvement (pain, hemorrhage), and nephritis (found less frequently). In 1990, the ACR developed criteria that potentially had higher sensitivity and specificity for the diagnosis of IgAV, which included isolated or predominant IgA vascular deposits and two or more of these clinical features: age 20 years or younger, GI involvement (colicky pain or hematochezia), upper respiratory tract infection prodrome, or hematuria or renal biopsy showing mesangioproliferative glomerulonephritis with or without IgA deposits. Long-term follow-up is important; renal impairment can be seen many years after the initial diagnosis in adults (fewer than 20% of children develop chronic renal failure 20 years after diagnosis). Nephrotic syndrome, hypertension, and renal failure at onset are associated with a poor outcome, and in adult patients, those who present with fever, purpura above the waist, and elevated ESR are significantly more likely to have IgA glomerulonephritis. A urinalysis is insufficient to determine the extent of proteinuria, and a 24-hour urine collection should be considered to evaluate the extent of renal involvement. In adult males over the age of 40, IgAV may be associated with malignancy and consideration of broad cancer workup may be warranted, particularly if constitutional symptoms such as weight loss and night sweats are present.

Histopathologic Findings

Skin biopsy in patients with IgAV demonstrates neutrophilic SVV restricted to the superficial dermis; usually the vascular damage induced is mild, but rarely the whole dermis may be involved. In a retrospective study of cases with IgAV, patients older than 40 years of age and found to have absent eosinophils on histopathologic examination demonstrated a threefold increased risk of renal involvement compared with those younger than 40 years with tissue eosinophilia.

Ancillary Studies

DIF shows isolated or predominant vascular IgA (Fig. 4.8) deposits from lesions less than 48 hours old.

URTICARIAL VASCULITIS

UV is also known as urticarial venulitis, hypocomplementemic or normocomplementemic UV, and hypocomplementemic UV syndrome.

Clinical Findings

Among all patients presenting with chronic urticaria, 20% or fewer will have UV. Most patients with UV are women (female:male ratio, 3:2 to 4:1) in their fourth or

FIG. 4.8
Vascular IgA deposition in a case of IgA vasculitis.

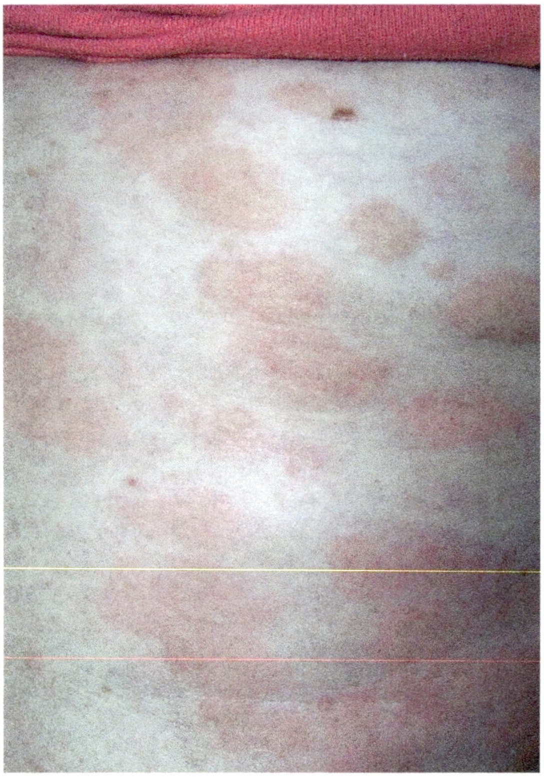

FIG. 4.9
Urticarial plaques caused by urticarial vasculitis.

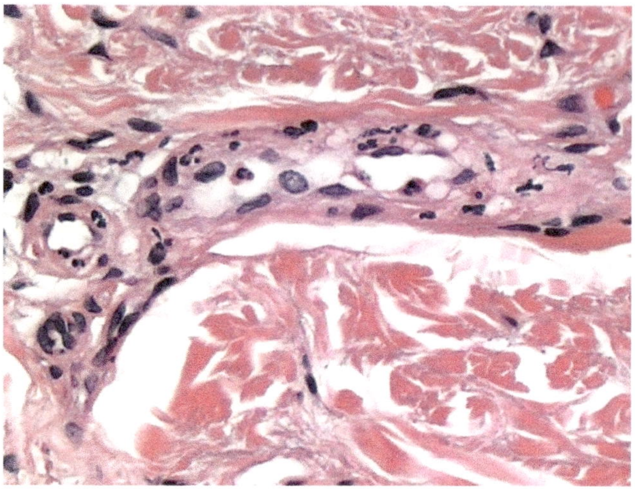

FIG. 4.10
Lesions of urticarial vasculitis do not have full-blown features of small vessel neutrophilic vasculitis. Instead, focal and mild perivascular neutrophilic infiltrates associated with nuclear debris are most often found.

fifth decade of life. Rather than pruritus, patients with UV have painful, tender, or burning papules and plaques (Fig. 4.9) affecting any cutaneous surface that persist longer than 24 hours and less than 72 hours and, in some cases, leave residual purpura or hyperpigmentation. Many patients with UV have systemic symptoms of low-grade fever, angioedema, arthralgias and arthritis, and abdominal pain. In addition, hypocomplementemia can be observed in 18% to 32% of patients. Patients with hypocomplementemic UV are mostly female and have more severe disease than those with normocomplementemic UV. The hypocomplementemic UV syndrome is defined by the presence of arthralgias or arthritis, glomerulonephritis, uveitis or episcleritis, recurrent abdominal pain, or obstructive lung disease. Up to 70% of UV patients with positive lupus band test results also have renal disease (e.g., membranoproliferative glomerulonephritis, focal necrotizing vasculitis). More than 50% of patients with hypocomplementemic UV will go on to meet criteria for SLE.

Histopathologic Findings

The criteria for the histopathologic diagnosis of vasculitis in UV are less rigorous because the infiltrates are sparse and vasculitis changes are focal and subtle. Typically, sparse perivascular and interstitial neutrophilic infiltrates are found with either focal small vessel neutrophilic vasculitis or focal perivascular neutrophilic nuclear debris without fibrin deposits and with or without extravasated RBCs. Minimal histopathologic criteria for the diagnosis of UV have been proposed, which are nuclear debris or fibrin deposits, with or without extravasated RBCs (Fig. 4.10). In addition, diffuse neutrophilic infiltrates are frequently found in hypocomplementemic UV, but dermal eosinophils are more common in normocomplementemic UV.

Ancillary Studies

DIF evaluation reveals vascular C3 or immunoglobulins, mostly IgM, in 47% of patients; however, vascular immunoreactants are found more frequently (87%–100%) in patients with hypocomplementemic UV. A positive lupus band test result (basement membrane zone deposits of C3 or immunoglobulin) is identified in 18% to 34% of all UV patients, most frequently in hypocomplementemic UV (70%–96%).

VASCULITIDES AFFECTING SMALL- TO MEDIUM-SIZED VESSELS

INFECTION-INDUCED AND SEPTIC VASCULITIS

Clinical Findings

About a quarter of all cases of cutaneous vasculitis are associated with infection, and all types of infectious

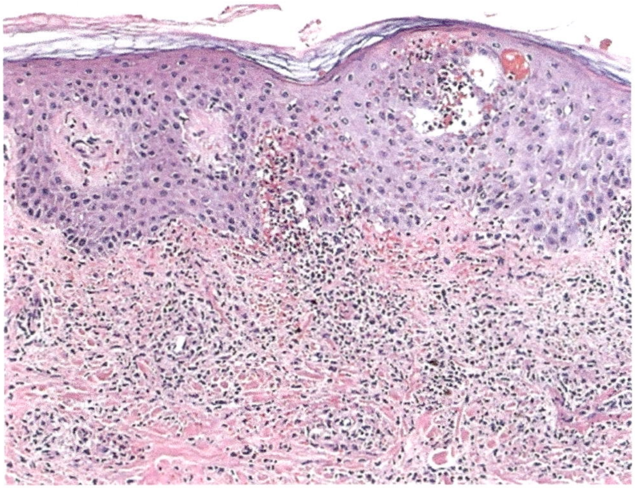

FIG. 4.11

Intracorneal and subepidermal pustules found in patient with small vessel vasculitis related to a bacterial infection.

agents (viruses, bacteria, fungi, protozoa, and helminths) have been associated with the development of vasculitis. Two well-known examples of infection leading to specific systemic vasculitis syndromes are infections caused by hepatitis B and hepatitis C viruses, which are strongly associated with the development of PAN and CV, respectively. Viral infection can be associated with localized cutaneous lesions showing lymphocytic or granulomatous muscular vessel vasculitis; varicella-zoster virus infection is the most frequent association. Infection-triggered CSVV is suspected to show a greater frequency of subcorneal, intraepidermal, and subepidermal neutrophilic pustules (Fig. 4.11), tissue neutrophilia, predominant IgA vascular deposits, and to have relatively fewer eosinophils and lymphocytes compared with idiopathic and drug-related CSVV. Patients with septicemia can present with cutaneous vasculitis. Acute vasculitis induced by septic states is often caused by infective endocarditis or infection with gonococci, meningococci, pseudomonas, staphylococci, streptococci, certain rickettsial infections, and other microorganisms. Clinical lesions are characterized by purpura (petechiae, ecchymoses, retiform morphology); vesiculopustules, often with dusky gray centers signifying necrosis; hemorrhagic bullae; and rarely, ulceration.

Histopathologic Findings

On biopsy, mixed neutrophilic small-to-medium vessel vasculitis with deep dermal and subcutaneous vessel involvement is found and associated with scant perivascular fibrin and no or little nuclear debris. In addition, fibrin thrombi, epidermal spongiosis, intraepidermal vesicles, and pustules are common in lesions of septic vasculitis. Organisms are rarely identified in skin lesions except in acute meningococcemia.

CRYOGLOBULINEMIC VASCULITIS

Cryoglobulinemic vasculitis is also known as essential CV.

Clinical Findings

Cutaneous vasculitis occurring in the presence of cryoglobulins is classified as CV. Cryoglobulins are cold-precipitating immunoglobulins that persist in the serum and resolubilize when rewarmed. There are three types of cryoglobulins: type I, monoclonal cryoglobulins comprise 10% to 15% of all cases and produce noninflammatory small vessel hyaline thrombi; type II, mixed monoclonal IgM RF, polyclonal IgG cryoglobulins are 50% to 60% of all cases; and type III, mixed polyclonal IgM (with RF activity) and IgG cryoglobulins are 30% to 40% of all cases. Type 1 cryoglobulinemia is associated with vasculopathy and not typically vasculitis. Mixed cryoglobulins (types II and III) are associated with connective tissue, hematologic malignancies, or infectious diseases, particularly hepatitis C infection. More than 50% of patients with hepatitis C have mixed cryoglobulins, with a lesser frequency of vasculitis. CV (mixed cryoglobulinemia with vasculitis) is characterized by the clinical triad of purpura triggered by cold exposure or prolonged standing, arthralgias, and weakness (asthenia). Other cutaneous manifestations include PAN-like lesions, ulcers, splinter hemorrhages, and palmar erythema. Systemic disease in CV includes glomerulonephritis, neuropathy, or pulmonary symptoms of hemoptysis and dyspnea. High titers of RF and low C4 levels are often observed in patients with CV, but not in patients with type 1 cryoglobulins.

Histopathologic Findings

In most cases, skin biopsy will show a small vessel neutrophilic vasculitis equally affecting superficial dermal and subcutis vessels and, in a minority of cases, neutrophilic muscular vessel vasculitis (PAN-like). Intravascular hyaline deposits can also be seen, particularly in ulcerative lesions. Reactive angioendotheliomatosis (lobular proliferation of capillaries harboring fibrin microthrombi) can be a sign of muscular vessel vasculitis.

Ancillary Studies

DIF demonstrates vascular immunoglobulins, mostly IgM, or complement deposits, in the majority of patients.

CONNECTIVE TISSUE DISEASE VASCULITIS

Clinical Findings

Approximately 12% of cutaneous vasculitis cases are associated with a CTD. Secondary vasculitis resulting from CTD should be considered in patients presenting with biopsy-proven cutaneous vasculitis who have signs and symptoms of dry eyes, dry mouth, arthritis, sclerosis, photosensitivity, or serologic evidence of ANA, RF, or anti-dsDNA, Ro, or La antibodies. Cutaneous vasculitis occurs frequently in patients with SLE, rheumatoid arthritis, and Sjögren's syndrome, and less commonly in those with dermatomyositis, scleroderma, and polychondritis. In general, CTD vasculitis shows more widespread organ involvement, and the caliber of vessels affected shows more variation compared with conventional CSVV. In addition, a minority of patients with CTD vasculitis have coexisting prothrombotic antiphospholipid antibodies, which can lead to the rapid evolution of vascular insufficiency with progressive tissue ischemia and infarction. Arterioles and postcapillary venules are the most commonly affected by vasculitis, manifested as purpura, vesiculobullous lesions, urticarial papules/plaques, and splinter hemorrhages (Fig. 4.12). One should suspect arterial involvement if cutaneous ulcers, nodules, digital gangrene, (necrotizing) livedo reticularis (Fig. 4.13), punctate acral scars, or pyoderma gangrenosum (PG)–like lesions are present; these patients have a higher probability of visceral vasculitis. CTD patients can also show pANCA (mostly) or cANCA by indirect immunofluorescence.

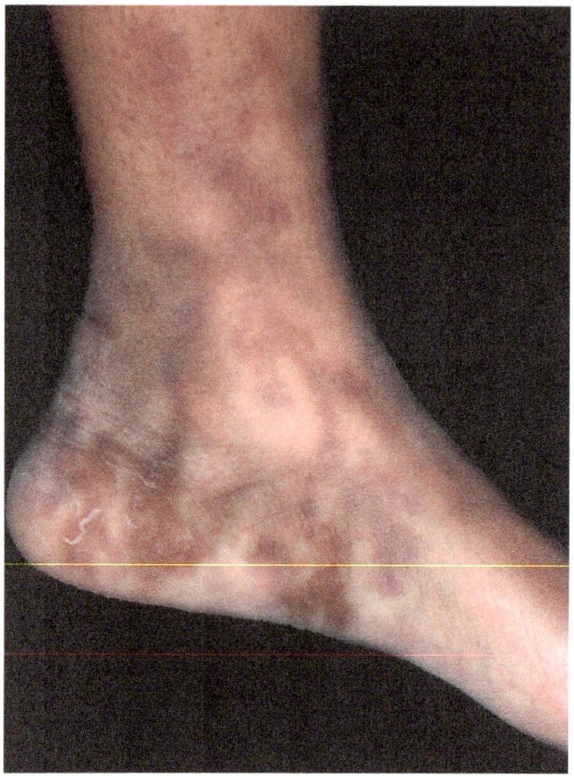

FIG. 4.13

Livedo reticularis.

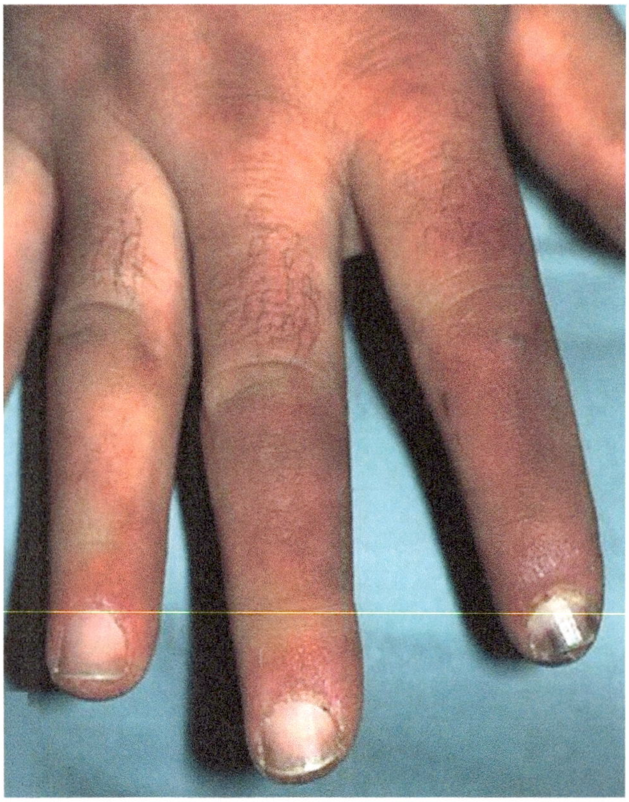

FIG. 4.12

Splinter hemorrhages, nail fold infarct, and digital cyanosis occurring in a patient with systemic lupus erythematosus. (Courtesy of Jörg Schaller, MD, Duisburg Germany.)

Histopathologic Findings

Skin biopsy shows a mixed, mostly small and muscular vessel neutrophilic vasculitis with lesions that can resemble PAN or typical CSVV. Chronic lymphocytic vasculitis with small or muscular vessel involvement is found in a minority of cases, mostly in patients with SLE and Sjögren's syndrome. This pattern of vasculitis is likely responsible for the slow, progressive occlusion of blood vessels (endarteritis obliterans) (Fig. 4.14) with end-organ ischemia found in some patients with CTD. Extravascular histologies can provide a clue to the diagnosis of CTD vasculitis such as the presence of interface dermatitis with dermal mucin deposition, which is found in lupus erythematosus and dermatomyositis; dermal or subcutaneous sclerosis in scleroderma; palisaded neutrophilic and granulomatosis dermatitis in rheumatoid arthritis or SLE; and neutrophilic urticarial dermatosis in SLE and Sjögren's syndrome. In general,

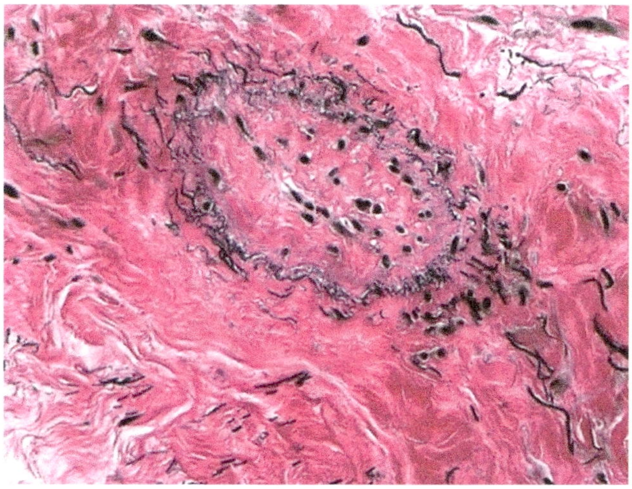

FIG. 4.14
Endarteritis obliterans identified in a small muscular vessel identified in the deep dermis of a biopsy of a punctate hand scar from a patient with systemic lupus erythematosus.

CTD-related vasculitis is a variant of immune complex vasculitis and will have a positive DIF study.

NODULAR VASCULITIS

Nodular vasculitis is also known as erythema induratum.

Clinical Findings

Patients presenting with painful ulcerated nodules over the lower extremities may have nodular vasculitis rather than cutaneous polyarteritis nodosa (CPAN). Nodular vasculitis (lobular panniculitis with vasculitis) was originally defined as erythema induratum (red, indurated plaques on the lower legs) associated with tuberculosis, the treatment of which leads to clearing of skin lesions. Other etiologic agents include drugs and nonmycobacterial infections associated with circulating immune complexes. Nodular vasculitis occurs in young to middle-aged women, who present with painful, tender, violaceous, indurated, and often ulcerated nodules affecting the calves, with less frequent involvement of the shins, ankles, thighs, and upper extremities. Healing of these lesions is often accompanied by scarring with hyperpigmentation.

Histopathologic Findings

Deep punch or excisional or incisional biopsy will demonstrate the presence of lobular panniculitis surrounding a central muscular vessel that is disrupted by a lymphocytic, neutrophilic, or granulomatous infiltrate. Accompanying this vasculitis are varying degrees of coagulative and caseous necrosis and granulomatous inflammation destroying the subcutis. In contrast, lesions of CPAN do not exhibit inflammation that extends past the adventitia of the artery to produce panniculitis. Polymerase chain reaction (PCR) studies have shown DNA fragments of mycobacteria in the lesions in those cases associated with mycobacterium tuberculosis.

ANCA-POSITIVE PRIMARY SYSTEMIC VASCULITIS

GRANULOMATOSIS WITH POLYANGIITIS, EOSINOPHILIC GRANULOMATOSIS WITH POLYANGIITIS, AND MICROSCOPIC POLYANGIITIS

Approximately 5% of all patients presenting with cutaneous vasculitis have PSV, less than 3% of which will affect predominantly small vessels of the skin and represent GPA, EGPA, or MPA. Histopathologically, small vessel neutrophilic vasculitis is the most prominent feature of the PSV. It can manifest as palpable purpura, pulmonary hemorrhage, mononeuritis, or glomerulonephritis of varying severity. ANCA, pANCA, or cANCA is identified in most cases, the level of which may vary with disease severity or activity and, in the case of cANCA, can predict relapse. However, in half of cases of GPA, cANCA levels may remain persistent despite adequate clinical response. ANCA-associated vasculitis can affect individuals of all ages, but mostly older adults in their 50s and 60s. Detection of serum cANCA, which is highly specific for PR-3, in a patient with active disease has a high sensitivity (≤80%) and high specificity (≤100%) for the diagnosis of GPA; in contrast, pANCA has less specificity for ANCA-associated vasculitis. The combined use of indirect immunofluorescence and antigen-specific assays for PR-3 and MPO increases the specificity and sensitivity for the diagnosis of ANCA-associated vasculitis in patients with a high pretest probability of vasculitis. By histopathologic and clinical criteria, palisaded and neutrophilic granulomatous dermatitis (also known as extravascular necrotizing [neutrophilic or "blue"] granulomatous inflammation) without asthma is more commonly identified in GPA compared to MPA and EGPA. Asthma, serologic and tissue eosinophilia, and eosinophilic-rich "red" necrotizing granulomas distinguish EGPA from GPA and MPA. MPA is differentiated from EGPA and GPA by the absence of granulomas, eosinophilia, and asthma. One-third to half of patients presenting with palisaded and neutrophilic granulomatous dermatitis have coexisting PSV; small vessel neutrophilic vasculitis is often found in the same sample, implicating a relationship between vasculitis and granulomatous inflammation. Rapid recognition of ANCA-associated PSV is critically important because life-threatening injury to multiple organs can develop quickly and is dramatically mitigated by immunosuppressive therapy.

GRANULOMATOSIS WITH POLYANGIITIS

GPA was previously known as Wegener's granulomatosis (pathergic granulomatosis).

Clinical Findings

GPA is defined as vasculitis with granulomatosis inflammation, and it has a predilection to affect the upper and lower respiratory tracts with necrotizing granulomatous inflammation and kidneys as glomerulonephritis. The disease is not evenly distributed among geographic areas, time intervals, or ethnic populations. Granulomatous lesions can affect any organ in the body, and generalized vasculitis occurs in a wide variety of sites, particularly the lungs. Fewer than 15% of patients with GPA present with cutaneous disease; however, 10% to 40% develop cutaneous disease during the course of the disease. Three categories of cutaneous disease exist in GPA: (1) palpable or nonpalpable purpura caused by small vessel neutrophilic vasculitis; (2) subcutaneous nodules, ulcers, and digital infarcts (gangrene) secondary to medium vessel vasculitis; and (3) polymorphic lesions consisting of rheumatoid papules (papules and nodules [necrotic over extensor surfaces, often the elbows]), PG-like ulcers (also known as malignant pyoderma) (Fig. 4.15), and gingival hyperplasia (strawberry gingivitis). Proposed criteria for the diagnosis of GPA include biopsy or surrogate marker (infiltrates or cavities) for granulomatous inflammation of the respiratory tract, biopsy-verified necrotizing vasculitis in small- to medium-sized vessels or biopsy or surrogate marker for glomerulonephritis or proteinuria and hematuria, or positive cANCA. Approximately 80% of patients with GPA are positive for cANCA. Patients with GPA should not have eosinophilia in blood and biopsy samples. Left untreated, GPA has a 1-year mortality rate of greater than 80%, and 75% undergo remission with a regimen of cyclophosphamide and glucocorticoids. Relapse, the most important clinical problem, occurs in up to 50% of patients by 5 years of follow-up.

Histopathologic Findings

On biopsy, three histopathologic patterns of inflammation can be found in cutaneous lesions of GPA, either alone (mostly) or together: (1) geographic ("pathergic") necrosis; (2) granulomatous extravascular inflammation (Fig. 4.16); and (3) neutrophilic, predominantly SVV and less commonly muscular vessel vasculitis. Up to 50% of cutaneous lesions show small vessel neutrophilic vasculitis. Authentic granulomatous vasculitis is exceptional and, if present, affects muscular vessels.

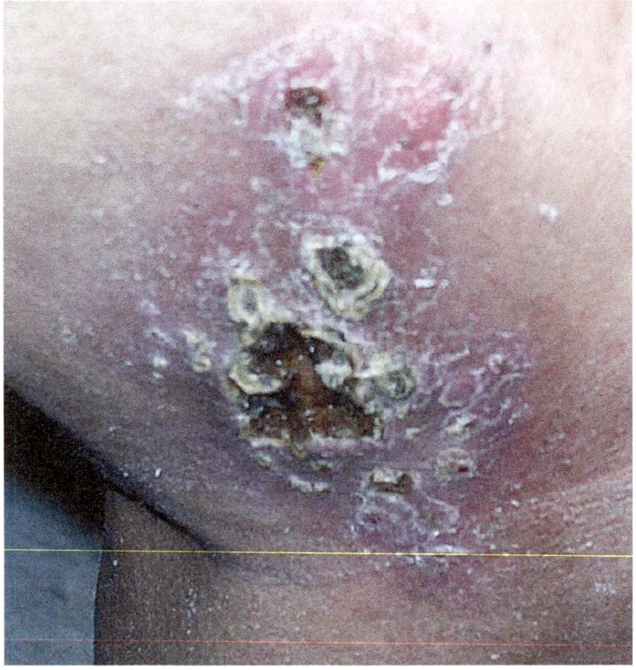

FIG. 4.15

Pyoderma gangrenosum–like ulcer over the medial aspect of knee in a patient with granulomatosis with polyangiitis.

EOSINOPHILIC GRANULOMATOSIS WITH POLYANGIITIS

Eosinophilic GPA was previously known as Churg-Strauss syndrome (allergic granulomatosis with asthma).

Clinical Findings

Eosinophilic GPA is characterized by the presence of asthma, usually of adult onset, and other allergic symptoms (allergic rhinitis), peripheral and tissue eosinophilia, and systemic vasculitis. Three phases have been described in EGPA. The first phase consists of persistent asthma and other atopic diatheses, the second phase starts with the onset and relapses of eosinophilia affecting one or more organs (e.g., eosinophilic pneumonia) and blood, and the third phase represents the development of systemic vasculitis. EGPA has been triggered by massive inhalation of particles, rapid steroid tapering, desensitization, or exposure to drugs such as leukotriene receptor antagonists. Compared with GPA, patients with EGPA have less frequent renal disease (<40%) and more

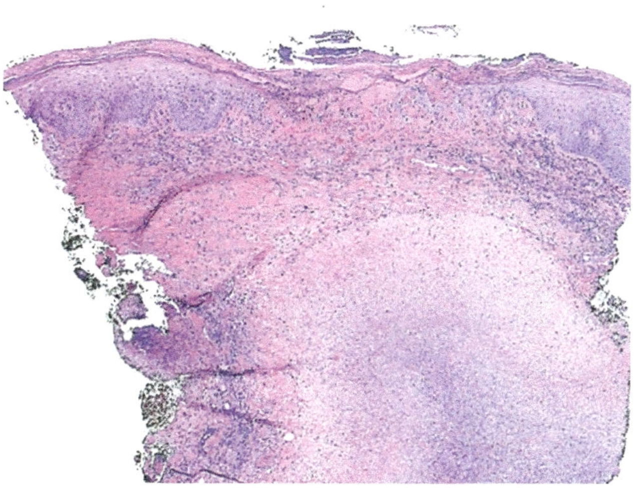

FIG. 4.16

Biopsy of pyoderma gangrenosum–like lesion showing palisaded and neutrophilic granulomatous dermatitis, "blue granuloma," in a patient with granulomatosis with polyangiitis.

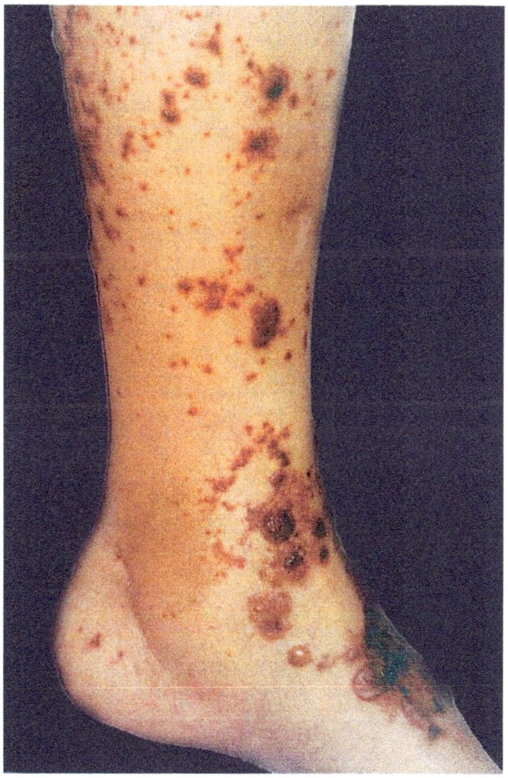

FIG. 4.17

Hemorrhagic vesicles with necrosis affecting the lower extremities in a patient with eosinophilic granulomatosis with polyangiitis.

frequent cutaneous (<80%), peripheral nerve (≤80%), and cardiac disease (≤50%). The skin manifestations of EGPA include palpable purpura, petechiae, ecchymoses, and hemorrhagic bullae (≤50%) (Fig. 4.17); dermal and subcutaneous papules and nodules often located on the scalp or symmetrically distributed over the extremities (elbows) (~30%); and urticaria or erythematous macules (≤25%) and livedo reticularis.

Histopathologic Findings

Cutaneous biopsy reveals three broad categories of changes, which can frequently be identified together: (1) vasculitis, mostly small vessel eosinophil-rich neutrophilic vasculitis affecting superficial and mid-dermal vessels and eosinophilic-rich neutrophilic muscular vessel vasculitis; (2) dermal eosinophilia; and (3) palisading neutrophilic and granulomatous dermatitis with abundant eosinophils and eosinophilic granules and debris coating degenerated collagen bundles ("red" granulomas) (Fig. 4.18).

MICROSCOPIC POLYANGIITIS

MPA is also known as microscopic polyarteritis or renal-dermal vasculitis syndrome.

Clinical Findings

MPA is defined as systemic neutrophilic SVV without extravascular granulomas or asthma. It is commonly associated with rapidly progressive renal disease (focal segmental necrotizing glomerulonephritis), skin involvement, and antibodies to pANCA (mostly MPO) (≤80%). The skin lesions found in MPA include palpable purpura and petechiae in more than three-quarters of patients, and in the remainder, splinter hemorrhages, nodules, palmar erythema, or livedo. The criteria for diagnosis of MPA are the findings of lack of biopsy or surrogate markers of granulomatous inflammation (e.g.,

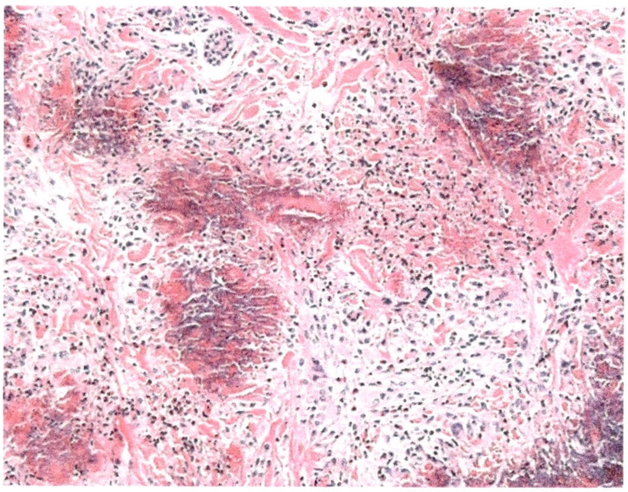

FIG. 4.18

Eosinophilic-rich debris forming the degenerated centers of "red" palisaded and neutrophilic granulomatous dermatitis found in papular and nodular lesions in patients with eosinophilic granulomatosis with polyangiitis.

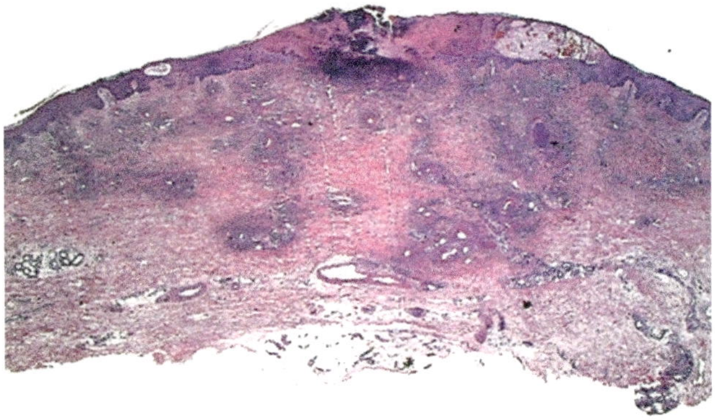

FIG. 4.19
Ulceration caused by extensive small vessel neutrophilic vasculitis in a patient with microscopic polyangiitis.

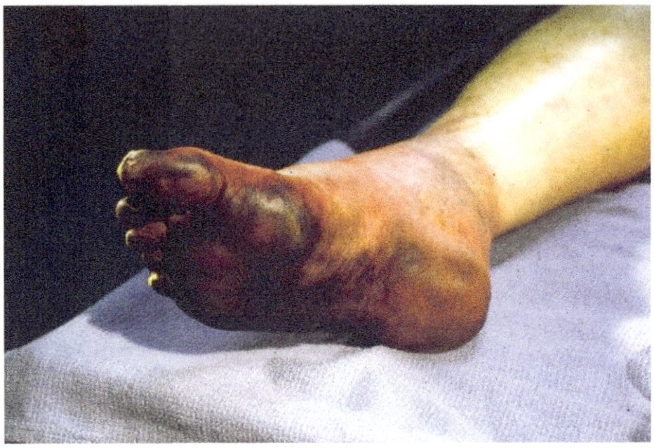

FIG. 4.20
Acral gangrene caused by cutaneous polyarteritis nodosa.

lung cavities or infiltrates of >1 month's duration), biopsy confirmation of neutrophilic SVV or glomerulonephritis with few or no immune deposits, and involvement of more than one organ system documented by biopsy or surrogate marker such as proteinuria and hematuria for glomerulonephritis.

Histopathologic Findings

Skin biopsy shows a small vessel neutrophilic vasculitis (Fig. 4.19). There are no distinct disease-specific findings.

VASCULITIDES AFFECTING PREDOMINANTLY MEDIUM-SIZED VESSELS

CUTANEOUS POLYARTERITIS NODOSA

CPAN is also known as cutaneous periarteritis nodosa or localized PAN.

Clinical Findings

Fewer than 3% of all patients presenting with cutaneous vasculitis have PAN (cutaneous or systemic with skin involvement). CPAN equally affects men and women of all ages, with a predominance between 40 and 60 years old. CPAN should be suspected in patients presenting with nodules, livedo, acral gangrene, or neuropathy. Typical skin manifestations of CPAN include painful 0.5- to 2-cm (lower much more frequently than upper extremity) nodules associated with livedo reticularis, ulcers, and rarely gangrene and digital necrosis. Of note, atrophie blanche (livedo vasculopathy) can be a manifestation of CPAN in patients who have no evidence of venous insufficiency and thrombophilia, and signs of mononeuritis multiplex. Exclusion of systemic disease is pertinent. A urinalysis with 24-hour urine protein and consideration of a renal angiogram to evaluate for stenoses/aneurysms may be warranted to evaluate for renal disease. CPAN follows a benign course in most patients. Patients with ulcers have more prolonged courses and associated neuropathy, and rare reports exist of patients who have progressed to systemic PAN after more than 15 years of follow-up. In some cases of CPAN, infectious causes can be found such as streptococcal infection or infectious hepatitis caused by hepatitis B virus. The severity of CPAN can be classified into three groups: class I, mild disease (nodular skin lesions, livedo reticularis, or mild polyneuropathy); class II, severe disease (prominent livedo; ulcers; pain; polyneuropathy; and constitutional symptoms of fever, malaise, and arthralgias); and class III, progressive systemic disease (necrotizing livedo, acral gangrene [Fig. 4.20], foot drop, progressive musculoskeletal involvement, positive autoimmune test results, and eventual visceral involvement).

Histopathologic Findings

Deep punch or excisional or incisional biopsy of the fascia will demonstrate neutrophilic muscular vessel vasculitis, which is located either at the dermal-subcutis junction where arteries bifurcate or within the subcutis. Repeated and deep biopsies accompanied by serial sections may be necessary to demonstrate the vasculitis because vessel involvement is segmental and focal. Older, advanced lesions exhibit vessel wall fibrosis, loss of the internal elastic lamina, and neovascularization of the adventitia (Fig. 4.21). In some patients, a lymphocytic infiltrate may be noted involving the medium vessels instead. These patients often present clinically with thinner papules/plaques or macules. The term macular lymphocytic arteritis or lymphocytic thrombophilic

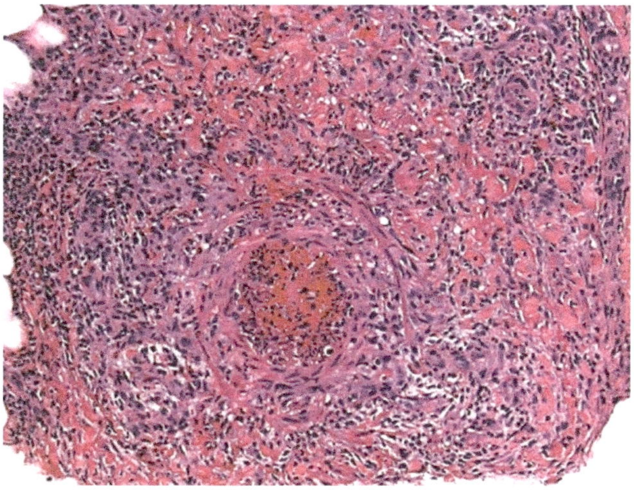

FIG. 4.21
Neovascularization of the adventitia associated with a thrombosed muscular artery lumen caused by cutaneous polyarteritis nodosa.

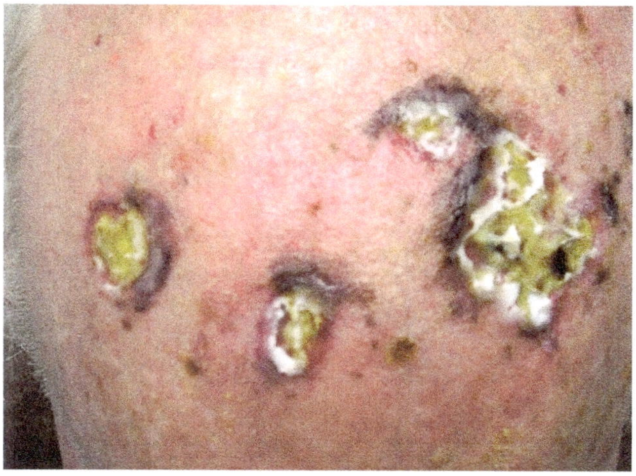

FIG. 4.22
Scalp ulceration secondary to giant cell arteritis

arteritis has been proposed for this presentation, which is likely a late-stage variant of CPAN.

VASCULITIDES AFFECTING PREDOMINANTLY LARGER VESSELS

GIANT CELL ARTERITIS

GCA is also called temporal arteritis. The superficial temporal artery runs in the temporoparietal fascia. It gives rise to smaller vessels that feed the skin, but GCA rarely involves the skin.

Clinical Findings

Occasionally, GCA will present with cutaneous disease (<1% of all cases). GCA is characterized by marked fair-skinned white female predominance, restriction to old age, and association with polymyalgia rheumatica. The clinical manifestations of GCA are attributable to ischemia secondary to endarteritis obliterans or exuberant systemic systems of malaise, weight loss, and fever caused by the release of inflammatory cytokines. Elevated CRP and/or ESR are often seen in GCA. The signs and symptoms of GCA include headache, jaw claudication, and visual and neurologic disturbances. The cutaneous signs consist of scalp tenderness, scalp blanching, decreased or loss of temporal artery pulses, or temporal artery thickening (cordlike). GCA can be complicated by scalp necrosis (Fig. 4.22), visual loss, gangrene of the tongue, and nasal septum necrosis. Less commonly, cutaneous nodules, ulcerations, and granuloma annulare-like eruptions distant from the head and neck region have been described. Accurate and timely diagnosis is important because serious morbidity, even death, may occur if proper treatment is delayed.

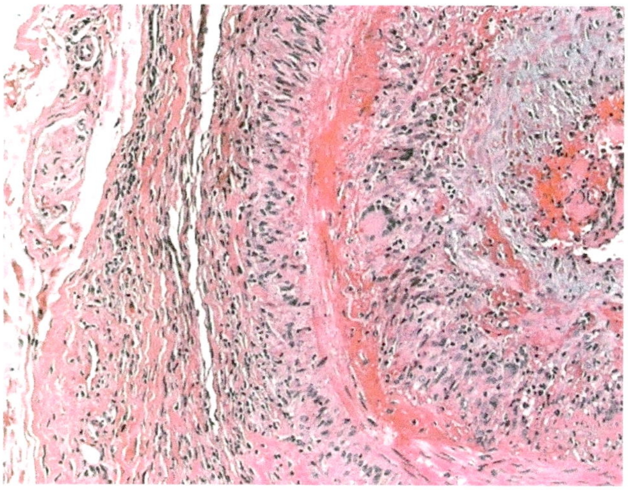

FIG. 4.23
Granulomatous muscular vessel vasculitis diagnostic of giant cell arteritis.

Histopathologic Findings

Skin biopsies that include muscular vessels of the subcutis or temporal artery biopsies demonstrate granulomatous muscular vessel vasculitis with giant cell–containing inflammatory infiltrate; the essential diagnostic features of GCA are segmental inflammation and disruption of temporal artery media and intima with fragmentation of the internal elastic lamina (Fig. 4.23). Late lesions exhibit segmental loss of the elastic lamina and a stenotic lumen secondary to replacement of the arterial wall and lumen by myointimal hyperplasia, myxomatous stroma, and scattered inflammatory cells.

OTHER MISCELLANEOUS VASCULITIDES

DRUG-INDUCED VASCULITIS

Clinical Findings

Approximately 20% of cases of cutaneous vasculitis represent an adverse drug eruption, and most will represent so-called hypersensitivity vasculitis (CLA) and exhibit a superficial dermal small vessel neutrophilic vasculitis (Fig. 4.2). Therapeutic agents from virtually every pharmacologic class have been implicated in the development of drug-induced vasculitis. The drugs most frequently associated with vasculitis are propylthiouracil, hydralazine, colony-stimulating factors, allopurinol, cefaclor, minocycline, d-penicillamine, phenytoin, isotretinoin, and methotrexate.

Manifestations of drug-induced vasculitis range from CLA to small vessel lymphocytic vasculitis to distinct vasculitic syndromes such as GPA, MPA, EGPA, and PAN. Patients may also present with concurrent drug-induced lupus erythematosus. Affected individuals may present with cutaneous involvement alone or life-threatening systemic involvement, which may result in severe and sometimes fatal illness. There are no significant differences in clinical presentation, serologic abnormalities, and pathologic findings compared with idiopathic vasculitides. However, in patients taking hydralazine, antibodies to ANA, dsDNA, histone, and pANCA may be observed. The interval between the first exposure and the appearance of symptoms for drug-induced vasculitis can be extremely variable (i.e., hours to years), with the vasculitis commencing after drug dosage increases and after rechallenge. Death has occurred in 10% of all published cases of drug-induced vasculitis, predominantly in patients with multiple organ involvement. Identifying the offending drug is the most important aspect of treatment because its discontinuation is followed by a rapid improvement of the vasculitis in many cases. Tissue eosinophilia is a histologic clue to a drug etiology.

One of the interestingly recognized agents inducing vasculitis is levamisole. Levamisole was originally introduced as an anthelmintic agent and later used in Behçet disease for immunosuppression, but because of its side effects, it has been withdrawn. More recently, levamisole has been added to cocaine to potentiate the stimulant effects. Affected patients had constitutional symptoms, arthralgia, leukopenia, agranulocytosis, and cutaneous vasculitis with purpuric lesions of the ears, nose, cheeks, and extremities. The lesions have bright red borders with central necrosis (Fig. 4.24). Despite the severe and dramatic clinical appearance of these lesions, they usually resolve spontaneously within a few weeks of drug discontinuation but can recur with subsequent contaminated cocaine misuse. pANCA is more common than cANCA in levamisole-associated vasculitis, and antihuman neutrophil elastase antibodies have been identified in affected patients.

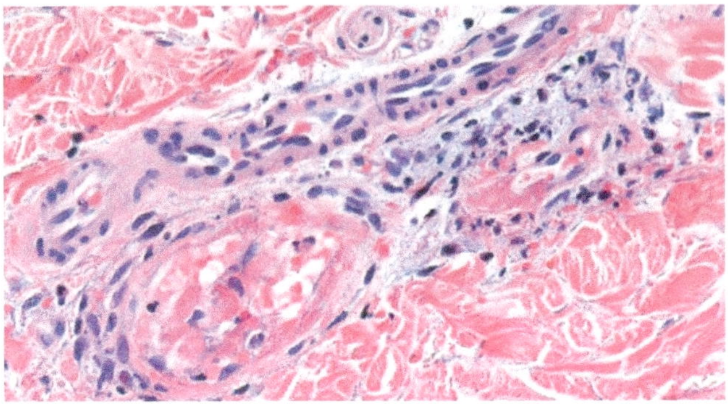

FIG. 4.24
Levamisole-induced vasculitis shows histologic signs of a vasoocclusive disorder and vasculitis.

Histopathologic Findings

Typically, H&E sections reveal LCV with variable degrees of vascular damage. It is often mild but may be severe with fibrinoid necrosis of vessel walls. Tissue eosinophilia is common and is a helpful clue. Drug-induced vasculitis may on occasion show features of a lymphocytic or granulomatous vasculitis with a predominant infiltrate of lymphocytes or histiocytes, respectively. A histologic clue to a drug reaction may be the presence of an additional inflammatory reaction pattern (e.g., spongiotic or interface dermatitis coexisting with vasculitis). In levamisole-associated vasculitis, vasoocclusion may also be observed, and patients with lupus anticoagulant antibodies have been reported.

PARANEOPLASTIC (MALIGNANCY-INDUCED) VASCULITIS

Clinical Findings

Paraneoplastic (lymphoproliferative-, myeloproliferative-, or carcinoma-induced) vasculitis represents fewer than 5% of all cases of cutaneous vasculitis. Paraneoplastic vasculitis should be suspected in patients with cutaneous vasculitis who present with recurrent purpura, hematologic abnormalities (cytopenia, monoclonal gammopathy, or immature blood cells), abnormal masses on imaging studies, hematuria, or failure to respond to corticosteroids. Malignancy-associated vasculitic syndromes can be grouped into three broad clinical categories: vasculitis-associated malignancies (true paraneoplastic vasculitic syndromes in which the vasculitis improves with extirpation or treatment of the tumor), vasculitis masquerading as malignancies (e.g., GPA with lung mass), and malignancies masquerading as vasculitides (e.g., emboli from an atrial myxoma, superficial migratory thrombophlebitis in pancreatic cancer). Most paraneoplastic cutaneous vasculitic syndromes are the result of a paraproteinemia secondary to lymphoproliferative disorders, typically cryoglobulins caused by lymphocytic lymphoma or Waldenström's macroglobulinemia. Perivascular IgA deposition may be noted in patients with an IgA monoclonal gammopathy.

CHRONIC LOCALIZED FIBROSING LEUKOCYTOCLASTIC VASCULITIS

Clinical Findings

Chronic localized fibrosing LCV is found in granuloma faciale, EED, IgG4-related disease, and some cutaneous inflammatory pseudotumors. Granuloma faciale is characterized by asymptomatic, slowly enlarging reddish-brown papules or plaques on the face of middle-aged adults, one-third of whom will have multiple facial site involvement; fewer than 10% will have extrafacial lesions (Fig. 4.25). EED is clinically denoted by symmetric, purple-red soft papules that evolve into firm, brown-yellow papules, plaques, or nodules located over extensor surfaces of extremities. EED occurs in systemically ill patients with CTD, infection, acquired immune deficiency, and hematologic abnormalities. IgA gammopathy is often present. IgG4-related disease most commonly presents on the head and neck with papules, plaques, and nodules with macules and bullae not typically being noted. Cutaneous inflammatory pseudotumors present as a solitary cutaneous nodule, which exhibits the histologic features that mimic either EED or granuloma faciale. The pathogenesis of these disorders is believed to be attributable to either systemic or local immune complexes producing recurrent vessel damage to the small, easily injured vessels of fibrosing granulation tissue.

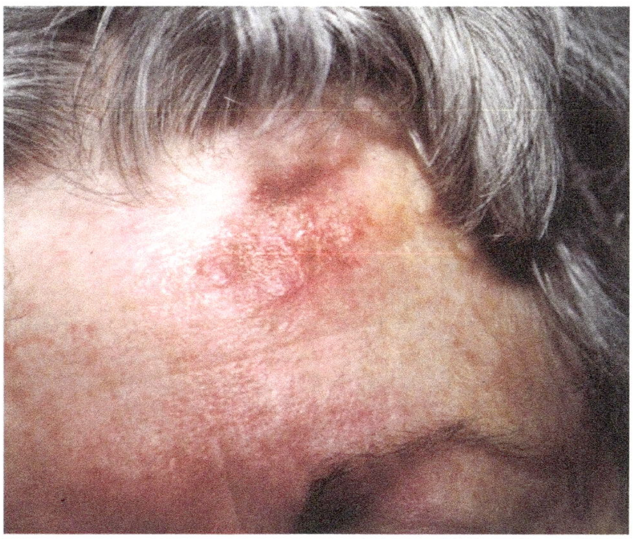

FIG. 4.25

Reddish-brown forehead plaque caused by granuloma faciale.

Histopathologic Findings

All of these disorders are characterized by small vessel neutrophilic vasculitis; patterned fibrosis; and dense nodular mixed, neutrophilic-rich inflammatory infiltrates (plasma cells, macrophages, lymphocytes, and granulocytes). Vasculitis is subtle in most cases with focal regions of nuclear dust or fibrin surrounding and within vessels; however, fibrosis is progressive, and mature lesions show granulation tissue with vertically oriented capillaries and horizontally arrayed collagen bundles and fibroblasts (lamellar fibrosis). In late lesions, lamellar, storiform, or angiocentric fibrosis is admixed with scattered macrophages with foamy or hemosiderin-laden cytoplasm (Fig. 4.4). Granuloma faciale has numerous eosinophils in its polymorphous infiltrate separated from the epidermis and adnexae by a grenz (clear) zone, but EED lacks a grenz zone and is predominantly neutrophilic. Proposed histopathologic diagnostic criteria for IgG4-related disease include a marked lymphoplasmacytic infiltrate, fibrosis (often with perivascular accentuation), and infiltration of IgG4+ plasma cells where the ratio of IgG4+ to IgG+ cells is greater than40%, and greater than 10 IgG4+ plasma cells/high-power field.

Ancillary Studies

DIF examination is variable and can show vascular and/or basement membrane zone complement and immunoglobulin deposits.

PSEUDOVASCULITIS

Because the clinical manifestations of vasculitis are protean and diagnosis is based on a constellation of clinical, histologic, imaging, and laboratory features, it is not surprising that nonvasculitis disorders can mimic vasculitis. Cutaneous pseudovasculitis represents a heterogeneous collection of disorders that are capable of simulating cutaneous vasculitis and can be broadly classified into diseases that produce hemorrhage, petechiae, purpura, and ecchymoses (Fig. 4.26) or vessel occlusion

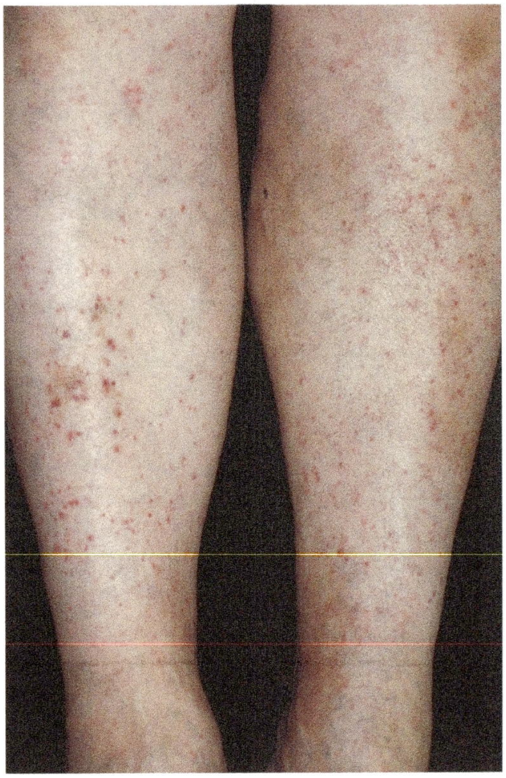

FIG. 4.26

Purpuric drug eruption caused by allopurinol. (Courtesy of Dr. Ko Ron Chen, Tokyo, Japan.)

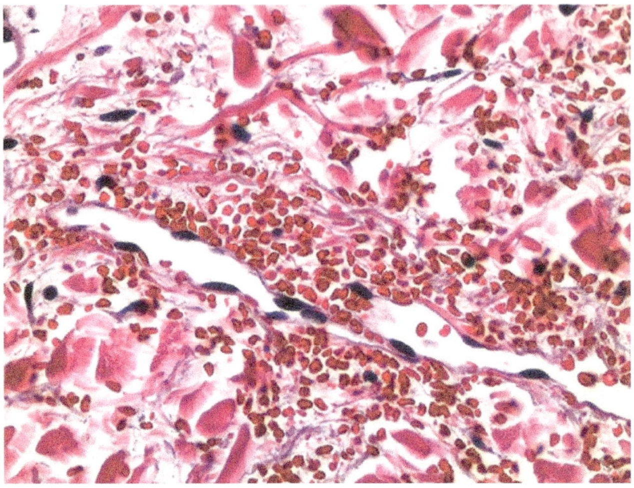

FIG. 4.27

Nonvasculitic inflammatory purpura: extravasation of red blood cells without evidence of vasculitis.

with resultant livedo, cyanosis, ulcers, digital necrosis, or gangrene. Overlap is common, but if present, one mechanism dominates. Hemorrhagic pseudovasculitis is caused by vessel wall dysfunction (incompetence), which can be related to diverse factors that include vessel wall deposition of metabolic substances (amyloid, calcium), nutritional deficiencies (scurvy), nonvasculitic inflammatory purpura (pigmented purpuric dermatitis; arthropod, viral, and drug reactions [Fig. 4.27 and Table 4.8]), degeneration of the vessel wall and supporting stroma (senile or solar purpura), direct vessel wall invasion of infective organisms, coagulation-fibrinolytic disorders (e.g., thrombocytopenia), and vessel wall trauma. Cyanotic-infarctive pseudovasculitis is caused by vasoocclusion by emboli, thrombi, or fibrointimal hyperplasia (endarteritis obliterans) and includes varied conditions such as purpura fulminans, Coumadin necrosis (Figs. 4.28 and 4.29), antiphospholipid antibody syndrome, cardiac myxoma, cholesterol embolization (Fig. 4.30), calciphylaxis, and radiation arteritis. Table 4.9 lists common, uncommon, and rare pseudovasculitic

TABLE 4.8

Pigmented Purpuric Dermatitis

Clinical Variants	Characteristic Features
Purpura annularis telangiectodes of Majocchi	Prominent telangiectasia
PPD of Schamberg	Prominent hemosiderotic pigmentation
PPD of Gougerot and Blum	Erythematous papules
Eczematoid-like PPD of Doucas and Kapetanakis	Eczematous and lichenified features
Lichen aureus	Localized lesion, usually on lower leg

Spectrum of clinical findings characterized by discrete purpuric puncta associated with histologic features of chronic lymphocytic infiltrates and superficial dermal hemorrhage

Differential Diagnosis of PPD:

- Stasis
- Drug reaction
- Bite reaction
- Solar purpura
- Mycosis fungoides

PPD, Progressive pigmentary dermatosis.

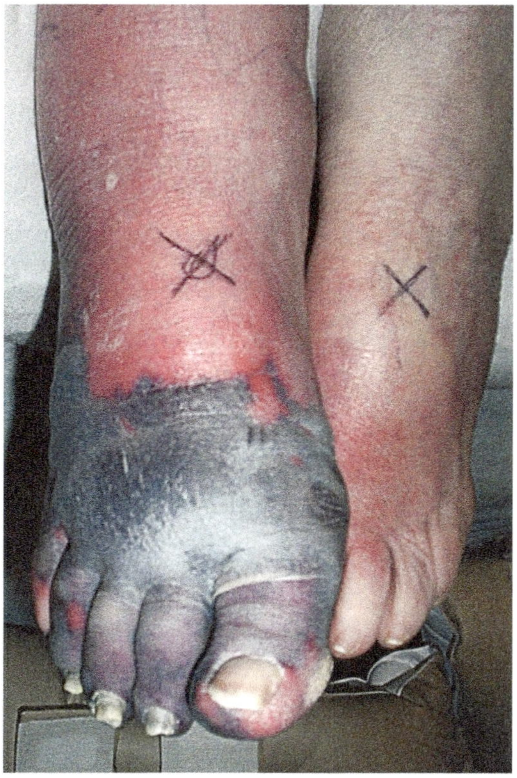

FIG. 4.28

Purpuric necrosis of feet in a patient with Coumadin (warfarin) necrosis.

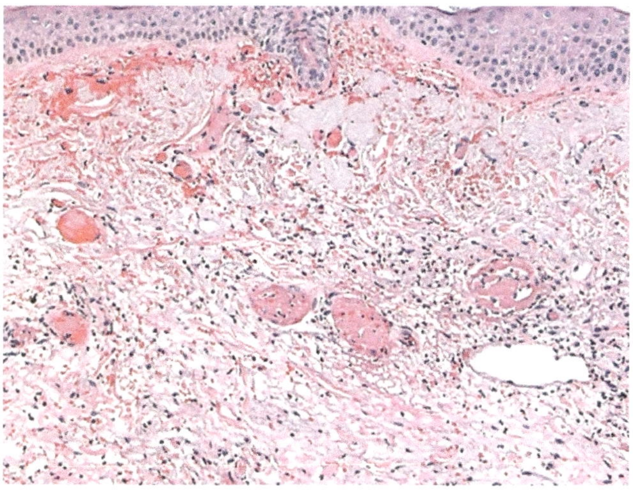

FIG. 4.29

Widespread noninflammatory small vessel thrombi characterize coagulation disorders such as Coumadin necrosis, disseminated intravascular coagulation, and purpura fulminans.

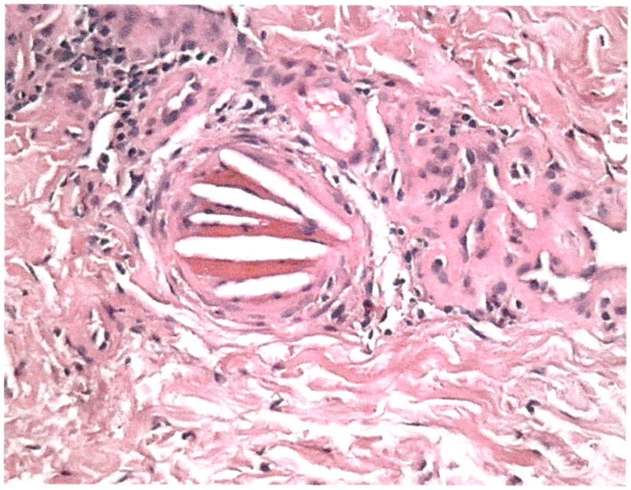

FIG. 4.30

Cholesterol emboli are identified by intravascular clefted spaces surrounded by multinucleated giant cells.

disorders. A delayed and inappropriate diagnosis of pseudovasculitis leads to incorrect management and exposure to potentially deleterious treatment modalities such as corticosteroids and cytotoxic agents. The diagnosis of a pseudovasculitic disorder requires a high index of suspicion and should always be part of the differential diagnosis of vasculitis. Skin biopsy is a crucial step in differentiating pseudovasculitis from authentic vasculitis; absence of histologic evidence of vasculitis, particularly after multiple biopsies, should direct evaluation and diagnosis toward a pseudovasculitis.

CUTANEOUS VASCULITIS—DISEASE FACT SHEET

Definition

- Inflammatory or immune-mediated destruction of dermal or subcutaneous vessels

Classification and Etiologic Associations

- Primary (idiopathic)
  - 40% CLA
  - 10% IgAV
  - <5% PSV (GPA, EGPA, GCA, MPA, and PAN)
- Secondary (known triggers, coexisting systemic disease)
  - 20% drugs
  - 20% infection
  - ~10% CTD vasculitis
  - <5% paraneoplastic vasculitis
  - Other systemic disorders (e.g., sarcoidosis, inflammatory bowel disease)
  - Cryoglobulinemic vasculitis
- Incidental (secondary to another pathologic process, e.g., trauma)

Incidence

- The annual incidence of biopsy-proven cutaneous vasculitis ranges from 39.6 per million to 59.8 per million.

Morbidity and Mortality

- Extracutaneous disease: <20%
- Chronic, debilitating disease: ~20%
- Fatal disease: <7%

Gender, Race, and Age Distribution

- All ages, sexes, and races are affected
- Adults ≫ children, females ≥ males
- Age range, 1 to 90 years
  - Adults: mean age, 47 years
  - Children: mean age, 7 years

TABLE 4.9

Mimickers of Vasculitis (Pseudovasculitis)

Relative Frequency	Pseudovasculitic Disorder	Mechanism
Common	Antiphospholipid antibody syndrome	Thrombosis
	Cholesterol embolization	Embolus
	Infective endocarditis	Infection and embolus
	Pigmented purpuric dermatitis	Hemorrhage
	Solar purpura	Hemorrhage
	Purpura fulminans	Thrombosis
	Warfarin necrosis	Thrombosis
	Livedo vasculopathy	Thrombosis
Less frequent than vasculitis	Hypothenar hammer syndrome (fibromuscular dysplasia)	Vascular trauma
	Scurvy	Hemorrhage
	Thrombotic thrombocytopenic purpura	Thrombosis
Rare	Amyloidosis	Vessel wall pathology
	Calciphylaxis	Vessel wall pathology
	Cardiac myxoma	Embolus
	Ergotamine and cocaine misuse	Vasospasm
	Angiotropic B-cell lymphoma	Intravascular proliferation/embolus

Signs Indicating the Possibility of Pseudovasculitis:

- Atherosclerosis, significant disease
- Nonconfirmatory biopsies for vasculitis
- Cardiac murmur
- Livedo reticularis
- Absence of inflammatory markers (e.g., normal ESR)
- Abnormal eating habits or chronic alcoholism
- Isolated vascular lesions on imaging studies

ESR, Erythrocyte sedimentation rate.
Adapted from Grau, R. 2002. Pseudovasculitis: mechanisms of vascular injury and clinical spectrum. Current Rheumatology Reports, 4(1), 83–89.

Clinical Findings

- In most patients, vasculitis occurs 7 to 10 days after exposure to a trigger such as a drug or infection, though review of medications over the last year is important
- In patients with vasculitis secondary to systemic disease, vasculitis develops after a mean interval of 6 months (range, days to years from the commencement of underlying disease)
- Duration of vasculitis depends on etiology; mean time, 28 months; median, 4 months; range, 1 week to >20 years
- Sites affected by vasculitis
  - Lower extremities, dependent areas, and regions covered by tight-fitting clothes (e.g., socks, collar) most frequently affected
  - Lower extremities ≫ upper extremities > trunk > head and neck
- Diverse morphology of vasculitic lesions, purpuric macules, and papules most common (see Cutaneous Vasculitis—Pathologic Features)

Radiologic Features

- Aneurysms or stenoses found in polyarteritis nodosa by arteriography
- Wall thickening, stenosis, and occlusion detected by duplex ultrasonography in GCA (temporal arteritis)

Prognosis

- Benign eruption in most patients (~60%) who will experience a single acute, self-limited episode of vasculitis that resolves in several weeks
- Minority (~20%) will have relapsing skin disease with symptom-free periods
- Fewer than 20% will develop chronic, unremitting skin and visceral disease that leads to death in about 5%

Treatment

- Empiric; tailor treatment to disease severity and risk for permanent organ damage
  - General care for all patients consists of avoidance of excessive standing, cold exposure, and tight-fitting clothing; rest; leg elevation; and antihistamines or NSAIDs for symptomatic relief
  - Mild skin disease: topical steroids, dapsone or colchicine (or both)
  - Moderate to severe skin disease: methotrexate, azathioprine, or prednisone
  - Systemic vasculitis: prednisone +/− cyclophosphamide, azathioprine, cyclosporine, mycophenolate mofetil, infliximab, or rituximab

CLA, Cutaneous leukocytoclastic angiitis; *CTD*, connective tissue disease; *EGPA*, eosinophilic granulomatosis with polyangiitis; *GCA*, giant cell arteritis; *GPA*, granulomatosis with polyangiitis; *IgAV*, IgA vasculitis; *MPA*, microscopic polyangiitis; *NSAID*, nonsteroidal antiinflammatory drug; *PAN*, polyarteritis nodosa; *PSV*, primary systemic vasculitis.

CUTANEOUS VASCULITIS—PATHOLOGIC FEATURES

Clinical Findings

- Diverse clinical morphologies
  - Most common
- Erythematous and purpuric macules
- Palpable purpura
- Hemorrhagic vesicles and bullae
- Nodules, dermal and subcutaneous
  - Less common
- Pustules
- Urticaria and annular lesions
- Ulcers
- Livedo reticularis
  - Infrequent or rare
- Splinter hemorrhages and nail fold infarcts (Bywaters lesions)
- Infarcts
- Digital gangrene
- Pyoderma gangrenosum–like lesions
- Palmar or digital erythema

Microscopic Findings

- Cutaneous morphology correlates with vessel size and extent of vascular bed affected
- Destruction of vessel wall by inflammatory cells associated with fibrin deposits and nuclear debris (leukocytoclasis) in acute vasculitis lesions
- Loss of elastic lamina and fibrosis in healed vasculitis lesions
- Varying degrees of extravasation of red blood cells, necrosis of skin, and ulceration
- Coexisting histologic findings identified in some cases are associated with specific vasculitic syndromes
  - Storiform fibrosis
  - Palisaded neutrophilic granulomatous dermatitis
  - Intra- and subepidermal pustules
  - Tissue eosinophilia
  - Tissue neutrophilia

Direct Immunofluorescence Findings

- Vascular immunoreactants (C3, IgM, IgG, or IgA) in >80% in biopsies of lesions <48 hours; C3 is frequent in lesions >48 hours old

Differential Diagnosis

- Pseudovasculitis
  - Purpuric (nonvasculitic) disorders
  - Vasoocclusive disorders

ACKNOWLEDGMENT AND APPRECIATION

This chapter was initially contributed by Drs. Al-Rohil and J. Andrew Carlson. It would not have been completed without the tremendous work, effort, help and mentorship that Dr. J. Andrew Carlson has provided through the years.

SUGGESTED FURTHER READING

Carlson, J. A. (2010). The histological assessment of cutaneous vasculitis. *Histopathology*, *56*, 3–23.

Carlson, J. A., & Chen, K. R. (2007). Cutaneous vasculitis update: Neutrophilic muscular vessel and eosinophilic, granulomatous, and lymphocytic vasculitis syndromes. *American Journal of Dermatopathology*, *29*, 32–43.

Carlson, J. A., Ng, B. T., & Chen, K. R. (2005). Cutaneous vasculitis update: Diagnostic criteria, classification, epidemiology, etiology, pathogenesis, evaluation and prognosis. *American Journal of Dermatopathology*, *27*, 504–528.

Chen, K. R., & Carlson, J. A. (2008). Clinical approach to cutaneous vasculitis. *American Journal of Clinical Dermatology*, *9*, 71–92.

Marzano, A. V., Vezzoli, P., & Berti, E. (2013). Skin involvement in cutaneous and systemic vasculitis. *Autoimmunity Reviews*, *12*(4), 467–476.

Russell, J. P., & Gibson, L. E. (2006). Primary cutaneous small vessel vasculitis: Approach to diagnosis and treatment. *International Journal of Dermatology*, *45*, 3–13.

Sais, G., & Vidaller, A. (2012). Cutaneous vasculitis. *Actas Dermo-Sifiliograficas*, *103*(8), 754; author reply 5.

Sunderkötter, C. H., Zelger, B., Chen, K. R., Requena, L., Piette, W., Carlson, J. A., Dutz, J., Lamprecht, P., Mahr, A., Aberer, E., Werth, V. P., Wetter, D. A., Kawana, S., Luqmani, R., Frances, C., Jorizzo, J., Watts, J. R., Metze, D., Caproni, M., Alpsoy, E., ... Jennette, J. C. (2018). Nomenclature of cutaneous vasculitis: Dermatologic addendum to the 2012 revised International Chapel Hill Consensus Conference Nomenclature of Vasculitides. *Arthritis & Rheumatology (Hoboken, N.J.)*, *70*(2), 171–184.

5 Blistering Skin Diseases

Julia S. Lehman

A blister is a fluid-filled space within or beneath the epidermis. Blisters may occur as a secondary event caused by factors such as trauma (e.g., friction, heat), infection (e.g., viral, bacterial), ischemia (e.g., occlusive vasculopathy), or inflammation leading to disruption of the dermal-epidermal junction (e.g., fixed drug eruption) or as a primary event in which a genetic mutation or immunologic event affects the structural integrity of the basement membrane zone (BMZ) (e.g., epidermolysis bullosa [EB] or pemphigoid, respectively).

APPROACH TO THE DIAGNOSIS OF BLISTERING DISEASES

Clinical Findings

Clinical findings are very helpful for accurate diagnosis of blistering skin diseases. Factors to consider include age of onset (e.g., bullous pemphigoid [BP] tends to affect elderly adults, while epidermolysis bullosa acquisita [EBA] is more common in middle-aged individuals), location, and distribution of the blisters (e.g., involvement of mucosal tissues is typical for pemphigus vulgaris [PV] but uncommon in pemphigus foliaceus [PF]), gross blister characteristics (e.g., large flaccid blisters are typical of pemphigus, while tense inflammatory blisters are seen in pemphigoid), arrangement of blisters (e.g., grouped or herpetiform pattern in dermatitis herpetiformis [DH]; annular or "cluster of jewels" pattern in linear IgA bullous dermatosis [LABD]), associated inflammatory background (e.g., the blisters of BP typically arise on an erythematous base, but those of porphyria cutanea tarda [PCT] are usually present on noninflamed skin), medical history (e.g., connective tissue disease, diabetes, associated malignancy), and recent medications (e.g., vancomycin-associated LABD, immune checkpoint inhibitor- or gliptin-associated pemphigoid).

Histopathologic Features

Identifying the mechanism of tissue split (e.g., spongiosis [Fig. 5.1] versus acantholysis [Fig. 5.2]) and determination of the microanatomic plane of the blister cavity are the first steps in the microscopic analysis of a vesiculobullous disorder. Spongiosis reflects intraepidermal edema, leading to stretching and breaking of intercellular connections between keratinocytes. The desmosomal connections between cells often become easily visualized (see Fig. 5.3). Acantholysis is a manifestation of loss of cell–cell adhesion between keratinocytes. Intercellular bridges disappear and individual keratinocytes change their shape from polygonal to round or oval and develop a smooth outer surface (see Fig. 5.2).

HISTOPATHOLOGIC FEATURES AND MECHANISM OF BLISTER FORMATION

Histopathologic Feature	Mechanism of Blister Formation	Example
Spongiosis	Intercellular edema leads to cell separation	Acute allergic contact dermatitis
Ballooning degeneration	Intracellular edema leads to cell death and vesicle formation	Herpesvirus infection
Acantholysis	Loss of cell-to-cell contact between keratinocytes mediated by genetic mutations or antibody blockage of adhesion molecules of the desmosomes	Pemphigus
Cytolysis	Physical trauma leads to cell–cell disruption or death	Heat, friction
Lichenoid or vacuolar interface reaction	Apoptosis of basal cells from interface reaction	Fixed drug eruption; graft-versus-host disease; immunotherapy
Basement membrane zone destruction	Genetic structural defects or immunologic events affecting proteins of the hemi-desmosomes of the basement membrane zone	Epidermolysis bullosa, bullous pemphigoid
Dermolysis	Sub-basement membrane zone disruption caused by structural defects, edema, or immunologic events affecting the superficial dermis	Dystrophic epidermolysis bullosa, polymorphous light eruption

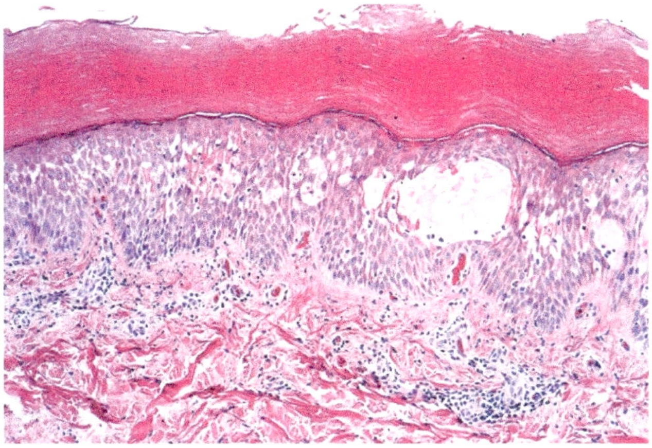

FIG. 5.1

Spongiotic blister. Edema separates keratinocytes, many of which are still connected to each other via intercellular bridges (desmosomes).

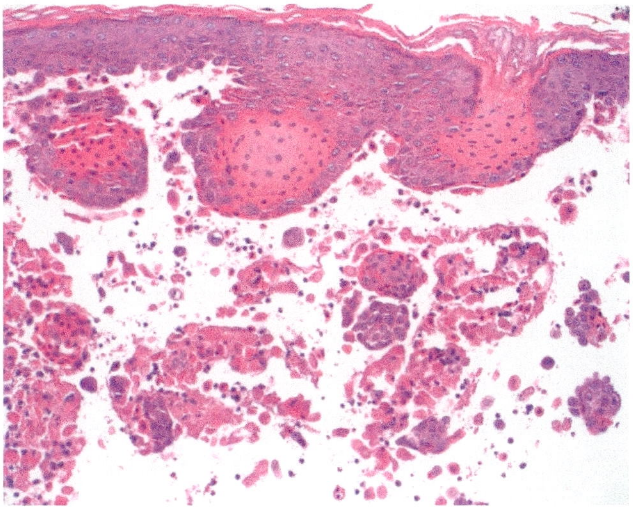

FIG. 5.2

Acantholytic blister. Loss of cell adhesion between keratinocytes has led to a change in their cell shape from polygonal to round or oval. Intercellular bridges are lost.

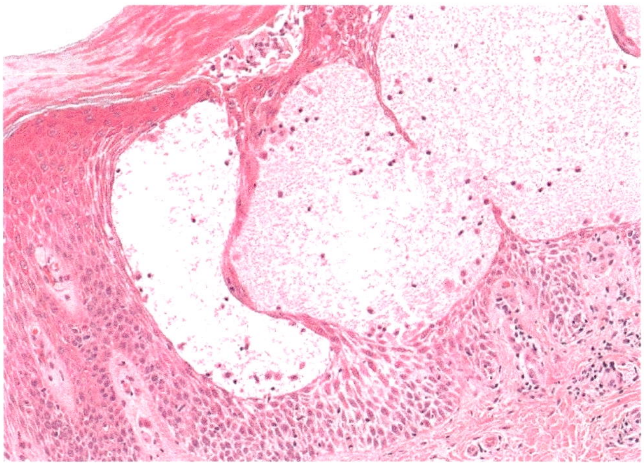

FIG. 5.3

Intraepidermal blister. Acute spongiotic dermatitis with multiple fluid-filled spaces within the epidermis.

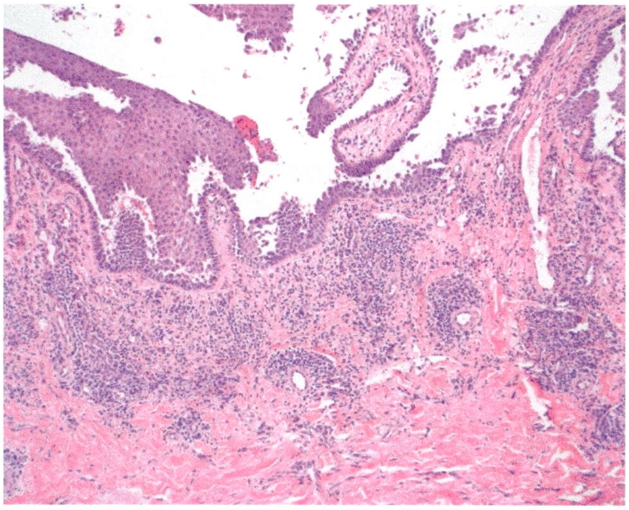

FIG. 5.4

Intraepidermal blister. Acantholytic subcorneal blister with split above the basilar layer.

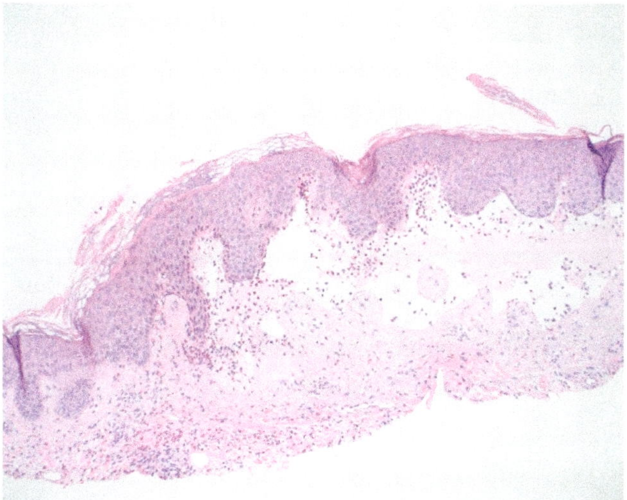

FIG. 5.5

Subepidermal blister. The epidermis has separated from the dermis, creating a blister cavity. The basal cell layer of the epidermis forms the bottom of the blister roof.

Regarding the microanatomic plane, blisters can be divided into intraepidermal (Figs. 5.3 and 5.4) and subepidermal (Fig. 5.5). However, one must be aware that blisters reepithelialize, and a biopsy of an older subepidermal blister may present with an intraepidermal split. Intraepidermal blisters can be further subclassified into subcorneal and suprabasilar. Assessment of an associated inflammatory infiltrate, if present, is also important because its composition (neutrophils, eosinophils, or both versus lymphocytes versus mast cells) and distribution pattern (papillary dermal abscesses versus diffuse bandlike) may provide useful clues to narrow the differential diagnosis. The detection of microorganisms or viral cytopathic changes may also provide specific evidence of the factors inciting blistering.

Ancillary Studies

Most autoimmune bullous dermatoses require direct immunofluorescence (DIF) for classification because the histopathology per se is often not specific. For the assessment of an immunobullous disorder by DIF, it is best to biopsy *perilesional* skin (i.e., adjacent to inflamed non-blistered skin). In biopsies that have compromised epidermis, evaluation of the follicular and eccrine epithelium for immunoglobulin deposition may contribute to the diagnostic sensitivity of DIF in bullous disorders with IgG or C3 linear or cell-surface immunoglobulin. For DIF, the biopsy specimen should be placed in a transport medium, such as Michel's medium, snap frozen in liquid nitrogen, or sent in saline-soaked gauze if delivery to the pathology laboratory performing DIF can be made within a few hours. There may be less background with nonfrozen saline–transported specimens. If a specimen is accidentally placed in formalin, there may be limited value in quickly removing it and putting it in Michel's medium. After 10 minutes of formalin exposure, skin biopsies of pemphigoid and DH can retain diagnostic DIF findings (longer for pemphigoid), but longer times in formalin will result in false-negative DIF or nonspecific nuclear staining simulating lupus. Pemphigus antibodies are degraded even after very transient exposure to formalin immersion.

Another testing method used to confirm a diagnosis of a bullous disorder of patients with circulating autoantibodies includes indirect immunofluorescence (IIF). With this technique, patient serum is incubated with various substrates including salt-split skin or primate esophagus and tagged with a fluorescent label. Salt-split skin substrate is generated by procuring normal mammalian skin and incubating it with 1 M NaCl. This procedure splits the BMZ at the level of the lamina lucida. Therefore, when patient autoantibodies localize to the epidermal side of the artifactual split, the pathogenic antibodies are directed against antigens above the lamina lucida, such as BP180, the immunologic target in BP. When patient antibodies localize to the dermal side, the pathogenic antibodies target antigens below the lamina lucida, such as collagen VII, the immunologic target in EBA or bullous lupus erythematosus. Rarely, there is a mixed epidermal and dermal pattern, which can occur in rare pemphigoid variants, such as laminin-332 pemphigoid, laminin γ1 pemphigoid, and others.

Correlation of histopathology and IF with the clinical presentation remains the gold standard for diagnosing autoimmune blistering disease. However, certain clinicopathologic features can be seen in multiple different disease entities. In these cases, additional laboratory testing may be required. For example, enzyme-linked immunosorbent assay (ELISA) is readily available for the detection of autoantibodies to the specific structural components of the hemi-desmosomes or desmosomes that are targeted in these disorders. In some patients, levels of antibody detected by ELISA correlate with disease activity and so can be helpful for disease activity monitoring. Immunoblotting and immunoprecipitation may offer more precise identification of autoantigens but are not widely available. Some of the main autoantigens that can be detected with these methods include BP180/COLXVII (BP, mucous membrane pemphigoid [MMP], pemphigoid gestationis [PG], LABD); BP230 (BP, PG, LABD); COLVII (EBA); laminin 332 (MMP); $\alpha6\beta4$ integrin (MMP); laminin γ1 chain (anti-p-200 pemphigoid); LAD-1 (LABD); desmoglein 1 (PV, PF, paraneoplastic pemphigus [PNP]); desmoglein 3 (PV, IgA pemphigus, PNP); desmocollin 1, 2, and 3 (IgA pemphigus); and tissue transglutaminase (DH).

INTRAEPITHELIAL BLISTERS

Characterizing the precise localization of the blister within the epithelium (corneal or subcorneal versus spinous cell layer versus within the spinous cell layer or immediately suprabasilar) helps to triage the differential diagnosis of intraepidermal blisters. Moreover, it is necessary to define the presence of acantholysis versus spongiosis or other features, such as dyskeratosis. Spongiotic disease processes (eczematous dermatitides) are described in more detail in Chapter 1 of this book but are briefly mentioned here. Understanding the clinical features, such as patient age, lesion morphology and anatomic distribution, and clinical course, helps to further refine the differential diagnosis.

DIFFERENTIAL DIAGNOSIS OF INTRAEPIDERMAL BLISTERS BY MICROANATOMIC LOCATION OF BLISTER

Corneal or Subcorneal Blister

- Miliaria crystallina
- Bullous impetigo
- Staphylococcal scalded skin syndrome
- Subcorneal pustular dermatosis
- Pustular psoriasis
- Acropustulosis of infancy
- Transient neonatal pustular melanosis
- Erythema toxicum neonatorum
- Acute generalized exanthematous pustulosis
- Pemphigus variants (especially pemphigus foliaceus, pemphigus erythematosus, and drug-induced pemphigus)

Spinous Cell Layer Blister

- Pemphigus variants
- Benign familial pemphigus (Hailey-Hailey disease)
- Keratosis follicularis (Darier disease)
- Transient acantholytic dyskeratosis (Grover disease)
- Spongiotic vesicles
- Viral (herpetic) dermatitis
- Friction
- Edema

Suprabasilar Blister
Pemphigus (especially pemphigus vulgaris and pemphigus vegetans)
Paraneoplastic pemphigus
Keratosis follicularis (Darier disease)
Benign familial pemphigus (Hailey-Hailey disease)
Transient acantholytic dyskeratosis (Grover disease)
Galli-Galli disease

INTRACORNEAL AND GRANULAR LAYER BLISTERS

MILIARIA

Miliaria reflects skin changes caused by blockage of the eccrine duct. The manifestations vary, depending on the level of blockage (intracorneal, intraepidermal, or intradermal).

Clinical Findings

Miliaria usually affects children, especially neonates but may also occur in adults. There is often a history of excessive perspiration and warm environments. Miliaria crystallina, which results from eccrine duct blockage within the stratum corneum, manifests as clear, small vesicles that tend to break easily, resulting in a collarette of scale. Miliaria rubra and miliaria profunda result from blockage of the acrosyringium (eccrine duct within the epidermis) in the mid to deep epidermis, respectively. Sweat leaks into the papillary dermis, leading to the development of small pruritic erythematous papules, often topped by microvesicles. This phenomenon typically occurs on the upper trunk and neck of children or adults. Intradermal blockage gives rise to inflamed pustules (miliaria pustulosa).

Histopathologic Features

Though rarely biopsied, the histopathologic features of miliaria crystallina include a noninflammatory subcorneal blister overlying the eccrine unit. Blockage of the duct lumen by keratinaceous debris may be observed. The ductal occlusive features in miliaria rubra are similar, but acrosyringeal spongiosis with inflammation is also observed. In well-developed lesions, there are subcorneal neutrophils and lymphocytes overlying the eccrine duct (Fig. 5.6). In miliaria pustulosa, there are more prominent subcorneal or intraepidermal microabscesses overlying the ductal unit.

Differential Diagnosis

The clinical presentation of miliaria is usually distinct, rarely requiring skin biopsy.

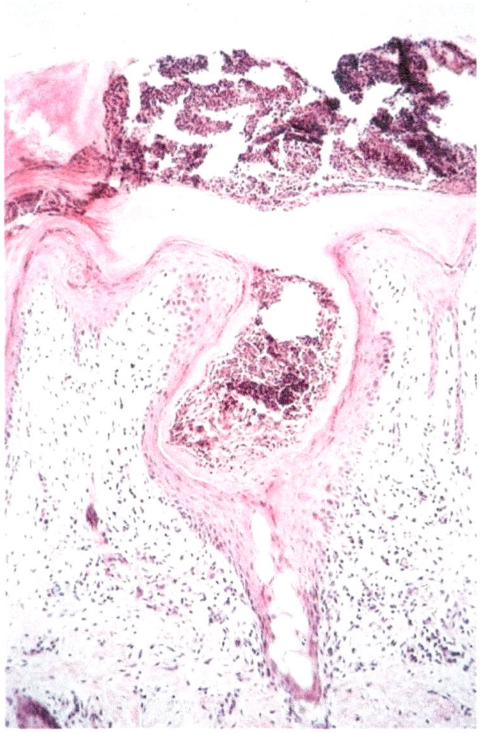

FIG. 5.6
Miliaria. Subcorneal pustule involving the ostium of the eccrine duct.

Prognosis and Treatment

Avoiding conditions that promote sweating (e.g., hot temperatures) facilitates resolution of the lesions. Lesions often resolve within a day of being in a cooler environment. Rarely, the anhidrosis associated with miliaria profunda can lead to heat exhaustion.

BULLOUS IMPETIGO

Clinical Findings

Bullous impetigo typically affects school-aged children and presents as vesicles containing cloudy yellow serous fluid. The blisters frequently break, resulting in superficial round erosions. The blister fluid dries as a honey-colored crust. Lesions tend to be distributed on exposed sites, such as the face (especially the perioral region) and upper extremities. Bullous impetigo is associated with a superficial infection by *Staphylococcus aureus* phage group 2, type 71, and its endotoxin cleaves desmoglein 1, an adhesion molecule in the desmosome and the target antigen in PF.

Histopathologic Features

Blisters may be subcorneal or intracorneal. Neutrophils are usually prominent, though early lesions may be noninflammatory. Clusters of bacteria may be observed on the skin surface.

Ancillary Studies

A Gram stain usually documents the presence of gram-positive cocci.

Differential Diagnosis

The identification of gram-positive cocci distinguishes bullous impetigo from other subcorneal bullous dermatoses. DIF study results are negative.

Prognosis and Treatment

There is usually a favorable response to topical or oral antibiotics, but recurrences may occur.

STAPHYLOCOCCAL SCALDED SKIN SYNDROME

Staphylococcal scalded skin syndrome (SSSS) is associated with infection from the same *S. aureus* phage group 2, type 71 that triggers bullous impetigo. Blistering is caused by proteolysis of desmoglein 1 by the *S. aureus* epidermolysin exotoxin.

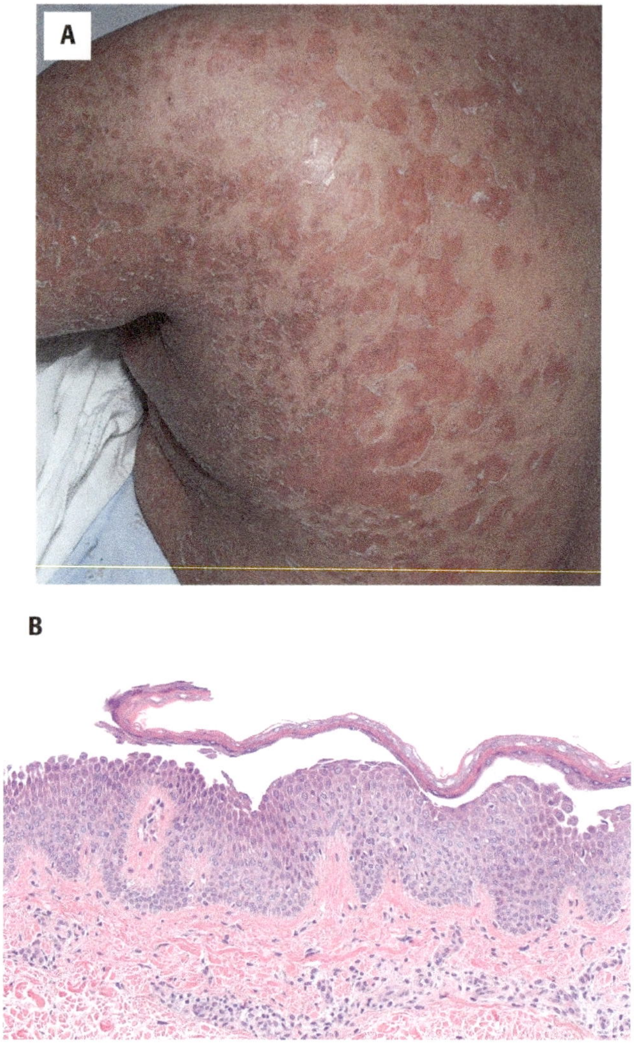

FIG. 5.7
Staphylococcal scalded skin syndrome. **A,** Flaccid blister. **B,** The stratum corneum is separated from the epidermis. There is no inflammation.

Clinical Findings

SSSS usually affects young children (neonatal period to younger than 5 years of age) or immunosuppressed adults or older children. Systemic symptoms include fever and malaise. The skin becomes inflamed and tender, and wrinkling and desquamation with denudation can be seen. The bullae, when intact, are large and flaccid (Fig. 5.7A). The blister expands with pressure into the adjacent nonblistered skin, known as the positive Nikolsky's sign. The mucous membranes are usually spared.

Histopathologic Features

When intact, blistering is seen at the level of the granular layer or just below. There is minimal, if any, dermal inflammation (Fig. 5.7B). Often, the blister is not intact, and the main clue to diagnosis is the absence of the granular layer and stratum corneum, with subtle acantholysis.

Ancillary Studies

Gram stain and DIF findings are negative.

Differential Diagnosis

Gram stains and DIF help distinguish SSSS from bullous impetigo or PF. Clinically, the differential diagnosis usually includes other desquamating conditions, such as Stevens-Johnson syndrome (SJS), toxic epidermal necrolysis (TEN), and pemphigus. TEN and SJS show interface dermatitis, with epidermal necrosis and a split at the BMZ.

Prognosis and Treatment

Antibiotics are needed to treat the infection. Supportive cares are required to restore fluid balance and promote wound healing.

ACROPUSTULOSIS OF INFANCY (INFANTILE ACROPUSTULOSIS)

Typically, acropustulosis of infancy affects black male infants, who develop small pruritic pustules on the palms and soles. Though lesions are rarely biopsied, microscopic features include a subcorneal pustule containing neutrophils admixed with eosinophils. Dyskeratotic keratinocytes may be noted. The clinical course is characterized by exacerbation in crops, often in the summer. There is spontaneous remission around age 2 to 3 years of age.

TRANSIENT NEONATAL PUSTULAR MELANOSIS

The disease has a predilection for black newborns who present at birth with flaccid, very transient vesicopustules that rupture within 1 to 2 days, leaving dark macules with a collarette of scale.

The lesions are located on the face, trunk, diaper region, palms, and soles. Histopathologically, intracorneal and subcorneal pustules are observed. The lesions are sterile. Gram stain results are negative. The process is self-limited and does not require specific treatment.

ERYTHEMA TOXICUM NEONATORUM

The lesions of this disease present from birth to 48 hours after birth as numerous asymptomatic small pustules associated with ill-defined, blotchy erythematous macules, papules, or plaques, most often on sites of pressure. On biopsy, there are subcorneal eosinophil-rich pustules, typically near a follicle. Biopsies of nonpustular areas will show perivascular or perifollicular eosinophils and papillary edema. The lesions clear spontaneously within a few days.

SUBCORNEAL PUSTULAR DERMATOSIS (SNEDDON-WILKINSON DISEASE)

Clinical Findings

Subcorneal pustular dermatosis (SPD) tends to present in intertriginous skin of middle-aged women, though it may affect children rarely. SPD typically manifests as small flaccid pustules that may form serpiginous plaques on erythematous or normal skin. The face, mucous membranes, palms, and soles are spared.

Histopathologic Features

Typically, there is a broad subcorneal pustule containing neutrophils and rare eosinophils. In contrast to acute folliculitis, the pustules are not follicular based and appear to sit on the top of the epidermis. Acantholytic cells are often seen within and at the edge of the blister. There is a mild neutrophil-rich perivascular dermal infiltrate, with exocytosis of neutrophils.

Ancillary Studies

DIF study findings are negative, and they are needed to exclude the subcorneal pustulosis variant of IgA pemphigus.

Differential Diagnosis

IgA pemphigus shows overlapping histopathologic and clinical features. Pustular psoriasis may present with similar microscopic findings but can be distinguished by the presence of psoriasiform hyperplasia and tortuous telangiectases in the dermal papillae. Acute generalized exanthematous pustulosis (AGEP) may show subcorneal pustules, but these are not as broad and prominent as those in SPD. The presence of scattered eosinophils favors AGEP, though these are not always present. Dermatophytosis should be excluded by fungal stains.

Prognosis and Treatment

SPD is chronic and relapsing but responds to dapsone. Patients should be evaluated for the presence of an IgA monoclonal gammopathy, which is often associated with SPD. Pyoderma gangrenosum; IgA myeloma; and systemic conditions such as rheumatoid arthritis, Sjögren syndrome, SAPHO (synovitis, acne, pustulosis, hyperostosis, osteitis) syndrome, Crohn's disease, and thyroid disease have been reported in association with SPD.

ACUTE GENERALIZED EXANTHEMATOUS PUSTULOSIS

AGEP is most often caused by a varied and ever-growing list of medications with beta-lactam antibiotics being a particularly common cause, but viral infections and exposure to mercury have also been reported to trigger AGEP. Patch testing may yield the development of erythema or pustules in approximately 50% of cases.

Clinical Findings

AGEP may occur at any age and is characterized by the development of an exanthem with small (less than 5 mm) nonfollicular pustules or blisters, often with urticarial changes (Fig. 5.8A). The skin eruption of AGEP typically arises within a few days of ingesting the culprit medication. AGEP frequently involves the intertriginous sites, and pruritus and a burning sensation are common. Oral mucosal and tongue erosions occur in 20% of cases. Patients are often febrile.

Histopathologic Features

Histopathologic features depend on whether erythema or a clinical pustule is sampled, though subcorneal pustules are typical, even in the erythematous lesions (Fig. 5.8B). Subtle acantholysis may be observed. Nearly all cases have spongiosis, and most have dyskeratosis. The dermis is edematous, with mixed inflammation including neutrophils and eosinophils, though the latter is variable. There may be evidence of mild vascular damage (endothelial cell swelling, purpura, and karyorrhectic debris).

Differential Diagnosis

Pustular psoriasis may be difficult to distinguish from AGEP, especially when a more established pustule of AGEP is sampled. The pustules tend to be located more superficially in the epidermis of pustular psoriasis, while they are lower in the epidermis or are variably located within the epidermis in AGEP. Additional features that favor AGEP over psoriasis include dyskeratosis, eosinophils in the pustules as well as in the dermis, a mixed neutrophil-rich superficial and mid to deep dermal infiltrate, erythrocyte extravasation, leukocytoclasis, prominent papillary dermal edema, vasculitis, and absence of tortuous dermal papillary vessels. The presence of mixed inflammatory reaction patterns (subcorneal pustules associated with mild interface dermatitis and mild vasculitis) also favors AGEP. Nondiscriminatory features include psoriasiform rete hyperplasia, Munro microabscesses, and follicular pustules. SPD usually has a broader pustule, with fewer mixed histopathologic features.

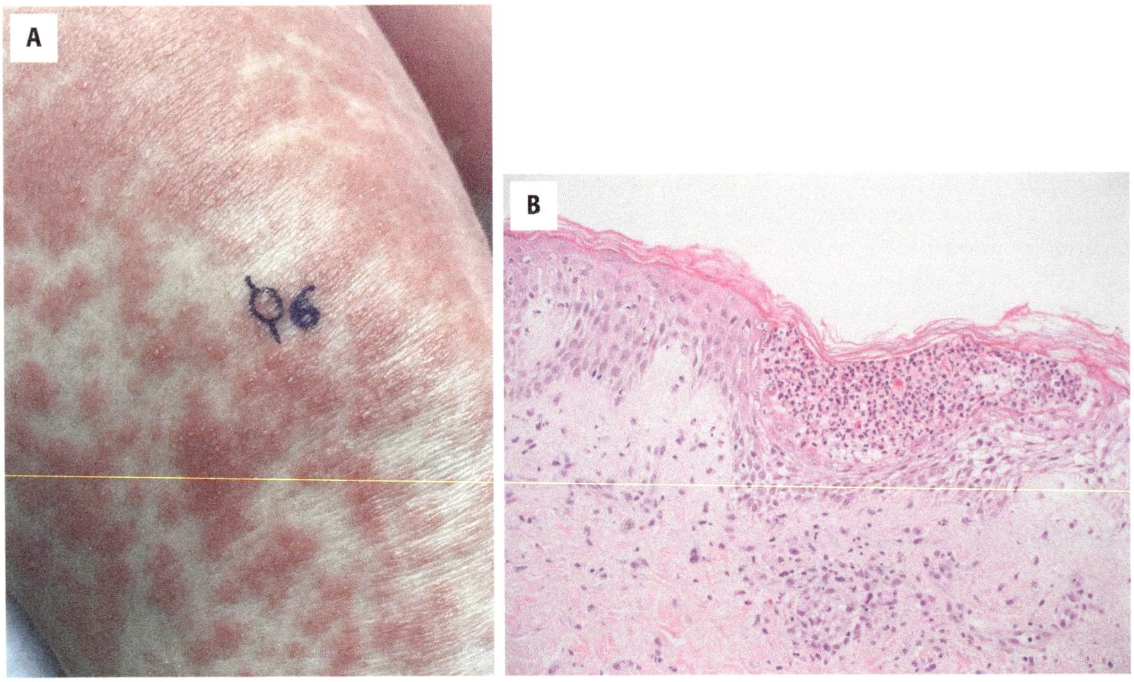

FIG. 5.8

Acute generalized exanthematous pustulosis. **A,** Clinical lesions include pustules on a morbilliform urticarial background. **B,** Aggregates of neutrophils are present in the stratum corneum.

Prognosis and Treatment

AGEP is self-limiting at 2 weeks after withdrawal of medication. Lesions heal with postinflammatory desquamation, which may offer a clue to the diagnosis.

INTRAEPIDERMAL BLISTER WITH SPONGIOSIS OR EDEMA

SPONGIOTIC DERMATITIS

Clinical Findings

An eczematous dermatitis may develop blisters as a result of excessive intraepidermal spongiosis leading to vesiculation, as in the setting of acute contact dermatitis or dyshidrotic eczema. The blisters are often associated with pruritic scaly erythematous or edematous patches and plaques. In conditions such as poison ivy, vesicles, juicy papulovesicular papules, and plaques are arranged in linear and geometric patterns. Dyshidrotic eczema often occurs in patients with atopic dermatitis but may be the clinical presentation of allergic contact dermatitis. Lesions of dyshidrotic eczema often start on the edges of the fingers as small "tapioca pudding" type vesicles, but with time, the blisters break, and the condition spreads to involve the palms and soles as scaly or hyperkeratotic patches or plaques.

Histopathologic Features

There is marked spongiosis with intraepidermal vesicle formation (see Fig. 5.1). The blister cavity contains serum and variable numbers of mixed inflammatory cells. In addition to spongiotic blister formation, there may be ballooning or reticular degeneration of keratinocytes. A variable perivascular and interstitial infiltrate is seen within the upper dermis. If the condition is caused by contact allergy, there may be numerous eosinophils in the dermis and often also epidermis (eosinophilic spongiosis). In addition, Langerhans cell aggregates may be present within the epidermis.

VESICULOBULLOUS BITE REACTIONS

Clinical Findings

Bullous reactions to arthropod bites may be seen at any age but are more common in children or in adults with an underlying hematologic malignancy. With this phenomenon, patients develop tense blisters of various sizes, usually on exposed parts of the lower extremities. The lesions are asymmetric, often with linear grouping. Fleas are more likely to cause bullous reaction, but chiggers, mosquitoes, and other insects can incite a bullous skin reaction. In some patients with scabies infestation, the skin manifestations can present with a generalized vesiculobullous or pustular eruption simulating an autoimmune bullous disorder such as pemphigoid.

Histopathologic Features

Intraepidermal blisters are caused by acute spongiosis or necrosis. There is usually a mixed superficial and deep dermal inflammatory infiltrate of lymphocytes and eosinophils, and hemorrhage is common (Fig. 5.9). A characteristic pattern may be a large intraepidermal blister centrally with smaller vesicles radiating off to each side as one moves further from the site of the bite. If there is a pustular reaction, this may be subcorneal simulating psoriasis. Arthropod bite blisters may also be subepidermal (see the following).

POLYMORPHOUS LIGHT ERUPTION

Clinical Findings

Polymorphous light eruption (PMLE) is a photodistributed reaction to ultraviolet (UV) light (ultraviolet A [UVA] and sometimes ultraviolet B [UVB]), characterized

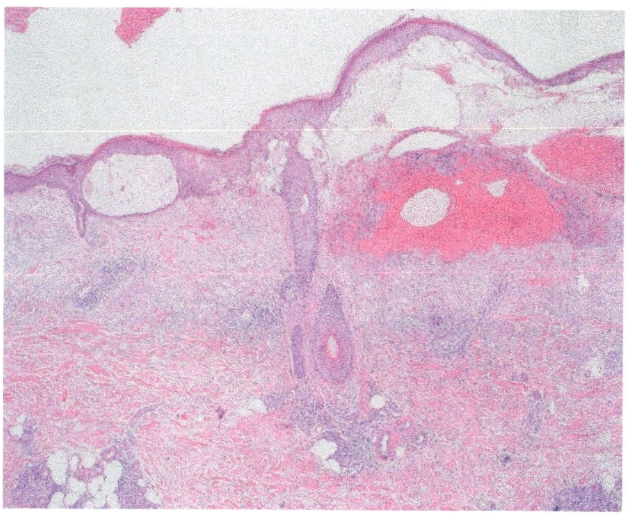

FIG. 5.9
Arthropod bite reaction, with exuberant dermal edema leading to subepidermal separation.

by a pruritic polymorphous eruption, including erythematous papules, eczematous papulosquamous lesions, and vesicles. The condition may occur in children but typically manifests in adults. The face, dorsal hands, and other chronically sun-exposed sites are classically spared because of immunologic "hardening" of these sites. A rare variant localized to the elbows or to the ears has been described. The eruption occurs with the first sun exposures of the early spring or summer season or during a sunny vacation in the winter season.

Histopathologic Features

The histopathologic findings are variable, paralleling the evolution in clinical morphology. There is usually an element of spongiosis and marked papillary dermal edema. There may be an intraepidermal spongiotic vesicle or a subepidermal separation resulting from severe dermal edema. In the dermis, there is a superficial and deep perivascular lymphocytic infiltrate which is sometimes accompanied by neutrophils and extravasated erythrocytes.

Prognosis and Treatment

The condition clears as tolerance develops but tends to recur with reexposure each spring and summer season. Treatment is not necessary, because the condition clears with sun avoidance or protection. Topical or systemic steroids may hasten the resolution. In refractory or predictably recurrent cases, hydroxychloroquine may be required to prevent flares. In addition, UV phototherapy may be used to harden the skin before anticipation of new UV exposure, as with a tropical vacation.

INCONTINENTIA PIGMENTI

Incontinentia pigmenti (IP) is an X-linked inherited disorder affecting a gene involved in NF-kappa B signaling that presents early in life in females; this condition is generally lethal *in utero* for males.

Clinical Findings

The rash of IP has three stages, each characterized by different morphologies: acute vesicular or urticarial, chronic verrucous, and chronic pigmented. Because skin is affected in a mosaic pattern, the lesions form swirled patterns and linear arrays on the unilateral trunk and extremities. The rash does not always progress from one stage to another and may present with later-stage features without having shown manifestations of an earlier stage. Extracutaneous manifestations are frequently seen and include ocular, dental, and central nervous system abnormalities.

Histopathologic Features

In the acute or vesicular stage, eosinophilic spongiosis with intraepidermal vesicles and microabscesses is characteristic (Fig. 5.10). Dyskeratotic keratinocytes near acrosyringia are often present. The epidermis shows variable acanthosis and papillomatosis, and the dermis shows variable pigment incontinence, depending on the stage.

Differential Diagnosis

The differential diagnosis includes eczema, autoimmune bullous disorders, or herpetic infection. To exclude the

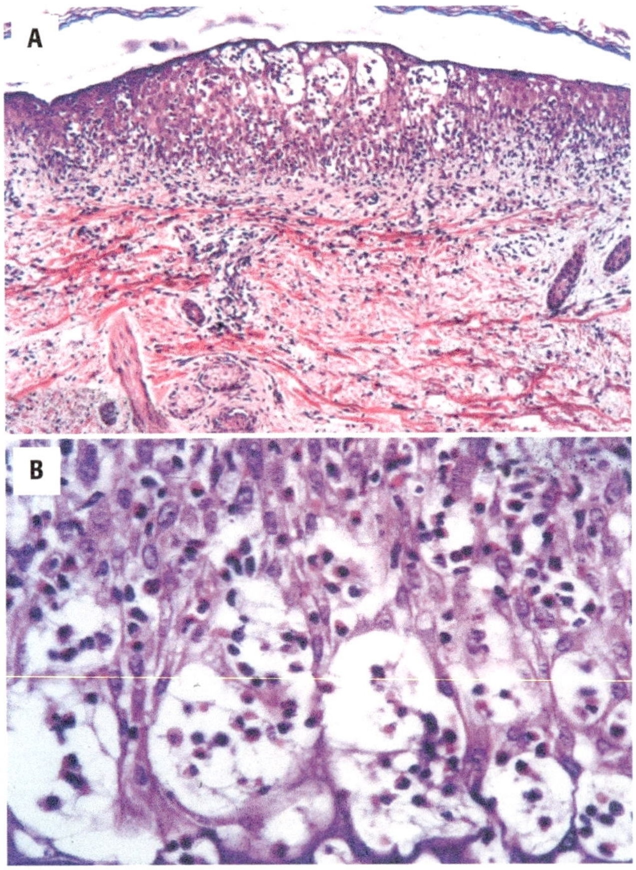

FIG. 5.10
Incontinentia pigmenti. **A,** Microvesicles within the epidermis. **B,** Eosinophilic spongiosis.

latter by DIF is helpful. The combination of eosinophilic spongiosis and the distinct pattern of dyskeratosis favor IP over allergic contact dermatitis and autoimmune bullous disorders.

Prognosis and Treatment

The vesicular stage is transient, but the condition is chronic, with the dyspigmentation persisting throughout adulthood.

INTRAEPIDERMAL BLISTER WITH ACANTHOLYSIS

PEMPHIGUS GROUP

Pemphigus is a group of blistering disorders caused by autoantibodies against components of the desmosome in the skin and/or mucous membranes. Acantholysis is a characteristic histopathologic feature, reflecting loss of adhesion of keratinocytes to each other from the sequelae of antibody binding to structural proteins, such as desmogleins. Unlike the intercellular separation that results from spongiosis, acantholysis imparts rounding up of the keratinocytes, and remnant desmosomes are not visible on light microscopy.

PEMPHIGUS VULGARIS

Clinical Findings

PV presents in the fourth to sixth decades of life and is rarely seen in children. The lesions are flaccid bullae on normal to slightly erythematous mucosa or skin. Breakage of the blisters results in large denuded or crusted erosions and erosive gingivitis (Fig. 5.11A). Generalized involvement may result in exfoliative erythroderma. The *mucous membrane dominant type* is caused by autoantibodies to desmoglein 3 (Dsg3) of the IgG4 subclass and presents with prominent involvement of mucous membranes but minimal cutaneous lesions, while the *mucocutaneous type* usually starts with mucosal disease and progresses to involve the skin over the course of weeks to months. In the latter, patients have both Dsg1 and Dsg3 antibodies. While the oral mucosa is most frequently affected, PV may also affect the nasopharyngeal, ocular, or anogenital mucosa. Precipitating factors include UV light, certain drugs, emotional stress, contact dermatitis, burns, radiation, infection, certain foods and nutritional factors, neoplasms, and, rarely, silicosis. Genetic factors are involved. Relatives of patients with pemphigus may be seropositive for Dsg3 autoantibodies even if asymptomatic. Extracutaneous associations include thymoma and myasthenia gravis.

SPECTRUM OF PEMPHIGUS DISEASES

Type	Clinical	Histopathology
Pemphigus vulgaris (PV)	Mucocutaneous type: mucosal erosions and flaccid blisters Mucosal dominant type: mucosal erosions with minimal skin disease	Suprabasilar acantholysis Eosinophils (variable)
Pemphigus vegetans (variant of PV)	Initially like PV; older lesions become papillomatous and hyperkeratotic, forming vegetations	Suprabasilar acantholysis Pseudoepitheliomatous epidermal hyperplasia Eosinophilic collections, sometimes with neutrophils, are frequent
Pemphigus foliaceus (PF)	Crusted and erosive scaly patches and plaques No mucosal involvement	Subcorneal acantholysis Eosinophilic spongiosis
Fogo selvagem	Variant of PF endemic in South America (Brazil)	Similar to PF
Pemphigus erythematosus	Localized variant of PF Photoexacerbated Involvement of malar region of face	Similar to PF
Drug-induced pemphigus	Clinical manifestations of PV or PF Drugs, especially penicillamine and captopril	Similar to PV or PF
Pemphigus herpetiformis	Grouped vesicles overlying elbows, knees, sacrum, upper back, mimicking dermatitis herpetiformis clinically	Similar to PV or PF
IgA pemphigus	Serpiginous or annular plaques with peripheral scale and pustules	Subcorneal pustule Intraepidermal neutrophils
Paraneoplastic pemphigus	Severe stomatitis, polymorphous skin lesions; morbilliform, bullous erythema multiforme like Associated tumor or Castleman disease, also often associated with lymphomatoid or hematologic malignancies	Lichenoid dermatitis with or without suprabasilar acantholysis and sometimes subepidermal blisters

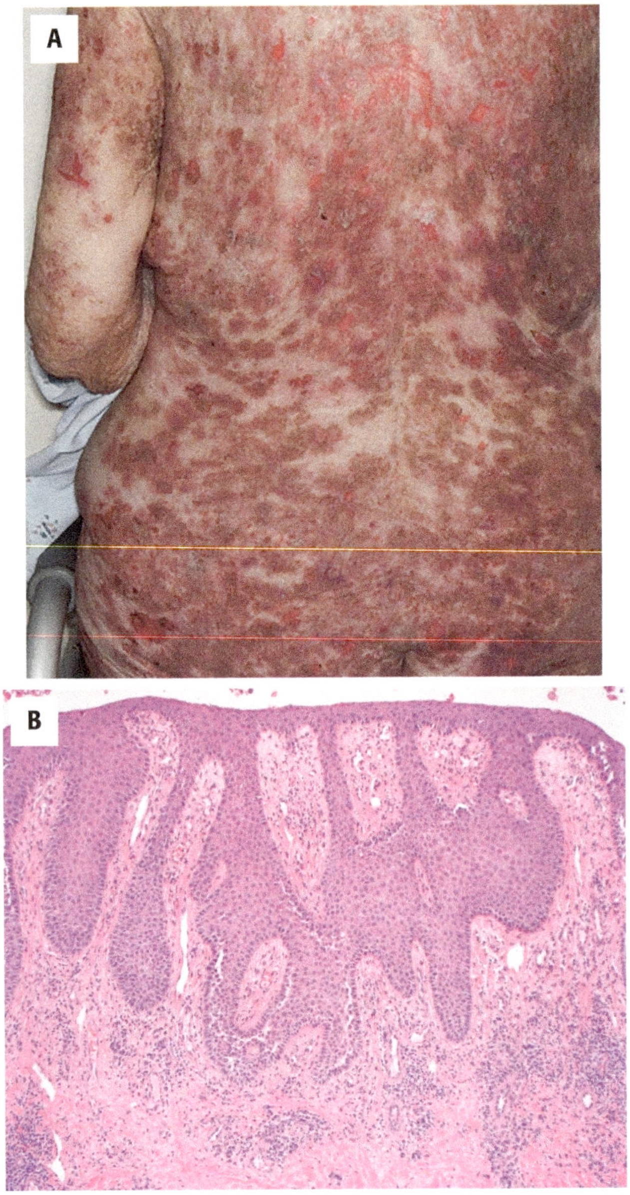

FIG. 5.11

Pemphigus vulgaris. **A,** Multiple erosions are present after rupture of flaccid blisters. **B,** Early lesion with acantholysis.

PEMPHIGUS VULGARIS—DISEASE FACT SHEET

Patient Group

- Onset typically in adults ages 40 to 60, rarely children

Site of Involvement

- Oral mucosa, head and neck, trunk, conjunctiva, intertriginous areas, nasal and anogenital mucosa

Clinical Findings

- Painful oral mucosal erosions common
- Flaccid blisters, positive Nikolsky's sign
- Large denuded weeping erosions on the skin

Prognosis and Treatment

- Chronic condition; can be fatal without treatment (loss of body fluids, malnutrition, and superinfection)
- Rituximab is FDA-approved and the treatment of choice for moderate to severe pemphigus
- Systemic corticosteroids, dapsone, intravenous immunoglobulin, and other immunosuppressive agents can be effective, and several clinical trials for new targeted therapies are underway
- Morbidity from chronic steroid/immunosuppressive therapy

FDA, Food and Drug Administration.

Histopathologic Features

Early lesions of PV may show eosinophilic spongiosis, and acantholysis can be subtle or even absent, particularly if clinicians select perilesional sites for biopsy (Fig. 5.11B). The histopathology of a fully developed PV blister is characterized by a suprabasilar and often also intraspinous acantholytic split (Fig. 5.12). Patients with autoantibodies exclusively to desmoglein 3 may have mostly suprabasilar acantholysis while those with autoantibodies to both desmoglein and 3 and 1 may have a combination of suprabasilar and intraspinous acantholysis. Acantholysis may extend into adnexal epithelium. When the basal cells detach from each other but adhere to BMZ, the resulting picture of solitary basal cells aligned along the base of the blister has been likened to "tombstones" (Fig. 5.13). Inflammation is usually minimal in an early blister, but a variable infiltrate of lymphocytes, eosinophils, and neutrophils, with or without crusting, may occur with established lesions.

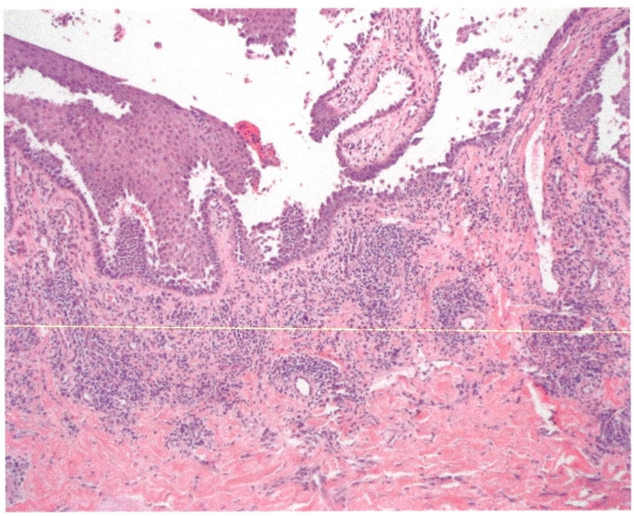

FIG. 5.12

Pemphigus vulgaris. Suprabasilar and intragranular acantholytic blister cavity with inflammatory cells.

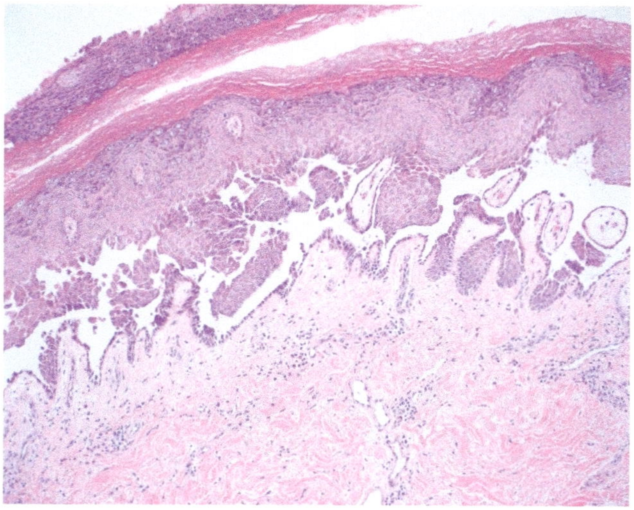

FIG. 5.13

Pemphigus vulgaris. Suprabasilar acantholysis leading to "tombstoning."

PEMPHIGUS VULGARIS—PATHOLOGIC FEATURES

Histopathologic Features

- Suprabasilar acantholytic blister
- Acantholysis extends down adnexal epithelium
- Eosinophils and neutrophils variably present

Ancillary Studies—Direct Immunofluorescence

- IgG, IgG4 (where available), and complement deposits (C3)
- Intercellular/cell-surface smooth or granular pattern
- Pathophysiology involves antibodies to DSG3 (desmoglein III [130 kD]) +/− DSG1

Differential Diagnosis

- Early lesions (see eosinophilic spongiosis)
- Blister: other types of pemphigus, herpetic infection
- Keratosis follicularis (Darier disease; dyskeratosis is more prominent in keratosis follicularis than PV)
- Benign familial pemphigus (Hailey-Hailey disease; acantholysis usually spares the follicles)
- Tissue artifact (usually lacks rounding up of cells, seen in true acantholysis)

Ancillary Studies

DIF typically shows IgG, IgG4 (where available), and C3 cell-surface membrane staining (Fig. 5.14A). Occasionally, this deposition is in a so-called punctate pattern. IIF also shows positive intercellular staining on monkey esophagus mucosa (Fig. 5.14B) but is negative on rodent bladder mucosa, because the latter lacks desmosomes. ELISA can be used to detect circulating desmoglein 3 and/or desmoglein 1 antibodies. Because antibodies are pathogenic, their titers can be used to follow the disease course in some patients. Sera rich in Dsg3 antibodies have greater sensitivity on monkey esophagus than sera rich in Dsg1 antibodies.

Differential Diagnosis

The differential diagnosis includes the various other intraepidermal blisters with acantholysis. A herpetic dermatitis shows viral cytopathic changes and tends to be associated with a denser mixed inflammatory cell infiltrate, often with necrosis or epidermal or follicular epithelium or secondary vasculitis in addition to acantholysis. PNP may be indistinguishable but typically shows lichenoid inflammation. If a patient has (or is suspected to have) an associated malignancy, one should exclude PNP with IIF against rat bladder epithelium or immunoprecipitation.

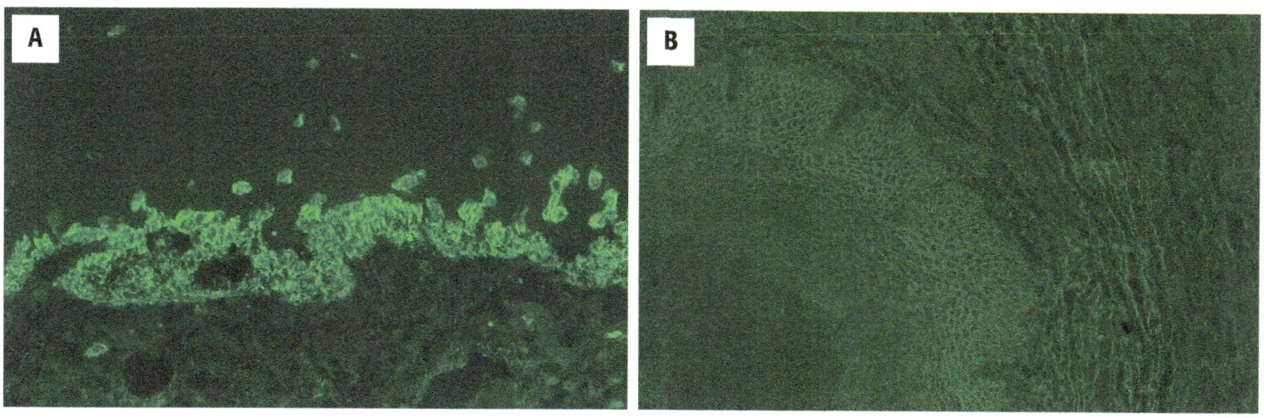

FIG. 5.14

Pemphigus vulgaris. **A,** Direct immunofluorescence shows deposition of IgG4 on the surface of epidermal keratinocytes. A similar pattern is seen with IgG and C3. **B,** Indirect immunofluorescence shows cell-surface deposition on monkey esophagus substrate with IgG.

Keratosis follicularis (Darier disease) differs from PV and other variants of pemphigus by the presence of *corps ronds* and *grains* (round and granular bodies), and negative DIF results. Isolated incidental acantholysis (e.g., acantholytic acanthoma) or transient acantholytic dyskeratosis (Grover's disease) should not be confused with pemphigus if attention is paid to the clinical context.

Although eosinophilic spongiosis, when present, can be a helpful clue to suspect pemphigus, it is neither sensitive nor specific for pemphigus.

Prognosis and Treatment

Without immunosuppression, the course of pemphigus can be fatal because of loss of fluids and secondary infections. Outcomes in PV have improved considerably with the widespread use of rituximab and systemic corticosteroids. Other steroid-sparing agents can also be used in pemphigus.

PEMPHIGUS VEGETANS

Clinical Findings

Pemphigus vegetans is a rare verrucous variant of PV, affecting intertriginous areas and oral mucosa. A *Neumann type* begins like PV, with the development of flaccid bullae, followed by peripheral pustules that evolve into hyperkeratotic verrucous vegetations. In the *Hallopeau type*, which tends to have a milder and sometimes self-resolving course, the primary lesion is a pustule, which evolves into verrucous vegetations studded with pustules.

Histopathologic Features

The histopathology is similar to that of PV except for the addition of pseudoepitheliomatous, often verruciform, epidermal hyperplasia and prominent intraepidermal collections of eosinophils, with or without neutrophils.

DIFFERENTIAL DIAGNOSIS OF EOSINOPHILIC SPONGIOSIS

Autoimmune Blistering Disorders

Pemphigus vulgaris
Pemphigus foliaceus
Bullous pemphigoid
Pemphigoid gestationis

Allergic Contact Dermatitis

Scabies infestation

Incontinentia Pigmenti

Drug Reaction

Ancillary Studies

DIF results are similar to those for PV.

Differential Diagnosis

Lesions of pemphigus vegetans need to be distinguished from other pseudoepitheliomatous processes, such as infections (e.g., blastomycosis) or iododermas (e.g., bromoderma). These microscopic mimickers can be readily differentiated with clinical correlation and DIF results.

PEMPHIGUS FOLIACEUS

Clinical Findings

PF typically affects young to middle-aged adults (30 to 50 years old) but may also rarely occur in children. Pemphigus erythematosus represents a subtype of PF that shares features of lupus erythematosus, such as photoexacerbation and the presence of circulating antinuclear antibodies. An endemic form called fogo selvagem exists in rural Brazil, while a distinct variant of endemic PF (EPF), El Bagre EPF, is found in Colombia. El Bagre EPF has features similar to the pemphigus erythematosus overlap subtype.

The scaly, crusted, and erosive well-demarcated patches and plaques of PF are predominantly located on the head and upper trunk (Fig. 5.15). Blisters tend to be flaccid but superficial. Often, only the annular periphery is blistered. Mucous membranes are usually not involved. Exfoliative erythroderma has been reported in severe cases. Precipitating factors include UV light, drugs, emotional stress, burns, radiation, or infection.

PEMPHIGUS FOLIACEUS AND FOGO SELVAGEM*—DISEASE FACT SHEET

Patient Group

- Adults. Fogo selvagem is seen in children.

Site of Involvement

- Usually localized to seborrheic areas of the face and trunk
- May be generalized
- No mucosal involvement
- El Bagre endemic pemphigus foliaceus (EPF) with ocular and eyelid involvement

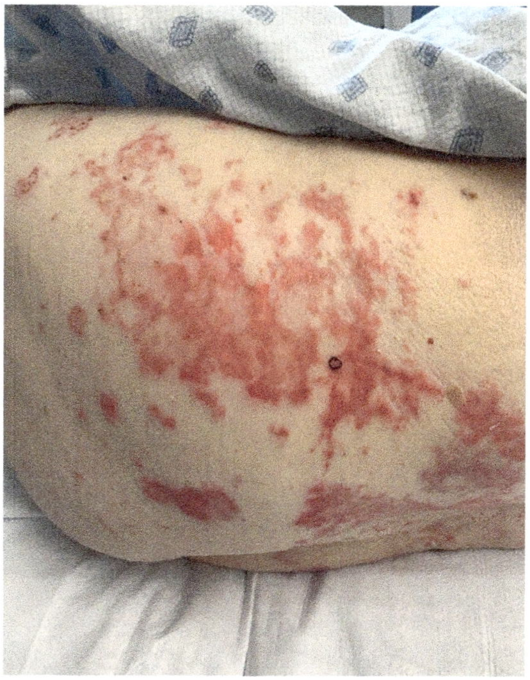

FIG. 5.15
Pemphigus foliaceus. Superficial erosions affecting the trunk.

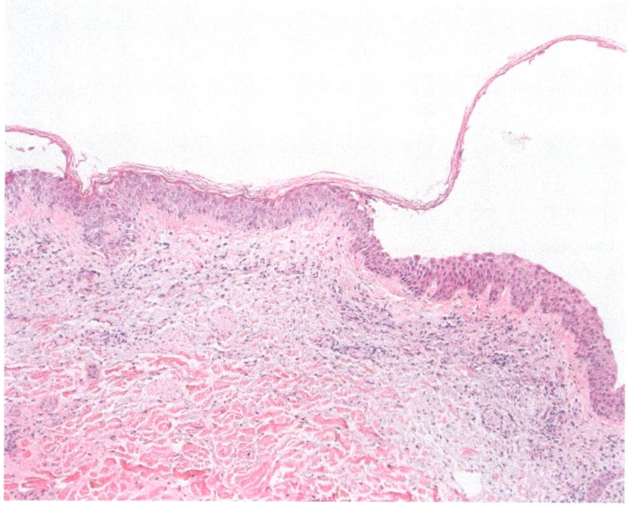

FIG. 5.16
Pemphigus foliaceus. Subcorneal split.

Clinical Findings

- ▸▸ Superficial vesicles with positive Nikolsky's sign
- ▸▸ Denuded skin, with collerette of residual blister, flaky puff pastry–like scale, exfoliative erythroderma

Prognosis and Treatment

- ▸▸ Better prognosis than pemphigus vulgaris
- ▸▸ Rituximab is the treatment of choice for moderate to severe PF, while corticosteroids and steroid-sparing agents are also effective

*Fogo selvagem is a form endemic to rural Brazil.

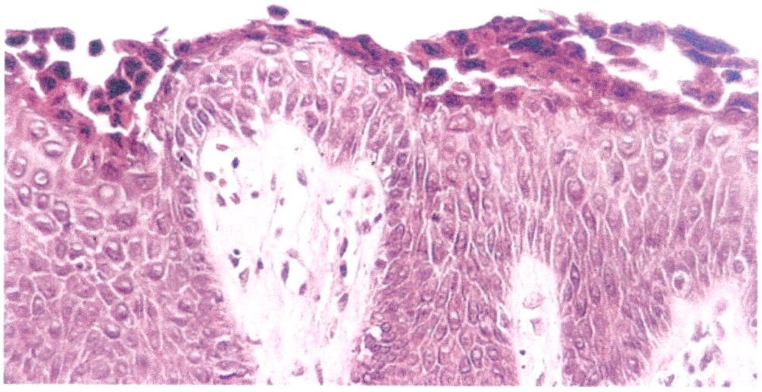

FIG. 5.17
Pemphigus foliaceus. Acantholysis in the granular cell layer with "missing" stratum corneum.

Histopathologic Features

If there is an intact intraepidermal blister, the split will be in the subcorneal layer (Fig. 5.16). Acantholysis typically involves the subcorneal or superficial layers of the epidermis but at times extends down to the follicular infundibulum. Acantholytic keratinocytes can be identified in the blister cavity or at the edge of the blister. In the absence of an obvious blister, it is important to carefully examine whether or not the stratum corneum may be focally missing and search for subtle evidence of acantholysis within the granular cell layer (Fig. 5.17). On occasion, no or only minimal acantholysis can be found. In those cases, the presence of neutrophilic or eosinophilic spongiosis may be the only clue to the diagnosis of PF, bearing in mind that PF is only one of several disease entities that may present histopathologically with eosinophilic spongiosis (Fig. 5.18). Initially,

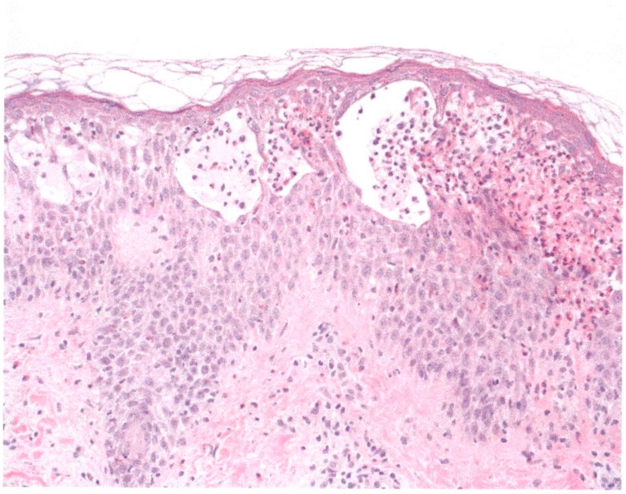

FIG. 5.18
Pemphigus foliaceus. Neutrophils in the granular cell layer.

PEMPHIGUS FOLIACEUS/FOGO SELVAGEM—PATHOLOGIC FEATURES

Histopathologic Features

- Intraepidermal vesicle in spinous or granular cell layer
- Acantholysis
- Eosinophilic or neutrophilic spongiosis

Ancillary Studies—Direct Immunofluorescence

- IgG, IgG4 (where available), and complement deposits (C3)
- Intercellular/cell-surface pattern
- Antibodies to meibomian gland BMZ and intercellular junction, tarsal muscle, and neurovascular structures around pilosebaceous structures of lids in el Bagre EPF
- Pathophysiology
- Autoimmune antibodies to desmoglein I (165 kD)

Differential Diagnosis

- Other types of pemphigus
- Pustular psoriasis
- Staphylococcal scalded skin syndrome or bullous impetigo

the process may have minimal inflammation, but often there is a perivascular lymphocytic infiltrate with neutrophils and eosinophils in the upper dermis. In some older lesions, there may be subcorneal pustules.

Ancillary Studies

DIF shows deposition of IgG, IgG4 (where available), and C3 on the cell surface of perilesional skin (Fig. 5.19). Although there is only a split superficially, immune conjugate deposition is often noted throughout the epidermis, which may be more prominent in the upper layers. IIF on monkey esophagus mucosa typically shows cell-surface membrane staining with IgG. This result can be reported as a titer because the amount of antibody will correlate with the disease activity, though it should be remembered that IIF titer determination is subjective. In up to 25% of DIF and 10% to 20% of IIF, the results may be negative or equivocal. In these instances, ELISA testing for desmoglein 1 autoantibodies can be diagnostically helpful.

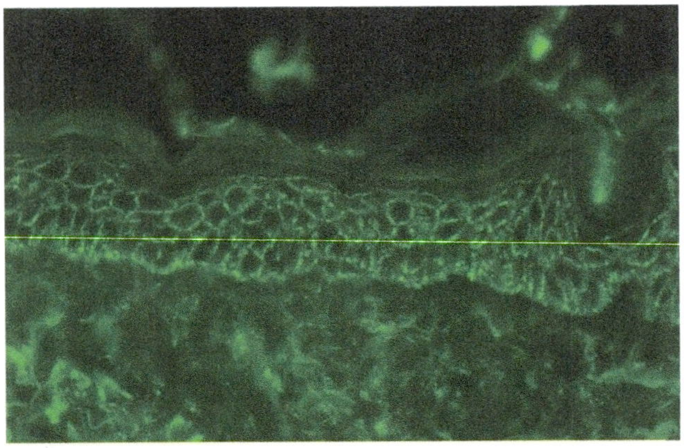

FIG. 5.19

Pemphigus foliaceus. Direct immunofluorescence shows deposits of IgG4 on the surface of epidermal keratinocytes. A similar pattern is seen with IgG and C3.

Differential Diagnosis

PF may be confused with SSSS, pustular psoriasis, and other variants of pemphigus microscopically. The distinction requires attention to associated clinical features and immunofluorescence studies.

Prognosis and Treatment

PF may respond to topical corticosteroid therapy, but often, systemic immunosuppressive agents are required to control the condition. PF has a better prognosis than PV.

PEMPHIGUS HERPETIFORMIS

Pemphigus herpetiformis (PH) is a rare variant of pemphigus that presents with a grouped or annular configuration of vesicles in a distribution that mimics that of DH. These pruritic herpetiform vesicles arise on the trunk and proximal extremities but tend to spare the oral mucosa. Histopathologically, eosinophilic or neutrophilic spongiosis with intraepidermal or subcorneal microvesicles is often seen. Acantholysis is minimal or absent. Immunopathologic features are heterogeneous. DIF often shows a pattern of superficial intraepithelial intercellular IgG, IgG4 (where available), and C3 deposition similar to PF, although a PV pattern may occasionally be seen. IIF shows cell-surface IgG. ELISA may demonstrate the presence of circulating desmoglein 1 antibodies most often but also desmoglein 3 antibodies. Desmocollin 1 is a targeted antigen in some patients with PH.

Patients with PH have a good prognosis with a good response to dapsone unless the process progresses to PV.

DRUG-INDUCED PEMPHIGUS

Clinical Findings

Certain drugs may trigger the development of pemphigus. Some patients experience a non-blistering prodrome eruption of morbilliform papules and macules, urticarial patches, or annular erythema. While the blisters of pemphigus tend to be more PF like, a combination of PV- and PF-like lesions can develop. Drug-induced pemphigus is usually caused by one of two chemically distinct drugs: thiol drugs (containing a sulfhydryl radical) and nonthiol drugs. Phenol drugs or combined phenol and sulfhydryl drugs may also induce pemphigus. Penicillamine is the most common culprit, and pemphigus may develop in approximately 7% of patients taking the drug for more than 6 months. Captopril is another common cause because it contains a sulfhydryl group similar to penicillamine. Thiol drugs account for 80% of drug-induced pemphigus. Other implicated medications include penicillins, cephalosporins, enalapril and nonsteroidal antiinflammatory drugs (NSAIDs).

Histopathologic Features

The histopathology of drug-induced pemphigus is similar to that of PV (suprabasilar or intraspinous acantholysis) and PF (subcorneal acantholysis). Features of both may be present in the same patient. Scattered eosinophils are expected.

Ancillary Studies

DIF results are similar to those of PV or PF.

Differential Diagnosis

Clinical information (drug history) is essential for distinction from non–drug-induced pemphigus.

Prognosis and Treatment

The condition often resolves with discontinuation of drug; however, it may not when triggered by nonthiol drugs. The nonsulfhydryl group medications impart features more similar to PV, and in this situation, the medications may unmask true, persistent disease.

IgA Pemphigus

There are three variants of IgA pemphigus: (1) *intraepidermal neutrophilic dermatosis*, (2) *SPD*, and (3) *pemphigus vegetans*, each of which has different clinical and pathologic presentations.

Clinical Findings

The *intraepidermal neutrophilic dermatosis* type of IgA pemphigus presents in children and adults. The distribution is concentrated on the trunk and proximal extremities, especially flexural sites. The lesions are polymorphous, ranging from vesicles or flaccid bullae to characteristic annular pustules with central crust (Fig. 5.20). The lesions may be pruritic. At times, there are only excoriated papules. The features of *SPD*-type IgA pemphigus are similar to those of Sneddon-Wilkinson SPD (see earlier section), and some have suggested that they are the same entity. The *pemphigus vegetans* type presents with intertriginous vegetative lesions or mucosal pustules, is very rare, and is also somewhat controversial.

In patients with IgA pemphigus, an associated monoclonal gammopathy or inflammatory bowel disease may be present. Cases with itchy excoriated papules similar to those of DH may be seen.

Histopathologic Features

Neutrophils are present within the epidermis, either throughout or preferentially in the upper epidermis. Aggregates of neutrophils may form an intraepidermal or subcorneal blister. There may or may not be associated acantholysis.

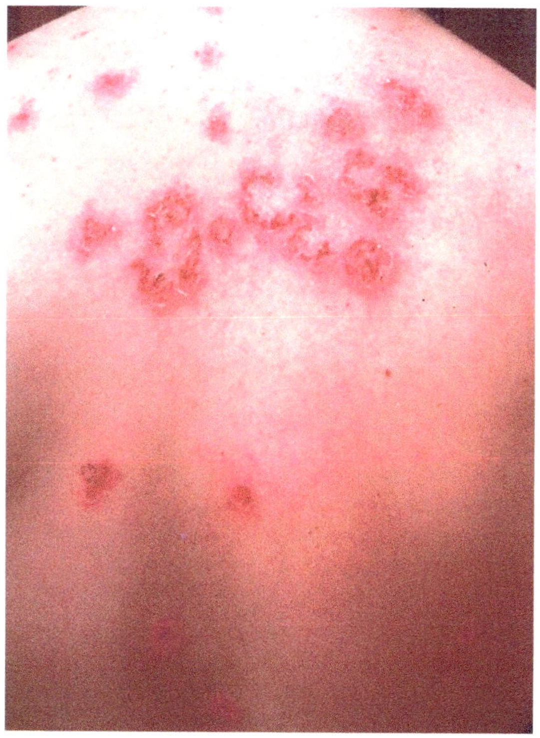

FIG. 5.20
IgA pemphigus. Annular erythema with pustules and crust.

Ancillary Studies

In *intraepidermal neutrophilic dermatosis*–type IgA pemphigus, DIF shows cell-surface IgA deposited throughout the entire epidermis. Rare cases with IgA and IgG have been reported. In *SPD*-type, cell-surface IgA deposits are concentrated in the upper epidermis. A subtype with atypical clinical presentations has both IgG and IgA deposited in either the upper or entire epidermis. In up to 50% of cases, IIF results with IgA may be negative. An IF assay using recombinant desmocollin-transfected COS-7 cells is more sensitive for diagnosis but is not widely available. ELISA and immunoblotting are less sensitive than a COS-7 assay. Immunoblotting studies may be helpful in documenting desmocollin 1 in the SPD variant.

Differential Diagnosis

PF and PV can be excluded by DIF, demonstrating IgG and not IgA cell-surface deposits. Sneddon-Wilkinson SPD will be identical clinically and histopathologically but will have a negative DIF result.

Prognosis and Treatment

The course is chronic, but patients may respond well to dapsone or colchicine. Severe cases may require systemic corticosteroids.

PARANEOPLASTIC PEMPHIGUS

Clinical Findings

PNP, an autoimmune bullous disorder mediated by both B- and T-cell immunity, is caused by a characteristic set of autoantibodies occurring in a patient with an associated malignancy or Castleman's disease. Its clinical manifestations include hemorrhagic mucositis with painful oral or perioral (Fig. 5.21) and conjunctival erosions and a polymorphous cutaneous eruption (vesicles, targetoid, lichenoid, or urticarial lesions). The most common associated diseases are chronic lymphocytic leukemia, non-Hodgkin lymphoma, and Castleman disease. Less frequently, it may be associated with solid malignancies, including melanoma, and in nonmalignant disease, including human immunodeficiency virus (HIV) disease, thymoma, and Waldenström macroglobulinemia. The term *paraneoplastic autoimmune multiorgan syndrome* (PAMS) is frequently used to highlight the multisystem involvement of the disease. In particular, associated immune-mediated pulmonary disease can be severe and contribute to increased mortality in affected patients.

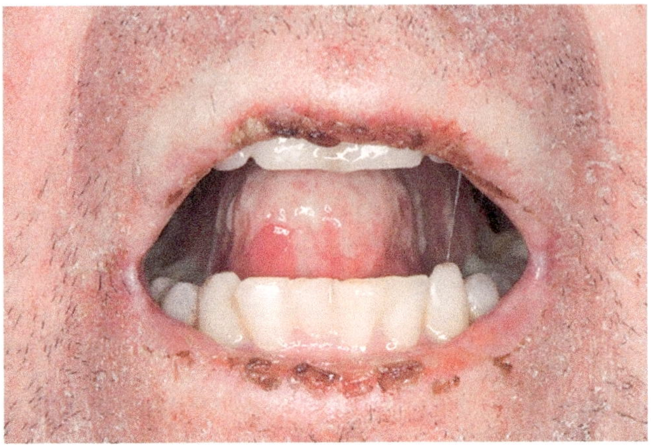

FIG. 5.21

Paraneoplastic pemphigus. Hemorrhagic stomatitis and submucosal blisters on tongue.

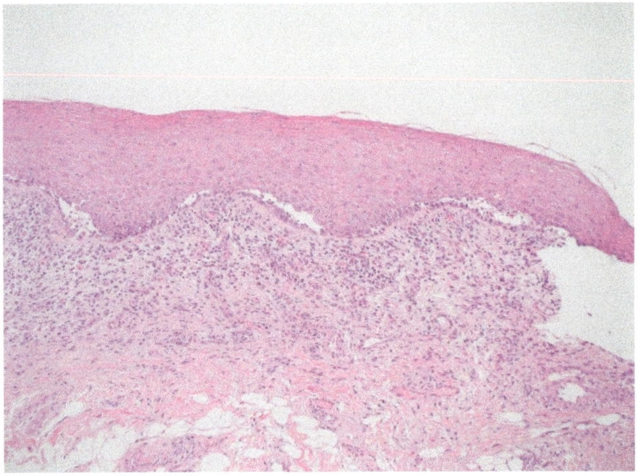

FIG. 5.22

Paraneoplastic pemphigus. Suprabasilar acantholysis associated with lichenoid dermatitis.

Histopathologic Features

PNP is histopathologically characterized by the presence of a mixed pattern of lichenoid dermatitis (often, erythema multiforme like) and an intraepidermal acantholytic blister (PV like; Fig. 5.22) and sometimes subepidermal blisters as there may be a wide spectrum of target antigens. The histopathologic features may vary depending on the site of the biopsy, time course of the lesion, and treatment regimen. In particular, patients treated with rituximab as part of their antineoplastic regimen frequently present with lichenoid dermatitis without acantholysis.

PARANEOPLASTIC PEMPHIGUS—DISEASE FACT SHEET

Patient Group

- Adults with malignant tumor (most often non-Hodgkin lymphoma), Castleman disease, or thymoma

Site of Involvement

- Oropharynx and conjunctiva
- Skin
- Lung (bronchiolitis obliterans)

Clinical Findings

- Painful mucosal erosions or ulcers, hemorrhagic mucositis
- Polymorphous skin lesions (blisters, plaques, erosions, targetoid lesions, lichenoid lesions)
- Associated malignancy during or after mucocutaneous disease

Prognosis and Treatment

- Dependent on underlying disease (e.g., thymoma or Castleman versus aggressive lymphoma)
- Treatment of underlying tumor
- Treatment of skin lesions with corticosteroids or steroid-sparing agents, selected carefully so as to balance treatment with the antitumor effects of host immunity

Indirect Immunofluorescence

- Serum autoantibodies that bind to cell surface of stratified squamous mucosa (monkey esophagus or urinary bladder)

Other tests

- ELISA for envoplakin antibodies
- Immunoprecipitation
- Serum antibodies that precipitate antigens of the following sizes:
  - 130 kDa: desmoglein 3
  - 160 kDa: desmoglein 1
  - 250 kDa: desmoplakin I
  - 230 kDa: bullous pemphigoid antigen I
  - 210 kDa: desmoplakin II (upper band of doublet); envoplakin (lower band)
  - 190 kDa: periplakin
  - 170 kDa: protease inhibitor α-2-macroglobulin-like-1
  - 500 kDa: plectin

Pathophysiology

- Autoantibodies to miscellaneous proteins (see above)

Differential Diagnosis

- Other lichenoid dermatitides (e.g., Stevens-Johnson syndrome, lichen planus)
- Other forms of pemphigus

Ancillary Studies

IMMUNOPRECIPITATION

PNP is associated with circulating antibodies directed against epithelial cell surfaces. These antibodies immunoprecipitate a complex of desmosomal proteins, which are known as the *plakin gene family*. They are intermediate filament–associated hemidesmosome/desmosomal proteins and can include desmoplakin I (250 kD), desmoplakin II (210 kD), BPAGI/BP230, HD1/plectin (500 kD), periplakin (190 kD), envoplakin (210 kD), and protease inhibitor α-2-macroglobulin-like-1 (170 kD) protein. Immunoprecipitation of these proteins represents the gold standard for the diagnosis of PNP. However, this test is not widely available and is expensive and cumbersome.

PARANEOPLASTIC PEMPHIGUS—PATHOLOGIC FEATURES

Histopathologic Features

- Interface or lichenoid dermatitis
- Intraepidermal acantholysis

Ancillary Studies

- Direct immunofluorescence
- IgG and C3 deposits on epidermal cell surface and along the basement membrane zone
- Scattered and clumped cytoid bodies with multiple conjugates; shaggy fibrinogen along the basement membrane zone (lichenoid tissue reaction)

DIRECT IMMUNOFLUORESCENCE

DIF usually shows IgG or C3 cell-surface membrane staining, similar to PV, thereby establishing a lesion in the pemphigus family. In addition to what is usually seen in PV, in PNP, there are often cytoid bodies with IgG, IgM, and C3, and fibrinogen deposits in a shaggy distribution along the BMZ.

INDIRECT IMMUNOFLUORESCENCE

IIF will be positive on both stratified and nonstratified epithelium, which is unique to PNP (different from PV). Demonstrating a positive IIF result to rat bladder transitional epithelium is an adequate screening test and, in the appropriate clinical setting, supports the diagnosis of PNP. While it is less expensive and easier to perform than immunoprecipitation, false-negative results may occur.

Differential Diagnosis

PNP may show overlapping clinical and histopathologic features with PV, erythema multiforme/SJS, and lichenoid dermatitis, including drug reactions and lichen planus. DIF and IIF studies are critical for the diagnosis. After DIF has established the presence of a pemphigus lesion, IIF studies against rat bladder epithelium, ELISA for envoplakin antibodies, or immunoprecipitation studies are required for definitive distinction of PNP from PV.

Prognosis and Treatment

Patients with PNP often do poorly, succumbing to complications of infection, of necrotizing tracheobronchitis and bronchiolitis obliterans, or of the underlying malignancy. The condition may respond to treatment of the associated malignancy. Patients with associated localized Castleman's disease or thymoma tend to improve significantly after surgical removal of the tumor.

KERATOSIS FOLLICULARIS (DARIER DISEASE)

Keratosis follicularis (Darier disease) is an autosomal dominantly inherited disorder with mutations in the *ATP2A2* gene, which encodes the sarcoendoplasmic reticulum calcium pumping ATPase type 2 (SERCA2). Sporadic or segmental cases may occur.

Clinical Findings

Keratosis follicularis (Darier disease) clinically presents with coalescing follicular papules with a greasy scale or crust (Fig. 5.23). These papules and plaques are distributed in seborrheic regions of the face, postauricular scalp, chest, and back. The palms and soles may be involved by keratotic papules. Often there is nail dystrophy. Oral whitish papules may present. Rarely, patients present with acne-like comedones. Neuropsychiatric comorbidities are associated with this condition.

Histopathologic Features

Characteristic for this entity is the combination of acantholysis (dyscohesive round keratinocytes with smooth cell surface, leading to intraepidermal cleft formation) and dyskeratosis (apoptotic keratinocytes with nuclear condensation) (Fig. 5.24). Two variants of dyskeratotic cells may be seen: *corps ronds* and *grains*. *Corps ronds* are large acantholytic keratinocytes in the spinous cell layer with a dark nucleus, perinuclear halo (clear space around the nucleus), and eosinophilic cytoplasm. *Corps grains* are small oval cells in the upper granular cell or corneal layer characterized by pyknotic nuclei with shrunken eosinophilic cytoplasm (Fig. 5.25). Rete hyperplasia in conjunction with acantholysis may result in villous projections of the underlying dermal papilla protruding into the blister cavity. Plugged follicles with typical changes of acantholytic dyskeratosis characterize the comedonal variant. Verrucous lesions on the hands, acrokeratosis of Hopf, can show papillomatosis.

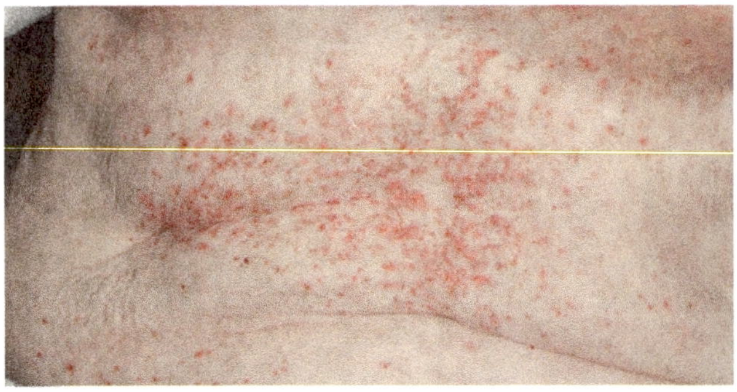

FIG. 5.23

Keratosis follicularis (Darier disease). Hyperkeratotic follicular erosive crusted papules on the chest.

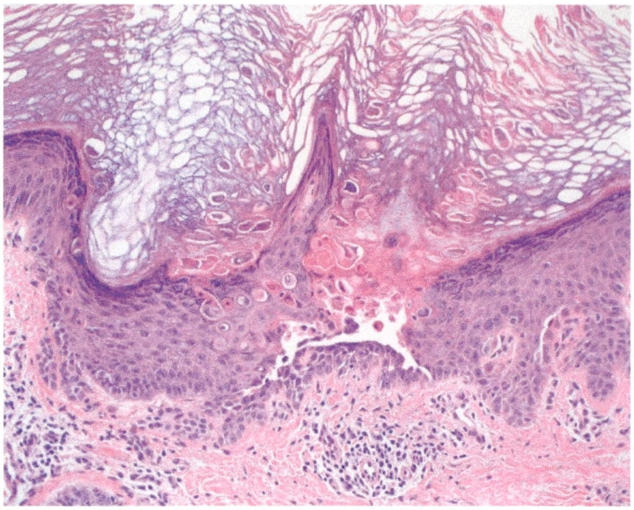

FIG. 5.24

Keratosis follicularis (Darier disease). Intraepidermal acantholysis associated with hyperparakeratosis. *Corps ronds:* large acantholytic keratinocytes with perinuclear halo.

Ancillary Studies

DIF result is negative in this condition.

KERATOSIS FOLLICULARIS (DARIER DISEASE)—DISEASE FACT SHEET

Patient Group

- Usually presents in second or third decade of life
- Hereditary (autosomal-dominant), sporadic, or segmental

Site of Involvement

- Oral mucosa
- Skin: seborrheic areas, palmoplantar, nails

Clinical Findings

- Greasy, crusted brown keratotic papules; rare comedones

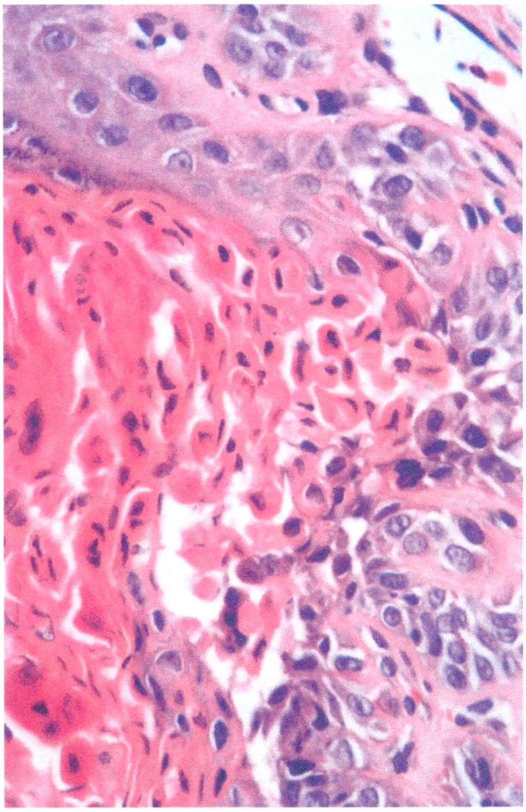

FIG. 5.25

Keratosis follicularis (Darier disease). *Corps grains:* pyknotic keratinocytes in stratum corneum with elongated dark nucleus and shrunken eosinophilic cytoplasm.

- Whitish mucosal papules and plaques
- Longitudinal red or white nail streaks

Prognosis and Treatment

- Lesions are prone to odiferous secondary infection
- Retinoids or CO_2 laser ablation can be effective

KERATOSIS FOLLICULARIS (DARIER DISEASE)—PATHOLOGIC FEATURES

Histopathologic Features

- Acantholysis
- Hyperkeratosis
- Dyskeratosis
- *Corps ronds* and *grains*
- Direct immunofluorescence
  - Negative
- Pathophysiology
  - Mutations in *ATP2A2*

Differential Diagnosis

- Pemphigus
- Transient acantholytic dyskeratosis (Grover disease)
- Benign familial pemphigus (Hailey-Hailey disease)

Differential Diagnosis

Transient acantholytic dermatosis (Grover disease) and incidental acantholysis (e.g., acantholytic acanthoma) are readily distinguished from Darier disease by clinical context. Warty dyskeratoma has a cup-shaped silhouette and is endophytic. The prominent dyskeratosis seen in keratosis follicularis (Darier disease) usually aids differentiation from acantholytic immunobullous disorders, though DIF can be helpful if there is ambiguity. Papular acantholytic dyskeratosis is possibly a *forme fruste* of keratosis follicularis that presents with papules limited to the male and female genitalia and genital crural intertriginous areas. This entity shares histopathologic features with keratosis follicularis.

Prognosis and Treatment

Keratosis follicularis is chronic and predisposes patients to secondary infection. Herpetic or bacterial superinfection can be life-threatening. Lesions may respond to retinoid therapy, antibiotics, steroids, or CO_2 laser.

BENIGN FAMILIAL PEMPHIGUS (HAILEY-HAILEY DISEASE)

This is an autosomal-dominant disease associated with mutations in *ATP2C1* encoding a Ca^{2+}-transport ATPase pump.

Clinical Findings

Benign familial pemphigus (Hailey-Hailey disease) is seen in adulthood and most frequently occurs at intertriginous sites (axillae, groin, and neck; Fig. 5.26A). More common than intact blisters are weepy or crusted, sharply marginated erosions with peripheral scale. The skin appears like wet tissue paper. Mucosal involvement is unusual.

Histopathologic Features

An intraepidermal blister caused by acantholysis involves the spinous layer and often, the entire thickness of the epidermis, leading to a "dilapidated brick wall"-like appearance (Fig. 5.26B). A well-formed blister may not be present. *Corps ronds* and *grains* occasionally manifest but are usually not prominent. Secondary

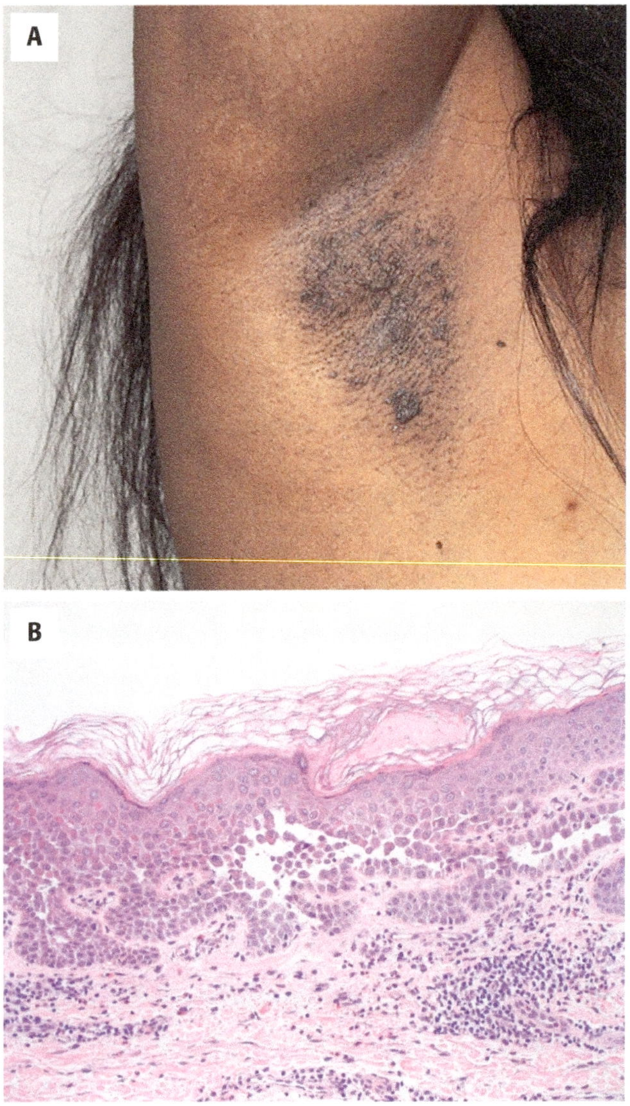

FIG. 5.26
Benign familial pemphigus (Hailey-Hailey disease). **A,** Hyperkeratotic plaques in intertriginous areas. **B,** Intraepidermal acantholysis.

inflammation may be seen but is not characteristic of the primary disease process.

Differential Diagnosis

Clinical correlation and DIF (negative in benign familial pemphigus) are necessary to distinguish it from other acantholytic disorders, such as acantholytic dermatosis of the genitocrural region or pemphigus.

Prognosis and Treatment

The course is chronic and recurrent, but lesions may be responsive to topical antibiotics, naltrexone, or CO_2 laser.

ACANTHOLYTIC DERMATOSIS OF THE GENITOCRURAL REGION

Also called papular acantholytic dyskeratosis, acantholytic dermatosis of the genitocrural region is histopathologically indistinguishable from benign familial pemphigus. Clinical features allowing differentiation of the former from the latter are the lack of familial association and the clinical anatomic distribution. As implied in its name, the disorder primarily affects the genital, perianal, and inguinal region. The clinical lesions appear as scaly papules and plaques. While an acantholytic intraepidermal blister may be suggested histopathologically, there is rarely true blister formation or erosions clinically.

TRANSIENT ACANTHOLYTIC DERMATOSIS (GROVER DISEASE)

Clinical Findings

Transient acantholytic dermatosis (Grover disease) is a pruritic condition that typically occurs in elderly adults, with a strong male predilection. The spectrum of lesions includes discrete erythematous papules with or without erosions and with small vesicles. Typically, the lesions are located on the chest and back, although they may also be found on the proximal extremities. The condition is exacerbated by heat, occlusion, and exercise.

Histopathologic Features

Acantholysis is seen with or without dyskeratosis and its presence may be subtle and may require multiple levels for visualization. There also may be spongiosis or an inflammatory cell infiltrate in the superficial dermis with lymphocytes and eosinophils (Fig. 5.27).

Differential Diagnosis

TRANSIENT ACANTHOLYTIC DERMATOSIS (GROVER DISEASE)—DISEASE FACT SHEET

Patient Group
- Middle-aged and elderly adults affected, especially white men
- Acquired (non-hereditary)

Site of Involvement
- Predilection for trunk

Clinical Findings
- Pruritic nonfollicular crusted papules
- Exacerbated by heat or sweat, occlusion

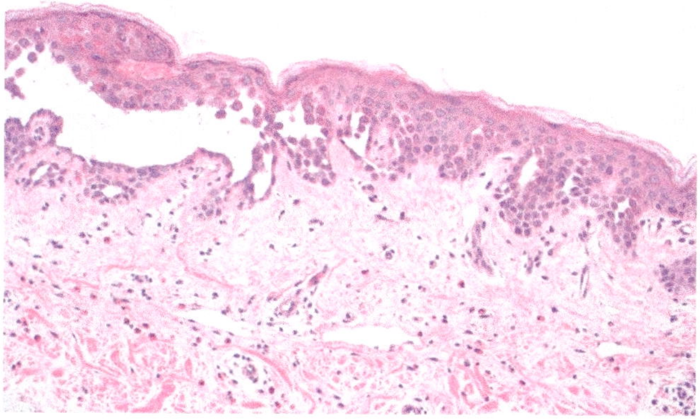

FIG. 5.27

Transient acantholytic dyskeratosis (Grover's disease). Focal intraepidermal acantholysis with dyskeratosis.

Prognosis and Treatment

- Avoidance of exacerbating factors (e.g., sweat, sunlight)
- Treatment of pruritus (topical corticosteroids, antihistamines, topical antibiotics)
- Retinoids to treat keratotic lesions

TRANSIENT ACANTHOLYTIC DERMATOSIS (GROVER'S DISEASE)—PATHOLOGIC FEATURES

Histopathologic Features

- Hyperkeratosis, parakeratosis, and acantholysis, often with dyskeratosis
- Mixed dermal inflammatory cell infiltrate, often with eosinophils
- May simulate keratosis follicularis (Darier disease) or pemphigus microscopically

Ancillary Studies

- DIF—negative
- Pathophysiology
- Etiology unknown

Differential Diagnosis

- Keratosis follicularis (Darier disease)
- Acantholytic acanthoma
- Incidental focal acantholytic dyskeratosis

The characteristic clinical findings and subtle focal nature of the histopathology help distinguish it from other acantholytic disorders. On occasion, a negative DIF result may help to exclude an immunobullous disorder.

Prognosis and Treatment

The condition is "transient" but may follow a chronic, protracted course. Avoidance of exacerbating factors, such as strenuous exercise, occlusion, and heat, is advised. Corticosteroids, antibiotics (for the antiinflammatory effect), phototherapy, or retinoids may offer some benefit.

GALLI-GALLI DISEASE

Galli-Galli disease is a rare form of Dowling-Degos disease wherein affected individuals develop intertriginous reticulated hyperpigmentation with scattered erythematous pruritic papules intermixed. Mutations in KRT5, POFUT1, and POGLUT1 have been observed in Galli-Galli disease. Microscopic features include rete elongation with keratinocyte hyperpigmentation, hypergranulosis with parakeratosis, and suprabasilar acantholysis

HERPETIC DERMATITIS

Clinical Findings

Herpesvirus infections may be caused by herpes simplex virus (HSV) or varicella-zoster virus (VZV). Infection with either agent can yield grouped or solitary vesicles on an erythematous base, which are variably hemorrhagic and crusted and may leave scarring. Skin manifestations of HSV or VZV infection often start with the development of very pruritic lesions on the face or scalp and disseminate in crops, resulting in lesions in different stages of evolution. Varicella infection used to be almost universal in childhood until the development of a highly effective childhood vaccination. When primary varicella zoster infection does occur, it is often accompanied by fever and may show features of central nervous system or pulmonary involvement, particularly in adults. After resolution, the virus remains dormant in ganglion nerves and can manifest at a later time—typically middle age to older adulthood—as herpes zoster, or shingles. These lesions are quite painful and are dermatomally distributed. The most common locations are on the forehead, associated with the trigeminal nerve; on the flank; along the thoracic nerve; and less likely down the upper or lower extremities. When these lesions clear, they may be associated with persistent painful neuralgia. If the lesions are not restricted to a dermatome, one should suspect an underlying immunocompromised state. In particular, disseminated zoster (defined by the presence of 10+ VZV lesions outside of the main affected dermatome) can be seen in patients with hematologic malignancy, iatrogenic immunosuppression, or HIV. Patients with HIV and zoster can rarely develop a chronic verrucous variant. HSV may be caused by serotype I or II, with the most common manifestation being the "cold sore," which develops around the mucocutaneous lip area. Lesions are provoked by sunlight, stress, or immunosuppression. The initial infection is often extensive and accompanied by fever, but the recurrence is usually limited in magnitude and discomfort. Genital herpes lesions typically arise on the penis, vulva, or perineum but may arise on the buttocks, thigh, or perianal area.

Histopathologic Features

Established lesions show epidermal necrosis that, if extensive, may result in an epidermal-dermal separation in a subepidermal plane. The blister cavity contains acantholytic cells and neutrophils (Fig. 5.28). The virally infected keratinocytes show intranuclear steel-gray inclusions, multinucleation, and balloon cell change epidermis and follicle. Necrotizing folliculitis and a lichenoid tissue reaction may be seen in prebullous lesions. The dermis shows a perivascular mononuclear inflammatory infiltrate. Endothelial cell swelling with necrotizing vasculitis often is seen, especially with VZV infection. In HIV-related infections, one may see verruciform epidermal changes or follicular involvement only. There are specific immunohistochemical stains targeting HSV and VZV, making it easy to confirm the diagnosis in cases where there is doubt.

Differential Diagnosis

The herpesvirus infections cannot reliably be distinguished from one another histopathologically with certainty. In addition, other viral infections showing reticular degeneration may enter the differential diagnosis and include orf, milker's nodules, smallpox, and vaccinia. These conditions usually do not confer the characteristic cytologic features of HSV or VZV infection, however.

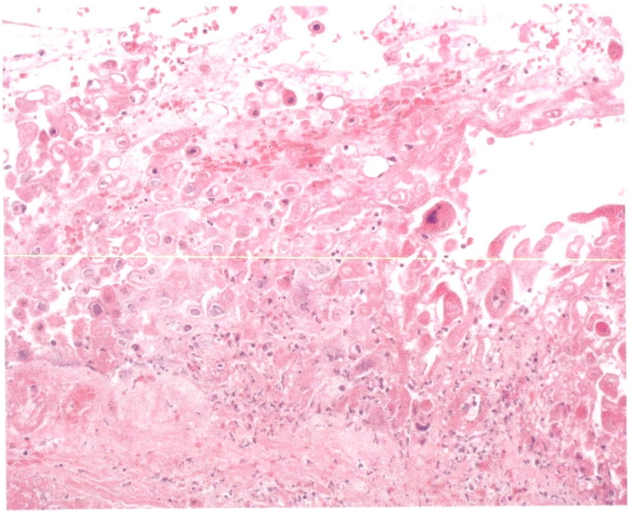

FIG. 5.28
Herpetic blister. Acantholytic keratinocytes with viral cytopathic changes.

Prognosis and Treatment

HSV is self-limiting, but recurrences are common, especially with stress, fatigue, or intense sun exposure. VZV is self-limiting but recurs in later adulthood as zoster. Herpes zoster infections are also self-limiting, but the pain may persist. Recurrences are rare. Granulomatous and lymphoid infiltrates may arise in chronic zoster scars. All of these infections may be treated with a variety of antiviral agents, such as acyclovir or valacyclovir.

INTRAEPIDERMAL BLISTER ASSOCIATED WITH EPIDERMOLYTIC HYPERKERATOSIS

There is a spectrum of lesions that may show the histopathologic feature of epidermolytic hyperkeratosis (EHK), ranging from keratoderma to the rare presentation of bullous congenital ichthyosiform erythroderma (BCIE). A vesicle may be seen within hyperkeratotic epidermis of such lesions. Vesicles in this setting result from intracellular edema and cell lysis ("epidermolysis" or "vesicular degeneration of the epidermis"). Intracellular edema is usually accompanied by the presence of clumps of granular material (representing dense aggregates of tonofilaments). Only in BCIE are blisters, skin fragility, and erosions clinically relevant.

EPIDERMOLYTIC HYPERKERATOSIS (BULLOUS CONGENITAL ICHTHYOSIFORM ERYTHRODERMA)

EHK, a condition characterized by abnormal keratohyalin granules, is caused by a defect in keratins 1 and 10, resulting in a distinct histopathologic presentation.

Clinical Findings

EHK manifests at birth as generalized erythroderma associated with vesicles and bullae. With time, the skin alterations progress to generalized verrucous hyperkeratosis, with prominent involvement of the flexural areas.

Histopathologic Features

The epidermis is acanthotic and hyperorthokeratotic, often with a verruciform architecture. The granular cell

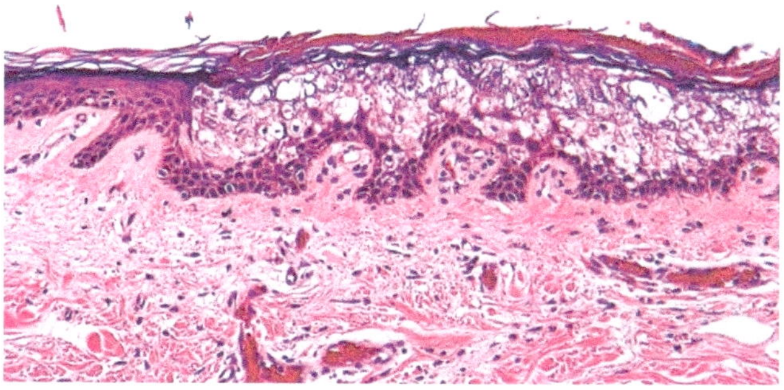

FIG. 5.29
Epidermolytic hyperkeratosis. Epidermis with granular and vacuolar changes in the upper layers.

layer is thickened because of a combination of increased amounts of abnormally formed large and irregularly shaped keratohyaline granules and variably sized perinuclear clear spaces within the keratinocytes of the stratum spinosum and granulosum (Fig. 5.29). There is reticulate light-staining material forming indistinct cell boundaries. Blisters are present within the epidermis. The keratinocytes surrounding an intraepidermal cleft are edematous.

Differential Diagnosis

The histopathologic changes are characteristic, but clinical correlation is important because features of EHK can also be found in keratodermas, acanthomas, or linear epidermal nevus.

Prognosis and Treatment

EHK follows a chronic course. An erythrodermic blistering presentation in early childhood typically changes to a verrucous, hyperkeratotic ichthyosiform phenotype. Retinoids or topical keratolytic therapy are often helpful in relieving some of the hyperkeratosis.

SUBEPIDERMAL BLISTERS

SUBEPIDERMAL BLISTER WITH NEUTROPHILS OR EOSINOPHILS

BULLOUS PEMPHIGOID

BP, the most common autoimmune subepidermal vesicular dermatitis, is associated with pathogenic autoantibodies to BP180 (also known as BPAG2 or type XVII collagen [COL17], a transmembranous protein) and autoantibodies to the BP antigen 230 (BPAG1, an intracellular component of the hemidesmosome).

Clinical Findings

BP typically affects elderly adults. Most patients are in the sixth through eighth decades of life. The clinical manifestations can be highly variable, including vesicular and nonvesicular lesions. During the nonbullous phase, patients tend to have generalized pruritus that can be associated with papular, eczematous, or urticarial lesions. The bullous stage manifests as blisters on normal or erythematous skin (Fig. 5.30). The blisters are tense with clear fluid before they erode and crust. The lesions preferentially affect flexural sites, the trunk, and the abdomen. There may be prurigo nodularis–like lesions (pemphigoid nodularis) or associated lichenoid lesions (lichen planus pemphigoides). Childhood pemphigoid is very rare. Infant pemphigoid affects the palms or soles and face preferentially, but in childhood BP, localized disease occurs on the genitalia, typically in girls. The oral mucosa is involved in 10% to 30% of patients with pemphigoid. Disease flares may be precipitated by UV light, radiation therapy, vaccination, or drugs (e.g., furosemide, NSAIDs). Between one-third and half of patients with BP may have neurologic disease, including cognitive impairment, stroke, Parkinson

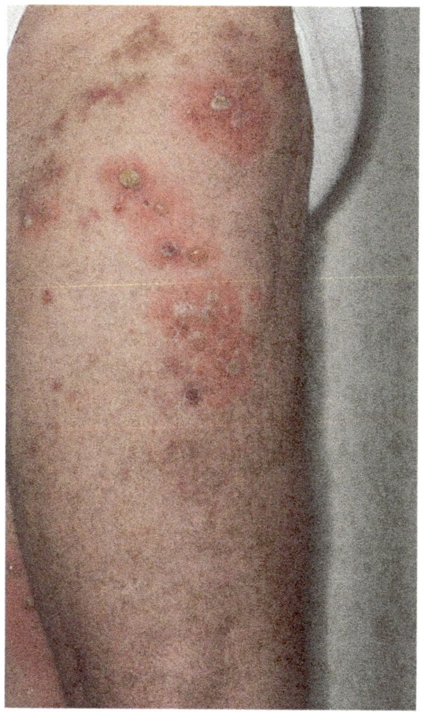

FIG. 5.30
Bullous pemphigoid. Multiple tense blisters on an erythematous base.

disease, or epilepsy. BP or BP-like lesions may develop in association with cancer therapy using checkpoint blockage inhibitors, and the clinical, microscopic, and immunologic features can be identical to those seen in idiopathic BP.

BULLOUS PEMPHIGOID—DISEASE FACT SHEET

Most common autoimmune blistering disorder

Patient Group

- ▸▸ Typically affects elderly adults but can occur at any age, including rarely infants and children
- ▸▸ Site of Involvement
- ▸▸ Widespread, trunk (lower abdomen), extremities, flexural sites; genital and acral sites in childhood variant
- ▸▸ May also be localized (often, to the lower extremities)
- ▸▸ Mucosal involvement present in a minority of affected patients

Clinical Findings

- ▸▸ Prodromal phase of erythema, urticaria, pruritus, or eczema
- ▸▸ Tense blisters on erythematous or normal skin, Nikolsky negative

Prognosis and Treatment

- ▸▸ Chronic disease with exacerbations and remissions
- ▸▸ Morbidity related to pruritus and superinfection of lesions
- ▸▸ Systemic corticosteroids are the treatment of choice but are associated with morbidity. High-potency topical steroids, steroid-sparing immunosuppressive agents, or tetracycline antibiotics with niacinamide are other options. Several clinical trials for new targeted therapies are underway

BULLOUS PEMPHIGOID—PATHOLOGIC FEATURES

Histopathologic Features

- ▸▸ Early lesions may show nonspecific changes of urticaria or dermatitis
- ▸▸ Dermal edema with eosinophil-rich mixed infiltrate
- ▸▸ Subepidermal vesicles with many eosinophils
- ▸▸ Eosinophilic epitheliotropism (i.e., eosinophils lining up at the basement membrane zone) and eosinophilic spongiosis are helpful clues

Ancillary Studies

Direct immunofluorescence

- ▸▸ Linear deposits of IgG, IgG4, and/or C3 at basement membrane zone (BMZ)
- ▸▸ Linear deposits of IgA are seen occasionally, particularly in patients with mucosal involvement
- ▸▸ Indirect immunofluorescence
- ▸▸ Linear IgG deposits at BMZ (70%)
- ▸▸ Salt-split skin preparations technique: "epidermal pattern" of IgG staining (deposits at blister "roof")
- ▸▸ Enzyme-linked immunosorbent assay: bullous pemphigoid (BP) serum with high reactivity to NC16 domain of BP180 (BPAG2)

Pathophysiology

- ▸▸ BP patients have circulating autoantibodies to extracellular noncollagenous (NC16) domain of BPAg2 (180 kD, type XVII collagen, COL17), a type II transmembrane protein that spans the lamina lucida and extends into the lamina densa; BPAg1 (230 kD), an intracellular component of the hemidesmosome; and a plakin family protein. BPAg2 (180 kD) contains the main pathogenic epitopes and is the primary target.

Differential Diagnosis

- ▸▸ Epidermolysis bullosa acquisita
- ▸▸ Linear IgA bullous dermatosis
- ▸▸ Mucous membrane pemphigoid
- ▸▸ Pemphigoid gestationis
- ▸▸ Anti–laminin $\gamma 1$ (p-200) pemphigoid

Histopathologic Features

During the nonbullous phase, the histopathologic findings may be indistinguishable from an allergic eczematous dermatitis with spongiosis and an urticarial tissue reaction, with superficial dermal mixed inflammatory cell infiltrate with eosinophils (Fig. 5.31). A clue to the diagnosis is the location of eosinophils immediately beneath the epidermis, tagging along the dermal-epidermal junction, or within a spongiotic epidermis (eosinophilic spongiosis; Fig. 5.32). If vesicles are clinically present, it is best to take a biopsy for microscopic analysis from the edge of the blister. One typically finds a subepidermal split associated with a polymorphous infiltrate composed of eosinophils admixed with neutrophils (Fig. 5.33). The density of the inflammatory cell infiltrate is variable. So-called cell-poor variants of BP may have minimal inflammation.

Ancillary Studies

- DIF studies of perilesional skin demonstrate the presence of fine linear deposits of IgG, IgG4, and/or C3 along the BMZ (Fig. 5.34A).

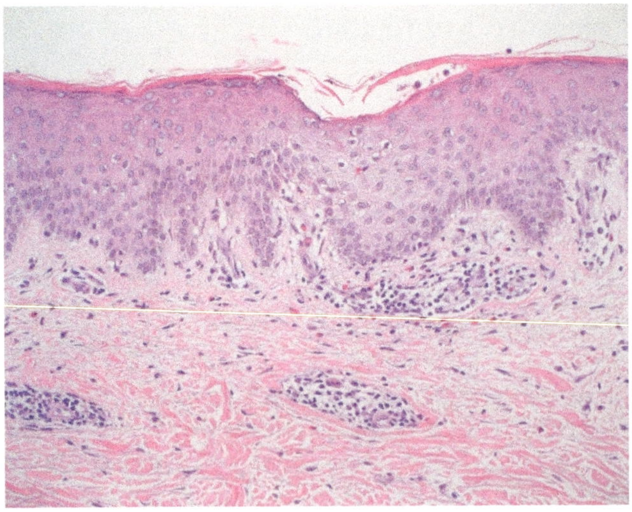

FIG. 5.31

Bullous pemphigoid. Early phase, with eosinophil tagging of the dermal-epidermal junction and focal spongiosis.

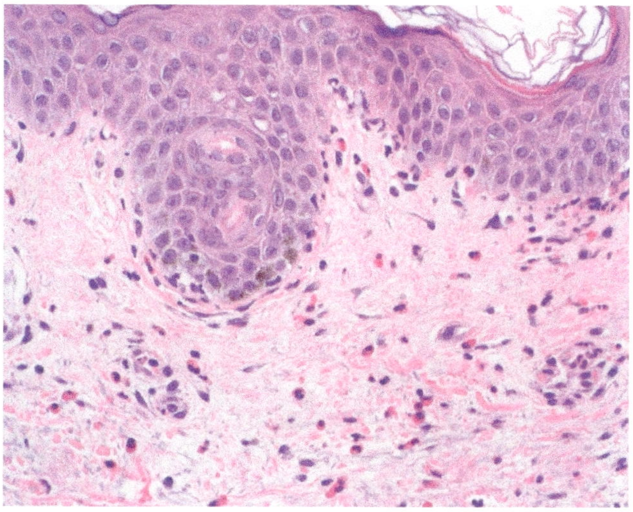

FIG. 5.32
Tagging of the dermal-epidermal junction with eosinophils.

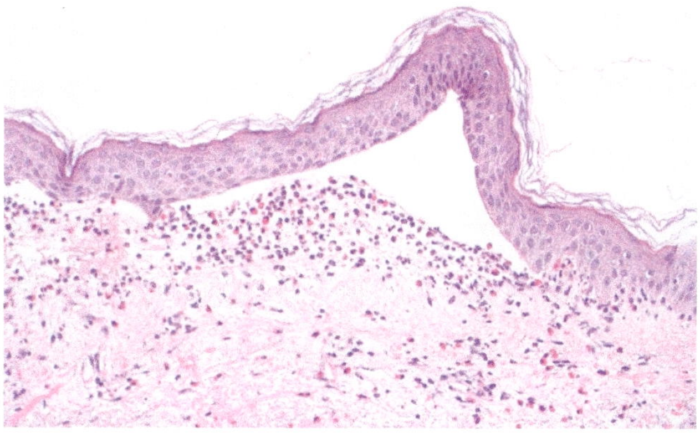

FIG. 5.33
Bullous pemphigoid. Eosinophil-rich subepidermal blister.

- IIF studies show linear deposition on monkey esophagus substrate (Fig. 5.34B) and epidermal pattern on salt-split skin substrate (Fig. 5.34C).
- Collagen type IV immunohistochemistry: staining on the blister floor.
- ELISA: BP serum with antibodies to NC16 domain of BP180; variable presence of antibodies to BP230.

Differential Diagnosis

The differential diagnosis is broad, especially if the histopathology of the urticarial phase of BP is included. After a subepidermal vesicular dermatitis is identified with a positive DIF test result, the main differential diagnosis is between cicatricial pemphigoid (CP) and EBA. BP can be distinguished from EBA by the salt-split skin technique. In BP, IgG is deposited on the blister roof (epidermal side of the split skin). In EBA, the immune deposits are located on the blister floor. ELISA is the definitive test to confirm BP but may miss up to 8% to 10% of cases, in which the antigen is exclusive to the typical NC16 region of BP180.

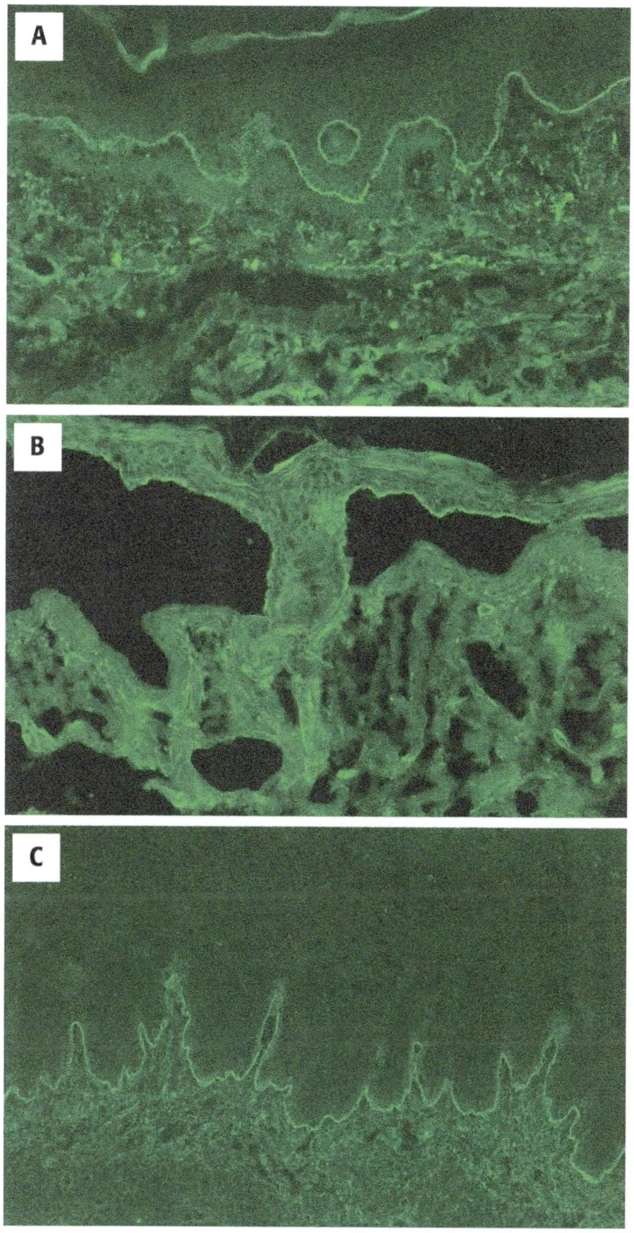

FIG. 5.34
Bullous pemphigoid. **A,** Direct immunofluorescence shows linear deposition of C3 at the dermal-epidermal junction. The same pattern is usually seen with IgG, with or without IgG4. **B,** Indirect immunofluorescence on salt-split skin shows linear deposition with IgG on the epidermal side of the artifactual blister. **C,** Indirect immunofluorescence on monkey esophagus substrate shows linear deposition with IgG.

Anti–laminin $\gamma 1$ (p200) pemphigoid is a subepidermal autoimmune bullous disorder with clinical features similar to BP but is instead associated with a neutrophil-rich subepidermal blister (similar to LABD and DH) and mixed or dermal deposition of IgG on salt-split skin IIF. The target autoantigen is a 200-kDa protein, which is identified as laminin $\gamma 1$ by immunoblotting or with ELISA, tests that are not widely available.

Prognosis and Treatment

BP is a chronic inflammatory disease with exacerbations and remissions. Systemic corticosteroids or other antiinflammatory/immunosuppressive agents are usually necessary. High-potency topical steroids have benefit with less morbidity. Tetracycline antibiotics combined with niacinamide can be quite effective in mild cases.

MUCOUS MEMBRANE PEMPHIGOID

MMP is a chronic autoimmune blistering disease caused by autoantibodies directed against components of the BMZ, including the subepithelial components, with predilection for mucosal surfaces and a tendency to heal with scarring (Fig. 5.35A). The term cicatricial pemphigoid (CP) was previously used synonymously with *mucous membrane pemphigoid* but is now reserved for cases in which there is evidence of scarring. Several tissue-bound antibodies to structural components of the BMZ have been identified, including antibodies to BP180, at times in conjunction with BP230. Other subtypes include laminin 332, which is composed of three subunits, $\alpha3\beta3\gamma2$ (previously termed epiligrin or laminin 5), collagen type VII, and $\alpha6\beta4$ integrin. CP is not considered a distinct disease entity but a clinical phenotype associated with a variety of different target antigens. The oral and conjunctival mucosa are most frequently involved by chronic painful erosions and adhesions. Other involved mucosal sites include the nasal cavity, pharynx, esophagus, larynx, and anogenital mucosa. The disease is associated with significant morbidity because of consequences of scarring. Conjunctival scarring may lead to blindness. Skin lesions develop in approximately one-quarter of patients with CP.

Anti–laminin 332 MMP is seen in up to approximately 20% of MMP patients, and about one-third of these patients have an associated malignancy, usually a solid tumor of the upper aerodigestive system. Patients with anti–laminin 332 tend to have prominent eye and mouth involvement. Additionally, the nasal and laryngeal mucosa are more frequently involved than in other subtypes. There is high mortality rate in patients presenting with blisters and cancer developing in close temporal proximity.

The histopathology and DIF findings of MMP and CP are similar to those of BP, inflammatory subtype, though often, there is a subepithelial split with fairly nonspecific inflammation (Fig. 5.35B). There are also variants with noninflammatory bulla. DIF frequently shows linear IgG, IgG4 (where available), and C3 but may also show IgA linear deposition. DIF of mucosal biopsies is more often positive than DIF of skin.

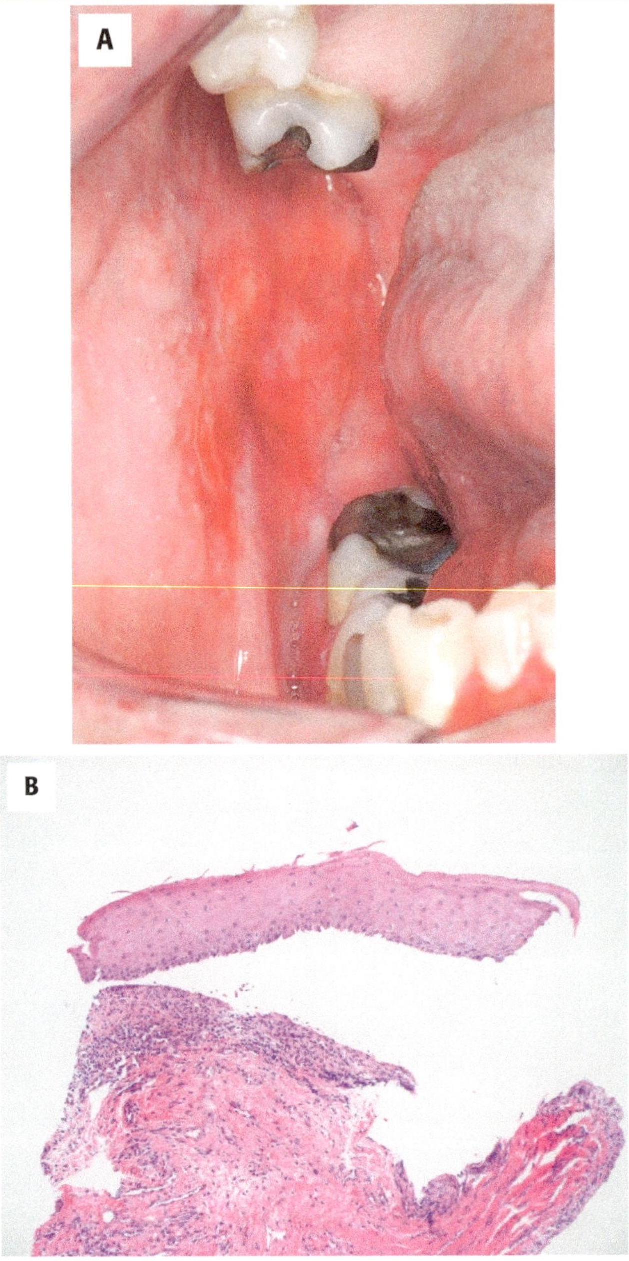

FIG. 5.35
Mucous membrane pemphigoid. **A**, Erosive mucositis. **B**, A complete submucosal split is observed. Associated inflammation can be variable.

Salt-split skin will show epidermal, dermal, or mixed pattern staining, depending on the target antigen. More than half of patients may have detectable circulating serum IgA autoantibodies. Combined IgA and IgG reactivity may be associated with more severe disease than in patients with isolated IgG. Immunoprecipitation or immunoblotting may be necessary to identify the pathogenic antibody target for patients with clinical MMP but with negative DIF results because this may allow documentation of autoantibodies to laminin 332 and prompt an investigation for malignancy.

PEMPHIGOID GESTATIONIS (HERPES GESTATIONIS)

Clinical Findings

Pemphigus gestationis presents with the abrupt onset of pruritic urticarial lesions on the trunk during late pregnancy or immediately postpartum. The cutaneous eruption rapidly progresses to a generalized pemphigoid-like picture (Fig. 5.36A). The mucous membranes, palms, and soles are typically spared. PG is associated with HLA-DR3 and HLA-DR4, and most patients have anti–human leukocyte antigen (HLA) antibodies.

PEMPHIGOID GESTATIONIS—CLINICAL FINDINGS

Patient Group
- ▸▸ Onset in second or third trimester
- ▸▸ Often flares up immediately postpartum
- ▸▸ Tends to be worse in subsequent pregnancies
- ▸▸ Unlike a clinical mimic, polymorphic eruption of pregnancy, can confer fetal risk, including prematurity or low birth weight

Site of Involvement
- ▸▸ Trunk, periumbilical early; extremities later

Clinical Findings
- ▸▸ Urticarial lesions and blisters
- ▸▸ Intense pruritus

Prognosis and Treatment
- ▸▸ Negligible maternal risk from lesions
- ▸▸ Risk of prematurity and bullous lesions in neonates
- ▸▸ Systemic corticosteroids are effective but may impact pregnancy

PEMPHIGOID GESTATIONIS—PATHOLOGIC FEATURES

Histopathologic Features
- ▸▸ Subepidermal blister
- ▸▸ Eosinophils, including eosinophilic spongiosis and eosinophilic epitheliotropism
- ▸▸ Dermal edema

Direct Immunofluorescence
- ▸▸ Linear deposits of C3 and often also IgG along basement membrane zone

Indirect Immunofluorescence
- ▸▸ Circulating antibodies in 25%, previously termed herpes gestationis (HG) factor
- ▸▸ Pathophysiology
- ▸▸ Autoantibodies to a variety of proteins, including BPAg2 (main epitope) and BPAg1, which activate the complement pathway

Differential Diagnosis
- ▸▸ Polymorphic eruption of pregnancy (pruritic urticarial papules and plaques of pregnancy)
- ▸▸ Drug reaction, eczema, allergic contact dermatitis
- ▸▸ Cholestatic pruritus of pregnancy

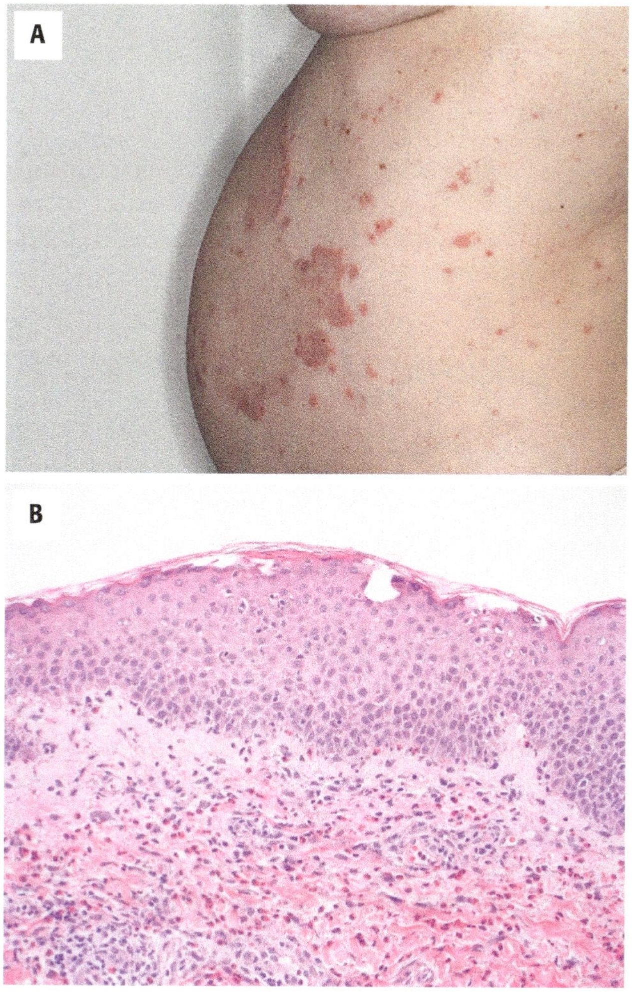

FIG. 5.36
Pemphigus gestationis. **A,** Tense blisters and erosions. **B,** Early changes include eosinophil tagging and eosinophilic spongiosis, with spongiosis.

Histopathologic Features

There is typically a subepidermal split with a mixed dermal infiltrate of lymphocytes and eosinophils (Fig. 5.36B). Eosinophils line up at the dermal-epidermal junction and are found within the blister cavity. Immunohistochemical staining on formalin-fixed paraffin-embedded tissue with C3d is reported to demonstrate linear positivity along the BMZ.

Ancillary Studies

DIF of perilesional skin shows a linear band of C3 along the BMZ. In salt-split skin specimens, staining is seen at the bottom of the epidermal fragment (blister roof). ELISA and immunoblotting can identify autoantibodies directed against BP180.

Differential Diagnosis

Clinically and histopathologically, PG needs to be primarily distinguished from the most common pregnancy-associated itchy eruption called polymorphic eruption of pregnancy (PEP; formerly, *pruritic urticarial papules and plaques of pregnancy* [PUPPP]). DIF studies are very helpful because no specific immune deposits are found in PEP. Other diseases that may clinically or histopathologically be confused with PG include drug reactions and eczema, especially allergic contact dermatitis. BP has similar histopathologic and IF features but typically presents in older patients.

Prognosis and Treatment

The clinical course is variable. Often there is spontaneous resolution, but the disease may flare up again, particularly at the time of delivery. Patients with PG may be at increased risk for other autoimmune diseases. For symptomatic treatment, corticosteroids are the treatment of choice.

POLYMORPHIC ERUPTION OF PREGNANCY (PEP; FORMERLY PRURITIC URTICARIAL PAPULES AND PLAQUES OF PREGNANCY)

Although not primarily a blistering disorder, PEP is described here because of the need to distinguish it from PG.

Clinical Findings

PEP manifests as pruritic urticarial papules and plaques during late term. The eruption usually begins in the abdominal striae, sparing the periumbilical area, face, palms, and soles, and spreads within a few days. Although spongiotic microvesicles may occur in PEP, fully developed blisters are rare. Occasionally, clinical lesions are annular or polycyclic.

Histopathologic Features

The histopathology is not distinct but can show spongiotic dermatitis with a mixed infiltrate of lymphocytes, neutrophils, and eosinophils associated and prominent dermal edema (Fig. 5.37).

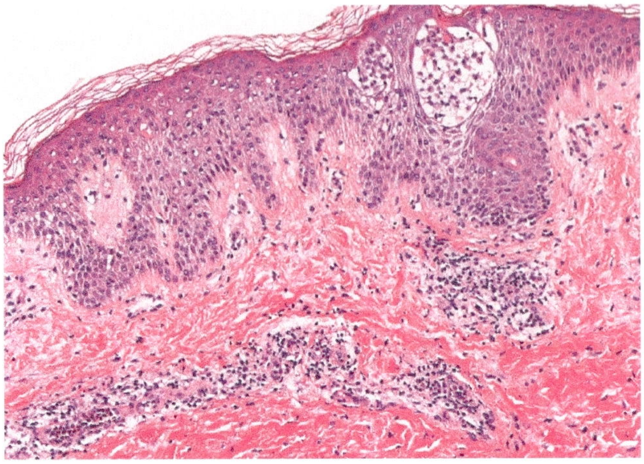

FIG. 5.37

Pruritic eruption of pregnancy (pruritic urticarial papules and plaques of pregnancy). Spongiosis with mixed inflammation.

Ancillary Studies

DIF study results are negative in PEP.

Differential Diagnosis

PEP is distinguished from PG by a combination of clinical and histopathologic findings. Periumbilical sparing, the lack of fully developed blisters, and a negative DIF test result permit a definite distinction.

Prognosis and Treatment

Topical or on occasion systemic steroids or oral antihistamines are often needed for symptomatic relief. The eruption usually resolves within 1 week after delivery.

LINEAR IgA BULLOUS DERMATOSIS—DISEASE FACT SHEET

Patient Group

- Usually adults in third decade of life or older
- May affect children, usually younger than 5 years of age (chronic bullous dermatosis of childhood)
- Patients receiving medications (e.g., vancomycin-induced linear IgA bullous dermatosis) or with underlying malignancy

Site of Involvement

- Trunk and extremities
- Mucosa

Clinical Findings

- Tense blisters and urticarial plaques
- Annular, polycyclic, and targetoid lesions
- "Cluster of jewels"

Prognosis and Treatment

- ▸▸ Chronic disease, with eventual remission common
- ▸▸ Treatment with oral dapsone or sulfapyridine, colchicine
- ▸▸ Cessation of drug for medication-induced disease

LINEAR IgA BULLOUS DERMATOSIS

Clinical Findings

LABD may be idiopathic or drug-induced most frequently. Infection, malignancy, and UV light–induced lesions may also be seen. Approximately half of the drug-induced cases are related to vancomycin. Children or adults may be affected. The disease in children has historically been referred to as *chronic bullous disease of childhood*. The disease manifests clinically as clear or hemorrhagic blisters on normal or erythematous skin (Fig. 5.38). The blisters may be discrete or arranged in a pattern ("cluster of jewels sign"). Vesicles may also form at the edge of annular lesions ("string of beads sign"). Crusts and erosion often develop. Rarely, prurigo-like lesions are seen. In children, the lesions tend to preferentially affect the abdomen, hands, feet, anogenital region, or perioral region. In adults, involvement of the trunk and extremities is most common. Oral mucosal involvement is common in both adults and children.

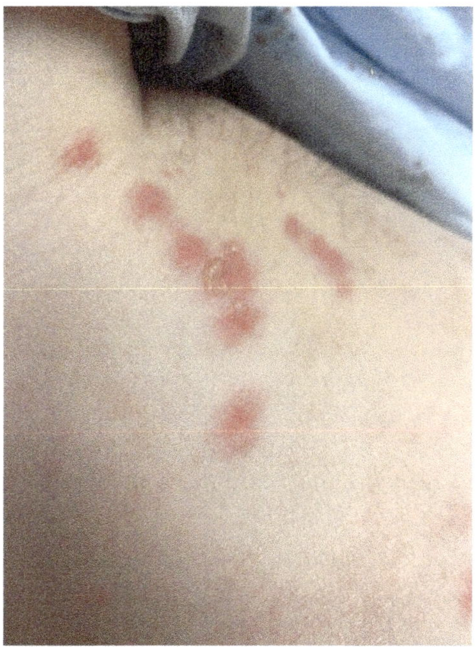

FIG. 5.38

Linear IgA bullous dermatosis. Intact vesicles arranged in an annular configuration.

Histopathologic Features

Early urticarial lesions may show neutrophilic microabscesses in the papillary dermis and clusters or strings of neutrophils at the dermal-epidermal junction (Fig. 5.39). The typical microscopic picture shows a neutrophil-rich subepidermal blister (Fig. 5.40), which may be multiloculated, and focal spongiosis may be seen. The number of polymorphonuclear cells and the proportion of neutrophils to eosinophils are highly variable.

Ancillary Studies

DIF studies of perilesional skin show linear deposits of IgA at the BMZ (see Fig. 5.41). IIF studies with IgA

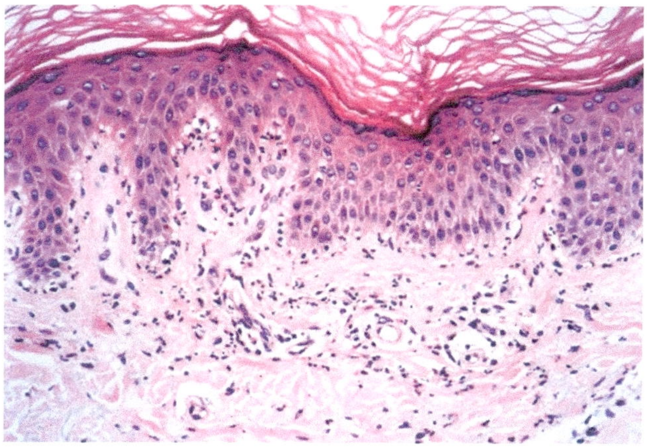

FIG. 5.39

Linear IgA bullous dermatosis. Urticarial phase with string of neutrophils along the dermal-epidermal junction.

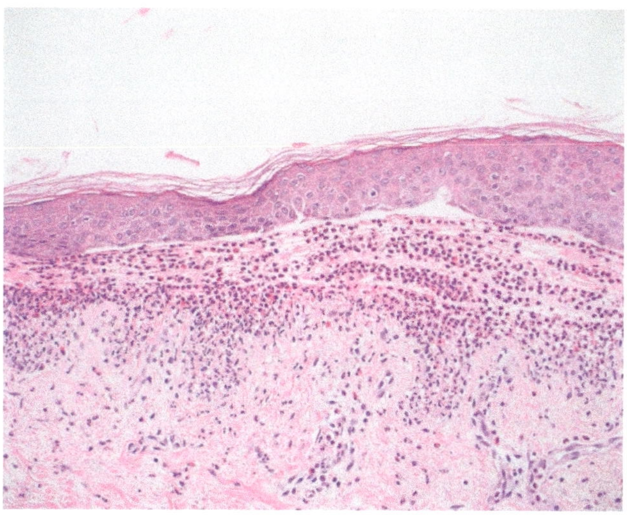

FIG. 5.40

Linear IgA bullous dermatosis. Subepidermal blister with polymorphonuclear cells.

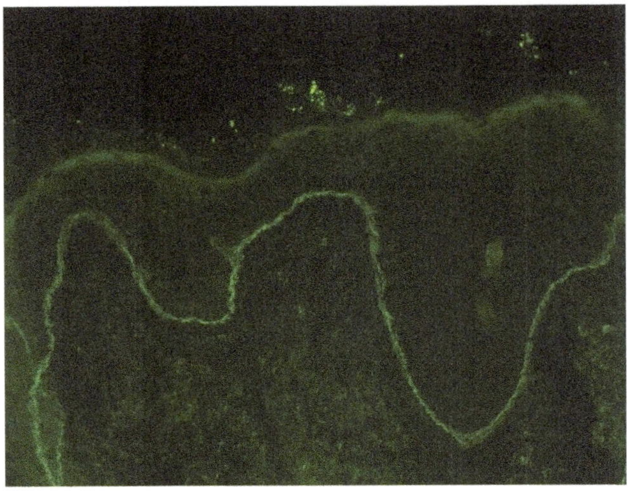

FIG. 5.41

Linear IgA bullous dermatosis. Direct immunofluorescence of perilesional skin reveals linear IgA deposits at the dermal-epidermal junction.

LINEAR IgA BULLOUS DERMATOSIS—PATHOLOGIC FEATURES

Histopathologic Features

- Neutrophilic papillitis with focal subepidermal clefting in early lesions
- Subepidermal blister with neutrophils and eosinophils in established lesions

Ancillary Studies

Direct Immunofluorescence

- Strong linear IgA deposits at basement membrane zone (BMZ)

Indirect Immunofluorescence

- Linear IgA deposits at the BMZ on monkey esophagus substrate
- Salt-split skin preparations: bind to the epidermal side (blister roof), and occasionally to the dermal side (blister floor), or both locations

Pathophysiology

- Autoantibodies to a variety of antigens in the lamina lucida and lamina densa
- Linear IgA bullous dermatosis (LABD) is a heterogenous disease resulting from autoantibodies directed to a variety of proteins (e.g., LABD97, 285 kD, 250 kD, collagen type VII, BPAg2, BPAg1, and 200-kDa laminin-γ1 chain)
- Lamina lucida type: target antigen is 97-kDa LAD-1 (LABD97) antigen represents a cleaved ectodomain of BPAg2
- Lamina densa-type: target antigens are dermal proteins, some of which bind to anchoring fibrils (comprised of collagen VII)

Differential Diagnosis

- Bullous pemphigoid, especially anti-200 pemphigoid
- Epidermolysis bullosa acquisita
- Dermatitis herpetiformis
- Arthropod bite blister

conjugate show linear deposition along the BMZ with monkey esophagus substrate and epidermal or, less frequently, dermal or mixed pattern with salt-split skin substrate.

Differential Diagnosis

LABD can be difficult to distinguish from BP or DH clinically and by routine microscopy. DIF studies are critical for the diagnosis. The presence of strong linear IgA supports a diagnosis of LABD. It is controversial whether the concomitant presence of linear IgG is compatible with LABD or should prompt reclassification as a form of pemphigoid.

Prognosis and Treatment

It is important to recognize and remove or replace inciting medications or treat any associated malignancy. Patients tend to respond well to dapsone or sulfapyridine, though corticosteroids and/or steroid-sparing immunosuppressive agents may be required.

DERMATITIS HERPETIFORMIS

Clinical Findings

DH, a gluten-sensitive dermopathy, is an autoimmune bullous dermatosis that is closely related to celiac disease. Both are associated with IgA autoantibodies to transglutaminase. Patients present with symmetric grouped (herpetiform) papules and vesicles, which tend to be intensely pruritic. There may be a spectrum of morphology, including urticarial plaques, papules, and erosions. There is a predilection for the extensor surfaces (e.g., elbows, knees). Other common sites include the buttocks, sacrum, face, and neck (Fig. 5.42). An unusual clinical manifestation is the presence of purpura and petechiae in this anatomic distribution. Most patients (90%) have an associated gluten-sensitive enteropathy. There may be overt celiac disease or subclinical manifestations of enteropathy, such as iron deficiency. DH may be associated with other autoimmune disorders, most commonly thyroid disease.

DERMATITIS HERPETIFORMIS—DISEASE FACT SHEET

Patient Group

- Association with gluten-sensitive enteropathy
- Preferred age group: third to fifth decade; rare in elderly, infants, or children

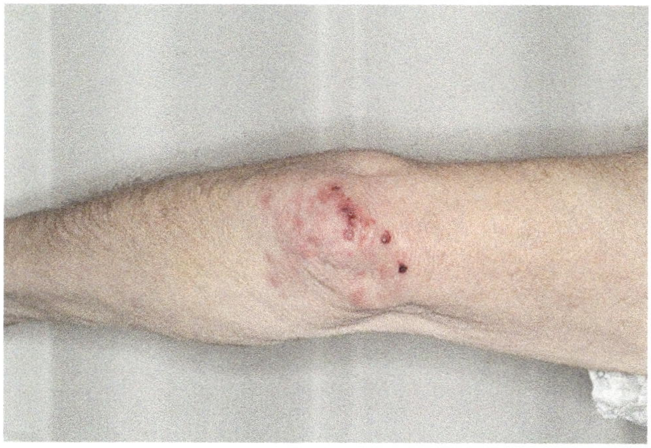

FIG. 5.42
Dermatitis herpetiformis. Small grouped pruritic vesicles and erosions on extensor surface.

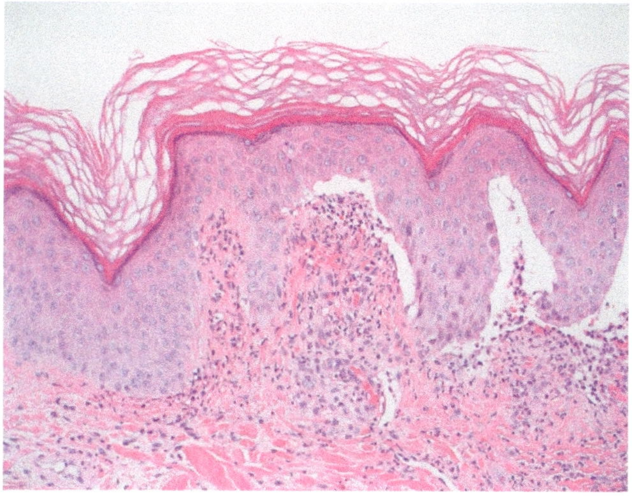

FIG. 5.43
Dermatitis herpetiformis. Neutrophilic microabscesses in papillary dermis, with subepidermal separation.

- Whites, male > female (female more common before age 20 years)
- 80% to 90% with human leukocyte antigen (HLA) DR3, HLA DQw2

Site of Involvement

- Symmetric distribution; preference for extensor surfaces
- Scalp, sacral region, shoulders

Clinical Findings

- Grouped (herpetiform) pruritic papules and small vesicles
- Urticarial plaques, consequence of pruritus such as erosions, postinflammatory pigment alteration

Prognosis and Treatment

- Dapsone and gluten-free diet are cornerstones of treatment

Histopathologic Features

Collections of neutrophils and, to a lesser extent, eosinophils are present within edematous dermal papillae (papillary microabscesses) of early lesions (Fig. 5.43).

DERMATITIS HERPETIFORMIS—PATHOLOGIC FEATURES

Histopathologic Features

- Neutrophilic microabscesses at tips of dermal papillae
- Subepidermal blister

Direct Immunofluorescence

- Granular IgA deposits in dermal papillae and along the basement membrane zone

Indirect Immunofluorescence

- Negative
- Indirect immunofluorescence with IgA on monkey esophagus substrate may be used to identify antiendomysial antibodies

Pathophysiology

- Autoimmune IgA antibodies

Differential Diagnosis

- Linear IgA bullous dermatosis
- Bullous lupus erythematosus
- Bullous pemphigoid

Subsequently, multilocular or unilocular subepidermal vesicles form. The blister cavity contains neutrophils, eosinophils, and fibrin. Perivascular lymphocytes may be present, occasionally with evidence of mild vascular damage in the superficial dermis. Biopsies submitted to evaluate for DH may show nonspecific findings, including scar or changes caused by scratching, yet may have diagnostic features of DH on DIF.

Ancillary Studies

DIF shows granular deposits of IgA in the dermal papillae and along the BMZ of perilesional skin (Fig. 5.44). Occasionally, IgM or C3 may also show this pattern. A rare manifestation of DH on DIF is the so-called fibrillary pattern, wherein fibrils rather than granules of IgA are present in the dermal papillae and along the BMZ. The optimal location for biopsy when DH is suspected is normal-appearing skin, located 1 cm away from skin lesions. IgA deposition tends to disappear after about 2 years of gluten avoidance, but it will not be altered with dapsone treatment. IIF may document antiendomysial IgA autoantibodies on monkey esophagus. ELISA may document the epidermal transglutaminase (eTG3) antigen, though this test is not widely available. This antibody cross-reacts with tissue transglutaminase (tTG3), the autoantigen of gluten-sensitive enteropathy, and can be useful in assessing bowel involvement and diet adherence. These tests are not 100% sensitive, so triggering a flare with a gluten challenge after 1 month of strict gluten avoidance is an accepted diagnostic option.

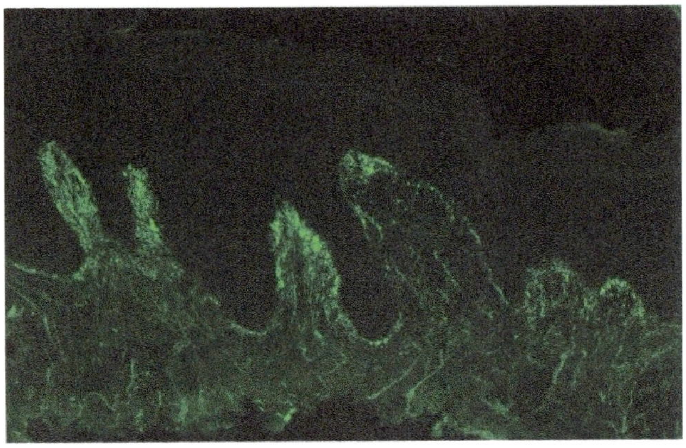

FIG. 5.44

Dermatitis herpetiformis. Direct immunofluorescence: Granular deposits of IgA in tips of dermal papillae and along the basement membrane zone.

Differential Diagnosis

Histopathologically, DH may be difficult to distinguish from LABD. Clinical context (e.g., history of vancomycin use versus gluten-sensitive enteropathy, anatomic distribution of lesions) and DIF findings (linear versus granular deposits of IgA) usually allow for a definitive diagnosis.

Prognosis and Treatment

The treatment of DH includes dapsone and a gluten-free diet. DH shows an association with Hashimoto thyroiditis. There is also an increased risk for enteropathy-associated intestinal T-cell lymphoma.

BULLOUS NEUTROPHILIC DERMATOSIS (SWEET SYNDROME)

Neutrophilic dermatosis refers to a sterile infiltrate of neutrophils which commonly presents with tender, bright red pseudo-vesicular or vesicular skin lesions. Neutrophilic dermatoses may herald the presence of malignancies, in particular leukemia and myelodysplastic syndrome; chronic inflammatory diseases, such as inflammatory bowel disease; drugs (e.g., granulocyte colony-stimulating factor); miscellaneous autoimmune diseases; and pregnancy.

Clinical Findings

The classic presentation of neutrophilic dermatosis is characterized by the development of tender erythematous

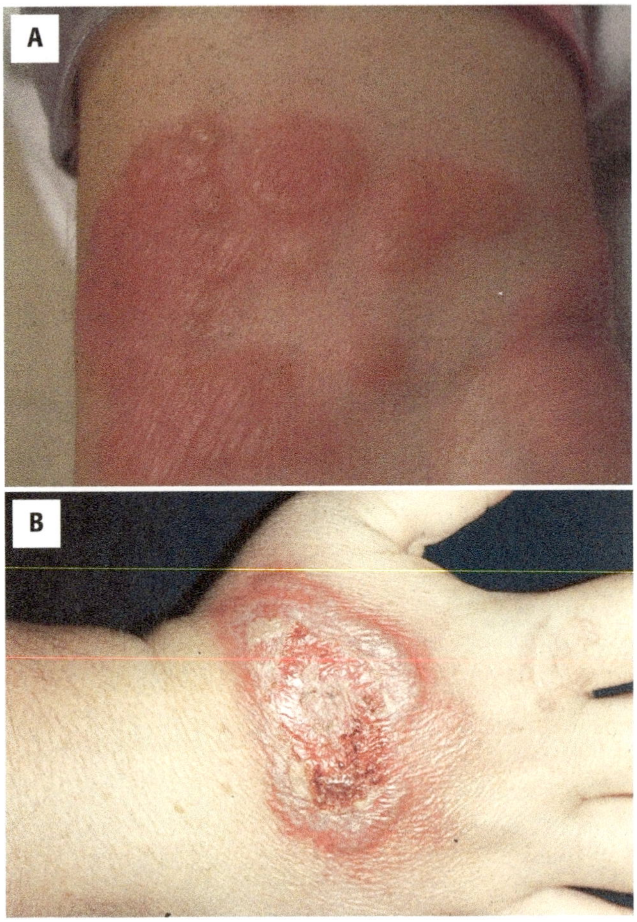

FIG. 5.45

Bullous Sweet syndrome. Erythematous urticarial plaques (**A**) and blister (**B**).

nodules and plaques on the skin, which may become bullous (Fig. 5.45), along with fever and leukocytosis. Skin lesions are typically found in the head and neck region and upper extremities.

Histopathologic Features

Lesions of bullous neutrophilic dermatosis are characterized by marked edema in the superficial dermis (Fig. 5.46), permitting separation of the epidermis from the dermis. Sheets of neutrophils are present in the dermis, and bystander vascular damage may be observed. A clue to distinction from vasculitis is that while there may be vascular damage, the damaged vessels are not the focal point of the inflammatory reaction.

Ancillary Studies

Special stains for microorganisms (in particular, a Gram stain) may be needed to evaluate for a possible cellulitis.

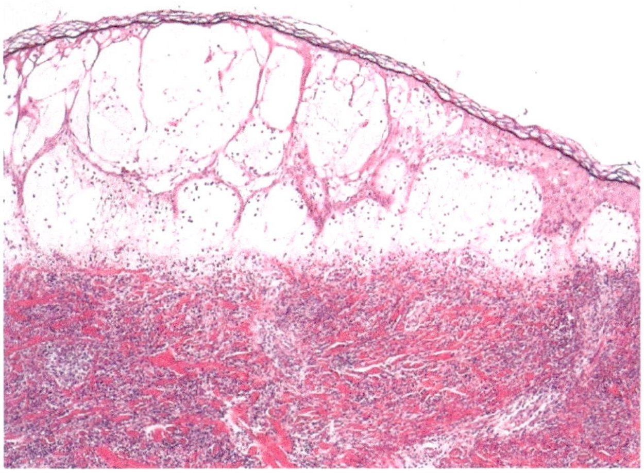

FIG. 5.46
Bullous Sweet syndrome. Subepidermal vesicular dermatitis with marked dermal edema and numerous neutrophils.

DIF is nonspecific in neutrophilic dermatosis, which is helpful when a distinction from an autoimmune bullous disorder is needed.

Differential Diagnosis

Neutrophilic dermatosis with or without a blister needs to be distinguished from an infection, which requires clinical correlation, special stains, and tissue cultures. If blood tests show a significant left shift among myeloid cells, there may be concern for leukemia, but the presence of a high proportion of mature neutrophils is reassuring against an acute myeloid leukemia. Other neutrophil-rich subepidermal vesicular dermatitides, such as LABD, can readily be distinguished from bullous neutrophilic dermatosis by DIF and clinical features. The differential diagnosis includes also pustular drug reactions and bullous lupus erythematosus.

Prognosis and Treatment

Clinical course can vary, depending on factors driving the process. The most effective treatment is oral corticosteroids.

BULLOUS LUPUS ERYTHEMATOSUS

Blisters may develop in the setting of acute, subacute, or chronic cutaneous lupus erythematosus. In this setting, the histopathology is that of vesicular lichenoid dermatitis (see below).

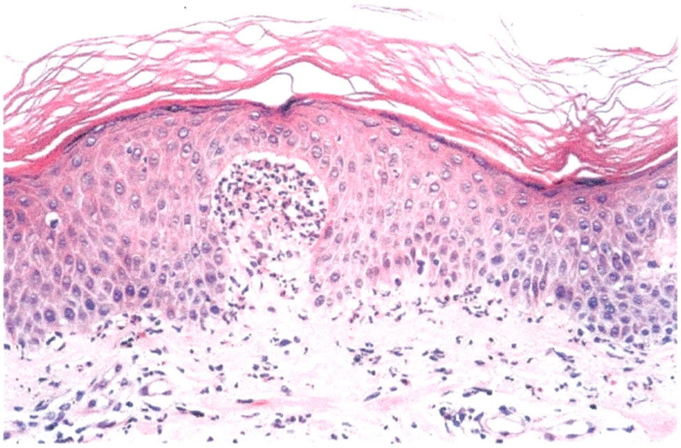

FIG. 5.47
Bullous lupus erythematosus. Clusters of neutrophils in the papillary dermis.

The term *bullous lupus erythematosus* in the strict sense is used to refer to a rare presentation of systemic lupus as a primarily blistering eruption histopathologically characterized by a subepidermal neutrophil-rich vesicular dermatitis. The histopathology shows overlap with inflammatory EBA, DH, and linear IgA dermatosis. Early lesions may show clusters of neutrophils in the papillary dermis without blister formation (Fig. 5.47). DIF reveals linear BMZ deposits of IgG, C3, and often IgA. Bullous lupus is mediated by autoantibodies to type VII collagen, as with EBA. These entities can be distinguished by the presence of photosensitivity and serologic or other evidence of lupus erythematosus in the former. In addition, bullous lupus is less likely to be associated with the formation of milia on healing.

ARTHROPOD BITES

Although arthropod bites commonly show intraepidermal edema (spongiosis) or mechanical disruption from the arthropod proboscis, the epidermis may be fairly unremarkable. However, dermal edema can be prominent and may lead to a subepidermal blister. Typically, other features of a hypersensitivity reaction (superficial and deep dermal perivascular lymphoeosinophilic infiltrate with variable evidence of vascular damage) are present (Fig. 5.48A), as may be abundant eosinophils and even flame figures (Fig. 5.48B).

LICHENOID INTERFACE DERMATITIS WITH SUBEPITHELIAL VESICULATION

Interface changes at the dermal-epidermal junction with levels of lichenoid inflammation may lead to separation of the epidermis from the dermis. This phenomenon may occur in any interface dermatitis, including graft-versus-host disease (Fig. 5.49), lichen

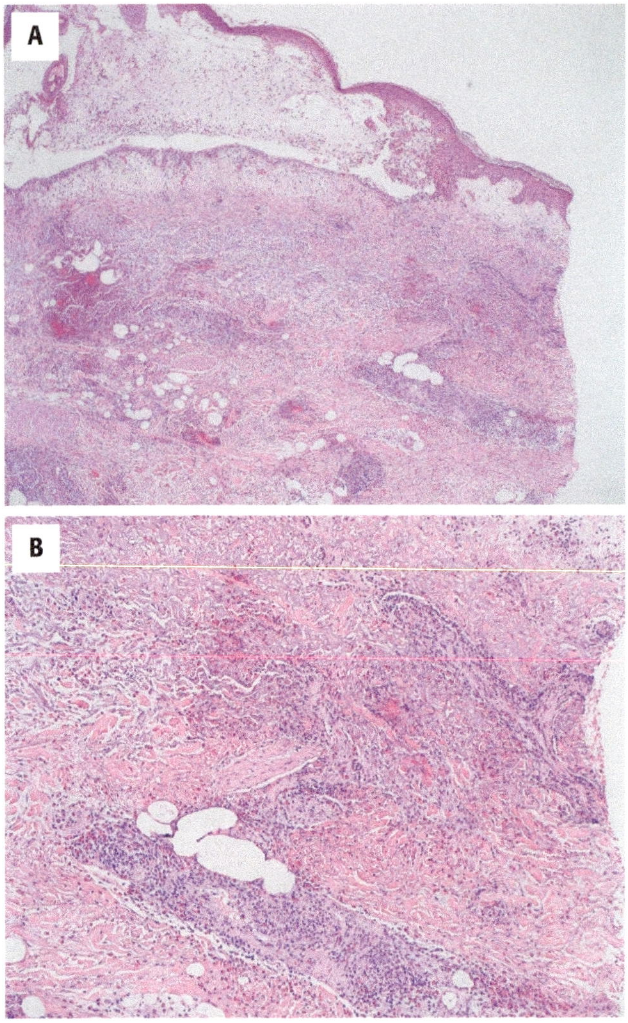

FIG. 5.48

Bullous arthropod bite reaction. **A,** Subepidermal blister. **B,** Many eosinophils in both the superficial and deep dermis, occasionally with flame figures.

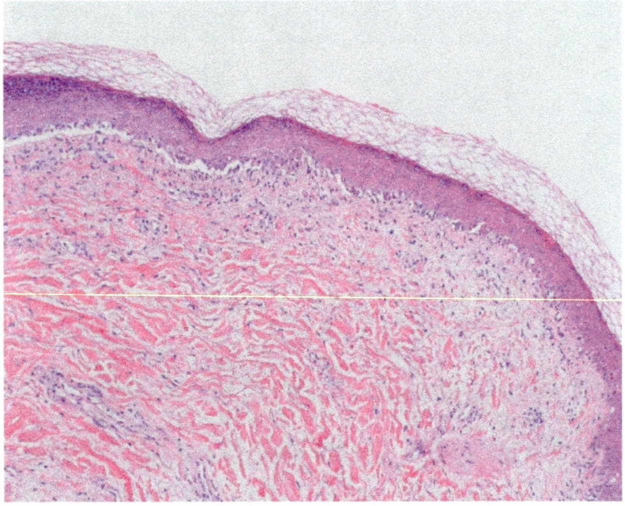

FIG. 5.49

Bullous graft-versus-host disease. Vacuolar interface changes with subepidermal separation.

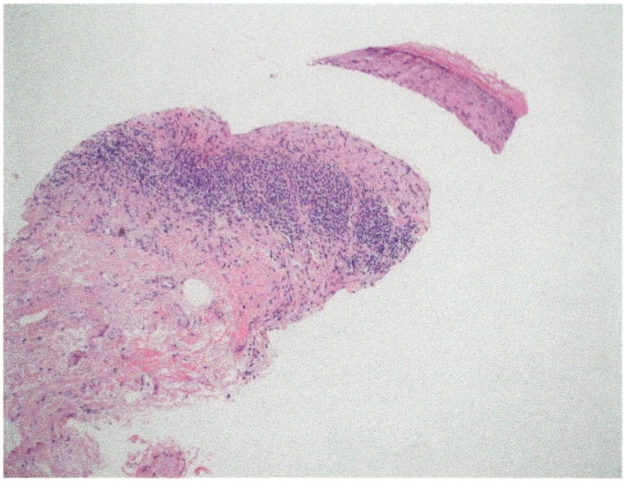

FIG. 5.50

Bullous vulvar lichen planus. Separation of epidermis from the dermis associated with lichenoid inflammation. Also, consider lichen planus pemphigoides, which shows linear deposition of IgG, IgG4, and C3 on direct immunofluorescence.

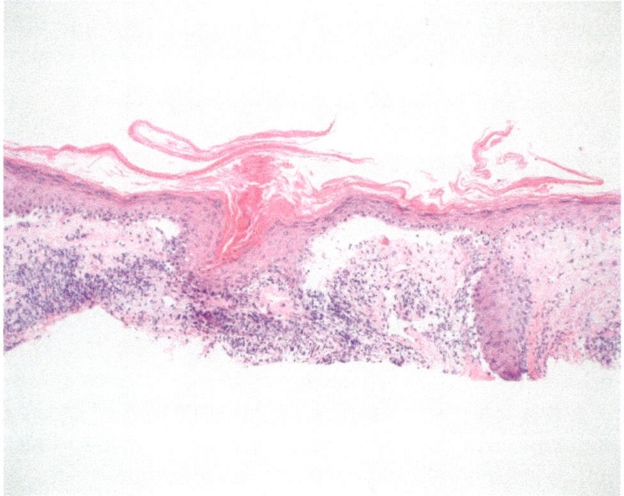

FIG. 5.51

Chronic cutaneous lupus erythematosus, discoid type. Brisk vacuolar interface inflammation with associated subepidermal separation, superficial perivascular lymphocytic inflammation, and follicular hyperkeratosis.

planus (Fig. 5.50), erythema multiforme, fixed drug reaction, lupus erythematosus (Fig. 5.51), and reactions observed in patients undergoing immunotherapy (e.g., checkpoint blockade inhibitors) for cancer. One may also include bullous lesions of mycosis fungoides, in which a dense neoplastic infiltrate of lymphocytes contributes to disruption of the dermal-epidermal junction. On occasion, PNP may lack detectable acantholysis in a biopsy sample and instead manifest as lichenoid vesicular dermatitis.

Histopathologically, clues to the presence of a lichenoid vesicular dermatitis are best found at the edge of a blister or at the base of the blister roof. There is a

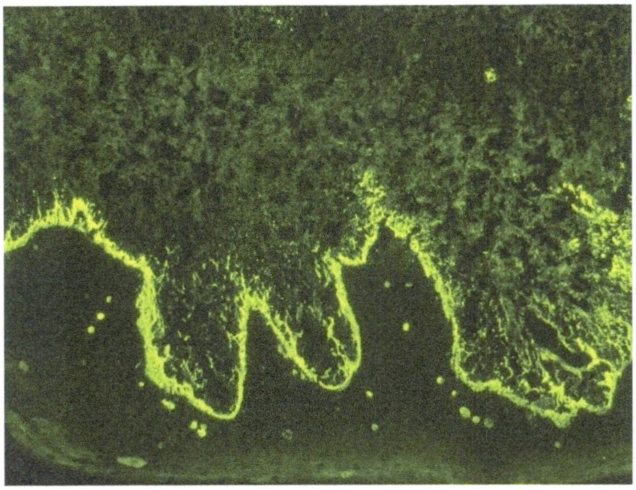

FIG. 5.52
Lichenoid inflammatory pattern. Direct immunofluorescence shows shaggy deposition of fibrinogen along the dermal-epidermal junction.

variably dense lymphocytic infiltrate at the dermal-epidermal junction associated with Civatte bodies, basal layer vasculopathy, or squamatization of the basal cell layer. Apoptotic keratinocytes or foci of necrosis may be seen at the dermal-epidermal junction or within the spinous cell layer.

To differentiate the various disease processes that may present as subepidermal vesicular lichenoid dermatitis, clinical correlation is paramount (e.g., status post–hematopoietic cell transplant, history of drug exposure, presence of other clinical lesions of lichen planus). There are also histopathologic clues that may help narrow the differential diagnosis (e.g., hyperchromatic atypical lymphocytes in mycosis fungoides, prominent granular cell layer and epidermal rete ridge saw-toothing in lichen planus, numerous eosinophils in a drug hypersensitivity reaction).

On DIF, a lichenoid tissue reaction characterized by scattered and clumped cytoid bodies with multiple conjugates, as well as shaggy fibrinogen along the BMZ, is typically seen (Fig. 5.52). DIF may also lend clues to lupus or PNP.

SUBEPIDERMAL VESICLE WITH NO OR ONLY MINIMAL INFLAMMATION

The spectrum of subepidermal vesicular dermatoses with minimal or no inflammation includes inherited and acquired EB, mechanical blisters, blisters related to physical trauma (e.g., heat, cold, friction), blisters related to depositions or metabolic disorders (e.g., amyloid, diabetes, porphyria, pseudoporphyria), TEN, or pauci-inflammatory variants of previously described processes (e.g., pauci-inflammatory BP or CP). Only diseases that have not previously been discussed are mentioned here.

EPIDERMOLYSIS BULLOSA ACQUISITA—DISEASE FACT SHEET

Patient Group
- May occur at any age but usually affects adults, ages 40 to 50 years
- Associated with increased rate of inflammatory bowel disease

Classic Presentation (65%)
- Skin fragility with erosions from minor trauma
- Blisters on noninflamed acral skin
- Healing with scars and milia
- Subclinical oropharyngeal and conjunctival involvement

Bullous Pemphigoid Like (25%)
- Tense blisters on erythematous base
- Widespread eruption involving trunk and extremities

Cicatricial Pemphigoid Like (10%)
- Mucosal involvement with erosions and scars

Prognosis and Treatment
- Often chronic, refractory disease, requiring oral corticosteroids and steroid-sparing immunosuppressive agents; potential for spontaneous remission

EPIDERMOLYSIS BULLOSA ACQUISITA

EBA is an immunobullous disorder with antibodies to type VII collagen, which is the major component of the anchoring fibrils of the dermal-epidermal junction. There are noninflammatory (i.e., mechanobullous) and inflammatory, and these manifestations may both be present in the same patient.

Clinical Findings

In the classic form of EBA, the skin is fragile, and blisters typically occur on noninflamed skin at trauma-prone areas, such as the dorsal aspects of the hands and feet (Fig. 5.53). The blisters tend to heal with atrophic scars. Associated milia and pigmentary changes are common. Although EBA is usually noninflammatory or pauci-inflammatory, the inflammatory variant simulating pemphigoid may occur. Patients may have concomitant inflammatory bowel disease.

Histopathologic Features

Skin biopsy of EBA shows a subepidermal blister with variable, usually minimal inflammation. If inflammation is present, it tends to be neutrophil-predominant, with an admixture of lymphocytes and eosinophils.

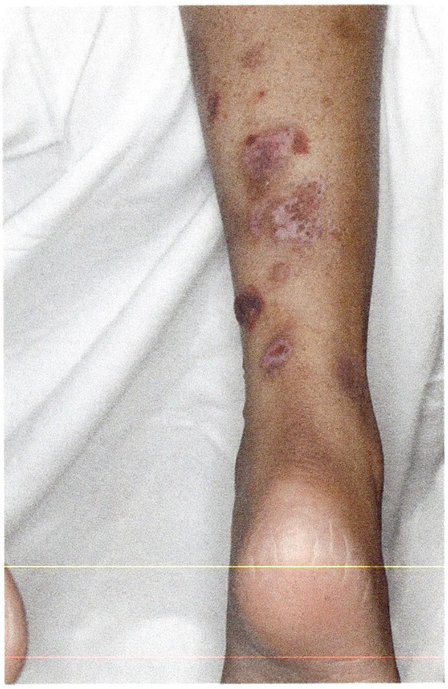

FIG. 5.53
Epidermolysis bullosa acquisita. Tense blisters with scarring.

Ancillary Studies

DIF of perilesional skin reveals IgG deposits in a continuous linear band along the BMZ. In salt-split skin preparations, the immune reactants are deposited on the dermal side of the blister (blister bottom). IIF with monkey esophagus substrate shows IgG deposition in a linear pattern. ELISA for collagen VII antibodies or immunoblotting is required for definitive differentiation of EBA from the pemphigoid variants with a dermal pattern on salt-split skin.

Electron microscopy (EM) can demonstrate a dermal-epidermal split and immunoglobulin deposition on anchoring fibrils at the level of the sublamina densa, though this technique is not typically pursued in clinical practice.

> **EPIDERMOLYSIS BULLOSA ACQUISITA—PATHOLOGIC FEATURES**
>
> **Histopathologic Features**
> - Classic variant: subepidermal noninflammatory or pauci-inflammatory blister; dermal fibrosis may be seen
> - Bullous pemphigoid–like variant: subepidermal blister with neutrophils and, to a lesser extent, eosinophils; eosinophilic spongiosis may be present
>
> **Ancillary Studies**
> - Direct immunofluorescence shows linear IgG (with or without C3) deposits at basement membrane zone
> - Indirect immunofluorescence salt-split skin preparations technique shows localization of IgG to blister base ("dermal pattern")
>
> **Pathophysiology**
> - Autoimmune antibodies to type VII collagen (290 kD)
>
> **Differential Diagnosis**
> - Bullous pemphigoid, cicatricial pemphigoid, or mucous membrane pemphigoid
> - Bullous lupus erythematosus
> - Linear IgA bullous dermatosis
> - Porphyria cutanea tarda
> - Pseudoporphyria
> - Congenital epidermolysis bullosa

Differential Diagnosis

Microscopic mimics of EBA include inherited dystrophic epidermolysis bullosa (DEB), BP, CP, porphyria, and pseudoporphyria, entities at all may show pauci-inflammatory subepidermal blistering on histopathology. Clinical and immunofluorescence findings are critical. In particular, DIF and IIF studies with salt-split skin preparations allow for a distinction of EBA from pemphigoid variants. Urine or serologic porphyrin studies, along with distinctive DIF findings, can differentiate EBA from porphyria variants.

Prognosis and Treatment

EBA is a chronic condition usually requiring systemic corticosteroids and steroid-sparing immunosuppressive agents. There is an association with inflammatory bowel disease, especially Crohn's disease.

PORPHYRIA CUTANEA TARDA

Porphyria is a metabolic disorder caused by deficiency or dysfunction of enzymes involved in the biosynthesis of heme. Several enzyme defects and clinical variants exist. All porphyria variants are inherited, including some forms of PCT, except for the acquired variant of PCT. PCT, the most common form of porphyria, predominantly affects the skin. It is associated with deficiency of uroporphyrinogen decarboxylase, which leads to accumulation of uroporphyrins.

Clinical Findings

PCT usually affects adults and manifests in men in their 40s and 50s, and women following menopause. PCT may be hereditary (enzyme deficiency in all tissues) or acquired (enzyme deficiency restricted to the liver). As

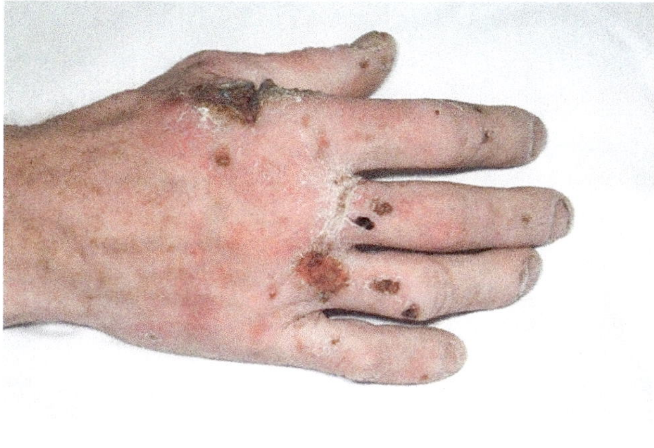

FIG. 5.54

Porphyria cutanea tarda. Small, eroded vesicles on the dorsum of the hands that heal with scarring and milia formation.

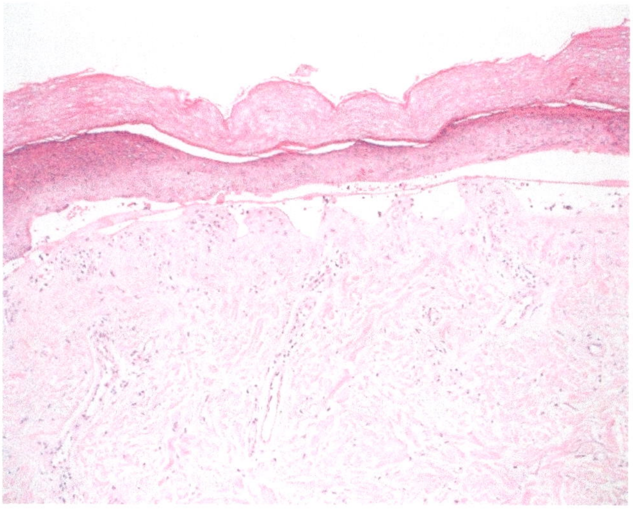

FIG. 5.55

Porphyria cutanea tarda. Noninflamed subepidermal blister. The dermal papillae are rigid ("festooning").

with other types of porphyria, PCT confers photosensitivity. Skin manifestations include blisters, erosions, milia, scars, hypertrichosis, and pigmentary alterations. The dorsal hands and forearms are commonly affected (Fig. 5.54).

Histopathologic Features

The classic histopathologic picture is that of a pauci-inflammatory subepidermal vesicle (see Fig. 5.55). Because of the deposition of glycoproteins in and around upper dermal vessels, the dermal papillae are rigid and give the impression of "festooning." There may be periodic acid-Schiff (PAS)–positive thickening of the BMZ and superficial vessels. Caterpillar bodies, which are eosinophilic, amorphous bodies at the base of the blister roof, are PAS positive and type IV collagen positive. Caterpillar bodies are a somewhat specific but not sensitive feature of PCT.

PORPHYRIA CUTANEA TARDA—DISEASE FACT SHEET

Patient Group

- Familial (early onset)
- Sporadic (adults in midlife), often associated with liver damage, secondary to alcohol abuse, hepatotoxic, estrogen-containing, or some recreational drugs, infection (such as hepatitis B or C infection), or other hepatotoxins

Site of Involvement

- Dorsal hands and forearms are most often affected

Clinical Findings

- Fragile skin with milia and scars
- Hypertrichosis
- Hyperpigmentation

Prognosis and Treatment

- Sun avoidance is the key to addressing photosensitivity
- Phlebotomy helps by reducing iron stores, which improves heme synthesis disturbed by ferroinhibition. Antimalarials are a second-line therapeutic approach.

PORPHYRIA CUTANEA TARDA—PATHOLOGIC FEATURES

Histopathologic Features

- Subepidermal blister
- Usually minimal or no inflammation
- Hyaline deposits around papillary dermal vessels
- Festooning (rigid papillae at blister base)
- Periodic acid-Schiff–positive and type IV–positive caterpillar bodies on blister roof
- Direct immunofluorescence deposits may be present in a thick, linear distribution at the dermal-epidermal junction or in a homogeneous perivascular pattern in the papillary dermis. This pattern of deposition is often seen with IgG and, variably, with other conjugates

Pathophysiology

- Hereditary or sporadic
- Decreased enzyme activity of uroporphyrinogen decarboxylase

Differential Diagnosis

- Epidermolysis bullosa acquisita
- Cell-poor bullous pemphigoid
- Pseudoporphyria

Ancillary Studies

A PAS stain may highlight perivascular deposition of glycoproteins and caterpillar bodies. DIF often shows thick linear deposition along the BMZ and around superficial dermal blood vessels with IgG and, variably, with other conjugates (Fig. 5.56).

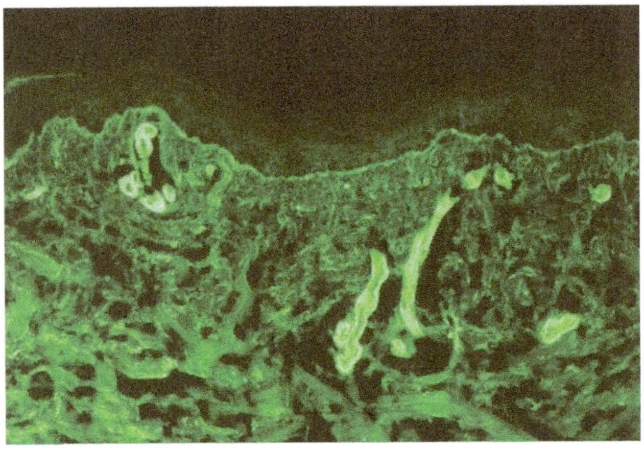

FIG. 5.56
Porphyria cutanea tarda. Direct immunofluorescence shows thick homogeneous IgG deposits around blood vessels in the superficial dermis, as well as along the basement membrane zone.

Differential Diagnosis

PCT needs to be distinguished from cutaneous involvement by other porphyrias, pseudoporphyria, and pauci-inflammatory variants of BP as well as EBA.

Prognosis and Treatment

PCT is a chronic disease. Avoidance of triggering factors (e.g., UV exposure, alcohol, estrogen use) is important. Phlebotomy is the first-line approach to treatment. Antimalarials may be beneficial because they accelerate porphyrin secretion and may also inhibit its synthesis.

PSEUDOPORPHYRIA

Pseudoporphyria refers to a clinical phenotype similar to that of PCT (skin fragility, blisters, and scarring with a predilection for the dorsal hands and forearms) that is not related to deficiency of enzymes in the porphyrin biosynthesis. Pseudoporphyria is usually associated with chronic renal insufficiency or a medication reaction from a variety of drugs, including NSAIDs (e.g., naproxen), diuretics (e.g., furosemide), antibiotics (e.g., nalidixic acid or tetracycline), retinoids, and others.

The histopathologic features are indistinguishable from PCT. Clinical context and biochemical analysis of stool or plasma samples with documentation of increased levels of porphyrin metabolites distinguish PCT from pseudoporphyria.

INHERITED EPIDERMOLYSIS BULLOSA

Inherited EB refers to a collection of heterogeneous disorders that have in common an inherited deficiency of critical structural proteins within or surrounding the BMZ. Clinically, patients experience mechanical fragility of the skin with frequent blister formation. There are numerous clinical phenotypes that correspond with the underlying genotype. Three major categories of inherited EB have been described based on the ultrastructural site within the skin where the split occurs: epidermolysis bullosa simplex (EBS), junctional EB (JEB), and dystrophic EB (DEB). In EBS, the ultrastructural level of the split is within the epidermis due to mutations in the keratin 5 or 14 gene. In JEB, the split occurs within the lamina lucida due to mutation of various proteins such as laminin 332 and BP180. In DEB, the split occurs in the sublamina densa due to mutations of type VII collagen. The classification has been updated to reflect improved recognition of the genetic underpinnings, extracutaneous associations, and range of clinical manifestations in EB variants. For example, intraepidermal EB has been divided into basal and suprabasal subgroups to accommodate additional EB subtypes that have been added. Some names have been altered (e.g., the Weber-Cockayne variant is now called localized EBS). A detailed discussion of the subtypes, structural abnormalities, and mutations is beyond the scope of this text.

Clinical Findings

All forms of inherited EB show mechanical fragility of the skin, with blisters easily induced by minor trauma. Scarring may occur in any subtype but is most often seen in variants with disruption located deeper microanatomically in the BMZ. Accordingly, it is uncommon in patients with localized EBS (formally called Weber-Cockayne variant) but almost always seen in recessive DEB (also called Hallopeau-Siemens type). There are associated extracutaneous conditions that further define the EB subtypes, including muscular dystrophy and pyloric atresia. Kindler syndrome is now included in the EB classification as a mixed type.

Histopathologic Features

Light microscopic analysis of lesions of inherited EB has a very limited role because it does not allow subclassification of the disease. However, it can document the presence of a pauci-inflammatory blister or reveal early features of skin fragility (Fig. 5.57A and B).

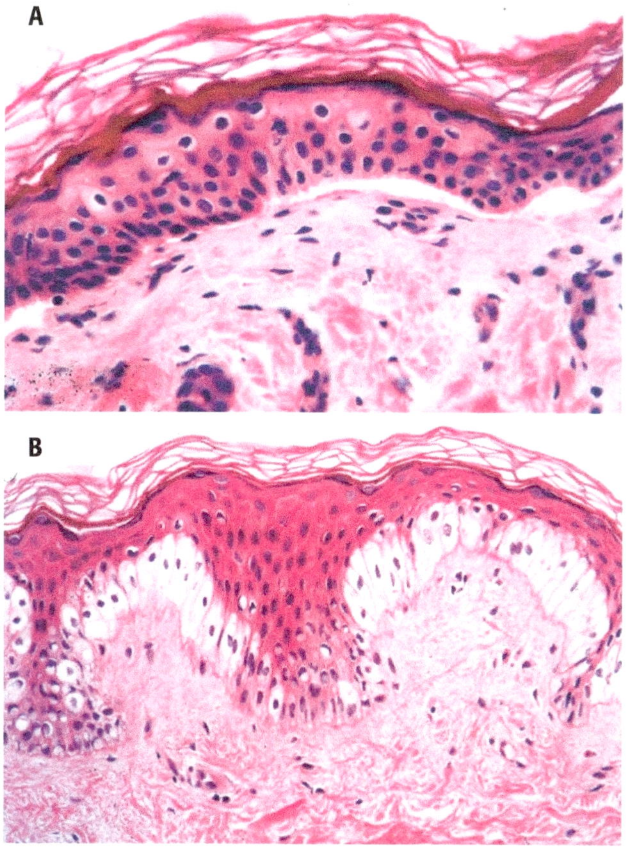

FIG. 5.57
Epidermolysis bullosa simplex. **A,** Noninflamed subepidermal blister. **B,** Pallor of basilar keratinocytes ("eraser effect").

Ancillary Studies

Ancillary studies, such as EM and immunofluorescence mapping (IFM), can help to determine whether a split is seen within the epidermis (e.g., intracytoplasmic within a basilar keratinocyte in the Weber-Cockayne variant of EBS), the lamina lucida (variants of JEB), or sublamina densa (variants of DEB). EM also allows assessment of the specific structures of the BMZ and sub-BMZ but is not offered in most laboratories. IFM is as reliable as EM for most of the EB when coupled with antibodies to the BMZ structures for localization of the blister plane (BP antigen, laminin-1, type IV collagen, and keratin 14), and with antibodies to some of the specific structures involved in the EB subtypes (laminin-332, type VII collagen, type XVII collagen, plectin, α6β4 integrin, and keratin 14). These markers will have diminished or absent staining in the recessive subtypes of EB. Since loss of the targeted antigen is the diagnostic finding, the presence of a reliable positive control showing normal staining is critical in performing IFM. After determination of the subtype with these studies, one should proceed to targeted DNA mutational analysis, because IFM is semiquantitative and does not have high enough specificity or sensitivity to accurately distinguish the EB subtypes. DIF should be performed to exclude an autoimmune subepidermal blistering process.

Prognosis and Treatment

Currently, treatment is mainly directed toward wound healing. However, gene- and cell-based therapies are being developed for more severe phenotypes. Patients with DEB are at increased risk for the development of aggressive squamous cell carcinoma.

MISCELLANEOUS OTHER INTRA- OR SUBEPIDERMAL BLISTERS

Blisters can be found in many other settings, such as nutritional deficiencies, diabetes, friction, coma, edema, vasculitis, and sepsis.

NUTRITIONAL DEFICIENCY SYNDROME BLISTERS

Nutritional deficiency syndromes, such as acrodermatitis enteropathica (AE), necrolytic migratory erythema (glucagonoma syndrome), and necrolytic acral erythema (associated with hepatitis C infection), may on occasion show blisters in addition to the erythematous papulosquamous lesions.

Histopathologically, there is variable psoriasiform epidermal hyperplasia, with epidermal pallor and parakeratosis (Fig. 5.58). In the blistering presentations, the

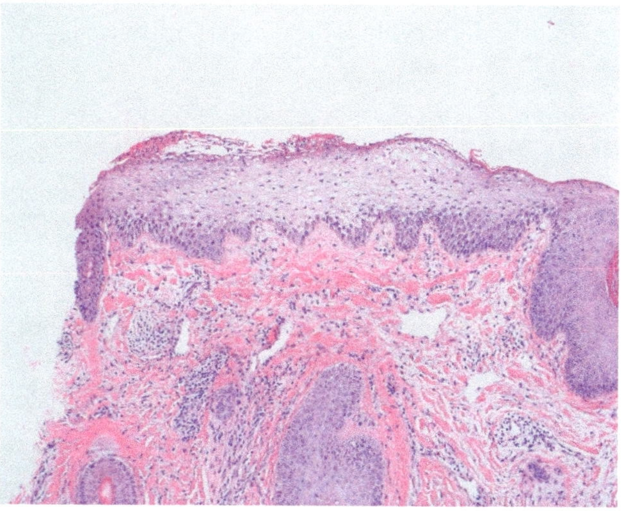

FIG. 5.58
Nutritional deficiency. There is pallor and necrosis of keratinocytes of the upper epidermis with intracorneal neutrophils and granular layer attenuation.

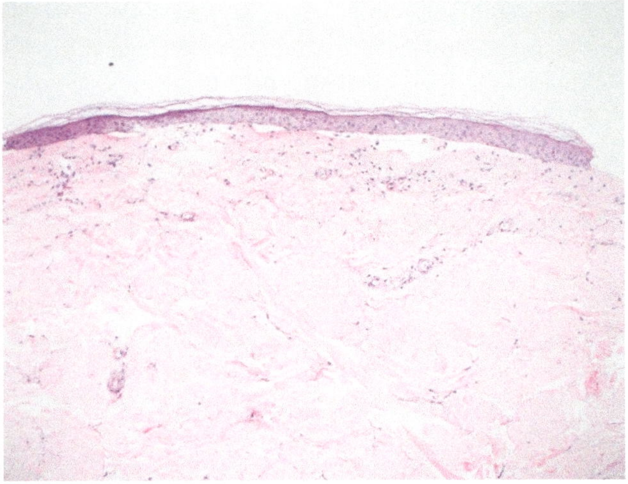

FIG. 5.59
Bullous diabeticorum. Pauci-inflammatory subepidermal separation.

split is usually intraepidermal, associated with intracellular edema and ballooning degeneration of keratinocytes of the upper half of the stratum spinosum. Subepidermal blisters may form if there is full-thickness necrosis. The clinical course varies with the condition. If the underlying systemic association or nutritional deficiency is corrected, there is a prompt resolution of the skin lesions.

BULLOUS DIABETICORUM

Blisters may arise in patients with poorly controlled diabetes mellitus. The blisters are usually large and tense, and they tend to arise spontaneously with a predilection for the lower leg, including the feet, toes, and hands.

Histopathologically, the blisters are pauci-inflammatory and may arise in an intraepidermal, subcorneal, or subepidermal plane (Fig. 5.59). There may be a mild lymphohistiocytic perivascular infiltrate associated with capillary wall thickening. The blisters tend to heal spontaneously but may recur.

BLISTERS CAUSED BY FRICTION

Clinical Findings

Friction blisters are usually seen on the soles, heels, and palms and are caused by external trauma, usually shearing forces (e.g., repeated friction, walking in ill-fitting shoes). The bullae may be flesh-colored or hemorrhagic.

Histopathologic Features

There usually is a noninflammatory intraepidermal blister associated with pallor of keratinocytes. The split is most often seen microscopically within the spinous cell layer. Inflammation is usually absent or minimal, though intracorneal neutrophils can be seen.

Differential Diagnosis

The diagnosis is usually apparent clinically, if the patient provides a history of trauma or if the anatomic distribution is suggestive. If there is an exaggerated response to friction, consideration may be given to the localized variant of EBS (Weber-Cockayne). Clinically, a friction blister may also be confused with EBA. Both EBA and EBS are histopathologically characterized by a subepidermal split.

Prognosis and Treatment

Friction blisters heal spontaneously with cessation of activity contributing to the skin trauma.

COMA BLISTERS

Tense blisters can develop in comatose patients, typically on otherwise normal skin exposed to pressure. If coma blisters are biopsied, a split may be seen within or, more commonly, beneath the epidermis. Inflammation is usually absent or minimal. A subtle but consistent histopathologic finding is basophilic sweat gland necrosis (Fig. 5.60A and B), which may be accompanied by perieccrine neutrophilic inflammation.

ACUTE EDEMA BLISTERS

Acute edema blisters are noninflammatory tense blisters which arise abruptly on the legs of patients with chronic dependent edema. Affected patients are often elderly or immobile. Microscopically, there is marked epidermal spongiosis or superficial dermal edema without well-defined bulla. There may be a sparse lymphohistiocytic infiltrate in dermis, associated with lymphatic dilation and fibrosis.

BLISTERS CAUSED BY HEAT OR COLD

Blisters may form in response to physical injury such as burns or freezing, including cryotherapy. Such lesions, particularly thermal burns, cause considerable morbidity. These blisters are typically subepidermal and associated with epidermal necrosis (Fig. 5.61). Depending on the degree of the burn, the dermal collagen may become

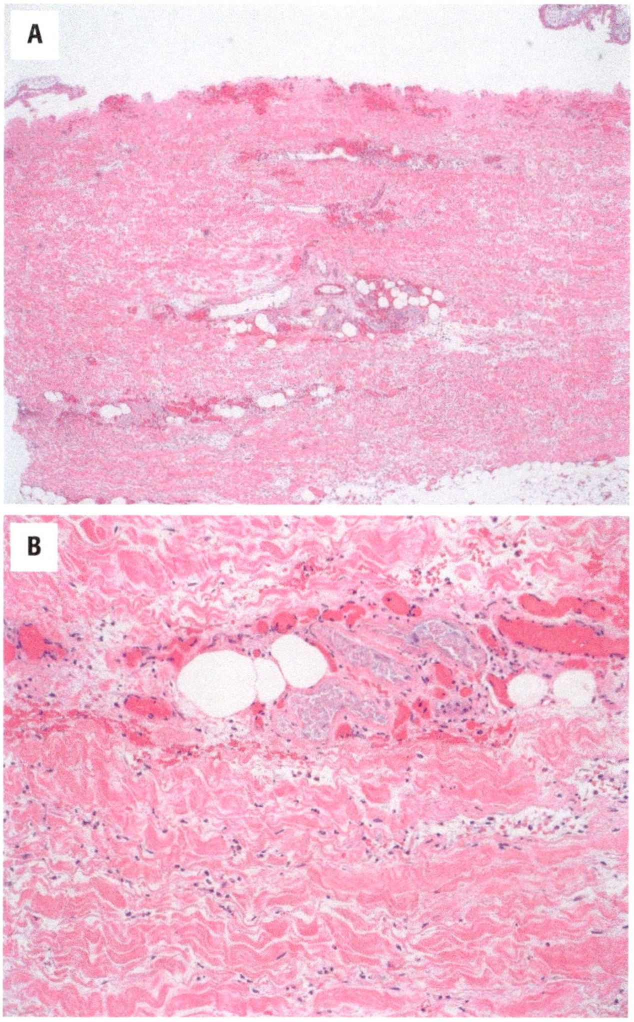

FIG. 5.60

Coma blister. **A,** Noninflammatory subepidermal vesicle with partial epidermal necrosis (pale keratinocytes with loss or reduced staining of nuclei). **B,** Necrosis of eccrine glands associated with vascular congestion.

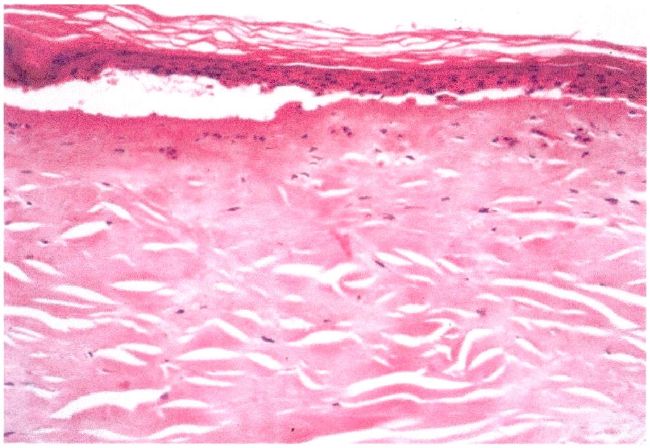

FIG. 5.61

Burn blister. Subepidermal vesicle with no inflammation.

hyalinized. Secondary infections represent a major complication of burn injuries. Blisters induced by electrical injury show alignment and elongation ("polarization") of keratinocytes.

BLISTERS CAUSED BY TOPICAL TREATMENTS

The topical anesthetic, eutectic mixture of local anesthetics (EMLA) composed of 2.0% lidocaine and 2.0% prilocaine in an oil and water emulsion, may induce blisters locally. Microscopically, these blisters impart upper epidermal pallor, spongiosis, destruction of the basal layer with basophilic granules, subepidermal clefting (Fig. 5.62), congestion with microthrombi, and extravasated erythrocytes in the papillary dermis. The changes may occur after approximately 15 minutes of application. Diagnosis is readily made based on clinical features.

Acute radiation dermatitis can lead to blistering via keratinocyte destruction (Fig. 5.63).

BLISTERS CAUSED BY VASCULITIS, VASCULOPATHY OR INFECTION

Ischemic necrosis to the skin may occur in the setting of vascular damage or occlusion, and this ischemia can contribute to subepidermal separation (Fig. 5.64).

BLISTERS ASSOCIATED WITH SUPERFICIAL DERMAL AMYLOID DEPOSITION OR SCLEROSIS

Blistering can occur in the setting of amyloidosis (Fig. 5.65) or lichen sclerosus. In both conditions,

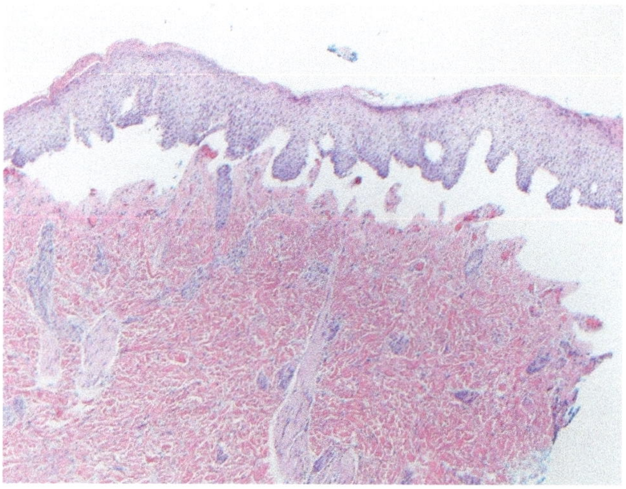

FIG. 5.62

Topical anesthetic blister. Pauci-inflammatory subepidermal vesicle. The epidermis shows pallor and mild spongiosis.

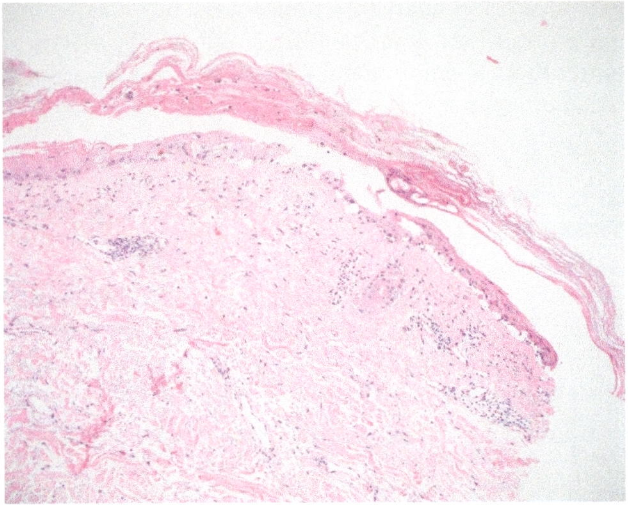

FIG. 5.63

Acute radiation dermatitis. Keratinocyte necrosis with vacuolar interface changes and minimal associated inflammation.

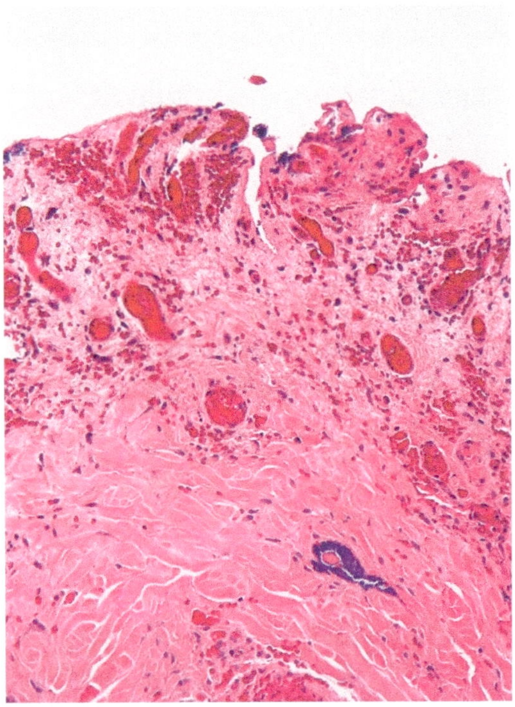

FIG. 5.64

Blister associated with staphylococcal sepsis. Clusters of cocci (septic emboli) are present within blood vessels. The skin surface is ulcerated (necrotic epidermis is sloughed off).

changes to the superficial dermis, either by deposition of amyloid or homogenization of the collagen, can make the epidermis more prone to shearing with minor trauma.

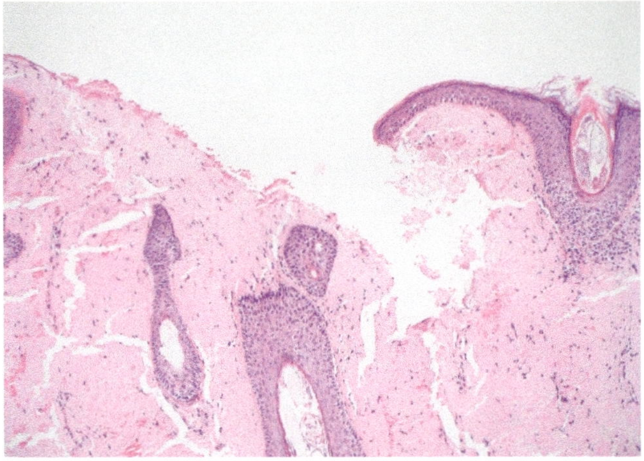

FIG. 5.65

Amyloidosis. Dermal deposition of amyloid, with shearing of the overlying epidermis.

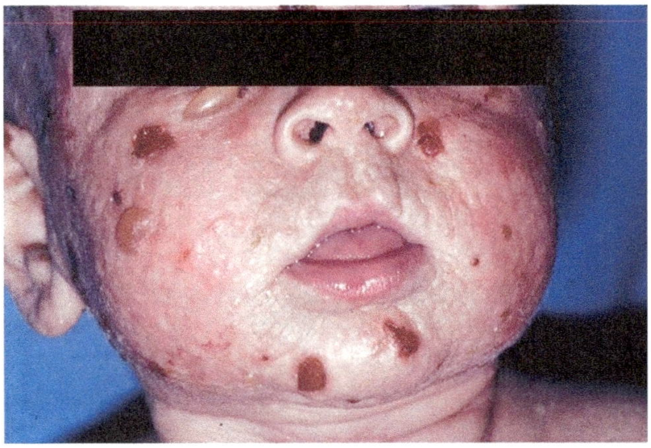

FIG. 5.66

Bullous mastocytosis. Blisters and crusts on the face.

BLISTERS ASSOCIATED WITH A SUPERFICIAL DERMAL NEOPLASTIC INFILTRATE

Blisters may also form in the setting of neoplastic infiltrates of the dermis (as with hematolymphoid or myeloid disorders; see bullous mycosis fungoides discussed above; and mastocytosis; Figs. 5.66 and 5.67) or the junction (as with malignant melanoma).

ACKNOWLEDGMENT

The author wishes to thank Dr. Klaus Busam and Dr. Jakki Junkins-Hopkins for writing the blistering skin disease chapter in the previous edition of this book.

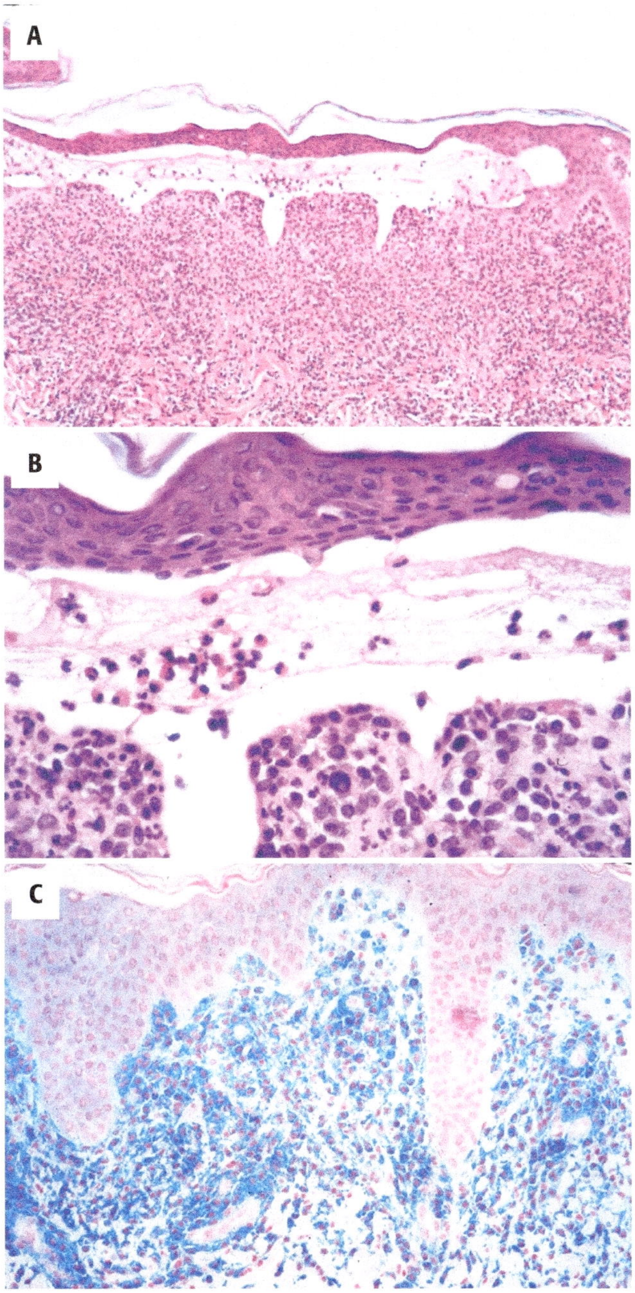

FIG. 5.67

Bullous mastocytosis. Subepidermal vesicle (**A**) with numerous mast cells in superficial dermis (**B**), which are metachromatic by Giemsa stain (**C**).

SUGGESTED FURTHER READING

Dasher, D., Rubenstein, D., & Diaz, L. A. (2008). Pemphigus foliaceus. *Current Directions in Autoimmunity*, *10*, 182–194.

Di Zenzo, G., Marazza, G., & Borradori, L. (2007). Bullous pemphigoid: physiopathology, clinical features and management [review]. *Advances in Dermatology*, *23*, 257–288.

Jordon, R. E. (2000). *Atlas of bullous disease*. Philadelphia: Churchill Livingstone.

Intong, L. R., & Murrell, D. F. (2011). Pemphigoid gestationis: Pathogenesis and clinical features. *Dermatologic Clinics*, *29*(3), 447–452.

Leger, S., Picard, D., Ingen-Housz-Oro, S., Arnault, J. P., Aubin, F., Carsuzaa, F., Chaumentin, G., Chevrant-Breton, J., Chosidow, O., Crickx, B., D'incan, M., Dandurand, M., Debarbieux, S., Delaporte, E., Dereure, O., Doutre, M. S., Guillet, G., Jullien, D., Kupfer, I., Lacour, J. P., ... Joly, P. (2012). Prognostic factors of paraneoplastic pemphigus. *Archives of Dermatology*, *148*(10), 1165–1172.

Montagnon, C. M., Tolkachjov, S. N., Murrell, D. F., Camilleri, M. J., & Lehman, J. S. (2021). Intraepithelial autoimmune blistering dermatoses: Clinical features and diagnosis. *Journal of the American Academy of Dermatology*, *84*(6), 1507–1519.

Montagnon, C. M., Tolkachjov, S. N., Murrell, D. F., Camilleri, M. J., & Lehman, J. S. (2021). Subepithelial autoimmune blistering dermatoses: Clinical features and diagnosis. *Journal of the American Academy of Dermatology*, *85*(1), 1–14.

Mihai, S., & Sitaru, C. (2007). Immunopathology and molecular diagnosis of autoimmune bullous diseases. *Journal of Cellular and Molecular Medicine*, *11*, 462–481.

Olasz, E. B., & Yancey, K. B. (2008). Bullous pemphigoid and related subepidermal autoimmune blistering diseases. *Current Directions in Autoimmunity*, *10*, 141–166.

Remington, J., Chen, M., Burnett, J., & Woodley, D. T. (2008). Autoimmunity to type VII collagen: Epidermolysis bullosa acquisita. *Current Directions in Autoimmunity*, *10*, 195–205.

Stanley, J. R., & Amagai, M. (2006). Pemphigus, bullous impetigo, and the staphylococcal scalded-skin syndrome. *New England Journal of Medicine*, *355*, 1800–1810.

Zhu, X., & Zhang, B. (2007). Paraneoplastic pemphigus. *Journal of Dermatology*, *34*, 503–511.

6 Mucinoses, Deposition Disorders, and Connective Tissue Alterations

Franco Rongioletti • Jacqueline M. Junkins-Hopkins • Luis Requena

This chapter includes cutaneous substances that may accumulate in abnormal amounts, such as mucin, as well as material deposits usually not present in the skin, either produced endogenously (e.g., porphyrins) or introduced as a foreign substance for lifestyle or cosmetic purposes (e.g., tattoo pigment, fillers). Deposits in the skin may be divided into broad groups: (1) calcium, osseous, and cartilaginous deposits; (2) hyaline deposits characterized by an eosinophilic, homogeneous, glassy appearance in hematoxylin and eosin (H&E)–stained preparations, which include amyloid, lipoid protein, colloid milium, porphyrins, and gout; (3) various pigmentary deposits, such as ochronosis, hemosiderin, tattoo pigment, and various metals; (4) substances used for cosmetic purposes; and (5) miscellaneous deposits, such as oxalate and polyurethane. The chapter also includes solar elastosis and pseudoxanthoma elasticum (PXE).

CUTANEOUS MUCINOSES

Dermal mucin is composed of acid glycosaminoglycans, particularly hyaluronic acid, and to a lesser extent chondroitin sulfate and heparin. They are normally present in the ground substance of the dermis and may abnormally accumulate either diffusely or focally in the dermis.

Cutaneous mucinoses can be divided into two groups: (1) primary cutaneous mucinosis, in which mucin deposition is the main histologic feature resulting in clinically distinctive lesions, and (2) secondary mucinosis, in which mucin deposition is not the principal but one of several other findings because it can be seen in conditions such as lupus erythematosus, scleroderma, dermatomyositis, Degos disease, and granuloma annulare.

The major primary mucinoses are generalized myxedema, pretibial myxedema, lichen myxedematosus, reticular erythematous mucinosis (REM), scleredema, papular and nodular mucinosis of connective tissue diseases, cutaneous myxoid cyst, cutaneous focal mucinosis, oral focal mucinosis, nodular mucinosis of the breast, and follicular mucinosis. Deposition of mucin in the dermis can also be seen in association with obesity, lymphedema, venous stasis, and occasionally after local radiation.

PRIMARY CUTANEOUS MUCINOSES—CLINICAL VARIANTS

Dermal

- Mucinoses with altered thyroid function
  - Thyroid dermopathy (pretibial myxedema)
  - Generalized myxedema
- Lichen myxedematosus (papular mucinosis)
  - Generalized/diffuse and sclerodermoid (scleromyxedema)
  - Localized
  - Atypical/intermediate
- Scleredema
- Reticular erythematous mucinosis
- Mucinosis of connective tissue diseases
- Cutaneous focal mucinosis
- (Digital) Myxoid cyst
- Mucocele of the lip
- Miscellaneous other variants (e.g., related to stasis, lymphedema or radiation)

Follicular

- Primary follicular mucinosis (Pinkus)
- Urticaria-like follicular mucinosis
- Secondary follicular mucinosis associated with cutaneous T-cell lymphoma

Clinical Findings

In *generalized myxedema* caused by hypothyroidism, the skin appears pale yellow because of the combined effects of edema, anemia, and carotenemia. The skin is cool, dry, coarse, waxy, and puffy, especially around the eyes, nose, and cheeks, and firm to touch. The face is often expressionless with a broad nose, swollen lips, and puffy eyelids.

Localized (pretibial) myxedema is most often associated with hyperthyroidism. It occurs in 3% to 5% of cases. It is one of three processes classically seen in Graves' disease, the other two being exophthalmos and thyroid acropachy (clubbing of the digits associated with subperiosteal new bone formation). Pretibial myxedema is usually a late manifestation of Graves' disease. Only rarely has it been reported preceding the diagnosis and occurring in the setting of Hashimoto's thyroiditis without thyrotoxicosis or hypothyroidism after treatment of Graves' disease and even in euthyroid patients.

In pretibial myxedema, typically, pink or yellow raised, nodular, waxy plaques and sometimes "tumors" develop, most frequently first on the anterolateral aspects of the lower leg but sometimes extending to the dorsum of the feet. In some patients, the skin is indurated with prominent hair follicle pores, giving rise to peau d'orange appearance. Infrequently, localized myxedema occurs on other sites such as the arms, shoulders, abdomen, neck, face, and even the ears. Pretibial myxedema is sometimes self-limiting, with involution occurring after a number of years.

There are two major forms of *lichen myxedematosus (papular mucinosis)*, a generalized/diffuse and sclerodermoid form also called scleromyxedema, and a localized form with several subtypes. However, there are also atypical or intermediate forms that include unusual or overlapping presentations of lichen myxedematosus. Criteria for scleromyxedema include a generalized papular and sclerodermoid eruption, dermal mucin with fibroblasts and fibrosis, monoclonal gammopathy, and absence of thyroid disease. It occurs equally in men and women and is seen most often in the third to seventh decades of life. Clinically, a widespread symmetric eruption of 2- to 3-mm, firm, waxy, closely spaced papules occurs on the hands, forearm, face, upper trunk, and thighs. Papules are commonly arranged in a linear fashion on an underlying sclerodermoid background, resulting in tethering and limitation of movement. The glabella is typically involved with deep longitudinal furrowing. Scleromyxedema is almost always associated with a monoclonal gammopathy (usually IgG-lambda) and with systemic manifestations (e.g., myositis, carpal tunnel syndrome, arthralgias, neurologic or neuropsychiatric dysfunctions).

In localized lichen myxedematosus, patients exhibit small, firm, waxy mucinous papules (or nodules and plaques produced by the confluence of papules) without sclerotic features, paraproteinemia, or systemic findings. The localized form has several variants, including discrete papular form of lichen myxedematosus lesions occurring at any site, acral persistent papular mucinosis, cutaneous mucinosis of infancy, and nodular mucinosis.

Self-healing juvenile cutaneous mucinosis can be considered as a peculiar variant of cutaneous mucinosis of infancy often associated with rheumatologic diseases. A pediatric cutaneous mucinosis that can be considered in the differential diagnosis is *cutaneous mucinosis of the infancy* which is the pediatric variant of localized lichen myxedematosus.

Reticular erythematous mucinosis is a photo-aggravated, erythematous reticulate, or plaque like eruption in the middle of the chest or back. This condition usually affects young to middle-aged women. Rarely, the face and arms are involved. The eruption is asymptomatic. Sunlight and hormonal influences exacerbate and induce mild pruritus. Its relationship with lupus erythematosus tumidus is controversial.

Scleredema (Buschke disease) is a rare primary mucinosis that presents with nonpitting indurated edema in the absence of any significant clinical abnormality of the overlying skin. The condition may occur at any age, but nearly 50% of cases develop in children and adolescents. It may be acute or insidious in onset and may be associated with late-onset diabetes mellitus. The most common presentation is acute, which predominantly affects children and is characterized by a rapid onset arising a few weeks after an infection, most often of the upper respiratory tract. Streptococcal infections are particularly implicated. Scleredema has also been described in human immunodeficiency virus (HIV) infection and has been reported in association with paraproteinemia. Patients present with nonpitting edema and dermal hardening mostly of the posterior and lateral aspects of the neck but also of the face, anterior neck, upper trunk, and upper limbs. Lesional skin is shiny and feels hard. Wrinkling is impossible. The face may be expressionless.

Mucin deposition as a specific clinical manifestation of lupus erythematosus occurs in up to 1.5% of dermatologic patients. *Papular and nodular cutaneous mucinosis associated with lupus erythematosus* presents as asymptomatic, flesh-colored, occasionally umbilicated papules and nodules on the neck, trunk, and upper limbs. Mucin deposition occurs most often in patients with the systemic variant, usually with diffuse antinuclear and anti-DNA antibodies, and is particularly associated with joint and kidney involvement, but it has been reported in subacute and discoid lupus erythematosus. Similar eruptions characterized by papules, nodules, and plaques have been described in dermatomyositis and scleroderma.

Digital myxoid pseudocyst (not a true cyst, although sometimes referred to as digital myxoid cyst) presents as a soft or fluctuant cystic nodule on the fingers, in particular the dorsal aspect of the distal interphalangeal and the metacarpophalangeal joints. Occasionally, lesions are multiple. Cutaneous myxoid pseudocysts may present at any age and are more common in females. They contain yellow, clear viscous fluid and are often painful or tender. Myxoid pseudocyst involving the proximal nail fold may be associated with longitudinal grooving of the nail.

Cutaneous focal mucinosis presents as an asymptomatic, usually solitary, benign dermal papule or nodule most commonly on the face, neck, trunk, or extremities of adults. The lesion is usually dome shaped, white, or flesh colored and sometimes has an erythematous halo.

Mucocoele of the lip, also known as *mucus extravasation phenomenon*, as it is a local reaction to extravasated mucin, occurs most frequently in the second or third decade as a dome-shaped normochromic or bluish-colored papule on the oral mucosa. The most common site is the lower lip.

Obesity-associated lymphedematous mucinosis and pretibial stasis mucinosis arise in patients with normal thyroid function, but a high body mass index, lymphatic insufficiency, and/or venous insufficiency. *Localized mucinosis* has been described associated with drug exposure including biologic therapy, after mechanical traumas, knee replacement and radiotherapy.

Pinkus' follicular mucinosis is a benign form of intrafollicular mucin deposition not associated with cutaneous T-cell lymphoma. Children and young adults present with one or several plaques of grouped follicular papules located on the face and scalp and associated with alopecia. Nodules, annular plaques, folliculitis, follicular spines, and acneiform eruptions have also been described.

Urticaria-like follicular mucinosis is a variant of follicular mucinosis in which there is a cyclic eruption of occasionally pruritic urticarial papules merging into plaques on the face, with background seborrheic dermatitis or rosacea-like changes. The neck and upper chest may be involved. The transient nature and absence of alopecia differentiate this from primary follicular mucinosis. The lesions wax and wane for a period that may span months to years.

Follicular mucinosis associated with folliculotropic mycosis fungoides. This form of follicular mucinosis tends to occur in older patients and is commonly associated with cutaneous T-cell lymphoma involving the hair follicles. In these cases, there may be widespread patches and plaques with alopecia, acneiform, or keratosis spinulosa-like lesions.

Histopathologic Features

Mucin presents as basophilic amorphous or granular material in H&E-stained sections (Fig. 6.1). Excess mucin disrupts the collagen fibers, giving them a frayed appearance. Mucin deposition may be associated with an increase in the density of fibroblasts.

GENERALIZED MYXEDEMA

There are subtle changes with only small interstitial, sometimes perivascular and perifollicular, deposits of mucin through the dermis. The epidermis may show mild hyperorthokeratosis with occasional follicular plugging. Fibroblastic proliferation is not a feature of primary generalized myxedema.

PRETIBIAL MYXEDEMA

Mucin deposition involves diffusely the mid and lower dermis (Fig. 6.2). The epidermis may be hyperkeratotic, with follicular plugging. Stellate fibroblasts are evident and referred to as mucoblasts, but they are not increased in number except perhaps for the more elephantiasic examples. There is a mild superficial perivascular chronic inflammatory cell infiltrate. Mast cells are often present.

SCLEROMYXEDEMA

There is a characteristic triad of diffuse mucin deposition in the upper or mid-dermis, prominent fibroblast proliferation, and increased collagen (see Fig. 6.3). A slight perivascular lymphoplasmacytic infiltrate is often seen in the superficial dermis. Mast cells and eosinophils are sometimes increased in number. With consequent fibrosis and dermal thickening, mucin deposits may become less evident. A granulomatous variant has been described. The histopathologic picture of the discrete type of localized lichen myxedematosus is not as characteristic as in scleromyxedema but is still recognizable. Mucin deposits are diffuse or focal, in the upper and mid-dermis with variable fibroblast proliferation and slight or absent fibrosis.

RETICULATED ERYTHEMATOUS MUCINOSIS

The deposits of dermal mucin in the upper or mid-dermis are small, and a mild or moderately pronounced lymphocytic infiltrate is present, predominantly around blood vessels and hair follicles

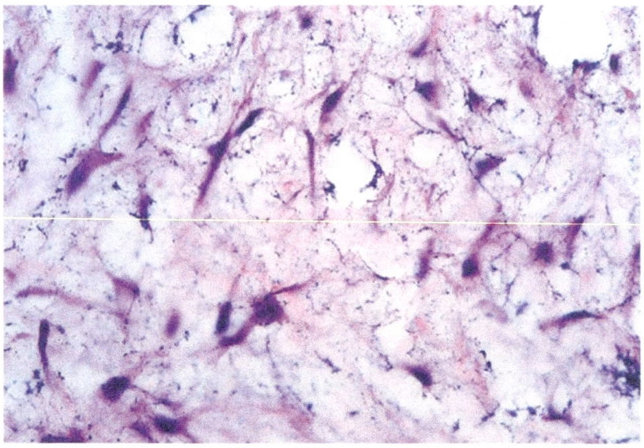

FIG. 6.1
Mucin. Edematous matrix with bluish granules and fibroblasts.

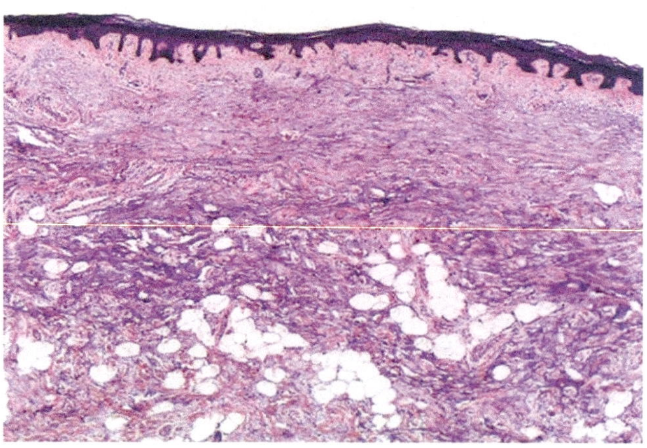

FIG. 6.2
Peritibial myxedema. Mucin deposition and fibroblasts in the dermis.

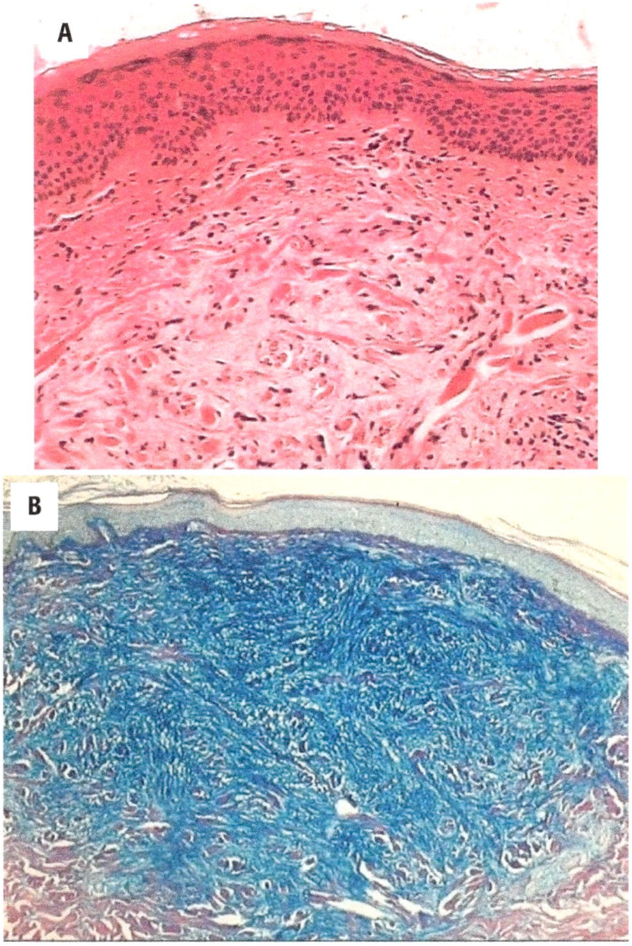

FIG. 6.3

Scleromyxedema. **A,** The characteristic triad of mucin, fibroblast proliferation, and fibrosis. **B,** Mucin deposition is stained with colloidal iron.

(Fig. 6.4). The relationship of REM with lupus erythematosus tumidus remains controversial, but the presence of clusters of CD123+ plasmacytoid dendritic cells supports the relationship of this process with lupus erythematosus tumidus.

SCLEREDEMA

There is a diffuse, variable interstitial deposition of mucin in the reticular dermis (Fig. 6.5). The reticular dermis is greatly thickened, often at the expense of the subcutaneous fat, because of swelling and separation of collagen bundles. Eccrine glands therefore become abnormally situated within the upper third or mid-dermis. Sometimes multiple biopsies are necessary for demonstrating mucin. Fibroblasts are in normal numbers. Inflammatory infiltrate is often absent.

PAPULAR AND NODULAR MUCINOSIS ASSOCIATED WITH LUPUS ERYTHEMATOSUS

Mucin is present in the papillary and upper reticular dermis with a diffuse pattern. A slight to moderately

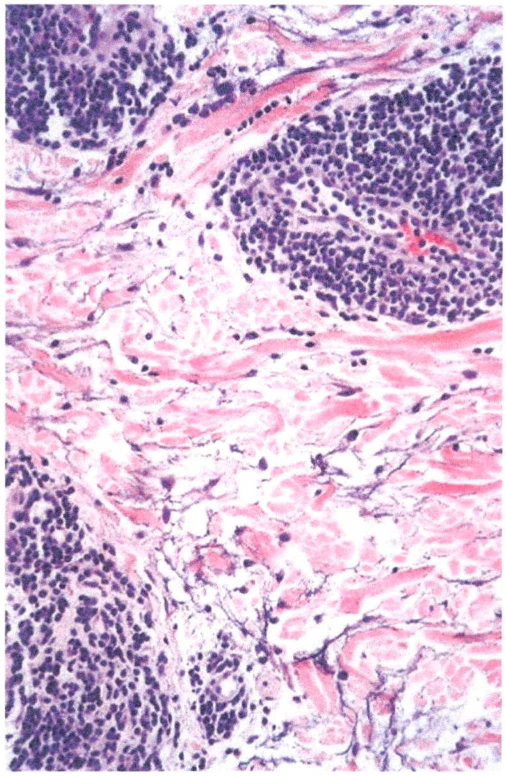

FIG. 6.4

Reticular erythematous mucinosis. Interstitial mucin deposition associated with perivascular lymphocytic infiltrate.

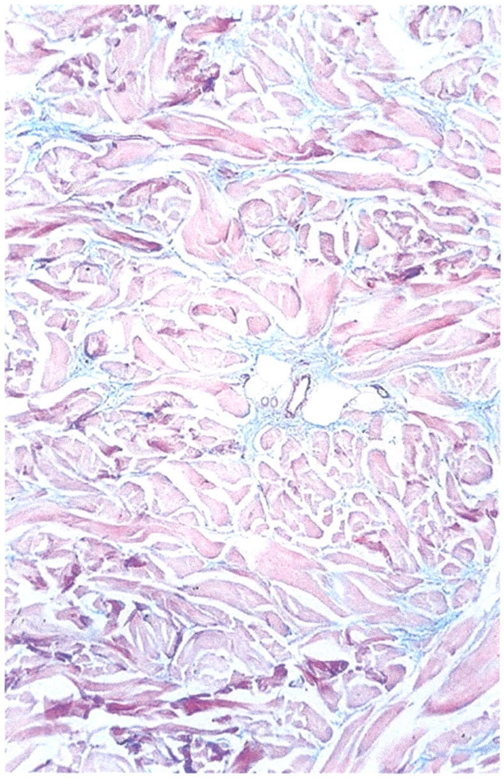

FIG. 6.5

Scleredema. Interstitial mucin deposition between fenestrated collagen highlighted by Alcian blue stain.

dense perivascular lymphocytic infiltrate is only occasionally present. The epidermis is normal, and no signs of interface dermatitis are present.

CUTANEOUS MUCOUS PSEUDOCYST (MYXOID PSEUDOCYST)

There is no "true" cyst with cyst lining. The lesion consists of a pool of mucin associated with spindle or stellate fibroblasts (Fig. 6.6). The overlying epidermis may be atrophic or hyperplastic and hyperkeratotic with a collarette surrounding the dermal pool of mucin.

MUCOCELE

A mucocele or mucous cyst results from rupture of the duct of a minor salivary gland. It most often affects the lip but may also develop in the buccal mucosa. Clinically, mucoceles are translucent or whitish cystic nodules. Histologically, there is a mucinous stroma but no epithelial-lined cyst. The associated inflammatory reaction varies greatly from a minimal infiltrate to granulation, tissue, fibrosis, and mixed inflammatory cells, including neutrophils and macrophages.

CUTANEOUS FOCAL MUCINOSIS

There is a focal accumulation of mucin in the dermis (Fig. 6.7). A slightly increased number of spindle cells and stellate fibroblasts with elongated cytoplasmic processes are often seen, sometimes containing conspicuous intracytoplasmic vacuoles. Collagen fibers are usually diminished in number. A mild perivascular chronic inflammatory cell infiltrate is often present in the adjacent dermis. Some cases are associated with epidermal hyperplasia.

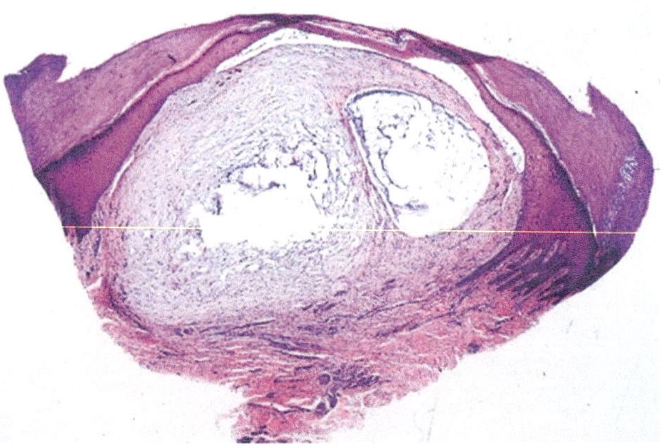

FIG. 6.6

Cutaneous myxoid cyst. Dermal nodule of mucin and fibroblasts flanked by the epidermis.

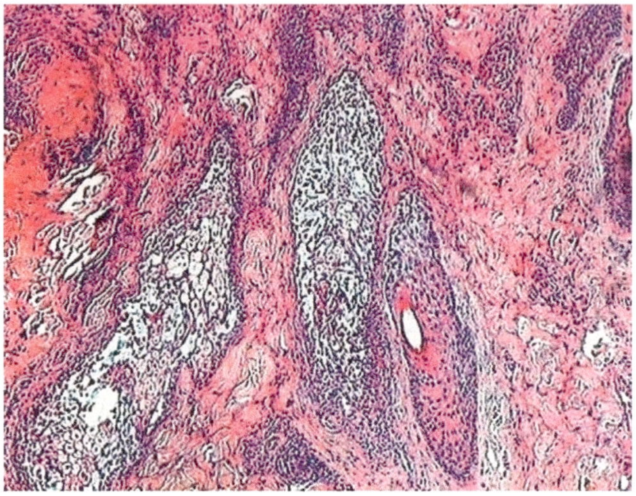

FIG. 6.7

Follicular mucinosis. Mucin accumulates within the follicular epithelium with some dissolution of cellular attachments.

FOLLICULAR MUCINOSIS

Mucin accumulates within the follicular epithelium and sebaceous gland with some dissolution of cellular attachments (Fig. 6.7). Sometimes the follicles are converted into cystic cavities containing mucin, inflammatory cells, and keratinous debris. A perifollicular infiltrate of lymphocytes, histiocytes, and eosinophils is seen.

SELF-HEALING JUVENILE CUTANEOUS MUCINOSIS

Self-healing juvenile cutaneous mucinosis is a rare disease affecting young individuals. It is characterized by the acute eruption of multiple papules and plaques or nodules, which may be associated with systemic symptoms. Two types of self-healing lesions occur: papules showing mucin deposition with mild inflammation and a small increase in fibroblasts and nodules showing deep mucinous areas associated with bands of fibrosis, multiple capillaries, fibroblastic proliferation, and gangliocyte-like giant cells in the fat. Knowledge of this entity is important to avoid overtreatment of a transient usually self-healing condition. Children affected with this condition may present associated rheumatologic diseases.

Ancillary Studies

SPECIAL STAINS

If one suspects mucin deposition because of light-blue staining between widely separated collagen bundles or empty spaces, special stains should be used, such as Alcian blue at a pH of 2.5 (Fig. 6.8) (negative at 0.5) or colloidal iron at least.

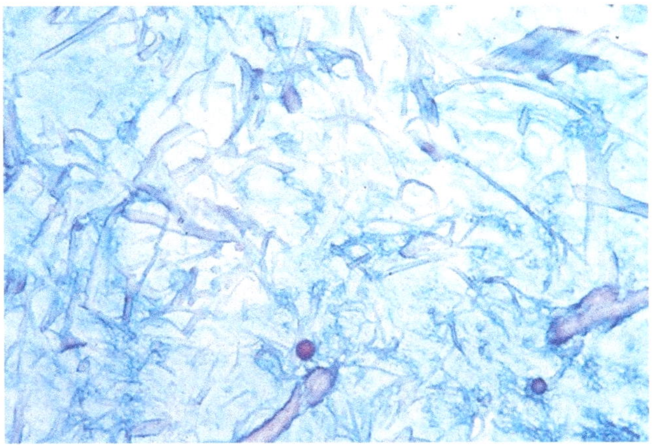

FIG. 6.8
Alcian blue highlights the myxoid matrix material.

IMMUNOFLUORESCENCE STUDIES

Immunofluorescence study results are usually negative in pretibial myxedema, REM, and scleredema. In lichen myxedematosus, there is immunoglobulin (IgG more than IgM) in the reticular dermis or just below the epidermis in about 35% of cases.

In papular and nodular cutaneous mucinosis of systemic lupus erythematosus (SLE), direct immunofluorescence (DIF) may show linear or granular immunoglobulin (IgG, IgM) deposits and complement at the dermal-epidermal junction.

Differential Diagnosis

Pretibial myxedema must be differentiated from pretibial mucinosis associated with venous stasis seen in patients without thyroid disease. In pretibial mucinosis, the excess mucin is localized to the thickened papillary dermis and is accompanied by angioplasia and siderophages.

The lack of acral calcification, absence of Raynaud's phenomenon, the papular component, and the absence of telangiectasia help to distinguish scleromyxedema from scleroderma. Scleromyxedema should also be distinguished from nephrogenic systemic fibrosis, also called nephrogenic fibrosing dermopathy. The latter is seen in patients with serious renal dysfunction, often with exposure to older gadolinium-based contrast agents, in the absence of face involvement (commonly seen in scleromyxedema) and paraproteinemia. The histologic findings are quite similar, but in nephrogenic fibrosing dermopathy, the fibroblast proliferation, fibrosis, and mucin deposition occur more deeply in the reticular dermis and subcutis; in scleromyxedema, they are usually confined in the superficial and mid-dermis. Elastocollagenous bodies are also a clue for nephrogenic systemic fibrosis.

Localized lichen myxedematosus of the discrete type may resemble granuloma annulare. However, in the latter, the cells accompanying the deposit of mucin are histiocytes arranged in a palisaded or interstitial pattern.

Reticular erythematosus mucinosis, Jessner lymphocytic infiltrate of the skin, and lupus erythematosus may share in common a perivascular and perifollicular lymphocytic infiltrate and increased mucin among collagen bundles. In Jessner lymphocytic infiltrate, the lymphocytic infiltrate is usually much denser than that in the reticular erythematosus mucinosis, and mucin is absent. Lupus erythematosus almost always shows vacuolar changes in the basal layer of the epidermis and follicular units, but vacuolar changes may be inconspicuous in the rare tumid lesions. Therefore, it may not be possible to distinguish between the tumid lesions of lupus erythematosus and reticular erythematosus mucinosis by conventional microscopy, although in lupus tumidus, the infiltrate is more conspicuous and mucin deposition is more prominent and deeply situated. Papular and nodular mucinosis associated with lupus erythematosus shows only a diffuse interstitial deposit of mucin in the reticular dermis in the absence of interface dermatitis or inflammatory dermal infiltrate. The presence of clusters of CD123+ plamocytoid dendritic cells in a dermal mucinosis supports the diagnosis of lupus erythematosus.

Early lesions of the myxoid cysts are sometimes confused with cutaneous focal mucinosis, but the sites of involvement are different.

Cutaneous focal mucinosis must be distinguished from superficial angiomyxoma, a benign myxoid cutaneous and subcutaneous lesion with a tendency for local recurrence. The latter can be distinguished by the presence of increased small vessels and scattered neutrophils in copious pools of mucin.

The differentiation between Pinkus' follicular mucinosis and mycosis fungoides–associated follicular mucinosis can be very difficult. Young age of the patient, a solitary lesion on the face or neck, and the absence of atypical epitheliotropic lymphocytes favor benign follicular mucinosis.

Prognosis and Treatment

Corticosteroids applied under occlusive dressings or delivered by intralesional injection may help in pretibial myxedema. Therapy for the associated hyperthyroidism does not improve the cutaneous lesions, and often localized myxedema develops after treatment has been instituted. Localized myxedema may clear spontaneously (average, 3.5 years).

In generalized myxedema, symptoms subside with thyroxine administration and recur if it is discontinued. Even areas of hair loss regrow with proper treatment.

Scleromyxedema is a disease with an unpredictable but usually progressive and disabling course, and the therapy is often disappointing. In addition to prednisone and chemotherapy, in particular, melphalan, which carries a high rate of potentially dangerous side effects, encouraging response to high-dose intravenous immunoglobulin, thalidomide, plasmapheresis, and autologous stem cell transplantation has been reported recently.

Localized lichen myxedematosus is a benign condition that does not require therapy. Topical steroids or calcineurin inhibitors may be of benefit. Spontaneous regression even after many years has been reported.

REM usually responds well to small doses of antimalarial drugs such as chloroquine. The lesions may clear spontaneously, even after 15 years.

Ultraviolet (UV) A-1 phototherapy seems a good treatment option for scleredema. No treatment is needed for scleredema associated with infection because it tends to resolve on its own. Regression in scleredema associated with diabetes or monoclonal gammopathy is more uncommon.

Therapy of papular and nodular mucinosis associated with lupus erythematosus coincides with that of the connective tissue disease. Only a few patients respond to antimalarials; the remainder require systemic corticosteroids. Intralesional corticosteroids have been useful for reducing large nodules and plaques.

Myxoid cysts can be surgically excised, but relapses are common. In contrast, focal dermal mucinosis usually does not recur.

There is no specific treatment for Pinkus' follicular mucinosis. A wait-and-see approach is recommended because many cases resolve spontaneously in 2 to 24 months. Topical, intralesional and systemic corticosteroids, psoralen plus ultraviolet A (PUVA), radiographs, dapsone, antimalarials, indomethacin, minocycline, oral isotretinoin, interferon alfa-2b, and UVA1 phototherapy have produced some beneficial effects.

DEPOSITION DISORDERS

HYALINE DEPOSITS

AMYLOIDOSIS

Amyloidoses comprise a spectrum of different disease processes that have in common the deposition of amyloid. Amyloid is morphologically defined as hyaline material with characteristic staining properties and ultrastructural features. It is not a single chemical substance. There are several types of amyloid, but all share the cross-β-pleated sheet configuration. Amyloid deposition in the skin may be a localized phenomenon (localized cutaneous amyloidosis) or represent a manifestation of systemic amyloidosis.

CLASSIFICATION OF AMYLOIDOSIS

Systemic Amyloidosis

- Primary systemic (plasma cell dyscrasia or myeloma associated)
- Secondary systemic (chronic inflammation or infection)
- Hereditary or familial

Localized Amyloidosis

- Primary cutaneous: macular, lichenoid, or nodular
- Secondary cutaneous: associated with tumors, such as basal cell carcinoma

Extracutaneous

- Endocrine
- Central nervous system

Clinical Findings

SYSTEMIC AMYLOIDOSIS

Systemic amyloidosis is classified into primary (usually associated with underlying plasma cell dyscrasia or neoplasm) and secondary (complication of chronic inflammatory disease or infection) forms. In systemic amyloidosis, deposits can be found in many organs. In primary systemic amyloidosis, skin involvement is seen in approximately one-third of patients. The lesions manifest as waxy papules and plaques. Hemorrhage is common. The lesions tend to affect the head and neck region, particularly the periorbital region (Fig. 6.9). The precursor of amyloid in primary systemic amyloidosis is a monoclonal immunoglobulin light chain, more frequently of lambda type (AL amyloidosis). In secondary systemic amyloidosis, skin involvement is rare. The amyloid in secondary systemic amyloidosis is not immunoglobulin but instead is derived from α-globulin called serum amyloid A (SAA), which is split into amyloid in chronic febrile conditions (AA amyloidosis).

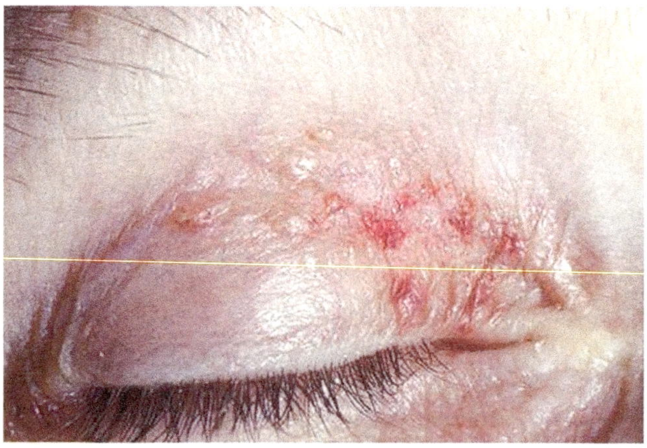

FIG. 6.9

Primary systemic amyloidosis with periorbital ecchymoses and waxy papules.

PRIMARY LOCALIZED CUTANEOUS AMYLOIDOSIS—DISEASE FACT SHEET

Patient Group

- Adults; usually otherwise healthy
- Macular variant often presents in young adulthood, more often in women
- Usually sporadic; rare familial cases
- May be associated with autoimmune disease

Site of Involvement

- Macular variant: usually upper back, scapula, or extremities
- Lichenoid variant: typically on extensor surfaces of extremities, especially shin
- Nodular variant: trunk or extremities

Clinical Findings

- Macular variant
  - Pruritic or asymptomatic hyperpigmented macules
  - Often become confluent and form a rippled pattern
- Lichenoid variant
  - Persistent pruritic papules and plaques
  - Scaly or hyperpigmented
  - Rippled pattern common
- Nodular variant (rare)
  - Single or multiple waxy nodule

Prognosis and Treatment

- The lesions are benign and extremely itching
- Treatment is directed at breaking the itch–scratch–itch cycle, for which topical steroids play an important role

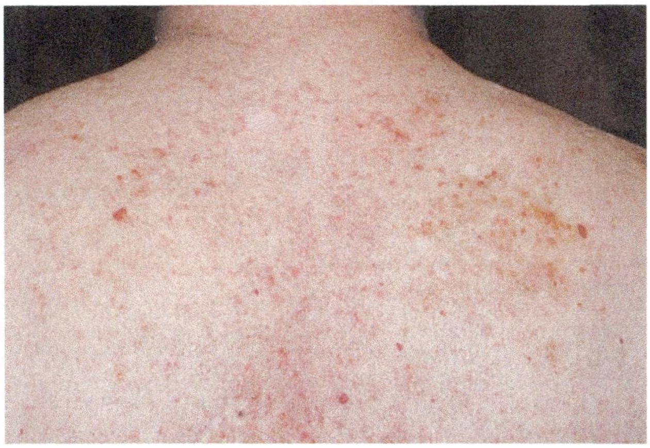

FIG. 6.10

Macular amyloidosis with hyperpigmented rippled macules.

CUTANEOUS AMYLOIDOSIS—PATHOLOGIC FEATURES

Histopathologic Features

- Homogeneous hyaline deposits

Ancillary Studies

- Positive staining with Congo red
- Apple-green birefringence by polarization after Congo red stain
- Metachromasia with crystal violet
- Characteristic fibrillary structures by electron microscopy
- Immunohistochemistry for cytokeratins

Differential Diagnosis

- Primary versus secondary localized cutaneous amyloidosis
- Primary versus secondary systemic amyloidosis
- Other hyaline deposits (e.g., colloid, lipoid proteinosis)
- Lichenoid dermatitis with clusters of Civatte bodies

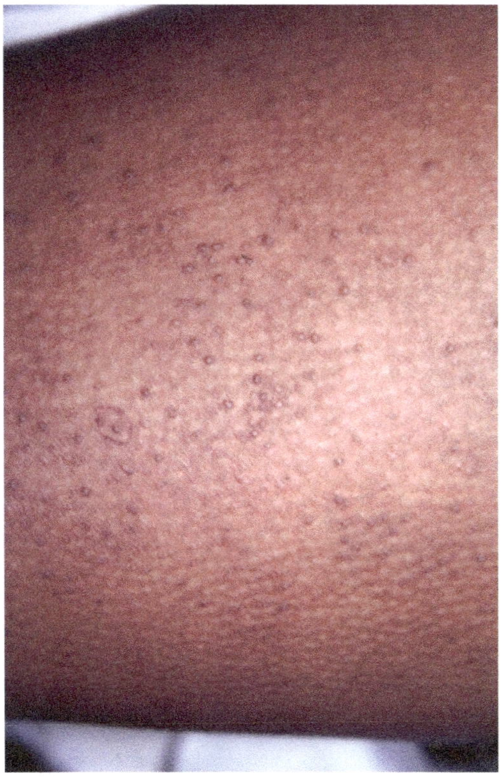

FIG. 6.11

Lichen amyloidosis with numerous small papules on the lower extremity.

LOCALIZED CUTANEOUS AMYLOIDOSIS

The spectrum of clinical variants of primary cutaneous amyloidosis includes macular (macular amyloidosis), papular (lichen amyloidosis), and nodular (primary nodular cutaneous amyloidosis) lesions. Whereas amyloid depositions in macular amyloidosis and lichen amyloidosis are of keratin type, in nodular amyloidosis, they are derived from the light chain of immunoglobulins. *Macular amyloidosis,* which is the most common form of localized cutaneous amyloidosis, is characterized by hyperpigmented macules and patches, most often on the trunk (Fig. 6.10). The lesions are often pruritic and tend to become confluent, often in a rippled pattern. In *lichen amyloidosis,* small, discrete, often pruritic waxy papules are present, typically on the lower extremities (Fig. 6.11). The nodular variant of primary localized amyloidosis is very rare (Fig. 6.12).

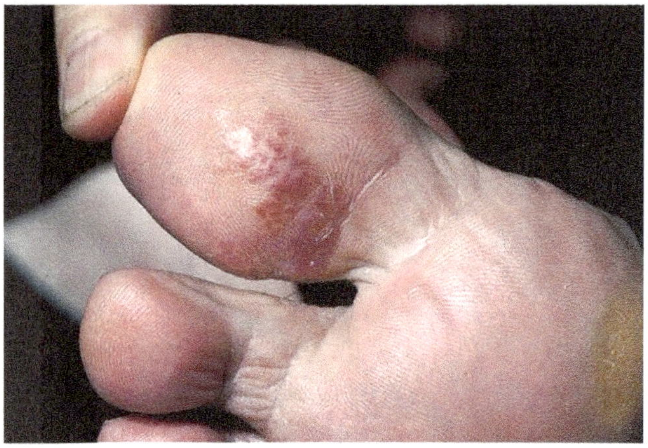

FIG. 6.12
Nodular amyloid with hemorrhagic nodules.

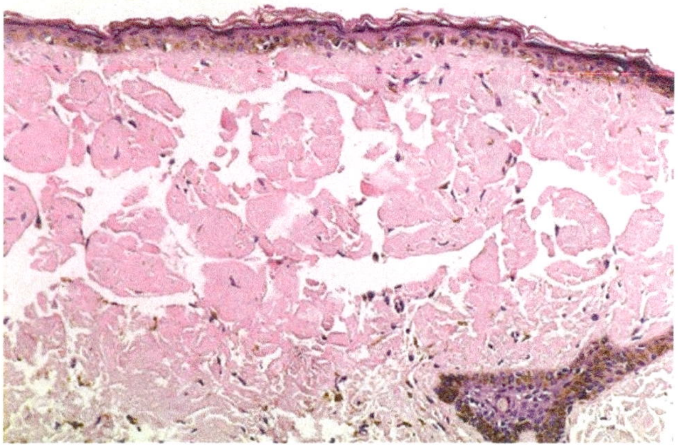

FIG. 6.13
Amyloid in dermis. Nodular aggregate of hyaline material with cracks.

Histologic Features

SYSTEMIC AMYLOIDOSIS

Nodular or plaque like areas of the dermis or subcutis are altered by the presence of hyaline material (Fig. 6.13). Clefts between hyaline fragments are common. Perivascular deposits may be seen in the subcutis (Fig. 6.14).

LOCALIZED CUTANEOUS AMYLOIDOSIS

In lichen amyloidosis or macular amyloidosis, multiple small globular deposits of hyaline material are present, typically confined to the papillary dermis (Fig. 6.15). Primary nodular amyloidosis is indistinguishable from nodular amyloid deposition secondary to systemic amyloidosis. Plasma cells may be present (Fig. 6.16). Some cases of nodular amyloidosis (amyloidoma) represent examples of primary cutaneous marginal B-cell lymphoproliferative disorder or insulin-derived localized amyloidosis.

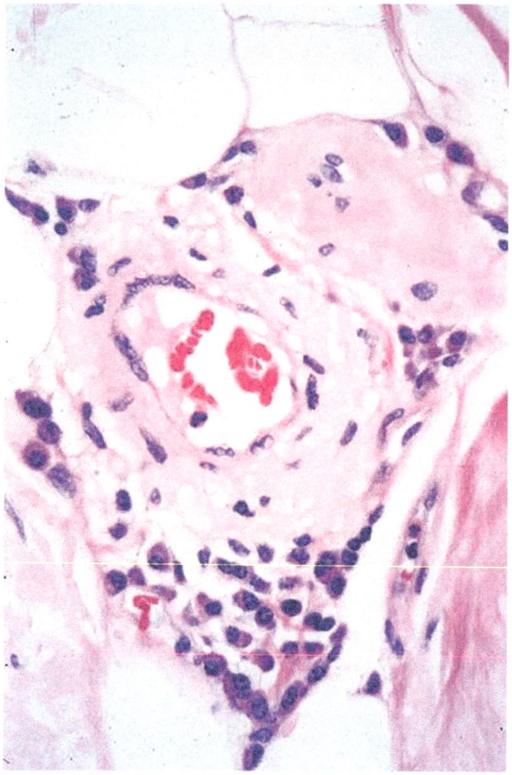

FIG. 6.14
Perivascular deposition of hyaline (amyloid) material, associated with plasma cells.

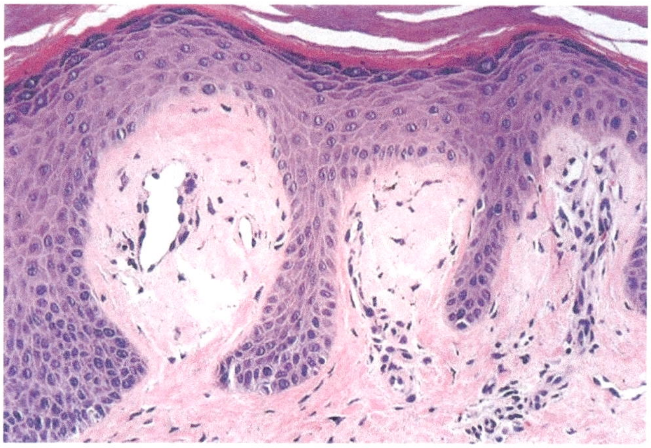

FIG. 6.15
Lichen amyloidosis. Small hyaline deposits in the papillary dermis.

Ancillary Studies

SPECIAL STAINS

Amyloid shows a number of diagnostically useful staining properties: it selectively stains with Congo red (see Fig. 6.16) and is apple-green birefringent when polarized. It is metachromatic with crystal violet and methyl violet. It gives yellow-green fluorescence with thioflavin T. After treatment with potassium permanganate, whereas

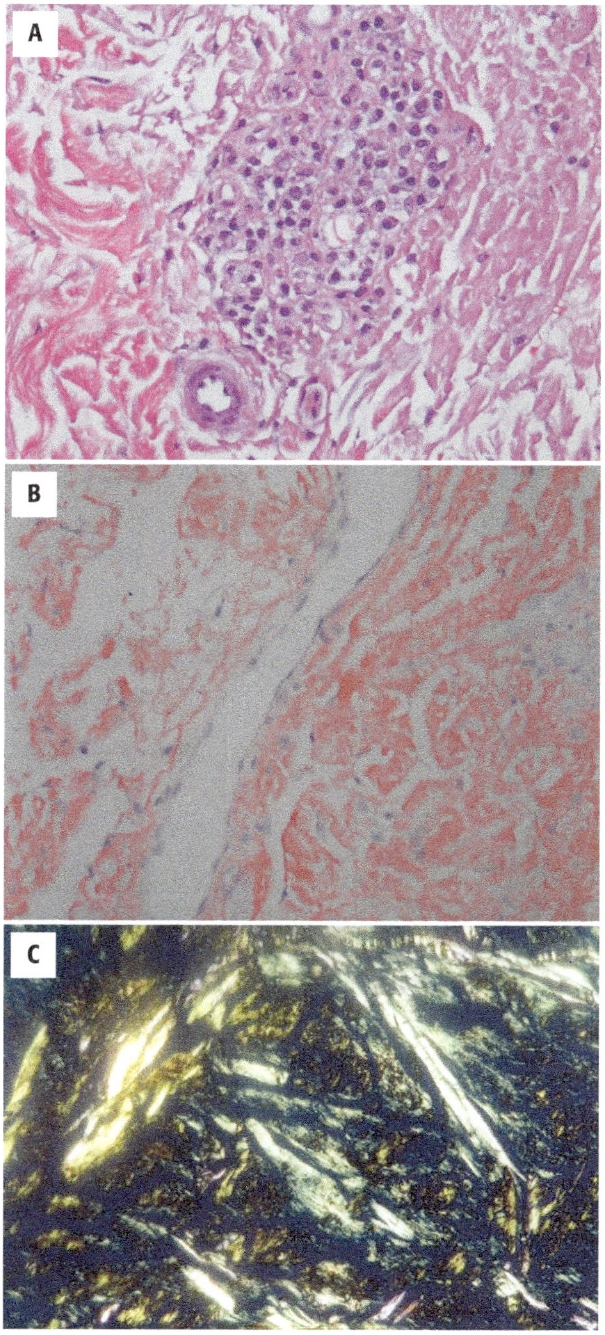

FIG. 6.16

Hyaline amyloid material associated with plasma cells. **A,** Pink appearance on hematoxylin and eosin stain. **B,** Orange color on Congo red stain. **C,** Apple-green birefringence with polarized light.

AA amyloid becomes nonreactive for Congo red stain, amyloid L is not affected by this treatment.

IMMUNOHISTOCHEMISTRY

Immunohistochemical stains for cytokeratins are helpful for the diagnosis of macular amyloidosis and lichen amyloidosis. Insulin-derived cutaneous amyloid is immunoreactive with anti-insulin antibodies.

ELECTRON MICROSCOPY

Amyloid shows characteristic ultrastructural features: It is composed of nonbranching filaments, 6 to 10 nm in diameter.

Differential Diagnosis

Amyloid deposits should be distinguished from other hyaline deposits. Such a distinction can usually be made with confidence with the help of special stains and clinicopathological correlation. The amount of hyaline material deposited in macular or lichenoid amyloid lesions may be subtle, and the lesions may be confused with lichen simplex chronicus or miscellaneous postinflammatory hyperpigmentary disorders.

Prognosis and Treatment

Localized cutaneous amyloidosis is a benign, often asymptomatic, sometimes pruritic condition. Treatment of localized cutaneous amyloid deposition is directed at breaking the itch–scratch–itch cycle. Topical steroids often help.

Systemic amyloidosis can be lethal if untreated. For patients with primary systemic amyloidosis, treatment with melphalan and autologous peripheral stem cell transfusions can significantly improve survival. For patients with secondary systemic amyloidosis, treatment of the underlying inflammatory process is critical to slow progression of amyloid deposition.

COLLOID MILIUM

A number of different clinical conditions are associated with colloid milium. We only describe here the classic variant. Classic adult-type colloid milium is characterized by numerous yellow-brown small papules occurring in older men with skin subject to chronic sun damage and repetitive trauma, particularly in farmers or outdoor workers. Histologically, nodular aggregates of hyaline material with clefts are seen (Fig. 6.17). The hyaline material of colloid milium is usually negative for Congo red and other stains positive for amyloid. Ultrastructurally, the filaments are ill-defined, short, and branching.

The distinction from amyloid can be very difficult as special stains for amyloid may be positive in colloid milium and electron microscopy is required for definitive diagnosis.

LIPOID PROTEINOSIS

Lipoid proteinosis (LP), also known as hyalinosis cutis et mucosae and Urbach-Wiethe disease, is a rare

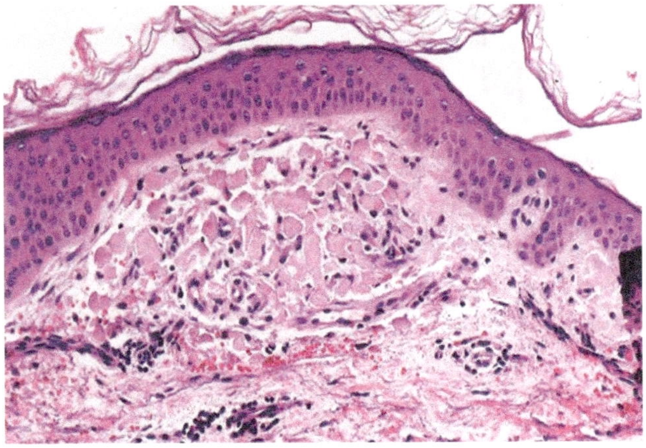

FIG. 6.17
Hyaline material of colloid milium.

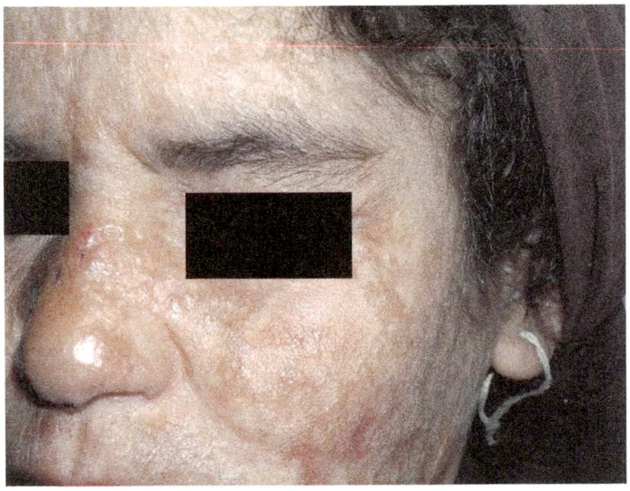

FIG. 6.18
Lipoid proteinosis. Thickened skin with waxy papules.

autosomal recessive disorder associated with reduced expression of the extracellular matrix protein 1 (*ECM1*) gene.

Clinical Findings

LP presents in early infancy with hoarseness followed by poxlike and acneiform scars and thickening of the skin and certain mucous membranes. Beaded eyelid papules (termed *moniliform blepharosis*) associated with waxy yellow papules and nodules are a classic presentation (Fig. 6.18). Hyperkeratosis or occasionally verrucous changes may appear in sites of friction. Extracutaneous features may include epilepsy and neuropsychiatric abnormalities.

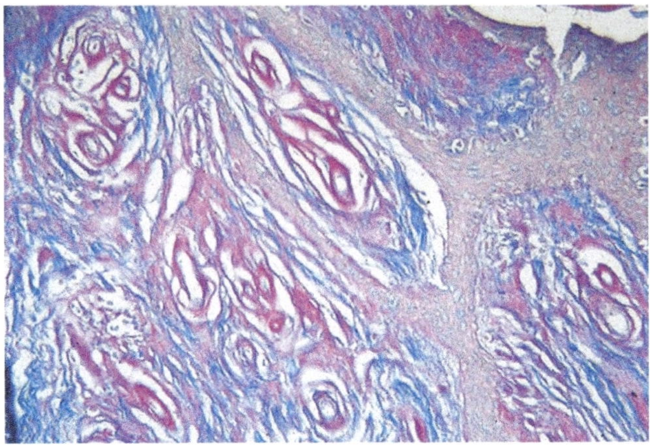

FIG. 6.19
Lipoid proteinosis with concentric deposits of periodic acid-Schiff-diastase–resistant material.

Histopathologic Features

The dermis is thickened, the upper half containing extracellular hyaline material deposited along the course of capillaries and concentrically around adnexal epithelia (Fig. 6.19). There is also progressive atrophy of the secretory sweat glands associated with increasing hyaline deposition. In verrucous lesions, the homogeneous bundles often are oriented perpendicular to the skin surface.

Ancillary Studies

The hyaline material is positive on PAS with diastase digestion (PAS-D), colloidal iron, and Alcian blue stain at a pH of 2.5 (see Fig. 6.19). Positive staining for laminin and type IV collagen is also seen.

Differential Diagnosis

The hyaline material in LP needs to be distinguished from hyaline material seen in porphyria (e.g., erythropoietic protoporphyria) and cutaneous amyloidosis. A helpful diagnostic clue is the presence of hyaline material around the eccrine coils in LP. Such material is usually absent around eccrine glands in erythropoietic protoporphyria. Stains for amyloid are helpful. In difficult cases, molecular studies documenting the presence of mutations in the *ECM1* gene allow a definitive diagnosis.

Prognosis and Treatment

Life expectancy of individuals with LP is normal, aside from the risks of respiratory obstruction. In general, patients with mutations in exon 7 of the *ECM1* gene tend to have milder upper respiratory tract abnormalities and less skin scarring or infiltration compared with patients with mutations in other parts of the *ECM1* gene, but neurologic features do not show any specific genotype–phenotype correlation. Mutational screening of the *ECM1* gene can aid in genetic counseling and prenatal diagnosis in families with known mutations. Although there have been many therapeutic trials in LP, only rarely have there been any sustained benefits. The benefit of therapeutic interventions, including oral steroids, oral dimethyl sulfoxide (DMSO), and intralesional heparin, is anecdotal. Oral retinoids, such as acitretin, have been used with some success, especially with improving vocal cord symptoms.

GOUT

Gout is a metabolic disease characterized by hyperuricemia, leading to deposition of urate crystals in and around joints, including the periarticular skin. In chronic gouty arthritis, massive deposits of urates occur (tophi).

Clinical Findings

The clinical course of gout passes through four stages: (1) asymptomatic hyperuricemia, (2) acute gouty arthritis, (3) intercritical gout, and (4) chronic tophaceous gout. The latter are urate crystal deposits, which eventually extend beyond the joint, into the surrounding tissues. The deposits range from less than 1 mm in size to the size of a baseball. They are yellow or cream in color and may break down, extruding the crystals.

Macroscopic Features

Grossly, the tophi deposits are chalky white and pastelike in consistency.

Histopathologic Features

Gouty tophi are deposited in the dermis and subcutaneous tissue. The morphologic appearance varies depending on whether the tissue has been processed routinely in formalin or has been fixed in alcohol (Fig. 6.20). The latter fixative preserves the sodium urate monohydrate deposits. When fixed in alcohol, the deposits are closely arranged brown, needle-shaped crystals that are doubly refractile under polarized light (Fig. 6.20). The characteristic negative birefringence is demonstrated with polarized light microscopy. The de Galantha stain is well suited to demonstrate the needle-shaped, doubly refractile crystals of the deposits. If fixed in formalin, the crystals usually dissolve, leaving behind amorphous light lavender to pale pink areas corresponding to the sites of crystal deposition. Within these acellular amorphous deposits, there is often a feathery appearance. The deposits are often associated with a foreign body granulomatous reaction. A sparse chronic inflammatory cell infiltrate can also be seen. Fibrosis is often present. Older lesions may develop calcification and ossification.

GOUT—DISEASE FACT SHEET

Patient Group
- Usually middle-aged men
- 20% of patients have family history

Site of Involvement
- Acute gout: in 75% of patients the first metatarsophalangeal joint is involved (podagra)
- Gout tophi: most common location is the skin overlying joints and the ear helix

Clinical Findings
- Acute arthritis with sudden attack of pain, swelling, tenderness, and erythema
- Cutaneous deposits (tophi) usually occur one decade after the first acute attack; tophi present as dermal or subcutaneous nodules

Prognosis and Treatment
- Directed at symptoms (pain relief for acute attacks)
- Directed at underlying cause (hypercalciuria) by xanthine oxidase inhibitors and dietary changes

GOUT—PATHOLOGIC FEATURES

Histopathologic Features
- Dermal or subcutaneous deposits of amorphous material with needlelike clefts
- Associated foreign body–type granulomatous reaction

Ancillary Studies
- Best seen with alcohol-based fixative
- Fine needlelike crystals under polarized light (fresh or alcohol-fixed material)
- Brown-black color on de Galantha stain

Differential Diagnosis
- Other foreign material
- Pseudogout (calcium pyrophosphate dehydrate crystals)

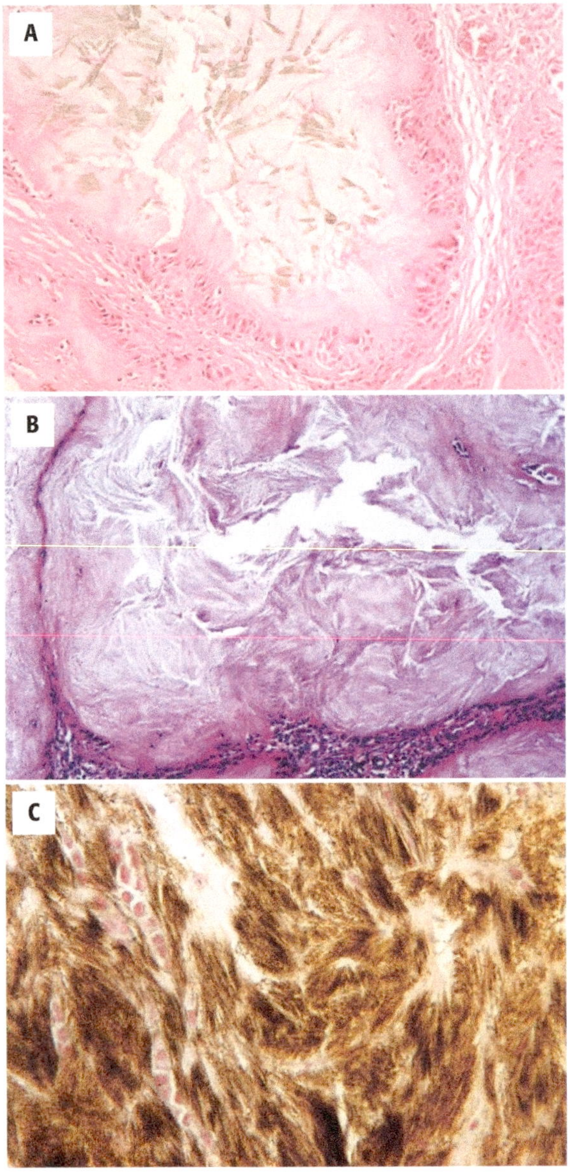

FIG. 6.20

Gout crystals. **A,** Crystals are visible after alcohol fixation. **B,** Amorphous material with feathery appearance after formalin fixation. **C,** The crystals are brown and have hay-stack-like appearance after alcohol fixation.

Differential Diagnosis

The differential diagnosis includes chondrocalcinosis (pseudogout) and rheumatoid nodules. Chondrocalcinosis is caused by deposition of calcium pyrophosphate crystals. These may be differentiated by assessing the morphology of the crystals. In pseudogout with polarized light, the crystals are rhomboid. In gout, they are needle shaped. Positive birefringent crystals of calcium pyrophosphate dihydrate crystal deposition are blue when parallel and yellow when perpendicular, in contrast to monosodium urate crystals of gout, which are yellow when parallel. Rheumatoid nodules occur on extensor surfaces of joints, similar to tophi, but histologically the multinucleated giant cells and histiocytes palisade around areas of fibrinoid collagen alteration, with neutrophilic debris.

Histopathologically, gout may be difficult to distinguish from injected triamcinolone because this also presents as pale-staining acellular material similar to gout. In contrast to gout, triamcinolone is more basophilic and has a foamy appearance. If there is extensive fibrosis, dystrophic calcification may ensue, simulating calcinosis cutis.

Needle-shaped crystals that are refractile under polarized light, indistinguishable from gout, have also been reported in cutaneous mucormycosis.

Prognosis and Treatment

Gout tophi may clear in response to treatment of the hyperuricemia. Surgical management is rarely necessary.

PORPHYRIA

Porphyria refers to a group of inherited or acquired disorders of enzymes involved in heme and porphyrin biosynthesis.

Clinical Findings

Porphyrias are generally grouped based on clinical presentation (acute or chronic) or predominant site or cells of the accumulation of heme precursors (hepatic or erythropoietic). Skin manifestations vary depending on the type of porphyria and are related to the accumulation of metabolic products in the skin. The most common form of porphyria with cutaneous manifestations is porphyria cutanea tarda (PCT) with reduced activity of uroporphyrinogen decarboxylase, which may be familial, sporadic (related to liver damage secondary to alcohol, infection, or cancer), or toxic (e.g., polychlorinated aromatic hydrocarbons). Cutaneous manifestations include mechanical skin fragility (blister formation), erosions, milia, scars, hypertrichosis, and areas of hyperpigmentation. Variegate porphyria and hereditary coproporphyria may have similar skin fragility

Histopathologic Findings

Porphyrin deposits in the skin manifest microscopically as hyaline material (Fig. 6.21A). In erythropoietic porphyria, this material is deposited in and around small blood vessels, forming perivascular hyaline cuffs (Fig. 6.21B). In PCT, the hyaline material is restricted to the vessel wall and immediate perivascular space without forming a noticeable cuff. In PCT, there is often a subepidermal blister. Perivascular hyalinized material results in

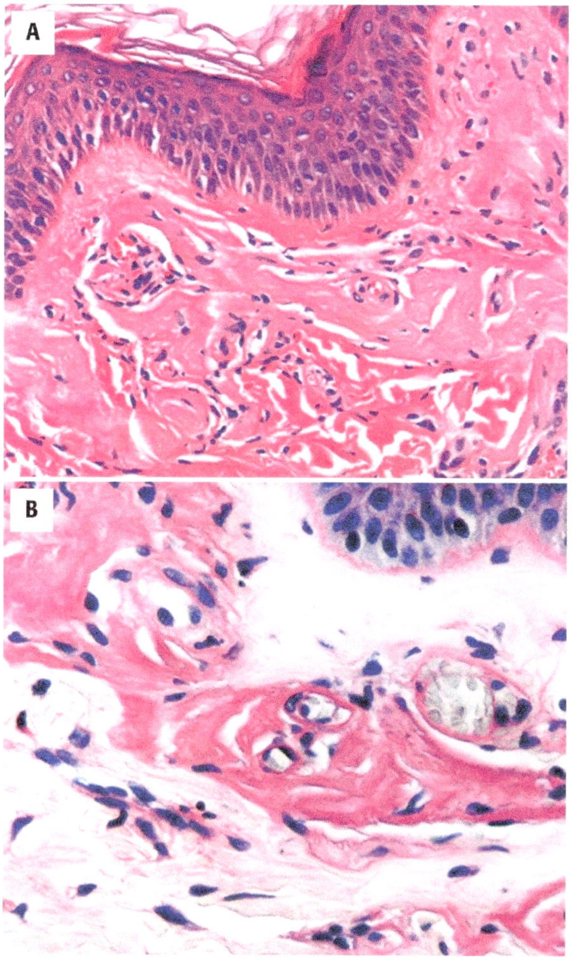

FIG. 6.21

Erythropoietic porphyria. **A,** Hyaline material in the dermis. **B,** Hyaline cuffs around small vessels, highlighted with a PAS stain.

firm dermal papillae protruding into the blister cavity (festoon). A distinctive feature of porphyrin deposits in the skin is the presence of "caterpillar bodies," or hyaline material deposited as elongated segmented globular structures in the basal layer of the epidermis, notably along the base of a blister roof, which represent fragments of collagen IV-positive fibers.

Ancillary Studies

The hyaline material is PAS-positive. DIF in porphyria usually reveals deposits of IgG and complement around dermal vessels and along the dermal-epidermal junction. Intravascular deposits of C5b-9 have been reported to be fairly characteristic for PCT.

Differential Diagnosis

Porphyrin deposits can be difficult to distinguish from lipid proteinosis. In contrast to lipid proteinosis, porphyrin deposits usually do not involve sweat glands. PCT needs to be distinguished from pseudo-porphyria by clinical information indicating a trigger by non-steroidal anti-inflammatory agents or other causes.

Prognosis and Treatment

The prognosis and treatment depend on the subtype of the porphyria.

CALCIUM, OSSEOUS, AND CARTILAGINOUS DEPOSITS

CALCIUM DEPOSITS

Historically, calcium deposits have been classified as idiopathic (etiology unknown), dystrophic (calcium deposited or inflamed in damaged tissue), or metastatic (associated with hypercalcemia).

Clinical Findings

There are various clinical presentations of calcium deposits. Deposits are commonly found at sites of trauma (e.g., auricular calcinosis, infantile calcinosis of the heel, dystrophic calcifications in scars or at injection sites) but may occur anywhere without a definable cause, as in subepidermal calcified nodules (solitary firm nodule, typically on the face, ears or digits) or in idiopathic scrotal calcinosis (usually multiple firm nodules). Some have suggested that the scrotal calcifications may be related to cysts.

Calcium deposits may also be a manifestation of systemic disease such as in metastatic calcifications of chronic renal failure and hyperparathyroidism, calciphylaxis, or autoimmune connective tissue disease. In calciphylaxis, there are progressive vascular calcification and ischemic necrosis of the skin. Calcification, Raynaud's phenomenon, esophageal dysmotility, sclerodactyly, and telangiectasia (CREST) is an example in which the presence of dystrophic calcifications has become part of the definition of a disease entity, which represents a variant of scleroderma. Calcium deposits are also often seen in dermatomyositis, especially juvenile onset.

Histopathologic Features

Calcium deposits are recognized by their intense basophilia. The deposits vary in size and shape (Figs. 6.22–6.24). In tumoral calcinosis, the deposits are large. Dystrophic calcification may be large or small. The deposits of subepidermal calcified nodule are small

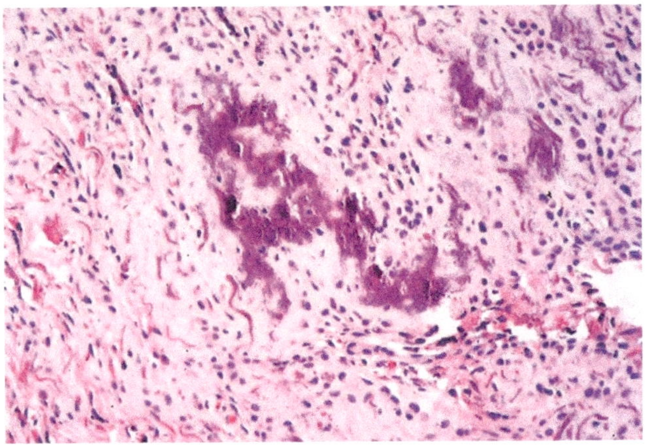

FIG. 6.22
Dystrophic calcifications.

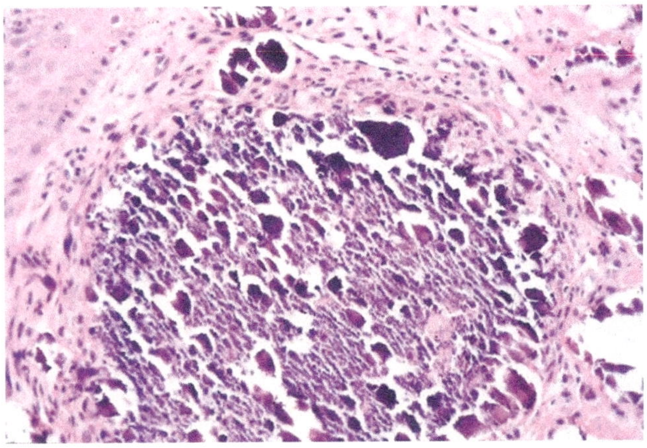

FIG. 6.23
Subepidermal calcinosis cutis.

and globular. Calcium salts may be found as isolated deposits or in association with tumors or cysts. In calciphylaxis (complication of chronic renal disease or secondary hyperparathyroidism), calcium deposits are found in the wall of blood vessels as well as in the soft tissue (Fig. 6.25). Early disease is subtle, with clues that include basophilic stippling in the fat or PXE-like elastic fiber calcification. Calcium deposits on the basement membrane around eccrine coils are a pathognomonic sign. Typically, there are also features of vascular occlusion (thrombi). Diffuse dermal angiomatosis may also be a clue to chronic renal disease and calciphylaxis.

Ancillary Studies

The presence of calcium salts can be confirmed by von Kossa's silver stain.

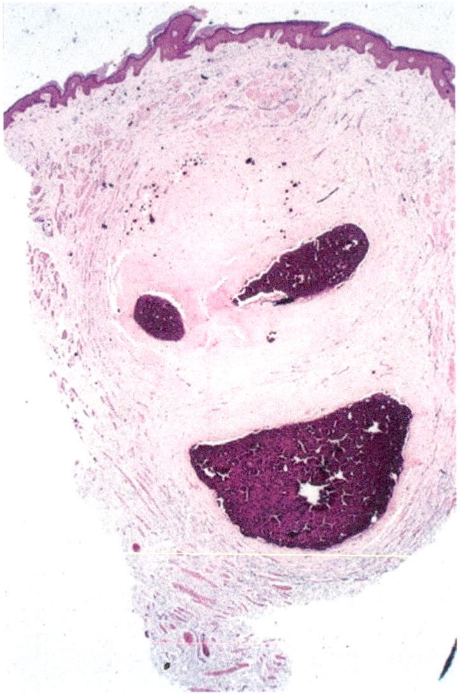

FIG. 6.24
Idiopathic scrotal calcinosis cutis.

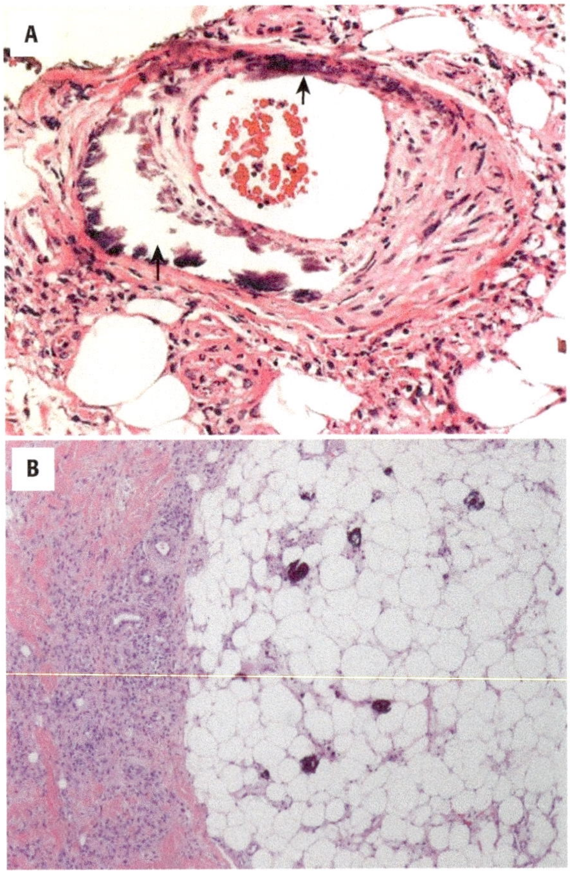

FIG. 6.25
Calciphylaxis. **A,** Calcium deposit in the arterial wall. **B,** Calcium deposits in fat.

Prognosis and Treatment

Isolated dystrophic deposits are inconsequential. Deposits in calciphylaxis or connective tissue disease may result in ischemic damage or functional impairment. Treatment is directed toward the underlying cause.

CUTANEOUS OSSIFICATION

Cutaneous ossification is usually categorized as either primary or secondary. In primary ossification, there is no preexisting lesion. Secondary ossification refers to metaplastic changes of a preexisting lesion.

Clinical Findings

Primary osteoma cutis may be solitary or multiple, hereditary (e.g., Albright's hereditary osteodystrophy), or acquired. A distinct clinical entity is the appearance of multiple miliary osteomas of the face, which may be related to a history of acne but can also present de novo. The well circumscribed button osteoma of the scalp and forehead is also clinically disctinct. Secondary metaplastic ossification may be associated with many different types of benign or malignant neoplasms (e.g., melanocytic nevi, basal cell carcinoma, squamous cell carcinoma, ossifying fibromyxoid tumor) or inflammatory reactions (folliculitis, surgical or acne scar).

Histopathologic Features

Cutaneous bone usually forms without a cartilaginous precursor by membranous (or mesenchymal) ossification. Spicules or nodular deposits of bone are present, usually with recognizable Haversian system and cement lines. Osteocytes are present in lacunae. Osteoblastic activity is only rarely seen. The stromal component is usually mature adipose tissue (Fig. 6.26), but on occasion one may see bone marrow or a few hematopoietic stem cells.

Differential Diagnosis

Bone is usually readily identified as such. Calcium deposits lack lacunae and osteocytes. Clinical correlation or ancillary studies may be necessary to determine the nature of an associated condition or tumor (e.g., hereditary osteodystrophy, solitary versus multiple osteomas, sarcomatoid carcinoma with metaplastic ossification versus osteosarcoma).

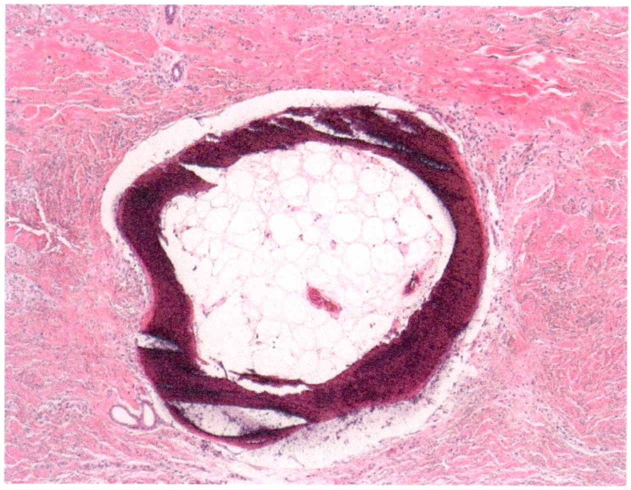

FIG. 6.26
Osteoma cutis. Bone with fatty marrow in the dermis.

Prognosis and Treatment

The bone formation per se is benign. Solitary or multiple osteomas may be removed by biopsy or curettage.

CARTILAGINOUS DEPOSITS

Cartilage may be deposited as part of a mesenchymal neoplasm (chondroma), in association with a hamartoma, or represent a metaplastic process.

PIGMENTARY DEPOSITS

Deposition of pigmented material may result from metabolic disorders (e.g., ochronosis or porphyria), incidental or deliberate exogenous introduction of pigment-containing compounds (e.g., mercury-containing creams, tattoos), or physiologic alterations secondary to trauma (e.g., hemosiderin).

OCHRONOSIS

Ochronosis refers to the deposition of ocher pigment (homogentisic acid) in the dermis. The classic setting is the occurrence in patients with alkaptonuria (endogenous ochronosis, an autosomal recessive disorder with deficiency of the enzyme homogentisic acid oxidase). However, similar compounds can be found after the intramuscular application of antimalarial drugs or the topical use of hydroquinone (exogenous ochronosis).

Clinical Findings

Early manifestations of the disease include dark discoloration of the urine and cerumen. Skin manifestations of alkaptonuria are rarely noted before the early teenage years. Skin discoloration is often bluish but may be yellow to brown. The classic bluish-gray discoloration is typically first noted on the helices of the ears and in the sclerae. In hydroquinone-induced lesions, hyperpigmentation is often associated with milium-like areas.

Histopathologic Features

Ocher (yellow-brown)–colored banana- or oddly shaped fibers are seen in the dermis (Fig. 6.27). Granular deposits may also be seen (intracellularly or extracellularly).

Prognosis and Treatment

In secondary ochronosis, discontinuation of the drug may lead to fading of the discoloration. Laser treatment may be applicable. There is no effective treatment for endogenous ochronosis. Some patients may benefit from high doses of vitamin C, which have been suggested to slow the buildup of pigment and the development of arthritis.

TATTOOS

Tattoos are exogenous pigments. Most, especially carbon tattoos, are readily recognized by routine H&E stains (Fig. 6.28). The pigment is usually localized. It may be deposited around vessels or adnexal structures extracellularly or within macrophages and fibroblasts. There may be associated inflammation, including granulomas as a manifestation of a hypersensitivity reaction to the pigment. On occasion, there may be pseudocarcinomatous epidermal hyperplasia or keratoacanthomas associated with a tattoo.

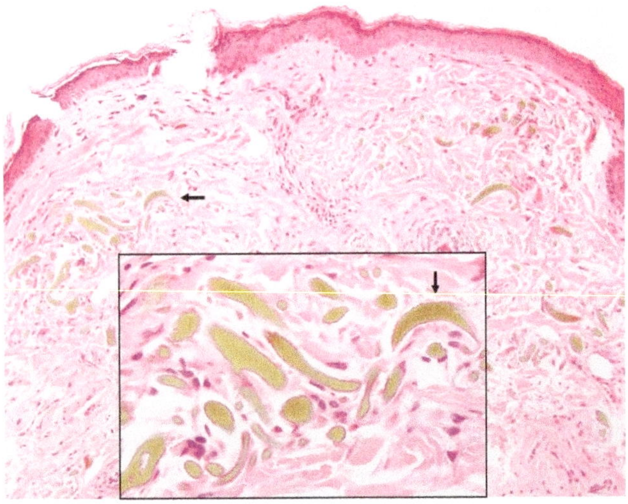

FIG. 6.27

Ochronosis with yellow-brown fibers in the dermis. Some are banana-shaped *(arrow)*. *Inset:* Close-up view of oddly shaped yellow fibers.

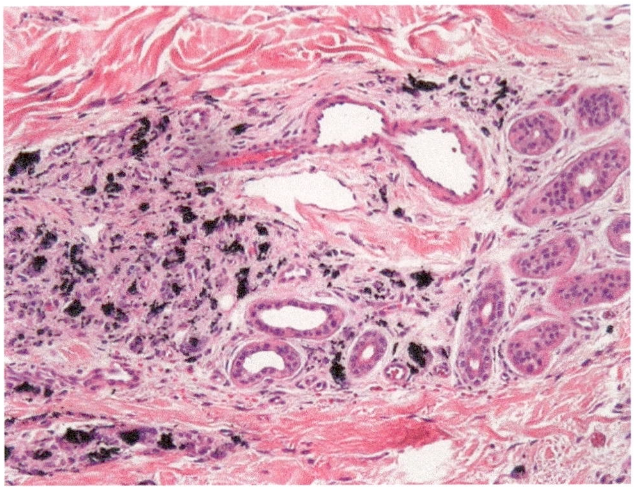

FIG. 6.28

Carbon tattoo. (Courtesy of Dr. K. J. Busam.)

HEMOSIDERIN PIGMENT DEPOSITION

Hemosiderin deposition may be localized (e.g., trauma-related hemorrhage) (Fig. 6.29) or diffuse, representing a manifestation of hemochromatosis. Localized hemosiderin pigment is often found in association with other features of trauma, such as scarring. The pigment appears as yellow-brown coarse granules on H&E-stained sections. It can be highlighted in blue by the Prussian blue reaction (Fig. 6.29).

MERCURY DEPOSITS

Mercury may be deposited in the skin by the topical application of mercury-containing ointments, resulting in slate gray pigmentation of the skin. This is now rarely seen because many such ointments have been taken off the market. Microscopically, mercury pigmentation is characterized by the presence of brown-black granules in macrophages around superficial dermal blood vessels as well as in linear bands along elastic fibers (Fig. 6.30).

ARGYRIA

Argyria refers to the deposition of silver salts. Historically, it has been related to the ingestion of silver-containing

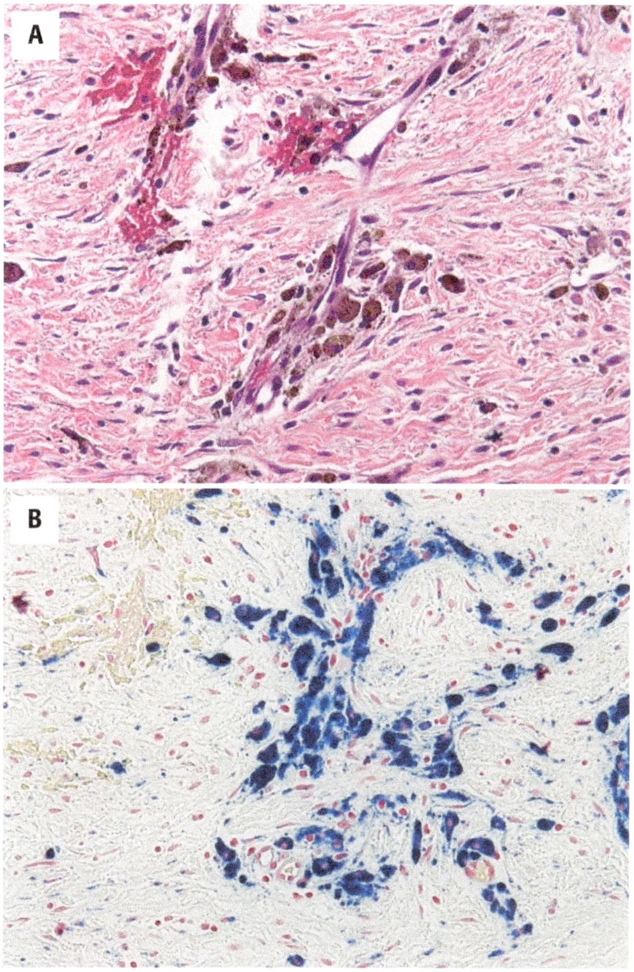

FIG. 6.29

Hemorrhagic scar with hemosiderin pigment. **A,** Hematoxylin and eosin stain shows coarse brownish-yellow granules. **B,** The granules turn blue with the Prussian blue reaction. (Courtesy of Dr. K. J. Busam.)

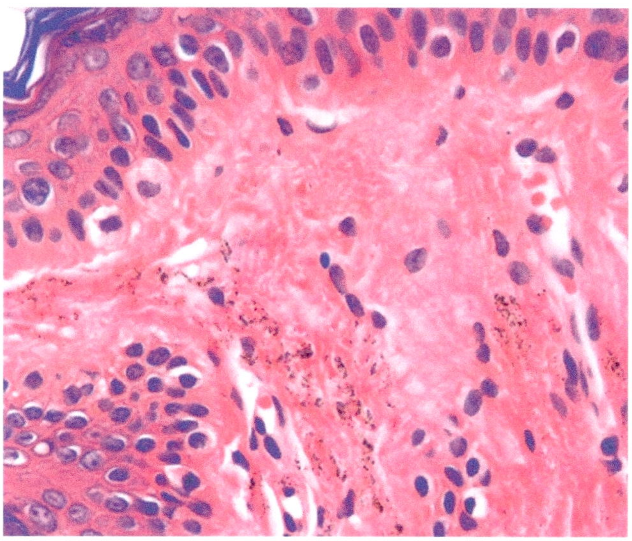

FIG. 6.30

Mercury. Brown-black granules in macrophages around superficial dermal blood vessels.

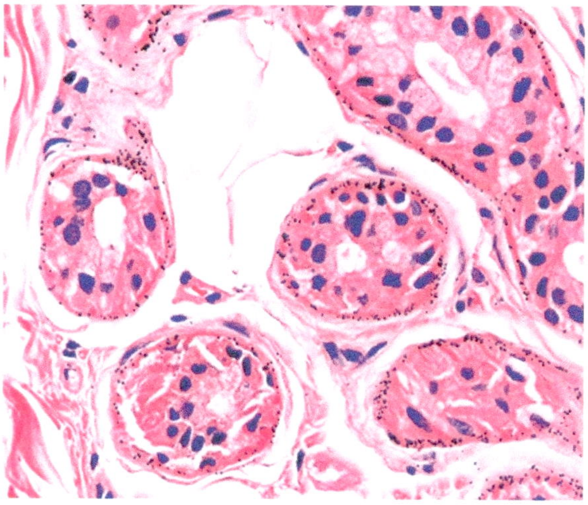

FIG. 6.31

Argyria. Pigmented granules around sweat glands.

compounds, their topical application to skin or mucous membranes, or due to trauma or prolonged topical exposure (e.g., silver-containing ear rings). Clinically, argyria manifests as blue-gray pigmentation, similar to cyanosis. It is usually most pronounced in sun-exposed areas of the body.

Histopathologically, small, brown, or black granules are seen, typically deposited around follicles, blood vessels, and sweat glands (Fig. 6.31). Deposits on elastic and collagen fibers characterize pseudo-ocronosis due to localized argyria (trauma related).

OXALOSIS

Oxalosis refers to the accumulation of oxalate crystals in tissues. There is hereditary (aka primary) and acquired oxalosis. Hereditary variants are related to enzyme defects. Acquired oxalosis may reflect increased intake (e.g., antibiotics, ethylene glycol, rhubarb leaves, enteric hyperabsorption), higher likelihood of crystal formation from metabolic acidosis, or reduced elimination of oxalate due to renal insufficiency. While primary oxalosis manifests clinically in the skin primarily with vasculopathic changes (e.g., livedo, acrocyanosis) related to crystal deposits in vessels, in acquired oxalosis calcium oxalate deposits may be found in the dermis or subcutis. Histopathologically, there is typically a granulomatous reaction to calcium oxalate deposits. The oxalate crystals manifest as thin rectangular crystals typically arranged in a rosette-like manner (Fig. 6.32). The crystals are birefringent under polarized light.

EXOGENOUS (FOREIGN) MATERIAL

A great variety of foreign material may be deposited in the skin. In hospital settings, suture (Figs. 6.33 and 6.34) granulomas are not uncommon scenarios.

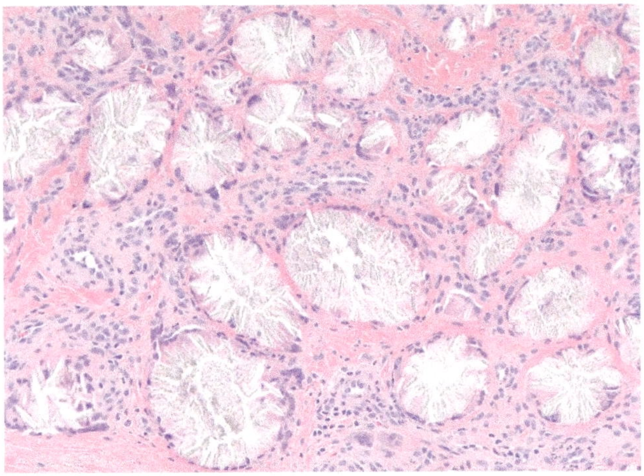

FIG. 6.32

Oxalosis. **A,** There is a granulomatous reaction to calcium oxalate crystals. **B,** The crystals are composed of rectangular-shaped needlelike structures arranged in a rosette-like fashion. **C,** The crystals are birefringent.

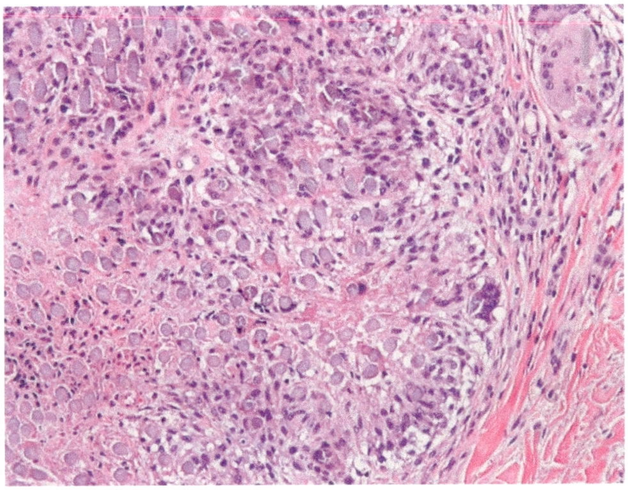

FIG. 6.33

Foreign body giant cell reaction to synthetic suture.

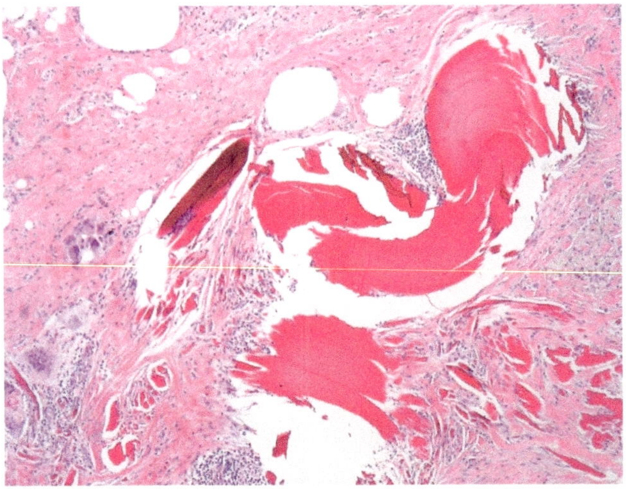

FIG. 6.34

Foreign body reaction to catgut suture.

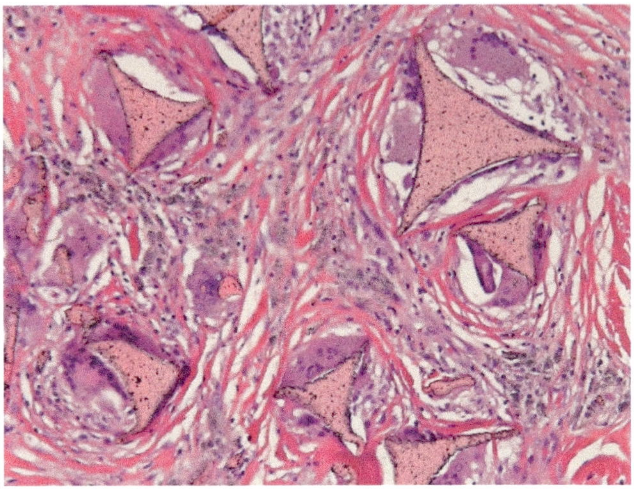

FIG. 6.35

Polyurethane granuloma. (Courtesy of Dr. K. J. Busam.)

On occasion, one may also see a granulomatous response to wound dressing material or a surgical sponge (Fig. 6.35). Other common foreign materials include wood splinters.

FILLERS AND IMPLANTS

A wealth of different materials has become available for cosmetic surgical procedures. Readers are referred to more specialized literature to learn about the microscopic features of various fillers and implants. In general, fillers can be subdivided into biodegradable and nonbiodegradable based on whether human enzymes can digest the filler material. The reactions seen in most cases independent of whether the material is biodegradable or nonbiodegradable substance is typically a granulomatous foreign body reaction with variable degrees of more acute suppurative inflammatory changes and eosinophils. Certain filler materials are highly recognizable, while in other cases, the material can only be recognized as a foreign substance.

CLINICAL FINDINGS

Erythematous papules, plaques, or nodules may occur in the area where the filler was injected, and in some cases, the filler may migrate resulting in these cutaneous manifestations at a site distant from the actual injection site. In severe cases, scarring and ulceration may occur. This is more likely in the case of nonbiodegradable fillers. The reaction may develop many years after injection, as can be seen with silicone. Inflammatory adverse events have also occurred at the sites previously injected with fillers after subsequent vaccination, such as post–COVID-19 vaccination. These reactions include edema, erythema, and granuloma formation. Fillers implicated in such reactions include hyaluronic acid, poly-L-Lactic acid microspheres, fluid silicone, polymethyl methacrylate (PMMA) microspheres, and poly-alkyl-imide (PAI).

Histopathologic Features

Some of the more common biodegradable fillers include human and animal collagens, hyaluronic acid, poly-L-lactic acid, and calcium hydroxylapatite. The collagens mainly result in an amorphous collagenous material with a foreign body granulomatous reaction. Hyaluronic acid gives a blue amorphous mucinous-appearing material (Fig. 6.36). It stains positively with Alcian blue. It may be present as an inert substance with no associated inflammation, but there is often an accompanying granulomatous reaction (Fig. 6.37). Poly-L-lactic acid appears as oval to elongated fusiform or spiky translucent particles in granulomas and foreign body giant cells. The particles are birefringent on polarizing microscopy. Calcium hydroxylapatite appears as blue-gray microspheres. These microspheres can be in giant cells or with an associated granulomatous reaction and sometimes cause dermal fibrosis. The material is nonbirefringent.

Some of the more common nonbiodegradable substances include paraffin, silicone, PMMA, and polyacrylamide gel (PAAG). Paraffin results in the well-known pattern of paraffinoma or sclerosing lipogranuloma. There are pseudocystic spaces with surrounding granuloma and scarring reaction. Paraffin is nonbirefringent. Silicone similarly results in the development of pseudocysts ("Swiss cheese-like appearance"), which contain the silicone material. There is accompanying granulomatous reaction. In PMMA, there are cystic spaces formed around translucent round microspheres which are nonbirefringent. There is usually an extensive granulomatous foreign body giant cell reaction (Fig. 6.38). With PAAG there is amorphous basophilic material with an accompanying granulomatous reaction. There are some filler materials which combine various substances and may present with some combination of the above features.

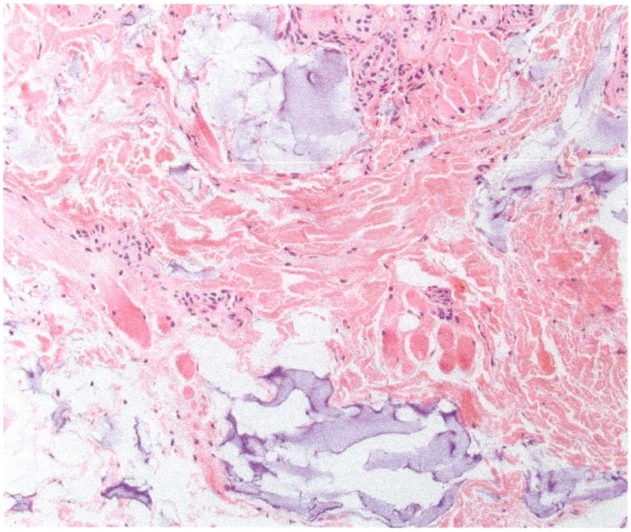

FIG. 6.36

Hyaluronic acid filler. Bluish material is dispersed in reticular dermis. There is no associated inflammatory reaction. (Courtesy of Dr. P Gerami.)

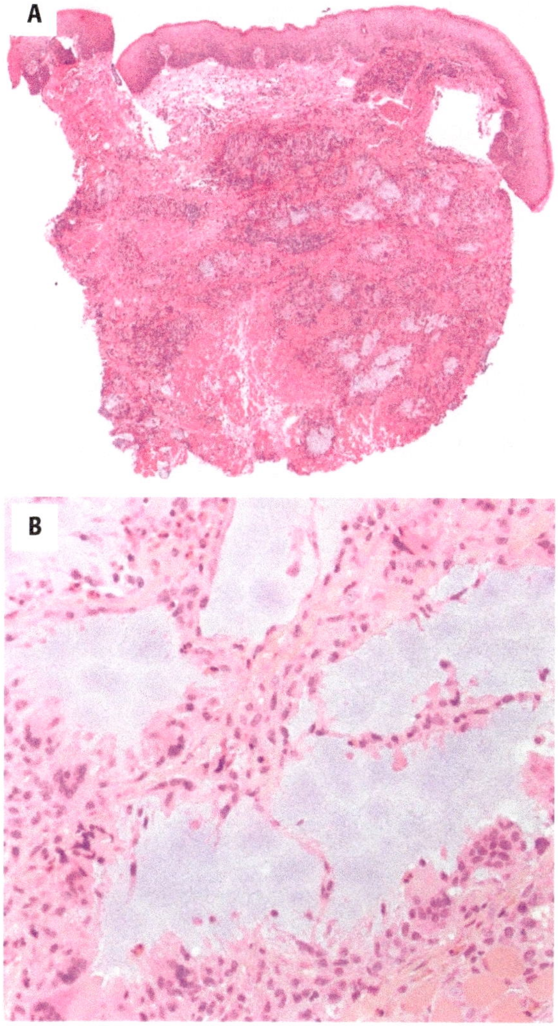

FIG. 6.37

Hyaluronic acid granuloma. **A,** The dermis is occupied by a nodular and diffuse infiltrate containing multinucleated giant cells surrounding deposits of light blue material. **B,** Aggregates of homogenous bluish material are surrounded by histiocytes, including foreign body–type multinucleated cells. (Courtesy of Dr. P Gerami.)

Differential Diagnosis

In most cases, the differential diagnosis is a foreign body reaction versus a possible infectious process. Recognizing the specific morphologic features of the foreign material and excluding infectious processes with

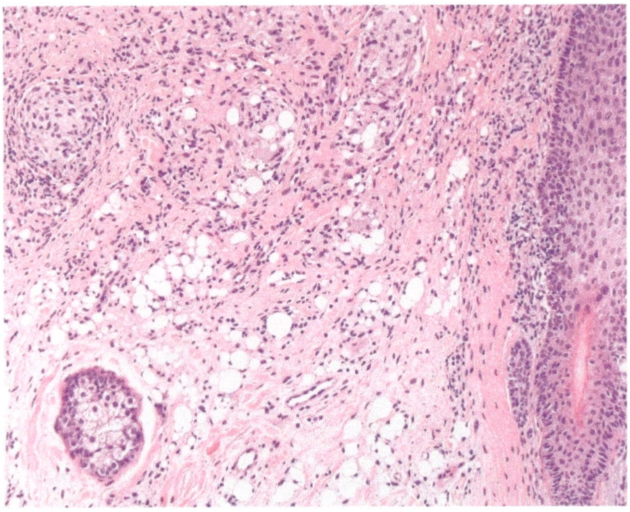

FIG. 6.38
Polymethyl methacrylate deposition manifesting as granulomatous reaction associated with microcystic spaces. (Courtesy of Dr. P Gerami.)

special stains for microorganisms and tissue culture usually resolve the dilemma.

Prognosis and Treatment

The inflammatory reaction is highly variable. In general, with the biodegradable substances, the reaction is more self-limited and tends to resolve over time, but in some cases, some permanent scarring may occur. With the non-biodegradable substances, the reactions may be more chronic and result in considerable disfiguring damage. Treatment options may include steroid injections or trying to remove the foreign material.

ALTERATIONS OF DERMAL CONNECTIVE TISSUE

SOLAR ELASTOSIS

Solar elastosis is a common finding of chronically sun-damaged skin.

Clinical Findings

Chronically sun-damaged skin appears dry and wrinkled with loss of tone. Occasionally, papular and nodular lesions may be present, often associated with telangiectasia, which may lead to clinical confusion with basal cell carcinoma.

Histopathologic Features

Pink collagen fibers are replaced by gray to metallic bluish fibers. They may coalesce to amorphous material (Fig. 6.39), especially on the head and neck regions.

Prognosis and Treatment

Solar elastosis is a marker of chronic UV damage to the skin. It is benign, but UV damage poses increased risk for the development of squamous cell carcinoma, and associated photoaging of the skin may result in cosmetic problems (wrinkles, atrophy). Treatment is directed at minimizing UV exposure (sun block, protective clothing).

PSEUDOXANTHOMA ELASTICUM

Pseudoxanthoma elasticum is an autosomal recessive disorder associated with inactivating mutations of the *ABCC6* gene. Its clinical manifestations reflect alterations of the elastic fiber network and predominantly affect the skin, eyes, and cardiovascular system.

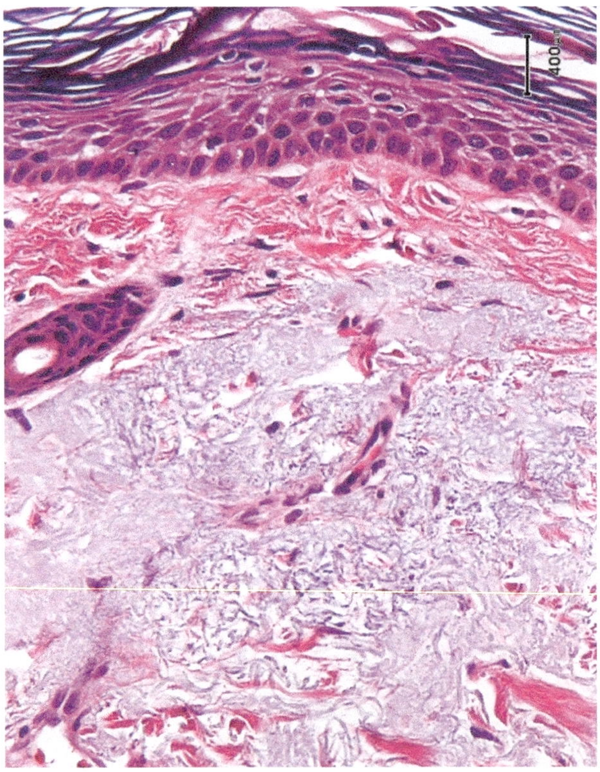

FIG. 6.39
Solar elastosis. (Courtesy of Dr. K. J. Busam.)

Clinical Findings

The skin findings are not present at birth but develop in childhood or adolescence. PXE affects the elastic network not only of the skin but also of the eyes and cardiovascular system, but not all patients develop problems in each organ site. Cutaneous lesions of PXE typically manifest as yellowish papules, especially on the neck and at flexural sites. The papules may coalesce to form cobblestone-like plaques. Extracutaneous findings include an angioid streak by fundoscopy and calcifications of midsized arteries. With more advanced disease, the soft cutaneous papules and nodules may become firm because of calcium deposits.

Histopathologic Features

Distorted fragmented calcified elastic fibers are present in the mid and deep reticular dermis (Fig. 6.40). They are best visualized by an elastic van Gieson stain.

Differential Diagnosis

The fragmented fibers of PXE should be distinguished from solar elastosis (basophilic amorphous fibers), late-onset focal dermal elastosis, and elastoderma, all of which show an increased density of normal-appearing elastic fibers in the dermis. PXE should also be distinguished from PXE-like papillary dermal elastolysis due to intrinsic and extrinsic aging in which the papillary elastic plexus is lost. PXE may be an incidental finding seen in surgical excisions, or as a features of early calciphylaxis.

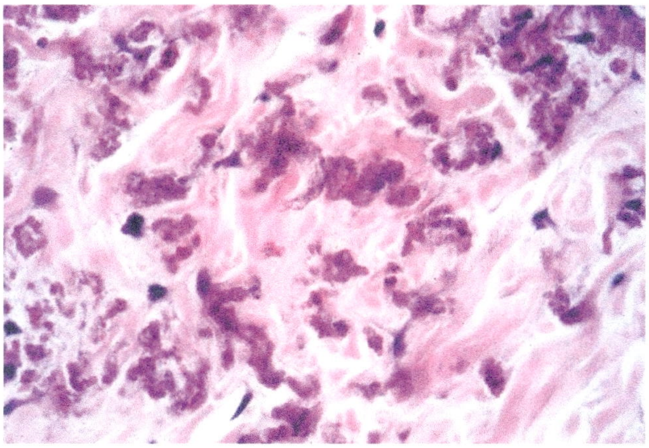

FIG. 6.40

Pseudoxanthoma elasticum with fragmented and clumped elastic fibers.

Periumbilical PXE, seen in multiparous obese women must be distinguished clinically from hereditary PXE.

Prognosis and Treatment

The cutaneous lesions primarily present a cosmetic problem. Significant morbidity may result from eye involvement, which may lead to progressive loss of visual acuity. Clinical management primarily involves monitoring disease progression (ophthalmologic examinations) and lifestyle adjustments with regard to potential cardiovascular complications.

SUGGESTED FURTHER READING

Alijotas-Reig, J., García-Gimenez, V., Velthuis, P. J., Niessen, F. B., & Decates, T. S. (2022). Inflammatory immune-mediated adverse reactions induced by COVID-19 vaccines in previously injected patients with soft tissue fillers: A case series of 20 patients. *Journal of Cosmetic Dermatology*, *21*(8), 3181–3187.

Clark, A., Kosik, G., Desrosiers, A., Tjarks, B. J., & Junkins-Hopkins, J. M. (2023). Localized argyria with pseudo-ochronosis: A report of two cases highlighting involvement of elastic fibers. *Journal of Cutaneous Pathology*, 50(9), 815–818. doi:10.1111/cup.14476.

Ferreli, C., Atzori, L., & Rongioletti, F. (2021). Obesity-associated lymphedematous mucinosis and stasis mucinosis. *Clinics in Dermatology*, *39*(2), 229–232.

Hamie, L., Haddad, I., Nasser, N., Kurban, M., & Abbas, O. (2021). Primary localized cutaneous amyloidosis of keratinocyte origin: An update with emphasis on atypical clinical variants. *American Journal of Clinical Dermatology*, *22*(5), 667–680.

Jin, M. F., Ali, N. S., Davis, D. M. R., Johnson, E. F., & Gibson, L. E. (2023). An update on long-term outcomes of pediatric follicular mucinosis over a 20-year period: A retrospective cohort study. *International Journal of Dermatology*, *62*(8), 1056–1059.

Molina-Ruiz, A. M., Cerroni, L., Kutzner, H., & Requena, L. (2014). Cutaneous deposits. *American Journal of Dermatopathology*, *36*, 1–48, 2014.

Park, H. J., Kim, W. S., Chae, S. W., & Choi, Y. J. (2023). Insulin-Derived Cutaneous Amyloidosis: A Possible Complication of Repeated Insulin Injections. *Annals of dermatology*, 35(Suppl 1), S71–S75. doi:10.5021/ad.20.207.

Requena, L., Cerroni, L., & Kutzner, H. (2012). Histopathologic patterns associated with external agents. *Dermatologic Clinics*, *30*, 731–748.

Rongioletti, F. (2006). Lichen myxedematosus (papular mucinosis): New concepts and perspectives for an old disease. *Seminars in Cutaneous Medicine and Surgery*, *25*, 100–104.

Rongioletti, F. (2020). Primary paediatric cutaneous mucinoses. *The British Journal of Dermatology*, 182(1), 29–38. doi:10.1111/bjd.18004.

Rongioletti, F (2022). New and emerging conditions of acquired cutaneous mucinoses in adults. *Journal of the European Academy of Dermatology and Venereology*: JEADV, 36(7), 1016–1024. doi:10.1111/jdv.17983..

Rongioletti, F., & Rebora, A. (2001). Cutaneous mucinoses. Microscopic criteria for diagnosis. *American Journal of Dermatopathology*, *23*, 257–267.

Santos-Juanes, J., Galache, C., Curto, J. R., Astudillo, A., & Sánchez del Río, J. (2004). Nodular primary localized cutaneous amyloidosis. *Journal of the European Academy of Dermatology and Venereology*, *18*, 224–226.

Vishwanath, T., Dhurat, R., Borawake, S., Joshi, A., Agrawal, S., & Ghate, S. (2019). Utility of Acitretin in Improving Quality of Life in Lipoid Proteinosis. *Annals of Indian Academy of Otorhinolaryngology Head and Neck Surgery*, 3(1), 49–53. doi:10.4103/aiao.aiao_4_19.

7 Nonneoplastic Disorders of Pigmentation

Kerith E. Spicknall • Ravi R. Ubriani • Loren E. Clarke • Michael E. Ming

This chapter describes key clinical and histopathologic features of relatively common or well-known nonneoplastic disorders of pigmentation. It is important to note that many pigmentary disorders will reveal normal, or only very minimally pathologic, findings on routine (hematoxylin and eosin) staining; melanin or iron stains may be necessary to detect diagnostic findings, although the results of special stains may also be nonspecific unless nearby unaffected skin is submitted together with affected skin for direct comparison.

CAFÉ-AU-LAIT MACULES

Clinical Findings

Café-au-lait macules are very common. Solitary lesions are seen in approximately 2.5% of neonates and up to 36% of school-age children. They are more common and more numerous in Black children than White children. Clinically, they appear as homogeneous light to dark brown completely macular lesions with well-defined borders that range in size from 1 mm to 20 cm or more in diameter (Fig. 7.1). Café-au-lait macules may be present at birth or manifest in the first few years of life; they increase in size proportionally as the child grows. They can be sporadic or part of a genetic syndrome, such as neurofibromatosis, Legius syndrome, or McCune-Albright syndrome; multiple lesions, especially if they are large in size or segmental in pattern, or lesions that are acquired after age 6 years, are unusual and should prompt evaluation for a genetic syndrome.

Histologic Features

Café-au-lait macules show an increase in melanin pigment within melanocytes and basal keratinocytes without proliferation of melanocytes.

Differential Diagnosis

Café-au-lait macules have a distinctive appearance and are usually easily recognizable on clinical examination, although they may be confused with lentigines, congenital melanocytic nevi, and postinflammatory hyperpigmentation. Café-au-lait macules can be differentiated from lentigines and melanocytic nevi by their lack of melanocyte proliferation and rete ridge elongation. Postinflammatory hyperpigmentation will reveal superficial dermal melanophages with or without inflammation. Histologically, café-au-lait macules are usually indistinguishable from freckles, although physical examination will easily distinguish the two diagnoses.

Prognosis and Treatment

Café-au-lait macules are benign lesions and do not require treatment. Bleaching agents and sun protection do not affect the appearance of these lesions. Laser surgery has been used to treat the cosmetic appearance of these lesions with variable success.

MELASMA

Clinical Findings

Melasma is a common acquired symmetrical hyperpigmentation of sun-exposed areas on the face found predominantly in women but may occasionally occur in men. It is most common in women of Hispanic and Asian descent. The pathophysiology of melasma is not well understood, but ultraviolet (UV) and visible light exposure, hormonal factors (contraceptives, pregnancy), and genetics may contribute. Melasma typically presents as well-defined hyperpigmented patches with scalloped borders. Three different patterns of pigmentation are commonly found: centrofacial (most common), malar, and mandibular. Wood's lamp examination has historically

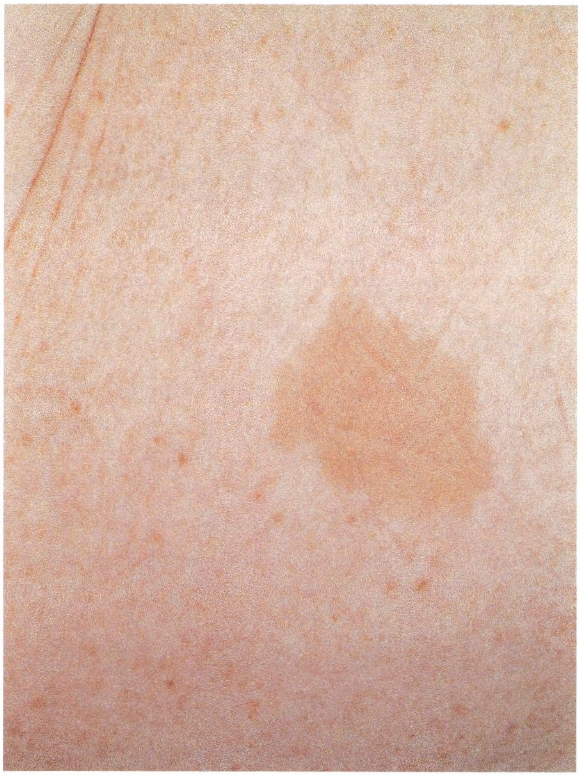

FIG. 7.1

Café-au-lait macule. A sharply demarcated, light brown patch with irregular borders.

been used as an aid in distinguishing epidermal from dermal melasma: in lesions with increased epidermal melanin, the contrast between affected and unaffected skin enhances with Wood's lamp examination. However, recent histopathologic studies have suggested that Wood's lamp examination may be inaccurate.

Histologic Features

Histologic comparison of affected to nearby unaffected skin may be necessary for diagnosis and to inform treatment and prognosis. Two histopathologic patterns have been recognized in melasma. In the first, melanin predominates within the epidermis, throughout all layers; in the second, melanin is found in the superficial dermis within macrophages (Fig. 7.2). In some patients with melasma, melanin deposition occurs within both the epidermis and dermis.

Differential Diagnosis

Melasma must be clinically distinguished from postinflammatory hyperpigmentation, drug-induced hyperpigmentation, and exogenous ochronosis. Clinically, a careful history of medications associated with hyperpigmentation, either systemic or topical; the absence of other primary lesions; and a history of worsening with sun exposure or during increased hormonal states such as pregnancy or while the patient is taking oral contraceptive pills help to distinguish melasma from other diseases.

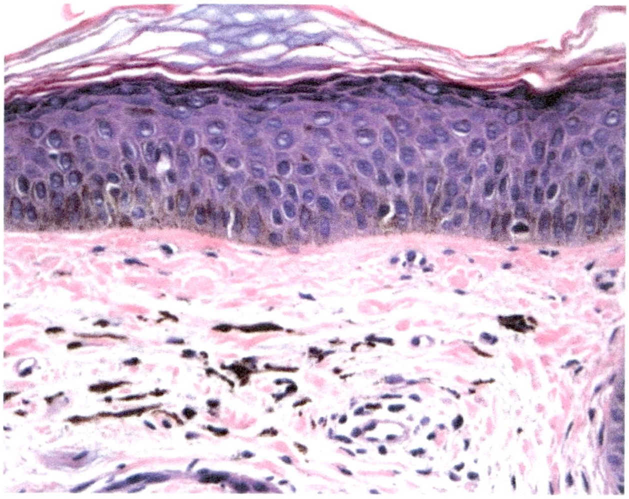

FIG. 7.2

Melasma. Both increased melanin deposition within the basal layer of the epidermis and pigment incontinence in the dermis can be seen.

Melasma may be histopathologically indistinguishable from postinflammatory hyperpigmentation. Microscopic examination may allow differentiation from certain drug-induced hyperpigmentation states that have distinctive features, such as the yellow-brown pigment seen in ochronosis.

Prognosis and Treatment

Strict photoprotection is required, including that which blocks visible light in addition to UV light. Topical bleaching agents including hydroquinone, oral tranexamic acid, and Q-switched lasers may be effective. Melasma, especially dermal melasma, is often recalcitrant to treatment and recurs when treatment is discontinued.

ACQUIRED DERMAL MACULAR HYPERPIGMENTATION

Lichen planus pigmentosus and ashy dermatosis (erythema dyschromicum perstans) are terms that have been used to describe disorders characterized by acquired patches of blue-gray-brown pigmentation on various anatomic sites that on histology reveal dermal melanophages with or without interface dermatitis. Because of considerable clinicopathologic overlap, some authors propose grouping these disorders together under the term "acquired dermal macular hyperpigmentation."

Clinical Findings

Ashy dermatosis is most commonly described in patients of Latin American descent but has also been reported in Asian and White populations. The age of onset is variable, and there is no gender predilection. No clear etiology has been established. Ashy dermatosis presents as asymptomatic ash-colored, blue-gray-brown macules and patches of variable size and shape (Fig. 7.3), sometimes with a narrow erythematous peripheral border. The lesions are symmetrically distributed, most commonly on the neck, trunk, and proximal arms. Lesions are usually slowly progressive and may persist for years.

Lichen planus pigmentosus preferentially affects adults with darker skin types and is considered by some to be a variant of lichen planus. It presents as blue-gray-brown macules and patches on sun-exposed and intertriginous sites; persistence is common, as are exacerbation and remission. Rarely, it is seen in association with other variants of lichen planus, although it is important to distinguish lichen planus pigmentosus from simple postinflammatory hyperpigmentation secondary to papular lichen planus.

Histologic Features

Superficial dermal melanophages are always seen. Epidermal atrophy, basal vacuolization, occasional colloid bodies, and an interface, lichenoid or perivascular, lymphocytic infiltrate may also be present (Fig. 7.4).

FIG. 7.3

Acquired dermal macular hyperpigmentation. Smooth brownish-blue patches on the face and neck of a patient with pigmented skin.

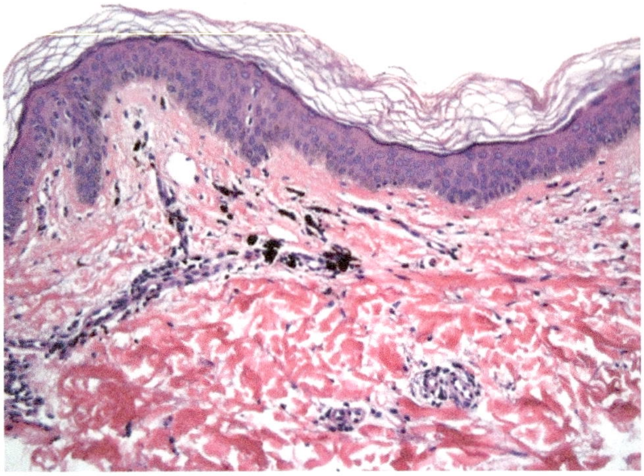

FIG. 7.4

Acquired dermal macular hyperpigmentation. There is pigment incontinence with numerous melanophages concentrated around vessels within the superficial dermis. A sparse perivascular inflammatory infiltrate is also present.

Differential Diagnosis

Lichen planus pigmentosus and ashy dermatosis must be distinguished from postinflammatory hyperpigmentation (including that seen after lichenoid eruptions), generalized fixed drug eruption, and pigmented contact dermatitis (Riehl melanosis); the histopathology of these conditions may overlap, so the distinction is clinical. The gray-blue hue of lichen planus pigmentosus and ashy dermatosis differs clinically from the brown hue seen in postinflammatory hyperpigmentation. The location of lesions and a careful drug history may be helpful in distinguishing lichen planus pigmentosus and ashy dermatosis from multiple lesions of a fixed drug eruption and lesions of drug deposition, the latter of which will also be histopathologically distinct, depending on the inciting drug. Exposure history and patch testing will distinguish lichen planus pigmentosus and ashy dermatosis from pigmented contact dermatitis.

Prognosis and Treatment

Treatment of lichen planus pigmentosus and ashy dermatosis is difficult and lesions tend to persist. Responses to clofazimine, dapsone, isotretinoin, bleaching agents, chemical peels, and lasers have been reported. There are occasional spontaneous remissions.

DRUG-INDUCED PIGMENTATION

Many drugs are associated with pigmentation of the skin. Medications commonly associated with pigmentary change include antineoplastic medications, antimalarial drugs, heavy metals, and hormones. Specific medications that are well known to cause pigmentation include amiodarone, azidothymidine, clofazimine, hydroxychloroquine, and minocycline. The clinical and histologic appearance of drug-induced pigmentation is variable, depending on the inciting agent, and an exhaustive description is beyond the scope of this chapter. Four of the more common or distinctive drug-induced pigmentations are described in detail here.

MINOCYCLINE-INDUCED PIGMENTATION

Clinical Findings

Minocycline is commonly used for acne and other inflammatory conditions. Long-term use of this tetracycline derivative can result in cutaneous pigmentation, which is thought to be the result of overproduction of melanin.

Three classic types of cutaneous pigmentation, and a very rarely reported fourth type, may be seen. Type I is a dark blue to black pigmentation that occurs on the face in areas of inflammation or previous scarring, such as in acne scars. Type II pigmentation is a blue to gray discoloration of previously normal skin (Fig. 7.5) that is most often seen on the anterior legs but that may also involve the arms. Type III is a diffuse muddy brown hyperpigmentation that is most prominent in sun-exposed areas. Type IV is blue-gray pigmentation within scars on the back.

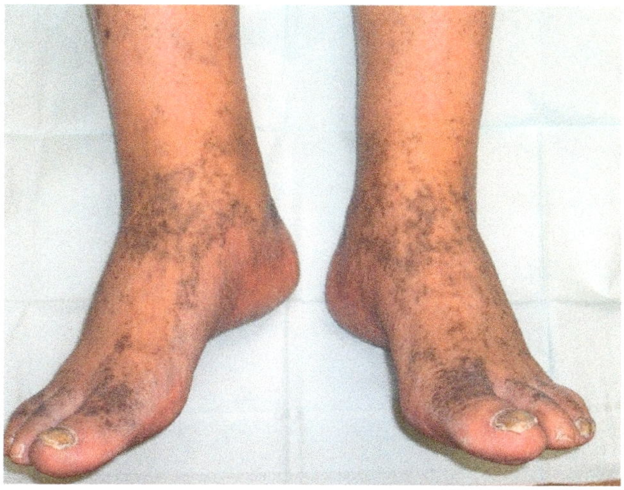

FIG. 7.5

Minocycline-induced pigmentation, type II. Gray-brown pigmentation on the dorsal feet.

Histologic Features

Each of the clinical types of minocycline pigmentation has distinctive histopathologic features (Fig. 7.6). Type I is characterized by aggregates of pigment-laden macrophages within the dermis which are labeled by Prussian blue stain, but melanin may also be present. Type II lesions also demonstrate macrophages containing pigment that is positive with iron stains and Fontana-Masson. The lesions in type III contain increased amounts of melanin within basal keratinocytes and within dermal macrophages. Type IV pigmentation reveals pigment in the dermis that is labeled by Fontana-Masson.

Ancillary Studies

A combination of histochemical stains helps classify the pigment based on its reaction with Prussian blue and Fontana-Masson stains (see the preceding discussion).

Differential Diagnosis

Clinically, types I and IV minocycline pigmentation can be confused with other drug-induced pigmentation such as that caused by amiodarone, exogenous ochronosis, and heavy metal exposure. Type II may overlap clinically and microscopically with hydroxychloroquine pigmentation. Type III must be distinguished from melasma and postinflammatory hyperpigmentation. In all cases, a careful exposure history is the most straightforward means of determining the correct diagnosis.

Prognosis and Treatment

After minocycline is discontinued, types I and II pigmentation will typically resolve over months to years but type III pigmentation persists indefinitely. Laser therapy has been used with some success in recalcitrant cases.

HYDROXYCHLOROQUINE-INDUCED PIGMENTATION

Antimalarials including hydroxychloroquine, chloroquine, mefloquine, quinacrine, and mepacrine may cause variable patterns of skin and mucosal pigmentation. Hydroxychloroquine is discussed here, as it is commonly used in dermatology practice and up to one-third of patients on the medication may be affected by pigmentation.

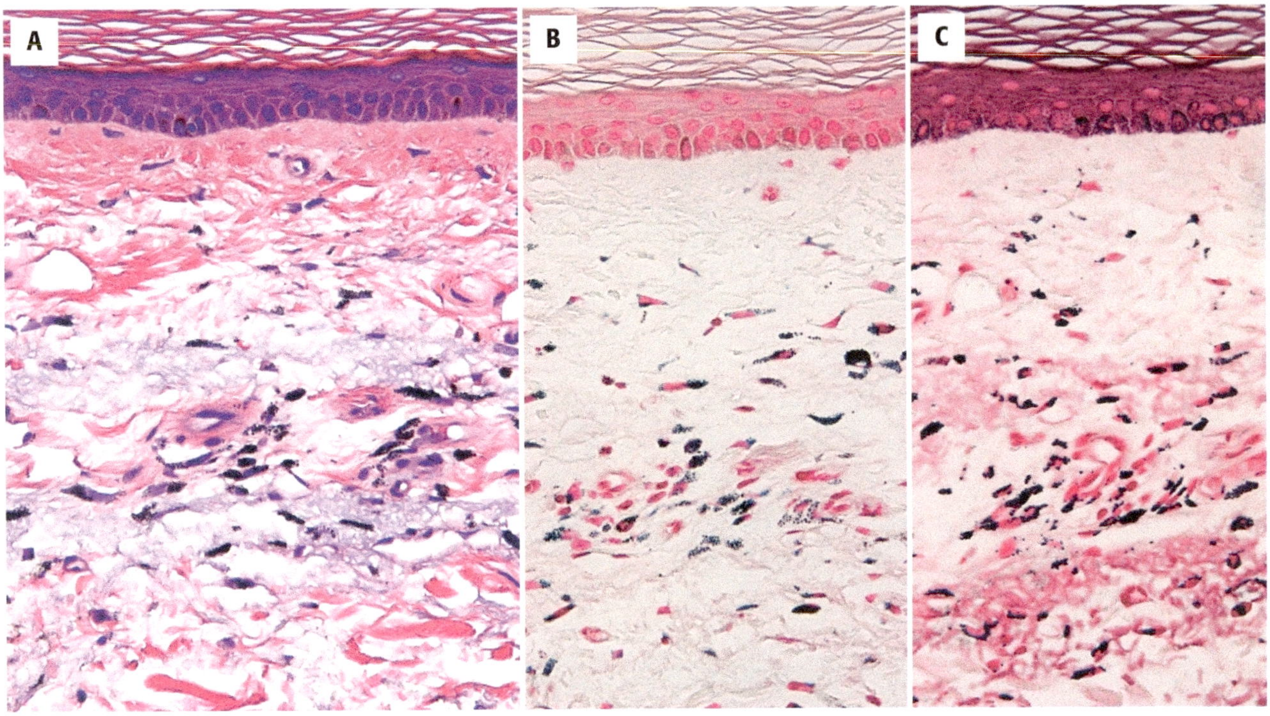

FIG. 7.6

Minocycline-induced pigmentation. **A,** Granular, dark brown or black pigment is present, both free within the dermis and within dermal macrophages. The pigment granules are highlighted by both the Prussian blue reaction (**B**) and Fontana-Masson (**C**).

Clinical Findings

Hydroxychloroquine may cause blue-gray to dark purple macules and patches on the head and shins (Fig. 7.7), typically after a cumulative dose of several hundred grams. Patients on antiplatelet and/or anticoagulation agents may be at higher risk of pigmentation than others.

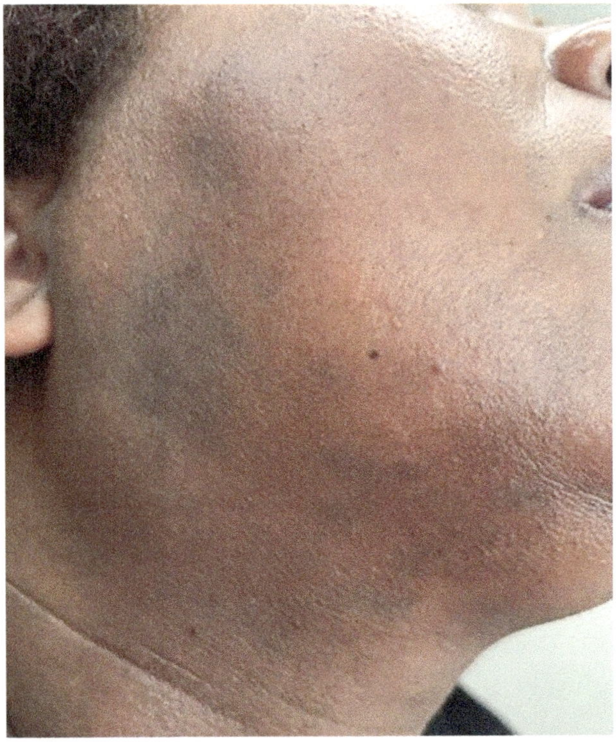

FIG. 7.7

Hydroxychloroquine-induced pigmentation. Brownish-blue smooth patches on the skin.

Histologic Features

There is yellow-brown pigment in the superficial dermis, both free and within macrophages (Fig. 7.8A).

Ancillary Studies

The dermal pigment is positive by both Prussian blue and/or Fontana-Masson stains (Fig. 7.8B and C).

Differential Diagnosis

Clinically and microscopically, hydroxychloroquine pigmentation is similar to type II minocycline pigmentation and must be distinguished by drug history.

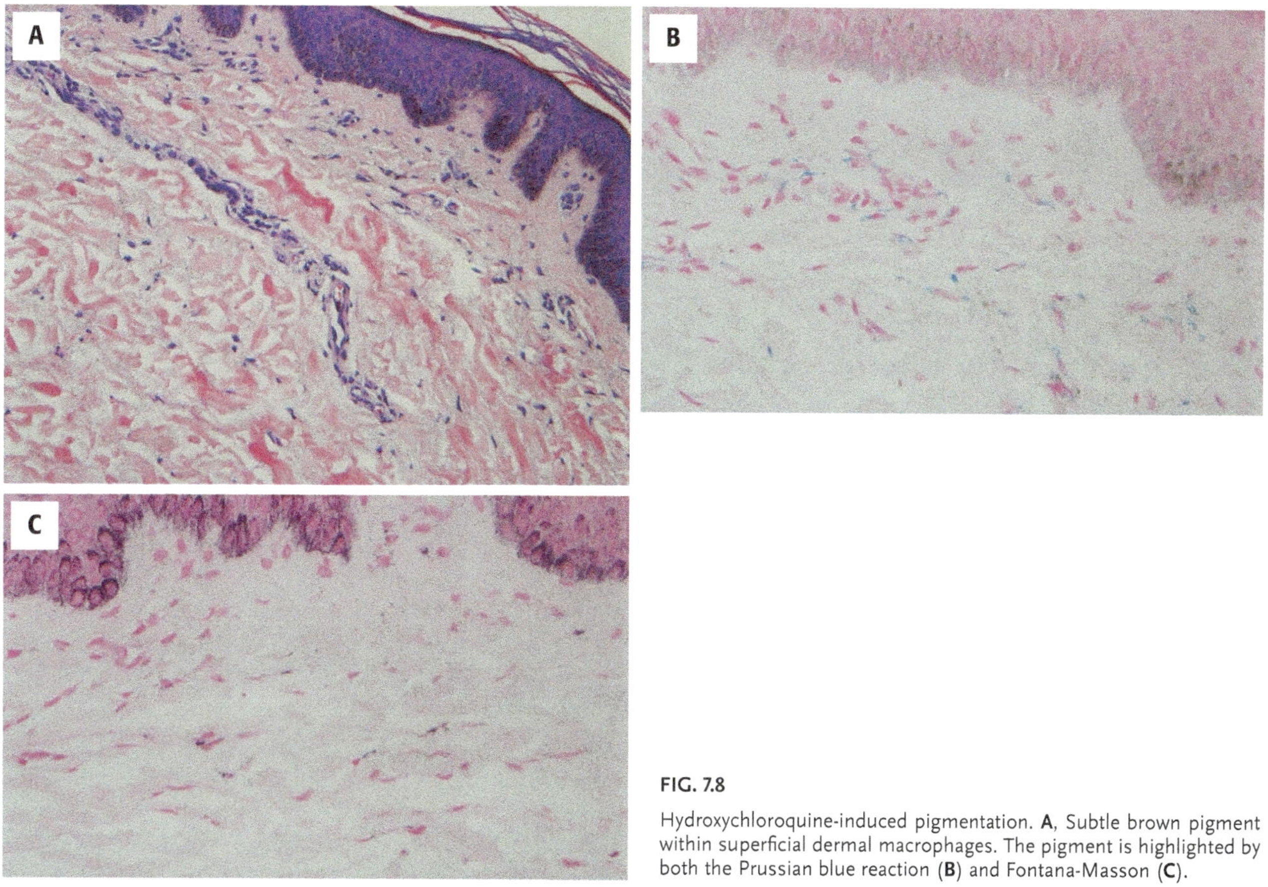

FIG. 7.8

Hydroxychloroquine-induced pigmentation. **A**, Subtle brown pigment within superficial dermal macrophages. The pigment is highlighted by both the Prussian blue reaction (**B**) and Fontana-Masson (**C**).

Prognosis and Treatment

Some improvement may occur if hydroxychloroquine is discontinued, although complete resolution is rare and improvement has also been reported even when the drug is continued.

AMIODARONE-INDUCED HYPERPIGMENTATION

Clinical Findings

Long-term continuous use of this antiarrhythmic agent can cause bluish-gray to purple pigmentation of photodistributed skin, most commonly the face. This condition is more common at higher doses of amiodarone.

Histologic Features

Yellow-brown lipofuscin pigment granules are present within dermal macrophages and endothelial cells.

Ancillary Studies

The granules are typically positive by periodic acid-Schiff (PAS) staining and in some cases stain with the Ziehl-Neelsen, Fontana, and Sudan black methods.

Differential Diagnosis

Other forms of drug-induced hyperpigmentation should be considered in the differential diagnosis, including minocycline hyperpigmentation, exogenous ochronosis, and heavy metal exposure. A careful history is usually sufficient to distinguish among these. Most patients who develop amiodarone hyperpigmentation have taken the drug continuously for at least 3 months.

Prognosis and Treatment

After discontinuation of amiodarone, the pigmentation fades in months to years in most cases, although some patients' hyperpigmentation never completely resolves.

IMIPRAMINE-INDUCED HYPERPIGMENTATION

Clinical Findings

Long-term use of imipramine, a tricyclic antidepressant, may result in slate-gray to blue to brown pigmentation of sun-exposed skin, typically the face (Fig. 7.9). The incidence is unknown but likely very rare. Typically, patients have taken imipramine for at least 2 years before changes in their skin color. Darkening of the iris has also been reported, although the mucous membranes are typically spared.

Histologic Features

Golden-brown globules of refractile pigment (Fig. 7.10) are present within macrophages and scattered among dermal collagen bundles.

Ancillary Studies

The pigment can be highlighted by the Fontana-Masson stain but is negative with Prussian blue stain.

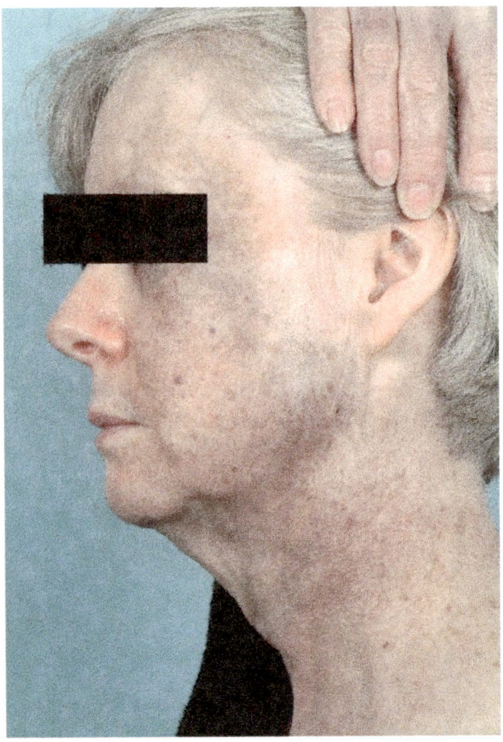

FIG. 7.9

Imipramine-induced pigmentation. Brown patches on the face, most prominently in sun-exposed areas, that occurred after initiation of imipramine.

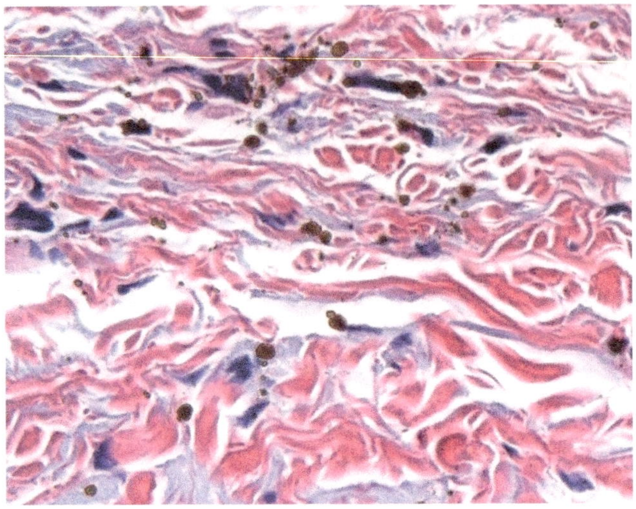

FIG. 7.10

Imipramine-induced pigmentation. Refractile gold-brown pigment globules are scattered throughout the superficial dermis.

Differential Diagnosis

Other forms of drug-induced hyperpigmentation should be considered in the differential diagnosis. As with other types of drug hyperpigmentation, the clinical history is usually sufficient to make the correct diagnosis.

Prognosis and Treatment

After discontinuation of imipramine, pigmentation may improve, although variably so. Laser therapy may be helpful.

POSTINFLAMMATORY HYPERPIGMENTATION

Clinical Findings

Postinflammatory hyperpigmentation is one of the most common types of hyperpigmentation and one for which clinical attention is often sought. A common consequence of a resolved inflammatory process in the skin, the resultant postinflammatory pigmentation is usually in the shape of the resolved active lesion. The pigment becomes more noticeable as the primary lesion fades. UV and visible light may worsen the pigmentation. Any inflammatory process can produce postinflammatory hyperpigmentation, but diseases characterized by a lichenoid infiltrate that damages the basal layer of the epidermis tend to produce the finding more often. Assuming that there is no recurrence of the primary

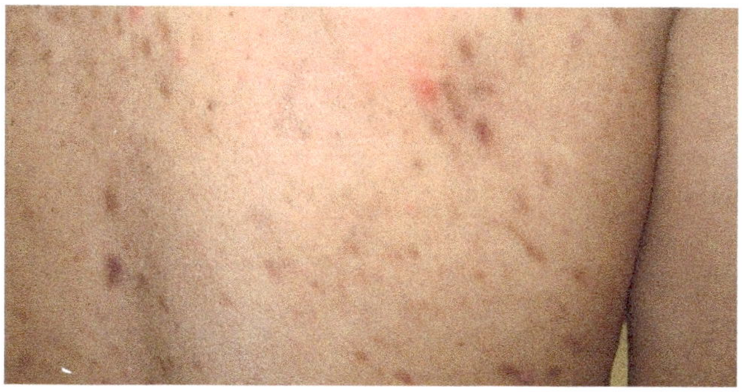

FIG. 7.11

Postinflammatory hyperpigmentation. Brown macules on the patient's back at the sites of previous inflammation from folliculitis.

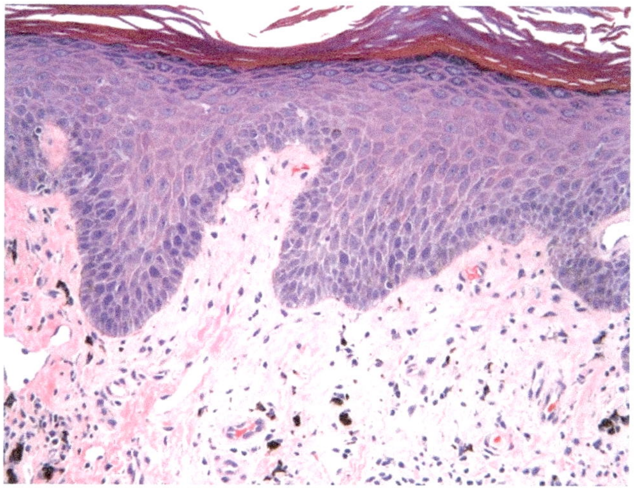

FIG. 7.12

Postinflammatory hyperpigmentation. Numerous melanophages and scattered mononuclear cells within the dermis in a patient with recent lichenoid drug eruption.

process, the postinflammatory pigmentation will resolve eventually over time, but it can take months or even years to completely fade. This process is much more common in darker-pigmented individuals. It shows no age or gender predilection.

The gross appearance of this lesion can be highly variable, depending on the morphology and distribution of the primary process. The color of the lesion is usually light to dark brown (Fig. 7.11) but can be gray or have a blue or red tinge.

Histologic Features

The lesions reveal dermal melanosis with or without an increase in epidermal melanin. Within the dermis, the melanin may be either free or contained within melanophages (Fig. 7.12). When increased epidermal melanin is present, it is concentrated within basilar keratinocytes. An inflammatory infiltrate, particularly one that is lichenoid, is often encountered within early lesions but may be absent in those of long duration. For prognostic reasons, comparison of affected hyperpigmented skin with unaffected skin may be helpful in order to localize the pigmentation.

Ancillary Studies

If there is concern about a regressed melanocytic lesion, an immunostain for a melanocyte differentiation antigen (SOX-10, microphthalmia-associated transcription factor [MITF]) may highlight any focal residual melanocytic neoplasm.

Differential Diagnosis

The diagnosis is usually straightforward because patients typically report a history of an inflammatory lesion at the site of increased pigmentation. When no such history can be obtained, the differential diagnosis may include melasma or erythema dyschromicum perstans, neither of which can be reliably excluded by microscopic examination alone. Clinicopathologic correlation can exclude the possibility of a regressing melanocytic lesion such as a nevus or melanoma.

Prognosis and Treatment

Postinflammatory hyperpigmentation tends to fade over time, resolving completely in many cases within 6 months, although in darker-pigmented individuals, and in cases where the pigment deposition is dermal, the lesions may take longer to resolve or be permanent. Chemical peels and laser treatment have resulted in variable success; potential benefits of treatment must outweigh the risk of treatment-induced postinflammatory hyperpigmentation.

DISORDERS OF DECREASED PIGMENTATION

Disorders that always result in decreased or absent pigmentation are described below. It is important to note that hypopigmented variants occur in many neoplastic, inflammatory, and infectious disorders, including mycosis fungoides, sarcoidosis, pityriasis lichenoides chronica, seborrheic dermatitis, tinea versicolor, and Hansen disease; these disorders are discussed in other chapters. The mechanism and histopathologic correlates of hypopigmentation in these variants are often not known.

VITILIGO

Clinical Findings

Vitiligo affects approximately 0.5% to 2% of the population with age of onset usually between 10 and 30 years old. There is no gender predilection, and it generally occurs in healthy individuals. Although it is known that depigmentation results from the loss of functional melanocytes, and vitiligo is now classified as an autoimmune disease, its pathogenesis is not known. Vitiligo is frequently associated with autoimmune thyroid disease, especially Hashimoto's thyroiditis.

The disease presents as well-demarcated macules completely devoid of pigment that are surrounded by normal skin (Fig. 7.13). They are more apparent in darkly pigmented skin; in individuals with lightly pigmented skin, a Wood's light may help to accentuate the pigment loss. The macules are usually asymptomatic but may occasionally itch or have an erythematous border and typically expand outward slowly over time. Markers of active, progressive vitiligo include Koebnerization, trichrome lesions, inflammatory lesions, and confetti-like depigmentation.

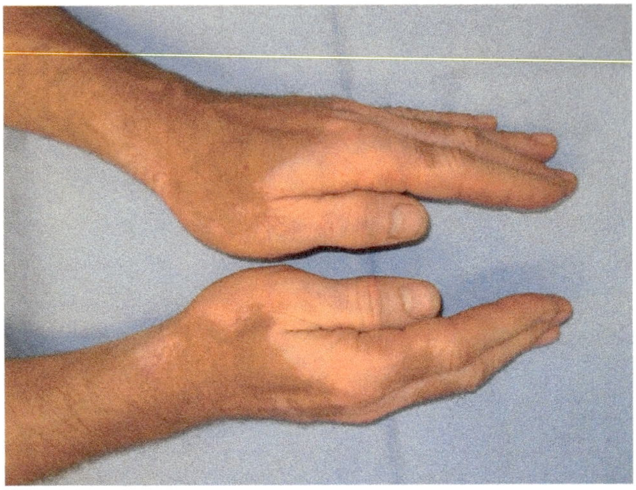

FIG. 7.13

Vitiligo. Sharply demarcated depigmented patches.

VITILIGO—DISEASE FACT SHEET

Patient Group

- 0.5% to 2% of the general population is affected
- Usual age of onset is 10 to 30 years
- Associated with autoimmune thyroid disease

Common Site of Involvement

- Face (periocular, periorificial)
- Extremities (hands, wrists, elbows, knees, ankles)
- Scalp: localized patch of white or gray hair (poliosis)

Clinical Lesional Appearance

- Depigmented (whitish) macules or patches
- Usually with discrete margins
- Lesions enlarge centrifugally

Clinical Subtypes

- Nonsegmental vitiligo
  - Generalized
  - Acral/acrofacial
  - Focal
  - Mucosal
  - Universal
- Segmental vitiligo
  - Monosegmental
  - Bisegmental
  - Plurisegmental
- Other mixed, rare, and unclassified types
- Chemical-induced vitiligo

Prognosis

- Clinical course is unpredictable
- Usually slow progression but may stabilize

Treatment

- Topical: corticosteroids, calcineurin inhibitors, JAK inhibitor
- Phototherapy
- Oral pulse dose corticosteroids
- Transplantation

Vitiligo is now classified as either nonsegmental or segmental. Nonsegmental vitiligo includes generalized, acral/acrofacial, and other variants and tends to progress slowly with time. Segmental vitiligo has a segmental pattern, often involves the head, and, after initial rapid onset, usually remains stable.

Chemical-induced depigmentation, indistinguishable from nonsegmental vitiligo in its morphology, pattern, and histopathology, is considered by some to be a variant of vitiligo. Similar to nonsegmental vitiligo, a symmetric distribution is common and sites that did not come into contact with the depigmenting chemical can be affected. Chemical-induced vitiligo is often caused by exposure to compounds that contain a phenol group, which may interfere with melanogenesis by causing melanocyte-specific autoimmunity. Monobenzyl ether of hydroquinone is one such chemical, which is used therapeutically to depigment normal skin in patients with extensive, treatment-resistant nonsegmental vitiligo. Spontaneous resolution may occur with removal of the offending agent but for lesions that require treatment, modalities similar to those used for vitiligo can be attempted, with a focus on UV therapy.

Histologic Features

The diagnosis of vitiligo is usually made based on clinical findings; thus histopathology is not needed.

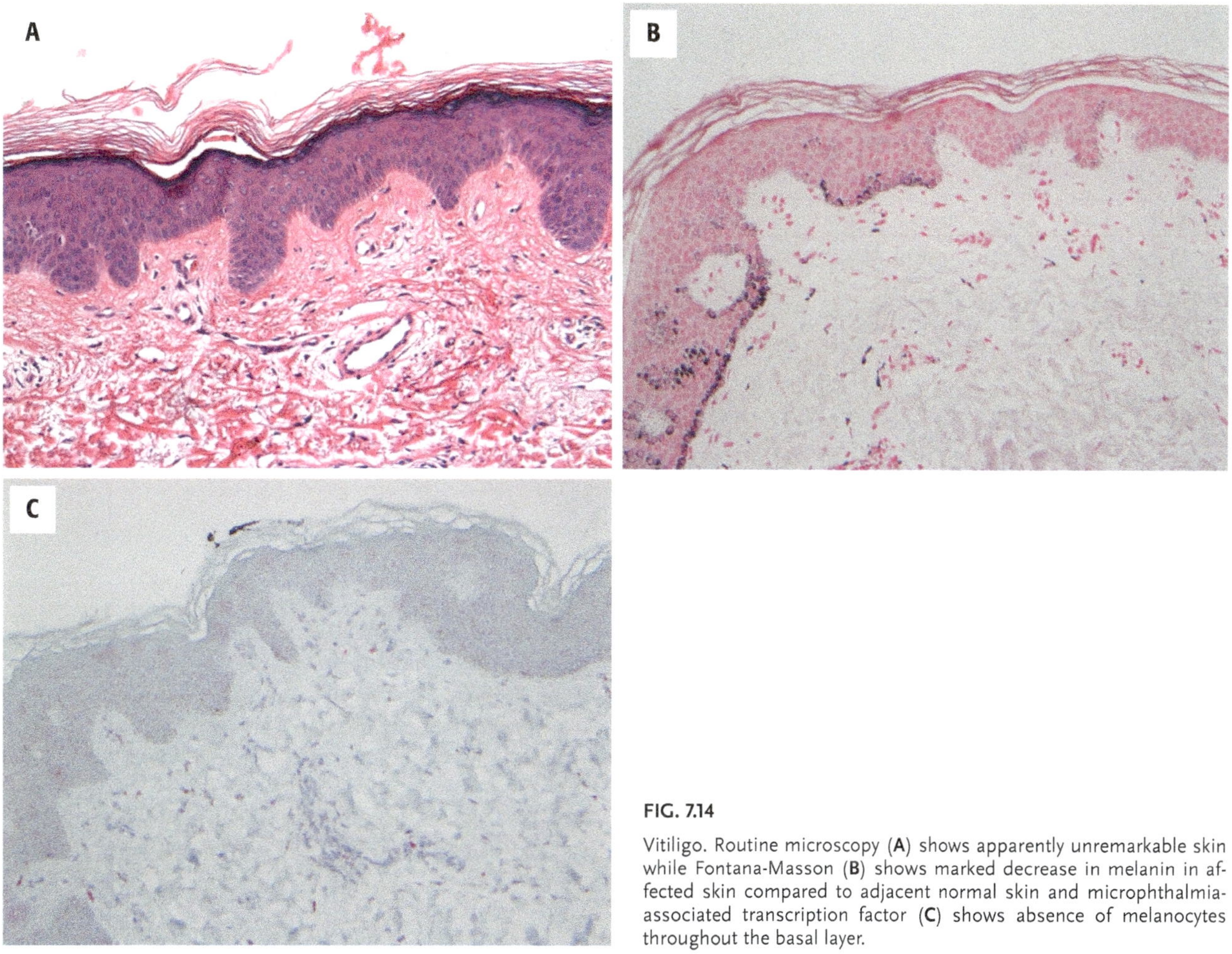

FIG. 7.14

Vitiligo. Routine microscopy (**A**) shows apparently unremarkable skin while Fontana-Masson (**B**) shows marked decrease in melanin in affected skin compared to adjacent normal skin and microphthalmia-associated transcription factor (**C**) shows absence of melanocytes throughout the basal layer.

In established lesions of vitiligo (Fig. 7.14), melanin and melanocytes are significantly decreased or absent. A sparse lymphocytic infiltrate may rarely be present in acute lesions, particularly near the advancing border.

VITILIGO—PATHOLOGIC FEATURES

Histologic Features

- Often, normal-appearing skin at scanning magnification
- Decrease to complete absence of melanin pigment and melanocytes in established lesions
- Rarely, a mild interface lymphocytic infiltrate

Ancillary Studies

- Fontana-Masson stain reveals marked decrease to complete absence of melanin
- Immunostains for melanocyte differentiation markers help assess density of melanocytes

Differential Diagnosis

- Chemical-induced vitiligo (indistinguishable)
- Hypopigmented mycosis fungoides (clinical correlation)
- Tinea versicolor (presence of fungal spores and hyphae)

Ancillary Studies

Histochemical stains for microorganisms, in particular fungal stains (Gomori methenamine silver, PAS with diastase digestion [PAS-D]), will exclude tinea versicolor.

Immunostains with antibodies to melanocyte differentiation antigens help assess the density of intraepidermal melanocytes. They typically reveal reduced or absent melanocytes in vitiligo lesions.

Molecular studies for *TCR* gene rearrangements may be helpful (albeit not decisive) for the distinction of vitiligo from hypopigmented variants of mycosis fungoides.

Differential Diagnosis

So long as depigmentation is not mistaken for hypopigmentation, the clinical diagnosis of vitiligo is usually straightforward. The clinical differential diagnosis of acquired generalized depigmented lesions includes chemical-induced vitiligo (sometimes referred to as chemical-induced leukoderma), discoid lupus erythematosus, scleroderma, lichen sclerosus (especially genital), and onchocerciasis; all of these disorders can be distinguished from vitiligo by history and clinical findings. The depigmented patches of albinism and piebaldism are present at birth, unlike vitiligo.

If lesions of vitiligo include prominent zones of hypopigmentation (as in trichrome vitiligo), then hypopigmented disorders may be considered, including hypopigmented mycosis fungoides, postinflammatory hypopigmentation, pityriasis alba, tinea versicolor, idiopathic guttate hypomelanosis, nevus depigmentosus, and Hansen disease; most of these are easy to distinguish from vitiligo by clinical morphology alone. It is important to note that acute vitiligo may rarely show exocytosis of CD8-positive lymphocytes that mimics hypopigmented mycosis fungoides; because loss of melanin and melanocytes may be incomplete in acute vitiligo, clinical course may be most helpful to distinguish the two diagnoses. While tinea versicolor and vitiligo may both reveal little or no pathology on scanning magnification, tinea versicolor will reveal many fungal elements in the stratum corneum at higher magnification.

Prognosis and Treatment

The course of vitiligo is unpredictable and there is no cure. The psychological effects of vitiligo can be profound; in some countries, there is a long-standing stigma associated with dyspigmentation. All patients may be counseled on use of camouflaging makeup. Early lesions may be more responsive to treatment than older lesions. Treatment is based on the subtype of vitiligo (nonsegmental vs. segmental) and presence or absence of active progression. Nonsegmental vitiligo may be treated with systemic steroids if rapidly progressive; topical steroids, topical calcineurin inhibitors, and UV therapy are used in stable patients. A topical JAK inhibitor was recently approved in the United States. In some cases where depigmentation is widespread, depigmenting agents are used on the remaining normally pigmented skin to achieve a uniform pigmentation pattern. Because segmental vitiligo has a short active phase before stabilization, transplantation is recommended.

PITYRIASIS ALBA

Clinical Findings

This disease mainly affects children. It typically manifests as ill-defined subtly scaly hypopigmented patches (Fig. 7.15) and is the most common type of hypopigmentation seen in children, with estimates that it affects about 5% of children. It appears most commonly on

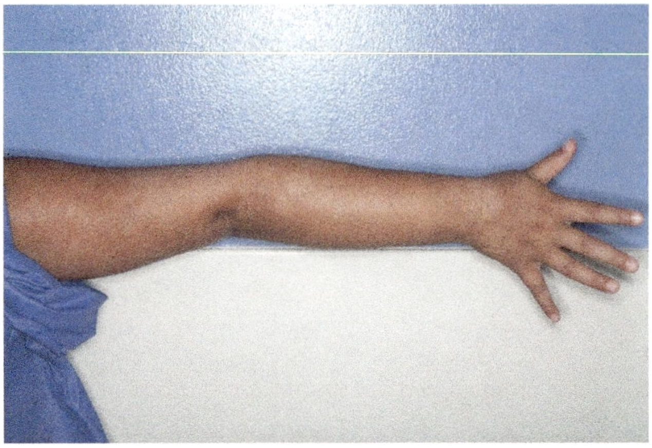

FIG. 7.15

Pityriasis alba. Hypopigmented patches with slight scale on the arm of a child.

the face, neck, or arms. Pityriasis alba is associated with an atopic diathesis.

The disease manifests as multiple symmetric 0.5- to 4-cm ill-defined patches, usually on the face, especially the cheeks. The lesions initially may appear erythematous before becoming hypopigmented with a fine scale. The hypopigmentation of the lesions is incomplete, as opposed to the depigmentation seen in vitiligo.

Histologic Features

Microscopic examination of lesions of pityriasis alba may show mild spongiotic dermatitis with a variable and irregular decrease of melanin in the epidermis. Melanocytes remain normal in number or are slightly decreased. Some authors have noted the appearance of follicular spongiosis and follicular plugging in early lesions.

Ancillary Studies

A PAS-D stain can help exclude tinea versicolor if the presence or absence of budding yeast or short hyphae is difficult to assess on hematoxylin and eosin-stained sections.

Differential Diagnosis

Pityriasis alba can be confused clinically with vitiligo, tinea versicolor, and hypopigmented mycosis fungoides. The presence of scale, and hypo-, rather than depigmentation, differentiates it from vitiligo; pityriasis alba will not reveal loss of melanocytes. Lesions of tinea versicolor affect the trunk and only rarely affect the face, unlike pityriasis alba; they will reveal microorganisms, either histologically or on potassium hydroxide preparation. Hypopigmented mycosis fungoides does not preferentially affect the face, as pityriasis alba does; histopathology of the two diagnoses may overlap.

Prognosis and Treatment

Pityriasis alba typically spontaneously remits by adulthood but may run a relapsing course of months or years before remission. It is especially noticeable in the summer when contrast between affected and normal skin is accentuated by tanning of the normal surrounding skin. Pityriasis alba can be distressing in darkly pigmented individuals, especially when it affects the face. Treatment with emollients may reduce scaling or dryness, but the hypopigmentation typically takes months or even years to resolve. Topical steroids, topical calcineurin inhibitors, and phototherapy are not uniformly effective.

HYPOMELANOTIC MACULES (ASH-LEAF SPOTS)

Clinical Findings

This skin finding is seen in tuberous sclerosis, which affects one in 6000 individuals. One-third of cases of tuberous sclerosis are familial, with the rest being the result of spontaneous mutations. Hypomelanotic macules, found in more than 80% of individuals with tuberous sclerosis, are often the earliest cutaneous finding of tuberous sclerosis (often present at birth) and expand in size and number with age. Up to 4% of normal individuals have this finding, but in large studies, no unaffected individual had more than three such lesions, and a large number of hypomelanotic macules should lead one to consider the diagnosis of tuberous sclerosis.

Classically, the lesion has one rounded edge and one sharp edge, as does the eponymous ash leaf (Fig. 7.16). They can be up to 12 cm in diameter. A Wood's light accentuates the appearance of these lesions. More than three of these lesions should prompt further consideration of the diagnosis of tuberous sclerosis.

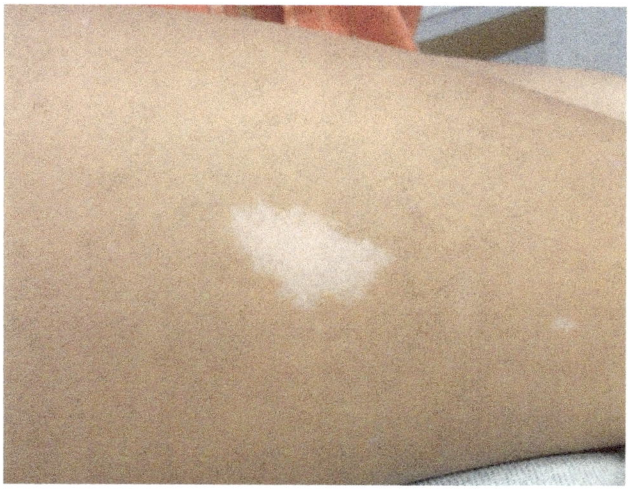

FIG. 7.16

Hypopigmented macule (ash-leaf spot). A hypopigmented patch on the thigh of a child with tuberous sclerosis shows retention of follicular pigment.

Histologic Features

Microscopic examination typically shows a normal or slightly decreased number of melanocytes but a reduction in the amount of epidermal melanin.

Differential Diagnosis

Hypopigmented macules can be confused with vitiligo, piebaldism, and nevus depigmentosus. Microscopically, whereas hypopigmented macules contain normal or only slightly decreased numbers of melanocytes, melanocytes are absent in piebaldism and fully developed cases of vitiligo. The distinction between hypomelanotic macules and nevus depigmentosus is difficult, as the histology is identical, as nevus depigmentosus is imprecisely named and reveals hypopigmentation rather than true depigmentation. Neurologic findings are not associated with any of the latter diagnoses; thus neurologic abnormalities should lead one to consider a diagnosis of tuberous sclerosis.

Prognosis and Treatment

The presence of more than three hypopigmented macules early in life should prompt clinical consideration of the diagnosis of tuberous sclerosis and further workup. Early diagnosis of the disease is crucial because of the need for monitoring and genetic testing.

POSTINFLAMMATORY HYPOPIGMENTATION

Clinical Findings

Postinflammatory hypopigmentation can follow resolution of the active lesions in many inflammatory skin

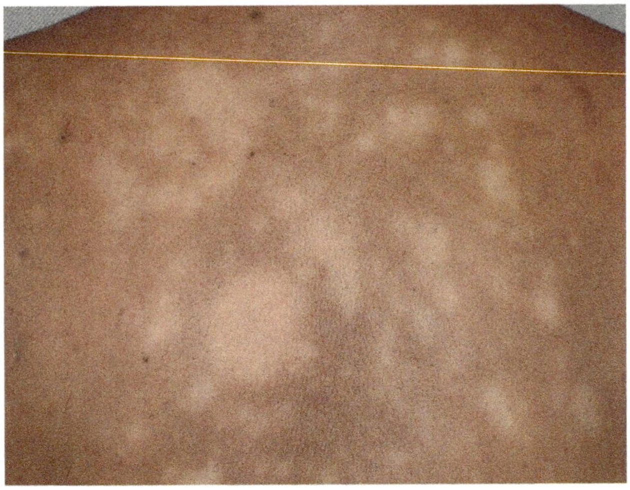

FIG. 7.17

Postinflammatory hypopigmentation. This patient had hypopigmentation after inflammatory process had resolved.

disorders (Fig. 7.17). After resolution of an inflammatory process in the skin, postinflammatory hypopigmentation in the distribution, pattern, and shape of the previous lesions may result. The lack of pigment becomes noticeable as the primary lesion fades. Assuming the primary process does not recur, postinflammatory hypopigmentation typically resolves over time, but it may take months or even years to completely fade.

The appearance is dependent on the morphology and distribution of the primary process. The lesion is a macule or patch with indistinct borders and a variable degree of hypopigmentation.

Histologic Features

The histopathology of postinflammatory hyperpigmentation is not well characterized, however, biopsies may be indicated in order to exclude active disease.

Differential Diagnosis

The diagnosis is usually obvious by the patient's report of a previous inflammatory lesion at the sites of hypopigmentation. When no such history can be obtained, the differential diagnosis includes pityriasis alba, hypopigmented tinea versicolor, hypopigmented mycosis fungoides, progressive macular hypomelanosis, and the hypopigmented lesions of Hansen disease. Histopathologic examination may be helpful to exclude active inflammatory or infectious disease.

Prognosis and Treatment

Assuming that the original inflammatory process does not recur, postinflammatory hypopigmentation will resolve slowly over time without any additional treatment, although months to years may be necessary for complete resolution.

SUGGESTED FURTHER READING

Bergqvist, C., & Ezzedine, K. (2020). Vitiligo: A review. *Dermatology, 236*(6), 571–592.

Harris, J. E. (2017). Chemical-induced vitiligo. *Dermatologic Clinics, 35*(2), 151–161.

Ko, D., Wang, R. F., Ozog, D., Lim, H. W., & Mohammad, T. F. (2023). Disorders of Hyperpigmentation. Part II. Review of management and treatment options for hyperpigmentation. *Journal of the American Academy of Dermatology, 88*(2), 291–320. doi:10.1016/j.jaad.2021.12.065.

Nahhas, A. F., Braunberger, T. L., & Hamzavi, I. H. (2019). An update on drug-induced pigmentation. *American Journal of Clinical Dermatology, 20*, 75–96.

Saleem, M. D., Oussedik, E., Picardo, M., & Schoch, J. J. (2019). Acquired disorders with hypopigmentation: a clinical approach to diagnosis and treatment. *Journal of the American Academy of Dermatology, 80*(5), 1233–1250.e10.

Wang, R. F., Ko, D., Friedman, B. J., Lim, H. W., & Mohammad, T. F. (2023). Disorders of Hyperpigmentation. Part I. Pathogenesis and clinical features of common pigmentary disorders. *Journal of the American Academy of Dermatology, 88*(2), 271–288. doi:10.1016/j.jaad.2022.01.051.

Alopecia

8

Nathaniel Evan Smith • Shawn E. Cowper

INTRODUCTION

Alopecia is one of the most challenging topics in dermatopathology. While the number of commonly encountered diagnoses is small, the histological overlap between entities can be substantial. In many cases, clinical correlation is required to reach a definitive diagnosis. Unfortunately, clinicians—an increasing number of whom may be nonphysicians—often have no specific training in the examination of alopecia patients and will simply obtain a shallow, 2- to 3-mm punch biopsy of the scalp and submit it with a diagnosis of "alopecia."

The problems do not end there. There are significant advantages to processing alopecia specimens in the transverse manner, but if this is not undertaken by the receiving laboratory, the diagnostic specificity may be impacted. Add to this the relative infrequency of alopecia biopsies received by dermatopathologists—many of whom are themselves intimidated by reading transversely cut specimens—and soon the formula for diagnostic mediocrity is complete.

The good news is that solutions to all these issues are available. While entire textbooks on alopecia can be consulted for additional background, the emphasis of this chapter is on practicality, not disease pathophysiology. The approach included in this chapter is one that teaches differentials through a systematic process of elimination that results in either a specific diagnosis or a differential that can often be resolved by the clinician. The emphasis is on primary alopecias; secondary alopecias, representing a minority of clinical cases, are not covered in depth in this chapter (Table 8.1).

As emphasized throughout this chapter, clinicopathological correlation is the formula for diagnostic success. If a specific diagnosis cannot be reached due to incomplete historical or clinical detail, there are practical tips provided for further clinical workup that can be provided in a diagnostic note. Inviting your contributor to be a part of the team will benefit everyone involved: patient, clinician, and pathologist.

BIOPSY COLLECTION AND PROCESSING

Collecting a biopsy sample is a statistical exercise. The goal is to take a small portion of tissue that will accurately

TABLE 8.1

Alopecias Covered in This Chapter

Cicatricial Alopecias	"Biphasic" Alopecias	Noncicatricial Alopecias
Lichen planopilaris	Androgenetic alopecia	Alopecia areata
Frontal fibrosing alopecia	Chronic traction alopecia	Noncicatricial alopecia of SLE
Fibrosing alopecia in a Pattern distribution	Alopecia areata (s)	Psoriatic alopecia
Central centrifugal cicatricial alopecia	**CONGENITAL ALOPECIA**	Sebopsoriasis/seborrheic dermatitis
Acne keloidalis	Temporal triangular alopecia	Acute telogen effluvium
Chronic cutaneous lupus erythematosus		Loose anagen hair syndrome
Dissecting cellulitis		Trichotillomania
Folliculitis decalvans		Fungal kerion (i)
End-stage cicatricial alopecia		Syphilitic alopecia (i)
		Postoperative pressure–induced alopecia (MD)
		TNF-inhibitor–induced alopecia (MD)

Definitions:
Cicatricial alopecia: clinical hair loss with destructive loss of the follicular unit.
Biphasic alopecia: clinical hair loss due to progressive shortening of anagen phase.
Noncicatricial alopecia: clinical hair loss without loss of the follicular unit.
Congenital alopecia: clinical hair loss present from birth.
i, Infectious; *MD*, iatrogenic; *s*, sometimes; *SLE*, systemic lupus erythematosus; *TNF*, tumor necrosis factor.

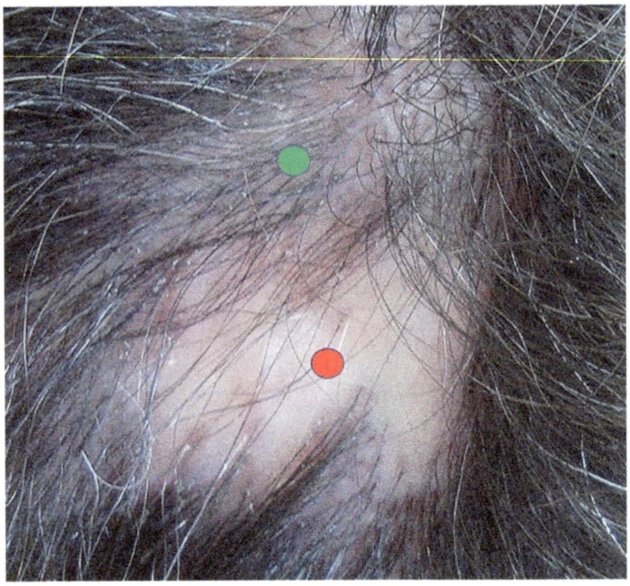

FIG. 8.1

Biopsy site selection. Avoid sampling where follicular markings are absent *(red)*. Instead, choose an area where erythema is present around hair follicles producing a shaft *(green)*. (From Miguel-Gómez, L., Rodrigues-Barata, A. R., Molina-Ruiz, A., Martorell-Calatayud, A., Fernández-Crehuet, P., Grimalt, R., et al. (2018). Folliculitis decalvans: Effectiveness of therapies and prognostic factors in a multicenter series of 60 patients with long-term follow-up. *Journal of the American Academy of Dermatology*, 79(5), 878–883, Fig. 1b.)

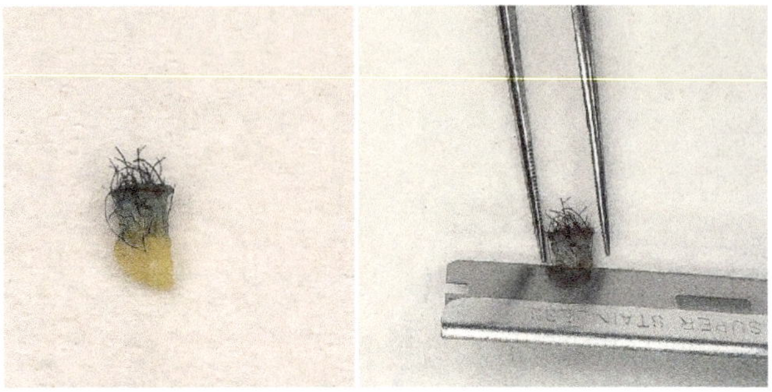

FIG. 8.2

A 4-mm punch biopsy specimen of scalp *(left)* with placement of knife for transverse sectioning *(right)*.

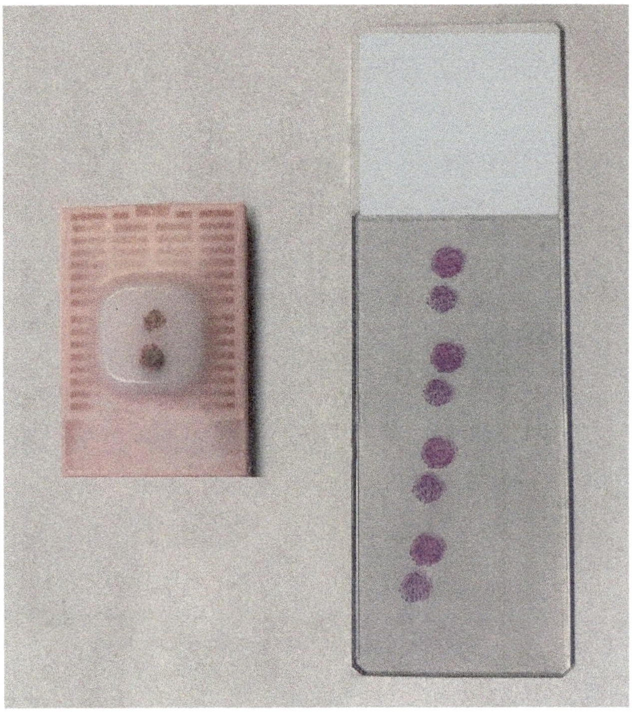

FIG. 8.3

Paraffin block after embedding of transversely sectioned scalp biopsy *(left)* with resultant glass slide *(right)*.

represent the pathological process so that definitive treatment can be planned. In alopecia workups, the target tissue is usually the scalp. Even though the loss of hair is often widespread, in most cases, the clinician will only perform a single punch biopsy. To maximize yield, a 4-mm (or larger) punch biopsy is recommended, and importantly, the punch instrument should be inserted to the hilt. This will ensure that the subcutis and hair bulbs are sampled. It is imperative that the sample be collected in an area of disease activity. In most cases, this will be a zone that contains some remaining hair shafts. Areas devoid of hair shafts should be avoided (Fig. 8.1).

The specimen is placed in fixative and delivered to a skin pathology laboratory familiar with transverse (horizontal/en face) alopecia biopsy preparation. Contrary to typical skin pathology biopsy specimens that are embedded and sectioned longitudinally (with skin on one end and subcutis on the other), alopecia samples are best cut transversely. A single cut along the midline of the specimen is preferred, with each of the resulting cylinders of skin embedded in paraffin on end (Fig. 8.2). After sectioning at the microtome, the tissue profiles visible on the glass slide will be discs representing cross sections of skin (Fig. 8.3). The tissue block is then sampled at multiple levels to ensure a representation of all follicles along their entire length, from their bulbs to the epidermis. Since the cut specimen is embedded en face in the midline, additional levels will expose the more superficial aspects of the biopsy half containing the epidermis and the deeper portions of the biopsy half containing the subcutaneous tissue. Six or more levels are usually adequate, and unstained recuts can be held at various levels in case additional stains are contemplated.

NORMAL HAIR FOLLICLE ANATOMY AND GROWTH CYCLES

Normal hairs of the scalp are of two types. The most numerous and largest hairs are the "terminal" hairs. These hairs are produced by follicles with their bulbs

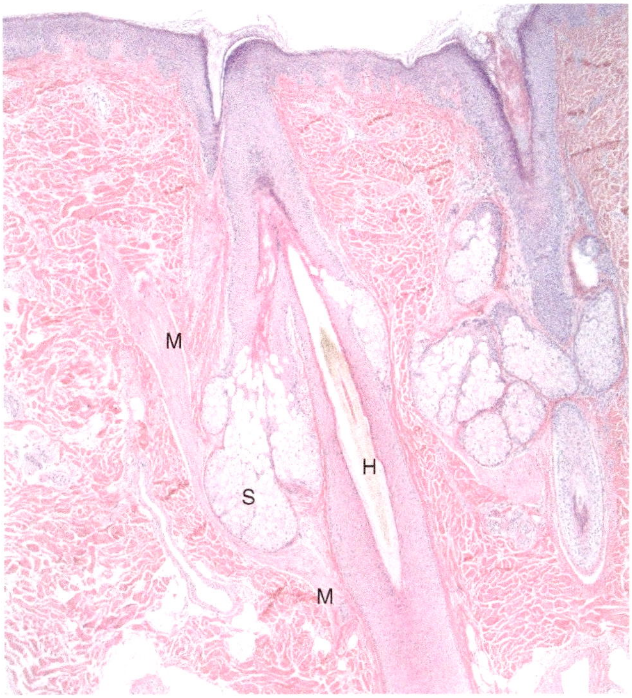

FIG. 8.4
Terminal follicle, perpendicular section, showing central hair shaft *(H)* with sebaceous lobules *(S)*, and pili arrector muscle *(M)* (Hematoxylin & eosin, ×40).

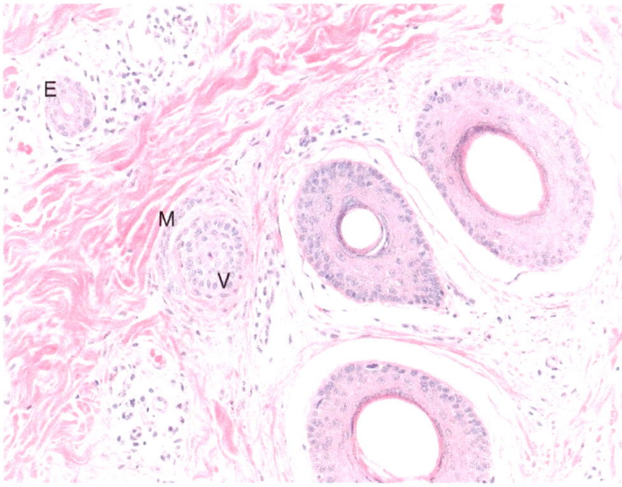

FIG. 8.5
Three terminal follicles *(right)* and one vellus follicle *(left)* in transverse section. Note the semicircular vellus mantle *(M)* around the vellus follicle epithelium *(V)*. The structure at the top left is an eccrine (sweat) duct *(E)* (Hematoxylin & eosin, ×200).

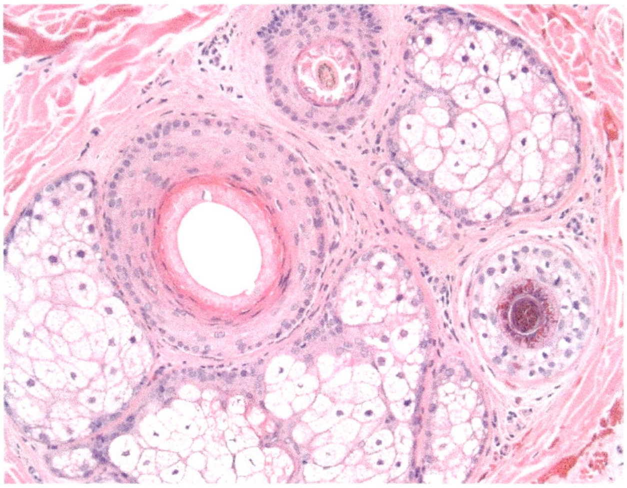

FIG. 8.6
One terminal follicle *(left)* and two vellus follicles *(top and right)* in transverse section, surrounded by sebaceous lobules (Hematoxylin & eosin stain, ×200).

anchored in the subcutis and are associated with full-size sebaceous lobules (Fig. 8.4). The other hairs, "vellus" hairs, are produced by a much smaller follicle that is anchored in the upper dermis and has an associated rudimentary sebaceous mantle rather than a sebaceous lobule (Fig. 8.5). The diameter of a terminal hair shaft is greater than 0.06 mm and that of a vellus shaft is less than 0.03 mm (Fig. 8.6). Hair shafts measuring between these sizes are sometimes observed and are termed "indeterminate."

In transverse section within the upper dermis, hair shaft epithelia are arranged in follicular "units" comprising 2–5 terminal hairs, up to two vellus hairs, and their associated sebaceous structures (Fig. 8.7). The average overall ratio of terminal to vellus hairs (T:V ratio) is 2:1, although variation within individual units is common. The follicular unit typically has an enveloping fibrous matrix that is slightly denser than the surrounding dermis. Units are arranged in a mostly orderly manner within the dermis, separated by dermal fibroconnective tissue that may contain vessels, nerves, eccrine ducts, and pili arrector muscles (Fig. 8.8). In the deeper dermis, the orderly bundled nature of the follicular unit is lost.

The density of follicular units averages about one per square millimeter of scalp surface area. A 4-mm punch biopsy of skin (12.6 mm^2) contains roughly 12 units. There is considerable variation in follicle unit density among ethnic groups, with Black patients typically manifesting a lower density than those of other groups (Fig. 8.9, Table 8.2).

Hair follicular epithelia undergo asynchronous cycles of growth and involution. These cyclic "phases" are termed anagen, catagen, and telogen. Each phase has characteristic histological features. The ratio of anagen to catagen and telogen phases can offer diagnostic clues to the alopecia workup.

Anagen phase typically lasts 2–7 years and is the period during which a hair shaft is actively produced (often referred to as "growth" phase). Anagen phase is always followed by catagen phase. Catagen phase

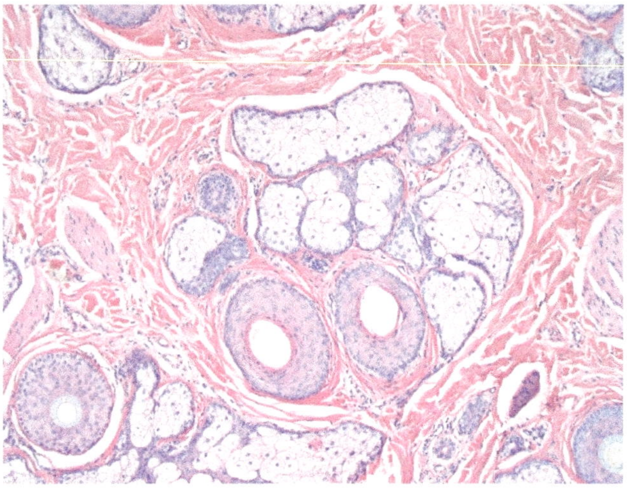

FIG. 8.7

One follicular unit *(center)* composed of two terminal follicles and one vellus follicle and associated sebaceous lobules in transverse section (Hematoxylin & eosin stain, ×100).

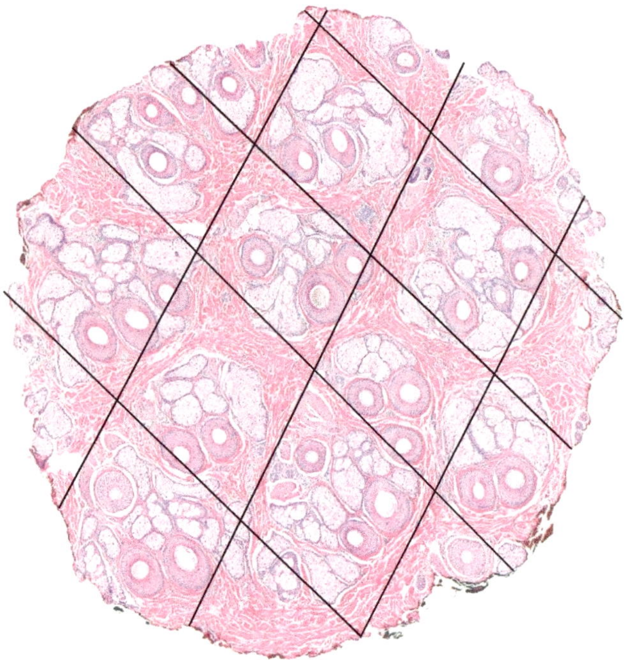

FIG. 8.8

A 4-mm transversely oriented punch biopsy of scalp with orderly arrangement of follicular units (Hematoxylin & eosin, low magnification).

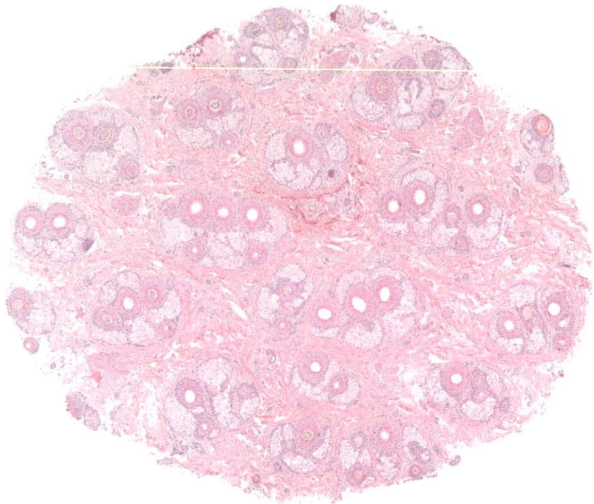

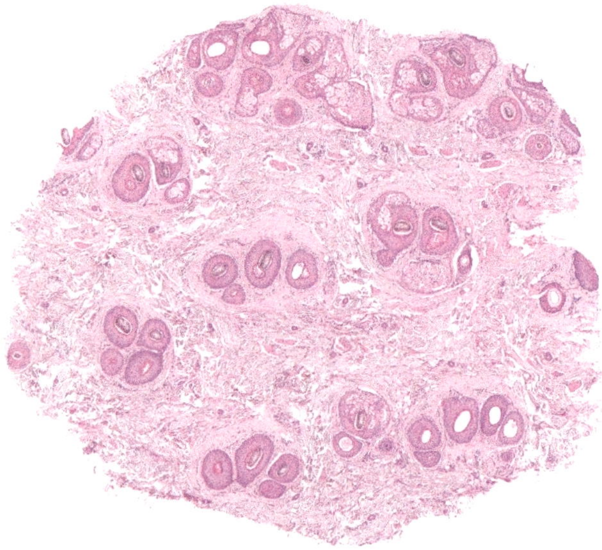

FIG. 8.9

A 4-mm transversely oriented punch biopsy of scalp. White patient *(top)* and Black patient *(bottom)* (Hematoxylin & eosin, low magnification).

is brief, lasting about 2 weeks. During catagen, the deep portion of the follicle undergoes apoptosis-mediated involution. Following catagen phase, a period of quiescence occurs. This phase, known as telogen, typically lasts about 2 months. During this period, the hair shaft produced by the most recent anagen phase is loosely anchored in the upper follicle and can be easily shed. Telogen ends when the next anagen phase begins.

Using the 2 year/2 week/2 month ratio outlined above as a "stereotypical" cycle, a normal census of follicles can be calculated. At any given time on the normal scalp, approximately 91% of follicles would be in anagen phase, with 2% in catagen and 7% in telogen phase (Fig. 8.10). Since catagen leads almost immediately to telogen, the two phases can be combined for practicality to generate a "telogen count." A normal telogen count is about 9% (2% + 7%). While there is individual variation, a telogen count greater than 20% is considered abnormal. As a rule of thumb, a 4-mm punch biopsy in transverse section may reveal one catagen phase follicle. More than one catagen follicle is a clue to increased follicular cycling.

TABLE 8.2

Variations in Normal Anatomy in White and Black Patients

	Terminal	Vellus	Total Hairs	Terminal Anagen	Terminal Cat/Tel	Telogen Count	Terminal: Vellus Ratio
	T	*V*	*T+V*	*TA*	*TCT*	*TCT/T*	*T:V*
4-mm PUNCH (12.6 mm²)							
White patients							
Deep dermis	33	0	33	28–33 (85%–100%)	0–5 (0%–15%)	6% (0%–15%)	At least 2:1
Superficial dermis	33	5	38 (19–59)				
Black patients							
Deep dermis	18	0	18	15–18 (85%–100%)	0–3 (0%–15%)	7% (0%–17%)	At least 2:1
Superficial dermis	18	3	21 (11–33)				
3-mm PUNCH (7.1 mm²)							
White patients							
Deep dermis	21	0	21	18–21 (85%–100%)	0–3 (0%–15%)	6% (0%–15%)	At least 2:1
Superficial dermis	21	1	22 (11–34)				
Black patients							
Deep dermis	10	0	10	8–10 (85%–100%)	0–2 (0%–15%)	7% (0%–17%)	At least 2:1
Superficial dermis	10	1	11 (5–17)				

Terminal hairs are greater than 0.06 mm diameter, bulbs in fat.
Indeterminate hairs are between 0.03 and 0.06 mm in diameter.
Vellus hairs are less than 0.03 mm in diameter (IRS as thick or thicker than shaft).

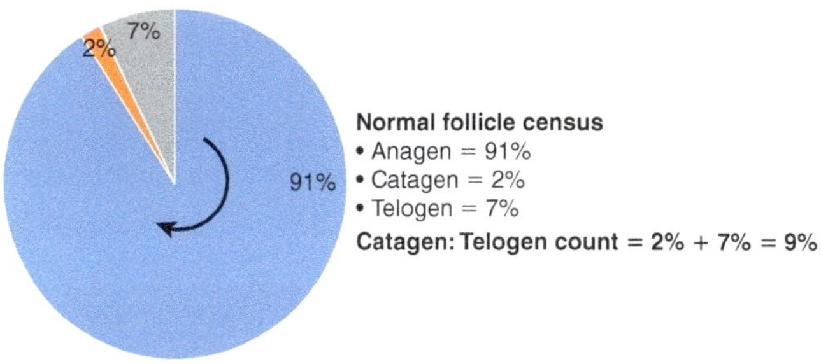

FIG. 8.10

While there is slight ethnic and individual variation, this chart illustrates the relative percentage *(census)* of anagen:catagen:telogen follicles on a normal scalp (assuming a 2-year:2-week:2-month cycle).

ANAGEN FOLLICLE ANATOMY

During growth phase, the follicular epithelium is represented in its fullest form. The deepest structure, residing in the subcutis, is the *follicular bulb* or "germ." The bulb consists almost entirely of an organized body of highly mitotically active basophilic matrical cells. This germinative body, when observed in transverse sections, forms a ring around a central mesenchymal papilla containing supportive vessels and nerve endings (Fig. 8.11). Maturing matrical cells grow parallel to one another, squeezed toward the epidermal surface through a sleeve of epithelium, the root sheath. The diameter of the hair shaft is dictated by the volume of the matrical cell mass. The bulbar matrix also contains pigment-producing melanocytes, and the density and type of melanin produced give the hair shaft its native color.

The germinative bulbar epithelium merges with (and is surrounded by) the root sheath epithelium. In the *suprabulbar zone*, the root sheath keratinocytes are glycogenated (pale to clear on hematoxylin and eosin [H&E]–stained sections) (Fig. 8.12). Maturation occurs from the perimeter of the root sheath and proceeds centrally, toward the emerging hair shaft. The outermost edge of the sheath is delineated by a thin anucleate glassy membrane (vitreous membrane) to which the most immature keratinocytes of the outer root sheath (ORS) are affixed. As the keratinocytes mature toward the hair shaft, a cornified zone containing bright red (trichohyalin) granules forms the inner root sheath (IRS). This IRS is adherent to the emerging nucleated hair shaft at this level of the hair follicle.

Continuing along the follicle toward the epidermis, the *isthmus* of the hair follicle begins as the suprabulbar trichohyaline granules vanish from the IRS. At this level, the extruding hair dissociates from the IRS, rapidly losing individual matrical cell nuclei, and emerging as a shaft of pigmented keratin. In histological sections, the hair shaft is often dislodged (Fig. 8.13). As the isthmus proceeds toward the surface, the ORS epithelium becomes less glycogenated and more keratinized, with a somewhat translucent IRS forming the inner keratinized

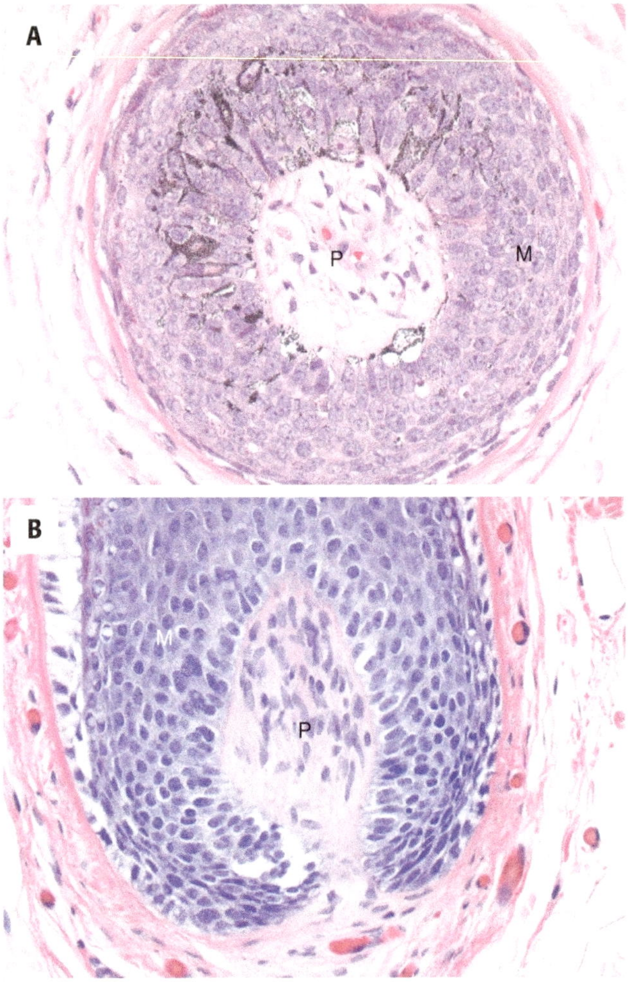

FIG. 8.11

Follicular bulb, transverse section (**A**) and perpendicular section (**B**). Basophilic matrical cells *(M)* surround the central mesenchymal papilla *(P)*. Matrical cells produce the keratin hair shaft. Darkly pigmented dendritic melanocytes are present in dark hair (Hematoxylin & eosin, ×400).

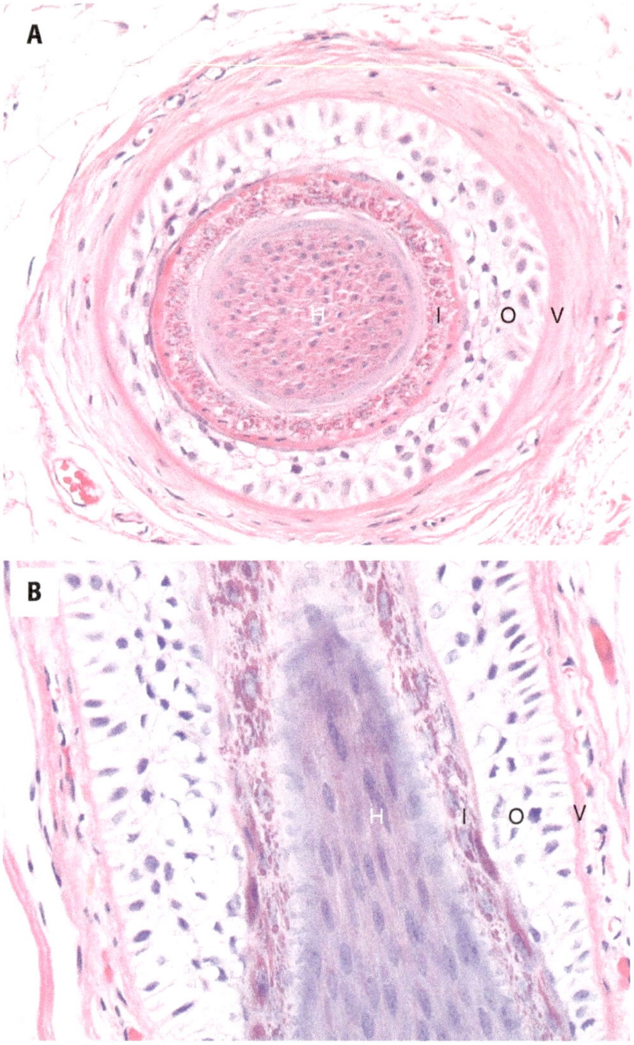

FIG. 8.12

Suprabulbar area, transverse section (**A**) and perpendicular section (**B**). From the center working outward there is a central nucleated hair *(H)* shaft surrounded by inner root sheath (I) containing trichohyaline granules. The outer root sheath *(O)* is glycogenated. Surrounding this is a thin, refractile vitreous membrane *(V)* (Hematoxylin & eosin, **A**, ×200 and **B**, ×400).

surface. In transverse sections, adjacent dermal eccrine coils are a helpful landmark at this level of the hair follicle. The cross-section of the hair shaft, now free-floating in the sleeve of root sheath epithelium, ranges from round to elliptical, the latter shape tending to form curlier hair (Fig. 8.14).

In the mid isthmus, the attachment point of the arrector pili muscle is encountered (Fig. 8.15). This useful anatomic landmark delineates the cycling portion of the follicle. Deep to the insertion point, the isthmus undergoes cyclic growth and involution. A pool of follicular stem cells located near the muscular insertion point facilitates the regrowth of deep follicle structures upon initiation of anagen. Destruction of this focus of follicular stem cells leads to loss of the entire follicular unit (a cicatricial alopecia).

In transverse sections, the deep border of full-sized sebaceous lobules serves as an anatomic landmark in the dermis suprajacent to the arrector pili muscles. Of diagnostic import, the IRS normally desquamates (Fig. 8.16) in the vicinity of this region of the isthmus. While the level of IRS desquamation shows slight variability from follicle to follicle, some cicatricial alopecias show premature desquamation of the inner root sheath (PDIRS) in most of the affected follicles (Fig. 8.17). This manifests as loss of the IRS in the deep isthmus, at (or deeper than) the eccrine coils. Confidence in identifying PDIRS is dependent on the number of follicles exhibiting this feature (more follicles = more confidence), the depth of the finding (deeper involvement = more confidence), and the experience level of the pathologist. In central centrifugal cicatricial alopecia (CCCA), PDIRS is considered the earliest identifiable histopathological finding.

Moving along the hair follicle toward the epidermis, the insertion of the sebaceous duct is encountered

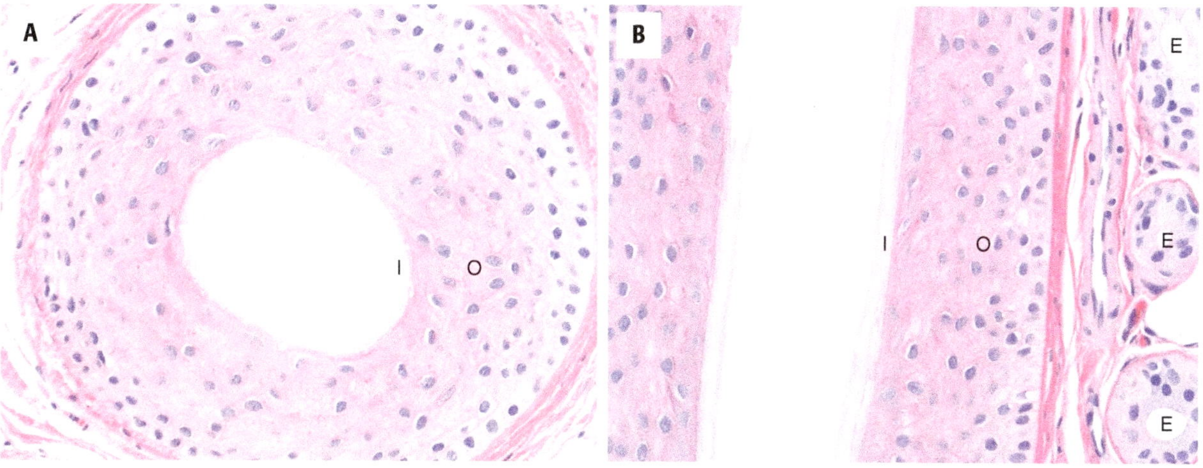

FIG. 8.13

Isthmus, transverse section (**A**) and perpendicular section (**B**). From the center working outward there is a central hair shaft (not pictured) surrounded by translucent inner root sheath *(I)*. The outer root sheath *(O)* becomes increasingly keratinized as the upper follicle is approached. Eccrine glands are noted in the adjacent dermis at this level *(E)* (Hematoxylin & eosin, ×400).

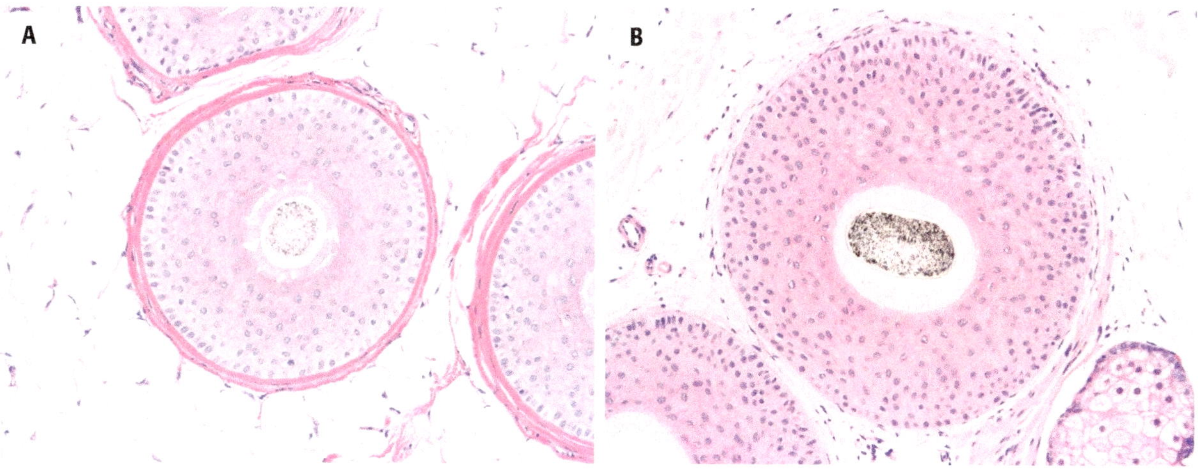

FIG. 8.14

Isthmus, transverse section, with central hair shaft with round cross-section (**A**) and elliptical cross-section (**B**) (Hematoxylin & eosin, ×200).

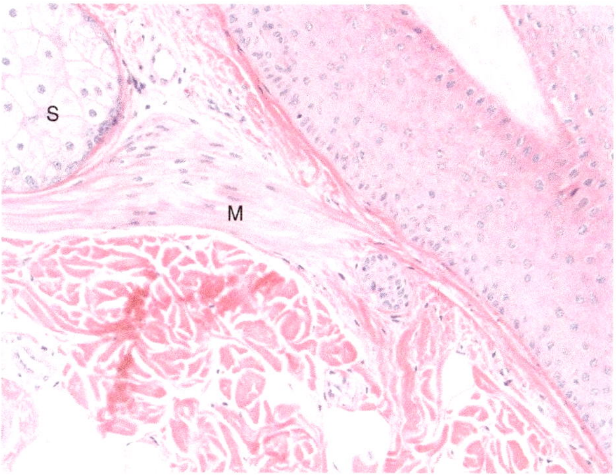

FIG. 8.15

Isthmus, perpendicular section, with attachment of the arrector pili muscle *(M)*. The attachment site on the isthmus epithelium marks the site of follicular stem cells needed for continued follicular cycling. The deep edge of a sebaceous lobule *(S)* is also noted (Hematoxylin & eosin, ×200).

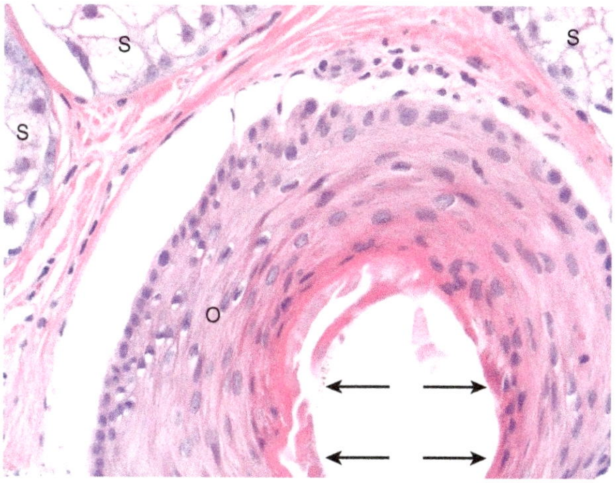

FIG. 8.16

Isthmus, transverse section. Desquamation of the inner root sheath *(arrows)* is noted at this level. The outer root sheath *(O)* remains intact. The deep edges of sebaceous lobules *(S)* are also noted (Hematoxylin & eosin, ×400).

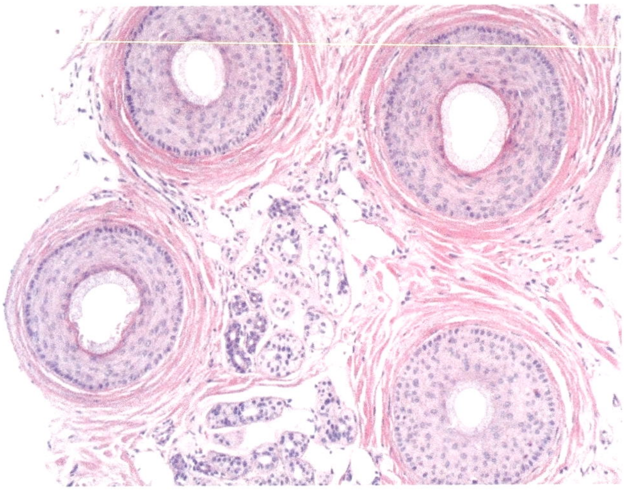

FIG. 8.17

A transverse section shows four follicles at the level of the eccrine coils. The inner root sheath of the bottom left follicle is prematurely desquamated. The top right follicle shows an earlier stage of this process with the junction between outer and inner root sheath becoming intensely eosinophilic. This biopsy is from a patient with central centrifugal cicatricial alopecia (Hematoxylin & eosin, ×100).

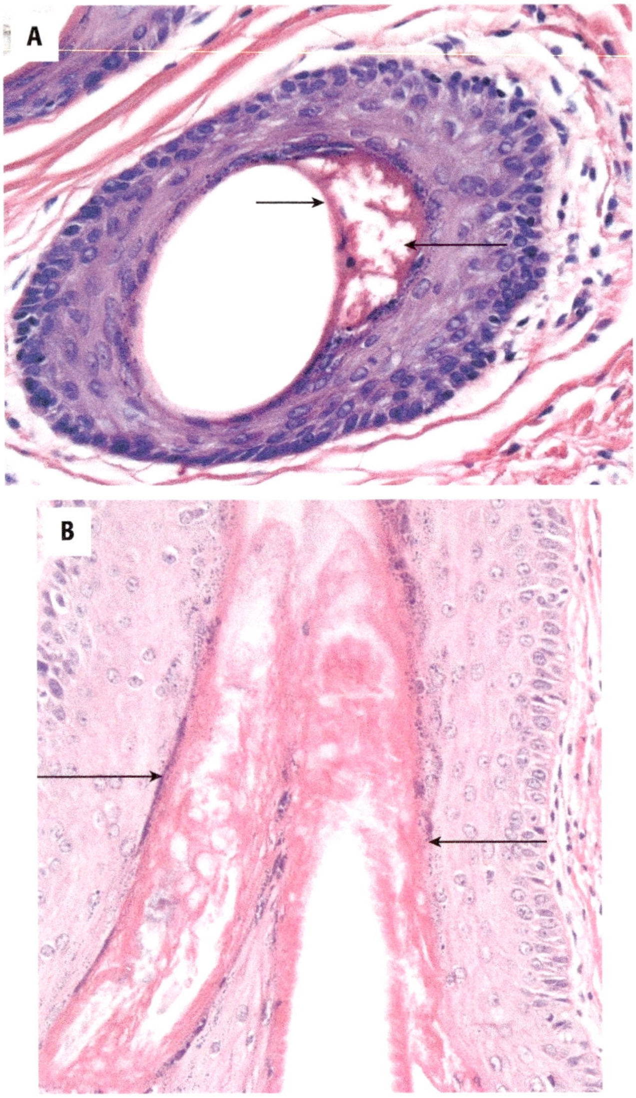

FIG. 8.18

Sebaceous duct entry point, transverse section (**A**) and perpendicular section (**B**). The shaft has been displaced. A few basophilic keratohyaline granules are noted in the surrounding epithelium. The sebaceous duct is denoted by a wavy eosinophilic cuticle *(arrows)* (Hematoxylin & eosin, **A**, ×400 and **B**, ×200).

(Fig. 8.18). The epithelium of the sebaceous duct displays a wavy eosinophilic cuticle that merges with the upper follicle epithelium. In transverse sections, the sebaceous lobules envelop the follicle epithelium at this level, and the innermost epithelium of the follicle begins to exhibit stippled basophilic keratohyaline granules.

The *infundibulum* is the region of follicular epithelium between the sebaceous duct and the epidermis. The sleeve-like infundibular epithelium contains keratinocytes that mature from the outer basement membrane toward the inner follicular lumen in a manner identical to that seen in the epidermis. Keratinocyte nuclear dissolution creates a continuous granular zone (composed of basophilic keratohyaline granules) and results in basket-woven orthokeratin that fills the gap between the emerging hair shaft and the epithelial luminal surface. This upper portion of the follicle, where the hair shaft emerges from the skin surface, is called the acrotrichium (Fig. 8.19).

CATAGEN FOLLICLE ANATOMY

Catagen is a 2-week period of follicular involution that occurs in the deeper (cycling) portion of the follicular epithelium following a period of anagen growth. Catagen follicles, constituting 1%–2% of the follicles present in a normal biopsy specimen, show characteristic histological features. The most important finding is keratinocyte apoptosis (Fig. 8.20). Involuting (apoptotic) keratinocytes rapidly diminish the volume of the isthmic epithelium. In transverse sections, as the ring of root sheath epithelium thins, the outer layer of keratinocytes affixed to the vitreous membrane squeeze together, with nuclei assuming a picket-fence or palisaded appearance (Fig. 8.21). The vitreous membrane thickens and wrinkles upon itself as the epithelial volume contracts (Fig. 8.22). In perpendicular sections, the contracting epithelium drags the follicular germ superficially, leaving a vascularized connective tissue streamer (or stela) in its wake (Fig. 8.23). The bulbar epithelial volume also contracts, with follicle matrix cells forming a small crescent around a relatively prominent mesenchymal papilla (Fig. 8.24). The upper portion of the hair shaft persists, anchored loosely just superficial to the arrector pili muscle insertion as a "club" hair (Fig. 8.25). Catagen is considered complete when active apoptosis is no longer detectable. Of note, apoptosis may occur unevenly within the same follicular epithelium.

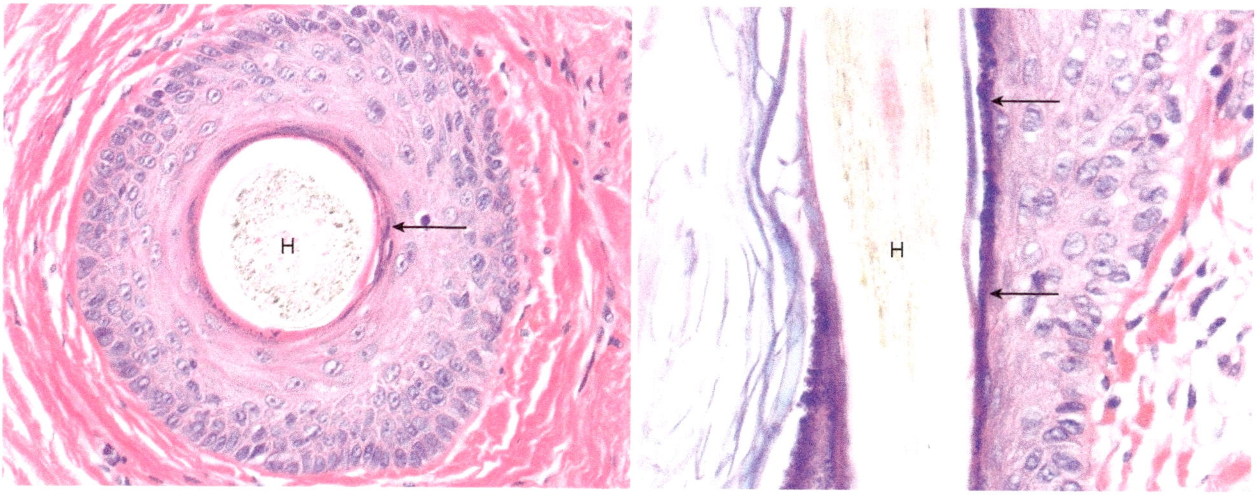

FIG. 8.19

Infundibulum, transverse section *(left)* and perpendicular section *(right)*. From the center working outward there is a central hair *(H)* shaft surrounded by epithelium that matures through a granular layer *(arrows)* in a manner identical to that seen in the epidermis (Hematoxylin & eosin, ×400).

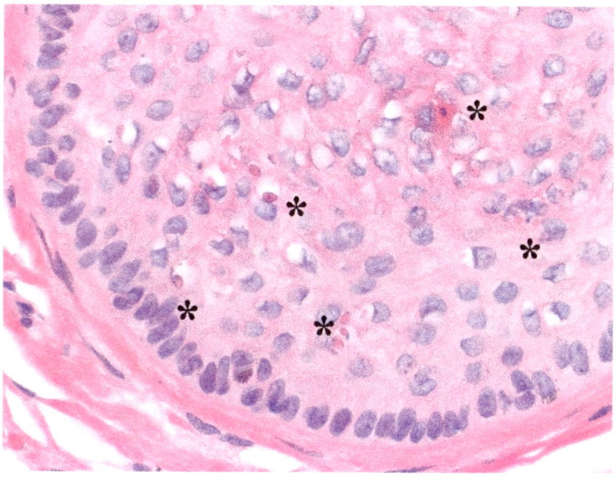

FIG. 8.20

Isthmus, catagen stage, transverse section. Apoptotic keratinocytes *(*)* signal catagen phase (Hematoxylin & eosin, ×600).

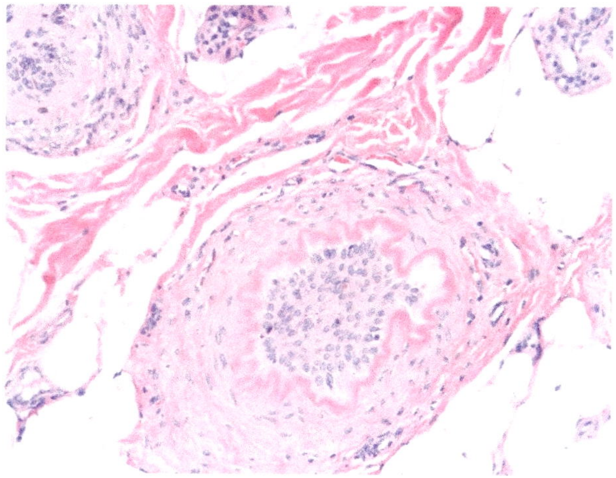

FIG. 8.22

Catagen phase follicles. As the outer root sheath involutes through apoptosis, peripheral basal keratinocytes align, and the surrounding vitreous membrane thickens (Hematoxylin & eosin, ×200).

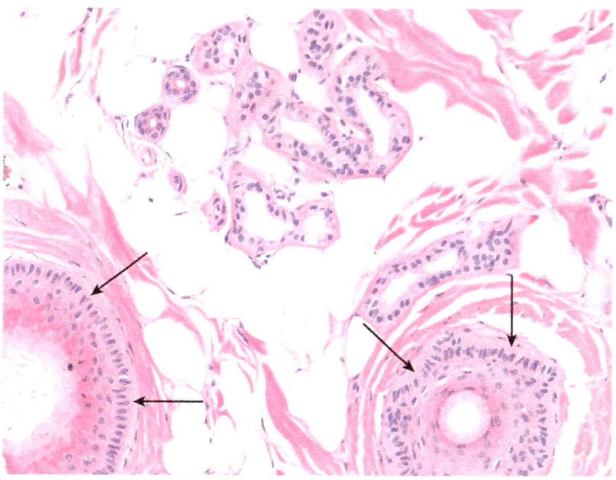

FIG. 8.21

Catagen phase follicles. Both follicles illustrate basal palisading *(arrows)*. The miniaturized follicle on the right also contains apoptotic keratinocytes. Eccrine coils are noted in the upper half of the image (Hematoxylin & eosin, ×200).

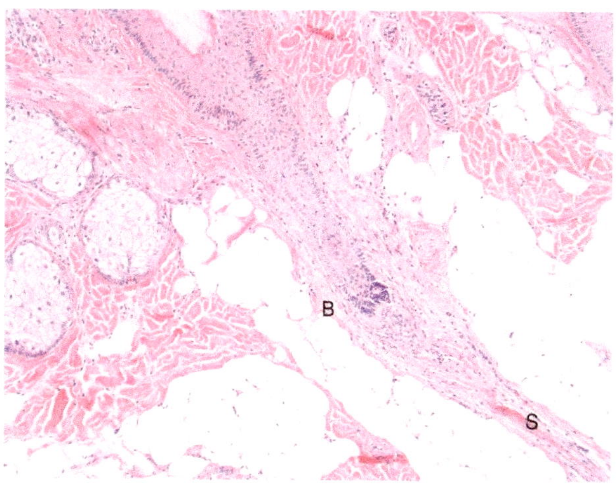

FIG. 8.23

Catagen phase follicle. The involuting isthmus drags the bulb *(B)* superficially, leaving behind a vascular streamer/stela *(S)* (Hematoxylin & eosin, ×100).

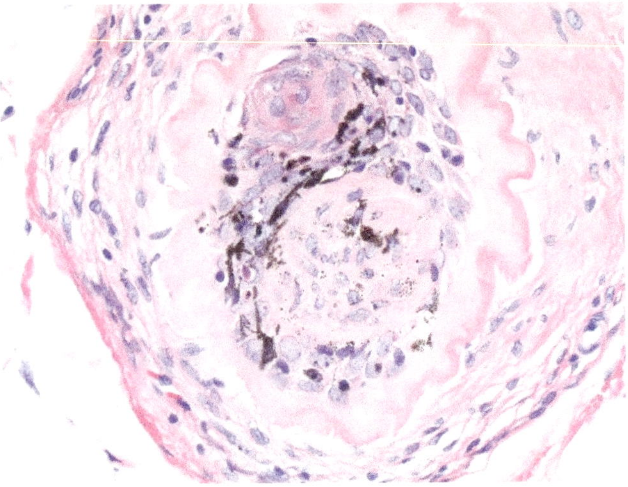

FIG. 8.24

Catagen phase bulb. The matrical volume contracts and the mesenchymal papilla appears relatively prominent (Hematoxylin & eosin, ×400). Compare to Fig. 8.11.

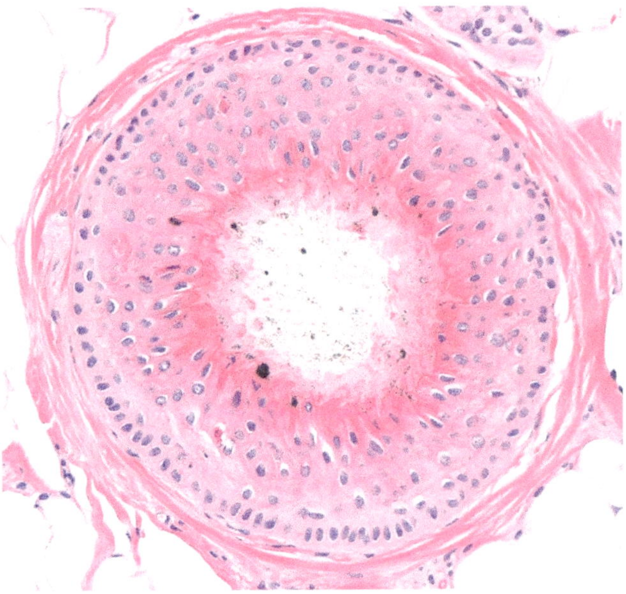

FIG. 8.25

Club hair. During catagen and telogen phases, the upper portion of the hair shaft from the previous anagen phase is loosely anchored in the upper follicular epithelium (Hematoxylin & eosin, ×200).

TELOGEN FOLLICLE ANATOMY

Upon the completion of catagen phase, the follicle enters a period of histological inactivity. During this period the telogen germ unit is affixed to the underside of the noncycling upper epithelium (Fig. 8.26). There is no evidence of apoptosis, and no hair shaft is produced. The residual club hair from the preceding anagen phase is loosely anchored in the upper follicle, from which it is eventually shed via gentle traction, combing, or brushing. In transverse sections, the palisaded keratinocytes

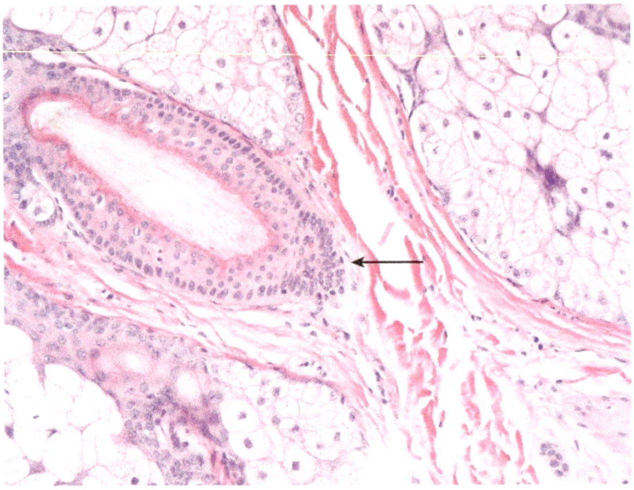

FIG. 8.26

The telogen germ unit *(arrow)*, representing the bulb for the next cycle of anagen, is affixed to the underside of the epithelium of the telogen club hair (Hematoxylin & eosin, ×200).

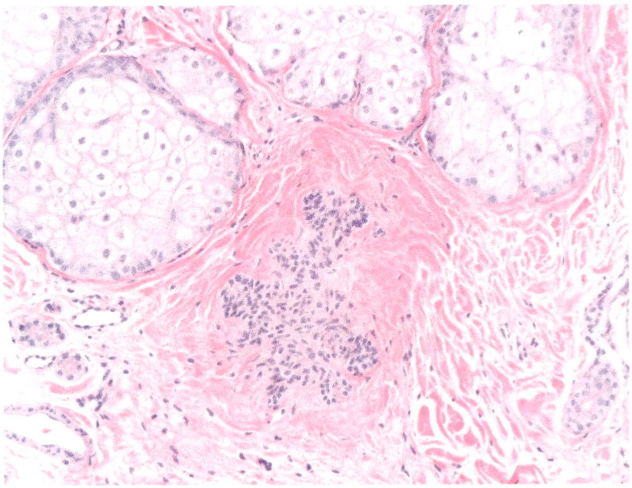

FIG. 8.27

Telogen phase follicle. The remaining epithelium from the isthmus, upon completion of apoptosis, remains quiescent until the next growth phase. Depending upon the level of the section, the epithelium may appear asterisk like when cut transversely (Hematoxylin & eosin, ×200).

remain evident around the epithelium, forming round to asterisk-like shapes (Fig. 8.27). The vitreous membrane is no longer thickened. Deep to the telogen germ unit, there is a fibrovascular streamer that extends into the subcutis, marking the location of the bulb during the previous anagen phase (Fig. 8.28).

THE RESUMPTION OF ANAGEN

Upon reinitiation of anagen, the isthmus is reconstituted between the base of the club hair and the surface of the telogen germ unit, propelling the germ along a pathway defined by the stela to its final location in the

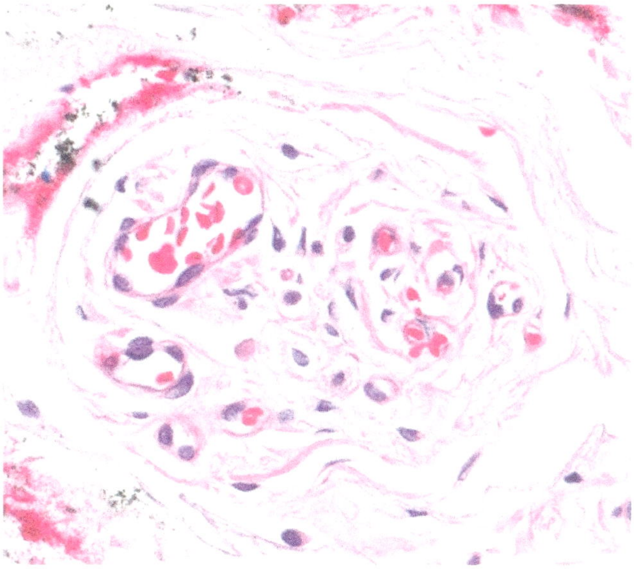

FIG. 8.28

After a catagen follicle has involuted, a streamer or stela, representing the nonepithelial supporting tissue of the follicle, marks the prior location of the previous anagen phase terminal follicle. This streamer, in cross-section, is one of recent origin (Hematoxylin & eosin, ×400).

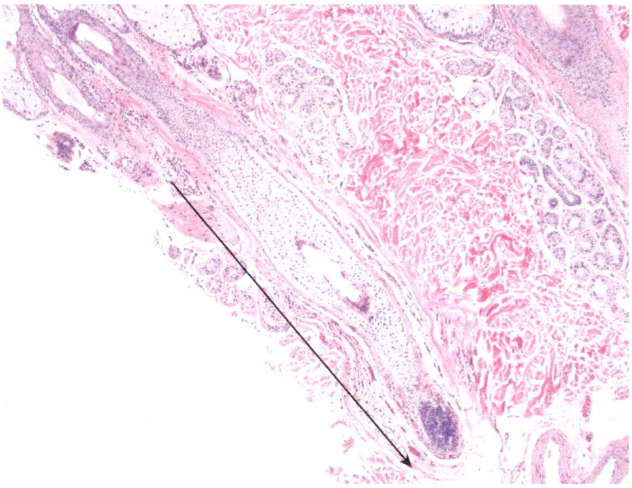

FIG. 8.29

The *arrow* shows the direction of growth of the new anagen follicle from its origin at the base of the previous telogen club hair (Hematoxylin & eosin, ×40).

subcutis. During this period, the isthmus grows to full size, the matrical cell mass expands, and the bulb begins to produce a hair shaft (Fig. 8.29).

AN ALGORITHMIC APPROACH TO DIAGNOSIS, WITH PATTERN CLUSTERS AND CRITICAL FIRST QUESTIONS

Dermatopathology is a team sport, with contributions made by the pathologist and the clinician. Each team member has strengths and biases. The goal of the pathologist is to evaluate the tissue without clinical bias, and the best way to do this is to initially bypass any submitted clinical history and images and go straight to tissue review. The outcome of this initial review is a list of histological differential candidates.

For alopecia evaluations, the histological differential can sometimes be narrowed to a single diagnosis. More commonly, however, a short list of diagnoses with identical or nearly identical features is generated. In this chapter, we refer to these short lists as "pattern clusters" (Table 8.3). Within these clusters, diagnoses may be further refined by careful attention to subtle histological clues and by reviewing any additional information provided by the clinician (e.g., alopecia distribution, photos, history, lab results). If further refinement cannot be accomplished, the pattern cluster remains a useful reporting aide that can guide further clinical and laboratory workup.

Properly classifying an alopecia into a pattern cluster is critical. A myriad of observations can be made while examining the various anatomic levels of a transversely sectioned alopecia specimen. A seasoned alopecia expert may simultaneously observe patterns of

TABLE 8.3

Pattern Clusters and Differentials

Pattern	Pattern Cluster Name	Diagnostic Differentials
CICATRICIAL		
1	LPP like	LPP, FFA, FAPD
2	Pauci-inflammatory cicatricial	CCCA, AK
3	CCLE	CCLE
4	Deep, mixed inflammatory	DC, folliculitis decalvans, fungal kerion
5	End-stage	Any cicatricial alopecia, end stage
BIPHASIC		
6	Biphasic	AGA, CTA, AA (some)
NONCICATRICIAL		
7	TTA	TTA
8	Peribulbar inflammation	AA, syphilis, noncicatricial alopecia of SLE
9	Collapsed sebaceous lobules	TAIA, sebopsoriasis, psoriasis
10	Uninflamed with trichomalacia	POPIA, TT
11	Normal	Normal, acute TE, hair shaft disorders, LAHS

AA, Alopecia areata; *AGA*, androgenetic alopecia; *AK*, acne keloidalis; *CCCA*, central centrifugal cicatricial alopecia; *CCLE*, chronic cutaneous lupus erythematosus; *CTA*, chronic traction alopecia; *DC*, dissecting cellulitis; *FAPD*, fibrosing alopecia in a pattern distribution; *FFA*, frontal fibrosing alopecia; *LAHS*, loose anagen hair syndrome; *LPP*, lichen planopilaris; *POPIA*, postoperative pressure–induced alopecia; *SLE*, systemic lupus erythematosus; *TAIA*, TNF-alpha inhibitor alopecia; *TE*, telogen effluvium; *TT*, trichotillomania; *TTA*, temporal triangular alopecia.

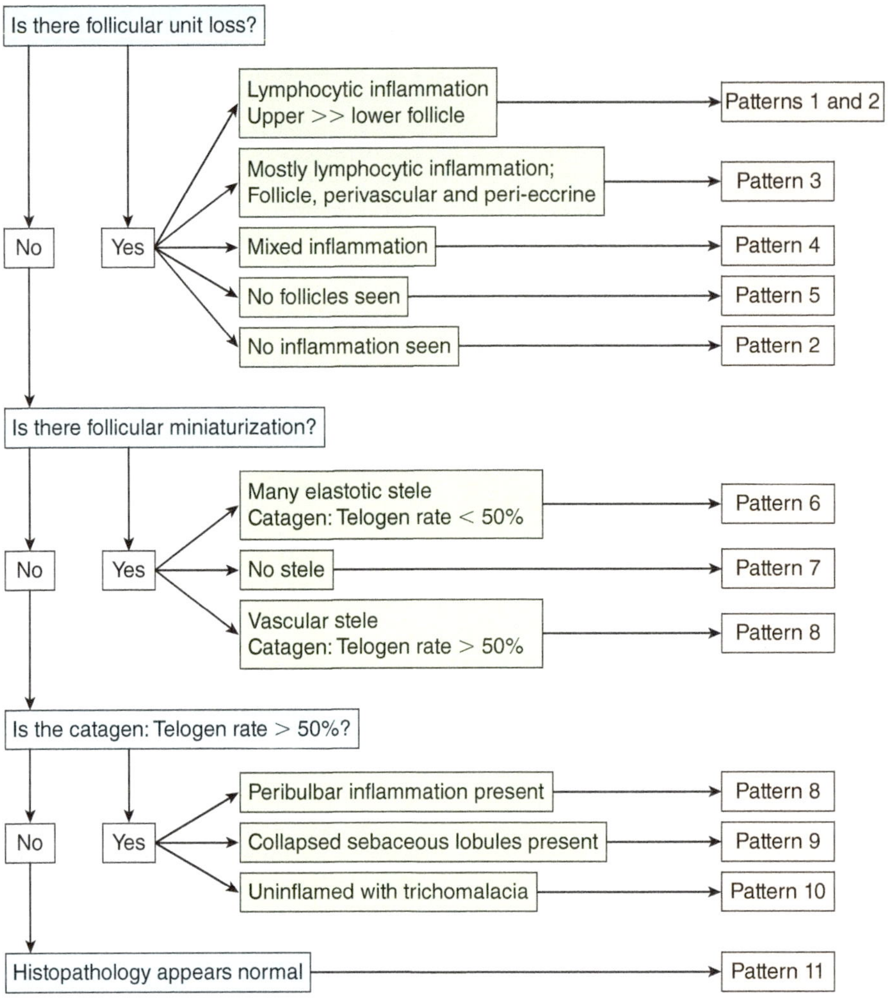

FIG. 8.30

Algorithmic approach to classifying common alopecias by histopathology.

inflammation, loss of sebaceous lobules, and follicular miniaturization and arrive nearly instantaneously at a final diagnosis.

Students and nonexperts are well-served by learning a systematic approach. One possible approach is outlined in Fig. 8.30. The first question that should be answered is: Is there loss of the follicular unit? Answering this first critical question correctly significantly narrows the differential possibilities. If there is loss of the follicular unit, the alopecia is considered "cicatricial" or "scarring." Loss of a follicular unit indicates that there will be no further growth of hair since the hair-producing apparatus is lost and cannot be recovered. There are numerous clues to help answer this first critical question, and these will be covered in the section on cicatricial alopecia below.

If the answer to the first question is "no," then the next question to ask is: Is there evidence of progressive follicular miniaturization? Progressive follicular miniaturization indicates shortening of the anagen (growth) phase over successive growth cycles. While not considered cicatricial, untreated alopecias in this category may contain follicles that have become so miniaturized that they produce no visible hair shaft. These alopecias—referred to as "biphasic" since they start out as noncicatricial and slowly become cicatricial—are covered in detail in the subsection on that topic.

The remaining alopecias, showing no loss of follicular units or evidence of miniaturization are termed "noncicatricial" and are covered in detail later in this chapter.

CICATRICIAL ALOPECIA OVERVIEW (PATTERNS 1–5)

As noted above, the first critical question to ask is: Is there loss of the follicular unit? This may seem like a simple question to answer; however, small sample size, poor orientation, and subtle findings may pose challenges to reaching a definitive conclusion. Thankfully, there are ancillary histological clues that may help support a diagnosis of subtle cicatricial alopecia.

Six general features to help the pathologist categorize an alopecia as cicatricial

(1) **Absence of the follicular unit.** In fully developed cicatricial alopecias, the follicle and sebaceous lobules are lost, becoming completely replaced by connective tissue matrix. This is recognized on low-magnification transverse sections by the presence of ovoid areas of dense, homogenous collagen lacking the usual fenestrations (gaps) seen in the surrounding normal dermis (Fig. 8.31). In our experience, sebaceous lobules are early casualties in inflammatory cicatricial alopecias that involve the upper follicular unit, leaving the follicle epithelium relatively well-preserved *without* sebaceous lobules (Fig. 8.32).

(2) **Circumferential fibroplasia.** Concentrically arranged fibroblasts in an "onion skin" arrangement may form around the upper follicular epithelium in transverse sections. The fibroplasia may exclude any surrounding chronic inflammatory infiltrate, pushing it away from the follicular epithelium (Fig. 8.33). In perpendicular sections, this circumferential fibroplasia may constrict the follicular epithelium into an "hourglass" shape (Fig. 8.34).

(3) **Dilated eccrine ducts.** In transverse sections, these are identified as dilated circular-shaped lumina lined by thin, cuboidal epithelium. The lumina may be empty or filled with a pink, homogeneous material (i.e., sweat) (Fig. 8.35). The cause of the dilation is not known.

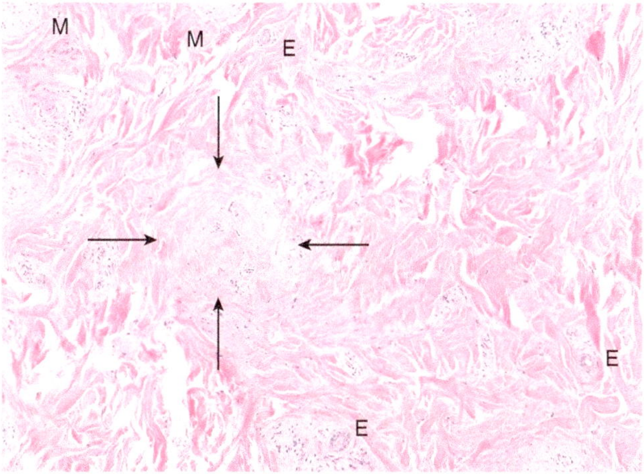

FIG. 8.31

Cicatricial alopecia, transverse section. No follicular units are identified in this profile, although eccrine *(E)* ducts and arrector pili muscles *(M)* indicate a mid-dermal location. All cicatricial alopecias are defined by eventual loss of the follicular unit. Sometimes the outline of the vanished follicular unit can be identified in the pattern of the dermal collagen *(arrows)* (Hematoxylin & eosin, ×40).

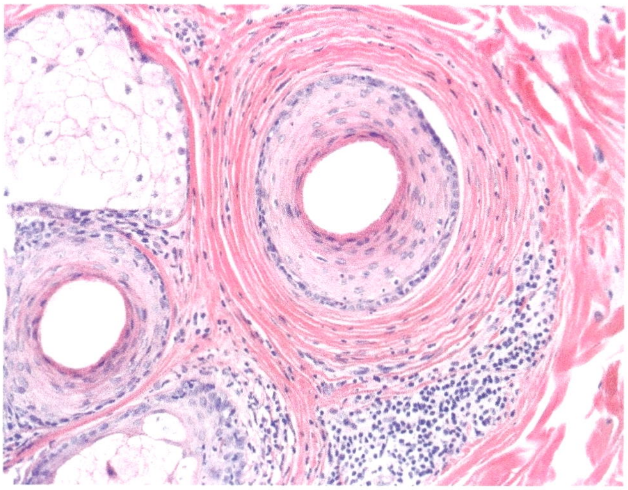

FIG. 8.33

Cicatricial alopecia, transverse section. Onion skin fibroplasia pushing back lymphocytes may be a feature of several cicatricial alopecias (Hematoxylin & eosin, ×200).

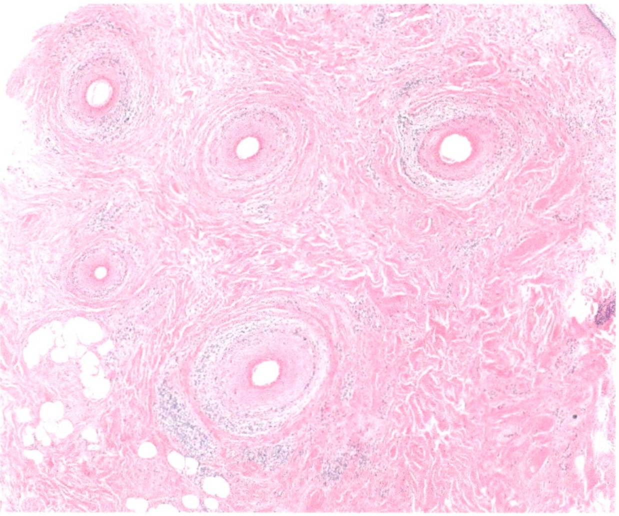

FIG. 8.32

Cicatricial alopecia, transverse section. Preserved follicular units despite absence of sebaceous lobules in a case of lichen planopilaris (Hematoxylin & eosin, ×40).

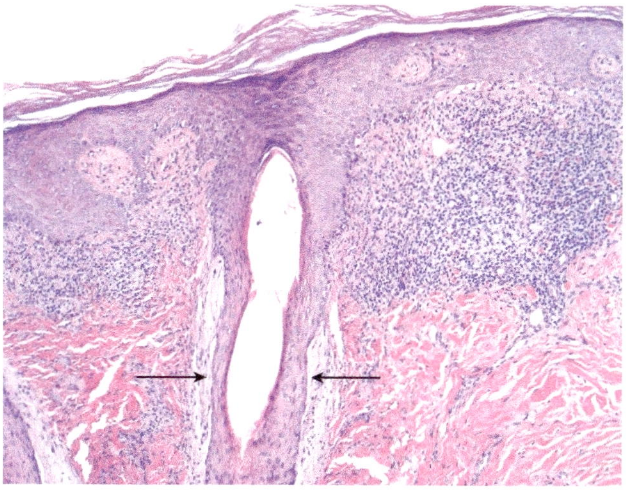

FIG. 8.34

Cicatricial alopecia, perpendicular section. Hourglass-like constriction of the upper follicular epithelium by encircling fibroplasia *(arrows)* in lichen planopilaris (Hematoxylin & eosin, ×100).

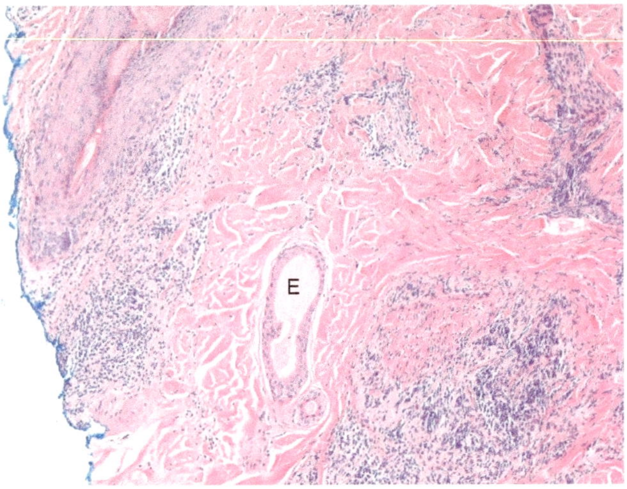

FIG. 8.35

Cicatricial alopecia, vertical section. Dilated eccrine ducts *(E)* are often seen in cicatricial alopecia. This is a case of chronic cutaneous lupus erythematosus (Hematoxylin & eosin, ×100).

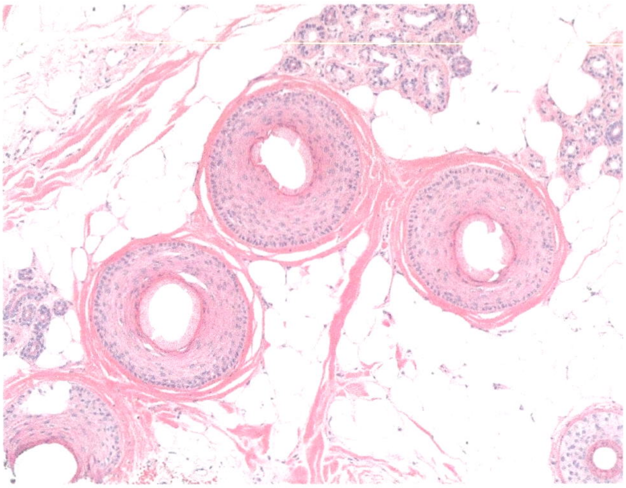

FIG. 8.37

Cicatricial alopecia, transverse section. Premature desquamation of the inner root sheath in central centrifugal cicatricial alopecia. The three central follicles show partial desquamation while the lower left one is fully desquamated (Hematoxylin & eosin, ×100).

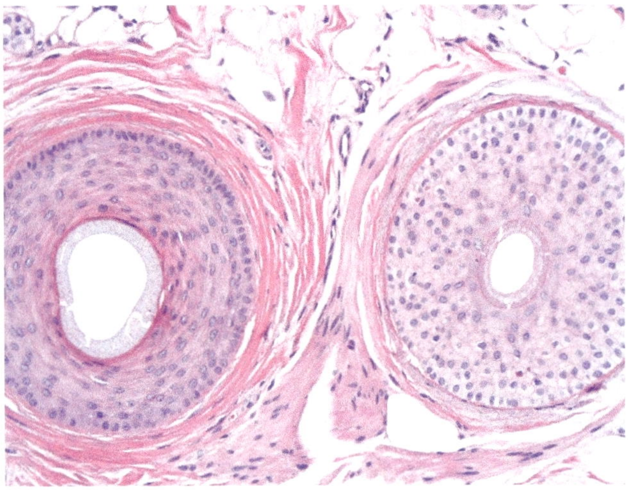

FIG. 8.36

Cicatricial alopecia, transverse section. Early premature desquamation of the inner root sheath starts as an intensely eosinophilic ring between the outer and inner root sheath *(left)*. For comparison, please note the adjacent unaffected follicle *(right)* in this example of central centrifugal cicatricial alopecia (Hematoxylin & eosin, ×200).

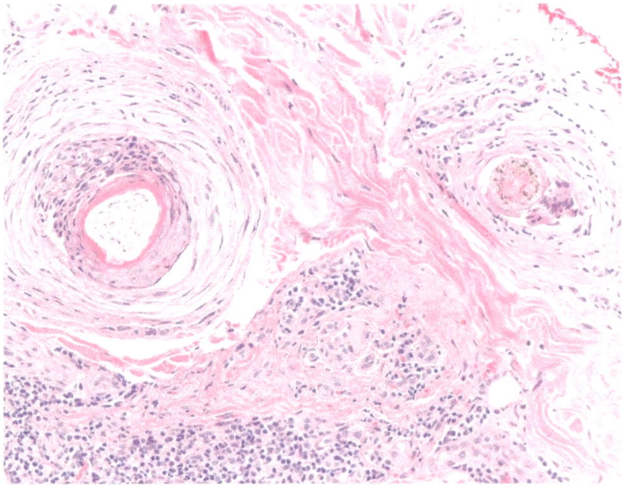

FIG. 8.38

Cicatricial alopecia, transverse section. Destruction of follicular epithelia can lead to "naked" hair shafts within the dermis. This typically triggers a granulomatous inflammatory response, as is seen in this case of lichen planopilaris (Hematoxylin & eosin, ×200)

(4) **Premature desquamation of the inner root sheath (PDIRS).** In transverse sections, the IRS is found in the isthmus and resembles a light pink homogenous ring directly abutting the hair shaft (Fig. 8.14). In a normal follicle, the IRS begins to "crumble" and fall off within the upper isthmus. Early in this process, the border between inner and ORS epithelium becomes more intensely eosinophilic (Fig. 8.36). *Premature* desquamation is identified when this "crumbling" and/or absence of the IRS is seen in the deep isthmus (i.e., at or below the level of the eccrine ducts) (Fig. 8.37).

(5) **"Naked" hair shafts.** Cicatricial alopecias may cause such rapid destruction of the follicular epithelium that the hair shaft becomes stranded within the dermis. Since keratin is immunogenic, a surrounding foreign body giant cell reaction is nearly always seen. Of note, the hair shaft may be inconspicuous, and the foreign body giant cell reaction may be the only clue to the presence of this phenomenon (Fig. 8.38).

(6) **Follicular epithelial fusion.** Follicular fusion may be seen in the superficial portions of the dermis. Histologically, this may resemble a pair of "eyes" or "goggles" as two individual follicular epithelia merge to form a single epithelial-lined structure. More than two follicles may fuse resulting in triads (Fig. 8.39), tetrads, or even higher numbers of grouped follicles. Clinically, this presents as polytrichia or "tufted" follicles (Fig. 8.40).

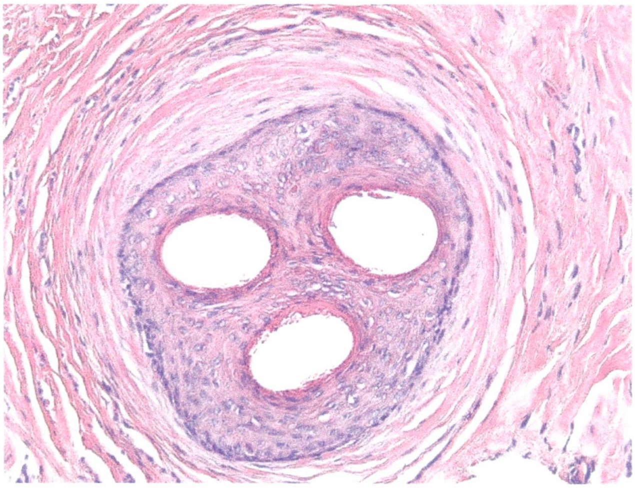

FIG. 8.39

Cicatricial alopecia, transverse section. The upper follicular epithelia may fuse into compound epithelia wrapped by encircling fibroplasia. This example is from a case of central centrifugal cicatricial alopecia (Hematoxylin & eosin, ×200).

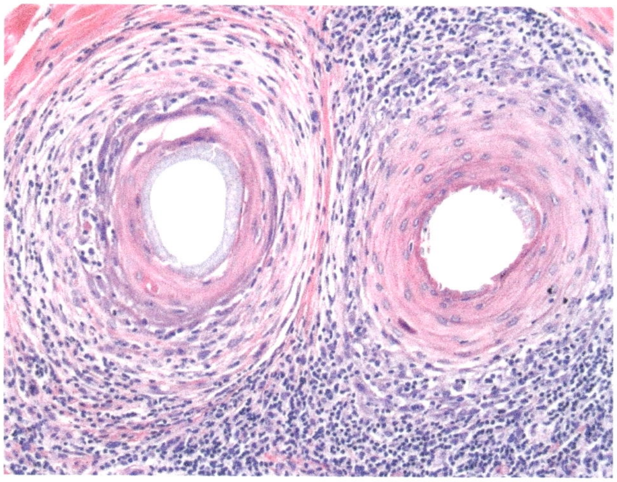

FIG. 8.41

Transverse section. Necrotic keratinocytes are seen predominantly along the basal (outer) portions of the epithelium in the lichen planopilaris pattern (Hematoxylin & eosin, ×200).

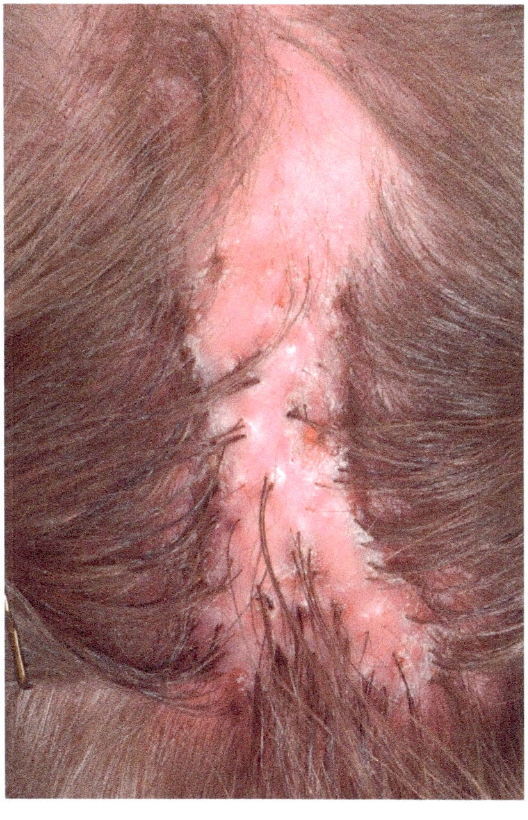

FIG. 8.40

Follicular fusion presents clinically as polytrichia or "tufted" follicles.

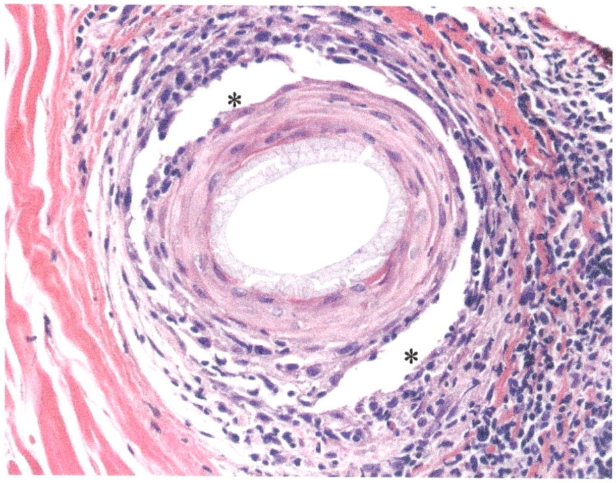

FIG. 8.42

Transverse section. Epithelial-dermal cleft formation (*) is a feature seen in the lichen planopilaris pattern, but not in central centrifugal cicatricial alopecia (Hematoxylin & eosin, ×200).

PATTERN 1: THE LICHEN PLANOPILARIS-LIKE PATTERN

Characteristics of the Pattern

Pattern 1 can manifest any (or all) of the six general features seen in cicatricial alopecias noted above. Pattern 1 is further characterized by a peri-infundibular and peri-isthmic lymphocytic inflammatory infiltrate with circumferential fibroplasia (see Fig. 8.33). The localization of the inflammatory response to these areas of the follicle effectively destroys follicular stem cells in the bulge region (near the attachment point of the arrector pili muscle). Interface changes in the form of necrotic keratinocytes and premature squamatization may be seen within the follicular epithelium (Fig. 8.41). Necrotic keratinocytes are seen predominantly along the basal (outer) portions of the epithelium. An exuberant reaction may result in profound epithelial thinning. Epithelial/dermal clefting (like that seen at the dermal-epidermal junction in lichen planus) is often present and is an important differentiating feature (Fig. 8.42). Interface change may also rarely be seen at the dermal-epidermal junction. Since many of the inflammatory changes are near the infundibular or superficial portions of the follicle, if the transverse sections are cut at a deeper level, the findings may be missed. Obtaining additional levels toward the epidermis may be revealing. If direct immunofluorescence (DIF) is performed, IgM-positive necrotic keratinocytes that have dropped into the dermis (Civatte bodies) will be highlighted.

Diagnoses Manifesting Pattern 1

Lichen planopilaris (LPP), frontal fibrosing alopecia (FFA), and fibrosing alopecia in a pattern distribution (FAPD) are histologically identical. All three of these diagnoses are distinguished based on clinical features.

Diagnoses With Similar Features

Pattern 2: CCCA/acne keloidalis (AK) and pattern 3: chronic cutaneous lupus erythematosus (CCLE).

Helpful Differentiating Features

HISTOLOGIC

LPP, FFA, and FAPD are histologically indistinguishable. CCLE, unlike the pattern 1 diagnoses, may have inflammation along the entire length of the follicle and typically presents with a concurrent deep perivascular and perieccrine inflammatory infiltrate. Increased dermal mucin may also be seen. CCCA lacks vacuolar change and is usually less inflamed than the pattern 1 diagnoses. CCCA displays PDIRS as its earliest finding, sometimes before inflammation is noted. Inflammation is present in pattern 1 (usually with loss of sebaceous lobules) before PDIRS appears. Follicular epithelial-dermal clefting is common in pattern 1 but is not present in CCCA. Follicular keratin plugging and a thickened basement membrane are common features in CCLE that are not typically present in pattern 1. DIF studies highlight Civatte bodies with IgM but do not show the linear deposition of immunoreactants seen in CCLE (see pattern 3 characteristics).

CLINICAL

Clinical correlation is the single most important factor differentiating between LPP, FFA, and FAPD. Clinically, LPP presents with patches of alopecia predominantly along the vertex and parietal areas of the scalp with perifollicular erythema, follicular hyperkeratosis, collarettes of scale, and tenderness (Fig. 8.43). Conversely, FFA presents as "band-like" alopecia along the hairline in a frontotemporal distribution (Fig. 8.44). The eyebrows are also affected in most cases. FAPD presents as accelerated cicatricial alopecia occurring exclusively in areas already involved by long-standing typical

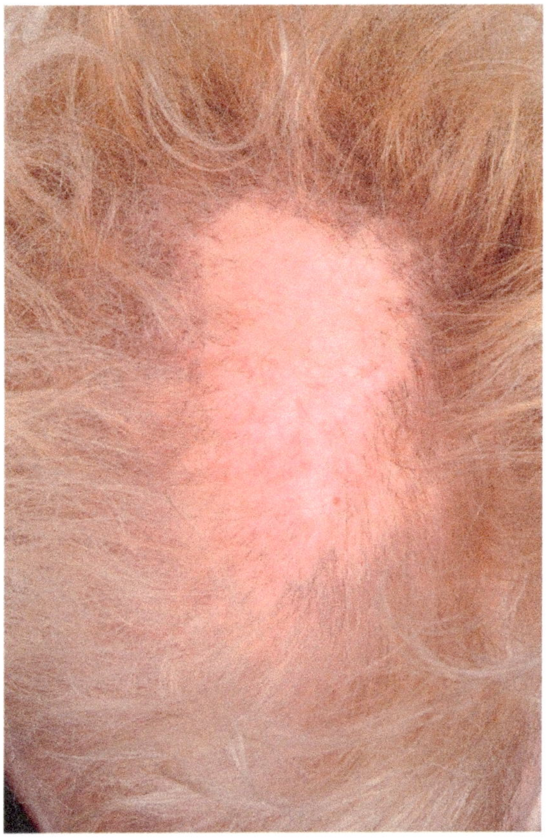

FIG. 8.43
Lichen planopilaris presents with patches of alopecia predominantly along the vertex and parietal areas of the scalp with perifollicular erythema, follicular hyperkeratosis, collarettes of scale, and tenderness.

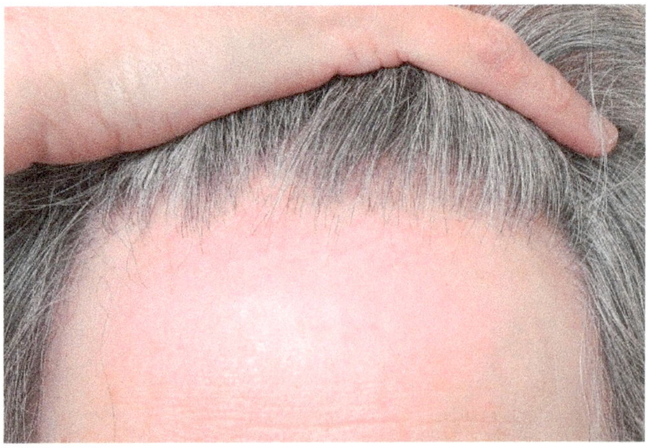

FIG. 8.44
Frontal fibrosing alopecia presents as "band-like" alopecia along the hairline in a frontotemporal distribution.

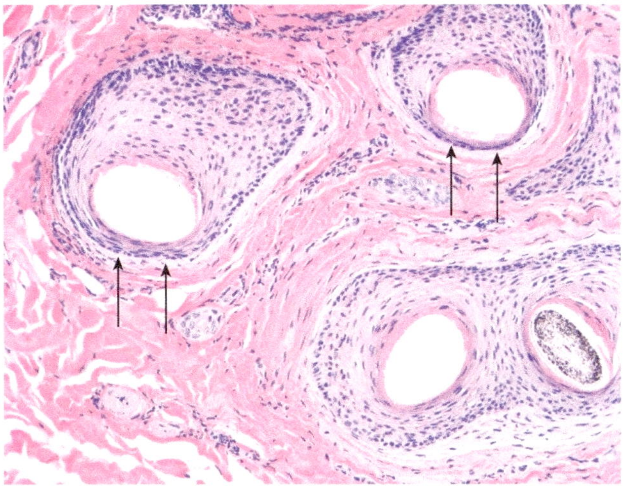

FIG. 8.45

Central centrifugal cicatricial alopecia, transverse section. The two non-fused follicles display eccentric epithelial thinning *(arrows)* (Hematoxylin & eosin, ×200).

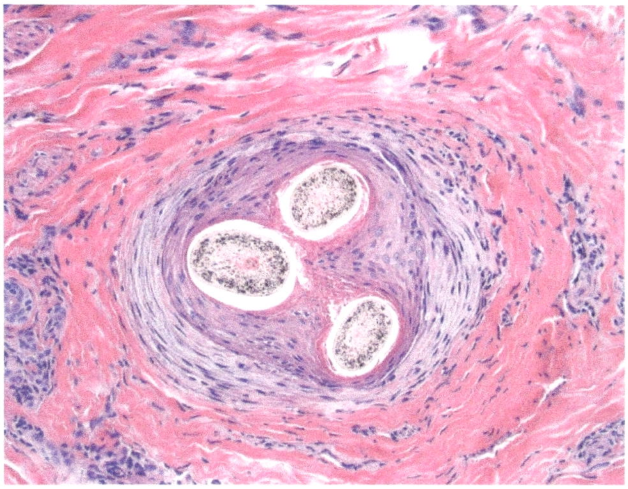

FIG. 8.46

Central centrifugal cicatricial alopecia, transverse section. Three fused follicles with encircling fibroplasia without an inflammatory cleft (Hematoxylin & eosin, ×200).

androgenetic alopecia (AGA). CCCA is typically seen in Black females. The alopecia has an initial presentation on the crown and subsequent hair loss expands outward (i.e., in a centrifugal pattern). CCLE most commonly presents as violaceous, disk-shaped lesions on the face, ears, and/or scalp.

PATTERN 2: THE PAUCI-INFLAMMATORY CICATRICIAL ALOPECIA PATTERN

Characteristics of the Pattern

Pattern 2 can manifest any (or all) of the six general features seen in cicatricial alopecias noted above. As the name implies, the inflammatory infiltrate is typically less prominent than that seen in other cicatricial alopecias. PDIRS is a characteristic feature of this pattern and, in its earliest stages, may be the only feature seen (see Fig. 8.37). As noted in the earlier discussion of normal anagen follicular anatomy, the IRS typically desquamates (sloughs) at the level of the sebaceous lobules in the mid-to-upper isthmic region. PDIRS is identified when desquamation is seen in horizontal sections deep to the location of the eccrine coils or within the adipose tissue. While nonspecific, eccentric follicular epithelial atrophy that barely contains the hair shaft may also occur (Fig. 8.45). Long-standing cases of the pauci-inflammatory pattern may show "naked hair shafts" with surrounding granulomatous inflammation (see Fig. 8.38). Even in the absence of significant inflammation, circumferential fibroplasia is still a feature in most cases, although epithelial/dermal clefting (as described in pattern 1) is not typical (Fig. 8.46).

Diagnoses Manifesting Pattern 2

CCCA and AK.

Diagnoses With Similar Features

Pattern 1: LPP/FFA/FAPD

Helpful Differentiating Features

HISTOLOGIC

The histological findings in AK overlap those seen in CCCA. As the name suggests, AK tends to produce masses of hypertrophic collagen around foci in which follicles have been destroyed, stranding naked hair shafts (Fig. 8.47). Otherwise, the distinction between the two entities is best made on clinical grounds. Pattern 1 diagnoses tend to manifest a more pronounced inflammatory infiltrate. PDIRS can be seen in pattern 1 but typically follows follicular inflammation and loss of sebaceous lobules. When PDIRS is identified in the absence of significant inflammation, especially if sebaceous lobules are intact, CCCA is more likely. Epithelial/dermal clefting is also less likely to be seen in CCCA when compared to pattern 1 (Fig. 8.42 versus Fig. 8.46). In biopsies with mild to moderate degrees of inflammation in which sebaceous lobules are lost *and* PDIRS is present, clinical correlation will be required to reach a confident diagnosis.

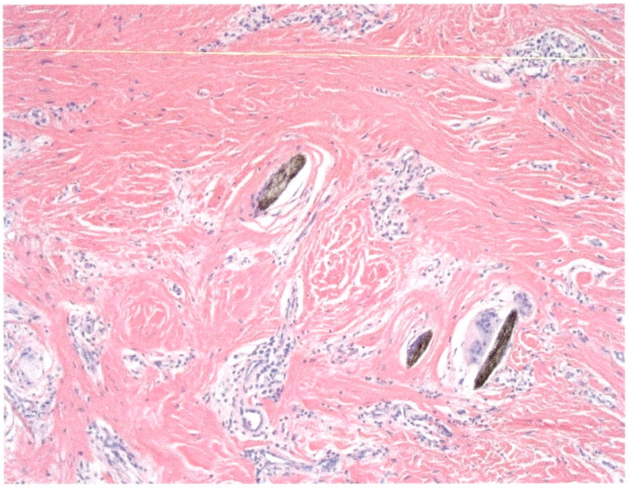

FIG. 8.47
Acne keloidalis, vertical section. Complete destruction of follicles with keloidal collagen surrounding naked hair shafts (Hematoxylin & eosin, ×100)

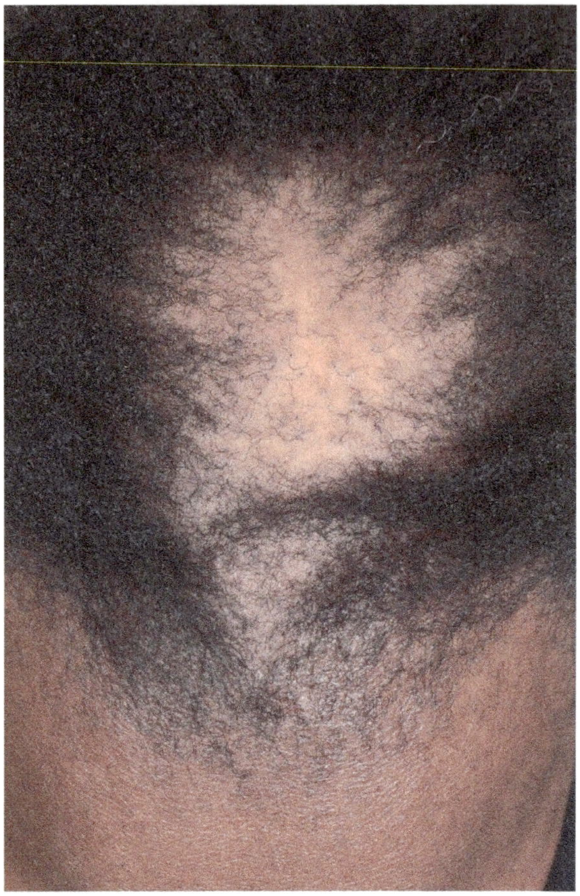

FIG. 8.48
Central centrifugal cicatricial alopecia is found nearly exclusively in Black women who present with cicatricial alopecia that begins on the crown or vertex scalp and progresses in an outward, radial (i.e., centrifugal) manner over time.

CLINICAL

Even though there are various histological findings that can favor CCCA/AK over LPP/FFA, correlation with clinical findings is often necessary to differentiate between these patterns. CCCA is found nearly exclusively in Black women who present with cicatricial alopecia that begins on the crown or vertex scalp and progresses in an outward, radial (i.e., centrifugal) manner over time (Fig. 8.48). AK presents as follicular papules and plaques on the occipital scalp and posterior neck, usually in young Black men (Fig. 8.49). The clinical presentation of pattern 1 diagnoses is discussed in detail in the preceding section of this chapter.

PATTERN 3: THE CHRONIC CUTANEOUS LUPUS ERYTHEMATOSUS PATTERN

Characteristics of the Pattern

Pattern 3 can manifest any (or all) of the six general features seen in cicatricial alopecias noted previously. The CCLE pattern typically comprises a peri-infundibular chronic inflammatory infiltrate, circumferential fibroplasia, and vacuolar interface change within the overlying epidermis and/or adnexal structures (Fig. 8.50). CCLE will also often have deep perivascular and perieccrine lymphocytic inflammation (Figs. 8.51 and 8.52), plasma cells (Fig. 8.53), and deep dermal mucin (Fig. 8.54). Eosinophils, not commonly observed in cutaneous lupus at other sites, may be present. A CD123 immunohistochemical stain may show clustered plasmacytoid dendritic cells (Fig. 8.55). Additional histological features in CCLE include follicular

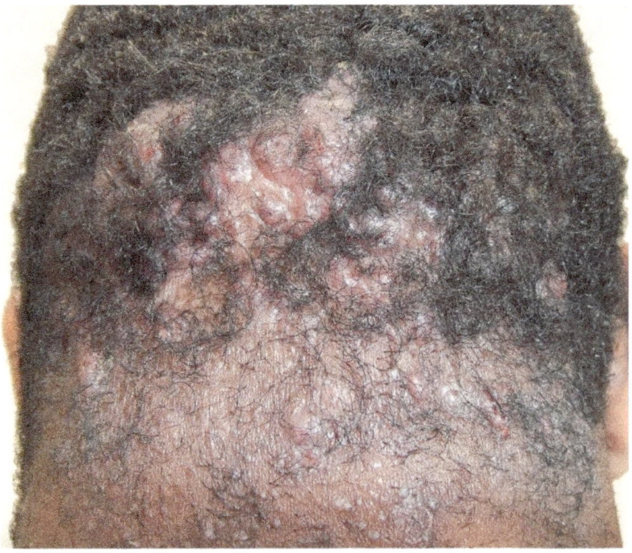

FIG. 8.49
Acne keloidalis presents as follicular papules and plaques on the occipital scalp and posterior neck, usually in young Black men.

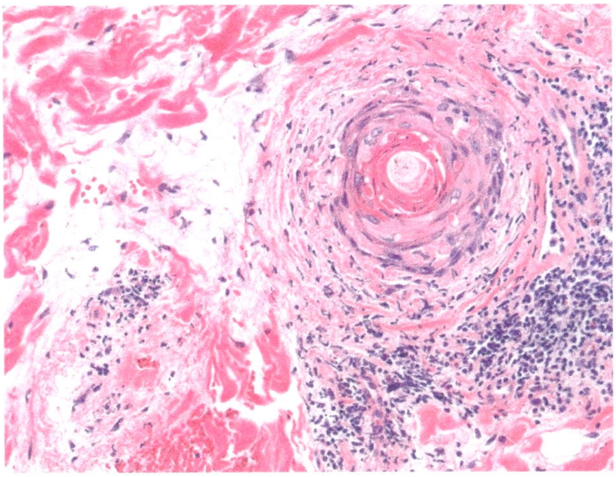

FIG. 8.50

Chronic cutaneous lupus erythematosus, transverse section. There is interface change associated with developing circumfollicular fibroplasia. Mucin is identifiable in the adjacent dermis (Hematoxylin & eosin, ×100).

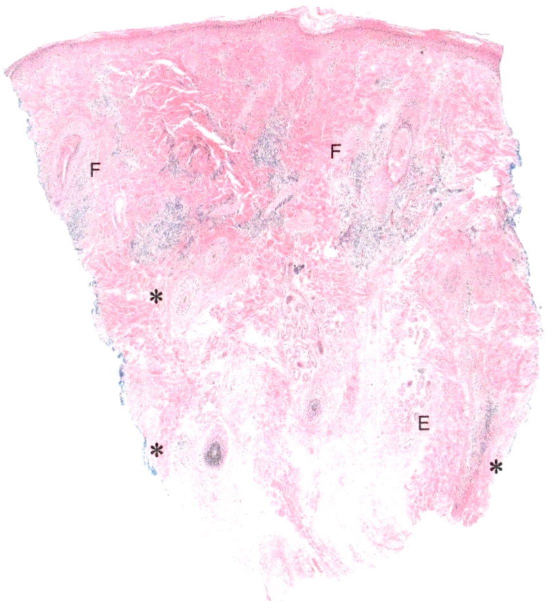

FIG. 8.51

Chronic cutaneous lupus erythematosus, vertical section. There is lymphocytic inflammation around follicles *(F)*, in the superficial and deep perivascular dermis *(*)*, and around eccrine units *(E)* (Hematoxylin & eosin, ×20).

keratin plugs (Figs. 8.56 and 8.57) and basement membrane thickening (Fig. 8.58) that can be highlighted by periodic acid-Schiff (PAS) staining.

DIF studies are sometimes used as an adjunct to histology in difficult cases (see below).

Diagnoses Manifesting Pattern 3

This pattern is highly specific for CCLE if all features are present.

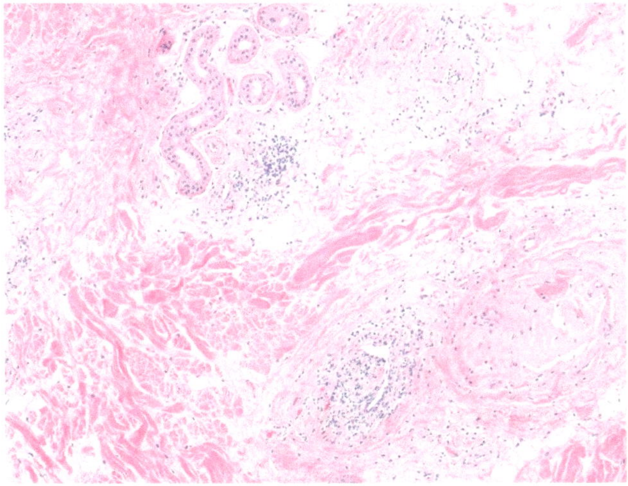

FIG. 8.52

Chronic cutaneous lupus erythematosus, transverse section. There is lymphocytic inflammation in the deep perivascular dermis and around an eccrine coil (Hematoxylin & eosin, ×100).

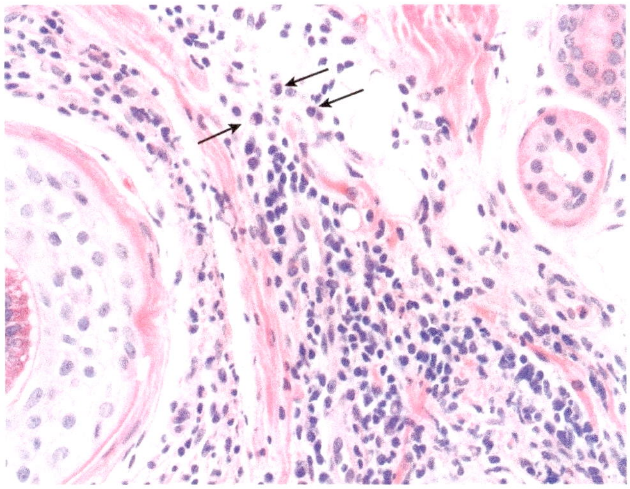

FIG. 8.53

Chronic cutaneous lupus erythematosus, transverse section. There is lymphocytic inflammation in the deep perifollicular dermis and around an eccrine coil. Plasma cells *(arrows)* are often in the infiltrate (Hematoxylin & eosin, ×400).

Diagnoses With Similar Features

Pattern 1: LPP, FPA, and FAPD.

Helpful Differentiating Features

HISTOLOGIC

CCLE most closely resembles the pattern 1 diagnoses histologically, with similarities likely arising from a related autoimmune pathway. Like pattern 1, inflammatory infiltrates gather in the region of the attachment of

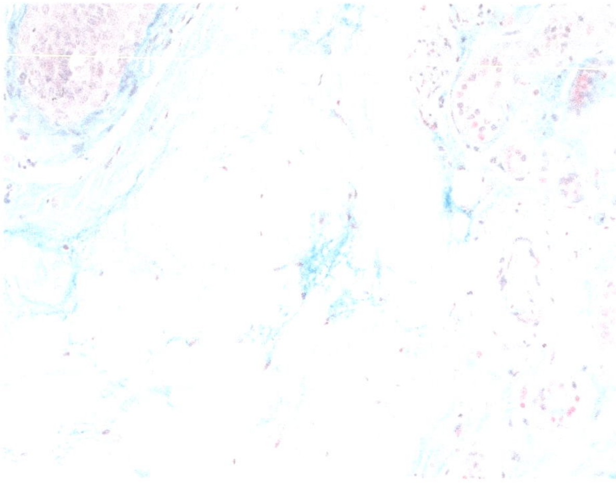

FIG. 8.54

Chronic cutaneous lupus erythematosus, transverse section. Deep dermal mucin is often identified (Alcian Blue, ×200).

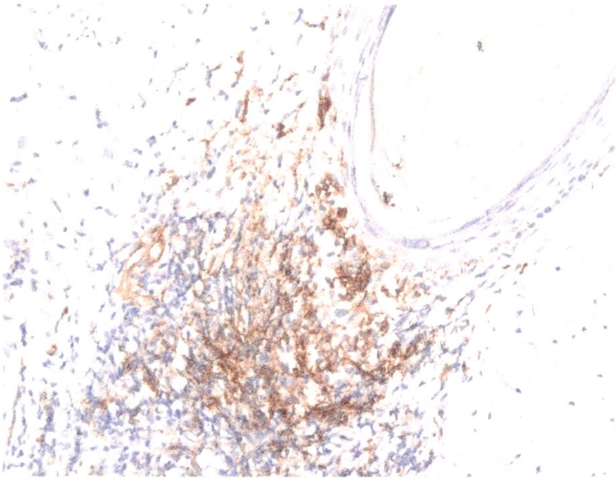

FIG. 8.55

Chronic cutaneous lupus erythematosus, vertical section. Clusters of plasmacytoid dendritic cells around a dilated follicle (CD123, ×200).

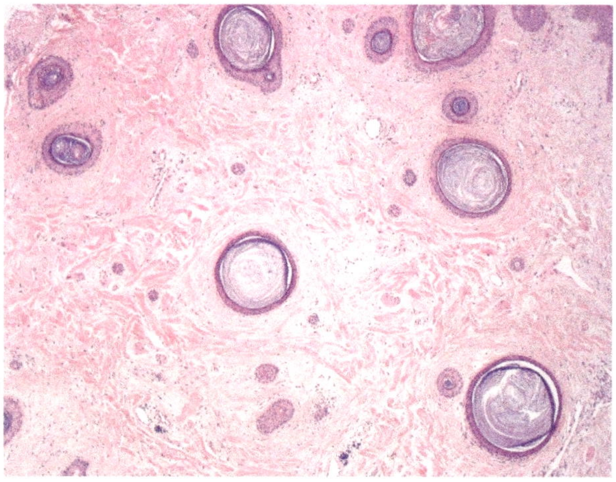

FIG. 8.56

Chronic cutaneous lupus erythematosus, transverse section. Dilated infundibula containing basket-woven orthokeratin (Hematoxylin & eosin, ×40).

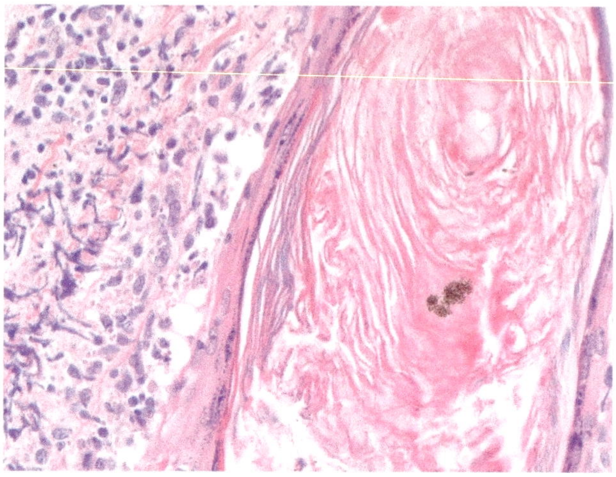

FIG. 8.57

Chronic cutaneous lupus erythematosus, vertical section. Thin-walled and dilated infundibulum containing basket-woven orthokeratin and surrounded by lymphocytes (Hematoxylin & eosin, ×40).

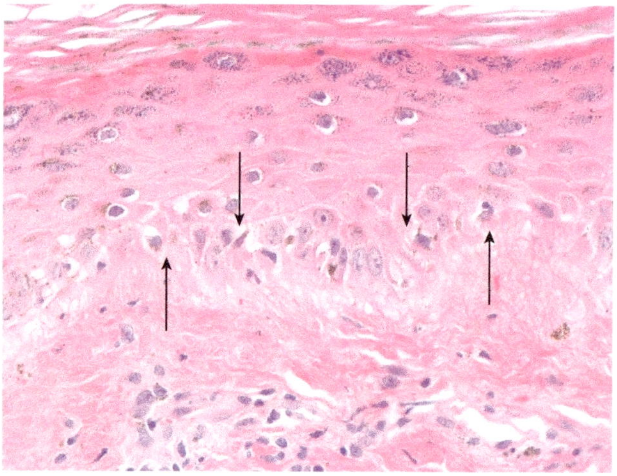

FIG. 8.58

Chronic cutaneous lupus erythematosus, vertical section. Thickened and indistinct dermal-epidermal junction *(arrows)* (Hematoxylin & eosin, ×200).

the arrector pili muscle to the follicular epithelium where there are abundant antigen-presenting Langerhans' cells in association with hair follicle stem cells. The inflammatory milieu also leads to sebaceous gland destruction. Unlike pattern 1 diagnoses, however, CCLE will often show deep perivascular and perieccrine lymphocytic inflammation, plasma cells, and deep dermal mucin. DIF studies are sometimes used as an adjunct to histology in difficult cases. On DIF, CCLE has granular and linear deposition of IgG, IgM, IgA, and C3 along the basement membrane of both the follicle and the epidermis, a pattern not seen in pattern 1 (Fig. 8.59).

CLINICAL

CCLE is a term that encompasses the cutaneous manifestations of multiple variants of lupus erythematosus,

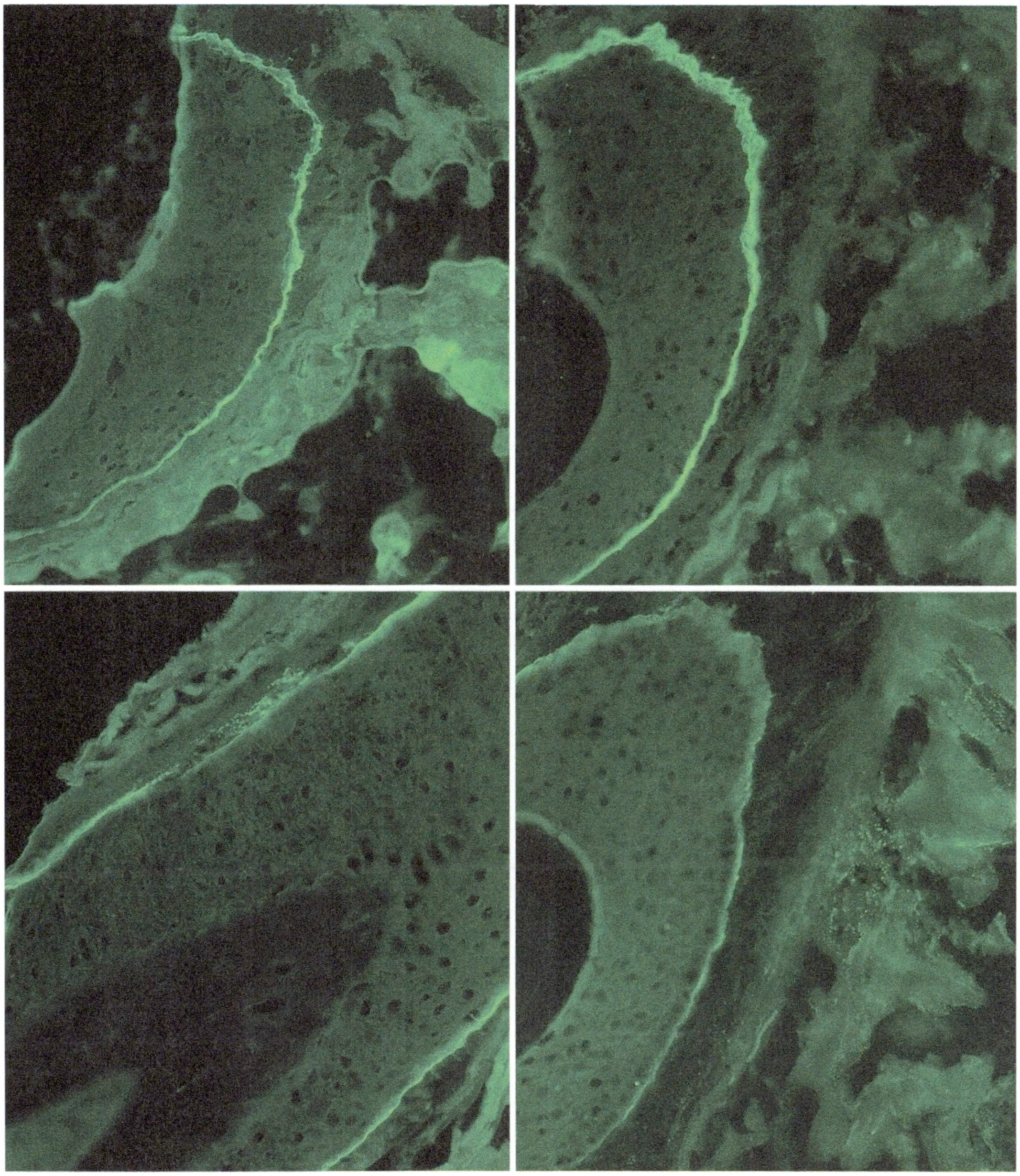

FIG. 8.59

Chronic cutaneous lupus erythematosus, vertical section. Direct immunofluorescence composite showing bright linear deposition of IgG *(top left)*, C3 *(top right)*, IgM *(bottom left)*, and IgA *(bottom right)* along the follicular basement membrane. (Image courtesy of Anjela Galan, MD.)

including discoid lupus erythematosus (DLE), lupus panniculitis, tumid lupus, hypertrophic lupus, and chilblain lupus. DLE comprises the vast majority of CCLE diagnoses and the two terms are often used synonymously. DLE presents with violaceous, disk-shaped lesions predominantly on the face, ears, and scalp with atrophic scarring, dyspigmentation, and follicular plugging (Fig. 8.60). Follicular ostia may be present in early disease but are subsequently lost with progression to scarring alopecia. Conversely, LPP presents with patches of alopecia predominantly along the vertex and parietal areas of the scalp with perifollicular erythema, follicular hyperkeratosis, collarettes of scale, and tenderness.

PATTERN 4: THE DEEP, MIXED INFLAMMATORY PATTERN

Characteristics of the Pattern

This pattern is characterized by a mixed inflammatory infiltrate that is frequently most dense in the subcutis, but often involves the infundibular/isthmic areas with progression over time (Fig. 8.61). The presence of numerous neutrophils and plasma cells is typical (Fig. 8.62). In addition, background lymphocytes, histiocytes, and edema may be seen (Fig. 8.63).

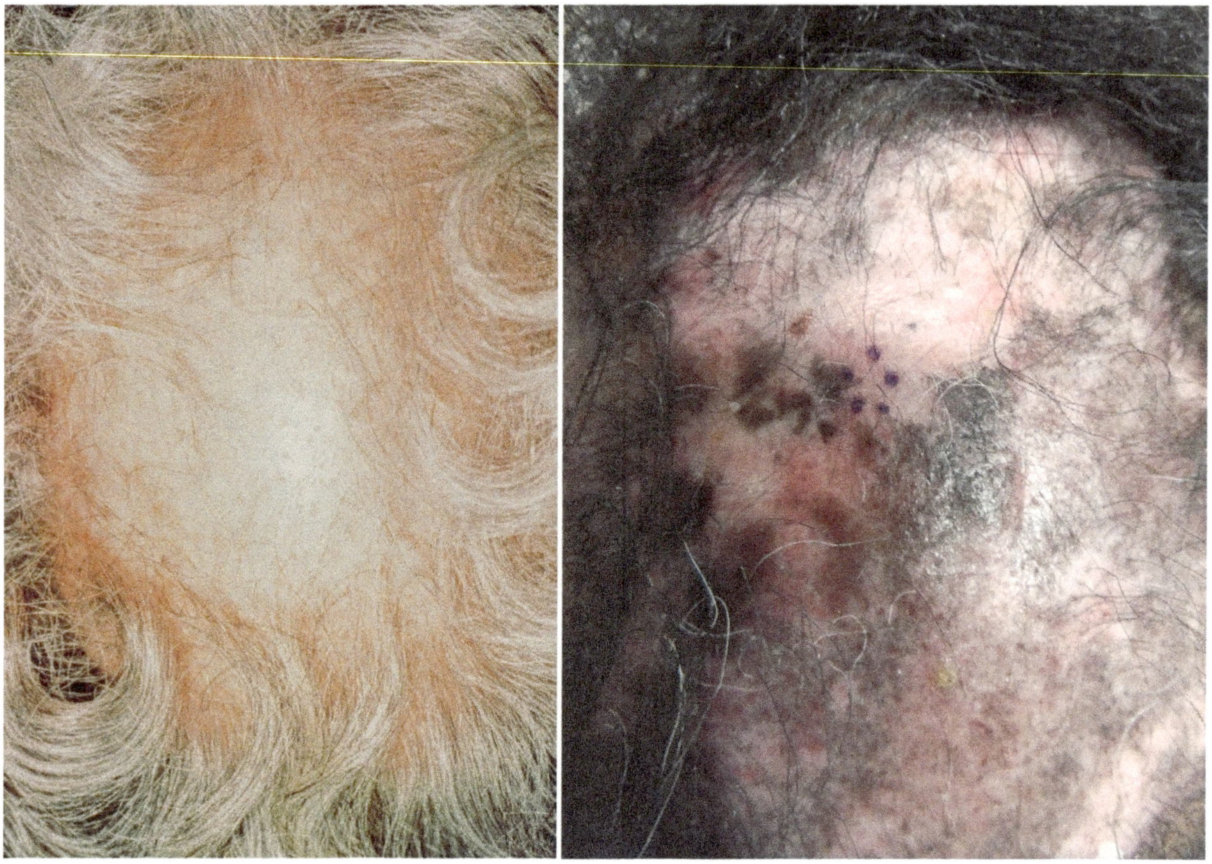

FIG. 8.60
DLE presents with violaceous, disk-shaped lesions predominantly on the face, ears, and scalp with atrophic scarring, dyspigmentation, and follicular plugging.

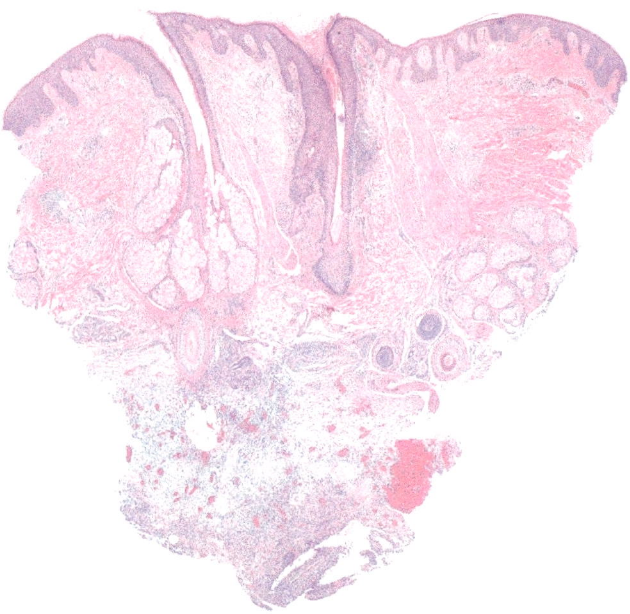

FIG. 8.61
Dissecting cellulitis, vertical section. There is a mixed infiltrate that is densest in the deep dermis and subcutis. The upper follicle and sebaceous glands may be spared until late in the disease (Hematoxylin & eosin, ×20).

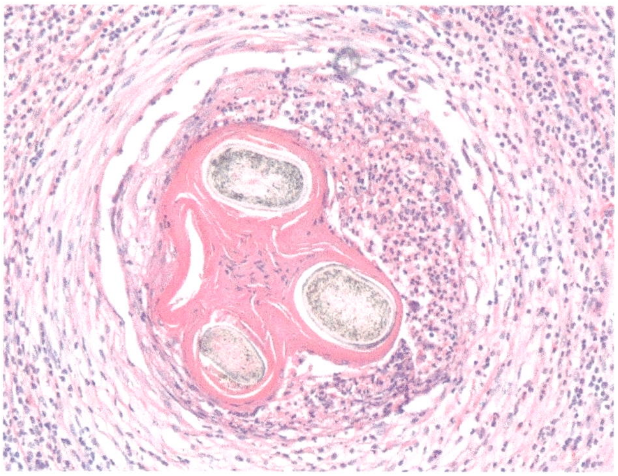

FIG. 8.62
"Folliculitis decalvans," transverse section. Follicular epithelium is destroyed by a mixed infiltrate dominated by neutrophils (Hematoxylin & eosin, ×200).

If follicular destruction involves the bulge zone, stem cells will be lost, and further follicular regeneration will not be possible. At that point, the process becomes cicatricial alopecia, and any of the six general features seen in cicatricial alopecias previously described may occur.

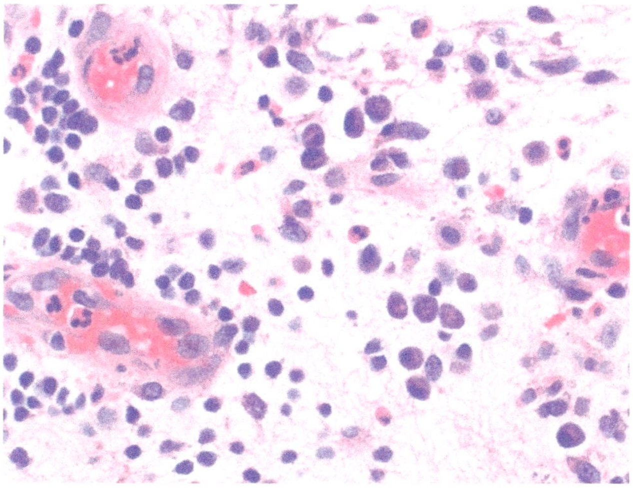

FIG. 8.63
In dissecting cellulitis there is a background of lymphocytes, histiocytes, and edema that may resemble granulation tissue (Hematoxylin & eosin, ×600).

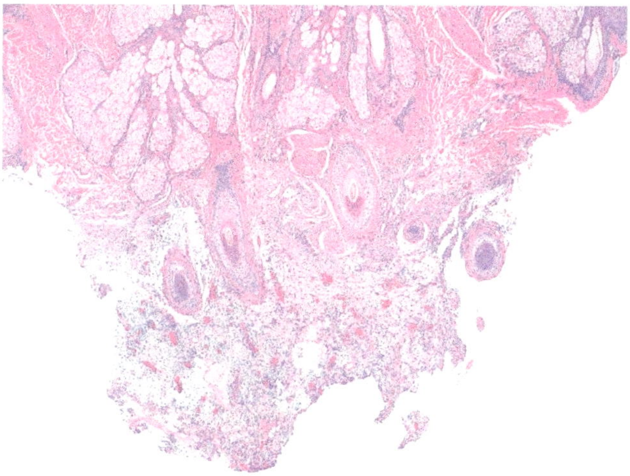

FIG. 8.64
Dissecting cellulitis, vertical section. There is a mixed infiltrate that is densest in the deep dermis and subcutis. Follicles tend to miniaturize, remaining superficial to the chronic inflammatory focus. Sebaceous glands may be spared until late in the disease (Hematoxylin & eosin, ×40).

Diagnoses Manifesting Pattern 4

Dissecting cellulitis (DC), secondary infectious alopecia, and "folliculitis decalvans."

Diagnoses With Similar Features

The other cicatricial alopecias are lymphocyte predominant, with rare to no neutrophils. For this reason, pattern 4 is highly specific.

Helpful Differentiating Features

HISTOLOGIC

Fluctuant lesions of DC typically display a deep mixed infiltrate, chiefly situated around the lower half of terminal follicles and extending into the subcutis. The associated edema and fibroplasia resemble deep granulation tissue. If inflammation is localized exclusively to the deeper dermis, miniaturized follicles will be noted with their bulbs placed just superficial to the infiltrate (Fig. 8.64). The overlying sebaceous lobules will be intact. Over time, the infiltrate involves the upper structures and destroys follicles and sebaceous lobules. Epithelial-lined sinus tracts may be seen in severe cases.

Infectious alopecias (bacterial folliculitis/abscess and fungal kerion) are technically secondary alopecias but may overlap clinically and histologically with DC. Bacterial and fungal stains and cultures are required to exclude infectious agents (Fig. 8.65).

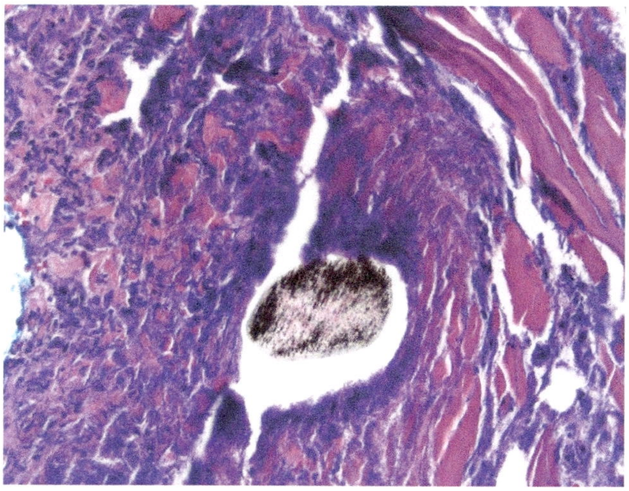

FIG. 8.65
This example of infectious alopecia shows a naked hair shaft surrounded by degranulated neutrophils. Culture studies revealed infection with the gram-negative bacillus, *Pseudomonas aeruginosa* (Hematoxylin & eosin, ×200).

The inflammation of "folliculitis decalvans" is typically most intense in the upper follicle, near the junction of the infundibulum and isthmus. Follicular epithelia are thinned and fused infundibula, sometimes with numerous shafts, are common (Fig. 8.66).

CLINICAL

The clinical pattern and history are usually very helpful in separating these disorders. Purulent discharge from the scalp should be appropriately cultured for bacterial and fungal organisms. Upon exclusion of an infectious process, consideration of the final two differentials can be entertained.

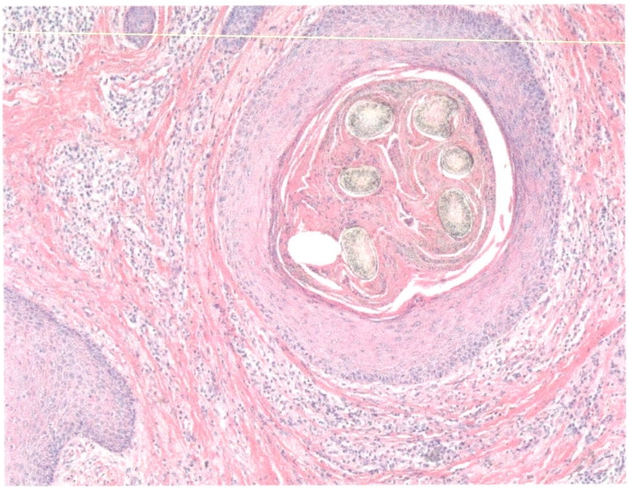

FIG. 8.66

"Folliculitis decalvans," transverse section. In this example, the fusion of multiple follicular epithelia has resulted in a compound follicle containing seven hair shafts. This number of fused follicles implies a neutrophil-driven cicatricial alopecia (Hematoxylin & eosin, ×100).

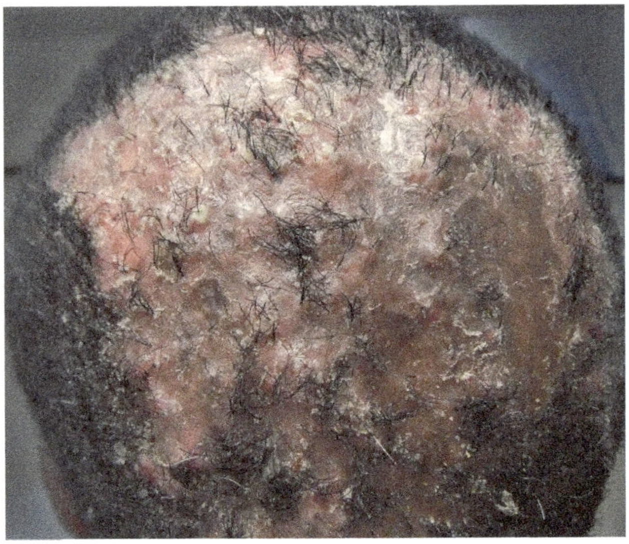

FIG. 8.67

Dissecting cellulitis presents as rapidly progressive, generally painless nodules on the top and posterior scalp that begin firm and become boggy and fluctuant.

DC presents as rapidly progressive, generally painless nodules on the top and posterior scalp that begin firm and become boggy and fluctuant (Fig. 8.67). Interconnection of the nodules through sinus tracts may occur, leading to purulent discharge upon pressure. Over time, permanent hair loss, fibrosis, and hypertrophic scarring ensue. Young Black men are most affected.

"Folliculitis decalvans" is a controversial entity, with some experts considering it a distinct disorder and others a variant form of CCCA or LPP. Typical cases consist of a highly inflammatory cicatricial alopecia with perifollicular pustules and papules localized chiefly to the posterior vertex scalp (Fig. 8.68).

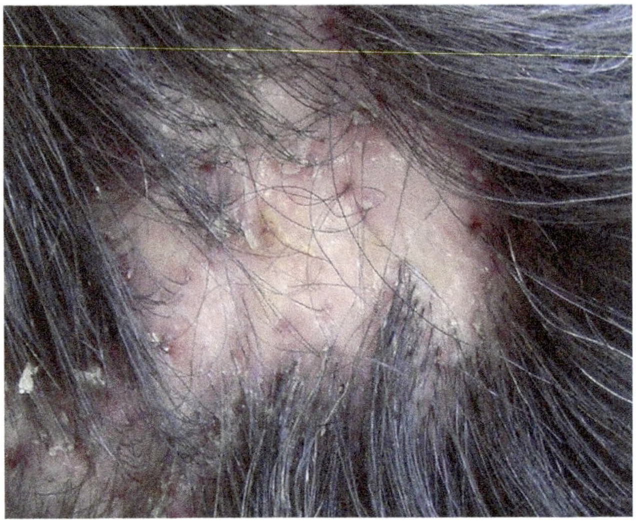

FIG. 8.68

"Folliculitis decalvans" consists of a highly inflammatory cicatricial alopecia with perifollicular pustules and papules localized chiefly to the posterior vertex scalp. (Miguel-Gómez, L., Rodrigues-Barata, A. R., Molina-Ruiz, A., Martorell-Calatayud, A., Fernández-Crehuet, P., Grimalt, R., et al. (2018). Folliculitis decalvans: Effectiveness of therapies and prognostic factors in a multicenter series of 60 patients with long-term follow-up. *Journal of the American Academy of Dermatology*, 79(5), 878–883, Fig. 1a.)

PATTERN 5: THE END-STAGE PATTERN

Characteristics of the Pattern

"End-stage alopecia" is the term applied when the degree of follicular unit destruction is so profound that a more specific histological diagnosis cannot be made. The pattern, representing the final stage of all cicatricial alopecias, is commonly seen because of poor biopsy site selection or sample inadequacy. The best use of time and resources upon receiving such a sample is to contact the clinician and explain the need for a new sample (with the possible inclusion of a second sample collected in Michel's solution if DIF studies are contemplated). The clinician should understand that the new sample must be collected from an area with preserved hair shafts, ideally in areas adjacent to disease activity. Proper site selection (see Fig. 8.1) and biopsy size are covered in the section on collecting and processing, early in this chapter.

The end-stage pattern displays circular to elliptical-shaped regions of dense fibrosis in regions of destroyed follicular units. There is typically a paucity of follicles (Fig. 8.69) and sebaceous lobules are absent. Focal hair shafts with a surrounding granulomatous response (Fig. 8.70) may be the only remaining indication that the skin was once "hair-bearing."

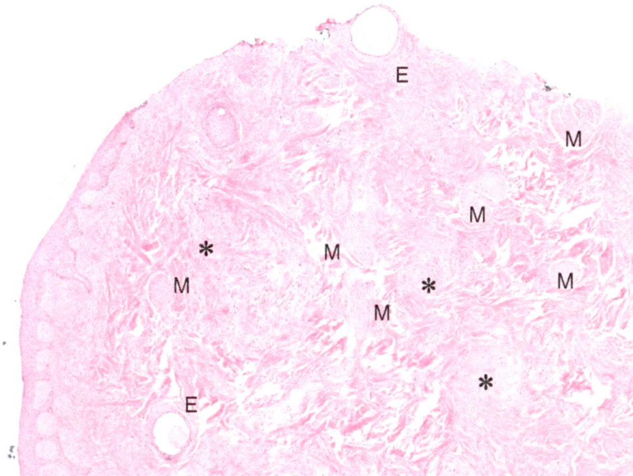

FIG. 8.69

End-stage cicatricial alopecia, transverse section. Foci of dense connective tissue *(*)* mark the sites of prior follicular units. There are two dilated eccrine ducts *(E)* and several background arrector pili muscles *(M)* (Hematoxylin & eosin, ×40).

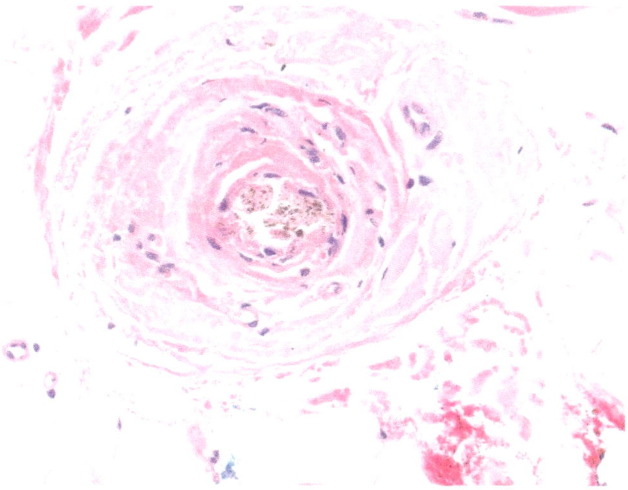

FIG. 8.70

End-stage cicatricial alopecia, transverse section. A naked hair shaft with scant inflammation may be the only histological evidence of that the skin was once hair-bearing (Hematoxylin & eosin, ×400).

Diagnoses Manifesting Pattern 5

The end-stage pattern is the common terminus of all cicatricial alopecias.

Diagnoses With Similar Features

Secondary alopecias due to trauma, burns, and some inflammatory conditions (such as morphea) will commonly result in complete destruction of follicular units and a pattern of "end-stage" alopecia. An in-depth discussion of secondary alopecias is beyond the scope of this chapter.

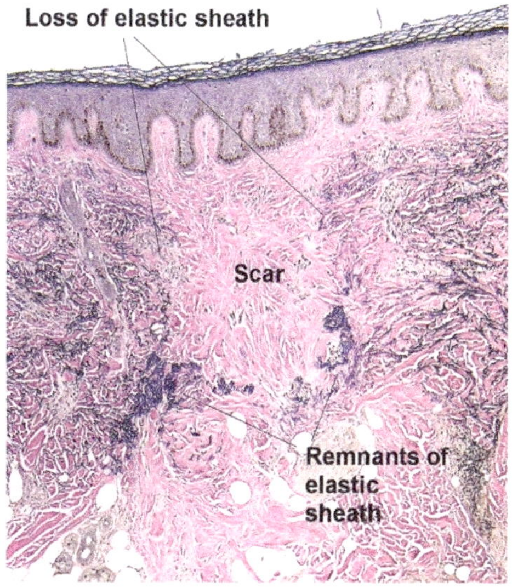

FIG. 8.71

Lichen planopilaris. Staining demonstrates loss of elastic fibers in superficial columnar pattern (Elastic van Gieson, ×200). (From Elston, C. A., Kazlouskaya, V., Elston, D. M. (2013). Elastic staining versus fluorescent and polarized microscopy in the diagnosis of alopecia. *Journal of the American Academy of Dermatology*, 69(2), 288–293. doi: 10.1016/j.jaad.2013.02.030, Fig. 1.)

Helpful Differentiating Features

HISTOLOGIC

Once a cicatricial alopecia reaches the end-stage helpful differentiating histological clues are typically absent. In the event a new sample cannot be collected, one potentially useful adjunct is to highlight the pattern and distribution of any remaining elastin fibers using the elastic van Gieson (EVG) stain and/or polarization microscopy. On EVG staining, pattern 1 diagnoses display superficial columnar or wedge-shaped areas of elastin fiber loss (Fig. 8.71). Conversely, CCCA shows widened fibrous tracts with focally interspersed intact elastin fibers (Fig. 8.72). The areas of elastin fiber loss in CCCA have also been described as "tree trunk-like." Lastly, CCLE has broad areas of elastin fiber loss both in a perifollicular and interstitial distribution reflecting the widespread inflammatory destruction of that entity (Fig. 8.73). If a sample collected in Michel's solution is available, DIF microscopy may prove helpful.

CLINICAL

End-stage alopecia presents as relatively nonspecific foci of extensive hair loss, lack of evident erythema/inflammation, and destruction of the follicular ostia.

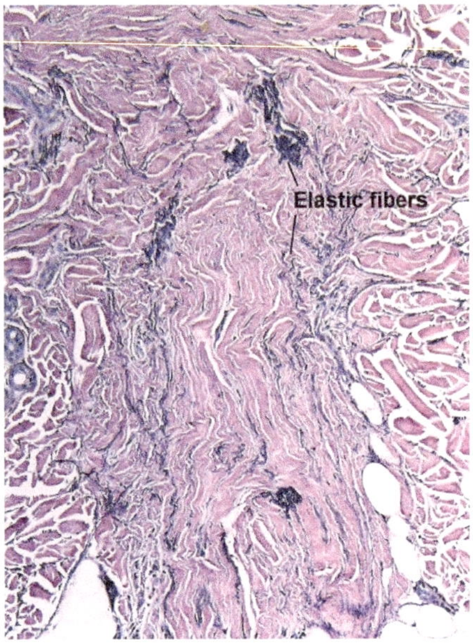

FIG. 8.72

Central centrifugal cicatricial alopecia. Staining demonstrates broad fibrous tract with retention of elastic fibers (Elastic van Gieson, ×200). (From Elston, C. A., Kazlouskaya, V., Elston, D. M. (2013). Elastic staining versus fluorescent and polarized microscopy in the diagnosis of alopecia. *Journal of the American Academy of Dermatology*, 69(2), 288–293. doi: 10.1016/j.jaad.2013.02.030, Fig. 2.)

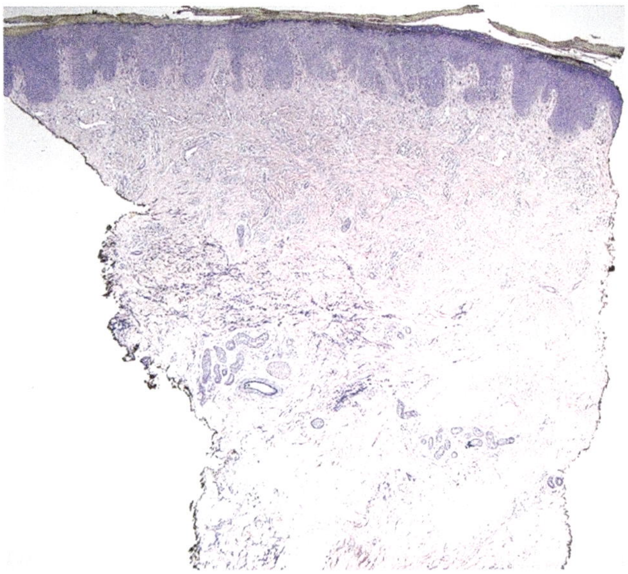

FIG. 8.73

Discoid lupus erythematosus. Diffuse perifollicular and interfollicular dermal fibrosis with loss of elastic staining (Elastic van Gieson, ×40). (From Fung, M. A., Sharon, V. R., Ratnarathorn, M., Konia, T. H., Barr, K. L., Mirmirani, P. (2013). Elastin staining patterns in primary cicatricial alopecia. *Journal of the American Academy of Dermatology*, 69(5), 776–782. doi: 10.1016/j.jaad.2013.07.018, Fig. 3B.)

Brocq's alopecia (pseudopelade of Brocq) is likely one of the various clinical patterns of end-stage cicatricial alopecia rather than a distinct clinical entity. The clinical pattern of Brocq's alopecia may be seen in end-stage LPP, CCLE, CCCA, and other forms of cicatricial alopecia. A diagnosis of end-stage alopecia should encourage a clinician to seek out additional biopsy sites if disease activity is still present.

"BIPHASIC" ALOPECIAS (PATTERN 6)

PATTERN 6: THE BIPHASIC PATTERN

Characteristics of the Pattern

This pattern is defined by the *absence* of stigmata of cicatricial alopecia (see "Cicatricial Alopecia Overview (Patterns 1–5)") and the *presence* of follicular miniaturization due to gradual shortening of the anagen phase (see "Normal Hair Follicle Anatomy and Growth Cycles"). Shortening of the anagen phase leads to a smaller and shallower follicular bulb. Rather than residing in the subcutis, the bulb may be found in the deep dermis (Fig. 8.74), mid (perieccrine) dermis (Fig. 8.75) or may become so superficial as to be nearly indistinguishable from surrounding normal vellus hairs. It is important to note that follicles are affected variably, and that full-size anagen follicles are commonly noted immediately adjacent to miniaturizd follicles (Fig. 8.76).

The gradual nature of the shortening of anagen phase is identifiable in the underlying fibrovascular stele, which mark the previous location of full-sized follicles (Fig. 8.77). Upon reinitiation of normal anagen, the bulb and regrowing isthmus expand along the pathway denoted by the stela. With anagen shortening, the deepest part of the stela will not be revisited by the miniaturized follicular bulb. In time, the abandoned fibrovascular stele become less vascular and more elastotic. The presence of these long-standing stele is strong evidence of a biphasic alopecia (Fig. 8.78).

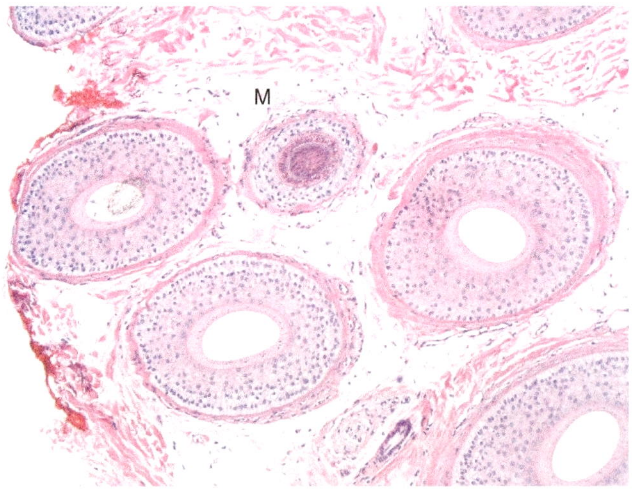

FIG. 8.74

Biphasic alopecia, transverse section. The bulb of a miniaturized *(M)* follicle is noted adjacent to several full-size terminal follicles (Hematoxylin & eosin, ×100).

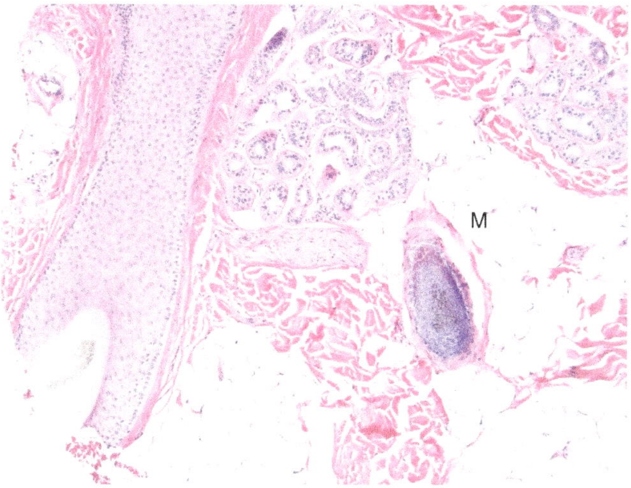

FIG. 8.75

Biphasic alopecia, vertical section. The bulb of a miniaturized *(M)* follicle is noted just deep to the eccrine coils. A full-size terminal follicle is noted on the left (Hematoxylin & eosin, ×100).

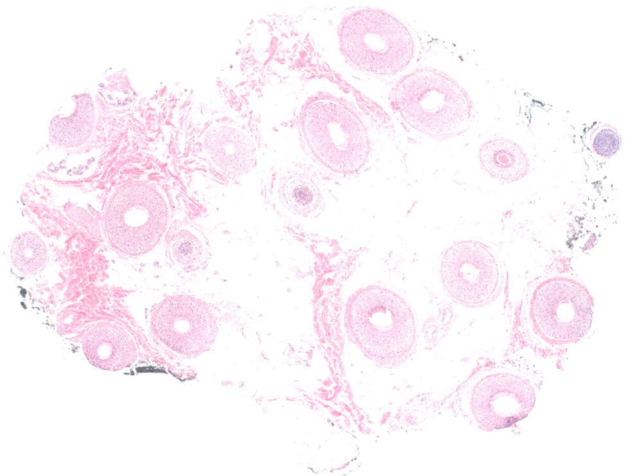

FIG. 8.76

Biphasic alopecia, transverse section. Follicles at the dermal subcutaneous junction showing variable size and depth (Hematoxylin & eosin, ×40).

One consequence of a miniaturized follicle is a proportionately smaller bulb with a smaller volume of follicular matrical cells. Since hair shaft caliber is proportional to the volume occupied by these cells, hair shafts become narrower, more translucent, and often less pigmented. These fine, translucent shafts are less evident clinically, and in late stages of the biphasic pattern, the anagen phase may become so short that these hair shafts barely emerge from their ostia before the next catagen phase begins.

In biphasic alopecias, sebaceous lobules remain intact but commonly become proportionately smaller with the follicles. Follicular cycling is normal or slightly increased (generally the catagen-telogen rate is below 50%). Inflammation is typically absent or nonspecific. The shift of the biphasic census is away from anagen phase, with catagen and telogen follicles representing larger proportions of the overall follicular population (Fig. 8.79 compared with Fig. 8.10).

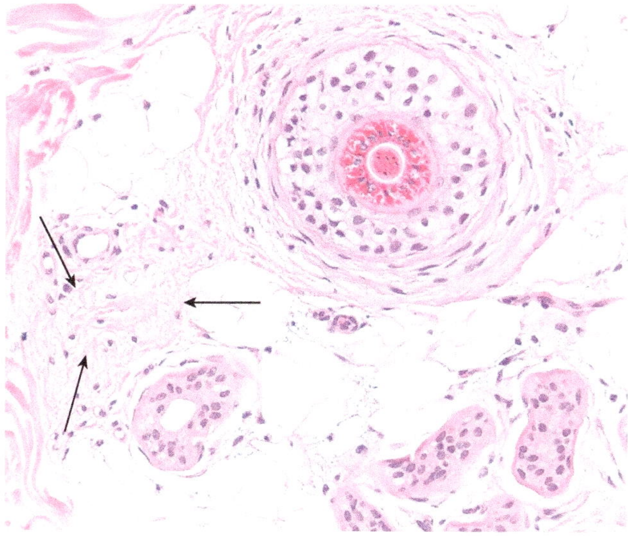

FIG. 8.77

Biphasic alopecia, transverse section. A miniaturized follicle is noted adjacent to an eccrine unit. An elastotic stela *(arrows)*, marking the location of a long since miniaturized follicle is apparent (Hematoxylin & eosin, ×200).

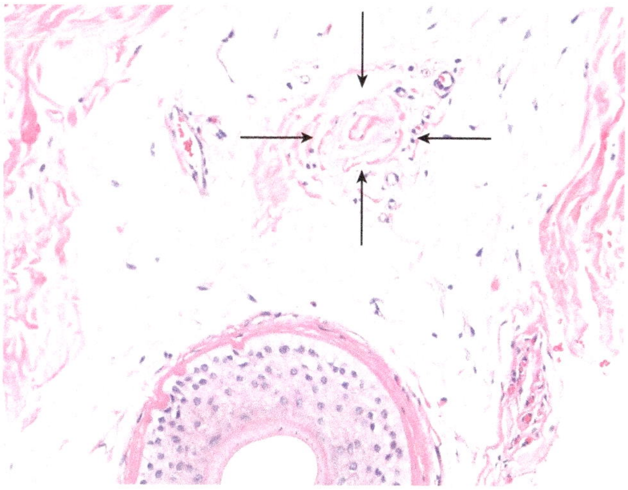

FIG. 8.78

Biphasic alopecia, transverse section. A terminal follicle is noted adjacent to an elastotic stela *(arrows)* (Hematoxylin & eosin, ×200).

Diagnoses Manifesting Pattern 6

AGA, chronic traction alopecia (CTA), and alopecia areata (AA) (some cases).

Diagnoses With Similar Features

Pattern 7: Temporal triangular alopecia (TTA), a congenital alopecia, displays numerous small follicles. As these follicles were never full size, they have not miniaturized and do not have underlying stele.

One important pitfall is that follicular miniaturization commonly occurs in cicatricial alopecias. Presumably, the

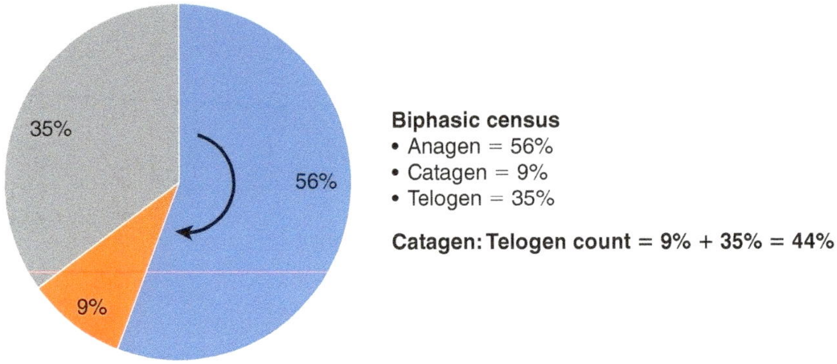

FIG. 8.79

In biphasic alopecias, anagen phase becomes progressively shorter. With follicles occupying significantly less cycling time in anagen, a larger proportion of follicles in the scalp census will be found in the fixed length catagen and telogen phases. If anagen phase is reduced to one-eighth of its normal duration, a telogen rate of 44% is achieved. This rate is within the range of values typically seen in biphasic alopecias (compare to normal scalp census, Fig. 8.10).

cyclic nature of ongoing disease activity in these conditions triggers anagen phase prematurely. This pitfall can be avoided by orderly application of the algorithm (see Fig. 8.30). The first question should always be: Is there loss of the follicular unit? If the answer is no, and miniaturization with stele is present, a biphasic alopecia should be suspected.

Helpful Differentiating Features

HISTOLOGIC

There is no histological feature that will reliably differentiate between AGA and CTA. Cases of AA that are devoid of the classic peribulbar lymphocytes may enter this histological differential (i.e., alopecia universalis), although AA is usually ensconced among the noncicatricial alopecias. The finding of nanogen hairs (see pattern 8), a few peribulbar lymphocytes (Fig. 8.80) and/or eosinophils, pigment within stele (Fig. 8.81), or a catagen rate greater than 50% should prompt consideration of AA. If miniaturization is noted and premature desquamation of the IRS (see Fig. 8.17) is present, the possibility of the earliest stages of CCCA should be entertained.

CLINICAL

The clinical pattern and history are critical in separating these disorders. If clinical information cannot be obtained, a diagnosis line of "noncicatricial alopecia with follicular miniaturization" with a note that includes the above diagnostic lineup may suffice.

AGA generally has a slow and progressive course, with stereotypical patterns in men and women (Figs. 8.82 and 8.83). In men, the frontal hairline (with bitemporal accentuation), as well as the parietal scalp, and the

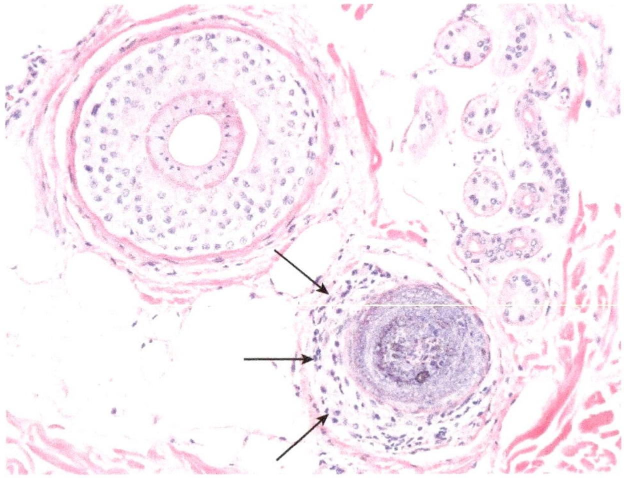

FIG. 8.80

Alopecia areata (AA), transverse section. A miniaturized bulb (adjacent to an eccrine unit) shows a few peribulbar lymphocytes *(arrows)*. Disease activity can wax and wane in AA, and peribulbar lymphocytes may be difficult to detect (Hematoxylin & eosin, ×200).

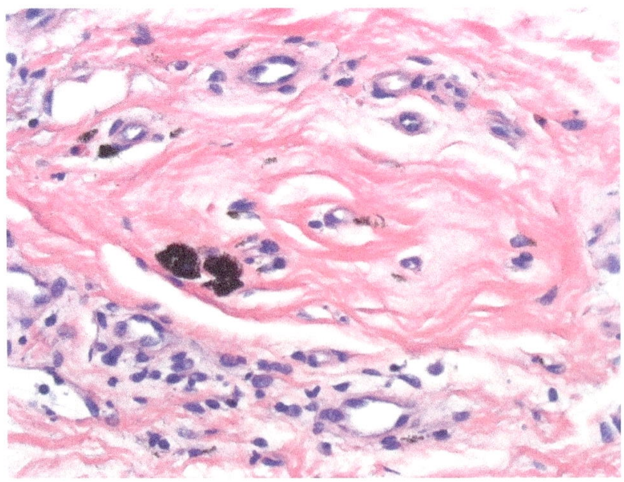

FIG. 8.81

Alopecia areata (AA), transverse section. A vascular stela with clumps of melanin pigment could signify AA (Hematoxylin & eosin, ×400).

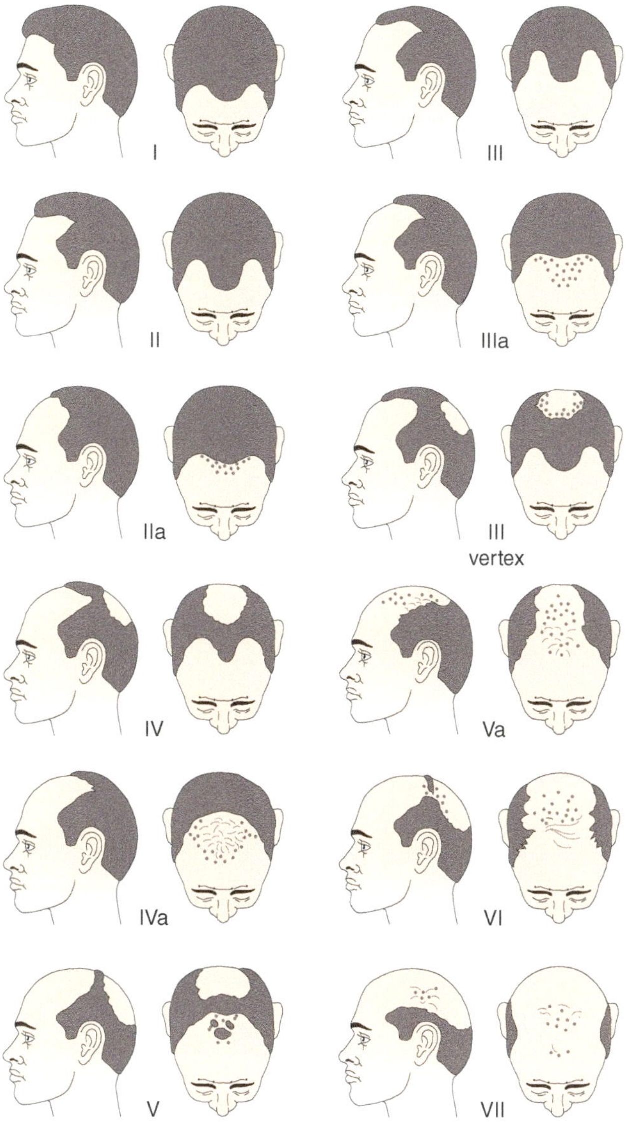

FIG. 8.82

The Hamilton classification system of male pattern baldness. (From Habif, T. P., Dinulos, J. G. H., Chapman, M. S., & Zug, K. A. (Eds.). Hair and nail disease. In *Skin disease: diagnosis and treatment*. Edinburgh: Elsevier. Fig. 20.1.)

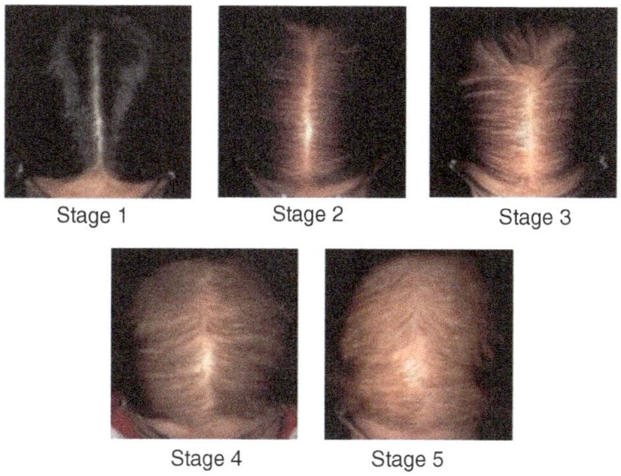

FIG. 8.83

The Sinclair scale for female pattern hair loss. (From Rudnicka, L., & Stefanato, C. M. (2024). Alopecias. In J. L. Bolognia, et al. (Eds.), *Dermatology* (5th ed.). Elsevier. Fig. 69.5.)

vertex area are involved. In women, the hair loss is more diffuse, affecting mostly the vertex and the mid-scalp, commonly with widening of the central part. Women present most commonly with diffuse hair loss and rarely have complete baldness, as opposed to men, in whom a rim of occipital hair may be the only hair remaining (Fig. 8.84).

CTA is most often caused by hairstyling techniques such as tight braiding, ponytails, cornrows, or the use of elastic hair bands. The alopecia is especially pronounced at the margin of tightly styled hair and, because of symmetry with bitemporal or frontal involvement, may closely resemble AGA clinically (Fig. 8.85). CTA may develop decades after tight hairstyling has stopped, so clinical questioning should always include prior hair styling practices.

Because clinical *and* histological patterns of AGA and CTA overlap, distinction between these two entities may not be possible.

PATTERN 7: TEMPORAL TRIANGULAR ALOPECIA

Characteristics of the Pattern

TTA is a congenital alopecia that is included here because of the histological finding of numerous small hair follicles that might suggest a "biphasic" alopecia. On transverse sections, the number of follicular units is normal and sebaceous lobules are unremarkable. However, the number of small/vellus follicles approaches 100% without an apparent reason. There is no significant inflammation and follicular cycling is normal. The critical finding is the *absence* of underlying stele, an indication that these follicles were *never* full-size (terminal) follicles (Fig. 8.86). TTA is hypothesized to occur when primary (congenital) vellus hairs are unstimulated by (or are unresponsive to) signals that initiate the first cycle of full anagen growth in the newborn.

Diagnoses Manifesting Pattern 7

This pattern is highly specific, although due to limitations of sampling and embedding, it may be difficult to prove the *absence* of stele in some samples.

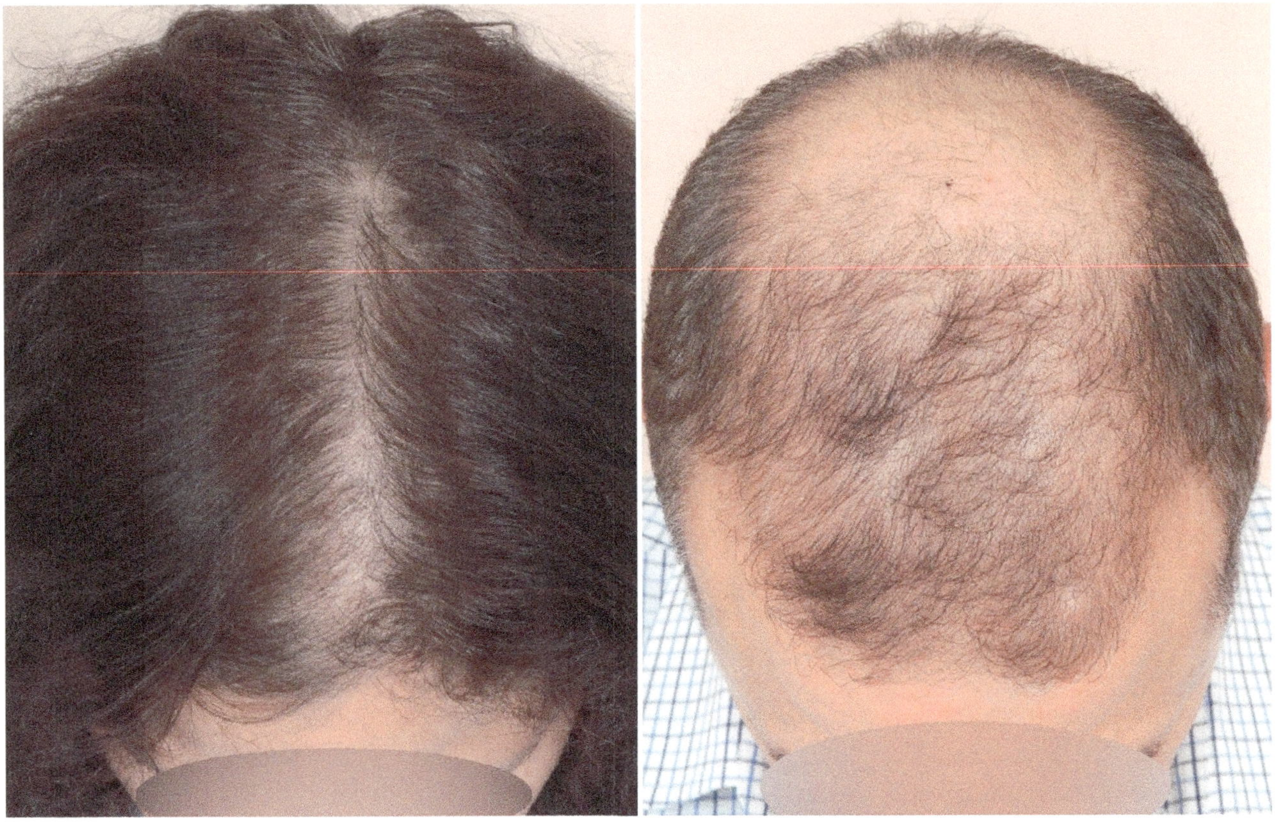

FIG. 8.84

Women with androgenetic alopecia present most commonly with diffuse hair loss and rarely have complete baldness, as opposed to men, in whom a rim of occipital hair may be the only hair remaining.

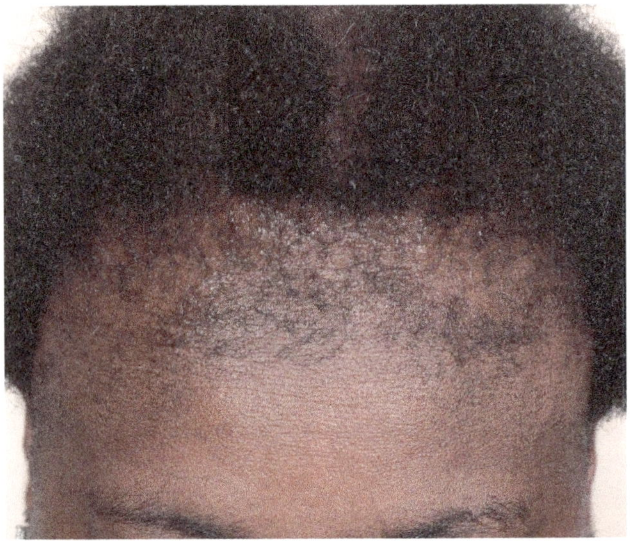

FIG. 8.85

Chronic traction alopecia is especially pronounced at the margin of tightly styled hair, and because of symmetry with bitemporal or frontal involvement, may closely resemble androgenetic alopecia clinically.

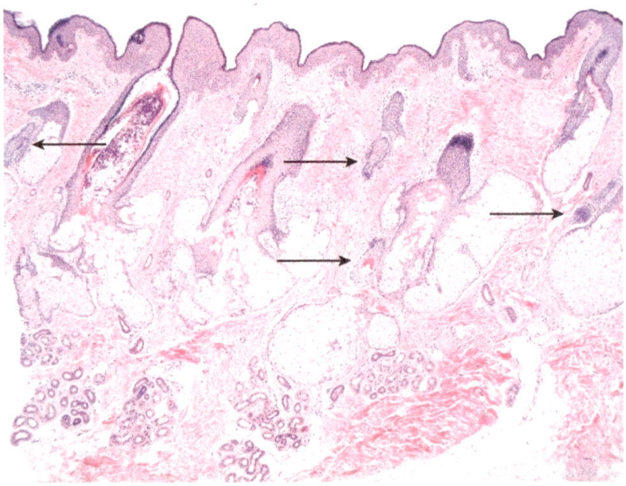

FIG. 8.86

Temporal triangular alopecia, vertical section. Multiple follicular units with no evident terminal follicles or stele. Several vellus follicles *(arrows)* are noted (Hematoxylin & eosin, ×40).

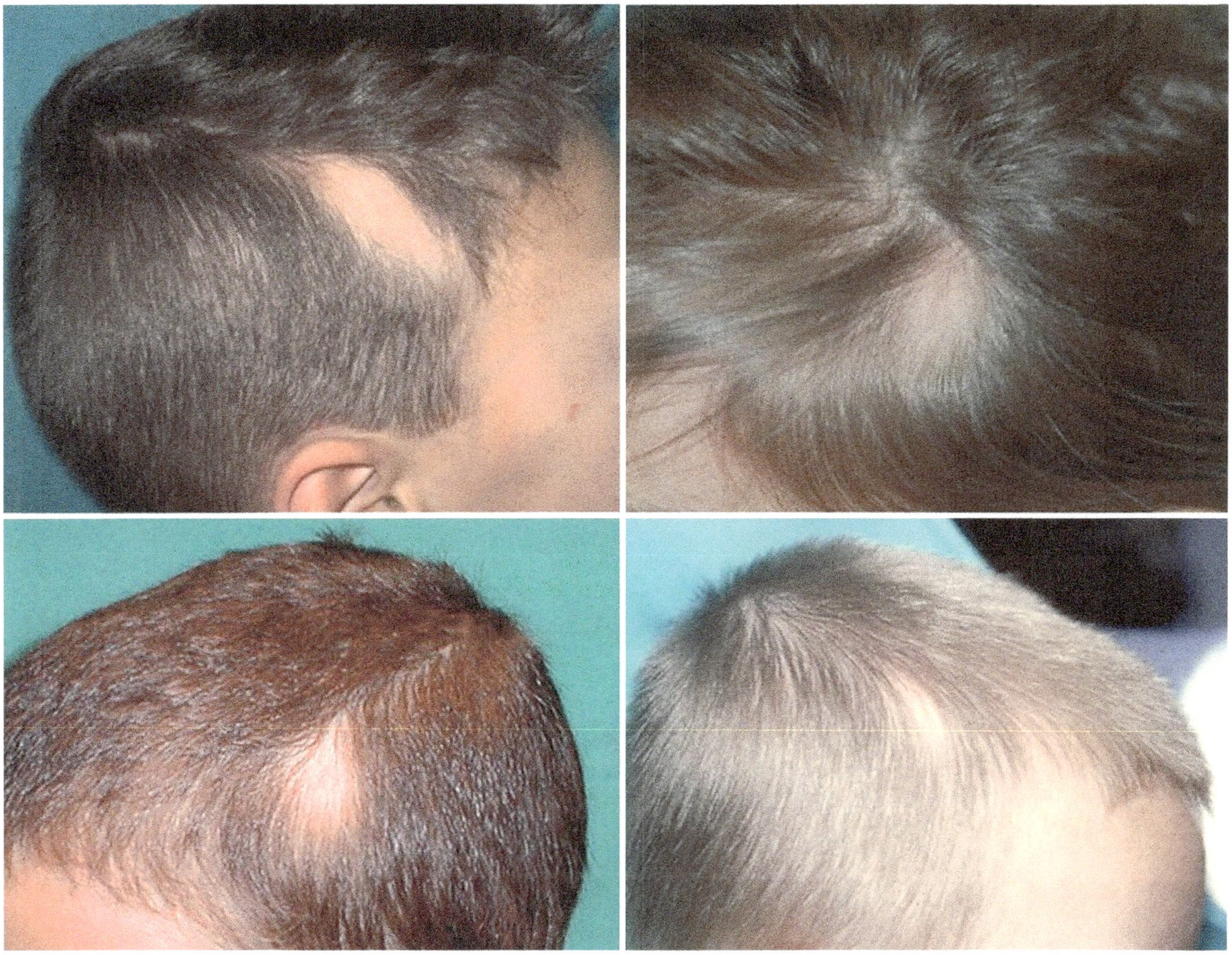

FIG. 8.87

Temporal triangular alopecia. Hairless triangular patches that may be unilateral or bilateral. (From Fernández-Crehuet, P., Vaño-Galván, S., Martorell-Calatayud, A., Arias-Santiago, S., Grimalt, R., Camacho-Martínez, F. M. (2016). Clinical and trichoscopic characteristics of temporal triangular alopecia: a multicenter study. *Journal of the American Academy of Dermatology*, 75(3), 634-637. doi: 10.1016/j.jaad.2016.04.053, Fig. 1.)

Diagnoses with Similar Features

Pattern 6: Biphasic alopecias contain truly miniaturized follicles, commonly with concurrent terminal or indeterminate follicles. Stele are seen in biphasic alopecias. Because of the presence of longtime hair thinning, solar elastosis is often observed in biphasic alopecias. As TTA is usually first noted in childhood, solar elastosis is not observed.

Helpful Differentiating Features

CLINICAL

As the histopathology is unique, it is important to corroborate with clinical findings. TTA is considered a congenital alopecia and is usually identified at birth or in the first decade of life. TTA appears as hairless triangular patches (Fig. 8.87) that may be unilateral or bilateral. Upon close inspection, fine vellus hairs can usually be seen. As the name suggests, these are usually noted in the temporal hairline, although exceptions to this location have been described.

NONCICATRICIAL ALOPECIA OVERVIEW (PATTERNS 8–11)

In contrast to the cicatricial alopecias noted earlier in this chapter, noncicatricial alopecia is clinical hair loss *without* histological loss of the folliculosebaceous unit. Many practitioners regard biphasic alopecias as noncicatricial alopecias, although histological and clinical findings justify classifying these diagnoses into a distinct subgroup, which, over many years, appears clinically and histologically cicatricial. Once the cicatricial and biphasic alopecias are eliminated by systematic application of

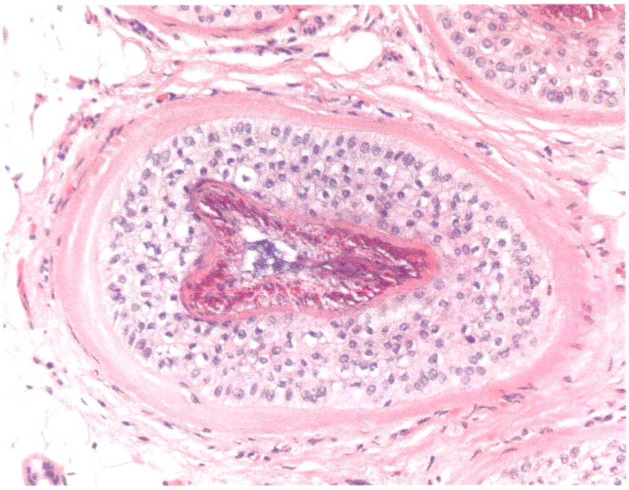

FIG. 8.88

Trichotillomania, transverse section. This follicular epithelium is distorted into a triangular shape by forceful removal of a well-anchored terminal anagen hair shaft (Hematoxylin & eosin, ×200).

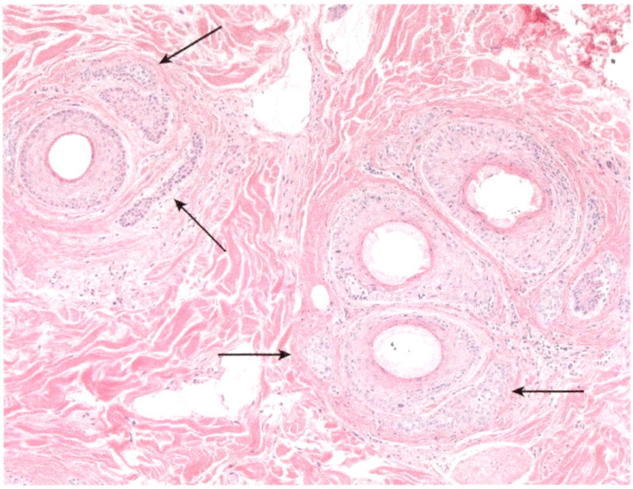

FIG. 8.89

Collapsed sebaceous lobules *(arrows)* may be a feature of some noncicatricial alopecias. They appear as unusually shaped, often crescentic or concentric epithelia around the upper hair follicles (Hematoxylin & eosin, ×100).

the algorithm (see Fig. 8.30), the diagnosis of a noncicatricial alopecia will apply.

Three general features to help the pathologist categorize alopecia as noncicatricial

(1) **Normal appearance.** The biopsy may look entirely normal on histological examination (see Fig. 8.8).

(2) **Miniaturized or distorted follicles.** As noted previously, follicular miniaturization is nonspecific. At this juncture in the algorithmic approach, cicatricial and biphasic alopecias have been eliminated, leaving noncicatricial alopecias. In some cases, the presence of follicular miniaturization may still be a helpful distinguishing feature among the remaining noncicatricial diagnoses. More importantly, follicular distortion, usually a result of external manipulation, is critical in a subset of the remaining diagnoses (Fig. 8.88).

(3) **Miniaturized or "collapsed" sebaceous lobules.** Like the follicular unit, sebaceous lobules are preserved in noncicatricial alopecias. However, they may also become miniaturized or "collapsed" (Fig. 8.89), leading to potentially important differential considerations.

PATTERN 8: THE PERIBULBAR INFLAMMATORY PATTERN

Characteristics of the Pattern

As is true in all noncicatricial alopecias, there are normal numbers of follicular units. The characteristic finding in this pattern is an inflammatory infiltrate conspicuously surrounding the follicular bulb. The analogy for this appearance is a lymphocytic "swarm

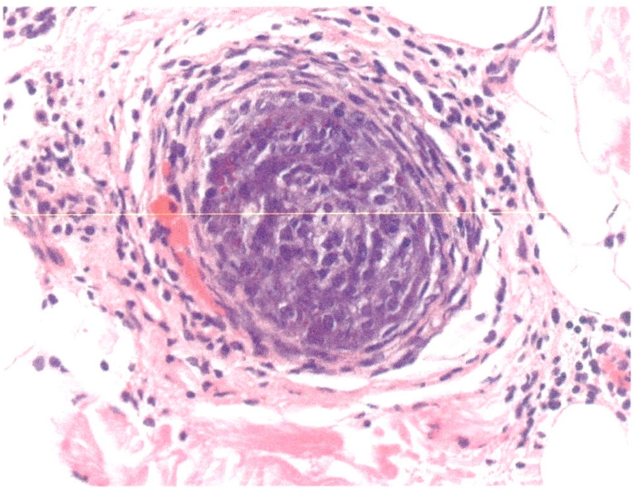

FIG. 8.90

Alopecia areata, transverse section. Lymphocytes encircle the bulb region and some entire the bulb epithelium. Matrical cells may become indistinct or blurry (Hematoxylin & eosin, ×400).

of bees" microscopically encircling the bulbar "hive" (Figs. 8.80 and 8.90). This pattern, classically used to describe AA, may occur in both syphilitic alopecia and noncicatricial alopecia of systemic lupus erythematosus (SLE). In most cases, other histological findings can be used to differentiate between these near look-alikes (see below).

The active peribulbar inflammation of pattern 8 leads to an abrupt shift from anagen to catagen:telogen phase, resulting in one of the most pronounced catagen:telogen shifts of any alopecia (typically between 50% and 100%) (Fig. 8.91). During the combined 8 weeks of catagen:telogen phase, shifted follicles are unable to incite inflammation (Fig. 8.92). If the

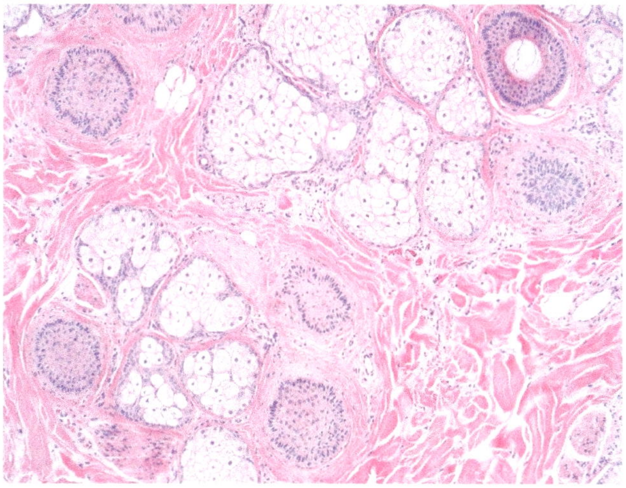

FIG. 8.91

Alopecia areata, transverse section. All of the follicles are in catagen phase, representing a 100% catagen:telogen count. Sebaceous lobules are uninvolved. No significant inflammation is noted in this section (Hematoxylin & eosin, ×100).

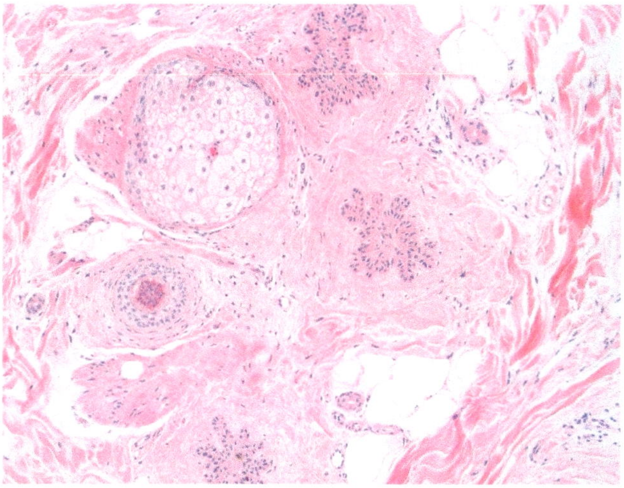

FIG. 8.92

Alopecia areata, transverse section. Following two weeks of catagen, all follicles will enter telogen phase for about 2 months before the next anagen phase occurs. During catagen and telogen phases, the follicles do not trigger an inflammatory reaction. This image shows three telogen follicles and one miniaturized "nanogen" follicle (left) (Hematoxylin & eosin, ×100).

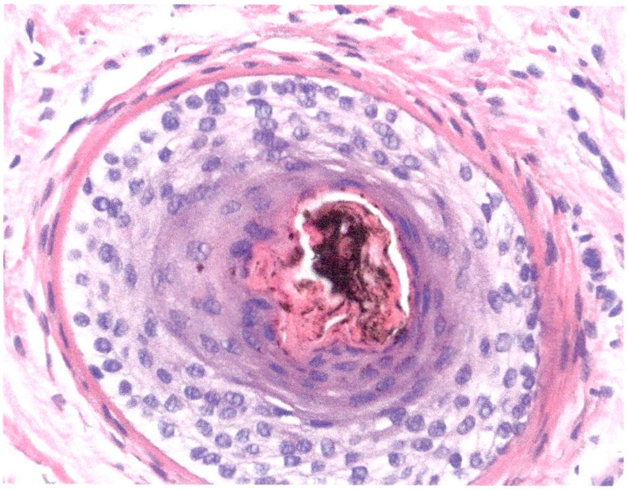

FIG. 8.93

A pigmented hair keratin cast within a transversely cut follicular lumen in alopecia areata (Hematoxylin & eosin, ×400).

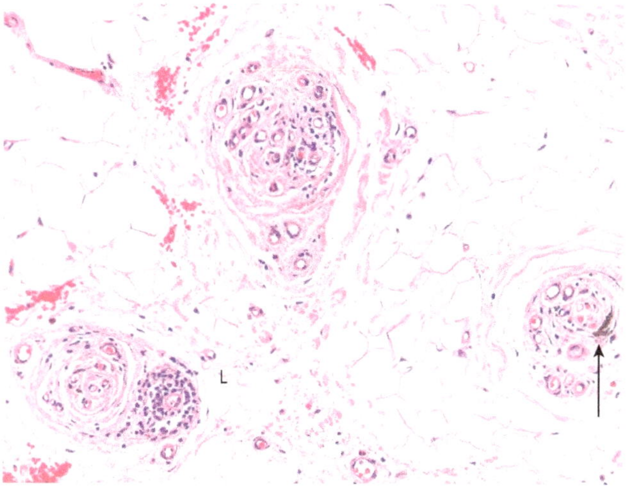

FIG. 8.94

Three recent vascular stele in a case of transversely cut alopecia areata. One contains lymphocytes *(L)* and the other contains pigment *(arrow)* (Hematoxylin & eosin, ×400).

condition persists or is untreated, peribulbar inflammation will recur upon the resumption of anagen, followed by a precipitous rebound into catagen:telogen.

The accelerated tempo of hair cycling that ensues can lead to dyssynchrony of the follicular cells, with secondary effects ranging from follicular miniaturization to the production of abnormal and distorted hair shafts (trichomalacia), to the spillage of matrical melanin (pigmented casts and pigmented stele) (Figs. 8.93 and 8.94), to the development of so-called nanogen (dwarf) follicles. Nanogen follicles, besides being small, may have overlapping characteristics of anagen, catagen, and telogen phases. In many cases, these follicles will be entirely or mostly filled with IRS keratin (Fig. 8.95) without production of a visible shaft.

Actively inflamed follicular bulbs may devolve into a disorganized conglomeration of cells with a less-crisp appearance than the normal follicular matrix. The presence of intrabulbar lymphocytes may contribute to this heterogeneous/cluttered appearance.

Diagnoses Manifesting Pattern 8

AA (most common), syphilitic alopecia, and noncicatricial alopecia of SLE.

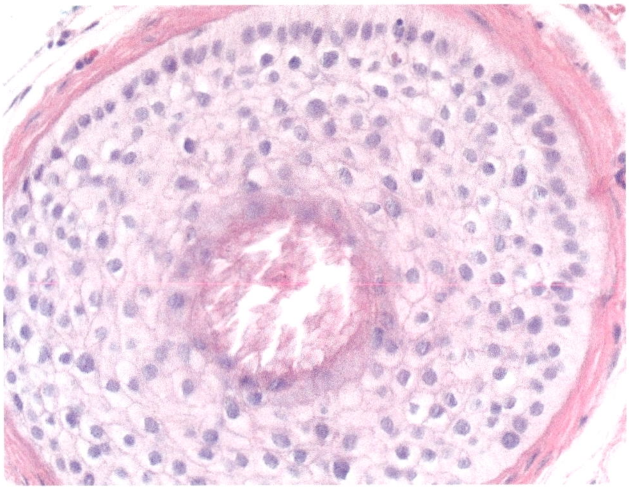

FIG. 8.95
A transverse nanogen follicle in alopecia areata. The outer root sheath is intact, and the inner root sheath spans the lumen of the follicle. No hair shaft is apparent (Hematoxylin & eosin, ×400).

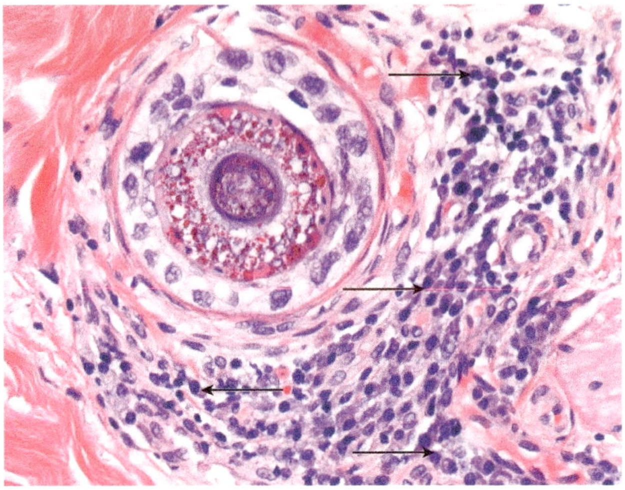

FIG. 8.96
Syphilitic alopecia, transverse section. When peribulbar inflammatory cells are dominated by plasma cells *(arrows)*, syphilis and systemic lupus should be considered (Hematoxylin & eosin, ×400).

Diagnoses With Similar Features

Trichotillomania (TT) may also display trichomalacia and pigment deposition. The catagen-telogen shift of TT is typically not as dramatic as that seen in AA. Peribulbar inflammation and miniaturization are absent in TT. Lastly, TT commonly shows dramatic follicular epithelial distortion, sometimes with intrafollicular hemorrhage and fractured hair shafts.

Helpful Differentiating Features

HISTOLOGIC

Syphilitic alopecia may appear nearly identical to AA. A helpful histological clue for syphilis not seen in AA is the predominance of plasma cells in the peribulbar infiltrate (Fig. 8.96). Eosinophils, commonly seen in the peribulbar infiltrate of AA, are not seen in syphilis. In addition, the infiltrate of syphilis may extend into the upper follicle and epidermis, where subtle interface changes can be seen (Fig. 8.97). Spirochete immunohistochemical staining is a useful adjunct in this setting (Fig. 8.98).

Like syphilis, the infiltrate of noncicatricial alopecia of SLE commonly contains plasma cells and extends into the upper portions of the hair follicle and to the dermal-epidermal junction. In SLE, the inflammatory infiltrate also extends into perivascular and perieccrine areas (Fig. 8.99), often with the deposition of interstitial dermal mucin.

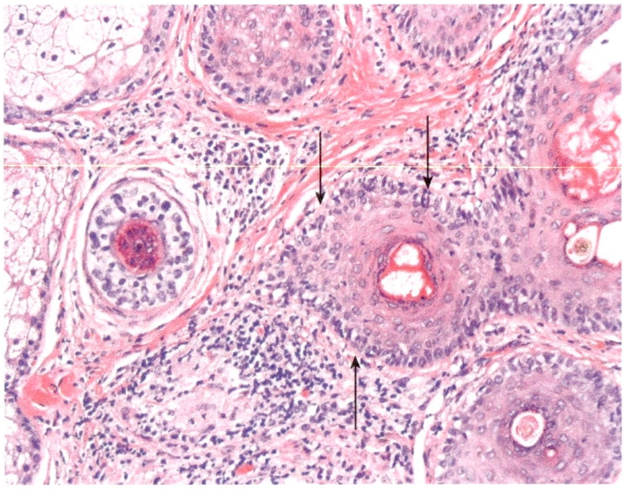

FIG. 8.97
Syphilitic alopecia with interface changes in the upper follicle. Plasma cells and interface changes *(arrows)* should prompt consideration of systemic lupus and syphilis (Hematoxylin & eosin, ×200).

CLINICAL

The classic presentation of AA is discrete, well-circumscribed patches of hair loss with preservation of follicular markings, although diffuse and band-like (ophiasis) patterns of hair loss may also occur (Fig. 8.100). Syphilitic alopecia manifests with a wide array of clinical presentations including papulosquamous lesions, patchy hair loss with a "moth-eaten" appearance (Fig. 8.101), and diffuse shedding resembling telogen effluvium (TE). Correlation with clinical history and serologies is useful for differentiating AA and syphilitic alopecia. The noncicatricial alopecia

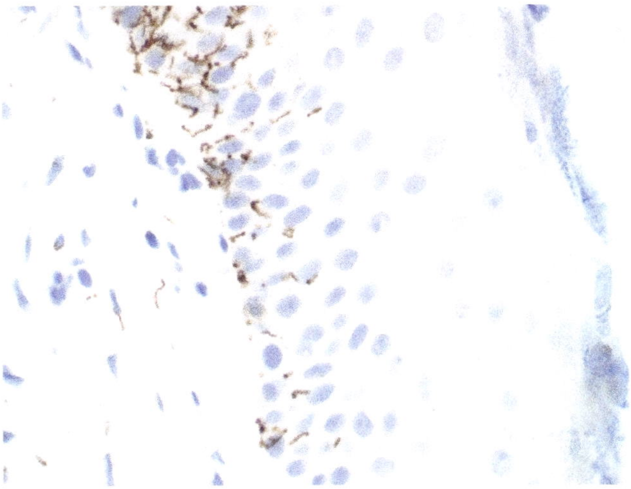

FIG. 8.98

Syphilitic alopecia with numerous organisms identifiable with an immunohistochemical stain directed against spirochetes (Spirochete IHC, ×600).

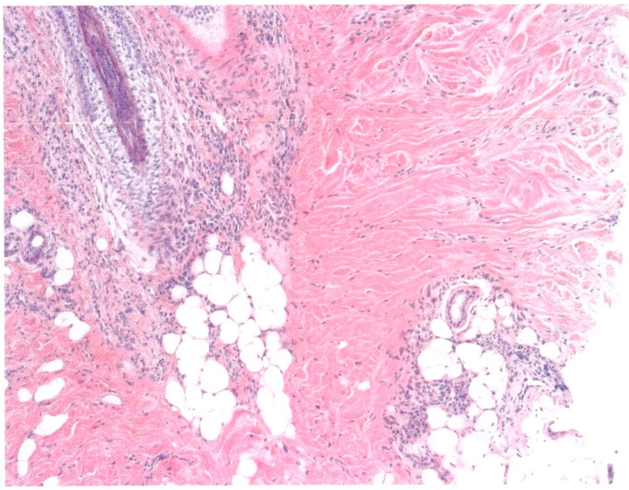

FIG. 8.99

Noncicatricial alopecia of systemic lupus, vertical section. There is follicular miniaturization and a perifollicular and perieccrine infiltrate of lymphocytes and a few plasma cells (Hematoxylin & eosin, ×100).

associated with SLE presents with patches of hair loss dispersed throughout the scalp, usually in a patient with known SLE. In challenging cases, correlation with antinuclear antibody (ANA) and other serologies can be helpful in making this distinction, although ANA testing can often be positive in both SLE and syphilis.

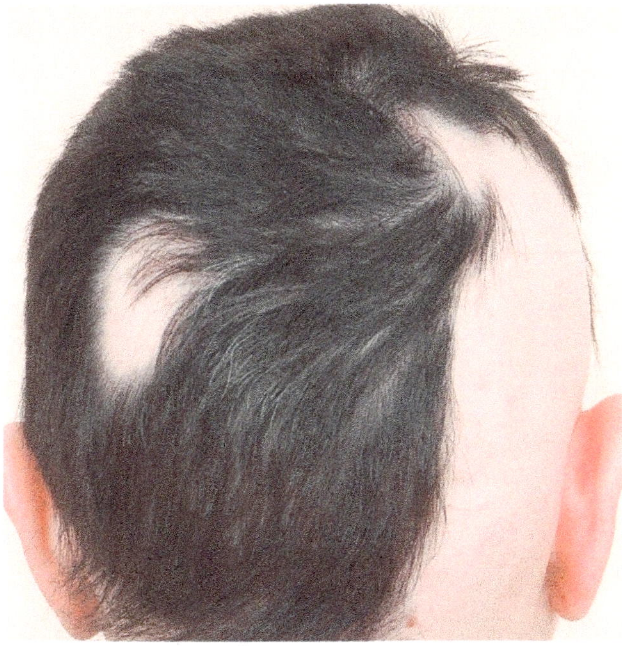

FIG. 8.100

The classic presentation of alopecia areata is discrete, well-circumscribed patches of hair loss with preservation of follicular markings, although diffuse and band-like (ophiasis) patterns of hair loss may also occur.

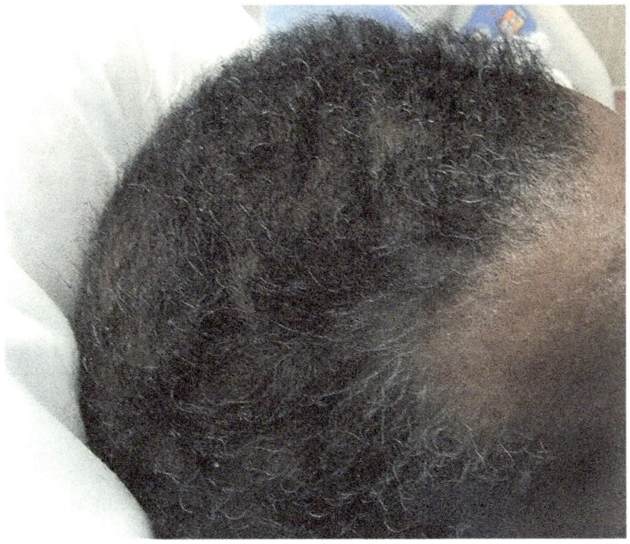

FIG. 8.101

Syphilitic alopecia manifests with a wide array of clinical presentations including papulosquamous lesions, patchy hair loss with a "moth-eaten" appearance, and diffuse shedding resembling telogen effluvium.

PATTERN 9: THE COLLAPSED SEBACEOUS LOBULE PATTERN

Characteristics of the Pattern

On horizontal histological sections, the most conspicuous features of pattern 9 is a marked catagen-telogen shift (>80%), diffuse follicular miniaturization, and atrophic/collapsed sebaceous lobules. The latter finding, the most specific histological feature, resembles "deflated balloons" abutting the isthmus portion of the follicle (Figs. 8.89, 8.102, and 8.103). A mild peribulbar inflammatory infiltrate with rare eosinophils may also be seen. Classic findings of conventional psoriasis may or may not be seen in the overlying epidermis. These include confluent

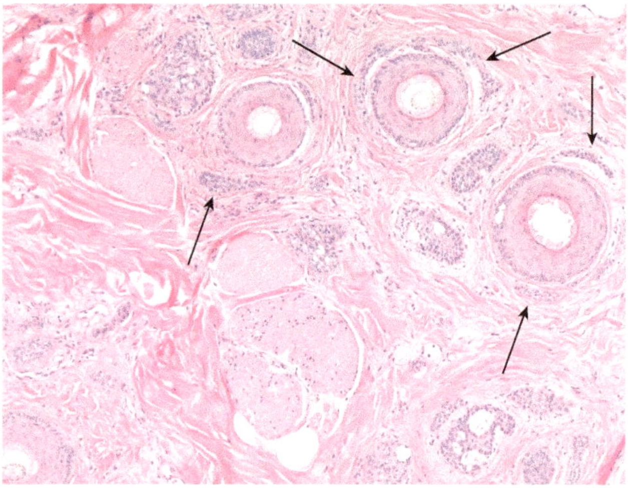

FIG. 8.102

Psoriatic alopecia, transverse section. Numerous sebaceous lobules collapse to thin crescent-shaped mantles *(arrows)* surrounding the upper follicles (Hematoxylin & eosin, ×100).

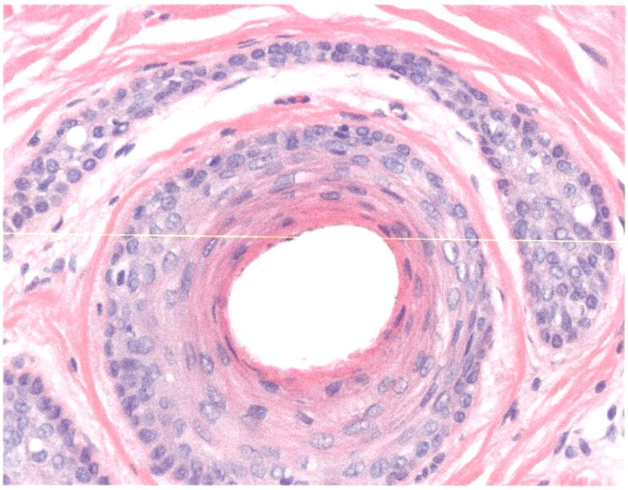

FIG. 8.103

Psoriatic alopecia, transverse section. A collapsed sebaceous lobule concentrically arranged around a follicle (Hematoxylin & eosin, ×400).

parakeratosis, neutrophils in the stratum corneum, regular acanthosis, and loss of the granular layer (Fig. 8.104).

Diagnoses Manifesting Pattern 9

Psoriasis, sebopsoriasis, tumor necrosis factor-alpha (TNF-α) inhibitor–associated alopecia.

Diagnoses With Similar Features

Pattern 8: AA, syphilitic alopecia, and noncicatricial alopecia of SLE.

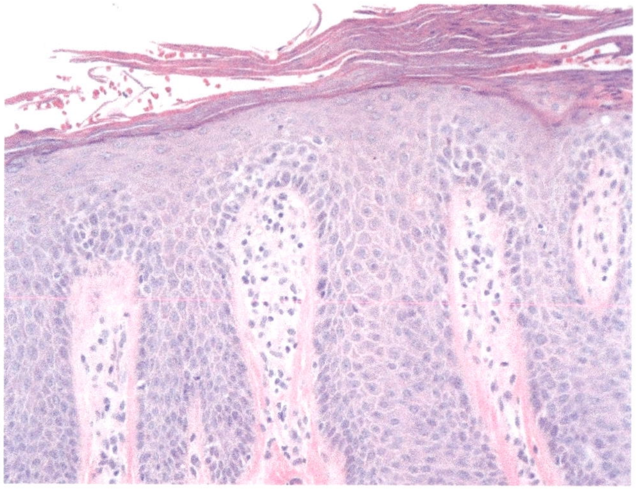

FIG. 8.104

Psoriatic alopecia, vertical section. The epidermis above psoriatic alopecia may or may not show the classic pattern of psoriasis seen here. There is psoriasiform epidermal hyperplasia, confluent parakeratosis, dilated capillary loops, and thinning of the supra-papillary plates (Hematoxylin & eosin, ×200).

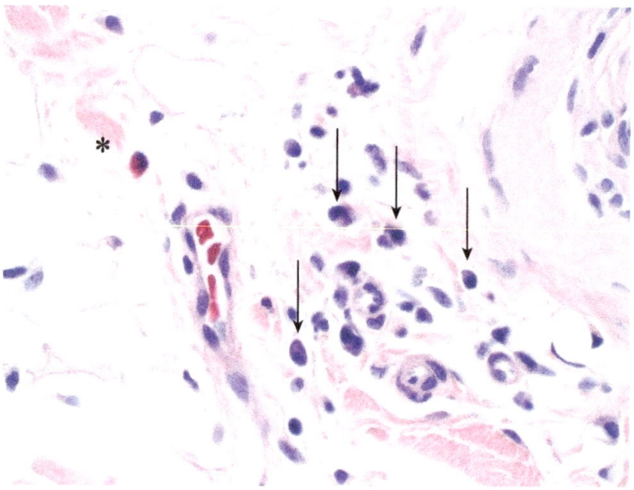

FIG. 8.105

TNF-alpha inhibitor–associated alopecia, transverse section. Contrary to other alopecias in pattern 9, TNF-alpha inhibitor–associated alopecia contains a dermal infiltrate of plasma cells *(arrows)* and eosinophils *(star)* (Hematoxylin & eosin, ×600).

Helpful Differentiating Features

HISTOLOGIC

Psoriasis and sebopsoriasis have identical histological features and are best differentiated clinically (see below). TNF-α inhibitor–associated alopecia presents with histological findings very similar to conventional psoriatic alopecia; however, there is typically a deeper inflammatory infiltrate that contains eosinophils and plasma cells (Fig. 8.105).

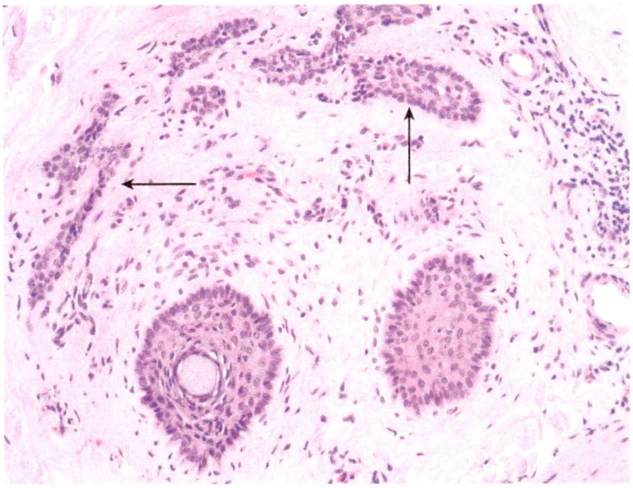

FIG. 8.106

Psoriatic alopecia, transverse section. The marked catagen:telogen shift and nearby lymphocytes could suggest alopecia areata. However, the collapsed sebaceous lobules *(arrows)* are a clue to the correct diagnosis (Hematoxylin & eosin, ×200).

Psoriatic alopecia may closely mimic AA given the marked catagen-telogen shift, diffuse miniaturization, and potential for a mild peribulbar inflammatory infiltrate (Fig. 8.106). In contrast to psoriatic alopecia, the sebaceous lobules retain their normal configuration in AA. The overlying epidermis in AA is also unremarkable when compared to the psoriasiform and other inflammatory changes that may be seen in psoriatic alopecia. Plasma cells are inconspicuous in both AA and classic psoriatic alopecia but are readily found in TNF-α inhibitor–associated alopecia.

CLINICAL

Psoriasis is a relatively common inflammatory dermatosis that presents as plaques of thickened skin with silvery scale. The scalp is involved in most cases. Alopecia typically occurs within a lesional plaque, but a more diffuse TE may also occur. Seborrheic dermatitis and so-called sebopsoriasis exist on a spectrum with psoriasis and may present with similar clinical and histological findings. Psoriasiform alopecia may also be seen in patients prescribed TNF-α inhibitors. These medications are commonly used in inflammatory bowel disease and autoinflammatory conditions but may be prescribed for psoriasis, further complicating the interpretation of biopsy specimens with this pattern. Clinically, these patients also present with alopecic plaques on the scalp that may be difficult to distinguish from psoriasis-related alopecia. Conversely, AA usually presents with round to oval areas of hair loss with relatively normal-appearing skin and intact follicular markings.

PATTERN 10: THE UNINFLAMED WITH TRICHOMALACIA PATTERN

Characteristics of the Pattern

As a noncicatricial pattern of alopecia, folliculosebaceous units are preserved. The defining histological findings in this pattern are pigment casts, trichomalacia, and an absence of inflammation. Pigment casts are irregular, darkly pigmented, amorphous to vermiform clumps of melanin pigment within the follicular lumen (and sometimes the stele) (Figs. 8.93 and 8.107). Trichomalacia is a similar phenomenon wherein distorted and ill-formed hair shafts are produced by traumatically disrupted and displaced matrical cells (Fig. 8.108).

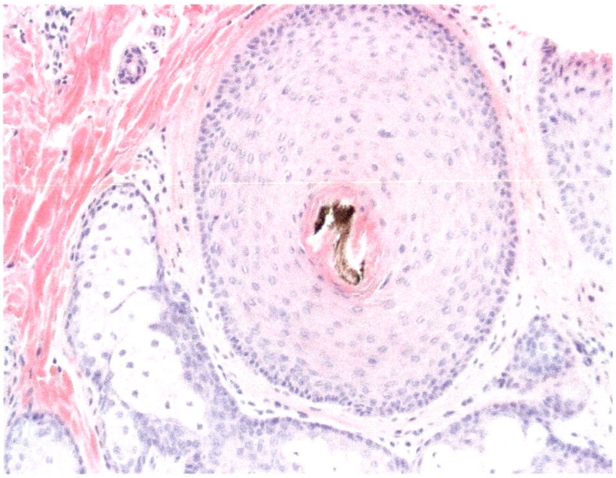

FIG. 8.107

Trichotillomania, transverse section. A pigmented cast within the upper follicle (Hematoxylin & eosin, ×200).

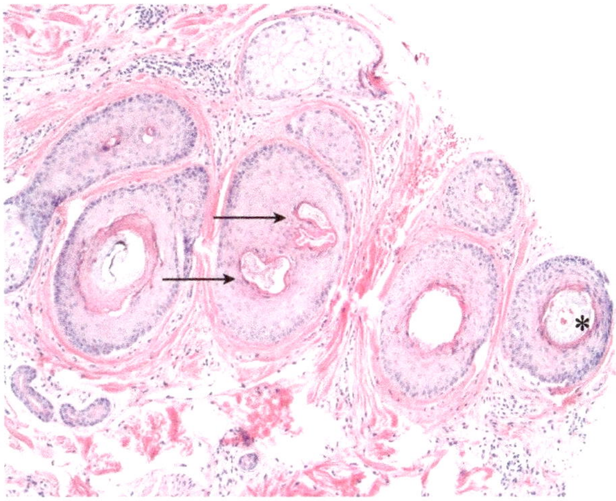

FIG. 8.108

Trichotillomania (TT), transverse section. Distorted follicular lumens, trichomalacia *(arrows)*, and intraluminal hemorrhage *(*)* are all features of TT (Hematoxylin & eosin, ×100).

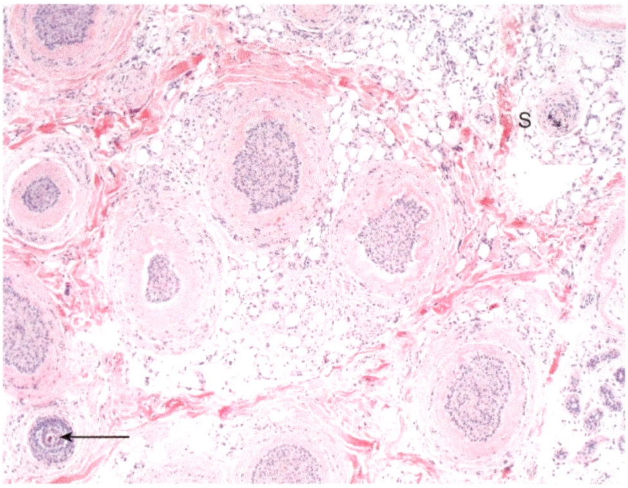

FIG. 8.109

Postoperative pressure–induced alopecia, transverse section. Nearly all follicles are in catagen phase. A pigmented cast is noted *(arrow)*. Pigment is also present in a stela *(S)* (Hematoxylin & eosin, ×40).

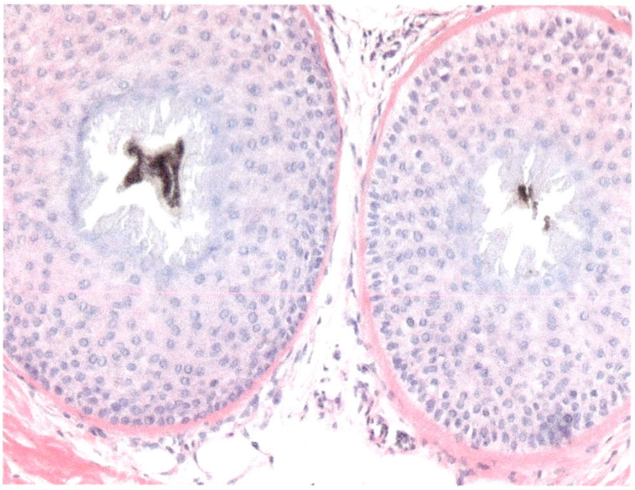

FIG. 8.110

Trichotillomania, transverse section. Two adjacent terminal follicles with fractured hair shafts and disrupted inner root sheaths (Hematoxylin & eosin, ×200).

The diagnoses in this pattern represent physical (traumatic) insults to the hair follicle, and thus, inflammation is minimal to absent. Since hair follicles have a limited histological repertoire to inflammatory and physical assaults, increased cycling, denoted by a shift from anagen to catagen-telogen phase is apparent in this pattern (Fig. 8.109). Upon entering catagen phase from anagen phase, *transiently* miniaturized "indeterminate" hairs may be noted. These can be recognized as such by their well-vascularized stele. Chronic follicular miniaturization with elastotic stele, as is typical of biphasic alopecia, is not a feature of this pattern.

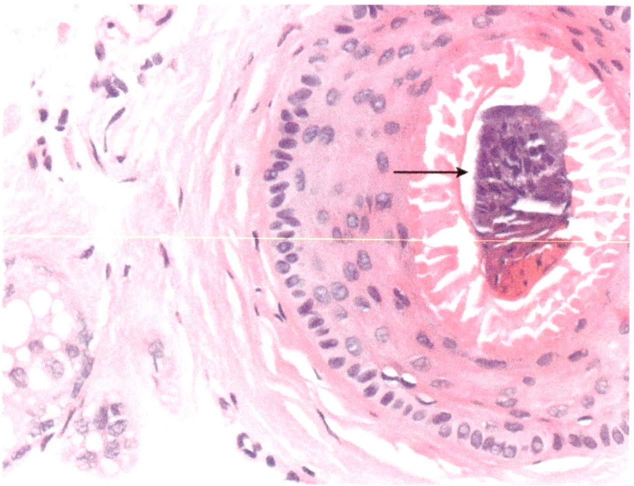

FIG. 8.111

Trichotillomania, transverse section. Matrical cells *(arrow)* have been displaced into the upper part of the isthmus by forceful pulling of the shaft. Note the adjacent sebaceous lobule (Hematoxylin & eosin, ×400).

Diagnoses Manifesting Pattern 10

TT and postoperative pressure–induced alopecia (POPIA).

Diagnoses with Similar Features

Pattern 8: AA may show histological overlap when pigment casts, trichomalacia, and increased cycling co-exist.

Helpful Differentiating Features

HISTOLOGIC

In TT, the traumatic removal of hair can cause "collapse" of the follicular lumen, the most common histological finding (see Fig. 8.88). The collapse can lead to follicles with unusual cross-sectional morphologies including hourglass shapes and triangles (Fig. 8.110). Translocation of matrical cells (Fig. 8.111) to any point along the follicular lumen, leading to trichomalacia and pigment casts, and dislocation of the sebaceous lobules to the lumen of the hair follicle, may also be seen. The so-called hamburger sign is a specific but rare histological feature that can be seen in TT. It consists of a relatively even longitudinal fracture of the hair shaft with entrapped red blood cells. Extravasated red cells around the follicular unit can also help support a diagnosis of TT in the presence of other features. This is a more specific finding when evidence of chronicity is seen (siderophages or deteriorating red cells). Lastly, red cells within the follicular lumen are strongly supportive of TT (Fig. 8.112).

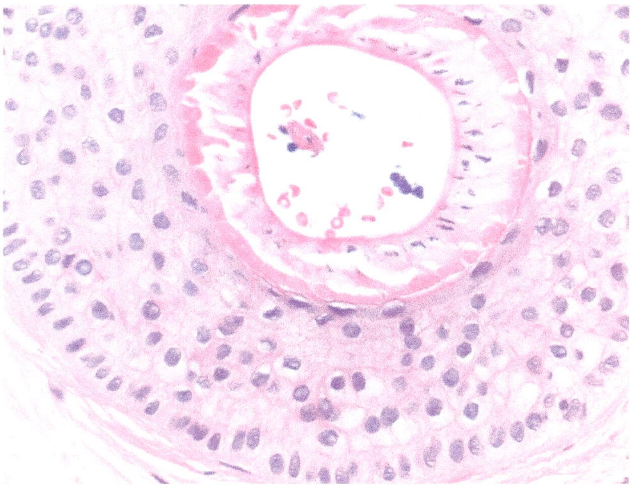

FIG. 8.112
Trichotillomania, transverse section. Red blood cells in the follicular lumen are a helpful indicator of trichotillomania (Hematoxylin & eosin, ×400).

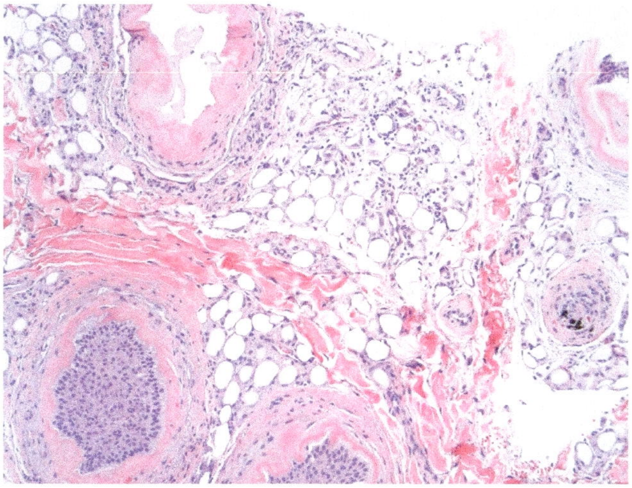

FIG. 8.113
Postoperative pressure–induced alopecia, transverse section. Follicles are in catagen phase. Fat necrosis and lipophages are noted (Hematoxylin & eosin, ×100).

POPIA shares many of the above histological features with TT but may show a more pronounced catagen-telogen shift (see Fig. 8.109). Extravasation of red cells, outside and within the follicular lumen, favors TT. POPIA may show subcutaneous fat atrophy (Fig. 8.113) with a sprinkling of inflammatory cells, as well as microthrombi. These features are not present in TT.

CLINICAL

TT is a psychiatric disorder characterized by repetitive pulling of the hair leading to irregular, patchy areas of alopecia. The prevalence in the general population is estimated to be 0.5%–2.0% with a 4:1 female predominance. Onset can occur at any age. In young children,

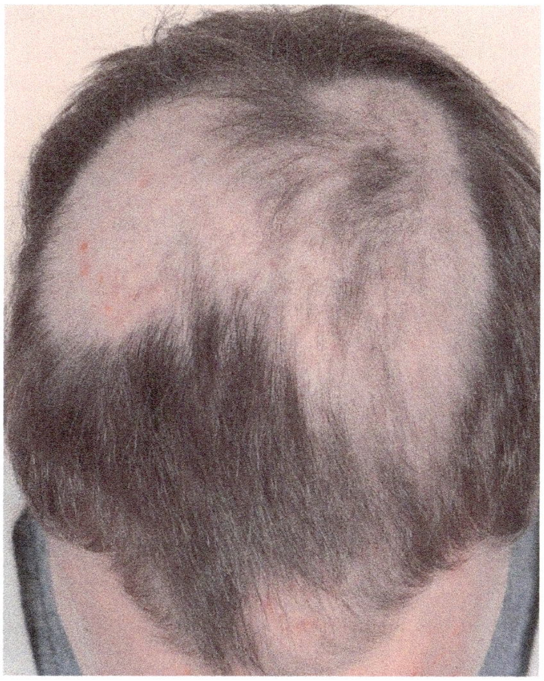

FIG. 8.114
In trichotillomania, irregularly shaped areas of alopecia are noted with broken hair shafts identifiable on close clinical examination.

the behavior is considered benign. Most cases develop in early adolescence and are chronic. Many cases are associated with anxiety, depression, obsessive compulsive disorder, or posttraumatic stress disorder. Onset in later life is often a sign of an underlying psychiatric disorder. Patients will often deny they pull their hair and may try to hide the behavior.

The scalp is the most common area of involvement in TT (~75% of cases) followed by the eyebrows. Irregularly shaped areas of alopecia are noted (Fig. 8.114). Broken hair shafts may be identifiable on close clinical examination. A hair-pull test is negative.

POPIA occurs with prolonged immobilization (e.g., postsurgery or injury) which leads to constant compression and subsequent alopecia in an area of hair-bearing skin. The alopecia occurs at a site of prolonged contact with a hard surface, as may occur during a lengthy surgical procedure. Clinically, the area of contact is well-demarcated and may closely resemble a solitary focus of AA. Close correlation with clinical and surgical history is required to make the diagnosis. In most cases, POPIA reverses over time.

PATTERN 11: THE "NORMAL" PATTERN

Characteristics of the Pattern

This pattern, as the name suggests, looks histologically normal. There is no loss of the folliculosebaceous architecture, no overt abnormality of follicular cycling, and no inflammation. Possible explanations for this pattern include (1) a hair shaft abnormality, (2) a nonrepresentative or inadequate biopsy, (3) recovering acute TE, and (4) absence of alopecia.

In cases of acute TE, normal asynchronously cycling follicles are abruptly jolted into catagen phase by a sudden change in the patient's medical status (e.g., severe illness, completion of pregnancy). Because follicles must pass through catagen and into telogen phase before the shaft is dislodged, clinical shedding appears late, often after the next cycle of anagen has commenced 8–10 weeks later. If a biopsy is conducted when shedding is underway, the proportion of follicles in catagen:telogen phase will be *lower* than 10% (and may be as low as 0%!). This can easily be overlooked unless a census of follicles is conducted (see "Normal Hair Follicle Anatomy and Growth Cycles").

The most useful next step when confronted with pattern 11 is to review the submitted clinical information. If this is incomplete, a phone call to the submitting clinician is required. Photography and a more detailed history will often narrow the differential possibilities (see below) although additional biopsy samples may also need to be considered if the sample is deemed to be nonrepresentative of a clinically apparent pathological process. Usually, a discussion with the clinician will suggest the next diagnostic steps.

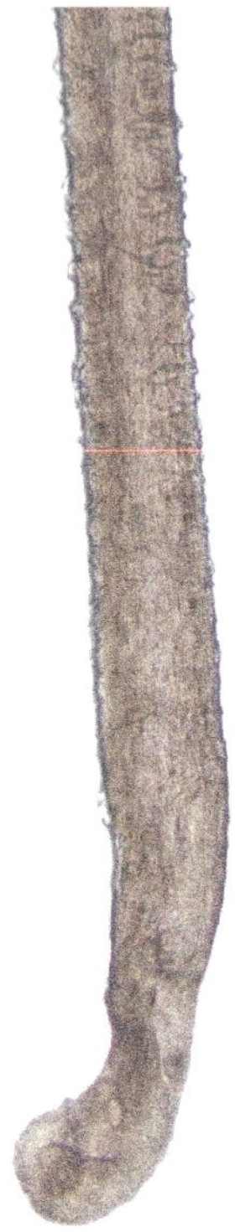

FIG. 8.115

Loose anagen hair syndrome, hair shaft mount. An anagen hair shaft displays ruffling of the adherent cuticle in the so-called fallen sock sign (×100).

Diagnoses Manifesting Pattern 11

Loose anagen hair syndrome (LAHS), hair shaft abnormalities, recovering acute TE, absence of alopecia.

Diagnoses with Similar Features

Subtle early biphasic alopecias may appear nearly normal histologically.

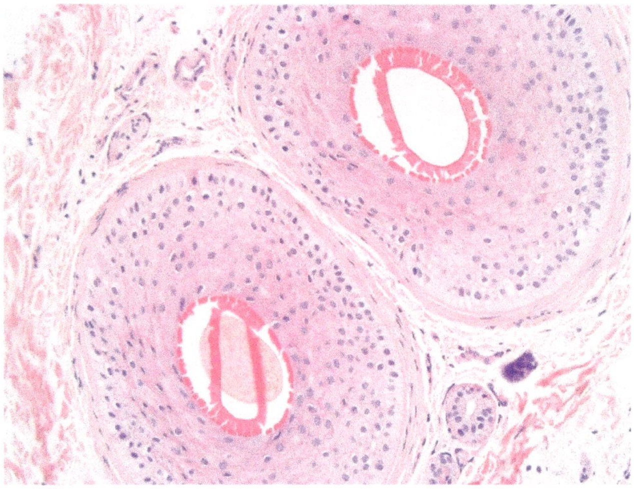

FIG. 8.116

Loose anagen hair syndrome (LAHS), transverse section. While not strictly necessary to diagnose LAHS, the inner root sheath of these follicles shows fracturing at the level of the isthmus (Hematoxylin & eosin, ×200).

Helpful Differentiating Features

HISTOLOGIC

Hair shaft fragility typically manifests as breakage after emergence of the shaft from the follicular ostium. Under these circumstances, the biopsy will likely appear normal. Examination of the hair shafts may reveal features that suggest the underlying disorder.

LAHS, best diagnosed by microscopic examination of an extracted anagen shaft, exhibits the classic pattern of the so-called fallen sock sign (Fig. 8.115). On histological examination of a tissue biopsy, subtle fracturing of the inner and/or ORS may be seen (Fig. 8.116).

Cases of acute TE may display a normal biopsy pattern as new anagen hairs dislodge the preceding telogen club hairs. The catagen:telogen count may appear lower than 10%.

CLINICAL

The clinical history is crucial in making sense of a histologically normal biopsy. If the clinician sees overt alopecia, the pattern of involvement should be elicited. Photography may prove useful. If no evident alopecia is seen by the clinician, yet the patient complains of loss, careful questioning for triggers of TE should be undertaken. Depending on the history, lab testing may be required. If hair breakage is observed or easy hair extraction is noted upon gentle traction, samples of affected shafts should be submitted for microscopic analysis.

NONCONFORMING PATTERNS

As with any attempts to systematize biological processes, there are always nonconformists.

Four possible explanations for findings that do not fit the above stereotypical patterns

(1) **Secondary and rare alopecias.** As noted earlier in this chapter, the preceding algorithmic approach covers nearly all alopecic conditions encountered in a typical dermatopathology practice. Secondary alopecias caused by neoplasms and other non-follicle-targeted inflammatory conditions are not covered here. Extremely rare conditions are also not included.

(2) **Clinical-pathological mismatches**. The mismatch of clinical history and histopathological findings should serve as an alert for a possible "mixed" alopecia. One common scenario is a patient presenting with rapid development of stereotypical AGA. The histopathological finding of follicular miniaturization confirms the diagnosis of AGA; however, the clinical history of rapid development precludes AGA as the sole cause. In this case, one should suspect AGA with superimposed acute TE. A telogen count of less than 10% may be the only histological finding to support the hypothesis, and if the sample is small, subtle changes in cycling may be difficult to detect.

(3) **Pathology mismatches.** Another trigger for possible "mixed" alopecias is the overlap of two or more of the patterns discussed in the preceding pages. If peribulbar lymphocytes are present along with distortion of follicular epithelia and intrafollicular hemorrhage, the common denominator among the patterns may be AA and concurrent TT. If collapsed sebaceous lobules are noted and background changes compatible with AGA are seen, consider a pattern 6 biphasic alopecia combined with a pattern 9 alopecia. In general, the simplest explanation is best, and careful consideration of the clinical presentation should prove helpful.

(4) **New and emerging alopecias**. The number of new biologic medications entering the market is stunning. In any setting in which alopecia does not conform to the patterns denoted above, inquiry about new medications may be informative.

ACKNOWLEDGMENTS

The authors and editors wish to thank Drs. Klaus Sellheyer and Wilma F Bergfeld who wrote the chapter on "non-neoplastic disorders of hair" of the two prior editions of this textbook. Some of the images that were contributed by them were retained in this new alopecia chapter.

SUGGESTED FURTHER READING

Banka, N., Bunagan, M. J., & Shapiro, J. (2013). Pattern hair loss in men: diagnosis and medical treatment. *Dermatologic Clinics*, *31*(1), 129–140. doi:10.1016/j.det.2012.08.003.

Bernárdez, C., Molina-Ruiz, A. M., & Requena, L. (2015). Histologic features of alopecias: Part II: Scarring alopecias. *Actas Dermo-Sifiliograficas*, *106*(4), 260–270. English, Spanish. doi:10.1016/j.ad.2014.06.016.

Bernárdez, C., Molina-Ruiz, A. M., & Requena, L. (2015). Histologic features of alopecias-part I: Nonscarring alopecias. *Actas Dermo-Sifiliograficas*, *106*(3), 158–167. English, Spanish. doi:10.1016/j.ad.2014.07.006.

Bolduc, C., Sperling, L. C., & Shapiro, J. (2016). Primary cicatricial alopecia: Other lymphocytic primary cicatricial alopecias and neutrophilic and mixed primary cicatricial alopecias. *Journal of the American Academy of Dermatology*, *75*(6), 1101–1117. doi:10.1016/j.jaad.2015.01.056.

Chanprapaph, K., Udompanich, S., Visessiri, Y., Ngamjanyaporn, P., & Suchonwanit, P. (2019). Nonscarring alopecia in systemic lupus erythematosus: A cross-sectional study with trichoscopic, histopathologic, and immunopathologic analyses. *Journal of the American Academy of Dermatology*, *81*(6), 1319–1329. doi:10.1016/j.jaad.2019.05.053.

Childs, J. M., & Sperling, L. C. (2013). Histopathology of scarring and nonscarring hair loss. *Dermatologic Clinics*, *31*(1), 43–56. doi:10.1016/j.det.2012.08.001.

Concha, J. S. S., & Werth, V. P. (2018). Alopecias in lupus erythematosus. *Lupus Science & Medicine*, *5*(1), e000291. doi:10.1136/lupus-2018-000291.

Doyle, L. A., Sperling, L. C., Baksh, S., Lackey, J., Thomas, B., Vleugels, R. A., Qureshi, A. A., & Velazquez, E. F. (2011). Psoriatic alopecia/alopecia areata-like reactions secondary to anti-tumor necrosis factor-α therapy: A novel cause of noncicatricial alopecia. *American Journal of Dermatopathology*, *33*(2), 161–166. doi:10.1097/DAD.0b013e3181ef7403.

Doytcheva, K., Tan, T., Guitart, J., Gerami, P., & Yazdan, P. (2018). Naked hair shafts as a marker of cicatricial alopecia. *American Journal of Dermatopathology*, *40*(7), 498–501. doi:10.1097/DAD.0000000000001075.

Elston, C. A., Kazlouskaya, V., & Elston, D. M. (2013). Elastic staining versus fluorescent and polarized microscopy in the diagnosis of alopecia. *Journal of the American Academy of Dermatology*, *69*(2), 288–293. doi:10.1016/j.jaad.2013.02.030.

Fung, M. A., Sharon, V. R., Ratnarathorn, M., Konia, T. H., Barr, K. L., & Mirmirani, P. (2013). Elastin staining patterns in primary cicatricial alopecia. *Journal of the American Academy of Dermatology*, *69*(5), 776–782. doi:10.1016/j.jaad.2013.07.018.

Gálvez-Canseco, A., & Sperling, L. (2018). Lichen planopilaris and frontal fibrosing alopecia cannot be differentiated by histopathology. *Journal of Cutaneous Pathology*, *45*(5), 313–317. doi:10.1111/cup.13112.

George, S. M., Taylor, M. R., & Farrant, P. B. (2015). Psoriatic alopecia. *Clinical and Experimental Dermatology*, *40*(7), 717–721. doi:10.1111/ced.12715.

Halley-Stott, R. P., Adeola, H. A., & Khumalo, N. P. (2020). Destruction of the stem cell Niche, Pathogenesis and Promising Treatment Targets for Primary Scarring Alopecias. *Stem Cell Reviews and Reports*, *16*(6), 1105–1120. doi:10.1007/s12015-020-09985-6.

Lee, C. N., Chen, W., Hsu, C. K., Weng, T. T., Lee, J. Y., & Yang, C. C. (2018). Dissecting folliculitis (dissecting cellulitis) of the scalp: A 66-patient case series and proposal of classification. *Journal der Deutschen Dermatologischen Gesellschaft*, 16(10), 1219–1226. doi:10.1111/ddg.13649.

Mirmirani, P., Uno, H., & Price, V. H. (2011). Abnormal inner root sheath of the hair follicle in the loose anagen hair syndrome: an ultrastructural study. *Journal of the American Academy of Dermatology*, 64(1), 129–134. doi:10.1016/j.jaad.2010.01.026.

Miteva, M., Romanelli, P., & Tosti, A. (2014). Pigmented casts. *American Journal of Dermatopathology*, 36(1), 58–63. doi:10.1097/DAD.0b013e3182919ac7.

Miteva, M., Torres, F., & Tosti, A. (2012). The "eyes" or "goggles" as a clue to the histopathological diagnosis of primary lymphocytic cicatricial alopecia. *British Journal of Dermatology*, 166(2), 454–455. doi:10.1111/j.1365-2133.2011.10578.x.

Nanda, S., De Bedout, V., & Miteva, M. (2019). Alopecia as a systemic disease. *Clinics in Dermatology*, 37(6), 618–628. doi:10.1016/j.clindermatol.2019.07.026.

Pratt, C. H., King, L. E., Jr, Messenger, A. G., Christiano, A. M., & Sundberg, J. P. (2017). Alopecia areata. *Nature Reviews Disease Primers*, 3, 17011. doi:10.1038/nrdp.2017.11.

Rebora, A. (2019). Telogen effluvium: A comprehensive review. *Clinical, Cosmetic and Investigational Dermatology*, 12, 583–590. doi:10.2147/CCID.S200471.

Siah, T. W., & Sperling, L. (2014). The histopathologic diagnosis of postoperative alopecia. *Journal of Cutaneous Pathology*, 41(9), 699–702. doi:10.1111/cup.12381.

Sperling, L. C., Knopp, E. A., & Cowper, S. E. (2012). *An atlas of hair pathology with clinical correlations* (2nd ed.). Boca Raton, FL: Informa Healthcare; CRC Press, Taylor & Francis.

Tan, T., Guitart, J., Gerami, P., & Yazdan, P. (2017). Eccrine duct dilation as a marker of cicatricial alopecia. *American Journal of Dermatopathology*, 39(9), 668–671. doi:10.1097/DAD.0000000000000747.

Cysts and Sinuses

9

Scott C. Bresler • Douglas R. Fullen

A cyst is a dilated, sac-like cavity lined by various types of epithelia. In most cases, cutaneous cysts are lined by one type of epithelium, most commonly stratified squamous epithelium. Infrequently, cutaneous cysts may have significant portions of more than one type of epithelium and have been given the appellation of "hybrid cysts." A pseudocyst, on the other hand, is a cystic cavity that lacks an epithelial lining.

The most common types of cutaneous cysts arise from adnexal structures (Fig. 9.1). In fact, follicular cysts arising from the infundibular (epidermoid cysts) or isthmus portions (trichilemmal cysts) of hair follicles account for the vast majority of cutaneous cysts. Rarely, cysts are developmental in nature and arise from sequestered tissue that has failed to migrate completely during embryogenesis. The common follicular cysts are lined by stratified squamous epithelium. In contrast, cysts derived from eccrine or apocrine ducts or glands have a double layer of cuboidal to columnar epithelium. Developmental cysts have more variability in the types of epithelia that constitute their cyst linings. It is not unusual to find either pseudostratified columnar and/or stratified squamous epithelium in the lining of branchial cleft or bronchogenic cysts. Hence, cysts can be classified based on the appendageal structure of origin, the type of epithelial lining in the cyst wall, or whether the cyst is or is not developmental in origin (Box 9.1).

The gross appearance of cysts is not specific and can overlap with some malignant cystic tumors of the skin,

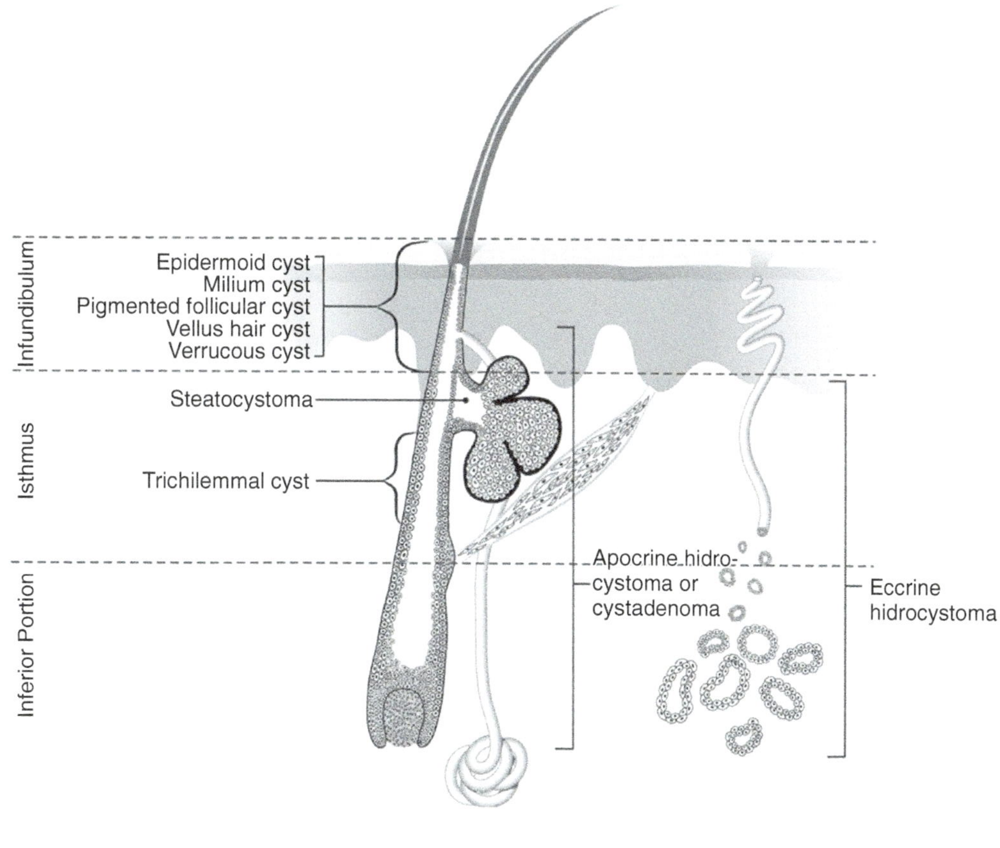

FIG. 9.1

Cysts derived from appendageal structures: schematic showing the origin of some cysts from various appendageal structures.

BOX 9.1

Classification of Cutaneous Cysts

Cysts Arising From Appendageal Structures

Infundibulum of terminal hair follicles—stratified squamous epithelium with an inner granular layer

- Epidermoid (infundibular type) cyst
- Proliferating epithelial (epidermoid) cyst
- Verrucous cyst
- Pigmented follicular cyst

Isthmus of terminal hair follicles—stratified squamous epithelium without an inner granular layer

- Trichilemmal (isthmus-catagen type) cyst
- Proliferating trichilemmal cystic tumor[a]
- Verrucous cyst (occasionally trichilemmal differentiation)

Infundibulum of vellus hair follicles—stratified squamous epithelium with a granular layer

- Milium
- Vellus hair cysts (solitary and eruptive variants)

Sebaceous duct—stratified squamous epithelium with an inner cuticular lining

- Steatocystoma (simplex and multiplex)

Eccrine duct/gland—cuboidal lining without apical snouting

- Eccrine hidrocystoma

Apocrine duct/gland—cuboidal lining with apical snouting

- Apocrine hidrocystoma/cystadenoma[a]

Multiple sites of origin

- Hybrid cyst

Cysts of Developmental Origin

Cysts lined by stratified squamous epithelium

- Dermoid cyst

Cysts lined by squamous and nonsquamous (columnar ciliated, pseudostratified columnar, or cuboidal) epithelium

- Branchial cleft cyst (predominantly stratified squamous or pseudostratified columnar ciliated)
- Bronchogenic cyst (predominantly pseudostratified columnar ciliated)

Thyroglossal duct cyst (predominantly stratified squamous)

- Thymic cyst (predominantly stratified squamous or pseudostratified columnar ciliated or columnar)
- Cutaneous ciliated cyst (predominantly columnar ciliated or cuboidal)
- Ciliated mucinous cyst of the vulva (predominantly simple columnar ciliated)
- Median raphe cyst (predominantly stratified or pseudostratified columnar)
- Omphalomesenteric duct cyst (gastric or intestinal columnar)

Cysts lacking a lining epithelium

- Pseudocyst of the auricle
- Digital mucous cyst
- Ganglion cyst
- Mucocele/mucous cyst of the oral cavity (most cases)
- Metaplastic synovial cyst

[a]Proliferating pilary cystic tumor and apocrine cystadenoma are discussed here for historic reasons and for the differential diagnosis, but they are cystic neoplasms.

as well as noncystic lesions. For this reason, excised cysts should be submitted for routine histology to render a definitive diagnosis and completely exclude malignant cystic tumors, such as cystic squamous cell carcinomas or nodulocystic basal cell carcinomas. Once a histologic diagnosis of a benign cyst is made, no further treatment is necessary except for cosmetic reasons or because of irritation from rupture or superinfection.

A sinus is a deep invagination or tract lined by epithelium or granulation tissue. As such, sinuses may be developmental in origin or arise secondary to an exuberant inflammatory reaction. The majority of sinus tracts encountered by dermatopathologists belong to the latter group. Sinus tracts are significant because of their propensity for recurrent infection and risk for malignancy arising secondary to long-standing chronic inflammation.

CYSTS DERIVED FROM APPENDAGEAL STRUCTURES

CYSTS ARISING FROM THE INFUNDIBULAR PORTION OF THE HAIR FOLLICLE

Cysts arising from the infundibular portion of terminal or vellus hair follicles have an epidermoid mode of keratinization and, therefore, keratinize through a granular layer like the epidermis. Epidermoid (infundibular) cysts, most verrucous cysts, and pigmented follicular cysts are types of cysts that originate from the follicular infundibulum of terminal hairs. Vellus hair cysts and most milia are derived from the infundibulum of vellus hair follicles.

EPIDERMOID (INFUNDIBULAR) CYSTS

Clinical Features

Epidermoid cysts are the most common cutaneous cysts, accounting for approximately 80% of all cutaneous cysts. These cysts arise in the dermis of hair-bearing skin, with a predilection for the head, neck, and trunk. Epidermoid cysts are usually solitary, slowly growing, and are typically 1 to 5 cm in diameter. A punctum, corresponding to the opening of the cyst to the skin surface, is often seen. Epidermoid cysts may be erythematous and tender, if ruptured or infected. Rarely, multiple epidermoid cysts are seen as a manifestation of Gardner syndrome or the basal cell nevus (Gorlin) syndrome. Treatment with BRAF inhibitors has also been associated with the development of epidermoid cysts in patients treated for advanced-stage malignant neoplasms, such as melanoma.

Epidermal inclusion cysts resemble epidermoid cysts but arise as a result of traumatic implantation of the epidermis, such as on the palms and soles, or on the vulva, where they may develop secondary to injuries during delivery or from ritual cutting.

Pathologic Features

Epidermoid cysts may show a connection to the surface epidermis. The cysts are lined by stratified squamous epithelium possessing an inner granular layer composed of keratinocytes containing keratohyaline granules (Fig. 9.2). The orthokeratin that fills the cyst cavity has a loose and laminated appearance. Occasionally, a few terminal hair shafts are present in the lumen. No adnexal structures are seen in the cyst walls.

Epidermoid cysts are prone to rupture, resulting in varying degrees of inflammation and scarring. When infected cysts rupture, a prominent mixed suppurative and foreign body granulomatous inflammatory response is elicited. Older lesions tend to have fewer neutrophils and more lymphocytes and plasma cells. In the absence of infection, a foreign body granulomatous reaction, composed of multinucleated foreign body giant cells and thin flakes of anucleate keratin, dominates the host response to ruptured epidermoid cysts (Fig. 9.3). The cyst lining may be obliterated by the inflammatory and scarring host response.

Secondary changes that may rarely be seen in epidermoid cysts include basal layer hyperpigmentation in dark-skinned individuals, acantholytic dyskeratosis, or epidermolytic hyperkeratosis (Fig. 9.4). Some epidermoid cysts have other types of epithelia, such as steatocystoma, trichilemmal cyst, or pilomatricoma, and are classified as follicular hybrid cysts (see below). Trichoblastic proliferations of follicular germinative epithelium may rarely be seen protruding from the lining of epidermoid cysts and must be distinguished from basal cell carcinoma arising in a cyst. Such lesions have been termed trichoblastic infundibular cysts or cystic trichoblastomas. Seborrheic keratosis-like proliferations emanating from the walls of infundibular cysts have also been described.

Differential Diagnosis

Milia are smaller (1 to 2 mm in diameter) than epidermoid cysts and arise in the superficial dermis. Pigmented follicular cysts have multiple pigmented hair shafts within their cyst cavities and rete ridges extending peripherally into the dermis from the lining epithelium, which are features not typical of epidermoid cysts. Trichilemmal cysts are readily distinguished from epidermoid cysts because of prominent eosinophilic keratinocytes in their cyst walls, absence of a granular layer, and dense eosinophilic orthokeratin filling the cyst cavity. Dermoid cysts

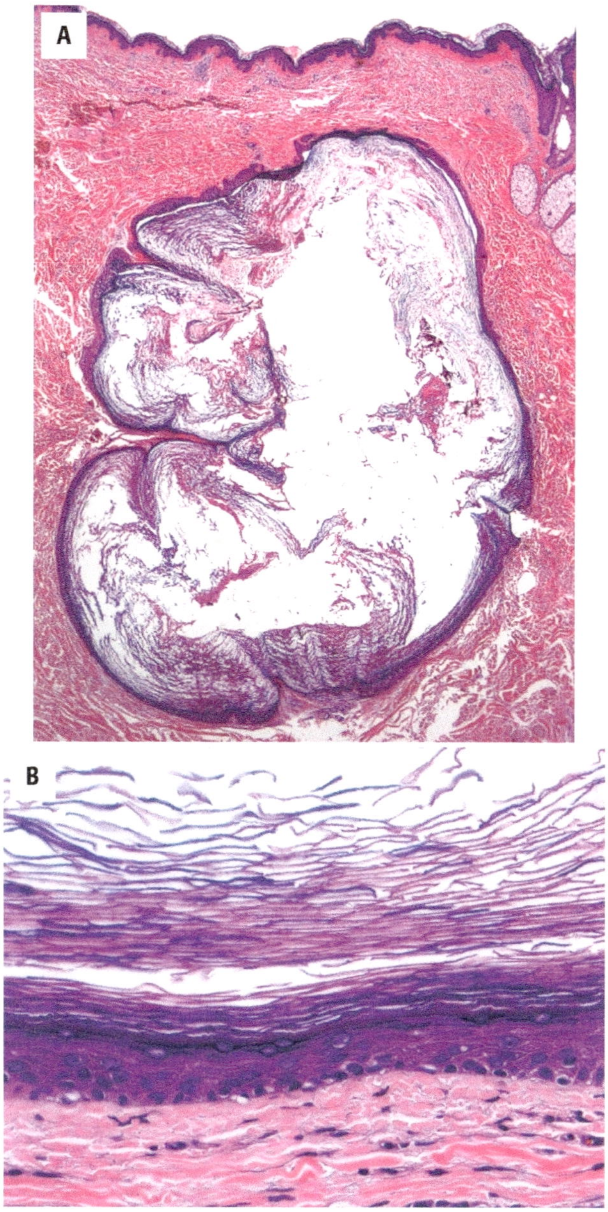

FIG. 9.2

Epidermoid cyst: microscopic features. **A**, Epidermoid cysts are located in the dermis and contain laminated keratin. **B**, The cyst lining has an inner granular layer composed of keratinocytes with keratohyaline granules.

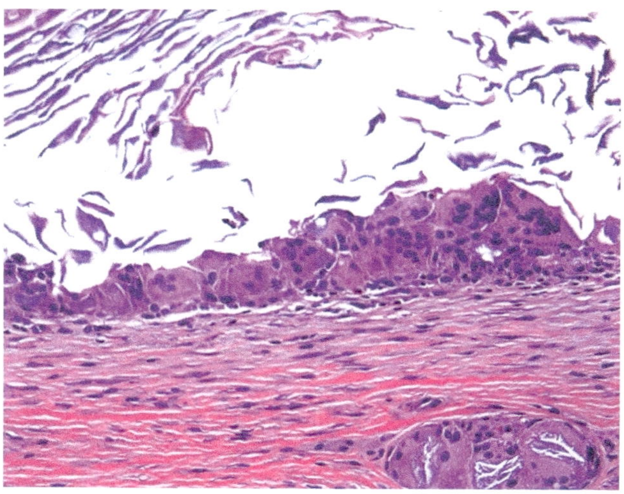

FIG. 9.3

Epidermoid cyst: microscopic features. A ruptured epidermoid cyst results in a foreign body giant cell reaction to extravasated keratin.

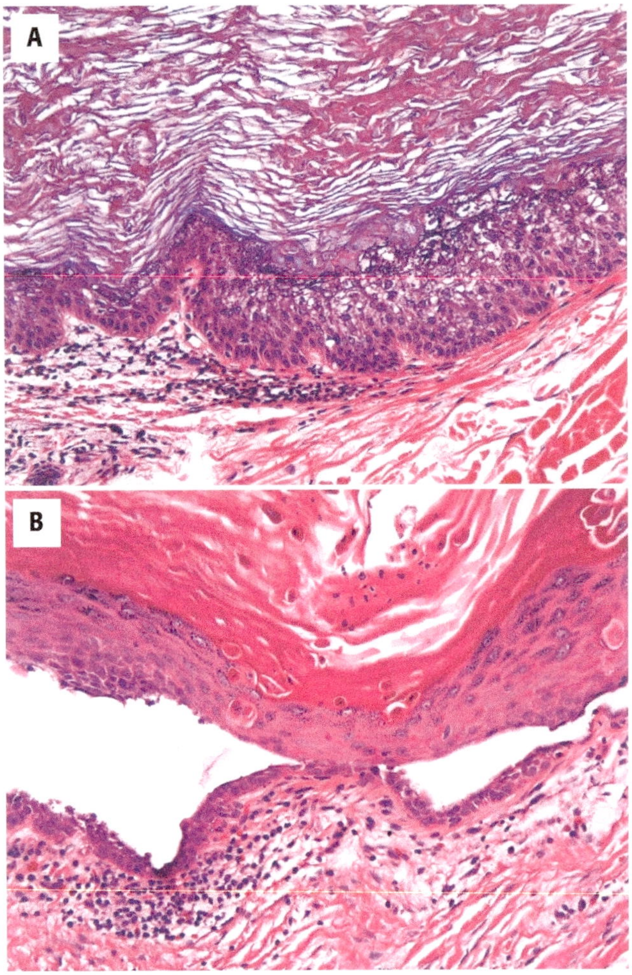

FIG. 9.4

Epidermoid cyst: unusual microscopic features. In rare instances, epidermoid cysts may have unusual secondary changes involving their cyst lining. **A**, Epidermolytic hyperkeratosis. **B**, Acantholytic dyskeratosis.

show an identical cyst lining and mode of keratinization to epidermoid cysts but differ by possessing adnexal structures within the cyst wall and several hair shafts in the cyst cavity. On rare occasions, carcinoma may arise in association with cysts. Some squamous cell carcinomas mimic a cyst in their superficial portion.

PROLIFERATING EPITHELIAL (EPIDERMOID) CYSTS

Clinical Features

Proliferating epithelial cysts is a term coined to encompass both proliferating epidermoid and trichilemmal cysts, the latter of which are discussed separately below. Proliferating epidermoid cysts arise from preexisting epidermoid cysts, akin to proliferating trichilemmal cysts that arise from trichilemmal cysts. In contrast to proliferating trichilemmal cysts, which have a strong predilection for the scalp, the majority (approximately 80%) of proliferating epidermoid cysts do not involve the scalp but rather are widely distributed, involving primarily the pelvic and anogenital regions, trunk, and upper extremities. Most tumors are well circumscribed and range from less than 1 cm to more than 10 cm in size. They are solid, solid and cystic, or cystic. The lesions occur in adults, and males are affected almost twice as often as females.

Pathologic Features

Most lesions show, at least focally, a cyst lining that keratinizes like the infundibulum of the hair follicle. The cyst epithelium shows varying degrees of acanthosis, papillomatosis, hypergranulosis, parakeratosis, and hyperkeratosis. A multilocular cyst may be seen in some cases. More solid areas of proliferating epithelium tend to radiate peripherally into the surrounding dermis and are composed of keratinocytes with abundant eosinophilic cytoplasm and sharp cytoplasmic borders. When keratinization is noted in the more solid lobules, keratinocytes with keratohyaline granules form a variably thick granular layer that separates the loose laminated keratin within the cyst lumen from the remainder of the stratified squamous epithelium (Fig. 9.5). Squamous eddies are commonly found. A foreign body giant cell reaction to extravasated keratin may be present. No cytologic atypia of keratinocytes or infiltrative peripheral growth patterns are seen.

Differential Diagnosis

Proliferating epidermoid cysts need to be distinguished from well-differentiated squamous cell carcinomas arising in an epidermoid cyst or growing in a cystic pattern thereby mimicking a proliferating cyst. Carcinoma is diagnosed by the presence of cytologic atypia or an infiltrative growth pattern at the periphery of the cystic lesion. Proliferating trichilemmal cysts differ from proliferating epidermoid cysts by the mode of keratinization, being trichilemmal in the former and epidermoid in the latter.

HUMAN PAPILLOMAVIRUS–RELATED FOLLICULAR CYSTS

Clinical Features

Human papillomavirus (HPV)–related follicular cysts encompass two groups of cutaneous lesions, verrucous

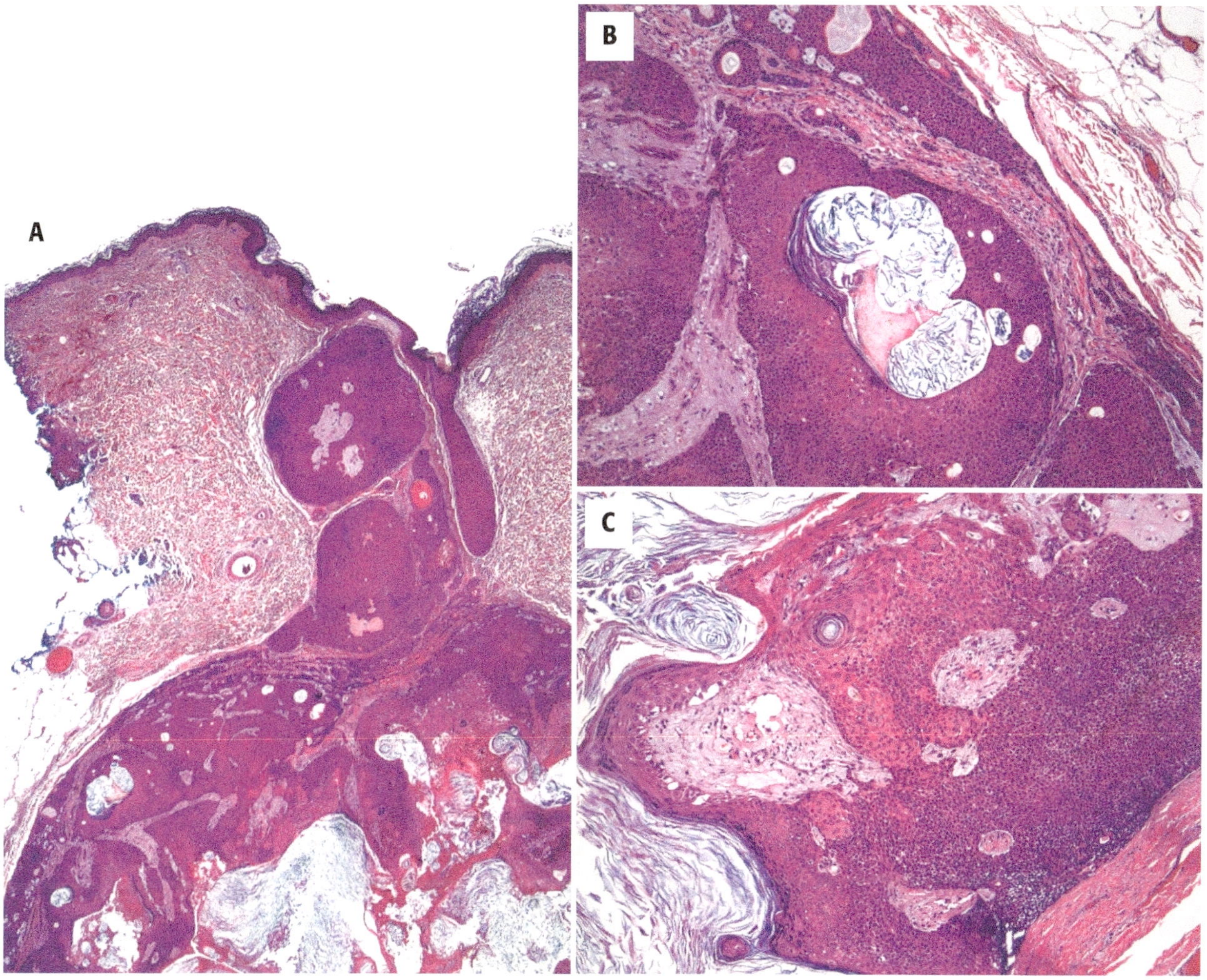

FIG. 9.5

Proliferating epidermoid cyst: microscopic features. **A**, A proliferating epidermoid cyst has cellular lobules of squamous cells that radiate peripherally from a central cyst but the periphery of the lesion is well circumscribed. **B**, Infundibular (epidermoid) keratinization occurs where cysts are formed. **C**, Small balls of keratinocytes (squamous eddies) are often seen in the cellular areas of the lesion.

cysts and HPV-infected palmar and plantar epidermal cysts. Verrucous cysts are rare epidermal cysts that are defined histologically by verrucous changes of their stratified squamous linings. These cysts have a predilection for the face, neck, trunk, and extremities of adults. Often the cysts appear inflamed.

Pathologic Features

Verrucous cysts are lined by stratified squamous epithelium with verrucous features (papillomatous hyperplasia, hypergranulosis with large basophilic keratohyaline granules, tiers of parakeratosis overlying papillomatous processes, and HPV-cytopathic changes) (Fig. 9.6). Whorls of squamous cells, or squamous eddies, are quite common.

Differential Diagnosis

Verrucous cysts differ from epidermoid cysts by having papillomatous hyperplasia and viropathic changes. Although verrucous cysts can have trichilemmal differentiation and thereby resemble trichilemmal cysts, verrucous cysts have papillomatosis and large, basophilic keratohyaline granules.

PIGMENTED FOLLICULAR CYSTS

Clinical Features

Pigmented follicular cysts are rare and present as solitary papules or nodules. They have a predilection for the

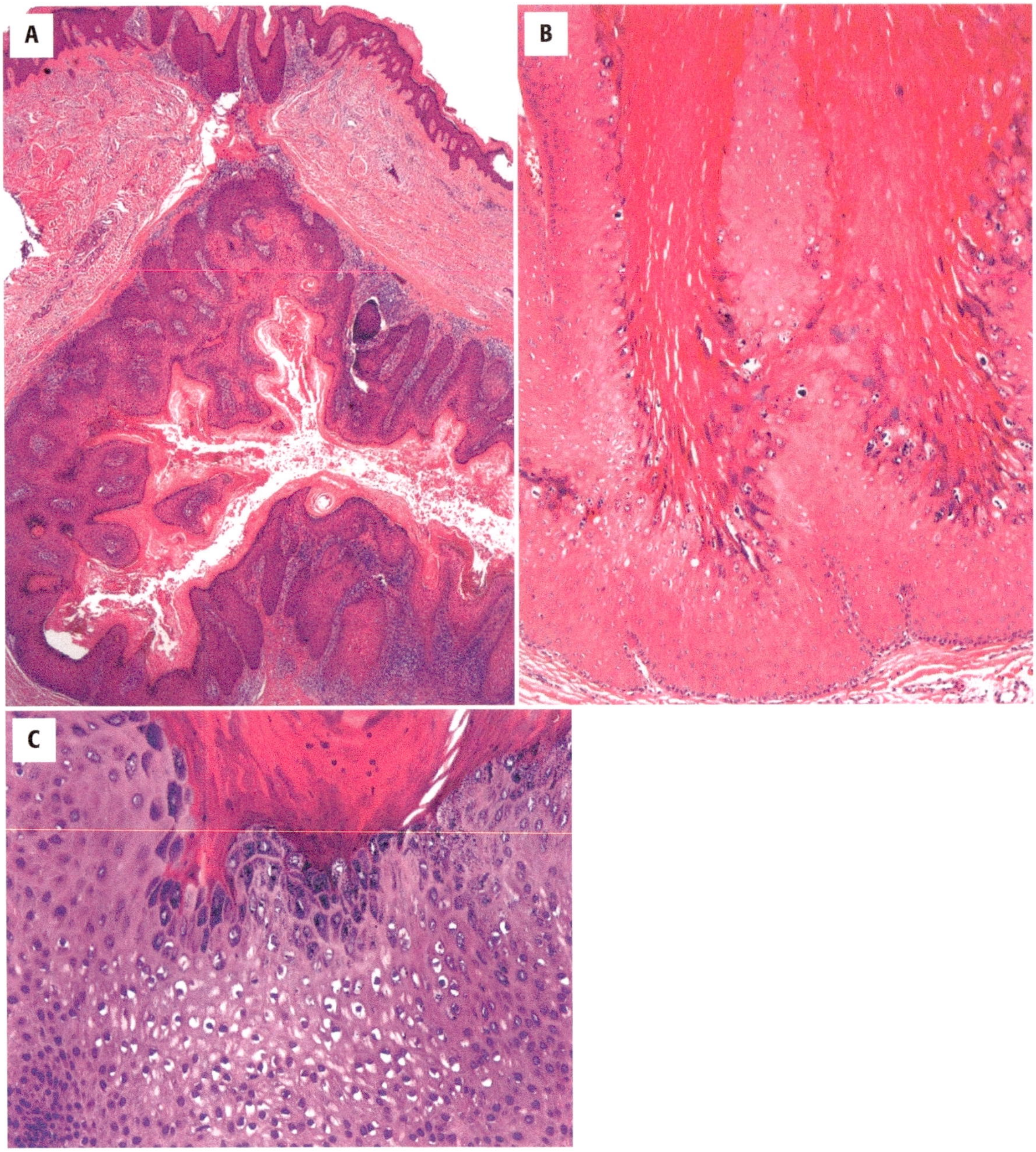

FIG. 9.6

Human papillomavirus (HPV)–related follicular cyst: microscopic features. **A**, Verrucous cysts are characterized by varying degrees of papillomatosis, acanthosis, and hypergranulosis. Most verrucous cysts have infundibular (epidermoid) keratinization. **B**, Occasionally, verrucous cysts can show trichilemmal keratinization. **C**, Viropathic changes of HPV are present in this HPV-infected plantar epidermal cyst.

head and neck of adults but can also arise on the trunk and rarely on the extremities. Males are more commonly affected than females. As a result of their dark brown or blue hue, the clinical differential diagnoses include hidrocystoma, melanocytic lesions such as blue nevus, dermatofibroma, or pigmented basal cell carcinoma.

Pathologic Features

Pigmented follicular cysts often connect via a small pore to the surface epidermis. They are lined by stratified squamous epithelium, often with a retained rete ridge pattern, that keratinizes through a granular layer. The keratin is loose and laminated. Essential to the diagnosis is observing several terminal-sized hair shafts within the cyst cavity. The pigmented hair shafts contain abundant melanin pigment (Fig. 9.7). Sebaceous lobules are not seen in the cyst wall.

Differential Diagnosis

Epidermoid (infundibular) cysts differ from pigmented follicular cysts by lacking both a rete ridge pattern in the

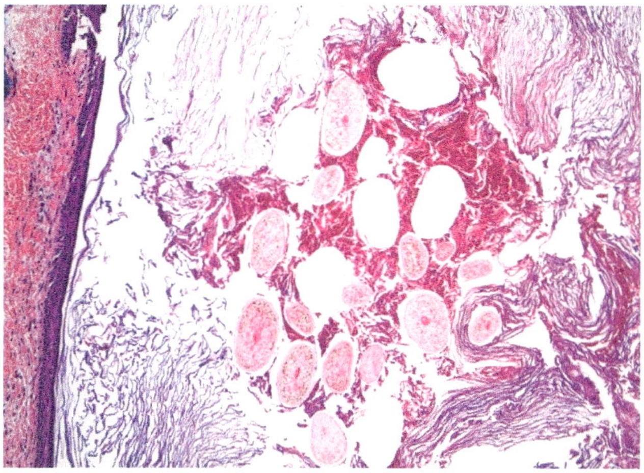

FIG. 9.7

Pigmented follicular cyst: microscopic features. Multiple, large-diameter, terminal hair shafts with medullary pigment and laminated keratin fill the cyst lumen.

cyst wall and multiple, pigmented hair shafts in the cyst cavity. Although eruptive vellus hair cysts have multiple hair shafts in the cyst cavity like pigmented follicular cysts, the hair shafts are of vellus type, that is, they are small in diameter and lack pigmentation.

MILIA

Clinical Features

Milia are small, 1 to 2 mm, white to yellow papules that are superficially located in the dermis. Primary milia arise de novo from the infundibular region of vellus hair follicles and present as multiple papules on the face. Infants and adults are primarily affected. Secondary milia result from scarring of the dermis caused by trauma, burns, an underlying subepidermal blistering disorder such as epidermolysis bullosa, cicatricial pemphigoid, or porphyria cutanea tarda, or following dermabrasion. Secondary milia may arise from a variety of adnexal structures, such as the infundibulum of vellus hair follicles, eccrine ducts, or implantation of the epidermis. They have a widespread distribution, occurring at sites exposed to trauma, burns, or scarring procedures, and can occur at any age. Very rarely, milia are seen in the Nicolau-Balus syndrome (milia, eruptive syringomas, and atrophoderma vermiculata) or in conjunction with trichoepitheliomas and cylindromas. Milia have also been reported in patients receiving BRAF inhibitor therapy.

Pathologic Features

Primary milia are small, thin-walled cysts in the papillary to upper reticular dermis. The cysts are lined by a thin layer of stratified squamous epithelium that keratinizes through a granular layer in an epidermoid mode (Fig. 9.8). Orthokeratin within the cyst cavities is loose and laminated. Milia lack multiple vellus hair shafts in their cyst cavities. These milia may be seen in continuity with the vellus hair follicles from which they arose in serial sections. Multiple levels may be necessary if a milium is suspected but not seen on the initial levels.

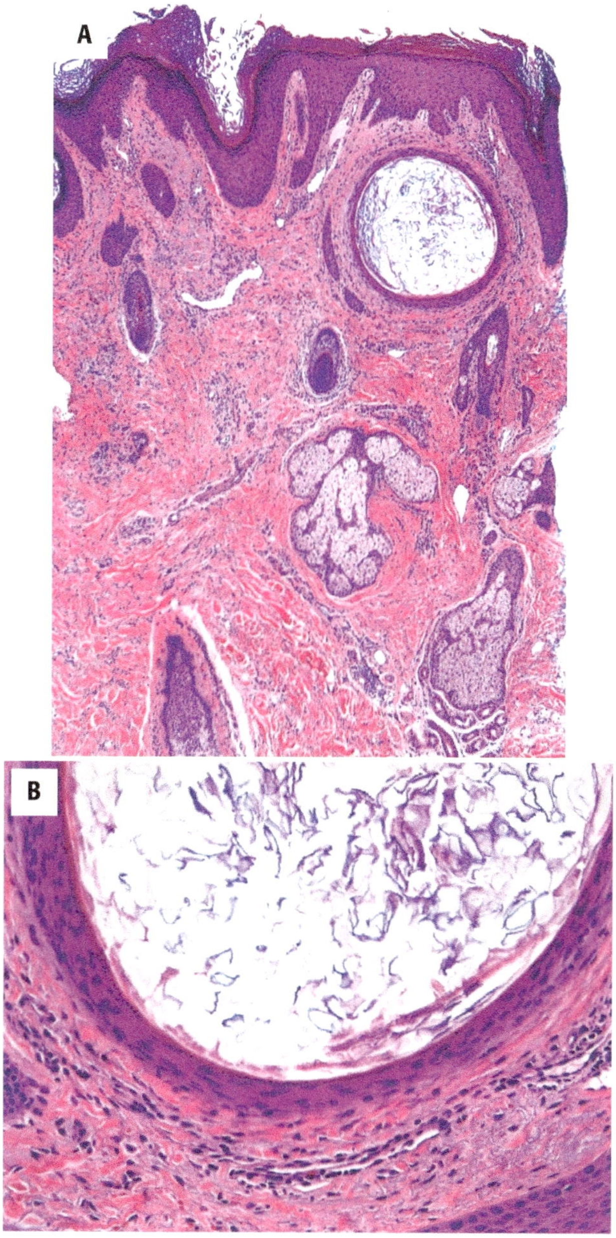

FIG. 9.8

Milium: microscopic features. **A,** A small cyst is located in the superficial dermis. **B,** The epithelial lining has a thin inner granular layer forming laminated keratin and is histologically indistinguishable from an epidermoid cyst.

Secondary milia have many of the same histopathological features as primary milia. In some cases, continuity with an underlying eccrine duct may be seen in serial

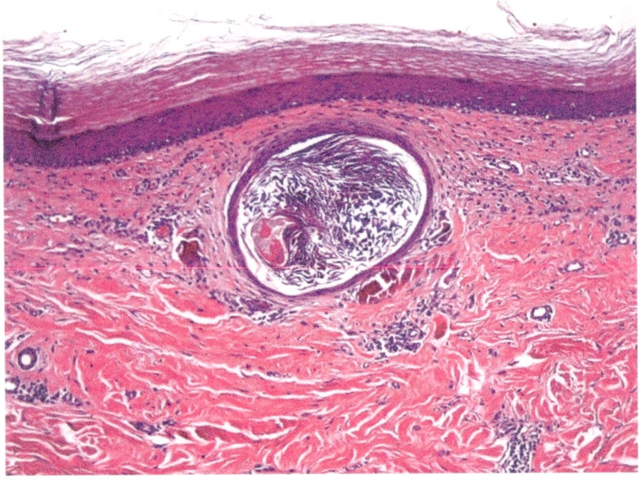

FIG. 9.9
Secondary milium: microscopic features. Milia may result from scarring processes, as in this example of a milium developing at a previous biopsy site.

sections. Scar in the dermis surrounding secondary milia is a typical feature (Fig. 9.9).

Differential Diagnosis

Epidermoid cysts are histopathologically indistinguishable from milia but are larger and more deeply seated in the dermis and subcutis. Vellus hair cysts, in contrast to milia, have multiple cross-sections of vellus hair shafts within their cyst lumens.

VELLUS HAIR CYSTS

Clinical Features

Vellus hair cysts may occur as sporadic, solitary lesions on a nonhereditary basis. More commonly, multiple, "eruptive" vellus hair cysts occur and in some cases are inherited in an autosomal dominant manner. The lesions develop abruptly as small, red, tan, brown, or black 1- to 4-mm papules. Central umbilication may be seen. Vellus hair cysts have a predilection for the trunk, especially the chest, abdomen, and extremities, but also can be found on the neck, face, and groin. Vellus hair cysts usually arise in the first four decades of life. The onset of familial cases is typically at an earlier age than sporadic cases, with most cases manifesting at birth or in early infancy.

Rarely, eruptive vellus hair cysts have been associated with steatocystoma multiplex, as a type of hybrid cyst.

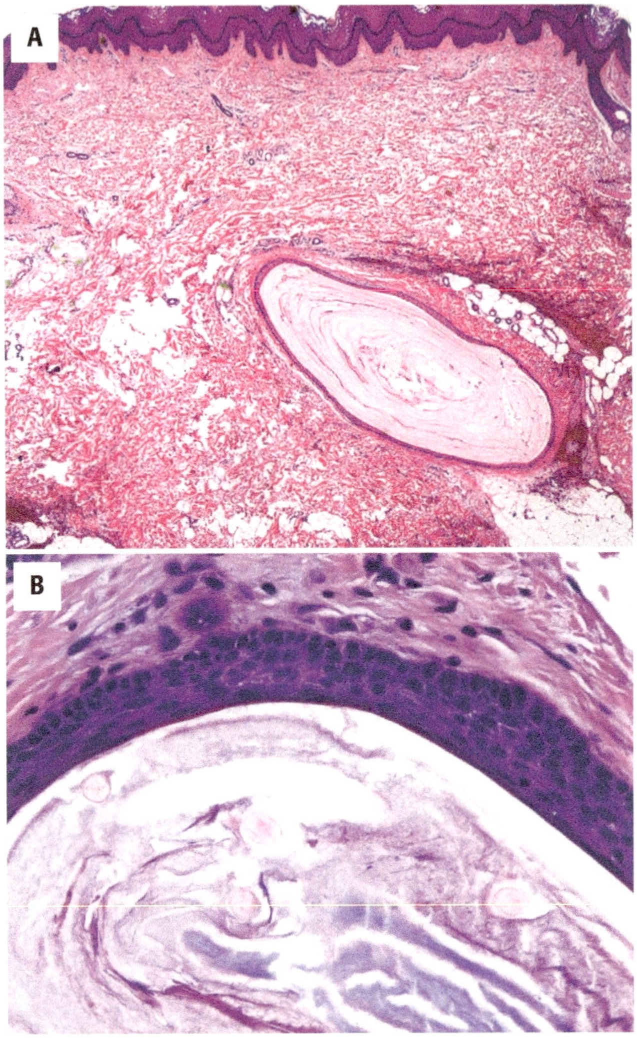

FIG. 9.10
Vellus hair cyst: microscopic features. **A**, Vellus hair cysts are located in the dermis. **B**, The cyst wall is composed of a thin layer of stratified squamous epithelium with an inner granular layer. Note the multiple, small-diameter vellus hair shafts and keratin within the cyst cavity.

A rare association exists between eruptive vellus hair cysts and pachyonychia congenita.

Pathologic Features

Vellus hair cysts present as small cysts in the upper to mid-dermis. A thin layer of stratified squamous epithelium possessing an inner granular layer forms the cyst lining. Orthokeratin within the cyst cavity has a loose and laminated appearance. Multiple vellus hairs, characterized by small caliber hair shafts that generally lack pigment, are admixed with the keratin within the lumen of the cyst (Fig. 9.10). Occasionally, telogen hair follicles, sebaceous lobules, and/or small slips of arrector pili muscle may be seen in the cyst wall.

Differential Diagnosis

Epidermoid cysts and milia show many features similar to vellus hair cysts but lack multiple, vellus-type hair shafts. Pigmented follicular cysts also share many similar features with vellus hair cysts but have terminal size hairs that contain pigment within the medullary portion of the shafts in their cyst lumens. Features that aid in distinguishing steatocystomas from vellus hair cysts are the presence of sebaceous lobules in the cyst wall of most cases and an undulating, eosinophilic inner lining in the former.

CYSTS ARISING FROM THE ISTHMUS PORTION OF THE HAIR FOLLICLE

Cysts arising from the isthmus portion of the hair follicle have a trichilemmal mode of keratinization. In this type of keratinization, large, eosinophilic keratinocytes in the inner layer of the cyst lining give rise to compact eosinophilic keratin without an intervening granular layer. Therefore this mode of keratinization resembles that seen in the outer root sheath of hair follicles or the sac around catagen follicles. Thus these cysts have been referred to as trichilemmal cysts, isthmus-catagen type of follicular cysts, or pilar cysts. Sebaceous cyst is an antiquated term that is best avoided.

TRICHILEMMAL (ISTHMUS-CATAGEN OR PILAR) CYSTS

Clinical Features

After epidermoid cysts, trichilemmal cysts are the second most common cutaneous cysts, accounting for approximately 10% to 15% of cysts in the skin. Approximately 90% of trichilemmal cysts occur on the scalp. These cysts arise in adulthood and women are more commonly affected than men. An autosomal dominant pattern of inheritance is common. The cysts are smooth, firm nodules, ranging from less than 1 cm to more than 5.0 cm in diameter. It is more common for an individual to have multiple trichilemmal cysts than a solitary cyst of the scalp. When trichilemmal cysts occur at sites other than the scalp, they are almost always solitary. Rarely, multiple trichilemmal cysts may occur as an organoid nevus distributed along the lines of Blaschko (trichilemmal cyst nevus or nevus trichilemmocysticus).

Pathologic Features

Trichilemmal cysts are lined by stratified squamous epithelium that generally lacks an inner granular layer, although it is not uncommon to find focal areas where keratinocytes possess occasional keratohyaline granules. Intercellular bridges between keratinocytes are absent within the epithelium of the cyst wall. One of the most characteristic features of trichilemmal cysts is the presence of an innermost layer of large keratinocytes with abundant eosinophilic cytoplasm that keratinizes abruptly. The orthokeratin that is produced is eosinophilic and densely packed. A common finding in trichilemmal cysts is palisading of the outermost layer of the epithelium, which tends to separate from the remainder of the cyst wall lining (Fig. 9.11). Adnexal structures are not observed in the cyst walls.

Trichilemmal cysts are prone to rupture, in which case a foreign body giant cell reaction is elicited in response to the extravasated keratin. Cholesterol clefts are usually admixed with the foreign body granulomatous reaction (Fig. 9.12). Calcifications occur in the cyst cavities of approximately 25% of cases. Occasionally, cysts may demonstrate areas of trichilemmal cyst and other areas of another type of cyst, such as an epidermoid cyst, resulting in follicular hybrid cysts.

Differential Diagnosis

Epidermoid cysts keratinize through a granular layer and produce loose and laminated keratin, in contrast to the absence of a granular layer and the presence of dense, eosinophilic keratin that occurs in trichilemmal cysts. The major histopathologic features that distinguish a proliferating trichilemmal cyst/tumor from a trichilemmal cyst are the presence of multiple, circumscribed squamous lobules, squamous eddies, some degree of nuclear atypia of squamous cells, and usually low mitotic activity in the former. Although the eosinophilic keratin of a pilomatricoma can resemble a trichilemmal cyst, in a pilomatricoma the keratin has clear nuclear spaces corresponding to shadow cells, and the epithelium, when present, is composed of uniform, basaloid matrical cells.

PROLIFERATING TRICHILEMMAL (PILAR) CYSTIC TUMORS

Clinical Features

Proliferating trichilemmal cystic tumors are almost always solitary lesions arising from a long-standing trichilemmal cyst in the dermis or upper subcutis. The vast majority of lesions occur on the scalp, most commonly in elderly women. These lesions can vary considerably in size and occasionally exceed 10 cm in diameter. A history of rapid enlargement of a preexisting nodule is usually elicited.

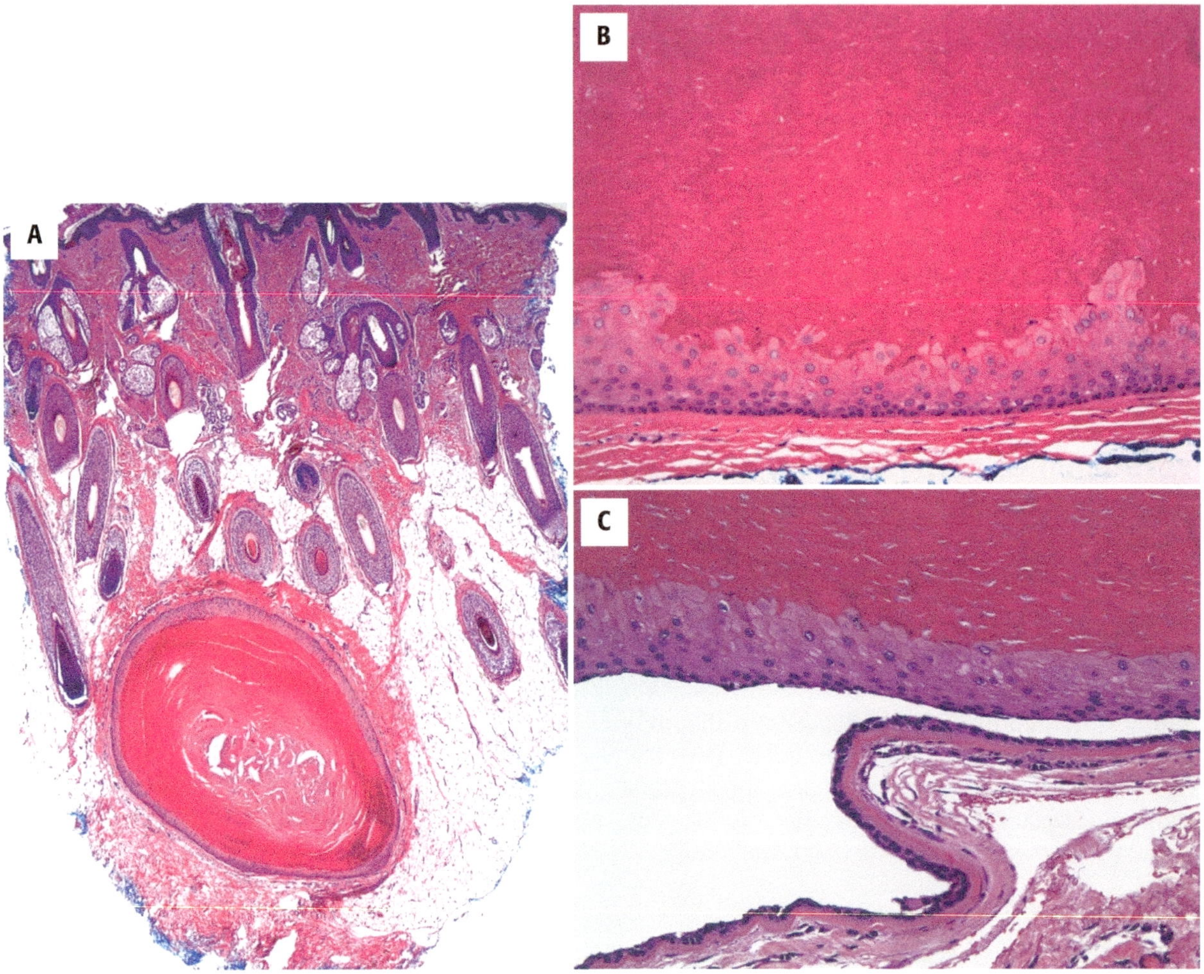

FIG. 9.11

Trichilemmal cyst: microscopic features. **A,** Trichilemmal cysts are located in the dermis and the cysts are filled with dense eosinophilic keratin. **B,** Trichilemmal keratinization occurs abruptly from large eosinophilic keratinocytes. **C,** The outer layer of trichilemmal cysts has a tendency to separate from the remainder of the cyst epithelium.

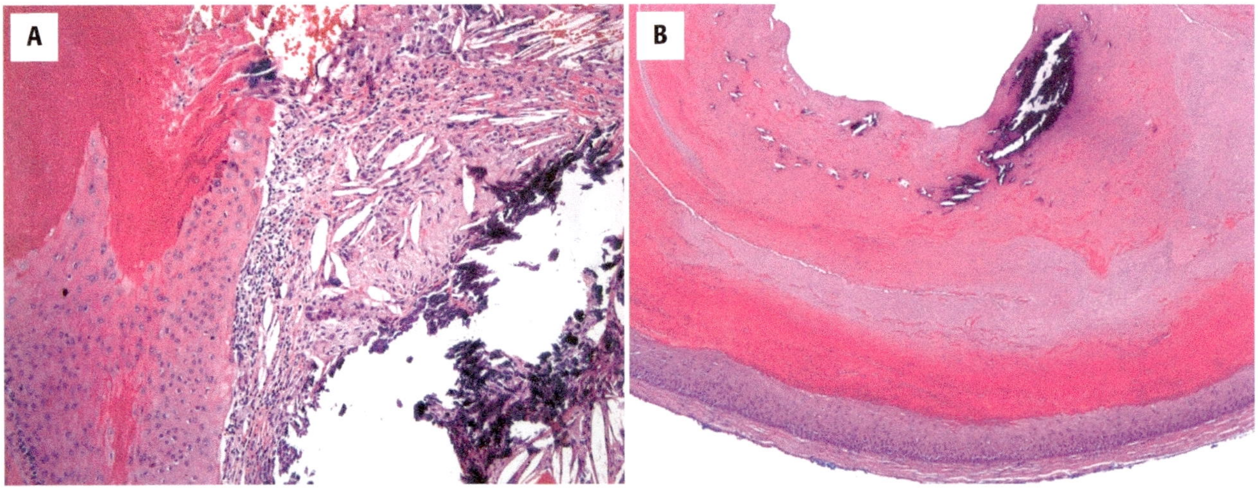

FIG. 9.12

Trichilemmal cyst: secondary microscopic features. **A,** A foreign body giant cell reaction is elicited to extravasated keratin from a ruptured trichilemmal cyst. **B,** Calcifications are a frequent finding.

Pathologic Features

Features typical of a trichilemmal cyst are present, but the epithelial layer is thickened, and the cyst is often multilobulated. Balls of squamous cells, or squamous eddies, are usually scattered through the lesion. Some mitotic figures may be seen in the proliferative areas of the lesion, but atypical mitoses are lacking. No significant cytologic atypia or infiltrative growth pattern at the periphery is seen (Fig. 9.13).

Differential Diagnosis

Trichilemmal cysts lack the complex multilobular architecture produced by the combination of solid and cystic squamous lobules that typify proliferating trichilemmal tumors. A malignant proliferating trichilemmal tumor can be diagnosed by its cytologic atypia and/or infiltrative growth pattern. Features diagnostic of malignancy may be focal, which is why it is prudent to completely remove partly biopsied lesions to exclude sampling

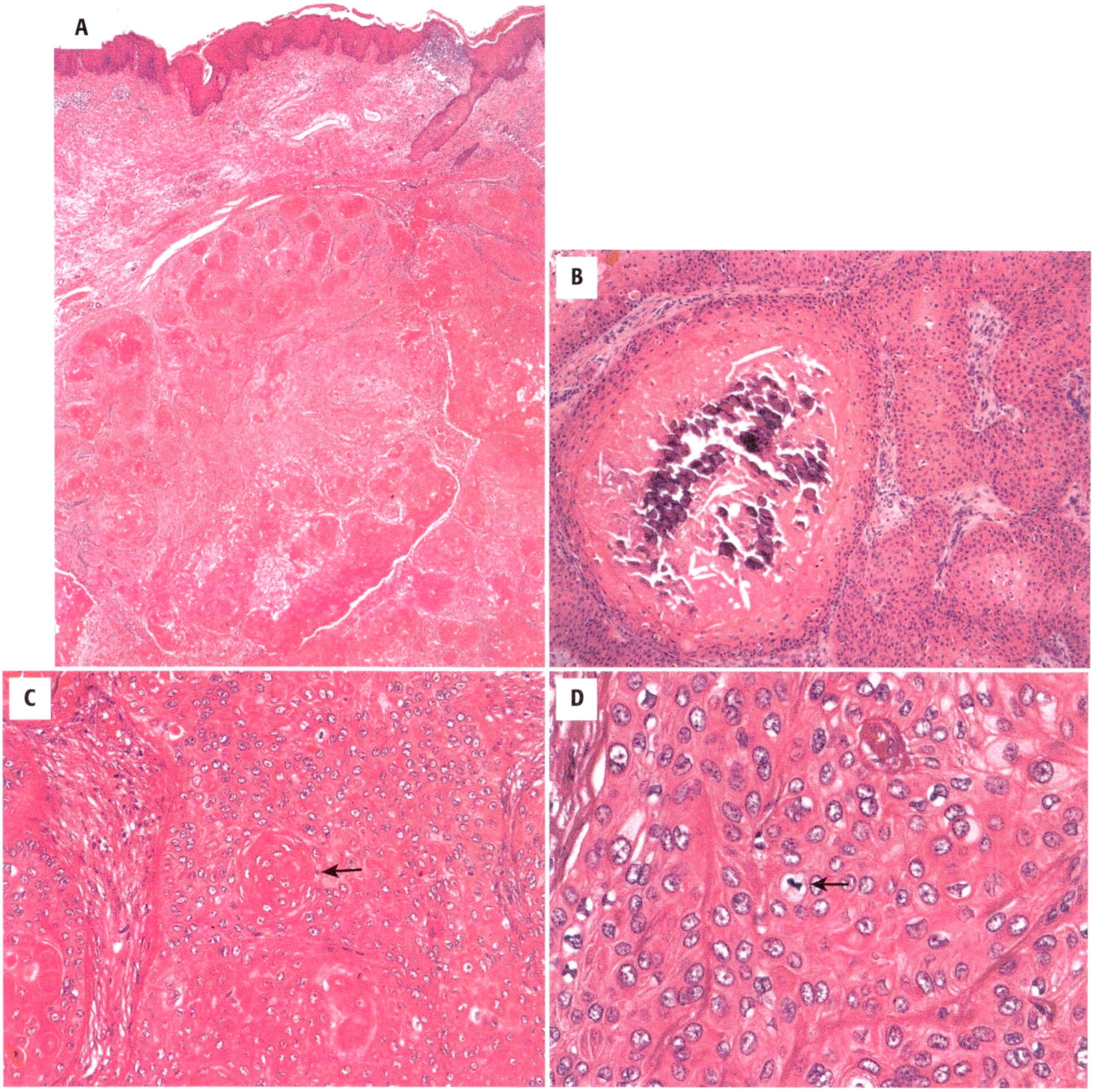

FIG. 9.13

Proliferating trichilemmal cystic tumor: microscopic features. **A,** The periphery of a proliferating trichilemmal cystic tumor is defined by circumscribed lobules of squamous cells with a pushing, noninfiltrative border. **B,** Evidence of a trichilemmal cyst can usually be found at least focally. **C,** Compact cellular lobules of squamous cells and scattered squamous eddies *(arrow)* comprise a variable portion of the lesions. **D,** Occasional mitotic figures *(arrow)* can be observed in the more proliferative zones of the lesion.

errors. Squamous cell carcinoma may resemble a proliferating trichilemmal tumor but lacks trichilemmal differentiation and is usually connected to the epidermis, although it can be cystic.

CYSTS ARISING FROM THE SEBACEOUS DUCT

Cysts derived from the sebaceous duct do not keratinize but rather have a thin stratified squamous epithelium with an inner cuticular lining that is deeply eosinophilic and has an undulating configuration. Steatocystomas are cysts derived from the sebaceous duct.

STEATOCYSTOMAS

Clinical Features

Steatocystomas most commonly present as multiple cysts (steatocystoma multiplex) in the second to fourth decades, especially around puberty, and arise sporadically or have an autosomal dominant pattern of inheritance. Less commonly, a solitary cyst (steatocystoma simplex) occurs, usually in adulthood. Females are affected slightly more often than males. The cysts present as firm, asymptomatic, flesh-colored to yellow papules or nodules that range from a few millimeters to several centimeters, with the majority in the 1- to 3-cm range. Lesions have a predilection for the arms, chest, axillae, and neck, but can also be found on the face, back, or groin region. Rare cases have been associated with Gardner syndrome, pachyonychia congenita, and various ectodermal dysplasias.

Pathologic Features

Steatocystomas arise in the dermis. The cysts are composed of a compressed, thin-walled stratified squamous epithelium without a granular layer. The most distinct feature of steatocystomas is the thin, compact, undulating, eosinophilic inner lining of the cyst wall. The cyst cavity is usually devoid of contents, although vellus hair shafts may occasionally be observed. Sebaceous lobules are found within or near the cyst wall in approximately two-thirds of all cases (Fig. 9.14). Occasionally, steatocystomas may be seen in conjunction with another type of cyst, such as an epidermoid cyst, resulting in a follicular hybrid cyst.

Differential Diagnosis

Milia and epidermoid cysts differ from steatocystomas by having a granular layer in the cyst wall and loose

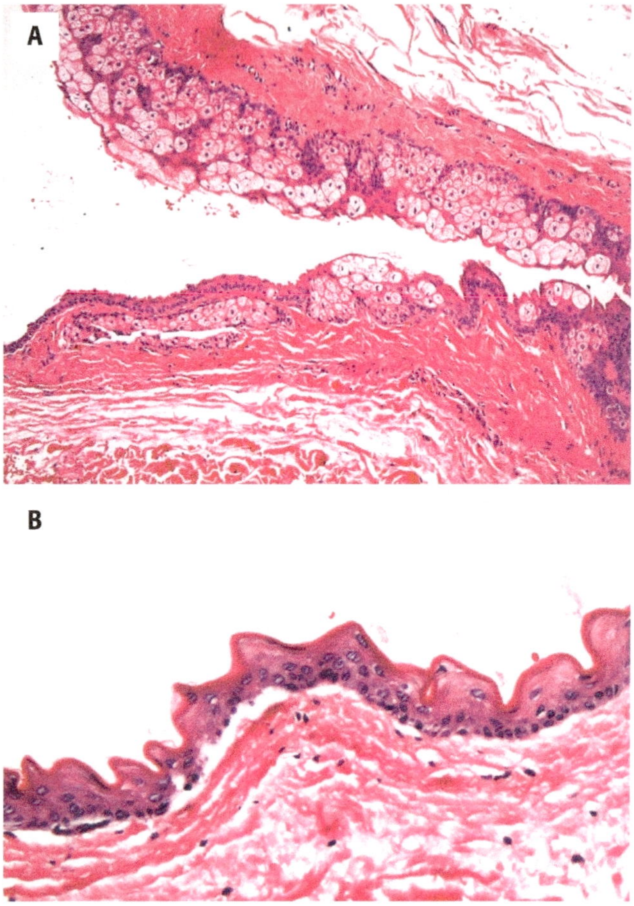

FIG. 9.14
Steatocystoma: microscopic features. **A,** Steatocystomas are dermal-based cysts with a thin cyst wall that often contains sebaceous glands. **B,** The hallmark of this cyst is the undulating, compact, eosinophilic inner layer corresponding to the cuticle of the sebaceous duct.

keratin in their cyst cavities and lacking an eosinophilic cuticle or sebaceous lobules in their cyst walls. Vellus hair cysts also lack the eosinophilic cuticle and sebaceous lobules that are seen in steatocystomas. Although both types of cysts can have vellus hairs in their cyst cavities, this feature is more prominent in vellus hair cysts.

FOLLICULAR HYBRID CYSTS

Clinical Features

Follicular hybrid cysts are rare cysts that are composed of two or more types of epithelial linings derived from the folliculosebaceous-apocrine unit. A variety of follicular hybrid cysts may be encountered, including epidermoid and trichilemmal cysts, epidermoid and matrical cysts, trichilemmal and matrical cysts, steatocystoma and epidermoid or dermoid cysts, steatocystoma and vellus hair cysts, and vellus hair and trichilemmal cysts. Gardner syndrome should be considered when a follicular hybrid cyst with epidermoid and matrical differentiation is encountered; these cysts are clinically indistinguishable from other cutaneous cysts. They are slightly more common in men than women.

Pathologic Features

Histopathologically, follicular hybrid cysts are characterized by an abrupt transition from one type of epithelial lining to another, with two or more types of epithelia being present. In the most common type of follicular hybrid cyst, that is, epidermoid and trichilemmal cyst, an abrupt transition is seen between the upper portion of the cyst, which keratinizes through a granular layer (epidermoid mode), and the lower portion of the cyst, which lacks a granular layer and keratinizes abruptly (trichilemmal mode). In Gardner syndrome, cysts show abrupt transition between epidermoid areas and matrical areas of keratinization, the latter consisting of a layer of uniform basaloid keratinocytes, resembling hair matrix epithelium, that gives rise to eosinophilic keratin with clear spaces where nuclei used to be, otherwise known as shadow or ghost cells (Fig. 9.15).

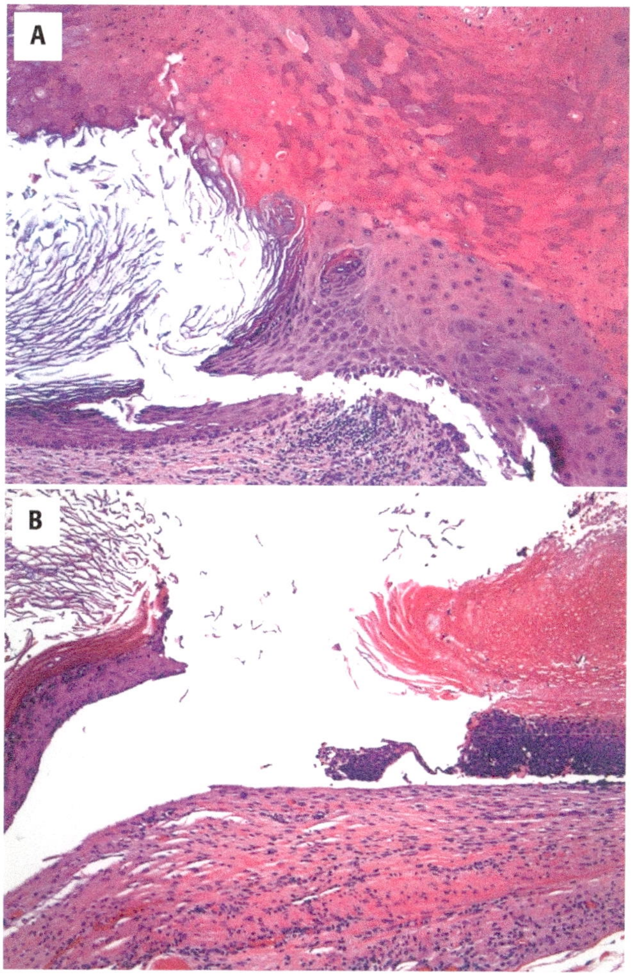

FIG. 9.15

Follicular hybrid cyst: microscopic features. **A,** This follicular hybrid cyst shows abrupt transition from epidermoid/infundibular *(left)* to trichilemmal/isthmus *(right)* differentiation. **B,** Abrupt transition between epidermoid *(left)* and matrical *(right)* differentiation is seen in this cyst from an individual with Gardner syndrome.

Differential Diagnosis

Hybrid cysts can be distinguished from pure cysts, such as epidermoid or trichilemmal cysts, by the presence of more than one type of epithelial lining. Dermoid cysts may closely resemble follicular hybrid cysts that combine features of steatocystoma and vellus hair cysts but lack the eosinophilic cuticular lining of a steatocystoma.

CYSTS ARISING FROM THE ECCRINE DUCT

ECCRINE HIDROCYSTOMAS

Clinical Features

Eccrine hidrocystomas are simple cysts that arise from eccrine ducts. These cysts are usually small (1 to 3 mm in diameter on average), translucent, cystic papules, which are more likely to be solitary than multiple. They often have a blue or blue-brown hue, leading to the clinical consideration of blue nevi or hemangiomas. There is a predilection for the face, especially the periorbital region, but the neck and trunk can also be affected. Solitary lesions are slightly more common in women, whereas patients with many lesions are almost always women. Patients with multiple eccrine hidrocystomas often notice fluctuation in the number and size of their cysts with changes in temperature, with a greater number and larger cysts in the summer compared to the winter.

Pathologic Features

The epithelium of eccrine hidrocystomas is typically two cell layers thick. The cells are cuboidal but occasionally may be flattened or attenuated (Fig. 9.16). The luminal cells are devoid of apical snouting, the hallmark of apocrine differentiation. A small amount of compressed fibrous stroma often invests the epithelial lining of these cysts. Normal eccrine glands or ducts are often observed near these lesions.

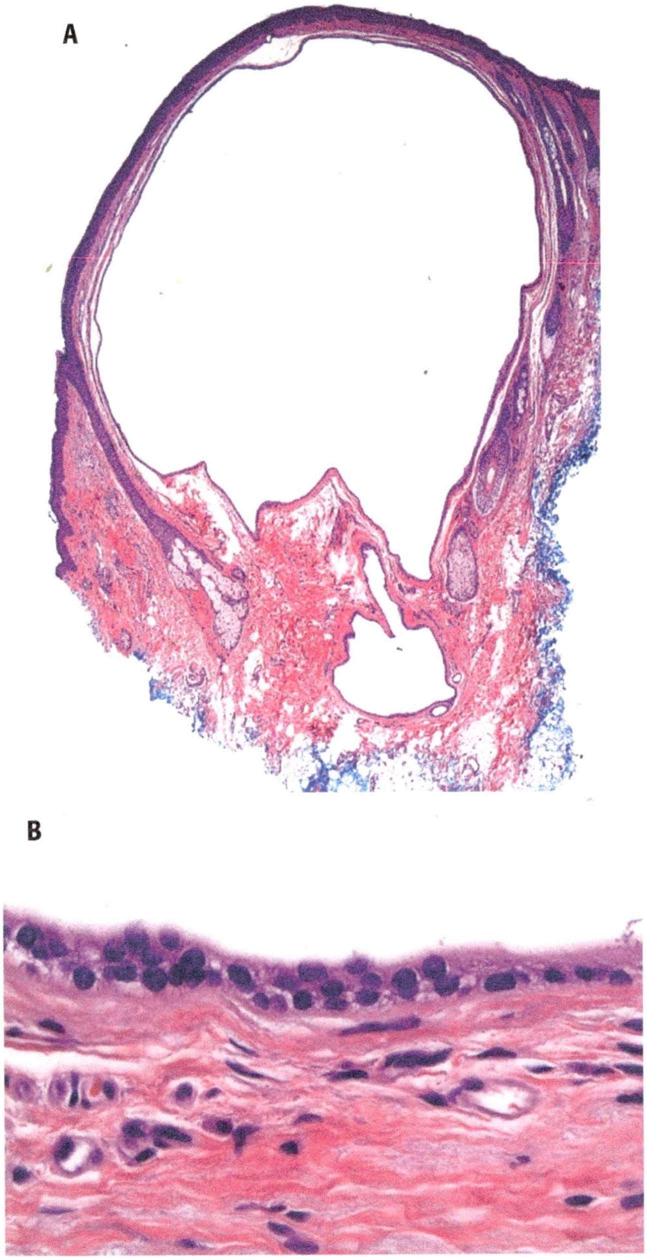

FIG. 9.16
Eccrine hidrocystoma: microscopic features. **A,** Eccrine hidrocystomas occur as unilocular cysts in the dermis. **B,** The epithelial lining consists of two layers of cuboidal cells.

Differential Diagnosis

In contrast to eccrine hidrocystomas, apocrine hidrocystomas have an inner columnar epithelial layer with apical snouts (apocrine decapitation secretion) and an outer layer of myoepithelial cells. Other cutaneous cysts are readily differentiated from eccrine hidrocystomas by lacking a double layer of cuboidal epithelial cell lining that defines the latter.

CYSTS ARISING FROM THE APOCRINE DUCT OR GLAND

APOCRINE HIDROCYSTOMAS/ CYSTADENOMAS

Clinical Features

Apocrine hidrocystomas/cystadenomas comprise a spectrum of apocrine gland lesions ranging from simple cysts (hidrocystomas) to complex cysts with solid and cystic areas (cystadenomas). These lesions are usually solitary, translucent, cystic papules or nodules, with most ranging from 0.3 to 1.5 cm, although occasional cases present as multiple lesions, and lesions measuring several centimeters have been reported. They have a predilection for the periorbital region of the face of adults. Other less common sites of involvement include the ears, scalp, neck, genital region, and upper trunk. Men and women are equally affected. These cysts may be skin-colored but often have a blue hue, leading to consideration of a blue nevus or hemangioma in the clinical differential diagnosis.

Pathologic Features

Apocrine hidrocystomas are composed of a cystic cavity lined by two cell layers. The distinctive feature of apocrine hidrocystomas is the inner cell layer, which consists of columnar epithelial cells with basilar nuclei, abundant eosinophilic cytoplasm, and apical snouts; this last feature is the hallmark of apocrine decapitation secretion (Fig. 9.17). Other areas of the inner cell layer of these cysts may have a cuboidal to flattened appearance, thereby resembling an eccrine hidrocystoma. The outer cell layer is composed of cuboidal to flattened and elongated cells, the latter representing myoepithelial cells.

Apocrine cystadenomas are more complex cysts than hidrocystomas, with proliferative foci that may have papillary, syncytial, or tubular architectural growth patterns (Fig. 9.18). These cellular areas may demonstrate slight cellular atypia and occasional division figures.

Differential Diagnosis

Eccrine hidrocystomas differ from apocrine hidrocystomas by having an epithelial layer of cuboidal to flattened cells that lack apical snouts (apocrine decapitation secretion). Other apocrine tumors are not readily confused with apocrine hidrocystomas/cystadenomas

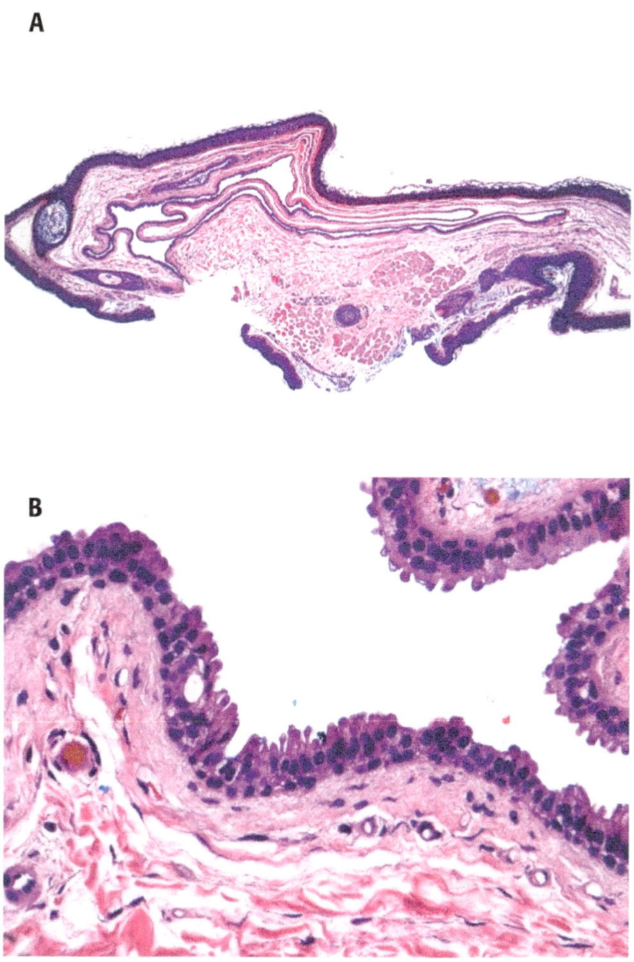

FIG. 9.17

Apocrine hidrocystoma: microscopic features. **A,** Apocrine hidrocystoma of the eyelid forms a unilocular cyst in the dermis. **B,** The diagnostic feature of this cyst is an inner layer of eosinophilic, columnar cells with apical snouts (decapitation secretion).

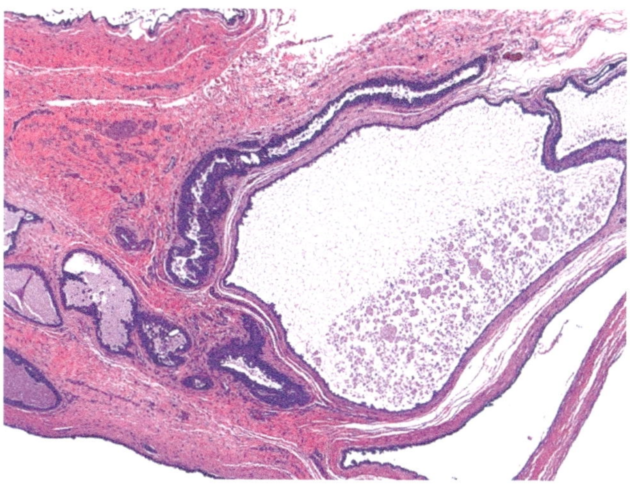

FIG. 9.18

Apocrine cystadenoma: microscopic features. An apocrine cystadenoma is a multilocular apocrine lesion with some solid areas of proliferative epithelium. In this example, papillary infoldings of epithelium are present in some areas.

because of their characteristic architectural patterns and clinical features.

DEVELOPMENTAL CYSTS

DERMOID CYSTS

Clinical Features

Dermoid cysts are usually present at birth or detected in early childhood. These cysts are derived from sequestered ectodermal tissue found at lines of embryonic closure, particularly the midline of the head and neck. The periorbital region, especially the eyebrows or lateral edge of the eyes, is the most common site. In this location, cysts do not typically extend into deeper tissues, especially within the cranial vault. Midline dermoid cysts involving the nasal dorsum or glabella account for approximately 3% of dermoid cysts. The major clinical significance of nasal dermoid cysts is that they may connect to the underlying central nervous system by a dermoid sinus tract; therefore these lesions are at risk for central nervous system infections and leakage of cerebrospinal fluid. Cysts can also occur along the midline of the scalp and neck, sternum, and perineum. Dermoid cysts are circumscribed, firm-to-rubbery nodules, ranging from 1 to 4 cm in diameter. Dermoid cysts can rupture, leading to inflammation and scarring.

Pathologic Features

Dermoid cysts have stratified squamous epithelium that keratinizes through a granular layer, that is, in an epidermoid mode, like epidermoid cysts. The cystic cavity contains loose, laminated orthokeratin. Multiple hair shafts are usually seen within the cyst lumen. The most helpful histological feature for diagnosis of a dermoid cyst is the presence of small pilosebaceous structures within the cyst wall and occasional hair shafts protruding into the cyst cavity (Fig. 9.19). Smooth muscle may also be seen in the cyst wall. Eccrine glands and occasionally apocrine glands may be identified in the vicinity of dermoid cysts. When a dermoid cyst ruptures, a foreign body giant cell reaction is elicited, and fibrosis may ensue. When infection supervenes, neutrophils infiltrate into the cyst and surrounding tissue.

Ancillary Studies

Nasal dermoid cysts should be evaluated by magnetic resonance imaging or computed axial tomography prior

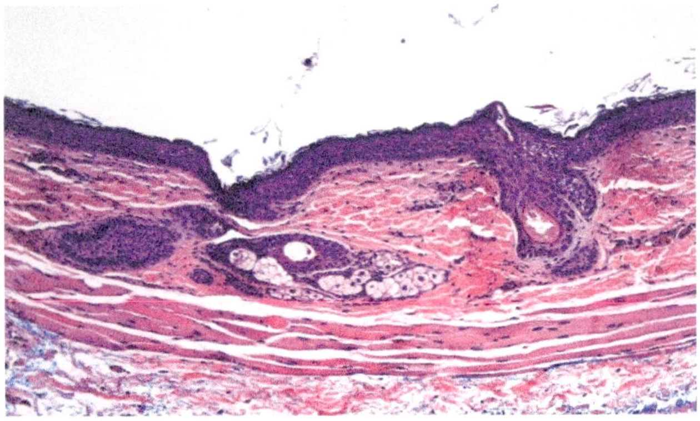

FIG. 9.19
Dermoid cyst: microscopic features. Dermoid cysts have a lining like an epidermoid cyst but have mature, small pilosebaceous units in their cyst walls.

to surgery to determine if the lesion communicates with the underlying central nervous system, necessitating neurosurgical intervention.

Differential Diagnosis

Dermoid cysts have multiple hair shafts in their cyst cavities and pilosebaceous structures with or without smooth muscle in their cyst walls, whereas epidermoid cysts lack these features. Dermoid cysts differ from vellus hair cysts by having multiple pilosebaceous structures in their cyst walls, while vellus hair cysts usually lack adnexal structures or contain only one vellus follicle in their cyst walls. In contrast to the eosinophilic cuticle lining of steatocystomas, dermoid cysts have keratinizing squamous epithelium resembling the follicular infundibulum.

BRANCHIAL CLEFT CYSTS

Clinical Features

Branchial cleft anomalies are rare and occur as cysts, sinuses, fistulas, and rarely skin tags. They arise because of incomplete migration of the corresponding branchial arch during embryologic development. The lesions occur in the skin or soft tissues of the head and neck. Lesions most commonly arise from the second branchial arch and are located at the anterior edge of the sternocleidomastoid muscle. In contrast, lesions that arise from the first branchial arch are located near the angle of the jaw. Third and fourth branchial arch anomalies are extremely rare and arise in the inferior neck.

Branchial cleft cysts are usually solitary, slowly enlarging flesh-colored nodules. The cysts may become erythematous and tender secondary to infection or rupture. Most of these lesions are diagnosed in the second and third decades of life.

Branchial cleft sinuses present as a small pit in the lateral neck in patients during the first 5 years of life. Sinuses may drain mucinous material or become infected and drain pus. Branchial cleft fistulas are less common than cysts or sinuses. Fistulas may connect to the oropharynx and/or the skin of the lateral neck, where they may also drain mucinous or purulent material.

Pathologic Features

Histopathologically, branchial cleft cysts are lined by stratified squamous and/or pseudostratified columnar epithelia, the latter of which is often ciliated (Fig. 9.20). The most helpful diagnostic feature is the presence of dense lymphoid tissue, often with discernible lymphoid follicles, within the cyst wall. Mucinous glands or cartilage may also be present in the cyst wall in occasional cases, but smooth muscle is absent.

Branchial cleft sinuses have stratified squamous epithelium that connects to the skin surface. The deeper aspects of the branchial cleft sinus may be cystic and lined by pseudostratified columnar or stratified squamous epithelium. Like branchial cleft cysts, lymphoid tissue invests the wall of branchial cleft sinuses.

Some branchial cleft anomalies have the configuration of skin tags. Cartilage is often present in the core of these lesions.

Differential Diagnosis

Branchial cleft cysts differ histopathologically from bronchogenic cysts by the presence of prominent lymphoid tissue and lack of smooth muscle in their cyst walls. Thyroglossal duct cysts have thyroid follicles in their cyst wall and, when infected, tend to have less lymphoid tissue compared to branchial cleft cysts. Thymic cysts can resemble branchial cleft cysts due to the presence of lymphoid tissue, but the lymphoid tissue is well organized into lobules separated by thin fibrous septae, and Hassall's corpuscles and cholesterol granulomas are present in thymic cysts.

BRONCHOGENIC CYSTS

Clinical Features

Bronchogenic cysts are rare cysts that develop from ectopic tracheobronchial remnants that have failed to

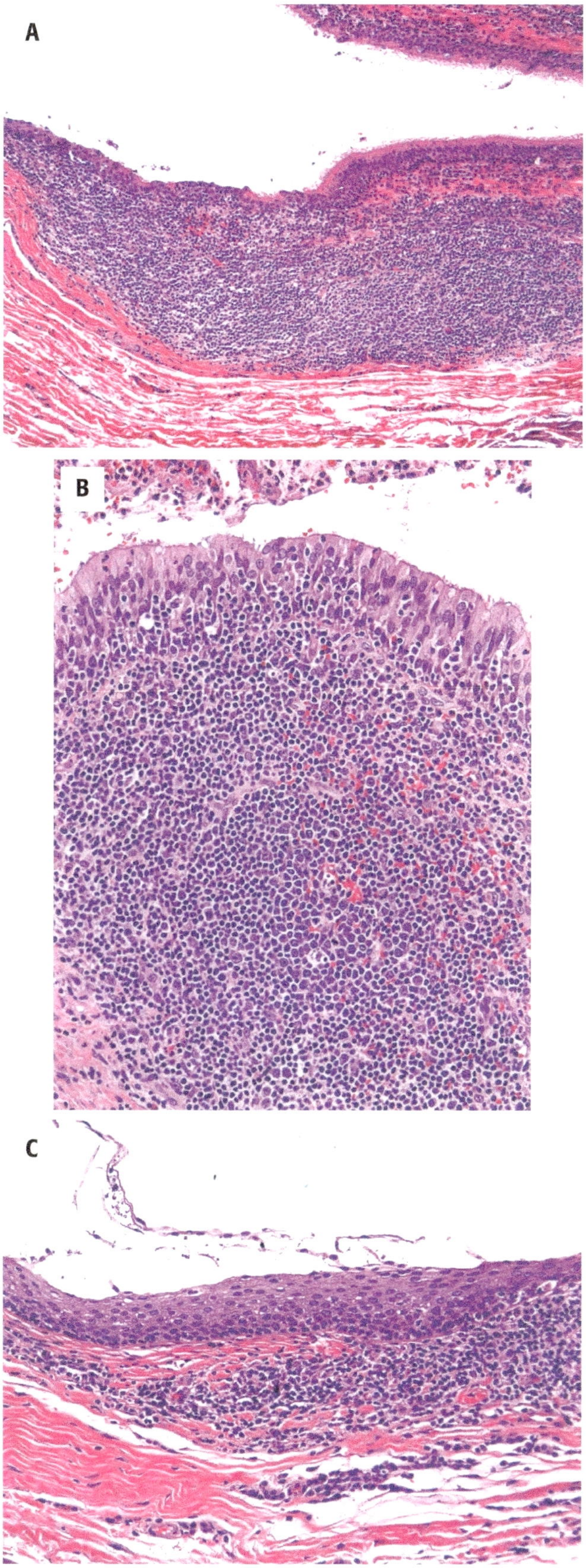

FIG. 9.20

Branchial cleft cyst: microscopic features. **A,** A branchial cleft cyst has prominent lymphoid tissue in its wall. The epithelial lining varies from ciliated pseudostratified columnar (**B**) to stratified squamous (**C**).

migrate completely during embryogenesis. They are usually present at birth or arise in infancy, although rarely cysts are not detected until adulthood. These lesions present as solitary cystic nodules, 0.3 to 6.0 cm in diameter, or draining sinus tracts. The midline of the lower neck near the suprasternal notch and the mediastinum are the most common locations. Bronchogenic cysts occurring on the upper trunk, neck, and chin have been reported. Males are affected about three times more often than females. White individuals are more commonly affected than Black patients.

Pathologic Features

The epithelial lining of bronchogenic cysts may consist of ciliated, pseudostratified columnar epithelium with mucin-secreting goblet cells, simple columnar, cuboidal, or occasionally stratified squamous epithelium. Some areas of the cyst lining may lack cilia. The cyst wall contains smooth muscle and mucous glands in over half of the cases. Cartilage can be seen in the cyst wall in a small percentage of cases (Fig. 9.21). Lymphoid follicles are typically absent from the cyst wall.

Differential Diagnosis

Considerable overlap in histopathological features exists between branchial cleft and bronchogenic cysts. The primary histopathological feature that distinguishes branchial cleft from bronchogenic cysts in most cases is the presence of prominent lymphoid tissue, often including lymphoid follicles, in the cyst wall of the former. The anatomical location of the cyst may prove most helpful in some cases where the histological diagnosis between a bronchogenic and branchial cleft cyst is uncertain. Thyroglossal duct cysts can have a similar cyst lining but differ from bronchogenic cysts by having thyroid follicles and lacking smooth muscle and/or cartilage in the vicinity of their cyst walls.

THYROGLOSSAL DUCT CYSTS

Clinical Features

Thyroglossal duct cysts arise from sequestered remnants of the thyroglossal duct that aid in the migration of the thyroid anlage from the base of the tongue to the anterior neck during embryogenesis. Thyroglossal duct cyst is the most common congenital cyst in the neck. Most cysts are detected in the first three decades of life. They present as slowly growing, 1- to 4-cm masses that move

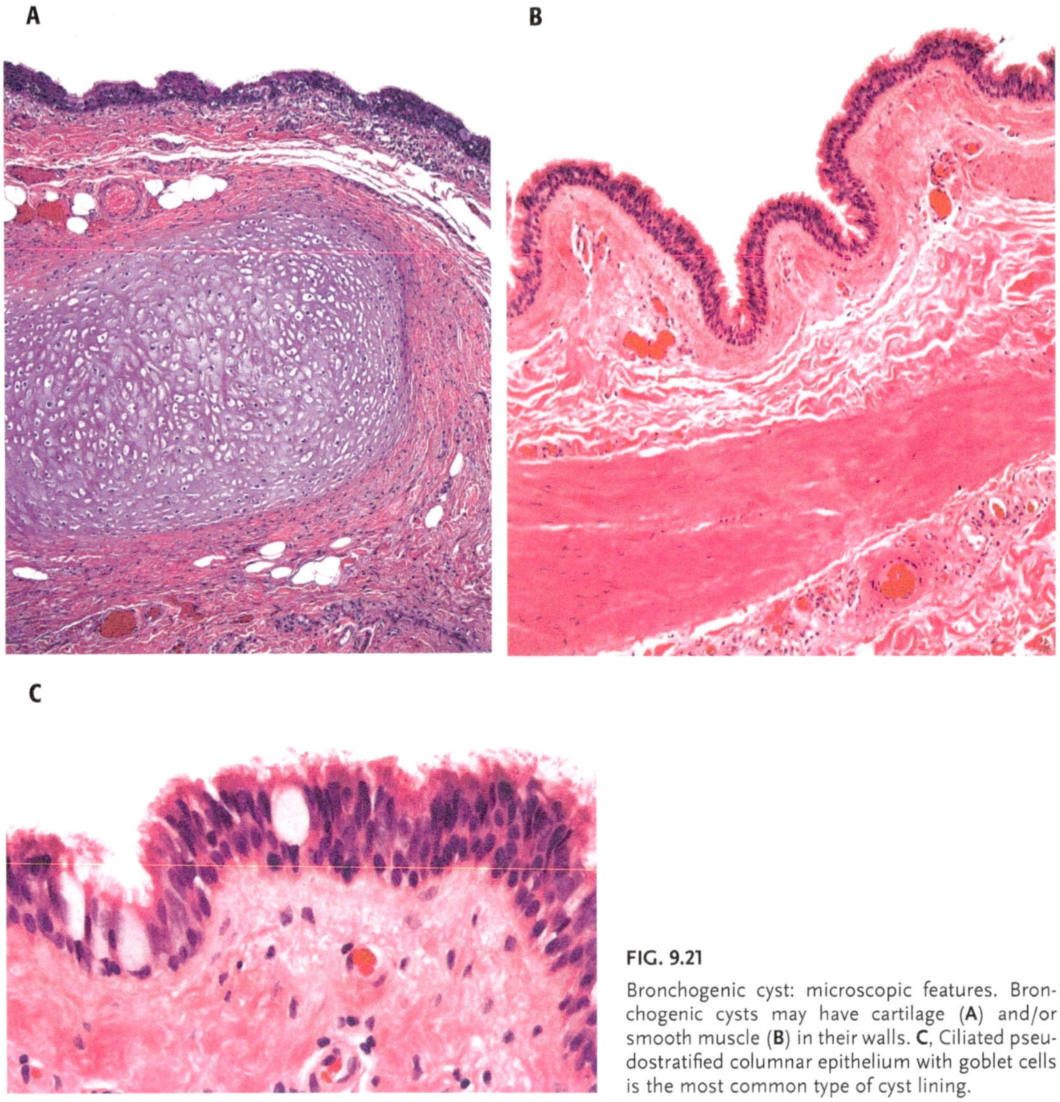

FIG. 9.21

Bronchogenic cyst: microscopic features. Bronchogenic cysts may have cartilage (**A**) and/or smooth muscle (**B**) in their walls. **C**, Ciliated pseudostratified columnar epithelium with goblet cells is the most common type of cyst lining.

during swallowing because of their connection to the underlying hyoid bone. The cysts may be tender due to secondary infection. Thyroglossal duct sinuses connect to the skin in the midline of the anterior neck and may drain clear fluid or pus. They are often associated with a deeper cyst. Approximately 1% to 2% of cases give rise to carcinoma in adulthood, with papillary thyroid carcinoma being the most common type.

Pathologic Features

Thyroglossal duct cysts occur in the subcutaneous tissue and only occasionally in the dermis. The cysts are lined by variously stratified squamous, cuboidal, and columnar epithelia, the latter of which is often ciliated. An important diagnostic feature is the presence of thyroid follicles in the cyst wall of most cases (Fig. 9.22). Cartilage and smooth muscle are lacking in the cyst wall. A remnant of the thyroglossal duct that connects to a portion of the hyoid bone may be detected in some cases. An inflammatory infiltrate is seen in cysts that are secondarily infected.

Differential Diagnosis

Branchial cleft cysts are distinguished from thyroglossal duct cysts by their location and absence of nearby thyroid tissue. In contrast to thyroglossal duct cysts, bronchogenic duct cysts do not have thyroid tissue but may have smooth muscle or cartilage in their cyst wall. Thymic cysts have abundant lymphoid tissue organized into lobules by thin fibrous septa, Hassall's corpuscles,

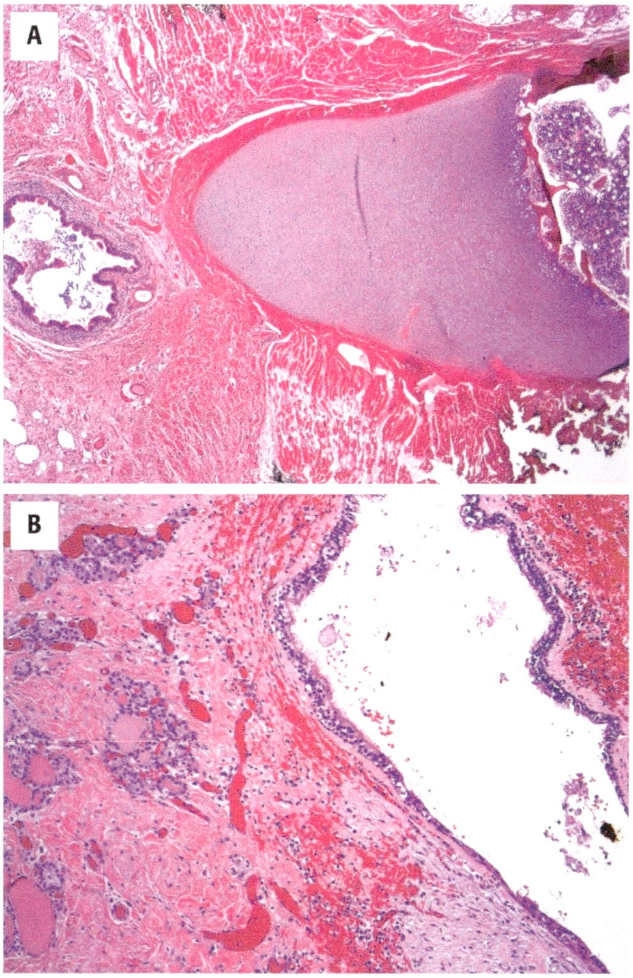

FIG. 9.22

Thyroglossal duct cyst: microscopic features. **A**, A thyroglossal duct cyst may be seen in the vicinity of a portion of hyoid bone with associated cartilage. **B**, Thyroid follicles *(left)* are seen adjacent to a thyroglossal duct cyst and are very helpful in its diagnosis.

and cholesterol granulomas, all features that are not observed in thyroglossal duct cysts.

THYMIC CYSTS

Clinical Features

Thymic cysts occasionally occur in the anterior cervical triangle of the neck, preferentially on the left side posterior to the lateral lobe of the thyroid gland. The cervical cysts are thought to arise from sequestered remnants of the third pharyngeal pouch due to an arrest in migration of the thymic anlage during embryonic development. Most cysts in the neck are detected during the first decade of life. Males are affected more often than females. The cysts present as solitary, painless, slowly growing masses that vary considerably in size, ranging from 2 to 15 cm in diameter. Rarely, large thymic cysts can produce obstructive symptoms, such as hoarseness, stridor, dyspnea, or dysphagia.

Pathologic Features

Most examples of thymic cysts are multilocular. Thymic cysts are lined by epithelium that may vary from stratified squamous to cuboidal to columnar or pseudostratified columnar. Some cells may possess cilia. The presence of associated thymic tissue, consisting of lobules of lymphoid tissue with intervening septa or follicles with Hassall's corpuscles, is diagnostic of this entity (Fig. 9.23). Cholesterol clefts and granulomas are additional common features that are helpful in the diagnosis of thymic cysts.

Differential Diagnosis

Branchial cleft cysts have prominent lymphoid tissue in their cyst wall, but the lymphoid tissue lacks the lobular architecture with thin fibrous septa, Hassall's corpuscles, or cholesterol granulomas seen in thymic cysts. Cystic thymomas, in contrast to thymic cysts, have proliferation of thymic epithelial elements. A lymph node can also enter the differential diagnosis if the cystic cavity of the thymic cyst is small or the lining is obliterated by secondary inflammation or fibrosis, but a careful search for Hassall's corpuscles and cholesterol clefts will lead to the correct diagnosis of a thymic cyst. Finally, metastatic cystic squamous cell carcinoma to a lymph node can resemble a thymic cyst. Careful examination for Hassall's corpuscles and their distinction from neoplastic squamous epithelium of squamous cell carcinoma can avoid a misdiagnosis of a malignant process.

CUTANEOUS CILIATED CYSTS

Clinical Features

Cutaneous ciliated cysts are rare cysts that arise almost exclusively on the lower extremities and buttocks of adolescents and young adult females. Exceedingly rare cases have been reported in males. Additional rare sites of involvement include the scalp, trunk, and perineal region. The lesions are solitary, 1 to 3 cm in diameter, cystic nodules that may be painful. The size of the cysts may increase during pregnancy under hormonal stimulation. The cysts are thought to arise from ectopic Müllerian rests, but ciliated metaplasia of sweat glands has also been proposed; the latter hypothesis accounts for rare reports in male patients.

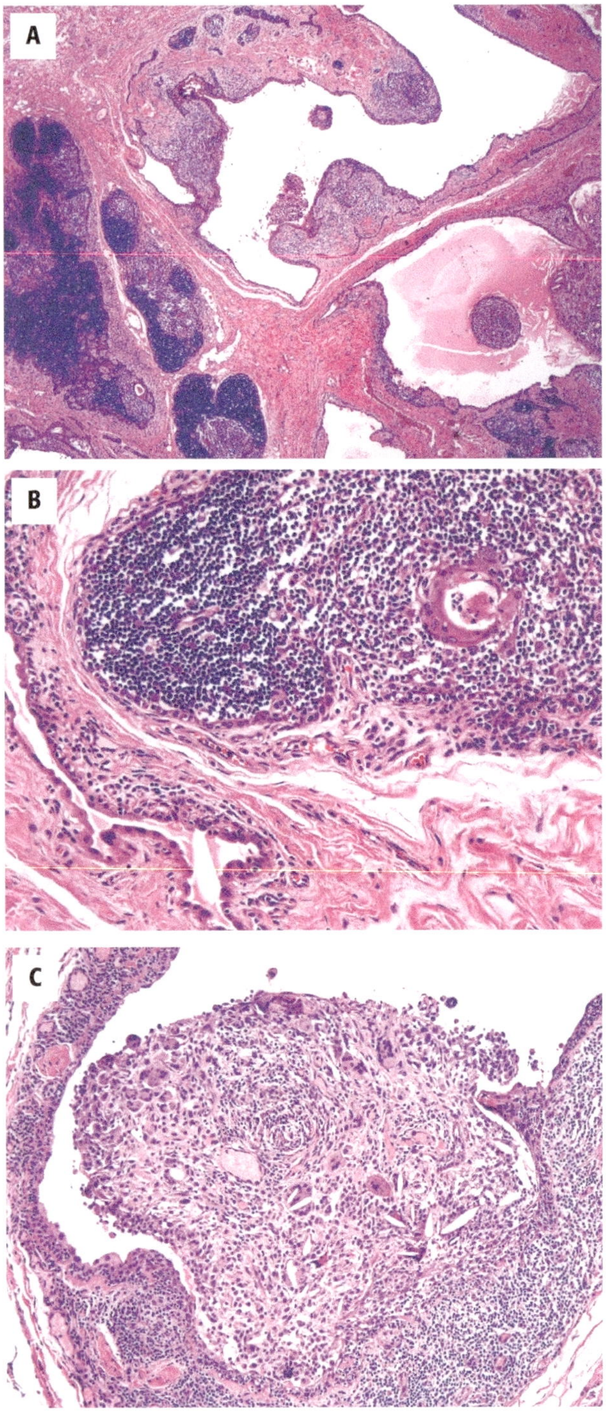

FIG. 9.23

Thymic cyst: microscopic features. **A**, Thymic cysts have cystic spaces associated with distinctly lobular arrays of lymphoid tissue. **B**, A Hassall's corpuscle *(upper right)* is present in the lymphoid tissue. **C**, Cholesterol granulomas are a common finding in thymic cysts.

Pathologic Features

The epithelial lining of cutaneous ciliated cysts ranges from cuboidal to simple columnar ciliated cells (Fig. 9.24). The nuclei are basally located. Sometimes foci of pseudostratified columnar or stratified squamous epithelium, the latter representing squamous metaplasia, are present. Papillary infoldings within the cyst lumen are quite common. There are no mucin-secreting goblet cells in the epithelium. The adjacent tissue lacks lymphoid tissue, adnexal structures, glandular elements, or smooth muscle. A dense rim of collagen may be tightly apposed to the cyst lining.

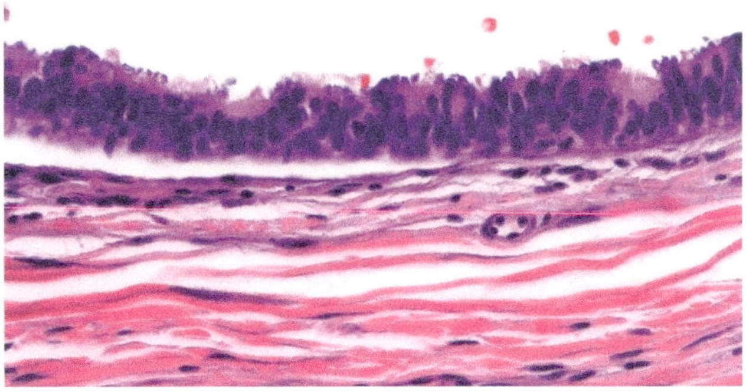

FIG. 9.24

Cutaneous ciliated cyst: microscopic features. Cutaneous ciliated cysts are lined by ciliated columnar epithelium.

Differential Diagnosis

The lower extremity location helps distinguish cutaneous ciliated cysts from other nonsquamous epithelial-lined cysts. From a histologic standpoint, the lack of other structures, such as smooth muscle, cartilage, thymic tissue, and lymphoid tissue, within the cyst wall of cutaneous ciliated cysts also aids in this distinction.

CILIATED MUCINOUS CYSTS OF THE VULVA

Clinical Features

Ciliated or paramesonephric mucinous cysts of the vulva occur in multiparous females, and most lesions are detected in the third and fourth decades of life. They are located on the vulva, particularly the superior aspect of the labium minus or vestibule. The lesions are solitary, 1 to 3 cm in diameter, and painful. Vulvar ciliated cysts are often related to pregnancy or the use of exogenous hormones. An origin from the urogenital sinus is generally accepted.

Pathologic Features

The epithelial lining of vulvar ciliated and mucinous cysts consists of columnar ciliated or cuboidal cells. The nuclei of cells are basally located. Mucin is often abundant in the apical cytoplasm of columnar cells. Squamous metaplasia of the cyst lining has been reported. Papillary infoldings within the cyst cavity may be observed. Lymphoid tissue, skin appendages, glandular elements, and smooth muscle are lacking in the cyst wall.

Differential Diagnosis

The major feature that distinguishes ciliated mucinous cysts of the vulva from cutaneous ciliated cysts is the mucin production in the former. In contrast to ciliated mucinous cysts of the vulva, the epithelial lining of mesonephric cysts is flattened, and mucin also is absent. Bartholin's gland cysts usually have transitional-type or stratified squamous epithelium.

MEDIAN RAPHE CYSTS

Clinical Features

Median raphe cysts are rare cysts that are located along the ventral surface of the penis anywhere from the urethral meatus to the anus in males. Most cysts are removed in young adults, but some are detected in infancy and early childhood. The cysts are solitary, usually asymptomatic, and range in size from a few millimeters up to 2.5 cm. A few pigmented cysts have been reported in the Japanese population. Some examples of median raphe cysts in the past have been misdiagnosed as apocrine cystadenoma. They most likely arise due to defects in the closure of the urethral or genital folds during embryogenesis.

Pathologic Features

Histopathologically, median raphe cysts are located in the dermis and lack connection to the overlying epidermis. The cyst lining ranges from pseudostratified columnar epithelium to a single cell layer. Some of the epithelial cells have clear cytoplasm. Mucin-producing cells can be demonstrated on occasion, as can prominent apical snouting of luminal cells consistent with an apocrine phenotype (Fig. 9.25). A rare case having cilia on the surface of scattered columnar cells has been reported. Squamous metaplasia may occasionally be observed. Rarely, melanin pigment has been present in the basal layer of the epithelial lining, corresponding to the rare, pigmented variant. Mucinous glands may be seen in the cyst wall; however, the cyst wall lacks lymphoid tissue, adnexal structures, cartilage, or smooth muscle.

A

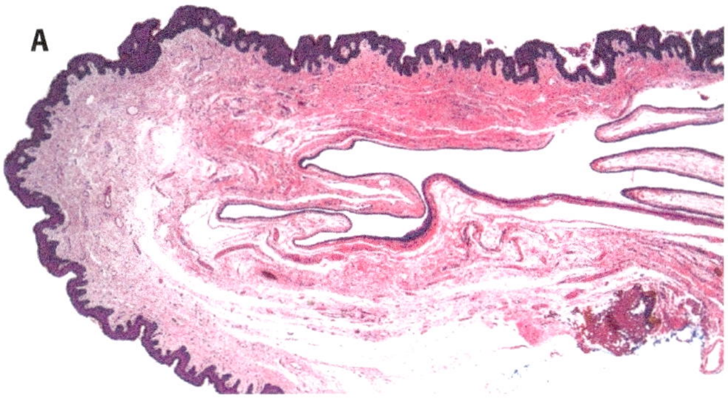

B

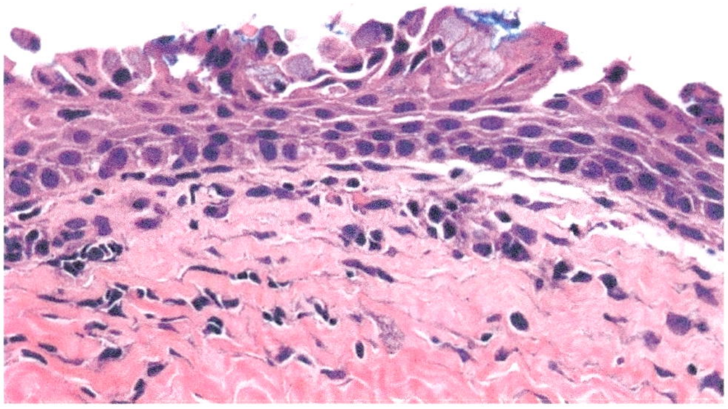

C

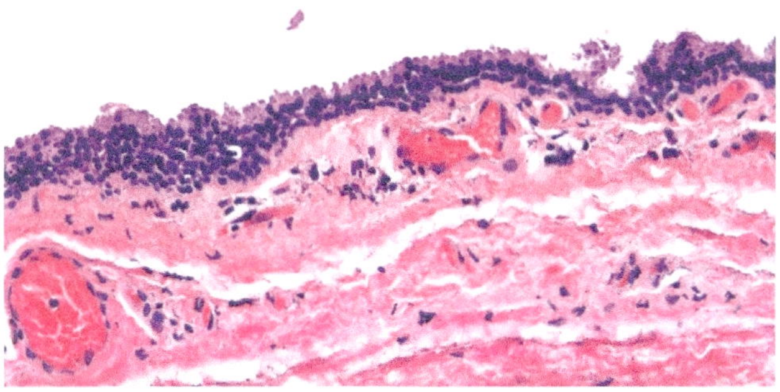

FIG. 9.25

Median raphe cyst: microscopic features. **A**, A median raphe cyst is present in the dermis. **B**, The epithelial lining is pseudostratified columnar. **C**, Apocrine decapitation secretion can be found in some median raphe cysts.

Differential Diagnosis

Epidermoid cysts can also involve the penis but have keratinizing stratified squamous epithelium, in contrast to median raphe cysts that only occasionally have foci of squamous metaplasia and have other areas of typical epithelium. Apocrine cystadenomas or hidrocystomas can closely resemble median raphe cysts with prominent apocrine change. In addition to the unique clinical features of a median raphe cyst, the presence of some areas with more typical pseudostratified columnar epithelium or mucin-producing epithelial cells aids in arriving at the correct diagnosis of a median raphe cyst rather than an apocrine hidrocystoma or cystadenoma.

OMPHALOMESENTERIC DUCT CYSTS

Clinical Features

Omphalomesenteric duct remnants are rare cutaneous lesions that present most commonly as erythematous cutaneous polyps, but also as subcutaneous cysts, sinuses, or fistulas, in the periumbilical region. Cysts or polyps vary from 0.2 to 2.0 cm in diameter. Most patients report drainage or discharge of serous, serosanguinous, bloody, mucoid, or purulent fluid. The lesions are usually detected in the first year of life but may not be removed until early adulthood. Males are more frequently affected than females. The cysts are unrelated to gravidity, maternal age, or premature birth. Meckel's diverticulum is a frequent underlying anomaly associated with omphalomesenteric duct cysts or polyps. Ileal prolapse may occur in the neonatal period and may be fatal in a minority of patients.

Pathologic Features

Regardless of whether the lesion is a polyp, cyst, or sinus, the histopathologic diagnosis is predicated on observing gastric (30% of cases), small intestinal (60% of cases), or colonic (10% of cases) mucosa lining a portion or the entire lesion (Fig. 9.26). Islands of pancreatic tissue may rarely be seen. An abrupt transition to hyperplastic, keratinizing squamous epithelium of the skin at the edge of polyps is commonly seen. Smooth muscle is often present in the cyst wall. Prominent numbers of blood vessels are in the adjacent stroma. A mixed inflammatory infiltrate in the adjacent stroma is common.

Differential Diagnosis

The presence of mature intestinal mucosa in a lesion from the periumbilical region is essentially diagnostic

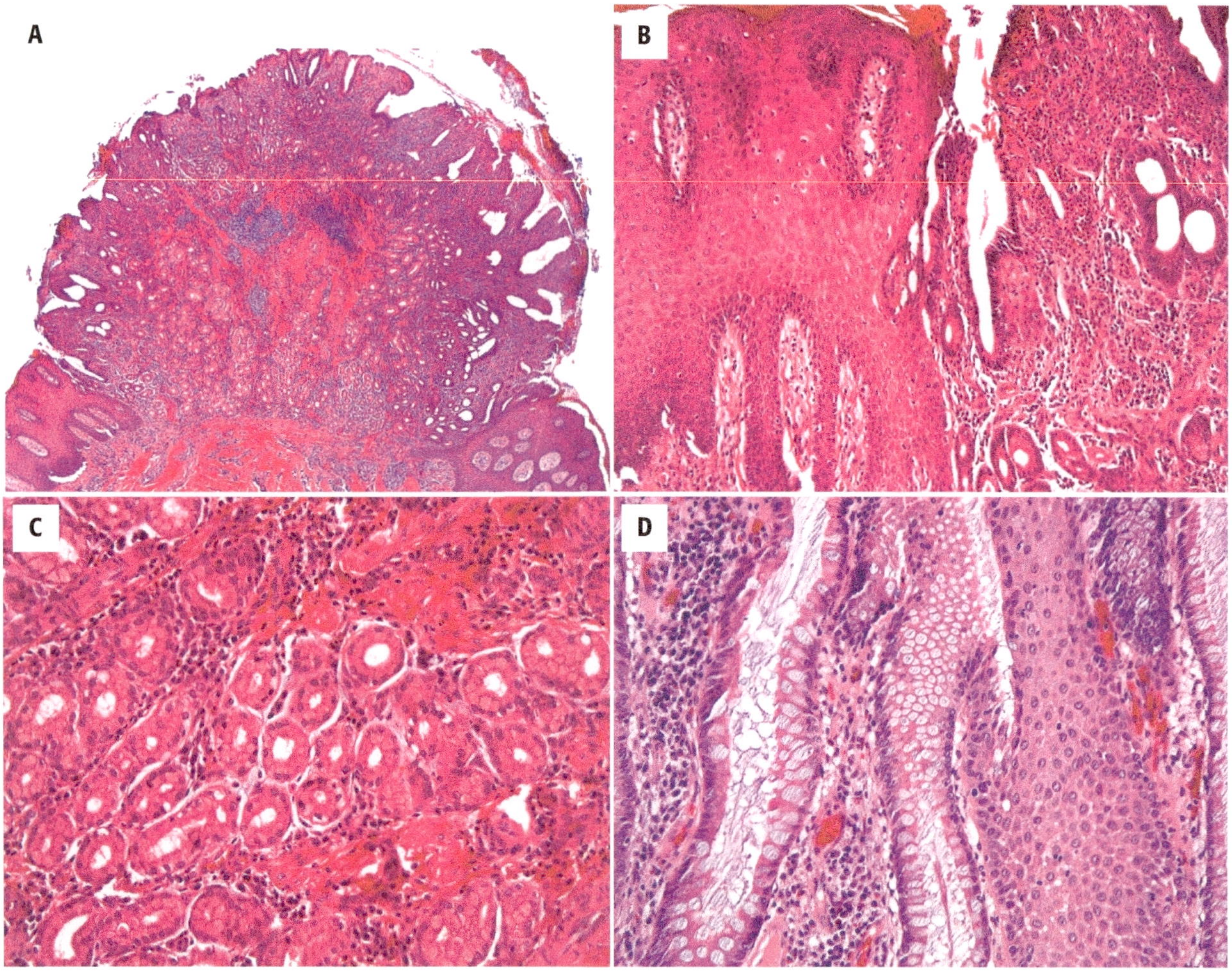

FIG. 9.26

Omphalomesenteric duct cyst: microscopic features. **A,** Omphalomesenteric duct polyps have a polypoid configuration from scanning magnification. **B,** An abrupt transition from the polyp to hyperplastic keratinizing squamous epithelium of adjacent skin is typical. Various types of gastrointestinal epithelium may line the polyp or cyst (**C,** gastric; **D,** colonic).

of an omphalomesenteric duct remnant. Umbilical pyogenic granulomas can produce a similar silhouette to omphalomesenteric polyps from scanning magnification, but the former is a vascular proliferation that lacks gastrointestinal mucosa. Urachal remnants can resemble omphalomesenteric remnants architecturally but differ by having transitional instead of gastrointestinal epithelium. Metastatic adenocarcinomas have more complex architecture, cytologic atypia, and mitoses compared to omphalomesenteric duct remnants.

PSEUDOCYSTS

PSEUDOCYSTS OF THE AURICLE

Clinical Features

Pseudocyst of the auricle is a rare, noninflammatory swelling of the external auricle due to the intracartilagenous collection of serous or serosanguinous fluid, with a predilection for the anterior upper half of the ear. The majority of lesions are 0.5 to 5 cm in diameter, asymptomatic, slowly evolving, solitary, and unilateral. Pseudocysts of the auricle occur more commonly in males and any age may be affected, although most cases are seen between the third and fifth decades. The etiology for this localized cystic degeneration of cartilage is not entirely clear, but local repetitive trauma or ischemic necrosis is currently favored.

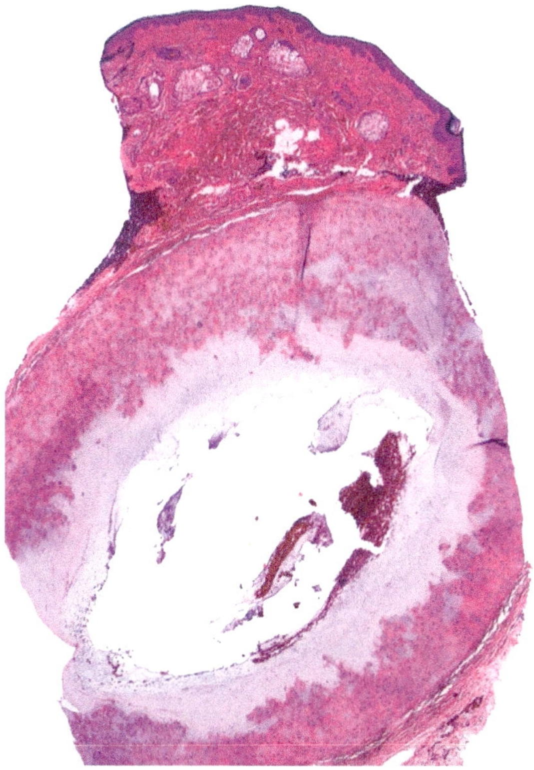

FIG. 9.27

Pseudocyst of the auricle: microscopic features. A pseudocyst forms as a cystic cavity without an epithelial lining within the auricular cartilage. Note the lack of inflammation around the cartilage.

Pathologic Features

A cystic space that lacks an epithelial lining is located within the cartilage (Fig. 9.27). The cartilage immediately adjacent to the cyst demonstrates hyalinizing degeneration and irregular thinning. Fibrous or granulation tissue may line portions of the cyst cavity. No inflammation is seen in the vicinity of the cyst. The overlying epidermis is normal.

Differential Diagnosis

Relapsing polychondritis is characterized by perichondral inflammation, whereas pseudocyst of the auricle lacks inflammation. However, an inactive lesion of relapsing polychondritis can be histologically indistinguishable from a pseudocyst of the auricle, but clinical features can readily distinguish the two disorders. Although chondrodermatitis nodularis helicis often has degeneration of cartilage, it lacks cystic degeneration typical of pseudocyst of the auricle and has prominent alteration of the overlying dermis and epidermis that is lacking in pseudocyst of the auricle. Traumatic perichondral or subperichondral hematomas have collections of blood around or within the cartilage rather than the acellular fluid that is present in pseudocysts of the auricle.

DIGITAL MUCOUS CYSTS

Clinical Features

Digital mucous cysts are located at the base of the nail on the dorsal aspect of the fingers and rarely the toes. These cysts do not connect to the underlying joint space. Another cyst, considered a variant of digital mucous cyst in the past, overlies the distal interphalangeal joint and connects to the underlying joint capsule; this type of cyst is better considered a ganglion cyst. Digital mucous cysts vary from soft and fluctuant to firm and dome-shaped cystic nodules. The cysts are usually solitary, range from 0.3 to 1.2 cm in diameter, and may be painful. Females are affected more than twice as often as males, and the lesions are seen primarily in adults, although occasional cases are seen in adolescents. The adjacent nail may be distorted.

Pathologic Features

Digital mucous cysts develop as papules or nodules on acral skin secondary to an accumulation of extracellular matrix material in the superficial dermis (Fig. 9.28). Occasional lesions have a verrucous surface. Some lesions are dominated by large cystic spaces that lack an epithelial lining. The extracellular matrix material is composed of weakly staining, bluish-gray mucin that expands the superficial dermis and compresses the dermal collagen at the periphery. Scattered stellate or spindled fibroblasts are present within the mucin. The mucin is well localized and usually near the epidermis, which often appears attenuated.

Differential Diagnosis

The characteristic location of digital mucous cysts should allow for easy distinction from other cutaneous mucinoses that enter the histopathologic differential diagnosis, such as focal cutaneous mucinosis, papular mucinosis, or a cutaneous myxoma.

GANGLION CYST

Clinical Features

Ganglion cysts are common and present as unilocular or multilocular cysts that arise in proximity to joints or tendon sheaths. The wrist is the most common site, especially the dorsal aspect, but ganglion cysts can also occur on the volar aspect of the wrist, dorsal foot, ankle, fingers, and toes. Most patients are young adults, and females are more commonly affected than males. Most cystic nodules are less than 2.0 cm in diameter, firm or soft and fluctuant, and often are mobile. Patients may complain of swelling or a mass, and occasionally pain and/or weakness. Spontaneous regression may occur in up to approximately 50% of cases. Recurrences are common, irrespective of the treatment option.

Pathologic Features

Ganglion cysts are characterized by unilocular or multilocular cystic spaces lined by a compressed fibrous wall. No epithelial or synovial lining is present (Fig. 9.29). Myxoid change is often present in the cyst wall. Mucin without accompanying spindled fibroblasts is identified within the lumen of most cysts.

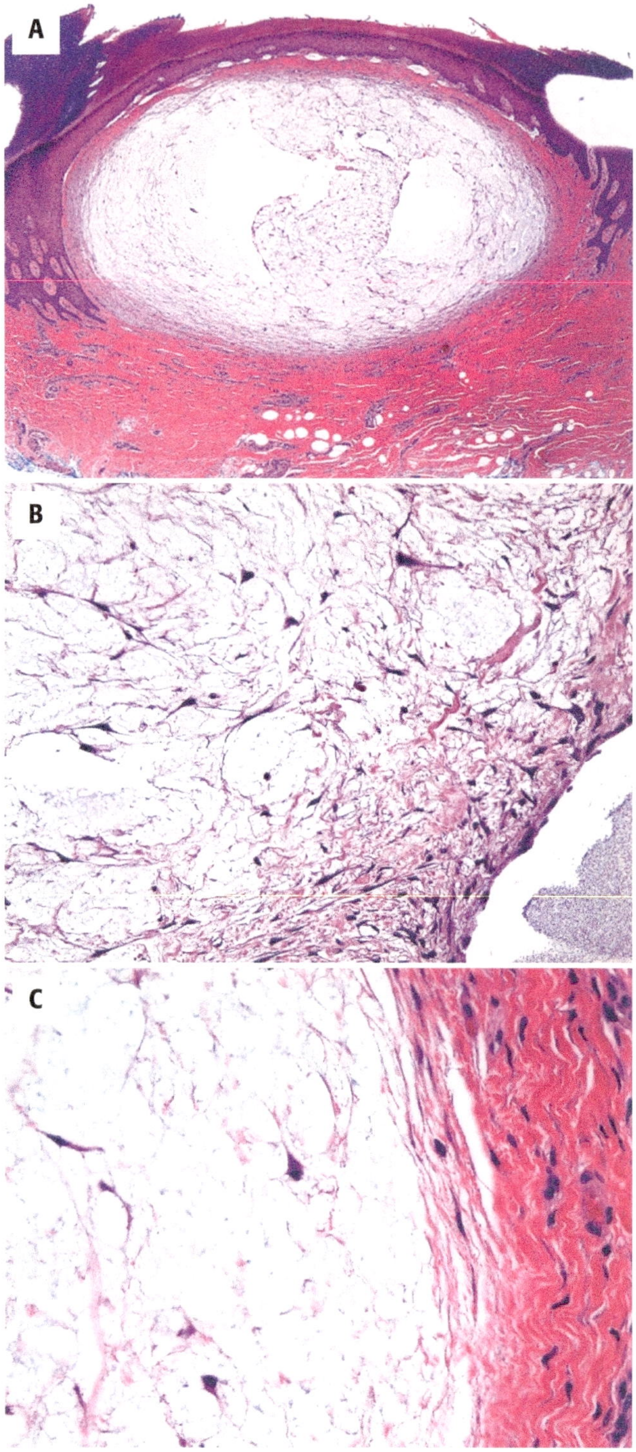

FIG. 9.28

Digital mucous cyst: microscopic features. **A,** A digital mucous cyst forms a circumscribed nodule in the superficial dermis on acral skin. **B,** Mucin is deposited between spindle and stellate cells or in cystic spaces *(lower right)*. **C,** The periphery of the lesion is well demarcated but an epithelial lining is absent.

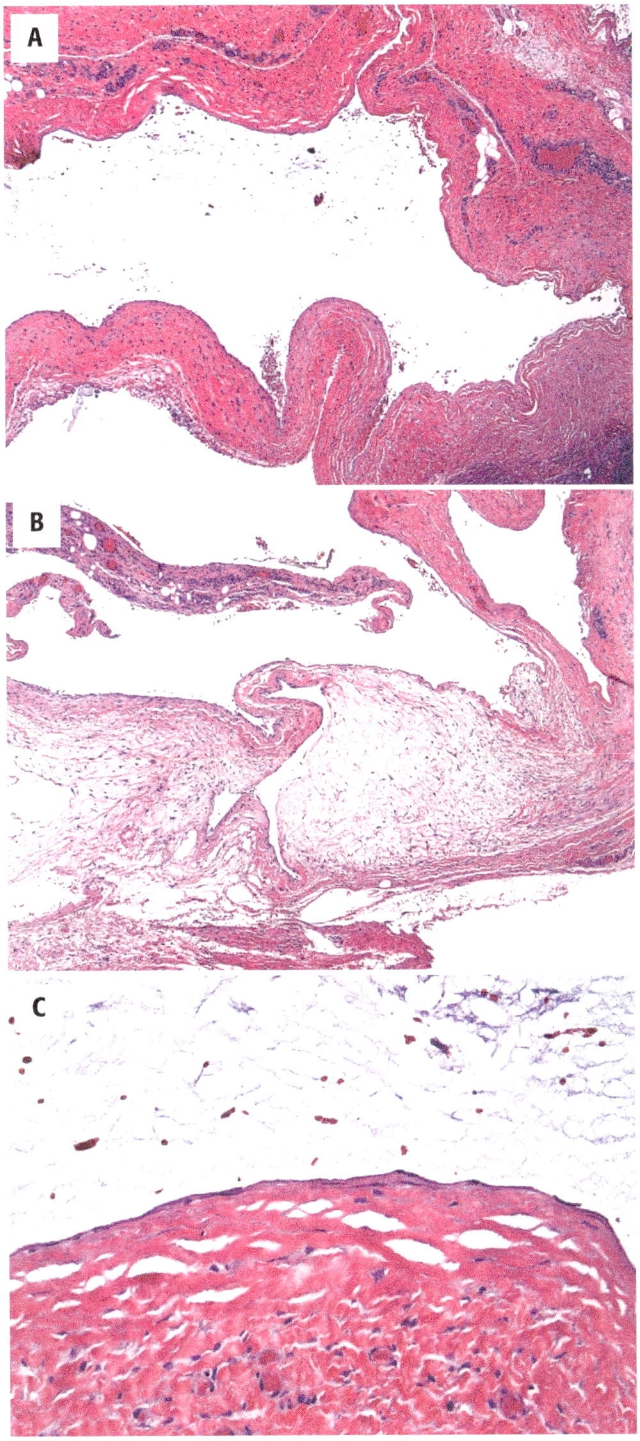

FIG. 9.29

Ganglion cyst: microscopic features. **A,** A ganglion cyst contains mucin and has a fibrous wall. **B,** Myxoid degeneration is often seen in the surrounding fibrous tissue. **C,** The cyst wall lacks an epithelial lining.

Differential Diagnosis

A digital mucous cyst generally has more spindled fibroblasts admixed with mucin in the cyst cavity and is usually superficial within the dermis when compared to a ganglion cyst. Cutaneous myxomas also have more spindle cells admixed with mucin than ganglion cysts and have an epithelial component in approximately one-third of cases. Metaplastic synovial cysts have villous projections extending into cystic spaces, merge with fibrous tissue at the periphery, and lack mucin within cystic spaces, in contrast to ganglion cysts.

MUCOCELES (MUCOUS CYST OF THE ORAL CAVITY)

Clinical Features

Mucoceles are very common cysts occurring in the oral cavity. They arise due to obstruction or minor trauma involving the superficial portion of a minor salivary gland duct. Mucoceles may be subclassified as mucous retention cysts, which are lined by epithelium, or extravasation mucoceles, which generally lack epithelium and are lined by inflamed granulation tissue. As extravasation mucoceles are much more common than mucous retention cysts, this entity is discussed under the category of pseudocysts.

The cysts are usually solitary, asymptomatic, bluish, translucent nodules that range from a few millimeters to several centimeters in diameter. Extravasation mucoceles have a predilection for the lower lip. Occasionally, mucoceles may involve the ventral surface of the tongue, floor of the mouth, buccal mucosa, and palate, in which case they are more likely to be of the retention cyst type. The majority of mucoceles occur in children and young adults. Rarely, mucoceles are associated with cheilitis glandularis.

Pathologic Features

Extravasation mucoceles demonstrate pale-staining bluish-gray mucin within the stroma of the submucosa. In early lesions, the stroma has granulation tissue admixed with inflammatory cells, especially neutrophils. In older lesions, histiocytes generally predominate and some, if not most, have a vacuolated appearance, leading to the term muciphages (Fig. 9.30). A variable number of lymphocytes, plasma cells, and neutrophils may also be present. Acini corresponding to an underlying salivary gland are a helpful clue to an extravasation mucocele where mucin is inconspicuous. In instances where a portion of the salivary duct remains, it may demonstrate squamous metaplasia. The overlying mucosa is usually intact but can occasionally be ulcerated.

Retention mucous cysts have a cystic cavity filled with mucin and lined by cuboidal salivary duct or metaplastic squamous epithelium. Periductal inflammation is slight to absent.

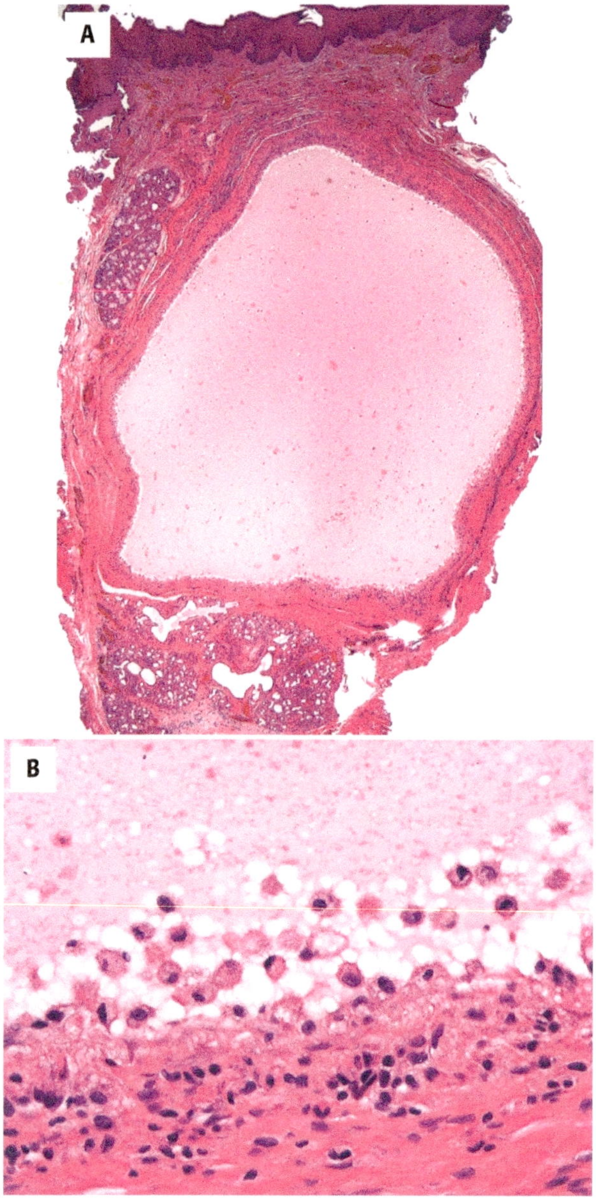

FIG. 9.30

Mucocele: microscopic features. **A,** A fluid-filled cyst underlying oral mucosa is typical of a mucocele. Note the minor salivary gland beneath the cyst, indicating that this cyst arose from the superficial portion of a salivary duct. **B,** Histiocytes with vacuolated cytoplasm (muciphages) result from ingested mucin. Note the absence of an epithelial lining.

Differential Diagnosis

In most instances, the location of the lesion, translucent clinical appearance, and conspicuous mucin accumulation does not cause diagnostic difficulties. When mucin is scarce and inflammation and granulation tissue are prominent in a mucocele, other inflammatory disorders enter the differential diagnosis, such as cheilitis granulomatosis or Crohn disease. Well-formed granulomas are not seen in extravasation mucoceles but are typical in cheilitis granulomatosis and Crohn disease.

METAPLASTIC SYNOVIAL CYSTS

Clinical Features

Metaplastic synovial cysts are pseudocysts of the skin that arise at sites of previous surgery or trauma. The lesions usually present as tender and erythematous papules or nodules. Most cysts are less than 1 cm in diameter. Essentially any age can be affected, although adults are more often affected than children. Most lesions are thought to represent suture granulomas prior to biopsy.

Pathologic Features

Metaplastic synovial cysts are dermal-based lesions, characterized by bulbous, villous projections of fibrous tissue into a central cystic cavity. The surface of the villous projections is variable, with hyperplastic areas lined by epithelioid cells, fibroblastic cells, and inflammatory cells bearing a striking resemblance to hyperplastic synovium, and some hypoplastic areas with a fibrinous or hyalinized appearance. The central cores of fibrous tissue forming the villous projections vary from dense to loose collagen, with small blood vessels and variable numbers of inflammatory cells and spindled fibroblasts (Fig. 9.31). The fibrous cores usually merge with scar at the periphery of the lesion. A fistulous tract connecting to the surface epidermis can be seen in many cases.

Differential Diagnosis

Digital mucous cyst is another pseudocyst in the differential diagnosis of a metaplastic synovial cyst, but the former lacks villous projections and is dominated by stromal mucin deposition with intermingled stellate and spindled fibroblasts. Ganglion cysts have mucin within cystic cavities, myxoid degeneration of the cyst wall, and generally lack the low-power architecture of bulbous villous projections into cystic spaces.

PITS AND SINUSES

LIP PITS

Clinical Features

Lip pits are exceedingly rare congenital anomalies that present as unilateral or, more commonly, bilateral depressions around the vermilion border, with a predilection for the lower lip. Most cases are inherited in an

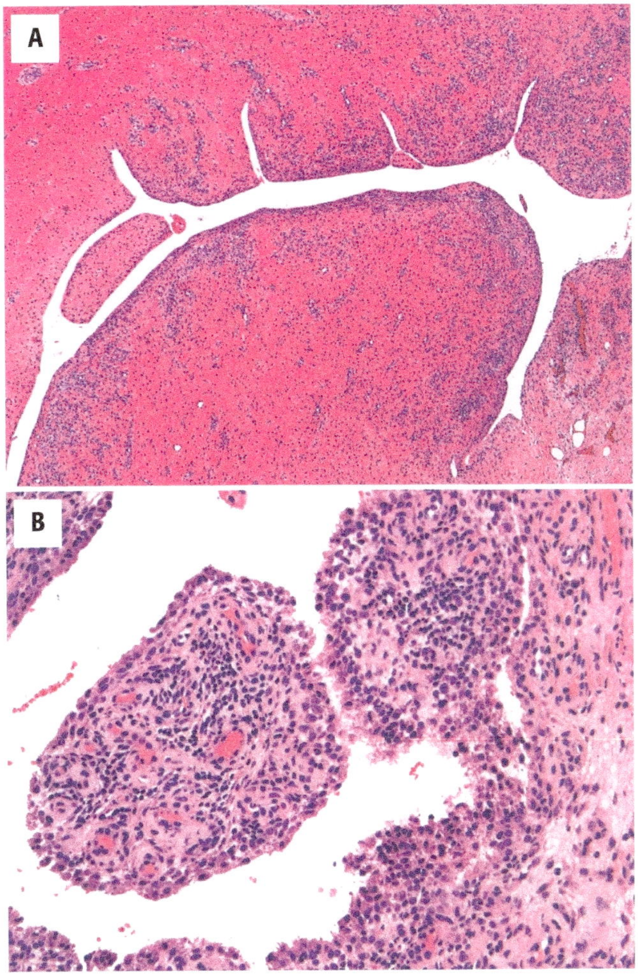

FIG. 9.31

Metaplastic synovial cyst: microscopic features. **A,** Villous projections of fibrous tissue into a cystic cavity are characteristics of metaplastic synovial cysts. **B,** The surfaces of some villous projections are composed of inflammatory or fibroblastic cells that resemble hyperplastic synovium.

autosomal dominant fashion (van der Woude syndrome) with variable penetrance. Females are affected approximately twice more often than males. Lip pits are closely associated with cleft lip and/or palate, as well as other congenital defects.

Pathologic Features

Microscopically, lip pits are characterized by invaginations of stratified squamous mucosa into the underlying submucosa (Fig. 9.32). These pits or channels are in continuity with the overlying squamous mucosa, which often has a heaped-up appearance. Rete ridges are seen along the length of the pit and tend to be long near the surface and short at the base of the pit. The underlying submucosa may contain thickened collagen.

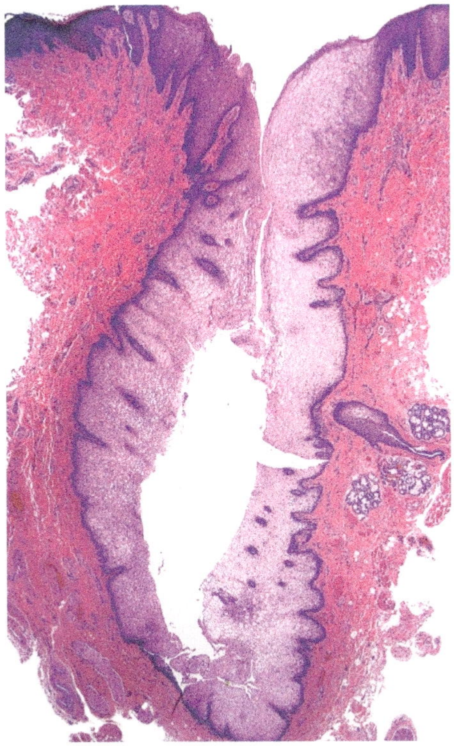

FIG. 9.32

Lip pit: microscopic features. An invagination of squamous mucosa is observed in a patient with van der Woude syndrome.

Differential Diagnosis

The histopathologic features, in conjunction with the location, should not cause a diagnostic dilemma.

SACRAL PITS

Clinical Features

Sacral pits or dimples are epidermal invaginations in the midline of the lumbosacral region. These lesions are common with the incidence estimated to be as high as 2% to 4% of the pediatric population. They are approximately four to five times more common in females than males and usually are detected in childhood. Occasionally, these lesions become infected. Sacral pits or dimples do not appear to be associated with a significant risk for underlying spinal dysraphism, although there is a low risk for a tethered spinal cord.

Pathologic Features

Sacral pits or dimples consist of stratified squamous epithelium in continuity with the epidermis that invaginates or protrudes into the underlying dermis (Fig. 9.33).

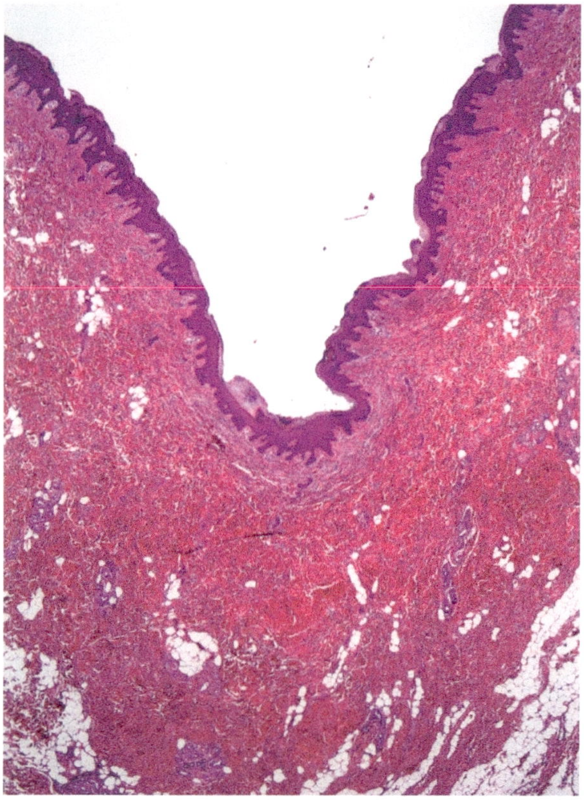

FIG. 9.33
Sacral pit: microscopic features. A shallow invagination of epidermis into the dermis characterizes the sacral pit or dimple arising in the midline of the sacrum.

Differential Diagnosis

The invaginations of sacral pits or dimples into the dermis are shallower than those seen in pilonidal sinuses or cysts, and rupture with associated suppurative and granulomatous inflammation, common in pilonidal cysts, is typically absent. Moreover, these lesions are usually removed at a younger age than pilonidal sinuses or cysts that are seen after puberty.

PILONIDAL SINUSES/CYSTS

Clinical Features

Pilonidal sinuses or cysts have a marked predilection for the sacrococcygeal region; rarely, pilonidal sinuses may occur in the axillae, genital region, umbilicus, or scalp. Most cases are acquired. They are usually detected in adolescents and young adults and are associated with hirsutism and obesity. Males are affected more than females at a ratio of 3 to 7:1. The lesions are often painful or tender and may have purulent discharge due to inflammation or superimposed infection. The sinuses or cysts probably arise secondary to perforating hair shafts. Rarely, squamous cell carcinomas can arise in a pilonidal sinus or cyst and, like those arising in scars, burns, or ulcers, are often aggressive tumors with a greater propensity for metastasis and risk of death compared to typical squamous cell carcinoma arising in the skin.

Pathologic Features

Pilonidal sinuses or cysts protrude into the deep dermis and often extend into the upper subcutis. Approximately one-half of cases show, at least focally, keratinizing stratified squamous epithelium lining a cyst or sinus tract in the dermis or subcutis. Granulation tissue and mixed inflammation, often composed of many neutrophils and variable number of lymphocytes, plasma cells, and histiocytes, result in response to superimposed infection or loss of integrity of the cyst lining. Multinucleated foreign body giant cells are found when extravasation of keratin and/or hair shafts occurs. In long-standing lesions, extensive fibrosis surrounds the sinus tract or cyst, and the inflammation is dominated more by lymphocytes, plasma cells, and histiocytes than neutrophils. An important diagnostic feature is the presence of multiple hair shafts within the cyst or sinus cavity or admixed with the inflammatory infiltrate in the surrounding dermis or subcutis (Fig. 9.34). Pseudoepitheliomatous hyperplasia, characterized by hyperplastic epithelium with sharp, pointed tips extending into the underlying dermis, occurs in some long-standing cases.

Differential Diagnosis

The combination of histopathologic features and typical location of this lesion usually lend to the correct diagnosis of pilonidal sinus or cyst. Other considerations in the differential diagnosis include infection, such as a furuncle secondary to *Staphylococcus* spp., hidradenitis suppurativa, a ruptured epidermoid cyst, or a fistulous tract associated with Crohn disease. Infection may need to be excluded with tissue stains and cultures but certainly can be superimposed on pilonidal cysts or sinuses. Crohn disease can be excluded by historical data and by absence of granulomas and presence of hair shafts in a pilonidal sinus or cyst. The sinus tract and hair shafts are generally longer in pilonidal sinuses than in epidermoid cysts.

A very important and often challenging issue is distinguishing between pseudoepitheliomatous hyperplasia and well-differentiated squamous cell carcinoma occurring in a long-standing pilonidal cyst or sinus. Pseudoepitheliomatous hyperplasia is characterized by

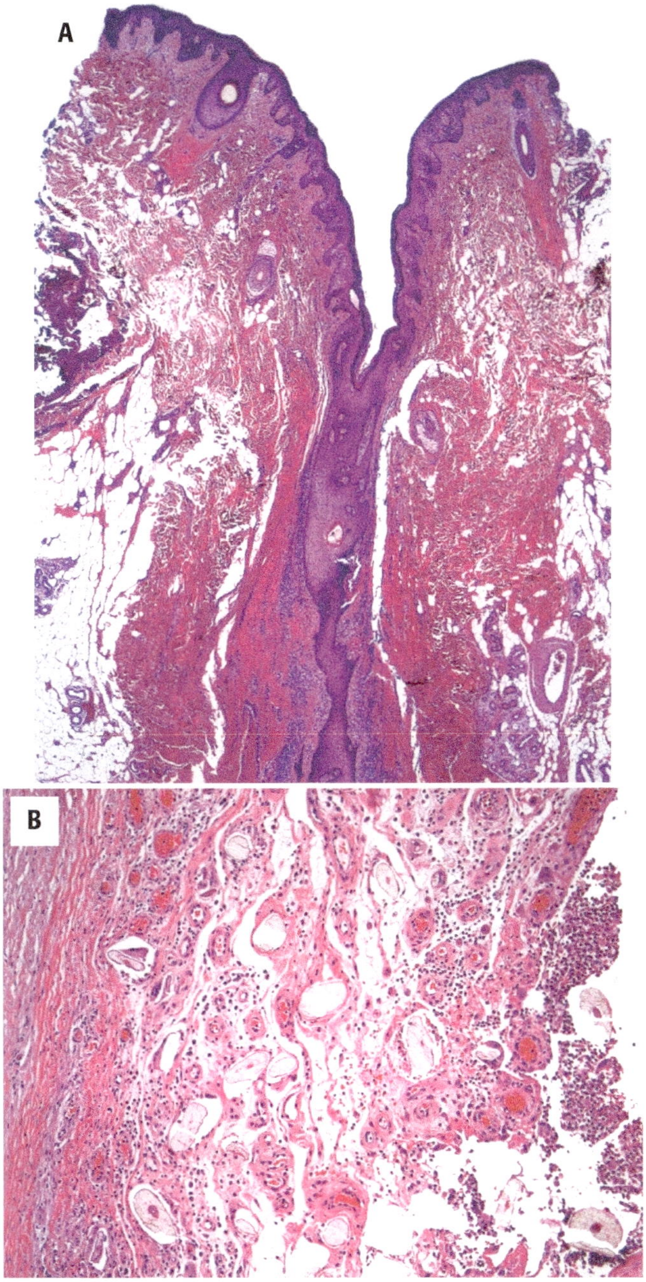

FIG. 9.34

Pilonidal sinus: microscopic features. **A,** The superficial aspect of this pilonidal sinus consists of an epidermal lining extending through dermis into subcutis. **B,** Rupture of a pilonidal sinus is associated with inflammation, scar, and a foreign body giant cell reaction to extravasated hair shafts.

irregular epidermal hyperplasia, maturation in upper levels of the epidermis, lack of significant cellular atypia, occasional mitoses, and most importantly sharply pointed epithelial strands projecting into the underlying dermis. In contrast, invasive squamous cell carcinoma has more irregular tumor islands infiltrating into the dermis, a greater degree of cellular atypia, atypical mitotic figures, and individual cell keratinization as well as keratin pearl formation.

CUTANEOUS DENTAL SINUS

Clinical Features

Dental sinus tracts present as suppurative nodulocystic lesions or draining sinus tracts in the skin that develop secondary to an underlying periodontal infection. Lesions often present as erythematous, firm to fluctuant nodules that may break down resulting in a draining sinus tract. Scar forms around the lesion with time and the center of the lesion may become depressed. Recurrent cysts and draining sinus tracts occur in response to local treatment without attention to the primary underlying periodontal process. The most common sites of cutaneous involvement include the chin or submental region and the mandibular or submandibular regions of the jaw. Most patients are adults, although children can also be affected. The gender distribution is equal. The clinical differential diagnoses include actinomycosis, infected epidermoid cyst, osteomyelitis, deep fungal or mycobacterial infection, foreign body reaction, or neoplasm. The correct diagnosis can usually be made by referral for dental examination and radiographs.

Pathologic Features

Most cases of dental sinus tracts have sinus tracts lined by granulation tissue lacking an epithelial lining. Suppurative inflammation and abscess formation are common. No sulfur granules composed of matted filamentous bacteria are seen.

Differential Diagnosis

Actinomycosis can resemble a dental sinus tract but differs by the presence of sulfur granules composed of a mat of filamentous bacteria, which are gram positive in a tissue Gram stain. Deep fungal infections are characterized by pseudoepitheliomatous hyperplasia, intraepithelial microabscesses, suppurative and granulomatous inflammation, and yeast forms on careful histologic inspection or in tissue stains for fungus. Mycobacterial infection has similar histologic features to deep fungal infections but has acid-fast bacilli confirmed in an acid-fast tissue stain. Infected epidermoid cysts usually have residual epithelial cyst lining or keratin debris admixed with the inflammation; these findings would also be true for nodulocystic acne, another consideration in the differential diagnosis.

Pseudoepitheliomatous hyperplasia can be present at the edge of a long-standing dental sinus tract and can raise the possibility of a well-differentiated squamous cell carcinoma (see pilonidal sinus for distinguishing histologic features).

SUGGESTED FURTHER READING

Bellet, J. S. (2013). Developmental anomalies of the skin. *Seminars in Perinatology*, *37*(1), 20–25.

Hörer, S., Marrakchi, S., Radner, F. P. W., Zolles, G., Heinz, L., Eichmann, T. O., Has, C., Salavei, P., Mahfoudh, N., Turki, H., Zimmer, A. D., & Fischer, J. (2019). A monoallelic two-hit mechanism in PLCD1 explains the genetic pathogenesis of hereditary trichilemmal cyst formation. *Journal of Investigative Dermatology*, *139*(10), 2154–2163.e5.

Jaworsky, C., & Murphy, G. F. (1989). Cystic tumors of the neck. *Journal of Dermatologic Surgery and Oncology*, *15*, 21–26.

Juárez, A., Rütten, A., Kutzner, H., & Requena, L. (2012). Cystic trichoblastoma (so-called trichoblastic infundibular cyst): A report of three new cases. *Journal of Cutaneous Pathology*, *39*(6), 631–636.

Kurban, R. S., & Bhawan, J. (1991). Cutaneous cysts lined by nonsquamous epithelium. *American Journal of Dermatopathology*, *13*(5), 509–517.

McGavran, M. H., & Binnington, B. (1966). Keratinous cysts of the skin. *Archives of Dermatology*, *94*, 499–508.

Requena, L., & Sáncez Yus, E. (1991). Follicular hybrid cysts. An expanded spectrum. *American Journal of Dermatopathology*, *13*(3), 228–233.

Tantcheva-Poor, I., Reinhold, K., Krieg, T., & Happle, R. (2007). Trichilemmal cyst nevus: A new complex organoid epidermal nevus. *Journal of the American Academy of Dermatology*, *57*(Suppl. 5), S72–S77.

Pediatric Dermatopathology 10

Sepideh Asadbeigi • Sharlene See

INTRODUCTION

While pediatric patients are subject to many of the same dermatoses seen in adults, this chapter focuses on conditions unique to or more typical of the pediatric population.

DISORDERS OF NEWBORNS AND INFANTS

ERYTHEMA TOXICUM NEONATORUM

Clinical Findings

Erythema toxicum neonatorum (ETN) is the most common pustular disease in neonates. Most children develop lesions within the first 48 hours of life, but lesions can also be present at birth. The condition evolves from small erythematous macules and papules to pustules and plaques. The pustules have a blotchy erythema which has been referred to as a "flea-bitten" appearance. The lesions clear spontaneously within a few days but may recur in the next few weeks.

Histopathologic Features

Microscopically ETN consists of subcorneal eosinophil-forming pustules. The eosinophilic pustules usually occur near the follicular units. The dermis shows perivascular or perifollicular eosinophils with papillary dermal edema.

Differential Diagnosis

The differential diagnosis includes mainly incontinentia pigmenti (IP) and transient neonatal pustular melanosis (TNPM). Both IP and ETN are associated with eosinophils, but IP shows dyskeratosis which is uncommon in ETN. TNPM is characterized by neutrophilic pustules, which are less common in ETN.

Prognosis and Treatment

ETN is usually benign and self-limiting. No treatment is necessary.

TRANSIENT NEONATAL PUSTULAR MELANOSIS

Clinical Findings

TNPM is a vesiculopapular rash mostly seen in darker skinned newborns. The process starts with pustules in a nonerythematous background, which rupture leaving behind hyperpigmented macules. These hyperpigmented spots resolve after a few weeks.

Histopathologic Features

Typically there are intraepidermal pustules with a predominance of neutrophils and some eosinophils.

Ancillary Studies

Gram stain to rule out a bacterial infection.

Differential Diagnosis

Erythema toxicum neonatorum: The lesions typically lack the background erythema seen in ETN. The predominance of neutrophils in TNPM helps to differentiate from ETN, which is predominantly eosinophilic.

Prognosis and Treatment

TNPM is usually benign and self-limiting. No treatment is necessary.

ACROPUSTULOSIS OF INFANCY

Clinical Findings

Acropustulosis of infancy is a recurrent but self-limiting vesiculopapular eruption that is mostly seen in infants. The lesions start as small and red areas on the palms and soles and evolve into pustules. They resolve with hyperpigmented spots. The lesions typically last for 7 to 10 days and then recur in 2 to 4 weeks. In most cases, the lesions resolve after the second or third year of life.

Histopathologic Features

There is usually a spongiotic epidermis with subcorneal or intraepidermal pustules. Those pustules contain mostly neutrophils and sometimes eosinophils. The dermis shows papillary edema and perivascular lymphocytic infiltration.

Ancillary Studies

Gram and periodic acid-Schiff with diastase digestion (PAS-D) stains to rule out infections.

Differential Diagnosis

The main differential diagnosis includes infectious etiologies such as impetigo or candida. Pustular psoriasis also needs to be considered. It is often accompanied by typical features of psoriasis vulgaris such as parakeratosis, thinning of the suprapapillary epidermis, and tortuous vessels in the papillary dermis. The pustules of ETN differ from acropustulosis because they contain mainly eosinophils.

Prognosis and Treatment

The process is self-limiting. However, the lesions can be extremely pruritic. Topical steroids or oral antihistamines are used to relieve symptoms. Dapsone is also used in more severe cases.

CONGENITAL EROSIVE AND VESICULAR DERMATOSIS

Clinical Findings

Congenital erosive and vesicular dermatosis (CEVD) is a rare condition that usually presents at birth. The eruption shows erythematous vesicles and erosions with crust formation. The lesions can be pruritic.

Histopathologic Features

Early lesions have perivascular inflammation with neutrophils and eosinophils, while later-staged lesions may show epidermal atrophy and scarring.

Differential Diagnosis

The viropathic changes need to be looked for to exclude herpetic dermatitis. IP differs from CEVD by an abundance of eosinophils and dyskeratosis. CEVD shows scarring, which is not commonly seen in IP.

Prognosis and Treatment

CEVD is usually benign and resolves spontaneously. Treatment is typically not necessary, but topical steroids are used to relieve symptoms and inflammation. The lesions may heal with a reticulate pattern of scarring.

SUBCUTANEOUS FAT NECROSIS OF NEWBORN

Clinical Findings

It is an uncommon disease that affects infants within the first few days of life. The lesions appear as hard and indurated nodules. These lesions can be fluctuant. Hypercalcemia is a common complication that happens in many patients. Some patients also show hyperlipidemia and thrombocytopenia. Numerous possible etiologies such as trauma during delivery, hypothermia, anemia, and asphyxia are suggested. The process resolves without treatment. However, in some patients, scarring and subcutaneous fat atrophy may persist.

Histopathologic Features

There is a lobular panniculitis with lymphohistiocytic infiltration and foreign body giant cells. The fat necrosis is basophilic and can form cystic areas (Fig. 10.1). Needle-shaped and refractile crystals in radial pattern are characteristic of this lesion. Foci of small calcification and granulomatous inflammation are also present. In older lesions, fibrotic replacement of fat cells is present.

Differential Diagnosis

Sclerema neonatorum is also associated with needle-shaped crystals, but they lack significant inflammation.

Prognosis and Treatment

Self-limited disease. No treatment is necessary. However, if hypercalcemia is severe, treatments such as hydration, calciuric diuretics, and bisphosphonates are administered.

SCLEREMA NEONATORUM

Clinical Findings

Sclerema neonatorum is a rare condition that usually affects ill and preterm neonates. Sclerema neonatorum is considered a sign of underlying fatal condition. The condition presents suddenly and progresses with hardening of the skin. The skin forms adhesion to subcutaneous tissue, muscle, and bone. Areas of induration and erythema can rapidly evolve.

Histopathologic Features

There are needle-shaped crystals, but there is no or limited associated inflammatory response or necrosis. The fibrous septa show thickening.

Differential Diagnosis

Subcutaneous fat necrosis of the newborn and post-steroid panniculitis need to be distinguished from sclerema neonatorum. All three conditions show needle-shaped crystals, but only subcutaneous fat necrosis and poststeroid panniculitis also shows fan inflammatory foreign body-type response.

Prognosis and Treatment

The prognosis depends on underlying condition and can cause mortality if the underlying condition is not treated. Usually, hospitalization in neonatal intensive care unit (NICU) is required.

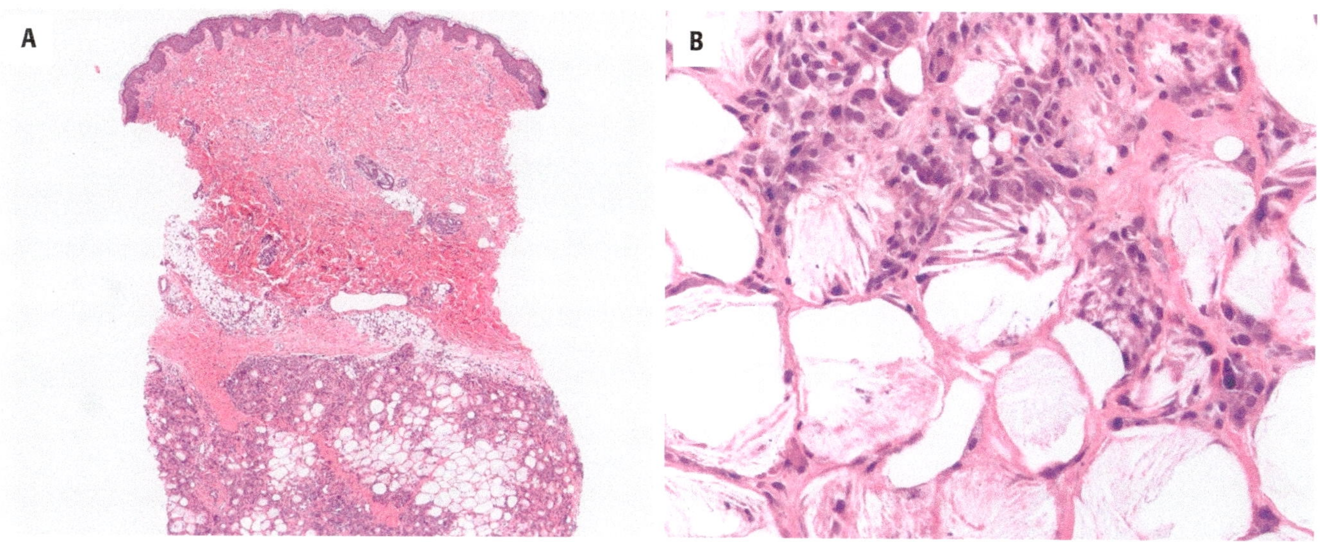

FIG. 10.1

A, Subcutaneous fat necrosis of a newborn. Lobular basophilic panniculitis with fat necrosis and granulomatous reaction. **B,** Fat cells show needle-like crystals with preserved outline.

HEREDITARY DISORDERS OF CORNIFICATION

ICHTHYOSIS VULGARIS

Clinical Findings

Ichthyosis vulgaris (IV) is an inherited condition caused by a mutation in the *FLG* (filaggrin) gene. The skin shows xerosis, scaling, hyperkeratosis, and erythema. The extremities are predominantly involved while skin folds are relatively spared. Patients may also show concurrent atopic dermatitis. The clinical onset typically occurs within the first year of life. In addition to xerosis and scaling, there is also hyperlinearity of the palms and soles.

Histopathologic Features

The main histopathologic finding is orthokeratosis of the stratum corneum. The stratum corneum is usually thicker than normal while the granular cell layer is significantly diminished.

Differential Diagnosis

Lamellar ichthyosis shows greater epidermal hyperplasia, which is not a feature in IV.

Prognosis and Treatment

There is considerable variability in disease severity, but the condition is inherited and lifelong. Therapeutic interventions such as daily application of topical keratolytics, such as lactic or glycolic acid emollients and urea, can improve the condition.

X-LINKED ICHTHYOSIS

Clinical Findings

X-linked ichthyosis (XLI), which is also known as steroid sulfatase deficiency or X-linked recessive ichthyosis, is an inherited skin disorder with xerosis and scaling. Patients present during the first few weeks of life with large scales that are loosely adherent. The lesions appear symmetrically and are widespread in the body, involving the extensor areas. The flexor surfaces are relatively spared.

Histopathologic Features

The histopathologic findings are mild. The epidermis shows orthohyperkeratosis, but the granular layer is preserved.

Prognosis and Treatment

There is no cure, but therapeutic modifications such as daily application of emollients, exfoliation, topical retinoids, topical keratolytics, and acitretin can improve the scaling.

LAMELLAR ICHTHYOSIS

Clinical Findings

Lamellar ichthyosis (LI) is an autosomal recessive disease, which presents at birth. The disease is caused by a mutation in the *transglutaminase 1* (*TGM1*) or the *ARCI* gene. The mutation causes accelerated epidermal proliferation and hyperkeratosis. Neonates are born with a collodion membrane. The skin develops generalized scaling. The scales are relatively large and form a mosaic pattern and are separated by cracks. The scalp may develop scarring alopecia. Some patients develop palmoplantar keratoderma. Nails can also show dystrophy. Thermoregulatory problems due to sweat gland dysfunction may occur. Also, stenosis of the auditory canal may lead to hearing impairment.

Histopathologic Features

Histopathologically there is compact hyperkeratosis and orthokeratosis with some increased mitoses. The granular layer is thickened. Some cases show focal parakeratosis (Fig. 10.2).

Differential Diagnosis

Nonbullous congenital ichthyosiform erythroderma (CIE): there are no distinct differences between these two, but nonbullous CIE shows a superficial inflammatory reaction, which is less common in LI.

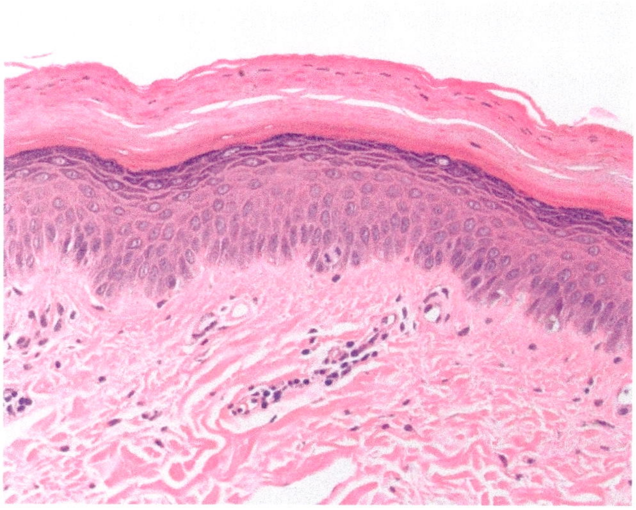

FIG. 10.2
Lamellar ichthyosis. Compact hyperkeratosis slightly thickened granular layer with focal parakeratosis.

Prognosis and Treatment

Although nonfatal, the disease is disfiguring. During the neonatal stage, the neonates are at an increased risk of infection. There is no cure but treatment modalities such as moisturizers, exfoliation, and oral retinoids are commonly used.

BULLOUS CONGENITAL ICHTHYOSIFORM ERYTHRODERMA

Clinical Findings

Bullous CIE or keratinolytic ichthyosis is a rare and autosomal dominant genodermatosis. A mutation in the keratin 1 and 10 genes is known to cause this condition. Bullous CIE presents as erythroderma with blistering in neonates and early childhood. As the patient ages, the blistering decreases but patients will develop ichthyosis.

Histopathologic Features

Histologically there is hyperorthokeratosis (Fig. 10.3). The epidermis is acanthotic with marked clumping of the keratohyalin granules. The upper epidermis also shows vacuolar degeneration (Fig. 10.3). The dermis can show a mild inflammatory reaction.

Molecular Studies

Genetic testing can confirm the keratin abnormality.

Differential Diagnosis

Epidermal nevi with features of Bullous CIE may also be seen. The clinical distribution helps distinguish whether you are dealing with a limited epidermal nevus or more widespread disease.

Prognosis and Treatment

Even though the skin appears thickened, the skin barrier is impaired. Treatment options include topical emollients,

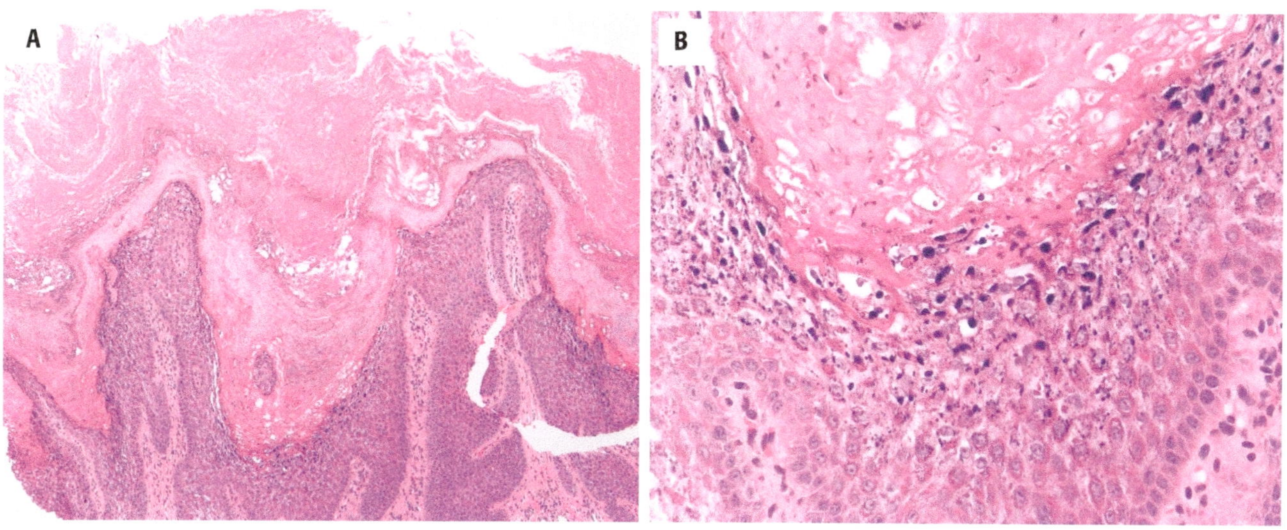

FIG. 10.3
A, Bullous congenital ichthyosiform erythroderma. Hyperorthokeratosis with acanthosis. **B,** Keratohyaline granules and vacuolar degenerative changes.

retinoids, and antibiotics in case of infections. Gentle debridement and exfoliation are also recommended.

NONBULLOUS CONGENITAL ICHTHYOSIFORM ERYTHRODERMA

Clinical Findings

Nonbullous CIE is a rare and autosomal recessive genodermatosis. It is similar to LI, and neonates present with a collodion membrane. The affected infants develop erythroderma and white scales after collodion membrane shedding. Palmoplantar keratoderma is also seen in some patients.

Histopathologic Features

There is hyperkeratosis and confluent parakeratosis. The epidermis shows psoriasiform proliferation. The dermis shows perivascular lymphocytic and neutrophilic infiltration.

Differential Diagnosis

Nonbullous CIE shows similar features as LI but displays more often a superficial inflammatory reaction.

Prognosis and Treatment

Nonbullous CIE is nonfatal, but infants may develop secondary infections and/or dehydration because of the impaired skin barrier. No cure is available, but emollients, exfoliation, oral retinoids, and topical keratolytics remain the primary therapeutic options for these patients. Topical antibiotics can be used in cases of infection.

ERYTHROKERATODERMIA VARIABILIS

Clinical Findings

Erythrokeratodermia variabilis (EV) is an autosomal dominant disorder, which usually presents at birth or within the first year of life. A mutation in the *Connexin 31* gene causes this inherited disease. The fixed lesions present as well-demarcated brown hyperkeratotic plaques. The migratory erythematous patches occur along the keratotic plaques. The hyperkeratotic plaques persist and progress over time.

Histopathologic Features

Histopathologically there is hyperkeratosis, orthokeratosis, acanthosis, and focal parakeratosis. The superficial dermis shows a perivascular lymphocytic infiltrate.

Prognosis and Treatment

EV is nonfatal but can worsen during childhood. The process mostly stabilizes during adulthood. There is no cure, but emollients, keratolytic agents, topical steroids, and topical and oral retinoids are used for symptomatic improvement.

PROGRESSIVE SYMMETRIC ERYTHROKERATODERMA VARIABILIS

Clinical Findings

Progressive symmetric erythrokeratoderma variabilis (PSEV) and EV are both autosomal dominant keratinization disorders with many similar findings. A mutation in the loricrin protein leads to PSEV. The disease presents with well-demarcated and symmetrical erythematous keratotic plaques. Approximately one-third of the patients show symptoms at birth. Both PSEV and EV are progressive and worsen over time. Both conditions stabilize during the adulthood.

Histopathologic Features

The histopathologic findings are nonspecific: orthokeratosis, hyperkeratosis, acanthosis, and a thickened granular layer.

Differential Diagnosis

In comparison to EV, the mitotic activity of keratinocytes is increased in EV patients.

Prognosis and Treatment

Similar to EV, PSEV is nonfatal but can worsen during childhood. The process mostly stabilizes during adulthood. There is no cure, but emollients, keratolytic agents, topical steroids, and topical and oral retinoids are used for symptomatic improvement.

NETHERTON SYNDROME

Clinical Findings

Netherton syndrome is a rare autosomal recessive genodermatosis. The syndrome affects the skin, nails, and the immune system. The gene responsible for this syndrome is *SPINK5*, which encodes the serine protease inhibitor LEKTI. Skin manifestations include ichthyosis. Neonates can show the symptoms at birth with a collodion membrane. The hair is brittle and shows trichorrhexis or a bamboo appearance.

Histopathologic Features

Histopathologically there is alternating parakeratosis and orthokeratosis. The parakeratotic foci have a diminished granular layer. The skin can show psoriatic-like changes with psoriasiform hyperplasia and neutrophilic abscess.

Differential Diagnosis

Netherton syndrome does not show thinning of the suprapapillary plates as seen in psoriasis.

Prognosis and Treatment

During infancy, some life-threatening complications, such as infection and dehydration, may arise. There is no cure, but multiple therapeutic strategies, such as antiseptic, emollients, and retinoid and keratolytic agents, are used to help with the symptoms. Other treatment options include intravenous immunoglobulins (IVIG) and narrow band ultraviolet B (NBUVB).

DIFFUSE AND FOCAL KERATODERMA

Clinical Findings

The palmoplantar keratodermas include a number of distinct entities resulting in hyperkeratosis of the palms and soles. There are three categories of keratodermas: diffuse, focal, and punctate. In the diffuse form, the palms and soles are involved. Focal keratoderma mostly involves the pressure foci. In punctate-type, small spots of hyperkeratosis appear on the palms and soles. This condition can be both acquired and hereditary.

Histopathologic Features

There are multiple forms of keratodermas, and they may have different presentations. The common feature they share is hyperkeratosis. Orthokeratosis is also found in many of the subtypes.

Prognosis and Treatment

Emollients, keratolytic agents, and topical retinoids are used for topical treatments. Oral retinoids are also used in more severe forms.

BULLOUS DISORDERS OF CHILDHOOD

EPIDERMOLYSIS BULLOSA SIMPLEX

Clinical Findings

Epidermolysis bullosa (EB) simplex is a subtype of a group of blistering disorders, which involve the skin and mucosa. A mutation in typically involving either *KRT5* or *KRT14* causes fragility of the skin, which can result in blisters. The disease is mostly dominantly inherited and exists in either localized or generalized forms. The localized form, also known as Weber-Cockayne, is the most common form of EB simplex. In this condition, the blisters mostly involve the hands and feet. Generalized EB simplex, also known as Koebner type, has a more generalized distribution and may involve the mucous membrane and nails. Dowling Mera is a generalized and severe form of EB simplex and is the most severe form it may take. It can cause severe thickening of the skin and the limiting of joint movement.

Histopathologic Features

The blisters are intraepidermal and occur within the basal layer. There may be degeneration of basal epidermal cells. The blisters mostly occur as a result of the fragility of the skin and friction. Hence, there is an absence of a significant inflammatory response in the epidermis or dermis.

Differential Diagnosis

Distinction from other forms of EB is mainly determined by the level of the blister with clinical and genetic correlation.

Prognosis and Treatment

Most patients have a normal life expectancy. The prognosis is variable. Avoidance of friction and pressure on the hands and feet can help with the lesions. However, the generalized severe type has a worse prognosis.

JUNCTIONAL EPIDERMOLYSIS BULLOSA

Clinical Findings

Junctional EB (JEB) is a form of EB, which is inherited and presents at birth. Associated mutations include *LAMA3*, *LAMB3*, *LAMC2*, and *COL17A1*. Patients present with generalized blisters and erosions, which occur in response to minor traumas. Nails and mucosa are also often involved. The blisters heal with scar formation of granulation tissue. The process can cause malnutrition and subsequent growth failure. There are two main types known as Herlitz JEB, which is more severe, and intermediate or the non-Herlitz form.

Histopathologic Features

The blister is subepidermal and has no to minimal inflammation because the lesions develop as a result of trauma. The basal cell layer is intact, which makes the split look clean and sharp. There is no epidermal necrosis.

Differential Diagnosis

Dystrophic epidermolysis bullosa: Scarring is more common in dystrophic EB, but since both blisters are subepidermal, distinction is typically made by correlation with clinical features, genetic testing, or immunomapping.

Prognosis and Treatment

The Herlitz form has a high rate of mortality and morbidity. The non-Herlitz form has a more favorable prognosis and some patients may survive to adulthood. The treatment includes lancing and draining the new blisters and protecting the skin from trauma and friction.

DYSTROPHIC EPIDERMOLYSIS BULLOSA

Clinical Findings

Dystrophic EB is a subtype of EB related to mutations in *COL7A1*. The distribution of disease is widely variable with some patients having more acral predominant disease and other patients having more widespread lesions. There are two subtypes of dystrophic EB: recessive and dominant. In both subtypes, the recessive subtype presents with milder symptoms. Nail dystrophy is also a common finding. Dermal scarring is present, which is a characteristic that differentiates its process from that of JEB.

Histopathologic Features

The microscopic findings are similar to JEB. Both entities show subepidermal blisters. However, dermal scarring and an associated inflammatory response is a more common finding in dystrophic EB and is rarely seen in JEB.

Differential Diagnosis

JEB: No scar formation or inflammatory response. Clinical correlation, genetic testing, and immunomapping are used for distinction.

Prognosis and Treatment

The prognosis for the recessive subtype of dystrophic EB is much better than that of its dominant form. That dominant subtype has a very severe and progressive course with significant morbidity and possible mortality. Additionally, patients with the autosomal dominant subtype are also more prone to developing invasive squamous cell carcinomas. Supportive care for both forms of dystrophic EB includes the same care used in all other EB disorders to relieve the symptoms and prevent further.

INFLAMMATORY SKIN CONDITIONS IN THE PEDIATRIC POPULATION

SPONGIOTIC AND/OR PSORIASIFORM DERMATITIS

The most prevalent epidermal and dermal inflammatory condition in children is atopic dermatitis. Atopic dermatitis can involve both pediatric and adult populations. The condition's histologic changes are very similar to the changes observed in the adult population, and this topic will be covered more comprehensively in other chapters. Other conditions most characteristic of the pediatric population will be covered in this chapter.

PITYRIASIS ALBA

Clinical Findings

Pityriasis alba is an atopy-related process most commonly seen in the pediatric population, between the ages of 3 and 16. Patients present with round to oval hypopigmented patches and fine scales. This disease is more common in individuals with darker skin and most patients report a history of atopy. The lesions are also mostly noticeable in patients with darker skin.

Histopathologic Features

The histopathologic findings are nonspecific. The epidermis may have some features of eczema such as mild hyperkeratosis with mild spongiosis and a perivascular lymphohistiocytic infiltrate. Parakeratosis may also be present. There may be irregular distribution of pigment in the basal layer, but melanocyte numbers are relatively normal.

Ancillary Studies

In contrast to vitiligo, immunohistochemistry for melanocyte differentiation antigens fails to reveal a marked loss in the density of junctional melanocytes. A PAS-D may be useful to rule out a fungal infection such as tinea versicolor.

Differential Diagnosis

When spongiosis is present, the differential diagnosis includes an eczematous dermatitis.

Prognosis and Treatment

Pityriasis alba has an excellent prognosis despite its relapsing nature. The treatment includes topical steroids, mild emollients, and calcineurin inhibitors. Phototherapy can be used in more severe cases.

JUVENILE PLANTAR DERMATOSIS

Clinical Findings

Juvenile plantar dermatosis is a chronic dermatitis of the feet in school-aged children. Most patients show symptoms during the winter. The process mostly involves the weight-bearing areas of soles. The skin can be pruritic or painful. The process also has an occlusive effect on skin.

Histopathologic Features

The epidermis shows psoriasiform hyperplasia and spongiosis. A confluent parakeratotic layer is usually present. A dense lymphohistiocytic infiltrate around the eccrine ducts and spongiosis around the acrosyringeal portion of eccrine glands are highly typical of this condition.

Differential Diagnosis

The differential diagnosis includes psoriasis. The latter shows less spongiosis and less perieccrine lymphocytic infiltration.

Prognosis and Treatment

Patients can improve symptoms by avoiding friction and wearing well-fitting shoes. Barrier creams, emollients, tacrolimus, and topical steroids can also be used.

HYPER-IgE SYNDROME

Job or hyper-IgE syndrome is an immune deficiency disorder that can affect several organs. The clinical and histologic presentation of patients with IgE syndrome is similar to atopic dermatitis, whose histologic presentation is discussed in other chapters.

GRANULOMA GLUTEALE INFANTUM

Clinical Findings

An uncommon form of irritant contact dermatitis which mostly occurs in infants under 1 year old. Patients often present with firm and erythematous nodules in convexities of the diaper area.

Histopathologic Features

The epidermis shows hyperkeratosis and parakeratosis. There is typically a mixed inflammatory infiltrate consisting of lymphocytes, histiocytes, eosinophils, neutrophils, and occasional plasma cells. While there may be dense perivascular inflammation, actual granulomas or multinucleated cells are not typical.

Ancillary Studies

A PAS-D or Gomori methenamine silver (GMS) stain may help exclude a fungal infection.

Differential Diagnosis

Granuloma gluteale is essentially a severe form of irritant contact dermatitis and mainly needs to be distinguished from other forms of eczema and fungal infections.

Prognosis and Treatment

It has an excellent prognosis. The condition is commonly treated with skin barrier, topical steroid, and antifungal if secondary infection is suspected.

INTERFACE/LICHENOID DERMATITIS

PITYRIASIS LICHENOIDES

Pityriasis lichenoides chronica (PLC) and pityriasis lichenoides et varioliformis acuta (PLEVA) are rare inflammatory diseases of unknown etiology, but they tend to affect children and young adults. Their clinical and histopathologic features are described in more detail in Chapter 1 of this book.

Clinical Findings

PLEVA typically presents abruptly with multiple erythematous papules, preferentially on the extremities. They become vesicular, hemorrhagic, and ulcerate. Most lesions are associated with itch.

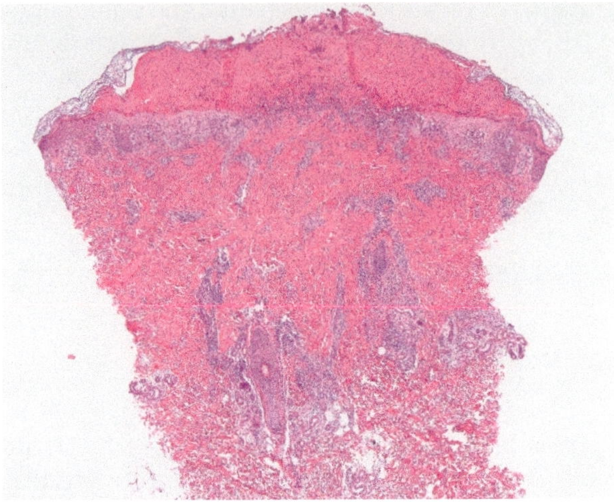

FIG. 10.4
PLEVA: Punch biopsy of an ulcerated hemorrhagic lesion associated with a lichenoid dermatitis.

Histopathologic Features

The histopathologic features of PLEVA depend on the stage of the evolution of the process. A fully developed hemorrhagic ulcerated lesion typically shows a hemorrhagic crust associated with lichenoid dermatitis with a wedge-shaped dermal inflammatory cell infiltrate (Fig. 10.4). PLC is characterized by focal parakeratosis and a variably cellular band-like lymphocytic infiltrate in the superficial dermis, which not uncommonly also involves the epidermis.

Differential Diagnosis

PLEVA needs to be primarily distinguished from lymphomatoid papulosis and bite reactions. The simultaneous presence of lesions at various stages of evolution and absence or low number of CD30-positive cells favors PLEVA. PLC in children may histopathologically closely simulate and be confused with mycosis fungoides (e.g., epidermotropism, lymphoid atypia). A predominant papular clinical presentation favors PLC. PLV and PLEVA are self-resolving processes. Residual hypopigmentation may last for a few years.

Prognosis and Treatment

Most lesions heal, but some ulceronecrotic lesions may be associated with scarring. Rarely, a severe acute febrile form of PLEVA may be associated with systemic disease and be potentially lethal. PLC is a chronic form of the disease with multiple papules at various stages of evolution and a tendency to relapse. PLEVA is often treated with erythromycin or doxycycline. Antihistamines may help reduce associated itch. Severe cases may require methotrexate or immune suppression.

LICHEN NITIDUS

Clinical Findings

Lichenoid disorder of the skin mostly affects children and young adults. The condition presents with small skin-colored papules which mostly involve upper extremities, trunk, genitalia, and buttocks. A Koebner phenomenon is usually present. Actinic lichen nitidus is a term used when the lesions appear on sun-exposed areas.

Histopathologic Features

Lichen nitidus shows a very characteristic feature referred to as a "claw and ball." There is a focal dense lymphohistiocytic infiltrate with epidermal collarette (Fig. 10.5). This pattern of elongated rete ridges gives a "claw" appearance around the inflammatory infiltrate and forms the edges of the lesion. Some cases show basal layer vacuolization. The overlying epidermis can show atrophy and parakeratosis. Multinucleated giant cells are often present. Red blood cells may be seen in hemorrhagic cases.

Differential Diagnosis

Diagnostic considerations may include lichen planus and lichen scrofulosorum. Lichen planus lacks the characteristic claw and ball morphology of lichen nitidus. Lichen scrofulosorum is associated with tuberculoid granulomas.

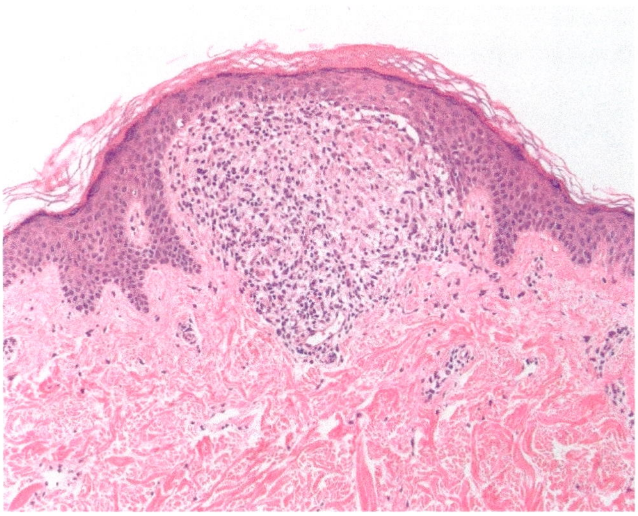

FIG. 10.5

Lichen nitidus. "Claw and ball" feature showing a dense lymphohistiocytic infiltration hugged by elongated epidermis.

Prognosis and Treatment

The prognosis is good and self-resolution happens in most cases. Treatment in patients with generalized lesions or prolonged course includes light therapy, topical steroids, or calcineurin inhibitors.

LICHEN STRIATUS

Clinical Findings

Lichen striatus is an uncommon and benign skin eruption that mostly affects children. The eruption starts with skin-colored to pink papules that can form linear bands over 1 to 2 weeks. The lesions affect the lines of Blaschko and mostly appear on extremities.

Histopathologic Features

Typically there is a lichenoid interface dermatitis (Fig. 10.6) accompanied by a superficial and deep perivascular and periadnexal lymphocytic infiltrate. Eosinophils and plasma cells are not commonly present.

Differential Diagnosis

Lichen striatus shows features overlapping with lichen planus at the dermoepidermal junction. However, the

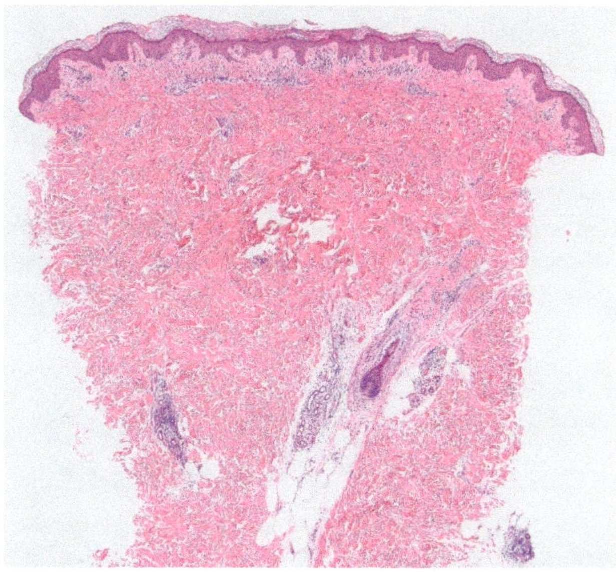

FIG. 10.6

Lichen striatus. The dermoepidermal junction shows vacuolar changes with lymphohistiocytic infiltration. There is also a deep perivascular and periadnexal infiltrate.

latter usually does not extend as deep into the reticular dermis as lichen striatus. Cutaneous lupus erythematous differs from lichen striatus by the presence of dermal mucin and basement membrane thickening. Lichen aureus is characterized by the presence of red blood cell extravasation and hemosiderin pigment.

PROGNOSIS AND TREATMENT

It is usually a self-limited process, and self-resolution happens in most cases within a year. For patients who experience pruritus or desire cosmetic treatment, a low- to mid-potency topical corticosteroid can be used.

NEONATAL LUPUS ERYTHEMATOUS

Clinical Findings

Neonatal lupus is a rare condition that is associated with passive transfer of maternal autoantibodies to the neonate. The antibodies involved are the same as those seen in Sjögren's syndrome (Ro/SSA or La/SSB). The rash appears at birth or within the first month of life. The rash can have different morphologies but in its most characteristic form shows annular lesions and can present with a similar pattern as that seen in subacute cutaneous lupus.

Histopathologic Findings

The microscopic presentation is similar to adult subacute lupus erythematous with interface changes. The DIF microscopy can show IgG deposition in a granular pattern.

Prognosis and Treatment

The prognosis for the skin lesions is good with resolution of symptoms after the first year of life. The most concerning cardiac manifestation is a result of damage to the cardiac conduction and AV block.

PAPULOSQUAMOUS CONDITIONS IN CHILDREN

INFANTILE GRANULAR PARAKERATOSIS

Clinical Findings

A rare and benign disorder of keratinization. It presents as red scaly papules or plaques. The most common involved sites are the intertriginous areas. This condition is associated with exposure to irritant agents and occlusion in folded areas.

Histopathologic Features

There is usually a thickened stratum corneum with parakeratosis. The hallmark feature is preservation of keratohyaline granules in the parakeratotic layer.

Ancillary Studies

A PAS-D or GMS stain may help exclude a fungal infection.

Differential Diagnosis

Atopic dermatosis, diaper dermatoses, or intertrigo: The preservation of the keratohyaline granules in the parakeratotic layer is distinct.

Prognosis and Treatment

Patients typically show a good response to topical steroid or retinoid therapy and removing responsible irritants.

PREDOMINANTLY PERIVASCULAR DERMATOSES

ANNULAR ERYTHEMA OF INFANCY

Clinical Findings

A benign hypersensitivity reaction that presents with varying-sized erythematous papules or annular plaques. These lesions evolve in infants and self-resolve with no scarring. The most common sites of involvement are face and extremities.

Histopathologic Features

Annular erythema of infancy shows a hypersensitivity reaction with dense perivascular lymphocytic infiltration and occasional eosinophils and plasma cells.

Ancillary Studies

A PAS-D or GMS stain may help exclude a fungal infection.

Differential Diagnosis

Other hypersensitivity reactions such as urticaria: The histology may be similar, and the distinction is mainly clinical.

Prognosis and Treatment

It is a self-resolving process, and no treatment is necessary

JUVENILE SPRING ERUPTION

Clinical Findings

Juvenile spring eruption presents as an abrupt papulovesicular rash which is triggered by sun exposure. The rash is considered one of the variants of polymorphous light eruption which arises in children.

Histopathologic Features

The histopathologic features are similar to polymorphous light eruption. The epidermis is mostly unremarkable. The dermis shows varying degrees of edema. Superficial and deep lymphocytic infiltration is a common histologic finding.

Differential Diagnosis

Lupus erythematous: shows interface dermatitis, a dermal mucin deposit, and periadnexal plasmacytoid dendritic cells, which are not routinely seen in juvenile spring eruption.

Prognosis and Treatment

Self-limiting process with healing without scarring. No treatment is necessary but topical steroids and antihistamines can be used when the lesions are pruritic.

ACTINIC PRURIGO

Clinical Findings

Actinic prurigo is also a form of photodermatosis that presents with pruritic rash in mostly sun-exposed areas. In severe cases, the lip and conjunctiva can also be involved.

Histopathologic Features

The histopathology is nonspecific, and clinical information is needed to make the diagnosis. The epidermis can show hyperkeratosis, acanthosis, and spongiosis. The dermis shows perivascular lymphocytic infiltration.

Differential Diagnosis

Juvenile spring eruption: shows fewer epidermal changes. The dermal edema is more prominent in juvenile spring eruption.

Prognosis and Treatment

Topical steroids and antihistamines are used to relieve symptoms. The main treatment is sun protection.

HYDROA VACCINIFORME

Clinical Findings

Hydroa vacciniforme is another type of photosensitivity disorder that presents with pruritic vesicles in sun-exposed parts of the body and is seen exclusively in children. The rash begins as vesiculopapular lesions which crust over time and leave a scar.

Histopathologic Features

The epidermis shows intraepidermal vesicles, spongiosis, and dyskeratotic changes. The dermis shows perivascular lymphocytic infiltration. Once the lesions crust, the biopsy shows confluent epidermal necrosis with a serous crust.

Differential Diagnosis

Other photosensitivity disorders: Intraepidermal vesicles and scarring are mostly seen in hydroa vacciniforme which are not common findings of other photosensitivity reactions.

Prognosis and Treatment

A self-limiting condition that remits by adulthood. However, scarring can be permanent. There are reports of a severe form of hydroa vacciniforme which can have systemic involvement. Like other photosensitivity reactions, sunblock and photoprotection are the main therapeutic management. Other treatments such as UVB and psoralen and ultraviolet A (PUVA) can be effective in some cases.

INFECTIOUS DISEASES WITH SKIN MANIFESTATIONS

VIRAL EXANTHEMS OF CHILDHOOD

VARICELLA

Clinical Findings

Chickenpox or varicella was one of the most common viral infections of childhood. However, its prevalence has decreased with vaccination. The process presents with fever and a vesicular rash. The vesicles tend to be pruritic.

Histopathologic Features

The diagnosis is mostly made based on clinical manifestations, polymerase chain reaction (PCR), and serology. It is uncommon to perform a biopsy in children. If a biopsy is performed, the histologic examination shows an intraepidermal blister. The blister has acantholysis and viral changes such as ballooning degeneration and nuclear or cytoplasmic inclusions. Other keratinocyte features include multinucleation, steel gray nuclei with peripheral margination of chromatin, and nuclear molding. Involvement of the hair follicle can also be present. The dermis shows perivascular lymphocytic infiltration. The histopathologic features of a herpetic dermatitis are illustrated in Chapter 3.

Ancillary Studies

For the distinction of different types of herpetic dermatitis from each other, immunohistochemistry can help support the diagnosis of varicella-zoster virus (VZV) (versus herpes simplex virus 1 [HSV1] or HSV2).

Differential Diagnosis

The main distinction is from other herpetic infections, which requires ancillary studies.

Prognosis and Treatment

The prognosis in children is good. The disease is usually self-limiting after 1 to 3 weeks. It can heal with a few scars. Adults show a more severe form of the disease and can even face life-threatening complications.

RUBEOLA

Clinical Findings

Rubeola or measles is a viral infection caused by the measles virus which presents with a fever and rash. The prevalence of measles has decreased after immunization became widespread but a recent spike has been seen due to some parents refusing vaccination for their children. Blue Koplik spots appear inside the mouth 24 hours before the rash stage. The rash is usually nonitchy and spreads all over the body, only sparing palms and soles.

Histopathologic Features

The diagnosis is mostly based on the clinical presentation, PCR, and serology. If a biopsy is performed, the epidermis shows syncytial epithelial giant cells. Perivascular lymphocytic infiltration is also present.

Prognosis and Treatment

A majority of patients do well however, about one-third of patients do have long-term complications. The treatment is supportive. Children diagnosed with measles should not be prescribed aspirin.

ERYTHEMA INFECTIOSUM

Clinical Findings

Erythema infectiosum or "fifth disease" is a viral infection caused by parvovirus B12. Its hallmark is the "slapped cheek" clinical appearance of the rash. A few days after the rash appears on the cheeks, it can spread to the extremities and trunk. The rash is generally nonpruritic.

Histopathologic Features

The diagnosis is made mostly on a clinical basis, PCR and serology, and a biopsy is rarely needed. The histology shows an urticarial pattern. The dermis shows perivascular inflammation with some eosinophils.

Prognosis and Treatment

In most cases, the disease is self-limiting and resolves after a few weeks. In some cases, complications may arise. The most common complication is aplastic crisis in patients with hematolytic blood disorders.

ROSEOLA INFANTUM

Clinical Findings

Roseola infantum or "sixth disease" is a viral infection caused by Herpesvirus 6 and, less commonly by Herpesvirus 7. It presents with a fever and rash. The disease has a classic presentation of a sudden onset high fever followed by a rash once the fever subsides.

Histopathologic Features

The histopathology is nonspecific and shows spongiotic changes in the epidermis with perivascular lymphocytic infiltration.

Prognosis and Treatment

The process is self-limiting and only supportive care might be needed.

UNILATERAL LATEROTHORACIC EXANTHEM

Clinical Findings

Unilateral laterothoracic exanthem is a rare rash in childhood that involves the trunk. The rash is typically present after viral infections and has been associated with different viruses. The eruption usually starts in the axilla and may remain isolated to one side of the body or eventually spread to the other side of the body.

Histopathologic Features

The histopathology is nonspecific and shows mild to moderate perivascular lymphocytic inflammation. The inflammatory cells surround the eccrine ducts without involving the secretary coils. The epidermis can show mild spongiosis.

Differential Diagnosis

Unilateral laterothoracic exanthem is more of a dermal process but foci of spongiosis may occur, which may lead to confusion with eczema. Clinical pathologic correlation is essential.

Prognosis and Treatment

It is a self-limiting condition. Supportive therapy is only used to alleviate the symptoms.

COVID TOES

Clinical Findings

The COVID-19 pandemic showed some distinctive skin manifestation among children. Inflammatory nodules in the toes and, less commonly, in the fingers have been reported. The lesions show similarity to perniosis. The symptoms include tenderness and a burning sensation.

Histopathologic Features

Histopathologically there is evidence of vascular damage with perivascular and perieccrine lymphocytic infiltration.

Prognosis and Treatment

The treatment is focused on pain control and in most cases, the COVID toes resolve after a few weeks.

GIANOTTI-CROSTI

Clinical Findings

Gianotti-Crosti or papular acrodermatitis of childhood is a skin eruption that primarily affects children. Gianotti-Crosti is a delayed immune response to a viral infection or more uncommonly can occur after vaccination. The clinical presentation starts with multiple symmetrical small papules or papulovesicles. The most common sites of involvement are extremities and buttocks, but the face can also be involved. Often there is a characteristic sparing of the trunk. The lesions can show positive Koebner phenomenon The process is benign but can be pruritic and lasts for a few weeks.

Histopathologic Features

If vesicular lesions are biopsied, the sections show extensive spongiosis with intraepidermal vesicle formation often containing Langerhans cells. The dermis shows marked edema and perivascular lymphohistiocytic infiltration. In nonvesicular lesions, acanthosis and moderate spongiosis are present. The dermis shows perivascular infiltration. In a small proportion of cases, lichenoid inflammation may be seen.

Ancillary Studies

Direct immunofluorescence is negative.

Differential Diagnosis

Some stages of the viral exanthem may be associated with spongiosis requiring clinical distinction from eczema. There may also be confusion with a drug reaction. The latter typically shows more dermal changes and may have more eosinophils.

Prognosis and Treatment

Usually benign and self-limiting skin eruption. No treatment is necessary but topical steroids can be given to alleviate the pruritus. Rare cases can have viral hepatitis with liver complications.

GRANULOMATOUS DERMATITIS ASSOCIATED WITH IMMUNODEFICIENCY AND PERSISTENT RUBELLA VACCINATION

Clinical Findings

Primary immunodeficiency in children may result in granulomatous skin lesions which can be one of the earliest symptoms of the disease. Other skin presentations include eczematous dermatitis, vasculitis, and erythroderma. Cutaneous granulomatous reactions are particularly common in patients with common variable immunodeficiency (CVID). Recent studies have shown that in some of these patients there is a persistent reaction to the rubella vaccine. In these cases, they have identified inactivated rubella vaccine viral particles in the center of the granulomatous reactions using specific immunohistochemical stains. Although the first cases of persistent rubella-induced granulomatous dermatitis were reported in patients with CVID, more recent studies showed the same reaction in patients with other inborn immune deficiencies.

Histopathologic Features

Histopathologically there is a dermal granulomatous reaction with a wide range of findings such as noncaseating, necrotizing, palisading, or tuberculoid granulomatous infiltration. Reported cases associated with rubella vaccination showed noncaseating granulomas or palisading granuloma with central necrobiotic collagen. The inflammatory reactions in cases of persistent rubella vaccine can be particularly destructive, with scarring and destruction of adnexa as well as suppurative inflammation (Fig. 10.7).

Ancillary Testing

IMMUNOHISTOCHEMISTRY FOR RUBELLA VIRUS

Immunofluorescence microscopy shows rubella vaccine capsid proteins. Reverse transcription (RT)-PCR and viral genomic sequencing for rubella virus RNA may help confirm the diagnosis.

Acid-fast bacilli (AFB) or Fite stains as well as cultures may help exclude a mycobacterial infection.

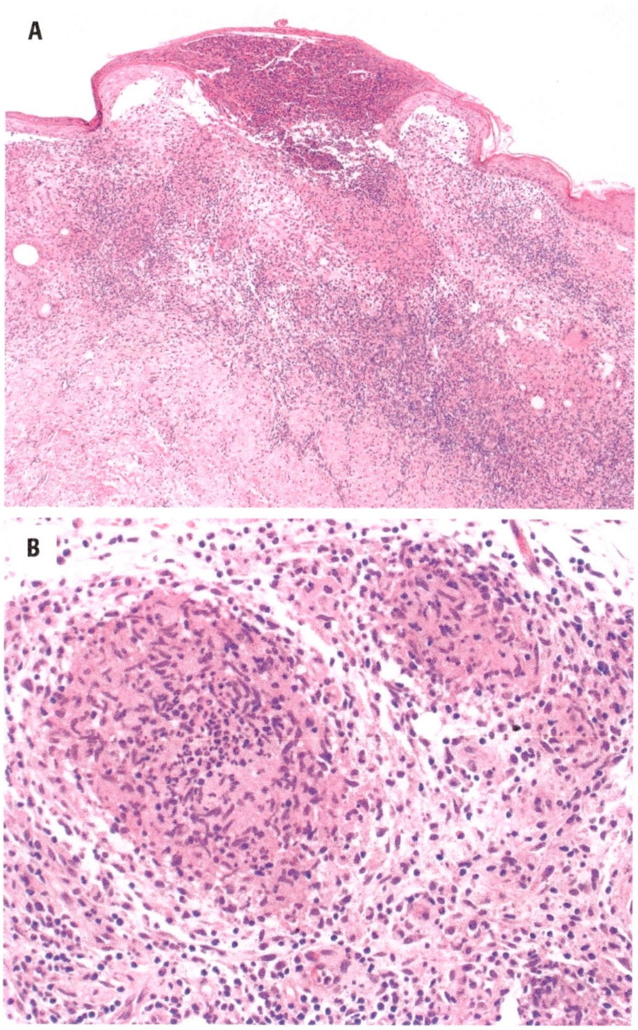

FIG. 10.7

A, Rubella virus-associated granulomatous dermatitis. Granulomatous dermatitis with associated suppurative inflammation as well as dermal scarring (lower left of image). **B,** Granulomas with central suppurative inflammation.

Differential Diagnosis

The differential diagnosis includes miscellaneous other granulomatous reactions of infectious or noninfectious etiology. Cultures, special stains, and clinical correlation are essential to establish the correct diagnosis.

MOLLUSCUM CONTAGIOSUM

Clinical Findings

A common skin infection which is caused by Poxvirus. This infection mostly affects children but can be seen in immunocompromised adults. Mollusca shows as tan, dome-shaped, and umbilicated papules which mostly appear on extremities sparing palms and soles. The lesions become ulcerated and inflamed.

Histopathologic Features

Histopathologic examination shows inverted lobules of hyperplastic epithelium with keratinocytes that contain eosinophilic intracytoplasmic inclusion. These inclusions are characteristic of molluscum contagiosum and called molluscum bodies or Henderson-Paterson bodies. The epidermis is often acanthotic. A mild to intense inflammatory response can be present. The findings are illustrated in Chapter 3.

Differential Diagnosis

The Henderson-Paterson bodies are very characteristics of molluscum and should not be confused with other diseases. On occasion, lesions may be densely inflamed and diagnostic features may not be visible on a partial biopsy sample.

Prognosis and Treatment

Self-limited but can show persistence which can be removed by curettage, cryotherapy, or a combination of salicylic acid and lactic acid, and imiquimod.

CONGENITAL RUBELLA

Clinical Findings

Rubella or German measles is a highly contagious viral infection that shows a maculopapular rash as the skin manifestation. Patients also present with fever and lymphadenopathy. Maternal infection during pregnancy can cause congenital rubella which results in fetal malformation syndrome. The infants present with "blueberry muffin" skin lesions.

Histopathologic Features

It is rare to see biopsies of skin lesions in congenital rubella. The diagnosis is mainly done based on serology and clinical information. If biopsy is performed, perivascular lymphohistiocytic infiltration is the main finding. No viral inclusions are present.

Differential Diagnosis

Other viral exanthems: the serology and clinical information will be used to narrow down the differential diagnoses.

Prognosis and Treatment

If the infection happens before 16 to 18 weeks of pregnancy, the risk of severe symptoms in fetus is very high. There is no cure for the syndrome.

EXANTHEMS OF CHILDHOOD RELATED TO BACTERIAL INFECTIONS

SCARLET FEVER

Clinical Findings

Scarlet fever is an infectious disease caused by *Streptococcus pyogenes* which mostly affects school-aged children. The skin rash starts with a blanching papular rash which coalesces into diffuse erythema which has a "sandpaper" texture.

Histopathologic Features

The diagnosis is made with clinical and serological findings and biopsy is not needed for diagnosis. The histologic findings are nonspecific. The epidermis shows spongiosis and parakeratosis. Edema, dilated vessels, and mild neutrophilic infiltrate.

Differential Diagnosis

Scarlet fever needs to be distinguished from various viral exanthems. Serologic and clinical findings are often needed for diagnosis.

Prognosis and Treatment

The prognosis is excellent with treatment. The treatment of choice is antibiotic (penicillin or amoxicillin).

CONGENITAL SYPHILIS

Clinical Findings

Syphilis is a sexually transmitted disease that can be transmitted congenitally from mother to fetus. Congenital syphilis can cause preterm or stillbirth. The causative organism is *Treponema pallidum*. Most infants are asymptomatic at birth and show clinical presentation within the first few months. The skin manifestation appears as a morbilliform erythematous rash which involves the posterior trunk, extremities, and soles. The lesions desquamate and crust over time, and if untreated, the lesions can scar and form gumma.

Histopathologic Features

The histopathologic changes are similar to infected adults. In primary syphilis, ulcer and lymphohistiocytic infiltration are present. Secondary syphilis can show psoriasiform changes. The dermis shows band-like lichenoid inflammation with many plasma cells. Perivascular and periadnexal infiltration is also present. Some cases show endothelial swelling and blood vessel proliferation. Granulomatous inflammation can be seen in later stages.

Ancillary Studies

Warthin-Starry stain and immunohistochemistry for Treponema *pallidum*.

Molecular Studies

PCR.

Differential Diagnosis

The presence of a lichenoid infiltrate with plasma cells helps to distinguish syphilis from psoriasis.

Prognosis and Treatment

Excellent prognosis if diagnosed and treated fast. Delayed diagnosis and treatment can lead to complications. Penicillin is the treatment of choice.

MISCELLANEOUS OTHER DISORDERS

VASOCCLUSIVE AND VASCULITIC CONDITIONS

KAWASAKI DISEASE

Clinical Findings

Kawasaki disease is an acute and systemic inflammatory disease that affects infants and young children and primarily involves the medium-sized arteries. The etiology is not fully understood, but an infectious process is suspected to trigger the onset. Patients present with fever followed by rash which can look morbilliform or maculopapular. Target-like lesions can be present in some cases. Changes in the oral cavity such as redness of lips, strawberry tongue, or injection of oral mucosa are present. Patients also show conjunctivitis, hands/feet swelling or erythema, arthritis, and lymphadenopathy.

Histopathologic Features

The skin shows severe edema and dilation of small vessels, and endothelial swelling, in superficial dermis. The smaller vessels show fibrin thrombi and patchy infarct.

Differential Diagnosis

Toxic shock syndrome does not show the vasculitis changes seen in Kawasaki disease.

Prognosis and Treatment

Typically, self-limiting within 4 to 8 weeks even without treatment. However, in severe cases, if untreated, patients can develop coronary artery damage during this time and eventual death. Patients are treated with steroids, antipyretics, and analgesics to control the fever and discomfort. Low-dose aspirin is used to reduce the clotting risk. IVIG is used as the treatment once the diagnosis is made.

DEPOSITION AND SCLEROSING DISORDERS

INFANTILE SYSTEMIC HYALINOSIS

Clinical Findings

This is a rare familial autosomal recessive disease resulting from mutations in capillary morphogenesis protein 2. The clinical features present by 6 months of life. The skin shows thickening and hyperpigmentation over bony prominences. Gingival hypertrophy, painful joint contractures, shiny and pearly facial papules, and perianal fleshy nodules are additional clinical features. These features and additional progressive symptoms such as diarrhea, malnutrition, and failure to thrive can lead to death within the first 2 years of life.

Histopathologic Features

The dermis and subcutaneous tissue show increase in thickness due to deposition of amorphous hyaline material. The dermis can show lack of elastic fibers and increase in fibroblasts.

Prognosis and Treatment

The disease may be fatal due to several multisystemic complications. The skin nodules can be treated with surgical procedures.

DISORDERS OF COLLAGEN AND ELASTIC TISSUE

PSEUDOXANTHOMA ELASTICUM

Clinical Findings

Pseudoxanthoma elasticum (PXE) is a rare autosomal dominant or recessive disease due to mutation of the *ABCC/MRP6* gene, which causes elastic fiber degeneration. The elastic tissue of the skin, eye, and blood vessels are mostly affected by this mutation. The skin becomes loose and wrinkled and shows yellow papules.

Histopathologic Features

The elastic fibers at mid-dermis show fragmentation and are short, clumped, and calcified (Fig. 10.8). The

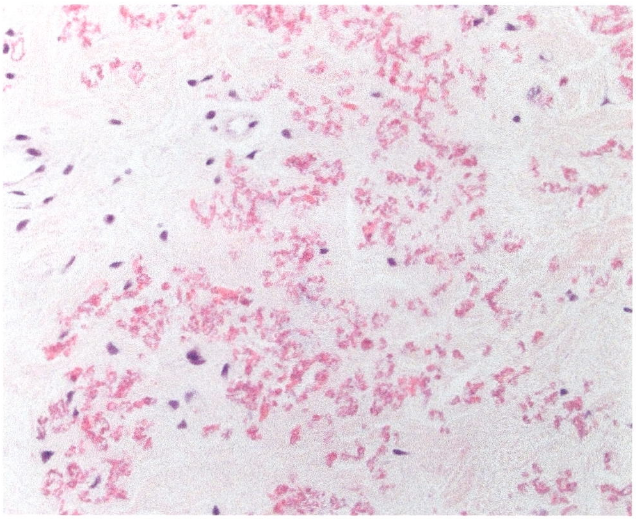

FIG. 10.8

Pseudoxanthoma elasticum. The elastic fibers in the dermis show fragmentation and are short, clumped, and calcified.

collagen fibers can show splitting and coiling. If vessels are involved, the internal and external laminae show elastic fragmentation.

Ancillary Studies

Verhoeff van-Gieson: Stains the elastin showing short fragmented elastic fibers.
Von Kossa: Stains the calcium deposits.

Differential Diagnosis

Cutis laxa shows loss of elastic fibers in more superficial dermis, remaining fibers are shortened and tapered rather than fragmented.

Prognosis and Treatment

Normal life expectancy but can have ocular or cardiovascular complications. Treatment is usually targeted toward symptoms.

CUTIS LAXA

Clinical Findings

Cutis laxa is a rare disorder of elastic tissue. It can be acquired or inherited. The skin looks loose, redundant, and prematurely aged. The skin manifestation appears at birth or early childhood.

Histopathologic Features

The elastic fiber density is decreased (Fig. 10.9). The elastic fibers are fragmented. Elastophagocytosis can be present. The acquired forms can start with inflammatory reaction.

Differential Diagnosis

PXE and PXE-like disorder.

Prognosis and Treatment

The prognosis depends on degree of systemic organ involvement. There is no treatment.

VASCULAR ANOMALIES

INFANTILE HEMANGIOMA

Clinical Findings

Infantile hemangioma is one of the most common vascular tumors in children. These benign tumors usually appear within the first few weeks of life, proliferate

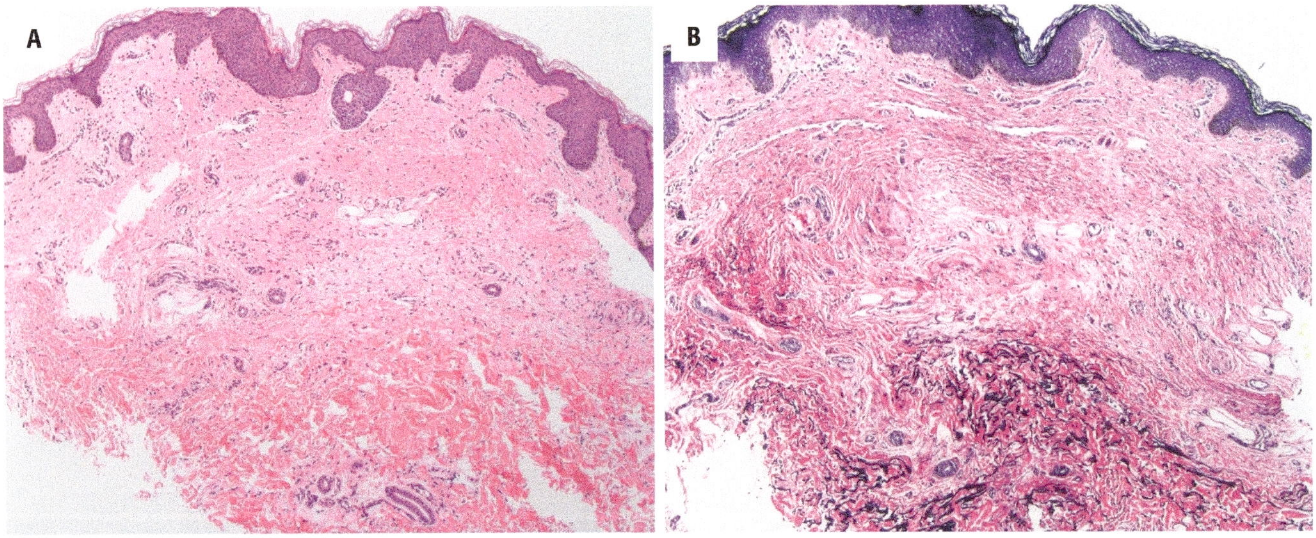

FIG. 10.9
Cutis laxa. **A,** There is a looser quality of the collagen fibers in the dermis. **B,** Verhoeff Van-Gieson stain highlights the decrease in elastic fibers in the dermis.

rapidly, have a stabilized phase, and then show involution. They can appear anywhere on the skin or occasionally in internal organs. Their appearance depends on the depth and location of the tumor. The superficial lesions show an erythematous papule, plaque, or nodule. The deep lesions have a bluish hue. If there are multiple lesions, screening for hepatic hemangiomas is recommended. Most lesions will have an involution phase after a few months. However, some lesions may not be completely resolved, and complications such as ulceration, obstruction, bleeding, and cosmetic concerns can occur.

Histopathologic Features

Histopathologically the lesions consist of a proliferation of variably sized capillaries (Fig. 10.10). Areas of dense cellularity and mitosis can be present, but the cells do not show any cytologic atypia. In later stages, fibroblasts and fat cells replace the vascular proliferation in later stages.

Ancillary Studies

Glucose transporter isoform 1 (GLUT1) and Lewis Y antigen stains are strongly positive.

Differential Diagnosis

Congenital hemangioma is negative for GLUT1 staining, while infantile hemangioma is positive. Pyogenic granuloma presents with a more lobular pattern and typically has a collarette.

Prognosis and Treatment

The overall prognosis is dependent on the size and location of the lesions. Most lesions involute. Lesions in cosmetically sensitive areas, larger lesions, or lesions without complete involution may require treatment. Topical propranolol is used for small and superficial lesions. Oral propranolol is used for lesions with higher risk of sequelae. More aggressive treatments such as laser, embolization, and surgery are used in patients with bleeding and in locations with more cosmetic concerns.

CONGENITAL HEMANGIOMA: RAPIDLY INVOLUTING CONGENITAL HEMANGIOMA (RICH) AND NONINVOLUTING CONGENITAL HEMANGIOMA (NICH)

Clinical Findings

Congenital hemangiomas are vascular neoplasms that start during the gestational phase and are present at birth. Rapid involution of the RICH subtype starts during the first weeks of life in contrast to NICH which does not involute. RICH is usually asymptomatic but may ulcerate and bleed.

Histopathologic Features

RICH shows small to large capillary lobules with well-formed and thin-walled vessels. The lobules are surrounded by dermal fibrosis (Fig. 10.11). Hemosiderin pigment can be present. Some vessels also show thrombosis. Some

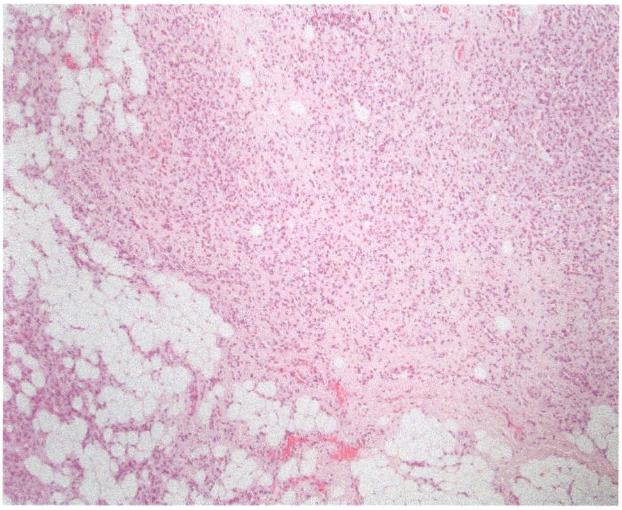

FIG. 10.10

Infantile hemangioma. Proliferation of capillaries of varying sizes.

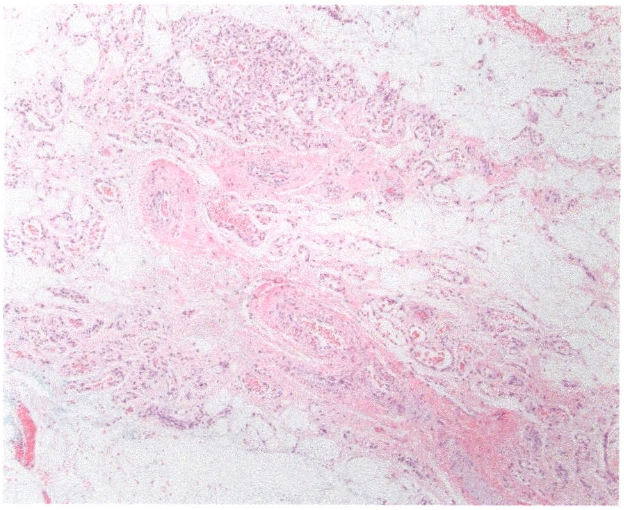

FIG. 10.11

Involuting infantile hemangioma.

lesions have a central convoluting zone. NICH shows dense fibrosis and the entire lobule can be thrombosed.

Ancillary Studies

GLUT1 and Lewis Y stains are negative in both RICH and NICH, and Wilms tumor protein-1 (WT-1) is positive.

Differential Diagnosis

Infantile hemangioma is more cellular and lacks the typical fibrotic septae separating the areas of capillary proliferation seen in RICH and NICH. Importantly the cells are positive for GLUT1 stain in hemangioma of infancy but negative in RICH and NICH.

Prognosis and Treatment

No treatment is necessary, but the secondary complication can be managed by pulse-dye laser therapy or topical becaplermin.

SUGGESTED FURTHER READING

Al-Rohil, R. N., & Selim, M. A. (2020). Inpatient pediatric dermatopathology. In M. Hoang & M. Selim (Eds.), *Hospital-based dermatopathology*. Springer, Cham. https://doi.org/10.1007/978-3-030-35820-4_19

Babu, N. A., Rajesh, E., Krupaa, J., & Gnananandar, G. (2015). Genodermatoses. *Journal of Pharmacy and Bioallied Sciences*, *7*(Suppl. 1), S203–S206. doi:10.4103/0975-7406.155903.

Boull, C., & Maguiness, S. M. (2016). Congenital hemangiomas. *Seminars in Cutaneous Medicine and Surgery*, *35*(3), 124–127. doi:10.12788/j.sder.2016.045.

Fraitag, S. (2021). New insights in paediatric dermatopathology. *Dermatopathology (Basel, Switzerland)*, *8*(4), 531–534. doi:10.3390/dermatopathology8040056.

Kahn, G., & Rywlin, A. M. (1979). Acropustulosis of infancy. *Archives of Dermatology*, *115*(7), 831–833.

Metze, D., Traupe, H., & Süßmuth, K. (2021). Ichthyoses—a clinical and pathological spectrum from heterogeneous cornification disorders to inflammation. *Dermatopathology*, *8*, 107–123. https://doi.org/10.3390/dermatopathology8020017

Phung, T. L., Wright, T. S. Pourciau, C. Y., & Smoller, B. R. (2017). *Pediatric Dermatopathology*. Springer, Cham. https://doi.org/10.1007/978-3-319-44824-4

Shields, B. E., Perelygina, L., Samimi, S., Haun, P., Leung, T., Abernathy, E., Chen, M. H., Hao, L., Icenogle, J., Drolet, B., Wilson, B., Bryer, J. S., England, R., Blumberg, E., Wanat, K. A., Sullivan, K., & Rosenbach, M. (2021). Granulomatous dermatitis associated with rubella virus infection in an adult with immunodeficiency. *JAMA Dermatology*, *157*(7), 842–847. doi:10.1001/jamadermatol.2021.1577.

Takeichi, T., & Akiyama, M. (2016). Inherited ichthyosis: Non-syndromic forms. *Journal of dermatology*, *43*(3), 242–251. doi:10.1111/1346-8138.13243.

Torrelo, A., & Hernández, A. (2008). Panniculitis in children. *Dermatologic Clinics*, *26*(4), 491–500, vii. doi:10.1016/j.det.2008.05.010.

Wagner, A. (1997). Distinguishing vesicular and pustular disorders in the neonate. *Current Opinion in Pediatrics*, *9*(4), 396–405. doi:10.1097/00008480-199708000-00015.

Wilson, A., & Murrell, D. F. (2022). Clinical features of chronic bullous dermatosis of childhood. *Clinical and Experimental Dermatology*, *47*(5), 873–881. doi:10.1111/ced.15059.

Section 2

Tumors of the Skin and Subcutis

11 Tumors of the Epidermis

Angela J. Wyatt • Klaus J. Busam

BENIGN TUMORS AND TUMOR-LIKE PROLIFERATIONS OF THE EPIDERMIS

The lesions described herein include noninfectious pseudoepitheliomatous epidermal hyperplasia, benign acanthomas and keratoses, and epidermal nevi. Epidermal proliferations associated with warts or deep fungal infections are described in the chapter on infectious diseases.

REACTIVE EPIDERMAL HYPERPLASIA WITH EMPHASIS ON PSEUDOEPITHELIOMATOUS HYPERPLASIA

Reactive epidermal hyperplasia is common. It may be associated with wound healing, infection, and miscellaneous inflammatory dermatoses, including lichen simplex chronicus (LLC) or prurigo nodularis. Epidermal hyperplasia may also be associated with a neoplastic process such as a dermatofibroma, melanocytic tumor or granular cell tumor, an inflammatory condition such as hypertrophic lichen planus, or a lymphoproliferative condition such as CD30-positive cutaneous anaplastic large cell lymphoma. Although most cases of benign reactive hyperplasia are easily distinguished from carcinoma, the diagnosis can be difficult, especially on partial superficial biopsies and/or associated ulceration with no clinical context. Reactive epidermal proliferation simulating carcinoma is referred to as pseudoepitheliomatous hyperplasia (PEH).

PEH is histologically characterized by irregular acanthosis of the epidermis, often with triangular-shaped and elongated thin epidermal rete ridges pointing into the dermis and squamatization of the basal layer (Fig. 11.1). Reactive nuclear atypia may be present manifesting as enlarged nuclei with smooth nuclear contours, an open chromatin pattern, and distinct nucleoli. Maturation of keratinocytes is maintained. PEH can affect the follicular infundibulum and acrosyringium and be associated with squamous metaplasia of the sweat duct.

Clinical and histologic context are important for the distinction of PEH from squamous cell carcinoma (SCC). PEH tends to be associated with a history of or histologic features of trauma (e.g., hemorrhage, subepidermal fibrin, ulcer, granulation tissue) or prior surgery (dermal fibrosis). Although PEH often blends into the background because of the similarity in nuclear features of its constituent keratinocytes to those of adjacent nonlesional epidermis, SCC has a distinct architecture and cytology, forming a discrete tumor with infiltrative growth, cytologic atypia, and disturbed maturation.

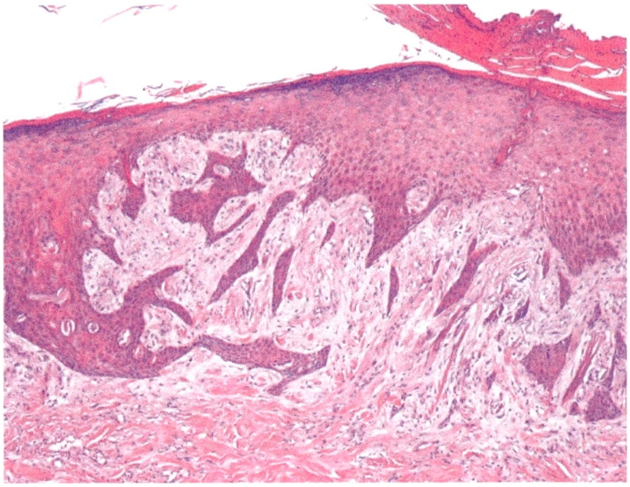

FIG. 11.1

Pseudoepitheliomatous hyperplasia. Irregular extension of elongated rete ridges is present at a healing biopsy site. The proliferative keratinocytes show normal maturation and lack atypia.

Other nonneoplastic squamoproliferative lesions that may mimic carcinoma include hypertrophic lichen planus and hypertrophic lupus erythematosus (LE). Their distinction from SCC is discussed later in this chapter.

KERATINIZING EPIDERMAL NEVUS

Clinical Findings

Epidermal nevi may be pink, flesh-colored, brown or gray, papillomatous or cerebriform, forming papules or plaques, at times in a linear configuration. They are frequently asymptomatic, although occasionally pruritic with erythema and hyperkeratosis as in the

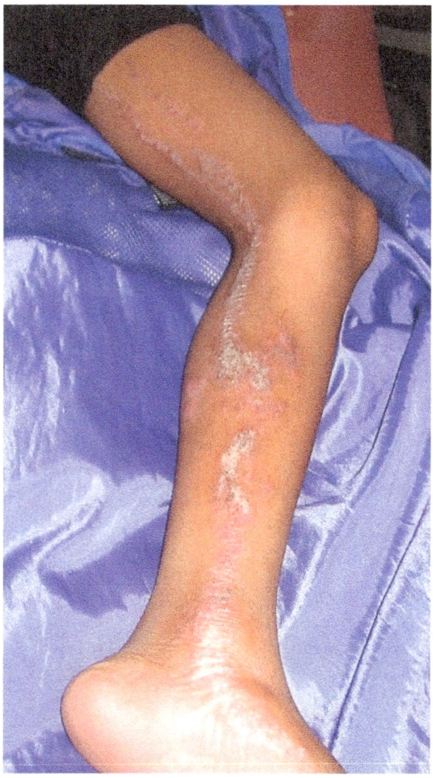

FIG. 11.2

Inflammatory linear epidermal nevus forming a linear keratotic lesion along the entire length of the leg.

inflammatory linear verrucous epidermal nevus (ILVEN). They can be present at birth. Most manifest during childhood and are noticeable by 10 years of age. These nevi are longitudinal on the extremities (Fig. 11.2) but transverse on the trunk, with a curvilinear, almost swirling configuration, following Blaschko's lines. They typically do not cross the midline. Secondary tumors such as trichoblastoma, keratoacanthoma (KA), and SCC have been reported to develop in association with epidermal nevi. Epidermal nevi may present as cutaneous lesions only or represent a part of syndrome (epidermal nevus syndrome). Cases of isolated epidermal nevi without a full developmental syndrome are the result of postzygotic mosaic mutations. The various histologic patterns are associated with specific mutations. For example, epidermal nevi with epidermolytic hyperkeratosis (EHK) are associated with mosaic mutations involving keratin 1 or 10, while epidermal nevi with acantholytic dyskeratosis as seen in Darier's disease are associated with ATP2A2.

EPIDERMAL NEVUS—DISEASE FACT SHEET

Definition

- Epidermal nevus represents a developmental malformation of the epidermis

Patient Group

- Usually manifests in childhood

Site of Involvement

- Extremities and trunk

Clinical Findings

- Warty papule or plaque
- May be linear or zosteriform

Clinical Variants

- Nevus verrucosus (localized wartlike lesion)
- Nevus unius lateralis (long linear unilateral lesion, usually on an extremity)
- Ichthyosis hystrix (large, often bilateral lesions on the trunk)
- Inflammatory linear verrucous epidermal nevus (persistent pruritic plaque composed of tiny confluent warty papules, usually on an extremity)
- Epidermal nevus with epidermolytic hyperkeratosis

Epidermal Nevus Syndromes

- Epidermal nevus is part of a syndrome, often with neurologic or musculoskeletal abnormalities

Prognosis and Treatment

- Epidermal nevus as an isolated skin lesion is mainly a cosmetic problem
- Treatment is often challenging depending on its size (surgery, medical)

EPIDERMAL NEVUS—PATHOLOGIC FEATURES

Histologic Features

- Epidermal hyperplasia with hyperkeratosis
- Absence of keratinocytic atypia
- May mimic any pattern seen in seborrheic keratosis
- May show features of epidermolytic hyperkeratosis
- May show acantholysis
- May show cornoid lamellae

Differential Diagnosis (Clinical History Is Essential)

- Seborrheic keratosis
- Verruca
- Nevus sebaceus
- Porokeratosis
- Focal acantholytic dyskeratosis

Histologic Features

All epidermal nevi share hyperkeratosis and epidermal thickening. Many different histologic patterns have been reported. The silhouette may be papillomatous (Fig. 11.3A), acanthotic, or a mixture thereof, often accompanied by hyperpigmentation of the basal cell layer. Any pattern associated with seborrheic keratoses (SKs) also may be found in epidermal nevi, including patterns of irritated and clonal SK (Fig. 11.3B). Features of EHK may be seen in an epidermal nevus (Fig. 11.4). An epidermal nevus with EHK demonstrates orthokeratosis and a thickened granular layer with enlarged

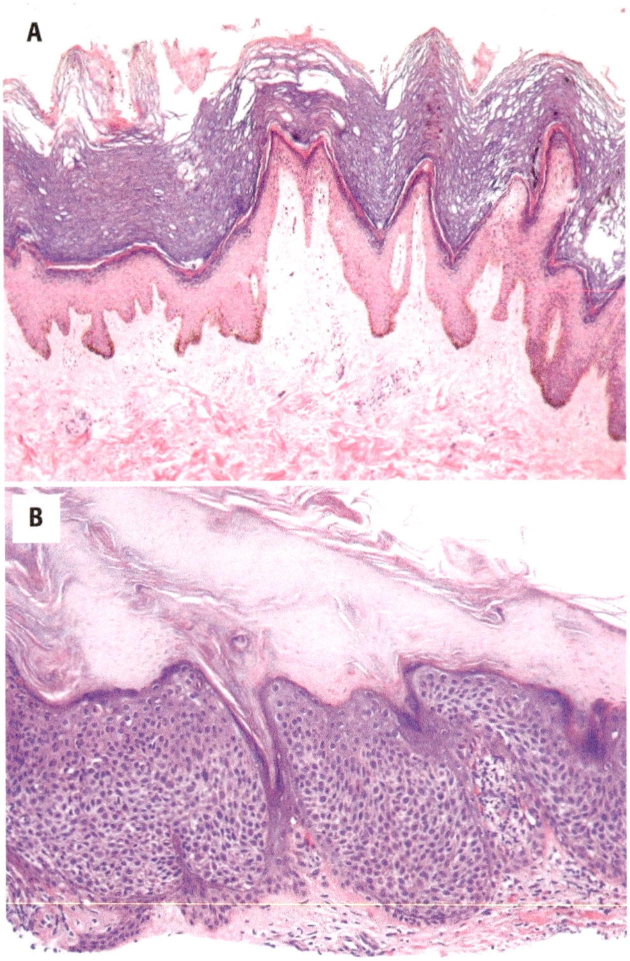

FIG. 11.3

A, Epidermal nevus with papillomatous epidermal hyperplasia and hyperkeratosis. **B,** Epidermal nevus with the pattern of an irritated "clonal" seborrheic keratosis.

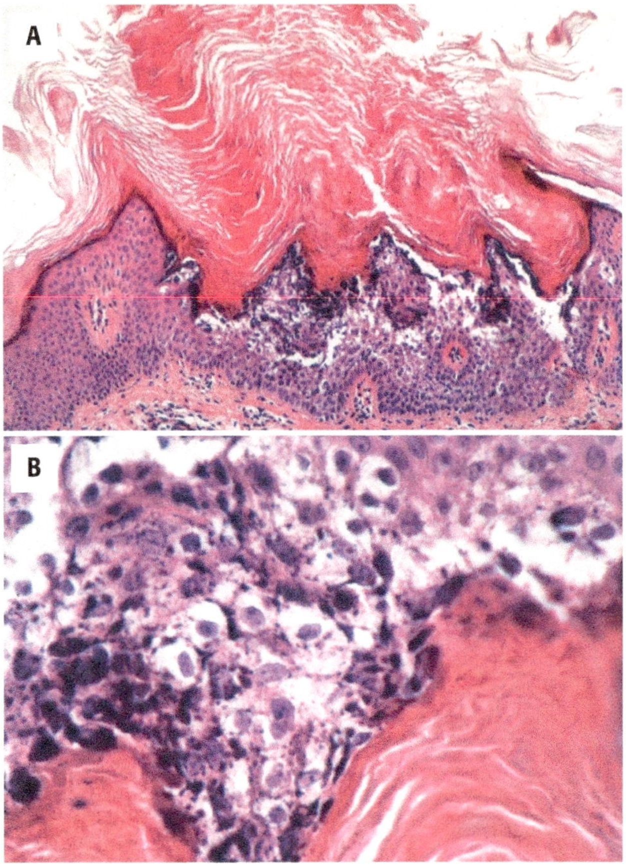

FIG. 11.4

Epidermal nevus with epidermolytic hyperkeratosis. **A,** Papillomatous silhouette associated with hyperkeratosis. **B,** Thickened granular layer with enlarged keratohyaline granules. The keratinocytes show perinuclear clearing and vacuolar change.

keratohyaline granules. Affected keratinocytes have perinuclear clearing and vacuolar change with indistinct cell borders.

ILVEN typically shows vertically and horizontally alternating parakeratosis with orthokeratosis (Fig. 11.5), which has been likened to a checkerboard. In addition to the psoriasiform epidermal hyperplasia, there is often a predominantly lymphocytic inflammatory cell infiltrate.

Differential Diagnosis

A keratinizing epidermal nevus is usually suspected based on the clinical picture, but nevus sebaceus may mimic it, and only histologic examination can differentiate the two. An epidermal nevus lacks the alterations of adnexal structures typically seen in nevus sebaceous. However, for adnexal structures to be of diagnostic value, a biopsy must include reticular dermis to visualize them. They may not be seen on a small superficial shave biopsy, in which case a reliable distinction between epidermal nevus and nevus sebaceus may not be possible.

Verrucous epidermal nevi may clinically mimic other linear conditions such as the verrucous stage of incontinentia pigmenti, lichen striatus, linear porokeratosis, or linear lichen planus. ILVEN may appear clinically and histologically identical to linear psoriasis. The overlapping features with linear psoriasis have led some physicians to propose that the two disorders are the same. However, the younger age of onset and the presence of peculiar histologic features, such as "checkerboard" parakeratosis, associated with ILVEN support the prevailing view of it as a distinct diagnostic entity. Histologically, an epidermal nevus can easily be confused with SK. Clinical context (e.g., long-standing lesion since childhood) and an adequate biopsy are critical in this regard.

Prognosis and Treatment

Localized or systemic epidermal nevi may be associated with underlying skeletal or soft tissue anomalies, which need to be evaluated by clinical workup. For the localized

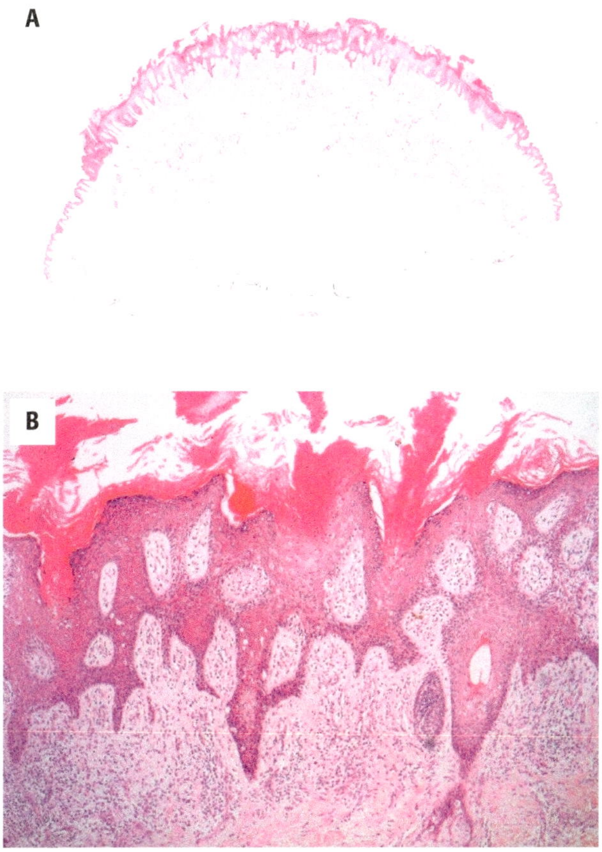

FIG. 11.5

Inflammatory verrucous epidermal nevus. **A,** Silhouette of a hyperkeratotic squamous proliferation. **B,** Psoriasiform epidermal hyperplasia is associated with alternating hyperorthokeratosis and parakeratosis and dermal inflammation.

epidermal nevus, reassurance is important for the patient and parents. Follow-up for any focal growth within the nevus is prudent because a secondary tumor may develop within the nevus, including basal cell carcinoma (BCC) and SCC. However, the development of a carcinoma in an epidermal nevus is a rare event. Most carcinomas are low grade and cured by simple excision. Intervention may also be sought by the patient or relatives for cosmetic reasons. Topical retinoids, cryotherapy, 5-fluorouracil, and chemical peeling agents have been used. Shave excisions also can provide an acceptable treatment result. To prevent recurrence, an excision should include the deep dermis, although this will leave a scar.

BENIGN ACANTHOMAS AND KERATOSES

SEBORRHEIC KERATOSIS

Clinical Findings

SKs are frequently encountered benign growths that begin to appear in early adulthood and become more frequent with age. They can be present anywhere on the body with the exception of mucosal membranes, palms, and soles. There is a predilection for the face, scalp, back, chest, and abdomen. The lesions typically present as sharply demarcated pink, tan, or brown stuck-on appearing papules or plaques (Fig. 11.6). Although generally smaller than 1 cm, larger plaques may occur. Follicular prominence is a helpful feature. Dermoscopy reveals the characteristic keratin-filled horn cysts.

Irritated and inflamed SKs (Fig. 11.7) may have a pink to erythematous halo, be indistinguishable from classic acanthotic SKs, or mimic squamous or BCC. Pruritus of SK is common. The rapid appearance of multiple irritated SKs is known as the sign of Leser-Trélat. This entity has been reported most commonly in association with gastrointestinal malignancies.

Pigmented SKs may clinically mimic melanoma or a melanocytic nevus. In particular, macular variants of pigmented SK may be confused with a lentigo or lentigo maligna.

SEBORRHEIC KERATOSIS—DISEASE FACT SHEET

Incidence
- Most common benign skin tumors in older individuals

Patient Group
- More common in White individuals than those with dark skin
- Frequency increases with age
- No gender predilection

Site of Involvement
- Anywhere but palms, soles, and mucosal surface

Clinical Findings
- Macule, papule, or plaque
- Flesh-colored, pink, red, or brown
- May blend with solar lentigo
- May appear warty or "stuck on"

Clinical Variants
- Dermatosis papulosa nigra (small facial lesions in dark-skinned individuals)
- Stucco keratosis (numerous flat keratotic lesions on dorsal distal extremities)

Clinical Relevance
- May be confused with melanoma, carcinoma, other tumors, or dermatoses
- May be cosmetic issue
- Irritated lesions may become superinfected

Prognosis
- Benign tumor, but squamous cell carcinoma may arise in association with it

Treatment
- Locally destructive therapy (e.g., cryotherapy)
- Surgical removal (shave biopsy, curettage, excision)

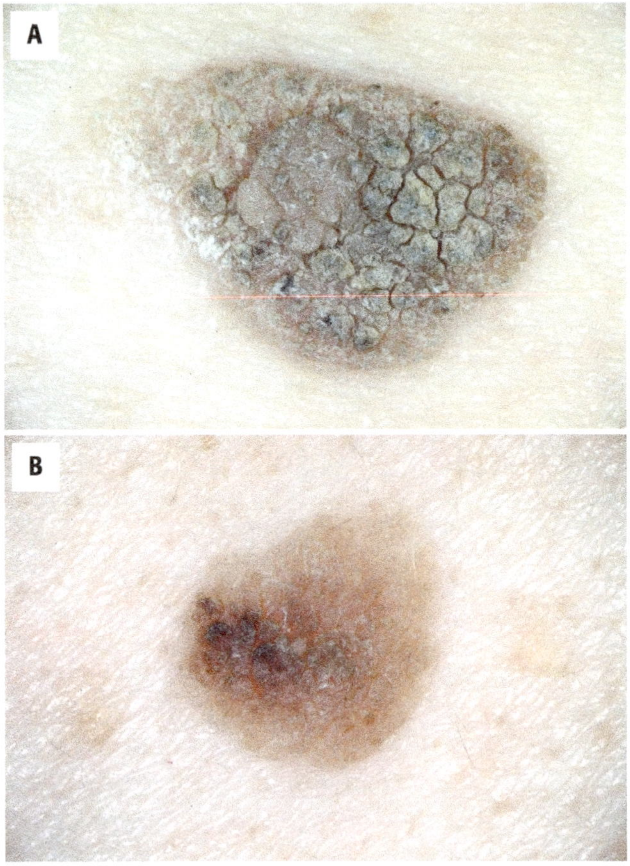

FIG. 11.6

A, Seborrheic keratosis presenting as brown warty "stuck-on" plaque. **B,** Seborrheic keratosis with variable papillomatous projections and pigmentation.

Dermatosis papulosa nigra is regarded by some as a variant of SK. Clinically, this is a distinct entity, which is only rarely biopsied. Multiple small (1–3 mm) light to dark brown dome-shaped papules are present on the face, neck, and upper chest. They are commonly encountered on these sun-exposed sites of women and begin to appear in young adulthood.

Stucco keratoses are considered another variant of SK, with numerous flat keratotic lesions present on the dorsum of the hands or feet, forearm, and/or ankle.

Histologic Features

There are many variations in the histologic appearances of SKs (Figs. 11.8–11.21). They may be flat, exophytic, or endophytic. SKs generally share the following features: basket-weave hyperkeratosis, presence of monotonous small cuboidal keratinocytes, anastomosing rete ridges, keratin-filled invaginations, and small horn cysts. The rete ridges may be widened and connect with each other in a broad acanthotic pattern or may be thin and elongated, forming a reticulate pattern. The surface may be papillomatous. Squamous eddies may be seen, and

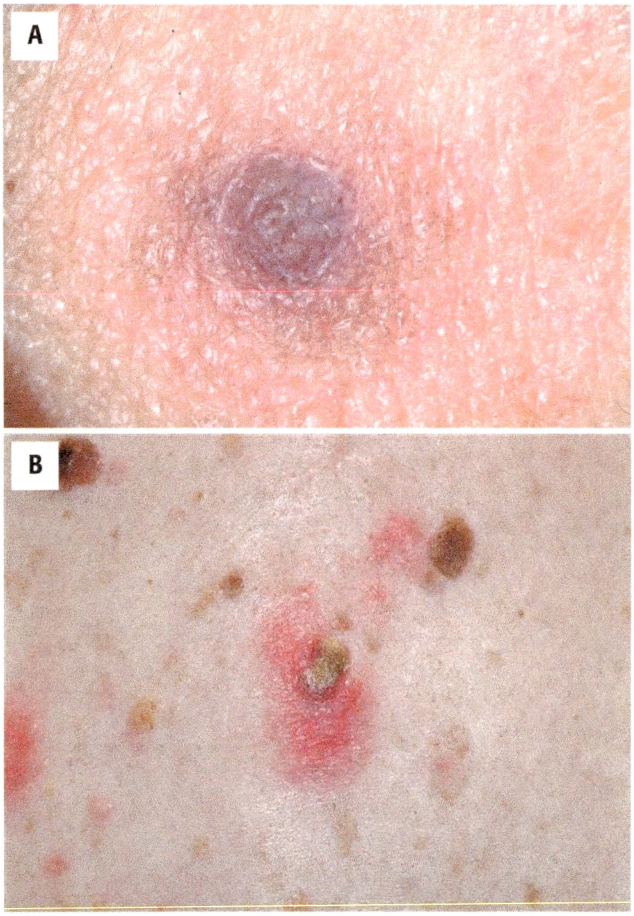

FIG. 11.7

A, Irritated seborrheic keratosis presenting as a red nodule. **B,** Irritated seborrheic keratosis: a crusted lesion with surrounding erythema.

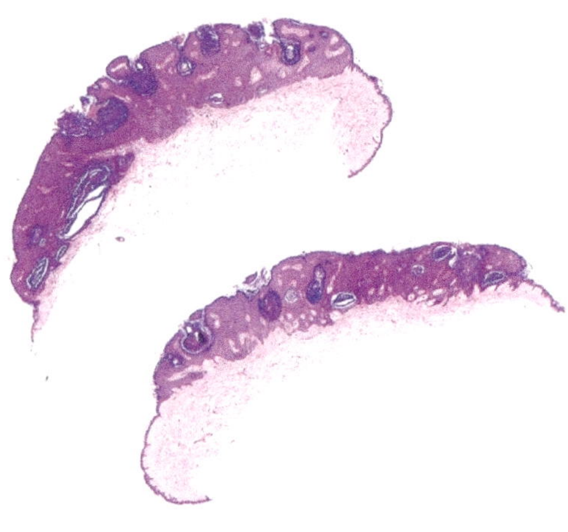

FIG. 11.8

Seborrheic keratosis. Scanning magnification shows an acanthoma forming a plaque. Horn pseudocysts are apparent.

mitoses may be present. The edges of the lesion tend to be sharply defined. An additional characteristic feature is the presence of a flat base or what has been referred to as "string sign," in which a straight line or string can be drawn across the base as opposed to the more infiltrative base of malignant tumors.

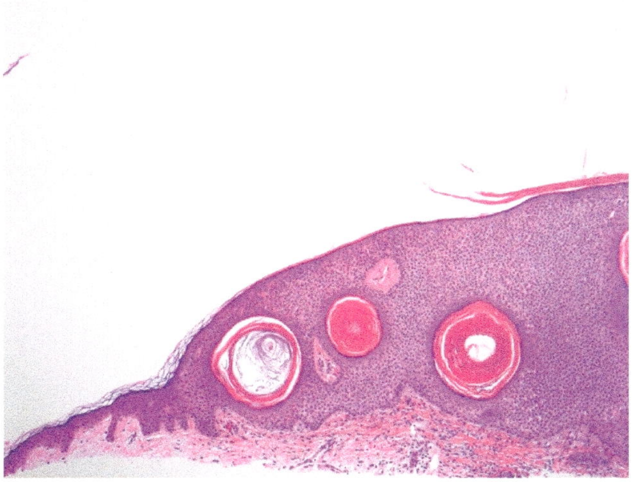

FIG. 11.9

Acanthotic seborrheic keratosis. Keratinocytes form a solid plaque of thickened epidermis.

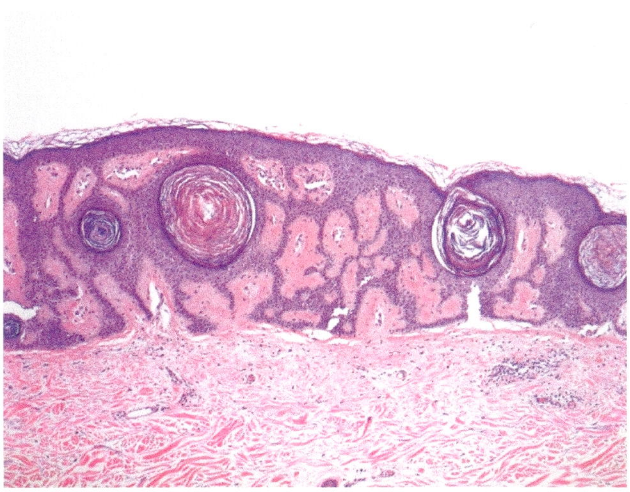

FIG. 11.10

Reticulated seborrheic keratosis. The rete ridges are thin and elongated.

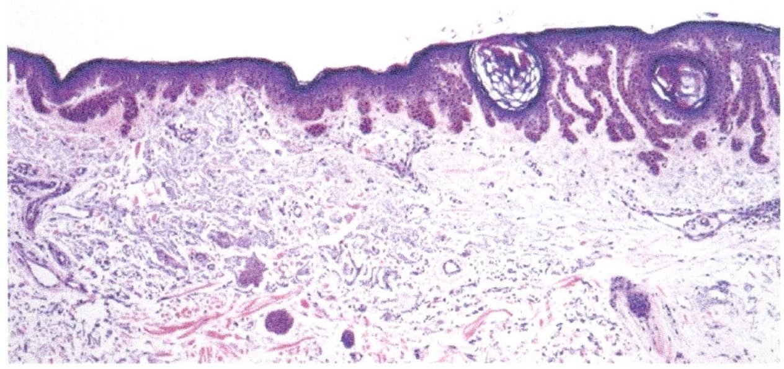

FIG. 11.11

Reticulated seborrheic keratosis. In this case, the features at the edge of the lesion are similar to a solar lentigo.

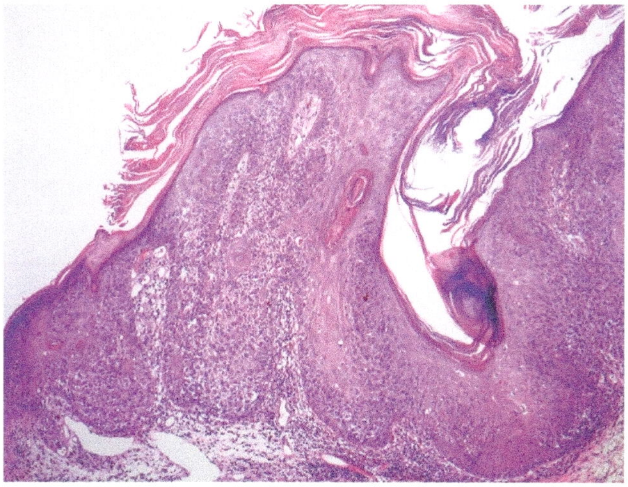

FIG. 11.12

Irritated seborrheic keratosis. Papillomatous and acanthotic growth pattern with spongiosis and inflammation.

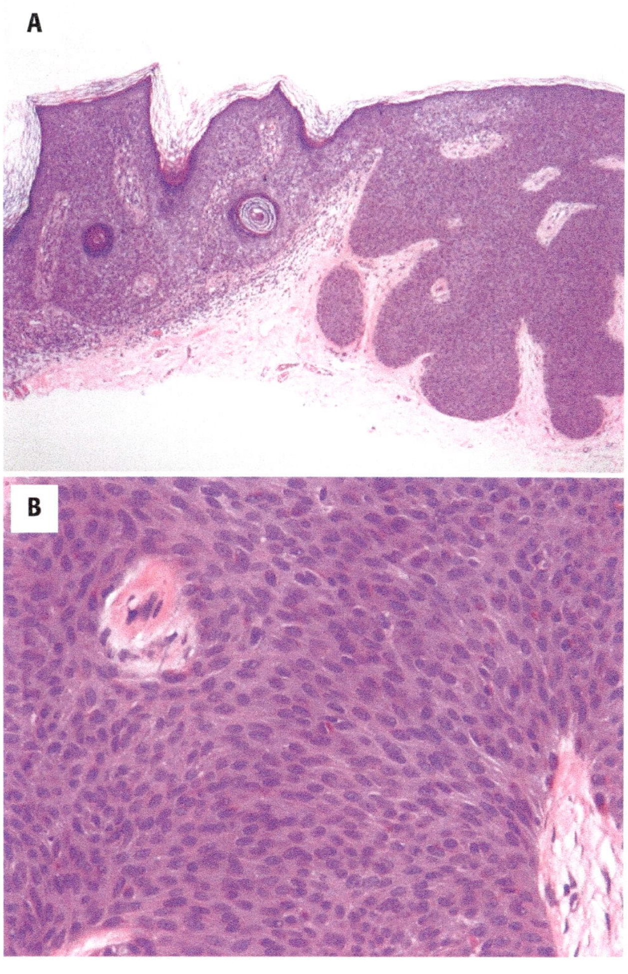

FIG. 11.13

A, Irritated seborrheic keratosis. One part of this keratosis grows outward and is inflamed. Another component grows inward and shows fusiform keratinocytes. **B,** Close-up view of the fusiform keratinocytes with small bland nuclei (same lesion as part **A**). Such fusiform keratinocytes are common in irritated seborrheic keratoses.

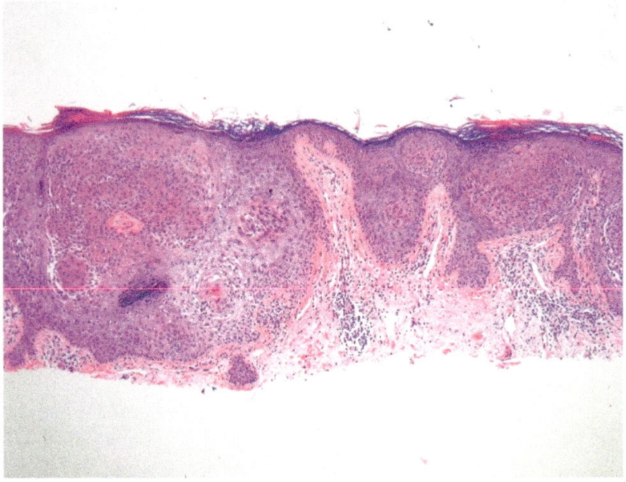

FIG. 11.14

"Clonal" seborrheic keratosis. This variant of an irritated seborrheic keratosis shows a nested or whorled arrangement of intraepidermal keratinocytes.

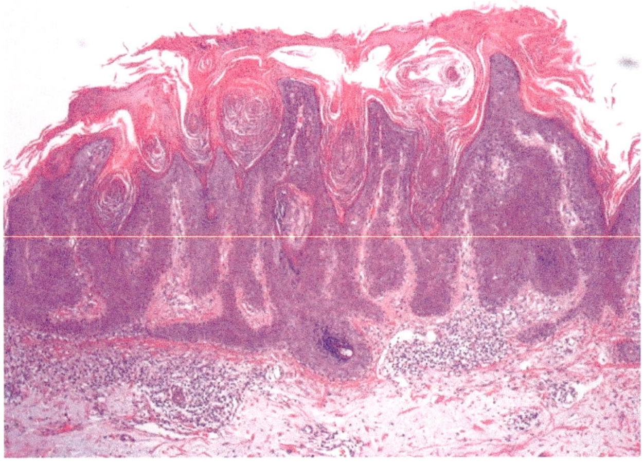

FIG. 11.15

Digitated seborrheic keratosis shows papillomatous outward projections simulating a verruca.

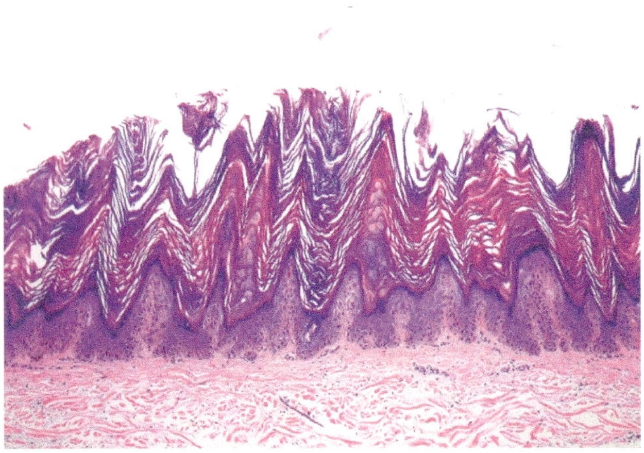

FIG. 11.16

Stucco keratosis. Small, sharply pointed papillomatous projections are seen with orthokeratosis and hyperkeratosis.

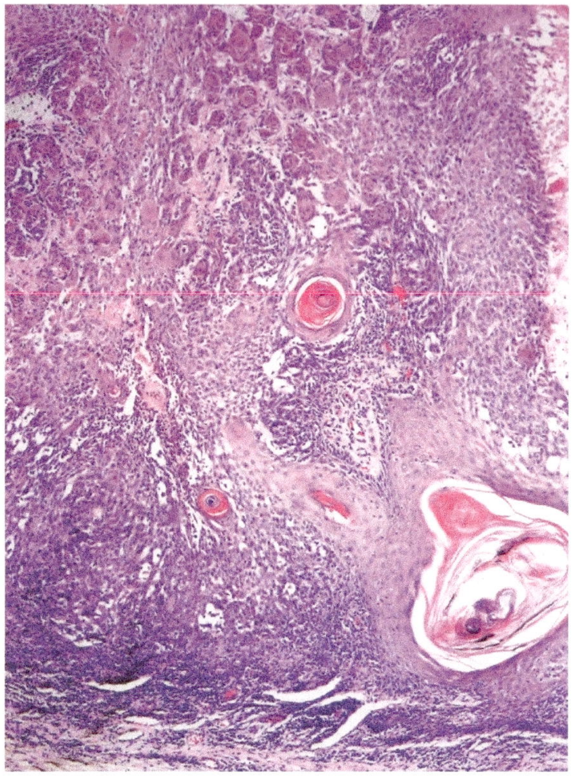

FIG. 11.17

Inverted follicular keratosis. The lesion has a smooth peripheral border and contains bland keratinocytes. An associated ectatic follicular infundibulum is seen. Many small keratinizing whorls of keratinocytes (squamous eddies) are seen.

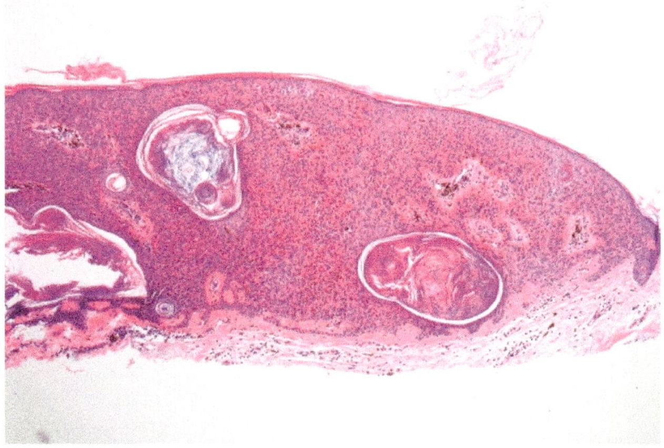

FIG. 11.18

Pigmented seborrheic keratosis. There is an increased amount of melanin pigment within lesional keratinocytes. This lesion shows an acanthotic pattern.

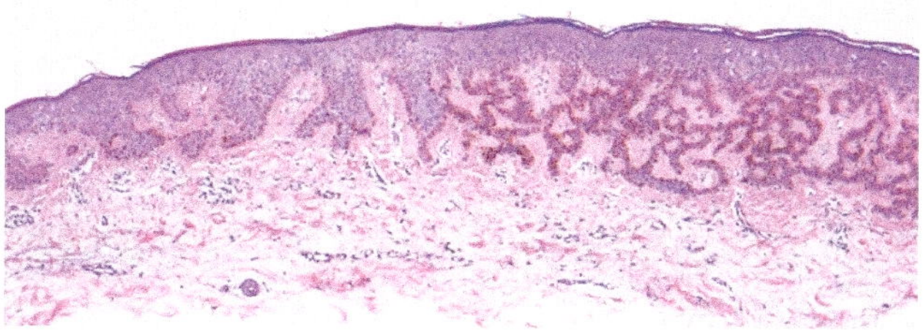

FIG. 11.19

Pigmented seborrheic keratosis with a reticulated pattern.

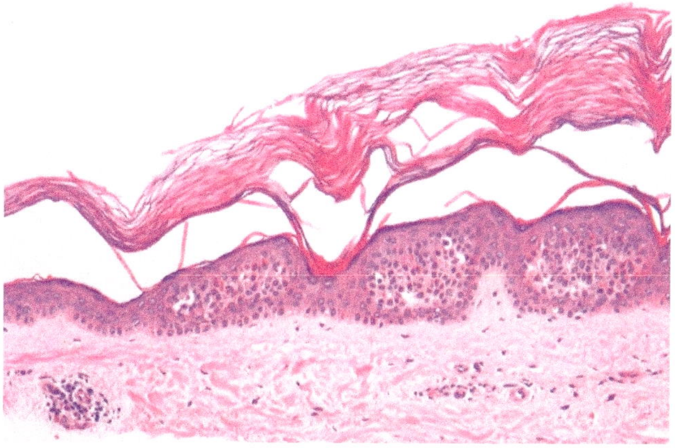

FIG. 11.20

Pigmented seborrheic keratosis with a "clonal," nested pattern.

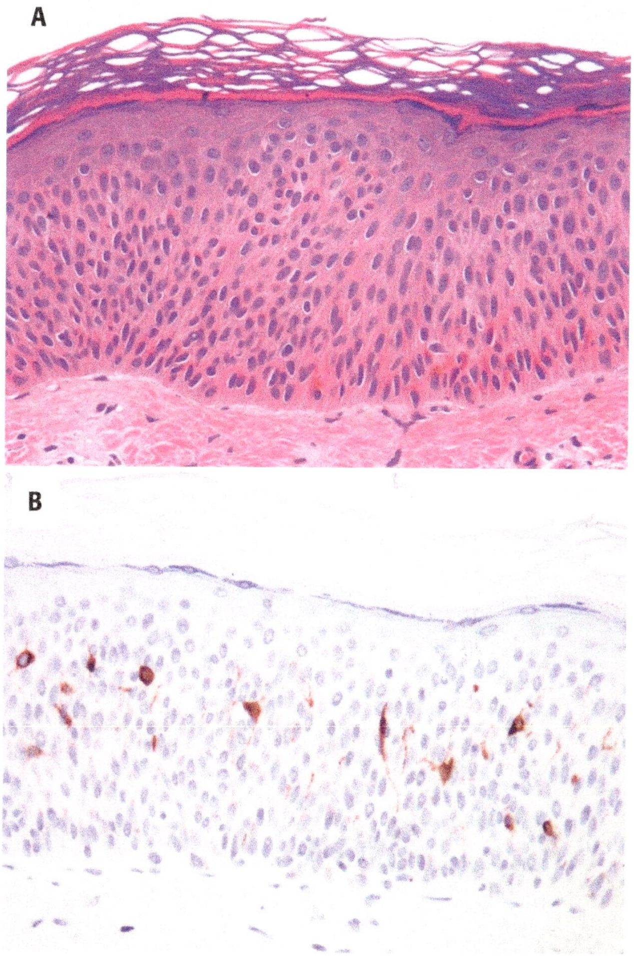

FIG. 11.21

A, Melanoacanthoma. There is a background of a pigmented seborrheic keratosis with a second population of scattered cytologically bland melanocytes in the spinous cell layer. **B,** Melanoacanthoma. The melanocytes are best seen on an immunostain for Melan-A, which highlights the cells' dendritic processes.

SEBORRHEIC KERATOSIS—PATHOLOGIC FEATURES

Histologic Features

- Hyperkeratosis (often orthohyperkeratosis, but parakeratosis may be present)
- Epidermal thickening
  - Acanthotic pattern
  - Reticulated pattern
  - Digitated or verrucoid pattern
  - "Clonal" intraepidermal nested pattern
- Cytologically bland small nuclei
- Presence of pseudohorned cysts
- May be inflamed
- May be pigmented
- May be pigmented and colonized by bland melanocytes (melanoacanthoma)
- May show features of irritation (spongiosis, hemorrhage)

Differential Diagnosis

- Epidermal nevus
- Nevoid hyperkeratosis of the nipple
- Actinic keratosis
- Verruca
- Squamous cell carcinoma
- Melanocytic lesions

The classic acanthotic SK is characterized by a raised plaque-like proliferation of cytologically bland small cuboidal keratinocytes with broad anastomosing rete ridges and circumscribed well-defined peripheral borders (see Figs. 11.8 and 11.9). Basket-weave hyperkeratosis and horn pseudocysts are usually present. The dermal papillae are often hypervascular. Vessels may be ectatic. Melanophages may be present.

In reticulated SKs, the rete ridges are thin, elongated, and often hyperpigmented (Fig. 11.10). At the periphery of the lesion, the features often resemble a solar lentigo (Fig. 11.11). Well-developed lesions show a delicate network of interconnecting thin epithelial strands.

Irritated SKs tend to have more foci of parakeratosis and associated inflammation than other SKs (Figs. 11.12 and 11.13). Spongiosis may be present or a lichenoid reaction pattern, in which case there may be prominent "squamatization" of the basal cell layer, wherein the basilar keratinocytes take on the appearance of spinous layer keratinocytes, carrying pinker cytoplasm. Pink globules, so-called Civatte bodies, also may be seen. The proliferating keratinocytes may be spindled (Fig. 11.13B) or at times show a nested "clonal" pattern (clonal SK) (Fig. 11.14). Reactive nuclear atypia may be present, characterized by enlarged nuclei with open chromatin pattern and a distinct nucleolus. Multinucleation of keratinocytes may also be found.

Hyperkeratotic variants of SK show a markedly thickened stratum corneum. The underlying epidermis often shows papillomatosis. These lesions may be quite exophytic. Occasionally, the excessive stratum corneum produces a cutaneous horn clinically.

Verrucoid, digitated, or stucco variants of SK show a papillomatous silhouette resembling a wart (Figs. 11.15 and 11.16). In contrast to a true wart, the stratum corneum of an SK is usually predominantly basket weave, the dermal papillae are less hypervascular, and viral cytopathic changes (koilocytes and enlarged keratohyaline granules) are lacking, but features more typical of SK (pseudohorned cysts, broad anastomosing rete ridges) may be present.

Inverted follicular keratosis (Fig. 11.17) is another variant of SK with a prominent endophytic epithelial proliferation, typically involving follicular infundibulum. There may be minimal orthokeratosis and keratin horn pseudocysts may be absent. Nests of brightly eosinophilic whorled collections of keratinocytes (squamous eddies) are characteristic (Fig. 11.17). The squamous eddies may constitute the bulk of the neoplasm. The lesion typically shows a lobular—that is, noninfiltrative—peripheral growth pattern.

The pigmented SK may come in any of the growth patterns described in the preceding but additionally has an increased amount of melanin pigment compared with the surrounding skin (Figs. 11.18–11.20). Melanin pigment may be present in keratinocytes or dermal macrophages. A slight increase in the number of junctional melanocytes is common in pigmented SKs. Macular variants of pigmented SK may at their periphery show features of or be contiguous with solar lentigines. A peculiar variant of pigmented SK is the melanoacanthoma, in which scattered, and at times numerous, solitary units of well-differentiated cytologically bland melanocytes with branching dendritic processes are dispersed in the spinous cell layer or acanthotic epidermis (see Fig. 11.21).

There are a number of different somatic mutations associated with SK, which include but are not limited to mutations in FGFR3, PIK3CA, RAS, AKT1, and epidermal growth factor receptor (EGFR).

Differential Diagnosis

Histologically, SK needs to be distinguished from other epidermal lesions, such as epidermal nevus, actinic keratosis (AK), SCC, verruca, clear cell acanthoma, acrochordon, nevoid hyperkeratosis of the nipple and areola, acanthosis nigricans, and LSC.

SEBORRHEIC KERATOSIS VERSUS EPIDERMAL NEVUS

Epidermal nevi and SK are best distinguished from each other by clinical history. Onset of the lesion in childhood supports a diagnosis of an epidermal nevus. SKs are fairly uncommon in patients before their late twenties.

SEBORRHEIC KERATOSIS VERSUS ACTINIC KERATOSIS

SK lacks the hyperchromatic, often enlarged, elongated, and overlapping nuclei of basilar keratinocytes typically associated with AK. Furthermore, whereas SK usually shows more prominent basket-weave hyperkeratosis, parakeratosis is more pronounced in AK.

SEBORRHEIC KERATOSIS VERSUS SQUAMOUS CELL CARCINOMA IN SITU

SCC may clinically and histologically mimic an irritated SK. Furthermore, SCC in situ (SCCIS) may arise in association with an SK (usually an irritated and inflamed SK). Attention to cytologic atypia and growth patterns is important. In irritated SK, the nuclei of keratinocytes are round to oval with a delicate chromatin pattern and smooth nuclear membranes. They lack the hyperchromatism, irregular nuclear membranes, and loss of polarity commonly seen in SCC. Scattered enlarged nuclei with an open chromatin pattern and small nucleolus or keratinocytes with multiple nuclei may be present in irritated SK. Their presence should not prompt a diagnosis of in situ carcinoma. Likewise, mitoses are not uncommon in SKs and should per se be interpreted as evidence of carcinoma.

SEBORRHEIC KERATOSIS VERSUS VERRUCA VULGARIS

SK and verruca vulgaris (VV) may show a similar silhouette at scanning magnification and can be difficult to distinguish from each other. SK may have prominent papillomatous exophytic projection of the epidermis; however, in SK, basket-weave orthokeratosis is often still prominent, and warts typically have compact hyperkeratosis and parakeratosis. Very pointed papillomatous projections of the epidermis with a thin long column of parakeratosis, hypervascular dermal papillae with dilated and tortuous capillary loops, and serum in the stratum corneum favor a verruca, but any of these features also occur in an SK on occasion. Viral cytopathic changes (raisinoid nuclei surrounded by a clear halo, koilocytes) are more definitive for the presence of a verruca. However, not all verrucae display histologically well-developed koilocytic changes. Nongenital SKs are usually negative for human papillomavirus (HPV), but HPV has been identified in a proportion of genital SKs.

SEBORRHEIC KERATOSIS VERSUS CLEAR CELL ACANTHOMA

SK may show focal clear cell features, but the remainder of the lesion shows typical features of SK. We reserve the term *clear cell acanthoma* for a small papule with the typical features described in the following to be uniformly present throughout the lesion.

SEBORRHEIC KERATOSIS VERSUS LICHENOID KERATOSIS

SKs may be associated with spongiotic or lichenoid patterns of inflammation or a mixture thereof. If the lichenoid inflammatory reaction is prominent throughout the entire lesion, one may also use the term *lichenoid keratosis.* (Many lichenoid keratoses represent nothing other than an inflamed lichenoid SK, in which case the distinction between an inflamed SK and a lichenoid keratosis is purely semantic.)

PIGMENTED SEBORRHEIC KERATOSIS VERSUS A KERATOTIC MELANOCYTIC LESION

Pigmented variants of SK need to be distinguished from melanocytic nevi and malignant melanoma. The presence of a melanocytic neoplasm is recognized by a significantly increased cellular density of solitary units or nests of melanocytes. Some SKs may show colonization or the presence of mild melanocytic hyperplasia within the lesion. This has also been referred to as melanoacanthoma.

1. *SK versus keratotic melanocytic nevus*. Melanocytic nevi may show an epidermal silhouette indistinguishable from an SK or they may collide with an SK. When the melanocytic proliferation is subtle, it may be overlooked on a quick review. At times, step sections are needed to identify a melanocytic nevus in a lesion, which at first glance has features of a pigmented SK.
2. *SK versus melanoma*. Similar to melanocytic nevi, some variants of melanoma have an SK-like epidermal silhouette and may be overlooked if the tissue is not examined at higher magnification. Furthermore, melanoma may collide with and colonize an SK. Thus it is prudent to examine a pigmented SK-like lesion at higher magnification for the possibility of an associated melanocytic neoplasm. The presence of cytologically bland melanocytes colonizing an SK (so-called melanoacanthoma) should not be mistaken for melanoma in situ. At times, one may also observe clear cell changes of basilar keratinocyte simulating a lentiginous melanocytic proliferation. If there is any doubt, an immunostain (e.g., SOX10) can clarify whether or not a melanocytic neoplasm is present.

PEDUNCULATED SEBORRHEIC KERATOSIS VERSUS ACROCHORDON

Clinically, pedunculated SKs may appear as skin tags. Histologically, these lesions differ from acrochordons by epidermal hyperplasia, hyperkeratosis, and other features, such as horn pseudocysts, if present.

SEBORRHEIC KERATOSIS VERSUS NEVOID HYPERKERATOSIS OF THE NIPPLE AND AREOLA

Clinical history is essential because histologically, the lesions show overlapping features of papillomatous epidermal hyperplasia and hyperkeratosis. The localization of the lesion to the nipple and areola (unilateral or bilateral) and associated hyperpigmentation are clinically characteristic.

SEBORRHEIC KERATOSIS VERSUS ACANTHOSIS NIGRICANS

Lesions of acanthosis nigricans rarely show epidermal hyperplasia and hyperkeratosis as prominent as seen in SK. The distinction, however, is best made clinically.

Prognosis and Treatment

SKs are benign lesions. They generally are only of cosmetic concern to the patient. Irritated SKs may be bothersome because of pruritus and are usually treated for this reason. Because SKs may clinically mimic a malignant tumor, they are usually biopsied to exclude other tumors in the differential diagnosis (e.g., carcinoma or melanoma). Management may involve a spectrum of options from observation to cryotherapy, electrodesiccation, or curettage.

VERRUCOUS KERATOSIS

Verrucous keratosis encompasses a spectrum of benign papillomatous squamous proliferative lesions. Often the term is used for papillomatous, verrucoid variants of SK. Some lesions reported as verrucoid keratosis are probably old warts lacking viral cytopathic changes. Verrucous keratoses are lesions commonly seen in patients undergoing BRAF inhibitor therapy.

LARGE CELL ACANTHOMA

Clinical Findings

Large cell acanthoma is a well-demarcated, slightly scaly, thin papule or brown patch on the sun-exposed areas of the head and extremities. The papule may be brown and flesh-colored and is more common in elderly individuals with a background of photodamage.

Histologic Features

There is usually slight hyperkeratosis of the stratum corneum and slight thickening of the epidermis with preservation of the granular layer. Within a circumscribed area of epidermis, there is a collection of enlarged keratinocytes with proportionately enlarged nuclei (Fig. 11.22). The lesional keratinocytes are approximately twice the size of normal and are found at all layers of the epidermis. Rete ridges are often bulbous. The nuclei are enlarged, but the chromatin pattern of the nuclei is delicate and similar to that of normal epidermal keratinocytes. No hyperchromatism or prominent nucleoli are present. Mitoses are only seen in the basal layer.

Differential Diagnosis

Clinically, this is not a very distinctive lesion, and most cases are submitted as SK, solar lentigo, pigmented AK, or Bowen's disease. Histologically, it may be confused with SCCIS. However, large cell acanthoma lacks the atypia and loss of polarity associated with SCCIS. Some pathologists view large cell acanthoma as a variant of solar lentigo or pigmented AK. Although one may question whether or not the presence of oversized albeit bland lesional keratinocytes warrants a designation as a distinct entity, there are reasons to discuss large cell acanthoma separately as is done in this chapter. The main reason is to draw attention to the fact that large nuclei may occur in a benign pigmented keratinocytic lesion. Recognition of this phenomenon should help avoid an erroneous diagnosis of SCCIS for such benign lesions.

Prognosis and Treatment

The lesion is benign and does not require treatment.

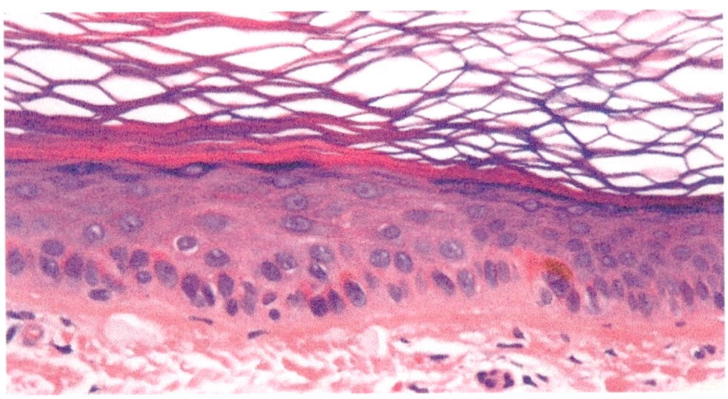

FIG. 11.22

Large cell acanthoma. The keratinocytes of large cell acanthoma enlarged nuclei compared with adjacent nonlesional keratinocytes. Hyperchromatism is lacking. There is good evidence of maturation. Pigmentation is common.

CLEAR CELL ACANTHOMA

Clinical Findings

Clear cell acanthoma is also known as pale cell acanthoma and Degos' acanthoma. It is a slowly growing, sharply demarcated, red or red-brown, dome-shaped papule (Fig. 11.23). Frequently, there is a thin, whitish, peripheral scale collarette. Usually less than 1 cm in diameter, the clear cell acanthoma tends to occur on the legs of middle-aged to elderly adults. These are often easily recognized on dermoscopic assessment become of the string of pearls–like pattern describing the presence of curvilinear or reticular pattern of glomerular or pinpoint-like blood vessels.

Histologic Features

Clear cell acanthoma is characterized by a contiguous collection of pale-staining keratinocytes, with a striking

CLEAR CELL ACANTHOMA—DISEASE FACT SHEET

Patient Group
- ▸▸ Adults

Site of Involvement
- ▸▸ Typically occurs on leg

Clinical Findings
- ▸▸ Pink papule with peripheral scale
- ▸▸ Usually biopsied to rule out basal cell carcinoma

Prognosis and Treatment
- ▸▸ Benign lesion
- ▸▸ Does not require further treatment

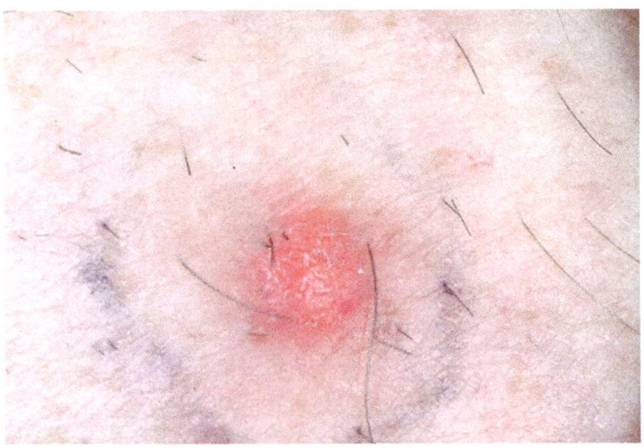

FIG. 11.23

Clear cell acanthoma. A circumscribed small erythematous papule (located on the thigh).

A

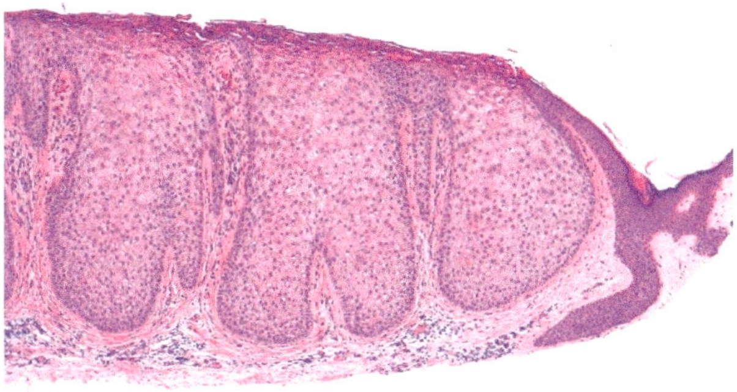

B

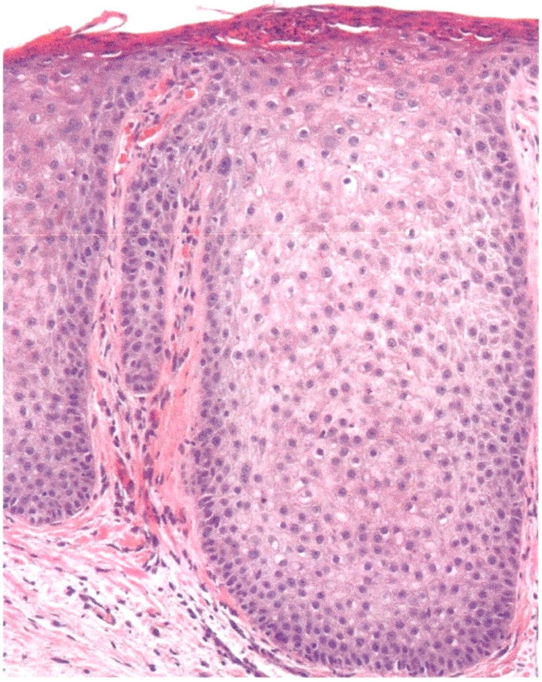

FIG. 11.24

A, Clear cell acanthoma: there is psoriasiform epidermal hyperplasia. Lesional keratinocytes differ in their pale cytoplasm from adjacent nonlesional epidermis. **B,** The surface is often eroded. Neutrophils are commonly seen within the lesion.

demarcation laterally from the normal epidermis (Fig. 11.24). These keratinocytes can stretch from the stratum granulosum down to but sometimes sparing the stratum basalis. Because of their expanded cytoplasm, the individual cells may appear larger than their adjacent normal counterparts, but the nuclear size remains fairly constant. There is typically loss of the granular layer, parakeratosis, and often neutrophils in the stratum corneum. This can often mimic a lesion of psoriasis vulgaris.

There is acanthosis, as the name implies, which extends across the top of the specimen like a band. Mild spongiosis, exocytosis of neutrophils, thinning of the suprapapillary plate, and papillary dermal edema are commonly seen. The adnexal epithelium is usually not involved. The parakeratotic stratum corneum may contain clusters of neutrophils. The surface of the lesion is not infrequently focally eroded. Periodic acid-Schiff stains with and without diastase will confirm cytoplasmic glycogen as the source of keratinocytic pallor.

CLEAR CELL ACANTHOMA—PATHOLOGIC FEATURES

Histologic Features

- Epidermal hyperplasia
- Clear or pale cell cytoplasmic change of lesional cells
- Collarette common
- Surface erosion common
- Intraepithelial neutrophils common

Differential Diagnosis

- Psoriasis
- Irritated seborrheic keratosis

Differential Diagnosis

The clinical differential includes dermatofibroma, hemangioma, and SK. Histologically, clear cell acanthoma may be confused with an irritated SK with clear cell changes. Without clinical context, some lesions of clear cell acanthomas may be confused with psoriasis because of the presence of neutrophils in the stratum corneum, psoriasiform epidermal hyperplasia, decreased or absent granular cell layer, and hypervascular dermal papillae.

Prognosis and Treatment

Clear cell acanthomas are usually biopsied to exclude other lesions, such as BCC. Biopsy frequently leads to complete removal. If there is a residual lesion and the patient wants it to be removed for cosmetic reasons, cryotherapy with liquid nitrogen is usually effective.

ACANTHOLYTIC ACANTHOMA

Clinical Findings

This is a solitary asymptomatic flesh-colored to tan, rough papule. It usually occurs on the trunk of older individuals, sparing palms, soles, and mucous membranes.

Histologic Features

There is orthokeratosis of the thickened stratum corneum. The epidermis shows irregular acanthosis with

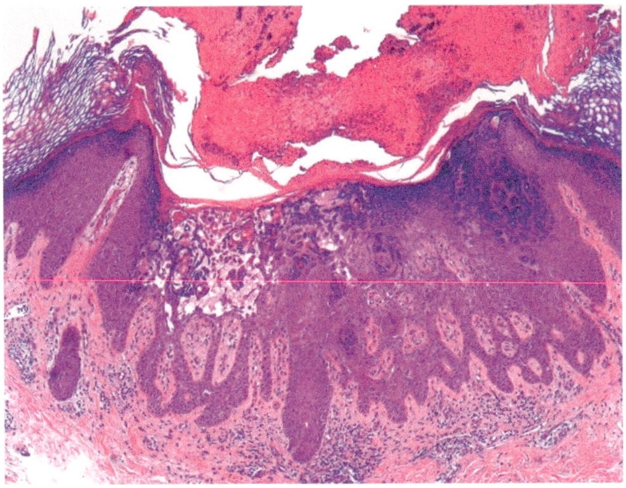

FIG. 11.25

Acantholytic acanthoma. An acanthoma with focal acantholysis.

hypergranulosis and papillomatosis. Acantholysis may affect any level of the epidermis but tends to be prominent in the inferior portion of the stratum spinosum (Fig. 11.25). The keratinocytes are loosely held together with foci of dyscohesion, in which the cells display a rounded surface lacking cell-cell contact through intercellular bridges.

Differential Diagnosis

Acantholytic acanthomas show features similar to Hailey-Hailey disease, pemphigus vulgaris, Grover's disease, or even Darier-White disease. The solitary nature of this acanthoma helps to distinguish it from those other conditions. It may also resemble a warty dyskeratoma, but the latter lesion has verrucoid features and is more endophytic.

Prognosis and Treatment

The lesion is benign. No treatment is necessary.

WARTY DYSKERATOMA

Clinical Findings

Warty dyskeratoma is a benign verrucous growth, usually on the head and neck of middle-aged and elderly people. It presents as a flesh-colored to brown, hyperkeratotic papule. This can occur as an isolated lesion or as multiple lesions.

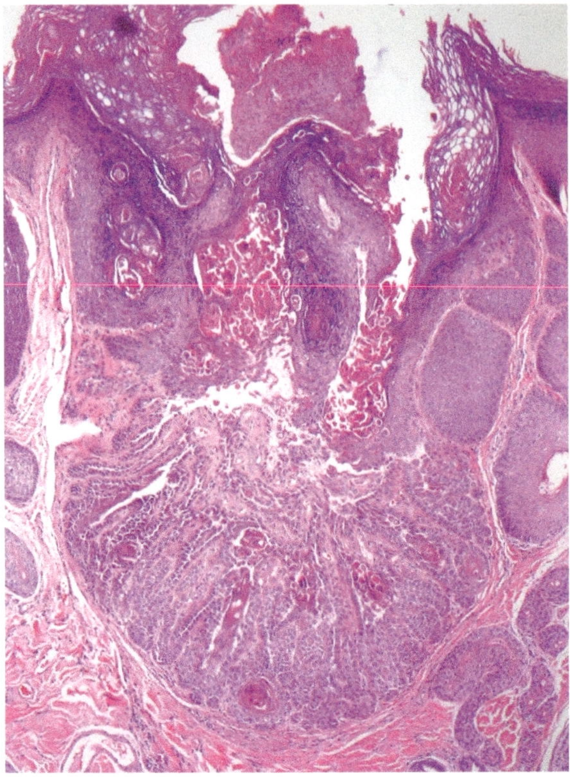

FIG. 11.26

Warty dyskeratoma. The outward growth is verrucoid. The inward-growing component shows suprabasilar acantholysis.

Histologic Features

A warty dyskeratoma typically shows a circumscribed, cup-shaped invagination of squamous epithelium with suprabasilar acantholytic clefts (Fig. 11.26). The center is filled with keratinous material. Dermal papillae covered by basal cell layer keratinocytes protrude like villi into a lacunar space created by acantholysis. The keratin plug may contain grains (dyskeratotic cells with hyperchromatic elongated nuclei and eosinophilic cytoplasm).

Differential Diagnosis

Most often this solitary lesion is clinically confused with VV. Histologically, warty dyskeratoma needs to be distinguished from acantholytic dermatoses (e.g., Darier's disease, Grover's disease) as well as acantholytic AK and SCC.

Prognosis and Treatment

This is a benign lesion, which has no relationship with HPV infection. No intervention is required. Complete removal is often achieved by the biopsy procedure.

BENIGN LICHENOID KERATOSIS (LICHEN PLANUS–LIKE KERATOSIS)

Clinical Findings

A lichenoid keratosis presents as a solitary, flesh-colored to tan, flat papule (Fig. 11.27). It has a predilection for the arms and upper chest in older women. It is typically biopsied to rule out BCC, which it may mimic clinically, or a melanocytic neoplasm. Lesions of lichenoid keratosis likely represent variants of SK or solar lentigo affected by a prominent lichenoid tissue reaction.

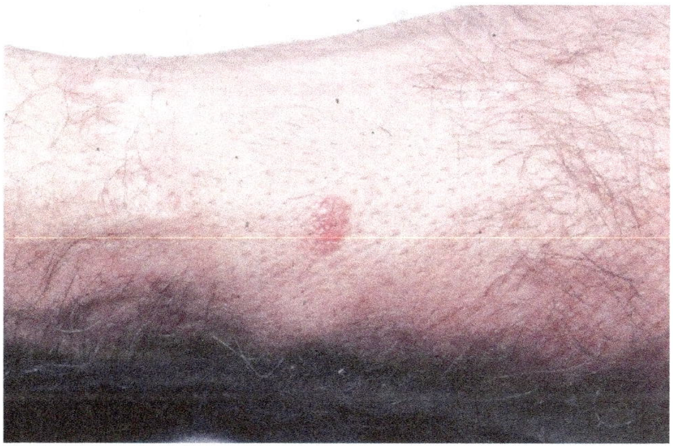

FIG. 11.27

Lichenoid keratosis presenting as a small erythematous plaque.

BENIGN LICHENOID KERATOSIS—DISEASE FACT SHEET

Patient Group
- Middle-aged or elderly individuals

Site of Involvement
- Chest but may occur anywhere

Clinical Findings
- Red papule
- Brown patch

Clinical Relevance
- May be confused with basal cell or squamous cell carcinoma
- May be confused with a melanocytic neoplasm
- May be confused with cutaneous T-cell lymphoma
- May be confused with a dermatitis

Prognosis and Treatment
- Benign lesion; often removed by shave biopsy
- Does not require further treatment except for cosmetic or symptomatic reasons
- Can be removed by locally destructive treatment (e.g., cryotherapy)

Histologic Features

There is considerable variation in the extent of epidermal hyperplasia and degree of associated inflammation, which is typically dense bandlike and predominantly composed of lymphocytes (Fig. 11.28). Parakeratosis is commonly seen, which can be a feature to help distinguish it from idiopathic lichen planus. As in lichen planus, wedge-shaped hypergranulosis, sawtoothing of the rete ridges with vacuolar degeneration, and squamatization of the basal keratinocytes are characteristic findings. Collections of eosinophilic globules, roughly the size of keratinocytes, are seen in the superficial papillary dermis adjacent to the dermal-epidermal junction (Fig. 11.29). These globules are known by many names, such as hyaline, cytoid, or Civatte bodies, and represent necrotic keratinocytes. The inflammatory cell infiltrate often contains melanophages, which may at times be dominant, especially when few other inflammatory cells are present, and thereby mimic a pigmented lesion. Care must be taken not to confuse clusters of lymphocytes or pigmented keratinocytes at the dermoepidermal junction, which may form "pseudonests" with bona fide melanocyte nests.

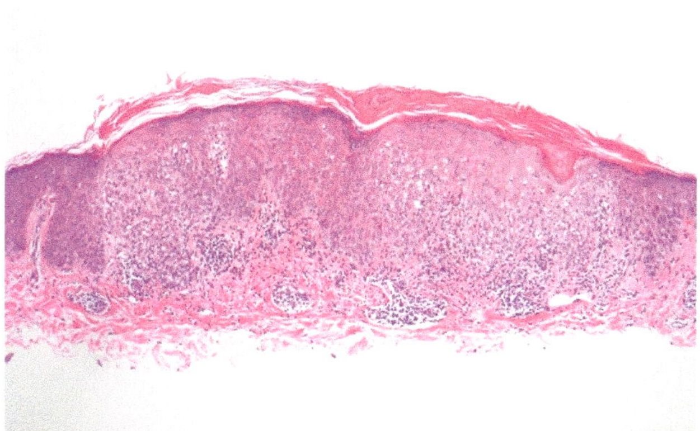

FIG. 11.28

Lichenoid keratosis. Epidermal hyperplasia is associated with a bandlike infiltrate of lymphocytes.

BENIGN LICHENOID KERATOSIS—PATHOLOGIC FEATURES

Histologic Features
- Epidermal hyperplasia (variable)
- Hyperkeratosis and parakeratosis
- Lichenoid inflammatory reaction with Civatte bodies
- Variable numbers of melanophages in the dermis

Differential Diagnosis
- Lichen planus (clinical correlation, e.g., mucosal lesions?)
- Lichenoid drug reaction (clinical history of new medication?)
- Inflamed or regressed melanocytic lesion (increased density of melanocytes, presence of melanocyte nests)
- Mycosis fungoides (lymphoid atypia, clinical findings)

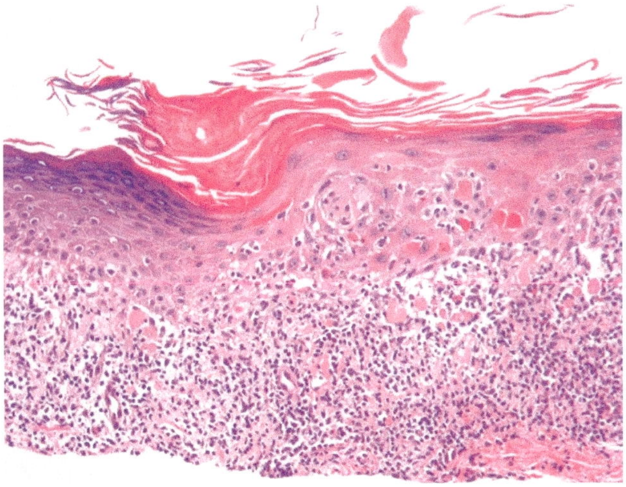

FIG. 11.29

Lichenoid keratosis. Several pink globules (Civatte bodies) are present at the dermal-epidermal junction and in the papillary dermis.

Differential Diagnosis

The clinical differential diagnosis includes BCC, Bowen's disease, irritated SK, postinflammatory hyperpigmentation, and melanocytic lesion. Rarely, if several papules are present, they may resemble a photodermatitis such as cutaneous lupus, polymorphous light eruption, or a photo-induced drug eruption. Histologically, the differential diagnosis includes lichen planus, an inflamed AK, and a regressed melanocytic lesion. Other entities with a lichenoid reaction pattern could also be considered, such as lichen striatus, keratosis lichenoides chronica, LE, lichenoid drug eruption, erythema multiforme, and mycosis fungoides (MF).

LICHENOID KERATOSIS VERSUS LICHEN PLANUS

The clinical history is of great help. For example, if a patient with no other cutaneous or mucosal features of lichen planus presents with a solitary red papule on the chest, which is thought to be a possible BCC and histologically shows features of lichen planus, the lesion is a lichenoid (lichen planus–like) keratosis. Histologically, lichenoid keratosis shows subtle features slightly different from lichen planus. In contrast to the latter, lichenoid keratosis is more likely to show parakeratosis and less likely to display prominent hypergranulosis.

LICHENOID KERATOSIS VERSUS INFLAMED ACTINIC KERATOSIS

A lichenoid keratosis is distinguished from an AK by the lack of hyperchromatic atypical basilar keratinocytes. This feature may be difficult or impossible to evaluate when a very dense inflammatory cell infiltrate obscures basilar keratinocytes. It is best to examine the periphery of the lesion. Whereas lichenoid keratoses often show features of solar lentigo or SK at their periphery, lichenoid AKs show typical features of AK away from the dense inflammation. Attention to the presence or absence of solar elastosis is also helpful: the lack of significant solar elastosis makes an AK less likely.

LICHENOID KERATOSIS VERSUS MYCOSIS FUNGOIDES

At times one may face the issue of having to distinguish a patch or plaque lesion of MF from a lichenoid keratosis (e.g., a patient with a history of MF may develop a lichenoid keratosis–like lesion). Lichenoid keratosis lacks the hyperchromatic lymphocytes with irregular nuclear contours typical of MF. Another helpful feature is the dermal stroma. In MF, the papillary dermis is often fibrotic, but it tends to be edematous in lichenoid keratosis. Furthermore, in lichenoid keratosis, there is often more pronounced epidermal hyperplasia than in MF. Civatte bodies are also a helpful clue. They are common in lichenoid keratosis but rare in MF.

LICHENOID KERATOSIS VERSUS A MELANOCYTIC LESION

The histologic features of an inflamed or regressed melanocytic lesion may at times overlap with a lichenoid keratosis. Clues to the correct diagnosis are clinical history (prior documentation of a nevus, which has "faded") and any histologic evidence of a residual melanocytic neoplasm (e.g., presence of melanocytic nests or focal significant increase in the number of solitary units of melanocytes). Caution is necessary not to mistake inflamed clusters of dyscohesive epithelial cells, lymphocytes, or melanophages as a junctional melanocyte nest (so-called "pseudo-melanocytic" nest). Immunostains for melanocyte differentiation markers may be helpful, but one needs to bear in mind that a slight increase in the density of solitary units of melanocytes along the dermal-epidermal junction may be seen in association with a lichenoid keratosis without implying the presence of a melanocytic neoplasm. Furthermore, especially when using antibodies against Melan-A or Mart-1, the interpretation of the staining result is not always straightforward. Strong labeling of melanocyte dendritic processes around keratinocytes or aberrant labeling of epithelial cells may lead to an erroneous overestimate of melanocyte density or false impression of nests. That pitfall can be avoided by using antibodies with nuclear labeling (e.g., SOX10).

LICHENOID KERATOSIS VERSUS BASAL CELL CARCINOMA

After tumor cell aggregates of BCC are identified, the distinction of lichenoid keratosis from carcinoma is straightforward. However, a diagnostic pitfall lies in the fact that BCC can sometimes be surrounded by features of lichenoid keratosis, and one may too quickly conclude based on initial levels that a lichenoid keratosis is present when in fact deeper sections of the biopsied tissue would reveal BCC. Careful attention to the size of the tissue sections (are they increasing from one level to the next, suggesting that the center of the tissue material has not been reached?) and subtle histologic clues (e.g., prominent stromal alterations, focally interrupted stroma) should prompt the pathologist to obtain additional levels to exclude BCC more definitively if it is clinically suspected and in initial levels may suggest a lichenoid keratosis.

Prognosis and Treatment

Lichenoid keratosis is usually biopsied to exclude other tumors, particularly BCC or melanocytic neoplasm. No further surgery is necessary after the diagnosis has been established. Lichenoid keratosis tends to resolve spontaneously and has reportedly involuted with topical corticosteroids.

POROKERATOSIS

Porokeratosis is a genodermatosis that includes a spectrum of squamous lesions histologically characterized by the presence of cornoid lamellae.

Clinical Findings

Porokeratoses usually form circular or oval lesions surrounded by a hyperkeratotic rim (Fig. 11.30). Several clinical variants are described. They include porokeratosis of Mibelli and disseminated superficial actinic porokeratosis (DSAP). The Mibelli type usually manifests in childhood. It typically begins as a small keratotic papule, which spreads peripherally and leaves an atrophic center surrounded by a keratotic rim. DSAP presents as numerous superficial small, annular, keratotic, red macules on sun-exposed areas of the skin, frequently the forearms and legs, affecting adults. Punctate, linear, reticulate, zosteriform, and many other variants of porokeratosis have been described. Porokeratoses have been associated with immunosuppression.

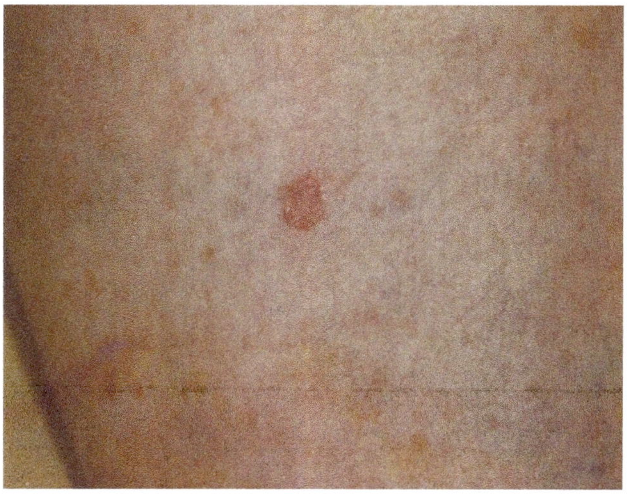

FIG. 11.30

Porokeratosis. A circular lesion with an atrophic center is surrounded by a hyperkeratotic rim.

POROKERATOSIS—DISEASE FACT SHEET

Patient Group and Site of Involvement
- Depend on clinical variant

Clinical Findings
- Erythematous annular lesion (papule or plaque) with a raised hyperkeratotic rim

Clinical Variants (Selected Examples)
- Mibelli (rare): plaque that appears in childhood, most often on the extremities
- Disseminated superficial actinic porokeratosis (most common form): thin papules, typically on the legs of adult women
- Punctate porokeratosis: isolated small papules in adolescents or young adults on palms and soles
- Linear porokeratosis: linear lesions in children that follow the lines of Blaschko

Prognosis and Treatment
- The lesions are benign; in rare instances, squamous cell carcinoma may arise in association with a porokeratosis
- Surgical removal
- Topical treatment with 5-fluorouracil, retinoids, or imiquimod; cryotherapy

Histologic Features

The presence of a cornoid lamella is the hallmark of porokeratosis. A cornoid lamella is a thin parakeratotic column overlying an area of epidermis with an absent or decreased granular cell zone and scattered dyskeratotic cells in the spinous cell layer beneath it (Figs. 11.31 and 11.32). In porokeratoses, cornoid lamellae are typically angulated, such that the inferior portion points away from the atrophic center of the lesion. Multiple cornoid lamellae may be present. The epidermis between

POROKERATOSIS—PATHOLOGIC FEATURES

Histologic Features

- Lamella (column of parakeratosis angulated to the center of the lesion, with loss of granular cell layer underneath the column)
- Center may be atrophic or acanthotic
- Lichenoid reactions common

Differential Diagnosis

- Squamous cell carcinoma
- Lichenoid keratosis
- Epidermal nevus

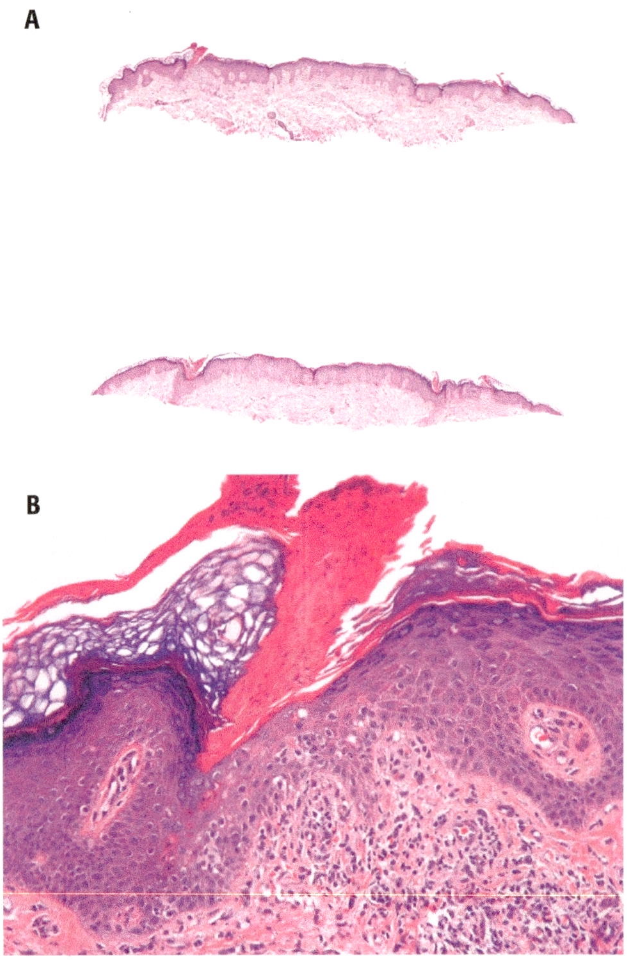

FIG. 11.31

Porokeratosis. **A,** Scanning magnification shows cornoid lamellae angulated toward the center of the lesion. **B,** A column of parakeratosis (cornoid lamella) is wedged into the epidermis at an angle. The underlying epidermis shows focal loss of the granular cell layer and dyskeratosis.

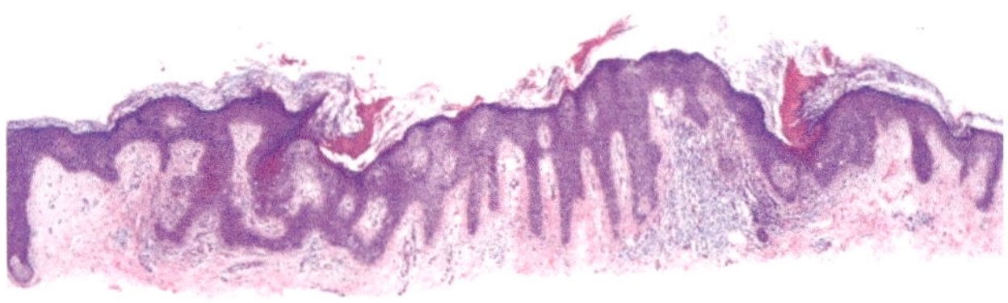

FIG. 11.32

Porokeratosis. Most porokeratoses show central epidermal atrophy, but this porokeratosis has a hyperplastic center. Associated lichenoid inflammatory reactions as seen here are common.

cornoid lamellae shows variable findings. It usually but not always shows some atrophy with overlying hyperkeratosis. In porokeratosis palmaris et plantaris disseminata, the orthokeratosis both in the center and periphery of the lesion is thicker than the parakeratotic column. The superficial dermis is often hypervascular and inflamed. A lichenoid inflammatory reaction pattern is seen commonly. It is important to be aware that if a lesion is not biopsied or sectioned in a manner in which the keratotic rim is captured in the sections the coronoid lamellae will not be seen histologically.

Differential Diagnosis

Cornoid lamellae are characteristic but not specific for porokeratosis. An isolated cornoid lamellae may be found in association with various neoplastic (keratoses, carcinoma) or hyperplastic (e.g., verruca) squamous proliferations. Clinical correlation and the lack of histologic features supporting an alternative diagnosis are important. Because the presence of a cornoid lamella is essential to establish a diagnosis, it is important for the clinician who suspects porokeratosis to take a biopsy across the edge of the peripheral rim.

Prognosis and Treatment

Porokeratoses are benign but may be complicated on rare occasions by the development of SCC. Porokeratoses may be treated by locally destructive therapy (cryotherapy) or topical reagents (e.g., imiquimod, retinoids, others).

INTRAEPIDERMAL SQUAMOUS "PRECURSOR" LESIONS: KERATINOCYTIC "DYSPLASIAS" AND SQUAMOUS CELL CARCINOMA IN SITU (NONINVASIVE CARCINOMA)

The development of SCC is similar to that of other carcinomas; it is an evolutionary process from a preinvasive to an invasive neoplasm. The histologic changes associated with the development of the intraepidermal neoplasm before stromal invasion have historically been referred to as "dysplasia," "intraepithelial neoplasia," or "in situ carcinoma." Although grading schemes have been proposed for dysplasias (mild, moderate, or severe dysplasia; low-grade versus high-grade "dysplasia"; or "intraepithelial neoplasia" grades I to III) and are accepted for precursor lesions of SCC at mucosal sites (e.g., cervical intraepithelial squamous neoplasia), there is currently no consensus for an analogous application of similar terms to cutaneous SCC.

When a squamous epithelial cell layer displays full-thickness atypia and disordered maturation, there is agreement among pathologists to designate such a lesion as SCCIS. There remains controversy, however, with regard to the best terminology for lesions lacking full-thickness atypia, especially concerning the continued use of the term AK (aka solar keratosis). Arguments have been made that AK represents nothing other than early SCC because features of AK are often associated with invasive SCC, and it is recognized that SCC can invade the dermis in the absence of full-thickness atypia of the overlying epidermis. However, many clinicians and pathologists, including the authors of this chapter, believe that the distinction of AK from outright SCC has clinical value and is beneficial for patients. Many AKs do not progress to invasive carcinoma. The vast majority of them do not require surgery for treatment, responding often to topical therapy or regress even spontaneously. To minimize harm to patients from indiscriminate surgical excisions, it seems prudent to continue to use the term *AK*, being aware of the imperfection of this terminology.

THE SPECTRUM OF ACTINIC KERATOSIS AND ACTINIC SQUAMOUS CELL CARCINOMA IN SITU

Clinical Findings

The term *actinic keratosis* was used by Pinkus, when he renamed in 1958 the same type of lesion, which had been identified earlier in 1926 by Freudenthal as *keratoma senilis.* The name *actinic keratosis* was chosen to describe the clinical phenomenon of a keratotic growth presumably related to sun rays, with no regard to histology or biology. It is now recognized that AK essentially represents a noninvasive epidermal keratinocytic neoplasia related to damage by sunlight or other radiation. As such, it represents the principal precursor lesion of cutaneous SCC. AK and lesions of actinic SCCIS (i.e., full-thickness epithelial atypia associated with a background of AK), if one attempts to make such a distinction, are common scaly, erythematous papules, patches, or plaques that are frequently encountered on sun-exposed sites such as the face, scalp, ears, and dorsal hands in middle-aged adults (Figs. 11.33 and 11.34). Most of the lesions are small, typically 2 to 6 mm in diameter. They are a mark of photodamage. AKs are usually seen in individuals with fair skin.

ACTINIC KERATOSIS (AKA SOLAR KERATOSIS)—DISEASE FACT SHEET

Patient Group

- ▸▸ Common in White individuals (>40% of adults in Australia)
- ▸▸ Common in elderly individuals

Site of Involvement

- ▸▸ Most often in head and neck region and upper extremities

Clinical Findings

- ▸▸ Erythematous lesion with scale

Prognosis and Treatment

- ▸▸ May progress to invasive squamous cell carcinoma
- ▸▸ Topical treatment (liquid nitrogen, 5-fluorouracil, imiquimod) or surgery

Histologic Features

There are several histologic variants of AK, but the unifying feature is that of keratinocyte atypia predominantly affecting the basal cell layer of the epidermis. There is also evidence of maturation of keratinocytes toward the skin surface and associated hyperkeratosis (Fig. 11.35). Basilar keratinocytes show enlarged, elongated, and hyperchromatic nuclei. There is often overlap of nuclei. The cytoplasm of the keratinocytes of the overlying spinous layer is often pale. Parakeratosis of the stratum corneum is commonly present.

In early lesions of AK, a basket-weave scale still overlies appendageal structures like follicles or the terminal portion of sweat ducts (Fig. 11.35), and the keratinocytes of skin appendages lack atypia. The change in the stratum corneum gives a picture of alternating horizontal parakeratosis with orthokeratosis, referred to as the "flag" sign. In later stages, atypical keratinocytes may populate the basal cell or suprabasilar layer of the follicular infundibulum (Fig. 11.36) or acrosyringium or populate the spinous cell layer of the epidermis (Fig. 11.37). The epidermis is usually thickened but may be thin and atrophic. The dermis underneath an AK is characterized by the presence of solar elastosis often accompanied by vascular ectasia. Solar elastosis may be so marked that it replaces or pushes away any normal-appearing collagen, filling the entire region of the papillary dermis. Many lesions of AK are inflamed.

The hyperplastic or hypertrophic variant of AK is usually found on the dorsal hands and forearms. This form of AK is characterized by irregular psoriasiform hyperplasia and often markedly thickened stratum corneum of

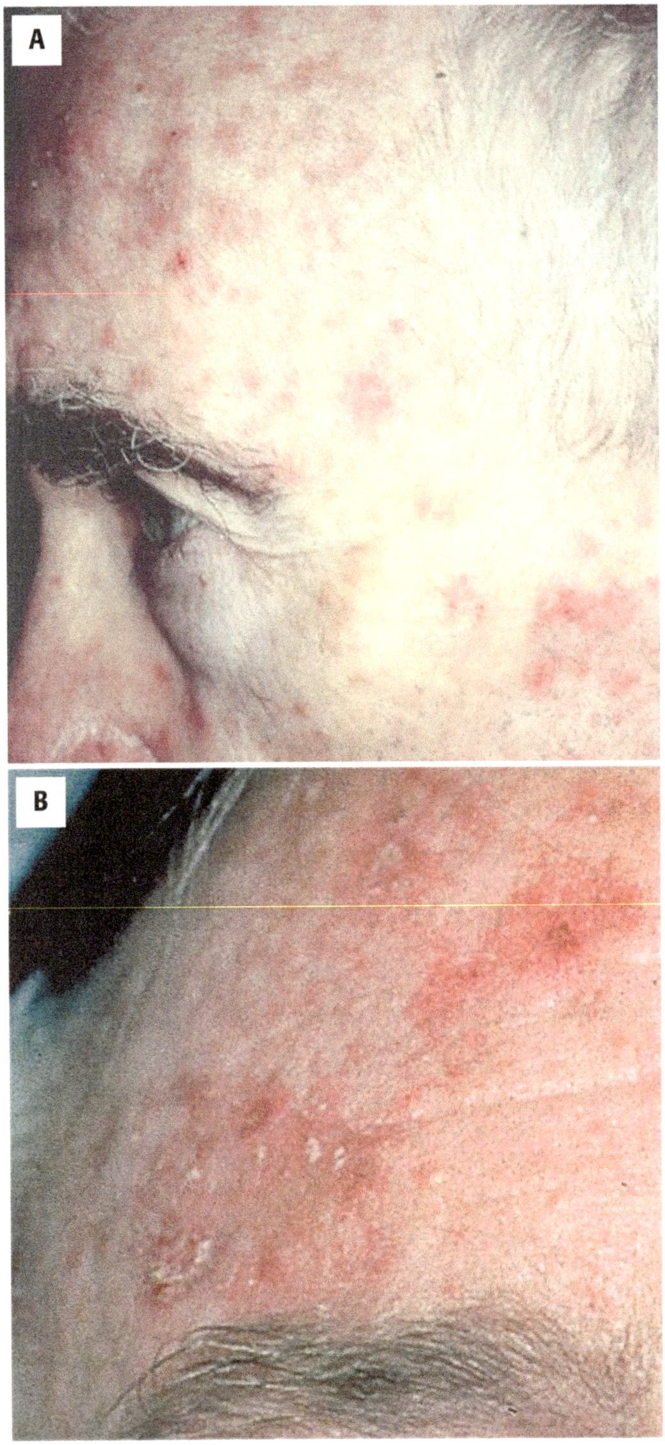

FIG. 11.33

Actinic keratoses. **A,** Multiple flat erythematous macules are present on the face. **B,** Large erythematous patch with variable scale on the forehead.

alternating orthoparakeratosis and hyperparakeratosis (Fig. 11.38). The presence of a prominent granular cell layer and stromal changes, such as dilated vessels in the papillary dermis, fibrosis, or hemorrhage, suggest that many of these lesions likely represent AK with superimposed features of LSC.

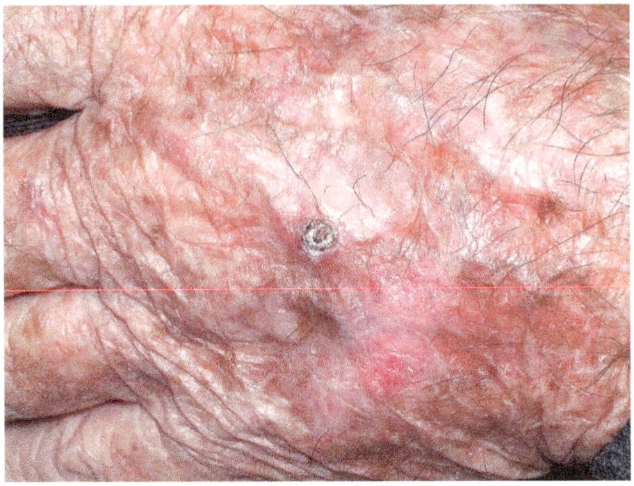

FIG. 11.34

Hypertrophic actinic keratosis on the dorsum of the hand.

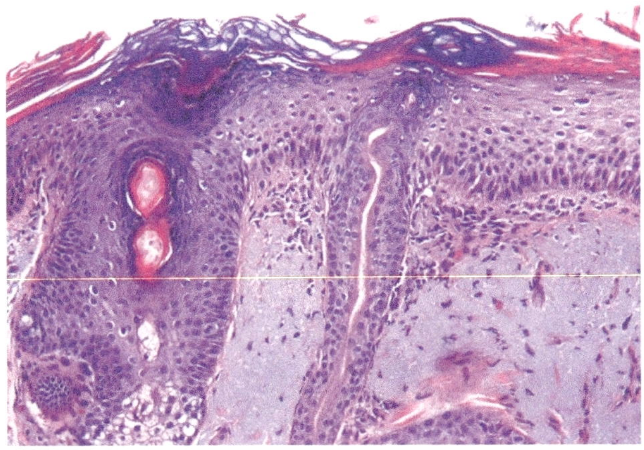

FIG. 11.35

Actinic keratosis. Basilar atypia of keratinocytes, parakeratosis, and solar elastosis are characteristic. In early lesions, adnexal structures lack epithelial atypia and parakeratosis.

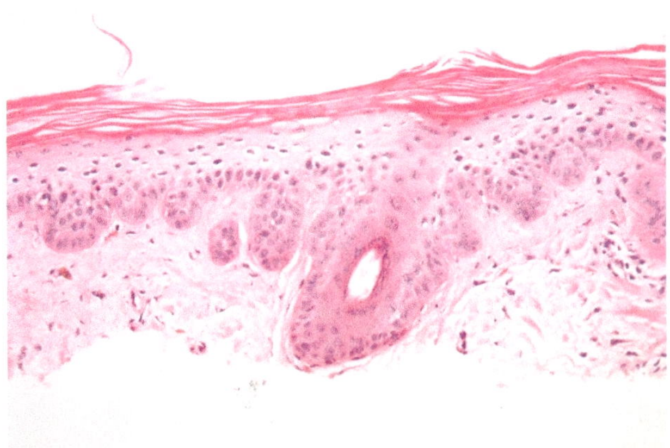

FIG. 11.36

Actinic keratosis. Basilar atypia is continuous and extends into follicular infundibulum. Maturing keratinocytes of the spinous cell layer show cytoplasmic pallor.

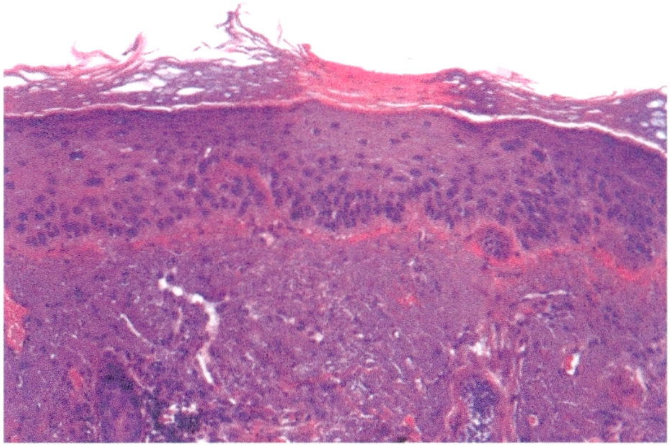

FIG. 11.37

Actinic keratosis with basilar and suprabasilar atypia of keratinocytes.

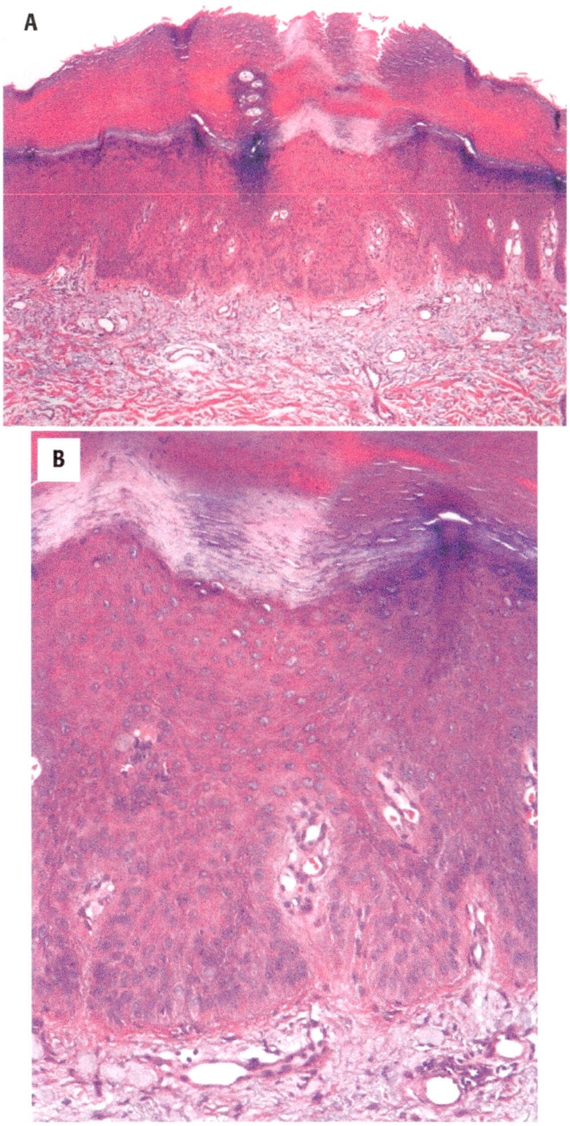

FIG. 11.38

Hypertrophic actinic keratosis. **A,** The epidermis and stratum corneum are thickened. The granular cell layer is focally prominent. **B,** Basilar keratinocytes show atypical hyperchromatic nuclei.

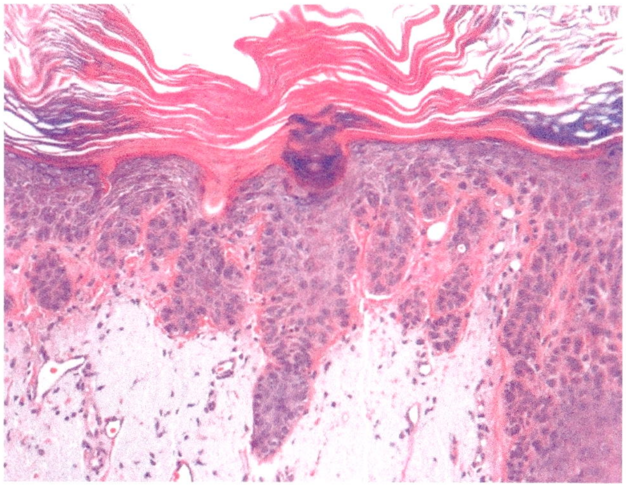

FIG. 11.39

Proliferative actinic keratosis. Thin extensions of rete ridge–like protrusions with atypical basilar keratinocytes are seen.

ACTINIC KERATOSIS—PATHOLOGIC FEATURES

Histologic Features

- Basilar keratinocytic atypia (hyperchromatic and elongate nuclei); suprabasilar atypia common, at least focally
- Alternating areas of parakeratosis and orthokeratosis (overlying appendages) in early lesions ("flag sign"); later lesions often have confluent parakeratosis
- Solar elastosis and variable inflammation
- Histologic variants: hypertrophic, acantholytic, proliferative, pigmented, lichenoid

Differential Diagnosis

- Squamous cell carcinoma
- Seborrheic keratosis
- Solar lentigo (versus pigmented actinic keratosis)
- Lentigo maligna (versus pigmented actinic keratosis)
- Chemotherapy effects

Proliferative AK is a variant of AK characterized by multiple downward, elongated rete ridge-like protrusions of atypical basilar keratinocytes (Fig. 11.39). Such protrusions often involve adnexal structures, which is why proliferative AK is thought to be more resistant to standard topical treatment than other types of AKs.

AK may be pigmented and associated with an increase in melanin pigment within epidermal keratinocytes (Figs. 11.40 and 11.41). Melanin pigment may also be present in macrophages within the superficial dermis. At times there is also a slight increase in the number of intraepidermal melanocytes as a manifestation of sun-induced melanocytic hyperplasia.

Lichenoid AKs have a bandlike, inflammatory infiltrate predominantly composed of lymphocytes. It is distinguished from benign lichenoid keratosis or lichen planus-like keratosis by the presence of actinic-type keratinocytic atypia (hyperchromatic and elongated

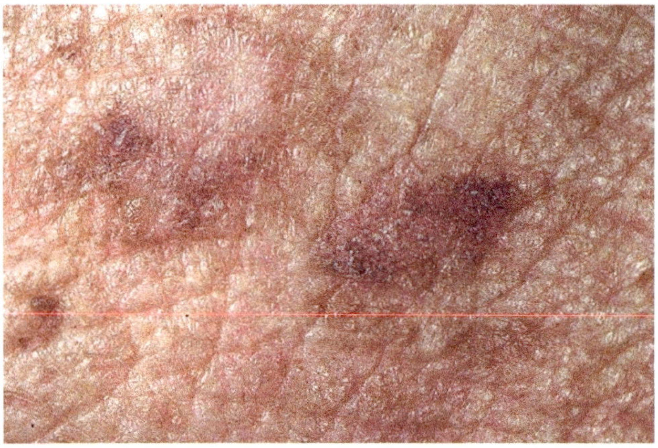

FIG. 11.40

Pigmented actinic keratosis. Brown scaly patch.

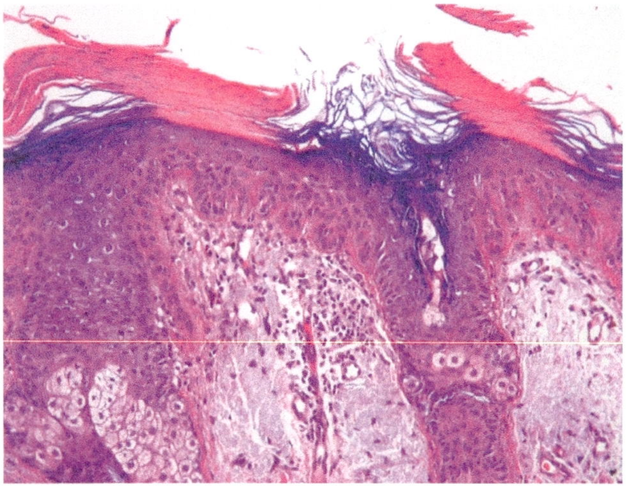

FIG. 11.41

Pigmented actinic keratosis. Actinic keratosis with an associated increase of melanin pigment deposition in keratinocytes. Pigmentation may also be related to the presence of melanophages or a melanocytic hyperplasia.

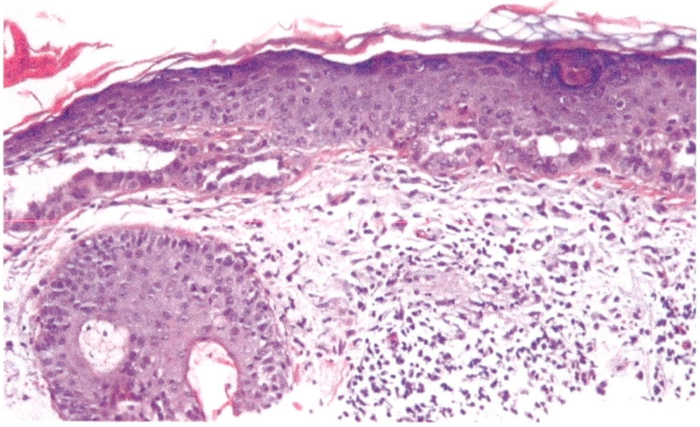

FIG. 11.42

Acantholytic actinic keratosis. Clefts are seen between basilar and suprabasilar keratinocytes reflecting intraepidermal acantholysis.

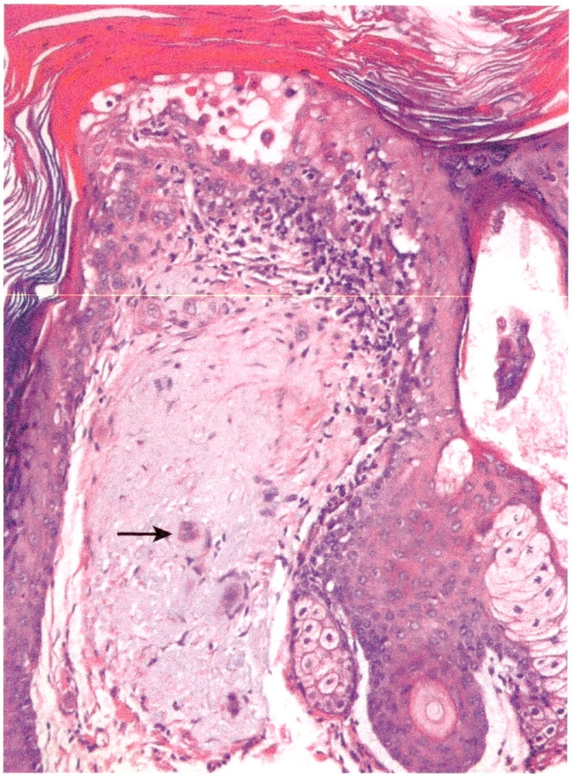

FIG. 11.43

Microinvasive squamous cell carcinoma. Isolated cells and small cell clusters of atypical keratinocytes are seen in the papillary dermis *(arrow)*. This microinvasive squamous cell carcinoma arose in association with an acantholytic actinic keratosis.

nuclei). Basal vacuolar change and Civatte bodies may be seen.

Acantholytic AK is characterized by the cellular dyscohesion. Clefts may be seen within the epidermis, especially between atypical keratinocytes of the basal cell layer and usually less atypical or normal maturing cells of the spinous cell layer (Fig. 11.42). Step sections are prudent when examining acantholytic AK because some of these lesions are associated with histologically subtle microinvasive SCC (Fig. 11.43).

Although keratinocytic atypia in AK starts and often remains confined to the basal cell and lower spinous cell layer, AKs may progress and in later stages contain foci with atypia also in the mid or upper spinous or even granular cell layer. When there is full-thickness atypia as well as abnormal maturation, we use the term *squamous cell carcinoma in situ* (Fig. 11.44). However, as straightforward as that seems, there is considerable latitude in how dermatopathologists deal with the histologic feature of full-thickness or "near full-thickness" atypia, when it is seen in a background of AK. Some pathologists may prefer to use the term *AK* or refer to them as "bowenoid AK." Others may report such lesions

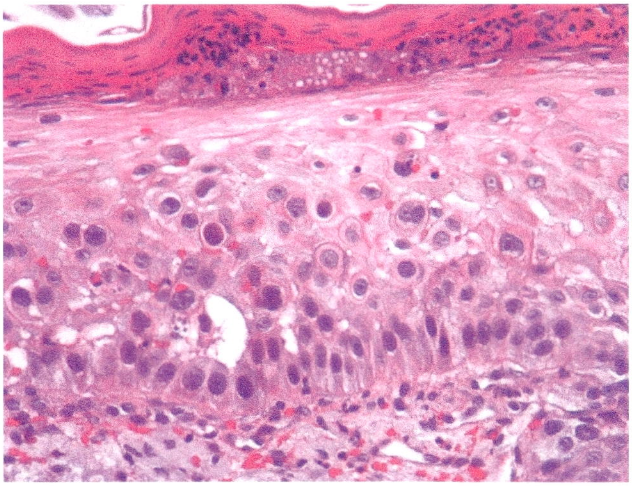

FIG. 11.44

Full-thickness epidermal atypia with loss of normal maturation indicates in situ (intraepidermal) squamous cell carcinoma. This feature was present in a background of an actinic keratosis.

as "AK with severe atypia," "AK with transition to SCCIS," or "SCCIS arising in a background of AK." In our opinion, there is no reason to believe that bowenoid AK is biologically anything other than SCCIS.

Differential Diagnosis

ACTINIC KERATOSIS VERSUS BENIGN KERATOSES

Clinically and histologically, the main differential diagnosis is from benign keratoses and invasive SCC. AKs differ from SKs by the presence of hyperchromatic enlarged basilar keratinocytes. AKs tend to have a parakeratotic stratum corneum in contrast with the common basket-weave stratum corneum of SKs. Pseudohorn cysts, which are often seen with SKs, are not a feature of AKs. Although the distinction of SK from AK is usually straightforward, it can at times be difficult on a small biopsy, because sun-exposed SKs may show focal actinic-type keratinocytic atypia, irritated SKs may contain enlarged nuclei, and SKs may collide with AKs.

Porokeratosis differs from AK by the lack of basilar keratinocytic atypia and the presence of cornoid lamellae. Likewise, lichenoid keratosis lacks the hyperchromatic nuclei of AKs. The distinction on a small biopsy, however, can be difficult because AKs also may be associated with a bandlike inflammatory cell infiltrate. If a lesion contains a noninflamed component, it is easier to establish a diagnosis. In lichenoid keratosis, the noninflamed component, which is often seen at the periphery of a lesion, tends to show features of SK or solar lentigo, but a lichenoid AK shows features of typical AK.

DIGITATED ACTINIC KERATOSIS VERSUS VERRUCA OF SUN-DAMAGED SKIN

A hypertrophic digitated AK may at times be difficult to distinguish from a verruca arising in chronically sun-damaged skin. A digitated AK is favored, if the squamous proliferation has a warty silhouette, but actinic-type epithelial atypia is present throughout the entire lesion and HPV cytopathic changes are absent. On occasion, a verruca may collide with an AK.

PIGMENTED ACTINIC KERATOSIS VERSUS SOLAR LENTIGO OR LENTIGO MALIGNA

Pigmented AK needs to be distinguished from solar lentigo and melanoma in situ. Solar lentigo lacks basilar hyperchromatic keratinocytes. Melanoma in situ is characterized by an increased and abnormal density and growth of intraepidermal melanocytes. It may collide with an AK.

ACANTHOLYTIC ACTINIC KERATOSIS VERSUS ACANTHOLYTIC SQUAMOUS CELL CARCINOMA OR BENIGN ACANTHOLYTIC LESIONS

The dermis underneath an acantholytic AK needs to be examined for possible invasive SCC. Single-cell invasion can be histologically subtle. Acantholytic AK does not only need to be distinguished from invasive SCC but also from other acantholytic lesions. Acantholytic acanthoma lacks the keratinocytic atypia of AK. Grover's and Darier's diseases also lack atypia and present with a distinct clinical picture.

ACTINIC KERATOSIS VERSUS CHEMOTHERAPY-INDUCED ATYPIA

Patients with photodamaged skin undergoing chemotherapy may develop lesions in the epidermis characterized histologically by keratinocytic atypia and abnormal maturation that can be confused with AK or SCCIS if the pathologist is unaware of the patient's history.

Prognosis and Treatment

The majority of AKs do not progress to invasive carcinoma. The likelihood of invasive SCC arising in a given AK has been estimated to range from 0.075% to 1% per lesion per year, but for a number of reasons, it is difficult to measure the incidence of this phenomenon with precision. Higher estimates (up to 20%, for untreated lesions over a period of 10 years) as well as lower estimates (0.025%) have been published in the literature for the progression of AK to SCC. However, when discussing the risk for SCC, one should bear in mind that many individuals with AKs tend to have multiple lesions, and the cumulative risk depends on the number of lesions and length of time they persist. Among persons with multiple AKs, the lifetime risk of developing at least one invasive SCC is likely in the range of 10%.

Most solitary or limited AKs and lesions of actinic SCCIS are treated with cryotherapy, which has the risks of pain, vesicle formation, infection, and postinflammatory pigmentary alterations. Multiple lesions or more widespread involvement usually warrants treatment with topical 5-fluorouracil, topical nonsteroidal antiinflammatory agents, or imiquimod. Photodynamic therapy may also be used for widespread involvement but seems to have efficacy only after debulking any hyperkeratotic scale. We report follicular involvement within an AK to our clinicians because topical treatment may be less effective.

Management problems sometimes arise from pitfalls in communication with clinicians related to nomenclature. Because some dermatopathologists refer to all AKs as *squamous cell carcinoma solar keratotic type*, a number of patients with lesions described herein as AK may unnecessarily undergo surgery even though the lesion could have been treated topically or even be observed. In the absence of a widely accepted consensus terminology, it is important for clinicians and pathologists to reach a mutual understanding of what is meant by the diagnostic terms they use for a patient's lesion.

If an initial superficial shave biopsy reveals evidence of SCCIS or an AK with worrisome features, such as acantholysis, and the base of the epidermis or lesion is not seen, it is best to communicate this to the clinician. The implication is that because of superficial sampling, associated invasive carcinoma cannot be excluded. A prudent approach to this problem would be to rebiopsy the site and include the superficial dermis in the tissue sample.

BOWENOID SQUAMOUS CELL CARCINOMA IN SITU (BOWEN'S DISEASE AND ITS VARIANTS)

SCCIS is histologically described as bowenoid when the keratinocytic atypia predominantly affects the spinous cell layer and is associated with loss of polarity. It is thought that many lesions of bowenoid SCCIS derive from preceding HPV infection. Numerous different types of HPVs have been detected in lesions of bowenoid SCCIS. Other etiologies include arsenic exposure and radiation.

Bowen's disease is a clinical term broadly referring to lesions of cutaneous SCCIS, although AKs, including AKs with focal full-thickness atypia, are generally discussed separately. A related clinical term is *erythroplasia of Queyrat*. It refers to SCCIS on the glans penis typically presenting as a well-demarcated erythematous, velvety thin plaque. Bowen's disease and erythroplasia of Queyrat represent clinical variants of SCCIS and not pathologic diagnoses.

The spectrum of precursor lesions with bowenoid keratinocytic atypia also includes bowenoid papulosis and epidermodysplasia verruciformis.

Clinical Findings

The clinical appearance is typically that of sharply demarcated erythematous, velvety, or scaly macules, papules, patches, or plaques (Fig. 11.45). Some lesions have a warty appearance, and some may be eroded. At times

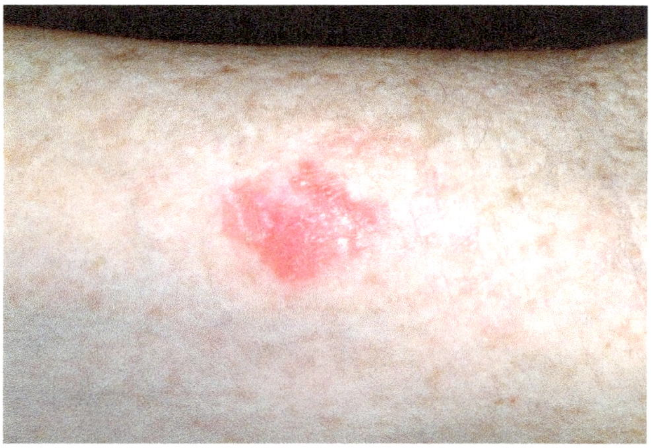

FIG. 11.45

Bowen's disease (squamous cell carcinoma in situ) presenting as an erythematous patch.

BOWEN'S DISEASE (SQUAMOUS CELL CARCINOMA IN SITU)—DISEASE FACT SHEET

Patient Group

- Primarily elderly White individuals
- Immunosuppressed individuals

Site of Involvement

- May occur anywhere
- Often involves sun-exposed areas of head and neck and extremities of fair-skinned individuals
- Non–sun-exposed sites more often affected in dark-skinned individuals

Clinical Findings

- Erythematous papule, patch, or plaque
- May be eroded (usually related to excoriation) or pigmented
- Usually arises de novo but may be associated with a verruca or keratosis

Prognosis and Treatment

- May locally recur or progress to invasive carcinoma if incompletely removed. (The risk for invasive carcinoma is <10%.)
- May regress spontaneously
- Can be treated topically (medically, e.g., imiquimod, or by cryotherapy)
- Surgical removal

the lesions may simulate the appearance of a superficial BCC, irritated keratosis, Paget's disease, or eczema. Pigmented variants exist (pigmented Bowen's disease), which may lead clinically to confusion with a melanocytic neoplasm.

Bowen's disease has a predilection for sun-exposed sites of fair-skinned older individuals, but lesions may develop anywhere and at any age, especially in the setting of immune suppression. It may develop de novo or in association with a preexisting lesion, such as an SK, verruca, porokeratosis, or a cyst. Bowen's disease is said to progress to invasive carcinoma in up to 8% of untreated cases. The risk for invasive carcinoma increases with age and immune suppression.

Bowenoid papulosis, which is often associated with HPV types 16 and 18, typically affects younger adults and tends to manifest as multiple hyperpigmented papules on the genitalia. Histologically, early lesions usually show mild atypia. More advanced lesions show features indistinguishable for bowenoid SCCIS. Epidermodysplasia verruciformis manifests as widespread fawn-colored flat warts, which may give rise to SCC.

Histologic Features

Bowen's disease is histologically SCCIS, that is, atypical keratinocytes at all layers of the epidermis ("full-thickness atypia") with loss of polarity (Fig. 11.46). "Classic" bowenoid SCCIS shows atypia first and foremost in the spinous cell layer in contrast to actinic-type SCCIS, in which atypia is first seen and often most pronounced at the basal cell layer.

Frequently, one sees a pagetoid pattern of isolated atypical keratinocytes or clusters thereof surrounded by normal nonneoplastic keratinocytes. The atypical keratinocytes typically have enlarged nuclei and less pink cytoplasm than the keratinocytes in AKs. Cytopathic features of HPV may be present (Fig. 11.47). Parahyperkeratosis and orthohyperkeratosis are common, but the stratum corneum of bowenoid SCCIS is usually not as thick as with AKs.

The degree of nuclear atypia is variable. It may range from subtle nuclear enlargement or hyperchromatism to keratinocytes with bizarre giant nuclei. An increase in the ratio of nucleus to cytoplasm is frequently seen. An important feature is the loss of normal polarity (maturation) of keratinocytes as they ascend to the stratum corneum. Mitoses and apoptotic bodies are often identified in the spinous cell layer. Some mitotic figures may be atypical. Associated inflammation is common and usually shows a lichenoid pattern. Bowenoid SCCIS may arise de novo or in association with a keratosis, typically an irritated and inflamed SK, or a verruca (Fig. 11.48).

Pigmented bowenoid SCCIS (pigmented Bowen's disease) is characterized by hyperpigmentation of keratinocytes (Fig. 11.49).

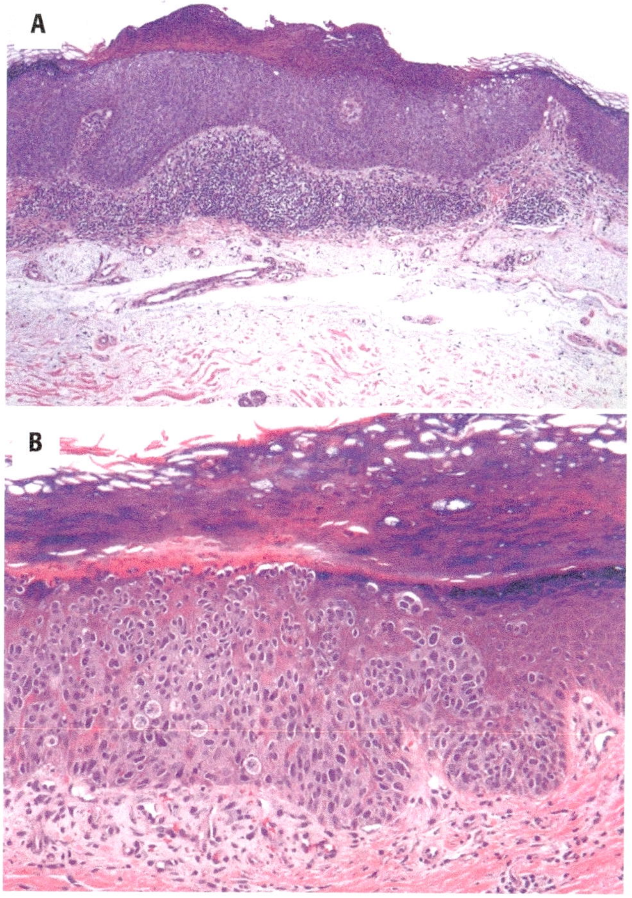

FIG. 11.46

Squamous cell carcinoma in situ, bowenoid pattern. **A,** Scanning magnification shows an intraepidermal squamous proliferation composed of keratinocytes with a higher nuclear to cytoplasmic ratio than the nonneoplastic epidermis, giving the carcinoma a darker appearance than the adjacent normal epidermis. There is associated inflammation. **B,** The basal cell layer shows bland keratinocytes. Atypical keratinocytes populate primarily the spinous cell layer.

BOWEN'S DISEASE (SQUAMOUS CELL CARCINOMA IN SITU)—PATHOLOGIC FEATURES

Histologic Features

- Keratinocytic atypia and loss of maturation in the spinous cell layer
- Pagetoid spread of tumor cells common
- Associated inflammation common
- Human papillomavirus cytopathic effects may be seen
- Pigmented variants show melanin pigment in keratinocytes or melanophages

Differential Diagnosis

- Irritated seborrheic keratosis
- Verruca
- Chemotherapy (systemic or topical)—induced atypia

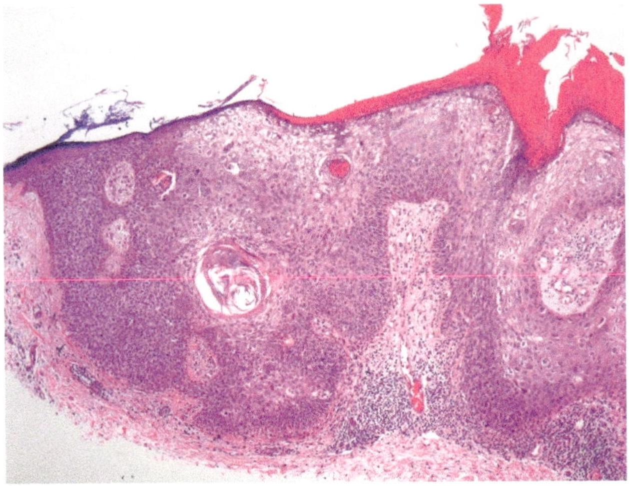

FIG. 11.47

Squamous cell carcinoma in situ, bowenoid pattern. Human papillomavirus cytopathic changes are seen in this lesion.

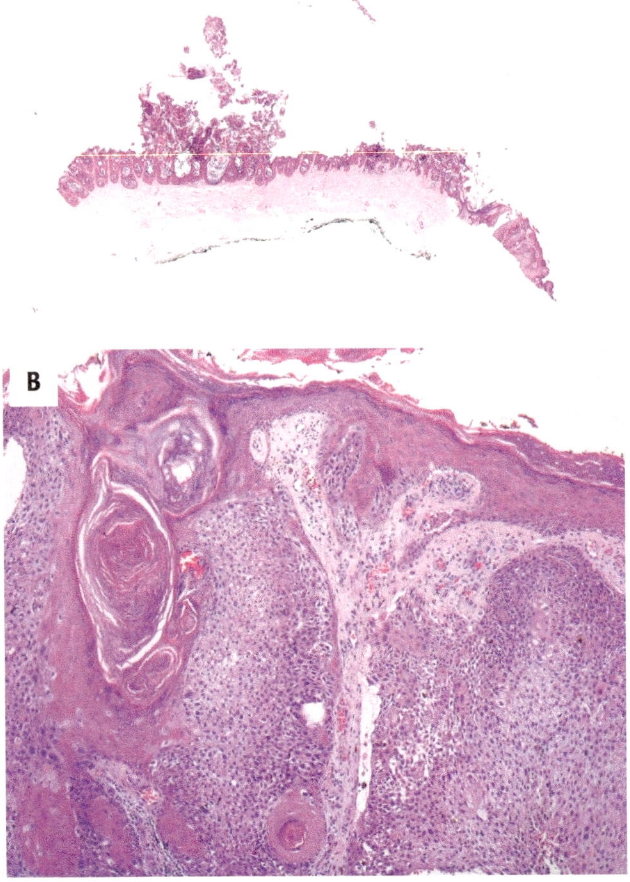

FIG. 11.48

Bowenoid squamous cell carcinoma arising in an irritated seborrheic keratosis. **A,** Scanning magnification reveals a broad seborrheic keratosis. At one edge, atypia is apparent. **B,** A close-up of this focus reveals squamous cell carcinoma.

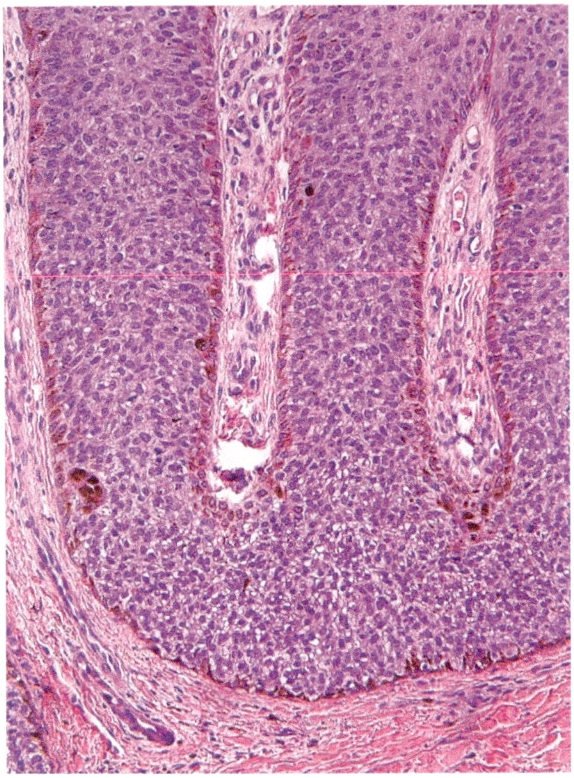

FIG. 11.49

Pigmented squamous cell carcinoma in situ, bowenoid type. There is an increase in melanin pigment deposition within keratinocytes.

Differential Diagnosis

Clinically, in nonmucosal skin, superficial BCC can mimic bowenoid SCCIS. On the genitalia, such a well-demarcated erythematous thin plaque can resemble inverse psoriasis or balanitis plasmacellularis (Zoon's balanitis). A more heaped-up appearance on the perineum or inguinal folds may also have the appearance of pemphigus vegetans or Hailey-Hailey disease. Extramammary Paget's disease as well as an eczematous dermatitis may clinically be indistinguishable from SCCIS.

Histologically, bowenoid SCCIS needs to be distinguished from other neoplasms with pagetoid spread of tumor cells, including melanoma in situ, Paget's disease, and intraepidermal sebaceous carcinoma (Fig. 11.50). Melanoma may be recognized by the presence of pigment or nests of melanocytes, Paget's disease by the presence of intracytoplasmic mucin, and sebaceous carcinoma by a clear vacuolated cytoplasm. If distinction by conventional histologic clues is not straightforward, immunohistochemical studies can be helpful. Bowenoid SCCIS is readily distinguished from melanoma in situ by immunohistochemistry (Fig. 11.50B). It is more difficult to distinguish immunohistochemically from Paget's disease due to overlap in protein expression. The distinction of bowenoid SCCIS from "bowenoid AK" is irrelevant because the latter is the actinic variant of SCCIS.

A

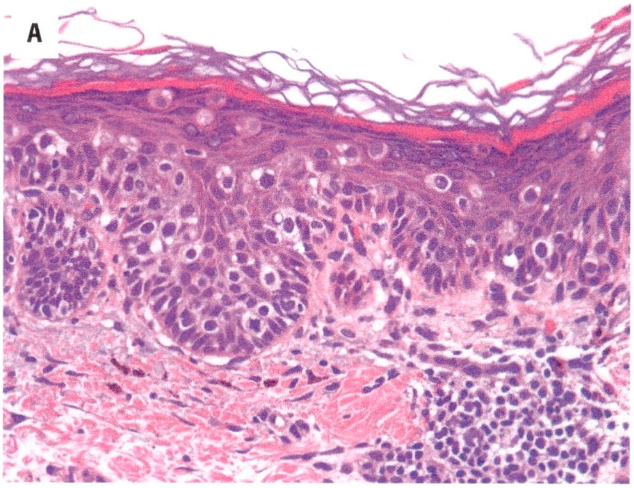

B

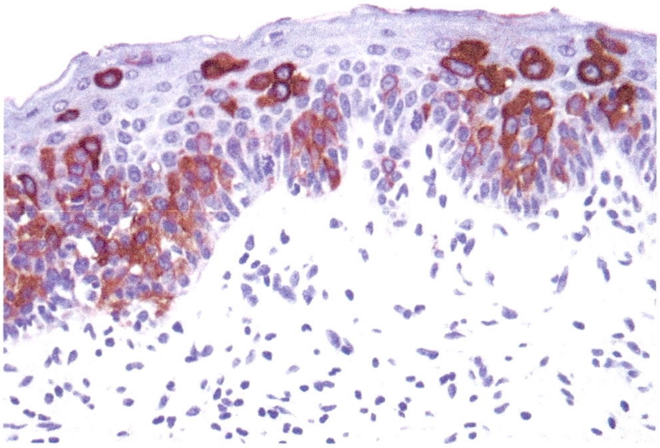

FIG. 11.50

A, Squamous cell carcinoma in situ with prominent pagetoid spread may be confused with other tumors (melanoma in situ, Paget's disease). **B,** Immunohistochemistry for cytokeratins AE1:AE3 confirms the epithelial nature of the tumor cells.

At times it may be difficult to distinguish SCCIS from invasive SCC. After an irregular infiltrative advancing border of the tumor is identified, the diagnosis of invasion seems certain. However, not every downward expansile growth represents invasive carcinoma. SCCIS may populate a preexisting keratosis or verruca and thereby extend below the level of the adjacent epidermis while still being confined to the intraepidermal compartment. SCCIS may also grow into adnexal structures, such as the infundibulum of the hair follicle, which should not be mistaken for stromal invasion (Fig. 11.51). Furthermore, lichenoid inflammatory reactions may disrupt the dermal-epidermal interface and lead to a false impression of superficial invasion.

Prognosis and Treatment

Complete removal is curative. Topical agents such as imiquimod may be considered. Electrodesiccation,

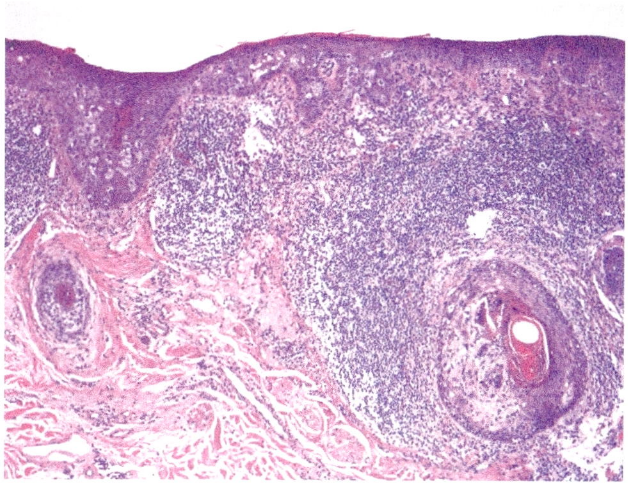

FIG. 11.51

Squamous cell carcinoma in situ may extend intraepithelially into adnexal structures. Such extension should not be confused with stromal invasion.

cryotherapy, curettage, excision, or Mohs micrographic surgery may be used depending on the extent of the lesion and its resistance to topical treatment. If a lesion is unresponsive to topical therapy, more definitive treatment with a surgical modality should be used.

VULVAR AND PERINEAL INTRAEPITHELIAL NEOPLASIA (VULVAR INTRAEPITHELIAL NEOPLASIA AND PAIN) OR DYSPLASIA

A different nomenclature is used for squamous precursor lesions at paramucosal sites, such as the vulva and perineum. They comprise a spectrum of HPV- and non–HPV-related squamous proliferations. Different categories of dysplasia or intraepithelial neoplasia are currently recognized and have been described in greatest detail for vulvar lesions: (1) low-grade lesions with minimal risk for cancer, (2) high-grade lesions (usually but not necessarily associated with HPV), and (3) squamous dysplasias defined more by abnormalities of differentiation than by nuclear atypia ("differentiated" or "simplex type" dysplasia).

Clinical Findings

Vulvar intraepithelial neoplasia (VIN) typically affects middle-aged women. Perianal dysplasia is more often seen in men. This type of dysplasia often arises in the setting of HPV infection but may be unrelated to it. Pruritus is a common symptom. The clinical appearance is highly variable and ranges from small macules or papules to keratotic plaques. The lesions may appear whitish (leukoplakia) or erythematous. Multiple lesions are common. HPV-associated lesions may display a verrucoid surface.

Histologic Features

LOW-GRADE DYSPLASIA (LOW-GRADE SQUAMOUS INTRAEPITHELIAL LESION)

This category of squamous lesions includes essentially exophytic as well as flat condylomas (Fig. 11.52). The condylomas may show typical viral cytopathic effects (e.g., koilocytes with resinoid nuclei, prominent keratohyaline granules) or lack diagnostic viral changes and have the histologic appearance of a hyperkeratotic papilloma or simulate an SK or acanthoma.

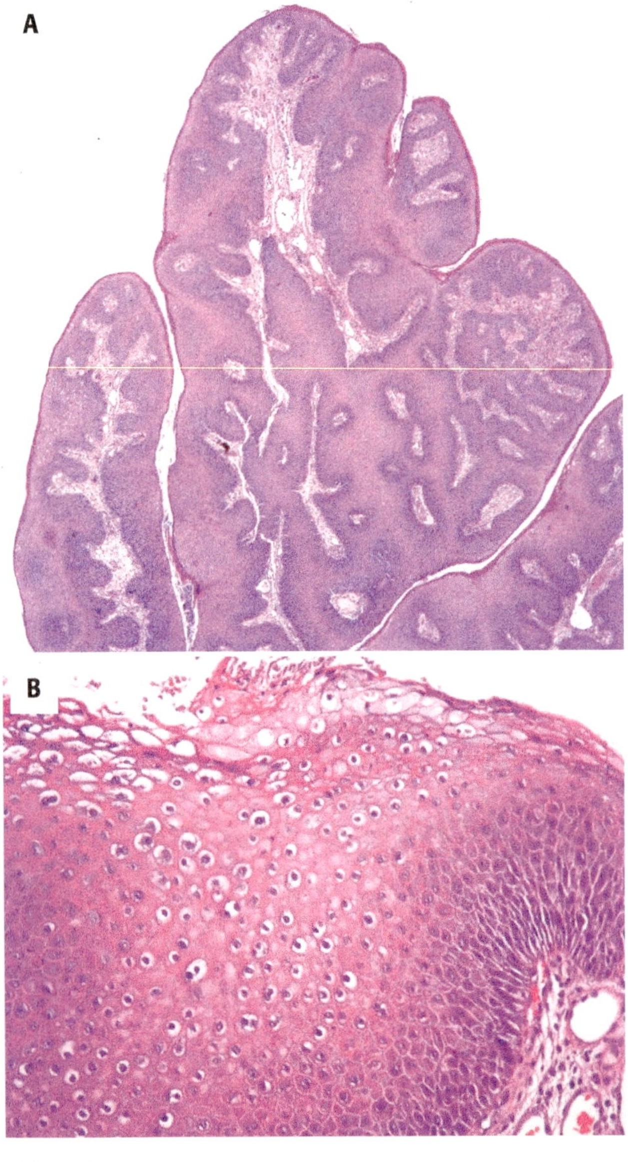

FIG. 11.52

Condyloma. **A,** A squamous papilloma is present. **B,** Human papillomavirus cytopathic effects are seen in the superficial portion of the lesion manifesting as epithelial cells with hyperchromatic resinoid nuclei surrounded by a clear space ("halo").

HIGH-GRADE DYSPLASIA (INTRAEPITHELIAL LESION GRADES II AND III)

This category of dysplasias includes squamous lesions that historically have been described as Bowen's disease, SCCIS, and bowenoid papulosis. Many but not all high-grade dysplasia lesions are associated with HPV, typically HPV 16 and 18 or other high-risk virus types. The lesions are characterized by the presence of keratinocytic atypia involving at least the lower two-thirds of the epithelium and often the entire thickness (Fig. 11.53). The degree of atypia is variable. Typically, the nuclei are enlarged and hyperchromatic. Abnormal mitoses may be present, and the epithelial surface is often covered by a thick layer of parakeratosis, although the latter features may be absent. Some high-grade dysplasias show more warty features with prominent features of HPV effects (koilocytosis), but others have a more basaloid appearance.

DIFFERENTIATED (SIMPLEX TYPE) OF DYSPLASIA

The clinical features of differentiated dysplasia have not yet been well described. Often the appearance of the lesion is that of a white (leukoplakia) or erythematous plaque (Fig. 11.54). Histologically, this type of

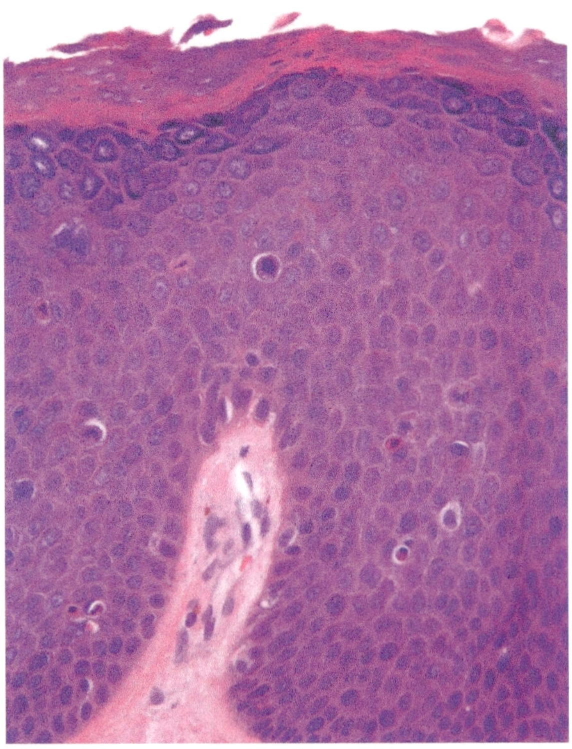

FIG. 11.53

High-grade squamous dysplasia (intraepithelial lesion). Full-thickness atypia and several mitotic figures are present.

VULVAR AND PERIANAL INTRAEPITHELIAL NEOPLASIA—PATHOLOGIC FEATURES

Histologic Features

- Epithelial atypia
- Abnormal maturation
- Variable hyperkeratosis
- Variable inflammation
- Variable features of human papillomavirus effect

Types and Grades of Dysplasia

- Classic vulvar and perianal intraepithelial neoplasia
  - I = Mild dysplasia: condyloma or flat lesion with epithelial atypia confined to the lower third of the squamous cell layer
  - II = Moderate dysplasia: epithelial atypia involving the lower and mid thirds of the squamous cell layer
  - III = Severe dysplasia: epithelial atypia involving more than two-thirds up to full thickness of the squamous cell layer (equivalent to squamous cell carcinoma in situ)
- Differentiated (simplex type) of dysplasia

Differential Diagnosis

- Inflammatory dermatoses (lichen planus, lichen simplex chronicus, eczema, psoriasis, tinea)
- Pseudoepitheliomatous hyperplasia secondary to trauma or infection

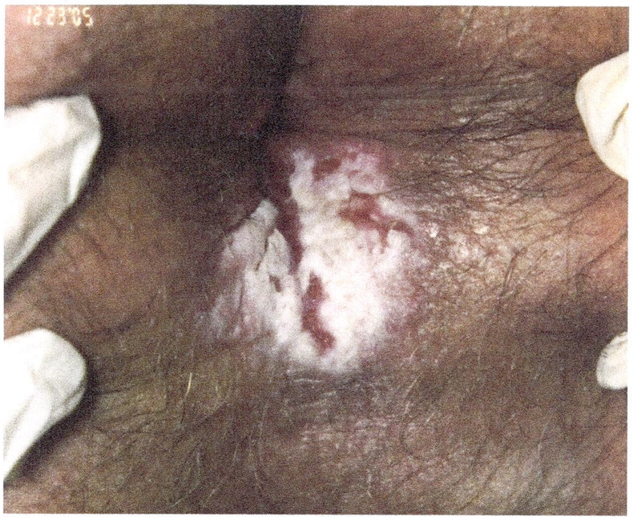

FIG. 11.54

Simplex type of dysplasia presenting as perianal leukoplakia.

dysplasia is characterized by abnormal cell maturation (Fig. 11.55). The rete ridges tend to be elongated. The basal cell layer typically shows pleomorphic or hyperchromatic nuclei. Above the basal cell layer, the keratinocytes are enlarged with abundant, dense, eosinophilic cytoplasm. Focal dyskeratosis is common. The overlying stratum corneum is usually thick and parakeratotic. Associated stromal changes of fibrosis and inflammation are variable. The spectrum of features of differentiated dysplasia includes lichen sclerosus–like lesions as well as lesions simulating LSC. The distinction of differentiated dysplasia from LSC is particularly

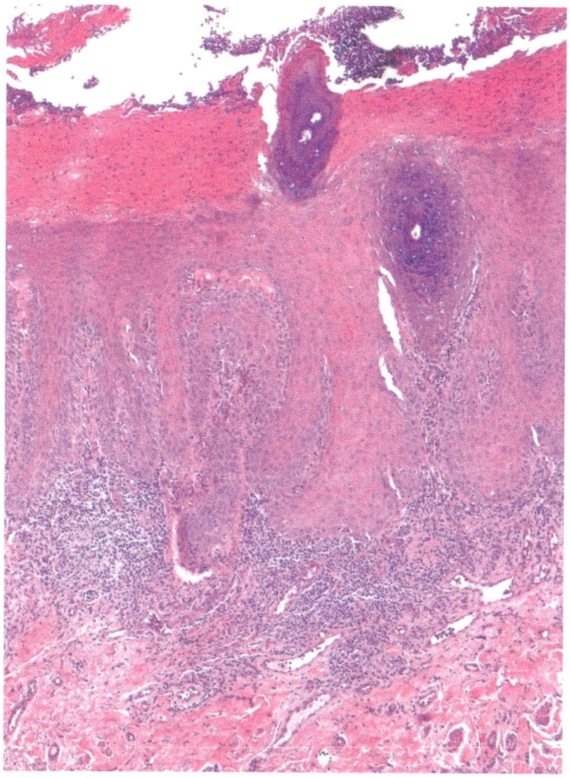

FIG. 11.55

Simplex type of squamous dysplasia. The lesion is characterized by marked hyperkeratosis and parakeratosis, broad rete ridges, basilar keratinocytic atypia, and abnormal maturation. Associated inflammation is common.

difficult because LSC may be superimposed on an area of dysplasia, and features of LSC are commonly seen at the periphery of tumors. Thus, when considering the diagnosis of LSC, it is important to search for an underlying reason for the patient's pruritus and correlate the biopsy findings with the clinical appearance of the lesion.

The simplex type of dysplasia is much less common than the previously described subtypes of dysplasia, but it is not infrequently identified at the periphery of the invasive component of many vulvar or perineal SCCs. One specific variant of differentiated vulvar intraepithelial neoplasia (DVIN) is that associated with lichen sclerosus. It is important to assess cases of lichen sclerosus for epithelial atypia because of the increased risk of DVIN. These lesions are most often mediated through a p53-associated pathway and are not related to HPV.

Differential Diagnosis

Clinically and histologically, paramucosal dysplasia needs to be distinguished from inflammatory dermatoses, such as atopic dermatitis with lichenification resulting from chronic scratching and rubbing, LSC, lichen sclerosus, candidiasis, or even lichen planus.

Prognosis and Treatment

In immunocompetent women, progression to frank invasion is rare, so therapy is usually at first conservative, including cryotherapy, podophyllin, podofilox (applied twice daily by the patient for three consecutive days each week), imiquimod (applied three nights a week by the patient), and topical caustic chemicals such as trichloroacetic acid.

For immunosuppressed women, a more aggressive destructive approach is used, which includes laser ablation, electrodesiccation, and excision. When electrodesiccation may be used, viral particles may be dispersed in the smoke plume. Thus such a procedure should be performed in conjunction with appropriate protective gear (mask and smoke evacuator).

ARSENICAL KERATOSIS

Clinical Findings

Arsenic was once commonly found in folk remedies such as Fowler's solution (potassium arsenite), which was historically used to treat psoriasis, as well as herbal remedies aimed at various ailments such as asthma and syphilis. Drinking water may also be contaminated with arsenic. More recently, intravenous arsenic trioxide has been used for acute promyelocytic leukemia. The most frequent cutaneous finding of chronic arsenic exposure is hyperpigmented macules, which may be quite hyperkeratotic. These thickened scaly lesions have a penchant for acral skin, giving the appearance of a keratoderma.

Histologic Features

There is usually significant orthokeratosis, although not compact. This hyperkeratotic stratum corneum is sometimes accompanied by acanthosis and papillomatosis. In early lesions, there is only mild keratinocytic atypia. More advanced lesions show features of SCCIS (Fig. 11.56).

Differential Diagnosis

Clinically, these may resemble a keratoderma or perhaps palmar plantar psoriasis. Thus a high index of suspicion is necessary on the part of the clinician. Histologically, an arsenical keratosis may resemble a hypertrophic AK or even a hyperkeratotic SK.

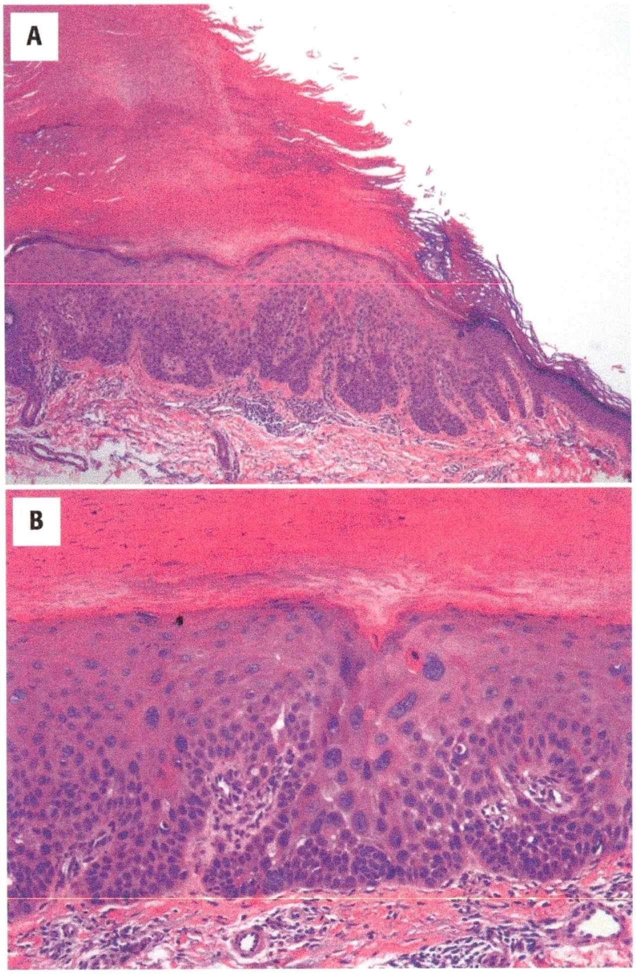

FIG. 11.56

Arsenical keratosis. **A,** Epidermal hyperplasia and hyperkeratosis. **B,** Keratinocytic atypia is present throughout the spinous cell layer (squamous cell carcinoma in situ).

Prognosis and Treatment

Oral retinoids such as acitretin and etretinate as well as intralesional 5-fluorouracil are used to manage patients with arsenical keratoses. Surveillance biopsies looking for transformation to SCC are also used. This condition is important to recognize because these lesions may evolve into cutaneous malignancies, such as SCCIS, SCC, and BCC. Chronic arsenic exposure is also associated with hepatocellular carcinoma, angiosarcoma of the liver, cirrhosis, and bladder cancer.

INVASIVE SQUAMOUS CELL CARCINOMA

Clinical Findings

Invasive SCC is, after BCC, the second most common type of skin cancer. It has a tendency to affect sun-damaged fair skin of older individuals and the skin of solid organ transplant recipients. It is also associated with chemical carcinogens or chronic wounds, such as nonhealing ulcers, burn scars, or sinus tracts. *Marjolin ulcer* is a term for SCC arising at the site of chronic inflammation, presenting as persistent ulceration. SCC can also be induced by ionizing radiation. When SCC is diagnosed in a child or young person, the possibility of a genodermatosis such as xeroderma pigmentosum should be considered. HPV plays a major role in the development of SCC of the penis, vulva, and perianal and periungual skin as well as at mucosal sites but can lead to SCC at any site, particularly in individuals with epidermodysplasia verruciformis. Recently, the development of well-differentiated SCC has become recognized as a cutaneous side effect of various new medications, such as the BRAF inhibitor vemurafenib or the antifungal agent voriconazole.

Invasive SCC may manifest as an erythematous, scaly papule to thin plaque. A thin (i.e., only superficially invasive) tumor may be clinically indistinguishable from any type of in situ carcinoma or AK. Thicker tumors typically present as an erythematous plaque, nodule, or ulcer (Figs. 11.57 and 11.58). The sites of predilection for SCC include the face, ears, scalp, and dorsal hands.

Histologic Features

Invasive SCC represents a carcinoma of epidermal origin that infiltrates the stroma of the dermis. An associated

INVASIVE SQUAMOUS CELL CARCINOMA (CONVENTIONAL TYPE)—DISEASE FACT SHEET

Incidence

- Approximately 1/1000 individuals (or 250,000 new cases per year) in the United States

Risk Factors

- Ultraviolet radiation
- Immunosuppression (organ transplantation, HIV)
- Ionizing radiation
- Infection (oncogenic human papillomavirus)
- Chemical carcinogens (e.g., arsenic)
- Chronic inflammation (e.g., Marjolin ulcer, burn scar)
- Genetic disorders of DNA repair (e.g., xeroderma pigmentosum)
- Fair skin complexion and light-colored hair
- Medication related (e.g., vemurafenib or voriconazole)

Patient Group

- Preferentially affects elderly individuals and men more often than women

Site of Involvement

- Head and neck most common but may occur anywhere

Clinical Findings

- Erythematous papule, patch, nodule, or plaque; may have scale; may be ulcerated

Prognosis

- Most superficial cutaneous squamous cell carcinomas are cured by surgery
- Unfavorable clinical parameters:
  - High-risk anatomic sites (ear, lip, eyelid)
  - Immunosuppression
- Unfavorable pathologic parameters
- Size (width) >2 cm; depth of invasion >4 mm; thickness >6 mm
- Lymphovascular or perineural invasion
- Poor differentiation

Treatment

- Surgery is the treatment of choice
- Nonsurgical modalities include radiation and laser therapy or chemotherapy

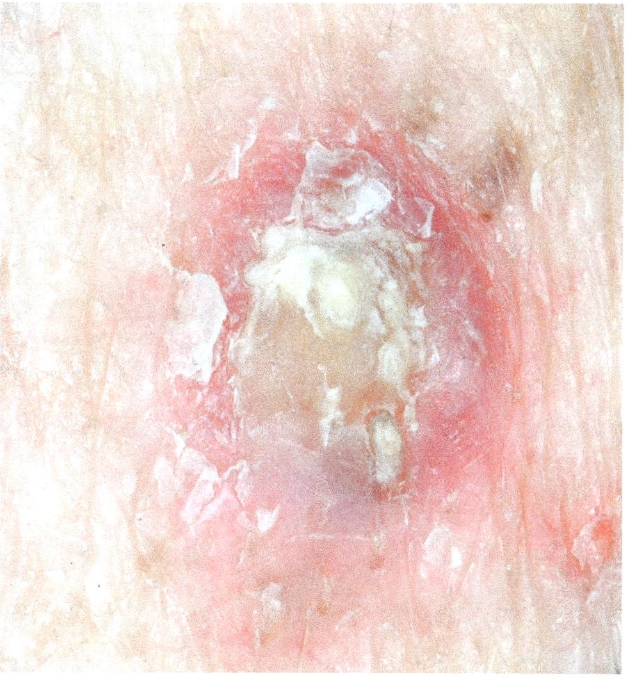

FIG. 11.57

Squamous cell carcinoma presenting as a keratotic erythematous plaque.

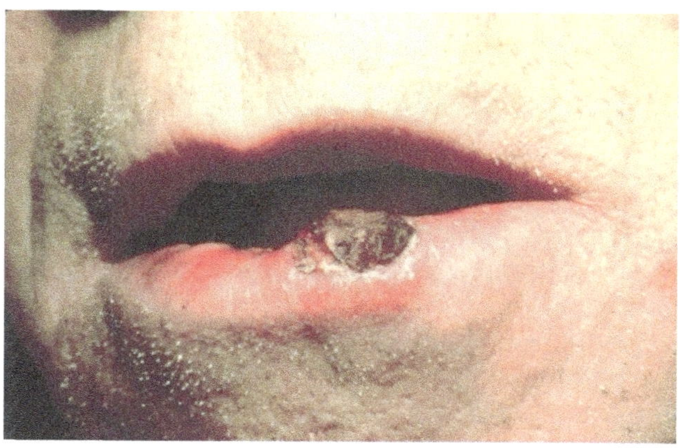

FIG. 11.58

Squamous cell carcinoma of the lip presenting as an ulcer.

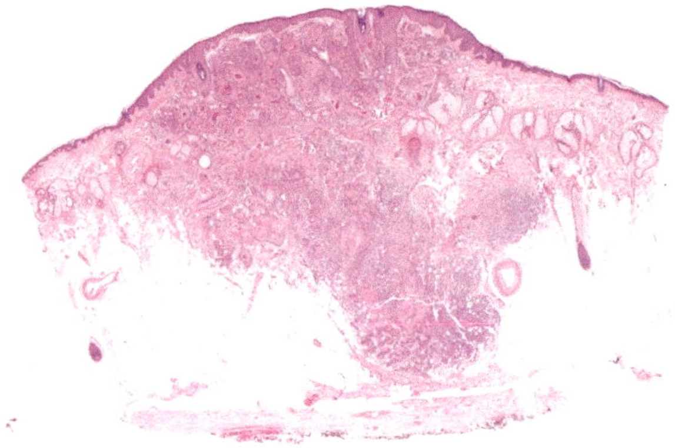

FIG. 11.59

Squamous cell carcinoma. Scanning magnification reveals a keratinizing tumor with an infiltrative growth pattern extending into the subcutis.

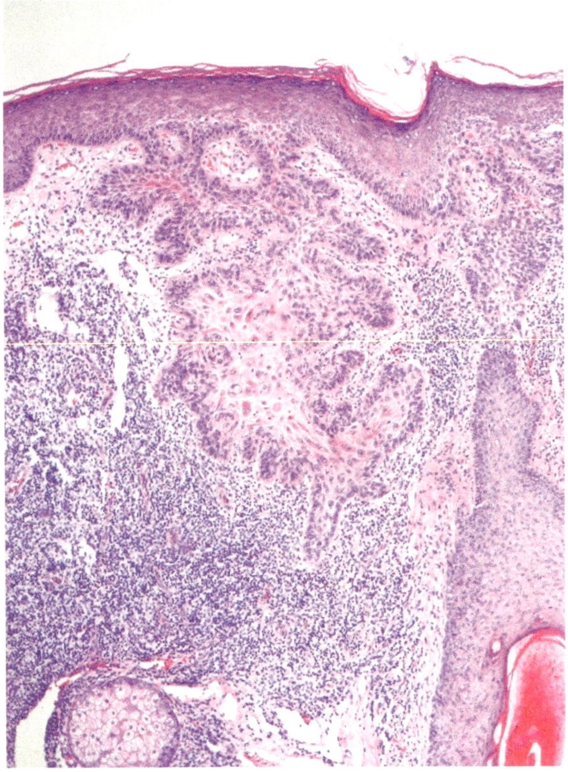

FIG. 11.60

Squamous cell carcinoma. Superficial invasion is recognized by an irregular scalloped outline of squamous protrusions with atypical cells growing downward into the dermis.

precursor lesion (AK, SCCIS) is often present but may not be detectable, for example, owing to ulceration. There is a spectrum of histologic features that has led to descriptions of various "types" of SCCs. They all have in common the fact that the silhouette of invasive SCC displays downward growth below the level of the adjacent or overlying epidermis (Fig. 11.59). The invasive front of the tumor typically shows an infiltrative (pointed and jagged) border (Figs. 11.60 and 11.61) except for verrucous carcinoma.

INVASIVE SQUAMOUS CELL CARCINOMA—PATHOLOGIC FEATURES

Histologic Features

- Infiltrative growth pattern
- Epithelial atypia (variable, from mild to marked)
- Keratinization (usually present except for poorly differentiated tumors)
- Variable stromal inflammatory reaction (from none to dense inflammation and desmoplasia)
- May be associated with a precursor lesion (actinic keratosis, Bowen's disease, verruca)

Ancillary Studies

- Immunopositive for cytokeratins, epithelial membrane antigen, p40

Differential Diagnosis

- Pseudoepitheliomatous hyperplasia (e.g., due to trauma, infection, granular cell tumor)
- Inflammatory dermatoses (e.g., hypertrophic lupus erythematosus, lichen planus)
- Miscellaneous keratoses (e.g., proliferative actinic keratosis, inverted follicular keratosis)
- Other malignant tumors (adnexal carcinomas, melanoma, sarcoma, lymphoma)

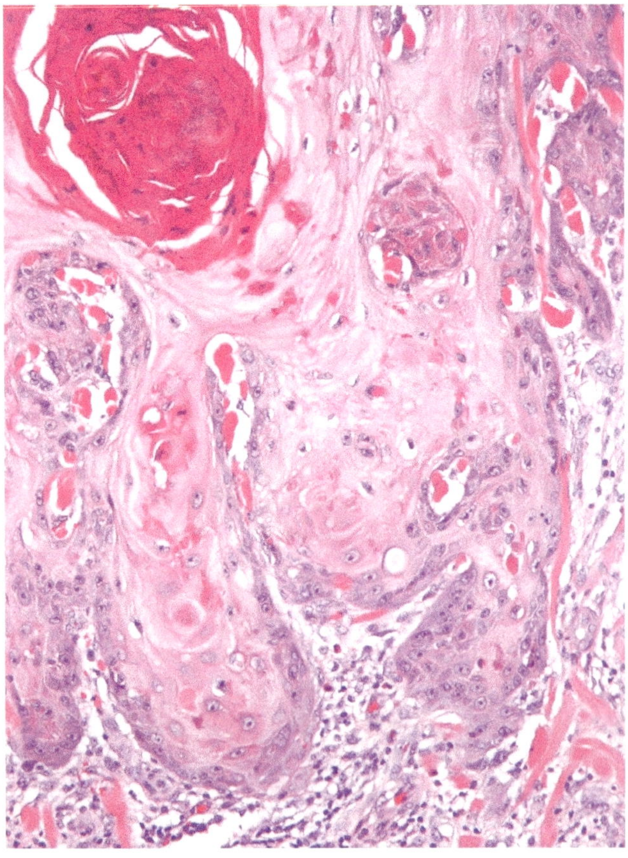

FIG. 11.61

Well-differentiated squamous cell carcinoma. Keratinization is predominant.

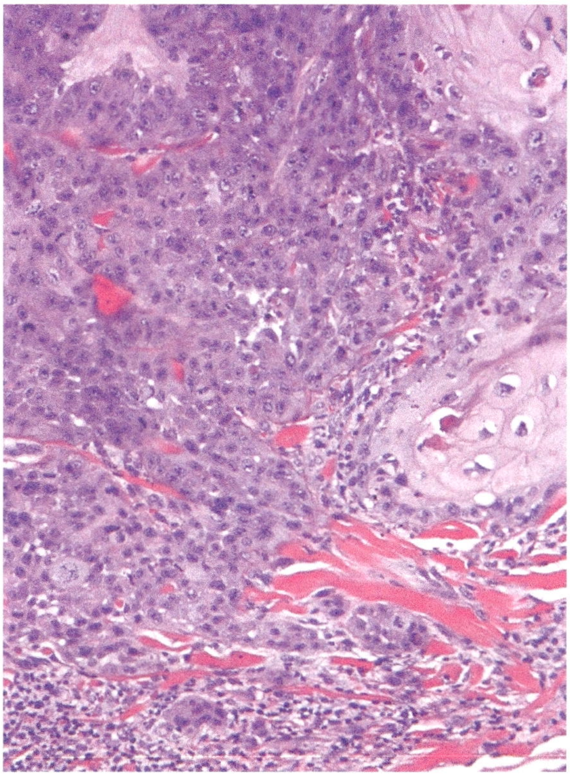

FIG. 11.62

Moderately differentiated squamous cell carcinoma. Only parts of the tumor show keratinization.

HISTOLOGIC VARIANTS* OF SQUAMOUS CELL CARCINOMA—PATHOLOGIC FEATURES

- Conventional SCC, not otherwise specified
- SCC with various phenotypes
  - Acantholytic
  - Clear cell
  - Basaloid
  - Warty
  - Desmoplastic
  - Spindle cell sarcomatoid
  - Lymphoepitheliomatous
- Verrucous
- Keratoacanthoma
- Biphenotypic tumors
  - Carcinosarcoma
  - Squamous cell carcinoma with a neuroendocrine component
  - Adenosquamous carcinoma
  - Basosquamous carcinoma

*The histologic variants are meant to describe the spectrum of microscopic appearances of cutaneous squamous cell carcinoma.

SCC is often graded somewhat subjectively based on the degree of differentiation and keratinization: well, moderately, or poorly differentiated. Well-differentiated tumors tend to have abundant pink cytoplasm, show only mild to moderate atypia, and tend to have well-developed keratinization (see Fig. 11.61). Moderately differentiated carcinomas fall in between and show at least in parts recognizable keratinization (Fig. 11.62). In poorly differentiated tumors, there is a high nuclear to cytoplasm ratio, the nuclei are markedly atypical or frankly anaplastic, and no or only minimal keratinization is recognized (Fig. 11.63). The term *undifferentiated* is used for tumors presumed to be SCC (e.g., based on a prior shave biopsy revealing more typical SCC at the same site) if no keratinization is identified under the light microscope throughout the entire tumor. Immunohistochemistry is usually necessary in this setting to exclude nonepithelial tumors (in particular melanoma or sarcoma).

Poorly or undifferentiated tumors may form solid spindle or epithelioid tumor cell aggregates (Fig. 11.63) but on occasion may show a growth pattern, in which most tumor cells are dispersed singly, permeating through stroma without forming discrete nodules. Invasive SCC may be associated with chronic inflammation and fibrosis in the dermis adjacent to the leading edge of the tumor, but the extent of the stromal changes is highly variable. Some invasive tumors may permeate through the dermis without a stromal reaction. This is particularly common for superficial invasion in the setting of marked solar elastosis. On the other end of the spectrum are tumors eliciting a prominent stromal, at times even desmoplastic, reaction. The composition of the inflammatory infiltrate is also variable. Lymphocytes are usually most prominent, but neutrophils, eosinophils, plasma cells, or granulomas may be seen.

The following paragraphs describe both common and selected rare histologic phenotypes of SCC. The discussion of various types of SCCs mainly serves to illustrate a spectrum of appearances of SCC as it may be helpful for the differential diagnosis. Few of these types represent a biologically distinct entity, such as verrucous carcinoma, with a clinical course different from conventional SCC.

CONVENTIONAL SQUAMOUS CELL CARCINOMA

This is the most common or classic type of SCC. If it occurs in chronically sun-damaged skin, it is often associated with features of AK. The carcinoma is characterized by a downward infiltrative growth of eosinophilic keratinocytes into the dermis (Figs. 11.60–11.62 and 11.64). The cellular aggregates may be broad, tongue- or sheetlike, thin (fingerlike), or lack of cohesive, breaking up into small clusters of cells or single cells. The degree of cytologic atypia is variable, from mild to severe. Inflammation may be sparse or dense, ranging in composition from lymphoplasmacellular to suppurative with intratumor neutrophilic abscesses (Fig. 11.65) or granulomatous. The silhouette of the lesion may be plaque like, wedge shaped, or crateriform.

Lesions with a crateriform silhouette may be termed *keratoacanthoma-like SCC*. They need to be distinguished from a KA. Although crateriform variants of

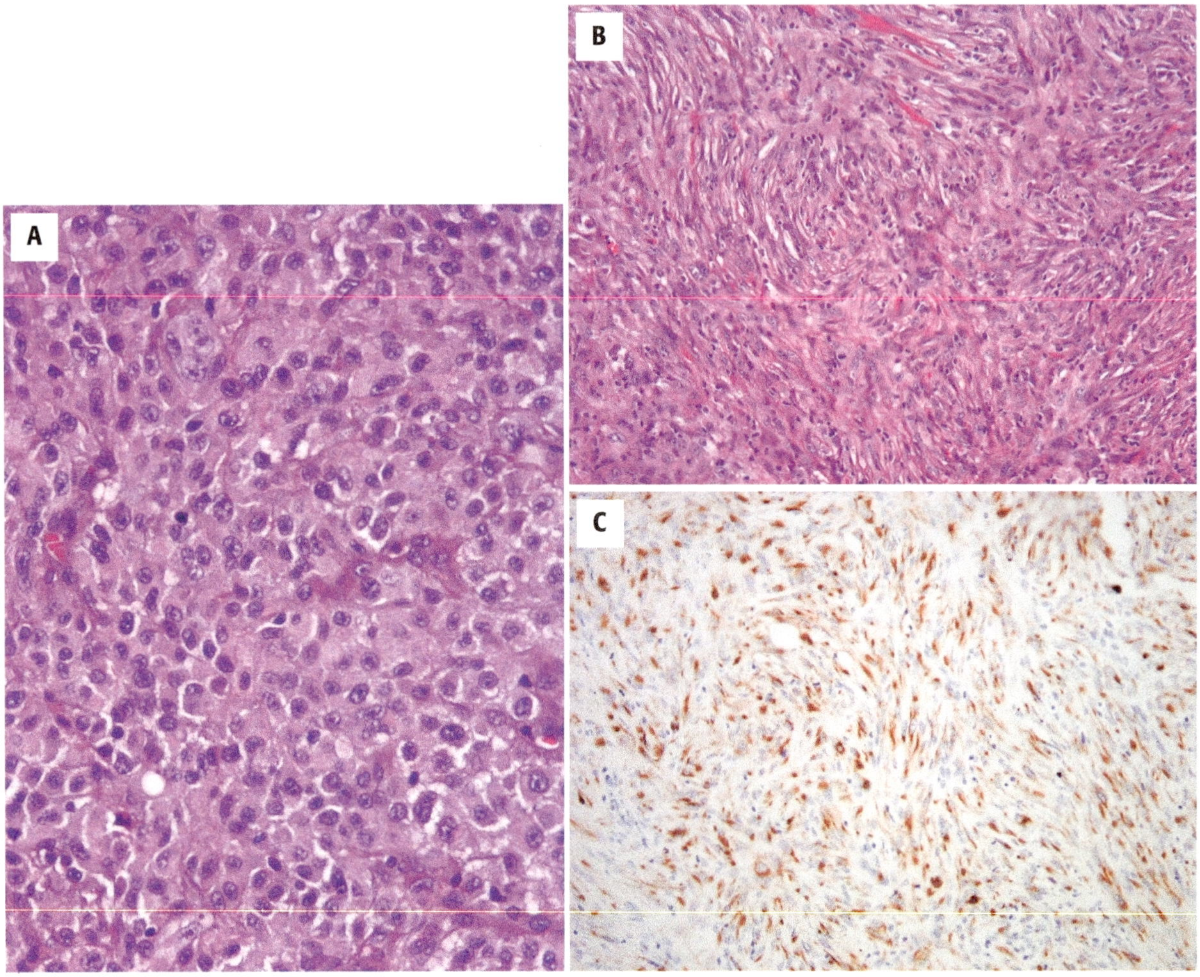

FIG. 11.63

A, Poorly differentiated epithelioid squamous cell carcinoma (SCC). Most of the tumor, such as the focus illustrated here, lacks keratinization. If no keratinization is seen whatsoever, one may use the term *undifferentiated* SCC. **B,** Poorly differentiated spindle cell SCC. **C,** The spindle cells are immunoreactive for AE1:AE3.

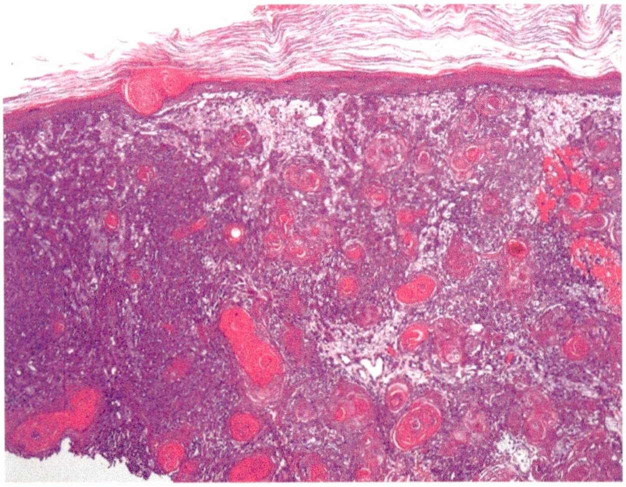

FIG. 11.64

Conventional invasive squamous cell carcinoma. The carcinoma shows prominent keratinization. It infiltrates the dermis without a stromal reaction. The overlying epidermis does not show more than basal cell layer atypia.

well-differentiated SCC share with KAs a cup-shaped silhouette, they display an unequivocally infiltrative growth pattern along the base and are composed of keratinocytes with marked cytologic atypia and abnormal maturation (Fig. 11.66). The presence of prominent AK at the lateral edges of a lesion may also favor a diagnosis of SCC over KA.

ACANTHOLYTIC SQUAMOUS CELL CARCINOMA

SCC may display prominent acantholysis, that is, marked disruption of cells with rounding up of the cell borders (Fig. 11.67). "Pseudoglandular" lumenlike structures may be present (pseudoglandular SCC), which may lead to confusion with adenosquamous carcinoma (Fig. 11.68). The tumor is usually recognized as SCC by adjacent foci of conventional SCC, with evidence of keratinization, or the presence of SCCIS. Single-cell infiltration is commonly seen in association with acantholytic SCC.

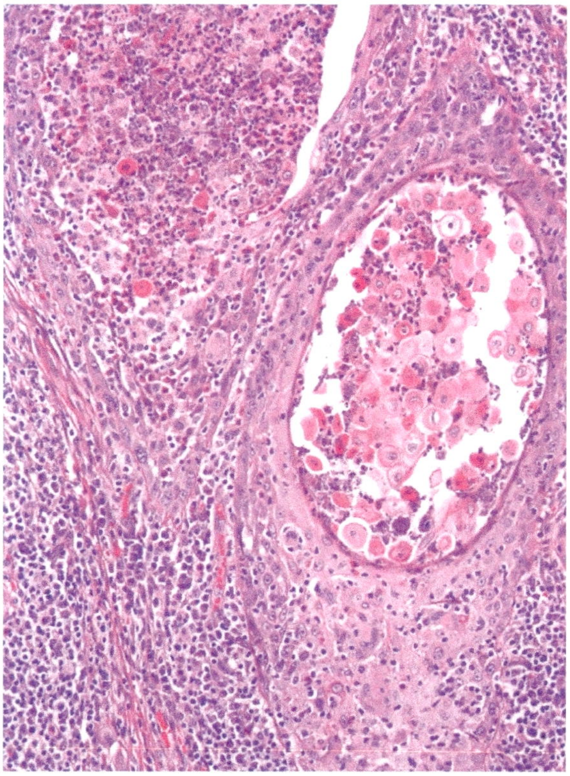

FIG. 11.65

Inflamed well-differentiated squamous cell carcinoma. Neutrophilic abscesses are present within the tumor.

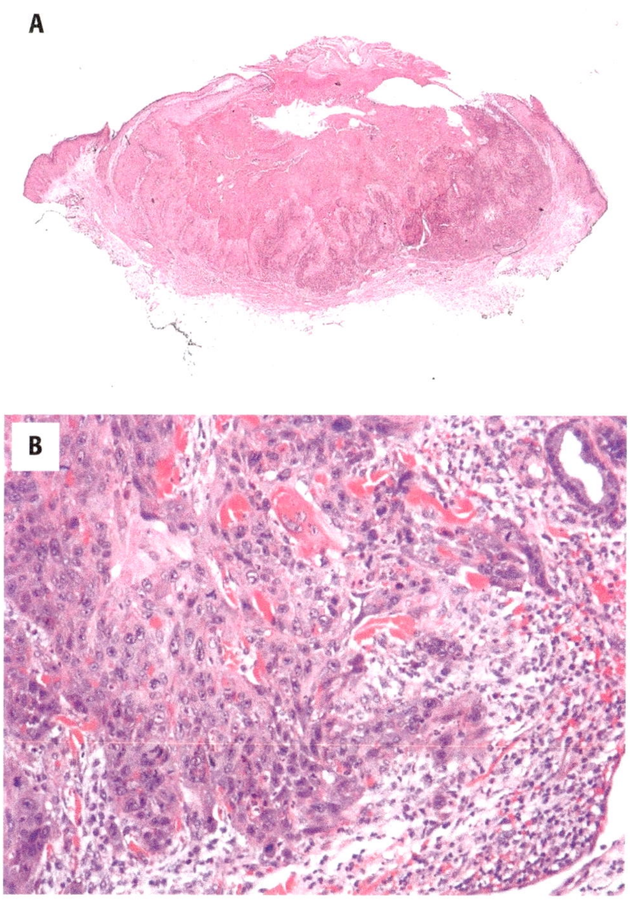

FIG. 11.66

Squamous cell carcinoma with a crateriform growth pattern. **A,** Scanning magnification shows a cup-shaped silhouette similar to keratoacanthoma. **B,** The tumor is a carcinoma because of its infiltrative growth and the presence of marked keratinocytic atypia.

CLEAR CELL SQUAMOUS CELL CARCINOMA

SCC may show partial or prominent clear or pale cytoplasmic staining related to the presence of glycogen (Fig. 11.69). Many lesions of SCCIS with clear cell changes display HPV cytopathic features. Recognition of clear cell features in SCC is important for the distinction from other clear cell tumors, such as clear cell sweat gland carcinoma, sebaceous carcinoma, trichilemmal carcinoma, balloon cell melanoma, and metastatic renal cell carcinoma.

BASALOID SQUAMOUS CELL CARCINOMA

Basaloid SCC usually arises in association with bowenoid SCCIS and is typically associated with HPV. It has a predilection for the anogenital or oral region. Basaloid SCC has a higher nuclear to cytoplasmic ratio and less pink cytoplasm than conventional SCC (Fig. 11.70). It needs to be primarily distinguished from BCC and basaloid adnexal carcinomas.

WARTY SQUAMOUS CELL CARCINOMA

Some SCCs have a digitated, that is, verrucoid, silhouette and may even show HPV cytopathic effects in association with features of conventional infiltrative

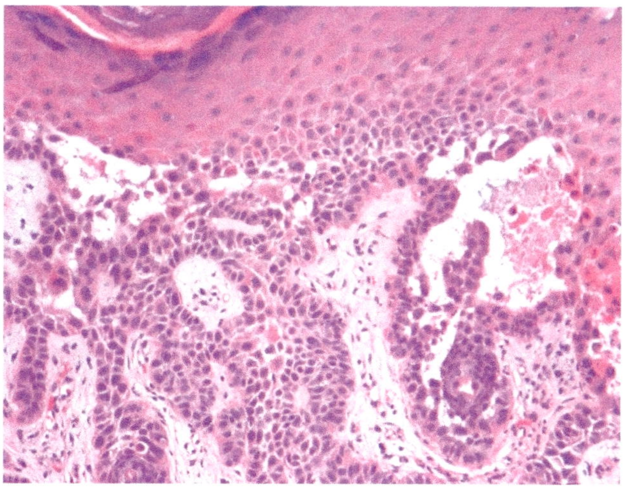

FIG. 11.67

Acantholytic squamous cell carcinoma is characterized by foci of lack of cohesion among tumor cells.

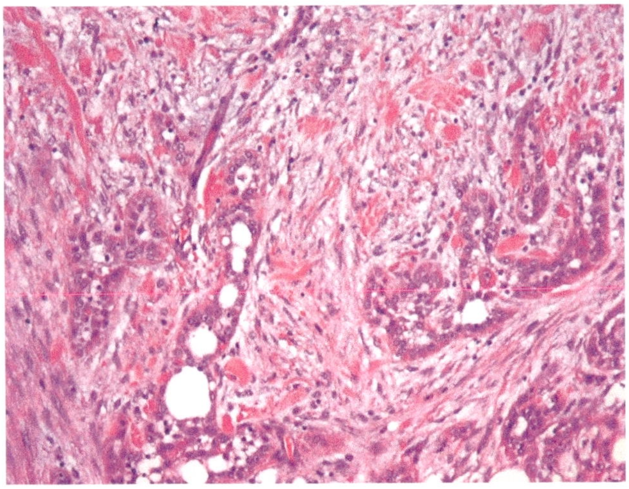

FIG. 11.68

Pseudoglandular squamous cell carcinoma. This invasive squamous cell carcinoma shows prominent pseudogland formation resulting from dyscohesion (acantholysis) of epithelial cells within cords and strands of invasive carcinoma.

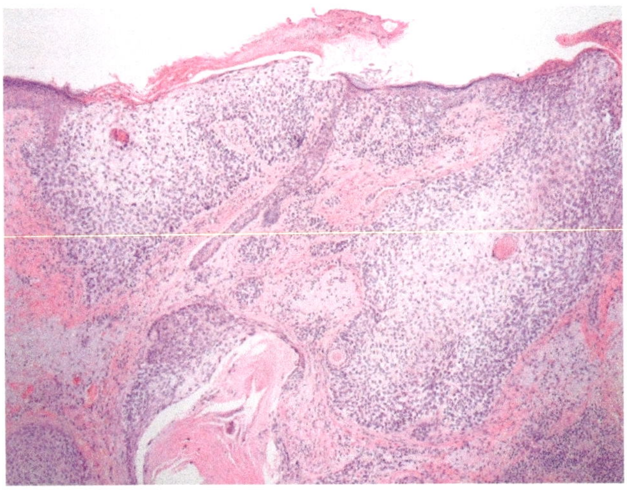

FIG. 11.69

Clear cell squamous cell carcinoma. This in situ and invasive squamous cell carcinoma is characterized by prominent clear cell features. The clear cytoplasm is caused by glycogen.

SCC (Figs. 11.70 and 11.71). This carcinoma needs to be distinguished from a true verrucous carcinoma. It differs from it by the presence of pointed tumor protrusions into the stroma or single-cell invasion as well as epithelial atypia.

DESMOPLASTIC OR SCLEROSING SQUAMOUS CELL CARCINOMA

SCC may on occasion be associated with a prominent desmoplastic stroma (Fig. 11.72). This is both of diagnostic and prognostic relevance. Prognostically, desmoplasia in a cutaneous SCC has been associated with a higher risk for recurrence. Diagnostically, if a desmoplastic SCC has a predominant spindle cell appearance,

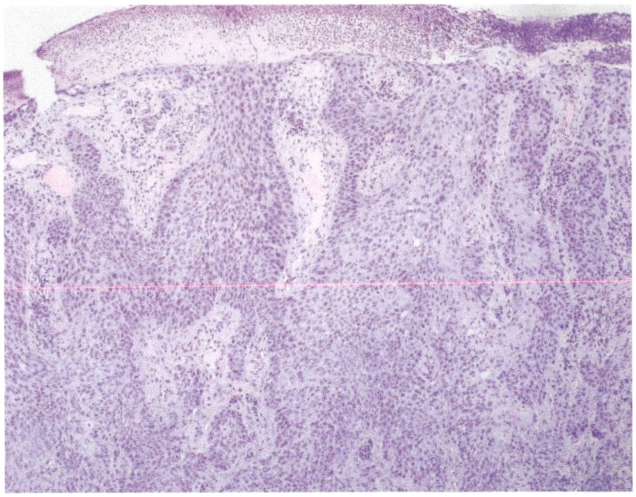

FIG. 11.70

Basaloid squamous cell carcinoma. The tumor cells have less pink cytoplasm.

this may lead to confusion with desmoplastic melanoma or desmoplastic leiomyosarcoma. When desmoplastic SCC contains thin cords of epithelioid tumor cells with small keratin cysts, it may simulate the appearance of a microcystic adnexal carcinoma (Fig. 11.72B) or a squamatized morpheaform BCC. SCC is best distinguished from microcystic adnexal carcinoma by the presence of marked cytologic atypia and associated typical features of SCC (e.g., presence of SCCIS or sheetlike aggregates of conventional invasive SCC).

SPINDLE CELL SQUAMOUS CELL CARCINOMA

Some variants of SCC are predominantly composed of spindle cells. If keratinization is poor (essentially a spindle cell variant of poorly differentiated SCC), the tumor may be confused with atypical fibroxanthoma, dermal sarcoma, or spindle cell melanoma (Fig. 11.73). Immunostains are typically necessary to confirm the epithelial origin of such tumors unless one can find foci of more typical SCC associated with the more poorly differentiated "sarcomatoid" component, or preceding it (prior biopsy findings).

ADDITIONAL RARE VARIANTS OF SQUAMOUS CELL CARCINOMA

The preceding list of morphologic appearances of SCC is not complete. Additional rare variants exist with unusual morphologic features, and additional terms are used, such as *pseudovascular* or *sarcomatoid SCC*. *Pseudovascular SCC* refers to an invasive carcinoma in which the tumor stroma is loose, allowing the tumor cells to form cystlike spaces mimicking vascular channels. It is a well-established "aggressive" variant of SCC at mucosal sites, such as the mucosa of the upper respiratory tract or esophagus. The prognostic significance of similar

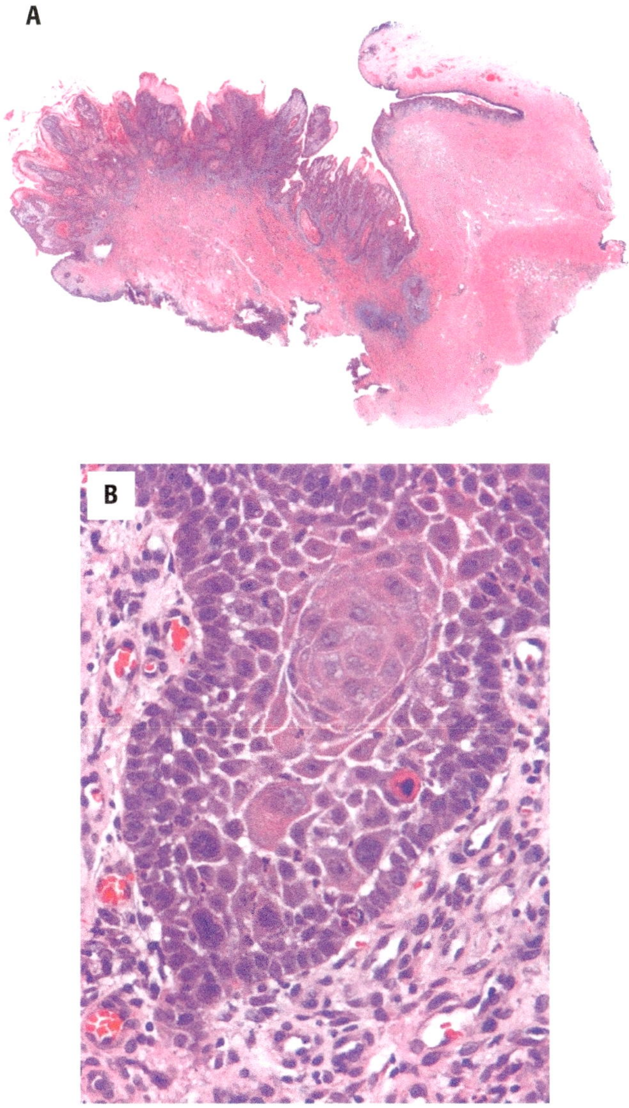

FIG. 11.71

Warty squamous cell carcinoma. **A,** This squamous cell carcinoma from the penis has a verrucoid exophytic silhouette. **B,** In contrast to verrucous carcinoma, the invasive component of warty squamous cell carcinoma shows pointed tongues and marked keratinocytic atypia similar to conventional squamous cell carcinoma.

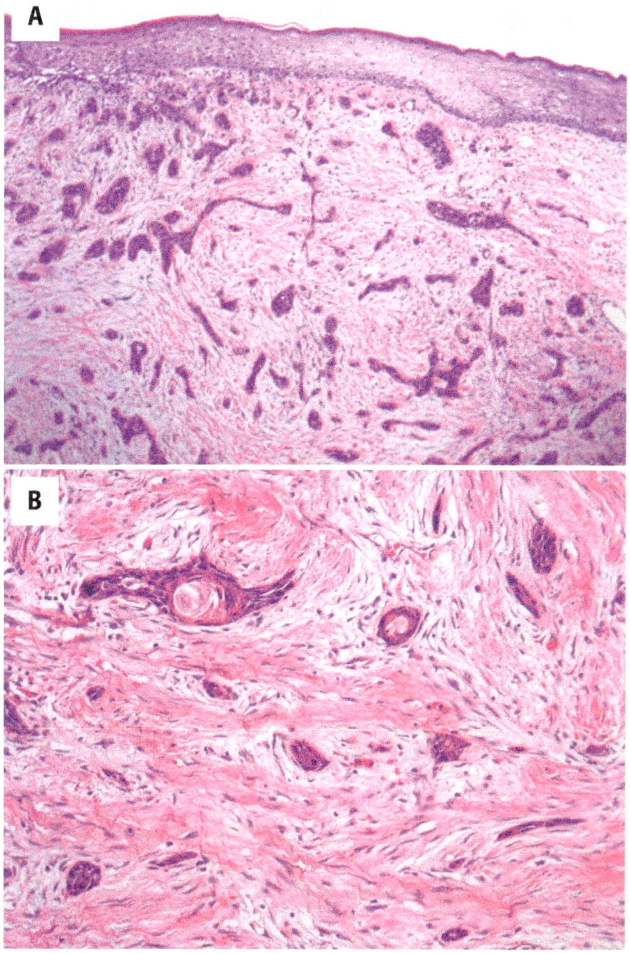

FIG. 11.72

Desmoplastic squamous cell carcinoma. **A,** Squamous cell carcinoma with desmoplastic stromal reaction (desmoplastic squamous cell carcinoma). This tumor is associated with prominent fibrosis. Its invasive component is composed of many thin tumor strands. **B,** When a desmoplastic squamous cell carcinoma contains strands of epithelium with small keratocytes, it may simulate the appearance of a microcystic adnexal carcinoma.

features in a cutaneous SCC, however, is unknown. The term *sarcomatoid SCC* may be applied to any poorly differentiated (epithelioid or spindle cell) SCC, which simulates histologically and thereby raises the differential diagnosis of a sarcoma.

SCC may have a deceptively subtle invasive pattern characterized by single-cell infiltration of the superficial dermal stroma (Fig. 11.74), which may be overlooked or dismissed as "inflammation" if the tissue is not examined carefully at higher magnification and not enough attention is paid to the cytologic features of the infiltrate. Such single-cell infiltrative patterns may occur in the setting of acantholytic AK or SCC, poorly differentiated epithelioid, or spindle cell sarcomatoid variants with or without stromal desmoplasia. Carcinoma cells are best recognized by their nuclear features (hyperchromatism, irregular-edged nuclear contours, or enlarged nuclear size compared with adjacent fibroblasts or inflammatory cells). Immunostains for cytokeratins (CK5/6, CK903, MNF116) or p40 are often necessary for definitive diagnosis.

Rare SCCs display lymphoepithelioma-like features, a histologic picture similar to nasopharyngeal carcinomas with basaloid epithelioid cells surrounded and infiltrated by a dense lymphocytic infiltrate (Fig. 11.75). In contrast to nasopharyngeal tumors, primary cutaneous lymphoepithelioma-like SCCs are negative for Epstein-Barr virus.

Rare poorly differentiated variants of SCC may be associated with Nuclear protein in testis (NUT) rearrangement. They typically show islands of squamous cells in the midst of poorly differentiated SCC and are commonly associated with an infiltrate of neutrophils.

A

B C

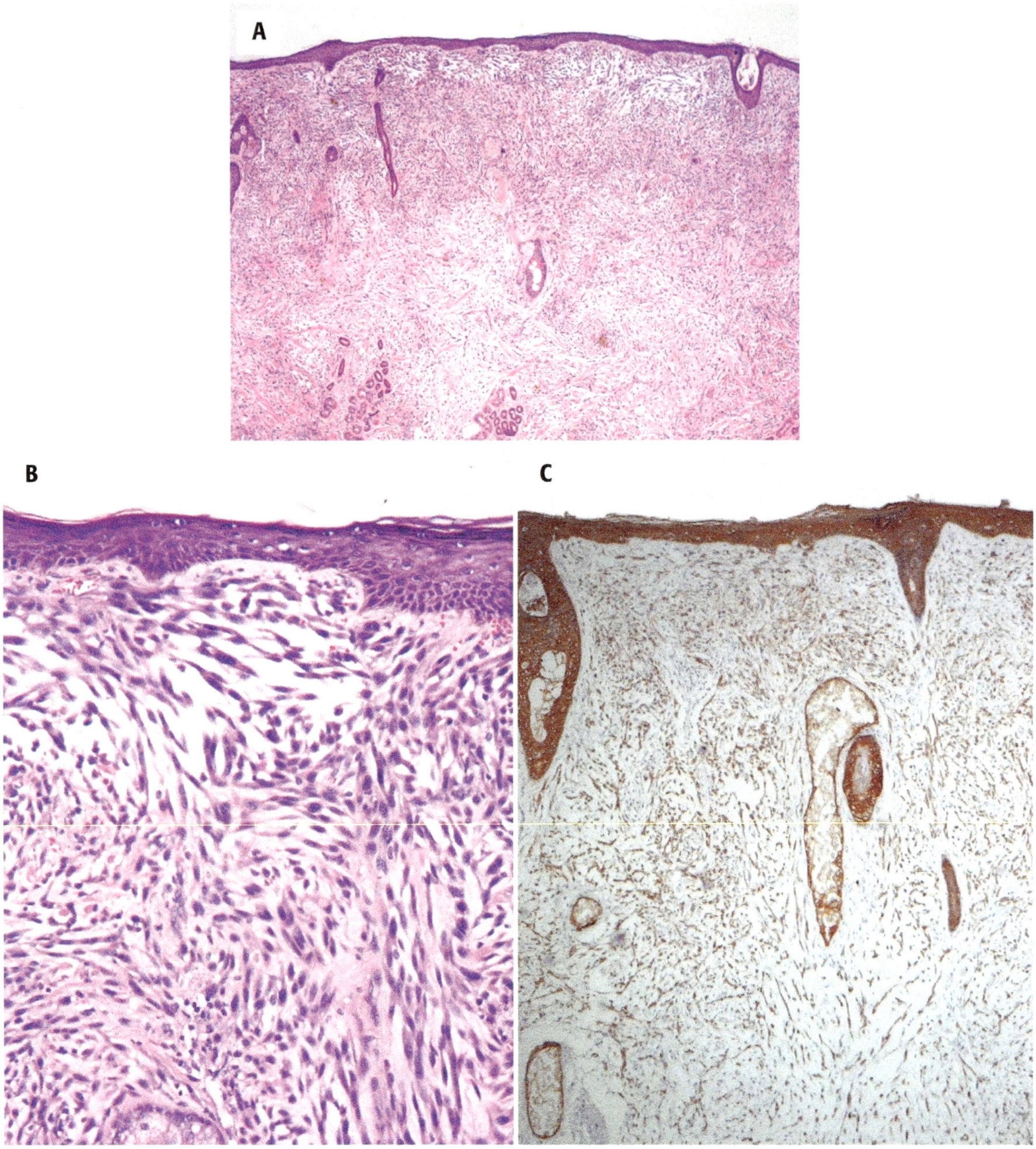

FIG. 11.73

Spindle cell squamous cell carcinoma. **A,** Scanning magnification shows an infiltrative spindle cell tumor extending from the dermal-epidermal junction to the subcutis. **B,** Close-up view of the fusiform tumor cells. **C,** The tumor is immunoreactive for cytokeratins (AE1:AE3).

VERRUCOUS CARCINOMA

Verrucous carcinoma is a flesh-colored to brown, hyperkeratotic plaque that may arise in association with or mimic a verruca (Fig. 11.76). It is characterized by the combination of an endophytic and exophytic profile. The outward-growing (exophytic) component often has a cauliflower-like verrucous silhouette with a thick layer of compact stratum corneum (Fig. 11.77). The endophytic component of verrucous carcinoma is characterized by downward bulbous growth of well-differentiated keratinocytes (Fig. 11.78) below the level of the adjacent nonneoplastic epidermis. The deep margin of this tumor pushes its way into the dermis as opposed to the infiltrating pattern of thin fingerlike projections with irregular outlines of more classic SCC. It is a defining feature of verrucous carcinoma that significant cytologic atypia is absent (Fig. 11.79). If a lesion shows features of verrucous carcinoma but does not extend below the level of the adjacent epidermis or squamous mucosa, it is best reported as noninvasive verrucous carcinoma.

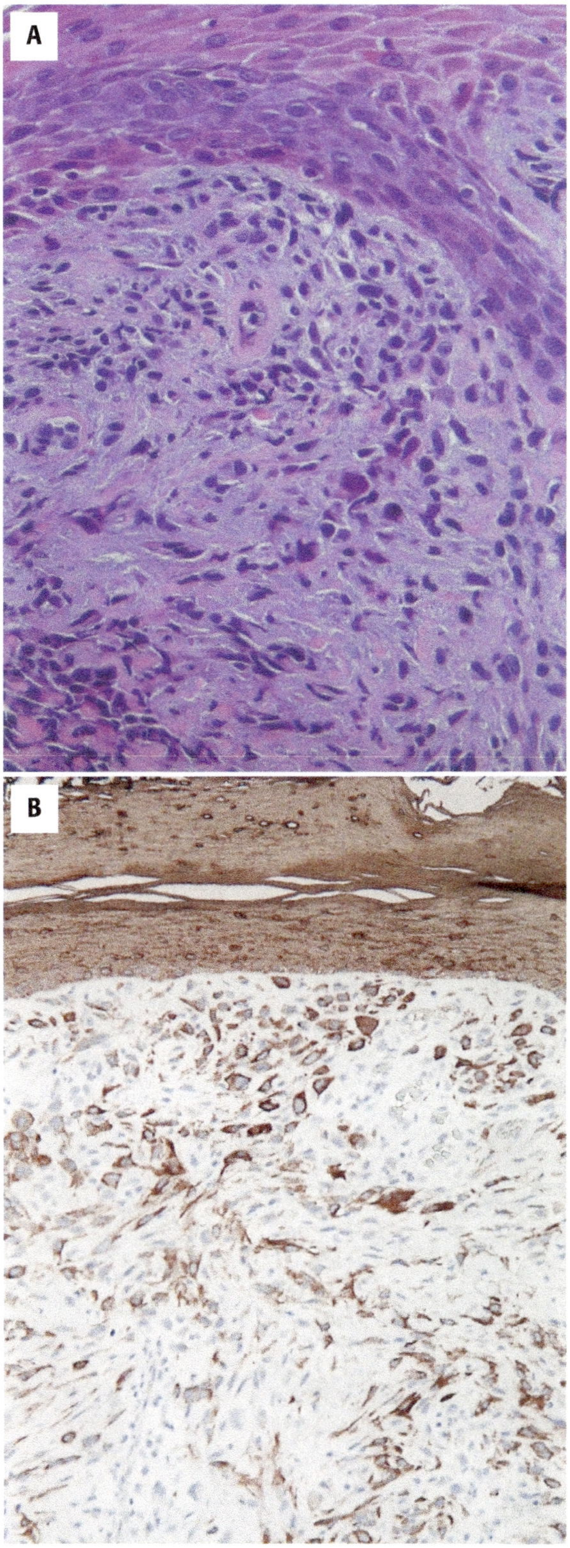

FIG. 11.74

Squamous cell carcinoma with single-cell infiltrative pattern. **A,** Solitary units of cytologically atypical cells are seen in the dermis. **B,** They are immunoreactive for 34BE12.

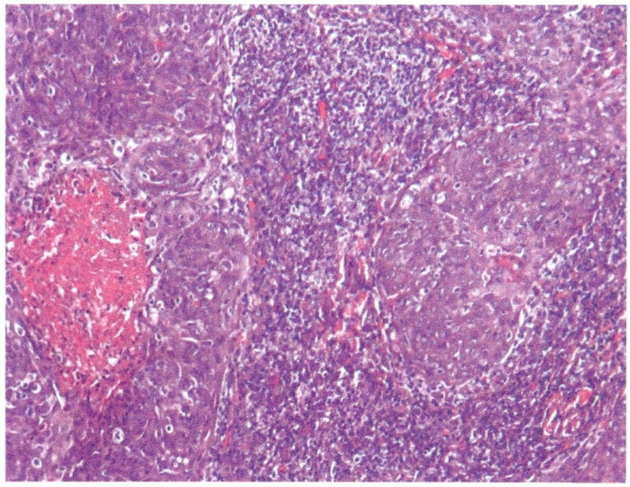

FIG. 11.75

Lymphoepithelioma-like squamous cell carcinoma. Poorly differentiated carcinoma is associated with a dense lymphocytic infiltrate.

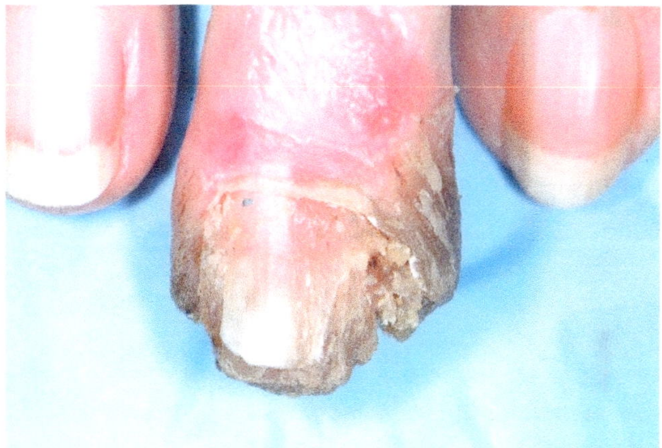

FIG. 11.76

Verrucous carcinoma of the distal finger, including the nail.

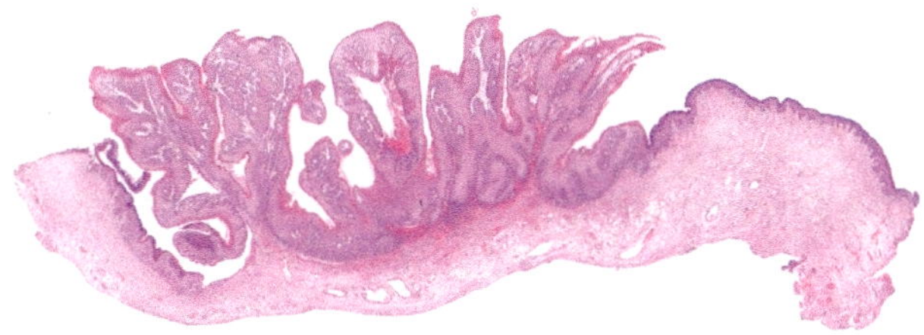

FIG. 11.77

Verrucous carcinoma. The tumor shows an exophytic cauliflower-like growth pattern.

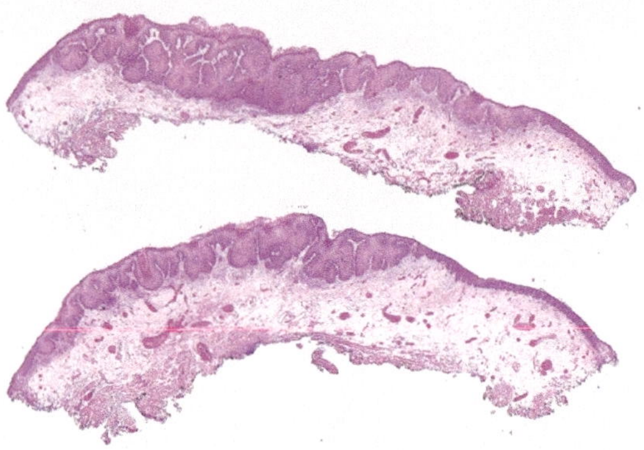

FIG. 11.78

The invasive tumor front has broad, fingerlike projections and extends below the level of the adjacent epithelium.

VERRUCOUS CARCINOMA—DISEASE FACT SHEET

Patient Group

- Middle-aged or elderly White individuals; men more often than women

Site of Involvement

- Oral mucosa (Ackerman tumor or florid oral papillomatosis)
- Anourogenital region (Buschke-Loewenstein tumor)
- Palmoplantar region (epithelioma cuniculatum)

Clinical Findings

- Usually slow growing
- Mucosal lesions may initially manifest as white patches (leukoplakia)
- Exophytic large cauliflower-like surface
- May ulcerate and fistulate

Prognosis and Treatment

- Low-grade tumor characterized by persistent local growth or local recurrences; metastases are very rare. (Metastases usually occur in the setting of a combined conventional well-differentiated and verrucous carcinoma [not a pure verrucous carcinoma].)
- Surgery is the treatment of choice
- Radiation therapy is an alternative option in selected cases

VERRUCOUS CARCINOMA—PATHOLOGIC FEATURES

Histologic Features

- Cauliflower-like exophytic silhouette is common
- Bulbous endophytic tonguelike projections
- Lack of epithelial atypia
- Normal maturation

Differential Diagnosis

- Verruca (smaller in size; presence of human papillomavirus cytopathic changes; lack of broad tonguelike invasive protrusions)
- Warty squamous cell carcinoma (presence of keratinocytic atypia; pointed invasive protrusions or focal single-cell invasion)
- Noninvasive verrucous carcinoma

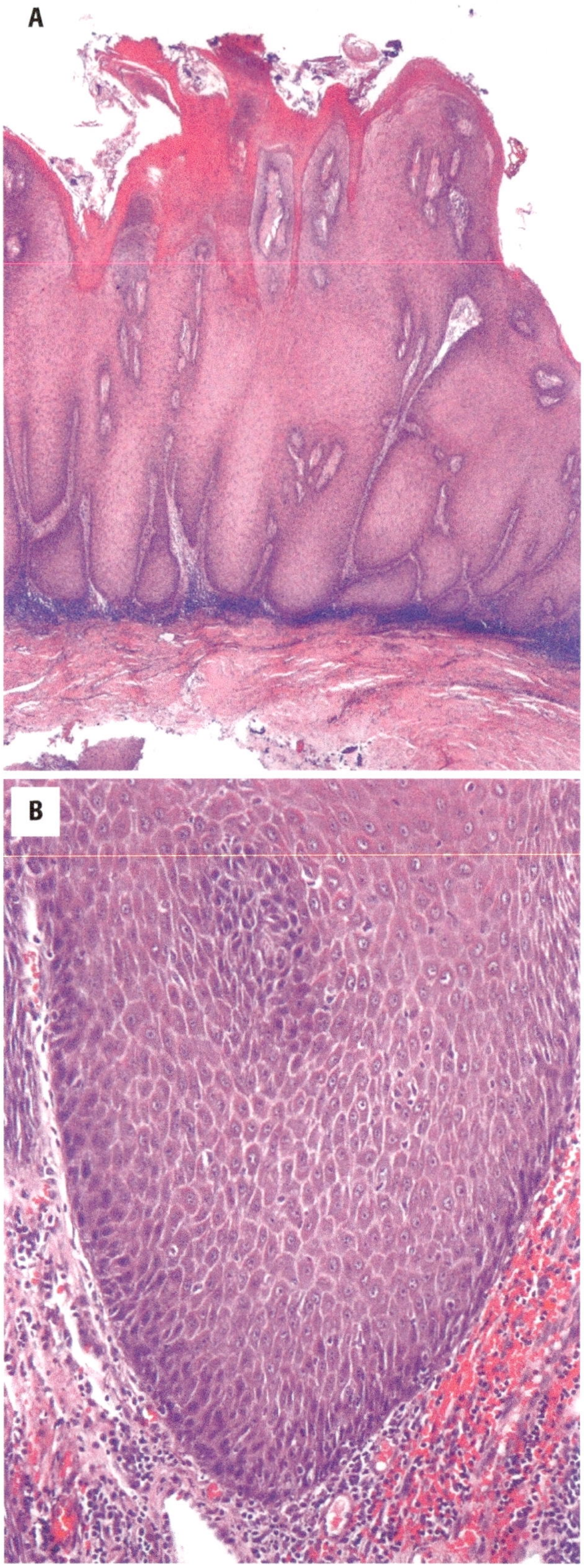

FIG. 11.79

Verrucous carcinoma. **A,** The invasive front is characterized by the presence of broad, bulbous tongues of well-differentiated squamous epithelium. **B,** Significant atypia is lacking. Keratinocytes show evidence of maturation and polarity.

KERATOACANTHOMA (SCC, KERATOACANTHOMA TYPE)

The term *keratoacanthoma* has been used for a spectrum of crateriform squamous proliferations ranging from benign, cup-shaped acanthomas to cup-shaped carcinomas. Based on the terminology used by the World Health Organization (WHO) on skin tumor classification, *KA* is to be regarded as a variant of SCC and accordingly grouped together with SCC in this chapter and used synonymously with SCC, KA type. However, we are cognizant of the fact that this may be an oversimplification and that not all squamoproliferative lesions historically placed into the spectrum of KA are bonafide carcinomas. Genomic studies have shown that while growing KAs may harbor some of the same oncogenic drivers as cutaneous SCCs while regressing KAs lack these oncogenic drivers.

Clinical Findings

A KA most commonly manifests as a solitary, flesh-colored or pink, firm papule or nodule with a central hyperkeratotic plug (Fig. 11.80). It tends to arise on sun-exposed areas of light-skinned, older individuals. The dorsal hands, arms, and forearms are the sites of predilection, although the face is most common. In elderly individuals, KAs also commonly occur on the lower extremities in association with venous stasis. Recently, KAs have been found to develop in patients treated with kinase inhibitors. KAs grow rapidly over a period of weeks to a few months but have a tendency to involute spontaneously after 3 to 6 months, leaving behind an atrophic scar.

Several clinical variants of KA have been identified. The Ferguson-Smith type consists of multiple, frequently ulcerated KAs. The Gryzybowski variant has numerous, generalized, small KAs. Witten and Zak typify multiple

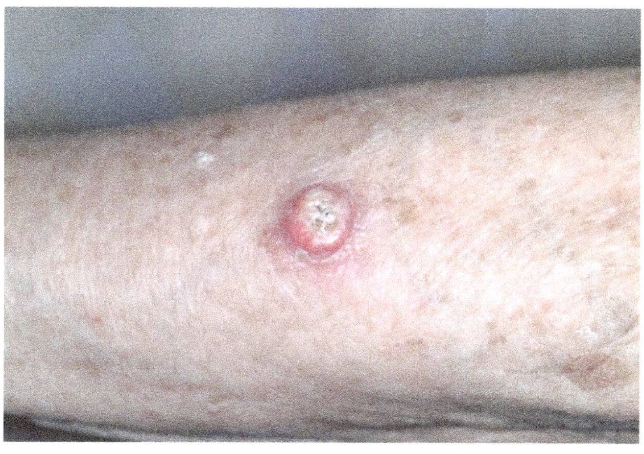

FIG. 11.80

Keratoacanthoma. A nodule with raised borders and central keratin plug.

familial KAs. Giant massive KA with a diameter of more than 5 cm has been reported. KA centrifugum marginatum (Fig. 11.81) is a large annular keratotic plaque with central clearing.

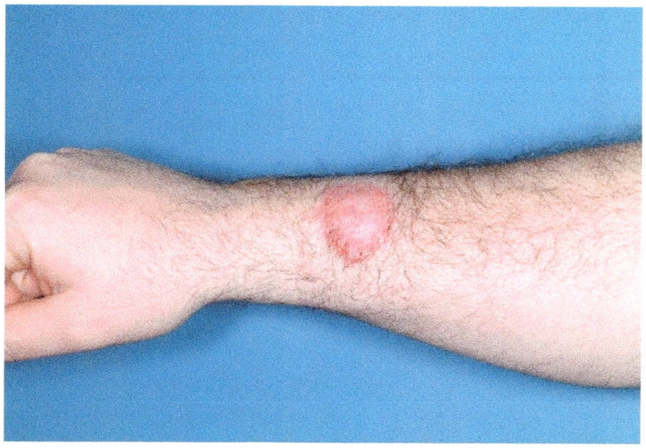

FIG. 11.81

Keratoacanthoma centrifugum marginatum. This variant of keratoacanthoma presents as a large plaque and heals centrally as it grows peripherally.

SCC, KERATOACANTHOMA TYPE (AKA KERATOACANTHOMA)—DISEASE FACT SHEET

Incidence

- Approximately 1 per 1000 per year in the United States

Patient Group

- Most commonly seen in elderly White individuals

Risk Factors

- Ultraviolet exposure, chemical carcinogens, human papillomavirus, immunosuppression, trauma
- Venous stasis (keratoacanthomas [KAs] of the lower extremity)
- Treatment with kinase inhibitor (e.g., vemurafenib)

Site of Involvement

- Usually sun-exposed areas

Clinical Findings

- Nodule with rolled borders and central keratin plug
- Rapid growth common
- May spontaneously involute
- Pathergy common (KA at sites of injury)
- Often a solitary lesion, but may present as multiple lesions
- Syndromes with KAs
  - Ferguson-Smith (multiple spontaneously regressing)
  - Gryzybowski (multiple nonregressing generalized eruptive)
  - Muir-Torre (associated sebaceous tumors and internal malignancy)

Prognosis and Treatment

- Usually indolent, but depending on size and location (e.g., subungual) can be locally destructive
- Surgery is the treatment of choice for solitary lesions
- Multiple lesions can be treated medically (e.g., intralesional methotrexate or systemic retinoids)
- Radiation therapy

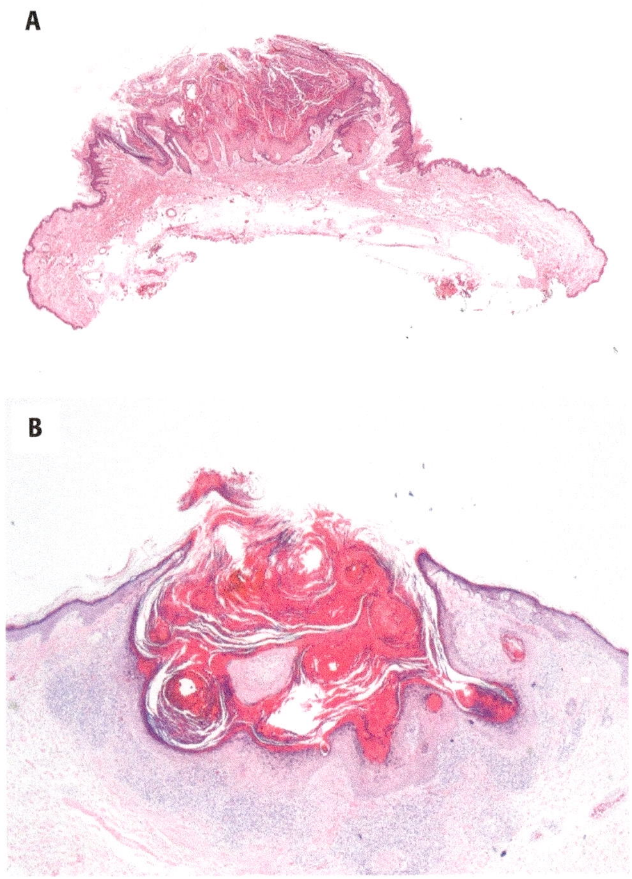

FIG. 11.82

A, Keratoacanthoma. A crateriform squamous proliferation is present with extensive hyperkeratosis. **B,** Keratoacanthoma associated with inflammation.

Histologic Features

The histologic findings may vary depending on the stage of the lesion. Early lesions often have verrucous changes. Scanning magnification of more well-developed lesions reveals a cup-shaped, squamous proliferation with a central keratin plug (Fig. 11.82). The squamous epithelium is usually acanthotic, pink, and glassy in the spinous layer with hypergranulosis. The adjacent epidermis often forms exophytic projections, resulting in a silhouette that has been likened to lips. The presence of high-grade nuclear atypia in the tumor or extensive AK in the adjacent epithelium favors a diagnosis of SCC. There is often an associated inflammatory reaction (Fig. 11.82B). The invaginated squamous epithelium typically has a lobulated expansile growth pattern with smooth borders. However, depending on the stage of evolution of the lesion and the extent of associated inflammation, the interface of the base of the lesion with the stroma may be disrupted and irregular, with entrapment collagen, elastic fibers, or both (Fig. 11.83). Intraepithelial clusters of neutrophils are commonly associated with KA (Fig. 11.83B). Later-stage regressed lesions may leave cystic changes with dermal fibroplasia.

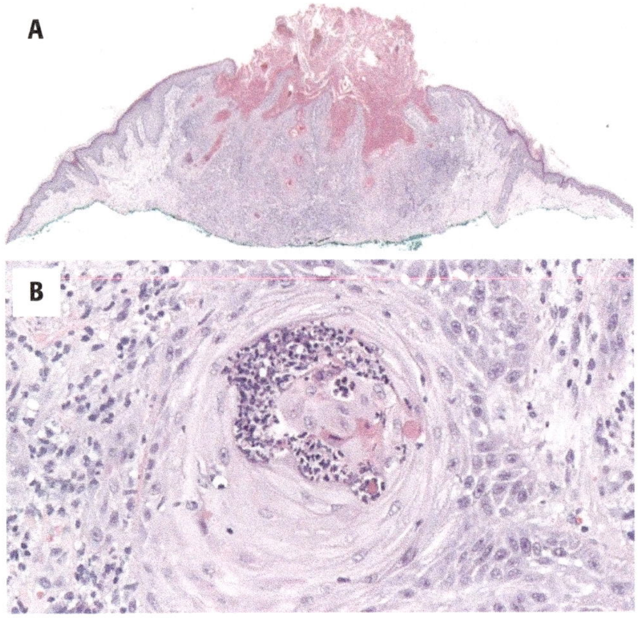

FIG. 11.83

Keratoacanthoma. **A,** Cup-shaped silhouette of the tumor with inflamed irregular periphery. **B,** The tumor cells display abundant eosinophilic cytoplasm and are associated with neutrophilic abscesses.

KERATOACANTHOMA—PATHOLOGIC FEATURES

Histologic Features

- Cup-shaped silhouette with central keratin plug
- Well-differentiated squamous epithelium with abundant pink cytoplasm
- Atypia is usually mild
- May have a smooth border at the base and/or jagged epithelial-stromal interface
- Inflammation is common

Differential Diagnosis

- Conventional squamous cell carcinoma with partial cup-shaped growth
- Pseudoepitheliomatous hyperplasia associated with infection, trauma, or bromoderma
- Verruca

The degree of cytologic atypia is variable but usually mild and limited to the basal cell layer. Keratinocytes with abundant bright eosinophilic cytoplasm are characteristic. Squamous eddies (groups of keratinized cells with a centrally swirled configuration) and intraepithelial neutrophilic microabscesses may be present within the deeper epithelial nests or tips of rete ridges. The dermis may demonstrate variable amounts of predominantly lymphocytic inflammation. KAs are usually superficial lesions but may extend into the deep dermis but not below the level of the sweat gland apparatus.

Regressed or involuting KAs appear flattened. At this stage, the lesional keratinocytes tend to have lost abundant bright eosinophilic cytoplasm. Atypia at the basal cell layer is diminished or absent. The base of the lesion is surrounded by inflammation and fibrosis.

Differential Diagnosis

The clinical history of a rapidly growing nodule usually helps with the diagnosis but is not specific. A fully malignant tumor may on occasion present with a similar history. KAs need to be distinguished from SCC, cysts, and warts. On small shave biopsies, KAs may also be confused with prurigo nodularis, hypertrophic AKs, deep fungal infection, or hypertrophic discoid LE.

The most important distinction is from a cup-shaped conventional SCC. A diagnosis of SCC should be made if a tumor shows an irregular, infiltrative growth pattern at the base and its constituent cells show marked cytologic atypia and abnormal maturation (loss of polarity).

COMBINED CARCINOMAS

A peculiar subset of tumors includes biphenotypic tumors with one component representing an SCC. Such tumors include carcinosarcoma, adenosquamous carcinoma, basosquamous carcinoma, and SCC with a neuroendocrine component (Merkel cell carcinoma ex-SCC).

CARCINOSARCOMA

Rare tumors show combined features of SCC and sarcoma (Fig. 11.84). The sarcomatous component may have the appearance of a fibrosarcoma, leiomyosarcoma, osteosarcoma, or rhabdomyosarcoma.

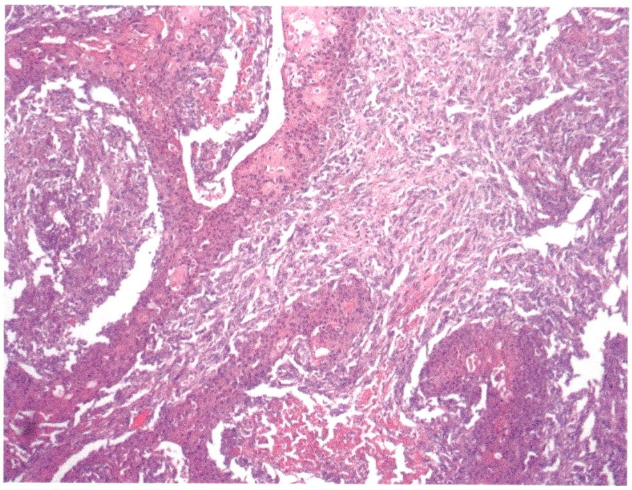

FIG. 11.84

Carcinosarcoma. The tumor has an epithelial component with features of squamous cell carcinoma as well as a keratin-negative malignant spindle cell component.

ADENOSQUAMOUS CARCINOMA

The term *adenosquamous carcinoma* refers to tumors with features of conventional SCC as well as glandular mucinous differentiation. The presence of mucin can be verified by a mucin stain. Depending on the location of an adenosquamous cell carcinoma in the dermis, the differential diagnosis includes porocarcinoma and mucoepidermoid carcinoma.

BASOSQUAMOUS CARCINOMA

The term *basosquamous carcinoma* is used for rare tumors with features of both basal cell and SCC. There is significant variability in how pathologists apply this term. The biologic behavior of combined squamous cell and BCCs is usually dictated by the predominant tumor component but overall more akin to SCC than a typical BCC.

MERKEL CELL (NEUROENDOCRINE) CARCINOMA EX–SQUAMOUS CELL CARCINOMA

Some tumors show a combined phenotype of SCC and neuroendocrine carcinoma (Fig. 11.85). They may start out as a combined tumor at the time of initial diagnosis, or the neuroendocrine component may develop later as a manifestation of tumor progression and transdifferentiation. In these tumors, the neuroendocrine component usually predominates and dictates the clinical course of the patient (similar to Merkel cell carcinoma without a squamous component). These tumors are negative for the Merkel cell polyomavirus.

Ancillary Studies

The vast majority of invasive SCC does not require special studies for diagnosis. However, immunohistochemistry represents a useful ancillary tool for the diagnosis of poorly differentiated and/or spindle cell tumors. Most SCCs are positive for AE1:AE3, but lack of staining for this marker does not exclude SCC. The most sensitive reagents for the diagnosis of poorly differentiated SCC are MNF116, p40, CK5/6, and 34BE12. One needs to keep in mind, however, that cytokeratins can also be expressed in some soft tissue tumors, such as epithelioid sarcoma or angiosarcoma, or melanoma.

Differential Diagnosis

The diagnosis of SCC is usually straightforward but can be difficult on small superficial biopsies or for poorly differentiated tumors. Superficially invasive SCC needs to be distinguished from its noninvasive precursor

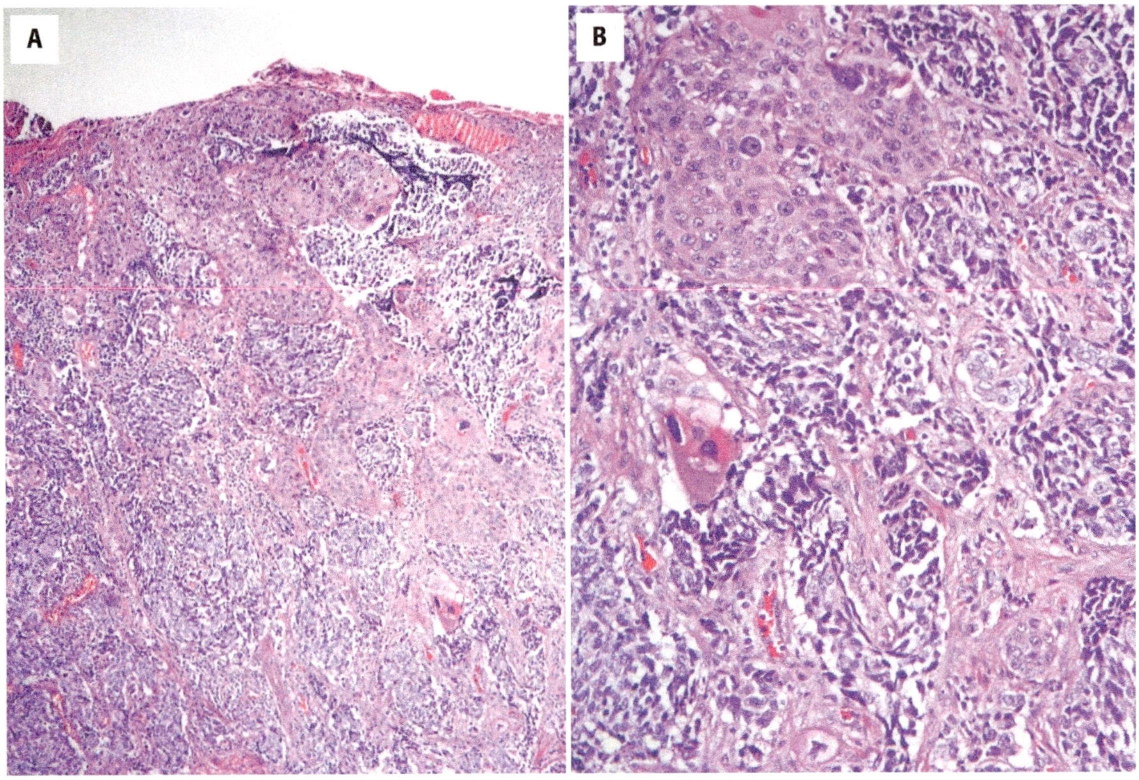

FIG. 11.85

Combined squamous and neuroendocrine carcinoma. **A,** In situ and invasive squamous cell carcinoma is associated with a malignant small cell tumor. **B,** The small cell neuroendocrine phenotype dominates in the invasive component.

lesions, benign keratoses, PEH associated with wound healing or infections, hypertrophic LE, metatypical BCC, miscellaneous adnexal tumors or carcinomas, sarcomas, melanoma, and large cell anaplastic lymphoma. On occasion, one may also need to distinguish a primary SCC from a metastasis of a cutaneous or extracutaneous SCC or tumor with squamous differentiation (e.g., bladder carcinoma).

INVASIVE VERSUS IN SITU SQUAMOUS CELL CARCINOMA

Invasion is present when the base of the lesions extends in an infiltrative pattern into the reticular dermis and there is a stromal reaction to the tumor. Abrupt maturation from basaloid cells to suprabasilar keratinocytes with abundant eosinophilic cytoplasm is common. The fingerlike extensions of invasive carcinoma tend to have jagged outlines. The "stromal response" typically manifests as peritumoral fibrosis and inflammation. "Early" superficial invasion may present as single-cell or small irregular cell cluster infiltration of atypical keratinocytes into the stroma.

The distinction of invasive from noninvasive SCC is not always straightforward. Not every endophytic growth represents bona fide invasion. In situ carcinoma, for example, may populate the intraepithelial component of a preexisting wart or endophytic keratosis or extend into and populate the adnexal epithelium (Fig. 11.86). Furthermore, rubbing and scratching of an in situ carcinoma may lead to superimposed features of prurigo nodularis.

The type of biopsy may also limit evaluation for invasion. If the base of a lesion with histologic features of SCCIS is transected, invasion cannot be excluded, and a reshave biopsy or excision (depending on the size of the clinical lesion and degree of clinical suspicion) may be necessary to exclude or document invasion. If invasion is suspected clinically, a biopsy deep enough to contain superficial dermis is necessary.

SQUAMOUS CELL CARCINOMA VERSUS PSEUDOEPITHELIOMATOUS HYPERPLASIA

PEH may closely mimic or be focally indistinguishable from SCC without proper context. It is important to know whether a biopsy was taken from the edge of an ulcer or after prior surgery or radiation. In PEH, an irregular proliferation of epidermal keratinocytes is seen in association with stromal reactive changes to trauma (hemorrhage, fibrin, edema, granuloma tissue, or fibrosis, depending on the age of the process) (see Fig. 11.1). The keratinocytes usually maintain polarity. Basilar keratinocytes may show reactive nuclear enlargement, but the nuclei usually show an open chromatin. Marked hyperchromatism and nuclear overlap are more typical

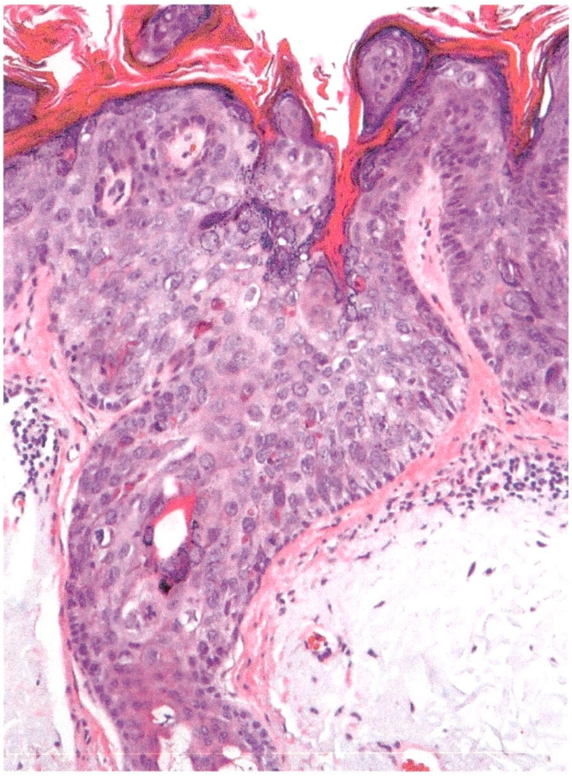

FIG. 11.86

Squamous cell carcinoma in situ populating the superficial portion of a hair follicle. This is not to be confused with invasion.

of carcinoma. The presence of broad squamous tongues or thin epithelial projections with scalloped contours lined by atypical keratinocytes with abrupt maturation and loss of polarity indicates the presence of carcinoma, especially if associated with a desmoplastic stroma. Likewise, single-cell infiltration of atypical keratinocytes into intact stroma (i.e., not fibrin) is usually diagnostic for invasive carcinoma.

Pseudoepitheliomatous features simulating SCC may also be encountered in inflammatory dermatoses, such as in the setting of hypertrophic LE (Fig. 11.87). The distinction from SCC is greatly facilitated after other features more typical of LE, such as keratin plugs, basement membrane thickening, periadnexal lymphocytic infiltrates, and dermal mucin deposition, are identified.

SQUAMOUS CELL CARCINOMA VERSUS METATYPICAL BASAL CELL CARCINOMA

On small superficial biopsies, a diagnosis of carcinoma may be readily apparent but not whether one deals with the top of an SCC or BCC with squamous metaplasia. The latter phenomenon is particularly common underneath an ulcer. Deeper levels may help by revealing in situ SCC or a component of more typical BCC. If no reliable distinction can be made, we recommend to state in the pathology report that review of additional tumor tissue is needed. If the patient is

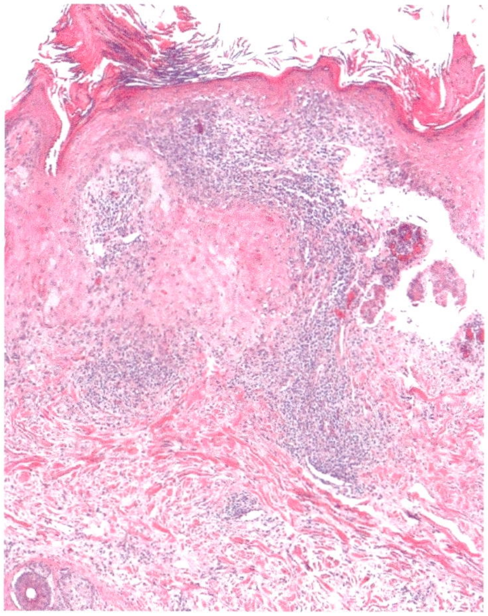

FIG. 11.87

Hypertrophic lupus erythematosus. There is a superficial squamous proliferation associated with an inflamed (lichenoid pattern) epidermis that shows variable thickness and keratin plugs.

treated by a Mohs surgeon, it would be prudent to submit the tumor debulk to a pathologist for definitive diagnosis and assessment of prognostic parameters of the tumor.

SQUAMOUS CELL CARCINOMA VERSUS ADNEXAL CARCINOMAS WITH SQUAMOUS DIFFERENTIATION

Adnexal carcinomas, such as porocarcinoma, may show features overlapping with SCC. A distinction is usually straightforward with a large enough tissue sample that permits detection of glandular/ductal differentiation. In difficult cases, ancillary studies (e.g., detection of YAP1 or NUT rearrangement) may be diagnostically helpful.

Because SCC may show clear cell changes, it can be confused with a trichilemmal carcinoma or sebaceous carcinoma. The presence of a broad intraepidermal (in situ) carcinoma component and detection of HPV favors a diagnosis of SCC.

SQUAMOUS CELL CARCINOMA VERSUS MELANOMA

Pigmented SCCIS with pagetoid spread may be confused with melanoma in situ. Spindle cell SCC may be confused with spindle cell melanoma. Immunohistochemistry usually permits a clear distinction. Melanomas are typically negative for cytokeratins. Most SCCs are negative for SOX10. A superficial shave biopsy of an amelanotic melanoma associated with pseudoepitheliomatous epidermal hyperplasia represents another pitfall: the pathologist may erroneously focus on the epithelial component and thus miss a subtle melanocytic tumor.

Spindle Cell Squamous Cell Carcinoma Versus Histologic Simulants

	SCC	Melanoma	AFX/UPS	Leiomyosarcoma
Cytokeratins, p40	+	−	−	−
S100P, SOX10	−	+	−	−
Actin	−	±	±	+
Desmin	−	−	−	±

+, usually positive; −, usually negative; *AFX*, atypical fibroxanthoma; *UPS*, undifferentiated pleomorphoc dermal sarcoma; *SCC*, squamous cell carcinoma.

SQUAMOUS CELL CARCINOMA VERSUS LARGE CELL LYMPHOMA

The phenotype of a poorly differentiated large cell SCC can also be simulated by an anaplastic lymphoma. Immunohistochemistry is definitive here. Anaplastic large cell lymphomas are usually positive for CD30 or T-cell markers. They are negative for cytokeratins. Confusion of CD30-positive large cell lymphoma with SCC may also occur on a superficial shave biopsy, because the lymphoma may induce florid PEH.

SQUAMOUS CELL CARCINOMA VERSUS SARCOMA

Poorly differentiated nonkeratinizing SCC may be confused with sarcomas. A spindle cell phenotype requires a different workup and diagnostic considerations than an epithelioid cell phenotype. When confronted by a malignant neoplasm arising in chronically sun-damaged skin, it is important to recognize that the presence of features of AK does not necessarily imply that the invasive tumor has to be an SCC. Features of AK may be adjacent to a sarcoma or melanoma. Therefore immunohistochemistry for epithelial and melanocytic antigens as well as markers favoring other tumors that are considered in the differential diagnosis is prudent.

When the predominant histologic phenotype is epithelioid, poorly differentiated SCC needs to be distinguished from solid epithelioid angiosarcoma as well as epithelioid sarcoma. Using cytokeratins alone will not be enough for a definitive diagnosis in this setting because both sarcomas are often keratin positive. In contrast to SCC, angiosarcoma also expresses vascular markers (FVIII, CD31, ERG, and CD34), and epithelioid sarcoma also commonly expresses CD34 or shows loss of staining for BAF-47.

Prognostic Features of Squamous Cell Carcinoma

Approximately 5% of patients with cutaneous SCC will have a local recurrence, and 2% to 3% of patients will die from SCC. Clinical stage (i.e., the presence or absence of regional or distant metastatic disease) is paramount for prognosis. For patients with clinical stage I disease (primary tumor with no evidence of metastasis), a number of clinical and pathologic features are relevant for the prognosis of cutaneous SCC.

CLINICAL FEATURES

Anatomic Site

SCCs arising from the lip or helix of the ear are more likely to metastasize than are those from other sites.

CLINICAL HISTORY

Patients with a history of radiation, rapid tumor growth, immunosuppression, or neurologic symptoms have a higher risk for recurrence and metastasis.

PATHOLOGIC FEATURES

Tumor Size, Thickness, and Depth of Invasion

The most important prognostic parameter for conventional SCC is related to tumor size, thickness, and anatomic levels of invasion. A size of more than 2 cm, thickness greater than 6 mm, and deep invasion into subcutis or skeletal muscle are prognostically unfavorable (Fig. 11.88). Size is measured clinically as the greatest horizontal diameter. Thickness reflects the distance from the top of the epidermis (or uppermost tumor under an ulcer) to the most deeply located invasive

Epithelioid Cell Squamous Cell Carcinoma Versus Histologic Simulants

IHC Marker	SCC	Melanoma	Epithelioid Sarcoma	Epithelioid Angiosarcoma
Cytokeratins, p40	+	−	+	+
S100 protein	−	+	−	−
ERG	−	−	−	+
BAF-47	+	+	−	+

−, negative; +, positive; *IHC*, immunohistochemistry; *SCC*, squamous cell carcinoma.

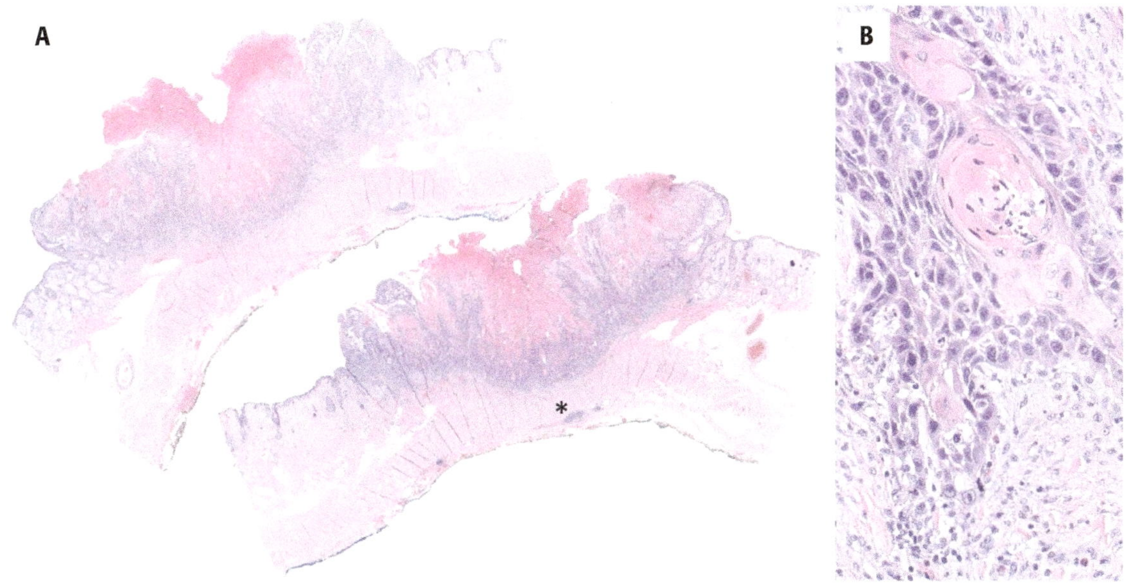

FIG. 11.88
High-risk cutaneous squamous cell carcinoma. **A,** Silhouette of the tumor. The squamous cell carcinoma measured more than 2 cm in horizontal dimension and more than 6 mm in depth of invasion. The tumor focally xtends into skeletal muscle (*). **B,** Cytology of the keratinizing tumor.

tumor cell. Depth of invasion refers to the distance of the tumor from the epidermal-dermal junction of the adjacent most superficial dermal papilla to the deepest point of invasion.

Tumors measuring less than 2 mm in depth rarely metastasize, but metastases occur in more than 15% of SCCs with a thickness greater than 6 mm. Likewise, tumors confined to the superficial dermis tend to be indolent, but the risk for metastasis increases (>12.5%) when tumors extend into muscle and bone.

Histologic Subtype

Some histopathologic variants are prognostically more favorable than others. Verrucous carcinoma and SCC KA type usually do not metastasize. However, one needs to bear in mind that conventional SCC may be associated with partial verrucous or keratoacanthomatous features and that the findings on a partial biopsy may not be fully representative. A final tumor classification can often only be made upon review of the completely excised tumor. While some histologic phenotypes such as desmoplasia and acantholysis have been reported to be associated with more aggressive behavior, the impact of these features on prognosis, after other parameters such as size and depth of invasion are taken into account, is not known. On the other hand, the combined phenotypes or SCC with neuroendocrine carcinoma or adenocarcinomas tend to be more aggressive.

Grades of Differentiation

Broders developed a grading scheme that has been associated with clinical behavior. In Broders' classification, grade 1 reflects a tumor with a ratio of differentiated to undifferentiated cells of 3 : 1. In grade 2, the ratio is 1 : 1. For grade 3, the ratio is 1 : 3, and grade 4 is assigned if no keratinization is seen. However, in real-life practice when pathologists grade an SCC, they often do not strictly apply Borders' criteria but make a quick assessment on whether a tumor shows prominent or only rare evidence of keratinization. Poor differentiation is thought to imply a higher risk for aggressive behavior, but the prognostic value of grade is limited in a multifactorial analysis taking thickness and depth of invasion into consideration.

Perineural Invasion

Perineural invasion is most commonly seen in SCCs of the head and neck region extending at least into the deep dermis (Fig. 11.89). The presence of perineural

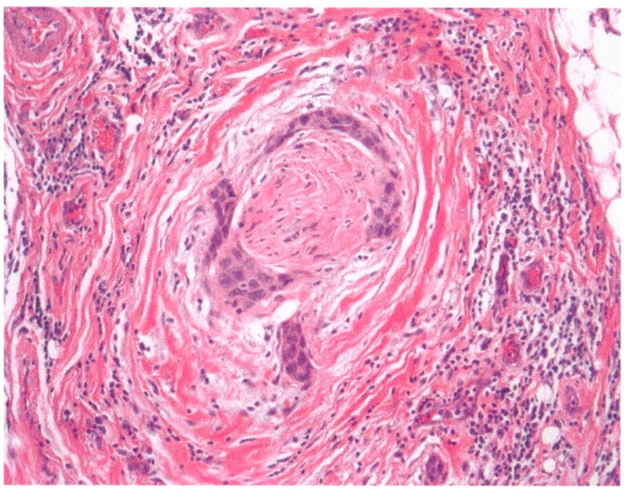

FIG. 11.89
Perineural invasion by squamous cell carcinoma.

invasion has been associated with a higher risk for local recurrence, which may be heralded by pain in the area supplied by the involved nerve. Some SCCs may grow extensively along small nerve bundles and extend far beyond the main tumor mass. This neurotropism can easily be overlooked by the unwary, especially on frozen sections. Recent data suggest that the caliber (and related anatomic level) or nerve involvement is relevant for prognosis. Perineural invasion of a small nerve in the mid-dermis with a caliber of less than 0.1 mm is much less significant for recurrence risk than involvement of a nerve in the deep subcutis with a caliber of more than 0.1 mm.

Vascular Invasion

It is intuitive that tumors with vascular invasion have a higher risk for metastasis, but data on added risk by lymphatic versus blood vessel invasion in association with SCC are limited.

STAGING OF SQUAMOUS CELL CARCINOMA

The staging of cutaneous SCC is problematic. Different staging systems have been proposed. According to the American Joint Committee on Cancer classification system of cutaneous tumors from 2010, for primary SCC, tumor size is the main parameter used for the tumor (T) classification. However, the T classification also takes into account tumor size "high-risk features" (perineural invasion, poor differentiation, location) and invasion of facial bones or skeleton. The number of regional lymph nodes (N) or distant metastases (M) is recorded. Although most useful for advanced head and neck cancers, the staging system is of limited value for the majority of cutaneous SCCs seen in most dermatology practices of dermatopathology laboratories. Most of those tumors are smaller than 2 cm in size (T1). An alternate staging system has been proposed, which distinguishes low- and high-risk settings within the group of patients with pT2 tumors (pT2a, tumor diameter >2 cm with one risk factor only; pT2b, tumor diameter >2 cm, with two or three risk factors) using the following parameters as risk factors: poor differentiation, perineural invasion, invasion beyond subcutaneous fact, and anatomically unfavorable sites. For patients with tumors larger than 2 cm in size, consideration may be given to staging by sentinel lymph node biopsy, especially in the head and neck region.

SQUAMOUS CELL CARCINOMA—ADVERSE PROGNOSTIC FINDINGS

Clinical Findings

- ▸▸ Tumor size >2 cm
- ▸▸ Immunosuppression
- ▸▸ Anatomic location on ear or lip

Histopathologic Findings

- ▸▸ Tumor thickness >6 mm
- ▸▸ Depth of invasion to deep subcutis, muscle, or bone
- ▸▸ Perineural invasion (nerve caliber >0.1 mm)
- ▸▸ Lymphovascular invasion
- ▸▸ Poor differentiation

US Staging Systems for Cutaneous Squamous Cell Carcinoma

	AJCC 7	AJCC 8 (Head Neck Only)	BWH
T1	Size ≤2 cm with <2 high-risk features	Size ≤2 cm	0 high-risk features
T2	Size >2 cm or any size with ≥2 high-risk features	Size ≥2 cm but <4 cm	T2a: 1 high-risk feature T2b: 2–3 high-risk features
T3	Tumor invades facial bone structures	Equal or greater than 4 cm > 4 cm or 1 high risk feature	All 4 high-risk features
T4	Tumor invades axial or appendicular skeleton or PNI of skull base	T4a: gross cortical bone invasion T4b: skull base invasion or foramen ovale involvement	Not applicable
High-risk features	• Depth >2 mm • PNI • Ear or lip location • Poor differentiation	• Invasion deep to fat or depth >6 mm • Minor bone erosion • PNI	• Poor differentiation • Size ≥2 cm • PNI • Deep tumor invasion (deeper than subcutis)[a]

[a]Excludes bone invasion, which implies T3.

AJCC, American Joint Commission on Cancer; *BWH*, Brigham and Women's Hospital; *cm*, centimeter; *PNI*, perineural invasion.

TREATMENT

A number of treatment modalities are used for SCC depending on the size and location of the lesion. They include electrodesiccation and curettage, excision, and Mohs micrographic surgery. Intralesional methotrexate or 5-fluorouracil are nonsurgical options for some tumors, in particular KAs. Topical imiquimod as well as topical and systemic retinoids may also be used in some cases of SCCIS. Pathergy-associated KAs may be widespread and a therapeutic challenge, particularly if a surgical modality is relied upon. The mainstay of treatment for invasive SCC is surgical excision (conventional or Mohs surgery). Electrosurgery or radiotherapy may be used in certain patients, who may not be good surgical candidates.

Lymph node examination is important, and some centers are evaluating the efficacy of sentinel lymph node biopsy, especially for large SCCs in the head and neck region. If perineural invasion is identified, local radiotherapy after excision of the tumor is a consideration, as well as imaging to assess for local extension or metastases. If lymphadenopathy is identified, sampling the lymph node either with fine-needle aspiration or open biopsy of the node should be performed. A multimodal approach to such a patient involves a team composed of the dermatologist and medical, surgical, or radiation oncologist. If distant metastases are present, chemotherapy may be used.

In the setting of immunosuppression in a solid organ transplant recipient, close work with the transplant team is critical. These patients develop cutaneous malignancies at an estimated 100-fold increase of the general population. Lowering their level of immunosuppression may be possible to curb progression and development of aggressive tumors. Oral retinoids such as acitretin in selected patients may also be beneficial. Unfortunately, cessation of the retinoid leads to development and progression of new lesions and, possibly, recurrence. There is hope that a newer agent, sirolimus, used to protect allografts may result in less frequent development of SCCs. Experience and data are limited with this drug, however.

PATHOLOGIST'S REPORTING OF SCC

For most shave biopsies of conventional SCC, it is sufficient to report the diagnosis, but if unusual findings are present (e.g., neurotropism or sarcomatoid spindle cell features) we recommend their documentation. If a small superficial SCC was meant to be excised completely by a shave procedure (shave removal), the margin status should be recorded. For excisions of larger tumors, the pathology report should include parameters relevant for prognosis and staging (e.g., tumor size, thickness, depth of invasion, perineural or lymphatic invasion) and the margin status. The degree of differentiation and various pathologic features, such as desmoplasia, acantholysis and sarcomatoid appearance, are additional parameters worth mentioning. Because perineural invasion of larger, more deeply located nerves likely implies a higher risk for local recurrence or morbidity than perineural invasion of small superficial dermal nerve twigs, we encourage pathologists to report the caliber and location of the involved nerve(s).

Unfortunately, from a perspective of ascertaining potentially relevant prognostic parameters for SCC and optimal staging of patients with such tumors, the current practice of dermatologic surgery often precludes precise tumor staging. Many invasive SCCs are diagnosed by shave biopsy, and the patients subsequently undergo Mohs surgery. Because many Mohs surgeons fail to produce pathology reports listing critical histologic parameters, such as depth of invasion or perineural invasion, prognostically relevant information often remains undocumented. Although we do not think that it is necessary to characterize in detail every superficial SCC, it would be good practice to examine the debulked portion of high-risk invasive carcinomas, that is, large tumors extending into the deep dermis or subcutis, histologically so that tumor size and the presence or absence of perineural invasion can be documented.

METASTATIC SQUAMOUS CELL CARCINOMA

Metastases from cutaneous SCC are rare, especially for the majority of small tumors limited to the dermis. Large and deeply infiltrative tumors of the head and neck region are the ones most likely to metastasize. Parotid nodes and cervical lymph nodes are commonly the initial sites of SCCs of the head and neck.

Metastases may also develop in the skin or soft tissues. Such tumors are usually rapidly growing and typically occur in the setting of a known large primary cutaneous or extracutaneous SCC. Rarely, the primary tumor location or its histologic features are unknown, or the corresponding slides are irretrievable for comparison. In these cases, it can be difficult to differentiate a new primary SCC from a metastasis. Features favoring a metastasis include rapid onset, lack of an in situ component (Fig. 11.90A), and the presence of vascular invasion. Additionally, lack of connection with the overlying epidermis and a dermal-based nodular growth pattern are seen with metastatic disease. However, these parameters are not absolute and can also be seen in a primary tumor, especially in a partial biopsy sample. Features supporting the primary nature of the tumor are the presence of a broad precursor lesion (SCCIS) associated with the invasive tumor and a stromal inflammatory or fibrosing reaction. However, small foci of intraepidermal carcinoma are not definitive for a primary tumor because metastatic SCC, similar to other carcinomas, may colonize the epidermis. Furthermore, some metastases are inflamed or affect the site of a scar.

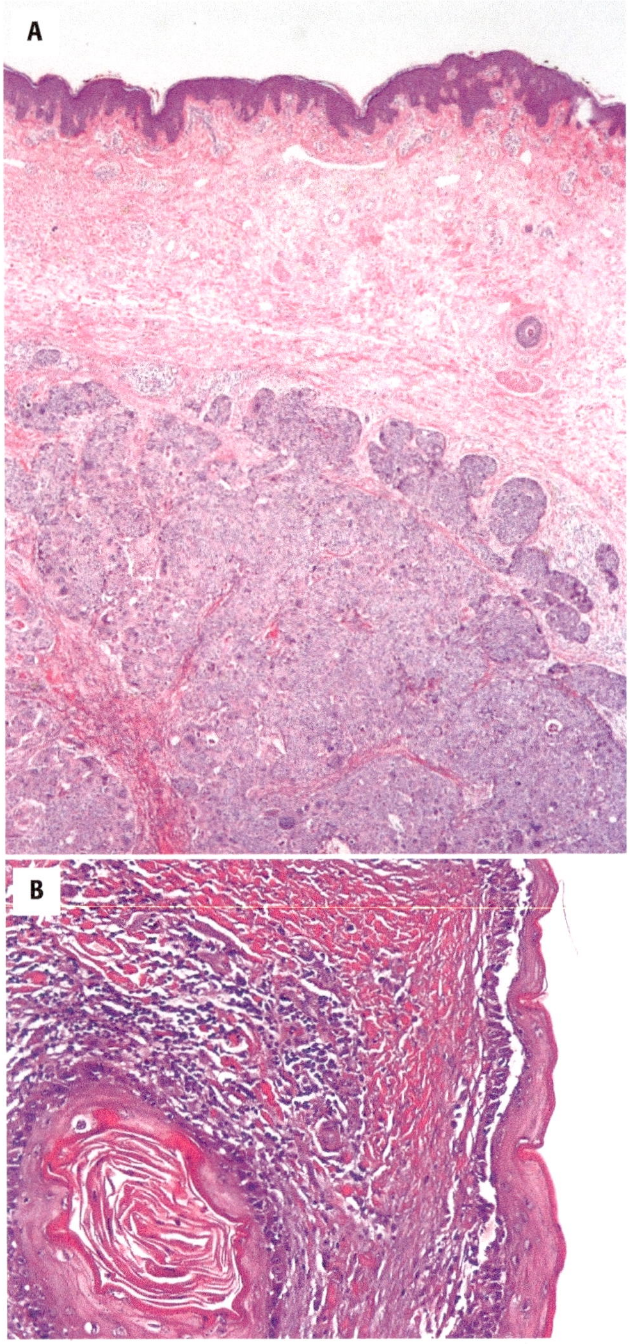

FIG. 11.90

Metastatic squamous cell carcinoma. **A,** Metastatic poorly differentiated squamous cell carcinoma in dermis with no connection to the epidermis. **B,** Metastatic cystic well-differentiated squamous cell carcinoma.

If the patient has a known extracutaneous (or prior cutaneous) SCC, review of the prior primary tumor is recommended to better assess whether the new lesion represents a metastasis (resembling the prior tumor) or more likely a new carcinoma if its appearance is significantly different.

Metastatic well-differentiated SCC may have a cystic appearance and be mistaken as a cyst, especially on a small partial biopsy (Fig. 11.90B). The presence of epithelial atypia in the cyst wall facilitates recognition of a

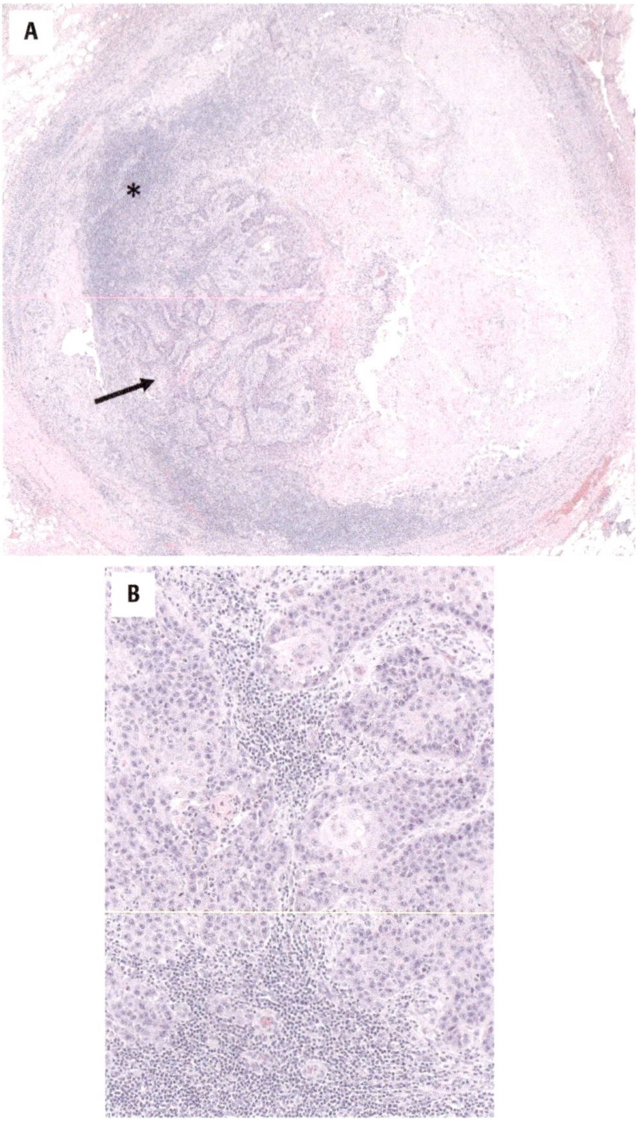

FIG. 11.91

Metastatic squamous cell carcinoma in lymph node (metastasis from tumor shown in Fig. 11.88). **A,** Squamous cell carcinoma *(arrow)* has replaced most of the lymphoid tissue *(*)*. **B,** Cytology of the squamous cell carcinoma.

cystic metastasis. However, most important for the correct diagnosis is knowledge of the clinical context (history of prior invasive SCC) and morphology of the primary tumor. Metastatic poorly differentiated SCC may also be confused with metastatic adnexal carcinomas, in particular metastatic porocarcinoma, which may show prominent squamous differentiation, and be epidermotropic (i.e., colonize the epidermis of the site to which it metastasizes). On a partial superficial biopsy, the glandular component of a porocarcinoma may not be sufficiently apparent for easy recognition.

Metastatic SCC in a lymph node (Fig. 11.91) usually does not pose a diagnostic challenge, unless the tumor is poorly differentiated. Determining the primary site of the metastatic SCC (skin versus head and neck versus other mucosal site), however, requires clinical correlation, because the morphology of the metastasis is usually not distinct. If the tumor has a basaloid appearance and there is no known regional high-risk primary cutaneous tumor, consideration needs to be given to the possibility of an HPV-related mucosal origin.

SUGGESTED FURTHER READING

Alam, M., & Ratner, D. (2001). Cutaneous squamous cell carcinoma. *New England Journal of Medicine*, *344*, 975–983.
Bander, T. S., Nehal, K. S., & Lee, E. H. (2019). Cutaneous squamous cell carcinoma: Updates in staging and management. *Dermatologic Clinics*, *37*(3), 241–251.
Butani, A., Arbesfeld, D. M., & Schwartz, R. A. (2005). Premalignant and early squamous cell carcinoma. *Clinics in Plastic Surgery*, *32*, 223–235.
Hafner, C., Hafner, H., & Groesser, L. (2014). Genetische Grundlagen seborrhoischer Keratosen und epidermaler Nävi [Genetic basis of seborrheic keratosis and epidermal nevi]. *Der Pathologe*, *35*, 413–423.
Kane, C. L., Keehn, C. A., Smithberger, E., & Glass, L. F. (2004). Histopathology of cutaneous squamous cell carcinoma and its variants. *Seminars in Cutaneous Medicine and Surgery*, *23*, 54–61.
Medeiros, F., Nascimento, A. F., & Crum, C. P. (2005). Early vulvar squamous neoplasia: Advances in classification, diagnosis, and differential diagnosis. *Advances in Anatomic Pathology*, *12*, 20–26.
Murphy, G. F., Beer, T. W., Cerio, R., Kao, G. F., Nagore, E., & Pulitzer, M. P. (2018). Squamous cell carcinoma. In D. E. Elder, D. Massi, R. A. Scolyer, & R. Willemze (Eds.), *WHO classification of skin tumours* (pp. 35–45). IARC, Lyon.
Schmitt, A. R., Brewer, J. D., Bordeaux, J. S., & Baum, C. L. (2014). Staging for cutaneous squamous cell carcinoma as a predictor of sentinel lymph node biopsy results: Meta-analysis of American Joint Committee on Cancer Criteria and a Proposed Alternative System. *JAMA Dermatology*, *150*, 19–24.
Schwartz, R. A. (2004). Keratoacanthoma: A clinicopathologic enigma. *Dermatologic Surgery*, *30*, 326–333.
Smoller, B. R. (2006). Squamous cell carcinoma: From precursor lesions to high-risk variants. *Modern Pathology*, *19*(Suppl. 2), S88–S92.
Waldman, A., & Schmults, C. (2019). Cutaneous squamous cell carcinoma. *Hematology/Oncology Clinics of North America*, *33*(1), 1–12.

12 Adnexal Tumors

Victor G. Prieto • Christopher R. Shea • Klaus J. Busam

Adnexal tumors are generally classified according to two principles: (1) benign versus malignant and (2) line of differentiation, referring to which normal cutaneous structure the lesion most resembles (hair follicle, apocrine or eccrine gland, or sebaceous gland). Although such a scheme might seem simple to apply, there is still considerable controversy on how best to classify many adnexal lesions. The historical nomenclature is sometimes confusing, with many different names for essentially the same type of tumor.

We recommend a pragmatic approach to the pathologist confronted with adnexal tumors. The most important issue is to distinguish benign from malignant tumors. In general, benign neoplasms are well-differentiated, circumscribed, and noninfiltrative. Malignant tumors tend to be infiltrative and to show cytologic atypia. However, there are exceptions to this rule. For example, on occasion, a malignant tumor may lack marked atypia and present with a nodular circumscribed adenoma-like growth, such as digital papillary adenocarcinoma.

Subclassification of malignant tumors is important when the tumor types being considered in the differential diagnosis greatly differ in biologic potential. Subclassification is much less relevant clinically when the biologic potential is more or less the same or the tumors are benign. However, we still recommend precise classification of benign tumors, when possible, for the sake of accuracy and because some such tumors may alert the clinician to the possibility of a genetic predisposition to internal cancers (e.g., sebaceous neoplasms and Muir-Torre syndrome [MTS]; fibrofolliculoma and Birt-Hogg-Dubé syndrome).

This chapter is not comprehensive. Rather, it provides an overview of common adnexal tumors and discusses important aspects of the differential diagnosis.

TUMORS WITH FOLLICULAR DIFFERENTIATION

FOLLICULAR HAMARTOMA (FOLLICULAR NEVUS)

This rare hamartoma is characterized by a locally increased number of mature hair follicles.

NEVUS COMEDONICUS

This rare hamartoma is characterized by numerous dilated hair follicles resembling acne comedones or small infundibular cysts.

BENIGN FOLLICULAR NEOPLASMS

DILATED PORE, PILAR SHEATH ACANTHOMA, AND TRICHOFOLLICULOMA

Dilated pore (of Winer), pilar sheath acanthoma, and trichofolliculoma typically present as a solitary small cyst, papule, or small nodule on the skin of the head and neck.

Dilated pore shares with infundibular cyst the presence of stratified squamous epithelium having a granular layer and containing loosely packed keratin. However, in contrast to a cyst, which has a flattened epithelial lining, rete ridges surround a dilated pore (Fig. 12.1). If the cyst lining epithelium is acanthotic, the term *pilar sheath acanthoma* (Fig. 12.2) is used.

Trichofolliculoma is characterized by a central, cystically dilated follicle, from which several small follicles with variable maturity radiate (Fig. 12.3).

INFUNDIBULOMA (TUMOR OF THE FOLLICULAR INFUNDIBULUM)

This uncommon, benign tumor is composed of a plate-like growth of keratinocytes with several points of attachment to the epidermis and the external root sheath of hair follicles (Fig. 12.4). Its cells may have basaloid features and simulate a superficial basal cell carcinoma (BCC) or the superficial portion of an infundibulocystic BCC. In contrast to bona fide BCC, infundibuloma has pale trichilemmal epithelium and lacks hyperchromatic nuclei, myxoid stroma, and peripheral clefting. Occasionally, infundibuloma may be difficult to distinguish from irritated endophytic seborrheic keratosis (SK).

TRICHOBLASTOMA AND TRICHOEPITHELIOMA

Trichoblastoma (TBL) and trichoepithelioma (TE) are benign follicular fibroepithelial tumors. Many contemporary

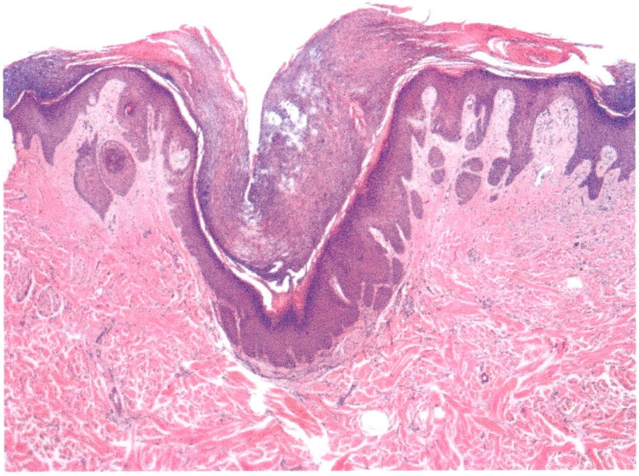

FIG. 12.1

Dilated pore. A central pore is present surrounded by infundibular epithelium of normal thickness.

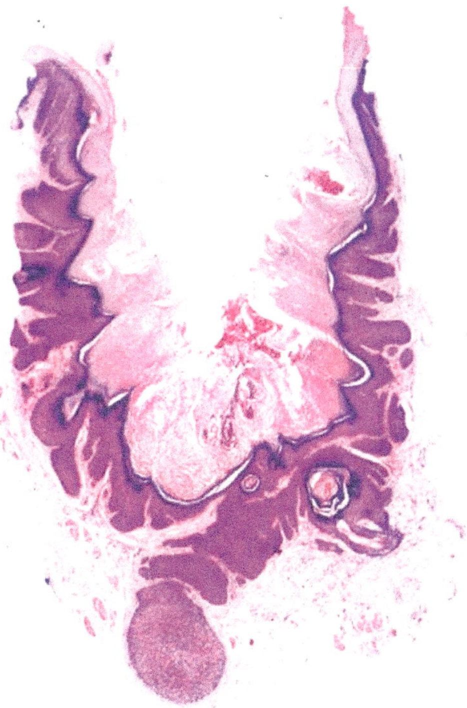

FIG. 12.2

Pilar sheath acanthoma. Cystic invagination lined by follicular infundibular type epithelium with epithelial hyperplasia.

dermatopathologists consider TE a superficial form of TBL. TE and TBL are grouped together in the 2018 World Health Organization classification of skin tumors. We share this view; therefore, we describe TE together with TBL herein. Because desmoplastic TE raises diagnostic issues different from TBL, it is discussed separately.

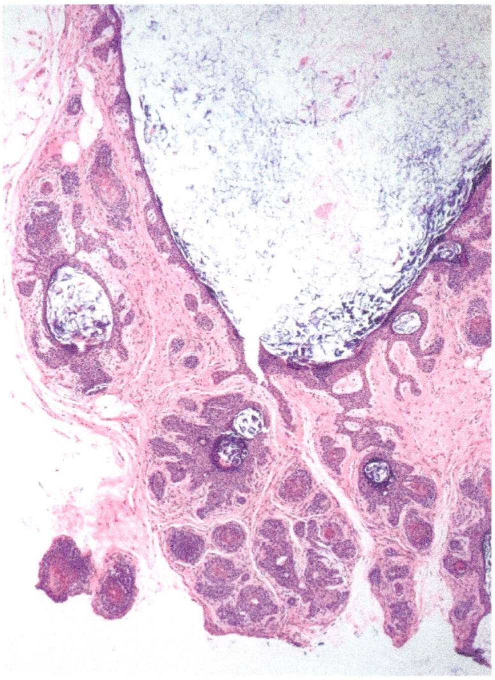

FIG. 12.3

Trichofolliculoma. A cystically dilated follicle is filled with keratin and surrounded by numerous secondary follicles.

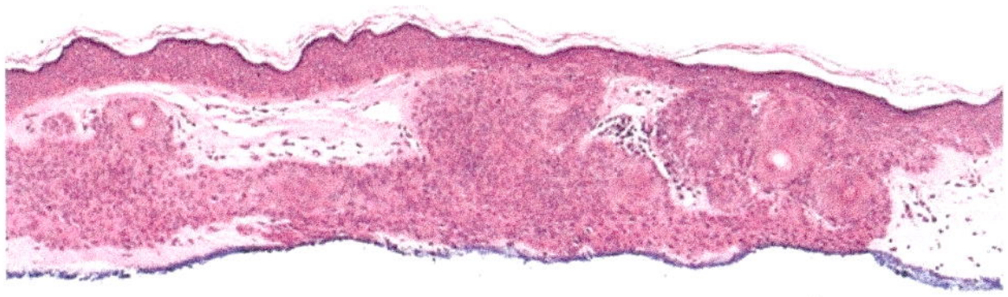

FIG. 12.4

Tumor of follicular infundibulum (infundibuloma). Aggregates of small keratinocytes show multiple connections to the epidermis and form a superficial dermal plaque.

Clinical Findings

TBL typically presents as a sporadic, solitary, flesh-colored, 2- to 8-mm papule on the face. Rarely, it may form a larger nodule (giant solitary TE). Uncommonly, multiple TBLs (Fig. 12.5) occur in families as an autosomal dominant condition or as part of the Brooke-Spiegler or Rombo's syndromes, with mutations of the *CYLD* or *PTCH1* genes. TBL is a common secondary neoplasm in nevus sebaceus (of Jadassohn).

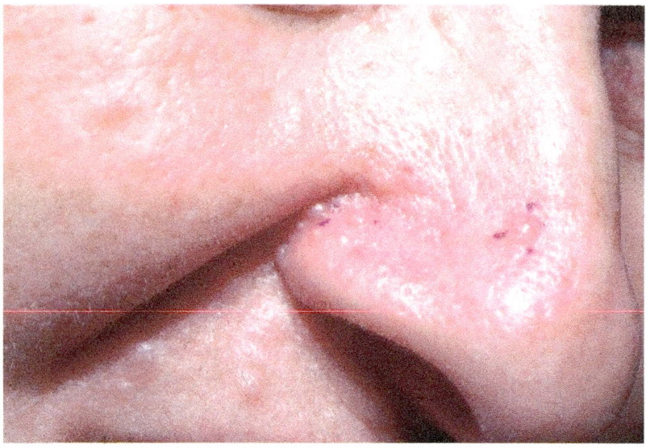

FIG. 12.5

Trichoblastoma. Multiple small skin-colored papules are present.

Histopathologic Features

TBL is a fibroepithelial tumor composed of basaloid epithelial cells with a cellular fibrous stroma distinctly different from the surrounding normal reticular dermis (Fig. 12.6A). Papillary-mesenchymal bodies (Fig. 12.6B), cuplike proliferations of basaloid cells engulfing fibroblasts, thereby recapitulating the follicular papilla, are characteristic. Mitotic figures or apoptotic bodies can be present, but they are not as frequent as in BCCs. Stromal calcifications are commonly present in TBLs.

Superficial TBLs (TEs) usually contain small keratocysts with infundibular keratinization and may form connections to the epidermis. More deeply located tumors usually lack epidermal connections and infundibular cysts.

TBL may be infiltrated by lymphocytes (so-called cutaneous lymphadenoma).

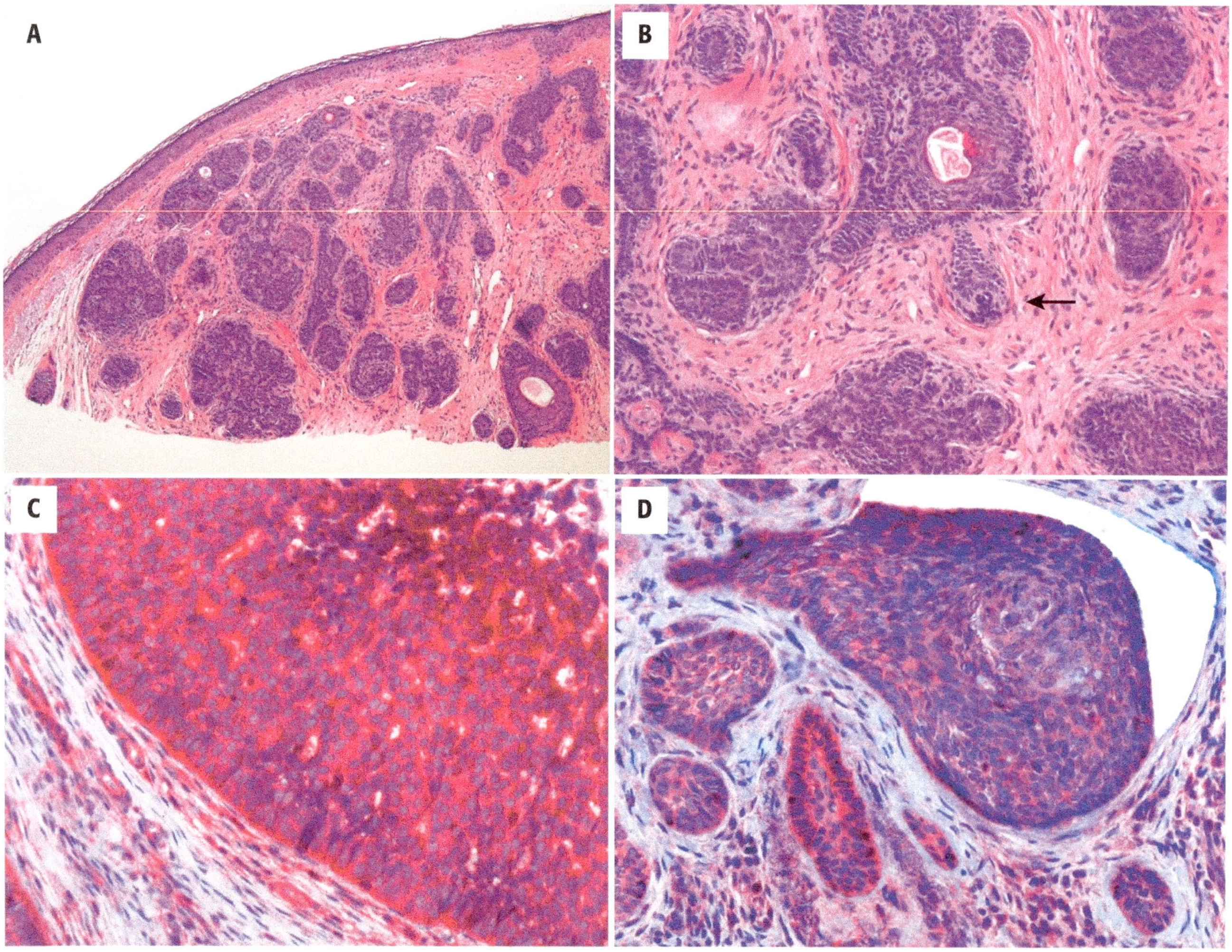

FIG. 12.6

Trichoblastoma. **A,** Groups of basaloid cells surrounded by fibroblasts forming a fibroepithelial lesion. **B,** The basaloid cells show follicular features, including papillary mesenchymal bodies *(arrow)*. **C,** Diffuse expression of PHLDA1. **D,** In contrast, basal cell carcinoma lacks PHLDA1 expression. (C and D courtesy of Dr. Luis Requena.)

Ancillary Studies

In keeping with TBLs' follicular differentiation, they usually contain Merkel cells, which express CK20. However, rare CK20-positive cells can also be seen in BCC. PHLDA1 is primarily expressed in TBL and usually not in BCC (Fig. 12.6C and D).

Differential Diagnosis

The main diagnostic distinction is from BCC. In contrast to BCC, the stroma of TBL shows a tight association with the basaloid epithelial cells. No clefts or retractions are present between epithelium and stroma, as is characteristic of BCC. Instead, TBL shows a distinct demarcation between its periepithelial stroma and the surrounding dermal collagen. TBL typically contains papillary mesenchymal bodies, which are usually absent in BCC. Mitotic figures and apoptotic bodies can occur in TBL but are not as common as in BCC. Certain stromal alterations, such as mucin or amyloid deposits, which are characteristic of BCC, would be unusual for TBL.

Trichoblastic proliferations simulating superficial BCC may occur as an inductive phenomenon along the dermal-epidermal junction overlying a dermatofibroma (Fig. 12.7) or along the follicular epithelial interface in association with a blue nevus.

DESMOPLASTIC TRICHOEPITHELIOMA

Clinical Findings

This tumor typically presents as a 2- to 9-mm, asymptomatic, slowly growing, indurated area, which may have an atrophic, depressed center (Fig. 12.8).

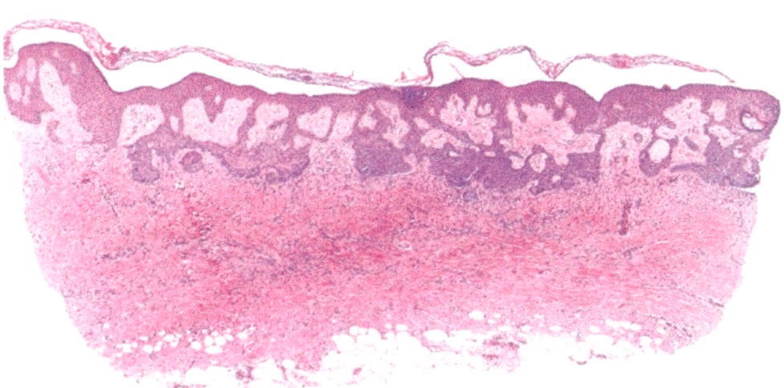

FIG. 12.7
Trichoblastic proliferation overlying a dermatofibroma.

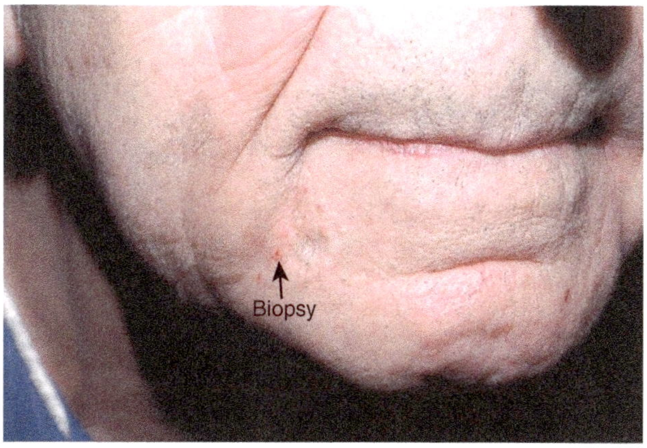

FIG. 12.8
Desmoplastic trichoepithelioma. A small indurated and indented skin-colored area is present.

Differential Diagnosis: Basal Cell Carcinoma Versus Trichoblastoma

	Basal Cell Carcinoma	Trichoblastoma
Papillary mesenchymal body	Usually absent	Usually present
Clefts	Between tumor and stroma	Between tumor stroma and surrounding normal dermis
Mitotic figures	Common	Rare
Mucinous stroma	Common	Rare
PHLDA1 expression	Rare	Usually present

Histopathologic Features

Desmoplastic or sclerosing TE is quite different microscopically from conventional TE or TBL. Although TBL usually forms a spherical nodule, the silhouette of desmoplastic TE is usually that of a superficial dermal plaque. This tumor is characterized by the triad of thin strands of basaloid epithelial cells, keratinous cysts, and a dense fibrous stroma (Fig. 12.9). Additional features may include foreign-body giant-cell reactions to keratin and calcifications. Focal papillary mesenchymal bodies may be present.

Ancillary Studies

CK20-positive Merkel cells are commonly associated with the tumor (Fig. 12.9C). PHLDA1 is reported to be primarily expressed in all types of TBL and TE but only rarely in BCC.

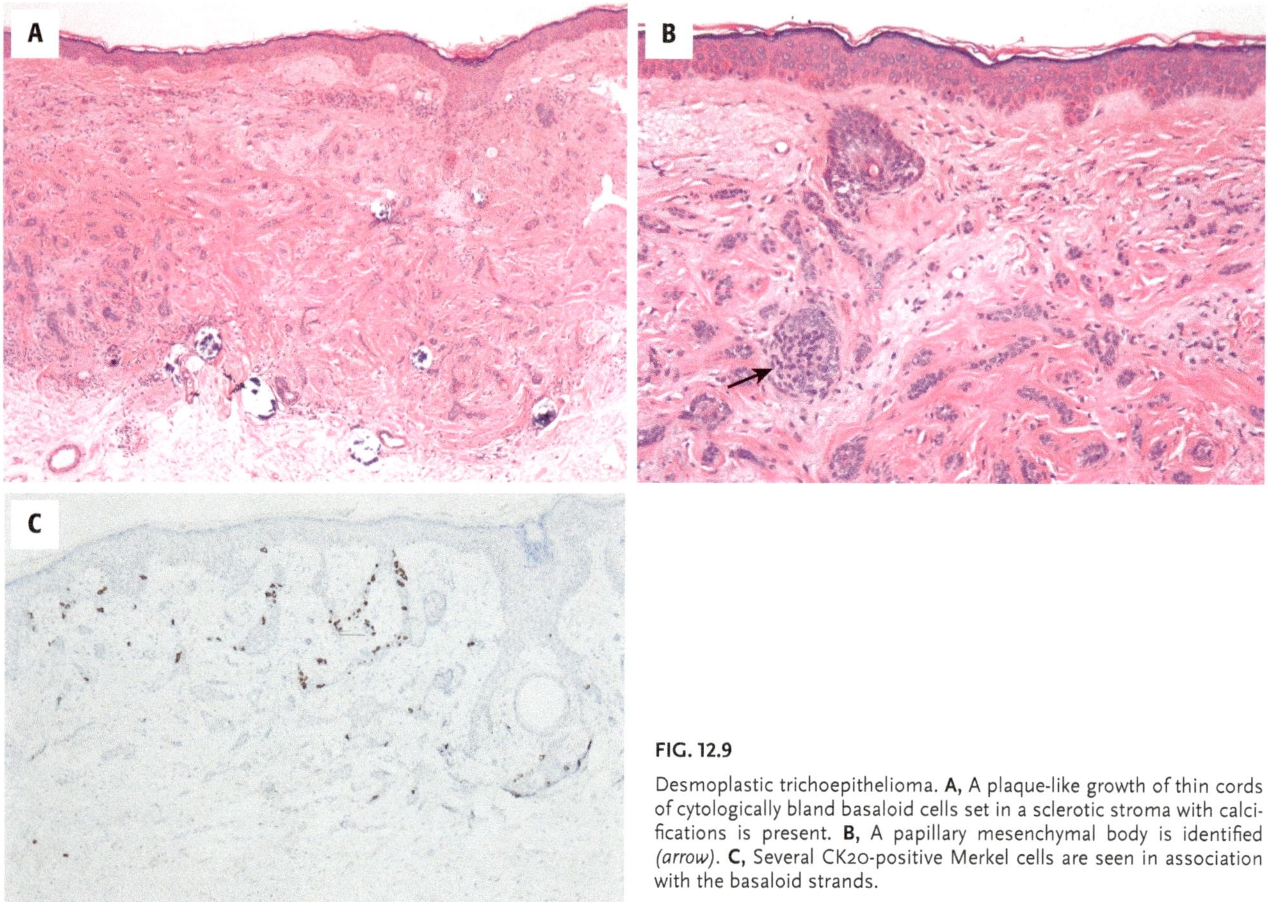

FIG. 12.9

Desmoplastic trichoepithelioma. **A,** A plaque-like growth of thin cords of cytologically bland basaloid cells set in a sclerotic stroma with calcifications is present. **B,** A papillary mesenchymal body is identified *(arrow)*. **C,** Several CK20-positive Merkel cells are seen in association with the basaloid strands.

Differential Diagnosis

Desmoplastic TE needs to be distinguished from morpheaform BCC and MAC. Morpheaform BCC tends to show greater asymmetry in its growth and to infiltrate more deeply. Furthermore, the degree of nuclear atypia and the number of mitotic figures or apoptotic bodies are higher in BCC. After one identifies foci of the characteristic features of BCC, such as sheets or small nodules of basaloid cells with peripheral palisading and retraction artifact, the diagnosis is straightforward. Another helpful feature is the presence of cytologically bland keratocysts, which are common in desmoplastic TE. Keratocysts may occur in infiltrative BCCs but rarely in morpheaform variants. If they are present, the tumor cells surrounding the cystic structures are atypical. A possible pitfall is the observation of perineural involvement in desmoplastic TE. Its presence per se does not necessarily imply a diagnosis of carcinoma.

Differential Diagnosis of Sclerosing Basaloid Tumors

	Desmoplastic richoepithelioma	Microcystic Adnexal Carcinoma	Sclerosing Basal Cell Carcinoma
Papillary mesenchymal bodies	Present	Absent	Absent
Keratin cysts	Common	Common	Usually absent
Atypia	Absent or mild	Absent or mild	Present
Mitotic figures	Absent or rare	Absent or rare	Common
Ducts or tubules	Absent	Usually present	Absent
CK20-positive cells	Common	Absent	Absent

MAC or syringoma may also be confused with desmoplastic TE, especially in a small superficial shave biopsy. The presence of papillary mesenchymal bodies excludes syringoma and MAC. On the other hand, if ductal differentiation is present, desmoplastic TE can be excluded. The identification of CK20-negative or chromogranin-positive Merkel cells in the tumor is also helpful to support follicular differentiation and to distinguish desmoplastic TE from syringoma (Fig. 12.9C). Microcystic adnexal carcinoma may show mixed follicular and glandular differentiation.

BASALOID FOLLICULAR HAMARTOMA

This entity is controversial. Some consider it a malformative proliferation. Others view it as a genuine neoplasm, but opinions vary again on whether it is a benign tumor distinct from TBL and TE, or an incipient infundibulocystic BCC. Basaloid follicular hamartoma may be an incidental histopathologic finding or may present clinically as a small papule. There are hereditary and nonhereditary, localized, and generalized variants.

Basaloid follicular hamartoma usually forms a small, dermal proliferation of thin, anastomosing strands and branching cords of basaloid cells, often adjacent to or attached to hair follicles. Small keratocysts may be present. The basaloid cells appear bland, and mitotic figures are absent or rare. Lesions reported as basaloid follicular hamartoma seem to span a spectrum of basaloid epithelial proliferations ranging from TBL, TE, and tumors indistinguishable from BCC (in particular, its infundibulocystic variants), to a subset of lesions for which a separate designation of basaloid follicular hamartoma may be reasonable.

TRICHOADENOMA

This rare tumor usually occurs on the face and is histopathologically characterized by a circumscribed, small, superficial dermal nodule of well-formed keratinous cysts (Fig. 12.10). In a small shave biopsy specimen, it may be difficult to render a definitive diagnosis of trichoadenoma, because MAC may show similar features in its superficial portion.

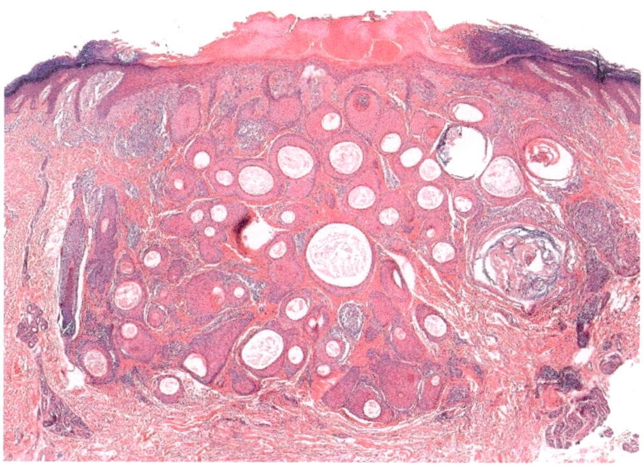

FIG. 12.10

Trichoadenoma. Numerous keratocysts are present in the dermis.

TRICHILEMMOMA

Clinical Findings

Trichilemmomas are solitary lesions typically present on the face of young individuals (Fig. 12.11). Most of them are sporadic, solitary lesions. Multiple lesions are a marker for Cowden's syndrome (CS; see the following).

Histopathologic Features

Trichilemmomas are usually small, circumscribed tumors composed of one or more lobules of cuboidal cells with central, round nuclei and light-pink or clear cytoplasm (Fig. 12.12). There is usually a small papular exophytic component, as well as an endophytic part extending into the upper reticular dermis. The lobules tend to connect to the epidermis or follicular infundibulum at several points. At the periphery of the lobules is a layer of columnar basaloid cells with nuclear palisading resembling cells of the follicular outer root sheath. They are usually surrounded by a hyaline, pink band representing thickened basement membrane. Clear-cell changes are common and reflect abundant cytoplasmic glycogen. Keratinization and squamous eddies may be present.

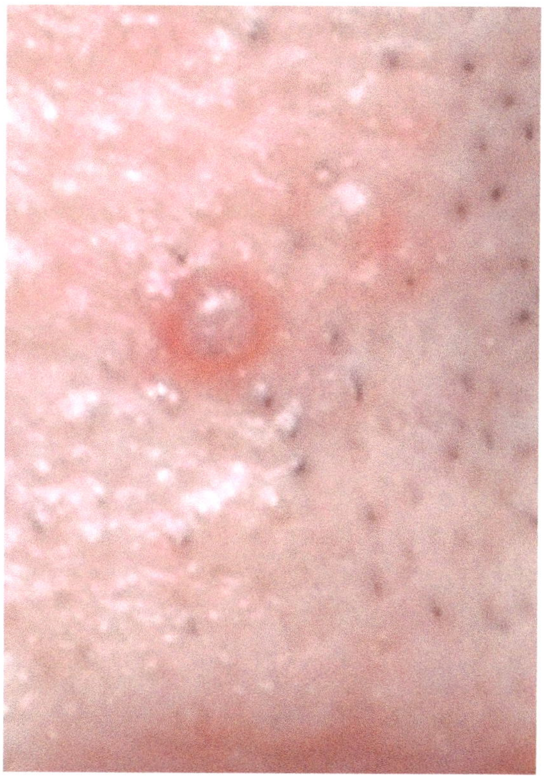

FIG. 12.11

Trichilemmoma. A small skin-colored papule is present.

A

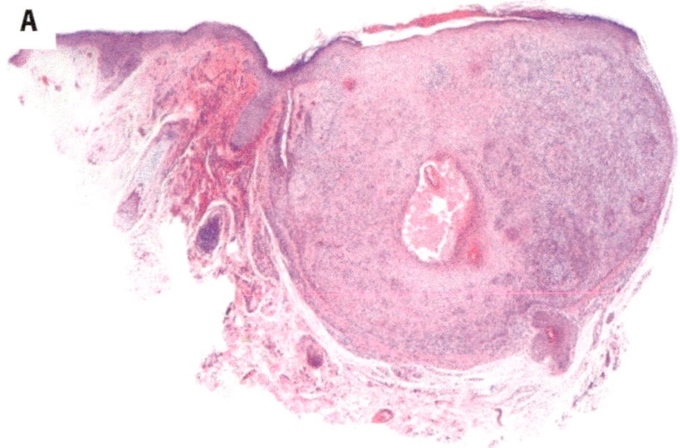

B

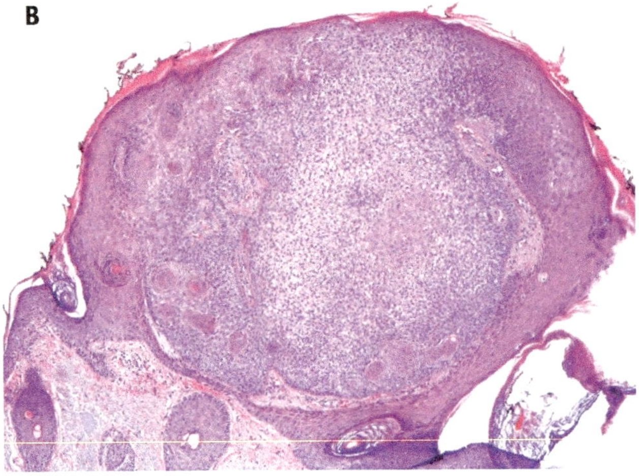

FIG. 12.12

Trichilemmoma. **A,** A superficial dermal nodule of small cuboidal keratinocytes with a lobular growth pattern is associated with a follicle. **B,** Clear-cell changes are common. Note also the dense pink membrane surrounding the base of the lobular proliferation.

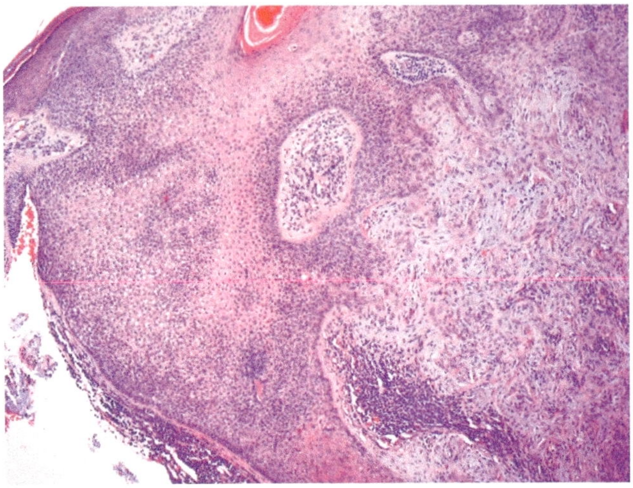

FIG. 12.13

Desmoplastic trichilemmoma. The periphery of the tumor shows features typical of trichilemmoma. In the center there is irregular epithelial growth with fibrosis.

Desmoplastic trichilemmoma is a variant showing a hyalinized or desmoplastic stroma (Fig. 12.13), in which the tumor cells often display an irregular and seemingly infiltrative growth pattern.

Ancillary Studies

Trichilemmoma expresses CD34.

Differential Diagnosis

Trichilemmoma shares many features with inverted follicular keratosis. However, the latter lacks hyaline membranes, and clear cell or basaloid features are less common. Trichilemmoma shows overlap with wart affecting a hair follicle, thereby inducing trichilemmal hyperplasia (so-called trichilemmal warts). Such warts typically have a papillomatous exophytic component (Fig. 12.14). On a partial superficial biopsy, trichilemmoma, especially when irritated and inflamed, may be confused with BCC or even squamous cell carcinoma (SCC). Attention to the bland cytology of the tumor cells should prevent this pitfall. In problematic cases, immunohistochemistry for CD34 can help because

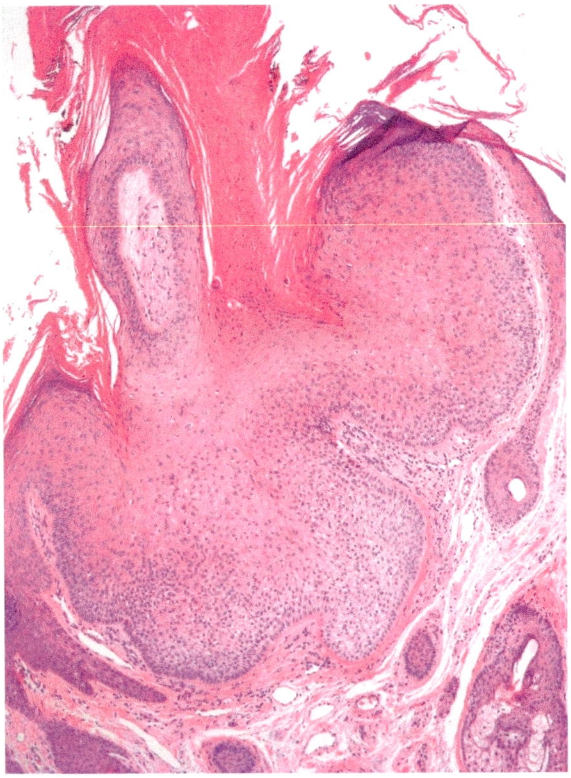

FIG. 12.14

Trichilemmal wart. An exophytic verrucous growth pattern is associated with a lobular perifollicular clear-cell proliferation at the base of the lesion.

strong labeling of a peripheral stromal cells is only seen in trichilemmomas, but not SCC, BCC, or trichilemmal carcinoma. Trichilemmoma differs from carcinoma by the lack of atypia and a benign (i.e., noninfiltrative) silhouette.

INVERTED FOLLICULAR KERATOSIS

Inverted follicular keratosis typically occurs on the central face in middle-aged individuals. It is clinically indistinct and often biopsied to rule out BCC or wart.

Typically, there is a wedge-shaped proliferation of keratinocytes with a lobulated, circumscribed, peripheral growth pattern. Coarse keratohyaline granules and whorls of squamous cells (squamous eddies) are usually present. Histopathologically, the differential diagnosis includes SCC and trichilemmoma. Inverted follicular keratosis lacks an infiltrative growth pattern and thereby differs from SCC. It differs from trichilemmoma by the lack of prominent peripheral palisading and of basement membrane thickening.

PILOMATRICOMA (CALCIFYING EPITHELIOMA OF MALHERBE)

Clinical Findings

Pilomatricoma usually manifests as a solitary, small (but rarely up to 5 cm), tan, firm nodule on the face or upper extremities, although it may occur in almost any hair-bearing area (Fig. 12.15). Most lesions arise during the first two decades of life, but they can also develop in elderly individuals. Familial occurrence is rare, particularly in association with myasthenia gravis or Gardner's syndrome.

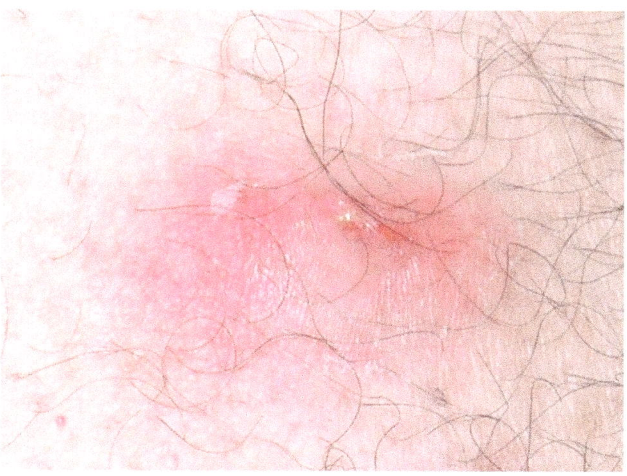

FIG. 12.15
Pilomatricoma. Erythematous firm nodule.

Histopathologic Features

Pilomatricoma tends to present as a well-circumscribed nodule in the dermis or superficial subcutis (or both) (Fig. 12.16). A typical pilomatricoma is composed of basaloid (matrical) cells with mitotic figures and "ghost" cells (polygonal, deeply eosinophilic cell remnants, with a centrally located clear area corresponding to the absent nucleus). There is often an associated foreign-body giant-cell reaction. Calcification is common, and ossification may occur. Some pilomatricomas contain melanophages in the stroma and dendritic melanocytes within the clusters of basaloid cells (pigmented pilomatricoma or melanocytic matricoma). The early (proliferative) stage of pilomatricomas has a higher proportion of basaloid cells (often with numerous mitotic figures). In a later stage, the basaloid component may be minimal or absent. Tumors in the proliferative stage have also been termed *proliferating trichilemmomas.*

Ancillary Studies

Pilomatricoma shows nuclear and cytoplasmic labeling for β-catenin.

Differential Diagnosis

Pilomatricoma must be distinguished from pilomatrix carcinoma. The main feature that helps in differentiating between them is the silhouette of the tumor. Whereas nodular, circumscribed lesions should be considered benign, infiltrative lesions may recur or, rarely, metastasize. Pilomatrix carcinomas typically show a high proportion of basaloid cells or features indistinguishable from SCC. Cytologic atypia and necrosis are often present in larger tumors.

On occasion, pilomatricoma must be distinguished from BCC, which may show focal matrical differentiation with ghost cells. Identification of classic features of BCC elsewhere in the tumor is helpful in this regard. Hybrid cysts of patients with Gardner's syndrome may show mixed features of pilomatricoma and other follicular cysts.

FIBROFOLLICULOMA AND TRICHODISCOMA

Clinical Findings

Both fibrofolliculoma and trichodiscoma occur as single or multiple, yellow-white papules, a few millimeters

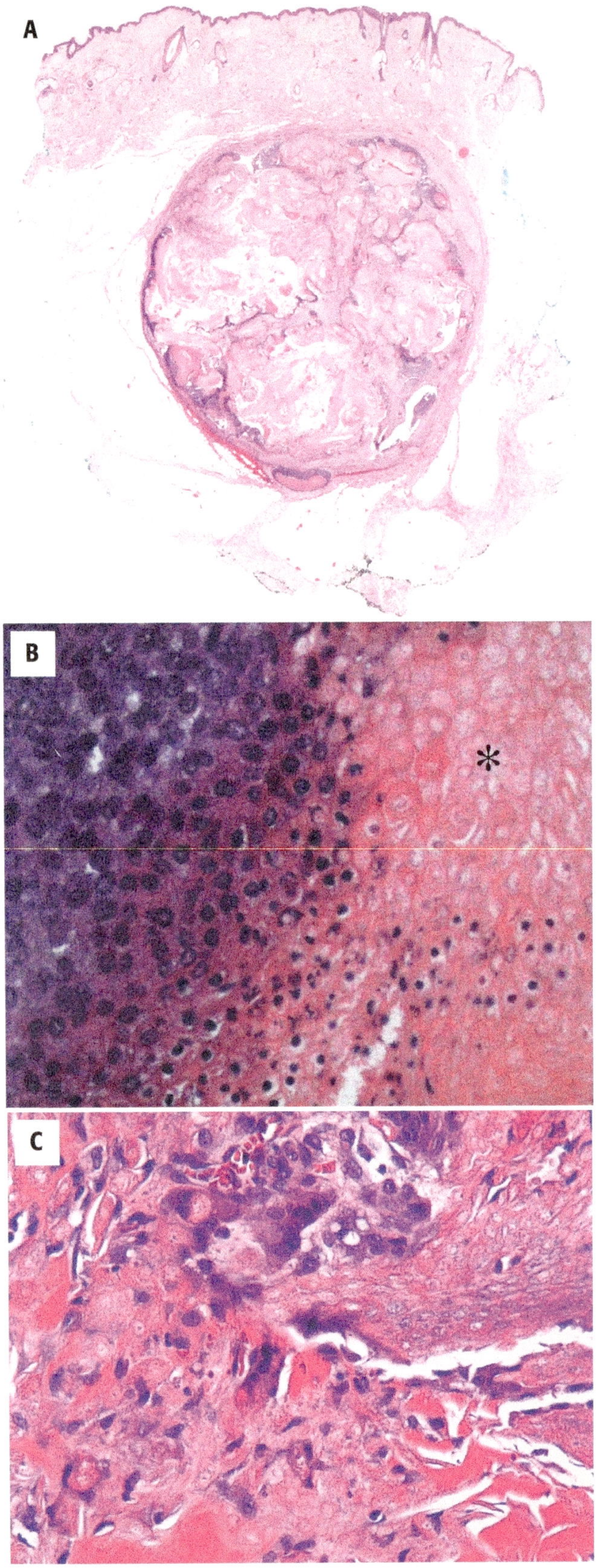

FIG. 12.16

Pilomatricoma. **A,** A circumscribed subcutaneous nodule is present. **B,** The tumor is composed of basaloid cells as well as "shadow" cells. **C,** Multinucleated giant cells are also common.

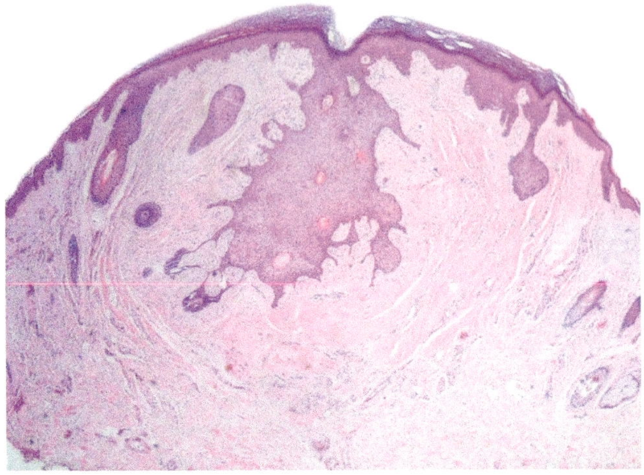

FIG. 12.17

Trichofolliculoma. Cords of epithelial cells emanate from the infundibular wall of a follicle and reach into a perifollicular stroma characterized by an increased number of fibroblasts, small capillaries.

in diameter, on the head and neck. Multiple lesions are associated with Birt-Hogg-Dubé syndrome (see the following).

Histopathologic Features

Fibrofolliculoma is composed of elongated, interlacing trabeculae of basaloid cells surrounded by fibromyxoid stroma. A dilated hair follicle may be present near the center of the lesion. Trichodiscoma typically appears as a perifollicular or parafollicular, elliptical, nonencapsulated, angiofibromatous stromal proliferation (Fig. 12.17).

TREATMENT OF BENIGN FOLLICULAR TUMORS

In general, no further surgery is necessary after an unequivocal diagnosis of a benign follicular tumor except for cosmetic reasons. Other than surgical excision, locally destructive modalities (laser, cryotherapy, or conservative surgery) are available to remove the lesion(s).

In doubtful, incompletely excised lesions—for example, when TBL is favored based on a small shave biopsy specimen, but BCC cannot entirely be ruled out—it seems prudent to recommend conservative complete removal of the lesion.

MALIGNANT NEOPLASMS WITH FOLLICULAR DIFFERENTIATION: BASAL CELL CARCINOMA

Many textbooks discuss BCC as an epidermal tumor, but we place it under adnexal tumors, because it predominantly displays follicular differentiation, and its differential diagnosis primarily involves other adnexal tumors.

BCC is a very common neoplasm. It mainly occurs on sun-exposed skin, in general in any hair-bearing area, but may also occur at sites with limited or no sun exposure. Patients with xeroderma pigmentosum, who have a diminished capability for repairing sun-induced mutations, develop a large number of both BCCs and SCCs early in life, as do patients with the nevoid BCC (Gorlin's) syndrome or Bazex-Dupré-Christol syndrome.

Mutations of the patched (*PTCH1*) gene are pathogenic in the majority of syndromic and sporadic BCCs.

Clinical Findings

The most common appearance is that of a papule or nodule, which may be eroded or ulcerated (ulcus rodens). Papules of BCC may clinically be confused with nevus, fibroma, or folliculitis. BCC may also manifest as an erythematous patch (Fig. 12.18), papule, nodule, or plaque (Fig. 12.19), often eroded, ulcerated (Fig. 12.20), or indurated (Fig. 12.21). It may be difficult or impossible to distinguish BCC clinically from Bowen's disease (SCC in situ) or irritated or lichenoid keratosis. Melanin pigment may be present (Fig. 12.22), and BCC may thereby simulate a melanocytic nevus or melanoma.

BASAL CELL CARCINOMA—DISEASE FACT SHEET

Incidence

- ▸▸ Approximately 900,000 new individuals with basal cell carcinoma (BCC) per year in the United States

Patient Group

- ▸▸ Occurs in all ethnicities but most often in fair-skinned people
- ▸▸ Usually in patients older than 40 years of age
- ▸▸ More often in men than in women (male:female ratio, 1.6:1)

Risk Factors

- ▸▸ Exposure to ultraviolet radiation
- ▸▸ Syndromes: nevoid basal cell carcinoma (Gorlin's) syndrome; Bazex-Christol-Dupré syndrome; xeroderma pigmentosum
- ▸▸ History of ionizing radiation treatment

Clinical Findings

- ▸▸ Flesh-colored, erythematous, or pigmented papule or nodule; may be ulcerated
- ▸▸ Indurated plaque (sclerosing BCC)

Prognosis

- ▸▸ Usually only local growth; may be locally destructive, with significant morbidity depending on location and size
- ▸▸ Exceedingly rarely can metastasize (preferred sites: lymph nodes, lung, and bones)

Treatment

- ▸▸ Surgical: saucerization, standard full-thickness excision, Mohs micrographic surgery, curettage with or without electrodesiccation, cryosurgery
- ▸▸ Medical: topical 5-fluorouracil, imiquimod; systemic vismodegib or sonidegib chemotherapy for metastatic or unresectable cutaneous disease
- ▸▸ Radiation

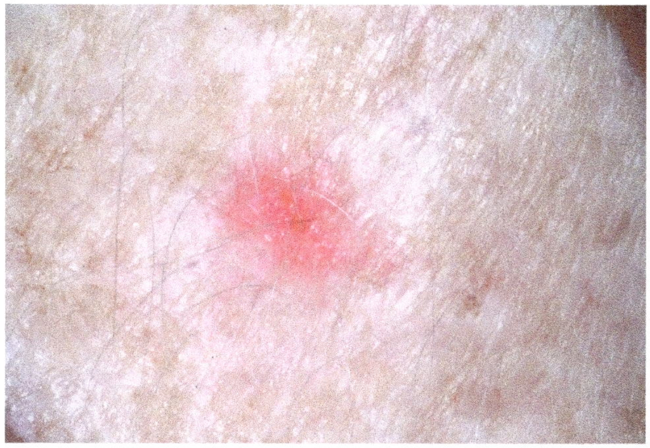

FIG. 12.18
Basal cell carcinoma, erythematous patch.

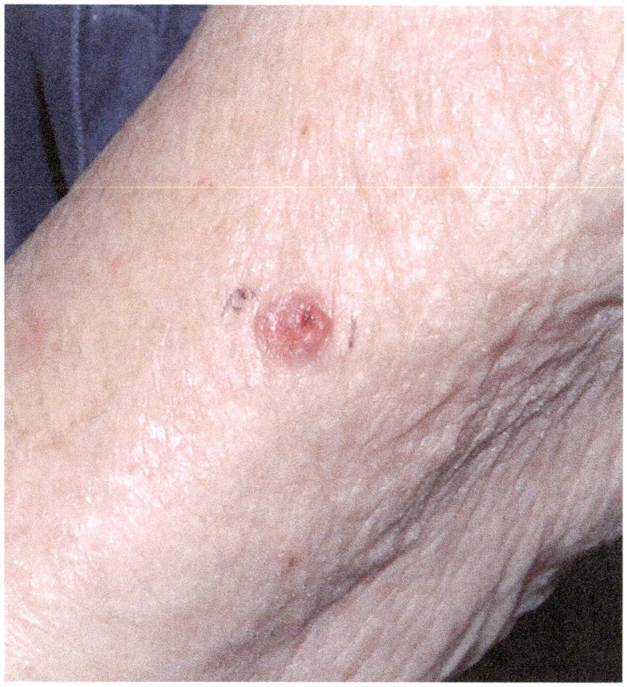

FIG. 12.19
Basal cell carcinoma, erythematous nodule.

Histopathologic Features

BCC is characterized by the presence of basaloid cells, peripheral palisading, mitotic figures, apoptotic bodies, myxoid stroma, and peritumoral clefting (Fig. 12.23).

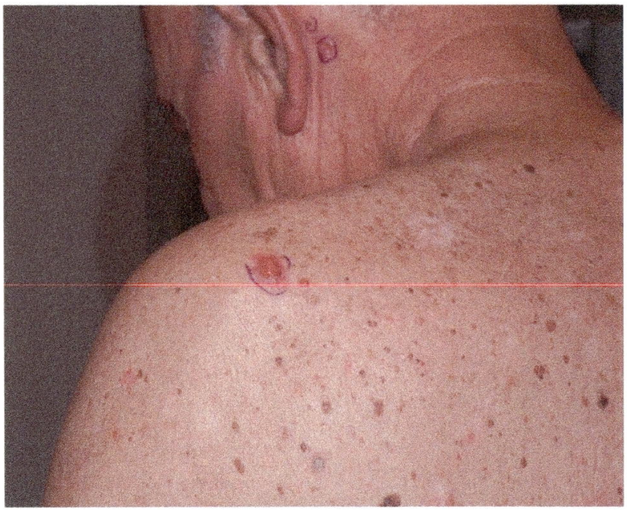

FIG. 12.20

Basal cell carcinoma, ulcerated plaque.

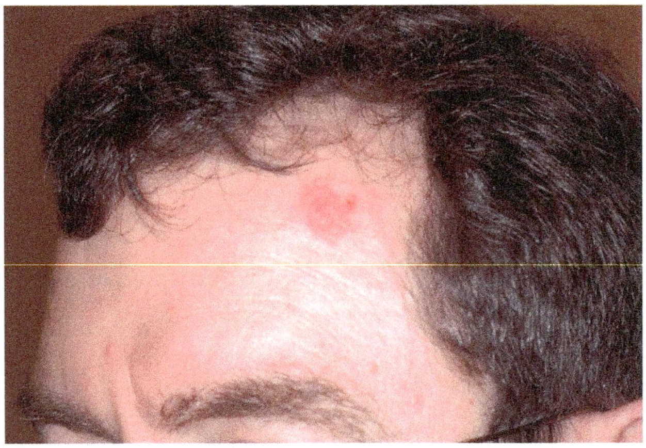

FIG. 12.21

Basal cell carcinoma, indurated erythematous patch.

The presence of myxoid stroma and peripheral clefting may be the most helpful features to distinguish BCC from other basaloid tumors, such as TBL. A number of secondary features may occur in BCCs, such as dystrophic calcifications, amyloid deposition, or inflammatory reactions with or without features of partial regression.

Several patterns of BCC have been described. The main clinical purpose is to distinguish those with circumscribed growth (nodular pattern), which are more easily excised with a negative margin, from infiltrative tumors, which are more likely associated with positive margins and local recurrences. One pattern may predominate or be present in pure form. Many times, however, a combination of patterns occurs. Furthermore, within these patterns, many additional variations may be noted (e.g., presence of melanin pigment, squamous metaplasia, stromal fibrosis). The main patterns include the following.

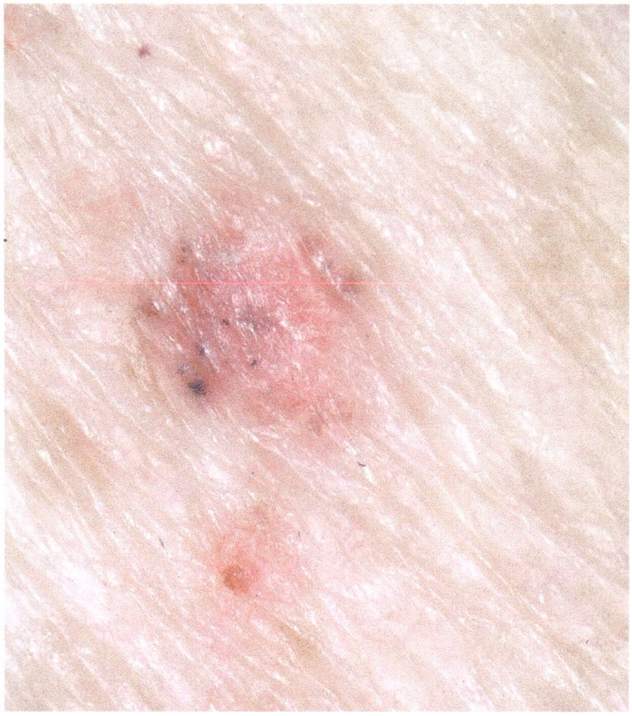

FIG. 12.22

Pigmented basal cell carcinoma. A plaque is present with erythema and brown pigmentation.

BASAL CELL CARCINOMA—PATHOLOGIC FEATURES

Major Diagnostic Criteria

- Basaloid cells with elongated hyperchromatic nuclei and scant cytoplasm
- Peripheral palisading
- Clefts between tumor and surrounding stroma
- Mucinous alteration of the surrounding stroma

Immunophenotype

- Positive for Ber-EP4, 34BE12, MNF116
- Negative with Cam5.2
- Melan-A often demonstrates melanocytes within the tumor

Differential Diagnosis

- Trichoblastoma
- Merkel cell carcinoma
- Squamous cell carcinoma with basaloid features
- Sebaceous carcinoma
- Microcystic adnexal carcinoma/sclerosing sweat duct carcinoma

SUPERFICIAL PATTERN

The superficial pattern exhibits aggregates of basaloid tumor cells attached to the epidermis or adnexal structures (Fig. 12.24). Such basaloid nests are typically multifocal and separated from each other by intervening areas of normal epidermis (skip areas). Measurement of the depth of invasion (similar to Breslow thickness) helps predict response to topical imiquimod therapy, with lesions thinner than 0.4 mm not recurring.

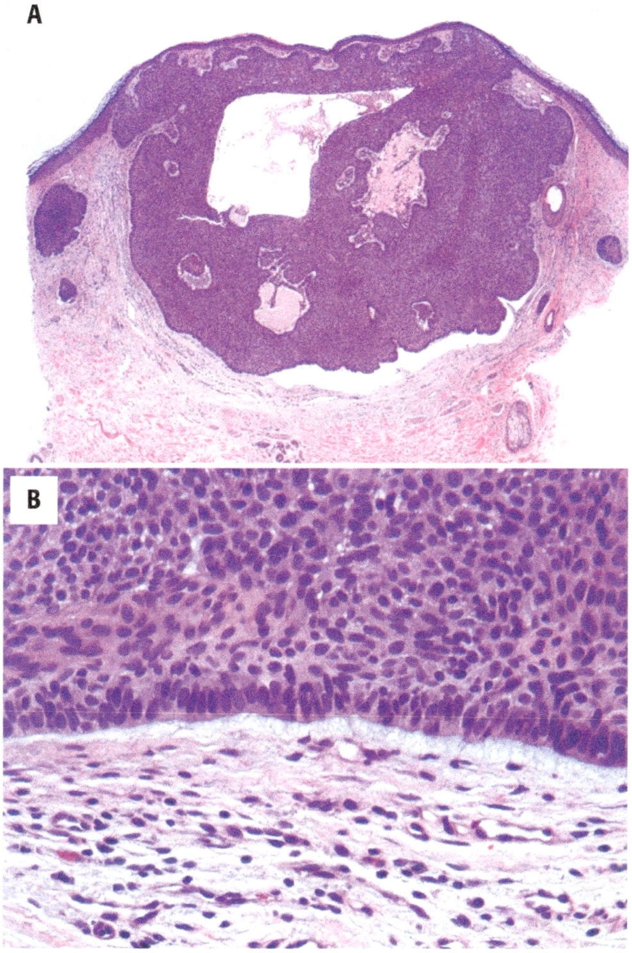

FIG. 12.23

Basal cell carcinoma. **A,** A nodular or nodulocystic tumor composed of basaloid cells is seen. **B,** At the periphery of the tumor nodule, basaloid cells form a picket fence or "palisading" arrangement. A cleft separates tumor from dermal stroma. The cleft is filled with mucinous material.

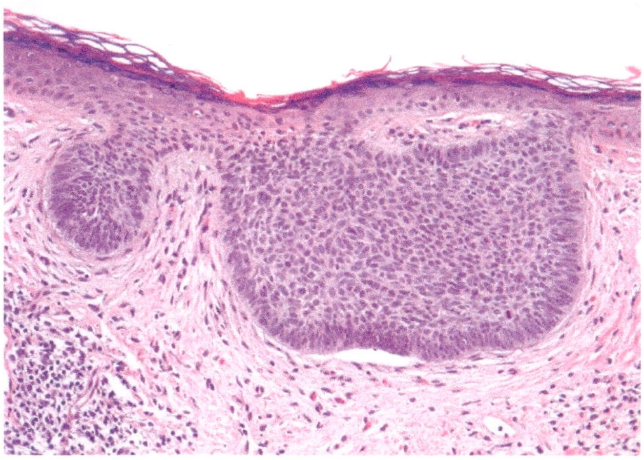

FIG. 12.24

Basal cell carcinoma, superficial pattern. Aggregates of basaloid tumor cells in the superficial dermis are connected to the epidermis. Typically, multiple such foci are present, separated from each other by "skip" areas of normal skin (in two-dimensional view).

NODULAR PATTERN

The nodular pattern exhibits nodular aggregates of tumor cells in the dermis, at least focally detached from the epidermis and involving the reticular dermis (Figs. 12.23 and 12.25). The nodules vary in size and shape. Some writers distinguish BCC with large dermal nodules from those with multiple small nodules (*micronodular pattern*) (Fig. 12.26). The actual size of these nests required to distinguish micronodular from nodular BCC is subjective. Some authors recommend considering micronodular lesions as those that have nests smaller than 0.5 mm in diameter; however, such a definition would include a majority of BCCs. We render a diagnosis of micronodular BCC when there are numerous similarly sized nests (occupying at least 25% of the base of the lesion) and these nests are smaller than a medium vessel (~0.2 mm).

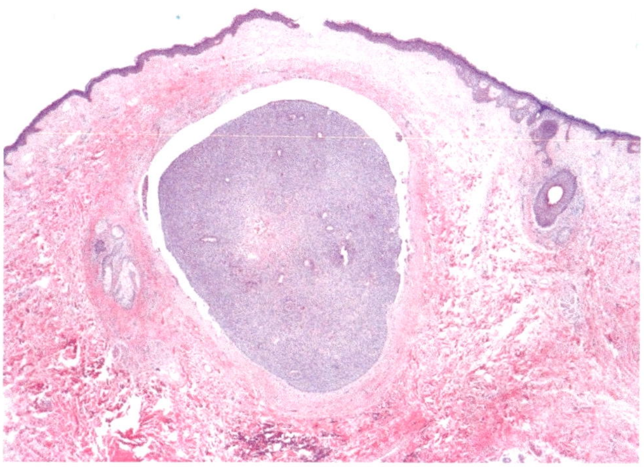

FIG. 12.25

Basal cell carcinoma, nodular pattern. A solid tumor nodule is present in the dermis.

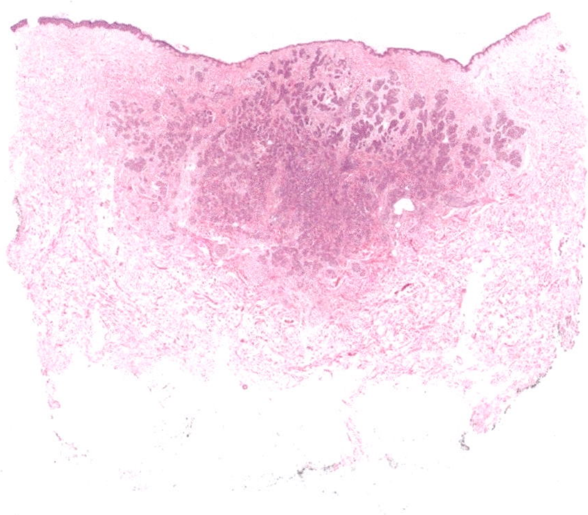

FIG. 12.26

Basal cell carcinoma, micronodular pattern. The tumor is composed of multiple small nodular aggregates of basaloid cells.

MORPHEAFORM AND INFILTRATIVE PATTERN

Although nodular BCCs are invasive carcinomas by definition, the term *infiltrative* is generally applied to a BCC with less or none of a solid nodular growth pattern, and composed predominantly of small, often irregularly shaped, cell aggregates, narrow strands of cells, multiple micronodules, or even single cells in the stroma. The haphazard distribution of such small tumor cell aggregates together with ill-defined interfaces with the surrounding stroma gives the tumor its infiltrative silhouette (Fig. 12.27). Not all infiltrative BCCs are morpheaform, which is associated with marked stromal fibrosis. We reserve the terms *morpheaform, sclerodermoid*, and *sclerosing* for BCCs that are associated with prominent fibrosis (Fig. 12.28). In this variant of BCC, the tumor cell aggregates are usually compressed into very narrow cords. Large solid nodules are usually absent or rare.

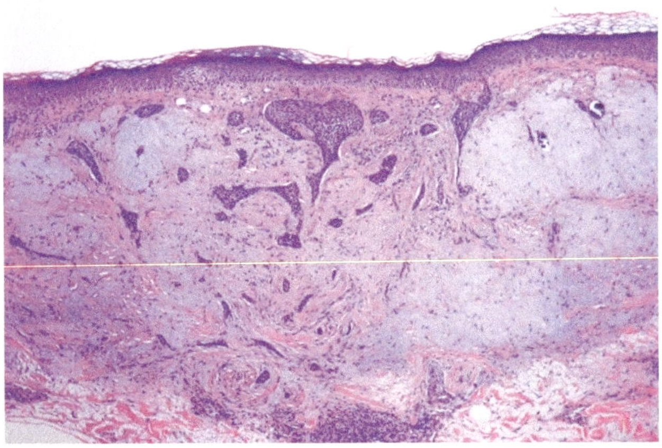

FIG. 12.27

Basal cell carcinoma, infiltrative pattern. Thin cords and oddly shaped aggregates of tumor cells are dispersed in a haphazard infiltrative pattern.

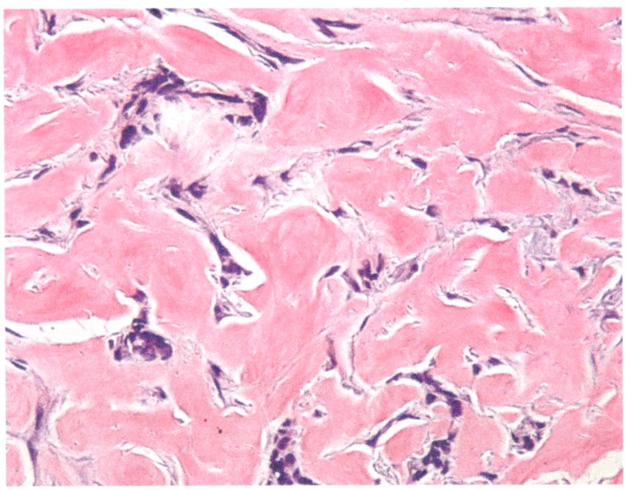

FIG. 12.28

Morpheaform basal cell carcinoma (BCC). This BCC shows an infiltrative growth pattern. Basaloid cords and strands are set in a densely fibrotic stroma.

FIBROEPITHELIOMATOUS PATTERN

The fibroepitheliomatous pattern is included here under BCC, bearing in mind that in its pure form it is most likely a variant of TBL. However, it can co-exist with more typical features of BCC. It is best reported as fibroepithelioma of Pinkus and conveyed to the clinician that this is usually an indolent neoplasm. Histopathologically it is characterized by cords and columns of basaloid cells with a fenestrated growth pattern associated with prominent fibroplasia (Fig. 12.29).

INFUNDIBULOCYSTIC BASAL CELL CARCINOMA

Infundibulocystic (aka *hamartomatous*) BCC is usually a small indolent lesion characterized by the presence of small keratocysts and bland basaloid cells, often arranged in small cords or a racemiform growth pattern (Fig. 12.30). This lesion has features intermediate between BCC and TBL, including immunohistochemical findings such as CD34 expression by the peritumoral stromal cells. It may be associated with conventional BCC (Fig. 12.30B). Multiple lesions of infundibulocystic BCC are frequent in patients with nevoid BCC (Gorlin's) syndrome.

Miscellaneous additional phenotypic variations of BCC exist, such as the following.

ADENOIDAL BASAL CELL CARCINOMA

BCCs may show a cribriform or pseudoglandular architecture (usually with an overall nodular growth pattern) associated with mucinous stroma, simulating adenoid cystic carcinoma (Fig. 12.31).

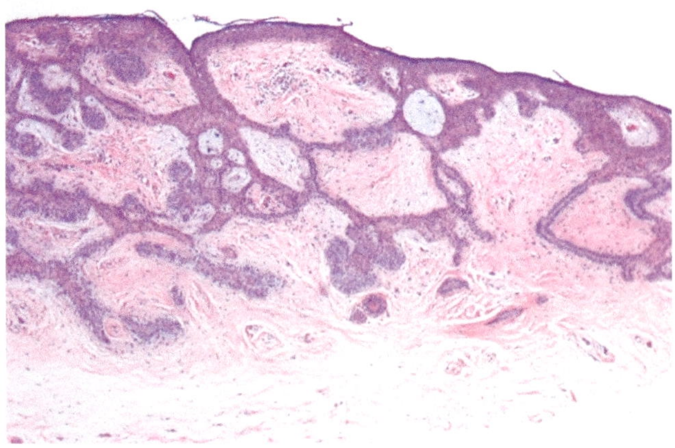

FIG. 12.29

Fibroepithelioma of Pinkus. Thin anastomosing cords of basaloid cells are present in association with a fibrous stroma.

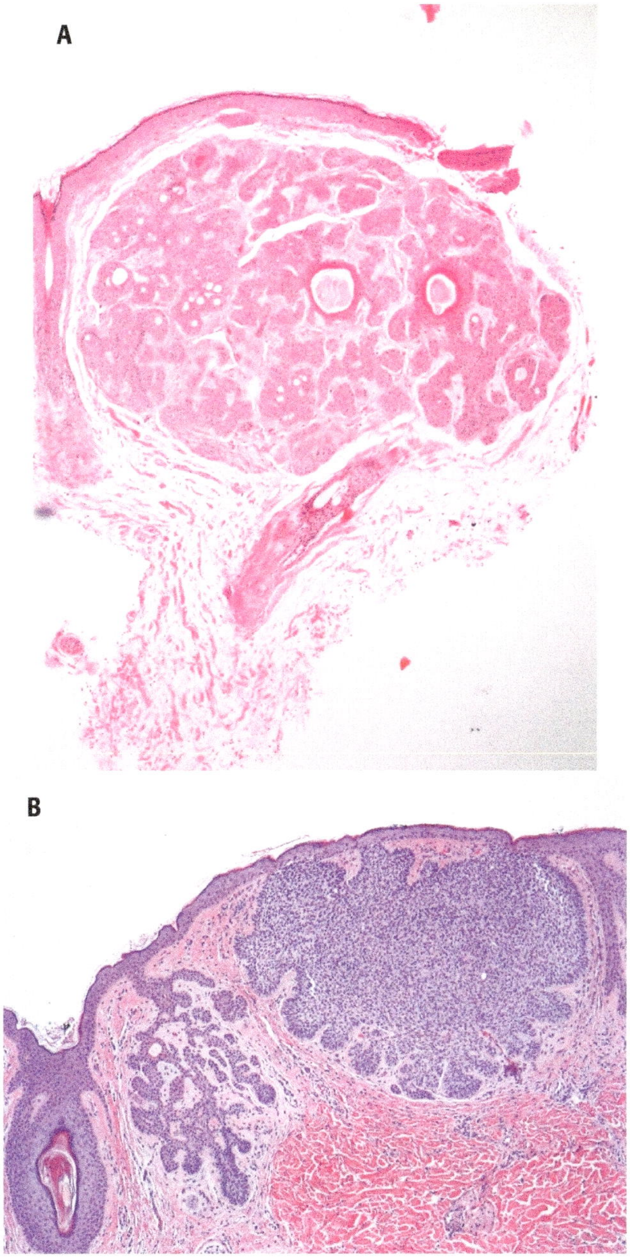

FIG. 12.30

Infundibulocystic basal cell carcinoma (BCC). **A,** A small nodule of cytologically bland basaloid cells is present with small keratocysts. **B,** A small hamartomatoid BCC component adjacent to a conventional BCC.

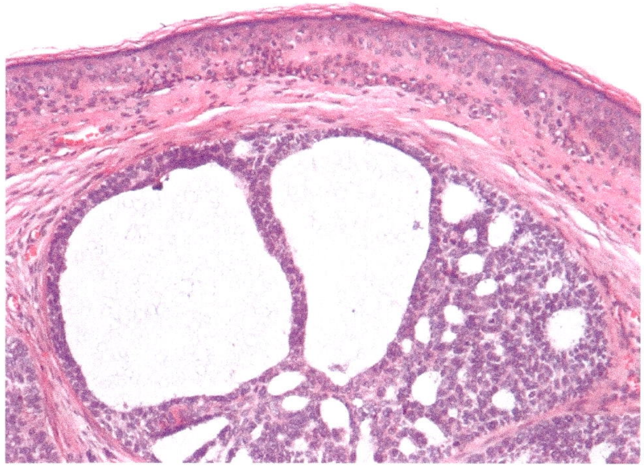

FIG. 12.31

Basal cell carcinoma with adenoidal features. Within the tumor nodule, a cribriform architecture is apparent.

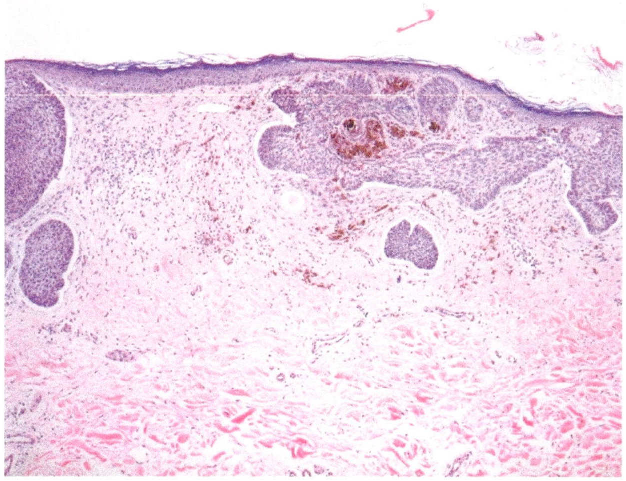

FIG. 12.32

Pigmented basal cell carcinoma. Melanin pigment is present in tumor cells as well as in macrophages.

PIGMENTED BASAL CELL CARCINOMA

Any pattern of BCC (most often superficial BCCs and nodular BCCs) can be pigmented. The histopathologic correlate of a clinically dark brown nodule is usually the presence of melanophages in the stroma (Fig. 12.32). However, melanin pigment may also be present in the carcinoma cells. On occasion, dendritic melanocytes are present within the tumor compartment. Collisions of BCC and melanocytic proliferations (most often nevi, at times melanoma, usually of lentigo maligna melanoma in situ type) may clinically simulate pigmented BCC.

BASAL CELL CARCINOMA WITH SQUAMOUS DIFFERENTIATION

At times, a BCC may show squamous differentiation, especially superficially underneath an ulcer. Squamous differentiation may also occur in deeper, infiltrative parts of the tumor, especially in recurrent tumors. BCCs with squamous differentiation are sometimes designated metatypical BCCs (Fig. 12.33). In a partial tissue sample, a squamatized BCC may be indistinguishable from SCC.

CLEAR-CELL BASAL CELL CARCINOMA

This BCC is characterized by the presence of tumor cells with glycogen-rich, clear cytoplasm (Fig. 12.34A).

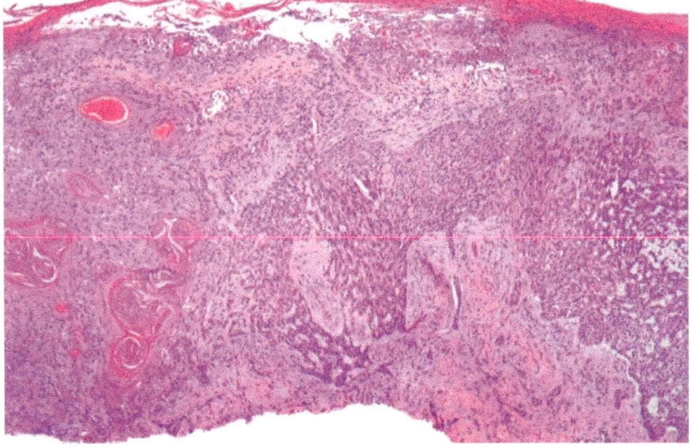

FIG. 12.33

Basal cell carcinoma with squamous differentiation (metatypical basal cell carcinoma). Parts of the tumor cell population have a pinker cytoplasm and are keratinizing.

GRANULAR-CELL BASAL CELL CARCINOMA

This BCC appears pink histopathologically because the tumor cells contain abundant, granular, eosinophilic cytoplasm (Fig. 12.34B and C). Because of its pink appearance, it may be confused with SCC. Ancillary studies, such as Berep4 and CD68 or NKI/C3, help to establish the correct diagnosis.

BASAL CELL CARCINOMA WITH ECCRINE DIFFERENTIATION

BCCs with focal eccrine duct formation are rare. More often, one can observe preexisting sweat ducts, which may be dilated, engulfed by BCC (Fig. 12.35). BCC with eccrine differentiation may have an aggressive behavior with distant metastases.

BASAL CELL CARCINOMA WITH SEBACEOUS DIFFERENTIATION

Sebocytes may become entrapped in a BCC (BCC may grow into and populate a sebaceous lobule). This should not lead to a diagnosis of sebaceous carcinoma.

BASAL CELL CARCINOMA WITH MATRICAL DIFFERENTIATION

Occasionally, a tumor with features otherwise typical of BCC shows focal "ghost" cells similar to bona fide pilomatrix tumors (Fig. 12.36).

BASAL CELL CARCINOMA WITH NUCLEAR PLEOMORPHISM

Occasionally, BCC shows marked nuclear pleomorphism (Fig. 12.37). To date, there is no evidence that this is a clinically significant finding.

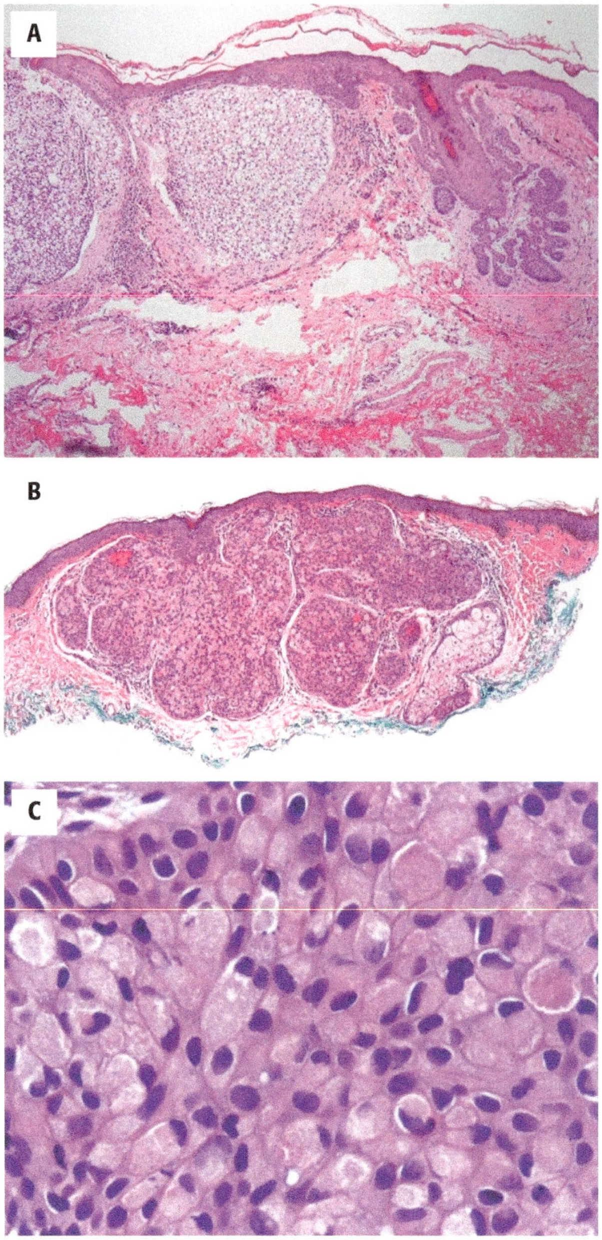

FIG. 12.34

Basal cell carcinoma (BCC) with clear-cell or granular cytoplasm. **A,** Part of this BCC shows a clear glycogenated cytoplasm. **B,** Granular cell variant of BCC with a pink appearance. **C,** The tumor cells have a granular cytoplasm.

COLLISION SCENARIOS

BCCs may collide with a number of epithelial and nonepithelial tumors. Common associations include BCC with SK (Fig. 12.38) and BCC with melanocytic nevus (Fig. 12.39).

BIPHENOTYPIC TUMORS

Rarely, a tumor may show features of both BCC and sarcoma (Fig. 12.40). Such tumors tend to be large and

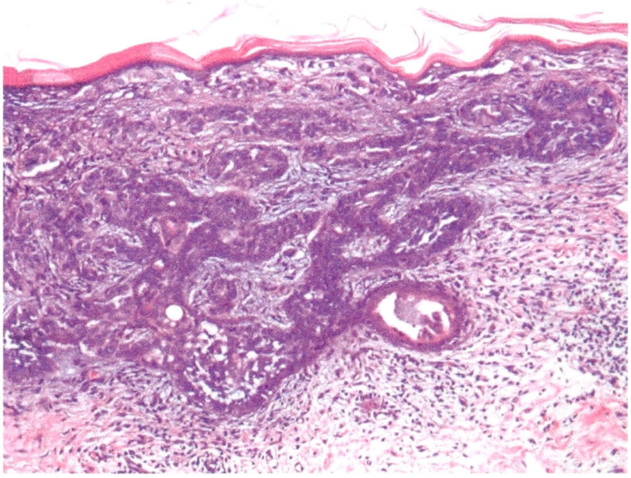

FIG. 12.35

Basal cell carcinoma (BCC) engulfing an eccrine duct. BCCs may contain ductal structures. Usually, as in this case, they are engulfed by the tumor, but occasionally, the tumor may show ductal differentiation.

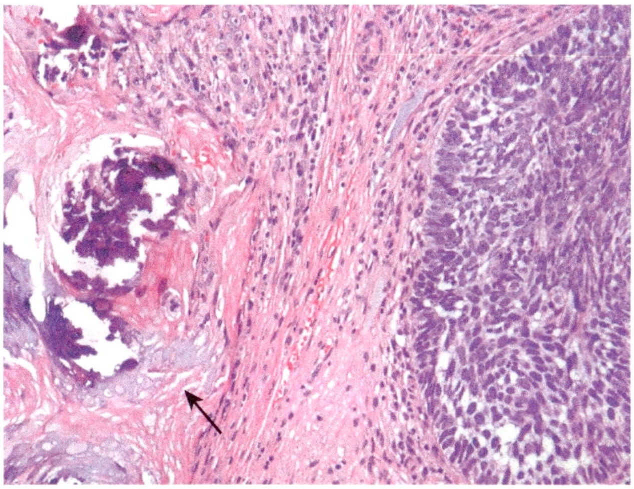

FIG. 12.36

Basal cell carcinoma (BCC) with matrical differentiation. A nodular BCC shows a focus of shadow cells *(arrow)*.

more aggressive. These tumors have been designated as carcinosarcoma, sarcomatoid BCC, or high-grade trichoblastic carcinosarcoma.

Ancillary Studies

Immunohistochemistry may on occasion be helpful for the distinction of BCC from its histopathologic mimics. BCC is usually immunoreactive for the following epithelial markers: 34BE12, MNF116, and Ber-EP4. They are usually negative with Cam5.2, epithelial membrane antigen (EMA), and CK7. Some BCCs are positive for chromogranin or synaptophysin.

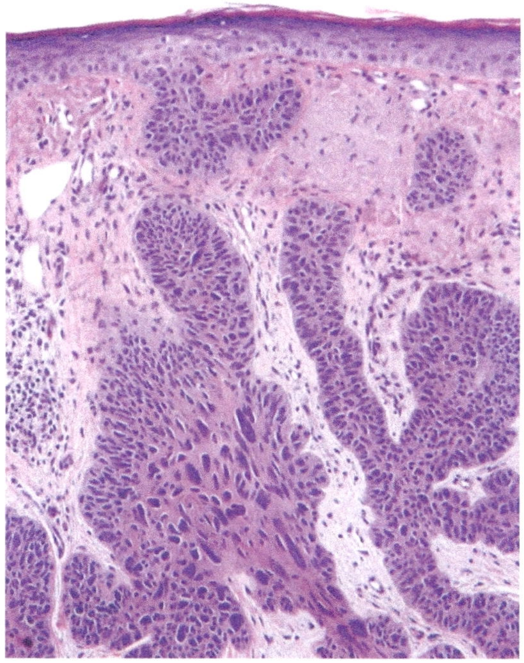

FIG. 12.37

Basal cell carcinoma (BCC) with pleomorphic features. This BCC contains tumor cells showing a greater degree of nuclear pleomorphism than usual.

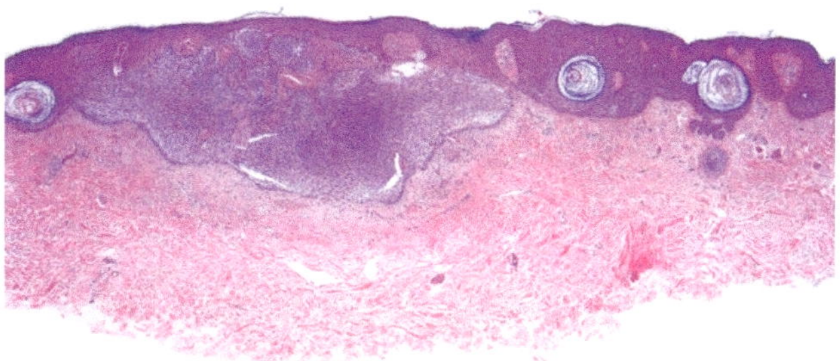

FIG. 12.38

Collision of a basal cell carcinoma and seborrheic keratosis.

Differential Diagnosis

The histopathologic diagnosis of BCC is usually straightforward. However, problems can arise from overlap with other basaloid epithelial neoplasms and from insufficient pathologic sampling.

BASAL CELL CARCINOMA VERSUS TRICHOBLASTOMA AND TRICHOEPITHELIOMA

In the differential diagnosis of BCC from TBL or desmoplastic TE, features that favor BCC include the lack of papillary mesenchymal bodies, presence of clefts

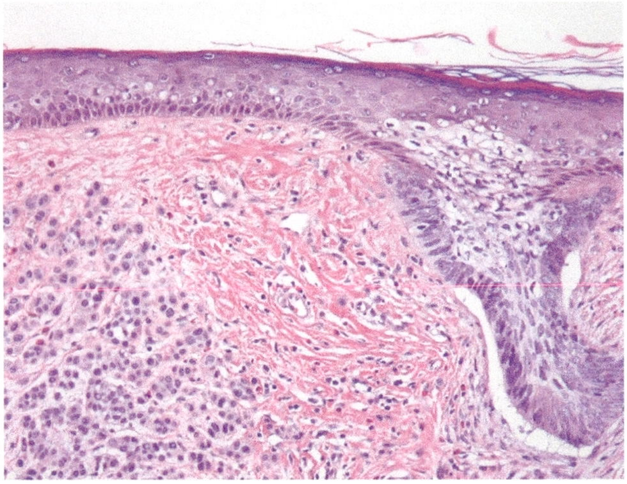

FIG. 12.39

Collision of a basal cell carcinoma with a melanocytic nevus.

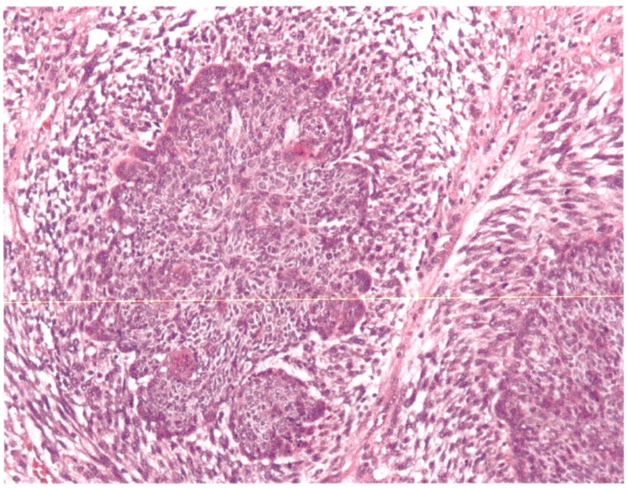

FIG. 12.40

Basal cell carcinosarcoma (sarcomatoid basal cell carcinoma [BCC]) is a biphenotypic tumor with an epithelial component in the appearance of a BCC and an associated malignant spindle cell component with mesenchymal features.

between tumor and immediately surrounding stroma, cytologic atypia, readily identifiable mitotic figures, and mucinous stroma (see also TBL and desmoplastic TE).

BASAL CELL CARCINOMA VERSUS SQUAMOUS CELL CARCINOMA

BCCs with squamous metaplasia may be difficult to distinguish from SCC, especially in a superficial shave biopsy specimen in which the squamous component predominates. At times, the BCC may only be fully diagnosable when more of the tumor is sampled and characteristic areas of BCC are identified. Likewise, biopsy of the deep portion of a recurrent BCC may reveal features of SCC. In these cases, the diagnosis of BCC rests on identification of areas of usual BCC in the same or prior biopsy. If an initial superficial biopsy does not permit reliable distinction between a squamatized BCC and SCC, it is best to acknowledge this uncertainty and defer final classification pending study of the excision specimen.

On occasion, collision tumors (BCC and SCC at the same site) or biphasic tumors ("true" basosquamous carcinomas) may occur that show veritable features of both BCC and SCC within the same tumor nodule. Biphenotypic carcinomas usually have a predominant basal-cell appearance on the initial biopsy but, with subsequent recurrences, the squamous component tends to dominate and dictate the clinical behavior.

BASAL CELL CARCINOMA VERSUS ADENOID CYSTIC CARCINOMA

BCCs with solid infiltrative or adenoidal patterns may be confused with adenoid cystic or basaloid sweat gland carcinoma. Identification of true tubule formation and attention to the overall growth pattern or immunohistochemistry are helpful. In contrast to BCC, adenoid cystic carcinomas are composed of both epithelial (CK7) and myoepithelial elements (p63, SOX10). Unlike BCC, they usually also express CD117 and MYB.

BASAL CELL CARCINOMA VERSUS MICROCYSTIC ADNEXAL CARCINOMA

Morpheaform BCC may be confused with a sclerosing basaloid proliferation of MAC. Sclerosing BCC tends to lack the keratocysts or small luminal structures within basaloid cells often seen in MAC and usually shows a higher degree of cytologic atypia.

BASAL CELL CARCINOMA VERSUS MERKEL CELL CARCINOMA

The most problematic diagnostic pitfall is the failure to recognize Merkel cell carcinoma (MCC), which may simulate the BCC both clinically and histopathologically. Attention to cytologic detail should allow for a distinction. The tumor cells of MCC show a salt-and-pepper chromatin pattern and many more mitotic figures and apoptotic bodies than BCCs. Moreover, MCC usually lacks the palisading arrangement of BCC. In difficult cases, immunohistochemistry for CK20 (positive in MCC; negative in BCC) allows for definitive diagnosis. Staining for chromogranin or synaptophysin is not as helpful, as a subset of BCCs shows focal expression of these neuroendocrine markers.

BASAL CELL CARCINOMA VERSUS "NO TUMOR SEEN"

Frequently, initial histologic sections of a clinically suspected BCC fail to reveal tumor cells. However, certain clues should prompt the pathologist to order deeper levels, which frequently reveal foci of tumor. In general, deeper levels are a prudent course of action if no histopathologic finding is identified that could explain the clinical lesion (usually that of a papule), such as a dermal melanocytic nevus, folliculitis, sebaceous hyperplasia, or fibrous papule. Clues to the possible presence of adjacent BCC include inflammation and fibrosis as well as "pseudocysts" (empty spaces from which tumor cells seemingly may have fallen out, a phenomenon also referred to as "stroma interrupted").

Prognosis and Treatment

BCC usually grows slowly. Some variants, such as infundibulocystic BCC, tend to be very indolent, with limited potential for tissue destruction over many years. Other so-called aggressive variants, which include infiltrating, morpheaform, and micronodular BCCs, may cause severe local tissue destruction.

Based on several clinical and pathologic features, patients with BCCs are often classified into low- and high-risk categories.

The vast majority of superficial and nodular circumscribed BCCs are curable by narrow excision, with no need for wide margins. For early, superficial lesions, local destructive modalities, such as cryotherapy, may be adequate. For facial lesions, surgery with frozen-section examination is the treatment of choice. Postoperative or intraoperative complete circumferential peripheral and deep margin assessment with frozen or permanent sections is critical for large and infiltrative lesions. Radiation therapy is also an option for patients who are reluctant or unable to undergo surgery or in the case of positive margins or extensive perineural invasion.

In very rare cases, usually after repeated local recurrences, large and deeply infiltrative BCCs may metastasize to lymph nodes or distant sites, such as the lung, and become lethal.

PATHOLOGIST'S REPORTING OF BASAL CELL CARCINOMA

The essential task for the pathologist is to diagnose the presence or absence of BCC in a biopsy specimen. Some clinicians may request subtyping of BCC. Knowledge of the subtype may be helpful, for example, for a Mohs surgeon to have a visual image of what to expect on frozen sections, especially if the slides of the prior biopsy are not readily available. On shave or saucerization excisions, it is also helpful to comment on the margin status. Otherwise, patients with a small BCC may undergo unnecessary subsequent excisions for tumors that had already been completely removed by the initial biopsy.

For an excision of a large BCC, in addition to the diagnosis and margin status, it also seems prudent to report the size of the lesion; to indicate which anatomic levels are involved (dermis only, subcutis, muscle, or bone); and to document the histopathologic pattern(s), the presence of perineural invasion, including caliber and location of the largest involved nerve, or the presence of squamous differentiation.

PILOMATRIX CARCINOMA

Clinical Findings

Pilomatrix carcinoma is a rare tumor of middle-aged and elderly individuals. The head and neck area or extremities are most often affected. The tumors may present as papules or nodules. They may be larger than 5 cm and are commonly ulcerated.

Histopathologic Features

The silhouette is asymmetric and infiltrative, with an overall lobular growth pattern. The tumors are composed of two major cell types: (1) basaloid cells with matrical features, arranged in lobules and sheets or cords and bands and (2) "ghost" or "shadow" cells as seen in pilomatricoma. Foci of necrosis are usually present (Fig. 12.41). Mitotic figures among basaloid cells are easily identified and may be numerous (areas with up to 10 mitotic figures per high-power field are not uncommon). The degree of nuclear atypia is variable. Some pilomatrix carcinomas show areas histopathologically indistinguishable from SCC.

Ancillary Studies

Pilomatrix tumors contain β-catenin mutations and show a distinct cytoplasmic and nuclear labeling of tumor cells (Fig. 12.42) in contrast to the membranous labeling of normal epidermis or SCCs.

Differential Diagnosis

Pilomatrix carcinoma differs from pilomatricoma primarily by its infiltrative growth pattern and the presence of cytologic atypia. Furthermore, pilomatrix carcinomas tend to be larger and are more likely to have necrosis and features of squamous metaplasia, simulating the appearance of SCC.

BCC, which may show focal matrical differentiation, differs from pilomatrix carcinoma (and pilomatricoma) by the presence of usual features of BCC, such as palisading nuclear arrangement, stromal mucin, clefts, or connections to the epidermis or nonneoplastic follicular structures.

SCC is best distinguished from pilomatrix carcinoma by the presence of a precursor lesion (SCC in situ), connection of invasive keratinizing tumor to the epidermis, and lack of ghost cells.

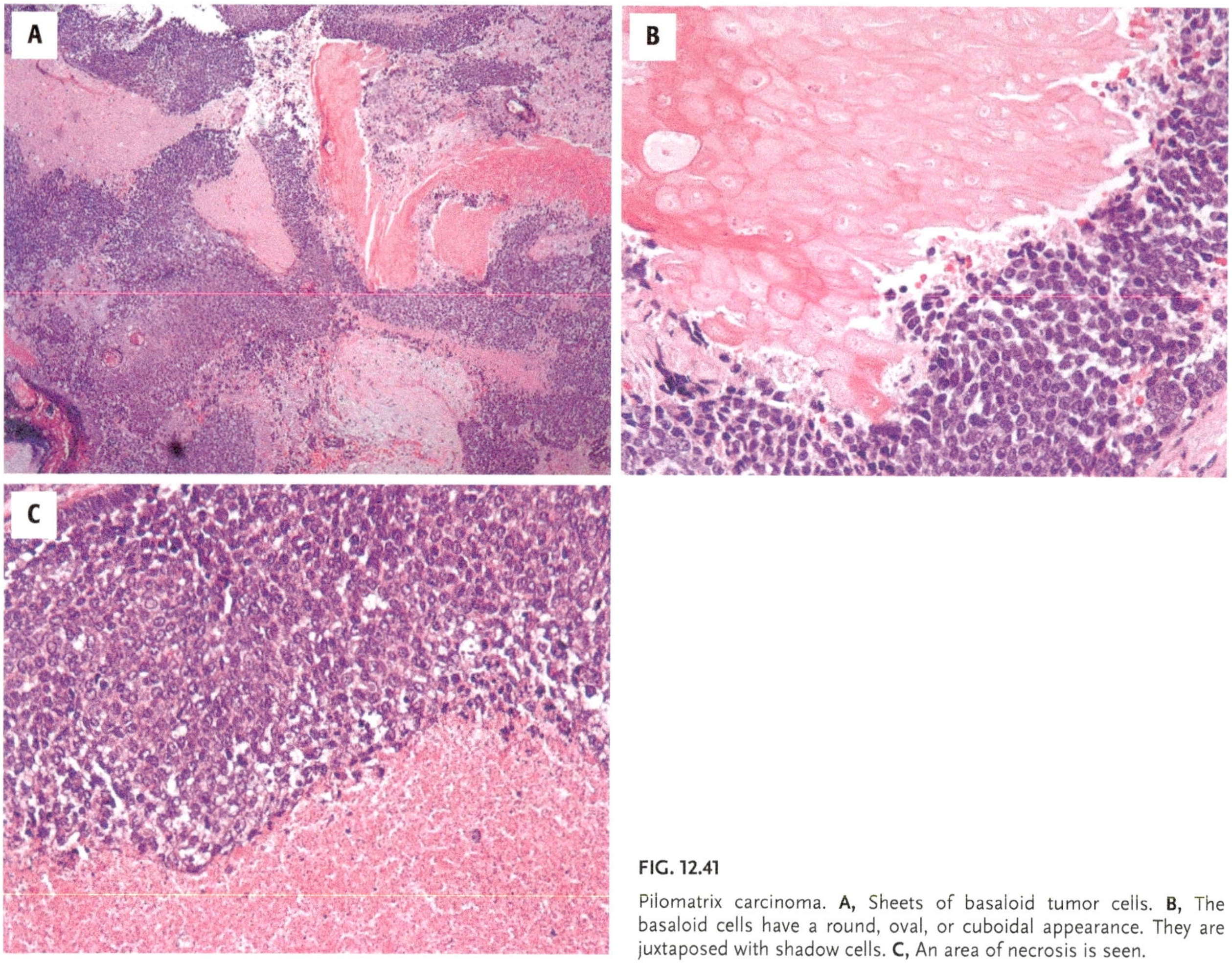

FIG. 12.41

Pilomatrix carcinoma. **A,** Sheets of basaloid tumor cells. **B,** The basaloid cells have a round, oval, or cuboidal appearance. They are juxtaposed with shadow cells. **C,** An area of necrosis is seen.

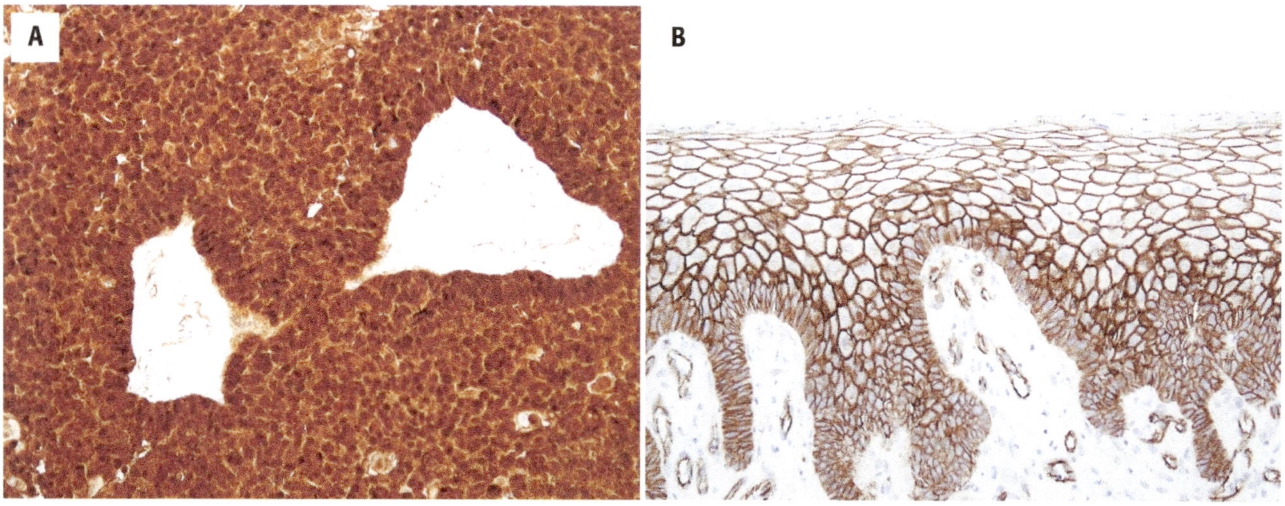

FIG. 12.42

A, Nuclear and cytoplasmic staining for β-catenin in pilomatrix carcinoma. **B,** Normal epidermis shows a membranous staining pattern.

Differential Diagnosis of Pilomatrix Tumors

	Pilomatricoma	Proliferating Pilomatricoma	Pilomatrix Carcinoma
CLINICAL FINDINGS			
Gender	F > M	F > M	M > F
Location	Head and neck, extremities	Head and neck	Head and neck, trunk, extremities
Size	Small (0.5–3 cm)	Medium (1–5 cm)	From 0.5 to >20 cm
HISTOLOGIC FEATURES			
Ulceration	Rare	Rare	Common
Growth pattern	Nodular	Nodular	Infiltrative
Shadow cells	Present	Present	Present
Basaloid cells	Variable	Prominent	Prominent
Atypia	None or mild	None or mild	Present
Squamous metaplasia	Rare	Rare	Common
Necrosis	Rare	Rare	Common
Mitotic figures	Present in basaloid cells	Present in basaloid cells	Present in basaloid and squamatized cells
Prognosis	Rare local persistence	Rare local recurrence	Frequent local recurrence Rare distant metastasis

F, Female; *M*, male.

Prognosis and Treatment

Pilomatrix carcinomas are slowly growing, locally aggressive tumors. They are usually curable by excision, but rare tumors metastasize to lymph nodes and visceral sites. There are too few published cases to establish prognostic parameters.

TRICHILEMMAL CARCINOMA

Trichilemmal carcinoma is rare, and an insufficient number of bona fide cases have been reported to allow a clear description of associated clinical and histopathologic features. Reported cases suggest a spectrum of papules and plaques clinically overlapping with basal cell and SCC. Trichilemmal carcinomas appear as infiltrative dermal tumors with outer root sheath differentiation, typically showing a clear, glycogen-rich cytoplasm. However, the presence of a clear cytoplasm is not distinctive because it can occur in several other neoplasms. For a superficial dermal, clear-cell carcinoma to be convincingly acceptable as a trichilemmal carcinoma, the tumor must either be associated with a benign precursor (trichilemmoma) or show continuity with the outer sheath epithelium of a coexisting hair follicle, with minimal or no intraepidermal extension. Otherwise, it is difficult and frankly arbitrary to distinguish a trichilemmal carcinoma from a clear-cell variant of squamous cell or BCC. Additional features suggestive of trichilemmal carcinoma include peripheral cell palisading and trichilemmal keratinization (i.e., absent or minimal granular cell layer, presence of dense keratin material). It is currently unknown whether the distinction of trichilemmal carcinoma from a clear-cell variant of SCC (which may colonize a hair follicle) is relevant for patient outcome.

NEOPLASMS WITH APOCRINE OR ECCRINE DIFFERENTIATION

Proliferations of the apocrine or eccrine gland apparatus exhibit ducts, that is, lumina lined by epithelial cells. The pathologist can confidently designate a glandular or ductal proliferation as apocrine if it exhibits the classic apocrine feature picturesquely described as epithelial snouting or decapitation secretion, or another manifestation of apocrine differentiation, such as the presence of plasmacytoid epithelial cells or mucin. However, lack of such features does not exclude apocrine differentiation. Because it is often difficult or impossible to distinguish apocrine from eccrine neoplasms histopathologically, and because this feature has no or little clinical relevance in the management of tumors, we place no emphasis on it in our presentation of glandular and ductal proliferations.

The main challenge is to distinguish benign adenomas from carcinomas. Most adenomas are well circumscribed and, if ducts are present, contain both an inner epithelial and outer myoepithelial cell layer. The latter can be highlighted by immunohistochemistry for p63 at times and also for SOX10 and SMA. Sweat gland carcinomas are usually infiltrative and display nuclear pleomorphism. However, there are exceptions. Some low-grade carcinomas (e.g., microcystic adnexal carcinoma, low-grade hidradenocarcinoma) may lack marked atypia and can only be recognized by a sufficiently large enough tissue sample to document infiltrative growth. Furthermore, some tumors may both be circumscribed and relatively bland, such as an adenoma-like digital papillary adenocarcinoma. While for tumors with ductal differentiation, the lack of a myoepithelial cell layer (immunohistochemically documented loss of p63) can be a clue to support the diagnosis of invasive carcinoma; some sweat gland carcinomas maintain myoepithelial cells throughout the invasive primary tumor and also in metastases, such as adenoid cystic carcinoma or digital papillary adenocarcinoma. Thus, while there are general guidelines for the distinction of adenomas from carcinomas, specific criteria for malignancy depend on the context of findings.

Significant insight has been gained over the past decade into molecular aberrations associated with sweat gland tumors. Some carry mutations. Other tumors have been found to harbor gene fusion. The detection of these aberrations by molecular methods (fluorescence in situ hybridization [FISH] or sequence analysis) or via the use of immunohistochemical surrogate markers can be useful for diagnostically challenging cases to distinguish one tumor type from a histopathologic mimicker. However, within certain lines of differentiation (e.g., poroid neoplasms), there is usually overlap in gene fusions between benign tumors and carcinomas, which is why other parameters, most importantly histopathologic findings, are needed to distinguish a benign from a malignant tumor.

Gene Fusions in Sweat Gland Tumors

Tumor Type	Gene Fusion	Frequency[1]
Poroma	*YAP1 fusions*	90%
	NUTM1 fusions	20%–80%
	WWTR1::NUTM1	Rare
Porocarcinoma	*YAP1::NUTM1*	60%
	YAP1::MAML2	8%
	YAP1::MAML3	Rare
Hidradenoma	*CRTC1::MAML2*	50%–75%
	CRTC3::MAML2	Rare
Hidradenocarcinoma	*CRCT1::MAML2*	Unknown
Mixed tumor	*PLAG1 fusions*	30%
	HMGA2 fusions	Unknown
Adenoid cystic carcinoma	*MYB::NFIB*	70%–80%
	MYBL1::NFIB	20%
Myoepithelioma	*EWSR1 fusion*	80%
	FUS fusion	20%
Secretory carcinoma	*ETV6::NTRK3*	>95%
	NFIX::PKN1	Rare
BNAC#	*BRD3::NUTM2B*	Unknown

BNAC, BRD3-NUT-rearranged adnexal tumor.
[1]The numbers provided are based on relatively small series and may not be accurate as more cases will be published.

HAMARTOMA AND NEVUS

ECCRINE NEVUS

This rare lesion is characterized by a circumscribed area of hyperhidrosis. Histopathologically, these lesions have localized increased number and size of eccrine glands. The variant called eccrine angiomatous hamartoma has, in addition to the eccrine glands, adipose tissue, and small capillaries.

APOCRINE NEVUS

An apocrine nevus exhibits an increased number of apocrine glands. It rarely occurs as a solitary lesion but is most often found as a component of nevus sebaceus.

BENIGN NEOPLASMS

ADENOMA (SPECTRUM OF APOCRINE OR ECCRINE ADENOMAS, WITH TUBULAR, CRIBRIFORM, PAPILLARY, MIXED, OR NOT OTHERWISE SPECIFIED PATTERNS)

Clinical Findings

These are clinically indistinct tumors, typically presenting as flesh-colored papules or nodules. Some may arise in association with nevus sebaceus.

Histopathologic Features

These are benign tumors with glandular differentiation (presence of ducts, lumina) (Figs. 12.43–12.45). They tend

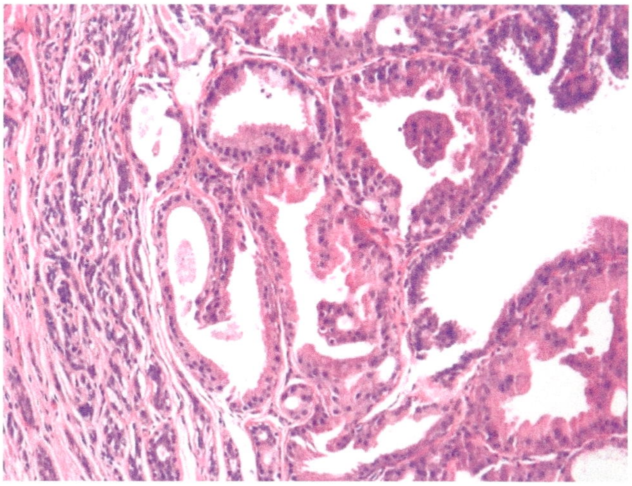

FIG. 12.43

Apocrine adenoma. The inner epithelial cells show abundant pink cytoplasm and apocrine-type secretion.

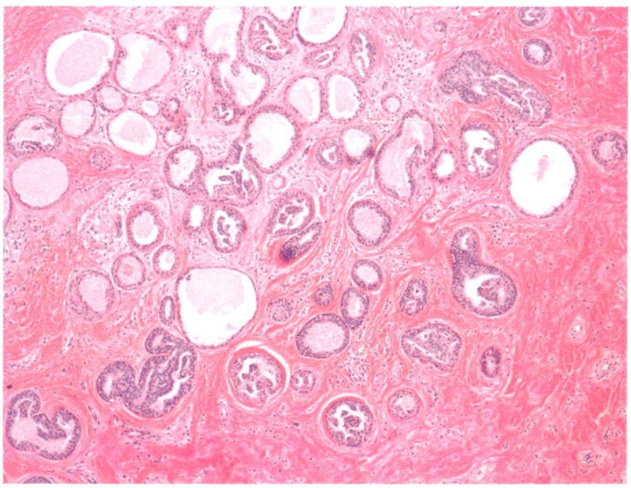

FIG. 12.44

Tubular and papillary adenoma. This adenoma shows a tubular and papillary pattern. The ductal structures are lined by two cell layers of inner duct epithelial and outer myoepithelial cells.

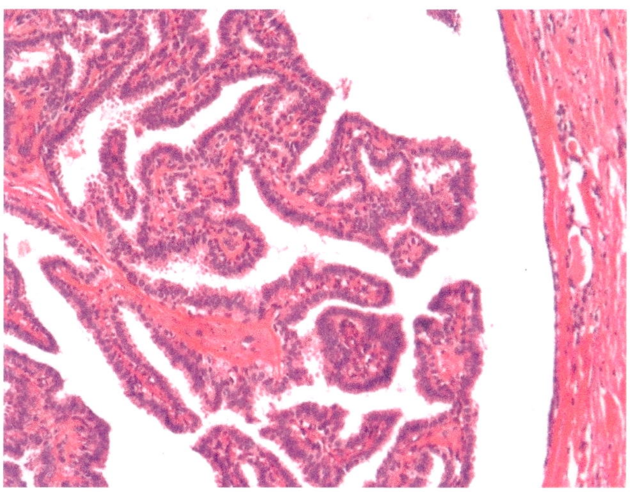

FIG. 12.45

Hidradenoma papilliferum. Papillary epithelial projections with a fibrovascular core are seen in a cystic lumen.

to be centered in the dermis and are well circumscribed. They may show tubular, cribriform, papillary, micropapillary, or mixed growth patterns and annotated accordingly. The ductal lining is bilayered, with luminal cuboidal secretory cells and peripheral cuboidal or flat myoepithelial cells. The epithelial cells may be small or large, cuboidal or flat. The cytoplasm may range from dense pink to a clear-cell appearance. Focal squamous or mucinous metaplasia may occur. The stroma of adenomas has various degrees of fibrosis and hyalinization. Lumina may be cystically dilated and contain secretory fluid or debris.

Adenomas can be further classified based on the predominant growth pattern (e.g., tubular, cribriform, papillary, or tubulopapillary adenomas). Tubular and papillary adenomas tend to be associated with *BRAFV600E* mutations. Subclassification of adenomas into tubular versus papillary or other is not clinically relevant. The important issue is simply to recognize them as benign neoplasms and not to confuse them with primary or metastatic carcinomas. Some subtypes of sweat gland adenomas, however, have become established entities with distinct clinical features (e.g., hidradenoma papilliferum, nodulocystic hidradenoma). They are worth discussing in further detail.

Differential Diagnosis

The important issue is to distinguish adenomas (circumscribed lesions) from well-differentiated adenocarcinomas. In the majority of cases, this distinction is straightforward because tubular and papillary adenomas tend to be relatively small and circumscribed, maintain a dual cell layer of epithelial and myoepithelial cells, and are cytologically relatively bland. Must ductal carcinomas are large, infiltrative, show nuclear pleomorphism and mitoses, and not uncommonly foci of necrosis. However, in some instances, such as digital papillary adenocarcinoma, a well-differentiated carcinoma may closely simulate an adenoma and maintain a dual epithelial and myoepithelial cell layer.

HIDRADENOMA PAPILLIFERUM

Clinical Findings

This lesion presents typically in the vulva and perianal region as a solitary papule or small nodule but may occur anywhere, especially along the "milk line."

Histopathologic Features

Hidradenoma papilliferum is a well-circumscribed dermal nodule composed of both solid and cystic regions.

The hallmark of this lesion is its papillary architecture, with a layer of luminal secretory cells surrounded by myoepithelial cells (Fig. 12.45). Occasionally, there are large cuboidal cells identical to those seen in apocrine metaplasia of mammary glands. Because identical lesions can occur in other anatomic locations, an alternative name for all of these lesions may be papillary apocrine adenoma.

Differential Diagnosis

In contrast with syringocystadenoma papilliferum, hidradenoma papilliferum does not show prominent plasma cell infiltrates.

HIDRADENOMA

Clinical Findings

Hidradenomas are solitary, skin-colored, or reddish papules or nodules (Fig. 12.46). They may be large, measuring up to 2 cm or more in diameter. They can occur at any anatomic location and any age.

Histopathologic Features

The tumor usually shows a predominantly solid nodular growth pattern (nodular hidradenoma) and often also a cystic pattern (nodulocystic hidradenoma) (Figs. 12.47–12.49). It is usually centered in the dermis and well-circumscribed, but large tumors may involve the subcutis. It is composed of lobules of uniform eosinophilic or clear, glycogen-rich cells. Ducts can be present throughout the lesion, some of them dilated and forming cystic areas filled with eosinophilic secretion.

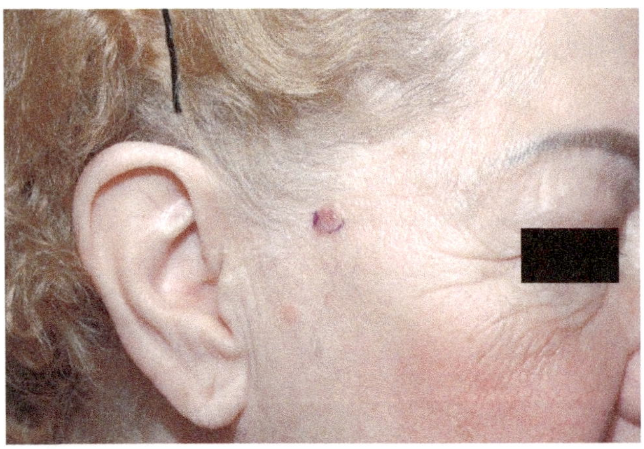

FIG. 12.46

Nodular hidradenoma. An erythematous nodular growth pattern is present.

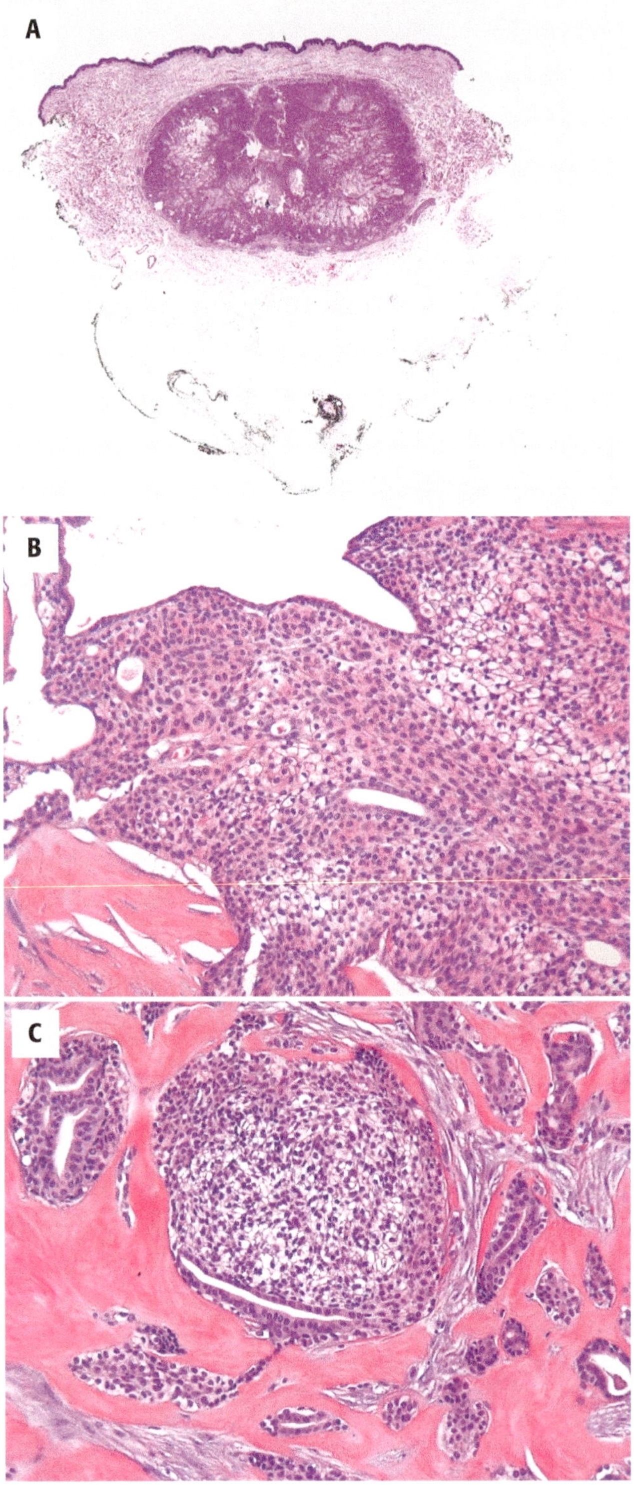

FIG. 12.47

Hidradenoma. **A,** Circumscribed dermal nodule. **B,** Cytologically bland epithelioid cells with eosinophilic or clear cytoplasm and associated ducts. **C,** Hyalinized fibrotic stroma within a hidradenoma.

The tubular lumina and cystic spaces are lined by cuboidal ductal cells or by columnar secretory cells. Nuclei are regular and slightly hyperchromatic. Mitotic figures are rare. Some areas may show squamous differentiation (keratin pearls). The stroma is fibrous and may show extensive hyalinization.

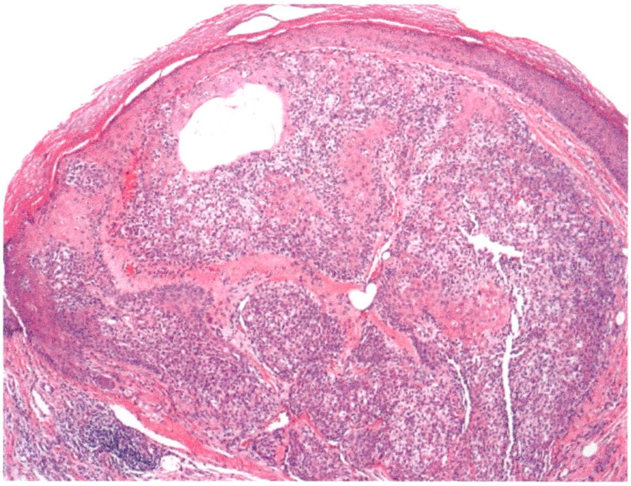

FIG. 12.48

Hidradenoma. Superficial dermal nodulocystic tumor with connections to the epidermis, clear-cell features, and squamous metaplasia.

Ancillary Studies

Ancillary studies are rarely needed for diagnosis, but immunostudies may be helpful on occasion to highlight glands when glands are sparse, which helps in the distinction of hidradenoma from other clear-cell tumors, such as trichilemmoma or renal cell carcinoma. Distinction of pauciglandular solid hidradenomas from myoepitheliomas and hidradenomas typically shows a mixture of CK7- or Cam5.2-positive epithelial as well as a subpopulation of calponin or smooth muscle actin (SMA)-positive myoepithelial cells. Immunostudies for CEA or BR-2 usually highlight ducts.

Hidradenomas have a chromosomal translocation t(11;19) associated with *CRTC1::MAML2* or *CRTC3::MAML2* gene fusions. MAML2 gene fusions are not specific for hidradenomas. They also occur in salivary gland tumors, such as mucoepidermoid carcinoma and Warthin tumor.

Differential Diagnosis

Hidradenoma must be distinguished from other benign adnexal tumors as well as hidradenocarcinoma and metastatic renal cell carcinoma. Hidradenoma may be confused with trichilemmoma or myoepithelioma

IMMUNOPHENOTYPE OF SWEAT GLAND TUMORS

- Usually positive with: Cam5.2, CK7, EMA
- Variably positive for: ER, PR, SMA, calponin, S100P, CEA, BR-2

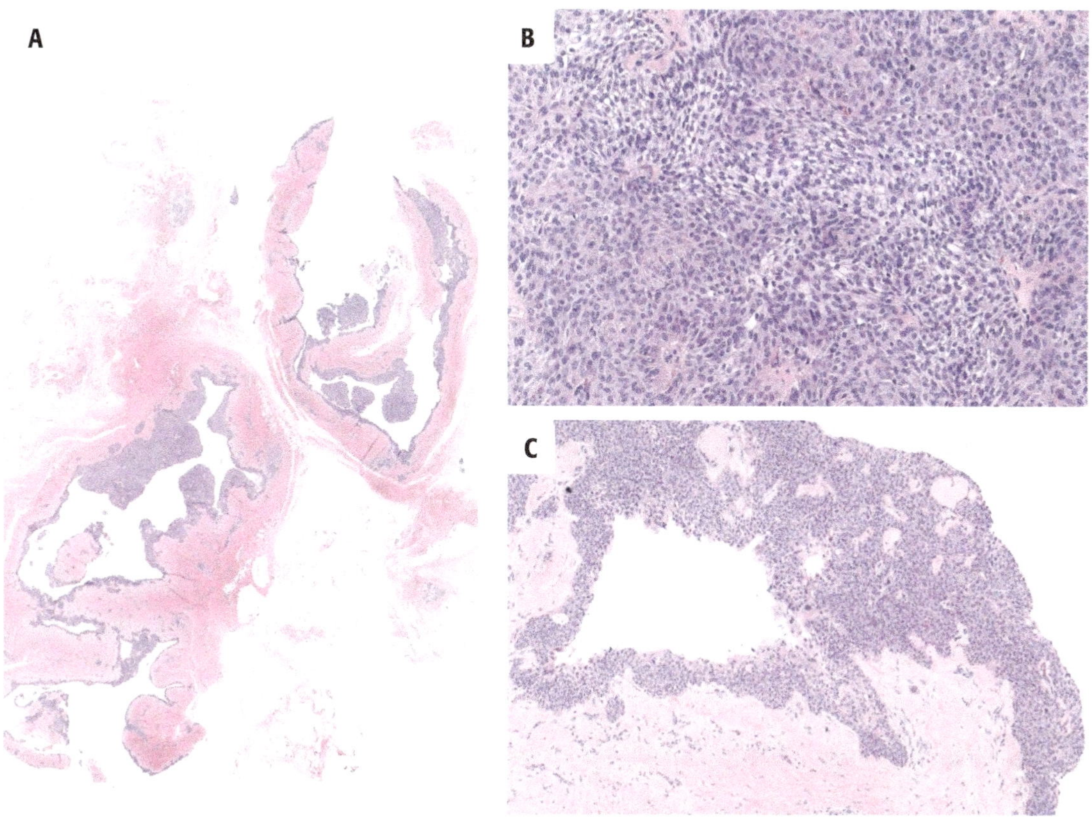

FIG. 12.49

Hidradenoma (acral). **A**, Nodulocystic tumor in subcutis. **B**, Solid areas within the tumor show bland nuclei with focal clear-cell features. **C**, The cyst-lining cells show secretory changes. The stroma is focally hyalinized. The tumor was associated with MAML2 rearrangement.

DIFFERENTIAL DIAGNOSIS OF CLEAR-CELL ADNEXAL TUMORS

Circumscribed, Noninfiltrative Dermal Nodules

- Hidradenoma (ducts and tubules; FISH positive for MAML2)
- Trichilemmoma (no ducts, but squamous eddies and prominent basement membrane; usually multiple connections to epidermis)
- Metastatic renal cell carcinoma, clear-cell type (no well-formed tubules; usually no connection to epidermis; hypervascular stroma; usually clinical history of prior tumor, IHC positive for Pax8)

Infiltrative Silhouette and/or High-Grade Atypia

- Hidradenocarcinoma (nodulocystic and infiltrative growth pattern with ducts; usually; FISH positive for MAML2)
- Trichilemmal carcinoma (association with follicle; clear-cell changes related to glycogen)
- Squamous cell carcinoma (associated intraepidermal precursor, i.e., in situ squamous cell carcinoma, keratinization, potentially positive for HPV)
- Basal cell carcinoma, clear-cell variant (growth pattern and cytology of basal cell carcinoma; positive for Ber-EP4)
- Sebaceous carcinoma (sebaceous differentiation; positive for adipophilin)
- Clear-cell adnexal carcinoma with comedo-necrosis
- Balloon-cell melanoma (positive for melanocyte differentiation antigens)

because of associated clear-cell changes. In contrast to hidradenoma, trichilemmoma shows peripheral palisading and lacks ducts. Hidradenoma differs from myoepithelioma by the predominance of epithelial over myoepithelial cells. Hidradenocarcinoma has an infiltrative silhouette and frequently shows cytologic atypia. Metastatic renal cell carcinoma of clear-cell type may have low-grade nuclear features and simulate a primary clear-cell tumor of the skin. Clinical history of prior renal cell carcinoma, the presence of a richly vascular stroma, and a high proliferative index (MIB-1 labeling index) of the epithelial tumor cells are clues to the diagnosis of metastatic clear-cell carcinoma.

SYRINGOMA

Clinical Findings

Syringomas usually present as multiple small, skin-colored papules (Fig. 12.50) around the eyelids, mostly in young women. Other locations include axillae, abdomen, and vulva.

Histopathologic Features

Syringomas are characterized by a small, circumscribed proliferation of small dermal ducts, some with cystic ectasia containing amorphous eosinophilic material (Fig. 12.51). Typically, there are at least two layers of flat

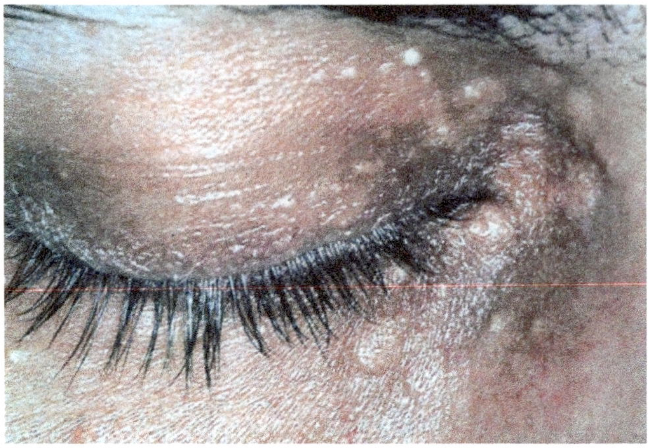

FIG. 12.50
Syringoma. Multiple skin-colored papules surround the eye.

or cuboidal cells. The nuclei are regular. Mitotic figures are absent or rare. Some ducts have a tennis racket or tadpole configuration. The cells often have an eosinophilic cytoplasm, but clear-cell change may occur.

Differential Diagnosis

The most important distinction is from MAC. Many MACs are readily diagnosable by the presence of infiltrating cords of basaloid cells and perineural invasion. However, some MACs in their superficial portion may be indistinguishable from syringoma. The only clue for the diagnosis may be tumor extension into the deep dermis or subcutis, or the detection of perineural invasion. The clinical description may also be helpful as syringomas often occur as multiple small papules, most commonly around the eyelids, while MAC is most commonly a single infiltrative plaque.

SYRINGOCYSTADENOMA PAPILLIFERUM

Clinical Findings

Syringocystadenoma papilliferum is a benign tumor that occurs most commonly on the scalp or face. About 40% of cases are associated with a congenital lesion, usually a nevus sebaceus. It is usually first noted at birth or in early childhood and consists of one or several yellowish papules, sometimes arranged linearly, and with reduced or absent hair growth. The lesions increase in size at puberty, becoming papillomatous and often crusted.

Histopathologic Features

Syringocystadenoma papilliferum is composed of papillae and ducts lined by cuboidal or columnar cells

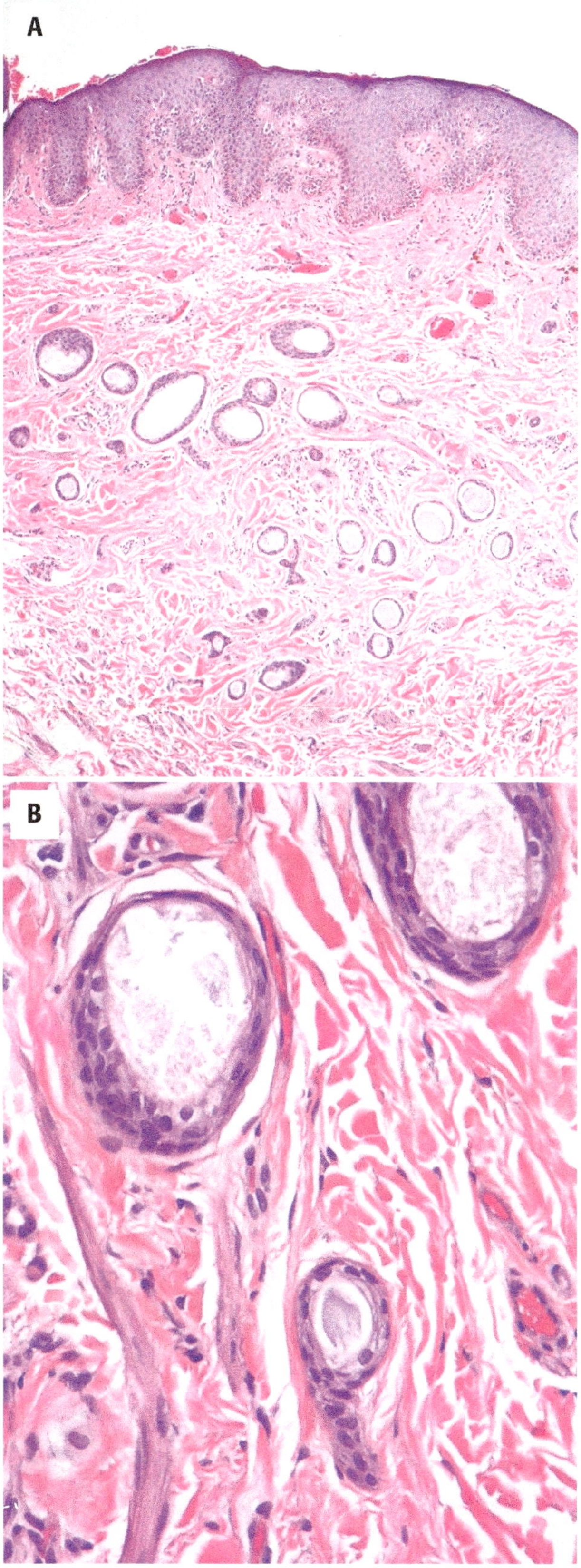

FIG. 12.51

Syringoma. **A,** Circumscribed small aggregate of small cysts and epithelial strands in the superficial dermis. **B,** Characteristic tadpole appearance.

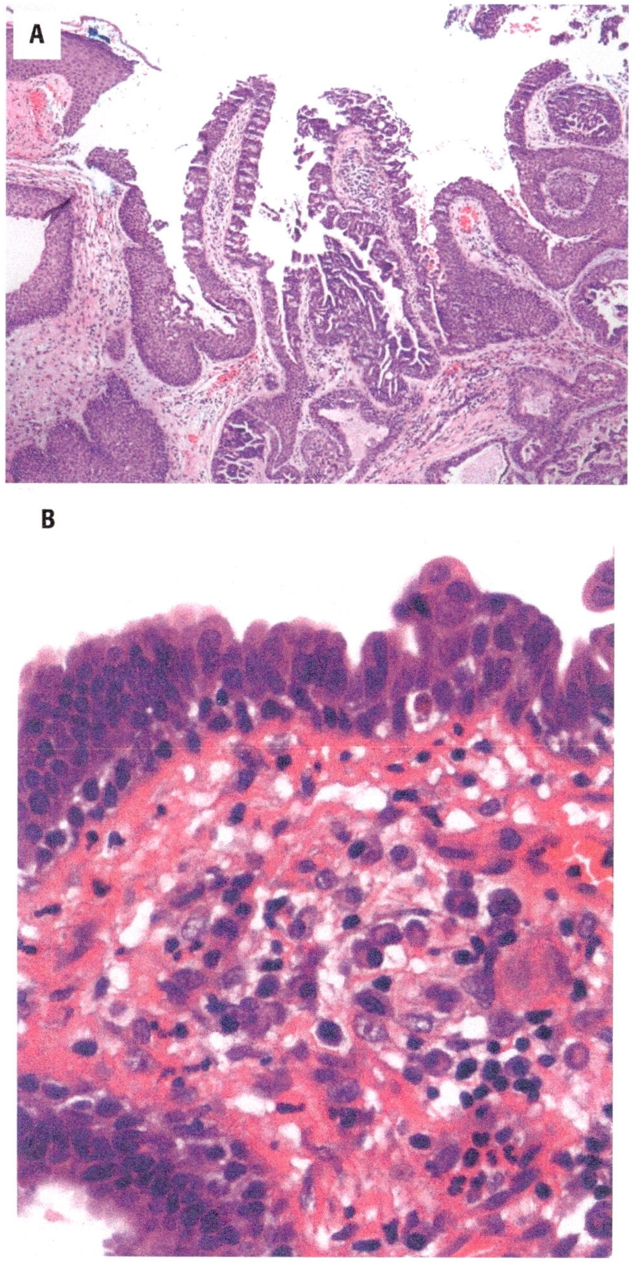

FIG. 12.52

Syringocystadenoma papilliferum. **A,** Papillary fronds project into a cystic lumen. They are lined by apocrine-type epithelial cells. **B,** Plasma cells in the stroma of the papillae are typical.

with abundant, basophilic cytoplasm, with an outer layer of myoepithelial cells. A connection to the overlying epidermis usually is present. The stroma characteristically contains plasma cells (Fig. 12.52). There may be a background of nevus sebaceous.

Differential Diagnosis

The main diagnostic issues are the distinction of syringocystadenoma from hidradenoma papilliferum and the detection of associated nevus sebaceous, because such lesions may give rise to secondary malignant neoplasms (see nevus sebaceous). Rarely, a carcinoma arises from a syringocystadenoma. It histopathologically manifests an infiltrative growth pattern.

SYRINGOFIBROADENOMA (OF MASCARÓ)

This solitary lesion is usually a hyperkeratotic nodular plaque of up to several centimeters in diameter, mainly on the extremities. Histopathologically, there are anastomosing cords of epithelial cells connected with the epidermis and usually containing ducts. The intervening stroma is slightly fibrous with abundant vessels.

THE SPECTRUM OF POROMAS

There is a spectrum of poromas, for which different names have been proposed. At times they were also referred to as *eccrine acrospiroma*, a term coined by Johnson and Helwig for a morphologically diverse group of tumors thought to differentiate toward (or originate from) the distal part of the sweat duct. Three categories were proposed: intraepidermal (hidroacanthoma simplex), juxtaepidermal acrospiroma (classic poroma), and intradermal (dermal duct tumor) acrospiroma. Lesions classified as poroid hidradenoma also belong to this group (equivalent to intradermal nodular poroma). The term *acrospiroma* is now rarely used anymore. Most pathologists prefer the terms *hidroacanthoma simplex* for intradermal tumors and *poroma* for juxta- and intradermal poroid tumors (classic poroma, poroid hidradenoma and dermal duct tumor).

HIDROACANTHOMA SIMPLEX

Clinical Findings

The lesion lacks distinct clinical features. It usually manifests as a small papule and is usually thought to be an SK.

Histopathologic Features

The lesion is characterized by slight acanthosis and hyperkeratosis. Nests of small cuboidal keratinocytes similar to the picture of a "clonal" SK are found (Fig. 12.53). Foci of ductal differentiation as opposed to the horn cysts of an SK are typically seen.

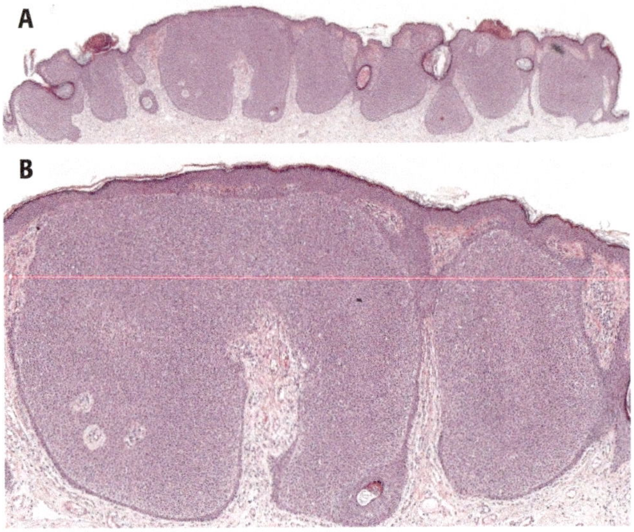

FIG. 12.53

Hidroacanthoma simplex (intraepidermal poroma). **A**, Multiple large nests of epithelial cells seen. **B**, The nests are composed of small cuboidal epithelial cells with bland nuclei. Occasional small lumina lined by ductal cells are present.

Differential Diagnosis

The main distinctions are from an irritated SK and, occasionally, Bowen's disease. In contrast to an irritated "clonal" SK, hidroacanthoma simplex shows lumen formation, at least focally. Immunohistochemistry for Brst-2 or CEA can facilitate the detection of lumina. Similar to irritated SK, hidroacanthoma with a nested or pagetoid pattern of keratinocytes within the epidermis differs from Bowen's disease by the lack of atypia.

POROMA

Clinical Findings

Poromas occur mostly on acral sites (feet, hands, fingers) in middle-aged individuals but can occur at any site, including the head and neck. They typically present as red, firm papules, usually greater than 2 cm in diameter (Fig. 12.54A). They are sometimes mistaken for pyogenic granulomas. Rarely, multiple papules are present. Poromas may be pigmented (Fig. 12.54B).

Histopathologic Features

Poromas tend to show a nodular silhouette. Broad, anastomosing trabeculae, composed of small cuboidal keratinocytes with uniform bland nuclei, connect to the epidermis (Fig. 12.55) and extend into the papillary

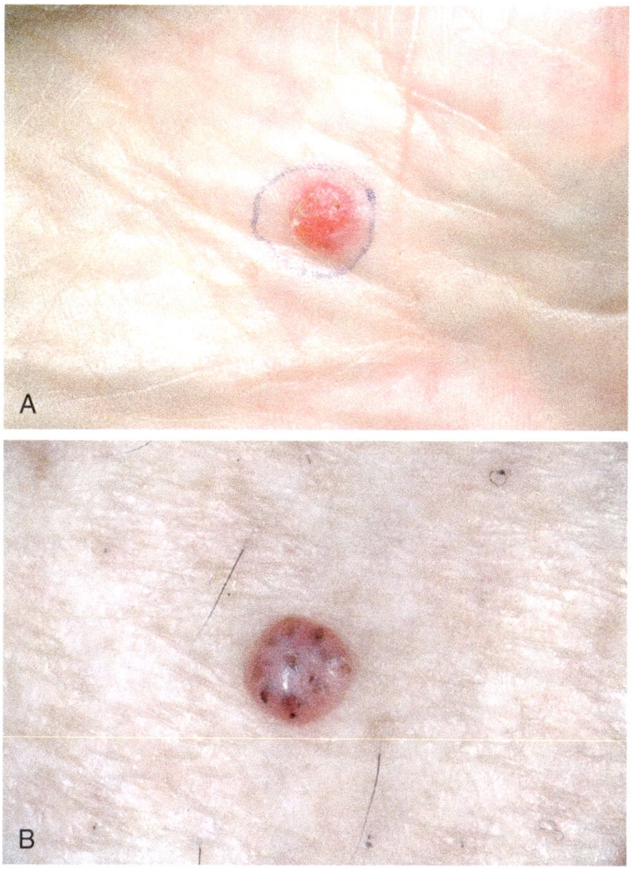

FIG. 12.54
Poroma. **A**, Erythematous papule. **B**, Pigmented poroma. Dome-shaped papule with brown dots.

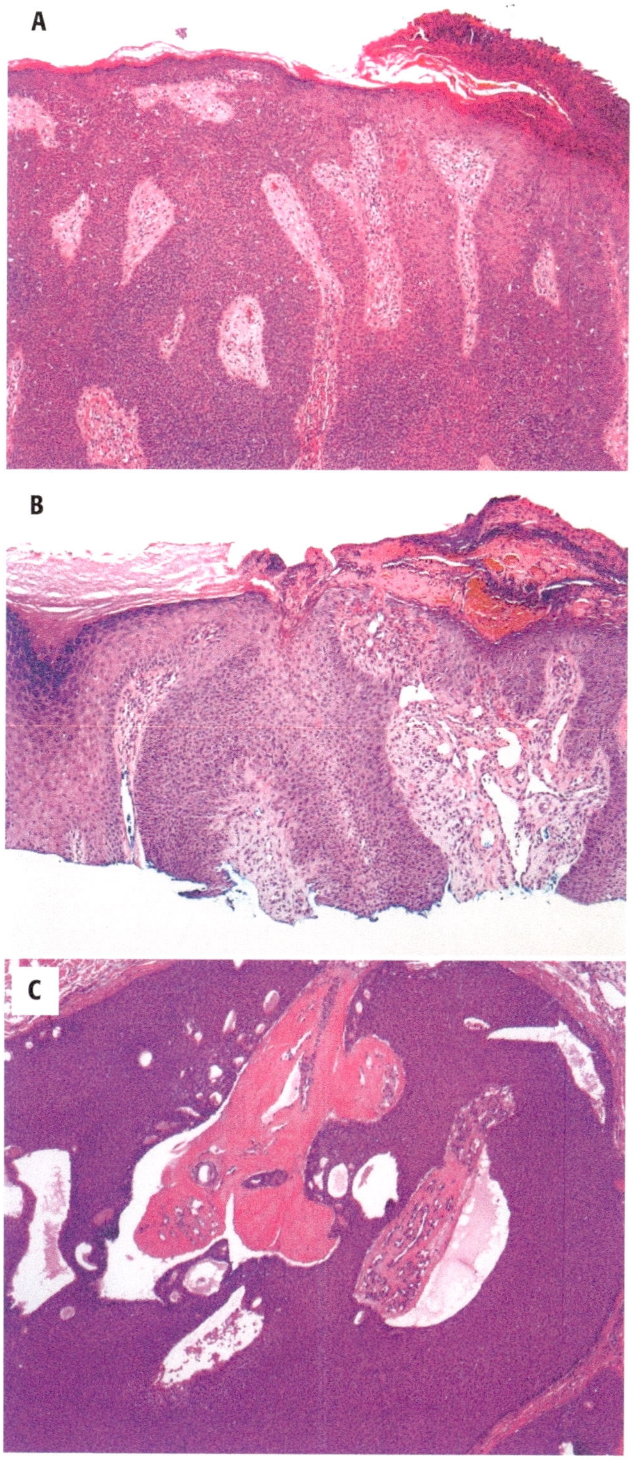

FIG. 12.55
Poroma. **A**, Broad anastomosing strands of small basaloid epithelial cells connected to the epidermis surround hypervascular papillae. **B**, Poroma with surface irritation. Poroma cells are juxtaposed to adjacent epidermal keratinocytes with more abundant eosinophilic cytoplasm. **C**, Intradermal nodular part composed of small cuboidal epithelial cells associated hypervascular and partly hyalinized stroma.

and reticular dermis. Small ducts are often present. In pigmented poroma, melanin may be present in keratinocytes or stromal macrophages (Fig. 12.56). The epithelial strands typically surround a hypervascular and variably edematous and/or fibrotic stroma. Polypoid or exophytic poromas may undergo trauma and surface ulceration and show reactive epithelial atypia.

Ancillary Studies

Poromas typically contain YAP1 and/or NUTM1 fusions. This can be documented by FISH or RNA sequence analysis. A more practical way for diagnostic purposes is immunohistochemistry for YAP1 and/or NUT. Nuclear immunoreactivity for NUT confirms the presence of a NUTM1 fusion. Immunohistochemistry for YAP1 using an antibody that recognizes C-terminal protein documents loss of labeling, if YAP1 is rearranged, while nuclear labeling would be preserved with an antibody to the N-terminal portion of YAP1.

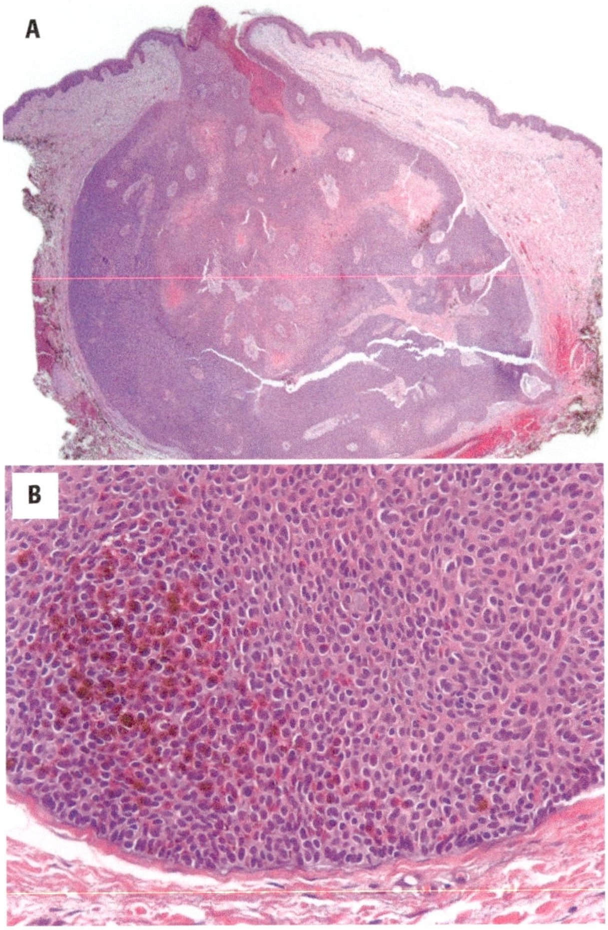

FIG. 12.56

Pigmented poroma. **A,** Circumscribed lobulated growth pattern of basaloid cells connecting to the epidermis. **B,** Melanin pigment is present in keratinocytes.

Differential Diagnosis

Poroma may be confused with an endophytic SK or BCC. Poroma should be considered when one encounters an endophytic, SK-like dermal tumor that lacks horn pseudocysts. In such cases, a careful search for small ductal lumina leads to a diagnosis of poroma. Immunohistochemical studies with anti-CEA may help by highlighting the presence of the ducts within the epithelial nests.

In contrast to BCC, poroma lacks peripheral palisading of nuclei and clefts between tumor cells and surrounding stroma. Most important, however, is the difference in cytology. Whereas poromas are composed of small, cuboidal cells with small nuclei showing a delicate fine or open chromatin pattern, BCC cells have elongated and hyperchromatic nuclei.

Poroma also needs to be distinguished from porocarcinoma, which may arise from or simulate features of poroma. Most porocarcinomas (also see the following) appear frankly malignant, with marked atypia and an infiltrative growth pattern. Focal epithelial atypia (not outright cytologic features of carcinoma) may occur in irritated poromas without apparent infiltrative growth and may lead to erroneous suspicion for carcinoma.

INTRADERMAL POROMA (DERMAL DUCT TUMOR AND POROID HIDRADENOMA)

Clinical Findings

The lesion presents as a clinically indistinct papule or nodule. The clinical suspicions range from cyst to BCC or adnexal tumor.

Histopathologic Features

While poroid hidradenoma displays a nodular or nodulocystic growth (Fig. 12.57), dermal duct tumor is characterized by multiple circumscribed micronodules of bland keratinocytes with poromoid features without any discernible connection to the epidermis (Fig. 12.58).

Differential Diagnosis

At scanning magnification, the tumor may be confused with nodular BCC. However, at higher magnification, the bland cytology of the tumor cells and lack of stromal changes associated with BCC usually allow distinction. Ancillary studies can assist in the diagnosis. The majority of poroid hidradenomas show nuclear labeling for NUT by immunohistochemistry.

SPIRADENOMA

Clinical Findings

Spiradenoma is usually a solitary, firm, intradermal nodule in young adults, around 1 to 2 cm in diameter. Occasionally, it presents as multiple lesions in a diffuse, linear, or zosteriform arrangement. It is one of the painful cutaneous tumors (BANGLE: *b*lue rubber bleb nevus, *a*ngiolipoma, *n*euroma, *g*lomus tumor [vascular], *l*eiomyoma, and *e*ccrine spiradenoma).

Histopathologic Features

One or several dermal circumscribed lobules of basaloid cells are present in the dermis, without connection to the

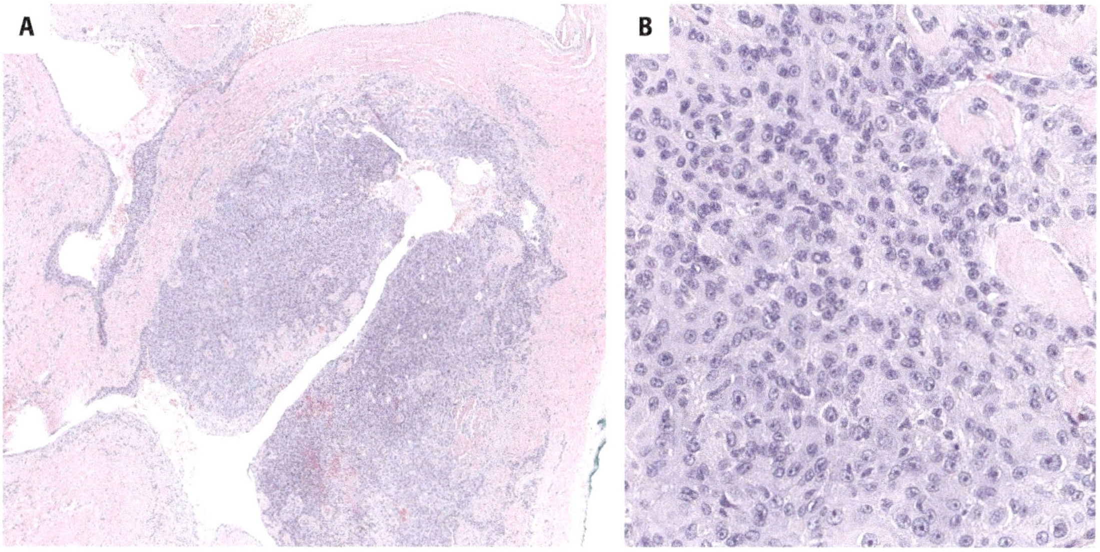

FIG. 12.57

Poroid hidradenoma. **A,** Nodulocystic growth. **B,** The tumor is composed of epithelial cells with little cytoplasm. Some of the stroma is hyalinized. The tumor carried a *YAP1::NUTM1* gene fusion.

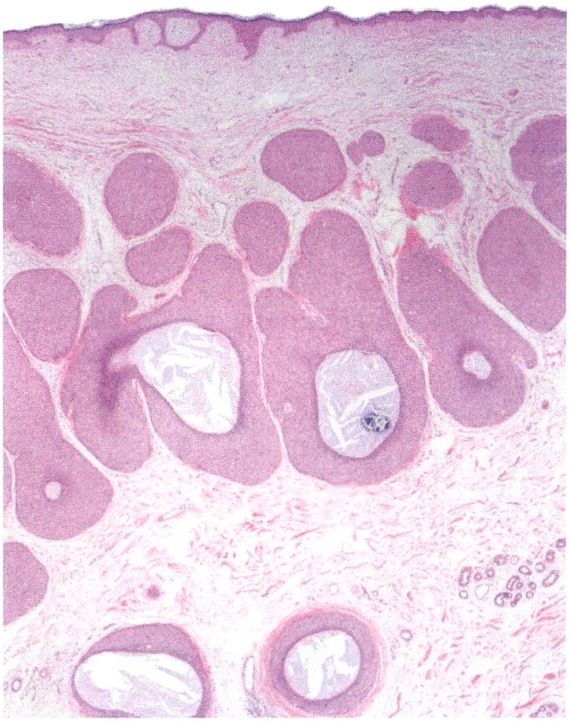

FIG. 12.58

Dermal duct tumor. Small nodular and nodulocystic aggregates of poroid tumor cells with no connection to the epidermis.

epidermis (Fig. 12.59). The nests are composed of two types of epithelial cells: one has a small, dark nucleus, mainly at the periphery of the cellular aggregates, while the second type of cell has a large, pale nucleus, sometimes located around small lumina with eosinophilic, periodic acid-Schiff (PAS)-positive, and diastase-resistant material. Occasionally, tumors contain cystic areas with

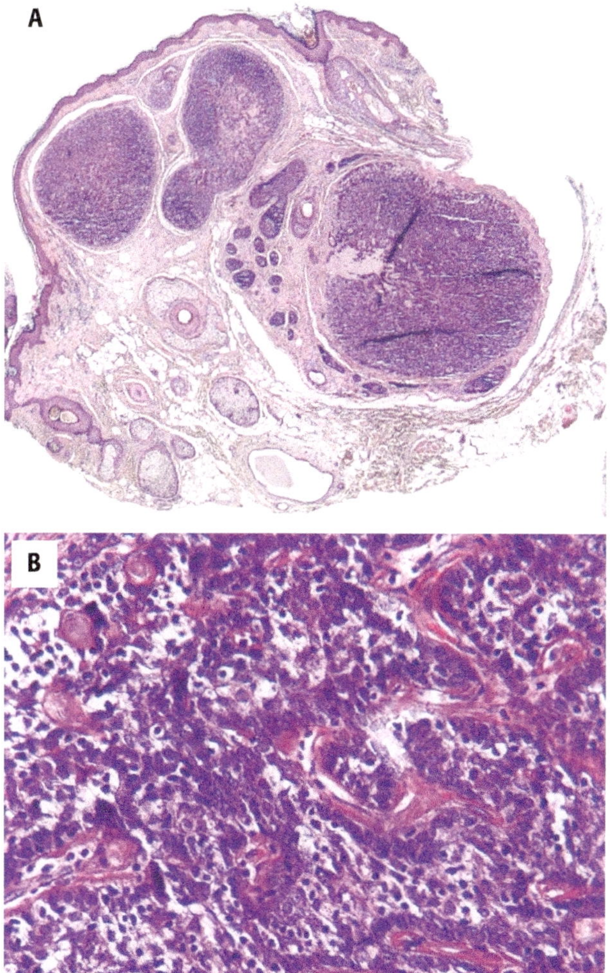

FIG. 12.59

Spiradenoma. **A,** Multinodular growth pattern. **B,** Two cell populations: small basaloid cells surrounding larger pale epithelial cells.

the same eosinophilic material. The intervening stroma may have some hyaline material. Some tumors show lymphocytic aggregates or prominent vascularity.

Differential Diagnosis

Spiradenoma differs from spiradenocarcinoma by its lack of atypia and infiltrative growth pattern. Cylindroma shows abundant basement membrane (eosinophilic) material around small clusters of basaloid cells in a jigsaw pattern. On rare occasions, an adenocarcinoma may arise in association with a preexisting spiradenoma (carcinoma ex spiradenoma; malignant eccrine spiradenoma; see the following).

CYLINDROMA

Clinical Findings

Cylindromas typically present as solitary small papules. They most often occur in the head and neck region of middle-aged or elderly women. Large tumors or multiple coalescing tumors may arise. An extreme variant of the latter is the phenomenon of a "turban tumor," which represents multiple nodules of cylindroma on the scalp and forehead (Fig. 12.60).

Histopathologic Features

At scanning magnification, there are usually multiple small islands of basaloid cells surrounded by pink, hyaline basement membrane material (Fig. 12.61). Cylinders of hyaline membranes are often present in the center of such islands. Two types of epithelial cells are usually present: (1) a peripheral cell with a large basophilic (dark-staining) nucleus and a tendency for palisading, and (2) a larger, centrally located, paler cell with a vesicular chromatin pattern.

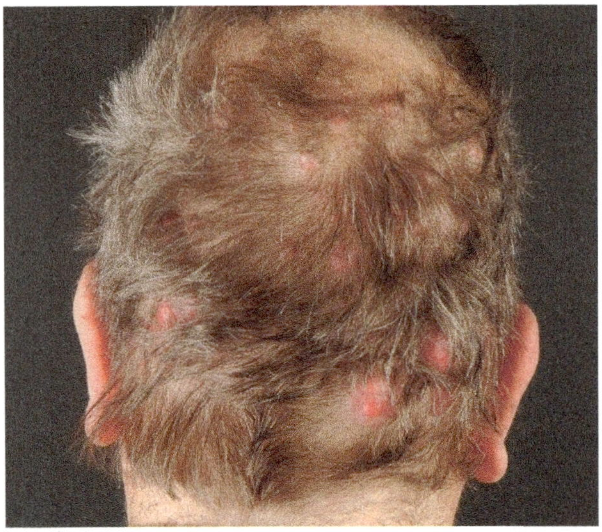

FIG. 12.60

Cylindromatosis (turban tumor).

Differential Diagnosis

Cylindroma may show overlap or even occur together with spiradenoma. The latter differs from the former by the lack of hyaline cylinders. Furthermore, spiradenoma tends to be more vascular and to show edematous and cystic stromal changes. Cylindroma also needs to be distinguished from adenoid cystic and BCC. BCC lacks the two cell types characteristic of spiradenoma. Adenoid cystic carcinoma differs from spiradenoma by the presence of cribriform growth, mucinous stroma, and

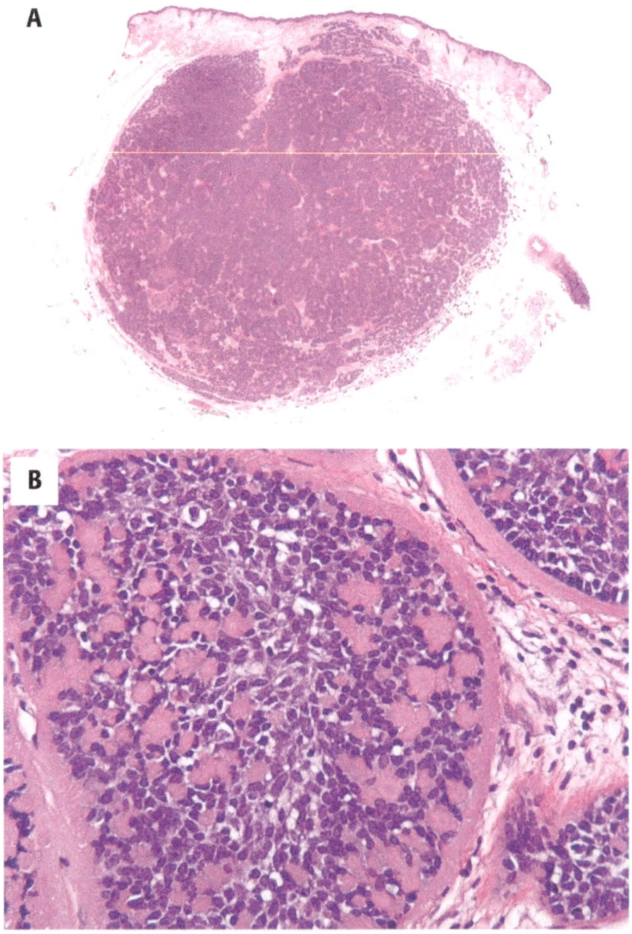

FIG. 12.61

Cylindroma. **A,** Dermal and subcutaneous nodules of basaloid cells. **B,** The tumor cells are bland, engulf cylinders of hyaline material, and are also surrounded by a hyaline membrane.

often more irregular growth. Furthermore, they often carry a gene fusion not found in spiradenomas.

BENIGN MIXED TUMOR (CHONDROID SYRINGOMA)

Clinical Findings

Benign mixed tumor or chondroid syringoma most often occurs on the head and neck in middle-aged or elderly individuals, slightly more frequently in men. The tumor typically manifests as a dermal or subcutaneous nodule. It may measure up to 3 cm in diameter. Some tumors may locally recur.

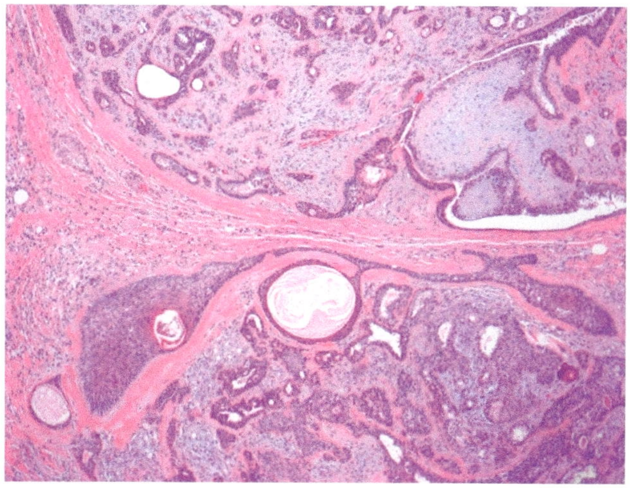

FIG. 12.62

Benign mixed tumor. A combination of ducts, keratocysts, myoepithelial cells, and myxoid stroma changes are present.

Histopathologic Features

The tumor manifests as a nodular or multinodular dermal or subcutaneous tumor with a well-circumscribed, lobulated peripheral border. The hallmark of all mixed tumors is the presence of divergent differentiation resulting in a combination of both epithelial duct (epithelial and myoepithelial) as well as mesenchymal components (Fig. 12.62). Epithelial cells may form ducts, cords, or solid sheets. Ducts typically show at least focal apocrine secretion. The intervening stroma has areas with fibrous, myxoid, or chondroid tissue. Some lesions may have squamous or sebaceous differentiation. Tumors with ducts placed in a prominent chondroid stroma may be designated as *chondroid syringomas* (Fig. 12.63).

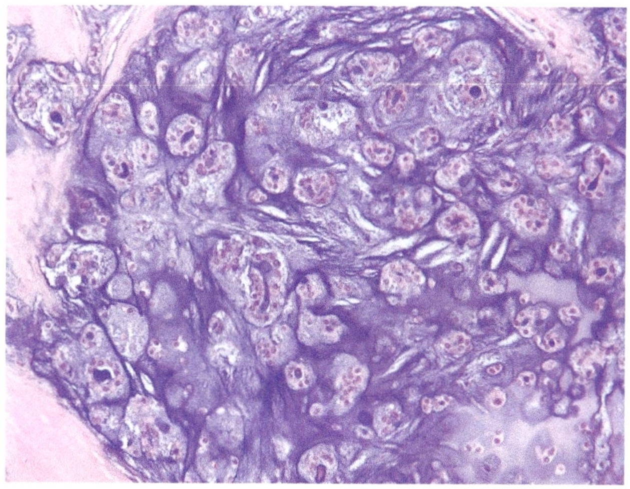

FIG. 12.63

Benign mixed tumor/chondroid syringoma. This variant shows a predominance of chondromyxoid matrix associated with clusters of epithelial cells.

Ancillary Studies

Immunohistochemically, mixed tumors show findings documenting the presence of both duct epithelial (positive for CK7) and myoepithelial (positive for p63 and SOX10) elements. The majority of cutaneous mixed tumors are immunoreactive for PLAG1.

Differential Diagnosis

Benign mixed tumors must be distinguished from malignant mixed tumors. The latter exhibit an infiltrative silhouette, atypia, and mitotic figures. The distinction between a benign mixed tumor with a prominent myoepithelial cell component, versus a myoepithelioma, is likely mainly semantic. If the myoepithelial cell component shows large nodules with atypia and mitotic figures, some pathologists may interpret such a finding as intratumoral (in situ) myoepithelial carcinoma. We do not use the term *carcinoma* in this setting because the presence of such features is of no clinical relevance or consequence. There is no evidence that such features are associated with an increased risk of recurrence.

In mixed tumors located on the cheek, the diagnostic considerations may include the superficial portion of a primary salivary gland mixed tumor rather than a primary sweat gland tumor. (The same is true for myoepitheliomas; see the following.) Because these tumors are histopathologically indistinguishable, diagnosis relies on knowledge of where the tumor is centered (deep parotid tissue versus dermis). Parotid tumors (myoepitheliomas or pleomorphic adenomas) with secondary involvement of the overlying epidermis require a different type of surgery than primary dermal tumors.

Benign mixed tumors with prominent chondroid matrix (chondroid syringoma) also may be confused with lesions of chordoma metastatic to the skin. Clinical history (history of chordoma), as well as careful attention to histopathologic features (physaliferous features of chordoma) and documentation of a myoepithelial component in mixed tumors (positive for SMA, calponin, p63, S100, SOX10), is helpful.

MYOEPITHELIOMA

Clinical Findings

This rare lesion may occur at almost any age and location. It is clinically indistinct, presenting as a dermal or subcutaneous nodule.

Histopathologic Features

Myoepitheliomas are well-circumscribed lesions in the dermis (and less commonly the subcutis). The hallmark is the predominance of myoepithelial cells that show considerable plasticity, with phenotypes ranging from fusiform to epithelioid. The cytoplasm may range from pink to pale or clear cell. The stroma may have a fibrous, hyalinized, or myxoid appearance (Fig. 12.64).

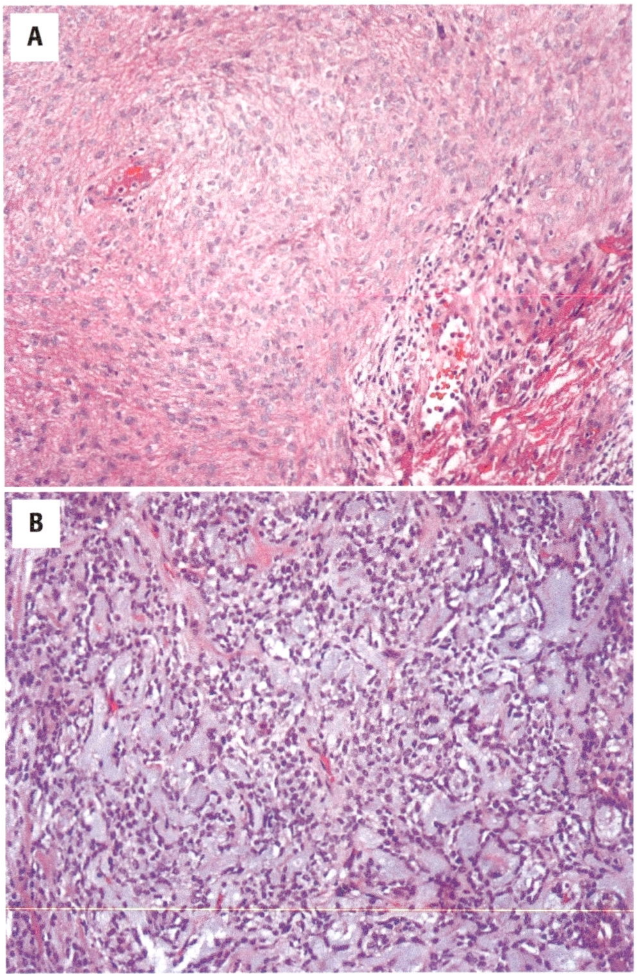

FIG. 12.64

Myoepithelioma. **A,** Myoepithelioma presenting as a pink dermal tumor with lobular growth. **B,** Myoepithelioma with myxoid features.

Ancillary Studies

Immunohistochemistry is often necessary to confirm the presence of myoepithelial differentiation. Myoepithelial cells express cytokeratins, S100 protein, EMA, actin, caldesmon, and calponin. They are associated with a range of genomic aberrations, typically gene fusions involving EWSR1 or FUS.

Differential Diagnosis

Chondroid syringoma or mixed tumor have both epithelial and myoepithelial components. Many reported cases of cutaneous myoepithelioma are merely myoepithelial-rich benign mixed tumors, in our opinion. We restrict the term *myoepithelioma* to tumors lacking prominent glandular epithelial differentiation. Myoepithelial carcinomas have an infiltrative growth pattern, display atypia, and show overlap with what is historically reported as malignant mixed tumor.

TREATMENT OF BENIGN GLANDULAR TUMORS

No further surgery is necessary after the biopsy diagnosis of a benign sweat gland tumor is established. Of course, additional surgery may be appropriate for a number of reasons, such as cosmetic concerns. Complete surgical excision is prudent if there is a chance that the biopsy may not be representative of the entire clinical lesion or if the clinical findings (large longstanding lesion with history of change) suggest the possibility of malignant transformation of a benign precursor lesion.

Complete surgical excision is also advised if no definite distinction between a benign or malignant tumor can be made, such as when a small superficial biopsy does not allow assessment of the growth pattern of a lesion (infiltrative versus noninfiltrative silhouette, superficial versus deep extension) required to distinguish an adenoma from a low-grade carcinoma. For example, a ductal adenocarcinoma or hidradenocarcinoma may simulate an adenoma or hidradenoma in its superficial portion, and MAC may be indistinguishable

SPECTRUM OF SWEAT GLAND CARCINOMAS

Low-Grade Tumors (Local Recurrences Common; No or Only Very Rare Metastases)

- Cribriform carcinoma
- Microcystic adnexal carcinoma
- Endocrine mucin-producing sweat gland carcinoma
- Pure mucinous carcinoma
- Secretory carcinoma

High-Grade Tumors (Risk for Metastases to Lymph Nodes, Lung, Bone)

- Porocarcinoma
- Ductal eccrine or apocrine carcinoma
- Hidradenocarcinoma
- Malignant mixed tumor
- Carcinoma ex spiradenoma
- Invasive extramammary Paget's disease
- Digital papillary adenocarcinoma

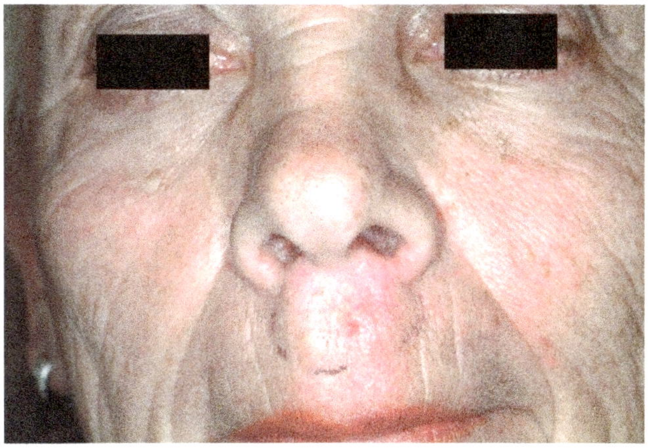

FIG. 12.65

Microcystic adnexal carcinoma presenting as an indurated plaque above the upper lip.

from syringoma. Some tumors, such as mixed tumors or myoepitheliomas, have a propensity for local recurrence or persistent growth and are probably also best treated by complete surgical excision upfront, to minimize the risk of continued growth and a less favorable long-term cosmetic result.

MALIGNANT NEOPLASMS

A broad group of malignant tumors has eccrine or apocrine differentiation, including low-grade tumors, which may be locally aggressive but rarely if ever metastasize, and high-grade malignant tumors with significant risk for metastasis to lymph node, viscera, and bone.

MICROCYSTIC ADNEXAL CARCINOMA (SCLEROSING SWEAT DUCT ADENOCARCINOMA)

Clinical Findings

The typical presentation is as a solitary firm plaque, on the upper lip, around the mouth, or involving the eyelid, usually affecting middle-aged individuals (Fig. 12.65).

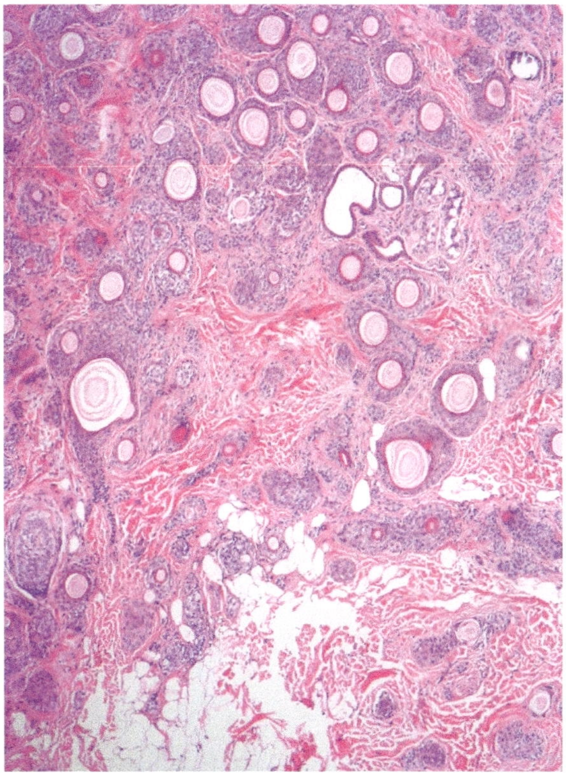

FIG. 12.66

Microcystic adnexal carcinoma. Appearance similar to a syringoma, but the tumor infiltrates deep dermis and superficial subcutis.

Histopathologic Features

The findings vary widely, from a tumor indistinguishable from syringoma (Fig. 12.66) except for its extension into the deep dermis or subcutis, to the picture of sclerosing sweat duct carcinoma (Fig. 12.67). The latter exhibits cords, ducts, and single cells dispersed in a sclerotic stroma. Many tumors have two components. The superficial one tends to have syringomatous features with keratocysts (at times simulating trichoadenoma). The second, deeper component has ducts and gland-like structures with a one- or two-cell-thick lining. Mixed follicular and glandular differentiation maybe seen. The cells are mainly cuboidal, with slightly hyperchromatic nuclei. Cytologic atypia and mitotic figures are uncommon. Perineural invasion is common.

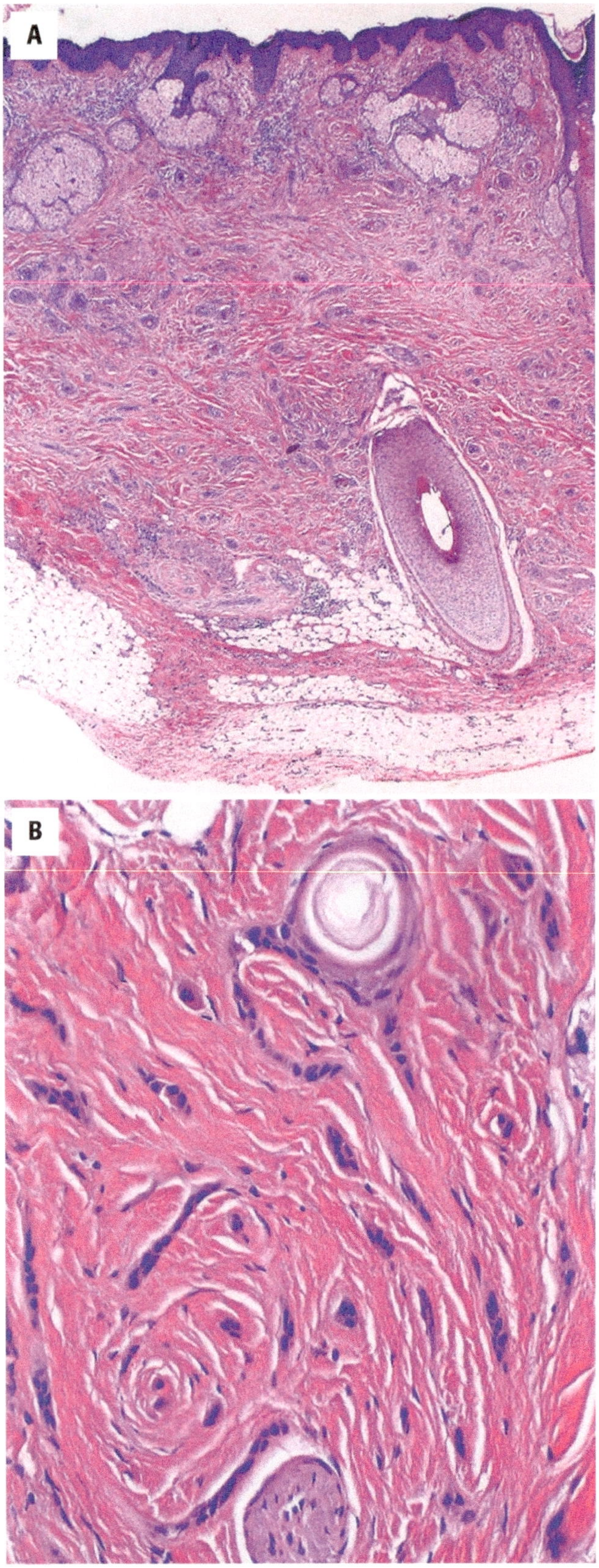

FIG. 12.67

Microcystic adnexal carcinoma. **A,** Diffuse infiltrative growth pattern. **B,** Compressed thin cords of basaloid epithelial cells in sclerotic stroma with rare small keratinocytes (sclerosing sweat duct tumor).

MICROCYSTIC ADNEXAL CARCINOMA—PATHOLOGIC FEATURES

Histopathologic Features

- Infiltrative silhouette, typically extending at least to the deep dermis, often into the subcutis
- Small keratocysts typically superficially
- May have a syringoma-like, bland cytologic appearance
- Sclerosing sweat duct appearance with compressed cords and strands of basaloid cells in a fibrotic stroma

Differential Diagnosis

- Desmoplastic trichoepithelioma
- Trichoadenoma
- Sclerosing basal cell carcinoma
- Infiltrative squamous cell carcinoma

Differential Diagnosis

Microcystic adnexal carcinoma may be confused with sclerosing BCC, desmoplastic TE, desmoplastic SCC, trichoadenoma, and syringoma. The key feature to distinguish MAC from syringoma is deep infiltration. MAC and trichoadenoma may look identical in their superficial portion, but trichoadenoma would lack any ductal or syringomatous component in its deeper component. The lack of papillary mesenchymal bodies but the presence of tubular structures or "tadpole"-like syringomatous structures exclude desmoplastic TE. Infiltrative morpheaform BCC usually shows some foci of more common BCC or tends to show overall more nuclear atypia and more numerous apoptotic bodies. Immunohistochemistry can aid detection of duct formation by tumor cells, as highlighted by CEA expression. In contrast with BCC, MAC expresses CK15. Anti-p63 highlights the peripheral cells in MAC while labeling most tumor cells in BCC.

The distinction is usually obvious when one examines the entire lesion but can be difficult or impossible based on the findings of a small superficial biopsy. If there is any diagnostic uncertainty, complete excision of the lesion is advisable.

Prognosis and Treatment

Microcystic adnexal carcinoma is usually low-grade neoplasm with risk for locally aggressive behavior and significant morbidity, if surgical treatment is delayed or unsuccessful. Complete surgical excision is best achieved using frozen section examination. Although cases of metastases have been reported, they are so rare that there is no role for sentinel lymph node (SLN) biopsy for patients with MAC. The role of postoperative radiation therapy is controversial.

POROCARCINOMA

Clinical Findings

Porocarcinoma may arise de novo or in association with a longstanding benign poroma. It typically presents as an ulcerated nodule (Fig. 12.68) or verrucous plaque on the lower extremities of elderly individuals, but it may also occur in the head and neck region or other sites. Invasive porocarcinoma is an aggressive tumor, frequently metastasizing to the skin, lymph nodes, lung, or bone.

POROCARCINOMA—DISEASE FACT SHEET

Patient Group
- Usually older patients

Site of Involvement
- May occur anywhere, often on extremities

Clinical Findings
- Erythematous patch, papule, nodule, or plaque
- May be ulcerated

Prognosis and Treatment
- Significant risk for metastasis (lymph node, skin, lung)
- Surgical excision and staging by sentinel lymph node mapping

POROCARCINOMA—PATHOLOGIC FEATURES

Histopathologic Features

Carcinoma ex Poroma
- Invasive carcinoma associated with a classic poroma

Carcinoma with No Recognizable Precursor Lesion
- Features of poroma (connections to epidermis with intraepidermal carcinoma, solid areas mixed with tubular or ductal growth pattern) but infiltrative growth pattern
- Variable degree of atypia, mitotic figures; variable incidence of necrosis, ulceration
- Squamous metaplasia (features indistinguishable in foci from squamous cell carcinoma) common

Ancillary Studies
- Tumor cells express epithelial markers (variable, depending on marker) by IHC
- Tumor cells may express NUT by IHC
- Molecular studies may reveal YAP1 or NUT fusion

Differential Diagnosis
- Benign poroma or poromatous hidradenoma (circumscribed growth, bland)
- In situ porocarcinoma (poroma with intraepithelial carcinoma but no stromal invasion)
- Hidradenocarcinoma (MAML2 fusion)
- Squamous cell carcinoma (SCC) with pseudoglandular features (acantholytic SCC)
- Adenosquamous carcinoma (primary or metastatic)

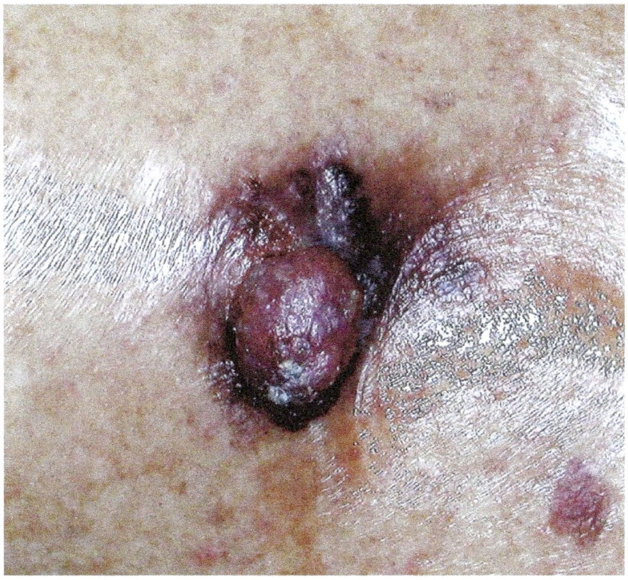

FIG. 12.68
Porocarcinoma. Ulcerated erythematous nodule with satellite lesion.

Histopathologic Features

The diagnosis is greatly facilitated for cases with a preexisting poroma (Figs. 12.69 and 12.70), especially for poorly differentiated invasive carcinomas. Such lesions have two distinct areas: a benign poroma, and a usually obvious carcinoma composed of pleomorphic tumor cells with variable duct formation. The carcinoma may be confined to the poroma (porocarcinoma in situ) or invade the surrounding stroma (invasive porocarcinoma). Porocarcinoma commonly populates the epidermis, resulting in a histopathologic appearance indistinguishable from SCC in situ. In the absence of a precursor lesion, porocarcinoma presents as adenocarcinoma with epidermal connection (Fig. 12.71). Squamous metaplasia is common and may contribute to the phenotype of an adenosquamous carcinoma. The peritumoral stroma may be fibrous, hyalinized, or myxoid. Cutaneous metastases may be epidermotropic.

Ancillary Studies

If the tumor has prominent squamous differentiation, immunostudies for CK7 or CEA can help highlight ductal differentiation. The detection of YAP1 or NUTM1 fusions by FISH or sequence analysis can be diagnostically helpful. Nuclear immunoreactivity for NUTM1 would support the presence of a gene fusion and in the right histologic context support the diagnosis.

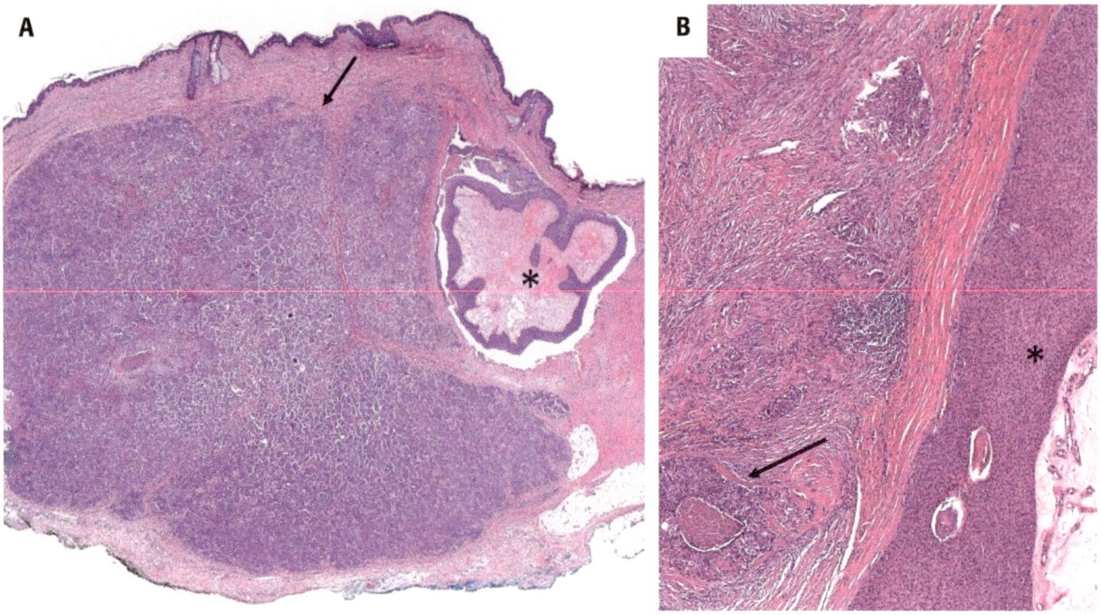

FIG. 12.69

Porocarcinoma associated with a poroma. **A**, A benign precursor poroma *(*)* is juxtaposed to an infiltrative tumor *(arrow)*. **B**, Cytologically bland poroid cells *(*)* are present adjacent to infiltrative tumor cells with atypia *(arrow)* in a desmoplastic stroma.

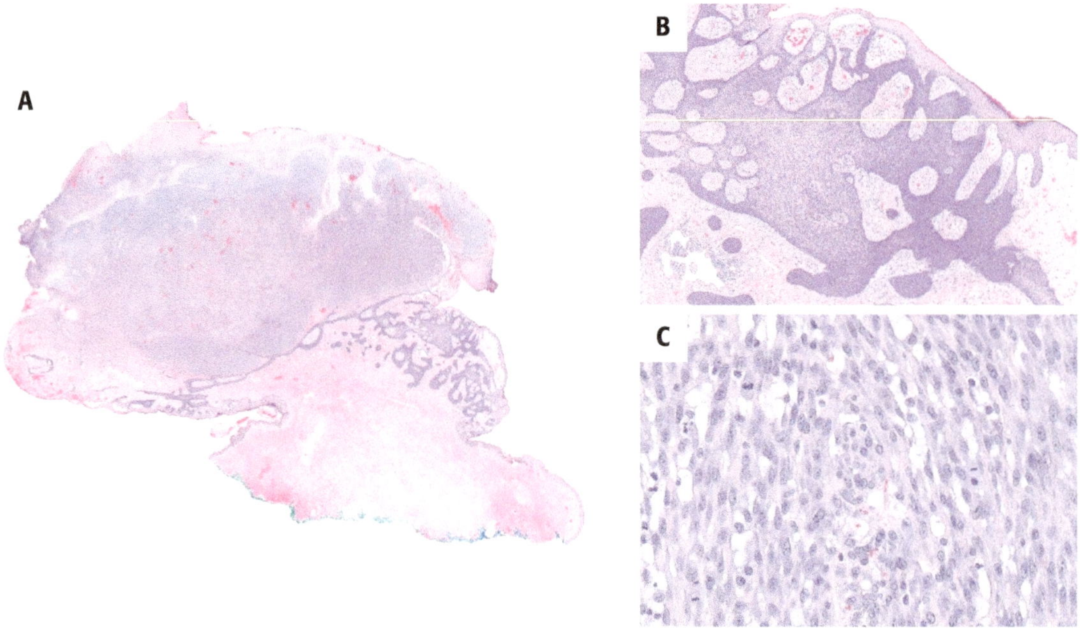

FIG. 12.70

Porocarcinoma associated with a poroa. **A,** There is an ulcerated poorly differentiated malignant tumor. **B,** The malignant tumor is flanked by a poroma. **C,** The malignant tumor is composed of undifferentiated spindle cells. They expressed epithelial markers. The tumor cells carried a *YAP1::MAML3* gene fusion.

Differential Diagnosis

On morphologic grounds, it may be difficult to distinguish a primary from a metastatic tumor. However, clinical correlation with a history of a prior porocarcinoma usually readily solves the problem. Porocarcinomas can display prominent squamous differentiation and simulate SCC. Conversely, SCC may simulate porocarcinoma if it shows pagetoid intraepidermal spread, colonizes adnexal structures, and shows acantholysis with pseudogland formation. The presence of bona fide neoplastic ducts is necessary for a diagnosis of porocarcinoma. Immunostudies may be helpful in difficult cases. Sebaceous

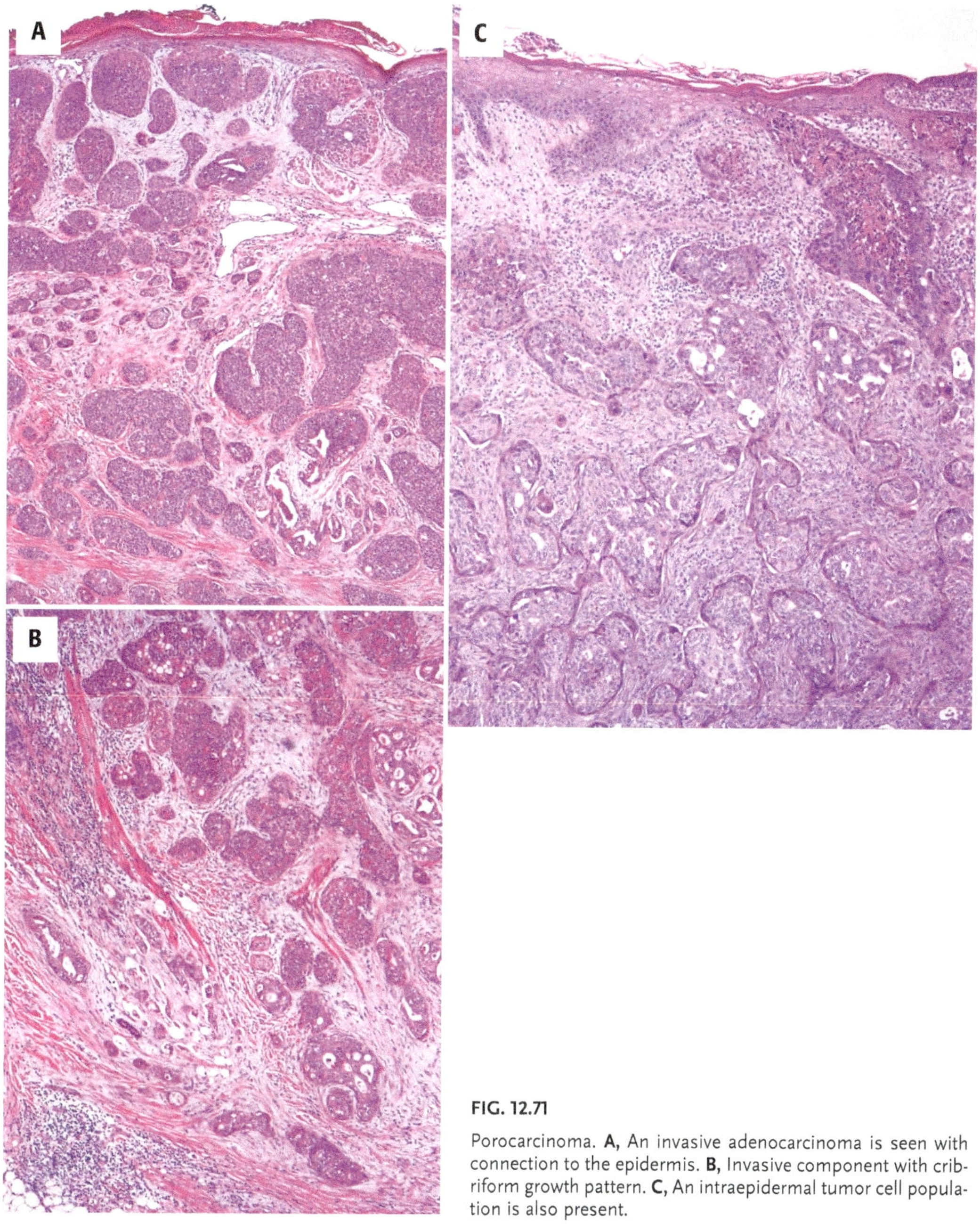

FIG. 12.71

Porocarcinoma. **A,** An invasive adenocarcinoma is seen with connection to the epidermis. **B,** Invasive component with cribriform growth pattern. **C,** An intraepidermal tumor cell population is also present.

carcinoma can also have pagetoid clear cells in the epidermis, but most sebaceous carcinomas are readily distinguished from porocarcinomas by more obvious sebaceous differentiation (nuclear scalloping, microvesiculated cytoplasm, lack of glycogen as assessed by PAS and PAS-diastase (PAS-D) stains, or immunoreactivity for adipophilin) and involvement of sebaceous lobules. Trichilemmal carcinoma also has clear cells but lacks eccrine ducts and may show trichohyaline granules.

Ductal (eccrine or apocrine) adenocarcinomas tend to show a more prominent and exclusive tubular or cribriform growth pattern than porocarcinomas. They are less likely to show solid "poroid" areas or components with squamous differentiation. Furthermore, they typically lack numerous connections to the epidermis. Poorly differentiated variants of porocarcinoma may be difficult or impossible to distinguish from poorly differentiated hidradenocarcinoma unless there is an associated benign precursor lesion (poroma or hidradenoma, respectively).

Prognosis and Treatment

Surgical excision is the treatment of choice. Porocarcinoma has a high risk of lymphatic spread, and cutaneous satellite and lymph node metastases are common. Therefore, SLN mapping and biopsy are appropriate for the staging of patients with porocarcinoma. Among distal sites of metastasis, the lung is often involved.

DUCTAL (ECCRINE OR APOCRINE) ADENOCARCINOMA (DE NOVO OR ARISING IN ASSOCIATION WITH AN ADENOMA)

Clinical Findings

The tumors typically manifest as a solitary nodule in the head and neck region or extremities of elderly individuals. Carcinomas ex adenomas usually manifest with a history of a longstanding nodule with a recent change in size and appearance.

Histopathologic Features

The tumors show an infiltrative silhouette (Fig. 12.72), usually involve the mid and deep dermis, and often extend into the subcutis. Focal connection to the epidermis, as well as intraepidermal pagetoid spread of tumor cells, may be present. The growth pattern may be tubular, cribriform, papillary, solid, or a mixture thereof (Fig. 12.72). The nuclear features are usually comparable to the intermediate nuclear grade of mammary duct carcinomas, but lower- and high-grade nuclear features may also be present. Apocrine duct carcinoma tends to show more abundant eosinophilic cytoplasm (Fig. 12.73) than eccrine carcinoma. Clear-cell changes may be present and predominate on occasion. Squamous metaplasia may also occur but is usually focal. The tumor stroma is sometimes at least focally sclerotic or hyalinized. The carcinoma may be associated with a concurrent or preceding precursor lesion (adenoma, not otherwise specified, or a specific adenoma, such as spiradenoma or cylindroma) (Figs. 12.74 and 12.75).

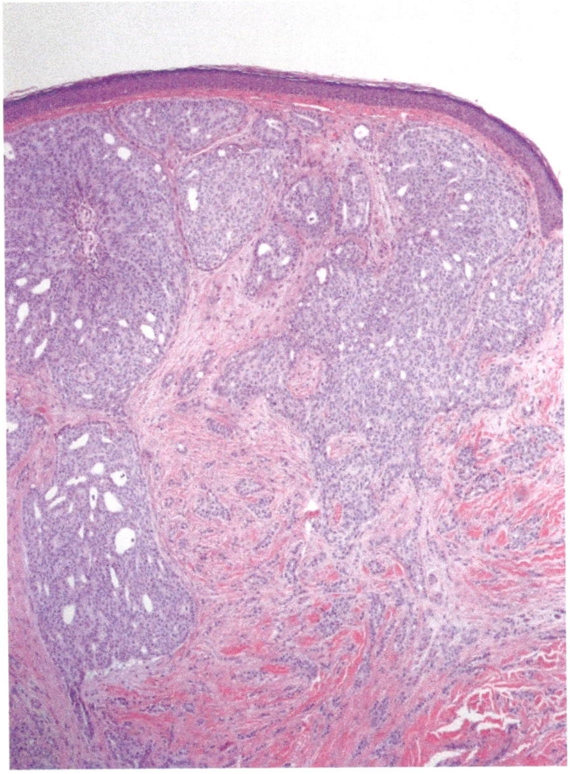

FIG. 12.72

Ductal carcinoma. Invasive adenocarcinoma with cribriform and tubular growth patterns.

Ancillary Studies

The tumor cells are immunopositive for Cam5.2 antigens, CK7, and variably for estrogen receptor (ER) and progesterone receptor (PR).

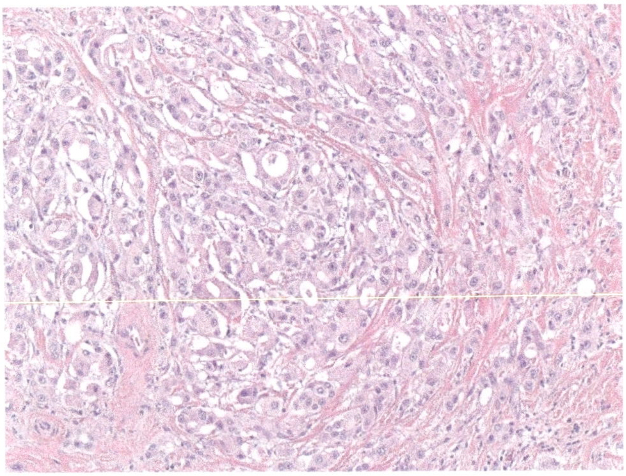

FIG. 12.73

Apocrine duct carcinoma. The tumor cells of this invasive adenocarcinoma display abundant pink cytoplasm.

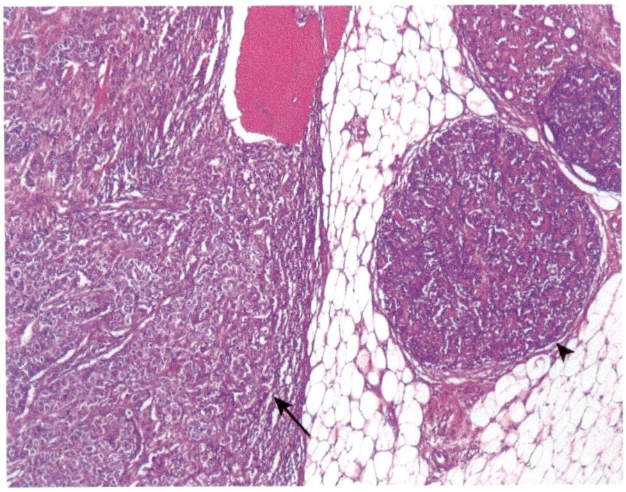

FIG. 12.74

Carcinoma ex spiradenoma. A poorly differentiated adenocarcinoma *(arrow)* is seen adjacent to a spiradenoma *(arrowhead)*.

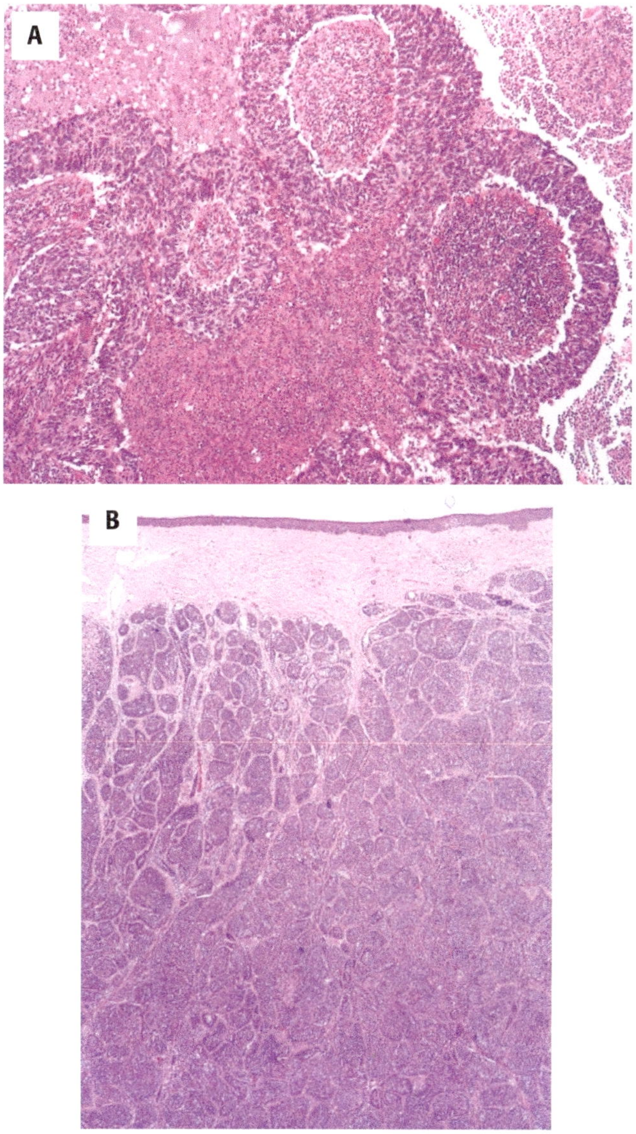

FIG. 12.75

Carcinoma ex cylindroma. A poorly differentiated adenocarcinoma is present (**A**) adjacent to nodule of cylindroma (**B**).

Differential Diagnosis

Ductal adenocarcinoma of sweat gland or duct origin must be distinguished from benign adenoma, and adenocarcinoma of extracutaneous sites metastatic to the skin. The distinction from adenoma is usually straightforward with an adequate biopsy sample, because of the presence of an infiltrative silhouette and cytologic atypia. Although a ductal eccrine or apocrine carcinoma can be readily identified as a primary sweat gland neoplasm if there is an associated precursor, it can be difficult or impossible to distinguish it from a metastasis without detailed clinical information. Immunohistochemistry does not allow a reliable distinction between sweat gland and mammary carcinoma. However, it may be helpful to distinguish sweat gland from others; that is, nonmammary extracutaneous adenocarcinomas, such as lung (positive for TTF-1) and colon (positive for CK20).

The histopathologic distinction of ductal adenocarcinoma not otherwise specified from other sweat gland carcinomas with ductal differentiation, such as hidradenocarcinoma or aggressive papillary digital adenocarcinoma, can be problematic. Diagnosis can be straightforward for well-differentiated tumors, but difficult or even impossible for more poorly differentiated carcinomas.

Prognosis and Treatment

Ductal eccrine or apocrine carcinomas tend to be high-grade adenocarcinomas with significant risk for lymph nodes and distant metastases. Surgical excision is needed. SLN mapping and biopsy are worth considering for staging for larger more aggressive appearing tumors. Individuals with metastatic ductal carcinomas may be treated analogously to patients with mammary carcinoma, and it is worth testing tumor tissue for receptors (ER, PR, Her2Neu).

DIGITAL PAPILLARY ADENOCARCINOMA

Clinical Findings

The tumor usually presents as a solitary mass in middle-aged men on the distal extremities, predominantly affecting the fingers and toes.

Histopathologic Features

The tumor usually involves both the dermis and the subcutis. It is composed of epithelial and myoepithelial elements. The silhouette of the lesion may be nodular or infiltrative. There is usually a combination of solid, solid cystic, cribriform, and tubular growth patterns (Fig. 12.76). Papillary projections into luminal spaces are common but occasionally are rare or absent. The stroma may be variably fibrotic. The spectrum of histopathologic appearances ranges from obvious carcinoma to adenoma-like tumors.

Differential Diagnosis

Digital papillary adenocarcinoma needs to be distinguished from a range of benign adnexal tumors that may affect the digits, such as poromas, tubular adenoma, hidradenomas, or cystadenomas.

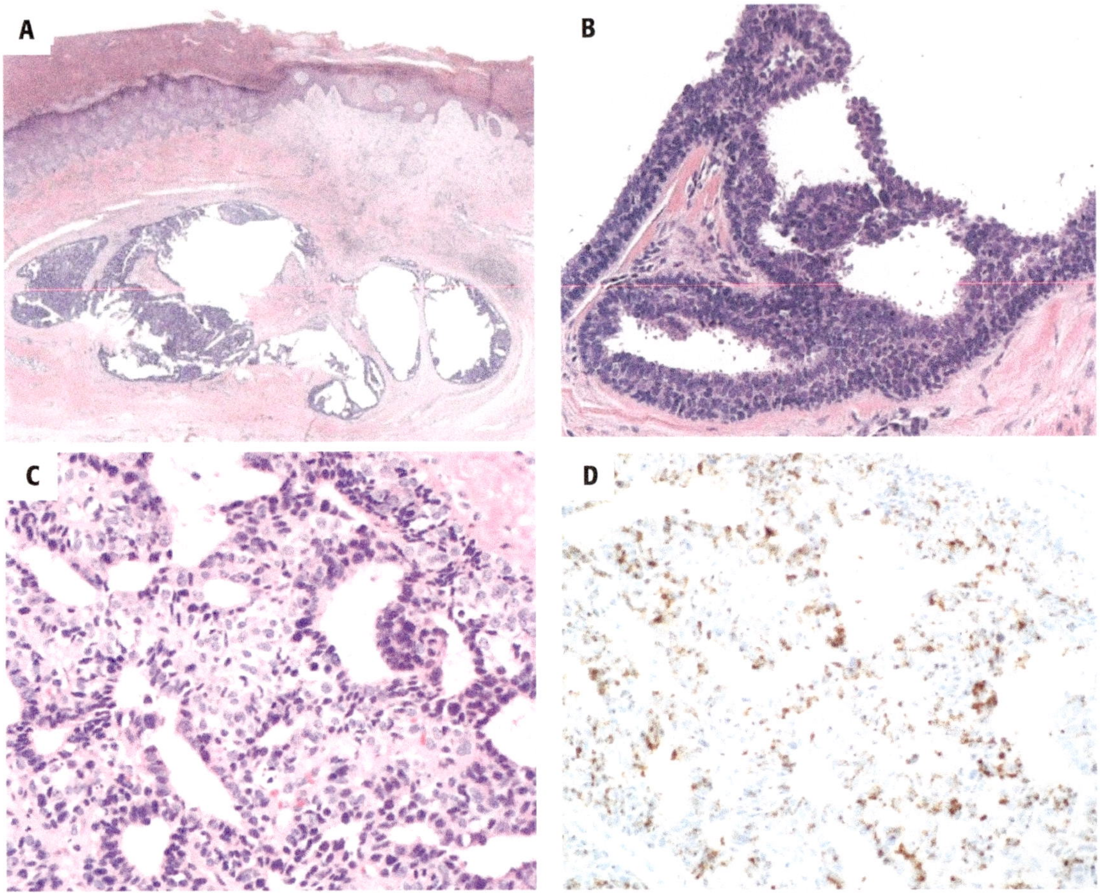

FIG. 12.76

Digital papillary adenocarcinoma. **A,** Nodulocystic tumor in dermis. **B,** Papillae are present. **C,** Tubular duct epithelial structures are associated with many myoepithelial cells, some of which show clear cell features. **D,** In situ hybridization for HPV42 is positive in the tumor cells.

Ancillary Studies

If the distinction is difficult, because of a partial biopsy and overlapping microscopic findings, ancillary studies may help. The vast majority of digital papillary adenocarcinomas are positive for HPV42 by in situ hybridization. Detection of distinct genomic aberrations, such as a *YAP1::NUTM1* or a MAML2-rearrangement by FISH or RNA sequence analysis, can help support the diagnosis of a suspected acral poroma (poroid hidradenoma) or nodular hidradenoma. For some poroid neoplasms, positive immunoreactivity for NUT may also be used as evidence against a digital papillary adenocarcinoma.

Prognosis and Treatment

Because of the high rate of recurrence of incompletely excised tumors and the possibility of metastasis, complete surgical excision is recommended for digital papillary adenocarcinomas. SLN biopsy has been found to be useful for staging and prognosis.

HIDRADENOCARCINOMA

Clinical Findings

The majority of tumors occur in the head and neck region or extremities as flesh-colored or reddish nodules. Larger tumors are often ulcerated.

HIDRADENOCARCINOMA—DISEASE FACT SHEET

Patient Group

- Usually older patients

Site of Involvement

- Predilection for head and neck

Prognosis and Treatment

- Low-grade carcinoma: may recur locally
- High-grade carcinoma: risk for metastases to lymph nodes and lung
- Surgical excision and staging by sentinel lymph node mapping

Histopathologic Features

The morphologic spectrum ranges from low-grade tumors (Fig. 12.77) with some features of a nodulocystic hidradenoma except for an infiltrative growth pattern, to obvious high-grade carcinomas with marked atypia, necrosis, and many mitotic figures (Fig. 12.78). The proportions of clear-cell changes, basaloid features, apocrine differentiation, or squamous metaplasia are highly variable.

HIDRADENOCARCINOMA—PATHOLOGIC FEATURES

Histopathologic Features

Carcinoma ex Hidradenoma

- Invasive carcinoma associated with typical hidradenoma

Carcinoma with No Recognizable Precursor Lesion

- Features of hidradenoma (nodulocystic growth component, clear-cell changes, myoepithelial component, squamous metaplasia) but with stroma infiltrative growth pattern or atypia (low- and high-grade variants depending on level of atypia)

Ancillary Studies

- Tumor cells express epithelial markers, with at least focal expression of ductal markers
- FISH for MAML2 rearrangement or RNA sequence analysis for gene fusion

Differential Diagnosis

- Benign hidradenoma (circumscribed growth)
- Porocarcinoma (associated poroma; YAP1, NUTM1 fusions) or digital papillary adenocarcinoma (positive for HPV42)

Differential Diagnosis

Hidradenocarcinoma may be confused with porocarcinoma; trichilemmal carcinoma; and squamous cell, sebaceous, or metastatic carcinoma. The presence of an associated hidradenoma or well-developed hidradenomatous appearance (nodulocystic growth pattern with clear-cell changes) helps distinguish it from a porocarcinoma. The presence of ductal structures distinguishes it from trichilemmal and SCC. The presence of cytoplasmic glycogen separates it from sebaceous carcinoma. Clinical history is most important to avoid confusion with a metastatic tumor. The fact that poro- and hidradenocarcinomas are associated with distinct genomic aberrations can be used for diagnostic purposes.

Prognosis and Treatment

Pleomorphic hidradenocarcinomas are high-grade tumors with risk for nodal and distant metastases (lung and bones). Surgical excision is needed, and SLN biopsy is appropriate for staging. Tumors with mild atypia simulating hidradenomas, but with an infiltrative growth pattern, tend to be less aggressive.

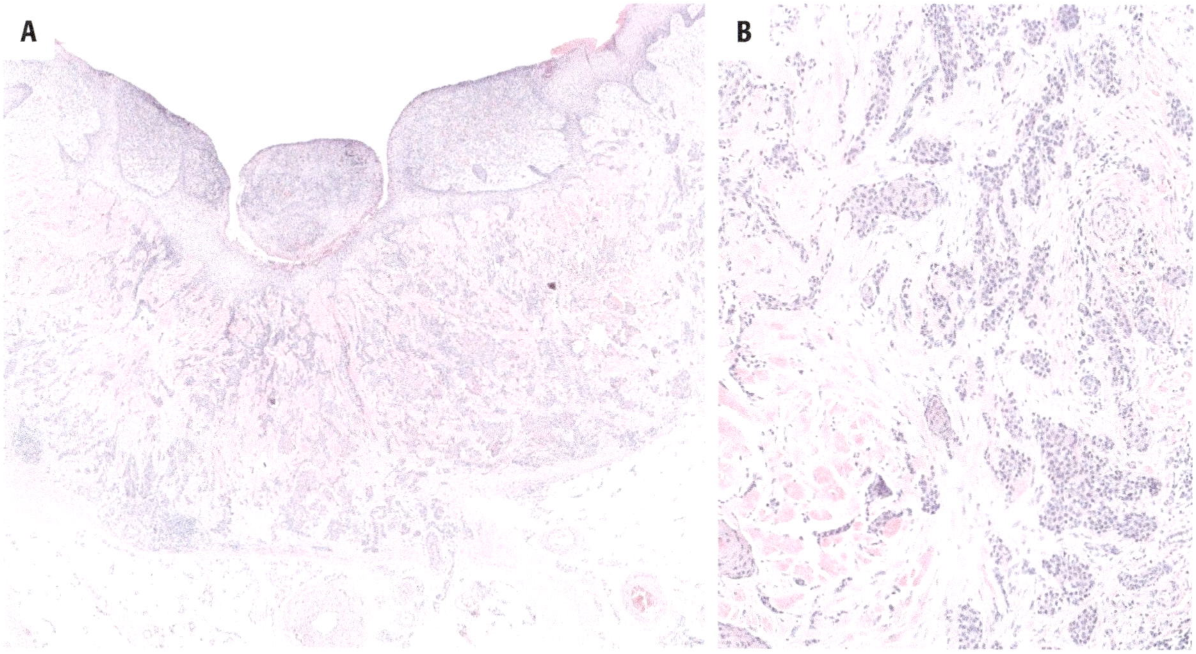

FIG. 12.77

Hidradenocarcinoma (low grade). **A**, The tumor presents as a broad plaque with infiltrative growth. **B**, The invasive tumor is composed of cords and nests of epithelial cells with basaloid and squamoid features. The tumor carried a *CRTC1::MAML2* fusion.

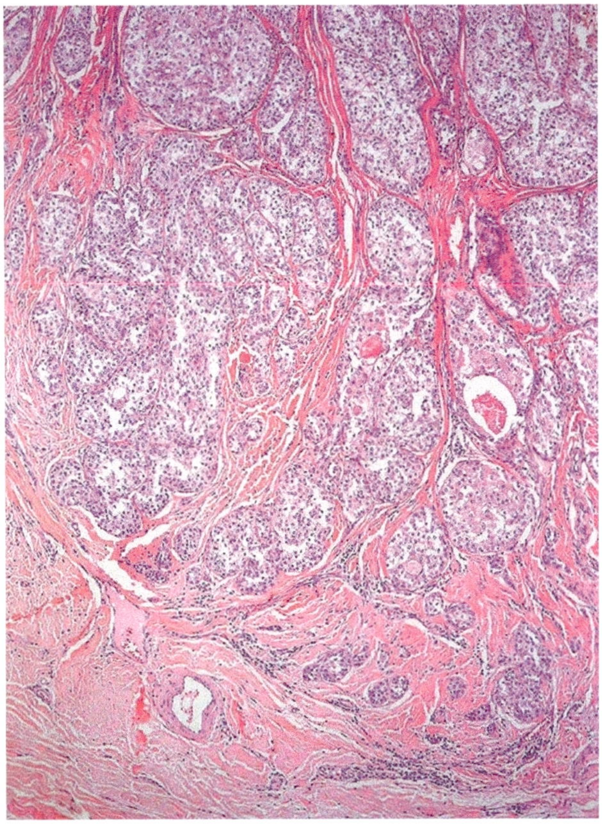

FIG. 12.78

Hidradenocarcinoma (high grade). Infiltrative adenocarcinoma with clear-cell features and marked atypia.

CRIBRIFORM CARCINOMA

Clinical Findings

Primary cutaneous apocrine cribriform carcinoma is a rare, primarily dermal neoplasm, more common in women in the fifth decade of life, mainly on the extremities, and measuring 1 to 3 cm.

Histopathologic Features

These are circumscribed, but nonencapsulated lesions composed of multiple, interconnected clusters of basaloid cells, with focal apocrine decapitation. Nuclei are large and pleomorphic. Tumor cells are arranged around small, open areas (i.e., cribriform pattern), throughout most of the lesion (Fig. 12.79).

Differential Diagnosis

The main differential diagnosis is with adenoid cystic carcinoma. Cribriform carcinoma has a more pinkish (less basaloid appearance) and lacks basement membrane material and perineural invasion. It is cytologically bland and mitoses are rare. In contrast to adenoid cystic carcinoma, it lacks myoepithelial elements. Rarely, there are metastases of carcinomas from other organs with cribriform patterns, such as the breast and salivary gland. They usually display a higher degree of atypia and mitoses. Clinicopathologic correlation will be necessary in such instances.

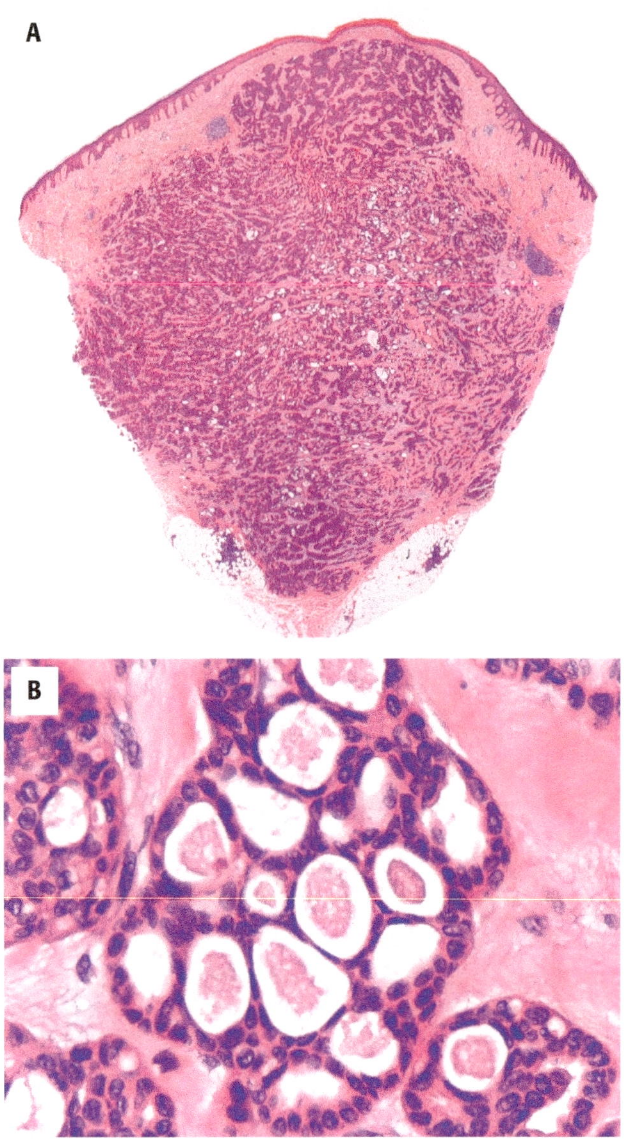

FIG. 12.79

Cribriform carcinoma. **A,** Relatively circumscribed lesion in the dermis. **B,** Notice the cribriform pattern and the focal apocrine differentiation. (Photographs courtesy of Dr. Luis Requena.)

Prognosis and Treatment

The cases described so far have behaved in a relatively indolent fashion, with only very rare local recurrences.

MUCINOUS ADENOCARCINOMA

Clinical Findings

Primary cutaneous mucinous apocrine carcinoma usually presents as a solitary papule, nodule, or plaque, typically affecting middle-aged or elderly individuals. It may occur anywhere but has a predilection to involve the head and neck region, in particular the eyelids and scalp. The tumors are usually slow growing.

Histopathologic Features

There is usually a mass rich in mucinous stroma involving the dermis and/or subcutis. Characteristically, well-differentiated tumor cells float in pools of mucin (Fig. 12.80). Pure mucinous carcinomas are mucin-rich and cell-poor throughout the entire mass. The nuclear grade of the tumor cells is low. As with mammary carcinoma, combined conventional and mucinous variants of sweat gland carcinomas exist, in which areas of pools of mucin with a few tumor cells coexist with solid, tubular, papillary, or cribriform growth patterns of conventional ductal adenocarcinoma with minimal or no mucinous stroma (Fig. 12.81). The nuclear grade of combined tumors is usually higher than that of pure tumors.

MUCINOUS CARCINOMA—DISEASE FACT SHEET

Patient Group

- Usually in elderly patients
- Male:female ratio, 3:2

Site of Involvement

- Most often in head and neck region, especially eyelids and scalp
- May occur at any site with apocrine glands

Clinical Findings

- Papule or nodule

Prognosis and Treatment

- Pure mucinous carcinomas are usually low-grade tumors
- Mixed mucinous carcinomas can metastasize

Differential Diagnosis

The main differential diagnosis is with mucinous adenocarcinoma metastatic to the skin. The two most common origins are the breast and gastrointestinal tract. Because of the similarities in morphology and immunohistochemical features, clinicopathologic correlation is essential in establishing the correct diagnosis. Both mucinous carcinomas of mammary and sweat gland origin tend to be strongly positive for CK7, ER, and PR.

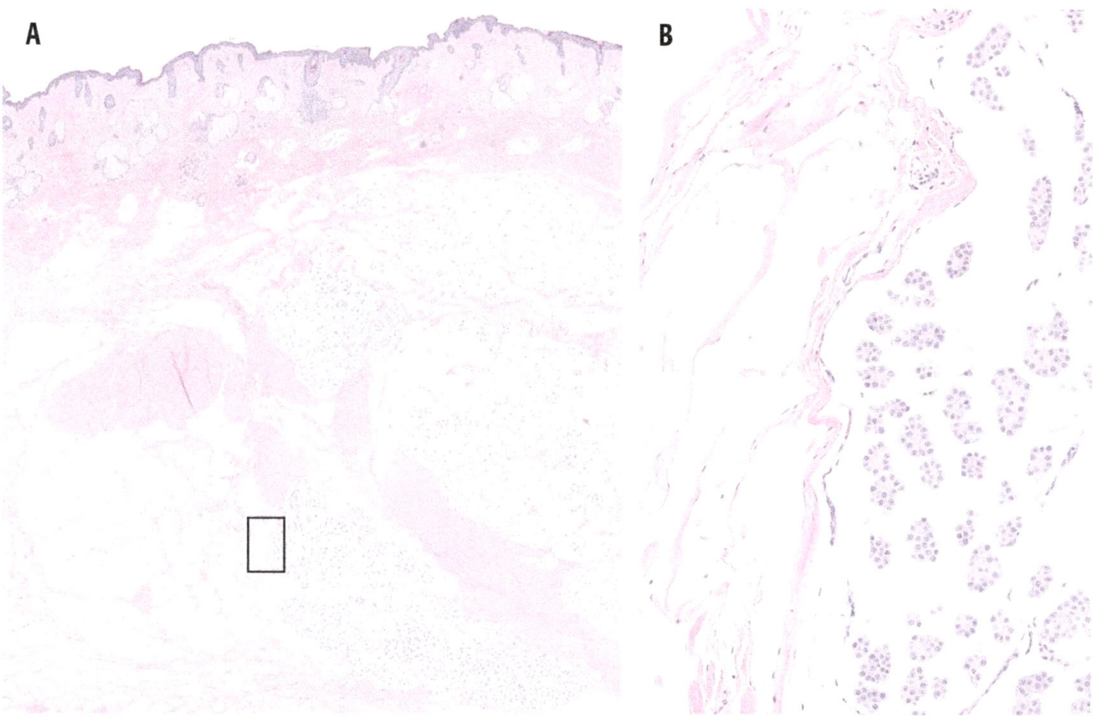

FIG. 12.80

Mucinous carcinoma. **A**, A tumor mass with abundant mucin and few tumor cells is present in the subcutis (stroma-rich, cell-poor). **B**, Bland epithelial tumor cells are seen in pools of mucin.

MUCINOUS CARCINOMA—PATHOLOGIC FEATURES

Histologic Features

- Pure mucinous carcinoma
  - Cytologically bland epithelial cells set in pools of mucin throughout the entire tumor
- Mixed or combined mucinous carcinoma
  - Part of the tumor looks like a pure mucinous carcinoma
  - Part of the tumor has a solid or tubular growth pattern with minimal if any mucin; it is often associated with more atypia and/or mitoses

Immunophenotype

- Positive for CK7, BR-2, CEA, Gata 3, p63
- Commonly positive for ER and PR
- Negative for TTF1, CK20

Differential Diagnosis

- Metastatic mucinous carcinoma from an extracutaneous primary (e.g., breast or stomach)

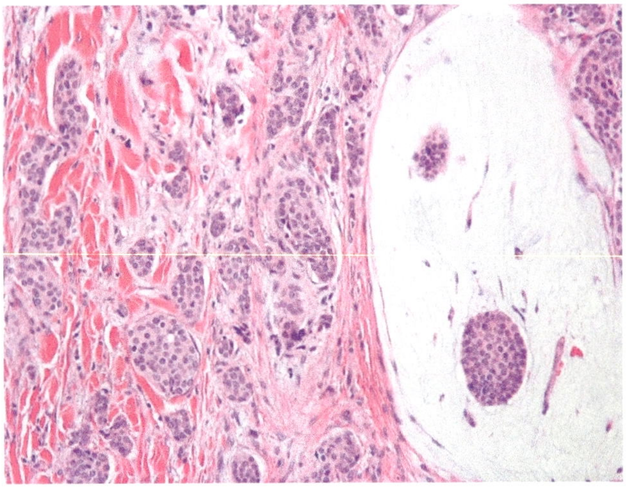

FIG. 12.81
Combined mucinous and conventional adenocarcinoma.

In a woman, metastatic mucinous mammary carcinoma is the leading concern. Metastases from mucinous breast tumors usually occur in the setting of a known primary breast cancer.

Prognosis and Treatment

This lesion has a tendency for recurrence. Metastases are very rare. If a primary cutaneous mucinous apocrine carcinoma metastasizes, it is usually a combined or mixed carcinoma with a nonmucinous component. We do not think that SLN biopsy is indicated for pure mucinous carcinomas, but it is worth considering as a staging procedure for tumors with a prominent nonmucinous component.

ENDOCRINE MUCIN-PRODUCING SWEAT GLAND CARCINOMA

This lesion is considered to be part of the spectrum of ductal lesions with mucinous stroma, with mucinous carcinoma representing the end with the most mucinous stroma.

Clinical Findings

This rare, low-grade sweat gland adenocarcinoma presents as a solitary, slow-growing plaque or cystic nodule, most often around the eyelid region in elderly women.

Histologic Features

It is relatively circumscribed, multinodular, with papillary and cribriform areas (Fig. 12.82). There is intra- or extracellular mucin deposition (or both). Cells are uniform, small- to medium-sized, and oval, with lightly eosinophilic to bluish cytoplasm (Fig. 12.83). Nuclei show neuroendocrine features (salt-and-pepper chromatin with inconspicuous nucleoli). Immunohistochemically, there is expression of CK7, estrogen, and progesterone receptors, as well as chromogranin and synaptophysin.

Differential Diagnosis

Endocrine mucin-producing sweat gland carcinoma may be confused with BCC or metastatic adenocarcinoma.

Prognosis and Treatment

Endocrine mucin-producing sweat gland carcinoma may occasionally recur, although distant metastases have not been reported so far.

EXTRAMAMMARY PAGET'S DISEASE

Paget's disease in general is an intraepidermal adenocarcinoma. Most lesions occurring on the breast represent colonization of the epidermis by mammary duct carcinoma (classic mammary Paget's disease). At extramammary sites, the presence of intraepidermal adenocarcinoma may represent a primary sweat gland carcinoma (extramammary Paget's disease [EPD]).

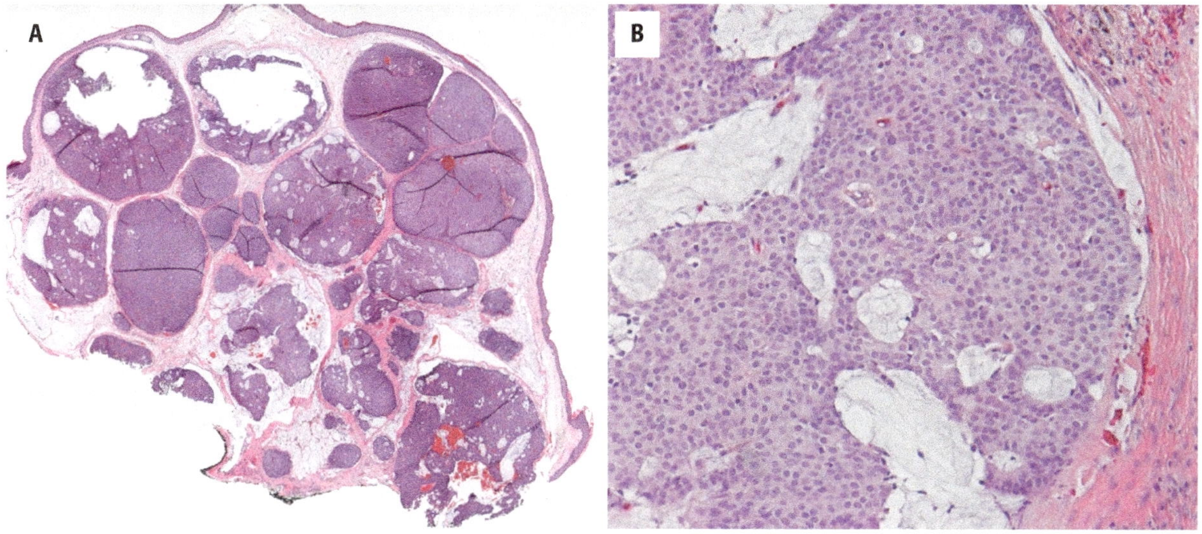

FIG. 12.82

Endocrine mucin-producing sweat gland carcinoma. **A,** Multinodular and focally nodulocystic basaloid tumor with mucin. **B,** Tumor cells with solid and cribriform growth pattern and low-grade nuclear features associated with mucin.

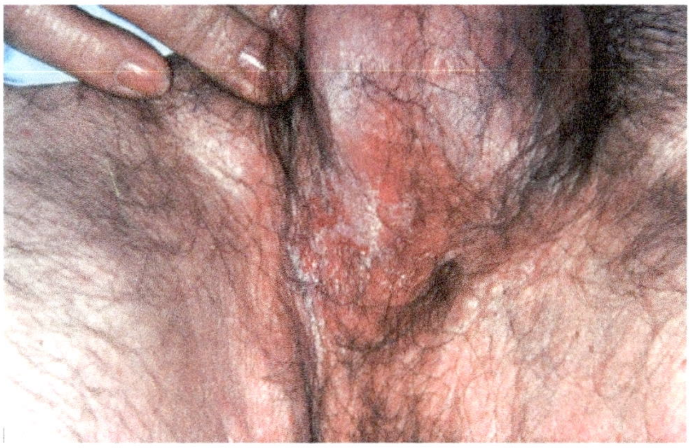

FIG. 12.83

Extramammary Paget's disease. Erythematous erosive changes of the scrotum and surrounding skin.

EXTRAMAMMARY PAGET'S DISEASE—DISEASE FACT SHEET

Patient Group
- Elderly adults

Site of Involvement
- Genital and perianal region
- Axilla, eyelid

Clinical Findings
- Erythematous patch or plaque
- May appear eczematous

Prognosis and Treatment
- Frequent local recurrence
- Risk for metastasis if associated with invasion

EPD usually represents a primary intraepidermal or intramucosal adenocarcinoma (primary EPD). It may also occur in the form of secondary involvement of the epidermis by an underlying or adjacent adenocarcinoma (sweat glands, anorectal glands), a phenomenon similar to mammary carcinoma (secondary EPD). Approximately 75% of EPD patients do not have an identifiable underlying adenocarcinoma. Primary intraepidermal or intramucosal EPD can become invasive and metastasize.

Clinical Findings

The most common location of EPD is the anogenital region followed by the axilla. It occurs mainly in elderly individuals as red, pruritic, eczematous-appearing patches and plaques with ill-defined peripheral growth (Fig. 12.83).

EXTRAMAMMARY PAGET'S DISEASE—PATHOLOGIC FEATURES

Histopathologic Features
- Intraepidermal epithelial cells with variable (none to abundant) amounts of cytoplasmic mucin distributed in a "buckshot" pattern
- Small glandular structures within the epidermis
- Possible associated epidermal hyperplasia
- May be associated with lichenoid inflammatory reaction

Immunophenotype
- Positive for Cam5.2, often CK7, at times CK20.
- Negative for melanocytic markers

Differential Diagnosis
- Melanoma in situ
- Squamous cell carcinoma in situ
- Intraepidermal sebaceous carcinoma
- Secondary Paget's disease from nearby adenocarcinoma

Histopathologic Features

The histology of EPD shows intraepidermal adenocarcinoma (Fig. 12.84). Tumor cells are characteristically distributed in buckshot pattern as solitary units of atypical epithelioid cells at all layers of the epidermis. Cytoplasmic mucin may be readily apparent or scant (Fig. 12.85). Intraepidermal ducts or glandular structures may be present. Occasionally, melanin pigment and/or melanocytic colonization is present in association with Paget's disease (Fig. 12.86). Such cases may mimic melanoma in situ. EPD may be associated with prominent epidermal hyperplasia (Fig. 12.87). The invasive component of EPD shows a morphologic spectrum similar to that of other ductal carcinomas of sweat gland or mammary gland origin (Fig. 12.88). The invasive ductal carcinomas associated with EPD tend to be high-grade tumors. Lymphatic spread is common.

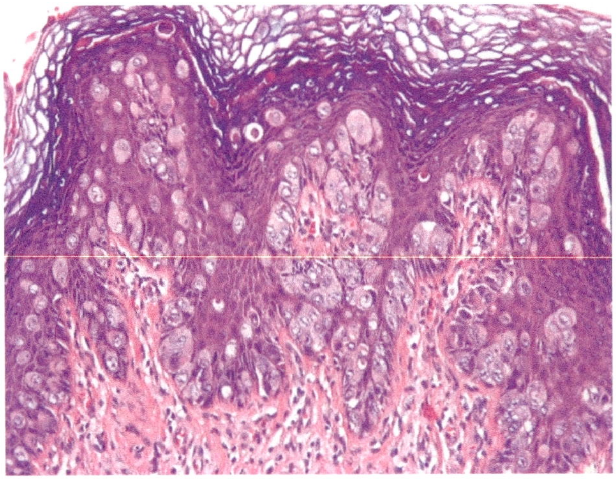

FIG. 12.84

Extramammary Paget's disease. Buckshot pattern of intraepidermal carcinoma cells.

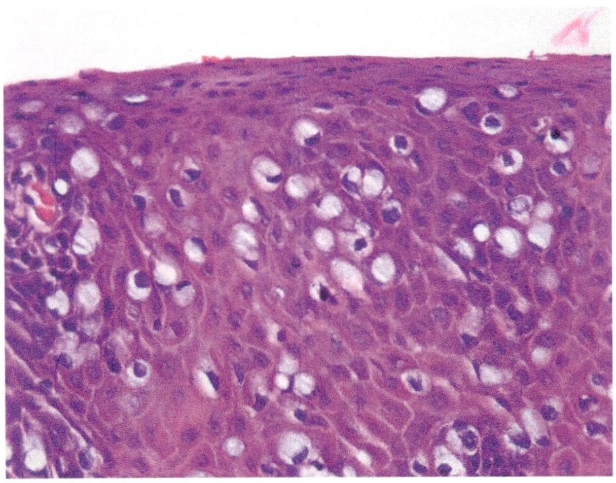

FIG. 12.85

Extramammary Paget's disease. Signet ring cells with cytoplasmic mucin.

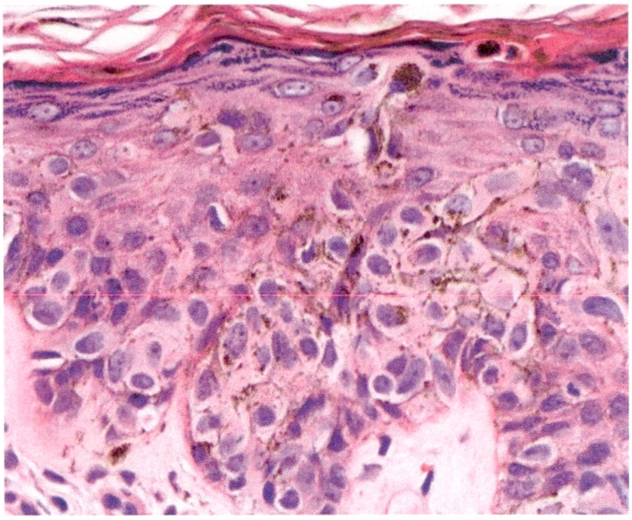

FIG. 12.86

Pigmented extramammary Paget's disease. There is an increase in melanin pigment within the epithelium.

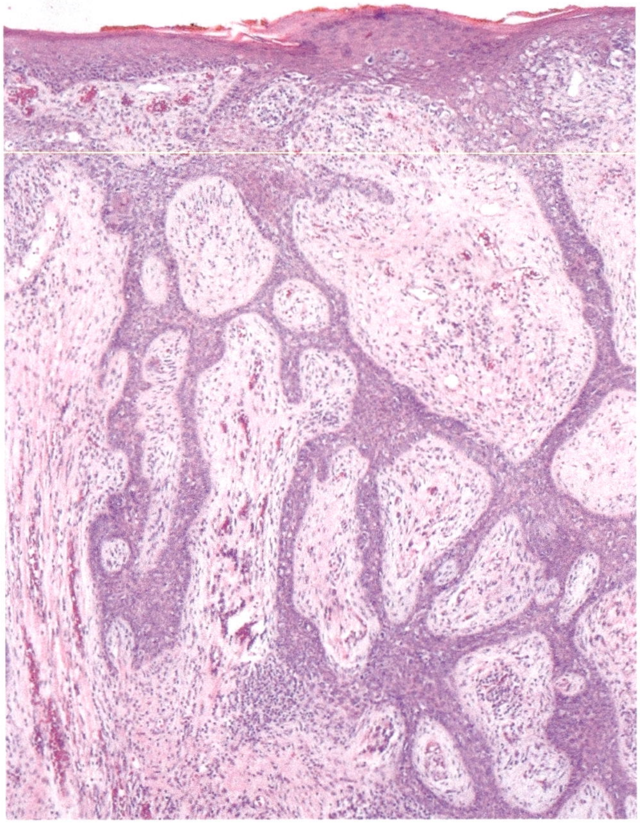

FIG. 12.87

Extramammary Paget's disease. In longstanding lesions, there may be marked epithelial hyperplasia and reactive stromal changes resulting in a fibroepitheliomatous appearance.

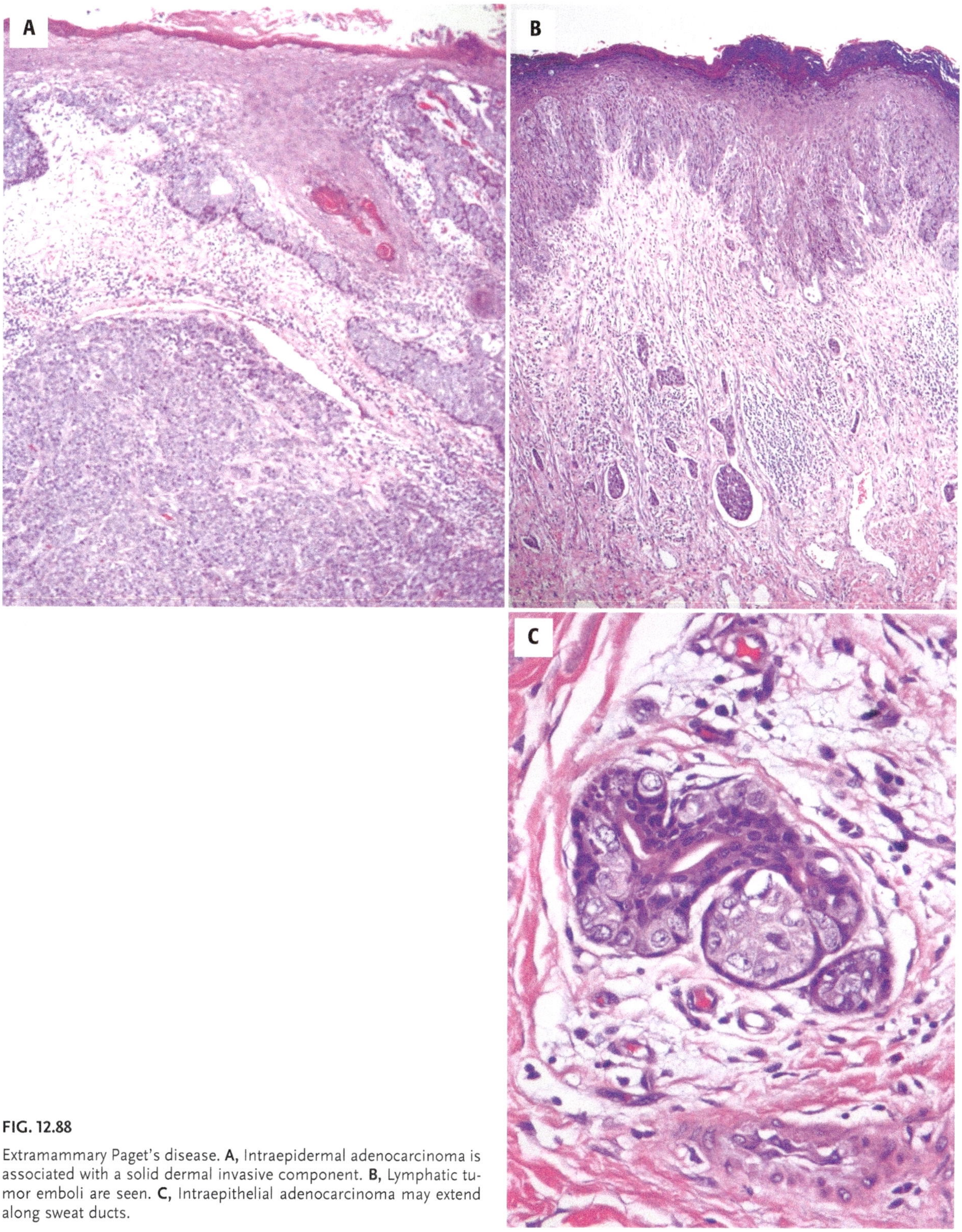

FIG. 12.88

Extramammary Paget's disease. **A,** Intraepidermal adenocarcinoma is associated with a solid dermal invasive component. **B,** Lymphatic tumor emboli are seen. **C,** Intraepithelial adenocarcinoma may extend along sweat ducts.

Ancillary Studies

The tumor cells of Paget's disease are positive for Cam5.2 (Fig. 12.89). The majority of EPD tumor cells express CK7, but some, especially in the anal region, may also express CK20. The large majority of EPD cases express also CEA, GCDFP15 (BR-2), and mucins.

Differential Diagnosis

Several intraepidermal lesions exhibit diffuse involvement by large, epithelioid cells at all layers of the epidermis (pagetoid extension). The main differential diagnosis is with melanoma and SCC (Bowen's disease). Melanocytes are readily recognized immunohistochemically by

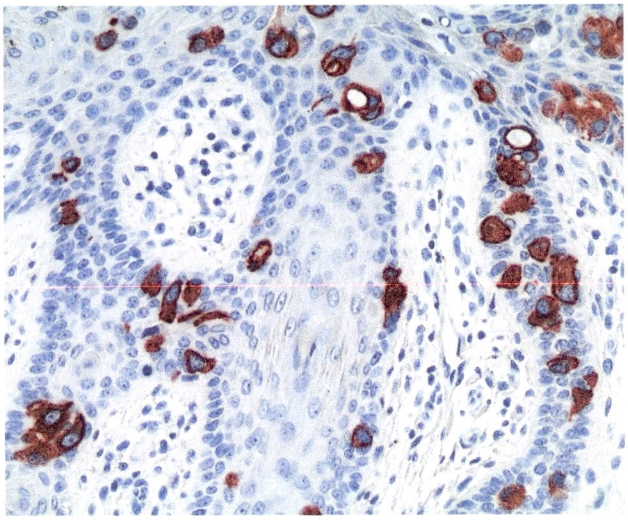

FIG. 12.89

Extramammary Paget's disease. The tumor cells are immunopositive with Cam5.2.

positive staining for Mart-1/Melan-A. SCC is usually negative with Cam5.2 but positive with AE1:AE3 or p40. Another differential diagnosis, primarily on the breast, is with Toker cells. These are large cells with clear cytoplasm located at all levels of the epidermis. Similar to EPD, Toker cells express CK7, low-molecular-weight cytokeratin, MUC1, and MUC5AC. In contrast to EPD, Toker cells show small, uniform nuclei with inconspicuous nucleoli.

Most primary EPD expresses CK7 but not CK20. However, primary anogenital EMPD may also express CK20, i.e., CK20 expression per se does not distinguish primary from secondary EMPD in the anogenital region.

Prognosis and Treatment

A significant number of cases of EPD recur after surgical excision. Some authors suggest using frozen sections (standard or Mohs surgery) to map the extension of EPD cells. The extent of the tumor is often underestimated clinically. Preoperative mapping of the area involved by tumor by taking several punch or shave biopsies helps to optimize the chances of obtaining a negative surgical margin. Invasive EPD has the potential to metastasize. Sentinel node biopsy may be considered as a staging tool but only for stromal-invasive tumors.

ADENOID CYSTIC CARCINOMA

Clinical Findings

This rare tumor most commonly occurs on the scalp and trunk.

Histopathologic Features

This lesion is identical to that seen in the salivary glands: cords and nests of basaloid cells with cribriform pattern containing mucinous or hyaline cylinders (Figs. 12.90 and 12.91). Well-formed glands are not prominent. Two layers of epithelium often surround ductal lumina (epithelial and myoepithelial cells). Perineural invasion may be present.

Ancillary Studies

The tumor cells of adenoid cystic carcinoma typically contain a glandular epithelial subpopulation, which is immunoreactive for CK7. Associated myoepithelial cells stain for SOX10 or p63. Other markers typically positive in adenoid cystic carcinomas include CD117 and EMA. Since many tumors are associated with MYB aberrations, immunohistochemistry or in situ hybridization of MYB can also be used in select cases to support the diagnosis.

Differential Diagnosis

Adenoid cystic carcinoma may be confused with an adenoidal variant of BCC. Clefts and the fibromyxoid stroma, which are commonly features of BCC, are uncommon in adenoid cystic carcinoma. BCC also differs from adenoid cystic carcinoma by possible epidermal connections (features of superficial BCC), infundibulocystic differentiation, and more frequent apoptotic bodies. Adenoid cystic carcinoma shows more, well-developed, ductal structures. Cylinders of myxoid or hyaline material are characteristic. In difficult cases, immunohistochemistry

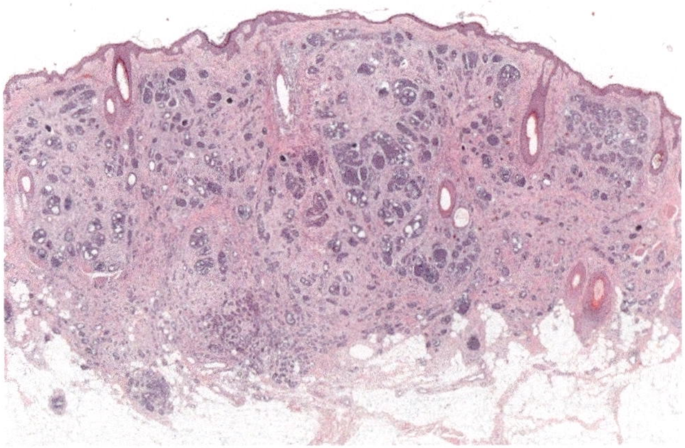

FIG. 12.90

Adenoid cystic carcinoma. Silhouette of infiltrative basaloid tumor in dermis and superficial subcutis.

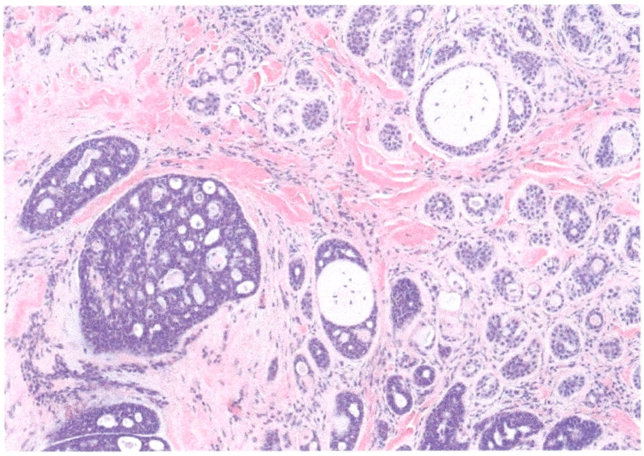

FIG. 12.91

Adenoid cystic carcinoma. Cribriform and tubular growth pattern with mucinous cylinders and focal pink hyaline material.

may be helpful or the documentation of a gene fusion (*MYB::NFIB*). In contrast with BCC, adenoid cystic carcinomas commonly stain for CK7 and EMA.

Prognosis and Treatment

Cutaneous adenoid cystic carcinoma generally behaves like a low-grade tumor, with potential for local recurrence. Metastases are exceedingly rare. Surgical excision is needed. Staging by sentinel node mapping and biopsy is not necessary.

HYALINIZING CLEAR-CELL CARCINOMA

Clinical Findings

Hyalinizing clear-cell carcinoma usually affects the minor salivary glands but can also rarely present as a skin tumor.

Histopathologic Features

Characteristically, the tumor is composed of tumor cells with pale to clear-cell cytoplasm dispersed as nests or cords in a hyalinized stroma (Fig. 12.92). The tumor is associated with a *EWSR1::ATF1* fusion.

Prognosis and Treatment

The tumor usually behaves as a low-grade neoplasm. Surgery is the treatment of choice.

SECRETORY CARCINOMA

Clinical Findings

Secretory carcinoma was first reported in the breast but can also affect salivary glands and skin.

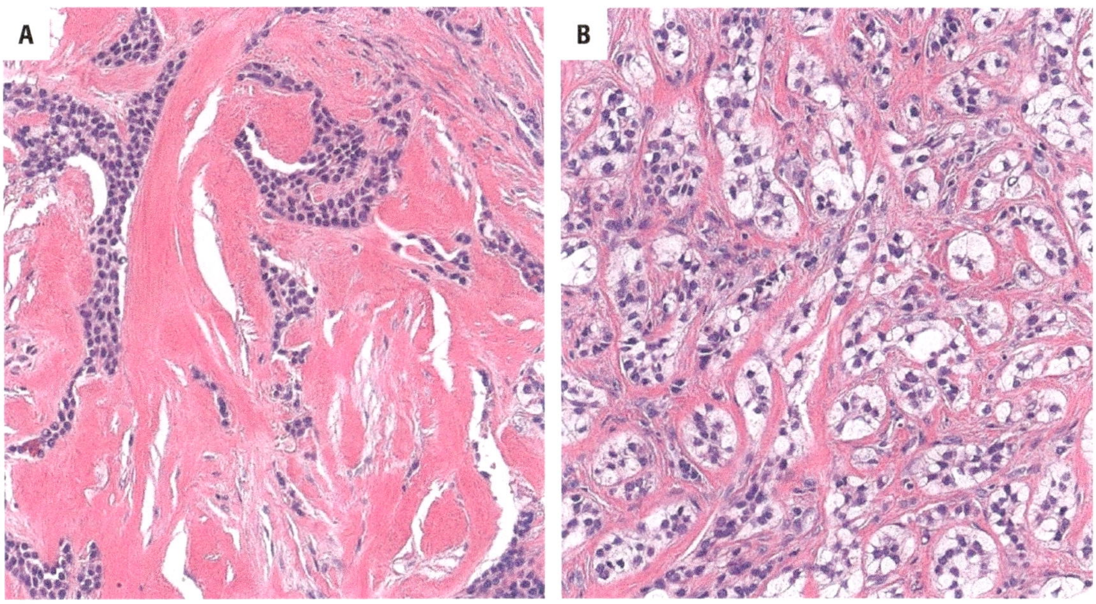

FIG. 12.92

Hyalinizing clear-cell carcinoma. **A,** Cords of basaloid tumor cells are seen in a hyalinized stroma. **B,** In other parts of the tumor, nests of clear cells were seen. The tumor had a *EWSR11::ATF1* fusion.

Histopathologic Features

The tumors may display a nodular or noduloinfiltrative growth. Within tumor nodules one may find solid, macro- and/or microcystic, tubular, follicular, or papillary architectures. The tumor cells are eosinophilic to pale and typically display vacuolated cytoplasm and monomorphic round to oval nuclei. Secretory (pink or mucinous) material is typically seen in the lumina of tubular or cystic structures (Fig. 12.93).

Ancillary Methods

The tumor cells are immunohistochemically positive for Ck7, Gata3, S100, SOX10, and pan-TRK. FISH or molecular studies can be used to document as associated gene fusion (most often involving *ETV6::NTRK3*).

Prognosis and Treatment

Secretory carcinoma of the skin is considered a low-grade neoplasm. Surgery is the treatment of choice.

MICROSECRETORY CARCINOMA

Microsecretory carcinoma is a relatively new category of salivary gland tumors, for which cutaneous analogs have

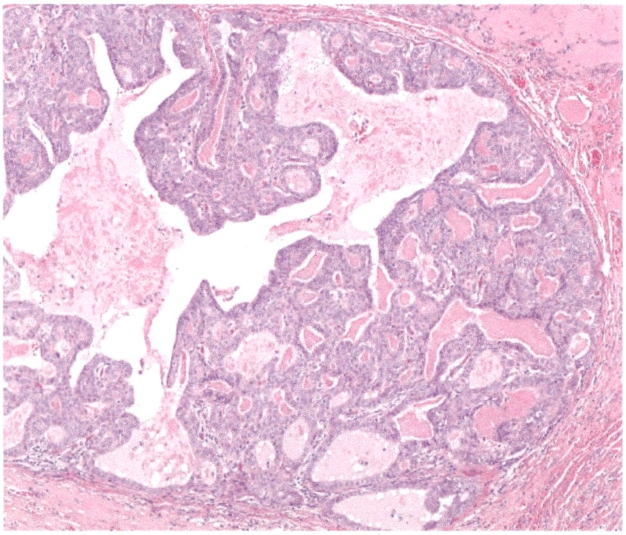

FIG. 12.93

Secretory carcinoma. There is a nodulocystic tumor with cribriform growth, low-grade atypia, and vacuolae rimming intraluminal secretory material.

also been reported. They display a microcystic growth pattern, stain for SOX10, and carry an MDF2C;;SS18 gene fusion. Among the reported cases, most are felt to be low-grade carcinoma, but a rare case with high-grade transformation has also been published.

CARCINOSARCOMA

Rare dermal and subcutaneous tumors of probable sweat gland origin show combined features of ductal adenocarcinoma and sarcoma. The sarcomatous component may show fibrous, cartilaginous, osseous, fatty, skeletal, or smooth muscle differentiation. Carcinosarcomas of sweat gland origin are thought to be high-grade malignant tumors.

MALIGNANT MIXED TUMOR

Clinical Findings

This is very rare tumor usually affects the extremities or head and neck region of an elderly patient.

Histopathologic Features

The diagnosis is best made when a histopathologically clearly malignant tumor (infiltrative growth pattern with cytologic atypia) is found in association with a precursor lesion (residual benign mixed tumor). Often, however, an associated precursor in which the diagnosis is more difficult cannot be identified. Typically, the tumor shows a combination of a malignant epithelial proliferation with features of an adenocarcinoma with focal mucinous alterations, usually in the stroma, but occasionally also within epithelial cells. Chondroid differentiation may be present.

Ancillary Studies

The tumor cells express cytokeratins and S100 protein. Positive staining for 4A4/p63 is common. Labeling for SMA or calponin may also occur.

Differential Diagnosis

In the absence of an associated precursor (benign mixed tumor), malignant mixed tumor may be confused with other tumors with a myxoid matrix, such as extraskeletal myxoid chondrosarcoma or epithelioid malignant peripheral nerve sheath tumor (MPNST). The distinction from chondrosarcoma is readily made by ancillary studies because the latter are immunonegative for cytokeratins and carry a characteristic translocation [t(9;22)]. Epithelioid MPNSTs are typically subcutaneous, more deeply located, and often associated with a nerve trunk and/or loss of INI1. In malignant mixed tumor, only the epithelium is malignant; in contrast, carcinosarcoma shows malignant features in both the epithelial and stromal components. Malignant mixed tumor shows overlap with myoepithelial carcinoma. We restrict the latter term for tumors entirely or predominantly composed of myoepithelial cells.

Prognosis and Treatment

Surgical excision is the treatment of choice. Most malignant mixed tumors are high-grade neoplasms with a propensity for spread to lymph nodes, lungs, and bone.

MALIGNANT MYOEPITHELIAL NEOPLASM

This rare tumor is histopathologically characterized by an infiltrative growth and variable degrees of cytologic atypia. Immunohistochemistry is usually necessary to document that the predominant tumor cell population shows myoepithelial differentiation (positive for S100 protein, SOX10, cytokeratins, EMA, calponin, SMA, or glial fibrillary acidic protein [GFAP])). Some pathologists distinguish low-grade from high-grade myoepithelial neoplasms. High-grade tumors are cytologically obviously malignant (pleomorphism, mitotic figures, and necrosis). Low-grade tumors show only mild atypia but have an infiltrative growth pattern. The term *myoepithelial carcinoma* may refer to nodular proliferations of "atypical" myoepithelial cells within otherwise benign mixed tumors. However, the use of the term *carcinoma* in this setting is controversial. Because such tumor nodules within an adenoma are not associated with an increased risk for recurrence or metastasis, we apply the term *carcinoma* only to myoepithelial tumors that show evidence of stromal invasion. Myxoid myoepithelial carcinomas may simulate the appearance of myxoid sarcomas.

METASTATIC SWEAT DUCT CARCINOMAS

High-grade sweat duct carcinomas frequently metastasize to regional lymph nodes, the skin, lung, and other sites. Without knowledge of the primary tumor, metastases may be confused with metastatic adenocarcinomas or adenosquamous carcinomas from extracutaneous sites.

If a patient is diagnosed with a high-grade sweat duct carcinoma, many cancer centers offer SLN mapping and biopsy for staging of patients. The workup of SLNs includes multiple (e.g., three) hematoxylin and eosin levels and at least one immunostudy for cytokeratins (Cam5.2 or CK7). Immunoprofiling of metastatic tumors for hormone receptor (ER, PR, Her2Neu) expression may be helpful for treatment protocols analogous to mammary carcinoma.

SEBACEOUS NEOPLASMS

The hallmark of all sebaceous lesions is the presence of sebocytes. They contain many lipid-rich vacuoles in their cytoplasms. On routine histology, these are seen as empty, small, clear, weblike spaces because the lipid content is dissolved during tissue processing. It is characteristic that the vacuoles impinge upon the nucleus, imparting a scalloped appearance. Although fairly characteristic, this morphology is not entirely restricted to bona fide sebaceous tumors. Other cell types, such as melanocytes (balloon-cell melanocytes), on epidermal or nonsebaceous adnexal epithelial cells, may also display on occasion clear-cell changes with weblike cytoplasms and even scalloped nuclei.

Ancillary IHC may be helpful in some cases. Strong staining with adipophilin strongly favors sebaceous differentiation. Strong positive staining with androgen receptor may also favor sebaceous differentiation, though it is less specific than adipophilin.

SEBACEOUS HYPERPLASIA

Clinical Findings

Sebaceous hyperplasia generally occurs on the face, usually in patients after 40 years of age. It rarely occurs in younger individuals. The most common locations are the forehead and cheeks as single or multiple, small, umbilicated papules. Because of their lipid content, lesions of sebaceous hyperplasia are soft and yellow.

Histopathologic Features

Sebaceous hyperplasia manifests histologically as sebaceous glands with increased numbers of sebaceous lobules, which are often enlarged. Typically, there is a dilated duct in the center of the lesion connected with the overlying epidermis, thus explaining the umbilicated clinical appearance (Fig. 12.94). Larger lesions may be composed of several hair units, containing more than one central duct opening to the epidermal surface.

Differential Diagnosis

Sebaceous hyperplasia should be distinguished from nevus sebaceus, rhinophyma, sebaceous adenoma, and carcinoma. In nevus sebaceus, there are typically associated epidermal hyperplasia, abnormally shaped hair follicles, and apocrine glands. Rhinophyma, in contrast to sebaceous hyperplasia, does not show multiple, enlarged sebaceous glands surrounding a single, dilated duct but rather has multiple hair follicles with prominent sebaceous glands. Sebaceous adenoma differs from sebaceous hyperplasia by the presence of an increased number of basaloid cells and tumorous expansion of sebaceous lobules. Sebaceous carcinoma shows atypia or an infiltrative growth pattern.

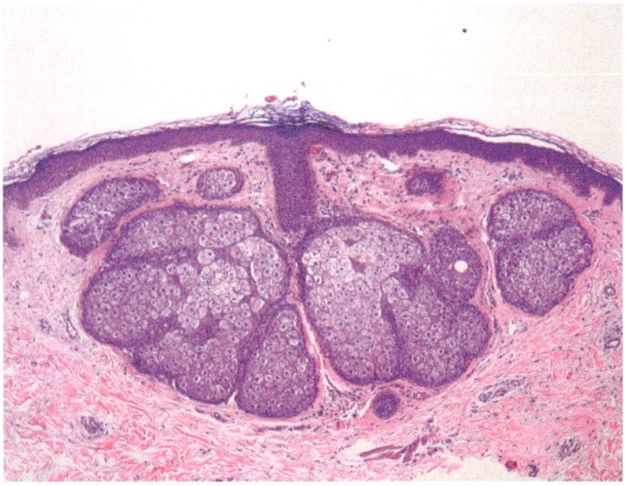

FIG. 12.94

Sebaceous hyperplasia. Multiple sebaceous lobules are associated with follicular infundibular epithelium.

Prognosis and Treatment

Sebaceous hyperplasia is a benign lesion. It is most often biopsied when it is clinically mistaken for another lesion, such as BCC. When sebaceous hyperplasia becomes a cosmetic issue, several destructive methods, such as cryotherapy, shaving, or electrodesiccation, are available.

SEBACEOUS TRICHOFOLLICULOMA (FOLLICULOSEBACEOUS CYSTIC HAMARTOMA)

Clinical Findings

Sebaceous trichofolliculoma is a well-circumscribed, solitary nodule on the face of middle-aged individuals.

Histopathologic Features

Sebaceous trichofolliculoma is composed of prominent sebaceous glands attached to a central, cystically dilated hair follicle. Rarely, hair shafts or apocrine glands are present around the cyst. The stroma is hypercellular, with spindle cells within a myxoid background very similar to the stroma of fibrofolliculoma or trichodiscoma. Because some of these lesions contain adipose or neural tissue, several authors propose to consider them as folliculosebaceous hamartomas.

Differential Diagnosis

Classic trichofolliculomas have small sebaceous glands and contain numerous hair shafts. Fibrofolliculomas show a more tortuous contour of the epithelial component. Sebaceous adenomas do not have a centrally dilated follicle.

Differential Diagnosis of Sebaceous Neoplasms

	Sebaceous Hyperplasia	Sebaceous Adenoma	Sebaceous Carcinoma
Silhouette	Noninfiltrative	Noninfiltrative	Infiltrative (solid or diffusely invasive)
Ratio of basaloid cells to sebocytes	Predominance of sebocytes	Proportional increase in basaloid cells common	Basaloid cells with atypia and mitotic figures
Atypia	Absent	Absent or mild	Present

Prognosis and Treatment

Sebaceous trichofolliculoma is a benign lesion that does not require therapy except for cosmetic reasons.

NEVUS SEBACEUS

Clinical Findings

Nevus sebaceus typically presents at birth or in early childhood as a solitary yellow-orange plaque on the scalp or face (Fig. 12.95). On hair-bearing areas, the partial or complete lack of terminal hairs within the lesion makes it particularly conspicuous. The tawny color is a gross clue to the presence of sebaceous differentiation. As with the normal sebaceous glands, the abnormal glands of nevus sebaceus are under androgenic control; thus, the lesions often become clinically more conspicuous at puberty, with development of a mammillated or pebbled surface and more intense orange hue. Lesions removed in the years before "sebarche" may show relatively small sebaceous glands.

Histopathologic Features

An increase in the number of sebaceous glands is common (Fig. 12.96). The glands may be aberrantly placed, such as inserting directly onto the epidermis rather than the hair follicle as usual. Follicles themselves may be reduced in number or abnormally shaped. The epidermis shows features of epidermal nevus with patterns varying from SK- to verruca-like hyperplasia. Another typical feature is the presence of an increased number of apocrine glands in the dermis and subcutis.

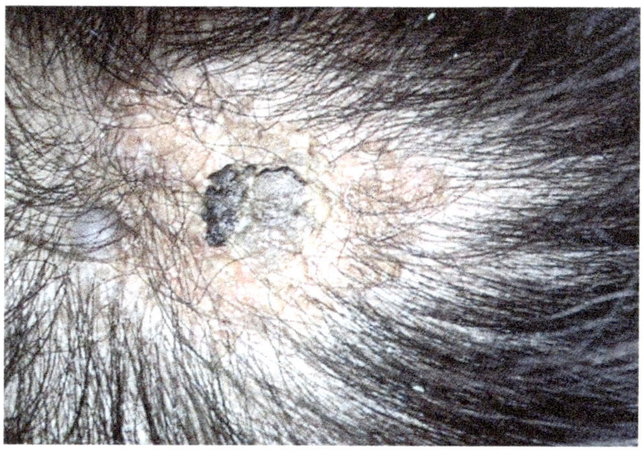

FIG. 12.95

Nevus sebaceous. Verrucous plaque on scalp.

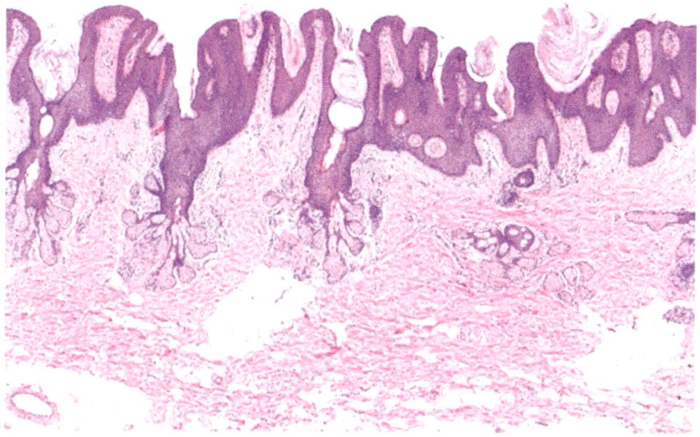

FIG. 12.96

Nevus sebaceous. Papillomatous epidermal hyperplasia overlying a dermis with altered "hamartomatous" sebaceous glands.

Secondary neoplasms may develop in association with nevus sebaceus, such as syringocystadenoma papilliferum, TBL, BCC, apocrine adenomas, or other adnexal tumors.

Prognosis and Treatment

Nevus sebaceus per se is benign. Complete surgical removal of nevus sebaceus is recommended for cosmetic reasons or to prevent development of secondary tumors.

SEBACEOUS ADENOMA

Clinical Findings

Sebaceous adenoma is a benign sebaceous tumor that usually occurs on the face of middle-aged individuals, particularly in patients with MTS. It is usually a raised papule or nodule, slightly firm, and yellow.

Histologic Features

Sebaceous adenomas are usually solid or cystic lesions, characterized by a well-circumscribed dermal growth of well-differentiated sebaceous lobules (Fig. 12.97). Generally, the number of sebocytes with vacuolated cytoplasm and scalloped nucleus predominates over the number of basaloid cells, similar to those seen at the periphery of normal sebaceous lobules. For tumors in which the proportion of basaloid cells is greater than the number of vacuolated sebocytes, some authors use the term *sebaceoma* (Fig. 12.98). Cystic sebaceous

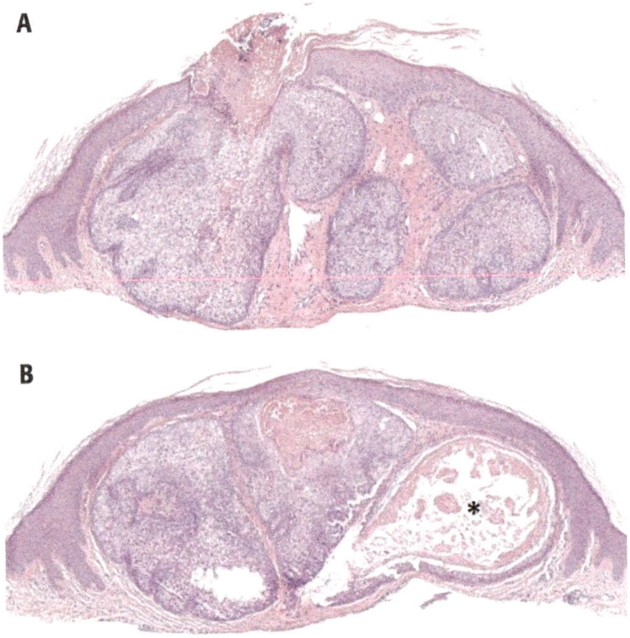

FIG. 12.97

Sebaceous adenoma. **A**, Expanded lobules of well-differentiated sebaceous epithelium directly connect to the epidermis. The cytologic features are bland. **B**, Part of this adenoma shows infundibular keratocystic features *(*)*.

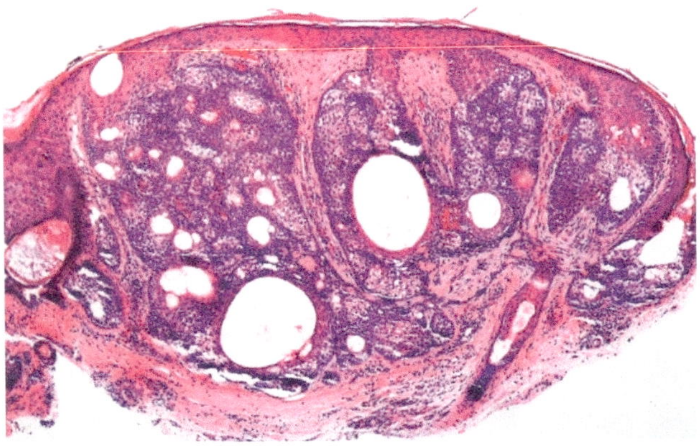

FIG. 12.98

Sebaceous adenoma. Expanded sebaceous lobules in the superficial dermis with an increase in number of basaloid cells. There is a predominance of basaloid cells. This tumor may also termed *sebaceoma.*

adenomas (Fig. 12.99) or adenomas with keratocystic features (Fig. 12.97), sometimes overlapping with keratoacanthoma, are typically associated with MTS.

Differential Diagnosis

Sebaceous adenoma is a superficial dermal tumor, which differs from sebaceous carcinoma by the lack of significant atypia or infiltrating growth.

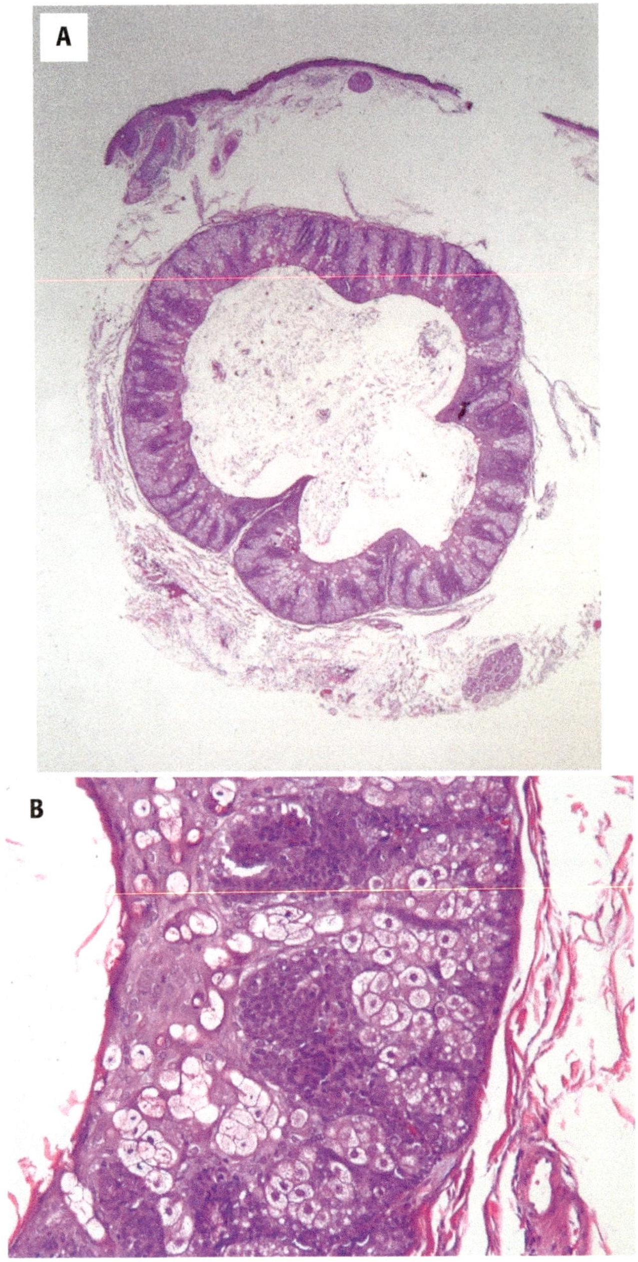

FIG. 12.99

Cystic sebaceous adenoma. **A,** Nodulocystic architecture; **B,** The tumor shows sebaceous differentiation. The cytology is bland.

Prognosis and Treatment

Sebaceous adenomas are benign tumors. They can only be distinguished from well-differentiated sebaceous carcinoma if the entire lesion is available for review to assess the growth pattern of the tumor (circumscribed or infiltrative). Therefore, superficial shave biopsies revealing a well-differentiated sebaceous tumor transected at the base require conservative, complete excision to allow a definitive diagnosis.

SEBACEOUS CARCINOMA

Clinical Findings

Sebaceous carcinoma typically occurs in elderly individuals in areas rich in sebaceous glands, such as the eyelid, ear, and other areas of the head and neck. It typically presents as a firm yellow or ulcerated reddish nodule. The tumors are generally divided into ocular and extraocular sebaceous carcinomas. Ocular sebaceous carcinomas are fairly well characterized, and some prognostic parameters have been established. By comparison, little is known about the much rarer extraocular tumors. A significant number of the latter patients have MTS.

Histopathologic Features

Sebaceous carcinomas may have an irregular diffusely or solid nodular invasive growth pattern (Figs. 12.100–12.104). They often extend into the deep reticular dermis and subcutis. Ulceration is common. The majority of tumors are composed of atypical and mitotically active basaloid cells and sebocytes with clear vacuolated cytoplasm. Usually, the proportion of basaloid cells predominates. Keratocysts, squamous metaplasia, and ductal structures are commonly present. Tumor cells may surround pools of secreted sebaceous material or keratinous debris. Depending on the proportion of typical sebocytes, sebaceous carcinomas may be classified as well, moderately, or poorly differentiated (Fig. 12.102). Squamous metaplasia may be present (Fig. 12.103). Pagetoid extension by tumor cells into the epidermis may occur (Fig. 12.104). The stroma surrounding the invasive tumor front often shows fibrosis and an inflammatory infiltrate with foreign body–type giant cells to keratinous or sebaceous material.

Ancillary Studies

Sebaceous carcinomas are immunoreactive for cytokeratins, EMA, adipophilin, and androgen receptor. The cytoplasmic vacuoles express adipophilin. The cytoplasm is also typically positive for PRAME. Particularly patients with MTS may show alterations in the expression of DNA mismatch repair enzymes (loss of nuclear staining). Commonly available IHC for mismatch repair genes include MLH1, MSH2, MSH6, and PMS2 (Fig. 12.105).

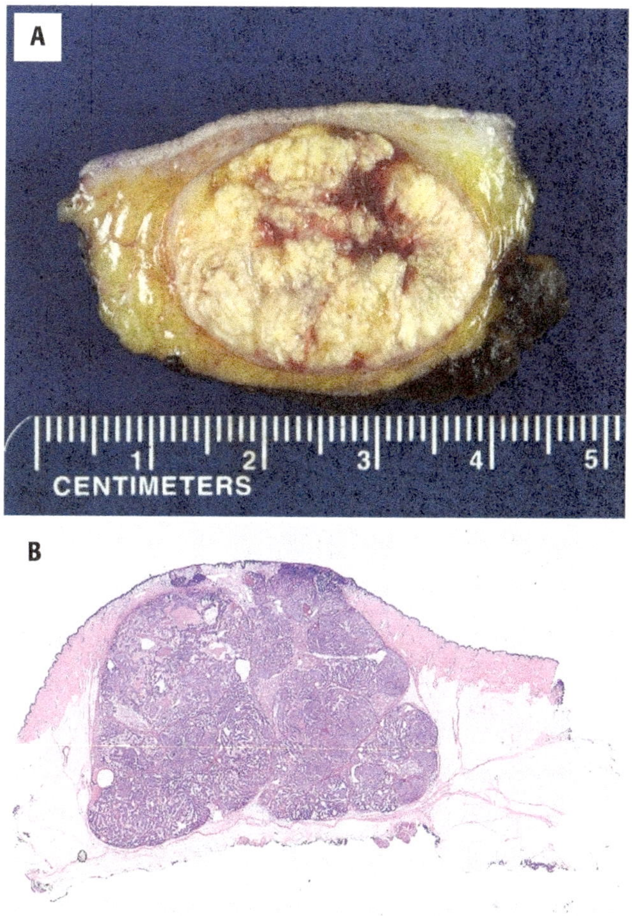

FIG. 12.100

Sebaceous carcinoma. **A,** Gross specimen. Nodular yellow tumor in dermis and subcutis. **B,** Large sebaceous tumor with a nodular silhouette.

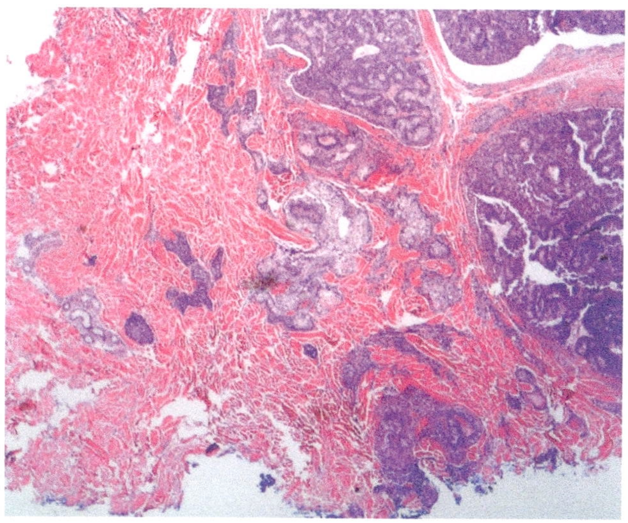

FIG. 12.101

Sebaceous carcinoma. Infiltrative growth pattern.

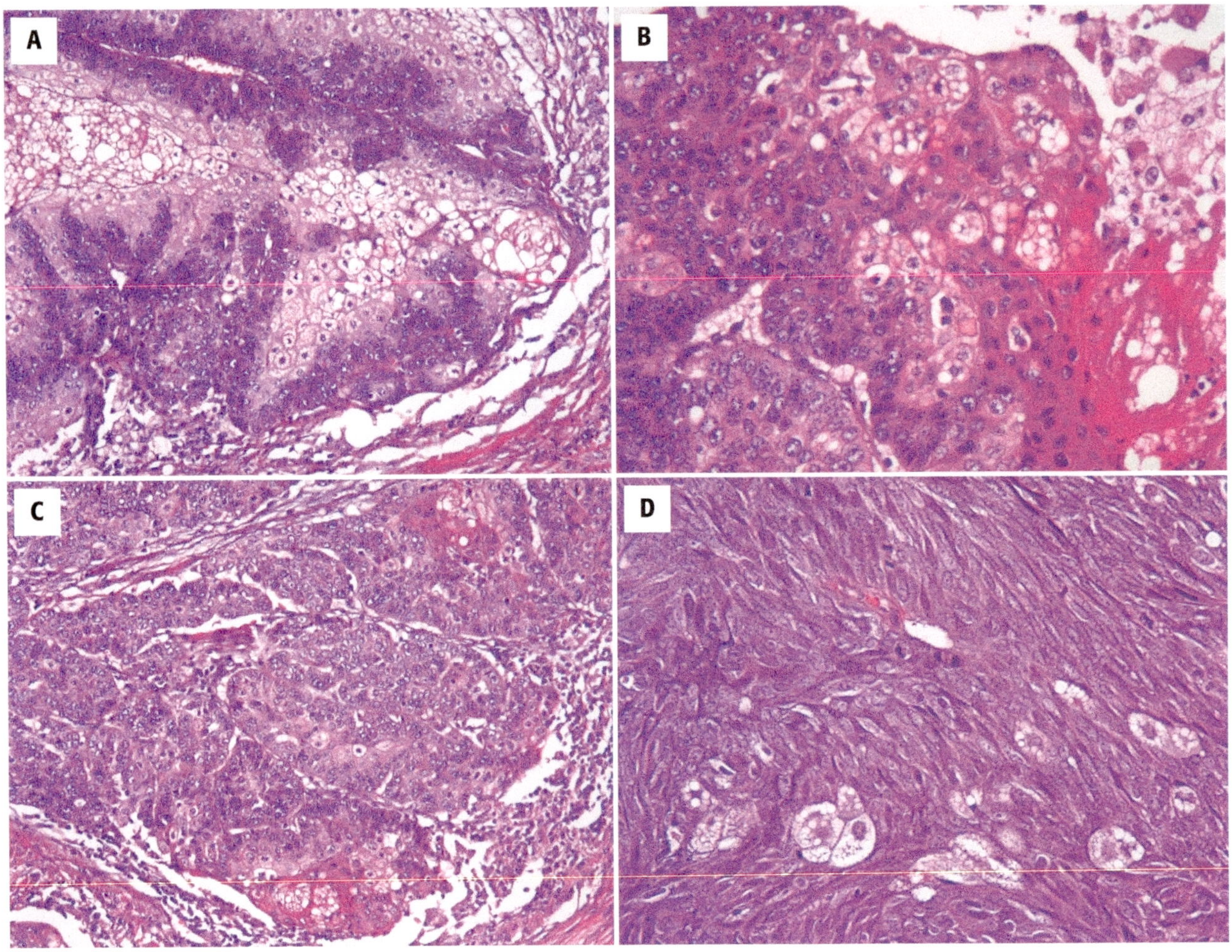

FIG. 12.102

Sebaceous carcinoma. **A,** Well differentiated. Sebocystic features predominate. **B,** Moderately differentiated. Sebocystic features are easily recognized but no longer predominate. **C,** Poorly differentiated. Sebocystic features are rare. **D,** Poorly differentiated. Spindle cell sarcomatoid features may be present.

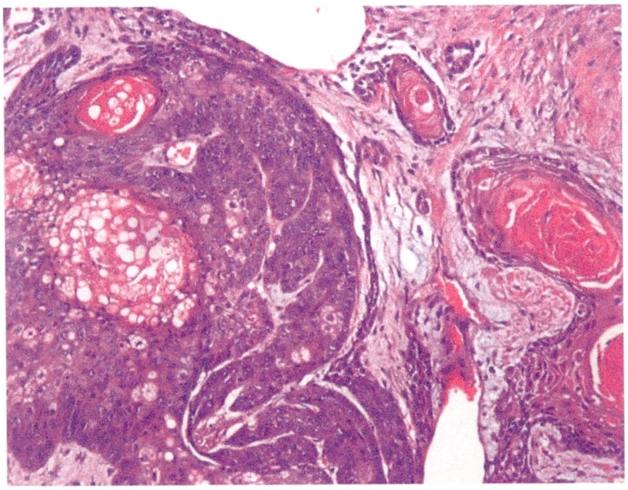

FIG. 12.103

Sebaceous carcinoma. Squamous metaplasia may be present.

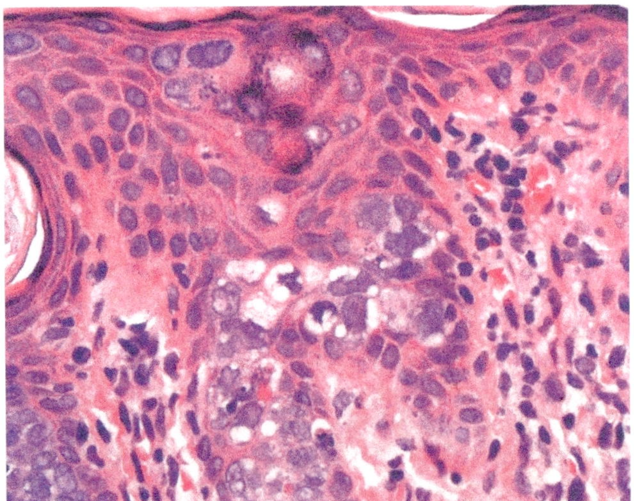

FIG. 12.104

Sebaceous carcinoma. Intraepidermal involvement may be seen.

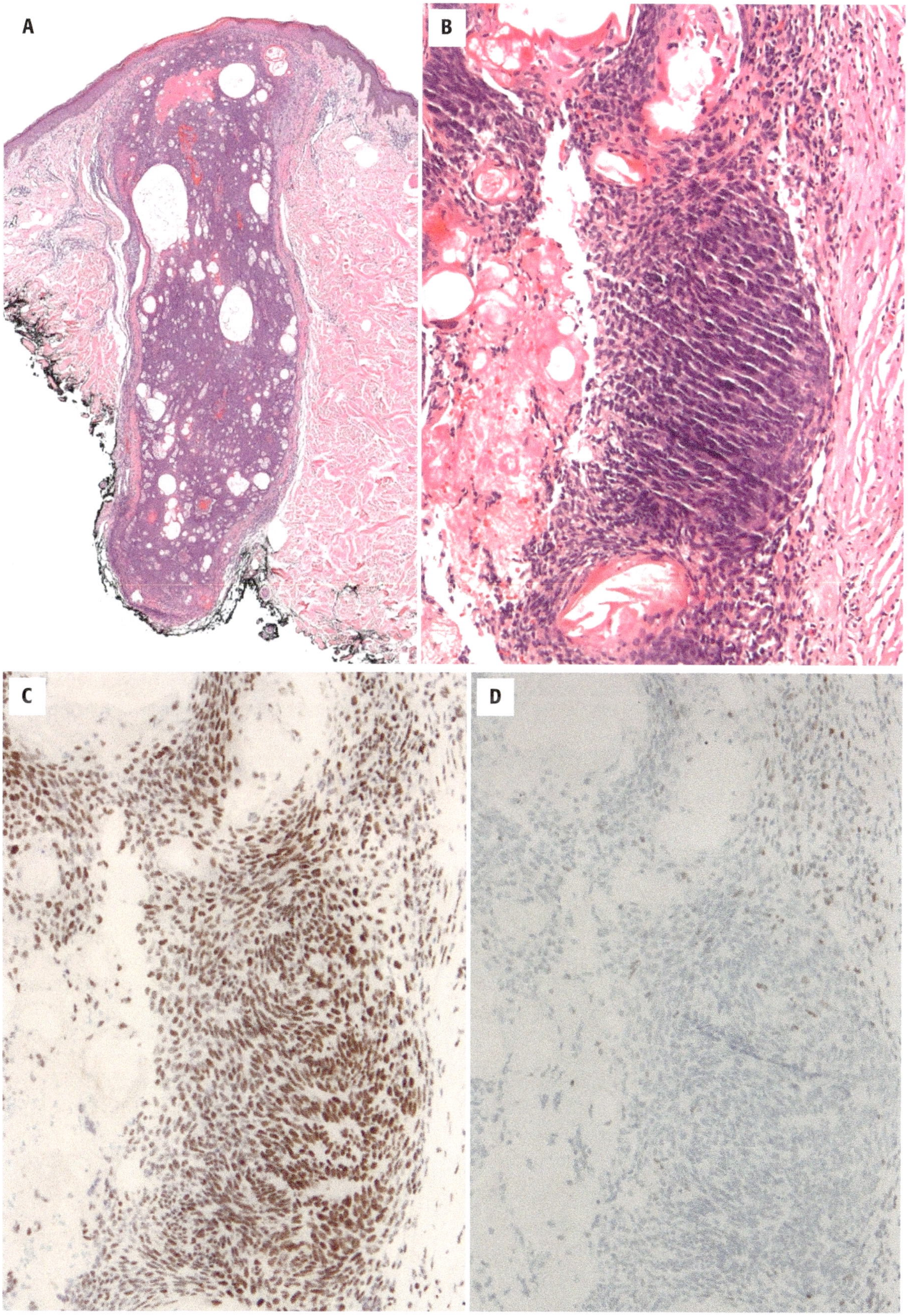

FIG. 12.105

Immunohistochemical testing of sebaceous tumor. **A,** Silhouette of a nodular sebaceous tumor from a patient with Muir-Torre syndrome. **B,** Edge of the tumor nodule (hematoxylin and eosin stain). **C,** Expression of MLH1 is retained. **D,** Expression of MSH6 is lost in the tumor cells.

Differential Diagnosis

Well-differentiated sebaceous carcinomas differ from sebaceous adenomas by their infiltrative growth pattern, deep extension, or atypia. Sebaceous carcinomas with prominent pagetoid intraepidermal or conjunctival mucosal involvement need to be distinguished from clear-cell variants of SCC (Bowen's disease), EPD, and melanoma. The distinction from melanoma and extramammary Paget's disease (EPD) is readily accomplished by immunohistochemical studies. Sebaceous carcinomas are negative for CEA or mucin (positive in EPD); they are also negative for melanocyte differentiation markers. The distinction of pagetoid sebaceous carcinoma from clear-cell squamous or BCC with secondary extension into sebaceous glands is more difficult. Detection of foci of typical BCC or SCC in situ is helpful in this regard. A careful search for bona fide sebaceous differentiation of the tumor (atypical, scalloped nuclei; cytoplasmic microvacuoles) is critical for establishing a diagnosis of sebaceous carcinoma.

A more problematic diagnostic issue is the distinction of poorly differentiated sebaceous carcinomas with minimal sebaceous differentiation from poorly differentiated sweat gland carcinomas with focal clear-cell changes. Whereas sweat gland carcinomas are more likely to show ductal differentiation, sebaceous carcinomas tend to be more basaloid and show keratinous material. Stains for glycogen or for CEA may help (positive in sweat gland tumors and usually negative in sebaceous tumors) or a profile of keratins (sweat gland tumors tend to be positive with Cam5.2 or CK7, but sebaceous tumors tend to be negative or only weakly positive for these keratins). Sebaceous tumors express EMA best. Expression of adipophilin is characteristic of sebaceous carcinoma and aids in its distinction from other carcinoma types. Clinical correlation may also help. Sweat gland carcinomas are much more likely to be associated with satellite metastases than sebaceous carcinomas. At times, a poorly differentiated adnexal carcinoma cannot be further classified into sebaceous or sweat gland origin. If that is the case, it is best to acknowledge it. There is no evidence to date that further subclassification has any impact on prognosis or clinical management for poorly differentiated adnexal tumors.

Prognosis and Treatment

Sebaceous carcinomas require surgical excision. Prognostic features have been established for ocular sebaceous carcinomas, with tumor size being the most important prognostic parameter. Little is known about the prognosis of extraocular sebaceous carcinomas. Although small case series of metastasizing extraocular sebaceous carcinomas have been published, it has been our experience that this scenario is very rare. The vast majority of well or moderately differentiated extraocular sebaceous carcinomas confined to the dermis or extending only into the superficial subcutis are cured by excision and do not seem to be significantly more aggressive than BCCs. Given the rare incidence of metastases, we do not recommend SLN mapping for extraocular tumors except for rare large carcinomas.

ADNEXAL CARCINOMAS

For some malignant epithelial neoplasms, it is difficult to determine the cell of origin or precise lineage of differentiation (e.g., follicular versus ductal). Two examples are mentioned here.

SQUAMOID DUCTAL ECCRINE SQUAMOUS CELL CARCINOMA

Clinical Findings

This rare tumor usually presents as a solitary nodule, occasionally ulcerated, in middle-aged or elderly individuals, more common in males, on the head and neck, and trunk.

Histopathologic Features

The tumor usually involves the dermis and superficial subcutis. It tends to be nodular, with an infiltrative border. The superficial areas show well-differentiated clusters of epithelial cells similar to standard SCC. Deeper areas contain cords with an associated desmoplastic stroma. There is frequent perineural and less frequently lymphovascular infiltration (Fig. 12.106).

Differential Diagnosis

Microcystic adnexal carcinoma also has biphenotypic superficial and deep components; however, the superficial one resembles a cystic lesion with follicular differentiation, in contrast to the compact clusters of squamous cells seen in squamoid ductal eccrine SCC. Standard ductal adenocarcinomas lack the superficial squamous area of the squamoid ductal eccrine SCC.

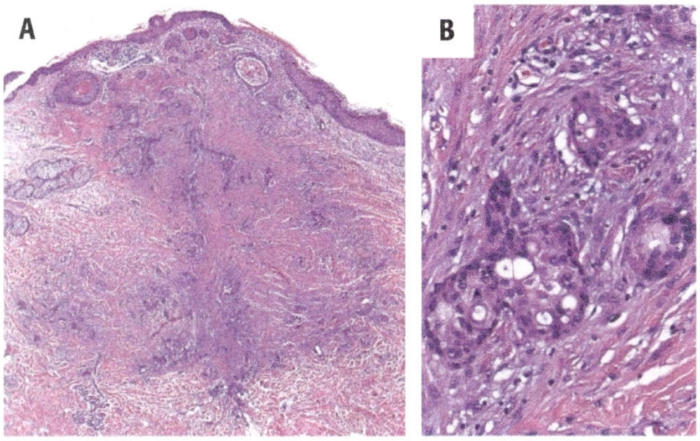

FIG. 12.106

Squamoid ductal eccrine squamous cell carcinoma. **A,** Poorly circumscribed lesion occupying the dermis. Uninvolved epidermis. **B,** High-powered view of the deeply located tumor clusters with ductal differentiation and desmoplastic stroma.

Prognosis and Treatment

This lesion can recur and occasionally metastasizes; thus, it requires complete surgical excision.

ADNEXAL CLEAR-CELL CARCINOMA WITH COMEDONECROSIS

Clinical Findings

This rare tumor usually presents in elderly individuals as a rapidly growing, solitary nodule on the head and neck, particularly the scalp. Due to its peculiar histopathologic features, it is placed here, after the more standard lesions.

Histopathologic Features

The tumor usually involves the dermis and superficial subcutis. It tends to be multilobular, with an infiltrative border. There are large clusters of squamous cells with central areas having clear cytoplasm and regions of comedonecrosis. There is no obvious duct formation. Immunohistochemistry reveals expression of EMA and CK17, with only rare cells expressing CEA (not associated with ductal structures).

Differential Diagnosis

SCC and other clear-cell adnexal tumors. They usually lack comedo-necrosis, or if there is necrosis display features (keratinization, duct formation) that help distinguish them from adnexal clear-cell carcinoma with comedo-necrosis.

Prognosis and Treatment

There is risk for local recurrence and metastasis. Complete surgical excision is the treatment of choice.

ADNEXAL NEOPLASMS ASSOCIATED WITH SYSTEMIC SYNDROMES

Adnexal tumors may be cutaneous manifestations of a systemic syndrome related to a germline mutation. A few of the more well-known syndromes are discussed herein.

GARDNER'S SYNDROME

Gardner's syndrome is a familial adenomatous polyposis syndrome caused by mutations in the APC gene. It is an autosomal dominant disease characterized by gastrointestinal polyps at high risk for malignant transformation and the presence of associated skin and soft tissue tumors. The most common skin lesion associated with Gardner's syndrome is a follicular cyst, including the typical infundibular cyst as well as "hybrid" cysts with mixed features of infundibular, trichilemmal, or matrical differentiation. Pilomatricoma is the one adnexal tumor associated with Gardner's syndrome. Soft tissue lesions typical of Gardner's syndrome include desmoid tumors, fibromas, lipomas, and osteomas. Patients with Gardner's syndrome are at increased risk for colon cancer and other cancers (e.g., thyroid, hepatobiliary malignancies).

XERODERMA PIGMENTOSUM

These patients have an impaired ability to repair the damage induced by ultraviolet radiation to the DNA because of deficient function of the nucleotide excision repair. There are at least seven genes associated with a DNA polymerase (XP-A to XP-G) and a different gene named XP variant (XP-V). These patients show from early age severe actinic damage with mottled cutaneous pigmentation and malignant neoplasms, including BCC (e.g., skin adnexal tumor), SCC, atypical fibroxanthoma, and melanoma.

NEVOID BASAL CELL CARCINOMA SYNDROME

The nevoid BCC syndrome (NBCCS, Gorlin's, or Gorlin-Goltz syndrome) is an autosomal dominantly inherited disease characterized by developmental anomalies, BCCs of the skin, and early onset extracutaneous neoplasms.

Although most BCCs occur sporadically, approximately 0.5% of BCC cases are attributable to NBCCS. Affected patients develop multiple tumors, ranging from a few to thousands of BCCs. They occur primarily on the face, neck, and upper trunk. Unlike sporadic BCCs, the tumors in NBCCS tend to occur early in life (usually between puberty and age 35 years). They may even occur in prepubescent children. At that young age, the tumors tend to be innocuous. Aggressive, locally destructive behavior is usually only seen in adults. Metastases are very rare. Other cutaneous findings in NBCCS include palmar or plantar pits, some of which may show BCCs.

A number of extracutaneous findings have been reported in patients with NBCCS. They include skeletal abnormalities, such as hypoplastic, fused, or bifid ribs; frontal bossing; or scoliosis. Odontogenic keratocysts of the jaws and calcifications of the falx cerebri or diaphragma sellae are characteristic findings. Many patients with NBCCS have characteristic coarse facial features with frontal bossing, macrocephaly, mandibular prognathism, and ocular hypertelorism.

Patients with NBCCS are at increased risk of developing miscellaneous tumors, such as medulloblastoma, meningioma, craniopharyngioma, cardiac fibroma, and bilateral calcified ovarian fibromas.

The susceptibility gene for NBCCS is the *PTCH* gene located on 9q22.3-q31; this tumor suppressor gene encodes for the receptor for the sonic hedgehog pathway.

Newer targeted therapies, such as vismodebig, are being recommended for some patients with this syndrome or else with multiple BCCs.

GENERALIZED BASALOID FOLLICULAR HAMARTOMA SYNDROME

Generalized basaloid follicular hamartoma syndrome (GBFHS) is an autosomal dominant disease characterized by the presence of multiple basaloid follicular hamartomas in association with hypotrichosis (sparse hair). As in NBCCS, multiple small papules develop in childhood. Unlike in NBCCS, there are no skeletal abnormalities, predisposition to tumors, tissue calcifications, or odontogenic keratocysts. Histologically, the lesions of GBFHS can be difficult to distinguish from infundibulocystic BCC or small lesions of TBL.

BAZEX'S SYNDROME (BAZEX-DUPRÉ-CHRISTOL SYNDROME)

Bazex's syndrome results from mutations in the *ACTRT1* gene. In this X-linked dominant disease, BCCs characteristically develop early in life, associated with congenital hypotrichosis, milia, facial hyperpigmentation, and follicular atrophoderma (icepick depressions).

This disease is not to be confused with the other Bazex's syndrome denoting acrokeratosis neoplastica (psoriasiform dermatitis associated with internal malignancy, especially SCC).

BROOKE-SPIEGLER SYNDROME, FAMILIAL CYLINDROMATOSIS, AND MULTIPLE FAMILIAL TRICHOEPITHELIOMAS

Brooke-Spiegler syndrome (BSS) is an autosomal dominantly inherited disease, with affected individuals developing a variety of skin appendage tumors, including cylindromas, TEs, spiradenomas, and hybrid spriadenocylindromas. Multiple familial trichoepithelioma (MFT) is characterized by TEs, and familial cylindromatosis (FC) is characterized by cylindromas as the only skin appendage tumor. All three conditions recently have been shown to be phenotypic variations of a single gene defect.

The skin lesions primarily occur in the head and neck region, cylindromas typically on the scalp, and TEs on the face. During the lifetime of a patient, the lesions may grow in size and cause considerable cosmetic harm and discomfort. The clinical phenotype of "turban tumor" refers to BSS or FC patients with cylindromas covering the entire scalp.

Rarely, carcinomas may arise in longstanding tumors. Malignant transformation of cylindromas and spiradenomas leads to ductal adenocarcinomas with potential for metastasis.

Malignant transformation of TEs or TBLs leads to BCCs (synonymous with trichoblastic carcinoma). In addition to tumors of skin appendages, BSS has also been infrequently associated with adenomas and adenocarcinomas of the salivary and parotid glands.

Patients with BSS, FC, and MFT have germline mutations in the *CYLD* gene located on chromosome 16q12-13. *CYLD* is a tumor suppressor gene that negatively regulates the nuclear factor κB signaling pathway.

COWDEN'S SYNDROME

Cowden's syndrome is an autosomal dominantly inherited disease characterized by cutaneous findings and benign and malignant tumors in various organ systems. A hallmark of the disease is multiple trichilemmomas, which typically manifest as rough keratotic papules on the face. In addition to trichilemmomas, patients with CS may have oral papillomas (cobblestone mucosa) and palmoplantar keratoses.

The commonest malignancy seen in this syndrome is breast carcinoma, with a lifetime risk of 25% to

50% in these patients. Benign breast lesions include fibroadenomas, adenosis, or microcysts. The risk for thyroid cancer is 10%, and for endometrial cancer it is 5% to 10%.

Lhermitte-Duclos disease (dysplastic gangliocytoma of the cerebellum) has also been reported to be a feature of CS. Ataxia and seizures are typical clinical manifestations of this disease.

The susceptibility gene for CS is phosphatase and tensin homolog (*PTEN*), a tumor suppressor gene located on 10q23.3.

MUIR-TORRE SYNDROME

MTS is an expression of Lynch's syndrome and is an autosomal dominantly inherited. It is defined by the presence of a sebaceous tumor in association with one or more visceral neoplasms. The spectrum of sebaceous tumors includes sebaceous adenoma and carcinomas. They may be solitary or multiple and precede, occur concurrently with, or follow the diagnosis of an internal cancer. The syndrome may manifest early in life, but most patients are in their sixth decade at the time of diagnosis. Sebaceous adenomas associated with MTS are often nodulocystic and commonly located on the trunk and extremities. MTS-associated sebaceous carcinomas typically have low biologic risk. Other skin lesions associated with MTS include keratoacanthomas and cysts.

Individuals with MTS are predisposed to developing visceral cancers. The majority (~50%) are adenocarcinomas of the colon followed by those of the endometrium (~25%). MTS-associated colonic carcinomas are typically proximal to the splenic flexure, occur a decade earlier, and tend to behave less aggressively than sporadic colorectal carcinomas.

The spectrum of internal tumors seen in MTS is identical to those in hereditary nonpolyposis colorectal cancer (HNPCC) families (hMSH2/hMLH1), and MTS is now considered to be a phenotypic variant of HNPCC (Lynch's syndrome). There may be germline mutations in various DNA mismatch repair genes (*MLH1, MSH2, PMS1, PMS2, MSH3,* and *MSH6*). The majority of affected patients show mutations of *MLH1* and *MSH2*.

Immunohistochemistry for Mismatch Repair Proteins

Microsatellite instability and altered mismatch repair protein expression have been found in skin tumors. Mutations are associated with loss of staining. Immunohistochemistry of sebaceous tumors with monoclonal antibodies to MLHL1, MSH2, MSH6, or PMS2 may be performed in the work-up of patients with HNPCC or MTS (Fig. 12.105). However, it lacks sensitivity and specificity for a robust screening method. Clinical criteria (age, number of sebaceous neoplasms, history of cancer, family history of Lynch's syndrome) provide a better guide for the need for further genetic testing and counseling.

BIRT-HOGG-DUBÉ SYNDROME

Birt-Hogg Dubé syndrome (BHDS) is an autosomal dominantly inherited disorder characterized by fibrofolliculomas, trichodiscomas, acrochordons, and a predisposition to renal tumors and pulmonary disease. The skin lesions typically appear in young or middle-aged adults and manifest as small, smooth, yellow-white papules on the face or upper trunk.

The most frequent pulmonary findings seen in BHDS patients include spontaneous pneumothorax, pulmonary cysts, and bullous emphysema. The predisposition to renal cell carcinoma in patients with BHDS has been well established, requiring careful monitoring of those at risk. The spectrum of renal tumors includes oncocytomas and chromophobe, papillary, and clear-cell carcinomas. Other tumors have also been described in patients with BHDS, such as medullary carcinoma of the thyroid, multiple angiolipomas, and parotid oncocytoma.

The affected gene, folliculin (*FLCN*), maps to chromosome 17p11.2. Patients with BHDS have germline mutations in *FLCN*, a putative tumor suppressor gene with unknown functions.

SUGGESTED FURTHER READING

Elder, D. E., Massi, D., Scolyer, R. A., & Willemze, R. (2018). *WHO classification of skin tumours* (4th ed.). Lyon: International Agency for Research on Cancer.

Kazakov, D. V., McKee, P., Michal, M., et al. (2012). *Cutaneous adnexal tumors.* Philadelphia: Wolters Kluwer Health/Lippincott Williams & Wilkins.

Macagno, N., Kervarrec, T., Sohier, P., Poirot, B., Haffner, A., Carlotti, A., Balme, B., Castillo, C., Jullie, M. L., Osio, A., Lehmann-Che, J., Frouin, E., & Battistella, M. (2021). NUT Is a specific immunohistochemical marker for the diagnosis of YAP1-NUTM1-rearranged cutaneous poroid neoplasms. *American Journal of Surgical Pathology, 45*(9), 1221–1227.

Macagno, N., Sohier, P., Kervarrec, T., Pissaloux, D., Jullie, M. L., Cribier, B., & Battistella, M. (2022). Recent advances on immunohistochemistry and molecular biology for the diagnosis of adnexal sweat gland tumors. *Cancers (Basel), 14*(3), 476.

Maisnam, D., & Dadzie, O. E. (2016). Adnexal tumors. In O. E. Dadzie & M. Mahalingam (Eds.), *Pearls and pitfalls in neoplastic dermatopathology* (pp. 129–197). Cambridge.

North, J. P. (2021). Molecular genetics of sebaceous neoplasia. *Surgical Pathology Clinics, 14*(2), 273–284.

Plotzke, J. M., Adams, D. J., & Harms, P. W. (2022). Molecular pathology of skin adnexal tumours. *Histopathology, 80*(1), 166–183.

Requena, L., & Sangueza, O. (2017). *Cutaneous adnexal neoplasms.* Springer.

Roberts, M. E., Riegert-Johnson, D. L., Thomas, B. C., Rumilla, K. M., Thomas, C. S., Heckman, M. G., & Purcell, J. U. (2014). A clinical scoring system to identify patients with sebaceous neoplasms at risk for the Muir-Torre variant of Lynch's syndrome. *Genetics in Medicine*, 16(9), 711–716.

Sekine, S., Kiyono, T., Ryo, E., Ogawa, R., Wakai, S., & Ichikawa, H. (2019). Recurrent YAP1-MAML2 and YAP1-NUTM1 fusions in poroma and porocarcinoma. *Journal of Clinical Investigation*, 129(9), 3827–3832.

Snow, J. T., Georgantzoglou, N., Green, D. C., Parra, O., LeBlanc, R. E., Yan, S., Sriharan, A., Momtahen, S., Winnick, K. N., Dimonitsas, E., Stavrianos, S., Lakiotaki, E., Korkolopoulou, P., Revelos, K., Guo, R., & Linos, K. (2022). Molecular analysis of NUT-positive poromas and porocarcinomas identifies novel break points of YAP1::NUTM1 fusions. *Journal of Cutaneous Pathology*, 49(10), 850–858.

Melanocytic Neoplasms 13

Klaus J. Busam

The histologic interpretation of pigmented lesions represents one of the most common and at times most difficult challenges in dermatopathology. This chapter introduces readers to basic aspects of the histologic diagnosis of melanocytic lesions.

LENTIGINES AND LENTIGO-LIKE LESIONS

SOLAR LENTIGO

Clinical Findings

The solar lentigo is a usually circumscribed pigmented macule ranging in color from tan to dark brown. It typically occurs on sun-exposed skin of older individuals (Fig. 13.1A). In contrast to freckles, solar lentigines persist in the absence of sunlight. Solar lentigines are often multiple. They may become confluent and large and clinically simulate a lentigo maligna.

Histopathologic Features

The solar lentigo is characterized by hypermelanization of basilar keratinocytes. Pigmentation is most pronounced at the tips of often elongated, club-shaped rete ridges (Fig. 13.1B). The density of junctional melanocytes is within normal limits but may be increased in chronically sun-damaged skin up to one melanocyte per three basilar keratinocytes. The stratum corneum may be normal or thickened. On occasion, particularly on the face, epidermal rete ridges may be short or effaced. Solar lentigines may be associated with a lymphocytic, often lichenoid inflammatory reaction, with scattered Civatte bodies or melanophages in the superficial dermis.

Differential Diagnosis

The most important distinction is between solar lentigo and lentigo maligna (melanoma in situ). However, solar lentigo also needs to be distinguished from benign melanocytic proliferations and miscellaneous pigmented epithelial lesions (macular seborrheic, lichen planus–like keratosis, or pigmented actinic keratosis). Seborrheic keratosis differs from solar lentigo by epidermal hyperplasia and hyperkeratosis. The lichenoid inflammatory reaction is more pronounced in a lichenoid keratosis. Solar lentigo differs from actinic keratosis by the lack of basilar keratinocyte atypia (e.g., hyperchromatic nuclei).

Benign melanocytic proliferations that may be confused with a solar lentigo include lentigo simplex and paucicellular lentiginous junctional nevus (also called "jentigo"). A lentigo simplex differs from solar lentigo by a definite increase in the density of solitary units of melanocytes within the lesion. The diagnosis of a junctional nevus requires identification of a junctional nest (group of three or more melanocytes). Solar lentigo may at times be difficult to distinguish from a histologically subtle ("early") evolving melanoma in situ of lentigo maligna type, especially if the solar lentigo occurs in the setting of background melanocyte hyperplasia of chronically sun-damaged skin. Clinical correlation (knowledge of the size and complexity of the lesion) and an adequate biopsy that permits assessment of a definite increase in melanocyte density within the lesion as compared with nonlesional background are paramount in such cases to arrive at the correct diagnosis.

Sampling errors may pose a pitfall. The clinician may have taken the biopsy from a paucicellular focus of an otherwise more cellular lesion. Furthermore, the cellular density may vary within a biopsy. Multiple levels and immunostains for melanocyte differentiation antigens may be necessary to document a subtle melanocytic proliferation, especially if the dermal-epidermal junction is blurred by a lichenoid inflammatory reaction. Knowledge of the clinical features of the lesion (size, complexity) greatly facilitates interpretation of subtle alterations.

LENTIGO SIMPLEX

Clinical Findings

A lentigo simplex (also called a nevoid lentigo) is a well-circumscribed pigmented macule. It is usually

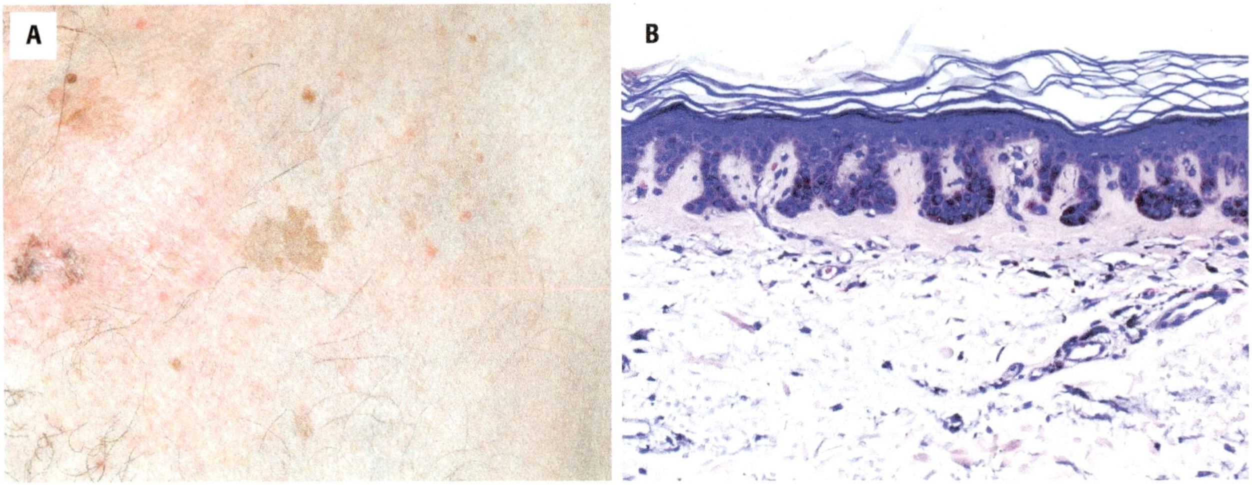

FIG. 13.1

Solar lentigo. **A,** Clinically, a slightly irregular brown macule is present. **B,** Histologically, slightly elongated rete ridges show basal layer hyperpigmentation. There is associated solar elastosis.

small (a few millimeters in diameter) and may occur anywhere on the body's surface. It is likely that some of these lesions represent the earliest stage in the evolution of lentiginous melanocytic nevi.

Reagents for the Immunohistochemical Detection of Melanocytes

Antigen	Antibody	Sensitivity (%)	Specificity (for Metastatic Melanoma)
S100 protein	Anti-S100P	>98	Low
SOX10	Anti-SOX10	>98	Intermediate
Glycoprotein 100	HMB-45	75	High
Melan-A/Mart-1	A103/M2-7C10	80	High
Tyrosinase	T311	80–90	High
MITF	C5/D5	80–85	Intermediate
TRP-1	TA99 (Mel-5)	90	High

MITF, Microphthalmia-associated transcription factor; *TRP*, tyrosinase-related protein.

Pigmented lesions with a lentigo simplex–like histologic picture occurring at mucosal or paramucosal sites have also been termed *labial and genital melanotic macules* (Fig. 13.2A). Genital lentigines are often associated with stromal melanophages. A lentigo-like lesion may be the histologic substrate of benign melanonychia striata or psoralen and ultraviolet A treatment-induced hyperpigmentation or may be seen in the epidermis overlying a dermal scar or dermatofibroma.

Various clinical scenarios have been described in which multiple lentigines can occur. In Carney's complex, for example, multiple lentigines and blue nevi are seen in association with melanotic schwannoma, myxomas, and endocrine disorders. Lentigines have also been described in Peutz-Jeghers syndrome, in patients with familial gastrointestinal stromal tumors, and as part of a paraneoplastic phenomenon (Peutz-Jeghers–like pigmented macules, usually in association with esophageal or intestinal adenocarcinomas).

Histopathologic Features

Lentigo simplex is histologically characterized by hyperpigmentation of basilar keratinocytes as well as an increase in the density of solitary units of melanocytes at the dermal-epidermal junction confined to the clinical correlate of a small and circumscribed macule (Fig. 13.2B). The melanocytes usually lack cytologic atypia. The nucleus of a melanocyte is usually smaller in diameter than the nucleus of a keratinocyte. On occasion, the melanocytes and their nuclei may be large and have an epithelioid appearance or spitzoid features (spitzoid lentigo). The presence of enlarged cells per se, that is, without an increase in cell density, should not lead to concern about melanoma or surgical intervention. Epidermal hyperplasia with elongation of rete ridges may be an associated histologic feature of lentigines. Some lesions show marked melanin pigment deposition in keratinocytes, melanocytes, or

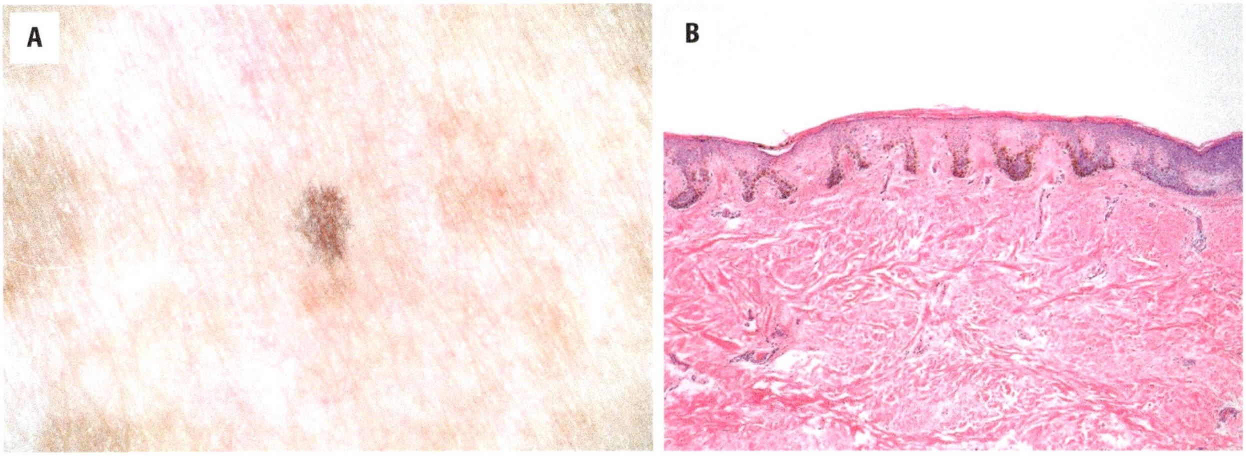

FIG. 13.2

Lentigo simplex. **A,** Clinically, a small dark brown macule is present. **B,** Histologically, the epidermal rete ridges are slightly elongated, associated with basal layer hyperpigmentation as well as a slight increase in the number of cytologically bland intraepidermal melanocytes.

superficial dermal macrophages and may represent a histologic correlate to what is clinically perceived as "ink spot" lentigo.

Syndromes With Lentigines

Laugier-Hunziker syndrome	Melanonychia, mucosal and cutaneous lentigines; sporadic; not associated with hamartoma or malignant tumor
Peutz-Jeghers syndrome	Mucosal (mostly oral, labial) and cutaneous lentigines; hamartomatous gastrointestinal polyps Autosomal dominant; mutation in *STK11/LKB1* gene
Carney complex	1. Cardiocutaneous type, also called LAMB syndrome (lentigines, atrial myxomas, mucocutaneous myxomas, blue nevi) 2. Multiple endocrine neoplasia–type pigmented nodular adrenocortical disease; pituitary adenoma; gonadal, thyroid tumors, and schwannomas Autosomal dominant; mutation in *PKAR1A* gene
Leopard syndrome	Lentigines Electrocardiographic abnormality Ocular hypertelorism Pulmonic stenosis Abnormality of genitalia Retarded growth, skeletal abnormalities Deafness Autosomal dominant; mutation in *PTPN11* gene

Differential Diagnosis

Lentigines need to be distinguished from solar lentigo; lentiginous nevi, including nevus spilus; but most importantly from in situ melanoma. A solar lentigo shares with a lentigo simplex the feature of hyperpigmentation of basilar keratinocytes. However, in contrast to a simple lentigo, a solar lentigo lacks an associated distinct increase in the cellular density of basilar melanocytes. Small lentiginous junctional melanocytic nevi may have only very few nests. Step sections may be necessary to reveal such nests and allow distinction of such nevi from a simple lentigo.

MISCELLANEOUS MELANOTIC MACULES

Hypermelanosis of basilar keratinocytes can be seen in a number of other lesions, such as Becker's nevus (hyperpigmentation associated with hypertrichosis and smooth muscle hamartoma) (Fig. 13.3), melasma, the pigmented macules of Albright's syndrome (associated with fibrous dysplasia and endocrinopathy), and café-au-lait macules.

MELANOCYTIC NEVI

Melanocytic nevi are benign proliferations of melanocytes. Historically, they have been classified by various clinical (e.g., congenital, acquired, blue) or microanatomic (e.g., junctional, compound, dermal) attributes or by eponyms (e.g., Spitz's, Unna's, Clark's). A detailed discussion of various terms and classifications is beyond the scope of this chapter. The main issue regarding the diagnosis of melanocytic nevi is their distinction from

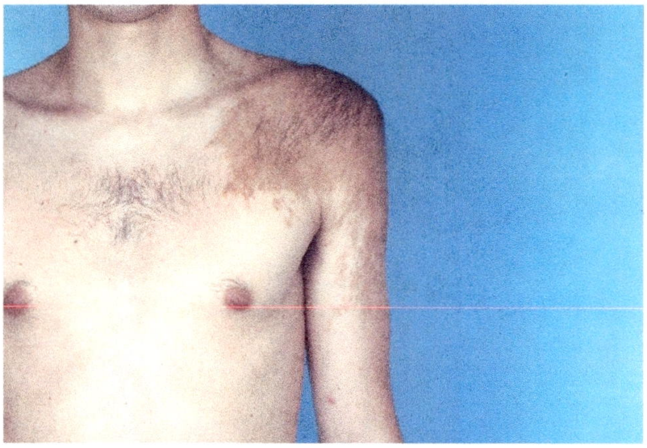

FIG. 13.3

Becker's nevus. There are unilateral hyperpigmentation and hypertrichosis of the left shoulder region.

melanoma. Recognizing variants of melanocytic nevi and familiarity with their spectrum of light microscopic appearances (e.g., pagetoid Spitz's nevus, acral nevus, recurrent nevus) serve to avoid confusion with melanoma. Recently, it has also become apparent that distinct molecular alterations are associated with different types of melanocytic nevi. The *BRAFV600E* mutation is frequently found in melanocytic nevi (ordinary acquired, "dysplastic," or nevi with superficial "congenital" pattern). *NRAS* mutations are frequent in congenital nevi, with the incidence increasing as the size of the congenital nevus increases and *HRAS* mutations are common in sclerosing Spitz nevi. *GNAQ* or *GNA11* mutations are typically associated with blue nevi.

CLASSIFICATION OF MELANOCYTIC NEVI—PATHOLOGIC FEATURES

Clinical Criteria

- Age of onset: congenital or acquired
- Anatomic site: acral, genital, conjunctival, other
- Color: blue nevus

Histopathologic Parameters

- Microanatomic involvement
- Junctional (intraepidermal only)
- Compound (dermal and intraepidermal)
- Dermal (intradermal only)
- Cell type
- Spindle and epithelioid cell nevus
- Pigmented spindle cell nevus
- Epithelioid cell nevus
- Balloon cell nevus
- Eponyms (selected examples)
  - *Unna's* nevus (ordinary melanocytic nevus)
  - *Miescher's* nevus (ordinary melanocytic nevus)–*Clark's* nevus (overlaps with dysplastic nevus)
  - *Spitz's* nevus (spindle and epithelioid cell nevus)
  - *Zitelli's* nevus (superficial congenital nevus)
  - *Mark's* nevus (superficial and deep congenital nevus)
  - *Myerson's* nevus (nevus with eczematous epidermal changes)
  - *Wiesner's* nevus (Spitz's nevus/tumor with loss of BAP1 nuclear labeling)
  - *Tieche's* nevus (common blue nevus)
  - *Ota's* nevus (nevus fuscoceruleus ophthalmomaxillaris)
  - *Ito's* nevus (nevus fuscoceruleus acromiodeltoideus)
  - *Sun's* nevus (nevus fuscoceruleus zygomaticus)

COMMON (TYPICAL OR ORDINARY) ACQUIRED MELANOCYTIC NEVI

Clinical Findings

Melanocytic nevi tend to be symmetric and have fairly sharp borders. They may be flat (Fig. 13.4) or raised (Fig. 13.5). Their color may be identical to the surrounding skin or differ from it (varying from pink or red to light or dark brown).

Histopathologic Features

Common or ordinary nevi are symmetric and circumscribed (Fig. 13.6). The melanocytes may populate the

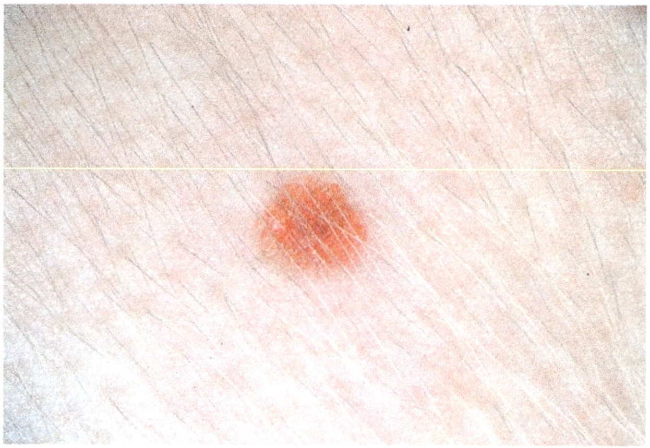

FIG. 13.4

Junctional melanocytic nevus. A circumscribed flat uniform brown macule is present.

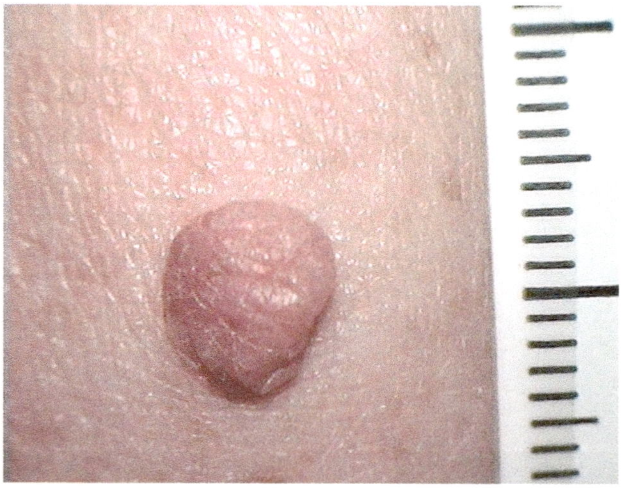

FIG. 13.5

Compound melanocytic nevus. A brown nodule is present.

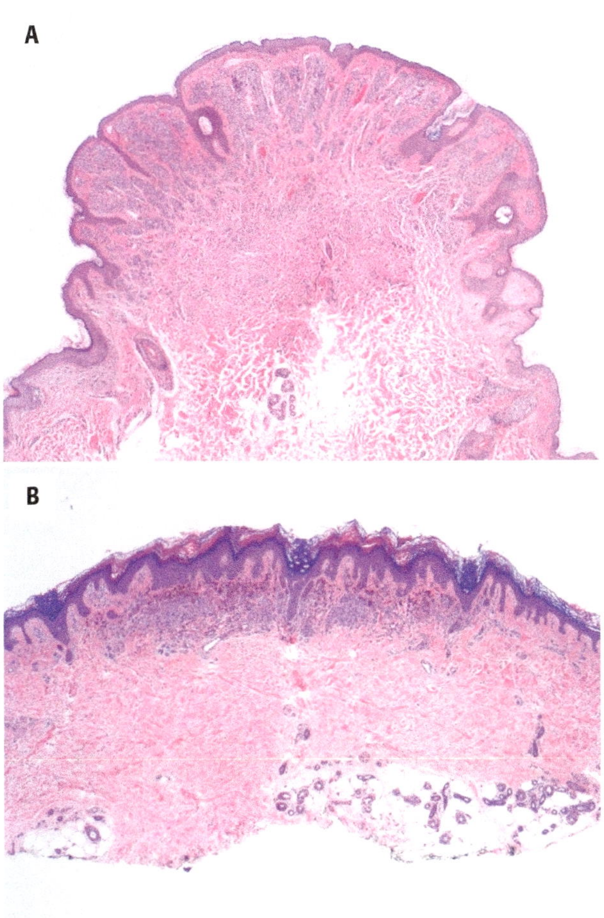

FIG. 13.6

Silhouette of an ordinary melanocytic nevus. **A,** Symmetric silhouette of an ordinary polypoid melanocytic nevus. **B,** Symmetric silhouette of an ordinary plaque-like melanocytic nevus.

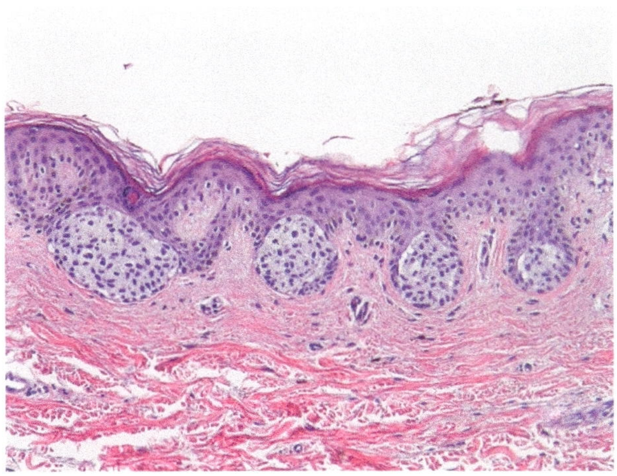

FIG. 13.7

Junctional melanocytic nevus. Nests of melanocytes are present at the dermal-epidermal junction.

epidermis as nests only along the dermal-epidermal junction (junctional nevus) (Fig. 13.7), as well as in the dermis (compound nevus) (Fig. 13.8), or be confined to the dermis without involvement of the overlying epidermis (intradermal melanocytic nevus). In ordinary

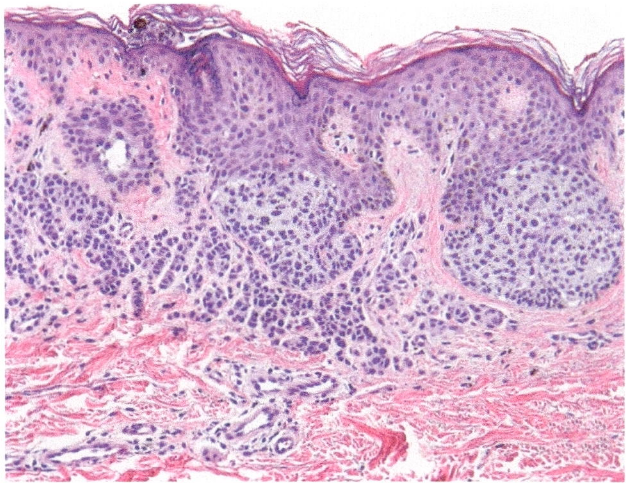

FIG. 13.8

Compound melanocytic nevus. Melanocytes are present at the dermal-epidermal junction and in the superficial dermis.

junctional and compound nevi, nests predominate at the dermal-epidermal junction and are preferentially positioned at or near the tips of rete ridges (see Fig. 13.7). Nevomelanocytes may be heavily pigmented or lack melanin granules by light microscopy. Melanocytic nevi may be associated with epidermal hyperplasia, which at times may have features of a keratosis (keratotic nevus). A melanocytic nevus may also incidentally collide with a seborrheic keratosis.

COMMON ACQUIRED MELANOCYTIC NEVUS—PATHOLOGIC FEATURES

Clinical Findings

- Usually small
- Circumscribed and symmetric; flat or raised
- Variable colors (pink, tan, brown) but usually uniform within a lesion

Histopathologic Features

- Usually small circumscribed and symmetric
- Junctional melanocytic proliferation, if present
  - Predominant nested pattern, rare solitary units of melanocytes
  - Most melanocytic nests are at tips of rete ridges
- Dermal nevus component
  - Evidence of maturation
  - Often "orderly" nested growth pattern
  - Often symmetric wedge or plaque-like growth pattern
  - Lack of marked nuclear pleomorphism and/or frequent mitoses
- Possible associated features
  - Epidermal hyperplasia with hyperkeratosis (keratotic nevus)
  - Spongiosis (eczematous nevus)
  - Papillomatous epidermal hyperplasia (papillomatous nevus)
  - Senescent atypia
  - Inflammation
  - Regression
  - Fatty metaplasia of the dermal stroma
  - Many others (e.g., calcifications, oncocytic changes)

Compound and dermal nevi typically show zonation with depth (so-called maturation) in the dermis. Such maturation may be manifest at the level of individual cells. Large epithelioid (type A) melanocytes tend to dominate in the superficial dermis (Fig. 13.9A). With descent into the reticular dermis, melanocytes tend to have less cytoplasm (type B cells) (Fig. 13.9B) and may become fusiform (type C cells) at the base of a lesion (Fig. 13.9C). Zonal changes (features of maturation) are not restricted to cell size and shape. The growth pattern of the melanocytes and their degree of pigmentation often change with microanatomic depth. Superficially, nests tend to be larger. With descent into the reticular dermis, they usually become smaller. At times, melanocytes at the

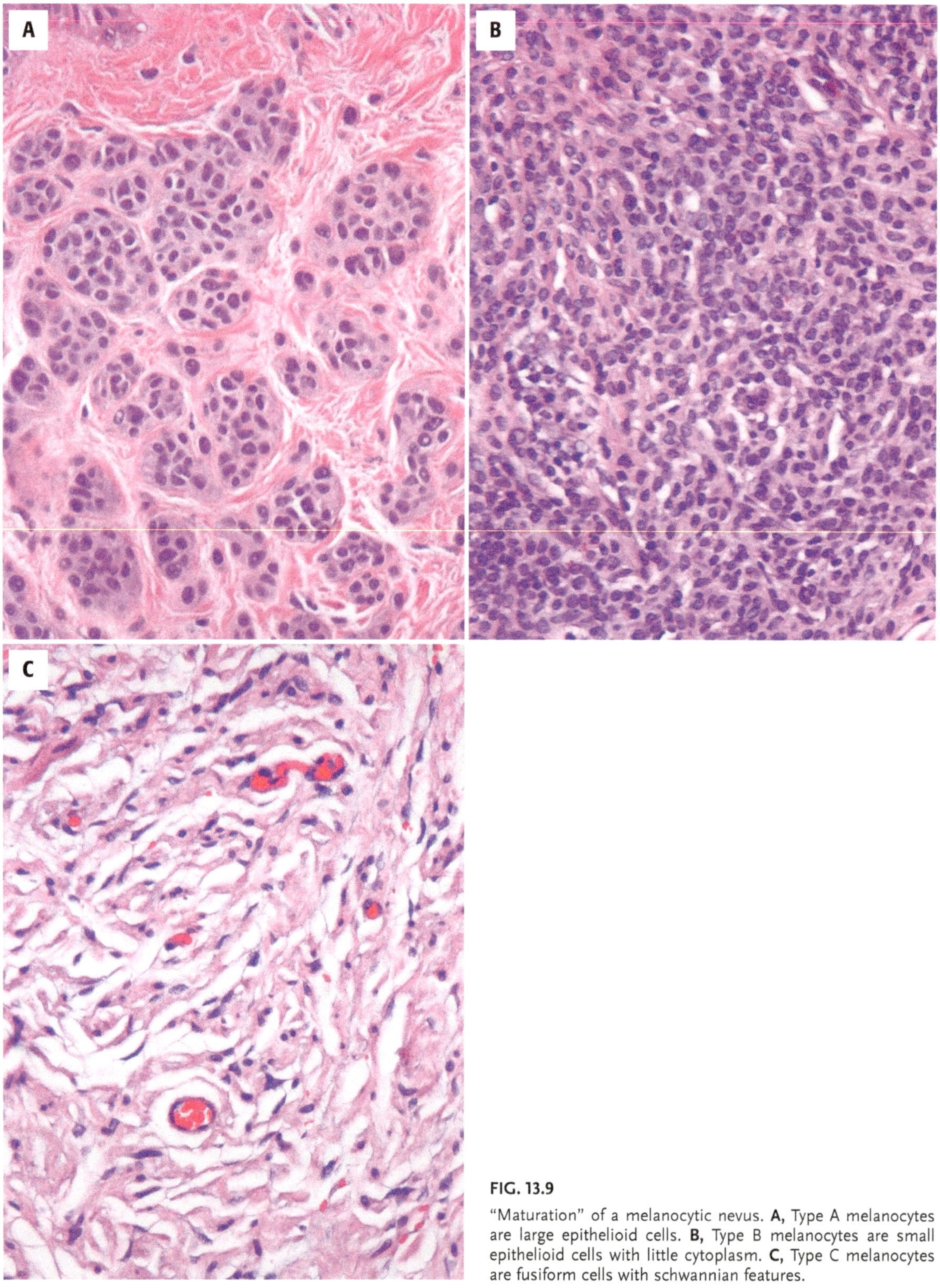

FIG. 13.9

"Maturation" of a melanocytic nevus. **A,** Type A melanocytes are large epithelioid cells. **B,** Type B melanocytes are small epithelioid cells with little cytoplasm. **C,** Type C melanocytes are fusiform cells with schwannian features.

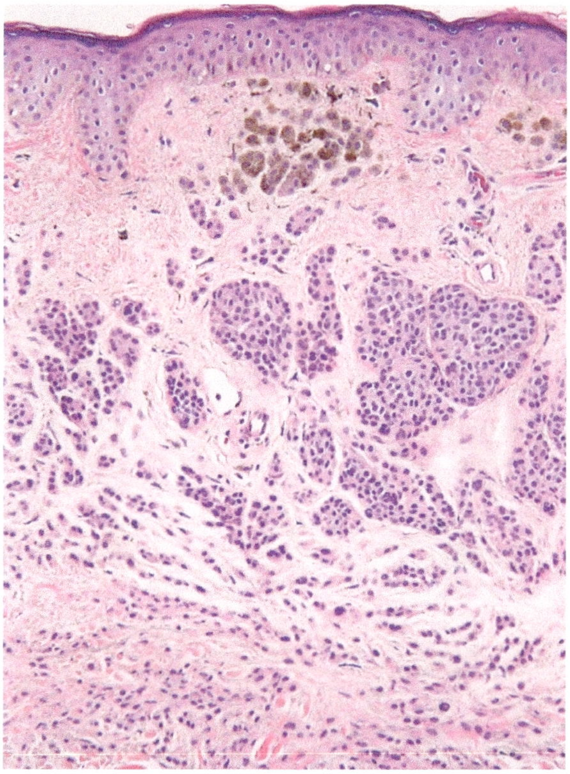

FIG. 13.10
"Maturation" of a melanocytic nevus. Superficial dermal melanocytes contain cytoplasmic pigment but not the cells in the deeper part of the nevus.

base of a nevus are dispersed as solitary units in the stroma. Intracellular melanin pigment tends to be more prominent in the superficial portion of a nevus than in its deep component (Fig. 13.10). The tendency for melanin pigment synthesis to be most visible superficially but disappear in the deeper component of melanocytic nevi has also been referred to as "biochemical" maturation. Exceptions to typical zonation exist (e.g., inverted type A nevus, with large pigmented epithelioid melanocytes in the mid- or deep dermis).

The full range of cytologic appearances from type A to type C melanocytes is seen only in a minority of nevi. Some nevi may be predominantly epithelioid in appearance; others fusiform with or without neural or schwannian differentiation (neuronevus or neurotized nevus) (Fig. 13.11). Neurotized nevi may show structures reminiscent of Wagner-Meissner corpuscles.

Mitoses are typically absent in common nevi. However, rare mitoses, especially in the superficial portion of a nevus, may occur. Several mitoses may be seen in benign growing nevi, especially in childhood, or in women of gestational age, especially during pregnancy. Nevi may rarely be ulcerated. Ulceration associated with benign nevi is usually secondary to trauma or excoriation.

Some dermal nevi are inflamed or may show features of regression (loss of melanocytes associated with various stromal changes, such as edema, fibrosis, hypervascularity, presence of melanophages). Inflammation is usually sparse but may be dense. Inflammation or regression at the periphery of a nevus may lead to a clinically depigmented or erythematous rim around a pigmented center (Fig. 13.12). Such nevi are referred to as "halo nevi." A halo phenomenon may occur in other types of nevi, such as dysplastic or Spitz's nevi. Another pattern of inflammatory process that may be found in association with a melanocytic nevus is that of spongiotic dermatitis. A melanocytic nevus with features of eczema is called a Myerson's nevus.

Various peculiar cytologic changes of melanocytes may occur in common as well as any other type of nevus, such as clear cell or balloon cell; oncocytic features; or prominent multinucleation, including Touton-type giant cell formation. Nevi may show fatty metaplasia (Fig. 13.13) or may be associated with calcifications. In some nevi, there is prominent cellular dyscohesion leading to the formation of "pseudovascular" spaces (Fig. 13.14).

Differential Diagnosis

Confusion of common nevi with melanoma is rare, except for cases of so-called nevoid melanoma (see the following). Dermal melanocytic nevi, in particular on the face, may be associated with an increase in the cellular density of solitary units of melanocytes in the overlying epidermis. Such a finding may raise concern about possible in situ melanoma, especially on a small shave biopsy. If the increase in number of intraepidermal melanocytes is limited to a small area of the center of the lesion, it is in keeping with a benign nevus. If the melanocytic proliferation involves the entire tissue sample and section margins, an additional biopsy or excision may be necessary to exclude in situ melanoma. Extensive ulceration may also pose a problem because it precludes evaluation of the part of the lesion that has been removed by trauma. Several mitotic figures in dermal melanocytes underneath an ulcer should not be dismissed as reactive but should prompt further examination of a lesion for other clues that may suggest melanoma.

Amelanotic melanocytic nevi may also be confused with various benign nonmelanocytic proliferations, such as neurofibroma, cellular neurothekeoma, or histiocytoma. The latter two entities are easily distinguished from melanocytic nevi by immunohistochemistry (IHC). Cellular neurothekeomas are negative for S100 protein. Histiocytomas are negative for melanocyte differentiation markers (e.g., Melan-A, tyrosinase). The distinction of a neurofibroma from a completely neurotized neurofibroma–like nevus can be very difficult. The presence of rare epithelioid cells or small nests

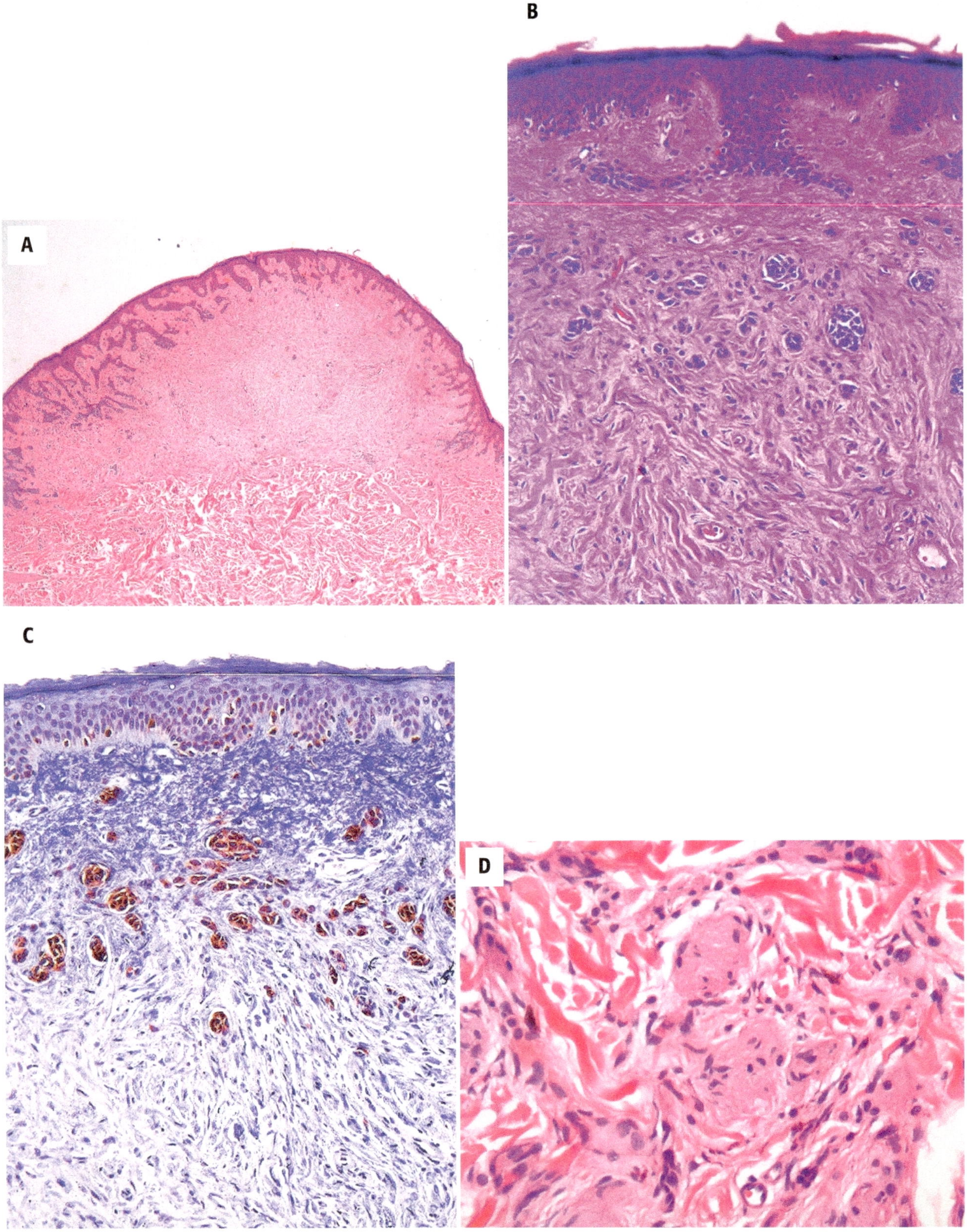

FIG. 13.11

Neuronevus. **A,** Silhouette of a compound melanocytic nevus with "neurotization" of its dermal component. **B,** Superficially, a mixture of nests of small epithelioid melanocytes and diffuse arrangement of fusiform melanocytes with schwannian features is seen. **C,** Only the epithelioid melanocytes are immunoreactive for Melan-A. The fusiform melanocytes are negative. **D,** Neuroid structures are present.

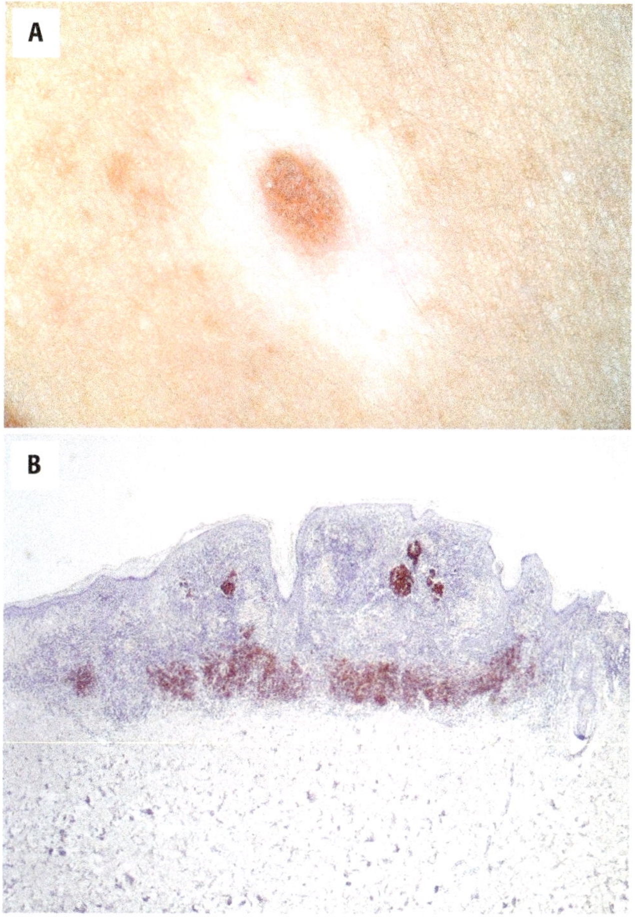

FIG. 13.12

"Halo" phenomenon. **A,** Clinically, a brown macule is surrounded by a hypopigmented rim. **B,** Histologically, the nevomelanocytes (stained immunohistochemically for Melan-A) are associated with a dense lymphocytic infiltrate.

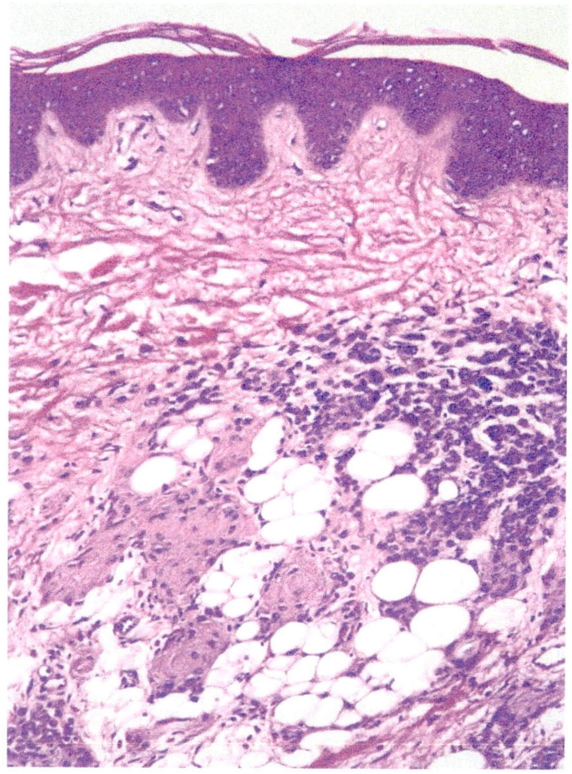

FIG. 13.13

Melanocytic nevus with fatty changes. Adipocytes are present in association with a dermal melanocytic nevus.

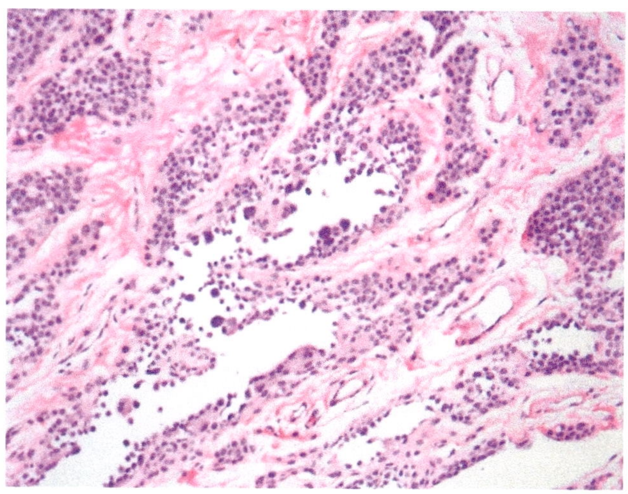

FIG. 13.14

Pseudovascular changes of a melanocytic nevus. Artifactual clefts are lined by melanocytes.

indicates a melanocytic nevus (Fig. 13.11B). Any immunoreactivity for melanocyte differentiation markers also favors a nevus except for pigmented neurofibromas.

DYSPLASTIC MELANOCYTIC NEVI

The concept and definition of the *dysplastic* melanocytic nevus (DMN; also called melanocytic nevus with architectural disorder and atypia) are controversial. In this section, we review some of the basic concepts. This type of nevus was first described in the context of the so-called *B-K mole* or *atypical mole syndrome,* which was later termed *dysplastic nevus syndrome.* The syndrome describes individuals at increased risk for melanoma with a skin phenotype characterized by the presence of numerous nevi, many of which are larger and more irregular than most ordinarily acquired nevi (Fig. 13.15). It was then recognized that such nevi also occur as solitary lesions or may be present in small numbers (Fig. 13.16). As such, this nevus type is a fairly common clinical finding. Estimates on the incidence of DMN in the population vary widely (2% to 50% of fair-skinned people). However, precise statistical data are problematic in this regard because of interobserver variation in the criteria used for classifying nevi as dysplastic. Most pathologists who use

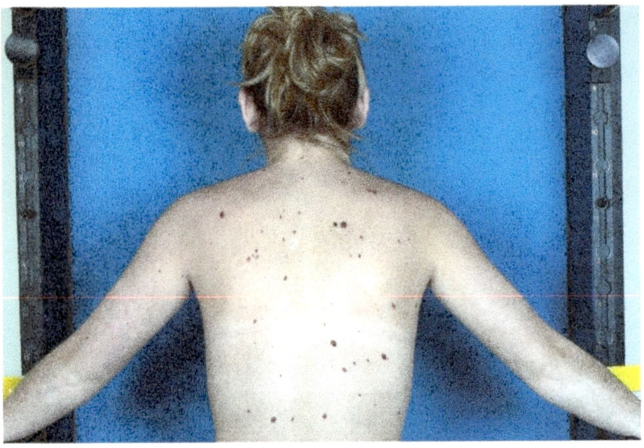

FIG. 13.15

Dysplastic nevus syndrome. A patient with numerous clinically irregular melanocytic nevi.

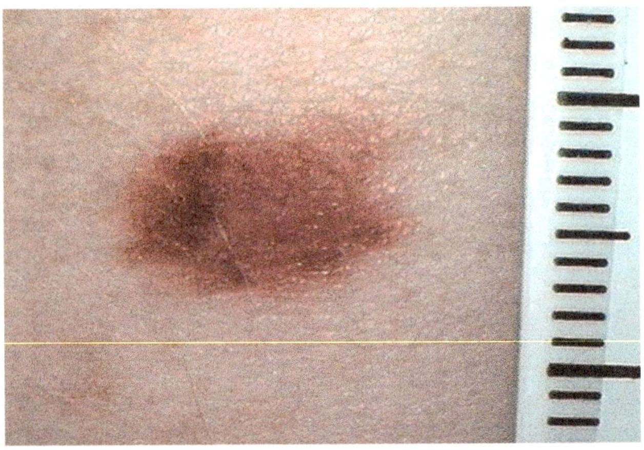

FIG. 13.16

Dysplastic nevus. Pigmented lesion with fuzzy borders and variations in colors and texture.

the term *dysplastic nevus* require both a certain set of architectural features as well as cytologic alterations for its diagnosis. Others, who tend to prefer the term *Clark's nevus,* pay attention primarily to architectural features. The latter approach has been criticized by advocates of the term *dysplastic nevus* with the argument that if cytologic atypia is not required for the diagnosis, the definition of the term becomes too broad, resulting in inclusion of many ordinary nevi, which commonly show a minor element of architectural disorder.

Some pathologists view the DMN not only as a marker of risk for melanoma in the context of the dysplastic nevus syndrome but also as a biologically "intermediate" stage lesion from banal nevi to melanoma (manifestation of tumor progression). The argument in favor of this viewpoint is that the histopathologic findings are often between banal nevi and melanoma, and that some ancillary test results are also at times intermediate. However, most dysplastic nevi do not significantly differ from ordinary nevi with regard to molecular or cytogenetic findings. Furthermore, and more importantly, epidemiologic studies have consistently shown that most dysplastic nevi are stable benign melanocytic neoplasms and that for any given lesion the risk for melanoma evolving in association with a dysplastic nevus is very low.

Clinical Findings

Clinically, dysplastic nevi tend to be larger than ordinary nevi and measure usually more than 4 mm in diameter (see Figs. 13.15 and 13.16). They often show variation in color (mixture of tan, brown, and pink) and have a slightly irregular or "fuzzy" periphery.

Histopathologic Features

Dysplastic nevi display both "architectural disorder and cytologic atypia" of melanocytes (Fig. 13.17). Frequently, there are associated stromal changes. *Architectural disorder* refers to the deviation of the growth pattern of melanocytes from an idealized prototypical "ordinary" nevus. It includes slight asymmetry, a lentiginous proliferation of solitary units of melanocytes along and focally in between elongated rete ridges, variation in the size and placement of junctional nests with fusion or bridging of nests (Figs. 13.17 and 13.18), or an irregular peripheral border, including a shoulder phenomenon (extension of the junctional melanocytic proliferation of a compound melanocytic nevus beyond the periphery of its dermal component) (Fig. 13.19). *Cytologic atypia* refers to nuclear alterations, such as nuclear enlargement, hyperchromasia, or the presence of prominent nucleoli. Stromal

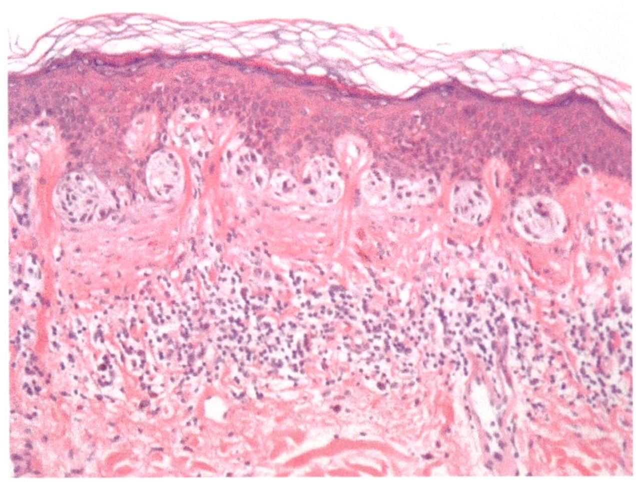

FIG. 13.17

Dysplastic nevus. Bridging and fusion of junctional nests of atypical melanocytes are apparent. There is associated dermal fibrosis and inflammation.

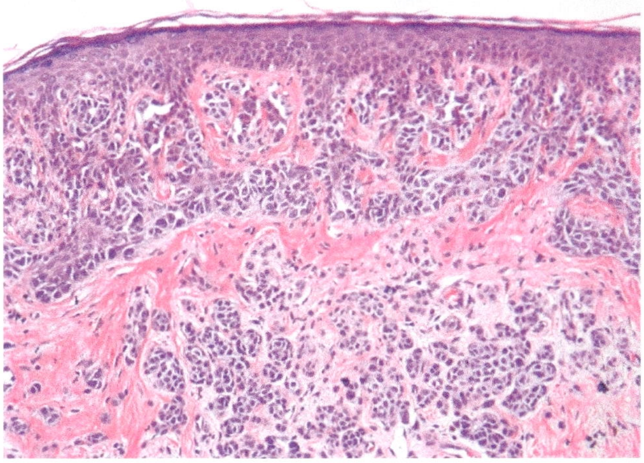

FIG. 13.18

Dysplastic nevus. There is architectural disorder (fusion of nests, confluence of single cells along the dermal-epidermal junction) and atypia (melanocytes with enlarged and hyperchromatic nuclei).

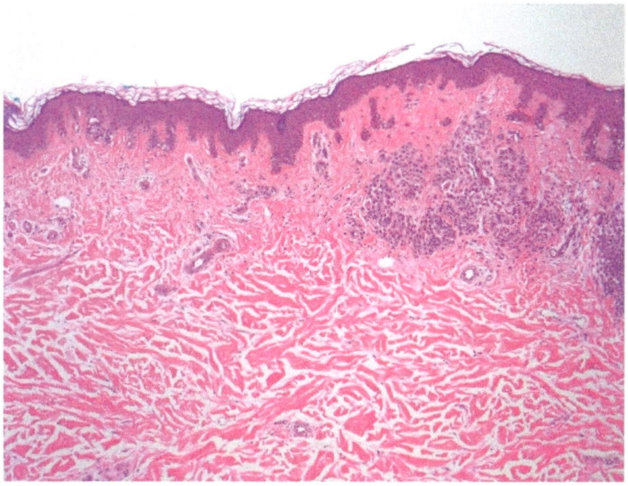

FIG. 13.19

"Shoulder phenomenon." The junctional melanocytic proliferation extends beyond the periphery of the dermal melanocytic nevus component.

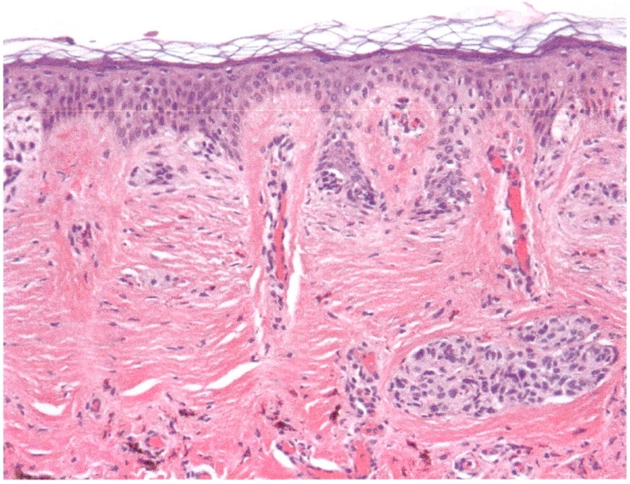

FIG. 13.20

Stromal changes associated with a dysplastic nevus. There is marked lamellar fibrosis in the superficial dermis.

DYSPLASTIC MELANOCYTIC NEVUS—PATHOLOGIC FEATURES

Clinical Findings

- ▸▸ Usually larger than most ordinary nevi
- ▸▸ Irregular borders or colors (not up to the level of melanoma)

Histopathologic Features

- ▸▸ Architectural disorder
  - Slight asymmetry
  - Slightly irregular border
  - Focal single-cell proliferation of melanocytes along and in between rete ridges
  - Variation in size and shapes of nests
  - Bridging or fusion of nests
  - Shoulder phenomenon
- ▸▸ Cytology
  - Enlarged nuclei
  - Hyperchromatic nuclei
  - Distinct nucleoli

Stromal Changes

- ▸▸ Lamellar fibrosis
- ▸▸ Inflammation

changes typically associated with dysplastic nevi include lymphocytic infiltrates, hypervascularity, or fibroplasia of the superficial dermis, which often shows a lamellar pattern (Fig. 13.20).

Naturally, there is a spectrum in the extent of such alterations. Some pathologists have attempted to grade the degree of cytologic and architectural atypia from mild to severe. Cytologic atypia is judged as mild if the nuclei of melanocytes are slightly hyperchromatic but overall similar in size to the nuclei of keratinocytes. A one- to twofold enlargement, often accompanied by other nuclear irregularities (irregular contours, nucleoli, hyperchromatism), is judged as moderate. A more than twofold increase in nuclear size associated with marked hyperchromatism or prominent nucleoli qualifies as severe atypia. However, architectural findings can also be used to assign a higher grade in spite of relatively small melanocyte nuclei. Such findings would include a high proportion of solitary units of melanocytes, clustering of solitary units of junctional melanocytes in between rete ridges, and focal pagetoid spread. In a two-tiered grading system, dysplastic nevi with moderate or severe atypia would be designated as high-grade lesions, while those with only slight atypia would be annotated as low grade.

The rationale behind grading dysplastic nevi is an attempt to separate slightly irregular but essentially banal nevi from those that might be confused with melanoma, that are possibly more likely to progress to melanoma, or that may be associated with a higher risk for melanoma. However, much of this exercise is currently still speculative, controversial, and of unproven benefit for patients. Moderately dysplastic nevi with positive margins usually do not progress to melanoma. However, a practical value of grading a DMN may be that it confers to the dermatologist some information about the pathologist's level of diagnostic certainty and concerns about the lesion, which may influence the need for obtaining a second opinion or the decision to perform a complete excision or not.

Instead of using a formal grading scheme, a pathologist may prefer to express their concerns about the level of certainty that the lesion is still a benign albeit atypical nevus or melanoma. If melanoma cannot be excluded, complete surgical excision is recommended.

Differential Diagnosis

The only distinction that really matters, of course, is the one between melanoma and nevus. Melanomas generally are more asymmetric and less circumscribed than dysplastic nevi. They show a more complex growth pattern along the dermal-epidermal junction with a greater distortion of the epidermis (loss of rete ridges or consumption of the epidermis). Pagetoid spread of intraepidermal melanocytes greatly facilitates the recognition of in situ melanoma. However, its presence is not entirely specific to melanoma. Focal pagetoid spread may occur in nevi, including dysplastic nevi, usually in the center of the lesion or in association with features of trauma. Prominent or chaotic pagetoid spread or pagetoid melanocytes at the periphery of a lesion indicate the presence of in situ melanoma. In contrast to most melanomas, the dermal component of a DMN shows evidence of maturation.

Because the features of the DMN overlap with melanoma and melanoma may be associated with a DMN, it may not be possible on a small partial biopsy to render a definitive diagnosis because some parameters cannot be evaluated (overall symmetry, features of the borders of the lesion). In such cases, it is best to defer the final diagnosis to the review of the completely excised lesion.

SPINDLE OR EPITHELIOID MELANOCYTIC (SPITZ) NEVI

According to the most recent World Health Organization (WHO) classification of melanocytic tumors, Spitz neoplasms are defined as melanocytic tumors with microscopic features historically attributed to Spitz nevi (e.g., plump epithelioid and/or spindle cells) and a distinct set of genomic aberrations, such as fusions involving *NTRK1*, *NTRK3*, *ROS1*, *RET*, *ALK*, *BRAF*, *MAP3K8*, or *MET* or activating point mutations in HRAS.

Clinical Findings

Spitz nevi preferentially affect the face and lower extremities of children and adolescents but may occur anywhere, as well as in adults. Often, they appear as red, pink, or flesh-colored dome-shaped papules (Fig. 13.21). Flat, pigmented, and fibrosing variants exist. Clinically, Spitz nevi may be confused with nonmelanocytic lesions, such as angiomas, pyogenic granulomas, fibromas, warts, or adnexal tumors.

Histopathologic Features

The hallmark of Spitz nevi is their composition of large plump spindle or epithelioid melanocytes (Fig. 13.22). Similar to other benign melanocytic nevi, they are typically

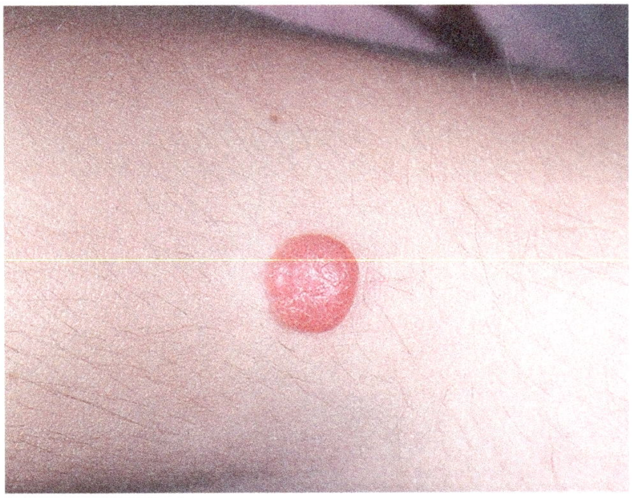

FIG. 13.21
Spitz nevus. A circumscribed dome-shaped red papule is present.

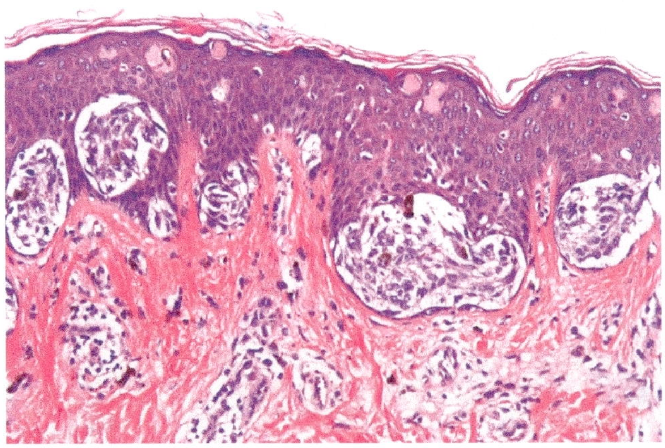

FIG. 13.22
Junctional Spitz nevus. Nests of large plump spindle and epithelioid melanocytes are present with clefts surrounding junctional nests. Dull pink globules ("Kamino" bodies) are also identified.

sharply circumscribed, display a symmetric growth pattern, and show evidence of maturation. Compound and dermal Spitz nevi are usually wedge shaped. Common associated secondary features include epidermal hyperplasia, dull pink globules (Kamino bodies) (Fig. 13.23) at the dermal-epidermal junction, stromal edema, and vascular ectasia. Scattered lymphocytic aggregates may be present. There is a spectrum of cytologic features from large epithelioid to spindle cells. Some lesions are predominantly epithelioid. Others may preferentially contain spindle cells. In many junctional or compound Spitz nevi, fascicles of spindle cells are arranged in tight fascicles parallel to epidermal rete ridges in a pattern that has been likened to hanging bananas (Fig. 13.24). Junctional

SPINDLE AND EPITHELIOID CELL MELANOCYTIC (SPITZ) NEVUS—PATHOLOGIC FEATURES

Clinical Findings

- Usually children and young adults
- Typical manifestation: pink papule on face or extremities

Histopathologic Features

- Architecture
  - Symmetric (often wedge shaped)
  - Sharp peripheral borders
  - Variation in size and shape of densely cellular nests
  - Pagetoid melanocytosis may be present
- Architecture
  - Large spindle and epithelioid cells with abundant pink cytoplasm
  - Evidence of maturation
  - Rare superficial dermal mitoses
- Secondary epidermal or stromal changes
  - Dull pink globules (Kamino bodies) present in many but not all cases
  - Vascular ectasia and edema
  - Lymphocytic infiltrate, variable
  - Stroma fibrosis, variable
  - Epidermal hyperplasia may be prominent

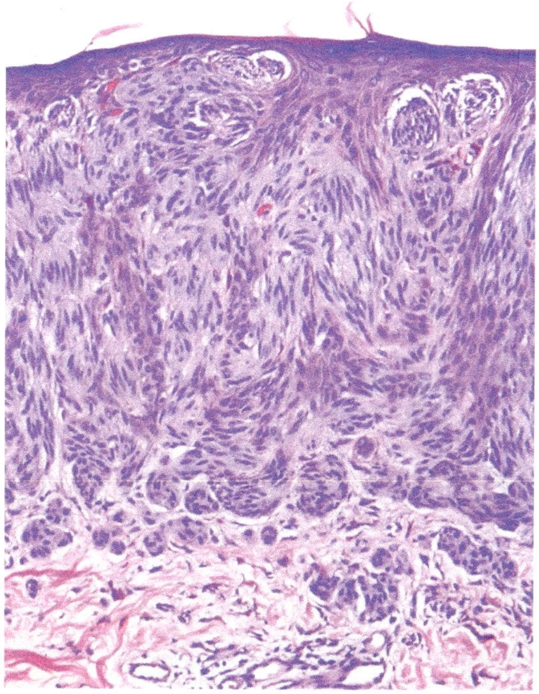

FIG. 13.24

Spitz nevus. Fascicles of fusiform melanocytes are present in association with elongated rete ridges.

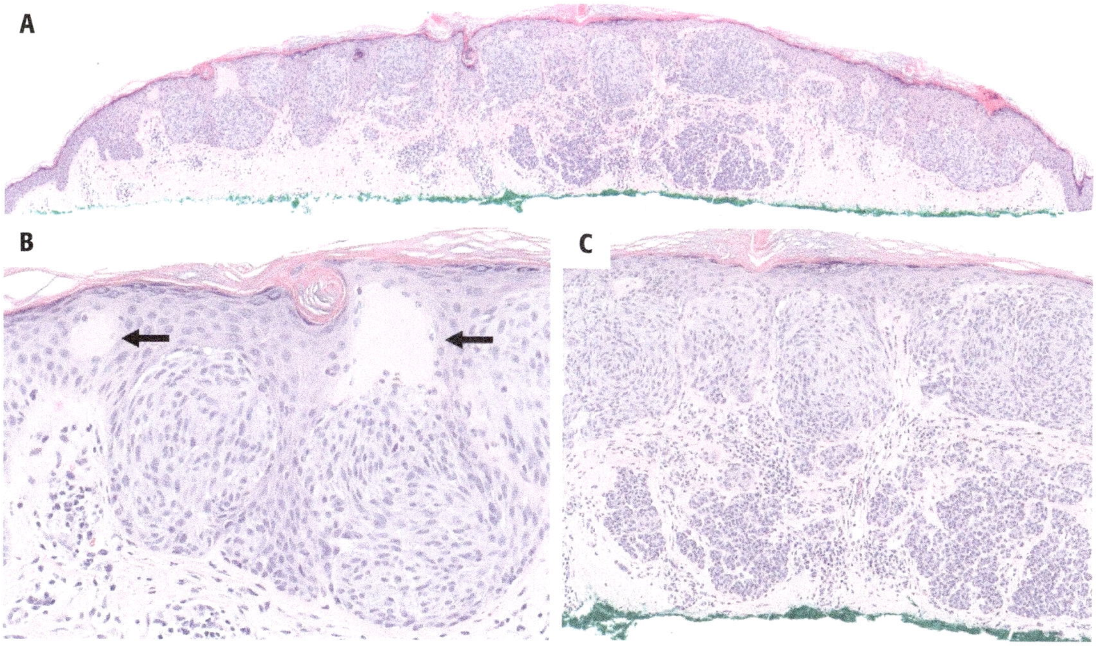

FIG. 13.23

Compound Spitz nevus. **A,** The lesion displays a fairly symmetric and circumscribed silhouette. **B,** Nests of fusiform melanocytes are associated with dull pink globules *(arrows)* at the dermal-epidermal junction. **C,** The dermal melanocytes show evidence of maturation.

nests of melanocytes often show "clefts." Mitoses may be found but are usually rare and limited to the superficial portion of densely cellular lesions. A number of histopathologic variants of Spitz nevus have been reported, including, but not limited to, desmoplastic, angiomatoid, myxoid, large epithelioid, pigmented spindle cell, and plexiform lesions.

Sclerosing or desmoplastic variants are associated with stromal fibrosis. Most of them are predominantly intradermal nevi, in which pleomorphic epithelioid melanocytes are dispersed as small nests, fascicles, and single cells in fibrous stroma (Fig. 13.25). At scanning magnification, these variants may resemble a dermatofibroma.

Many Spitz nevi are amelanotic or paucimelanotic. However, heavily pigmented variants thereof exist with various proportions of spindle to epithelioid melanocytes. The so-called *pigmented spindle cell nevus* represents one pole of the spectrum of such pigmented nevi (Fig. 13.26A). It is cytologically characterized by a

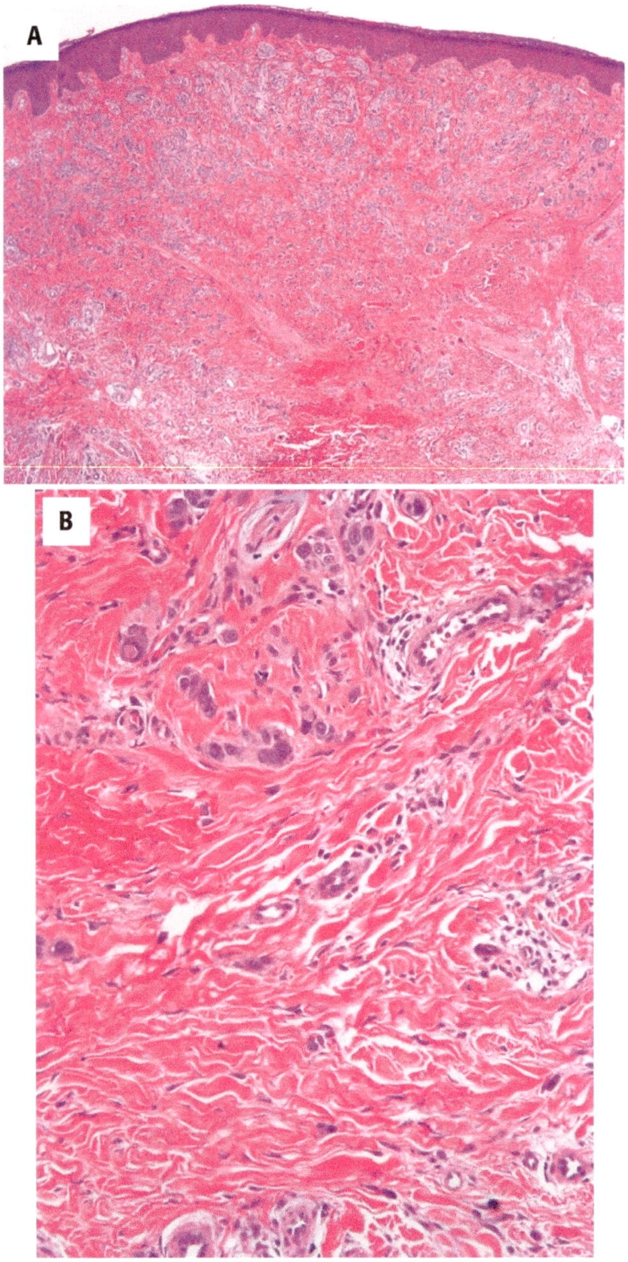

FIG. 13.25

Sclerosing Spitz nevus. **A,** Wedge-shaped intradermal melanocytic nevus. **B,** Plump spindle and epithelioid cells, some with enlarged nuclei, are embedded in fibrotic dermis.

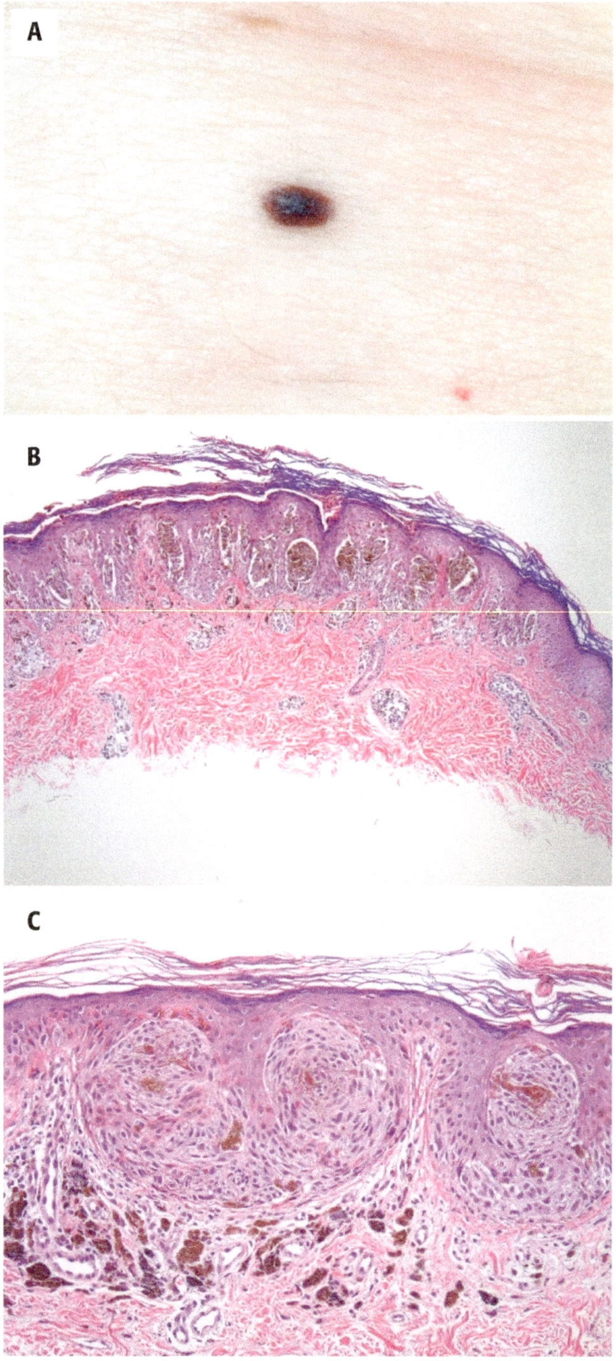

FIG. 13.26

Pigmented spindle cell nevus. **A,** A small dark circumscribed melanocytic nevus is seen. **B,** Histologically, it is composed of many nests of melanocytes at the dermal-epidermal junction surrounded by clefts, and associated with epidermal hyperplasia and hyperpigmentation. **C,** The nests are composed of slender pigmented fusiform melanocytes.

predominant composition of heavily pigmented slender fusiform melanocytes (Fig. 13.26B and C). The lesions are usually small, symmetric, and sharply circumscribed. There are typically densely cellular nests at the dermal-epidermal junction. The epidermal rete ridges tend to be hyperplastic. Melanin pigment is often present in the cytoplasm of keratinocytes at all layers of the epidermis, including the stratum granulosum and corneum (not to be confused with melanocytes). Pagetoid melanocytes may be found, especially in the center of the lesion. Dull pink globules (Kamino bodies) are frequently seen. The nevi may be inflamed and associated with many melanophages in the superficial dermis.

While historically Spitz nevi have been subclassified based on morphologic features (e.g., angiomatoid, tubular, myxoid, verrucous, spindle cell, or large epithelioid cell Spitz nevus), more recently, proposals for different variants of Spitz nevi (and related atypical tumors or melanomas) are based on molecular aberrations. Some of the genomic findings correlate to some extent with microscopic features, but there is a range of phenotypes that can be seen with each aberration. Examples of genomic-microscopic associations include NTRK3 fusions in some pigmented spindle cell nevi (Fig. 13.27). Spitz nevi with ALK fusions tend to display intersection fascicles of spindle cells (Fig. 13.28). Those with NTRK1 fusions may display rosette-like arrangements of melanocytes (Fig. 13.29) or show evidence of hypermaturation (Fig. 13.30). There is a wide range of microscopic appearance of Spitz nevi with ROS1 fusions (Fig. 13.31). Spitz neoplasms with BRAF fusion tend to contain large pigmented and atypical epithelioid cells (Fig. 13.32).

While sequence analysis is the most robust method for documenting the presence of a Spitz-related gene fusion, it is not practical for most dermatopathology laboratories. Sometimes IHC may serve as a surrogate marker for a gene fusion, because the fusion leads to overexpression of the respective protein. Antibodies currently (2023) available for the identification of Spitz gene fusions include ALK, pan-NTRK, and ROS1. Positive IHC results can help support the presence of a bona fide Spitz neoplasm (Figs. 13.30 and 13.31). However, the documentation of a gene fusion only helps for placing a melanocytic neoplasm into the group of Spitz tumors. The distinction of a Spitz nevus from Spitz melanoma depends on microscopic findings and the detection of other aberrations.

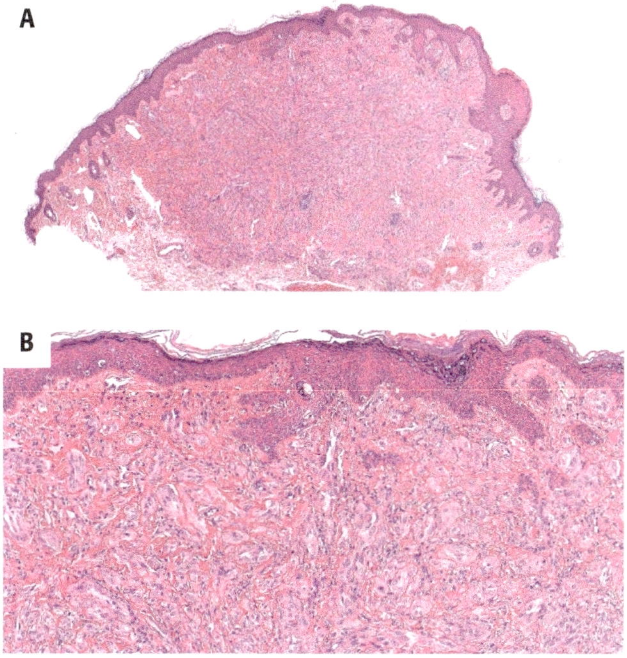

FIG. 13.28

Spitz nevus with ALK fusion. **A,** Silhouette of a relatively circumscribed tumor. **B,** Predominantly intradermal proliferation of amelanotic plump spindle cells forming fascicles that intersect.

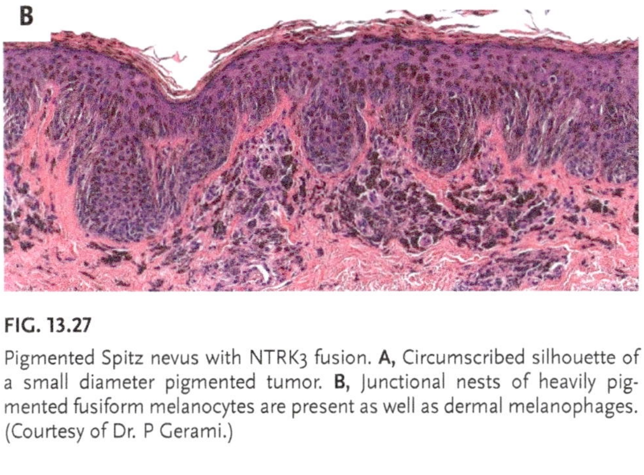

FIG. 13.27

Pigmented Spitz nevus with NTRK3 fusion. **A,** Circumscribed silhouette of a small diameter pigmented tumor. **B,** Junctional nests of heavily pigmented fusiform melanocytes are present as well as dermal melanophages. (Courtesy of Dr. P Gerami.)

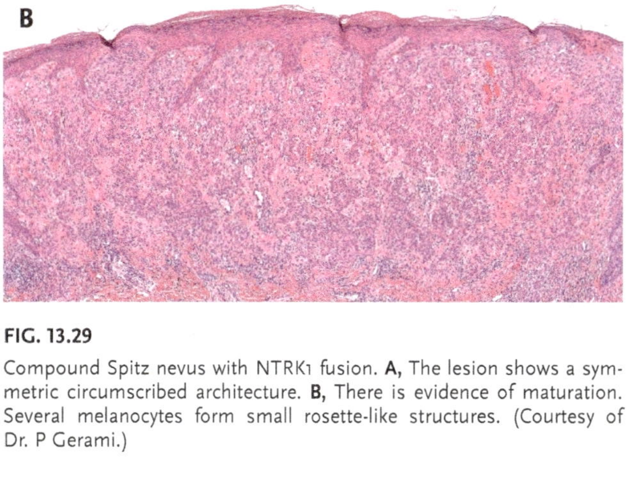

FIG. 13.29

Compound Spitz nevus with NTRK1 fusion. **A,** The lesion shows a symmetric circumscribed architecture. **B,** There is evidence of maturation. Several melanocytes form small rosette-like structures. (Courtesy of Dr. P Gerami.)

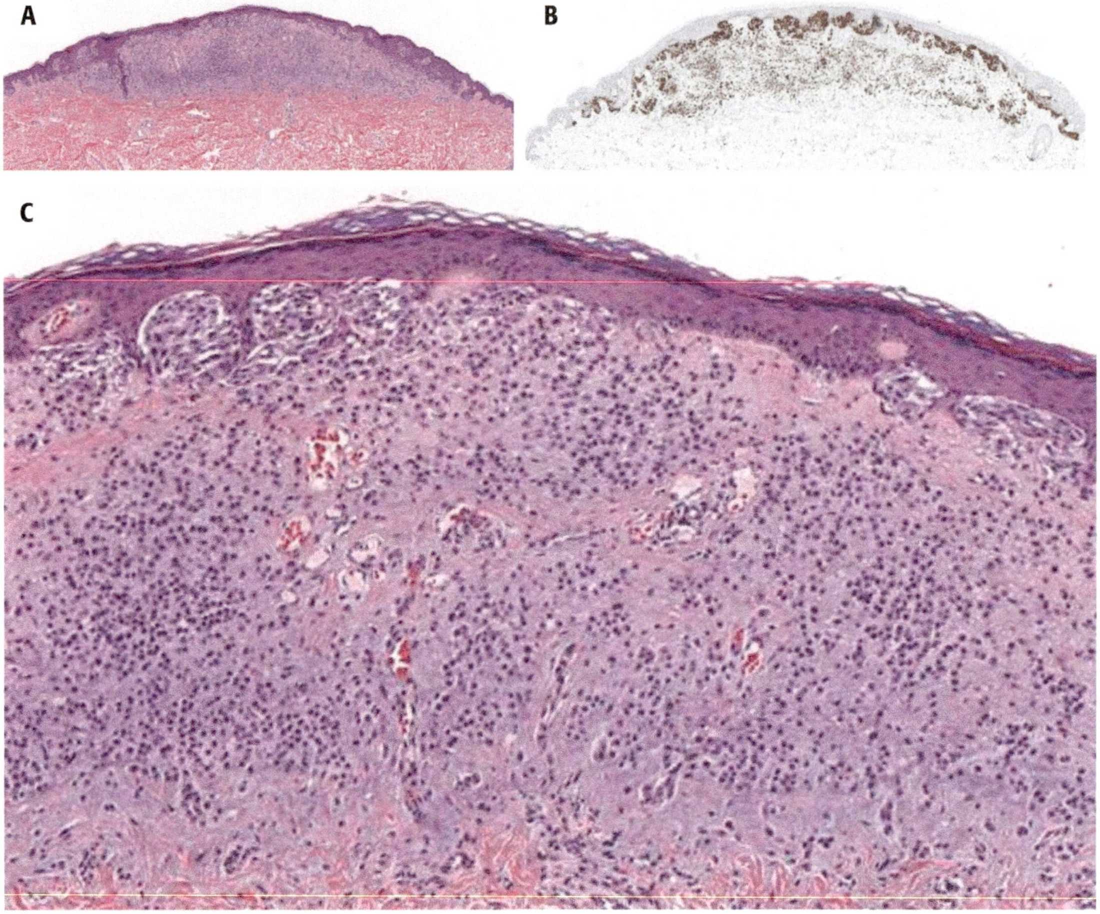

FIG. 13.30

Compound Spitz nevus with NTRK fusion. **A,** The lesion shows a symmetric circumscribed silhouette. **B,** All tumor cells are immunoreactive for pan-NTRK. **C,** The melanocytes show features of maturation and are associated with a slightly myxoid stroma.

A brief comment is also needed to Wiesner's or BAP1-inactivated nevi. They show overlap with epithelioid Spitz nevi and have historically been grouped together with Spitz nevi. However, the current WHO guidelines recommend excluding these spitzoid (Spitz-like) lesions from the category of "true" Spitz neoplasms because they are usually associated with *BRAF* or less commonly with *NRAS* mutations. The presence of multiple BAP1-associated tumors in a single patient may reflect a BAP1 germline mutation and in some instances be associated with a cancer syndrome. On rare occasions, melanoma may arise in association with a BAP1-loss nevus.

Differential Diagnosis

There is a body of literature on the difficulty of distinguishing atypical or unusual variants of Spitz nevi from Spitz's nevus–like melanomas. This is reflected in diagnostic errors as well as proposals for diagnostically indeterminate or intermediate-grade categories, such as atypical Spitz tumor or Spitz melanocytoma. For the differential diagnosis between Spitz nevus and "spitzoid" melanoma, the following light microscopic features favor melanoma: large size, asymmetry, complex growth pattern, presence of mitotic figures in deep dermal melanocytes, atypical mitotic figures, thinned epidermis with effaced rete ridges ("consumption of the epidermis"), lack of maturation, and absence of Kamino bodies. However, none of these features is specific to melanoma. Each of them can also be seen in nevi or *borderline* Spitz melanocytomas. Likewise, features more often found in Spitz nevi than melanoma, such as Kamino bodies, may also be present in fully malignant tumors. However, melanomas tend to show only rare and small Kamino bodies. Numerous large Kamino bodies strongly favor a benign lesion.

In distinguishing a Spitz nevus from melanoma, it is important to realize that some pagetoid spread of melanocytes is acceptable for the diagnosis of a Spitz nevus as long as the other features of the lesion favor a benign melanocytic proliferation. Pagetoid spread of melanocytes in Spitz nevi is usually focal, at or near the center of the lesion, and often associated with ascent of melanocytic nests rather than only solitary units. Pagetoid

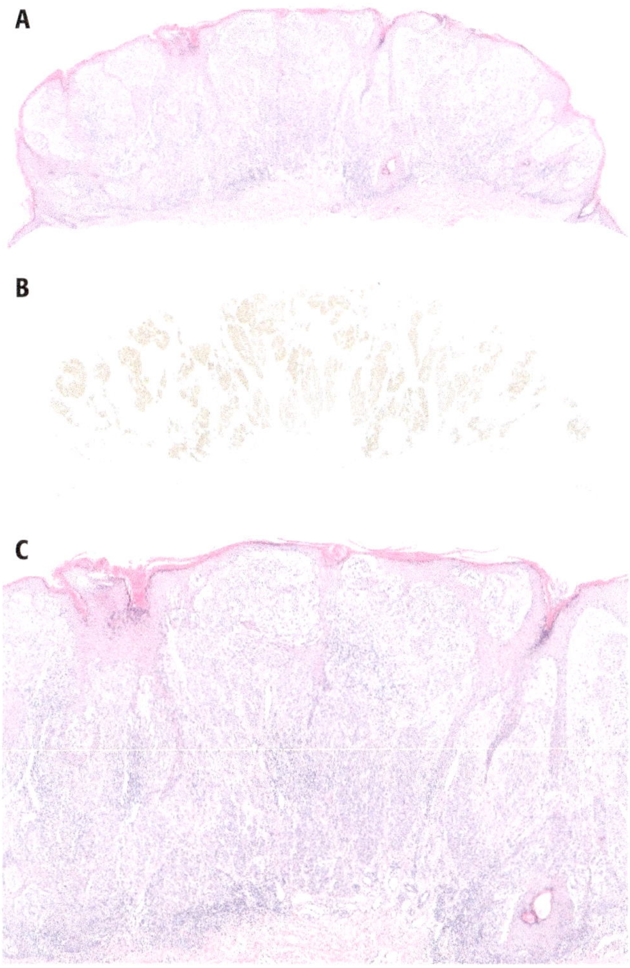

FIG. 13.31

Compound Spitz nevus with ROS1 fusion. **A,** There is a compound melanocytic proliferation with circumscribed architectur. **B,** The tumor cells are immunoreactive for ROS1. **C,** The tumor cells display spitzoid cytology and evidence of maturation.

spread may on occasion be more than focal and readily apparent throughout the lesion (pagetoid Spitz nevus) (Fig. 13.33).

If a pathologist is not comfortable making a distinction between an unusual or atypical variant of Spitz nevus and melanoma, it is best to acknowledge the diagnostic difficulty, consult with other pathologists, or use ancillary studies that may assist in the distinction of Spitz nevus from melanoma. At times, even expert consultants may also not be able to establish an unequivocal diagnosis or agree with each other. Furthermore, results from ancillary studies may not be definitive and conflict with each other, if several different tests are used. In that case, a pragmatic decision needs to be made. Spitzoid melanocytic proliferations with ambiguous findings that are associated with interobserver variability or controversy may be descriptively reported as atypical Spitz tumor or spitzoid melanocytic tumor of uncertain malignant potential (STUMP). For such tumors, conservative complete excision is prudent practice.

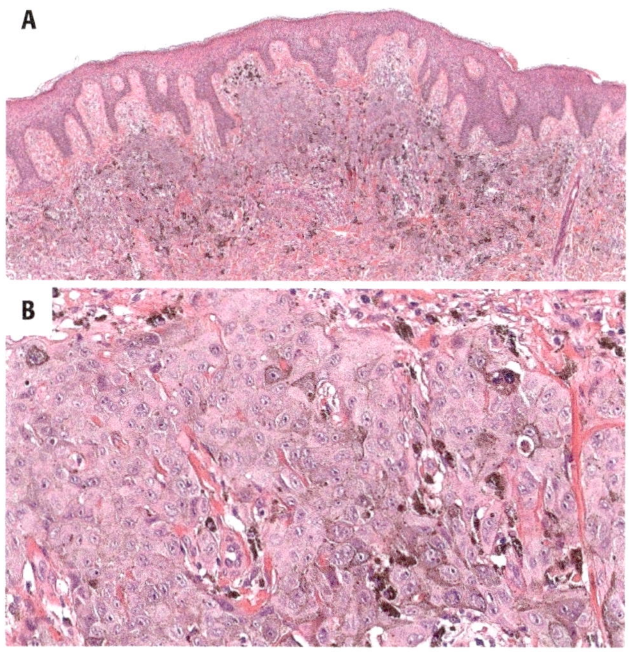

FIG. 13.32

Atypical Spitz tumor with BRAF fusion. **A,** The lesion shows predominantly intradermal growth of pigmented melanocytes. **B,** The tumor cells display large epithelioid atypia and form irregular sheetlike aggregates. (Courtesy of Dr. P Gerami.)

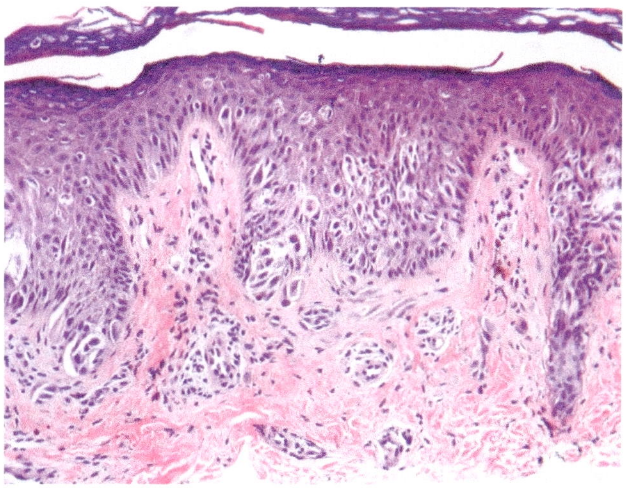

FIG. 13.33

Pagetoid Spitz's nevus. This spindle and epithelioid melanocytic nevus from an 8-year-old child shows many melanocytes above the basal cell layer.

When several pathologists strongly suspect melanoma and/or results from ancillary tests favor melanoma, most surgeons and patients opt for a surgical management algorithm as for melanoma. This may include sentinel lymph node (SLN) biopsy.

If a lymph node biopsy is performed and contains metastatic melanoma (i.e., not a nodal nevus or false-positive isolated immunoreactive cells but dense clusters of atypical or mitotically active melanocytes in the subcapsular sinus or nodal parenchyma), there should be no more doubt about the malignant nature of the primary tumor draining to this node. However, we caution against reclassifying a primary lesion of atypical Spitz tumor as melanoma, if only small deposits of cytologically not obviously malignant melanocytes are detected in the SLN draining such a lesion. Such deposits could represent benign/indolent nodal nevomelanocytes. Current evidence does not suggest that microscopic deposits of tumor cells in the SLN of a patient with a primary atypical Spitz tumor have significant prognostic significance.

Arguing that the binary division of Spitz nevus versus Spitz melanoma may be too simplistic, the category of Spitz melanocytoma has recently been proposed as a third option for reporting Spitz neoplasms. A Spitz melanocytoma is defined as an intermediate-grade neoplasm that shows microscopic and genomic aberrations in between a classic Spitz nevus and Spitz melanoma. For example, a tumor may display atypical microscopic findings (some asymmetry, mitoses), harbor a Spitz-fusion and some deletions of p16, but lack other segmental copy number changes typical of melanoma. Spitz melanocytomas are thought to be indolent neoplasms and do not require more than complete surgical excision for treatment.

The most informative ancillary testing is determining whether the lesion truly belongs to the Spitz family at the genomic level or contrastingly is a *BRAF* or *NRAS*-mutated neoplasm with some spitzoid features. One way to address this question is IHC for BRAFV600E. A positive result is diagnostic for the presence of a BRAFV600E mutation. This does not warrant a diagnosis of melanoma but excludes a Spitz nevus/tumor. Fluorescence in situ hybridization (FISH) and IHC studies for ROS1, ALK, or NTRK can yield positive results in support of a Spitz pathway but require guidance by microscopy, which is imperfect. Next-generation sequencing (NGS) studies are the most comprehensive method to assess the molecular pathway associated with melanocytic tumors. Unfortunately, most panels have limited fusion coverage. If novel or uncommon fusions are suspected, whole transcriptome mRNA sequencing is the preferred method. While determining the genomic lineage of the tumor does not give a malignant or benign diagnosis, it does inform the pathologist regarding how they should modify their criteria for assessing if the tumor is benign or malignant.

Other ancillary techniques include comparative genomic hybridization (CGH) or FISH to look for clonal segmental chromosomal copy number aberrations that may be more typical of melanoma. NGS or targeted sequencing for a TERT promoter mutation (TPM), which is also more typical of melanoma, can also be helpful. IHC for PReferentially expressed Antigen in MElanoma (PRAME), which is more frequently expressed in melanoma than benign melanocytic tumors, can also be used. Ancillary techniques when used in conjunction with the morphologic interpretation can be helpful, but one must be aware of possible false-positive or false-negative results. None of the tests should be used as stand-alone tests.

Amelanotic Spitz nevi without a junctional component may be confused with nonmelanocytic lesions, such as reticulohistiocytoma and cellular neurothekeoma. IHC usually permits a clear distinction. Spitz nevi are positive for S100 protein and Melan-A/Mart-1; reticulohistiocytoma and cellular neurothekeoma are melanocyte differentiation markers.

CONGENITAL MELANOCYTIC NEVI

Clinical Findings

By definition, the term *congenital nevus* implies the presence of a melanocytic lesion at birth. Such nevi tend to be larger (Fig. 13.34) than most ordinarily acquired nevi. They have arbitrarily been classified according to their size as small (less than 1.5 cm), medium (1.5 to less than 20 cm), and giant (20 cm or larger). Congenital nevi may occur in context with neurocutaneous melanosis, a syndrome in which melanocytic nevi are associated with leptomeningeal melanocytosis or melanoma. Congenital nevi, especially large variants, represent primarily a cosmetic problem, but there is also a risk for the development of melanoma. Published data have likely exaggerated this risk because of referral bias and misdiagnosis of atypical melanocytic proliferations arising in congenital nevi as melanoma. Most dermal or subcutaneous nodules that develop within congenital nevi, especially giant congenital nevi, are clinically indolent and represent so-called cellular or proliferative nodules. Patients with giant bathing trunk nevi may also have leptomeningeal melanocytosis and be at risk for the development of an intracranial melanocytoma or melanoma.

Histopathologic Features

Congenital melanocytic nevi may or may not have a papillomatous epidermal silhouette. Their superficial portion is similar to acquired nevi. However, congenital nevi typically show infiltration of melanocytes into the reticular dermis (Fig. 13.35). Melanocytes may even be present in the subcutis or deep soft tissues in a perivascular or interstitial distribution. In congenital nevi, melanocytes are more often seen involving adnexal

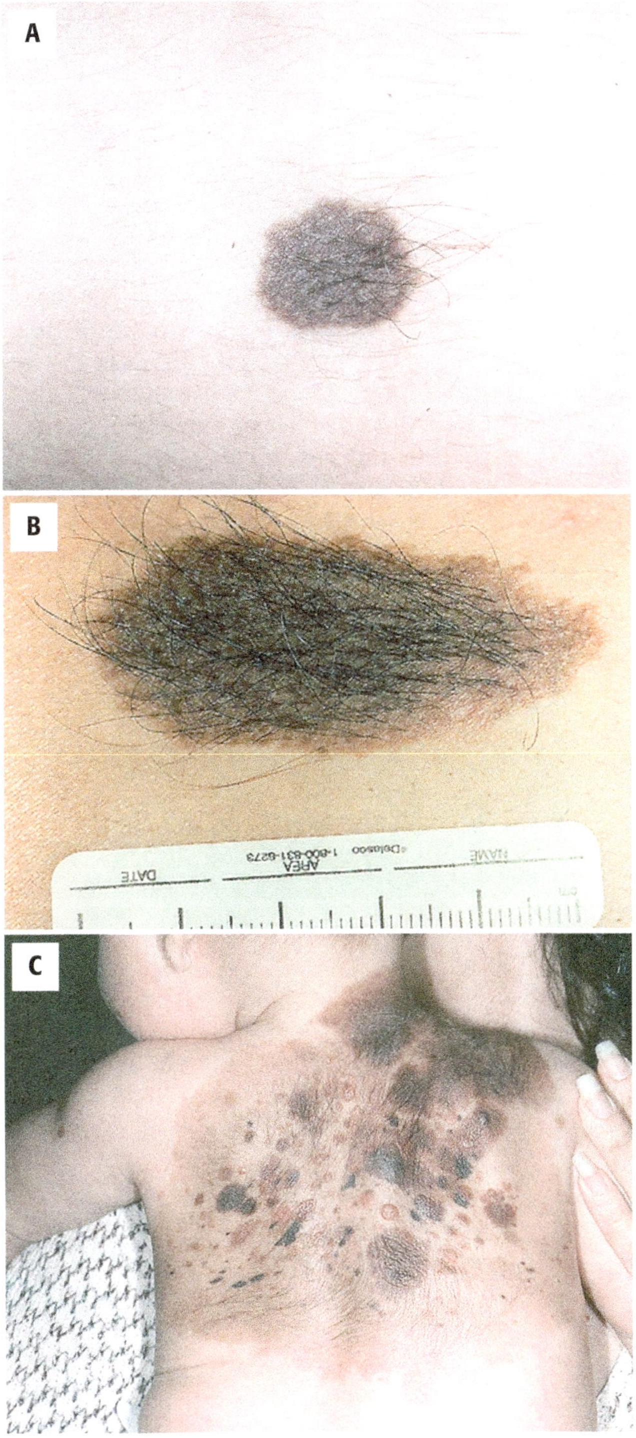

FIG. 13.34

Congenital melanocytic nevus. **A,** Small congenital nevus. **B,** Medium-sized congenital nevus. **C,** Giant hairy nevus.

structures (eccrine ducts, folliculosebaceous units) than in acquired nevi. Involvement of smooth muscle and peripheral nerve trunks may also be found. In some congenital nevi, melanocytes are present in the walls of blood vessels. Large congenital nevi may show prominent schwannian or neurofibromatous features and contain heterologous elements such as cartilage.

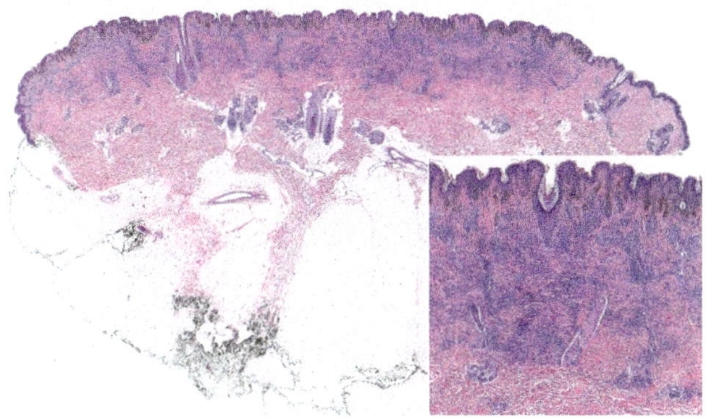

FIG. 13.35

Congenital melanocytic nevus. Broad plaque-like compound melanocytic proliferation extending into the reticular dermis. Involvement of adnexal structures by melanocytes is seen *(inset)*.

CONGENITAL MELANOCYTIC NEVUS—PATHOLOGIC FEATURES

Clinical Findings

- Present at birth or clinically apparent in early childhood
- May be large (giant nevi)

Histopathologic Features

- Silhouette
  - Symmetric
  - Sharp peripheral borders
- Junctional component
  - Similar to common nevi but may be broader
  - Possible pagetoid melanocytes
- Subepithelial component
  - Evidence of maturation
  - Frequently involves reticular dermis, may extend into subcutis
  - Patterns of stromal involvement: diffuse, interstitial, or perivascular
  - Adnexal involvement is common
  - Nerve involvement may be seen
  - Schwannian differentiation may be prominent
  - Cellular or proliferative nodules may be present
  - Heterologous elements may be present in large nevi

Cellular or proliferative nodules may develop in congenital nevi, especially giant congenital nevi. They manifest as areas of high cellular density that typically blend with the surrounding nevus component. Mitotic figures may be present (proliferative nodule). The melanocytes in these nodules may be fusiform or epithelioid. Cellular spindle cell nodules may have a primitive mesenchymal or sarcomatoid appearance. They may not be uniformly immunoreactive for melanocyte differentiation antigens or even S100 protein.

On exceedingly rare occasions, sarcomatoid nodules with histologic and immunohistochemical features indistinguishable from a sarcoma, such as a rhabdomyosarcoma, may arise in a giant congenital nevus.

Differential Diagnosis

The distinction of congenital nevi from acquired nevi is best made clinically. Although large and deep congenital nevi are histologically distinctive, many features associated with small congenital nevi may also be seen in acquired nevi. Confusion with in situ melanoma is possible because benign pagetoid melanocytes may be found in congenital nevi. Attention to clinical and histologic context (young age; nevus with otherwise benign features, including cytologically bland melanocytes with evidence of maturation) is needed to avoid a diagnostic error. In situ melanoma is best recognized by the presence of cytologically atypical pagetoid melanocytes and asymmetric extension of such cells peripherally beyond the dermal nevus component.

With regard to the dermal or subcutaneous component, congenital nevi may contain areas of high cellular density without (cellular nodules) or with mitotically active melanocytes (proliferative nodules) that need to be distinguished from melanoma (Fig. 13.36). Characteristically, melanoma displays a sharp demarcation between its cytologically atypical cells and the adjacent bland nevus cell population (Fig. 13.37). In contrast, cellular or proliferative nodules tend to mature and blend with the surrounding nevus cells. Cellular or proliferative nodules are usually composed of epithelioid melanocytes, but some nodules are almost exclusively composed of fusiform melanocytes.

When congenital nevi show prominent differentiation along schwannian lines and contain heterologous elements, they may also be referred to as *neurocristic hamartoma*. However, the latter term has generated some

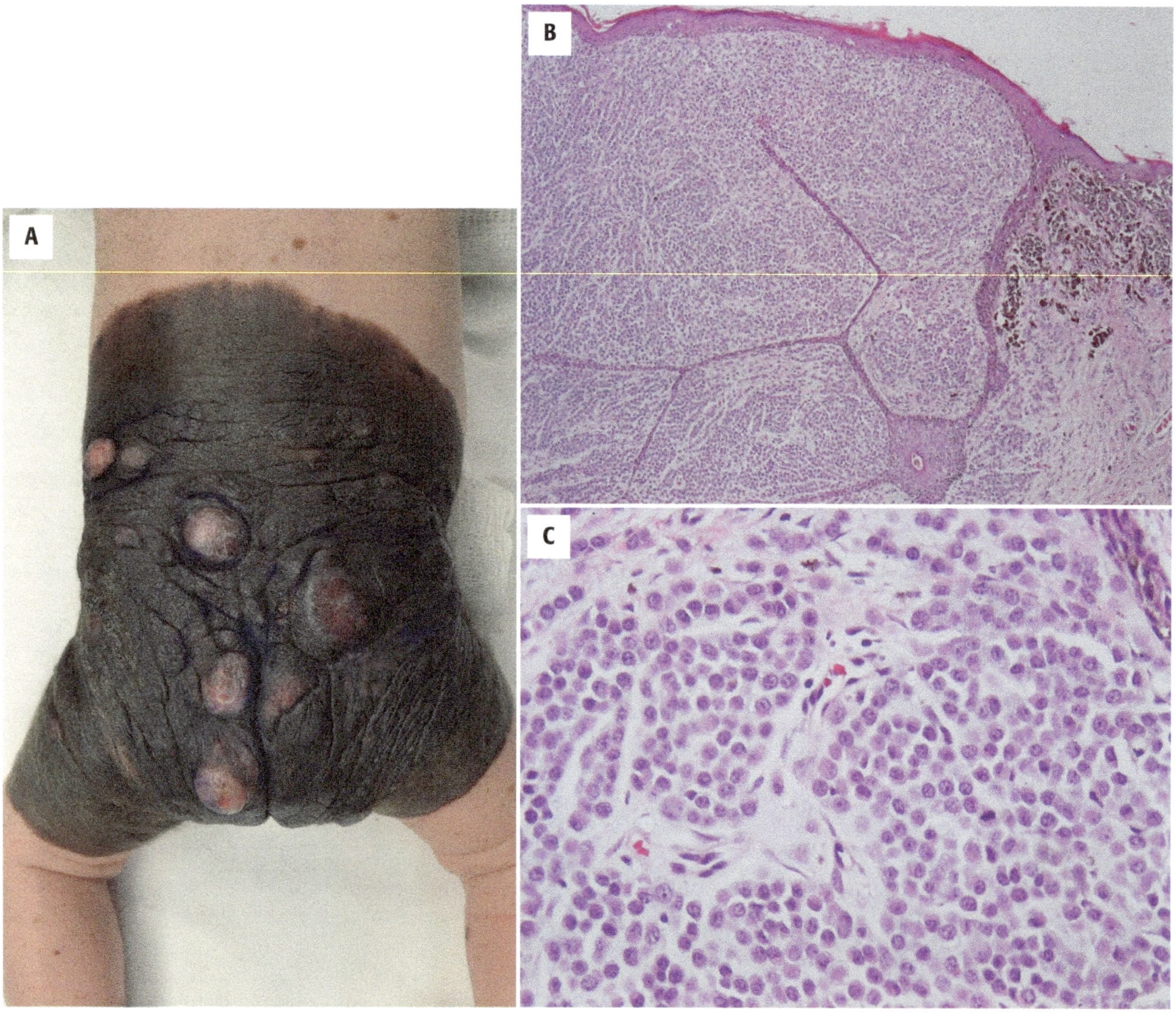

FIG. 13.36

Proliferative nodule in a giant congenital nevus. **A,** Giant congenital melanocytic nevus with nodules. **B,** Histologically, at the site of a nodule, there is a nodular proliferation of epithelioid melanocytes. **C,** Some melanocytes are seen in mitosis.

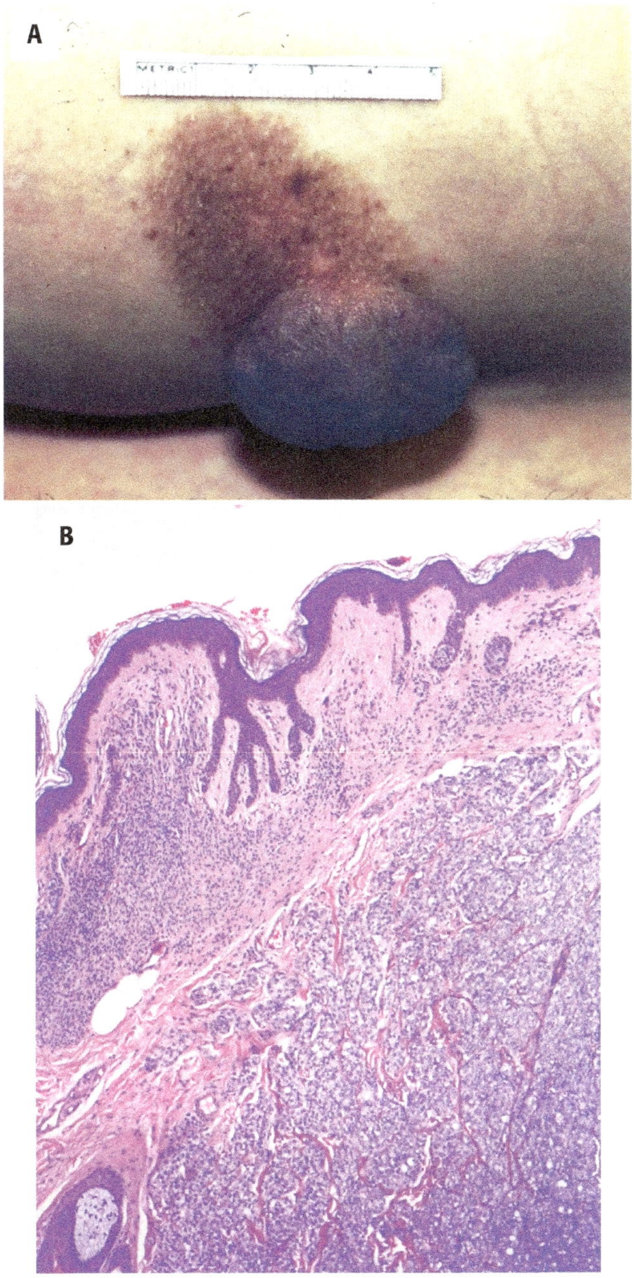

FIG. 13.37

Melanoma arising in association with a congenital nevus. **A,** A polypoid nodule is present in association with a medium-sized congenital nevus. **B,** Superficially, bland nevomelanocytes are present. Underneath is a dermal melanoma composed of atypical epithelioid tumor cells.

confusion because it has been used in the literature for a spectrum of melanocytic proliferations, including large blue nevi, combined nevi, neurotized nevi, and congenital nevi with and without heterologous elements.

Cytogenetic analysis may be helpful for the distinction of cellular or proliferative nodules from malignant melanoma. Benign proliferations in congenital nevi either lack chromosomal copy number changes or display whole chromosome gains, in contrast to malignant melanomas, which tend to display a mix of gains and losses at several chromosomes.

BLUE NEVI AND DERMAL MELANOCYTOSES

Clinical Findings

Blue nevi comprise a spectrum of melanocytic lesions characterized clinically by a bluish appearance (Fig. 13.38). A blue nevus (BN) may be present at birth or appear later in life. Preferred locations are the head and neck region, buttock, and dorsum of the wrist or foot. Most BNs are small and circumscribed lesions (Fig. 13.38). However, unusual clinical variants exist, which may clinically present as large nodules (cellular BN) or plaques (plaque-type BN) (Fig. 13.39) or as targetoid lesions (targetoid BN). Extracutaneous occurrence has been reported at various sites, including conjunctival,

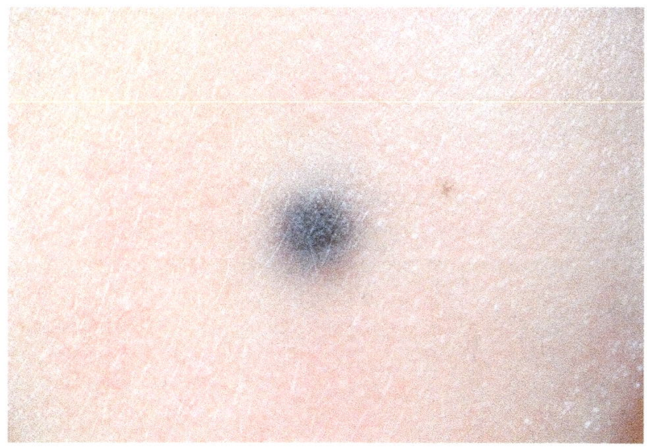

FIG. 13.38

Common blue nevus (BN). Common BN presenting as a small bluish papule.

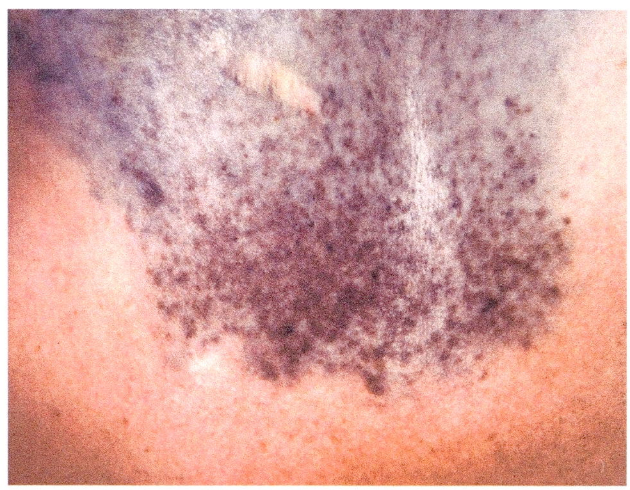

FIG. 13.39

Plaque-type blue nevus (BN). Rare plaque-type BN presenting as a large pigmented bluish-brown plaque with mottled pigmentation.

oral, or sinonasal mucosa; the gastrointestinal or urogenital tract; and lymph nodes. Leptomeningeal melanocytosis or intracranial lesions reported as melanocytoma represent lesions in the spectrum of BN-like melanocytic proliferations.

The related dermal melanocytoses usually manifest clinically early in childhood and tend to be flat lesions of brown-bluish discoloration. The Mongolian spot typically affects the lumbosacral region, the nevus of Ota (nevus fuscoceruleus ophthalmomaxillaris) involves the segment of skin innervated by the first and second branches of the trigeminal nerve, and the nevus of Ito (nevus fuscoceruleus acromiodeltoideus) is present on the shoulder or upper arm. Acquired and congenital variants of dermal melanocytoses exist, which may manifest with an unusual anatomic distribution.

Histopathologic Features

Both BN and dermal melanocytosis are characterized by the presence of dendritic or fusiform melanocytes in the dermis or subcutis. Variable numbers of melanophages may be present. Except for combined or collision lesions, BNs lack a junctional melanocytic proliferation. In dermal melanocytoses, the melanocytes are dispersed as solitary units and separated from each other by abundant intervening stroma (Fig. 13.40). BNs represent localized melanocytic proliferations (Fig. 13.41), in which the lesional cells are more closely apposed to each other and may even form fascicles or nests. There is a spectrum of light microscopic appearances of lesions classified as BN. The typical "common" BN (Fig. 13.41) is an intradermal proliferation of slender fusiform and dendritic pigmented melanocytes, which are often associated with melanophages and variable degrees of dermal fibrosis. Often, they are found in association with a hair follicle. Variations may be seen with regard to size, intralesional stromal fibrosis, pigmentation, cellularity, cellular composition (presence of another nevus-type component), cytology (e.g., epithelioid

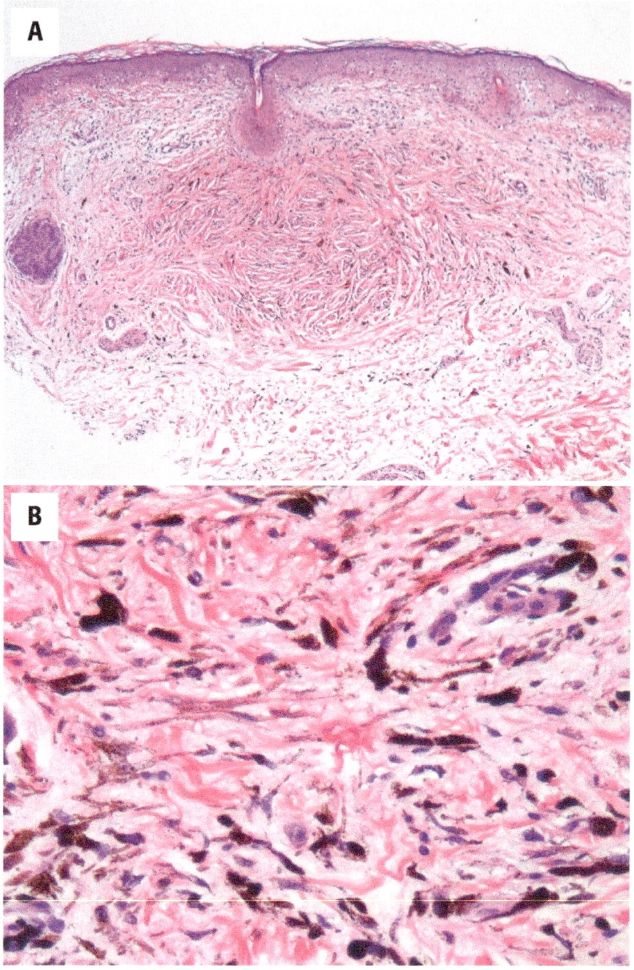

FIG. 13.41

Common blue nevus. **A,** A perifollicular pigmented lesion is present associated with mild dermal fibrosis. **B,** It is composed of pigmented fusiform and dendritic melanocytes as well as macrophages.

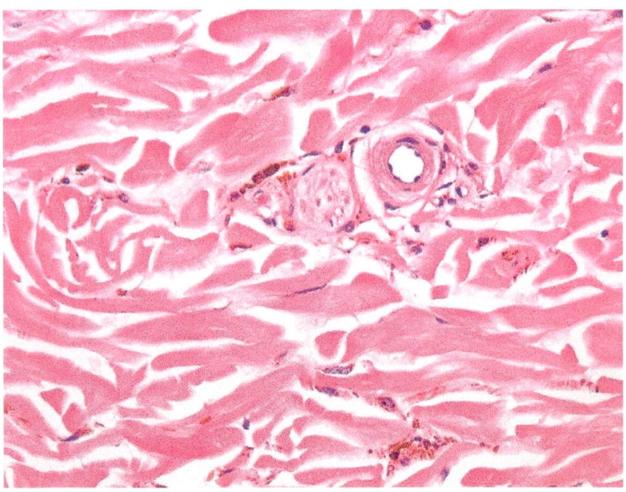

FIG. 13.40

Melanocytosis. Scattered and widely spaced isolated fusiform melanocytes and melanophages are seen in the dermis.

COMMON BLUE NEVUS—PATHOLOGIC FEATURES

Clinical Findings

- Bluish or gray to black appearance
- Usually small papule
- Common sites include dorsum of foot, wrist, and head

Histopathologic Features

- Usually oval-shaped lesion in reticular dermis
- Slender fusiform and dendritic melanocytes, usually heavily pigmented
- Melanophages are common
- Stromal fibrosis is common
- Periadnexal growth is common
- Nerve involvement may be seen

versus spindle versus dendritic cells), and growth patterns. Accordingly, a number of subtypes of BN have been proposed that reflect this spectrum (e.g., sclerosing BN, hypo- or amelanotic BN, epithelioid BN [EBN], cellular BN). On rare occasions, a BN may be associated with a benign trichoblastic proliferation (similar phenomenon as with superficial trichoblastic proliferations and dermatofibromas). BN may be large and present as diffuse dermal or subcutaneous pigmented plaque (plaque-type BN).

The sclerosing BN is characterized by prominent stromal fibrosis (Fig. 13.42). It usually has an overall low cellular density. However, some larger lesions may display a combination of hypo- and hypercellular areas (Fig. 13.43). Hypo- or amelanotic BN lacks readily detectable melanin pigment and may be confused with a dermatofibroma. The classic cellular BN shows a circumscribed nodular growth pattern (Fig. 13.44). Bulging tonguelike extensions of densely cellular sheets into the deep dermis or subcutis may be present. Often a biphasic pattern is seen, characterized by the presence of common BN-like areas juxtaposed with more densely cellular paucimelanotic or amelanotic nested or fascicular aggregates of melanocytes with pale cytoplasm (Fig. 13.44). Cystic degeneration may occur in large lesions (Fig. 13.45).

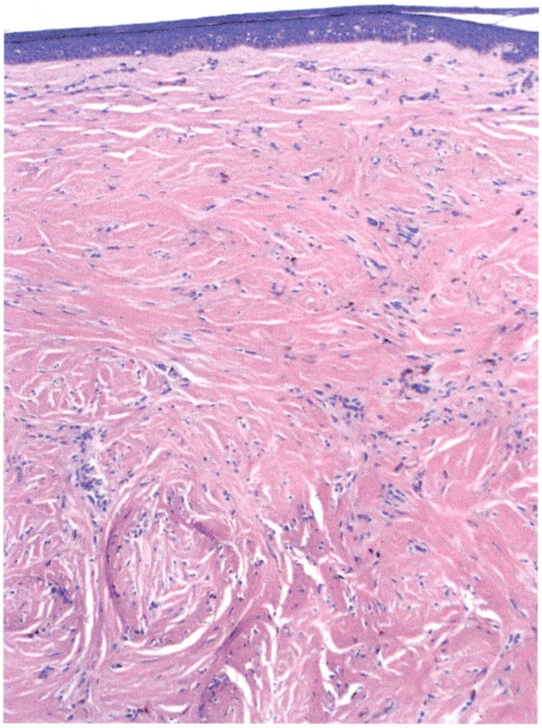

FIG. 13.42

Sclerosing blue nevus (BN). A paucimelanotic BN is seen with prominent dermal fibrosis.

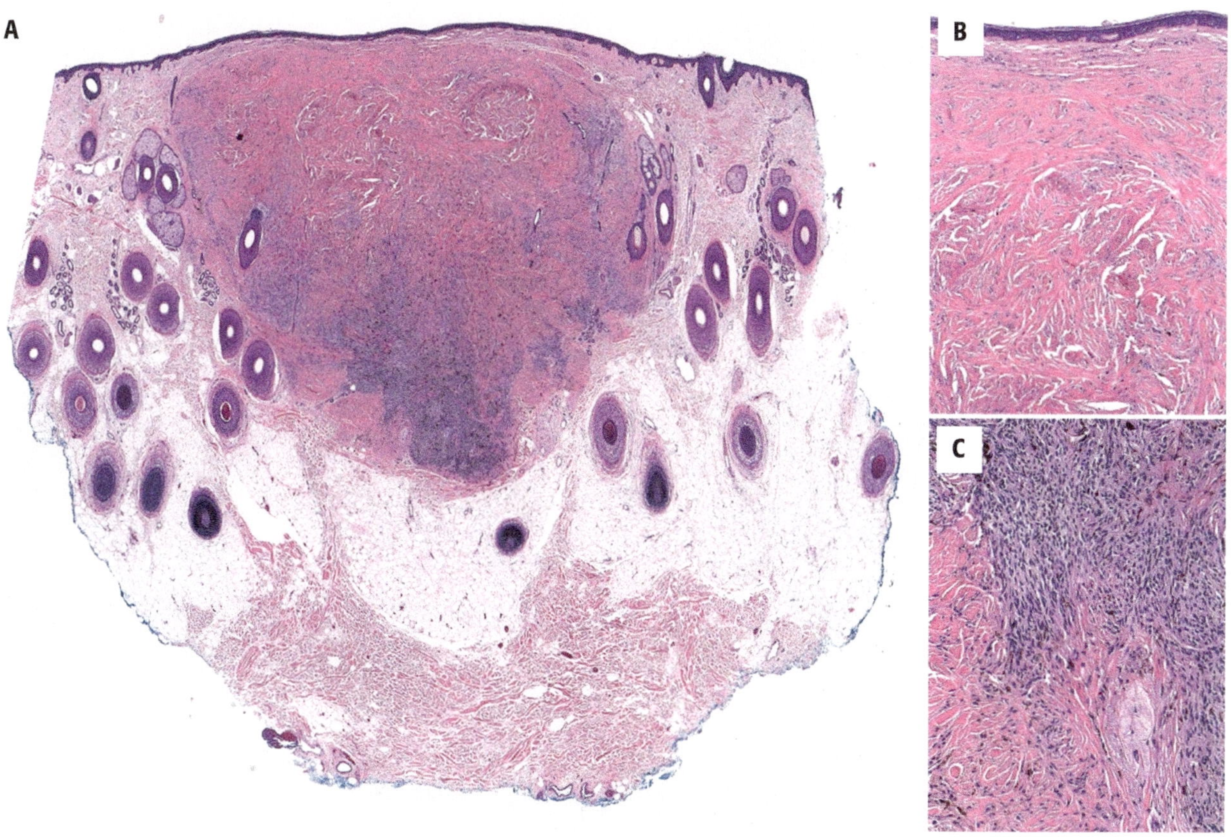

FIG. 13.43

Sclerosing blue nevus with cellular areas. **A,** Nodular melanocytic nevus involving the dermis and subcutis of the scalp. **B,** The superficial part of the lesion is sclerosing. **C,** The deep part is cellular.

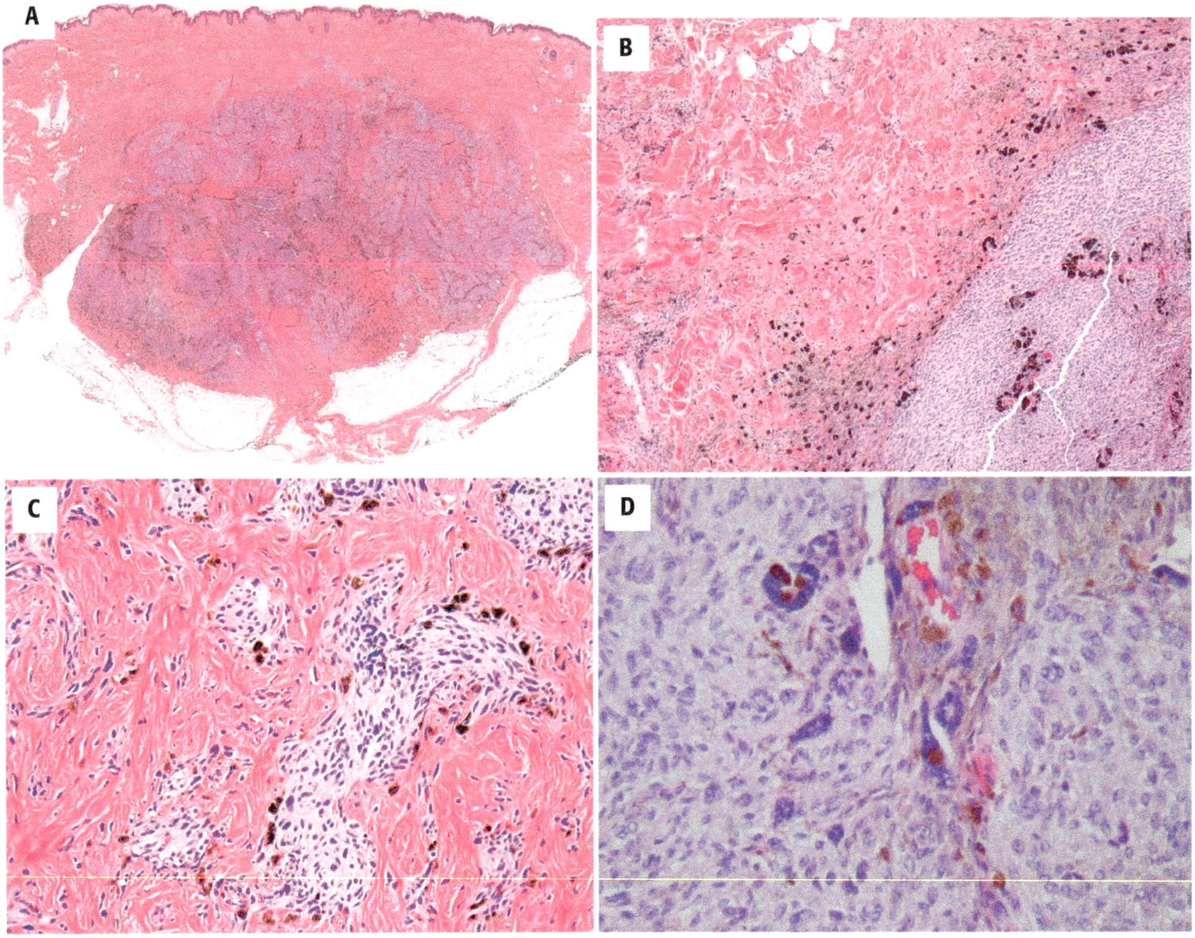

FIG. 13.44

Cellular blue nevus (BN). **A,** Biphasic cellular nodule in the dermis. **B,** Densely packed groups of pale spindle cells adjacent to paucicellular fibrotic area with conventional BN-like features. **C,** Aggregates of cytologically bland pale melanocytes with surrounding fibrotic stroma. **D,** Cellular area with multinucleated melanocytes.

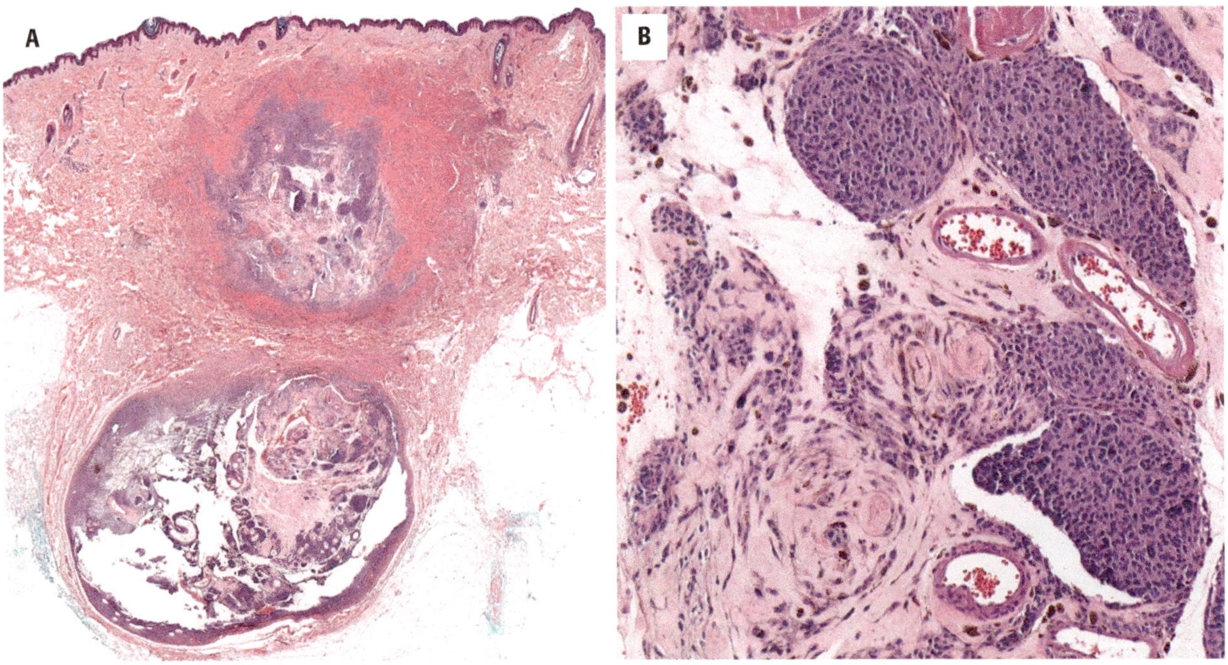

FIG. 13.45

Cellular blue nevus. **A,** Nevus with central cystic degeneration. **B,** Cytologically bland clusters of melanocytes, stromal edema, and hyalinized vessels.

CELLULAR BLUE NEVUS—PATHOLOGIC FEATURES

Clinical Findings

- Sacral region or buttock, foot, and scalp are most commonly affected
- Onset usually in childhood
- Well-circumscribed gray-blue nodule

Histopathologic Features

- Localized to reticular dermis
- Nodular expansile growth patterns of cellular aggregates
- Often bulging extensions seen at the base of the lesion
- Biphasic pattern common with cellular nodules in a background of features of common BN
- Alveolar pattern may be seen (fascicles of spindle cells compartmentalized by fibrosis)
- Monophasic fascicular pattern

Differential Diagnosis

- Melanoma arising in association with a BN
- Clear cell sarcoma
- Metastatic melanoma
- Nerve sheath tumor

Multinucleation of melanocytes in cellular blue nevi is a common finding.

The plaque-type BN broadly infiltrates dermis and often deeper soft tissue (Fig. 13.46). It may have an appearance that except for the area of involvement and clinical size is indistinguishable from a common BN. However, not uncommonly, larger long-standing lesions contain variably cellular nodules.

The EBN is characterized by the predominance of epithelioid melanocytes (Fig. 13.47). Their nuclei usually show an open chromatin pattern with or without a small distinct nucleolus.

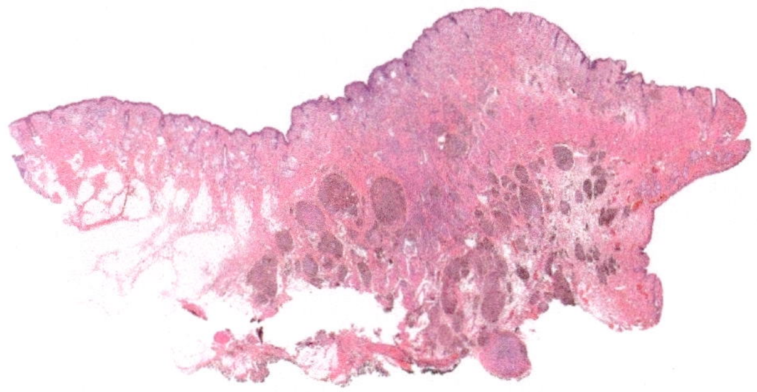

FIG. 13.46

Plaque-type blue nevus (BN) with cellular nodules. BN grows in a broad plaque-like pattern in the skin and soft tissue. Multiple cellular nodules are seen.

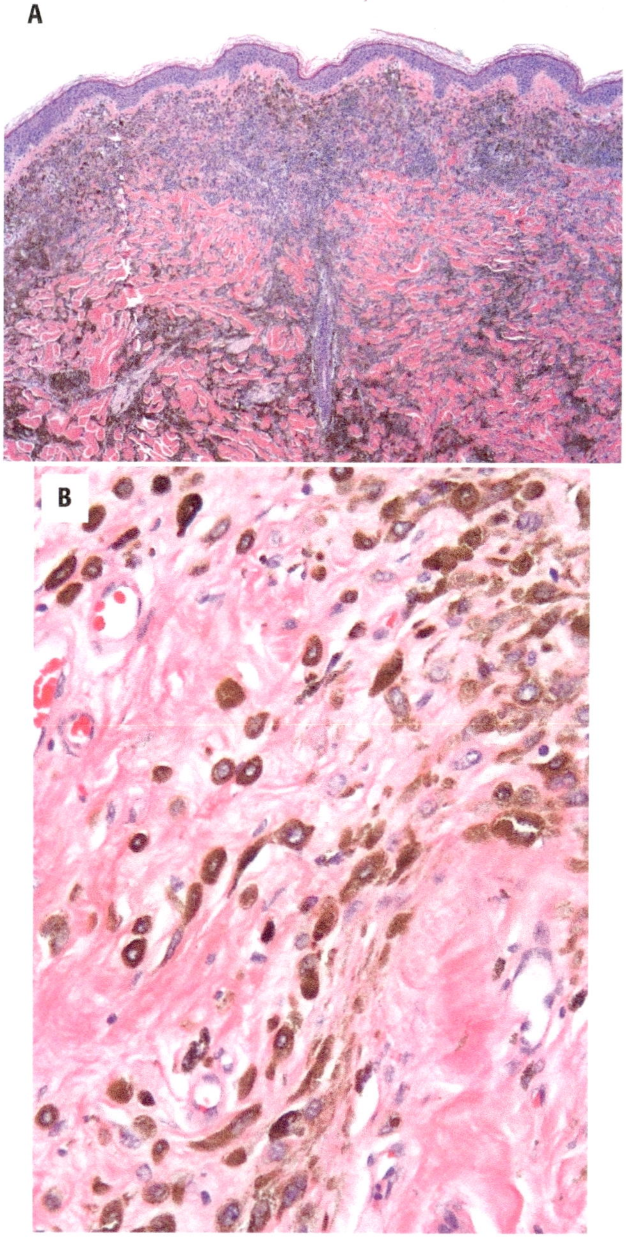

FIG. 13.47

Blue nevus with epithelioid cell features. **A,** Pigmented compound melanocytic nevus with congenital pattern. **B,** The nevus is composed of many pigmented epithelioid melanocytes; some cells display bipolar dendritic processes.

Differential Diagnosis

Primary melanoma may arise in association with or histologically mimic a BN, usually a cellular BN. Metastatic melanoma may also be similar to a BN. The diagnosis of melanoma is straightforward if the histopathologic appearance is that of an obvious malignant tumor (necrosis, atypia, mitoses, infiltrative growth), but it can be difficult when mitoses are rare and the degree of atypia is low. Attention to the presence of aggregates or sheets of atypical epithelioid melanocytes with mitotic figures is important to recognize melanoma arising in a cellular BN. Melanoma may also be suspected if there is a large expansile area of fascicular (sarcomatoid) growth with lack of fibrous stroma. Monophasic amelanotic variants of cellular BN may be confused with a sarcoma.

Melanoma metastatic to skin may have a BN-like clinical and microscopic appearance. For the diagnosis of such a metastasis, clinical context is essential. Most BN-like melanoma metastases occur in the setting of a known prior cutaneous or ocular melanoma. Histopathologically, such lesions usually contain atypical epithelioid melanocytes with at least a rare mitotic figure.

The differential diagnosis of BN also includes *pigmented epithelioid melanocytoma* (PEM), a usually heavily pigmented melanocytic neoplasm containing large epithelioid melanocytes with open chromatin pattern and distinct nuclei ("fried egg" appearance) along with fusiform melanocytes and melanophages (Fig. 13.48). In contrast to most BN, PEM tends to be associated with epidermal hyperplasia and is more likely to have junctional nests. Lesions of PEM are associated with a range of molecular changes, including alterations in PRKAR1A or PRKCA fusions, which differ from BN. Blue tumors with *CYSLTR2* mutations are particularly prone to be confused with PEM. Loss of immunoreactivity for PRKAR1A can help support the diagnosis of PEM, but molecular analysis permits the most precise classification of blue tumors and their mimics. PEM is often referred to as an "intermediate-grade" neoplasm. If correctly diagnosed, that is, not confused with a PEM-like melanoma, it is associated with an indolent clinical course. Small tumor deposits have been found in SLN of patients with PEM, but this does not seem to affect the good prognosis associated with this tumor. It is not recommended for individuals with a PEM to undergo an SLN biopsy unless there is suspicion for a PEM-like melanoma.

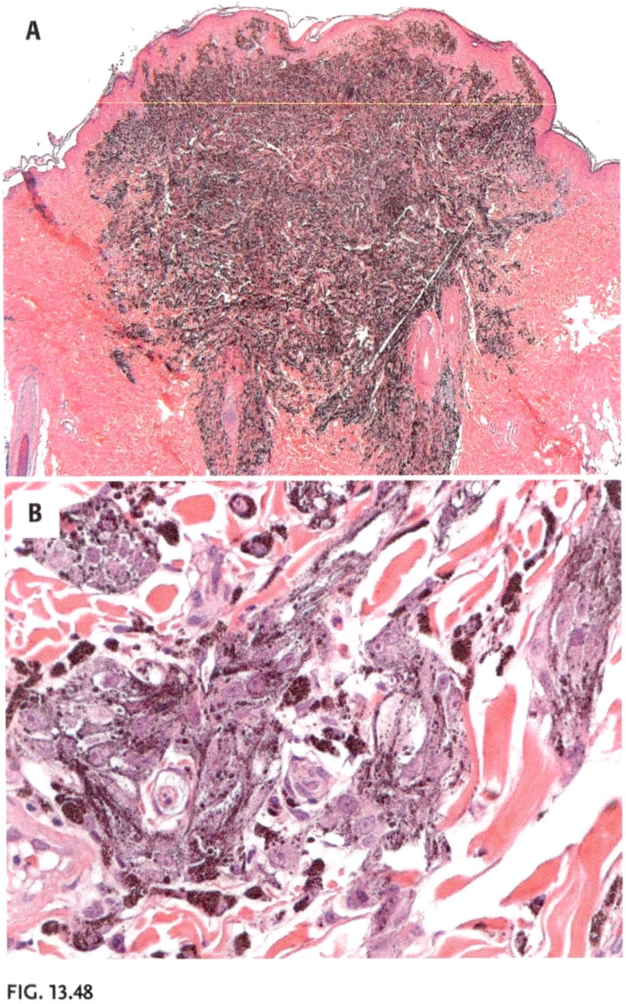

FIG. 13.48
Pigmented epithelioid melanocytoma. **A,** Cellular hypermelanotic melanocytic proliferation with epidermal hyperplasia. **B,** Lesional melanocytes contain large round to oval nuclei with open chromatin pattern.

Ancillary cytogenetic studies can be helpful for the distinction of BN from melanoma and other pigmented neoplasms. Copy number changes are commonly found in melanomas arising in association with BN. Mutation analysis may assist in distinguishing BN from other pigmented melanocytic or soft tissue tumors. Mutations in *GNA11* or *GNAQ* would support a diagnosis of BN. However, these mutations are not found in all BN. Recently some melanocytic nevi with features overlapping with BN have been found to carry PRKCA or PRKCB gene fusions. The term BLUF nevus (blue fusion n) has been proposed for them.

MELANOCYTIC NEVI OF SPECIAL ANATOMIC SITES

The spectrum of histologic features of melanocytic nevi depends to some degree on the anatomic site. Knowledge of the spectrum of site-dependent features is important when one weighs the significance of various findings for the final diagnosis.

Nevi at flexural sites, including the axilla, umbilicus, and groin, for example, may have large nests or great variation in the size and shape of nests (Fig. 13.49). Cellular dyscohesion of nevomelanocytes may be seen. Often there is a complex pattern of associated epidermal hyperplasia. Similar features may also be present in nevi of the genital region, where nests may greatly vary in size and shape and display complex growth patterns. Additional complexity and diagnostic confusion may be related to superimposed inflammatory or fibrosing changes from conditions, such as lichen sclerosus. Likewise, nevi of the ear may show a complex growth pattern and associated features secondary to irritation.

Nevi at acral sites, especially on the palms and soles, may show discrete columns of melanin pigment in the stratum corneum (Fig. 13.50). There may be ascent of cytologically bland melanocytes as solitary units of nests into the mid- and upper epidermis. Thus pagetoid spread of melanocytes (pagetoid melanocytosis) per se is not sufficient for a diagnosis of melanoma in situ at an acral site if the lesion otherwise shows features of a

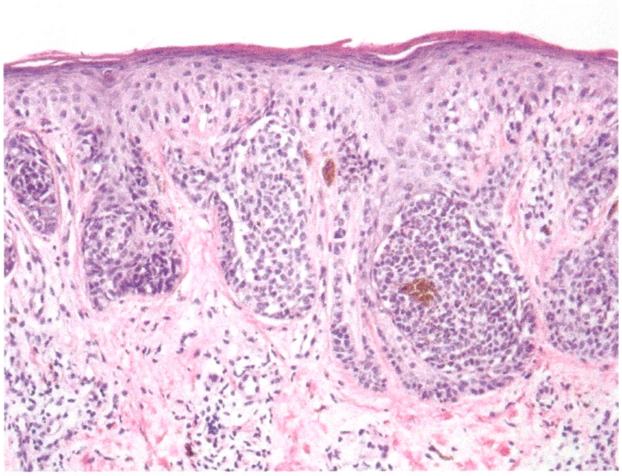

FIG. 13.49

Melanocytic nevus of flexural site. A compound melanocytic nevus is present with many large nests and variation in the size and shape of nests.

benign nevus. In acral nevi, melanocytes may be dispersed prominently along eccrine ducts.

NEVUS SPILUS OR SPECKLED NEVUS

Clinical Findings

The nevus spilus or speckled lentiginous nevus is a lightly pigmented macular lesion (ranging from less than 1 cm to greater than 20 cm in size) that contains dark speckles (Fig. 13.51A) that may be flat or raised. It may be present at birth but more commonly develops in childhood, with a predilection for the trunk and extremities. These lesions are the result of mosaic-activating point mutations in *HRAS*.

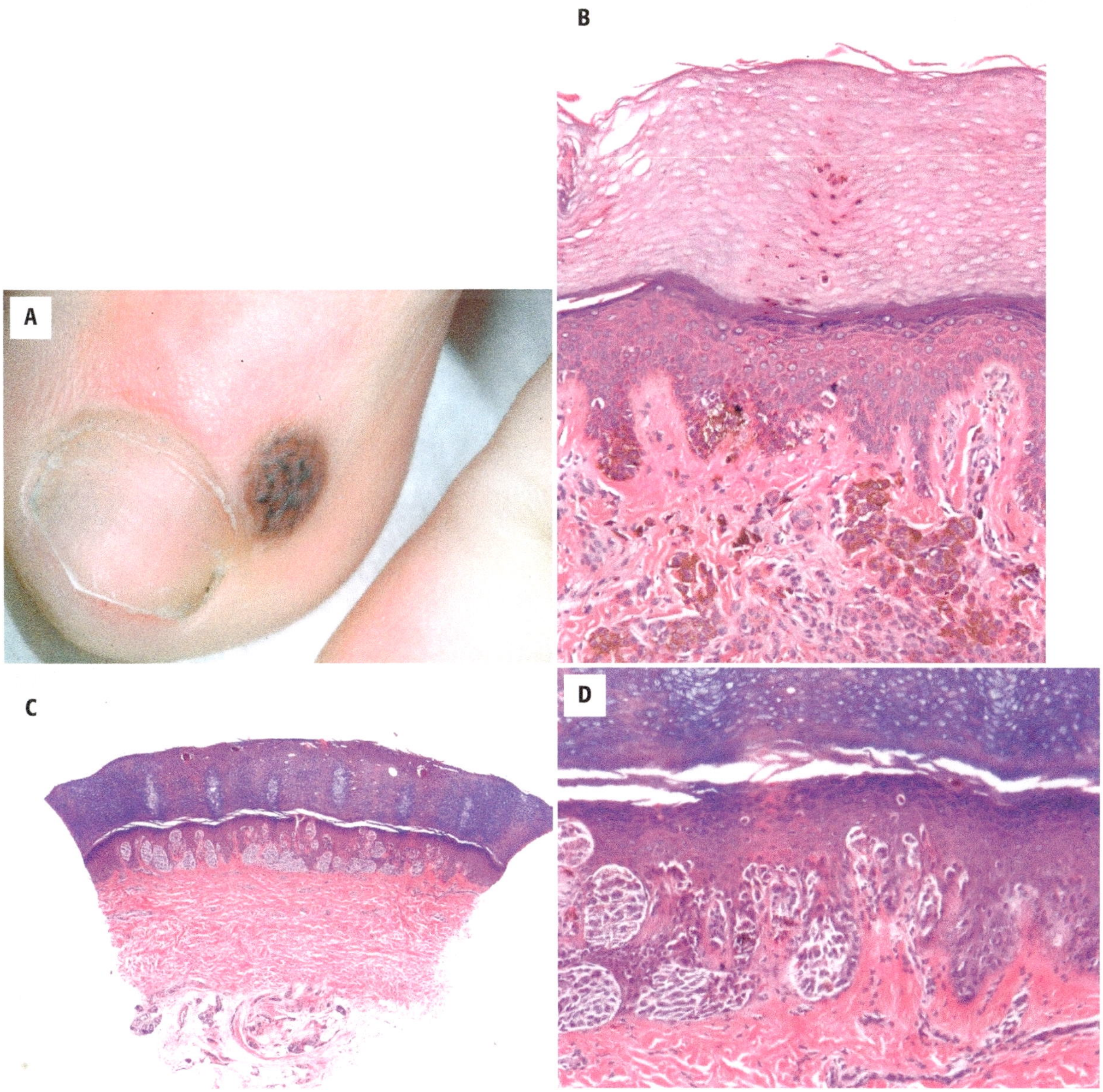

FIG. 13.50

Melanocytic nevus of acral skin. **A,** A circumscribed pigmented macule is seen near the toenail. **B,** Silhouette of nevus with predominant nested pattern and sharp lateral demarcation. **C,** A compound melanocytic nevus with superficial dermal pigmentation is present. A vertical column of melanin pigment is seen in the stratum corneum. **D,** Pagetoid spread of cytologically bland melanocytes may be seen in an acral nevus.

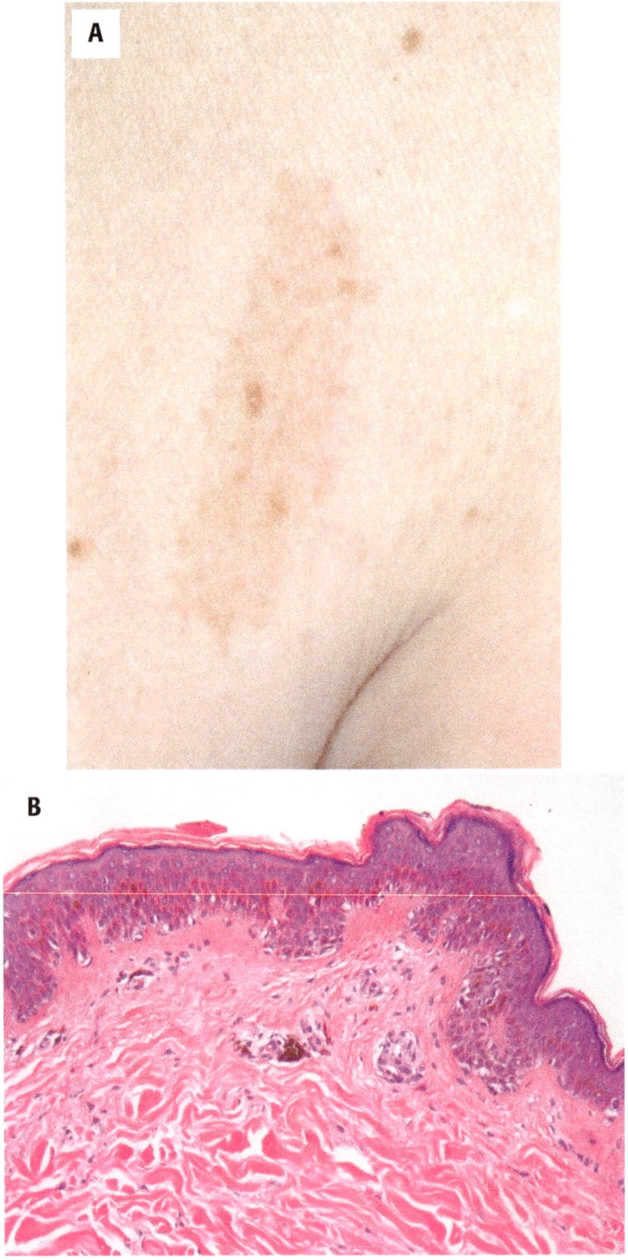

FIG. 13.51

Nevus spilus. **A,** A light brown macular lesion is present with darker brown spots within it. **B,** There is a focus of a lentiginous melanocytic proliferation in a background of basal layer hyperpigmentation.

Histologic Features

The tan macular component is histologically characterized by basal layer hyperpigmentation, often accompanied by a slight increase in the density of solitary melanocytes (similar to a lentigo). The histologic correlate of the clinically darker speckles may be that of a lentigo simplex, lentiginous junctional (Fig. 13.51B), compound, or intradermal melanocytic nevus. Various histologic types of nevi may be represented within the dark spots of speckled nevi.

ACRAL MELANOCYTIC NEVUS—PATHOLOGIC FEATURES

Clinical Findings

- Any age
- Usually small (except for dysplastic or congenital acral nevi)
- Benign dermoscopic patterns (e.g., furrow pattern)

Histopathologic Features

- Symmetric and circumscribed
- Predominant nested growth pattern
- Pagetoid melanocytes may be present
- Inflammatory stromal changes are uncommon

MISCELLANEOUS OTHER MELANOCYTIC NEVI

Additional types of melanocytic nevi have been described, which are uncommon. Two such types are briefly presented here: the deep penetrating nevus (DPN) and the desmoplastic nevus.

DEEP PENETRATING NEVUS

In its classic manifestation the DPN is a dome-shaped dark papule. Histopathologically, it is characterized by a wedge-shaped silhouette (Fig. 13.52). It often extends into the deep dermis and may involve the subcutis. The melanocytes of a DPN may be large and epithelioid or fusiform in appearance. They are often pigmented. Melanophages are present in variable numbers. Lesional melanocytes often display a plexiform growth pattern. Enlarged and hyperchromatic nuclei may be present, some with pseudoinclusions. A few mitotic figures are not uncommon. DPN often has mutations in β-catenin with associated nuclear labeling by IHC (Fig. 13.52C). DPN needs to be distinguished from blue nevi and DPN-like melanomas. The latter are typically more asymmetric and display more atypia and mitoses.

DESMOPLASTIC (SCLEROSING) MELANOCYTIC NEVUS

A nevus may be termed *desmoplastic nevus* when a compound or intradermal benign melanocytic proliferation is associated with prominent dermal fibrosis. There is a spectrum of lesions because there are different types of melanocytic nevi (e.g., ordinary acquired nevus [Fig. 13.53], congenital nevus, acral nevus) with stromal sclerosis. Well-recognized variants of the desmoplastic nevus include the desmoplastic Spitz nevus with large epithelioid cells and the sclerosing BN, which is composed of slender fusiform and dendritic cells. The main significance of a sclerosing nevus is

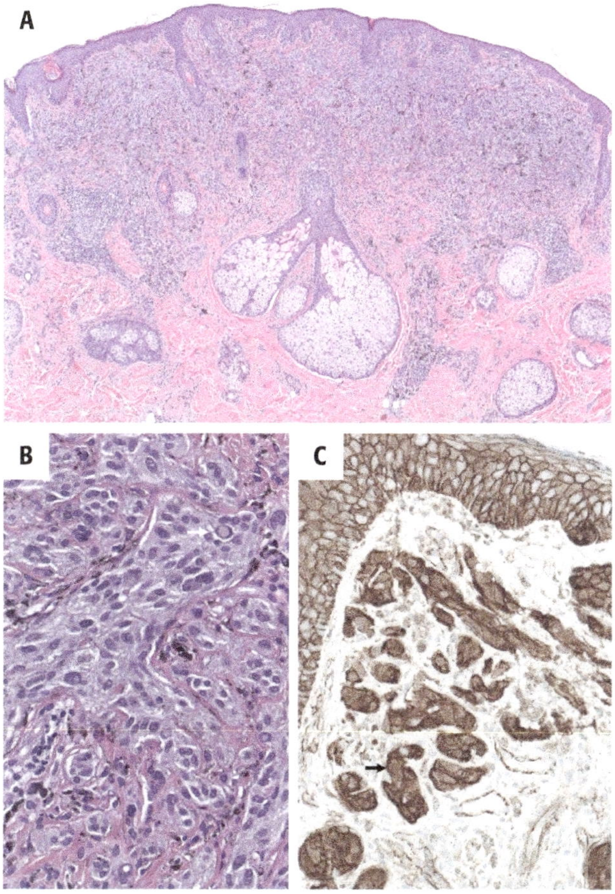

FIG. 13.52

Deep penetrating nevus. **A,** Pigmented melanocytic nevus with a wedge-shaped silhouette. **B,** Pigmented spindle and epithelioid melanocytes for fascicles and nests. Some nuclei are enlarged and have cytoplasmic pseudoinclusions *(arrow)*. **C,** The melanocytes show nuclear labeling for β-catenin *(arrow)*.

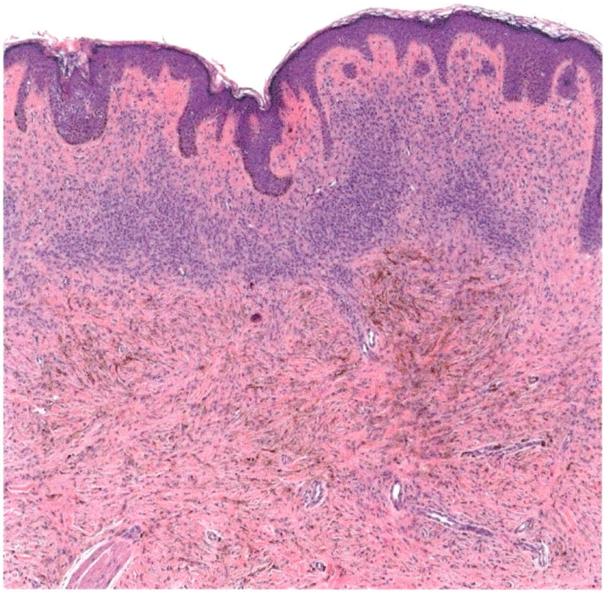

FIG. 13.53

Combined ordinary and blue nevus (BN). A compound melanocytic nevus is present. Its superficial component shows conventional features. Its deeper component shows features of a BN.

SCLEROSING MELANOCYTIC NEVUS—PATHOLOGIC FEATURES

Clinical Finding

- Often thought to be a dermatofibroma or scar

Histopathologic Features

- Symmetric and circumscribed
- Benign junctional melanocytic proliferation, if present
- Extent in depth usually confined to superficial dermis
- Maturation usually apparent (larger cells and cell clusters superficially)
- Lack of mitotic figures in dermal melanocytes

Variants

- Common nevus with sclerosis
- Congenital nevus with sclerosis
- Sclerosing blue nevus
- Sclerosing Spitz nevus

Immunophenotype

- Most are positive for Melan-A/Mart-1 (in contrast with desmoplastic melanoma)
- Sclerosing Spitz nevi are strongly positive for p16

Cytogenetic or Molecular Studies

- Sclerosing blue nevi may carry *GNA11* mutation
- Sclerosing Spitz nevi may carry *HRAS* mutation, gain of 11p, or fusions

Differential Diagnosis

- Desmoplastic melanoma
- Dermatofibroma
- Desmoplastic cellular neurothekeoma

potential confusion with desmoplastic melanoma (DM). Sclerosing nevi are distinguished from melanoma by a usually symmetric silhouette. Mitotic figures are usually absent. In contrast with DM, most sclerosing nevi are small, symmetric superficial dermal lesions. They tend to be diffusely immunoreactive for Melan-A but show minimal staining for Ki-67. Desmoplastic Spitz nevi tend to be strongly positive for p16. Although lymphocytic aggregates are a clue to the diagnosis of DM, they can also be found in association with a sclerosing nevus. In a difficult case, ancillary cytogenetic or molecular studies may help establish a definitive diagnosis. An isolated gain in 11p would support a diagnosis of a desmoplastic Spitz nevus. Sclerosing blue nevi tend to harbor a *GNA11* mutation. A high mutation burden and *TP53* or *NF1* mutations would support a diagnosis of DM.

COMBINED NEVI (MELANOCYTIC NEVI WITH PHENOTYPIC HETEROGENEITY)

Melanocytic nevi may show combined features of two or more separate nevus types within the same lesion. Such nevi are commonly referred to as *combined nevi*.

Any admixture of melanocytic phenotypes may occur in the same lesion. Examples include a BN (Fig. 13.54), large epithelioid cell nevus (aka clonal nevus, inverted type A nevus) (Fig. 13.55), a DPN (Fig. 13.56), a BAP1-inactivated epithelioid cell nevus (Fig. 13.57), or balloon cell nevus (Fig. 13.58) associated with an ordinary acquired or congenital nevus. The inverted type A nevus is probably related to the DPN and likely represents an early superficial variant thereof.

When a morphologically distinct population of melanocytes is found separate from the nevus background, one should consider the possibility not only of a combined nevus but also of melanoma arising in the dermal component of a melanocytic nevus or a melanoma with phenotypic heterogeneity. Although malignant transformation of a nevus without involvement of the dermal-epidermal junction is rare, it does occur in congenital and acquired nevi. Melanoma needs to be suspected if there are cytologically atypical epithelioid cells forming expansile nodular aggregates and mitotic figures are identified. In contrast, a combined nevus is favored if the cytologically different component shows overall features of a nevus (lack of or only minimal atypia, good evidence of maturation) and blends with the other nevus component.

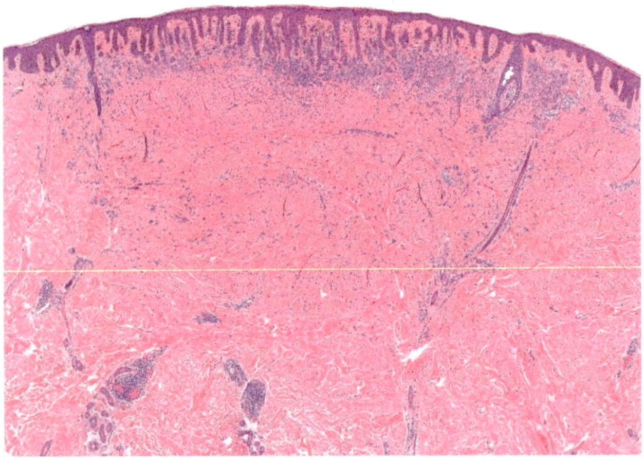

FIG. 13.54

Combined nevus with a sclerosing component. The nevus shows conventional features superficially and desmoplastic features in its deeper component.

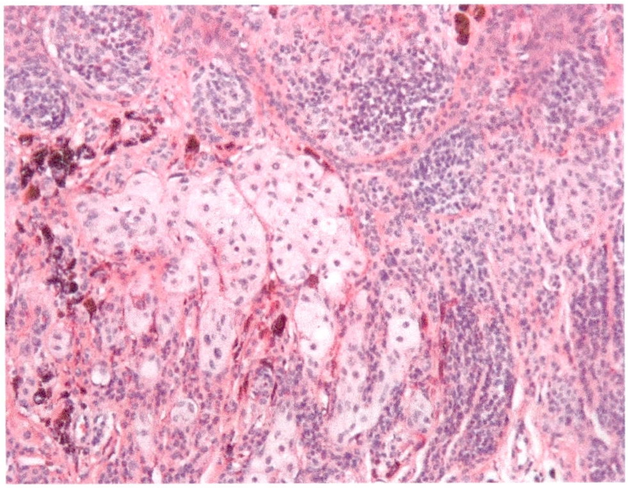

FIG. 13.55

Combined melanocytic nevus with conventional small and pigmented large epithelioid melanocytes.

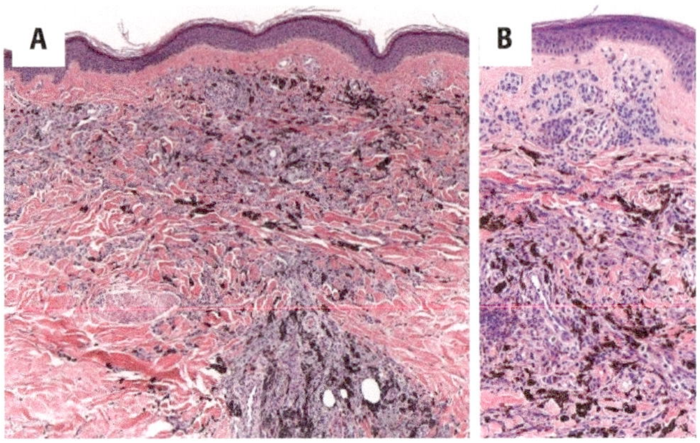

FIG. 13.56

Combined ordinary and deep penetrating nevus. **A,** Most of the lesion shows features of a deep penetrating nevus. **B,** Focally, there is a small ordinary dermal nevus situated above the deep penetrating nevus cell population.

RECURRENT OR PERSISTENT MELANOCYTIC NEVUS—PATHOLOGIC FEATURES

Clinical Finding

- Repigmentation at the site of a scar

Histopathologic Features

- Intraepidermal melanocytes overlying the scar may show architectural disorder, including pagetoid melanocytosis
- An associated dermal nevus component may be present within the scar
- Hyperpigmentation is common within melanocytes and keratinocytes
- Intraepidermal melanocytes peripheral to the scar show a predominant nested pattern as expected for a junctional nevus

RECURRENT OR PERSISTENT MELANOCYTIC NEVI

Melanocytic nevi may clinically "recur" at the site of a prior biopsy. Such a recurrence is usually because of growth of melanocytes left behind from an incompletely removed nevus. Histologically the junctional or intraepidermal growth pattern of recurrent or persistent nevi may show features overlapping with those of in situ melanoma (pseudomelanoma), such as the presence of pagetoid spread, confluent nests at the dermal-epidermal junction, and a predominance of solitary units of melanocytes (Fig. 13.59).

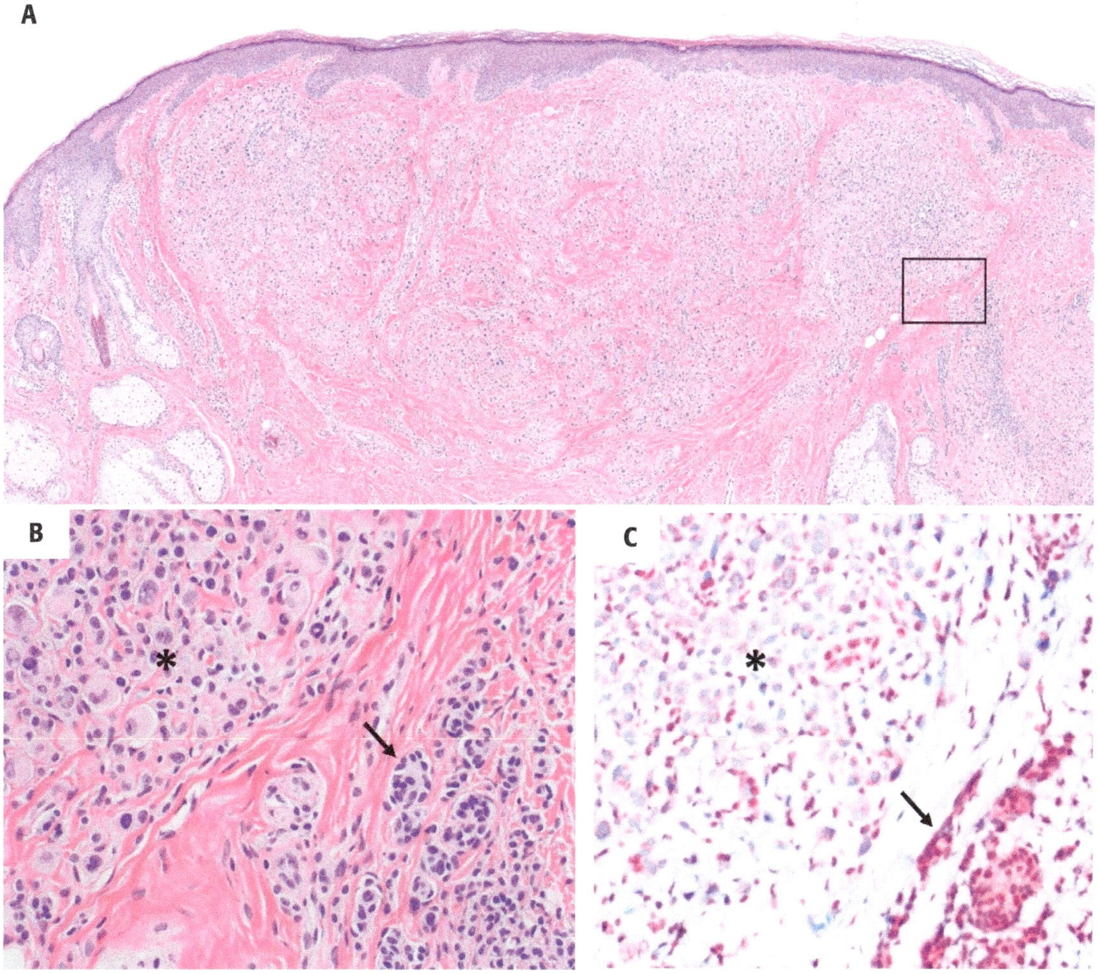

FIG. 13.57

Combined BAP1-inactivated melanocytic nevus. **A,** Silhouette of a nevus that is associated with mild fibrosis. **B,** There is a dual population of melanocytes with large epithelioid cells *(*)* and ordinary small epithelioid cell features *(arrow)*. **C,** The large epithelioid melanocytes *(*)* lack nuclear BAP1 expression, while it is retained in all other cells, including the ordinary nevus cells *(arrow)*.

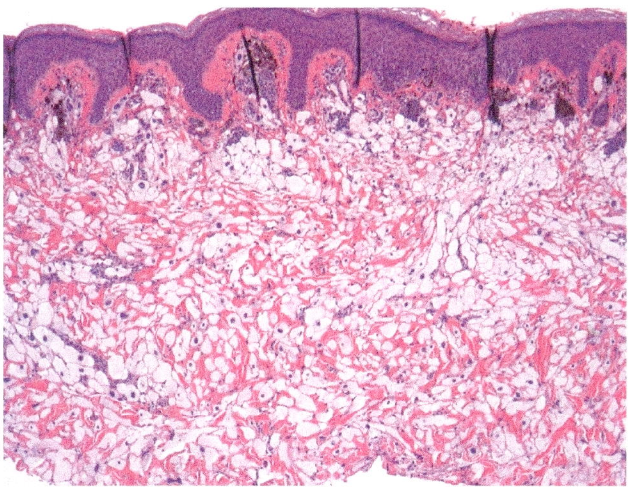

FIG. 13.58

Compound nevus with a balloon cell population. A predominant population of melanocytes with abundant clear cytoplasm ("balloon cells") is associated with pigmented small epithelioid melanocytes. The lesion was clinically congenital.

In a recurrent or persistent nevus phenomenon, the atypical melanocytic growth pattern is restricted to the epidermis overlying the scar. An unequivocally benign nevus component is commonly present adjacent to or underneath the atypical proliferation. Furthermore, the melanocytes of recurrent nevi usually lack marked cytologic atypia. In contrast, in situ melanoma at the site of a scar (from a previously biopsied nevus or melanoma) usually extends significantly beyond the area of the dermal scar with an ill-defined peripheral border. In difficult cases, it is helpful to review the prior biopsy because what is reported to have been a prior benign or atypical nevus may represent an in situ melanoma that was not recognized as such.

PRIMARY MELANOMA

The number of people who develop melanoma continues to increase. The reported incidence in the White population has more than tripled over the past 20 years.

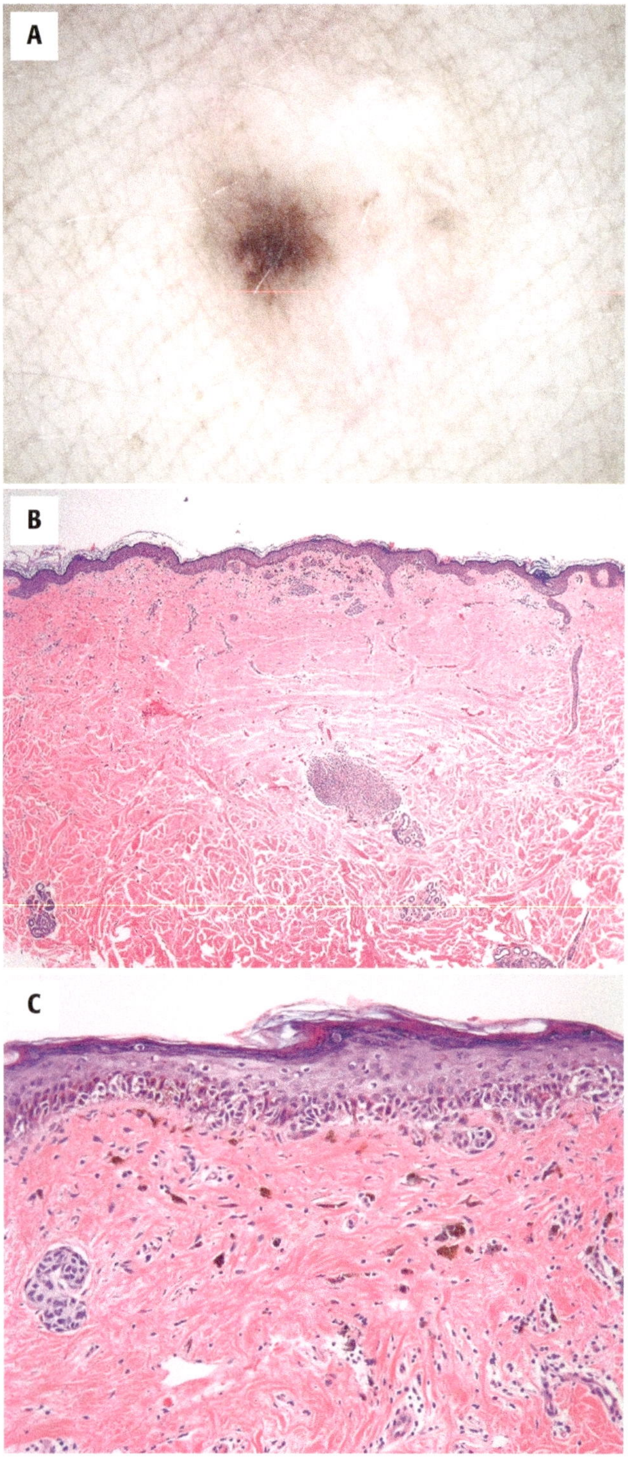

FIG. 13.59

Recurrent melanocytic nevus. **A,** Pigmentation is seen within a scar of the site of a previously biopsied nevus. **B,** Histologically, a melanocytic nevus is present in association with a dermal scar. **C,** The junctional melanocytic proliferation shows architectural disorder.

Approximately 76,000 new cases of invasive melanoma are estimated to be diagnosed in the United States during 2014. There is emerging evidence for multiple different pathways that can result in melanoma, with both genetic and environmental factors.

MELANOMA—DISEASE FACT SHEET

Incidence

- Approximately 99,780 new invasive melanoma cases estimated in the United States for 2022
- Fifth most common cancer in women; sixth most common in men (North America)
- Most common cancer in White women aged 25 to 29 years

Risk Factors

- Family history of melanoma
- Numerous melanocytic nevi
- Fair skin
- Ultraviolet exposure
- Age older than 50 years
- Tanning bed use
- Genodermatoses: xeroderma pigmentosum or familial atypical mole syndrome

Clinical Warning Signs for Melanoma: ABCDE Rule

- **A**symmetry
- **B**order irregularity
- **C**olor variegation
- **D**iameter (greater than 6 mm)
- **E**volving (change of a pigmented lesion)

The risk for developing a melanoma is increased if there is a family history of melanoma or a clinical phenotype of numerous nevi, especially numerous atypical nevi. Melanomas are more common in fair-skinned individuals with sun sensitivity and a history of excessive sun exposure. The risk for melanoma increases with age. Other risk factors include DNA repair defects (xeroderma pigmentosum), a history of melanoma, and immunosuppression.

Clinical Findings

Melanoma is clinically suspected if a preexisting mole is changing or a new pigmented lesion appears that shows worrisome features, such as large size, variability in colors, surface texture, or irregular peripheral borders (Fig. 13.60) or if it is symptomatic (itch, pain, tenderness, bleeding). Although the clinical impression is a good guide for the diagnosis, especially in well-developed lesions, there are many exceptions, and the accuracy of the clinical diagnosis is less than perfect (≈60%). Histopathologically, unequivocal melanoma may be clinically confused with a benign or atypical nevus or even a keratosis. If no pigment is visible clinically (amelanotic melanoma), other tumors, such as basal cell carcinoma (BCC), may be suspected instead of melanoma. Likewise, a clinically complex pigmented lesion suspected to be melanoma may be histologically banal (e.g., a macular pigmented seborrheic keratosis or solar lentigines).

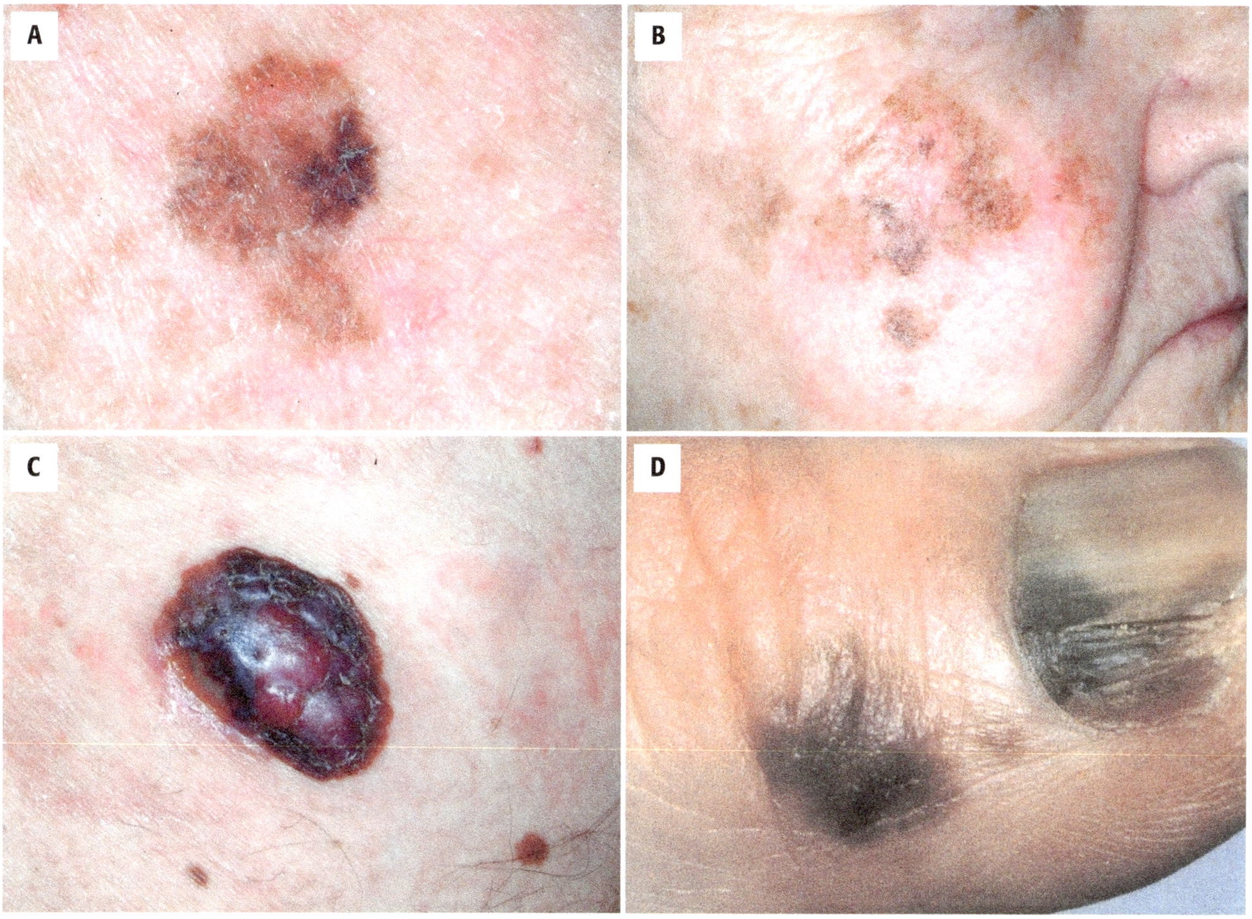

FIG. 13.60

Clinical appearance of conventional melanoma types. **A,** Asymmetric complex silhouette of a melanoma from the trunk (superficial spreading melanoma). **B,** Asymmetric complex macular pigmented lesion on the face (lentigo maligna). **C,** Nodular melanoma. **D,** Acral melanoma.

Histopathologic Features: General Considerations for the Diagnosis of Melanoma

Microscopic examination and clinicopathologic correlation represent the gold standard for the diagnosis of melanoma. Among experienced pathologists, assessment of melanocytic lesions is fairly accurate and reliable in the majority of cases but cannot be expected to be perfect in every case. Diagnostic controversy may arise when melanoma closely mimics a nevus or the biopsy sample is small and incomplete and displays only subtle and/or ambiguous features.

A diagnosis of melanoma is usually not based on a single microscopic finding but on a constellation of clinical and histopathologic parameters. The proportional weight of various features for the diagnosis depends on the degree to which they are developed and the clinical context. Pagetoid spread of melanocytes, for example, is a finding commonly associated with in situ melanoma (*de novo* or associated with a melanocytic nevus). If in a clinically acquired and changing, previously nontraumatized melanocytic lesion of an adult pagetoid melanocytes are prominent, cytologically atypical, and displayed in a chaotic pattern, the diagnosis of intraepidermal melanoma is certain. In a different clinical and/or histopathologic context, however, pagetoid spread per se may not be sufficient for a diagnosis of melanoma. A benign or atypical melanocytic nevus may show pagetoid spread of usually bland melanocytes near the follicular infundibulum secondary to irritation or at the site of prior trauma or surgery. Furthermore, acral, congenital, and Spitz's nevi may display some pagetoid melanocytosis.

In many cases, assessment of the silhouette and gestalt of a lesion (comparing it with stored mental images of previously observed nevi and melanomas) is diagnostic for an experienced pathologist. For didactic (and for beginners, also practical) purposes, however, a stepwise approach is presented here to discuss various diagnostic features. Scanning magnification allows assessment of the overall symmetry of a lesion. The more complex and asymmetric a lesion is, the more likely it represents melanoma (Fig. 13.61). A thick primary ulcerated tumor with dense sheets of mitotically active

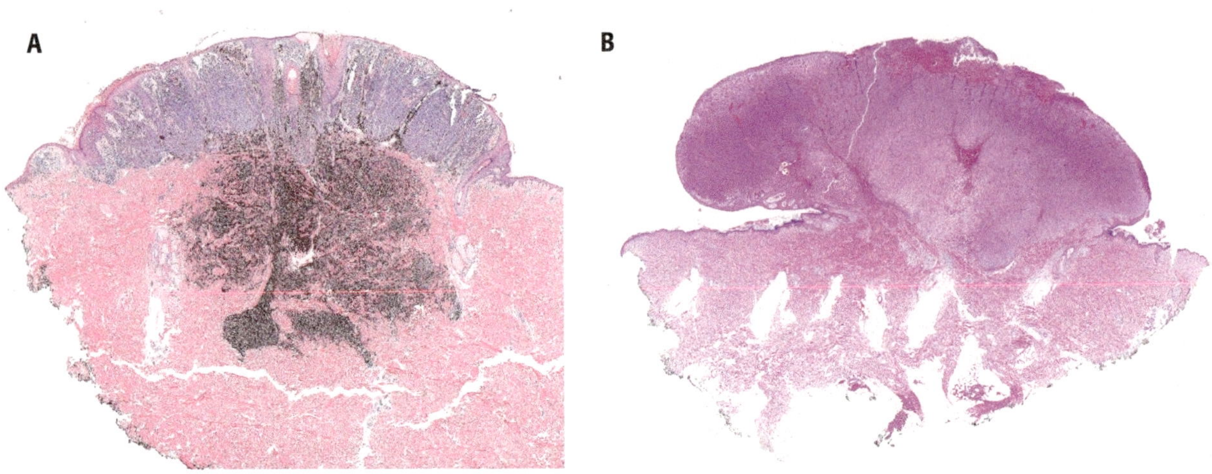

FIG. 13.61
Melanoma. **A,** Complex infiltrative silhouette. **B,** Densely cellular polypoid nodular with broad ulceration.

atypical melanocytes is readily apparent as malignant and unlikely to be confused with a benign melanocytic nevus. Most of the time, however, pathologists need to interpret thinner tumors, which requires systematic analysis of parameters outlined in the following to distinguish them from melanocytic nevi.

For lesions with an intraepidermal melanocytic proliferation (with or without an associated dermal component), it helps to determine first whether or not criteria for melanoma in situ are met. A different approach is needed for melanomas lacking an intraepithelial component.

SYNOPSIS OF CONVENTIONAL MELANOMAS—PATHOLOGIC FEATURES

Superficial Spreading Type

Clinical Findings

- Intermittent sun damage: most common on the trunk and extremities
- Individuals aged 20 to 50 years
- May arise de novo or in association with melanocytic nevi

Histopathologic Features

- Nests and single-cell scatter of melanocytes within the epidermis

Lentigo Maligna Type

Clinical Findings

- Chronic sun damage: most common on head and neck and arms
- Fair-skinned older people (mean age at diagnosis, 65 years)
- Usually de novo; rarely associated with nevus
- Usually slowly growing

Histopathologic Features

- Predominance of solitary units of melanocytes at the dermal-epidermal junction

Nodular Type

Clinical Findings

- Most common on trunk and legs
- History of rapid growth
- May arise de novo or in association with melanocytic nevus

Histopathologic Features

- Invasive melanoma with no or minimal in situ component
- If in situ melanoma is present, it does not extend peripheral to the invasive tumor

Acral Type

Clinical Findings

- Most common melanoma in individuals with darker skin
- Palms and soles; subungual
- Usually de novo but may be associated with a melanocytic nevus

Histopathologic Features

- Most often displays a lentiginous pattern with a predominance of solitary units of melanocytes along the dermal-epidermal junction

DIAGNOSIS OF CONVENTIONAL PRIMARY CUTANEOUS MELANOMA—PATHOLOGIC FEATURES

- Silhouette: asymmetry
- Borders: usually ill-defined
- Size: usually, but not always greater than 4 mm in diameter
- Intraepidermal melanoma component
  - Irregular pagetoid spread or broad lentiginous junctional proliferation
  - Predominance of solitary units of melanocytes
  - Markedly irregular disposition of melanocytes
  - Complex and oddly shaped junctional nests
  - Marked confluence of melanocytes along the dermal-epidermal junction
  - Marked dyscohesion of melanocytes
  - Cytologic atypia of melanocytes (variable)
- Dermal or subcutaneous melanoma component
  - Complex asymmetric growth pattern
  - Lack of maturation or only minimal maturation
  - Expansile nodules
  - Oddly shaped nests
  - Mitotic figures may be present
  - Cytologic atypia of melanocytes (variable)
- Stromal changes
  - Lichenoid inflammatory reaction may be present
  - Fibrosis and dermal regression may be present
- Associated surface epiphenomena
  - Ulceration or "consumption of the epidermis" (obliteration or effacement of rete ridges) is more often seen with melanomas than with nevi

Histopathologic Features for the Diagnosis of Melanoma In Situ

The majority of cutaneous melanomas begin as intraepidermal melanocytic proliferations with or without an associated melanocytic nevus. As a general rule, in situ melanoma is characterized by a broad irregular proliferation of atypical melanocytes within the epidermis. Solitary units of melanocytes tend to dominate over nests, at least focally. They tend to fill the spaces between rete ridges. Melanocytes may be present at the mid- or upper spinous cell layer (pagetoid spread). At one end of the spectrum, pagetoid spread may be well developed (pagetoid in situ melanoma) (Fig. 13.62). At the opposite extreme, few or no pagetoid cells may be noted, and melanoma cells are primarily distributed as solitary units along the dermal-epidermal junction (lentiginous pattern) (Figs. 13.63–13.65). Overlap of these patterns in the same lesion is common.

DIFFERENTIAL DIAGNOSIS OF PAGETOID MELANOCYTOSIS—PATHOLOGIC FEATURES

- ▸▸ Irritated (rubbed or scratched) nevus
- ▸▸ Recurrent or persistent nevus (prior surgical trauma)
- ▸▸ Acral nevus
- ▸▸ Congenital nevus
- ▸▸ Spitz nevus
- ▸▸ Melanoma in situ

Other features that help identify in situ melanoma are the presence of solitary units of melanocytes extending into epithelial structures of adnexa (follicular infundibulum or eccrine duct), marked confluence or nests along the dermal-epidermal junction, and dyscohesion of cells within often large and irregularly shaped cell aggregates along the dermal-epidermal junction. There are often secondary epidermal (e.g., effacement of rete ridges with thinning of the epidermis, also referred to as consumption of the epidermis) or dermal stromal alterations (e.g., lichenoid inflammatory reaction). Cytologic atypia of melanocytes may be prominent but is at times only mild, especially in lentiginous melanomas of chronically sun-damaged skin or at acral or mucosal sites. In the majority of cases, analysis of the architecture of the lesion, in particular the growth pattern of melanocytes, is the key to the diagnosis. On occasion, in particular with small and paucicellular lesions, the presence of cytologic atypia may carry more weight for judging the nature of a lesion. A useful ancillary tool for melanoma in situ and its margin assessment is IHC for PRAME (Fig. 13.64). Strong diffuse staining of the melanocytes supports the diagnosis of melanoma. However, approximately 10% of melanoma in situ lesions are negative for PRAME, and on occasion, benign proliferations may aberrantly express PRAME.

Differential Diagnosis of Melanoma In Situ

When pagetoid spread is noted, especially in association with features of an associated melanocytic nevus, one needs to bear in mind that it may be related to trauma, nevus type, or anatomic site.

Lentiginous melanoma in situ needs to be distinguished from solar lentiginous melanocytic hyperplasia, lentigo simplex, and atypical lentiginous junctional melanocytic nevi. The recognition of a lentiginous melanoma is straightforward if one deals with the excision of a large irregular junctional melanocytic proliferation of a clinically suspected melanoma. It can be very difficult or impossible, however, on a partial biopsy if one does not know the size of the lesion.

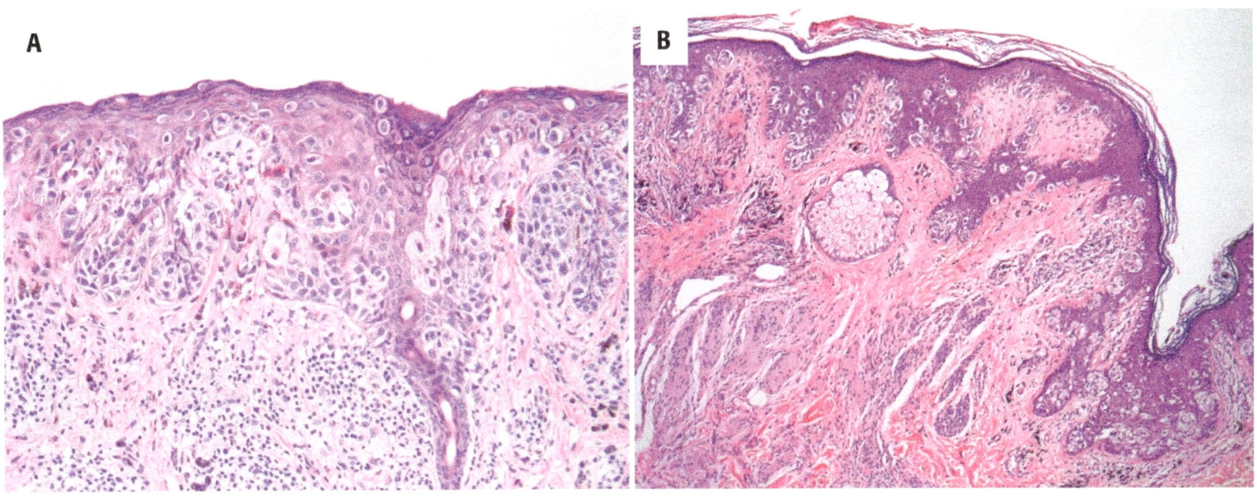

FIG. 13.62
Melanoma in situ, pagetoid pattern. **A,** De novo pagetoid melanoma in situ associated with inflammation. **B,** Pagetoid melanoma in situ arising in association with a melanocytic nevus.

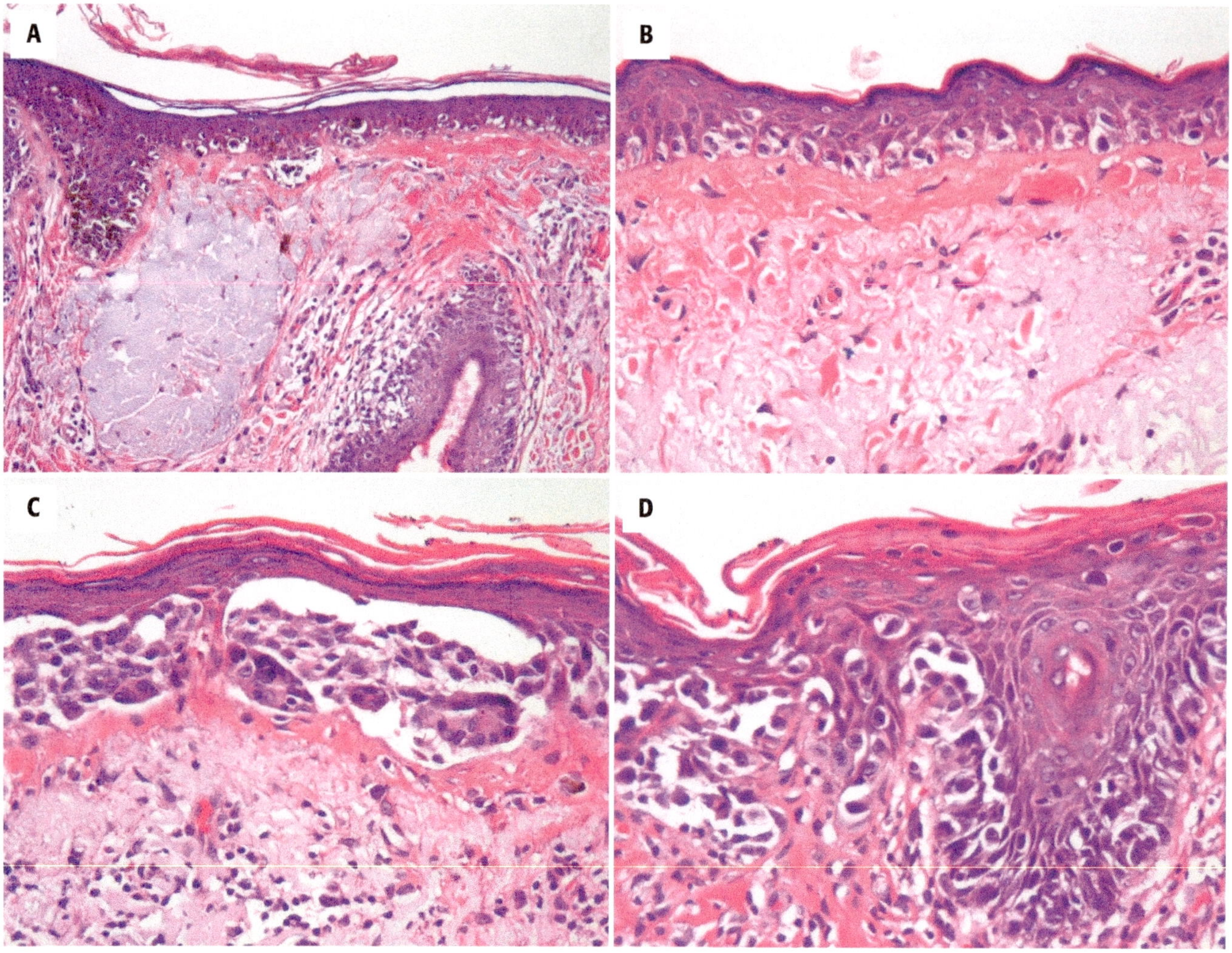

FIG. 13.63

Melanoma in situ, lentiginous pattern. **A,** An atypical proliferation of solitary units of melanocytes is present along the dermal-epidermal and infundibular dermal junctions. **B,** Solitary units of melanocytes predominate along the dermal-epidermal junction. Epidermal rete ridges are effaced. There is marked solar elastosis. **C,** However, nests of melanocytes are also seen. Some melanocytes are multinucleated. **D,** Focally pagetoid intraepidermal spread of melanocytes is present. **A** to **D** are different foci from the same melanoma.

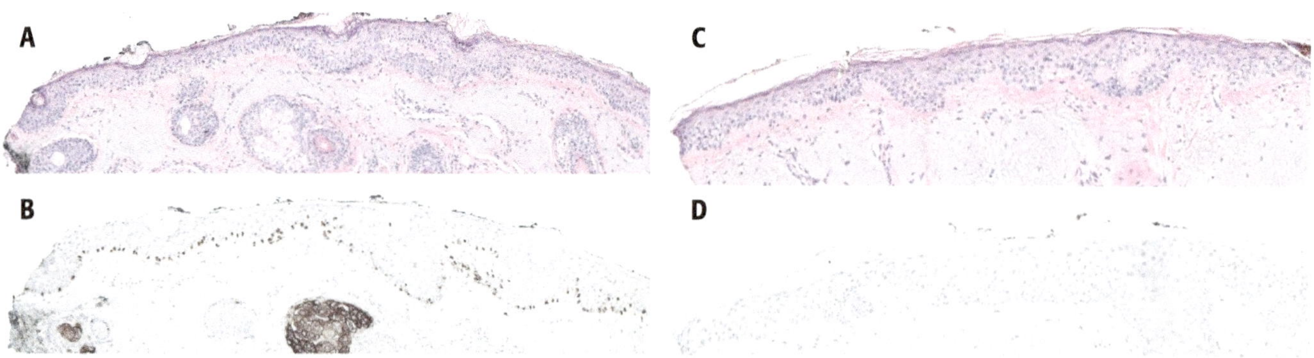

FIG. 13.64

Staged excision of melanoma in situ. **A,** Margin section involved by melanoma in situ with a low cell density at the dermoepidermal junction (hematoxylin and eosin [H&E]). **B,** An immunostain for PRAME performed on the same section highlights and more easily documents the presence of melanoma in situ. **C,** Margin section negative for melanoma (H&E). **D,** An immunostain for PRAME is completely negative, thereby confirming the absence of melanoma in situ.

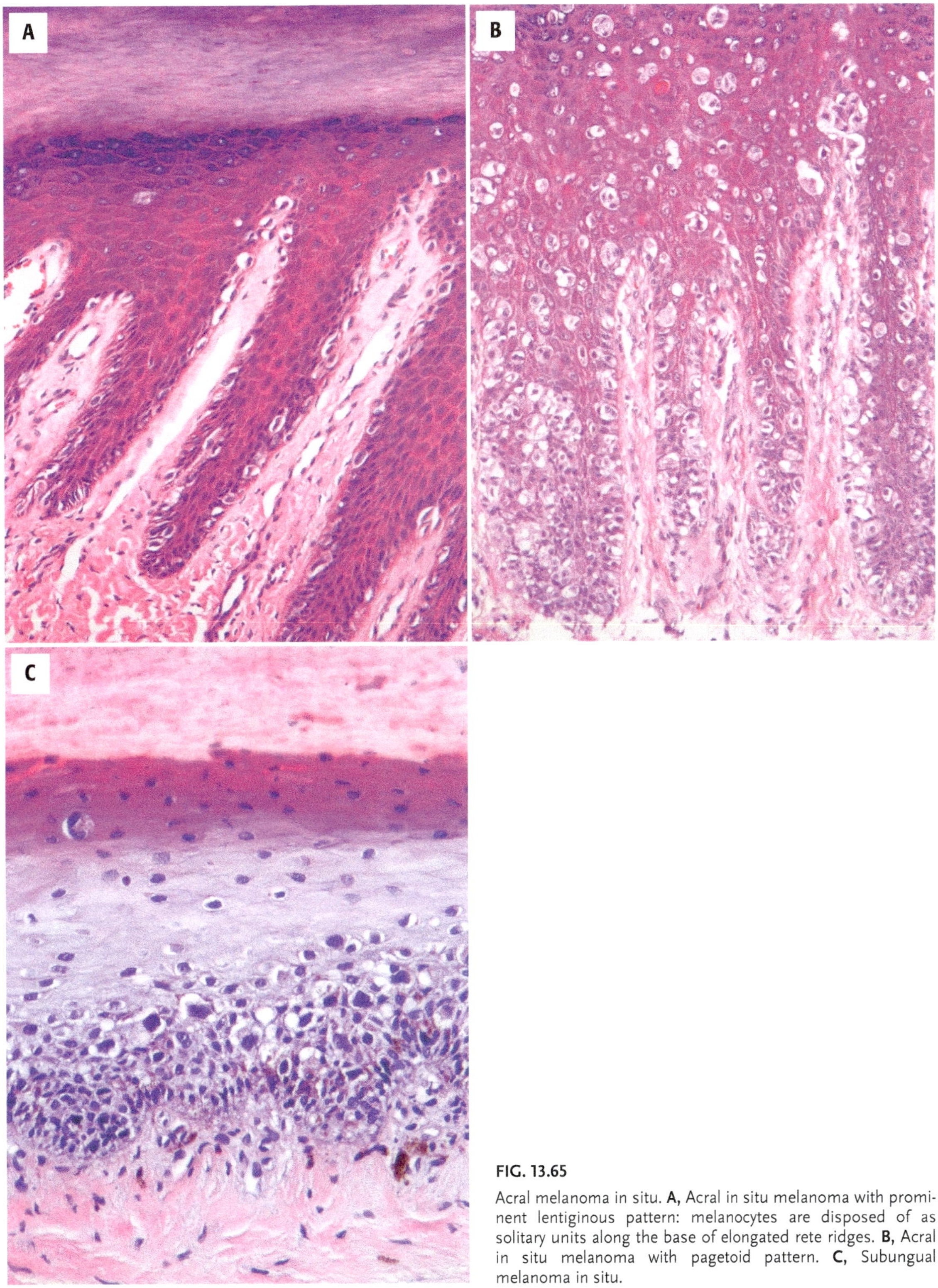

FIG. 13.65

Acral melanoma in situ. **A,** Acral in situ melanoma with prominent lentiginous pattern: melanocytes are disposed of as solitary units along the base of elongated rete ridges. **B,** Acral in situ melanoma with pagetoid pattern. **C,** Subungual melanoma in situ.

The distinction of a lentiginous melanoma in situ of chronically sun-damaged skin (*lentigo maligna* melanoma in situ) from solar melanocytic hyperplasia is best accomplished by comparing the lesional cell density and atypia of melanocytes with a reference (control) biopsy of clinically "normal" skin. Too often, such a "control" biopsy is not available. In this instance, a reference for "normal" skin may be found in negative margins of an excision or other anatomically matched additional biopsies (e.g., for BCC) from the same patient. If no reference is available, the presence of confluent melanocytes at the dermal-epidermal junction favors melanoma.

The distinction of an atypical lentiginous junctional melanocytic nevus from in situ melanoma can be problematic as well. A lentigo maligna melanoma in situ may display a predominant nested growth pattern and in foci be indistinguishable from a lentiginous junctional dysplastic nevus. Clinical features (size, location, complexity to the clinical eye, or dermoscopically assisted visual examination) are important for the correct diagnosis. Flat lesions associated with an atypical lentiginous junctional melanocytic proliferation located in the head and neck region of elderly individuals with chronic sun damage are more often than not in situ melanomas. A diagnosis of a melanocytic nevus can still be made if the lesion has been present for some time, is small and circumscribed, and its histology shows nests predominating over solitary units of melanocytes. A diagnosis of in situ melanoma is favored if solitary units predominate, become confluent at the dermal-epidermal junction, and show an ill-defined border. In the absence of an associated dermal melanocytic nevus component, involvement of adnexal epithelium (proliferation of melanocytes along the infundibular dermal junction or along terminal sweat ducts) also favors melanoma over a junctional nevus. The presence of several multinucleated cells (starburst giant cells) favors in situ melanoma but is in itself not specific because it may also be seen with nevi. The presence of skip areas (seemingly normal or solar lentigo–like areas separating the junctional melanocytic proliferation in a two-dimensional view) is diagnostically useful because it is much more frequently seen in association with a lentigo maligna than a lentiginous nevus (but beware of the possibility of two adjacent nevi). Diffuse immunoreactivity of the melanocytes for PRAME favors melanoma in situ.

Histopathologic Features for the Diagnosis of Invasive Melanoma

If a diagnosis of in situ melanoma has been established and there is an associated dermal melanocytic component, the issue is whether the dermal melanocytes represent a nevus, invasive melanoma, or perhaps a mixed population of melanoma and nevus. The issue of invasion may be readily apparent if the dermal component is deeply infiltrative with an asymmetric growth pattern. Furthermore, the presence of atypical mitotically active melanocytes in the dermis cytologically similar to the in situ melanoma component makes a diagnosis of invasive melanoma (Fig. 13.66) straightforward.

Differential Diagnosis of Primary Invasive Melanoma

If a lesion is recognized as melanocytic in origin, the main differential diagnosis is between primary cutaneous melanoma and a melanocytic nevus. Melanoma may simulate the growth pattern of or arise in association with any kind of nevus. The differential diagnosis of various problems, such as the distinction of superficial spreading melanoma from a dysplastic nevus or a sclerosing nevus from DM, is discussed in more detail under the respective nevus or melanoma subtype.

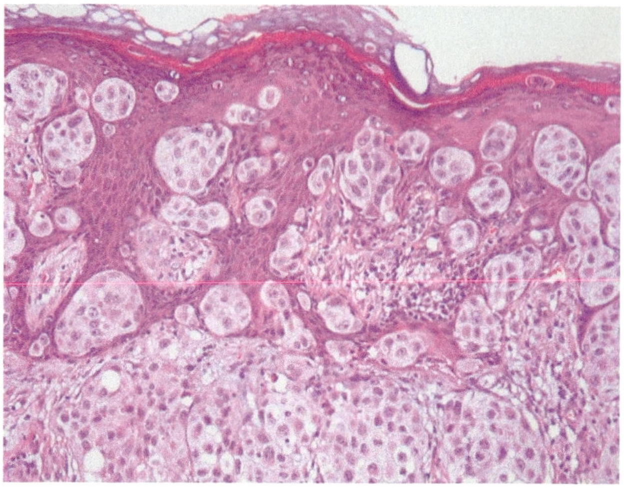

FIG. 13.66

Invasive melanoma. Melanocytes in the dermis resemble intraepidermal melanoma cells. The dermal melanocytes lack an orderly nested pattern and diffusely infiltrate the dermis.

In situ melanoma may erroneously be interpreted as invasive tumor when it colonizes adnexal structures and expands within them (Fig. 13.67). Another problem of potential over- or underestimation of the extent of invasion may occur when a melanoma arises in association with a melanocytic nevus. The distinction is easy if there is marked difference in the cytology and growth patterns between melanoma and nevus (Fig. 13.68). The recognition and measurement of invasion, however, can be very difficult when the invasive tumor lacks marked atypia and maintains a nested growth pattern and displays "pseudomaturation" (a change in cell size from top to bottom of the lesion).

If a lesion is amelanotic, primary melanoma may be confused with a number of benign or, more often, malignant nonmelanocytic tumors. Benign tumors, which may be misinterpreted as melanoma on routine hematoxylin and eosin (H&E)–stained sections, include foam and giant cell-poor xanthogranuloma or fibromas incidentally associated with a nevus (they may be misdiagnosed as DM). Malignant tumors, which may show overlap with melanoma, include poorly differentiated carcinomas, miscellaneous sarcomas, and anaplastic large cell lymphoma. Immunohistochemical studies usually allow a definitive determination of the line of differentiation and have rendered confusion of a primary melanoma with a malignant nonmelanocytic tumor an uncommon event.

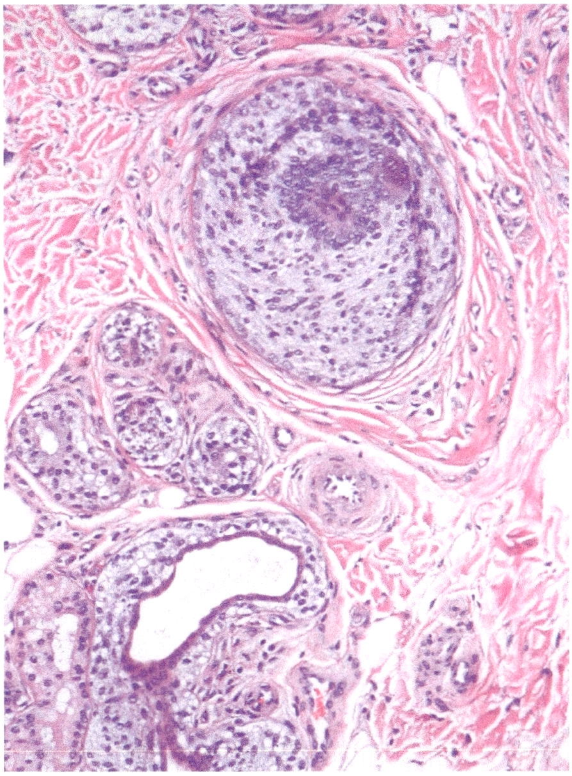

FIG. 13.67
In situ melanoma mimicking invasive melanoma. Melanoma cells are confined to the epithelial site of the basement membrane within the sweat gland apparatus and a hair follicle.

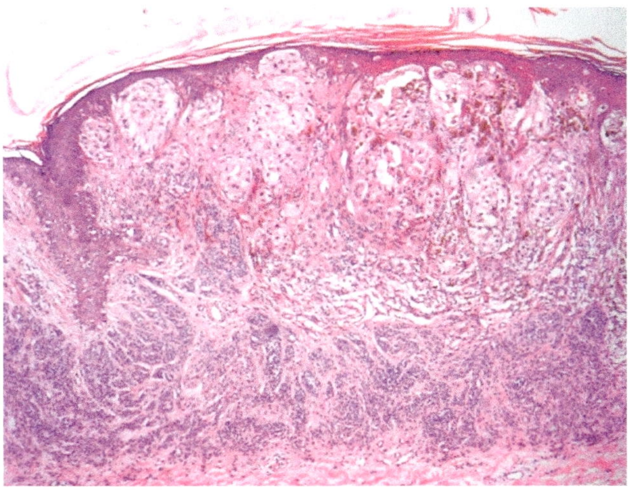

FIG. 13.68
Melanoma arising in association with a nevus. There is a clear distinction between the cytology of the melanoma and nevus cells.

Histopathologic Parameters Relevant to Prognosis

A number of histopathologic features have been identified that correlate with patient outcome. Although it is impossible to precisely predict the clinical outcome for an individual person, prognostic parameters are relevant for clinical trials to stratify patients into risk groups to better identify potential effects from surgical or medical treatment modalities (versus the natural history of the disease). Risk assessment is also relevant for decisions on the extent of clinical workup and follow-up, and for the affected patients for plans for their life. For the care of an individual patient, it is important to realize that statistical data are probability scenarios for patient populations with certain characteristics. They do not predict a particular individual's fate. There is always hope for survival against the odds. Likewise, there is no guarantee for individual good outcome in spite of favorable statistical data.

Tumor thickness has been established as the most powerful among the currently available predictors in many multivariate analyses of large cohorts. The ulceration status and presence or absence of satellite lesions are also prognostically relevant. Other parameters that have been reported to correlate with prognosis include lymphovascular and/or perineural invasion, tumor mitotic rate (TMR), and the pattern of tumor-infiltrating lymphocytes. In the most recently revised melanoma staging system of the American Joint Committee on Cancer (AJCC) (2018), only tumor thickness and ulceration are used as parameters for the T classification. The presence of satellites affects the N classification.

TUMOR THICKNESS

Tumor thickness is measured with an ocular micrometer according to Breslow as the greatest vertical distance (expressed in millimeters) between the deepest invasive melanoma cells and the granular cell layer of the overlying epidermis. If the overlying epidermis is ulcerated, the base of the ulcer is taken as a reference point. When there is an associated melanocytic nevus or in situ melanoma within an adnexal structure, the measurement should not include the nevus or in situ melanoma but be limited to what can be recognized unequivocally as invasive melanoma.

ULCERATION

Ulceration is detected as a tumor-related defect in the skin surface. The epidermis is missing, and there is a stromal inflammatory and granulation tissue–type reaction. Ulceration because of a prior surgical procedure or focal excoriation should not be designated as tumor ulceration. In tumor-induced ulceration, the epidermis adjacent to the ulcer is often effaced and thinned.

MICROANATOMIC (CLARK) LEVEL

Clark levels are no longer required for reporting but are explained here nonetheless for historic reasons and educational purposes. They indicate which microanatomic compartments are involved by melanoma. Clark level I represents intraepidermal or in situ melanoma

(Fig. 13.69A). Clark level II reflects partial invasion of the papillary dermis (Fig. 13.69B). Clark level III refers to melanomas that fill or expand the papillary dermis (Fig. 13.69C). When invasive melanoma has entered the reticular dermis and tumor cell aggregates are completely surrounded by reticular dermal collagen, a Clark level IV is assigned (Fig. 13.69D). Melanomas invading the subcutaneous fat or deeper (e.g., muscle or bone) are of Clark level V (Fig. 13.69E).

TUMOR MITOTIC RATE

TMR is measured as the number of mitotic figures of melanoma cells per millimeter squared of invasive

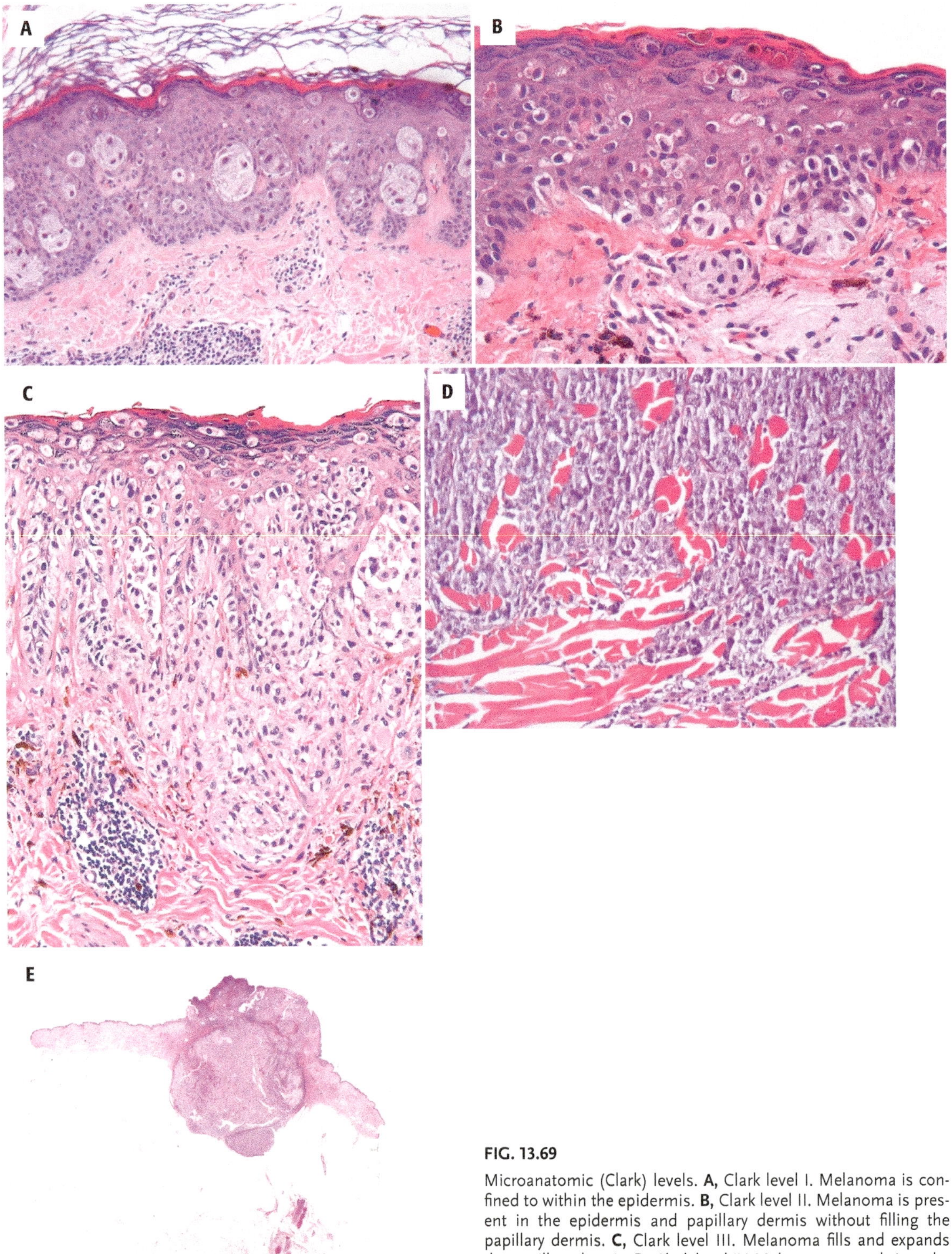

FIG. 13.69

Microanatomic (Clark) levels. **A,** Clark level I. Melanoma is confined to within the epidermis. **B,** Clark level II. Melanoma is present in the epidermis and papillary dermis without filling the papillary dermis. **C,** Clark level III. Melanoma fills and expands the papillary dermis. **D,** Clark level IV. Melanoma extends into the reticular dermis. Coarse reticular dermal collagen bundles surround melanoma cells. **E,** Clark level V. Melanoma extends into subcutaneous adipose tissue.

tumor. For practical purposes, invasive melanoma is scanned for mitotic figures, and the mitotic count is started at an area where mitoses can easily be spotted (mitotic hot spot). Using a 40× objective, additional randomly chosen high-power fields in the area of invasive melanoma are then examined for tumor cells in mitosis until an area of 1 mm^2 is covered. With many current microscopes, this implies examining five high-power fields. However, it is best to calibrate one's own microscope for the area examined at high power and to verify how many high-power fields are necessary to cover 1 mm^2. TMR is worth reporting, because it is used in several prognostic models.

LYMPHATIC OR BLOOD VESSEL INVASION

Lymphovascular invasion is diagnosed by the presence of intravascular tumor deposits that cannot be attributed to "artifacts" from using an unclean knife or pushing tumor tissue into empty spaces during cutting. Unequivocal vascular invasion is present if tumor cells within a vascular lumen are intimately admixed with blood cells, focally adherent to the vessel wall (Fig. 13.70), or, in the case of large blood vessels, seen within the vessel wall (Fig. 13.71). Vascular invasion is an uncommon finding in primary melanomas. It is usually seen in association with large tumors. A related term is *angiotropism*, which refers to the cuffing of vessels by melanoma cells. Its presence is also an adverse prognostic feature.

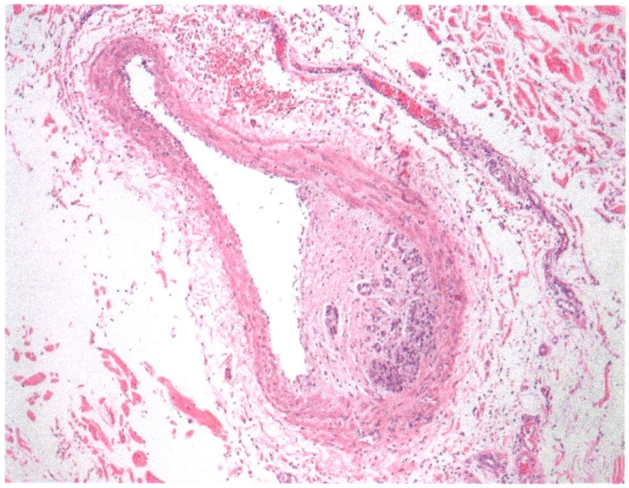

FIG. 13.71
Blood vessel invasion. Tumor cells are present in the wall of a blood vessel.

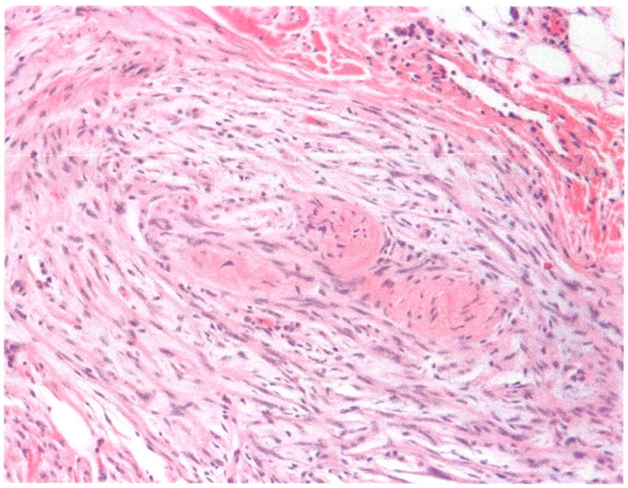

FIG. 13.72
Nerve involvement. A peripheral nerve is invaded and surrounded by fusiform melanoma cells.

NERVE INVOLVEMENT

Melanoma may involve the sheath of a nerve (perineural invasion) or extend into the nerve (endoneurial invasion) (Fig. 13.72). Nerve involvement should not be regarded as proof of malignant melanoma. It can be seen in congenital or neurotized acquired ordinary and blue nevi. *Nerve involvement* is often used synonymously with *neurotropism*. Some pathologists, however, use the term *neurotropism* to indicate the presence of a neuroma-like growth pattern and line of differentiation by a melanoma or nevus. Neurotropic lesions typically show involvement of multiple nerve bundles.

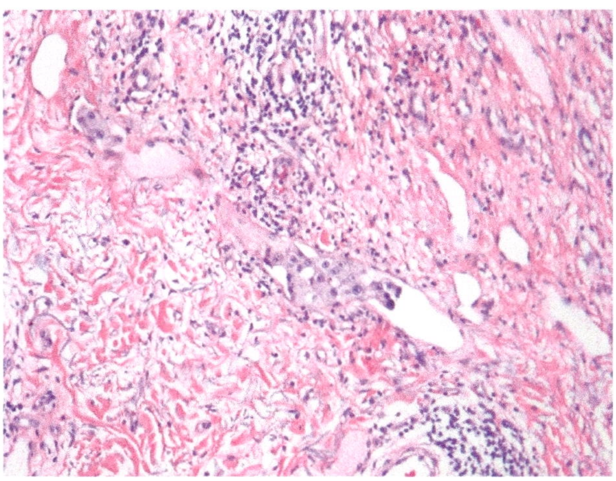

FIG. 13.70
Lymphatic invasion. Clusters of melanoma cells are present in a lymphatic channel.

SATELLITES OR LOCOREGIONAL CUTANEOUS METASTASES

Satellites are locoregional melanoma metastases that may be clinically apparent (Fig. 13.73) or only be seen under the microscope (microscopic satellites) as tumor cell aggregates away from the main invasive tumor mass (not artifactually separated by the plane of section by regression) (Fig. 13.74).

TUMOR-INFILTRATING LYMPHOCYTES

Several studies have suggested that the presence of a "brisk" infiltrate of lymphocytes infiltrating melanoma

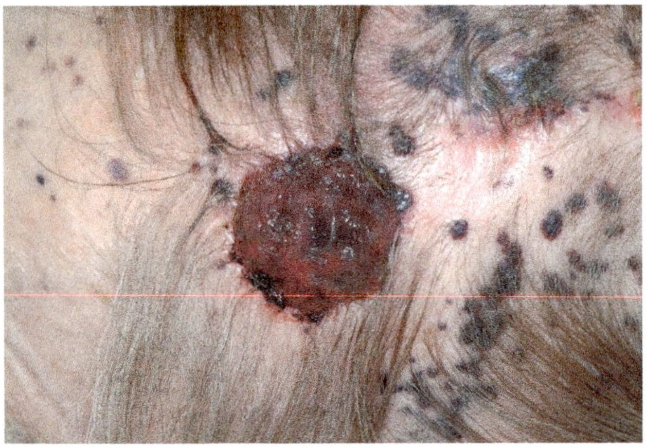

FIG. 13.73
Melanoma with satellites, clinical. A primary melanoma nodule of the scalp is surrounded by many small satellite nodules.

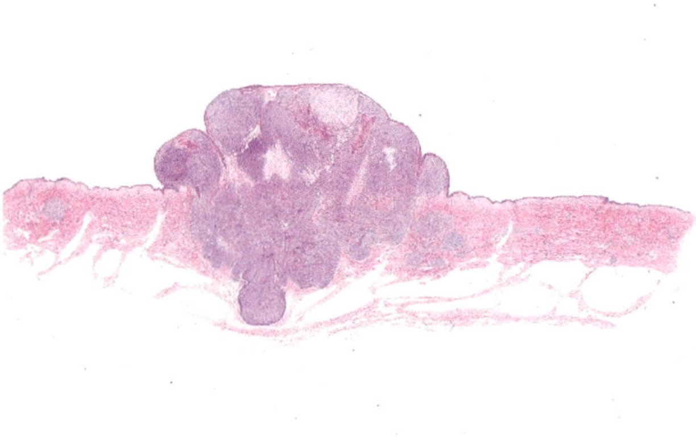

FIG. 13.74
Melanoma with satellites, histology. A primary melanoma is seen as well as melanoma nodules in the dermis separate from the main tumor mass.

is associated with a more favorable outcome. A brisk infiltrate is defined as a dense infiltrate of lymphocytes that involves either diffusely the entire invasive tumor or at least surrounds and disrupts the entire advancing periphery of invasive melanoma (Fig. 13.75). Any lymphocytic infiltrate short of these features is classified as "nonbrisk." (Most melanomas have a nonbrisk infiltrate.) If there are no lymphocytes or lymphocytes that do not infiltrate and disrupt the tumor, they are designated as absent.

REGRESSION

Regression refers to features that suggest a loss or disappearance of melanocytes, generally assumed to be related to immunologically mediated tumor cell death. Regression is best recognized if there is an area within a melanoma that suddenly lacks melanocytes within the dermis or epidermis in the absence of a prior biopsy. Histopathologic traces of regression include various stromal alterations, such as inflammation, edema or fibrosis, hypervascularity, and melanophages (Fig. 13.76).

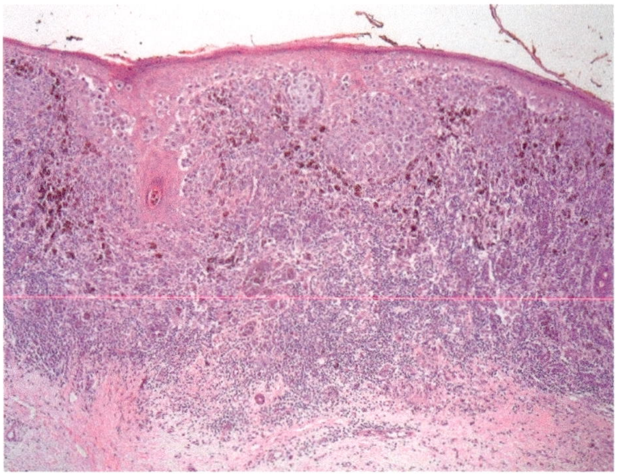

FIG. 13.75
Tumor-infiltrating lymphocytes. The invasive front of the melanoma is surrounded and infiltrated by lymphocytes.

A

B

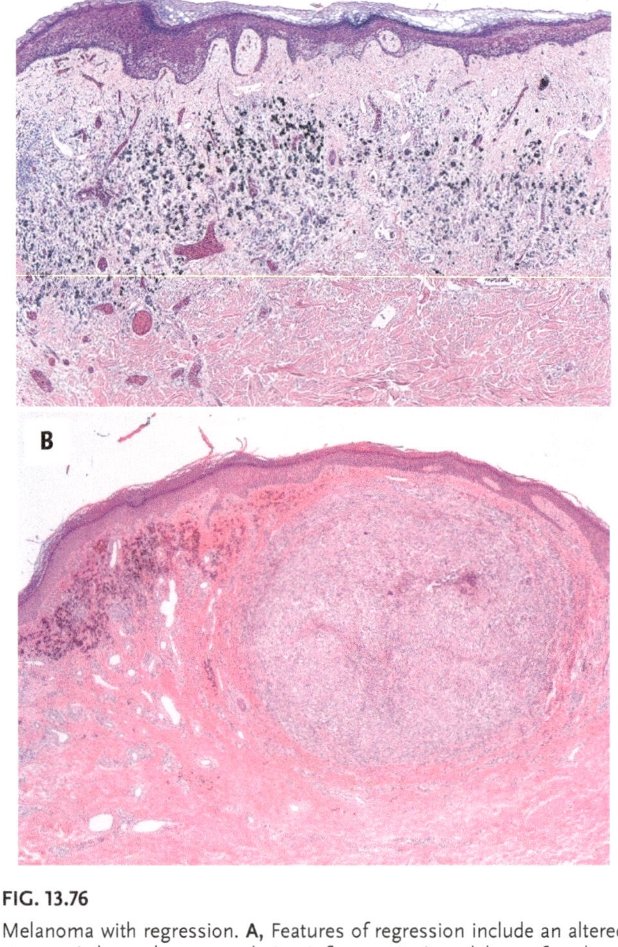

FIG. 13.76
Melanoma with regression. **A,** Features of regression include an altered stroma (edema, hypervascularity, inflammation) and loss of melanocytes. **B,** Primary nodular melanoma with adjacent features of regression.

On occasion, the entire tumor may be regressed, and only the silhouette of a presumed regressed melanocytic lesion can be found. There is significant interobserver variability in the assessment of regression. The main significance of reporting regression lies in the fact that if in situ melanoma is found together with features of regression, associated invasive melanoma can no longer be excluded. It is important to realize, however, that not every focus of regression implies regressed melanoma. It may also represent a regressed nevus component. Regression with melanophages may also be associated with nonmelanocytic tumors, such as a BCC. Furthermore, not every cluster of melanophages or lymphocytes implies regression. Melanophages may simply be associated with increased melanin pigment production and pigment release.

COMMON (CONVENTIONAL) VARIANTS OF MELANOMA

Cutaneous melanomas have historically been classified into four major types: superficial spreading, lentigo maligna, acral lentiginous, and nodular. The first three types are classified by the growth pattern of the intraepidermal (in situ) melanoma component. Superficial spreading melanoma is characterized by prominent intraepidermal pagetoid spread of melanoma cells (pagetoid in situ melanoma) or the presence of many well-formed junctional melanocyte nests. This type of melanoma is commonly associated with melanocytic nevi. Melanomas of lentigo maligna and acral lentiginous types show a predominance of solitary units of melanocytes at the dermal-epidermal junction (lentiginous melanoma). Lentigo maligna is associated with marked solar elastosis and usually affects the head and neck region. Acral lentiginous melanomas occur by definition at acral sites. Nodular melanoma is an invasive melanoma without or only a minimal detectable in situ component.

There has been much debate about the validity of this classification scheme and to what extent the dominant histologic growth pattern is a reflection of anatomic site. Because this historical classification scheme lacks prognostic value and there is overlap in histopathologic findings (e.g., lentigo maligna or acral melanomas may also show pagetoid growth patterns) as well as significant interobserver variability, many pathologists do not use this classification in their daily practice.

Melanomas have also been classified by growth phases for prognostic purposes. The so-called *radial* growth phase refers to a flat peripheral spread of melanoma and is said to lack competence for metastasis. The so-called *vertical* growth phase reflects invasive downward growth and indicates the ability to metastasize. In this concept, radial and vertical growth phases are not entirely synonymous with in situ and invasive melanoma. Radial growth phase is said to include intraepidermal (in situ) melanomas with isolated small solitary units or clusters of melanocytes in the papillary dermis without mitotic figures and compact dermal tumor cell aggregates larger in size than the largest junctional melanocytic nest. The concept of radial and vertical growth phases has been incorporated into some prognostic models but has been questioned by others on practical grounds because of limited interobserver reproducibility. Furthermore, it is of questionable value because some melanomas said to be confined to the radial growth phase were found to have metastasized to distant sites, and many melanomas said to be in the vertical growth phase are cured by simple excision. Reporting growth phases is not recommended for routine practice.

It has become apparent that melanomas are genetically heterogeneous and associated with different molecular signatures (e.g., driver mutations, gene fusions, mutation burden). The molecular profiles depend on anatomic site and the mode of sun damage and correlate to some degree with histopathologic patterns. *BRAFV600E* mutations, for example, are common in "superficial spreading" melanomas arising in association with nevi of skin with intermittent sun exposure, but they are rare in tumors of chronically sun-damaged skin or acral or mucosal sites with limited or no sun exposure. *KIT* mutations occur primarily in acral, mucosal lentiginous, and heavily pigmented melanomas. *GNAQ*, *GNA11*, or *SF3B1* mutations are typical of uveal melanomas and melanomas arising in association with blue nevi. *NRAS* mutations are commonly found in nodular melanomas or melanomas arising in congenital melanocytic nevi. Mutation analysis of melanomas is becoming increasingly important for selecting patients for various treatment regimens targeting specific mutations. With scientific advances and an increased role of molecular pathology for diagnosis and treatment, the WHO classification of melanocytic tumors has been revised to take into account not only histopathologic findings but also the mode of sun exposure and associated genomic aberrations.

UNCOMMON PATHOLOGIC VARIANTS OF MELANOMA

A number of uncommon and unusual histologic variants of melanomas have been described. Separating them from conventional melanomas mainly serves to remind pathologists of the morphologic heterogeneity of melanomas and to point out diagnostic pitfalls.

SPINDLE CELL MELANOMA

Melanomas with predominant spindle cell morphology comprise a spectrum of tumors (Fig. 13.77). If associated with a fibrous stroma throughout the invasive component, they are designated DM. If intraneural or perineural invasion is prominent and a neuroma-like growth pattern is present, the term *neurotropic melanoma*

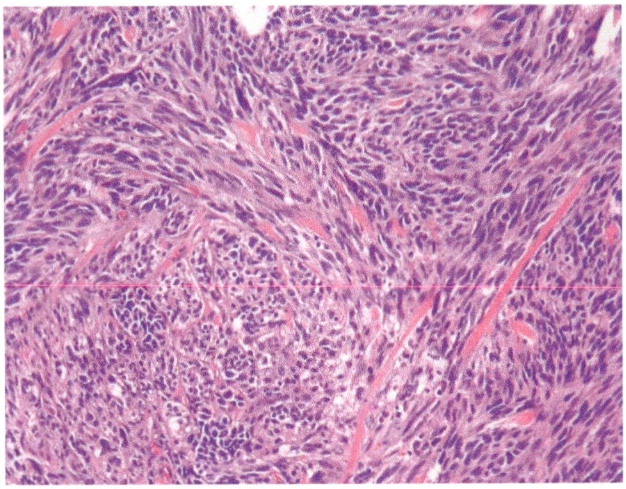

FIG. 13.77

Spindle cell melanoma. The tumor is composed of atypical fusiform melanocytes without any significant intratumoral fibrosis (nondesmoplastic melanoma).

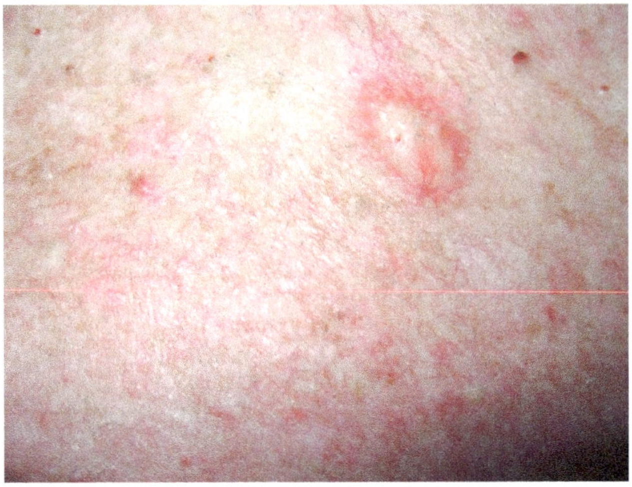

FIG. 13.78

Desmoplastic melanoma. A flesh-colored nodule is seen, which was clinically thought to be a keloid but represented histologically as desmoplastic melanoma.

(NM) may be applied. Spindle cell melanoma (SCM) may be desmoplastic or neurotropic, both or none of the above (SCM, not otherwise specified). Some SCMs are heavily pigmented. Most of them, however, are amelanotic or paucimelanotic. The main diagnostic problem related to amelanotic SCMs is their potential confusion with various types of sarcomas or sarcomatoid carcinomas.

DESMOPLASTIC MELANOMA

Clinical Findings

DM constitutes fewer than 4% of invasive melanomas. It typically occurs in the head and neck region of elderly individuals. However, DM may occur at any site, including mucosal sites, and may affect young adults. The clinical presentation is usually indistinct. Frequently, it manifests as a slightly erythematous or skin-colored nodule suspected to be a keloid or dermatofibroma (Fig. 13.78). DM differs from conventional melanoma in its clinical course by a higher propensity for local cutaneous or subcutaneous recurrences and less frequent metastases to regional lymph nodes. Distant metastases typically appear first in the lung. Evidence has also emerged that desmoplasia may be a favorable prognostic finding, especially for patients with tumors measuring more than 4 mm in thickness.

Histopathologic Features

DM is characterized by the dispersion of usually amelanotic fusiform melanocytes in a prominent fibrous stroma, which gives the tumor a pink appearance at scanning magnification (Figs. 13.79 and 13.80). The associated in situ melanoma component typically displays a predominantly basilar lentiginous growth

UNCOMMON VARIANTS OF CUTANEOUS MELANOMAS—DISEASE FACT SHEET

- Desmoplastic melanoma (pure and mixed)
- Neurotropic melanoma
- Nevoid melanoma
- Spitz melanoma
- BLUE melanoma
- Rare tumors with peculiar morphologic features (e.g., balloon cell, myxoid, rhabdoid)
- Sarcomatoid (undifferentiated) melanoma

DESMOPLASTIC MELANOMA—PATHOLOGIC FEATURES

Clinical Findings

- Usually older patients but may occur in younger individuals
- Usually chronically sun-damaged skin of head and neck, but may occur anywhere
- Often confused with a scar or fibroma
- Regional lymph nodes rarely involved

Histopathologic Features

- In situ melanoma:
  - Present in approximately two-thirds of cases
  - May involve follicles
- Invasive melanoma:
  - Usually amelanotic spindle cell
  - Pure: fibrous stroma-rich; tumor cell-poor
  - Mixed: paucicellular fibrosing areas admixed with areas with no or little desmoplasia
  - Nerve involvement: common
  - Patchy lymphocytic infiltrates: common
  - Cytologic atypia: variable; hyperchromatic spindle cells are often seen

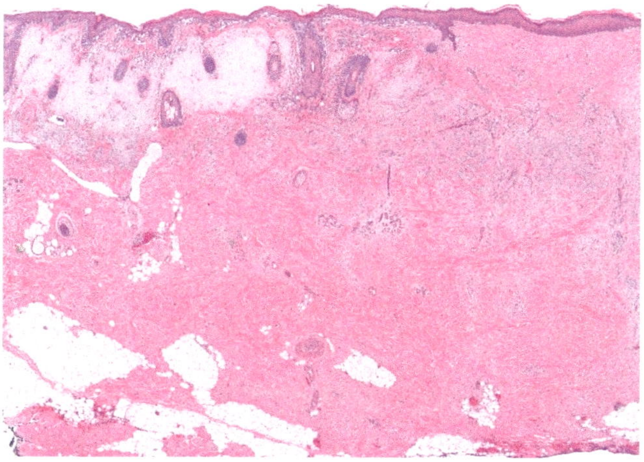

FIG. 13.79
Desmoplastic melanoma (DM). Silhouette of a DM shows a diffuse fibrosing process in the dermis and subcutis. There is associated in situ melanoma.

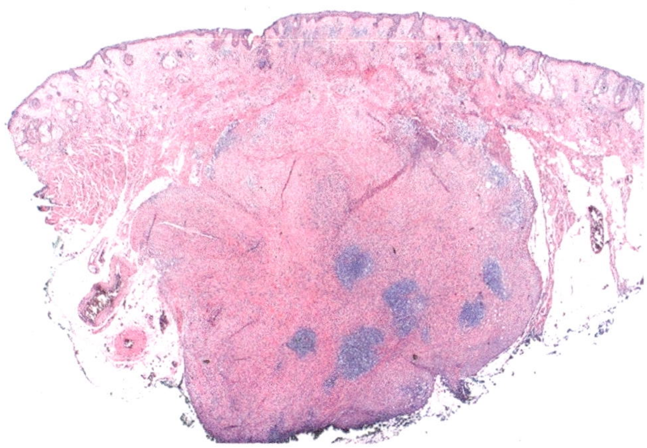

FIG. 13.80
Desmoplastic melanoma (DM). This DM shows nodular fibrosing pattern. Clusters of lymphocytes are commonly seen in association with DM.

pattern (lentigo maligna). In approximately one-third of the cases, no associated in situ melanoma component can be detected. When DM is diagnosed, the majority of tumors have already invaded the reticular dermis. Extension into the subcutis with replacement of the fat by fibrous tissue is common. Patchy lymphocytic aggregates and perineural or intraneural invasion are commonly associated with DM (Fig. 13.80). Pure DM displays the microscopic picture of a paucicellular fibrosing spindle cell proliferation throughout the entire tumor (Fig. 13.79). If desmoplasia is only a partial feature of an otherwise conventional melanoma, the tumor is classified as a mixed DM (Fig. 13.81).

The degree of cytologic atypia of the tumor cells in a DM is variable. Melanocytes may be relatively bland,

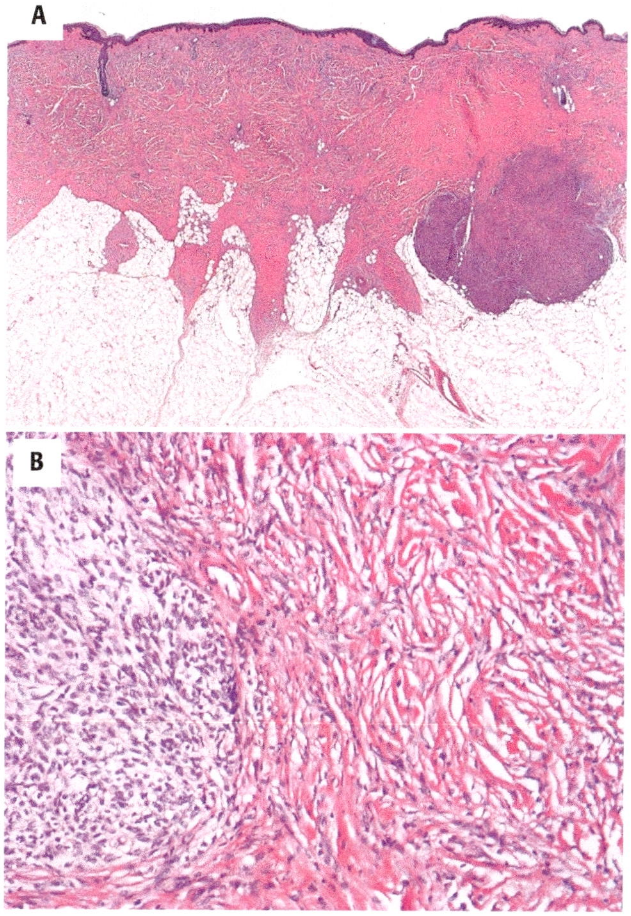

FIG. 13.81
Mixed desmoplastic melanoma. **A,** Infiltrative fibrotic tumor with cellular nodule. **B,** Solid melanoma nodule without intratumoral fibrosis adjacent to paucicellular desmoplastic tumor component.

mimicking the appearance of fibroblasts or Schwann cells. However, usually at least scattered pleomorphic melanocytes with large hyperchromatic nuclei are present. At times, pleomorphic cells predominate. Some cases can closely simulate a neurofibroma and have been referred to as neurofibroma-like DM.

Differential Diagnosis

DM continues to be misdiagnosed and constitutes a significant part of medical malpractice claims related to melanoma. The most problematic diagnostic pitfall is to mistake a DM for a dermal scar or fibroma. It is prudent to perform IHC for S100 protein or SOX10 for any unusual or otherwise unexplained scarlike dermal spindle cell proliferation of chronically sun-damaged skin of the head and neck region (Fig. 13.82). IHC is also useful to assess and measure the extent of invasive DM in previously biopsied cases of lentigo maligna.

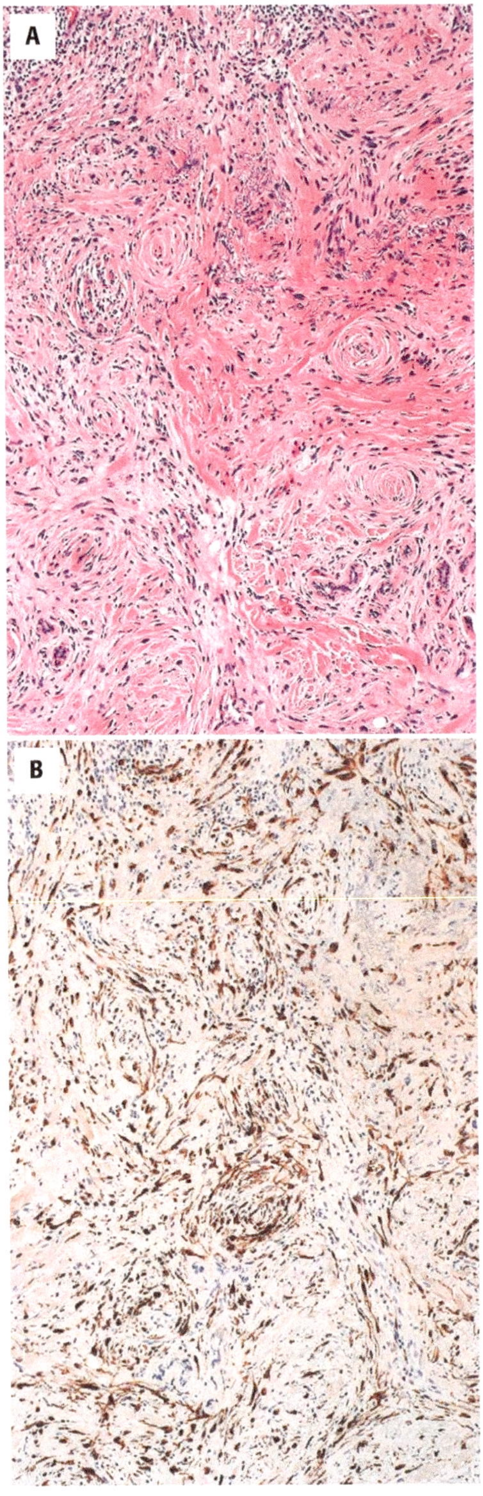

FIG. 13.82
Desmoplastic melanoma. **A,** The tumor has an inflamed scarlike appearance. **B,** The tumor cells are positive for S100 protein.

DM also needs to be distinguished from fibrosing (sclerosing) melanocytic nevi and nonmelanocytic tumors (e.g., dermatofibroma, neurofibroma, spindle cell carcinomas, or sarcomas with desmoplasia). DM differs from a sclerosing nevus by a number of features, such as associated in situ melanoma (if present), asymmetric silhouette, larger size, deep infiltration, and presence of cytologic atypia and mitotic figures as well as the common association with patchy lymphocytic aggregates. Furthermore, DM is usually immunopositive only for S100 protein, SOX10, and neurotrophin receptor p75, but desmoplastic nevi are often positive for A103, p16, and sometimes also HMB-45. Distinction of DM from nonmelanocytic tumors is usually readily achieved by strong and diffuse immunostaining of DM for S100 protein or SOX10. In difficult cases, molecular studies may help.

DIFFERENTIAL DIAGNOSIS: SCLEROSING NEVUS OR DESMOPLASTIC MELANOMA—PATHOLOGIC FEATURES

Features Favoring Melanoma

- Silhouette
  - Asymmetry
  - Infiltrative, usually extending into deep dermis or subcutis
- Associated melanoma in situ
  - Usually lentiginous junctional pattern, may be folliculotropic
- Cytology
  - Nuclear atypia, such as hyperchromasia
  - Some lesions may be deceptively bland
- Stromal changes
  - Patchy lymphoid aggregates
  - Fibrosis, occasionally with myxoid changes
- Immunohistochemistry
  - Lack of staining for Melan-A, gp100, tyrosinase, MITF, p16

MITF, Microphthalmia-associated transcription factor.

NEUROTROPIC MELANOMA

The term *neurotropic melanoma* refers to variants of invasive melanoma with frequent invasion of the perineurium or endoneurium of nerve trunks at the periphery of the main tumor mass (Fig. 13.83). NMs are usually amelanotic. They may also show desmoplastic features (desmoplastic and NM) but do not need to do so. Some NMs lack any or show only minimal intratumoral fibrosis. NMs may show a traumatic neuroma–like pattern. On occasion, an epithelioid cell melanoma shows prominent nerve involvement.

A neurotropic SCM may be difficult to distinguish from a nerve sheath tumor (malignant peripheral nerve sheath tumor [MPNST]). Although both melanoma and MPNST are positive for S100 protein and SOX10, immunostaining for these markers may nonetheless be helpful. As a general rule, whereas most MPNSTs stain only weakly and focally for S100 protein or SOX10, most melanomas are strongly and diffusely immunoreactive. Anatomic location is also important. The majority of sporadic (i.e., outside of the clinical setting of neurofibromatosis occurring) malignant spindle cell tumors with schwannian features in the superficial soft tissue of the head and neck region turn out to be

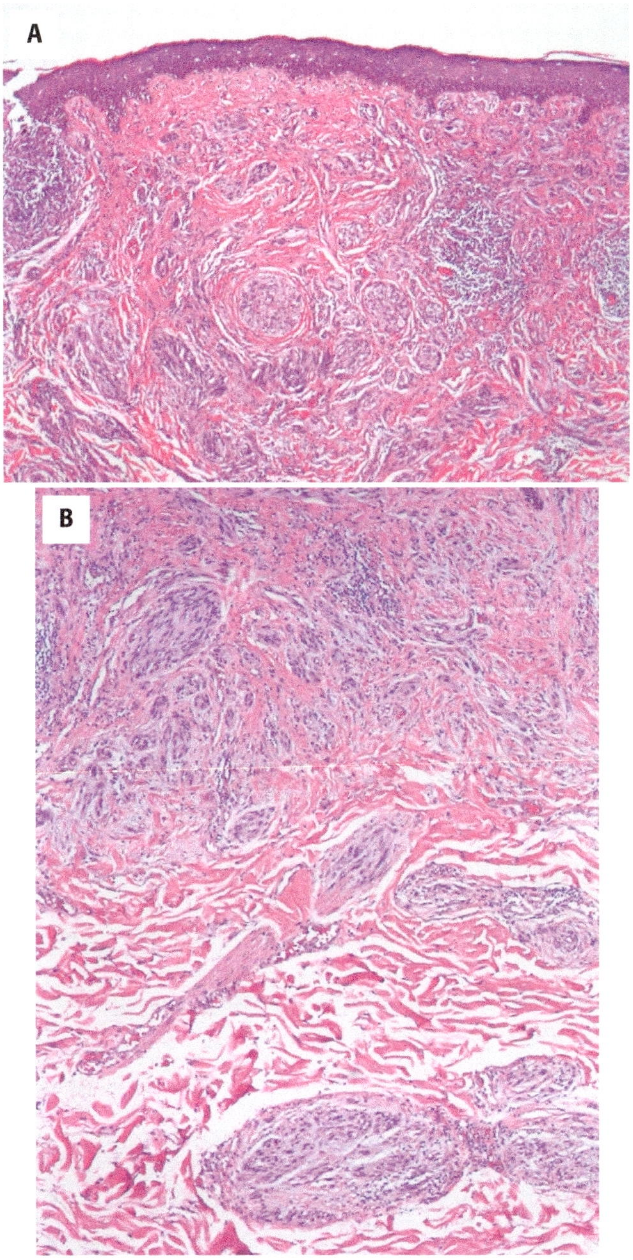

FIG. 13.83

Neurotropic melanoma. **A,** Spindle cell melanoma with plexiform growth pattern. **B,** Several nerve trunks at the periphery of the tumor are involved by melanoma.

melanomas. Deep soft tissue and paraspinal location favors MPNST.

NEVOID MELANOMA

Nevoid melanoma is a variant of nodular melanoma. One may describe nevoid melanoma as a melanocytic proliferation, which at first glance looks like a nevus. A well-developed in situ melanoma component is usually absent. Long, thin, elongated epidermal rete ridges surrounding expanded dermal papillae densely populated by melanocytes are a clue (Fig. 13.84). Some lesions simulate the appearance of a papillomatous nevus (Fig. 13.85). The "puffy shirt" sign is often mentioned as a "low power clue" to the diagnosis of nevoid melanoma. It refers to the presence of rows of dermal papillae packed with and expanded by a dense population of melanocytes surrounded by elongated rete ridges forming collarettes. Other microscopic clues to the diagnosis of nevoid melanoma include limited maturation, the presence of mitoses, or expansile aggregates of atypical intradermal melanocytes. Naturally, there is a wide spectrum of melanomas that are reported as "nevoid." The term *nevoid melanoma* serves to emphasize the diagnostic challenge or pitfall. Nevoid melanoma represents a diagnostic pitfall, but not a prognostically distinct variant of melanoma. Tumors designated as nevoid melanoma tend to behave like other conventional invasive melanomas if adjusted for various histologic prognostic parameters. Most lesions of nevoid melanomas likely arise from common acquired or small congenital nevi.

SPITZ MELANOMA

Historically the term spitzoid melanoma has been used for melanomas simulating and/or misdiagnosed as Spitz nevus (Figs. 13.86 and 13.87). Recently the terms spitzoid and Spitz melanoma have been separated and refined by including molecular findings. The WHO currently recommends the term Spitz melanoma for melanomas with spitzoid microscopic features and verified Spitz molecular pathway (Spitz genomic fusion or *HRAS* mutation) (Fig. 13.88). The term spitzoid melanoma is used for melanomas with some Spitz-like cytology, but non-Spitz molecular aberrations (e.g., *BRAF, NRAS, NF1* mutations).

It is currently unclear whether Spitz melanomas in adults have a different prognosis than conventional melanomas. However, preliminary experience suggests that melanocytic tumors with a verified Spitz-associated genomic fusion and Spitz cytomorphology tend to have a relatively indolent course compared to conventional melanomas. Usually only rare bulky tumors with obviously malignant (high-grade) histopathology are associated with recurrences. The prognostic difference between Spitz and conventional melanomas is more recognized in children.

With the knowledge of a Spitz-associated genomic fusion, the microscopic threshold for establishing a diagnosis of malignant melanoma (as opposed to atypical Spitz tumor or melanocytoma) is relatively high. In our experience, atypical melanocytic tumors with BRAF or MAP3K8 fusions are the ones most likely to qualify as melanoma. Histopathologic findings supporting a diagnosis of Spitz melanoma include marked pleomorphism; sheetlike or expansile nodular growth without

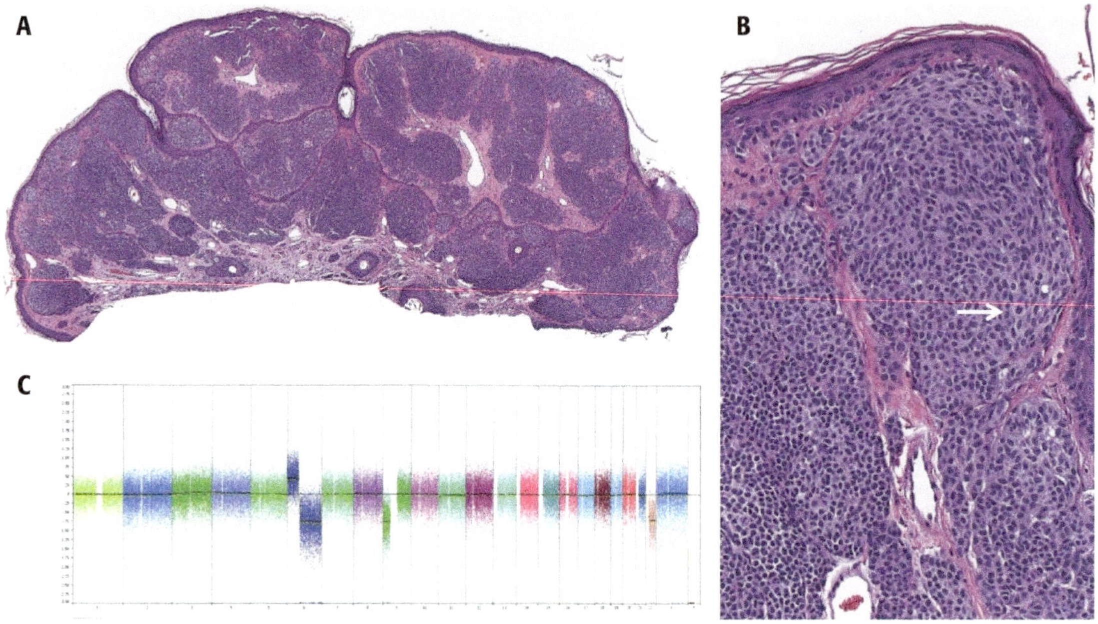

FIG. 13.84

Nevoid melanoma. **A,** The silhouette of the lesion is nevoid. There is no apparent intraepidermal melanoma. The tumor cell density is high and thin elongated rete ridges are present. **B,** Expansile aggregates of dermal melanocytes with mitotic figures *(arrow)*. **C,** Cytogenetic (single nucleotide polymorphism [SNP] array) analysis reveals chromosomal copy number aberrations typical of melanoma.

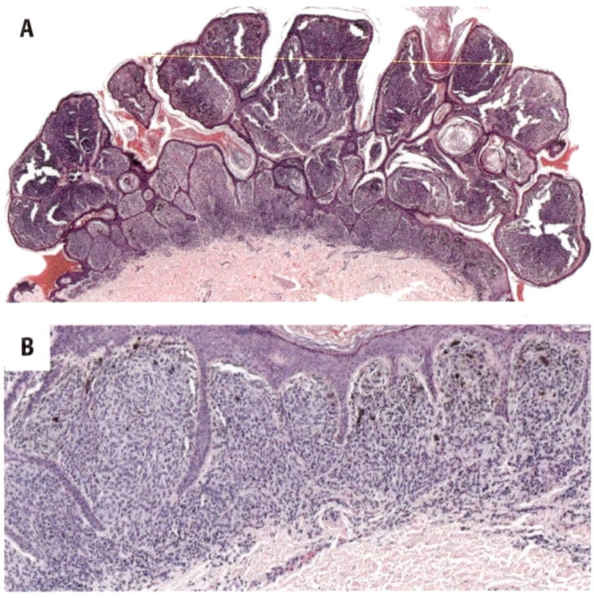

FIG. 13.85

Papillomatous nevoid melanoma. **A,** The tumor has papillomatous projections. They are densely packed with melanocytes. **B,** The dermal papillae are filled and expanded by tumor cells. Rete ridges form small collarettes. Rows of such collarettes of densely packed dermal papillae have been referred to as "puffy short sign."

maturation; and mitotic figures, including atypical mitoses, or mitoses near the deep aspect of the tumor. Cytogenetic studies with FISH or CGH showing multiple clonal segmental copy number aberrations typical of melanoma such as homozygous deletions of 9p21 as well as TPM analysis may also yield evidence to support a diagnosis of melanoma.

It should be kept in mind that 40% to 50% of atypical Spitz tumors may show involvement of regional lymph nodes with an SLN biopsy, but metastases beyond the node are very rare.

NEVOID MELANOMA—PATHOLOGIC FEATURES

Clinical Findings

- Usually small papule (submitted as nevus; rule out atypia)

Histopathologic Features

- Nevus-like silhouette
- Lack of obvious features of in situ melanoma
- Nested growth pattern
- Incomplete maturation
- Focal expansile nests of melanocytes with atypia
- Mitotic figures
- Thin elongated rete ridges
- Densely packed dermal papillae ("puffy shirt sign")

Ancillary Test Results

- Immunohistochemistry
  - Diffuse immunoreactivity for PRAME
  - Loss of p16 expression
- Cytogenetics
  - Positive melanoma FISH test
  - Segmental copy number variations by CGH or SNP array

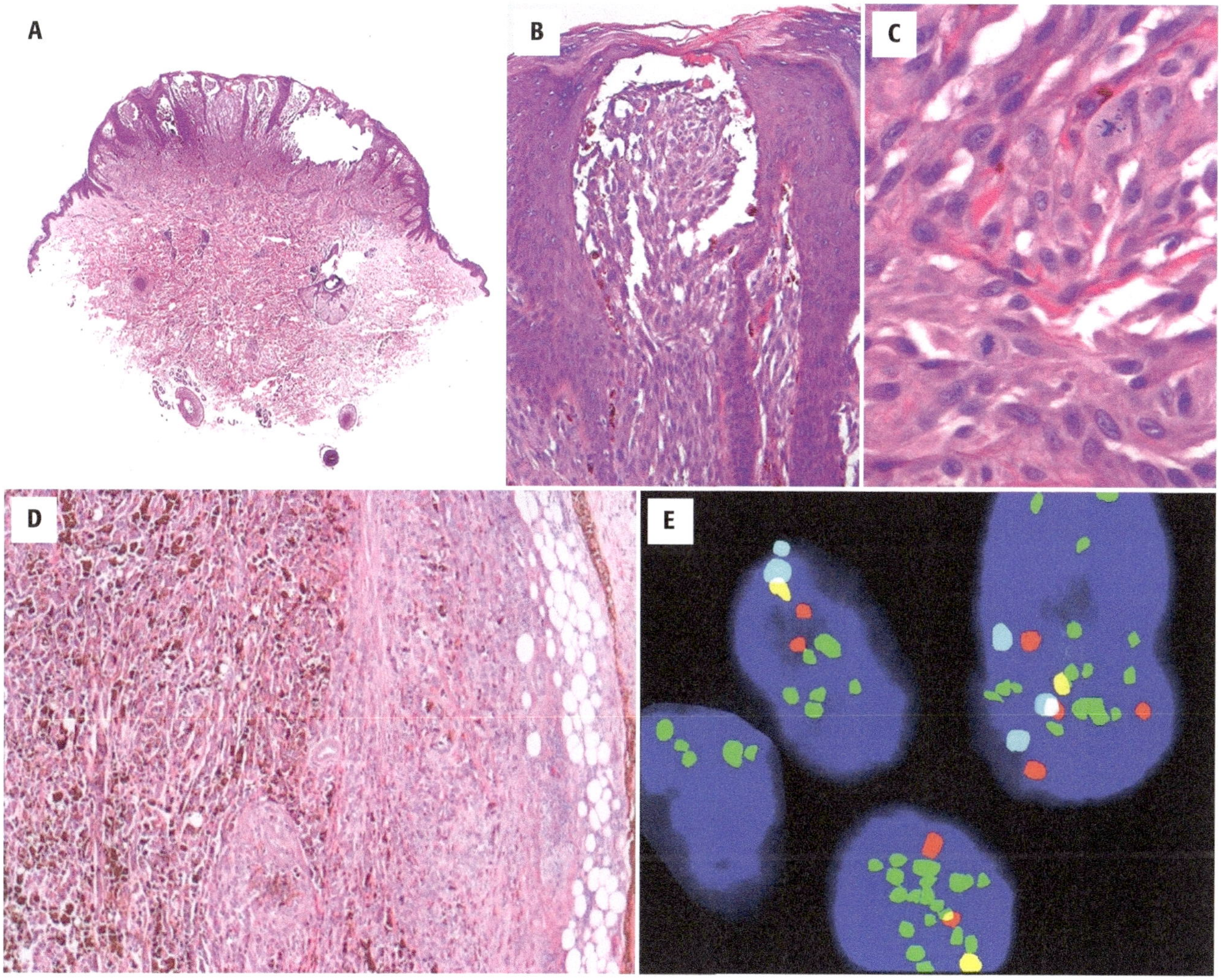

FIG. 13.86

Spitzoid melanoma. **A,** Circumscribed papule with nevoid silhouette. **B,** Pigmented spindle cells are present with clefts between the tumor fascicles and epidermis. **C,** Mitotic figures are present in epithelioid melanocytes at the base of the tumor. **D,** Regional lymph node metastasis. **E,** Copy number gains documented by fluorescence in situ hybridization.

BLUE MELANOMA (MALIGNANT BLUE TUMOR)

Melanoma may arise in association with a BN or share a molecular driver with blue nevi (Fig. 13.89). Historically, such lesions have been designated *malignant blue nevus*. Such melanomas are usually heavily pigmented and lack an intraepidermal component. This rare variant of melanoma can be diagnosed readily if a pleomorphic and mitotically active melanoma cell component with or without necrosis is immediately adjacent to a benign (usually cellular) BN. Recognition of tumors with less atypia and without necrosis as malignant is more difficult. Malignant transformation of a cellular BN is typically heralded by the emergence of sheets of epithelioid cells (Fig. 13.89), often, but not always, associated with an increased mitotic index. Rare cases exist, however, in which a reliable distinction between early melanoma and cellular BN with atypical features cannot be made on morphologic grounds alone. Loss of BAP1 would favor melanoma, but it is not lost in all melanomas. Cytogenetic studies can be very helpful. Most melanomas associated with a BN carry copy number gains or losses, especially affecting chromosome 6.

Although BN-like melanomas with high-grade features (pleomorphism and necrosis) tend to behave aggressively, there is a range of low- to intermediate-grade BN-like melanomas characterized by repeated local subcutaneous recurrences with rare distant metastases, which may occur many years after the diagnosis of the primary tumor.

Although melanoma simulating BN is usually thought of as a scenario in which a tumor mimics a cellular BN, melanoma may also mimic the features of an EBN. EBN-like melanoma is recognized by cytologic atypia, lack of maturation, absence of mature dendritic melanocytes, the presence of lymphocytic aggregates, mitotic figures, or ancillary cytogenetic studies.

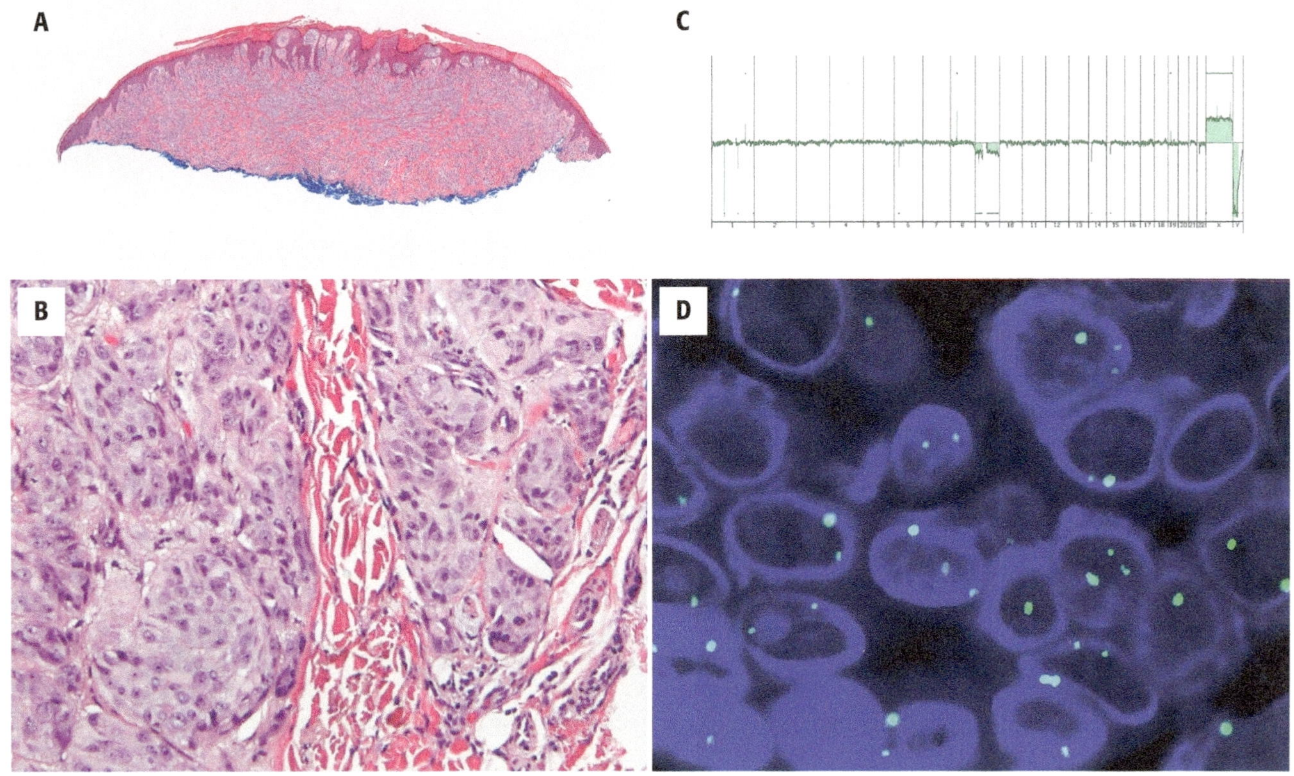

FIG. 13.87

Spitzoid melanoma of childhood. **A,** This spitzoid melanocytic proliferation is from a 2-year-old child. **B,** The tumor cells are cytologically atypical. **C,** Comparative genomic hybridization reveals loss of chromosome 9. **D,** Fluorescence in situ hybridization documents homozygous deletions of p16 on 9p (only the signal of the centromeric probe is seen; no signal of the p16 probe is identified in any nucleus).

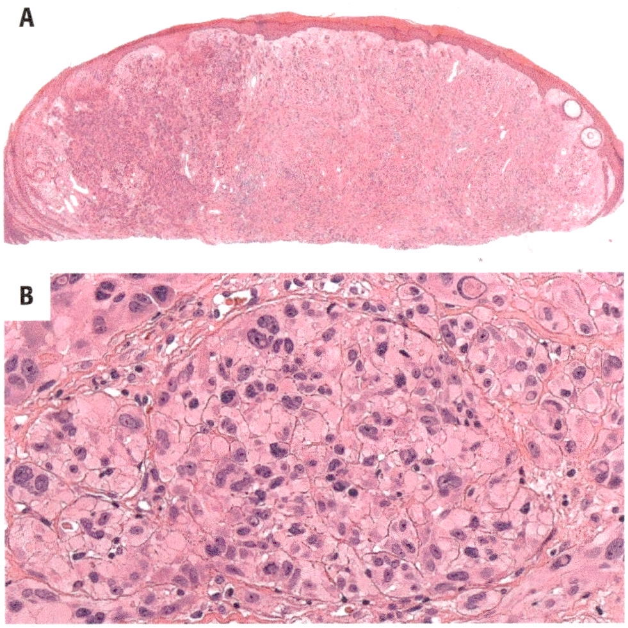

FIG. 13.88

Spitz melanoma. **A,** The tumor is asymmetric, densely cellular, and associated with consumption of the epidermis. **B,** Sheets of markedly atypical large epithelioid tumor cells are present. The tumor harbored a *MAP3K-UPL3* gene fusion. (Courtesy of Dr. P Gerami.)

MELANOPHAGE-RICH MELANOMA (AKA PIGMENT-SYNTHESIZING MELANOMA)

Some melanomas are associated with numerous melanin pigment–laden macrophages, giving the lesions a very dark appearance. Historically, some of these melanomas have been termed *animal-type melanoma* in reference to darkly pigmented melanocytic tumors in animals, such as in horses. We discourage the use of the term *animal-type melanoma* for a number of reasons. There is no solid evidence that melanophage-rich melanomas behave differently from other melanomas if adjusted for other prognostic markers.

RARE MELANOMAS WITH PECULIAR MICROSCOPIC FEATURES

SMALL CELL MELANOMA

Small cell variants of melanoma have been described that are histologically characterized by hyperchromatic

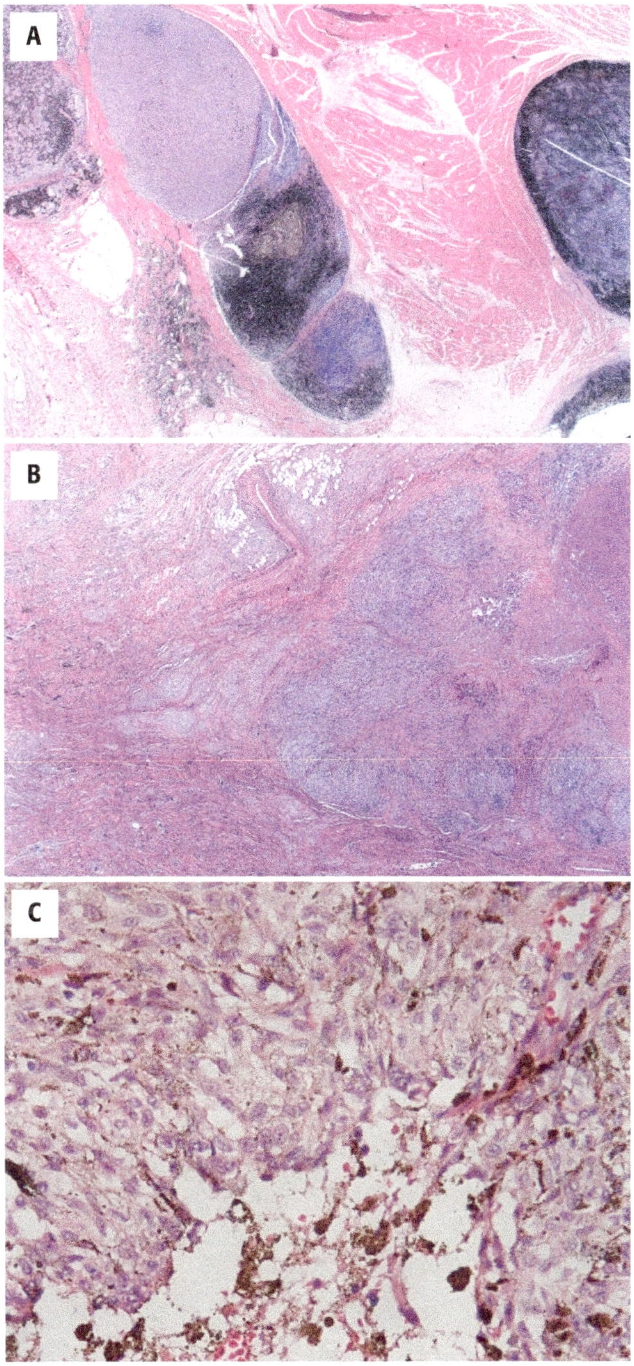

FIG. 13.89

Melanoma arising in association with a blue nevus (BN). **A,** Large nodules of melanocytes are present with focal necrosis and melanosis. **B,** The nodules are present in a background of BN. A transition from ordinary to cellular BN and melanoma is seen. **C,** The melanoma is characterized by the presence of large atypical epithelioid melanocytes and focal necrosis.

cells with little or no cytoplasm (Fig. 13.90). Knowledge of this histopathologic phenotype is relevant for potential confusion with neuroendocrine carcinoma, Ewing sarcoma, or neuroblastoma. The use of IHC should avoid potential diagnostic errors.

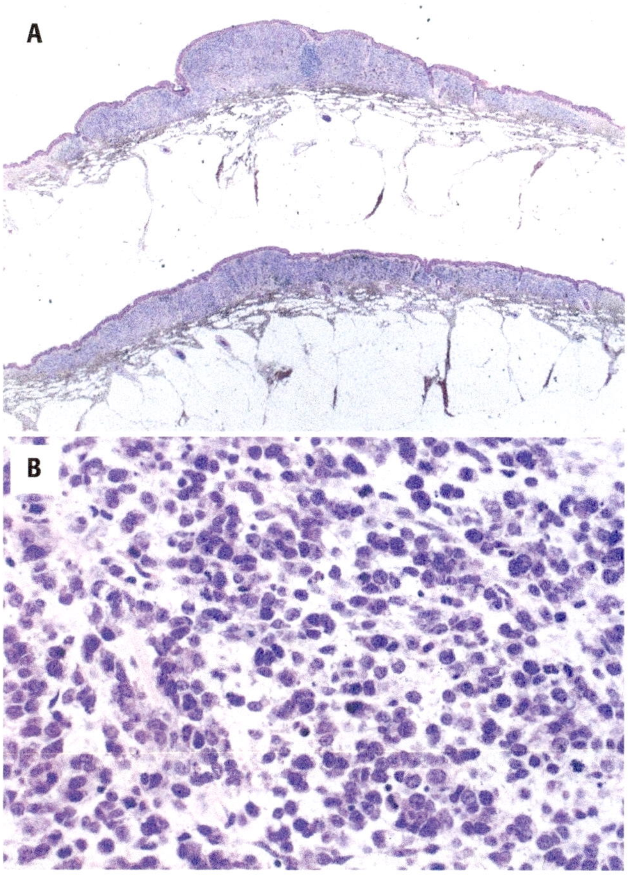

FIG. 13.90

Small cell melanoma. **A,** Silhouette of a small cell melanoma arising in a congenital nevus. **B,** Small hyperchromatic melanocytes are present with numerous mitoses and individually necrotic cells. This melanoma occurred in a 4-year-old child who developed lung metastases.

BALLOON CELL MELANOMA

A peculiar histologic appearance of melanoma may be the presence of large epithelioid cells with abundant clear cytoplasm (Fig. 13.91). Primary balloon cell melanomas are usually recognized as such but may on rare occasions lead to confusion with other primary cutaneous clear cell tumors. Knowledge of this morphologic phenotype of balloon cells is primarily relevant for the differential diagnosis and workup of metastatic clear cell tumors (melanoma versus metastatic renal or adrenocortical carcinoma or foamy histiocytes). There is no known prognostic significance associated with balloon cell changes in primary or metastatic melanoma.

SIGNET RING CELL MELANOMA

Melanoma can also manifest with signet ring cell morphology (Fig. 13.92). This is of no prognostic significance but relevant for the analysis of metastatic or mucosal signet ring cell tumors to bear in mind that

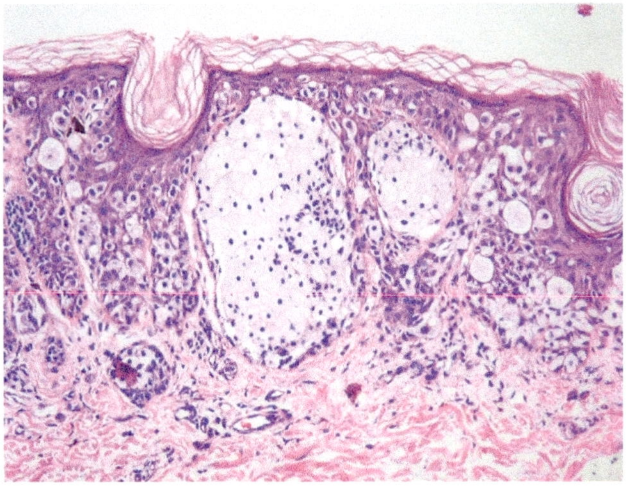

FIG. 13.91

Balloon cell melanoma. Melanoma with large pale epithelioid melanocytes ("balloon" cells).

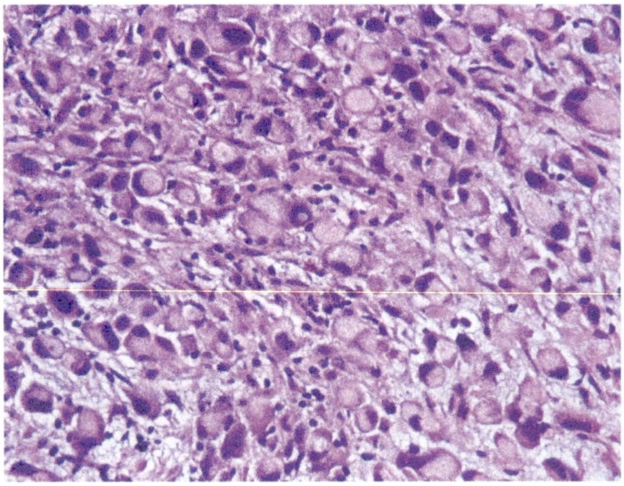

FIG. 13.92

Signet ring cell melanoma. Melanoma with eccentric nuclei and cytoplasmic vacuole giving rise to a signet ring appearance.

melanoma needs to be considered in the differential diagnosis.

RHABDOID MELANOMA

Rhabdoid melanomas are characterized by the presence of large plasmacytoid epithelioid tumor cells, often with eccentrically located nuclei and abundant pink cytoplasm. Such tumors may be confused with other rhabdoid neoplasms.

CLEAR CELL SARCOMA (MELANOMA OF SOFT PARTS) AND RELATED TUMORS

This tumor has historically been classified as sarcoma but is discussed here because its tumor cells show evidence of melanocytic differentiation and the need to distinguish it from cutaneous melanoma.

Clinical Findings

Clear cell sarcoma (CCS) usually arises in deep soft tissues closely associated with facial or tendoaponeurotic structures but may extend into the subcutis or even dermis. On rare occasions, the tumor may be centered in the dermis. It typically affects adolescents or young adults with a predilection for the distal extremities, but it may occur at many anatomic sites. The majority of patients eventually die of metastatic disease.

Histopathologic Features

Nest or fascicles of tumor cells infiltrate fibrous tissues (Fig. 13.93). The tumor cells may be pale (clear cell features) or pink and fusiform or epithelioid in appearance. Multinucleate "wreath-type" giant cells are often seen at the periphery of the tumor.

Primary tumors often lack marked pleomorphism. CCS may be indistinguishable from cutaneous melanoma. It is typically positive for S100 protein, gp100, and Melan-A.

On rare occasions, a melanoma of soft parts may be dermal based (Fig. 13.94) and even be associated with a junctional growth of melanocytes.

Differential Diagnosis

CCS can be confused with primary or metastatic cutaneous melanoma as well as cellular blue nevi and Spitz

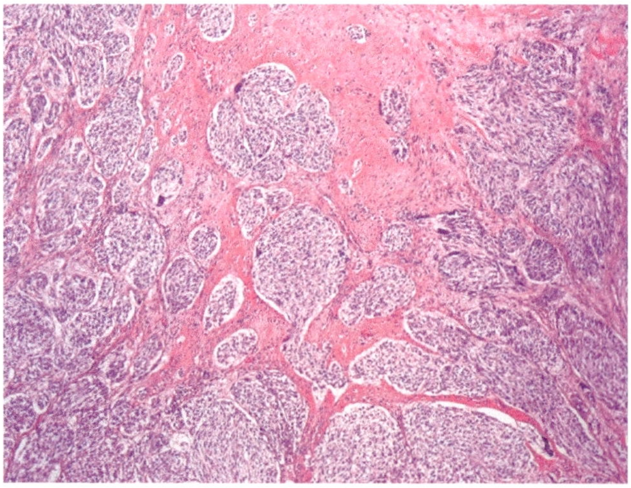

FIG. 13.93

Clear cell sarcoma. Nests and fascicles of melanoma cells are present in deep tendinous tissue.

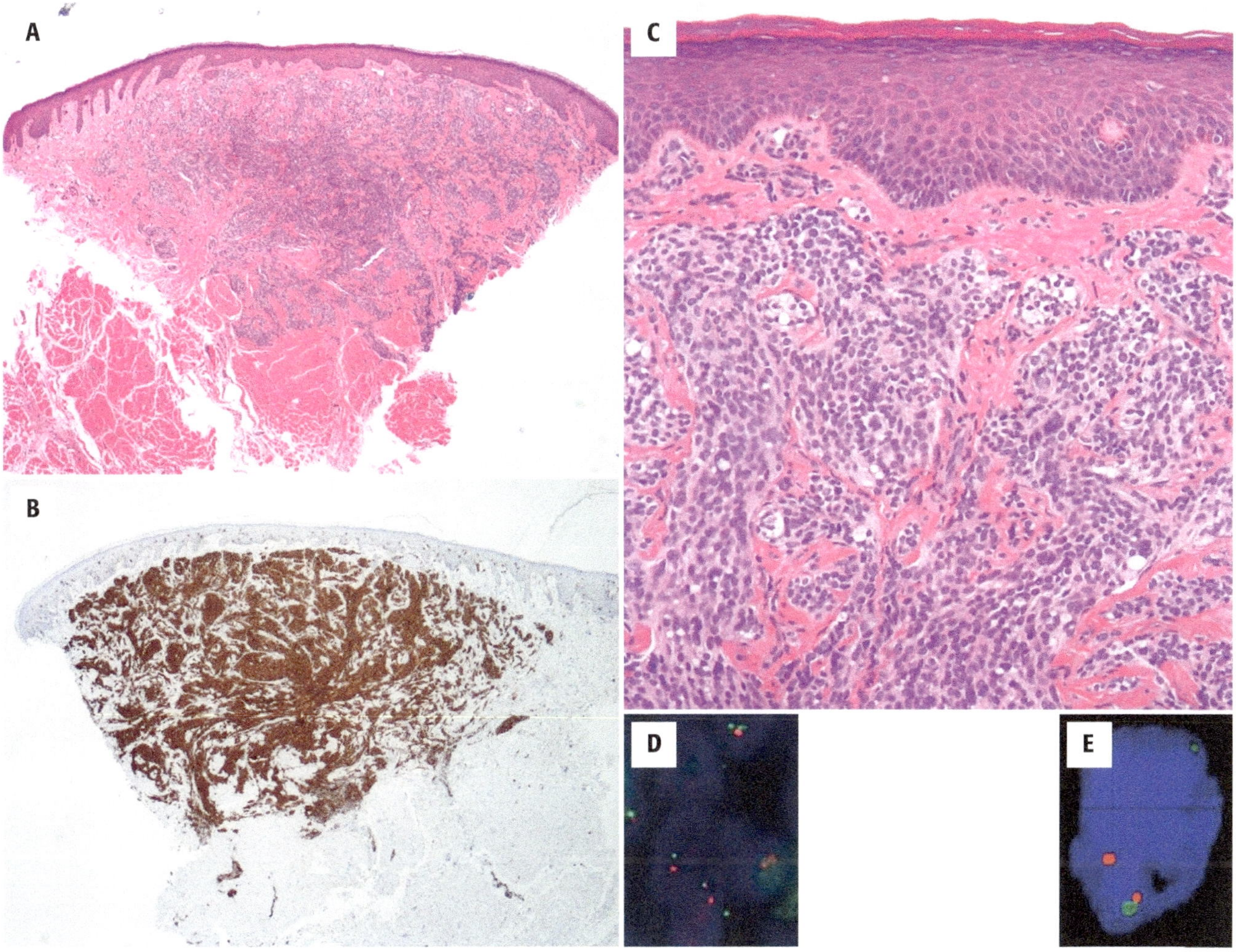

FIG. 13.94

Dermal clear cell sarcoma. **A,** Dermal-based tumor. **B,** The tumor cells are immunoreactive for Melan-A. **C,** Nests and fascicles of cells are seen, some with clear cytoplasm. Fluorescence in situ hybridization documents rearrangement of *ATF1* (**D**) and *EWSR1* (**E**).

tumors. Its deep location and lack of an associated intraepithelial component are very helpful for the distinction from primary cutaneous melanoma. The presence of many wreath-like giant cells is a diagnostic clue. Metastases from cutaneous melanoma are usually more pleomorphic than melanomas of soft tissue. If an unequivocal distinction is needed, cytogenetic studies can be definitive (Fig. 13.94). In contrast with cutaneous melanoma, CCS is associated with a distinct set of gene fusions between EWSR1 and ATF1, CREB1, or CREM. Approximately 90% of CCS have an EWSR1::ATF1 fusion. There are also other related soft tissue tumors. They display melanocytic differentiation and harbor gene fusions, such as CRTC1::TRIM11, MED15::ATF1 or CREM::MITF.

UNDIFFERENTIATED (SARCOMATOID) MELANOMA

Undifferentiated or dedifferentiated melanomas are melanomas with limited or no expression of melanocyte differentiation antigens, including S100P and SOX10. Clues to the diagnosis are usually clinical context, such as a prior history of melanoma, especially in the case of undifferentiated metastatic melanoma, and molecular studies documenting the presence of a UV signature mutation profile and a driver mutation typical of melanoma. It is important to distinguish undifferentiated melanoma from sarcoma, because patients with undifferentiated melanomas respond to melanoma therapy.

MELANOCYTIC TUMORS OF UNCERTAIN MALIGNANT POTENTIAL OR BORDERLINE LESIONS

Although the histopathologic assessment of melanocytic tumors by an experienced pathologist yields a reliable diagnosis in the majority of cases, there are occasional lesions in which it is best to acknowledge that one simply does not know for sure whether a tumor is a melanoma or not. There are different ways to express one's uncertainty. Terms such as *melanocytic tumor of uncertain malignant potential* or *borderline lesion* are ways to paraphrase a pathologist's inability to distinguish a nevus from melanoma. This is not necessarily a diagnostic failure from lack of experience or knowledge but at times is the most honest assessment of what can reliably be said about an unusual tumor by light microscopic analysis.

Because the depth of experience varies (seeing a daily high volume is not necessarily as critical as getting follow-up or cytogenetic verification on difficult cases) as well as one's willingness to admit that one does not know, such cases are usually controversial. When one faces diagnostic controversy and uncertainty, we advocate a pragmatic approach. A second opinion from a respected colleague is prudent practice. As long as melanoma cannot be excluded with certainty (i.e., several experienced pathologists consider melanoma), diagnostic uncertainty and/or controversy should be acknowledged and the tumor in question should be completely excised. If sufficient tumor tissue is available for ancillary studies, we recommend proceeding with further characterization of the tumor, when possible and feasible, because the test results may permit a definitive classification. If ancillary tests favor melanoma, a more compelling case can be made that a diagnostically problematic tumor is a malignant melanoma.

MELANOCYTIC PROLIFERATIONS ASSOCIATED WITH EPITHELIAL TUMORS

Occasionally, a nevus or melanoma may arise intimately admixed with an epithelial tumor. This may be in the setting of a teratoma or neurocristic hamartoma (congenital nevus with heterologous elements) or as a collision scenario, such as with a seborrheic keratosis, squamous cell carcinoma (SCC), or BCC. When a nevus or melanoma collides with another epithelial tumor, it may populate and colonize it. We regard *squamomelanocytic* and *basomelanocytic* tumors as histologic patterns, which usually reflect a collision phenomenon, such as the collision of a cutaneous melanoma metastasis with BCC (Fig. 13.95). One must be careful not to overinterpret florid reactive pseudoepitheliomatous epidermal hyperplasia associated with melanoma as evidence of SCC and melanoma. True transdifferentiation of a melanoma to an epithelial phenotype is exceedingly rare.

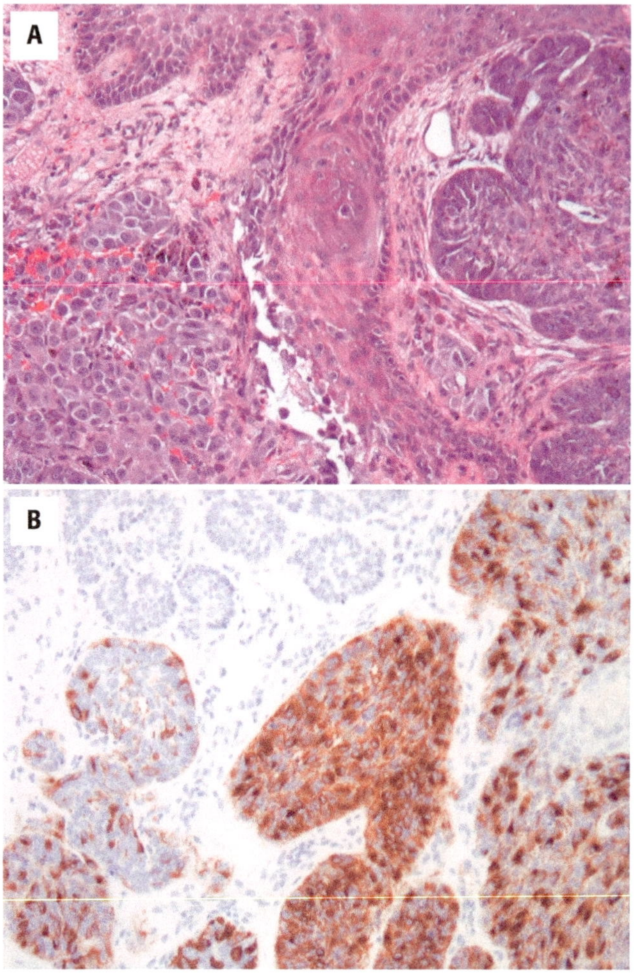

FIG. 13.95

Basomelanocytic tumor. **A,** Melanoma has metastasized to the site of basal cell carcinoma (BCC) (collision phenomenon). **B,** An immunostain for gp100 (HMB-45) demonstrates that the BCC has been colonized by melanoma cells, simulating the pattern of what has been referred to as *basomelanocytic tumor.*

METASTATIC MELANOMA

Metastases occur in approximately one-third of patients with primary invasive cutaneous melanoma. The pattern of spread is unpredictable. Any site of the body may be involved. Melanoma can spread to distant sites hematogenously as well as through lymphatic channels. The site of initial metastasis is of prognostic significance. Patients with regional lymph node metastasis who undergo lymphadenectomy have a 5-year survival rate ranging from 20% to 50%. The survival rate for patients presenting with distant metastases involving visceral sites is only 5%. Initial metastases to lymph nodes, the skin, and soft tissues are much more common than metastases to visceral sites. Metastases are generally divided into locoregional and distant.

LOCOREGIONAL METASTASES (AMERICAN JOINT COMMITTEE ON CANCER STAGE III DISEASE)

Locoregional metastases include tumor deposits in lymph nodes draining the site of the primary tumor (Figs. 13.96 and 13.97) and metastases in the skin (Fig. 13.98) or soft tissue located between the primary

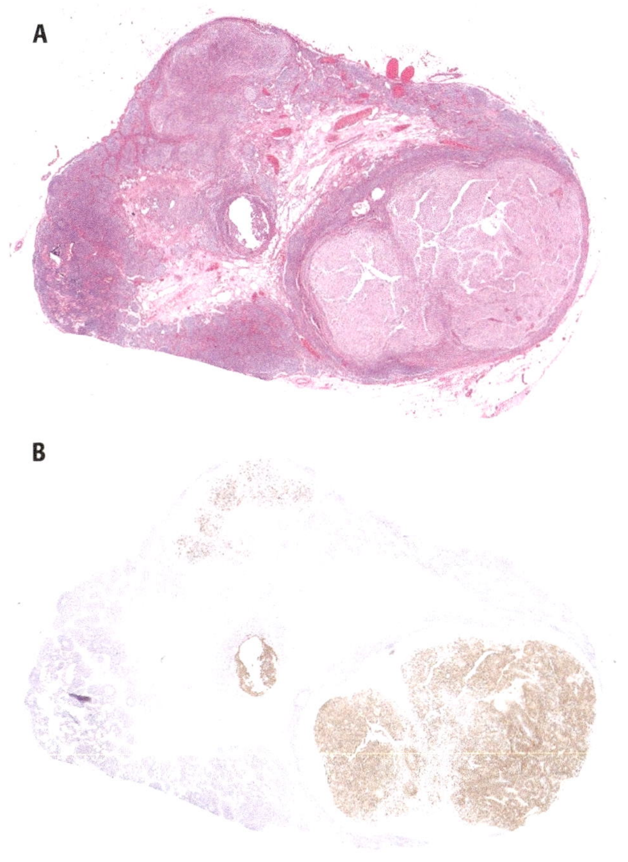

FIG. 13.96

Melanoma metastatic to a lymph node. **A,** Silhouette of a lymph node with nonpigmented metastatic tumor deposit. **B,** The tumor cells are immunoreactive for Melan-A.

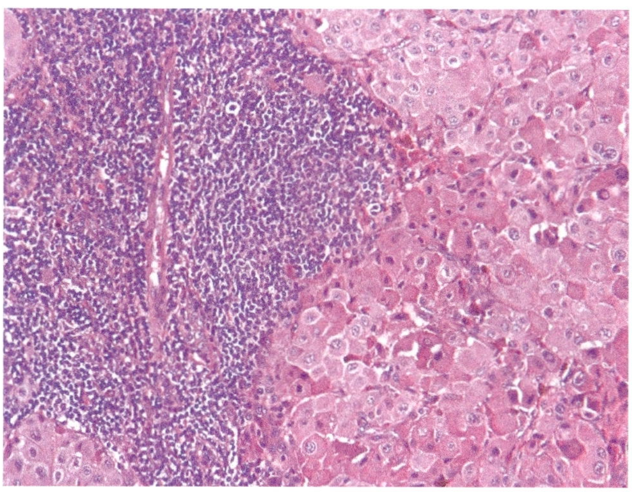

FIG. 13.97

Melanoma metastatic to lymph node. Atypical pigmented tumor cells are present.

tumor and the regional lymph node. Historically, the latter have been divided into satellite and in-transit metastases. Metastases confined to a defined radius, such as less than 2 cm from the primary tumor, were classified as satellites. If they were found farther away, they were designated in-transit tumors. Because biologically and prognostically satellite and in-transit metastases imply the same process, their distinction is arbitrary and unnecessary.

SENTINEL LYMPH NODE BIOPSY

SLN mapping and biopsy have become standard procedures in the United States and Australia for most patients with a primary cutaneous melanoma that is at least 1 mm thick. The procedure is also routinely offered to patients whose tumor measures slightly less than 1 mm in thickness but is ulcerated or mitotically active. The widespread use of SLN biopsy has been criticized because to date no overall survival benefit has been demonstrated, and there is associated risk for iatrogenic morbidity as well as the financial cost to society. Advocates of SLN biopsy argue that trials addressing potential therapeutic benefits are still ongoing and that the procedure at the very least provides prognostic information. We see a role for SLN biopsy for patients willing to participate in clinical trials. In the context of a trial, stratifying patients by risk for recurrence is critical. Otherwise, differences in survival attributable to therapeutic intervention may not become apparent. However, we also understand that patients may want the most accurate prognostic information for themselves irrespective of the purposes of a clinical trial.

Because the status of the SLN is a powerful predictor of outcome, its careful pathologic examination is important. For best results, the SLN is to be bisected in the plane of the hilum along the longitudinal axis of the node. Most pathology laboratories examine multiple H&E-stained sections and immunostains. In our experience, three H&E-stained sections and two immunostains (for S100 protein and Melan-A/Mart-1 or gp100 [HMB-45]) suffice. More levels and more immunostains may yield additional rare cases of single-cell metastases, but to date, there is no evidence to suggest that results from a more extensive analysis justify the added time and cost. In fact, evidence is emerging that usually only those metastases that are clinically "relevant," that is, of prognostic significance, are detectable by routine H&E stains. Contrary to initial hopes, results from additional step sectioning or polymerase chain reaction analysis for tyrosinase have not improved prognostic models.

Different laboratories have a different approach to the workup of SLNs. Some use only H&E stains. Others use three or more antibodies. We take a pragmatic approach. In our laboratory, we examine one H&E-stained and one immunostain (usually for Melan-A, unless the tumor is known to be negative for Melan-A). If metastatic tumor (Fig. 13.97) is found, we order an immunostain for *BRAFV600E* to help assess treatment options. In select cases, such as with unclear or uncertain findings on initial sections, additional levels and

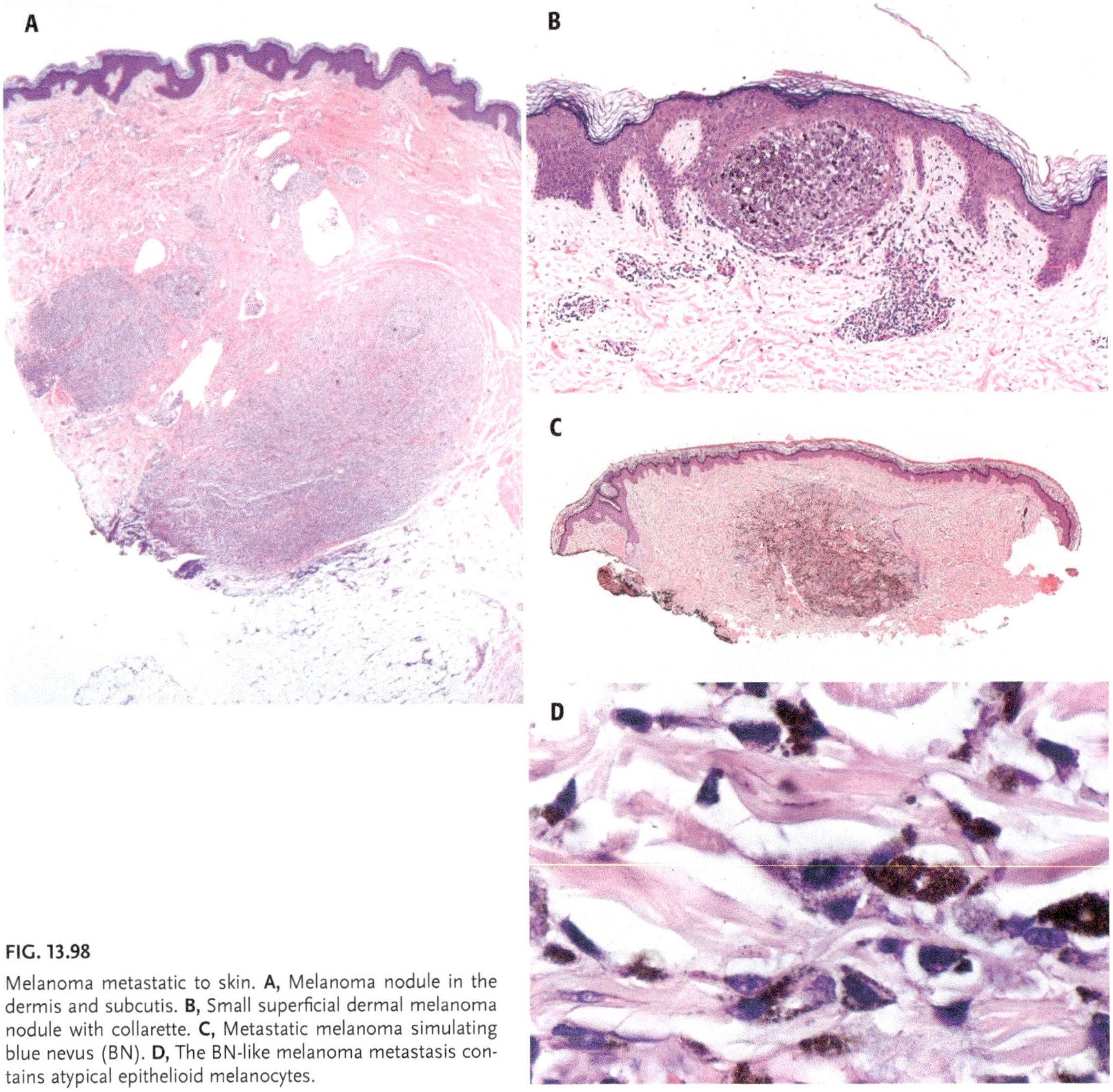

FIG. 13.98
Melanoma metastatic to skin. **A,** Melanoma nodule in the dermis and subcutis. **B,** Small superficial dermal melanoma nodule with collarette. **C,** Metastatic melanoma simulating blue nevus (BN). **D,** The BN-like melanoma metastasis contains atypical epithelioid melanocytes.

immunostains (e.g., SOX10/Melan-A or PRAME/Melan-A) may be requested. With this or similar approaches, metastases are detected in SLNs in approximately 15% to 20% of patients. In most cases, an immunopositive tumor has a clear-cut histologic correlate on H&E-stained sections. Rare cases exist, however, in which single-cell or micrometastases are only seen on immunostains. There are currently conflicting data about the significance of rare isolated immunoreactive tumor cells. Caution is necessary to recognize "false-positive" results because of technical reasons (e.g., overstaining, with labeling, e.g., of mast cells).

DISTANT METASTASES (AMERICAN JOINT COMMITTEE ON CANCER STAGE IV DISEASE)

Any metastasis beyond the regional lymph nodes and the area drained by them is a distant metastasis, which includes skin, soft tissue, distant lymph nodes, and viscera. The site of initial metastasis affects prognosis. Patients presenting with nonvisceral metastases have longer survival periods than those with visceral tumor deposits. Among visceral metastases, evidence suggests that patients with pulmonary metastases live longer than those with other visceral metastases.

Melanoma can metastasize to any site and in unexpected patterns. However, as a general rule, it can be said that the most common first sites of visceral metastases are the lung (15% to 20%), liver (15% to 20%), and brain (10% to 20%) followed by bone and intestine.

Differential Diagnosis of Metastatic Melanoma

METASTATIC MELANOMA SIMULATING OTHER NEOPLASMS

If a patient has a known primary melanoma and presents with a pigmented metastasis, the diagnosis of metastatic melanoma is straightforward. If the metastasis is amelanotic, the situation may be more challenging because melanoma may assume a great variety of histopathologic appearances and mimic a number of primary or metastatic nonmelanocytic tumors, such as lymphoma, carcinoma, or sarcoma. In the absence of melanin pigment, immunohistochemical studies for melanocyte differentiation antigens are helpful. Immunostains may not be necessary, of course, if the primary tumor is available for review and the morphology of the invasive primary tumor and metastatic tumor deposit match. However, melanoma metastases may look different than the primary tumor. Furthermore, some patients have other malignant tumors that may complicate the clinical situation and assessment of the origin of metastatic disease.

Lentiginous Melanocytic Proliferations

	Solar Lentigo	Lentigo Simplex	Lentiginous Nevus	Lentiginous Melanoma In Situ
Size	Small (<4 mm)	Small (<4 mm)	Variable	Variable; often large
Borders	Regular	Regular	Regular	Irregular
Density of MC	Normal or slightly increased	Slightly increased	Increased	Significantly increased
Confluence of MC	Absent	Absent	May be present	Common
Melanocytic nests	Absent	Absent	Present	Variable
Pagetoid MC	Absent	Absent	Absent	Common
Solitary units of MC along adnexa	Absent	Absent	Rare	Common
Atypia of MC	Rare	Rare	Rare	Common
Multinucleated melanocytes	Absent	Absent	Rare	Common
Skip areas	Absent	Absent	Usually absent	Common
Epidermal rete ridges	Normal or slightly elongated	Normal or slightly elongated	Normal or elongated	Normal or effaced

MC, Melanocyte.

When melanoma assumes an undifferentiated or unusual morphology, a major pitfall arises if melanoma is not being considered in the differential diagnosis, especially in the absence of a known primary melanoma. Such unusual amelanotic variants include spindle cell features (to be distinguished from sarcoma or sarcomatoid carcinoma), signet ring cell features (to be distinguished from adenocarcinoma), balloon or clear cell morphology (to be distinguished from renal cell or adrenocortical carcinoma), and myxoid or giant cell features (to be distinguished from sarcomas). A panel of immunomarkers addressing possible alternative tumor types usually allows a definitive diagnosis.

Immunohistochemistry for the Distinction of Melanocytic Tumors from Histologic Simulants

Marker	Melanoma	Carcinoma	Sarcoma	Lymphoma
S100P	+	− or +−[a]	− or +[b]	−
SOX10	+	−	− or +[b]	−
T311, HMB-45, M2-7C10	+	−	−	−
A103	+	− (+)[c]	−	−
Cytokeratins	− (+)[d]	+	− or +[e]	−
Muscle markers	− (+)[f]	− (+)[g]	− or +[h]	−

[a]Some carcinomas, such as myoepithelial carcinomas, are positive for S100 protein.
[b]Follicular dendritic cell tumors are positive for S100 protein; malignant nerve sheath tumors or alveolar soft part sarcomas may be positive for S100 protein; malignant nerve sheath tumors may be positive for SOX10.
[c]Adrenocortical carcinomas may be positive with A103.
[d]Some melanomas express cytokeratins (e.g., Cam5.2).
[e]Some sarcomas, such as epithelioid sarcomas and angiosarcomas, express cytokeratins.
[f]Some spindle cell melanomas may be positive for smooth muscle actinic or desmin.
[g]Muscle markers may be positive in some sarcomatoid carcinomas as well as in spindle cell melanomas.
[h]Muscle markers are positive in leiomyosarcomas or other myogenic and myofibroblastic sarcomas.

DIFFERENTIAL DIAGNOSIS: SPITZ NEVUS OR MELANOMA—PATHOLOGIC FINDINGS

Histopathologic Features Favoring Melanoma

- Asymmetric silhouette
- Large size (>1 cm) with ulceration
- Complex growth pattern with oddly shaped or large expansile cell aggregates
- Consumption of the epidermis
- Lack of maturation
- Mitotic figures, especially in the deep portion of the lesion
- Apoptosis or necrosis of melanocytes
- Marked nuclear atypia (enlarged nuclei with irregular contours, hyperchromasia)
- Lack of dull pink globules

Ancillary Test Results Favoring Melanoma

- Segmental gains or losses of multiple different chromosomes
- TERT promoter mutations, numerous mutations
- Strong and diffuse PRAME expression
- Complete loss of p16 expression
- Positive gene expression profile

METASTATIC MELANOMA OF UNKNOWN PRIMARY TUMOR

Approximately 5% to 10% of patients with metastatic melanoma present without a clinically apparent primary tumor (by history, clinical examination, and review of prior biopsies). Two-thirds of them have metastatic disease in lymph nodes (especially in the axilla, groin, or neck). It is generally believed that this phenomenon is related to complete regression of a cutaneous melanoma. Before a diagnosis of unknown primary tumor can be established, potential extracutaneous primary sites need to be excluded, such as the eye; oropharyngeal, nasopharyngeal, or anogenital mucosa; and soft tissue. When melanoma manifests as metastatic disease in the liver, strong consideration needs to be given to a primary choroidal melanoma. The diagnosis of metastatic melanoma in the absence of a known primary tumor is straightforward if the tumor is pigmented and occurs at a site, such as the lung or liver, where one would not expect a primary melanoma to occur. If a tumor is nonpigmented, immunohistochemical studies usually allow one to confirm the presence of a melanocytic differentiation. At most sites, such as the parenchyma of lymph nodes, brain, or lung, the metastatic nature of the disease is readily apparent. However, if a melanoma nodule occurs in the skin, squamous mucosa, soft tissue, or leptomeninges, the distinction of a primary from a metastatic tumor nodule can be difficult solely on morphologic grounds.

PRIMARY CUTANEOUS MELANOMA VERSUS METASTATIC MELANOMA TO THE SKIN

The distinction of primary from metastatic melanoma has obvious prognostic significance. If a large melanoma nodule is present in the subcutis with uniformly pleomorphic cells, numerous mitotic figures, and necrosis, one can assume the presence of metastatic disease if no associated nevus component is identified and the superficial dermis and epidermis are entirely normal without features of regression or prior biopsy. A small deep dermal or subcutaneous melanoma nodule is also readily identified as metastatic (Fig. 13.98A), especially if lymphatic tumor emboli are identified. The situation is different with small superficial dermal melanoma nodules in close proximity to the epidermis (Fig. 13.98B), when a metastatic melanoma nodule mimics a nevus (Fig. 13.98C and D), or when the metastatic tumor also involves the epidermis (epidermotropic metastatic melanoma) (Fig. 13.99).

A number of features need to be evaluated for the distinction of a primary melanoma from a superficial dermal metastasis. If a melanoma nodule is associated with a precursor (a broad in situ melanoma component or melanocytic nevus), this represents very strong evidence in favor of a primary melanoma (on very rare

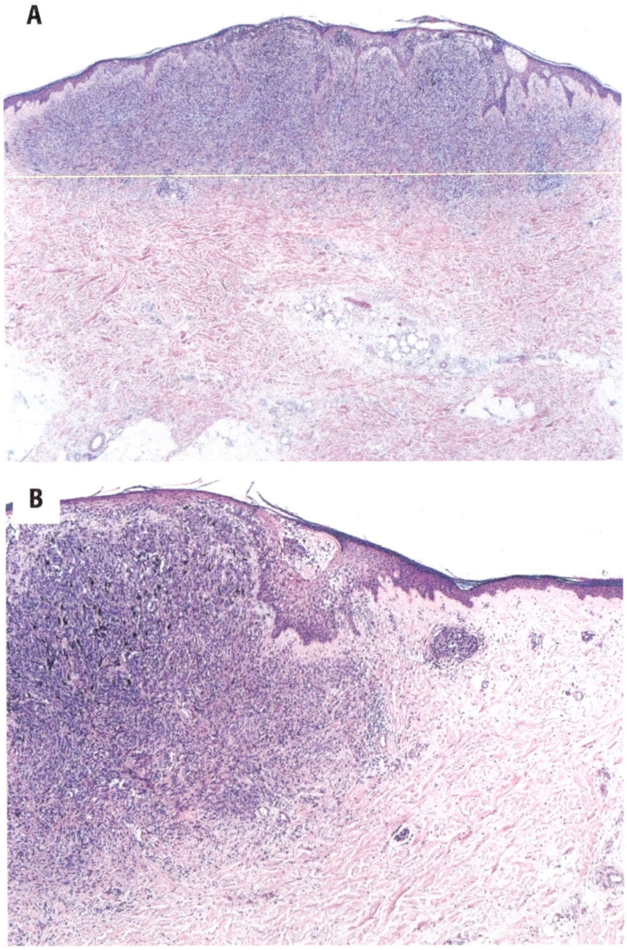

FIG. 13.99

Epidermotropic metastatic melanoma to the skin. **A,** Melanoma is present in the epidermis and dermis. The greatest horizontal dimension of the dermal component exceeds that of the intraepidermal melanoma. **B,** Lymphatic tumor emboli are present.

DIFFERENTIAL DIAGNOSIS: PRIMARY MELANOMA OR DERMAL MELANOMA METASTASIS—PATHOLOGIC FEATURES

Features Favoring Primary Melanoma

Clinical Findings

- No history of prior melanoma
- History of long-standing lesion that has changed

Histopathologic Features

- Major criteria
  - Intraepidermal melanoma extends beyond the perimeter of the dermal melanoma
  - Associated melanocytic nevus
- Minor criteria
  - Associated stromal changes (inflammation, fibrosis, features of regression)
  - Low mitotic index
- Marked phenotypic heterogeneity of tumor cells
- Absence of lymphatic tumor emboli
- Associated inflammation, fibrosis, or features of regression

occasions, a melanoma may metastasize to the site of a nevus or melanoma biopsy site). In the absence of a precursor, other parameters provide some guidance. Most metastases do not involve the overlying epidermis. If there is an intraepidermal component, it is usually small. Its width tends to be narrower than the greatest horizontal diameter of the dermal melanoma nodule. If the metastasis is very superficial, the overlying epidermis may be thinned, and the tumor may be surrounded by an epidermal collarette. Lymphatic tumor emboli are more likely to be found in association with metastatic tumors than primary melanomas.

At scanning magnification, a dermal melanoma metastasis is suggested by a small, at times oddly shaped, nodule of homogeneously atypical melanocytes. Mitotic figures tend to be more commonly seen in metastases than in primary tumors. Primary melanomas generally display more heterogeneity in the size and shape of nuclei and texture of the cytoplasm than metastatic tumors, which tend to be more uniform. There is typically more fibrosis and inflammation associated with primary tumors compared to metastases. These guidelines are not absolute. Clinical correlation is paramount. In the absence of a known prior melanoma, one should hesitate in establishing a diagnosis of metastatic disease if only a single superficial dermal melanoma nodule is found. Although the vast majority of primary melanomas arise at the dermal-epidermal junction, not all of them do. Some represent primary dermal melanomas. They may have developed from a dermal melanocytic nevus. It is a different story with large subcutaneous melanomas with necrosis. Even in the absence of a history of melanoma, they can be assumed to be most likely metastatic except for rare primary melanomas arising in soft tissue.

PRIMARY MELANOMA OF SOFT TISSUE (CLEAR CELL SARCOMA) VERSUS METASTATIC MELANOMA TO SOFT TISSUE

Primary malignant melanocytic tumors may present in soft tissue, which includes CCS and other fusion-associated tumors. When CCS occurs in the expected clinical setting (young patient, distal extremity), consideration is usually given to this diagnosis, especially if the tumor is found in association with deep tendinous tissue. A diagnostic problem typically arises when this tumor presents at an unusual site, such as the axilla, in which case it may be mistaken for metastatic melanoma. Metastatic melanomas tend to be more pleomorphic than primary melanoma of soft parts. However, because of morphologic overlap, molecular studies are usually needed for a definitive diagnosis.

MELANOCYTIC NEVUS VERSUS NEVOID METASTASIS

Metastatic melanoma may not only be confused with primary melanoma but even with melanocytic nevi. Variants of dermal metastases have been described, which are difficult to distinguish from nevi, at least at scanning magnification. Such melanoma variants include BN-like metastases that have been associated with cutaneous as well as choroidal melanoma. Metastatic melanoma simulating BN should be considered, especially in a patient with a known primary pigmented melanoma if a BN-like proliferation appears suddenly and shows histologically unusual features, such as rare mitoses, epithelioid cell atypia, and associated inflammation. An immunostain for MIB-1 may be helpful to confirm the presence of an increased proliferative index. On rare occasions, small melanoma metastases may also mimic amelanotic epithelioid cell nevi. Fortunately, the clinical setting (history of melanoma, sudden appearance of multiple dermal nodules) usually strongly favors metastatic disease. In problematic cases, ancillary cytogenetic studies may help because BN lacks chromosomal gains or losses, but the latter are common in melanoma, especially metastatic melanoma. BN-like melanoma metastases may not only derive from primary cutaneous but also uveal melanoma. Loss of labeling for BAP1 may be a clue for metastatic uveal melanoma. Diffuse labeling for PRAME can also help distinguish a nevoid melanoma metastasis from a nevus.

NODAL NEVUS VERSUS METASTATIC MELANOMA

Benign nevomelanocytes may be present in lymph nodes. They are usually small and confined to the fibrous tissue of the lymph node capsule or fibrous trabeculae traversing through the node (Fig. 13.100). When they are pigmented, they are easily found. Amelanotic small nodal nevus cells are often best recognized with immunohistochemical stains (Fig. 13.101). Nodal nevus

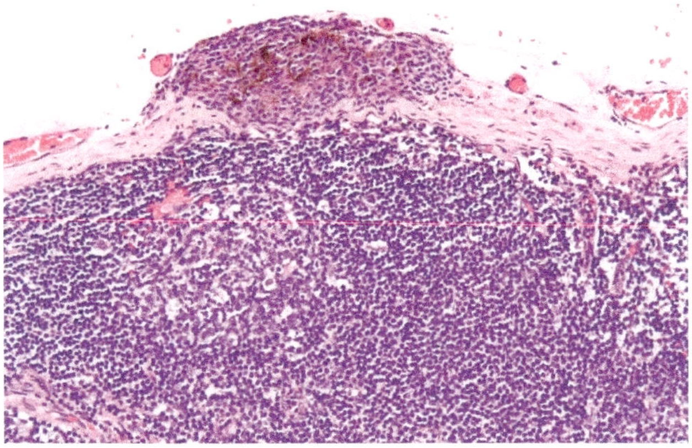

FIG. 13.100
Melanocytic nevus in lymph node. Small nodal nevus with cytologically bland pigmented melanocytes in the lymph node capsule.

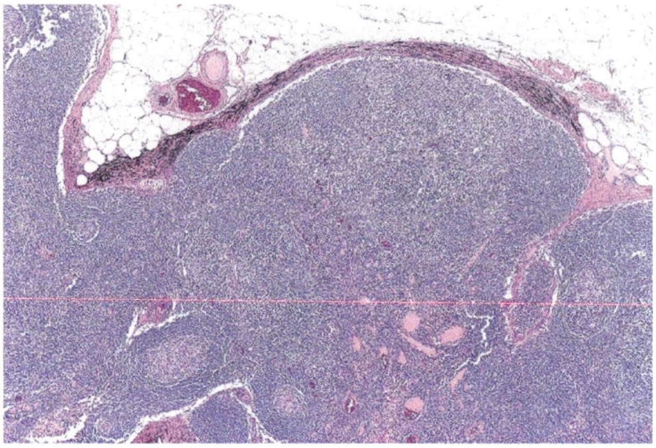

FIG. 13.102
Capsular nodal blue nevus. Slender pigmented melanocytes are seen in the lymph node capsule.

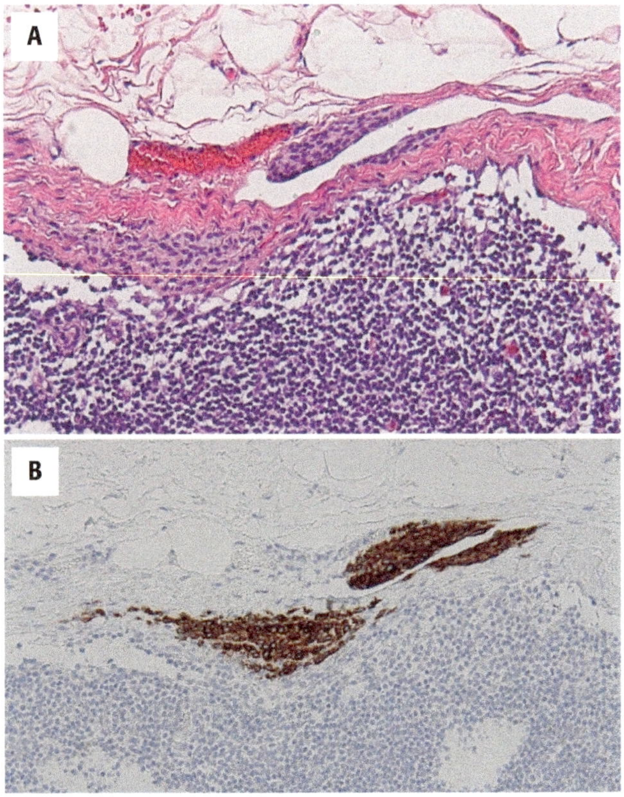

FIG. 13.101
Melanocytic nevus in lymph node. **A,** Cytologically bland small amelanotic melanocytes in the lymph node capsule and around intracapsular channels. **B,** The melanocytes are highlighted immunohistochemically using the anti–Melan-A antibody A103.

cells may be pigmented or amelanotic, epithelioid, or fusiform in appearance. They may have the appearance of a BN (Fig. 13.102), including cellular BN. Rarely, a nodal nevus may extensively involve the fibrous tissue around and within a lymph node (Fig. 13.103). At times, nodal nevomelanocytes may also be present in the subcapsular sinus or lymph node parenchyma (Fig. 13.104). This is usually in the context of a well-developed capsular nodal nevus. Nodal nevi may be confused with metastatic melanoma, especially small microscopic subcapsular melanocyte aggregates in SLNs of patients with an established primary cutaneous melanoma (Fig. 13.105). For the distinction of nodal nevus from metastatic melanoma, one needs to look at the location and cytology of the cells and compare them with those of the primary invasive melanoma.

Nevi are predominantly confined to fibrous tissue of the node. Small metastases are typically located in the subcapsular sinuses. However, exceptions exist. Melanoma metastases may be confined to the lymphatic channels of the lymph node capsule or be present in the center of a node (Fig. 13.106). Rare nevi may involve subcapsular sinuses. Finding a nodal nevus in a lymph node, however, does not end the search for metastatic melanoma: on occasion, melanoma may coexist with a nodal nevus (Fig. 13.107).

After assessing the location of the melanocytes and their growth pattern within the lymph node, attention to cytologic features is important. Nodal nevomelanocytes are cytologically bland and lack mitotic figures. Metastatic melanoma cells tend to display cytologic atypia and mitoses. In difficult cases, comparison of the nodal melanocytes with the invasive tumor cells of the primary melanoma is essential. Immunostains are of limited value. They mainly highlight melanocytic differentiation and facilitate recognition of the cells. Nodal nevomelanocytes are usually immunoreactive for S100 protein, SOX10, Melan-A, tyrosinase, and microphthalmia transcription factor. Sometimes, nonmelanocytic cells may show immunoreactivity for Melan-A/Mart1. A dual label of SOX10/Melan-A can help distinguish true melanocytes from false-positive cells. Although most nodal melanocytes tend to be negative for gp100, some (e.g., nodal blue nevi) are immunoreactive with HMB-45.

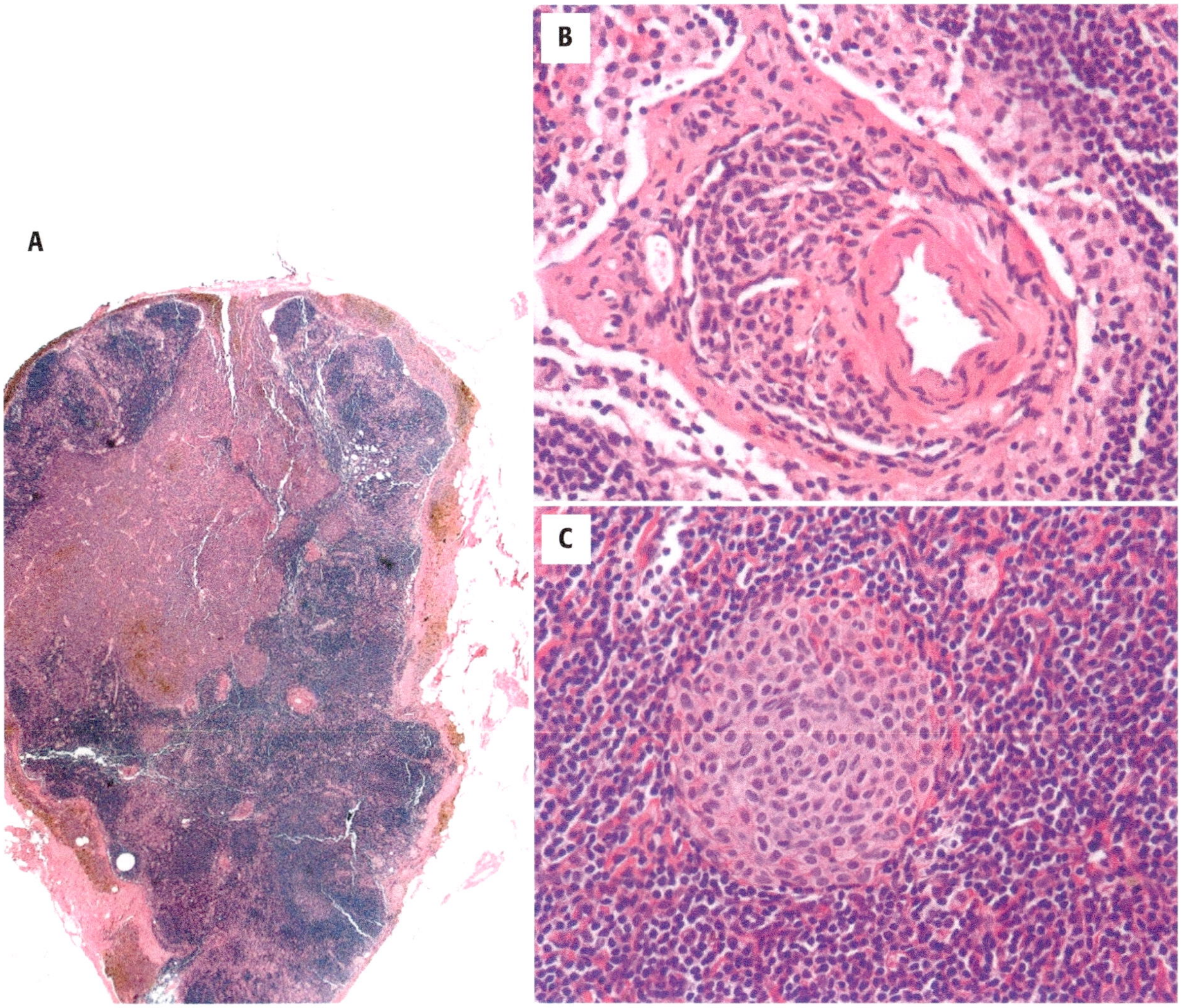

FIG. 13.103

Large nodal melanocytic nevus in fibrous tissue and nodal parenchyma. Incidental large nevus found during an axillary node dissection in a patient with breast carcinoma. **A,** Melanocytes are present in the capsule and extend into the nodal parenchyma. **B,** The melanocytes are cytologically bland; some are clustered around small vessels in fibrous trabeculae. **C,** An occasional nest of melanocytes is completely surrounded by lymphocytes.

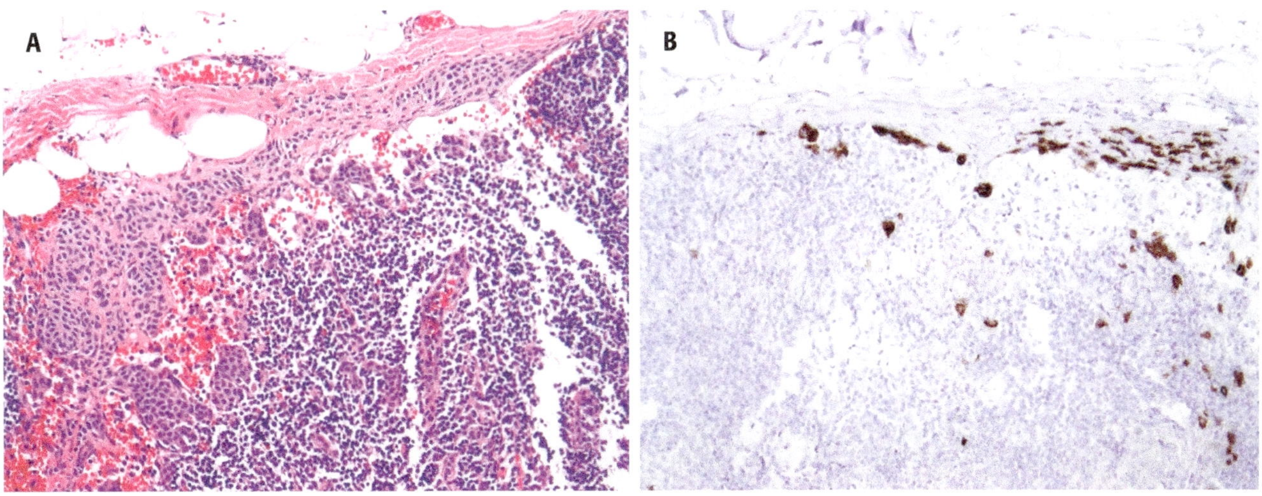

FIG. 13.104

Sentinel lymph node with intracapsular and subcapsular nodal nevomelanocytes. **A,** Cytologically bland small amelanotic epithelioid melanocytes are present in the capsule of a sentinel lymph node from a woman with breast cancer. Similar melanocytes are also present in the node beneath the capsule. **B,** Another focus of intranodal melanocytes in the same node highlighted by an immunostain for Mart-1.

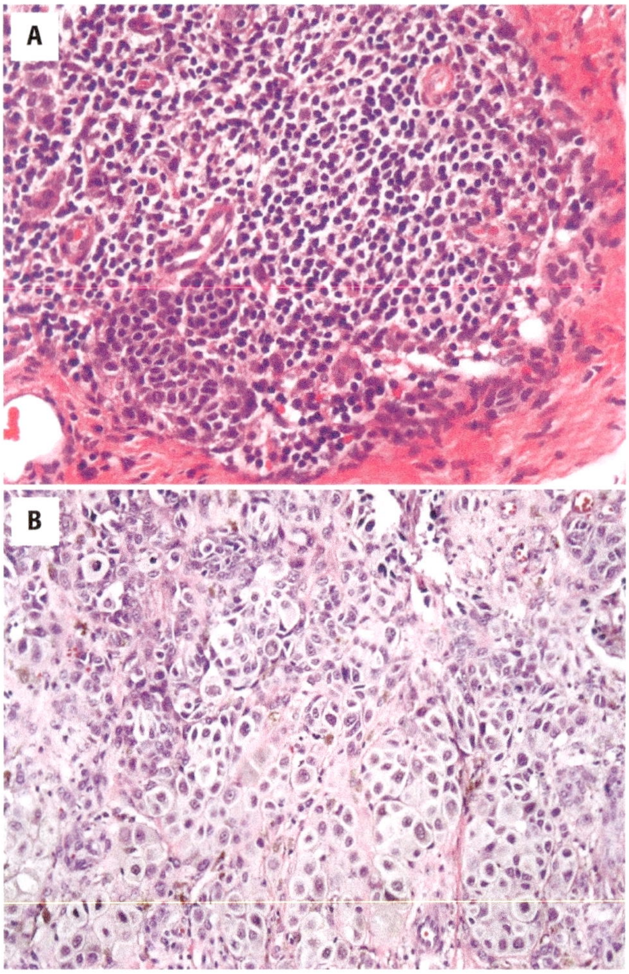

FIG. 13.105

Sentinel lymph node with a small subcapsular nodal nevus. **A,** Cytologically bland amelanotic small epithelioid melanocytes are present beneath the lymph node capsule. **B,** Their cytology differs markedly from the atypical pigmented large epithelioid melanocytes of the patient's primary invasive melanoma.

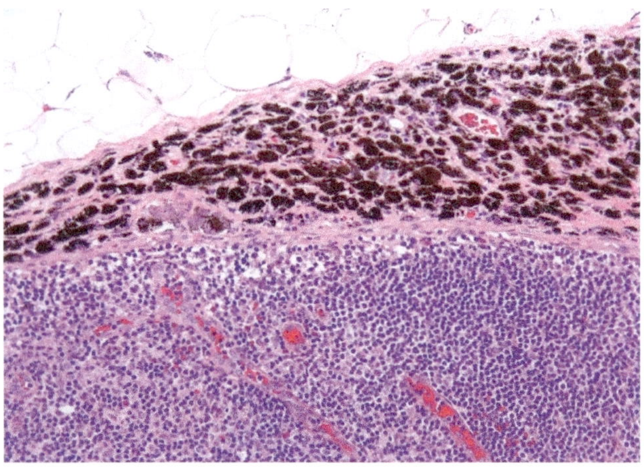

FIG. 13.106

Intracapsular metastatic melanoma associated with capsular melanosis. Metastasis is present in a capsular lymphatic channel. There is capsular nodal melanosis.

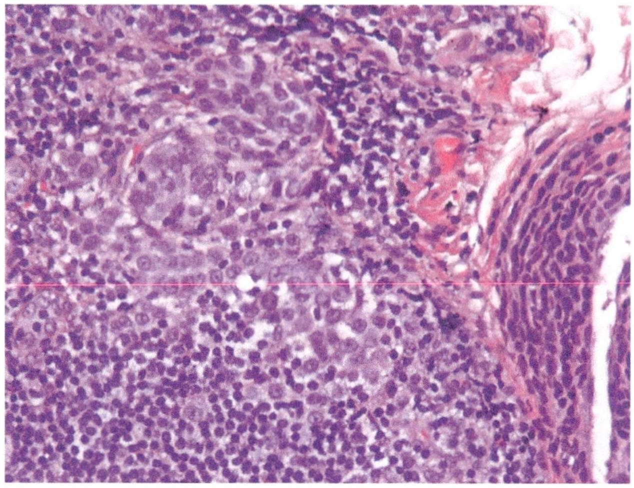

FIG. 13.107

Sentinel lymph node with metastatic melanoma adjacent to a nodal nevus. A subcapsular melanoma metastasis is present as well as an intracapsular nevus component.

Thus labeling for HMB-45 per se is insufficient evidence for malignancy. Likewise, lack of staining for gp100 does not prove the presence of a nevus because one-third of melanoma metastases are negative for this antigen. IHC for PRAME has been found to be very useful for the distinction of nodal nevi from metastatic melanoma. Nodal nevi should be negative for PRAME. Nearly 90% of metastatic melanomas are positive for PRAME. Thus immunoreactivity of nodal melanocytes strongly favors melanoma. If a nodal melanocyte deposit is cellular enough, FISH for copy number gains or losses may also be of diagnostic value, especially for PRAME-negative cases.

DIFFERENTIAL DIAGNOSIS—NODAL NEVUS OR METASTATIC MELANOMA—PATHOLOGIC FEATURES

Features Favoring Melanoma

Location of Nodal Melanocyte Aggregates

- Intraparenchymal or within lymphatic spaces

Cytology of Tumor Deposits

- Atypia (enlarged nuclei with hyperchromatism or prominent nucleoli)
- Mitotic figures
- Similarity to tumor cells of the primary tumor

Immunophenotype

- Positive for PRAME
- Strongly positive for gp100 (except for nodal blue nevi)

Cytogenetic Studies

- Chromosomal copy gains or losses by FISH

FISH, fluorescence in situ hybridization; *MIB* (antibody clone against the proliferation antigen Ki-67).

MELANOSIS ASSOCIATED WITH METASTATIC MELANOMA

Metastatic melanoma may be associated with prominent intratumoral or peritumoral melanosis characterized by dense collections of melanophages in soft tissue. This is most often seen in partly necrotic melanoma and is likely caused by release of melanin pigment from dying tumor cells but can also occur in association with small dermal melanoma metastases. Prominent peritumoral melanosis may pose a diagnostic pitfall if a biopsy samples only melanophages and fails to capture viable tumor cells.

Diffuse cutaneous or generalized melanosis is a rare complication of end-stage metastatic melanoma. It is clinically characterized by slate blue to gray discoloration of the skin. Histologically, there is increased melanin pigment deposition in the dermis and subcutis, primarily in macrophages, but it can also be found in other cells, such as fibroblasts or as free melanin. There may or may not be hyperpigmentation of the overlying epidermis.

Ancillary Studies

FONTANA-MASSON STAIN

The Fontana-Masson stain for documenting the presence of melanin pigment still has value for the evaluation of primary pigmentary disorders. However, because of inferior sensitivity compared with immunohistochemical methods, it is currently rarely used to assess the melanocytic origin of an amelanotic primary or metastatic tumor.

ELECTRON MICROSCOPY

Historically, electron microscopy has been useful to detect melanosomes as evidence of melanocyte differentiation of amelanotic tumors. However, the availability of numerous melanocyte markers for immunohistochemical assessment of melanocyte differentiation has largely rendered electron microscopy irrelevant (and too costly) for the evaluation of melanocytic tumors.

IMMUNOHISTOCHEMISTRY

IHC is most often used to establish the line of differentiation (melanocytic or not) but may also be used to assess biologic parameters (proliferation, mitosis) or to determine the mutation status.

Immunohistochemistry for Melanocyte Differentiation
IHC aids primarily in the distinction of amelanotic primary or metastatic melanocytic tumors from nonmelanocytic mimics. It also facilitates the recognition of microscopic deposits of melanocytes in lymph nodes. Furthermore, IHC can help to better assess the density and growth pattern of primary melanocytic tumors when melanocytes are poorly visible because of suboptimal histology or dense inflammation. A number of reagents are currently available for the detection of proteins associated with melanocyte differentiation. They include monoclonal antibodies HMB-45 (to detect glycoprotein 100), A103 (to detect Melan-A), M2-7C10 (to detect Mart-1), T311 (to detect tyrosinase), and D5 (to detect microphthalmia-associated transcription factor). A positive reaction with these antibodies leads to cytoplasmic staining of melanocytes, except for D5. A positive result for microphthalmia-associated transcription factor is obtained once nuclear staining is observed. For primary melanomas, antibodies for Melan-A/Mart-1 are helpful for the distinction of amelanotic epithelioid nodular melanoma from poorly differentiated carcinoma or epithelioid sarcoma. For spindle cell melanomas, especially DM, anti-S100P and/or SOX10 are the most important markers for diagnosis. For the detection of metastatic tumors, S100 protein has the greatest sensitivity, but one needs to be aware of the limitations in specificity (dendritic cells and miscellaneous other cell types). Primary or metastatic tumors that are histologically compatible with melanoma and strongly immunoreactive for anti-S100P, although negative for epithelial, myoepithelial, or dendritic cell markers, are usually melanomas even if the tumor cells fail to stain for the more specific melanocyte differentiation antigens. Although the combination of S100 protein, SOX10 and Melan-A/Mart-1, or gp100 strongly supports melanocytic differentiation, positive staining for melanocyte differentiation antigens alone does not always imply that the tumor is a bona fide melanocytic tumor. Positive staining with A103, for example, may be seen in adrenocortical tumors. Positive staining for miscellaneous melanocyte markers is a hallmark of angiomyolipomas and related tumors (perivascular epithelioid cell tumors, or as PEComas). PEComas, however, tend to be negative for S100 protein or SOX10.

Occasionally, a patient with a history of melanoma develops a pleomorphic tumor morphologically compatible with melanoma that is negative for S100 protein and any other melanocyte marker. Although the rare possibility of a second malignancy (e.g., undifferentiated sarcoma) needs to be considered, such tumors may represent un- or dedifferentiated metastatic melanoma, especially if present within a lymph node. Other synchronous or metachronous metastatic lesions in such patients may display focal bona fide melanocytic differentiation.

Immunohistochemistry to Assess Cell Growth
Antibodies are also available to highlight cells in mitosis. The most commonly used marker is pHH3. IHC

using MIB-1 can detect the proliferation marker Ki-67. Mitotic or proliferation markers are most often used as a soft parameter for the distinction of nevus from melanoma. When assessing cell proliferation for diagnosis, one needs to bear in mind that growing nevi (e.g., nevi of childhood or during pregnancy) may be mitotically active and display an increased Ki-67 labeling index but are benign. Furthermore, some melanomas grow slowly and may display a labeling index for Ki-67 of less than 5% or lack a detectable mitotic figure.

Immunohistochemistry to Document Genetic Changes

IHC can also assist in assessing genetic changes of a tumor. The antibody VE1, for example, recognizes the mutant protein *BRAFV600E*. It is a highly specific antibody. Positive labeling implies in the vast majority of tumors the presence of the *BRAFV600E* mutation. IHC for mutation analysis is most beneficial when there is insufficient or suboptimal material for conventional molecular methods (e.g., a few tumor cells in a lymph node) (Fig. 13.108). IHC for ALK, ROS1, or NTRK can function as a surrogate marker for gene fusions and support the presence of a Spitz neoplasm. IHC for BAP1 has also become important. Loss of nuclear labeling of BAP1 implies an adverse prognosis in uveal melanoma. Loss of nuclear labeling also defines a particular subset of melanocytic nevi with BAP1 inactivation. Loss of BAP1 can also support a diagnosis of blue melanoma.

OTHER IMMUNOHISTOCHEMISTRY TO DISTINGUISH NEVI FROM MELANOMA

IHC for PRAME can be a useful ancillary test for the distinction of nevi from melanoma, since most (approximately 80% to 90%) of melanomas diffusely express PRAME, while most nevi are negative for only focally positive for PRAME. However, an occasional nevus

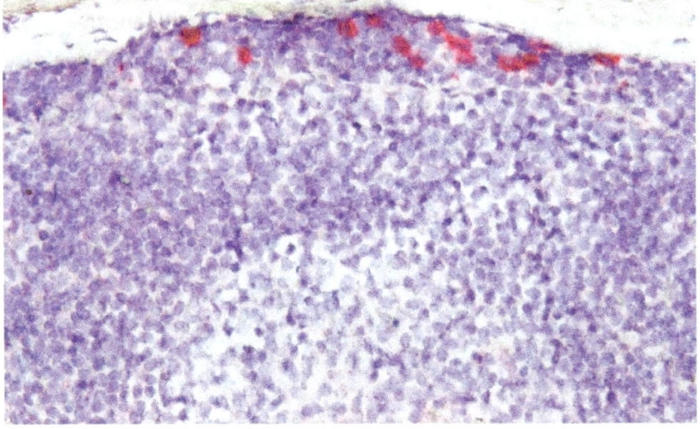

FIG. 13.108

Immunohistochemical stain for *BRAFV600E*. Isolated metastatic tumor cells in the lymph node are immunoreactive for VE1 (anti-*BRAFV600E*).

may display unexpected diffuse PRAME expression and melanomas can be PRAME-negative; IHC for p16 IHC can help. If a tumor with microscopic features suspicious for melanoma, for example, is completely negative for p16 and diffusely positive for PRAME, it is more likely a melanoma than a nevus.

Next-Generation Sequencing

NGS studies have emerged as a useful ancillary method for evaluation of melanocytic tumors. It is particularly useful when knowledge of the associated molecular driver is diagnostically very important, such as for the distinction of Spitz tumors with characteristic genomic aberrations from spitzoid melanomas with conventional mutations. Other diagnostic roles for sequencing analysis include the detection of *GNAQ* or *GNA11* mutations (e.g., for the distinction of an amelanotic sclerosing BN from DM).

Once the genomic class of a tumor is identified, another sequencing test that can be utilized to assist in determining if a melanocytic tumor is malignant or not is sequencing through NGS or a more targeted sequencing approach to assess for TPMs. Mutations in TERT promoter can also be diagnostically useful, since they are more common in melanomas than in melanocytic nevi.

Mutation analysis plays an important role for treatment decisions by selecting patients with tumors most likely to respond to therapy targeting molecular pathways. Common mutations in melanoma involve *BRAF*, *NRAS*, *KIT*, and *GNAQ/GNA11*.

BRAF encodes a serine/threonine protein kinase downstream of the epidermal growth factor receptor (EGFR) and the RAS family of small G proteins. It is mutated in approximately 40% to 60% of melanomas. There are different *BRAF* mutations. Most melanomas have a V600 mutation. About 70% to 85% of them are *V600E* mutations, in which a thymidine at nucleotide 1799 on exon 15 is replaced by adenine, resulting in the substitution of glutamic acid for valine at residue 600. Another not infrequent mutation is *V600K*. In this mutation, adenine is replaced by lysine. The incidence of the *V600K* mutation ranges from 5% to 30% of patients with *BRAF* mutations.

NRAS is an isoform of the RAS family of GTPase proteins involved in cell growth and differentiation. Activating mutations of *NRAS* have been identified in 15% to 20% of melanoma samples. The most common mutations are located in exon 2 at codon 61. *NRAS* mutations tend to occur in nodular melanomas and melanomas of sun-damaged skin. They are usually mutually exclusive of *BRAF* mutations.

GNAQ and *GNA11* encode for α subunits of G protein–coupled receptors. Mutations result in constitutive activation. Somatic mutations in *GNAQ* or *GNA11* are found in approximately 80% of uveal melanomas. They are also present in many BN and melanomas associated with BN. The most common mutation affects exon 5 (Q209).

KIT is a cell surface receptor tyrosine kinase that is involved in a number of intracellular signaling pathways, including MAP kinase and PI3K. *Kit* mutations tend to occur in some acral and mucosal melanoma.

CYTOGENETIC AND MOLECULAR STUDIES

Cytogenetic analysis is a value ancillary diagnostic tool for the assessment of diagnostically controversial melanocytic tumors with ambiguous or unusual light microscopic features. The main methods useful for analysis of archival material include array CGH, single nucleotide polymorphism (SNP) array, and FISH. CGH and SNP arrays detect copy number changes throughout the genome, thereby permitting a more comprehensive assessment. FISH targets individual chromosomes or specific regions within a chromosome. FISH requires much less tissue for analysis and permits visual analysis of subpopulations within a heterogeneous tissue mix.

The rationale for using cytogenetics for the diagnosis of melanocytic tumors is based on the fact that the vast majority of melanomas harbor clonal segmental chromosomal copy number aberrations. However, there are exceptions to the rule and inherent limitations to the method. Although the presence of multiple gains or losses of different chromosomes argues against a diagnosis of a benign melanocytic nevus, the detection of a copy number change, especially an isolated change, should not be regarded as proof of malignancy. A Spitz nevus, for example, may harbor a gain in 11p. Furthermore, there are reader errors and problems related to polyploidy.

While CGH and SNP arrays are more comprehensive, for small superficial lesions cytogenetic evaluation may only be amenable by FISH. A number of FISH probes are currently available for the diagnosis of melanoma. The so-called "melanoma FISH test" initially used four probes targeting *Ras*-responsive element-binding protein-1 (RREB1) on 6p25, *myeloblastosis* (MYB) on 6q23, *cyclin D1* (CCND1) on chromosome 11q, and centromeric enumeration probe control for chromosome 6 (CEP6) (Fig. 13.109). Additional probes have in the meantime been added to improve sensitivity and specificity. They include the probe targeting CDKN2A(p16) on 9p21 and the probe for MYC on 8q24. Using FISH

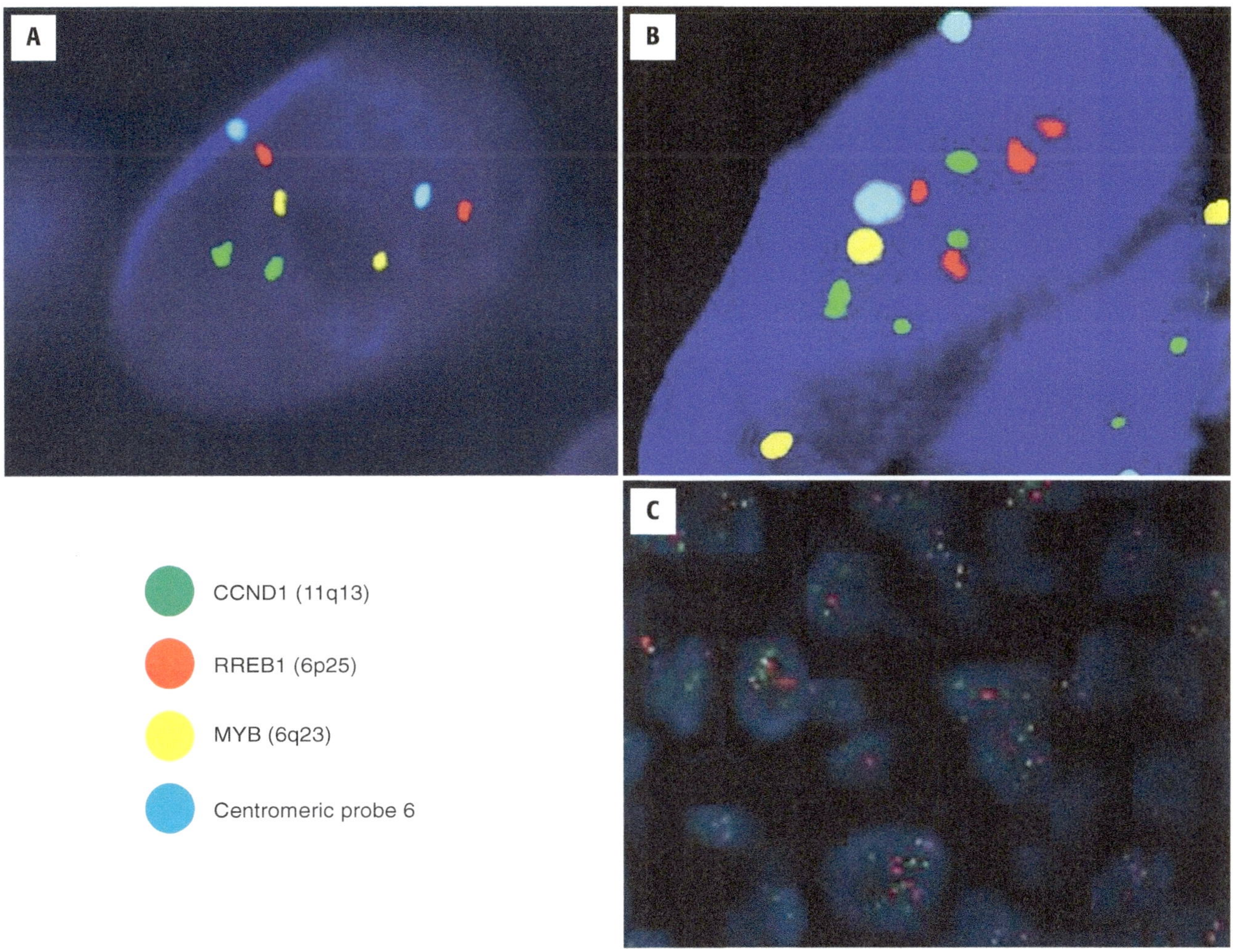

FIG. 13.109

Fluorescence in situ hybridization analysis (four-color assay). **A,** Normal melanocyte with two signals of each probe per nucleus. **B,** Melanoma cell nucleus with two signals of each 6cent and 6q but copy gains of 11q and 6p. **C,** Many tumor cells show copy number aberrations.

for the distinction between nevus and melanoma has a sensitivity of 85% and specificity of 90% to 95% for histologically obvious noncontroversial lesions. Its predictive value in a prospective setting of ambiguous lesions is likely significantly lower.

Pitfalls associated with the FISH analysis include false-negative results (a melanoma with no copy number changes or changes at chromosomes not measured by the FISH test) and potentially false-positive results, usually related to reader error ("cherry-picking" of atypical nuclei, polyploidy) or a rare benign tumor that just happens to have enough copy number changes of a chromosome in the test sample that meets the test cut-off value. With progress in scientific methods we anticipate that next generation sequence analysis will replace to a large extent cytogenetic studies, since it can provide information on both mutations, gene fusions and genomic aberrations.

PATHOLOGY REPORTING OF MELANOMA

PRIMARY CUTANEOUS MELANOMA

A pathology report of melanoma should clearly state the diagnosis, identify the patient and site of involvement by melanoma, and document the status of the margins. If melanoma is limited to the epidermis, it should be specified as in situ melanoma. If melanoma is invasive, as a minimum, the features needed for staging the tumor (thickness, the presence or absence of ulceration, and satellites) should be listed. The reporting of additional features, such as tumor mitotic rare, is encouraged, since they may factor into prognostic models. For the margin status, it generally suffices to report that the margins are negative or positive. However, if melanoma is seen within less than 1 mm of a margin (or diffusely infiltrative, desmoplastic neurotropic within less than 2 mm), it seems prudent to document this for considerations of additional surgery or in the case of desmoplastic melanoma radiation therapy. If a margin is positive and the precise location of the positive margin matters, attempts should be made to provide information on the area of the skin excision involved by tumor.

METASTATIC MELANOMA

In addition to the usual patient identifiers, the pathology report should specify the anatomic site as well as tissue type (e.g., lymph node, brain, subcutaneous adipose tissue) involved by melanoma. If a regional lymph node is positive for melanoma, the current AJCC staging system requires documentation on whether or not metastatic melanoma extends into extranodal soft tissue. One may also comment on the tumor volume (rare solitary melanocytes versus bulky intranodal tumor deposits). Studies are currently underway to evaluate how this information can best be standardized and what its relevance might be for clinicians with regard to their decision on whether or not to remove additional nodes. When several lymph nodes are removed, the total number of positive nodes and negative nodes should be reported.

PROGNOSIS

The prognosis of a patient affected by melanoma depends on the clinical stage.

CLINICAL STAGES I AND II

For those with localized primary melanoma, the histologic features of the primary melanoma, in particular tumor thickness, presence of ulceration, TMR, and level of invasion, are relevant parameters to assess a patient's risk for recurrence. Host factors such as age and immuvnocompetence are also important.

Melanoma Staging

Clinical Stage	Pathologic Findings	5-Year Survival Rate (%)
0	Melanoma in situ	100
IA	Thickness: <0.8 mm and no ulceration	≥95
IB	Thickness: 0.8–1.0 mm or ≤1.0 mm and ulcerated Thickness: 1.01–2.0 mm, nonulcerated	89–91
IIA	Thickness: 1.01–2 mm, ulcerated Thickness: 2.01–4 mm, nonulcerated	77–79
IIB	Thickness: 2.01–4 mm, ulcerated Thickness: ≥4 mm, nonulcerated	63–67
IIC	Thickness: >4 mm, ulcerated	45
III	Regional lymph node metastasis[a]	25–70
IV	Distant skin, subcutaneous, or nodal metastases or visceral metastases	<20

[a]Subcategories IIIA, B, and C exist. Within stage III, the prognosis is best for nodal micrometastasis (metastasis detected only by microscopic examination) associated with a nonulcerated primary tumor (stage IIIA). It is worst for patients with multiple positive nodes, grossly positive nodes, extension of metastatic tumor into extranodal soft tissue, and satellites.

Adapted and modified from Balch, C. M., Gershenwald, J. E., Soong, S. J., Thompson, J. F., Atkins, M. B., Byrd, D. R., et al. (2009). Final version of 2009 AJCC melanoma staging and classification. *Journal of Clinical Oncology: Official Journal of the American Society of Clinical Oncology*, 27(36), 6199–6206.

Patients with thin primary tumors (Breslow thickness less than 1 mm) have an estimated 5-year survival rate of 90% to 95%, depending on the presence or absence of histologic ulceration and a Clark level of greater than III.

The 5-year survival rate for patients with intermediate-thickness melanoma (1.01 to 4 mm) is 60% to 90%. It is 65% to 70% for a more than 4-mm-thick primary tumor without ulceration and approximately 45% if the tumor is ulcerated.

Clinical Stage III

Regional lymph node metastasis is associated with a 5-year survival rate of 13% to 69%. The odds for survival depend on the number of nodes involved and extent of disease (micrometastasis versus macrometastasis). Regional cutaneous or soft tissue metastases (also known as in-transit or satellite lesions) are associated with a 30% to 50% 5-year survival rate. The prognosis is worse (reduced 10% to 30% 5-year survival) if both regional cutaneous and nodal metastases are present.

Clinical Stage IV

The prognosis for distant metastatic disease is generally poor, with 5-year survival rates of less than 20%. The prognosis depends on the numbers and sites of metastases as well as on host factors.

SURGICAL MANAGEMENT

BIOPSY AND EXCISIONS OF MELANOCYTIC NEVI

Although shave biopsies are suitable for small pigmented lesions, especially if located in the face or if the suspicion for melanoma is low, they are to be discouraged for large and clinically complex-appearing lesions. Although in many cases a definitive diagnosis can be made on a shave biopsy, partial biopsies carry the risk of sampling errors as well as suboptimal diagnostic evaluation because important histologic parameters, such as symmetry or circumscription of the peripheral border of a lesion, may not be evaluable.

After a melanocytic nevus is diagnosed histologically, it does not need to be excised except for specific requests by patients for cosmetic reasons or concerns about its biology, for example, if the diagnosis is not entirely certain because of sampling issues (too small a biopsy to distinguish nevus from melanoma) or for other reasons (unusual morphology that is difficult to interpret). Margins for such excisions may be as narrow as possible.

Primary Melanoma

Malignant melanomas should be completely excised surgically. Recommendations for the optimal width of an excision for a primary cutaneous melanoma (Fig. 13.110) should be viewed as guidelines, not as dogmatic rules. They are clinical measurements and increase the odds for a negative histopathologic margin. They have been revised repeatedly at various times with a trend toward more conservative surgery.

Current guidelines recommend a 5-mm margin for in situ melanoma and at least a 1-cm margin for invasive melanoma. For the benefit of the patient, compromises may be necessary. The desire for a "save" surgical margin should be weighed against the potential harm from tissue loss for the patient in a cosmetically sensitive area. A narrow margin is acceptable at times, especially for a more sharply demarcated tumor or when a wider margin leads to unnecessary morbidity. For a patient with a melanoma near the eyelid, for example, a suboptimal

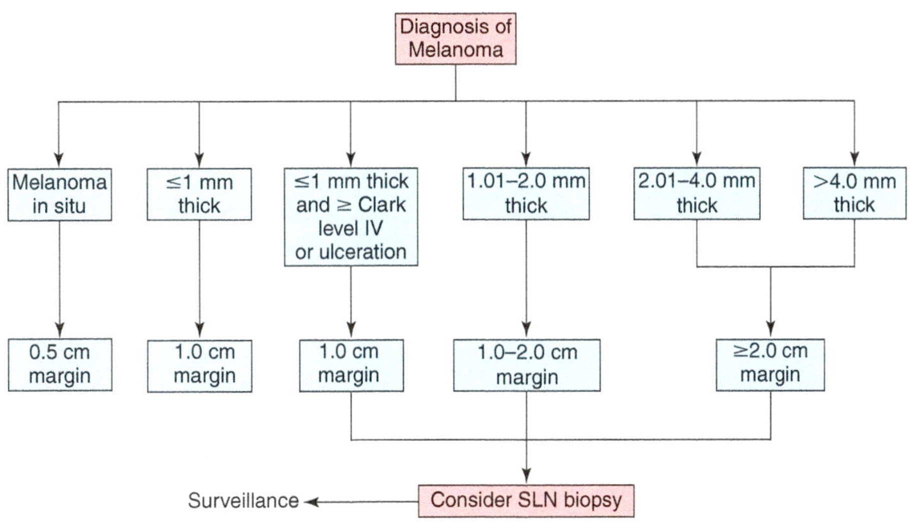

FIG. 13.110
Treatment algorithm for primary cutaneous melanoma. *SLN*, Sentinel lymph node.

margin may be preferable to potential complications or disfiguring from wider surgery.

A number of dermatologic surgeons attempt to excise primary melanomas, especially of the lentigo maligna type, using frozen section for margin assessment. We discourage the use of frozen sections for margin status assessment of melanocytic tumors because of the inherent difficulty of interpreting frozen section material. However, in exceptional circumstances, especially in a laboratory that can produce high-quality frozen sections, frozen section analysis may be appropriate or prudent, such as for margin control in the region of the facial nerve, to avoid increased risk of nerve injury from a second operation at that site.

Sentinel Lymph Node Mapping and Biopsy

SLN mapping and biopsy are currently routinely performed as a staging procedure for most patients with a primary melanoma of AJCC 2018 stage pT1B or higher (i.e., the melanoma measures at least 0.8 mm in thickness or), but less than pT4. SLN biopsy may also be performed on patients with thin or thick melanomas (pT1A or PT4), but this practice is controversial.

Management of Metastatic Melanoma

The role of surgery in the management of metastatic melanoma is primarily to obtain tissue for diagnostic and staging purposes, to relieve tumor burden, or to assess treatment responses. Pathologists play an important role in documenting pathologic features associated with response or resistence to treatment, such as the percentage of viable tumor versus necrosis, and the extent of fibrosis and inflammation.

NONSURGICAL TREATMENT OPTIONS

Various nonsurgical therapies are being offered for primary and metastatic lesions of melanoma. Topical agents, such as imiquimod or radiation, may be used for the management of lentigo maligns when surgery may not make sense (e.g., comorbidity). Radiation may also be used for primary or locally persistent melanomas when a negative surgical margin cannot be achieved, especially in the head and neck region.

Medical treatments of metastatic melanoma have for decades been disappointingly ineffective. However, this is no longer the case. Targeted therapy and novel immunologic approaches have led to significant improvements in managing metastatic disease. The most significant recent advances include targeted therapy for melanomas with *BRAFV600* mutations and immunotherapy (checkpoint blockade inhibitors).

SUGGESTED FURTHER READING

Ackermann, A. B., Massi, D., & Nielsen, T. (1999). *Dysplastic nevus*. Philadelphia: Ardor Scribendi.

Barnhill, R. L., Piepkorn, M., & Busam, K. J. (2004). *Pathology of melanocytic nevi and malignant melanoma* (2nd ed.). New York: Springer.

Busam, K. J., Gerami, P., & Scolyer, R. (2018). *Pathology of melanocytic tumors*. Philadelphia: Elsevier.

Costa, S., Byrne, M., Pissaloux, D., Haddad, V., Paindavoine, S., Thomas, L., Aubin, F., Lesimple, T., Grange, F., Bonniaud, B., Mortier, L., Mateus, C., Dreno, B., Balme, B., Vergier, B., & de la Fouchardiere, A. (2016). Melanomas associated with blue nevi or mimicking cellular blue nevi: Clinical, pathologic, and molecular study of 11 cases displaying a high frequency of GNA11 mutations, BAP1 expression loss, and a predilection for the scalp. *American Journal of Surgical Pathology*, *40*, 368–377.

Elder, D. E., Bastian, B. C., Cree, I. A., Massi, D., & Scolyer, R. A. (2020). The 2018 World Health Organization classification of cutaneous, mucosal, and uveal melanoma: Detailed analysis of 9 distinct subtypes defined by their evolutionary pathway. *Archives of Pathology and Laboratory Medicine*, *144*, 500–522.

Massi, G., & LeBoit, P. (2004). *Histologic diagnosis of nevi and melanoma*. Darmstadt: Steinkopff Verlag.

Swetter, S. M. (2008). *Malignant melanoma*. http://emedicine.medscape.com/article/1100753-overview @Refs:Scolyer, R. A., Rawson, R. V., Gershenwald, J. E., Ferguson, P. M., & Prieto, V. G. (2020). Melanoma pathology reporting and staging. *Modern Pathology*, *33*(Suppl. 1), 15–24.

Thompson, J. F., Scolyer, R. A., & Uren, R. F. (2006). Surgical management of primary cutaneous melanoma: Excision margins and the role of sentinel lymph node examination. *Surgical Oncology Clinics of North America*, *15*, 301–318.

Yeh, I., & Busam, K. J. (2022). Spitz melanocytic tumours - a review. *Histopathology*, *80*(1), 122–134.

Soft Tissue Tumors

14

Jennifer Ko • Darya Buehler

TUMOR-LIKE REACTIONS THAT MIMIC CUTANEOUS MESENCHYMAL TUMORS

DERMAL SCAR AND KELOID

Clinical Findings

The most frequently encountered soft tissue lesion is a dermal scar, which is commonly seen in a re-excision or may be associated with other trauma or a ruptured cyst. Hypertrophic scar and keloid are exuberant scarring reactions resulting in a cosmetically or functionally burdensome nodule. Susceptible individuals are younger, often of African descent, and have familiar predisposition. Keloids are often multifocal and commonly occur on the head and neck and upper trunk; the ear is an especially common site.

Histopathologic Features

Dermal scars are composed of a variably cellular proliferation of bland fibroblasts in a collagenous stroma. As the scar becomes more organized, the cellularity decreases, and the fibroblasts tend to be arranged parallel to the epidermis and be associated with extravasated erythrocytes (Fig. 14.1A). The fibroblasts are accompanied by reactive thin-walled capillary vessels that tend to run perpendicularly to the overlying epidermis. Hypertrophic scar shows increased cellularity and is often accompanied by prurigo nodularis-type changes. In contrast to the keloid scar, hypertrophic scars are generally limited to the site of injury.

Keloids are characterized by widely spaced fibroblasts that extend beyond the site of injury associated with prominent thick and glassy collagen fibers, and less conspicuous vasculature (Fig. 14.1B).

Differential Diagnosis

The appearance of hypertrophic scar can be indistinguishable from superficial and desmoid fibromatosis. Fibromatosis tends to have long, multidirectional sweeping fascicles as opposed to shorter, more loosely arranged fascicles of a scar arranged parallel to the epidermis. The vasculature of fibromatosis consists of uniformly distributed, slender, or gaping vessels in contrast to the perpendicular arrangement of the reactive vessels in a scar. Desmoid fibromatosis may occasionally contain keloidal collagen fibers mimicking keloid scars; in this setting, identification of β-catenin alteration by immunohistochemistry (IHC) or molecular profiling is very helpful. Malignant tumors, most importantly sarcomatoid carcinoma including spindle cell squamous cell carcinoma (SCC) and desmoplastic melanoma, may also present with a scar-like appearance due to abundance of desmoplastic stroma. These scar-like tumors tend to have more uniformly collagenous background and a somewhat "dirty" low power look resulting from the cytologic atypia of the embedded tumor cells and some degree of chronic inflammation that often accompanies these tumors. Careful attention to clinical (no history of trauma; clinical suspicion for tumor) and histopathologic (sun-damaged skin, associated atypical intraepidermal melanocytic proliferation or epidermal atypia) context is needed to avoid overlooking the presence of a desmoplastic carcinoma or melanoma.

Prognosis and Treatment

Ordinary scars may need revision for cosmetic reasons. The treatment of hypertrophic scars and keloids is challenging as they are very prone to local recurrence. Current literature supports a combination of treatment modalities including intralesional corticosteroid injections as first-line therapy, alone or in combination with 5-fluorouracil (5-FU) or bleomycin, pressure and occlusive silicone gel therapy, adjuvant laser and cryotherapy, and excision of keloids with adjuvant radiation therapy for recalcitrant lesions.

MYCOBACTERIAL PSEUDOTUMOR

Clinical Findings

Mycobacterial spindle cell pseudotumor (MSP) is a rare reactive tumor-like process composed of spindled

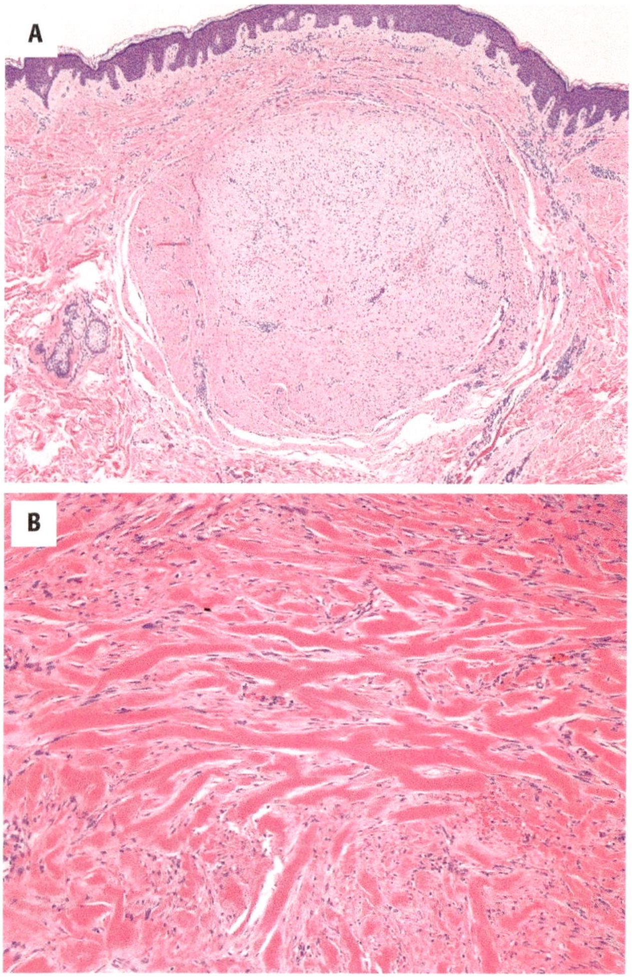

FIG. 14.1
Dermal scar. **A,** Hypertrophic scar showing a nodular proliferation of fibroblasts in the superficial dermis with attenuation of rete ridges. **B,** Keloid scar showing broad, glassy collagen fibers.

histiocytes containing acid-fast mycobacteria. It most often occurs in the skin and lymph nodes and, rarely, other sites in immunocompromised individuals. In the skin, it occurs as one or multiple papules or nodules.

Histopathologic Features

Cytologically bland fibroblastic spindled cells are arranged in sheets or a vaguely storiform pattern and admixed with sparsely scattered foam cells, epithelioid histiocytes, inflammatory cells, and multinucleated giant cells (Fig. 14.2A and B). Clumps of intracellular mycobacteria may produce eosinophilic, granular cytoplasm. Lesional cells are positive for CD68 and may variably coexpress smooth muscle actin (SMA), desmin, muscle-specific actin, and CD34, in keeping with fibroblastic/myofibroblastic phenotype. Acid-fast bacilli are highlighted with Ziehl-Neelsen special staining, within spindled cells and epithelioid histiocytes and giant cells (Fig. 14.2C).

Differential Diagnosis

Histopathologic mimics of mycobacterial pseudotumor include inflammatory myofibroblastic tumor (IMT), nodular Kaposi sarcoma, and benign fibrous histiocytoma (FH). If the clinical context is suggestive, special staining for acid-fast bacilli is a prudent practice for myofibroblastic or fibrohistiocytic lesions with an inflammatory component. IMT can be distinguished based on identification of anaplastic lymphoma kinase (ALK) protein expression or *ALK* gene rearrangements. Benign FHs, especially deep benign FH, may be difficult to separate from MSP and require a high index of clinical suspicion and confirmatory staining for acid-fast bacilli. Nodular Kaposi sarcoma (discussed elsewhere in this book) expresses vascular markers like CD31 and ERG (ETS family-related gene) and is positive for human herpesvirus 8 (HHV-8).

Prognosis and Treatment

Patients typically experience symptom resolution with appropriate antimycobacterial therapy.

ERYTHEMA ELEVATUM DIUTINUM

Clinical Findings

Erythema elevatum diutinum (EED) is a vasculitis that occurs mostly in middle-aged patients as bilateral, symmetric, erythematous, purpuric, brown or yellow plaques, papules or nodules on the backs of the hands, or other extensor surfaces, overlying joints. Lesions are firm and can be otherwise asymptomatic, painful, or cause a burning or itching sensation, which can worsen after cold exposure. Arthralgias may occur, and there is an association with a host of underlying diseases including autoimmune disease, inflammatory bowel disease, human immunodeficiency virus (HIV) infection, and malignancy.

Histopathologic Features

Lesions of EED evolve over time. Newer lesions show a leukocytoclastic vasculitis with mixed diffuse dermal inflammatory infiltrate that includes numerous neutrophils. Later lesions form mass-like nodules of hyalinized fibrosis with an angiocentric storiform arrangement of plump fibroblasts, hypertrophic endothelial cells that may contain residual foci of leukocytoclastic vasculitis, neutrophilic debris, and plasma cells (Fig. 14.3A–C).

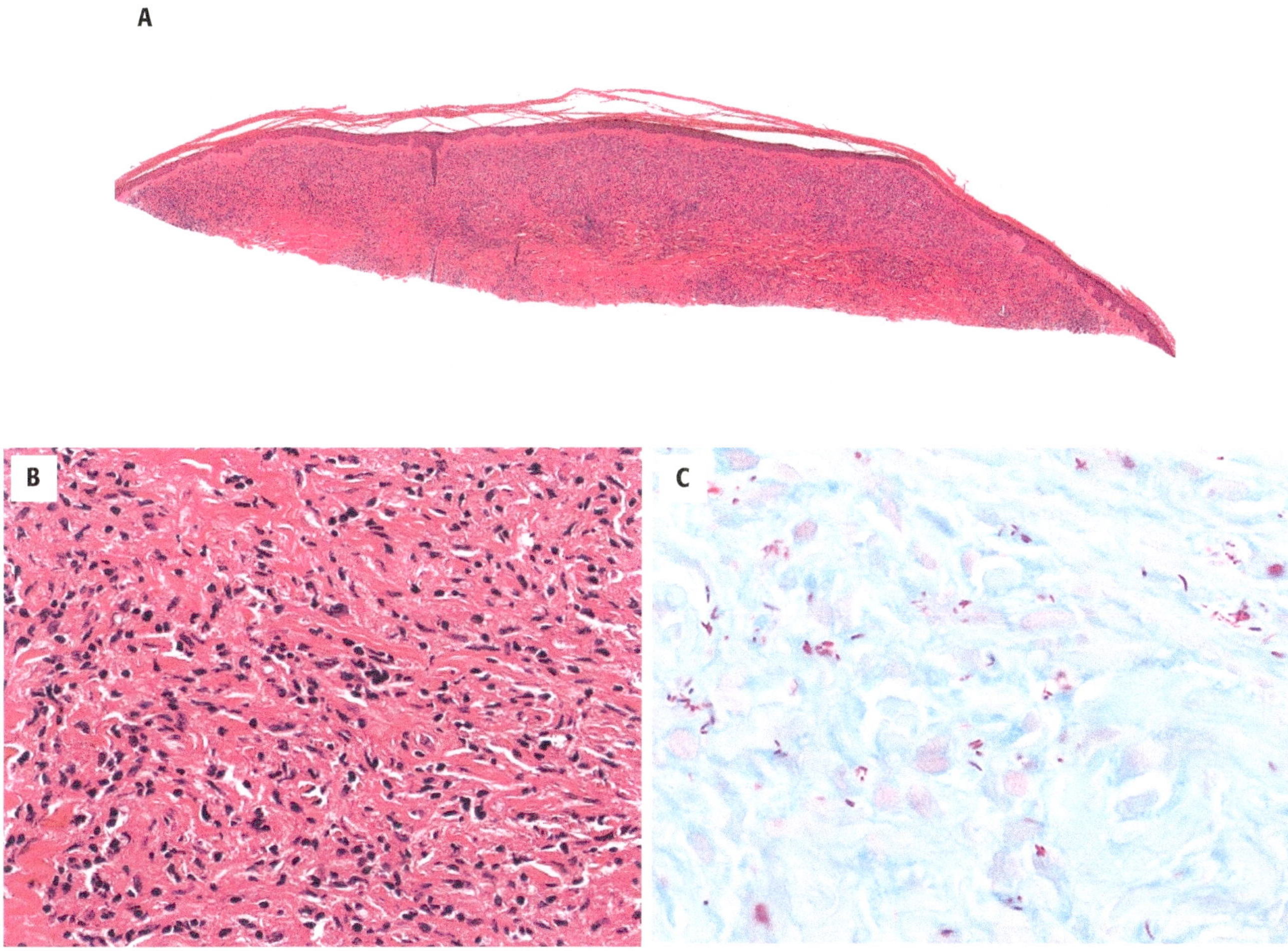

FIG. 14.2
Mycobacterial pseudotumor. **A,** A cellular infiltrate in the upper dermis with a narrow grenz zone. **B,** Spindled histiocytes with granular eosinophilic cytoplasm growing in a vaguely storiform pattern. **C,** Slender mycobacterial bacilli highlighted by Ziehl-Neelsen stain.

The nodules are typically separated from the overlying epidermis by grenz zone.

Differential Diagnosis

Later-stage EED lesions can clinically and histopathologically mimic spindle cell neoplasms (SAMS) ("pseudotumoral EED"). The differential diagnosis in this context includes dermatofibroma (DF), IMT, superficial nodular fasciitis, and, as the lesions evolve and become more sclerotic, dermatofibrosarcoma protuberans (DFSP), sclerosing perineurioma, and sclerotic fibroma/storiform collagenoma. None of these lesions present as multiple nodules in the characteristic distribution or contain significant neutrophils or leukocytoclasis. EED lacks the epidermal hyperplasia and peripheral collagen trapping seen in DFs. It is negative for CD34, in contrast to DFSP and sclerotic fibroma, and negative for ALK, in contrast to the IMT. Myxoid stroma and fascicular growth seen in nodular fasciitis are not characteristic of EED. Sclerosing perineurioma can be readily distinguished by epithelial membrane antigen (EMA), claudin-1, or glucose transporter 1 (GLUT1) immunostaining.

Prognosis and Treatment

EED may spontaneously clear or may become chronic and progressive, lasting 5 to 25 years. Medications to limit progression include dapsone and other immune modulators, nonsteroidal antiinflammatory drugs (NSAIDs), and tetracycline. EED is difficult to treat, and lesions often recur after discontinuation of treatment.

SILICON AND FILLER GRANULOMAS

Clinical Findings

Virtually any injectable or prosthetic foreign material can elicit an inflammatory, foreign body response.

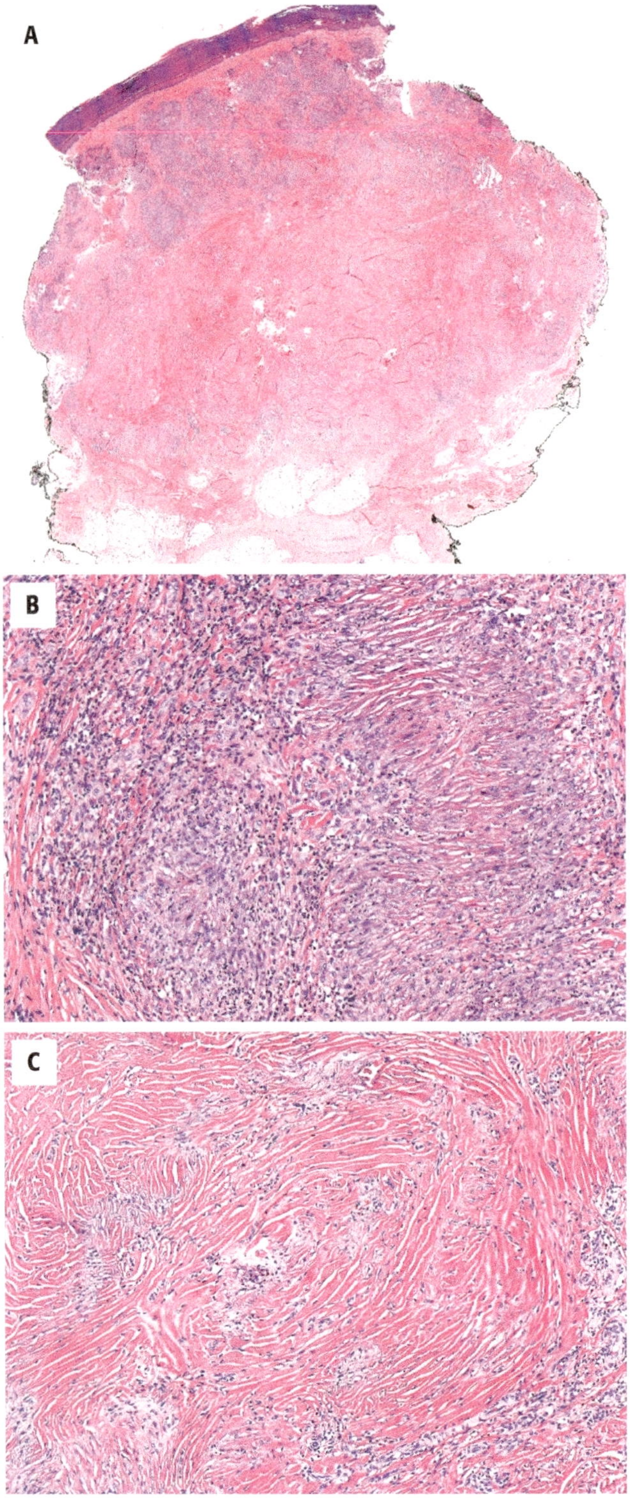

FIG. 14.3

Erythema elevatum diutinum (EED). **A,** Dense dermal inflammatory infiltrate with a grenz zone. **B,** Early EED with a mixed diffuse dermal inflammatory infiltrate with leukocytoclastic vasculitis and numerous neutrophils. **C,** Late EED showing a mass-like storiform fibrosis admixed with hypertrophic vessels and residual inflammatory cells.

Silicone was one of the first materials with widespread use but was banned as an injectable in 1982 due to adverse effects such as migration to distant sites including lymph nodes and lungs. However, silicone is still commonly used in breast implants, and granulomas have been reported after rupture or presumed leakage. Additionally, injectable materials used in nonsurgical facial rejuvenation procedures can cause an inflammatory reaction. The most common presentation in the skin includes papules and/or nodules, often with erythema, edema, and, at times, ulceration. Silicone granulomas may occur 10 to 15 years after injection with a high rate of incidence.

Histopathologic Features

Early granulomatous nodules, of all etiologies, are composed of a mixture of macrophages/histiocytes, giant cells, lymphocytes, neutrophils, and eosinophils surrounding the foreign material. With time, lesions become larger and deeper and may move inferiorly with gravity. Mononuclear cells remain, including histiocytes, lymphocytes, plasma cells, and giant cells (Fig. 14.4A). Silicone granulomas contain numerous multivacuolated histiocytes representing empty spaces where silicone is lost during tissue processing; these multivacuolated histiocytes closely resemble lipoblasts and for this reason can mimic liposarcoma (Fig. 14.4B).

Select esthetic materials and their chemical ingredients and unique histologic findings are presented in Table 14.1.

Differential Diagnosis

Silicone granulomas can contain histiocytes, which phagocytose silicone materials and resemble lipoblasts. This finding, in combination with fibrosis and empty spaces in tissue, can raise the possibility of atypical lipomatous tumor/well-differentiated liposarcoma (ALT/WDL) or atypical pleomorphic lipomatous tumor. However, the combination of histiocytes, foreign body giant cells, and foreign material or acellular spaces makes the diagnosis relatively simple; and, even when the patient denies cosmetic procedures or surgery, the diagnosis can be suggested.

Prognosis and Treatment

The primary treatment of foreign body granulomas caused by fillers is intralesional corticosteroid injections, which typically resolve the issue. Minocycline combined with oral or intralesional steroids is also effective in treating widespread lesions.

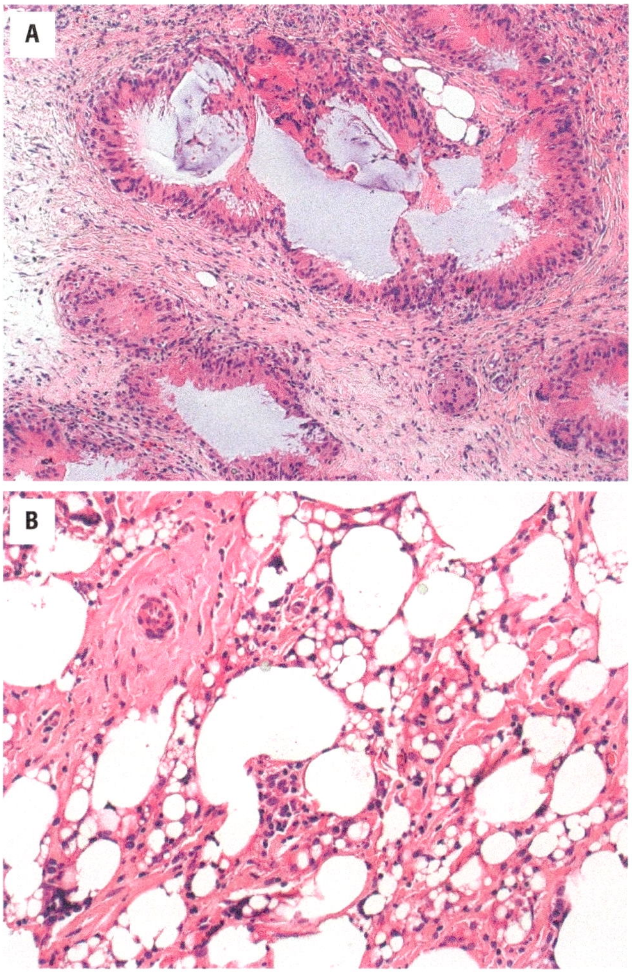

FIG. 14.4

A, Filler granuloma with an irregularly shaped foreign material surrounded by giant cell reaction. **B,** Silicone granuloma showing numerous multivacuolated histiocytes that closely resemble lipoblasts; silicone droplets are washed away during processing.

MASSIVE LOCALIZED LYMPHEDEMA

Clinical Findings

Massive, localized lymphedema (MLL) is a mass-forming variant of chronic lymphedema that occurs in morbidly obese individuals due to chronic lymphatic obstruction by excessive adipose tissue. The most common presentation is of a very large, superficial pedunculated mass affecting medial thigh, anogenital region, abdomen, and arms. Like other forms of chronic lymphedema, MLL can rarely give rise to angiosarcoma, but most cases are completely benign and come to surgical attention due to size and discomfort to the patient. The impressive clinical presentation may lead to a mistaken diagnosis of ALT/WDL.

Histopathologic Features

MLL is an ill-defined fatty mass composed of lobulated adipose tissue expanded by edematous and fibrotic connective tissue stroma. The overlying dermis merges imperceptibly with the mass and shows various degrees of stromal edema, fibrosis, lymphangiectasia, and reactive lymphatic and capillary vascular proliferation; chronic inflammation and lymphoid aggregates may be present. The expanded interlobular connective tissue septa contain reactive myofibroblasts that can show significant nuclear atypia and closely mimic ALT/WDL (Fig. 14.5A and B). However, true lipoblasts or any significant degree of nonlipomatous spindle cell component are not seen in MLL.

TABLE 14.1

Esthetic Granulomas

Chemical Ingredient	Product(s)	Histologic Features
Silicone	Silikon 1000, Silskin, Adatosil 5000	Empty vacuoles surrounded by histiocytes and giant cells with intracytoplasmic vacuoles
Polydimethylsiloxane/polyvinyl pyrrolidone	Bioplastique	Translucent jagged structures within cystic spaces surrounded by foreign body cells and fibrosis
Bovine collagen	Zyderm, Zyplast	Plane eosinophilic, amorphous, thick acellular bundles with perivascular and interstitial mixed inflammation
Bovine collagen/polymethylmethacrylate microspheres (PMAA)	Artecoll, Arteplast, Artefill, Metacril	Diffuse and nodular granulomatous inflammation surrounding cystic spaces with central round translucent nonbirefringent microspheres
Hyaluronic acid/polyhydroxyethylmethacrylate (HEMA)/ethylmethacrylate (EEMA)	Dermalive, Dermadeep	Diffuse and nodular granulomatous inflammation surrounding cystic spaces with central round translucent nonbirefringent polygons +/-calcification
Hyaluronic acid (nonanimal)	Restylane, Juvaderma, Perlane	Mononuclear cells and eosinophils with foreign body cells surrounding basophilic, Alcian blue-positive foreign material
Polyacrylamide gel (PAAG)	Aquamid	Palisaded, mononuclear cells and eosinophils with foreign body cells surrounding necrotic tissue, necrobiosis and basophilic foreign material
Poly-L-lactic acid	Newfill, Sculptra	Granulomatous inflammation with long spiky translucent birefringent bodies in giant cells

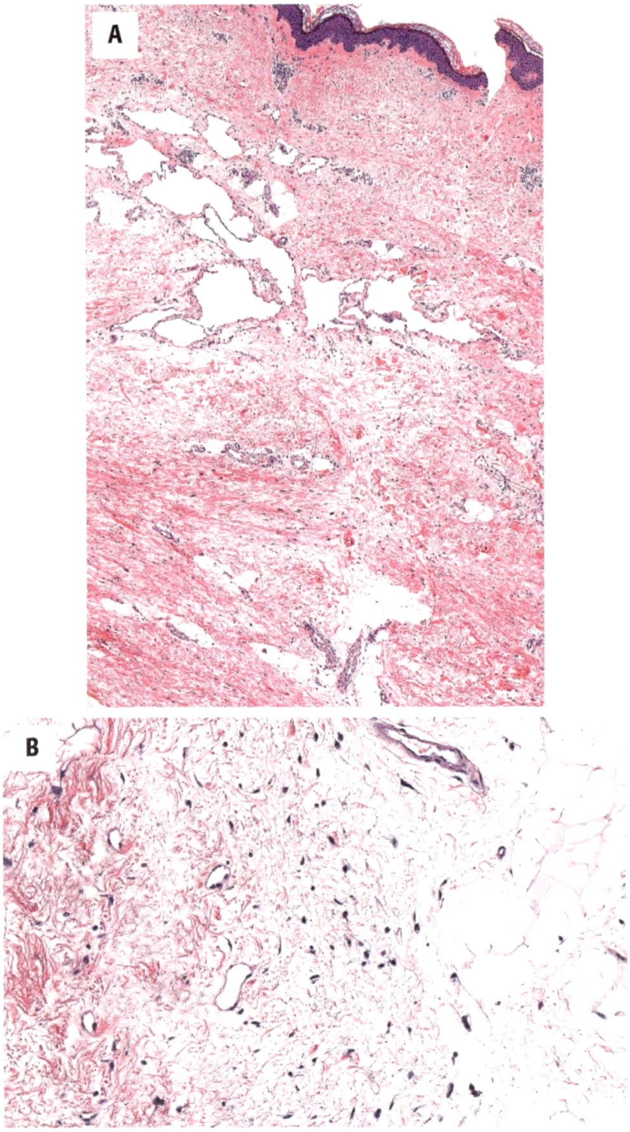

FIG. 14.5
Massive, localized lymphedema. **A,** The dermis shows stromal edema, fibrosis, atrophy of the sweat glands, and lymphangiectasia. **B,** The expanded interlobular septa contain reactive atypical myofibroblasts mimicking atypical lipomatous tumor/well-differentiated liposarcoma.

Differential Diagnosis

The distinction from ALT/WDL can be established based on the following features: (1) superficial location, which is rare in ALT/WDL; (2) ill-defined boundaries with the dermis, which is almost always involved in MLE in contrast to the sharply demarcated border in superficial ALT/WDL; (3) preservation of lobular fatty architecture at scanning magnification in MLE; and (4) dermal edema and a reactive-type capillary proliferation, which often is located at the periphery of fatty lobules in MLE and is highly uncharacteristic of ALT/WDL. Fluorescence in situ hybridization (FISH) testing for *MDM2* gene amplification can help in diagnostically challenging cases. Atypical spindle cell and pleomorphic lipomatous tumor (ASCPLT), a member of tumor family with Rb1 loss (discussed later in this chapter), can be distinguished from MLE based on the sharp border with the dermis, the presence of CD34-positive spindle cell component, lipoblasts, absence of reactive vascular proliferation, and loss of Rb1 expression by IHC.

ISCHEMIC FASCIITIS

Clinical Findings

Ischemic fasciitis also known as atypical decubital fibroplasia is a subcutaneous mass-like reactive process that occurs at the sites of intermittent pressure-induced ischemic tissue injury. The lesion typically affects dependent sites overlying body prominences such as hips, sacrum, elbows, scapula, or shoulders. Classically described in elderly, debilitated, and immobilized patients, ischemic fasciitis is now being increasingly recognized in younger patients without the classic comorbidities.

Histopathologic Features

Ischemic fasciitis shows a characteristic zonal pattern histologically, with area of central fibrinoid necrosis surrounded by loose myxoid and vascular stroma containing proliferation of reactive myofibroblastic cells including ganglion-like myofibroblasts resembling those seen in proliferative fasciitis. The misleading feature is a rather significant degree of nuclear atypia and hyperchromasia seen in these reactive myofibroblasts raising the possibility of a sarcoma (Fig. 14.6). Older lesions may show predominantly collagenous background. While clonal alterations have been detected in some cases, ischemic fasciitis is regarded as a reactive pseudotumor.

Differential Diagnosis

Myxofibrosarcoma, dermal pleomorphic sarcoma undifferentiated pleomorphic sarcoma, or sarcomatoid/spindle SCC are the key diagnostic considerations. The latter can be distinguished by the appropriate immunophenotype, but the distinction from a primary cutaneous sarcoma is based on the recognition of the characteristic zonal pattern and clinical context.

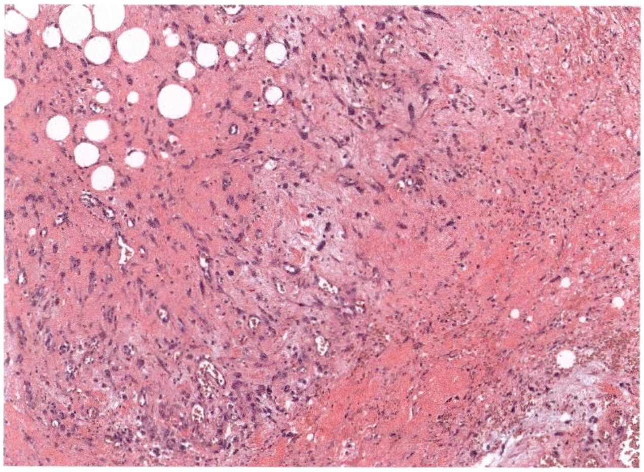

FIG. 14.6

Ischemic fasciitis. An area of central fibrinoid necrosis is surrounded by loose myxoid and vascular stroma containing reactive myofibroblasts with mild nuclear atypia.

REACTIVE VASCULAR PROLIFERATIONS

REACTIVE ANGIOENDOTHELIOMATOSIS

Clinical Findings

Reactive angioendotheliomatosis (RAE) is a rare, self-limited cutaneous vascular proliferation that typically occurs in middle-age to older patients with various co-existing systemic diseases including connective tissue disease, hypercoagulable states, cryoglobulinemia, hematopoietic disorders, end-stage liver and kidney disease, smoking, and natural and iatrogenic immunosuppressive states. The pathogenesis is thought to result from activation of proangiogenic factors related to tissue ischemia. Lesions present as multiple coalescing, erythematous (at times purpuric) macules, nodules, and plaques, some with ulceration, which tend to involve the extremities. Localized lesions are related to severe atherosclerotic peripheral vascular disease, arteriovenous fistulas, calciphylaxis, macromastia, and obesity. Diffuse dermal angiomatosis is a subset of RAE usually associated with vascular disease/atherosclerosis. The clinical course is variable, with the majority regressing or stabilizing spontaneously.

Histopathologic Features

Histopathologically, lesions show a multifocal proliferation of closely packed dermal capillaries in a lobular and/or diffuse pattern wrapping around dermal vessels and skin appendages. The diffuse growth pattern (diffuse dermal angiomatosis) is a particularly worrisome pattern at scanning magnification as it shows a diffuse proliferation of slitlike vessels dissecting dermal collagen that closely resembles an infiltrative pattern of angiosarcoma. The extension into the subcutis is limited and typically involves the periphery of the fat lobules resembling septal panniculitis (Fig. 14.7A and B). Microthrombi and reactive, fasciitis-like dermal reaction may be present. The capillaries are cytologically banal, although they may show normal mitotic figures, and are invested by pericytes (Fig. 14.7C). Intracapillary/intravascular histiocytosis, mainly seen in patients with rheumatoid arthritis, has been recently classified within the spectrum of RAE. This histologic vascular reaction may be mechanistically related to a response to localized or diffuse luminal occlusion by intravascular histiocytes with resultant reduced oxygenation. The clinical course is variable, with the majority regressing or stabilizing spontaneously with improvement of the underlying problem.

Two other distinctive clinical forms of RAE are recognized:

- Acroangiodermatitis (or acroangiodermatitis of Mali) is a superficial, often symmetric reactive capillary vascular proliferation in the setting of venous insufficiency, amputation stumps, or following cardiac bypass surgery. Clinically, this lesion presents as brown macules, papules, or confluent plaques that can mimic Kaposi sarcoma (this lesion used to be called kaposiform angiodermatitis). Microscopically, the superficial dermis shows reactive capillaries in a somewhat lobular configuration in a background of edema, extravasated red blood cells, and hemosiderin deposits (Fig. 14.7D).
- Stewart-Bluefarb syndrome is a similar cutaneous reaction in response to AV shunting and resultant tissue ischemia in the setting of underlying arteriovenous malformation (AVM) or arteriovenous fistula.

Differential Diagnosis

The principal differential diagnosis is with patch stage Kaposi sarcoma and cutaneous angiosarcoma. Well-formed capillaries, microthrombi, and pericytic layer are not usually seen in Kaposi sarcoma; likewise, a spindle cell proliferation with intracytoplasmic hyaline globules and plasma cells are not typical of RAE. HHV8 immunostaining is typically negative in RAE. Cutaneous angiosarcomas are expected to show endothelial multilayering and overt cytologic atypia. An immunohistochemical stain for SMA to highlight the pericytic layer surrounding the capillaries is helpful as neither Kaposi sarcoma nor angiosarcoma has pericytic investment.

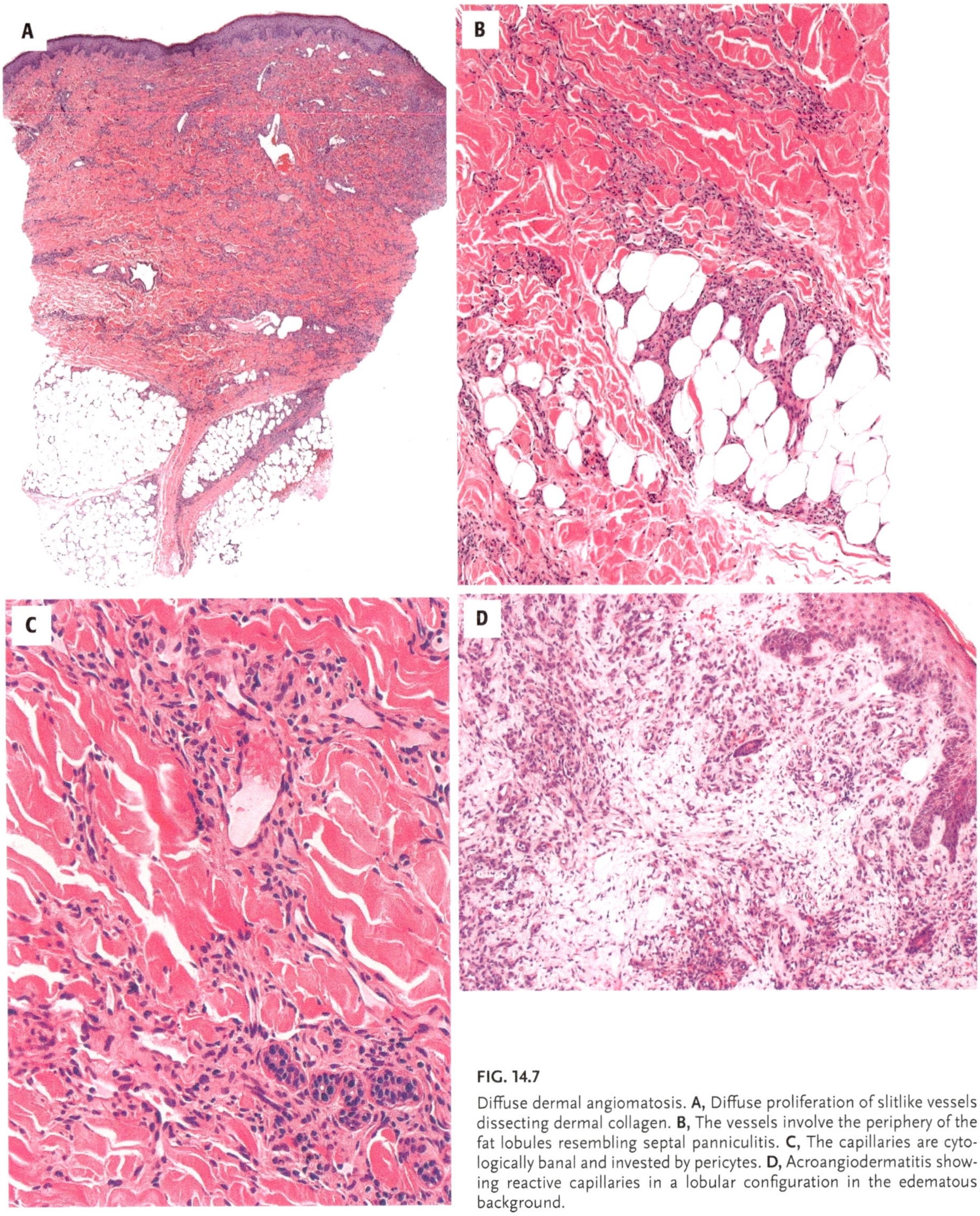

FIG. 14.7

Diffuse dermal angiomatosis. **A,** Diffuse proliferation of slitlike vessels dissecting dermal collagen. **B,** The vessels involve the periphery of the fat lobules resembling septal panniculitis. **C,** The capillaries are cytologically banal and invested by pericytes. **D,** Acroangiodermatitis showing reactive capillaries in a lobular configuration in the edematous background.

Prognosis and Treatment

Treatment centers around identifying and treating the underlying disease that is causing vascular compromise and can be augmented by systemic antibiotics for infectious complications, and corticosteroids to attenuate neoangiogenesis. Compression garments and surgical relief of occlusions are also helpful.

INTRAVASCULAR PAPILLARY ENDOTHELIAL HYPERPLASIA (MASSON TUMOR)

Clinical Findings

Intravascular papillary endothelial hyperplasia presents as an erythematous or violaceous small nodule, most often on the head and neck and hands and feet.

Histopathologic Features

Intravascular papillary endothelial hyperplasia is a pattern of organization of an intravascular thrombus or, rarely, a hematoma. It can occur in a thrombosed vein or in any vascular lesion with dilated vessels and slow blood flow. At scanning magnification, papillary endothelial hyperplasia is usually confined to the boundaries of the vessel from which it originates, although it may extend into adjacent soft tissue. The lesion consists of variably sized papillary structures lined by a single layer of plump endothelial cells. The papillary structures contain fibrin, which gets replaced by collagen over time. The endothelial cells can show mild atypia and normal mitotic figures. The lesion is confined by the wall of the affected vessel and does not have infiltrative growth (Fig. 14.8A and B).

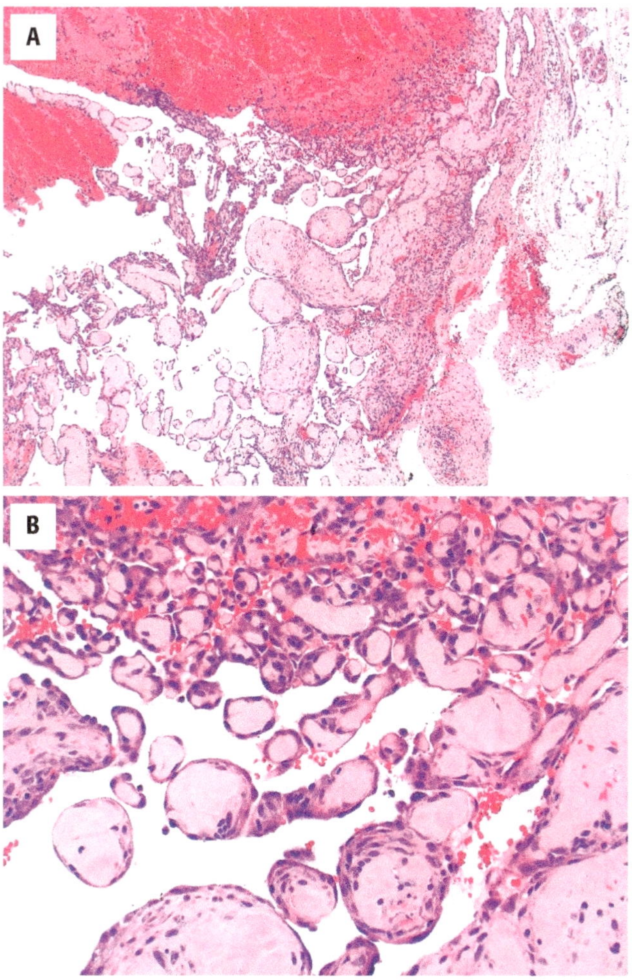

FIG. 14.8

Papillary endothelial hyperplasia (Masson tumor). **A,** An architecturally complexed lesion confined by the boundaries of the precursor vessel. **B,** Papillary structures lined by a single layer of plump endothelial cells with mild atypia.

Differential Diagnosis

Because of the complex papillary architecture, intravascular papillary endothelial hyperplasia can be mistaken for a well-differentiated angiosarcoma, especially in small samples. Key distinguishing features include well-circumscribed appearance at low power, lack of true tissue infiltration, endothelial multilayering, overt nuclear atypia and atypical, mitotic figures.

REACTIVE VASCULAR LESIONS AFFECTING SUN-DAMAGED SKIN: VENOUS LAKE AND ACQUIRED ELASTOTIC HEMANGIOMA

Clinical Findings

Venous lake presents as a violaceous papule in the sun-damaged skin, usually on the lips, and can clinically mimic mucocele, melanoma, or angiosarcoma. Acquired elastotic hemangioma occurs on the sun-damaged skin of the arms and neck of older patients as a slowly growing erythematous plaque.

Histopathologic Features

A venous lake is an ectatic vein in the superficial dermis resulting from a lack of stromal support due to chronic solar damage. The vessel is lined by bland attenuated endothelium without atypia (Fig. 14.9A). Acquired elastotic hemangioma consists of a bandlike proliferation of well-formed capillary vessels in the upper reticular dermis, with a narrow grenz zone (Fig. 14.9B). The blood vessels are lined by bland, slightly hobnailed endothelial cells without atypia or mitotic activity. Background skin shows solar elastosis and chronic inflammation.

Differential Diagnosis

A venous lake is readily recognizable and rarely mimics other lesions. Thrombosed venous lake with papillary endothelial hyperplasia may resemble angiosarcoma. The bandlike growth pattern and background solar elastosis help to distinguish acquired elastotic hemangiomas from other vascular tumors. Kaposi sarcoma and low-grade angiosarcoma are the only clinically relevant mimics. Kaposi sarcoma can be distinguished based on a more infiltrative growth pattern, irregular vessels, a spindle cell component, the presence of plasma cells in the inflammatory infiltrate, and HHV8 latent antigen 1 expression by IHC. Cutaneous angiosarcomas are more

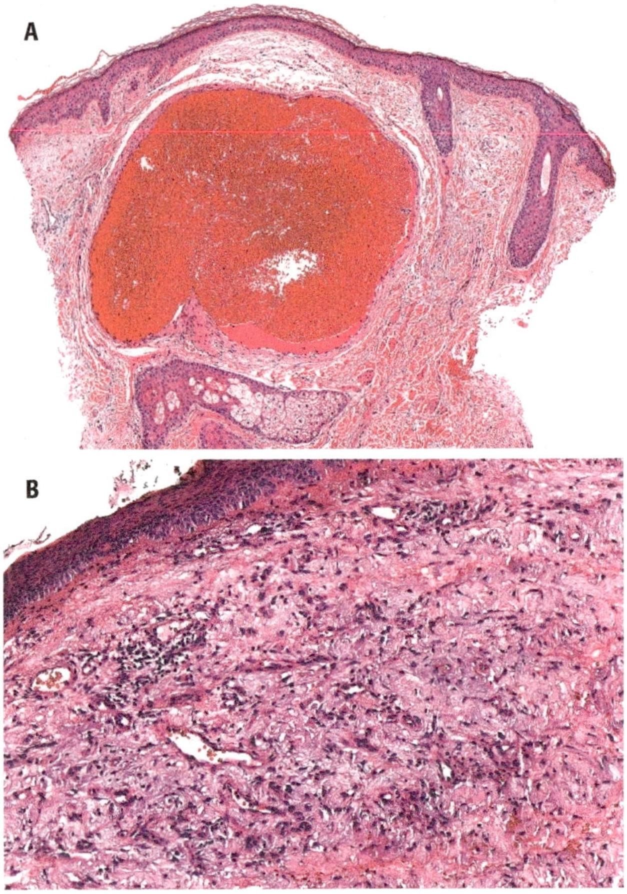

FIG. 14.9

A, Venous lake. A single dilated vein in the superficial dermis in the background of solar damage. **B,** Acquired elastotic hemangioma. A bandlike proliferation of cytologically bland capillary vessels in the reticular dermis in the background of solar damage.

architecturally complex lesions with an infiltrative growth pattern and greater nuclear atypia. Radiation-associated atypical vascular lesions (AVLs) may appear similar morphologically (see below) but can be readily ruled out on clinical grounds.

BACILLARY ANGIOMATOSIS

Clinical Findings

Bacillary angiomatosis (BA) is a rare reactive vascular proliferation caused by infection with gram-negative bacteria *Bartonella henselae* or *B. quintana*. Disease is spread by cat bites/scratches or via fleas and lice. BA effects children and adults of both genders who are immunocompromised, almost always in the setting of AIDS but can rarely occur in immunocompetent patients after major local trauma. It occurs anywhere on the skin as widely distributed, variably sized, erythematous to violaceous papules and nodules. BA is associated with fever, lymphadenopathy, nausea/vomiting/anorexia, and chills and sweats.

Histopathologic Features

BA is an exuberant dermal and subcutaneous lobular capillary proliferation admixed with neutrophils, lymphocytes and histiocytes, and cellular debris. BA may contain a peripheral collarette simulating pyogenic granuloma at low power. At high power, the capillaries are lined by plump, epithelioid endothelial cells that may obscure the lumina and contain pericytes. Pale and smudgy amphiphilic granular material representing bacterial colonies may be present (Fig. 14.10A and B). The gram-negative intracellular organisms may be demonstrated by Warthin-Starry, Giemsa, or Gomori methenamine silver (GMS) stain.

Differential Diagnosis

Owing to the lobular configuration and epithelioid morphology, BA resembles both pyogenic granuloma

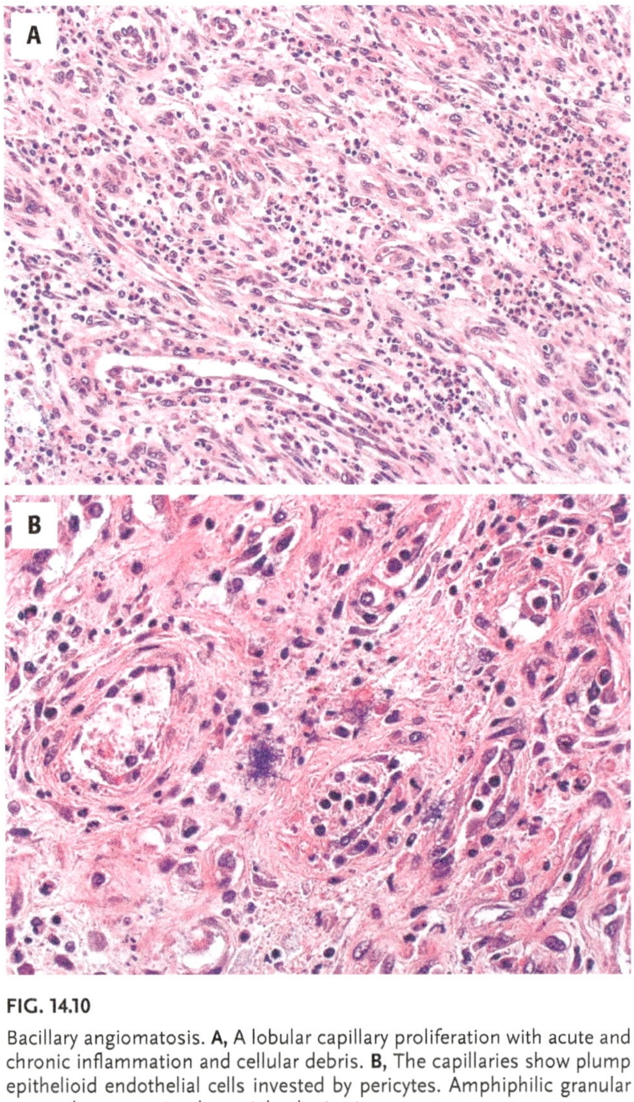

FIG. 14.10

Bacillary angiomatosis. **A,** A lobular capillary proliferation with acute and chronic inflammation and cellular debris. **B,** The capillaries show plump epithelioid endothelial cells invested by pericytes. Amphiphilic granular material representing bacterial colonies is present.

and epithelioid hemangioma. Knowledge of the clinical history is extraordinary helpful due to the almost exclusive association of BA with AIDS. Morphologically, BA can be distinguished from epithelioid hemangioma by the presence of the amphophilic clusters of organisms and neutrophil and karyorrhexis-rich background inflammatory infiltrate, as opposed to eosinophil-rich chronic inflammation seen in epithelioid hemangioma. Pyogenic granulomas lack the epithelioid endothelial cells and amphophilic granular material of BA.

Prognosis and Treatment

Systemic disease and/or internal organ involvement can become life threatening. Treatment includes antibiotics, continued for 3 to 6 months to prevent recurrence. Most lesions respond to treatment within days or weeks.

FIBROBLASTIC AND MYOFIBROBLASTIC TUMORS

ANGIOFIBROMA AND FIBROUS PAPULE

Clinical Findings

Angiofibromata are a clinically heterogenous group of related lesions with similar histopathologic features that present as solitary or multiple firm, flesh-colored papules, or nodules. Fibrous papule is a solitary, acquired lesion of adults that occurs on the central face, especially the nose, and can be confused clinically with basal cell carcinoma (BCC) or melanocytic nevus. Syndromic facial angiofibromas (so-called adenoma sebaceum) manifest in childhood as numerous small papulonodular lesions on the central face, especially the nasolabial fold, and are most often associated with tuberous sclerosis and sometimes other syndromes such as Birt-Hogg-Dubé or multiple endocrine neoplasia (MEN) type 1. Pearly penile papules present as crops of angiofibromas, primarily the coronal margin and sulcus in up to 10% of young healthy adults, and may be mistaken for warts. Acquired digital fibrokeratomas and periungual fibromas (discussed below) are a variant of angiofibroma with a topographic predilection for fingers and toes, especially the nail region.

Histopathologic Features

Angiofibromas are dome-shaped paucicellular lesions characterized by proliferation of spindled to stellate fibroblasts and occasional multinucleated cells embedded in a variably collagenous stroma containing thin ectatic vessels (Fig. 14.11A and B). The overlying epidermis may be variably hyperkeratotic and show a collarette. Histologic variations have been described referring to differences in cell density and cytology of the fibroblasts, including cellular, epithelioid, granular, pigmented when the lesion contains overlying melanocytic hyperplasia and pigmented macrophages, pleomorphic, and clear-cell variants. Pleomorphic fibrous papule contains multinucleated giant cells resembling pleomorphic fibroma. Clear-cell fibrous papule is distinctive as it contains numerous clear cells resembling foamy macrophages or epithelial neoplasms with clear-cell morphology (Fig. 14.12A and B).

Differential Diagnosis

Characteristic collagenous paucicellular stroma containing ectatic vessels seen in all angiofibroma variants is the most helpful histologic clue to the correct diagnosis. Fibrofolliculomas/trichodiscomas are tumors of

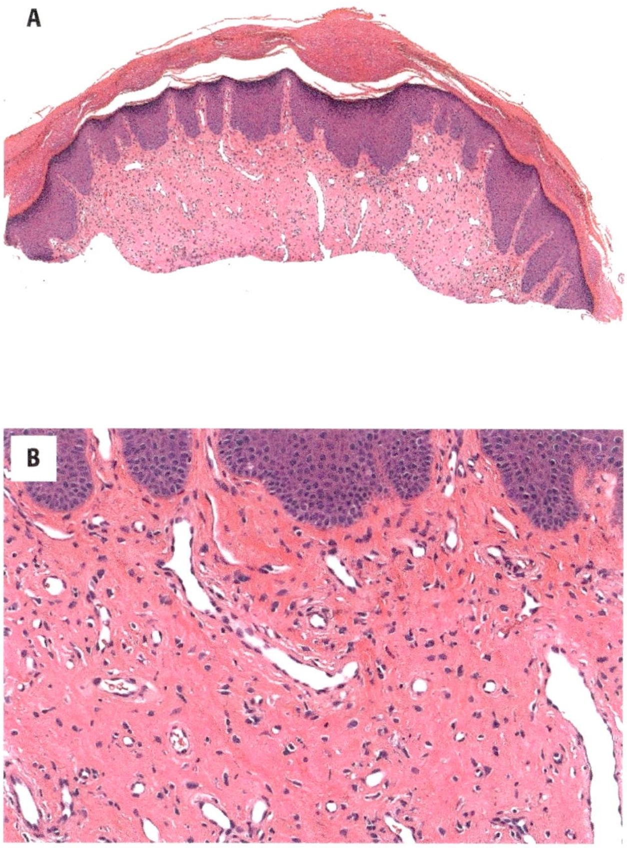

FIG. 14.11

Angiofibroma. **A,** A dome-shaped paucicellular lesion with hyperkeratosis. **B,** Spindled to stellate fibroblasts are dispersed in a collagenous stroma containing ectatic vessels.

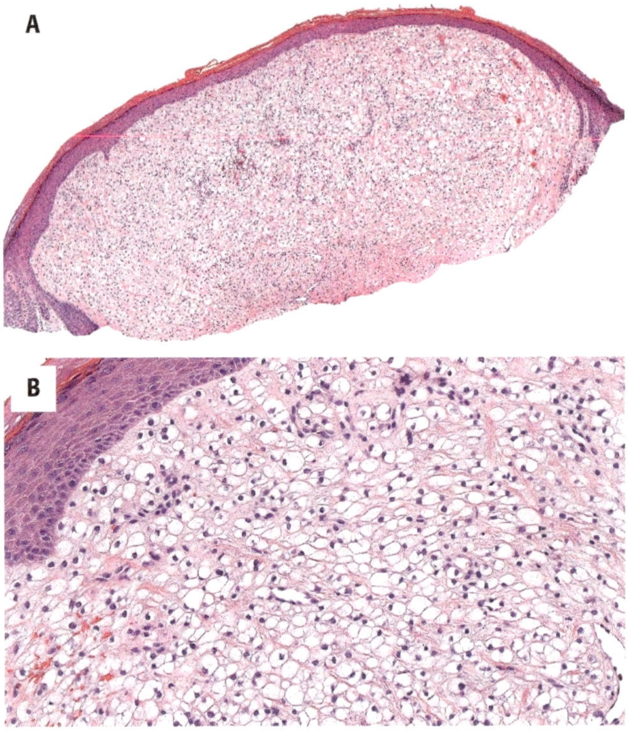

FIG. 14.12

Clear-cell fibrous papule. **A,** A dome-shaped paucicellular lesion with an epidermal collarette. **B,** The lesion consists of epithelioid cells with clear cytoplasm resembling histiocytes.

perifollicular mesenchyme that can be confused with angiofibromas. The stroma in these two tumors tends to be more myxoid, with more slender fibroblasts. An epithelial component is present in the form of a folliculosebaceous collarette surrounding the fibroblastic proliferation in a trichodiscoma and a proliferation of follicular mantle epithelium in a fibrofolliculoma. Epithelioid, cellular, and clear-cell fibrous papules may need to be distinguished from melanocytic and epithelial tumors by application of melanocytic and epithelial markers. Superficially sampled pigmented angiofibromas can raise concern about the possibility of an associated lentigo or lentigo maligna. Careful attention to the cellular density and distribution of melanocytes as well as clinical correlation is important. The differential diagnosis of acral fibrokeratomas and periungual fibromas is discussed below.

Prognosis and Treatment

Angiofibromas are benign lesions usually treated for cosmetic reasons by simple excision, ablative laser, or cryotherapy, and in the setting of syndromic lesions, application of topical sirolimus or topical or systemic mammalian target of rapamycin (mTOR) pathway inhibitors.

ACQUIRED DIGITAL FIBROKERATOMA (ACRAL FIBROKERATOMA) AND PERIUNGUAL FIBROMA

Clinical Findings

Acquired digital fibrokeratoma, also known as acral fibrokeratoma or acquired periungual fibrokeratoma, is a benign tumor that typically occurs on fingers and toes and less often, palms and soles, of adults, more often men, as a flesh-colored, slow-growing, small (typically <5 mm) firm nodule, although occasionally it may present as a large pedunculated polyp or fingerlike projection. It may occur in an immunosuppressed host. The overlying epidermis is hyperkeratotic such that the lesion can clinically resemble a cutaneous horn or a verruca. Acquired periungual fibrokeratoma is an anatomic variant of acquired digital fibrokeratoma arising from the proximal nail fold or nailbed and producing the characteristic "garlic clove" appearance. Periungual and subungual fibroma also arises in the setting of tuberous sclerosis complex (TSC) as variably sized, multilobulated nodules affecting multiple fingers or toes and disfiguring the nail (Koenen tumor).

Histopathologic Features

Acquired digital fibrokeratoma has a polypoid silhouette, with a variably acanthotic and hyperkeratotic epidermis and an epidermal collarette. The dermis is hypocellular and contains small, spindled fibroblasts and

ACQUIRED DIGITAL FIBROKERATOMA—DISEASE FACT SHEET

Clinical Findings

- ►► Acquired digital fibrokeratoma
  - Small nodules on hands and feet of adults
- ►► Acquired periungual fibrokeratoma
  - Proximal nail fold with a "garlic clove" appearance
- ►► Periungual fibroma of tuberous sclerosis
  - Lobulated disfiguring nodules on multiple fingers or toes

Histopathologic Features

- ►► Acquired digital fibrokeratoma and periungual fibrokeratoma
  - Polypoid silhouette
  - Hyperkeratotic epidermis with an epidermal collarette
  - Bland fibroblasts and collagen fibers parallel to the long axis
  - A pseudonail appearance
- ►► Periungual fibroma of tuberous sclerosis
  - Circumscribed lesions with attenuated epidermis
  - Myxoid stroma containing stellate fibroblasts

Differential Diagnosis

- ►► Acrochordon
- ►► Superficial acral fibromyxoma
- ►► Supernumerary digit

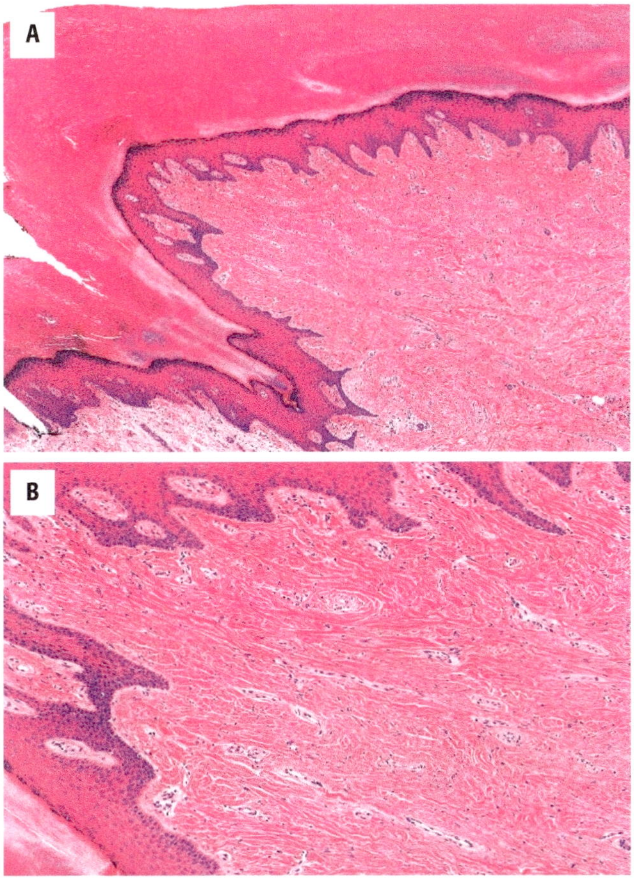

FIG. 14.13

Acquired digital fibrokeratoma. **A,** A polypoid hypocellular lesion with acanthotic and hyperkeratotic epidermis and an epidermal collarette. **B,** The dermis contains spindled fibroblasts and dense collagen fibers that run parallel to the long axis of the polyp.

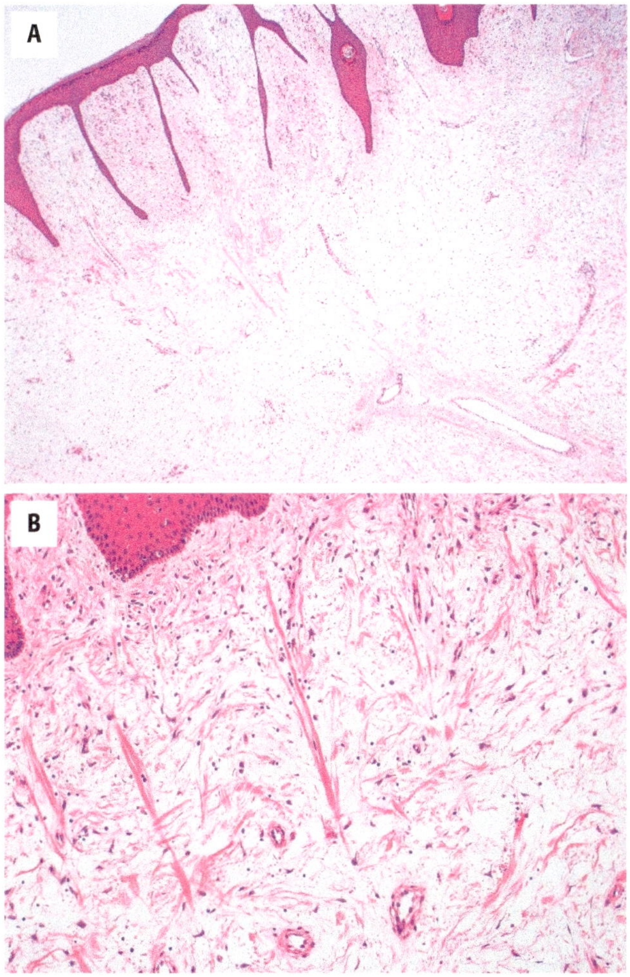

FIG. 14.14

A and **B**, Periungual and subungual fibroma of tuberous sclerosis forming a circumscribed lesion with attenuated epidermis and myxoid stroma containing stellate, bland fibroblasts.

dense collagen that runs parallel to the long axis of the polyp and blends with the normal dermis at the base (Fig. 14.13A and B). A pseudonail appearance may be present. Adnexal or neural structures are not seen. Large periungual and subungual fibromas of tuberous sclerosis present as multiple circumscribed lesions with attenuated epidermis and more vascular and myxoid stroma containing stellate fibroblasts (Fig. 14.14A and B).

Differential Diagnosis

The principal diagnostic considerations are other polypoid fibroepithelial lesions. Acrochordon is not acral and does not show the hyperkeratosis and vertically oriented dense collagen. Superficial acral fibromyxoma (SAF, described below) shows a more striking cellularity, CD34-positive fascicular architecture, and myxoid stroma. There is a loss of Rb1 expression by IHC. A supernumerary digit (rudimentary polydactyly) occurs on the fifth digit and can be distinguished by the presence of hyperplastic nerve bundles at the base of the lesion.

Angiofibroma or fibrous papule (discussed above) is a histologically related lesion but with a predilection for the central face.

Prognosis and Treatment

Acquired digital fibrokeratoma is benign and can be treated by excision or laser ablation; in the setting of tuberous sclerosis, topical rapamycin or sirolimus or systemic mTOR pathway inhibitors may be used. Periungual fibromas of tubular sclerosis tend to locally recur.

DERMAL PLAQUE-LIKE FIBROBLASTIC PROLIFERATIONS THAT MAY RESEMBLE PLAQUE-LIKE DFSP

There are three distinctive, plaque-like dermal lesions that likely arise from a dermal fibroblastic precursor.

These lesions overlap clinically (well-circumscribed plaques in children and young adults) and morphologically (short monotonous fascicles of bland fibroblastic cells predominantly in the dermis). All three lesions are benign, cured by simple excision and typically do not require re-excision unless a better cosmetic outcome is desired. Distinguishing this lesion from plaque-like DFSP is the most important task to ensure appropriate patient management.

DERMATOMYOFIBROMA

Clinical Findings

Dermatomyofibroma manifests as a flesh-colored or hypopigmented, slowly growing painless plaque on the upper trunk or head and neck of young adults, more often females. The clinical presentation may resemble DF or granuloma annulare.

Histopathologic Features

Dermatomyofibroma is composed of bland fibroblastic/myofibroblastic cells that are arranged in fascicles with a strikingly parallel orientation to the overlying epidermis (Fig. 14.15A and B). The parallel arrangement of fascicles is key to the diagnosis. The tumor is usually restricted to the reticular dermis but may show limited involvement of the upper subcutis like DFs. The individual tumor cells are monotonous with elongated vesicular nuclei and faintly eosinophilic cytoplasm resembling superficial fibromatosis, but in contrast to fibromatosis, they do not destroy adnexal structures or vessels. Elastic stain, if performed, will highlight preserved and somewhat thickened intercellular elastic fibers. By IHC, the spindle cells inconsistently express SMA, more so in early lesions, and may be variably positive for CD34, although most cases are either negative or fail to show the diffuse, strong pattern of CD34 expression seen in DFSP. Desmin and S100 are negative.

DIFFERENTIAL DIAGNOSIS—DERMATOFIBROMA VERSUS DERMATOFIBROSARCOMA PROTUBERANS

Dermatofibroma	Dermatofibrosarcoma Protuberans
Epidermal hyperplasia with or without follicular induction	Normal or attenuated epidermis
Relatively circumscribed or stellate	Deeply infiltrative
Heterogenous cell population (fibroblasts, histiocytes, dendritic cells, giant cells; foamy histiocytes	Monotonous fibroblasts in a storiform pattern
Collagen trapping at the periphery	Diffuse infiltration with incorporation of adipocytes
Minimal infiltration into subcutis along fibrous septa in cellular DF	
IHC: Conventional DF: CD34 usually negative	CD34 diffusely positive
CD68/163, factor XIIIa positive	
Cellular DF: variable SMA, desmin, CD34 negative except the lesion periphery	SMA, desmin consistently negative
Deep DF: variable SMA, desmin, CD34	
Molecular: *PRKC-B* and *PRKC-D* fusions	*COL1A1::PDGFRB*, *COL6A3::PDGFD* fusions

DF, Dermatofibroma; *IHC*, immunohistochemistry; *SMA*, smooth muscle actin.

A

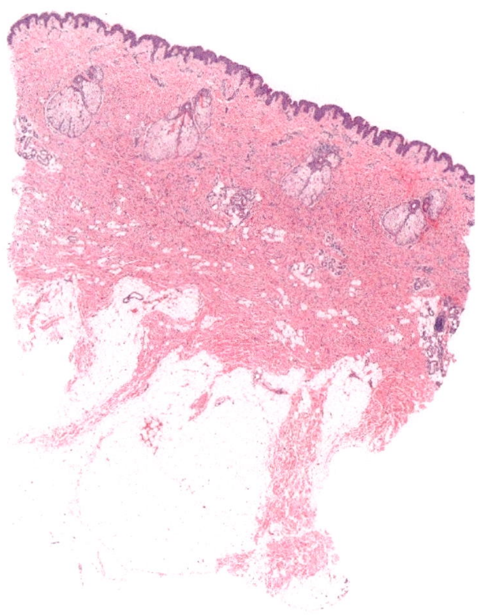

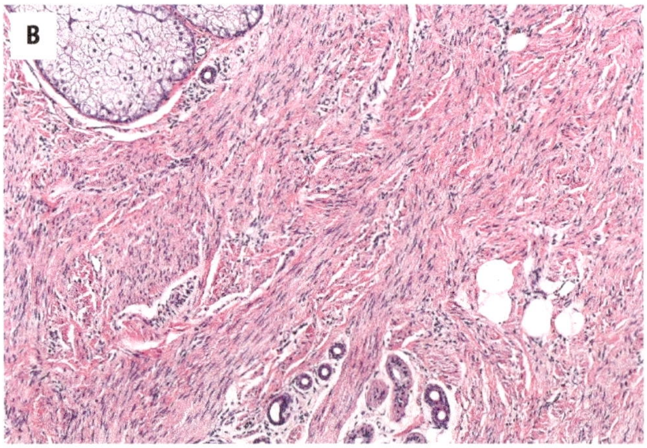

FIG. 14.15

Dermatomyofibroma. **A,** A modestly cellular infiltrative lesion restricted to the reticular dermis. **B,** Bland myofibroblastic cells arranged in fascicles that run parallel to the epidermis. The growth is nondestructive with preservation of dermal elastic fibers and adnexal structures.

Differential Diagnosis

The differential diagnosis of dermatomyofibroma includes fibroblastic connective tissue nevus (FCTN), DFSP, pilar leiomyoma, superficial fibromatosis, dermal scar, DF, and fibrous hamartoma of infancy (FHI). It should be noted that variable degrees of CD34 and SMA expression may be observed in all these lesions with exception of DFSP, which is usually devoid of SMA staining unless it forms myoid nodules. Thus, the morphologic appearance, notably, the parallel arrangement of the characteristic bland slender fascicles, and, perhaps, the presence of thickened intralesional elastic fibers by Verhoeff elastic or MOVAT stains are more helpful in the diagnosis of dermatomyofibroma than the immunoprofile. Additional distinguishing morphologic features are listed below:

- Plaque-stage DFSP shows greater cellularity, storiform rather than fascicular growth pattern and a diffusely infiltrative architecture incorporating subcutaneous adipocytes; difficult cases may be tested for *PDGFB* gene rearrangements or other rare fusions.
- DFs show storiform growth pattern, a polymorphous cellular composition including fibroblastic cells, histiocytes, and factor XIIIa–positive dendritic cells, and a characteristic collagen trapping at the periphery. The fascicles of cellular FH are cellular and plump in appearance, have a stellate rather than parallel configuration, and often show mild nuclear atypia and mitotic activity.
- Dermal scars can be confused with dermatomyofibroma because of the parallel arrangement of spindled cells. Dermal scars usually show evidence of epidermal injury with effacement of the normal rete peg architecture and reactive vasculature oriented perpendicularly to the overlying epidermis. Keloidal collagen, if present, is not typical of dermatomyofibroma. Adnexal structures are not spared in a scar.
- Superficial fibromatosis (Dupuytren's contracture) may show cytologic overlap with dermatomyofibroma, but the infiltrative, nodular growth pattern and the clinical setting (tendons on the palmar surfaces of hands and feet with or without contractures) is quite distinct. While it is tempting to also consider desmoid-type fibromatosis, the latter usually presents as a larger, subcutaneous mass-forming lesion and nuclear expression of β-catenin. It is exceedingly rare for desmoid-type fibromatosis to occur in the dermis or present as a plaque-like lesion.
- FHI (discussed below) is a mostly subcutaneous, mass-like lesion of infants and young children showing a triphasic architecture with nodules of immature mesenchymal cells, fascicles of bland spindle cells that run in all directions, and adipose tissue.
- Distinction from a FCTN (discussed in the following) may be truly difficult as clinical and histologic appearance overlaps significantly. FCTN is composed of haphazardly arranged bundles of bland spindle cells involving the dermis and subcutaneous tissue in contrast to a more orderly arrangement and somewhat greater cellularity of spindle cell fascicles in dermatomyofibroma. Conspicuous presence of adipocytes within the reticular dermis and epidermal papillomatosis is more typical of FCTN. FCTN express CD34 and typically lack SMA immunoreactivity, but this immunophenotype overlaps with that of dermatomyofibroma.

FIBROBLASTIC CONNECTIVE TISSUE NEVUS

Clinical Findings

FCTN is a rare benign cutaneous proliferation of CD34-positive fibroblastic or myofibroblastic cells. It typically appears during the first decade of life, although it may affect a wide age range. The lesion presents as a solitary, slowly growing firm plaque on the trunk, extremities, and head and neck area and is more common in female patients.

Histopathologic Features

FCTN is a poorly circumscribed plaque-like proliferation of bland fibroblastic fascicles growing in an irregular, ramifying pattern through the reticular dermis and entrapping adnexal structures (Fig. 14.16A and B). The overlying epidermis often shows papillomatous hyperplasia. Another distinctive feature is the presence of adipocytes very superficially in the reticular dermis. Extension into the subcutis is not uncommon but usually occurs along the fibrous septa. Cytologically, the cells show features of bland fibroblasts or myofibroblasts with oval tapering nuclei and pale amphophilic cytoplasm. There is no cytologic atypia or mitotic activity. Most fibroblastic connective tissue nevi express CD34, although it is usually patchy and variable in intensity.

Differential Diagnosis

The differential diagnosis of FCTN includes plaque-like DFSP, dermatomyofibroma, pilar leiomyoma, and occasionally fibromatosis. DFSP can be distinguished based on the presence of storiform rather than fascicular growth pattern and diffuse, strong CD34 immunoreactivity.

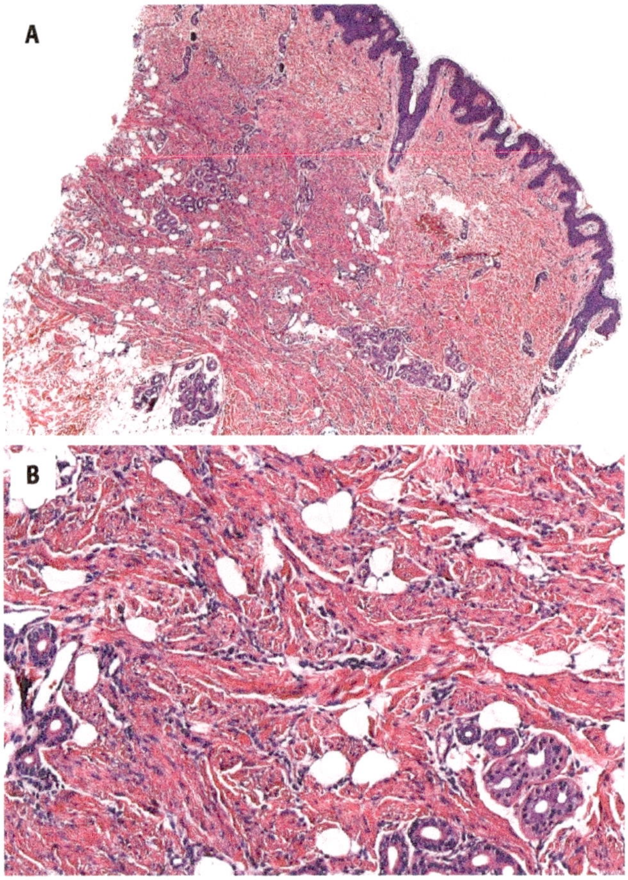

FIG. 14.16

Fibroblastic connective tissue nevus. **A,** Plaque-like fibroblastic fascicles growing in a ramifying pattern through the reticular dermis, with papillomatous hyperplasia of the epidermis. **B,** Bland fibroblasts or myofibroblasts with oval tapering nuclei and pale amphophilic cytoplasm entrapping adnexal structures and incorporating adipocytes high in the dermis.

Prognosis and Treatment

The available data suggest that FCTN does not recur and does not metastasize and thus does not require a complete excision unless indicated for cosmetic reasons.

PLAQUE-LIKE CD34-POSITIVE DERMAL FIBROMA

Clinical Findings

Plaque-like CD34-positive dermal fibroma originally described as "medallion-like dermal dendrocyte hamartroma" presents as congenital or acquired reddish to brownish annular plaques that can resemble DF, plaque-like DFSP. The overlying skin can be wrinkled and atrophic. These lesions often occur during the first decade of life but can affect any age group and are slightly more prevalent in women.

Histopathologic Features

A bandlike proliferation of bland, spindled fibroblasts in the upper dermis, with an overlying grenz zone is typical. The distinctly bandlike proliferation occupying reticular dermis is striking at scanning magnification, although this feature is less appreciable in small biopsies (Fig. 14.17A and B). The spindle cells in the superficial dermis may be arranged perpendicular to the epidermis while the deeper layers can be arranged in a storiform pattern, although this feature is inconsistent. In contrast to dermatomyofibroma, there is a paucity of intralesional elastic fibers. In contrast to the FCTN,

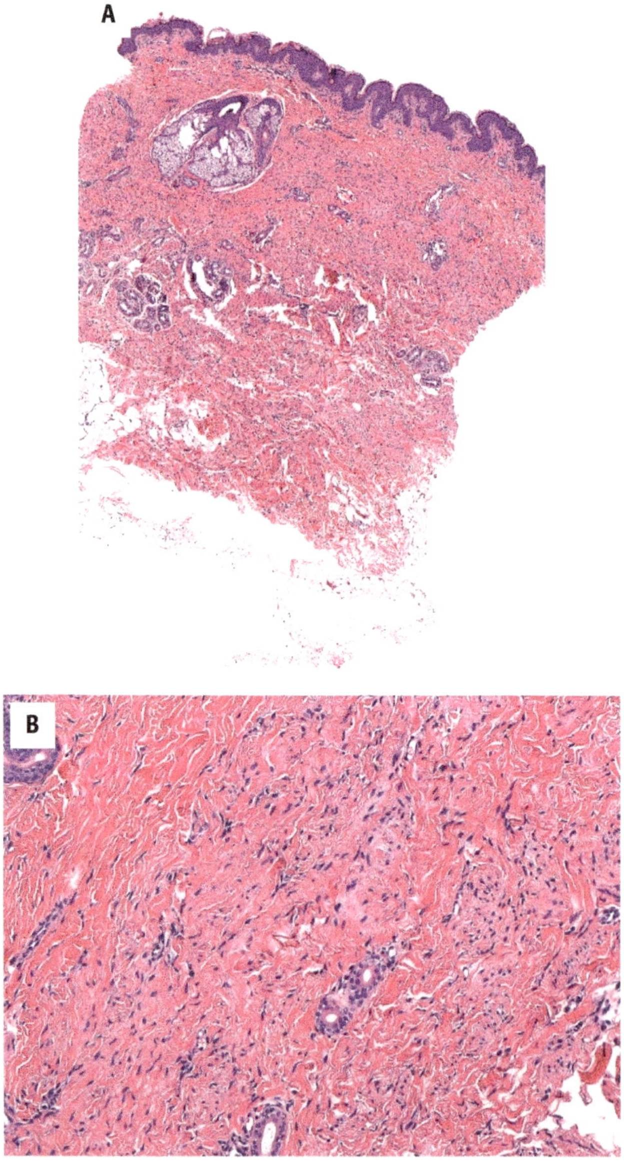

FIG. 14.17

Plaque-like CD34-positive dermal fibroma. **A,** A bandlike fibroblastic proliferation in the upper dermis, with an overlying grenz zone. **B,** Bland fibroblastic spindle cells limited to the reticular dermis.

extension into the subcutis is rare, occurring in congenital/early childhood examples. Dilated small vessels and mast cells may be observed. The lesional cells show no atypia or mitotic activity and diffusely express CD34 and fascin.

Differential Diagnosis

Plaque-like CD34-positive dermal fibroma shares many features with FCTN and may in fact be the same entity. The differential diagnosis includes dermatomyofibroma and plaque-like DFSP. Plaque-like DFSP can be distinguished based on an ill-defined margin and greater cellularity. In challenging cases, molecular genetic analysis for *PDGFB* or rare other fusions implicated in DFSP pathogenesis may be employed.

SUPERFICIAL FIBROMATOSIS

Clinical Findings

Superficial fibromatosis presents as slow-growing multinodular soft tissue masses or flexion contractures at acral sites; based on location, superficial fibromatosis is known as palmar (Dupuytren's contracture), plantar (Ledderhose's disease), and penile (Peyronie's disease). Palmar and plantar fibromatosis presents as a diffuse thickening or a nodule and is frequently bilateral. Peyronie's disease usually manifests as a plaque-like induration on the dorsal or lateral penis. Palmar fibromatosis typically affects older adults with male predilection while patients with plantar and penile fibromatosis are younger (second to third decade). There is an autosomal dominant inheritance pattern with variable penetrance, and synchronous or metachronous development of other lesions is common. There are variably strong clinical associations with epilepsy, diabetes mellitus, and alcoholic liver disease, the mechanism of which is unknown. Knuckle pads and pachydermodactyly are also regarded as forms of superficial fibromatosis.

Histopathologic Features

Superficial fibromatoses are multinodular, somewhat circumscribed but unencapsulated masses that invariably show an infiltrative edge with the tendon or adjacent soft tissue. They are composed of cellular yet completely monotonous and bland-appearing long fibroblastic fascicles with tapered nuclei with vesicular chromatin, undulating nuclear membranes and pinpoint nucleoli, and pale eosinophilic cytoplasm in a collagenous stroma (Fig. 14.18A and B). Typical highly parallel, wavy, and refractile collagenous fibers of the affected tendon or fascia can be seen between the cells. Occasional multinucleated giant cells are noted, and the mitotic figures can be quite conspicuous, especially in plantar lesions in younger individuals. The vessels are regular and evenly spread and may show perivascular inflammation or red cell extravasation. The cells are variably positive for SMA in a fibroblastic pattern, and negative for CD34, desmin, neural markers, and cytokeratin. In contrast to the desmoid fibromatosis, the nuclear expression of β-catenin is weak and inconsistent, as superficial fibromatoses lack *CTNNB1* or *APC* mutations that drive the former. Instead, reported abnormalities in superficial fibromatoses show gains of whole chromosomes 7 and 8 and abnormalities

---

FIBROMATOSIS—DIFFERENTIAL DIAGNOSIS

Superficial Fibromatosis

- Mass or flexure contraction at acral sites in adults (palmar, plantar, penile)
- Autosomal dominant with variable penetrance
- Association with diabetes mellitus, alcoholic liver disease, epilepsy
- Fascicles of monotonous fibroblasts infiltrating tendon or fascia
- Occasional multinucleated giant cells
- Negative for β-catenin (*CTNNB1*) mutations
- Rare nuclear β-catenin expression
- High risk of local recurrence

Desmoid Fibromatosis

- Infiltrative mass deep in the subcutis, skeletal muscle, mesentery, viscera
  - Sporadic (>80%) due to somatic activating *CCNB1* exon 3 mutations
  - Familial (2%–3%) due to inactivating *APC* mutations in familial adenomatous polyposis
  - Other mutations in Wnt/β-catenin pathway
  - Typical nuclear β-catenin expression
- Sweeping fascicles of bland fibroblasts with infiltrative border
- Regular slitlike or gaping vessels with perivascular red blood cells
- Hyalinized areas, keloidal collagen, perilesional lymphoid aggregates
- High risk of local recurrence

Inclusion Body Fibromatosis

- Polypoid dermal nodules on phalanges of fingers or toes
- Infants and very young children
- Cytologically bland fibroblastic cells in fascicles or whorls in deep dermis and subcutis
- Round eosinophilic intracytoplasmic inclusions composed of actin filament
- Negative nuclear β-catenin
- High risk of local recurrence

Differential Diagnosis

- Hypertrophic scar
- Fibroma of tendon sheath
- Plexiform myofibroblastoma

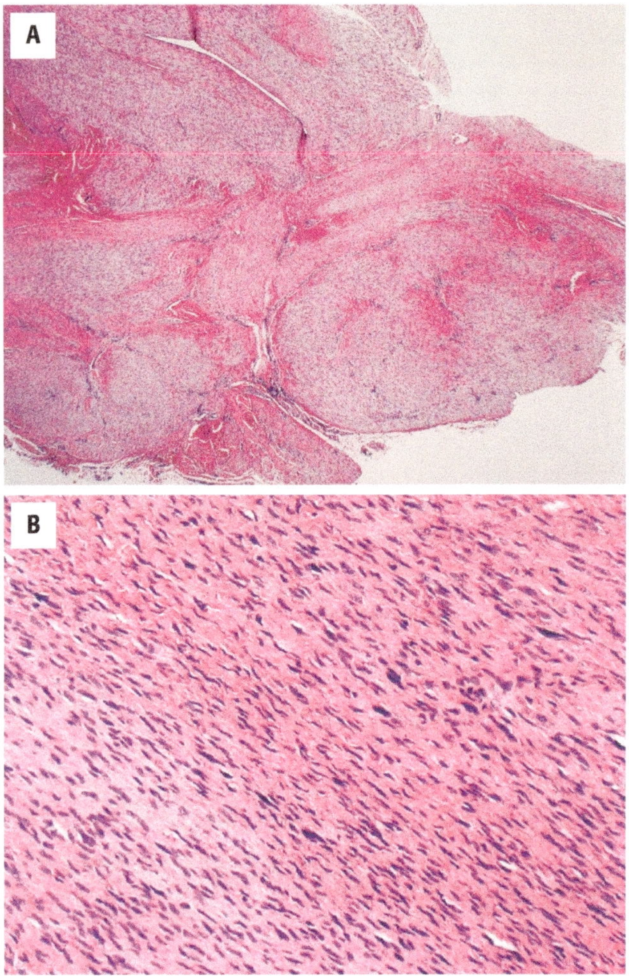

FIG. 14.18
Superficial fibromatosis. **A,** A multinodular, unencapsulated mass with an infiltrative border with the adjacent tendon. **B,** Cellular fascicles of completely monotonous eosinophilic fibroblastic cells with tapered nuclei, undulating nuclear membranes, and pinpoint nucleoli. The refractile collagenous fibers of the affected tendon or fascia can be seen between the cells.

involving 14q11.2 and 7p14.1. Immunohistochemistry is hardly ever needed for the diagnosis of superficial fibromatosis.

Differential Diagnosis

Fibroma of tendon sheath is a circumscribed, minimally infiltrative lesion that is typically less cellular, lacks prominent fascicular growth pattern, often shows loose, fasciitis-like arrangement of fibroblasts in a myxoid background—a feature not seen in superficial fibromatosis. The vessels in fibroma of tendon sheath are more prominent at the periphery where they have a distinctive crescentic appearance. Fibromas of tendon sheath often have *USP6* gene rearrangement. Distinguishing superficial fibromatosis from a scar such as from prior injury or in the setting of a ruptured ganglion cyst can be problematic, but the clinical history and the location on the plantar/palmar surface is very helpful. Fibromatosis tends to have long, multidirectional sweeping fascicles as opposed to shorter, more loosely arranged fascicles of a scar arranged parallel to the epidermis. The vasculature of fibromatosis consists of uniformly distributed, slender, or gaping vessels in contrast to the perpendicular arrangement of the reactive vessels in a scar. Plaque-like dermal proliferations that include FCTN, dermatomyofibroma, and CD34-positive plaque-like dermal fibroma are composed of fascicles that are individually very similar to fibromatosis; however, the clinical presentation and the location of all these lesions are completely different, and none forms a mass-like nodule or a contracture. The presence of individual adipocytes within the lesion is uncharacteristic of superficial fibromatosis. On occasion, plantar fibromatoses may be cellular and mitotically active enough to mimic an acral fascicular sarcoma such as synovial sarcoma (SS) or clear-cell sarcoma; these lesions can be distinguished based on the characteristic immunophenotype (cytokeratins, EMA, melanocytic marker expression) and unique molecular alterations.

Differential Diagnosis

Superficial fibromatoses are indolent, but recurrences are very common following surgical resection. A variety of nonsurgical approaches has been employed do delay progression and reduce pain including intralesional corticosteroids, percutaneous needle fasciotomy, radiotherapy, and shockwave therapy.

INCLUSION BODY FIBROMATOSIS

Clinical Findings

Inclusion body fibromatosis (IBF) also known as infantile digital fibroma/fibromatosis or Reye's tumor is a benign fibroblastic proliferation that affects the dorsal or the lateral distal phalanx of fingers or toes. These lesions present as polypoid or dome-shaped painless dermal nodules and almost always occur in infants or very young children; adult cases are exceptionally rare.

Histopathologic Features

Histologically, IBF is an ill-defined, uniform proliferation of cytologically bland, plump fibroblastic cells arranged in short fascicles or whorls and extending into the deep dermis and subcutis. The scanning appearance may resemble hypertrophic scar or superficial fibromatosis; however, at high magnification, the cytoplasm contains small round eosinophilic inclusions (actin myofilaments) that are separated from the nucleus by a clear zone and can be mistaken for red blood cells (Fig. 14.19A and B). The inclusions can be highlighted by trichrome staining (Fig. 14.19C) or picked up by myofibroblastic stains like SMA, caldesmon, or calponin.

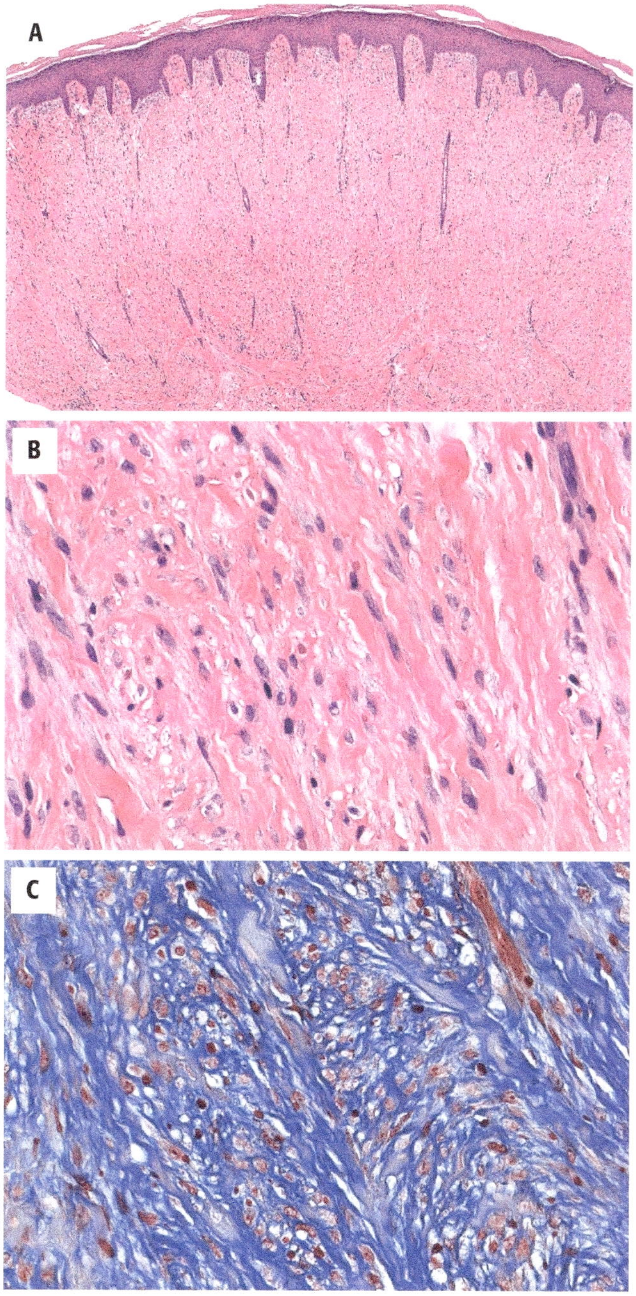

FIG. 14.19

Inclusion body fibromatosis. **A,** A uniform proliferation of plump, cytologically bland fibroblastic cells arranged in short fascicles. **B** and **C,** The cytoplasm contains small round eosinophilic inclusions that can be highlighted by trichrome stain.

Differential Diagnosis

Both superficial palmoplantar fibromatosis and hypertrophic scar can look very similar, but these lesions lack the characteristic eosinophilic inclusions.

Prognosis and Treatment

IBF is benign but characterized by rather high local recurrence rate following surgery (up to 74%); the current treatment approach is conservative with watchful waiting as many lesions stabilize or regress over time; intralesional steroid injections or surgical excision is recommended in cases with significant functional or cosmetic interference.

DESMOID FIBROMATOSIS AND GARDNER FIBROMA

Clinical Findings

Desmoid fibromatosis is an infiltrative myofibroblastic proliferation that occurs deep in the subcutaneous tissue, skeletal muscle, visceral sites, and bone that, despite its bland histologic appearance, has the significant potential for locoregional recurrence. This lesion most often occurs sporadically due to recurrent somatic activating mutations in exon 3 of *CCNB1* gene (>80%), or in association with familial adenomatous polyposis (FAP) syndrome with inactivating *APC* gene mutations (2%–3%) or other mutations that lead to Wnt/β-catenin pathway activation. Desmoid fibromatosis very rarely affects the skin. Gardner fibroma is a benign fibrous soft tissue tumor that occurs in patients with FAP syndrome and desmoid fibromatosis and can be the first manifestation of this disorder as often it presents in childhood (median age, 5 years). Gardner fibroma is a solitary, firm, fibrous mass in the superficial or deep soft tissue of the back, the paraspinal region and sometimes the abdomen, head and neck or mesentery where it overlaps with desmoid fibromatosis.

Histopathologic Features

Desmoid fibromatosis is composed of very bland myofibroblasts arranged in long, sweeping fascicles. The tumor nuclei are evenly spaced and slender, with tapered ends, and have characteristically pale chromatin to the extent that the nuclei of adjacent endothelial cells may appear dark in comparison. Regularly distributed slitlike or gaping vessels are seen throughout the lesion and often show perivascular edema, inflammatory cells, or extravasated red blood cells. Keloid-like collagen deposition is common to a point that some cases of fibromatosis are indistinguishable from a scar in limited biopsy material. Peripheral lymphoid aggregates are another common and very helpful feature. Mitotic activity is absent or sparse, and there is no necrosis. Hyalinized areas are strikingly hypocellular and can be difficult to differentiate from normal connective tissue or a scar (Fig. 14.20A–C). Consistent with its myofibroblastic phenotype, fibromatosis shows variable, typically weak immunoreactivity for SMA and desmin, and it is almost always negative for CD34. Nuclear staining for β-catenin is supportive of a diagnosis of desmoid fibromatosis but the interpretation of this stain can be problematic, since even a "negative" result retains a considerable level of membranous staining which can be difficult to distinguish from bona fide nuclear staining. At the molecular level, fibromatosis harbors either mutations in exon 3 of *CTNNB1* or inactivating alterations of the *APC* gene, including mutation, chromosome 5q allelic loss, or both. A subset of *CTNNB1* and *APC* wild-type cases have recently been shown to harbor large intragenic deletions in *CTNNB1*. Accordingly, molecular testing for both *CTNNB1* and *APC* mutations/alterations might be necessary to confirm the diagnosis in difficult cases. Gardner fibroma is a hypocellular lesion composed of haphazardly arranged thickened collagen fibers with characteristic cracking, and very sparce, cytologically banal fibroblasts entrapping nerves, muscle, and adipose tissue at the periphery, very similar in appearance to nuchal fibroma (discussed below). Gardner fibroma differs from desmoid fibromatosis by the absence of active fibroblastic proliferation; however, hyalinized areas of desmoid fibromatosis can look very similar. Approximately 60% to 70% of Gardner fibromas express β-catenin, and the lesion can be positive for CD34.

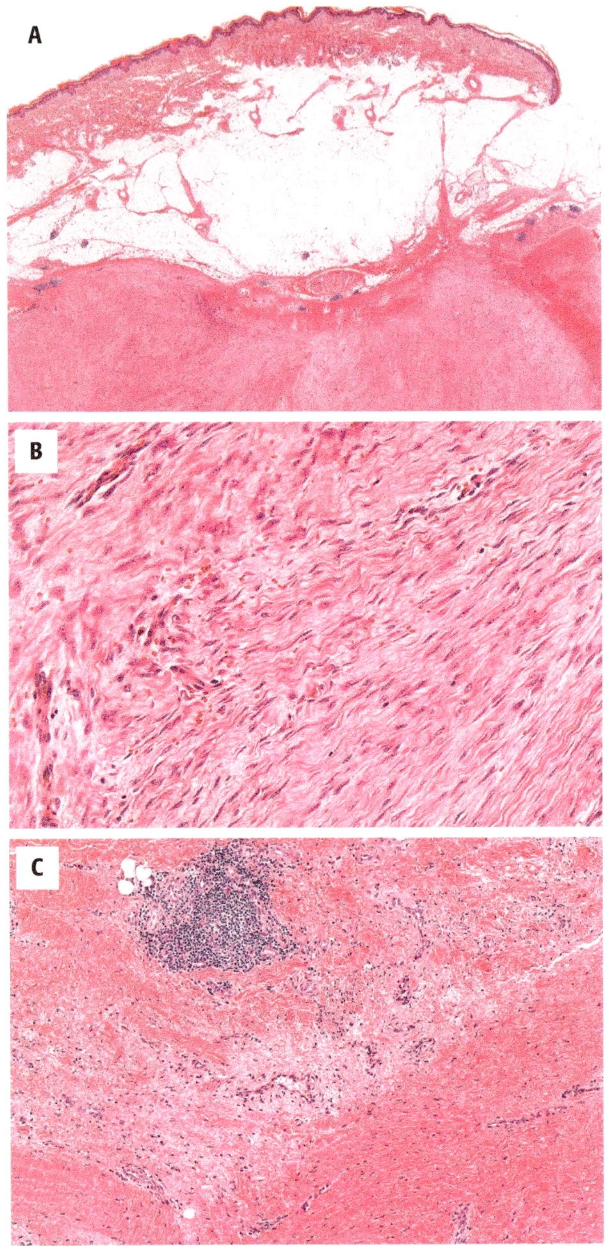

FIG. 14.20

Desmoid fibromatosis. **A,** A deep-seated subcutaneous mass with an infiltrative border. **B,** Bland myofibroblasts arranged in long, sweeping fascicles, with evenly spaced and slender tapered nuclei, separated by regular slitlike vessels. **C,** Hypocellular hyalinized zones may be difficult to distinguish from the normal connective tissue. Peripheral lymphoid aggregates often present.

Differential Diagnosis

The most challenging differential diagnosis of desmoid fibromatosis is superficial fibromatosis and hypertrophic or keloid scar as these three lesions can be virtually indistinguishable on histologic grounds alone. It is worth remembering that desmoid fibromatosis hardly ever involves dermis or superficial subcutaneous tissue, and therefore reactive vasculature and papillary dermal and epidermal alterations are uncharacteristic. Fibromatosis tends to have long, multidirectional sweeping fascicles as opposed to shorter, more loosely arranged fascicles of a scar arranged parallel to the epidermis. The vasculature of fibromatosis consists of uniformly distributed, slender, or gaping vessels in contrast to the perpendicular arrangement of the reactive vessels in a scar. Identification of β-catenin alteration by IHC or molecular genetic testing for confirmatory features of fibromatosis (i.e., exon 3 mutations in *CTNNB1* or alterations of the *APC* gene) can be pursued in challenging cases. FHI can be distinguished based on the following features: (1) triphasic lesional architecture (fibromatosis-like fascicles, adipose tissue and nests of primitive basophilic mesenchymal cells set in myxoid stroma); (2) intermingling appearance of all three components with large amount of adipose tissue between fibroblastic cells rather than solid, mass-like appearance with a broad edge of fibromatosis; and (3) lack of β-catenin alterations. Another lesion that can closely mimic desmoid fibromatosis at the level of subcutis is plexiform myofibroblastoma (discussed below); the latter lesion is more uniformly plexiform and lacks β-catenin gene alterations. Gardner fibroma needs to be distinguished from nuchal fibroma (discussed below), a histologically similar lesion with a completely different presentation as a sporadic solitary lesion in the neck region of middle-aged adults, unrelated to FAP. A helpful histologic clue in distinguishing these two very similar lesions is the presence of traumatic neuroma-like changes in the latter and lack of β-catenin alterations. Hyalinized desmoid fibromatosis and Gardner fibroma may look very similar and, arguably, represent a histologic spectrum.

Prognosis and Treatment

Desmoid fibromatosis was traditionally treated with surgery, but those cases often showed positive margins (32% to 75%) and up to 40% of cases recurred locally. Most importantly, the margin clearance in desmoid fibromatosis is a poor predictor of recurrence, and therefore aiming for an R0 resection may produce a potentially disfiguring result with little long-term benefit. Recent studies showed no difference in event-free survival and long-term disease control between patients undergoing surgery and those managed conservatively, and some patients paradoxically fare worse if managed by initial surgery than if managed non-surgically. Thus, the current consensus approach to the initial management of fibromatosis in most patients is active surveillance, with CT/MRI at 3- to 6-month intervals over 1 to 2 years. Many such patients will experience stabilization or regression of their disease requiring no further surgical intervention, whereas patients who show a persistent progression or significant morbidity can be selected for active treatment (surgery, radiation, or medical management). This approach prevents overtreatment of desmoid fibromatosis and excessive morbidity from surgical intervention. Gardner fibroma is benign and is cured by simple excision; however, it is strongly associated with concurrent or subsequent development of desmoid fibromatosis and therefore should prompt identification of FAP.

PLEXIFORM MYOFIBROBLASTOMA

Clinical Findings

Plexiform myofibroblastoma is a distinctive benign superficial fibroblastic/myofibroblastic neoplasm with predilection for truncal locations (back, chest wall, axilla, abdominal, and pelvic region) in children and young adults. The tumors vary in size (average 2.7 cm, range from 0.6 to 8 cm) and present as an ill-defined nodule, mass, or plaque-like lesion. Rare cases are multifocal.

Histopathologic Features

Plexiform myofibroblastoma is composed of fascicles of bland fibroblastic/myofibroblastic cells with oval or elongated nuclei and palely eosinophilic cytoplasm resembling fibromatosis. The lesional cells grow in a distinctly plexiform, infiltrative pattern through the subcutaneous fibroadipose tissue and reticular dermis. There is no significant atypia or mitotic activity. The stroma within the fascicles can be collagenous, myxoid, fasciitis-like, or show focal keloidal hyalinization (Fig. 14.21A–C). By IHC, most cases express SMA, consistent with myofibroblastic differentiation, and approximately half are positive for CD34 and desmin. S100 and β-catenin (nuclear expression) are consistently negative. Molecular studies to date show rare *FGFR2* mutations.

Differential Diagnosis

Desmoid fibromatosis shows some overlap. The key distinguishing feature of plexiform myofibroblastoma is a consistently plexiform growth pattern present throughout the lesion in contrast to the confluent, mass-like growth with broad pushing margin of fibromatosis, and the absence of *CTNNB1* (β-catenin) and *APC* gene alterations. Plexiform fibrohistiocytic tumor (PFHT, described below) shares the clinical presentation as a superficial mass in young adults and a distinctly plexiform growth pattern with infiltration of deep subcutis at scanning magnification. However, PFHT is not a purely fibroblastic tumor; the nodules of PFHT containing pale histiocytoid cells admixed with osteoclast-type giant cells are at least focally present in most cases. PFHT is often positive for CD68 in the histiocytoid component and is negative for CD34.

Prognosis and Treatment

Plexiform myofibroblastoma is benign and rarely recurs even in marginally excised cases, despite an infiltrative growth pattern.

NUCHAL-TYPE FIBROMA

Clinical Findings

Nuchal-type fibroma (NTF) is an uncommon benign fibrocollagenous lesion that presents as an ill-defined, fixed mass in the posterior neck of adult patients, more often in men. Very rarely, it occurs at extra-nuchal locations and is often associated with diabetes mellitus or a repetitive trauma.

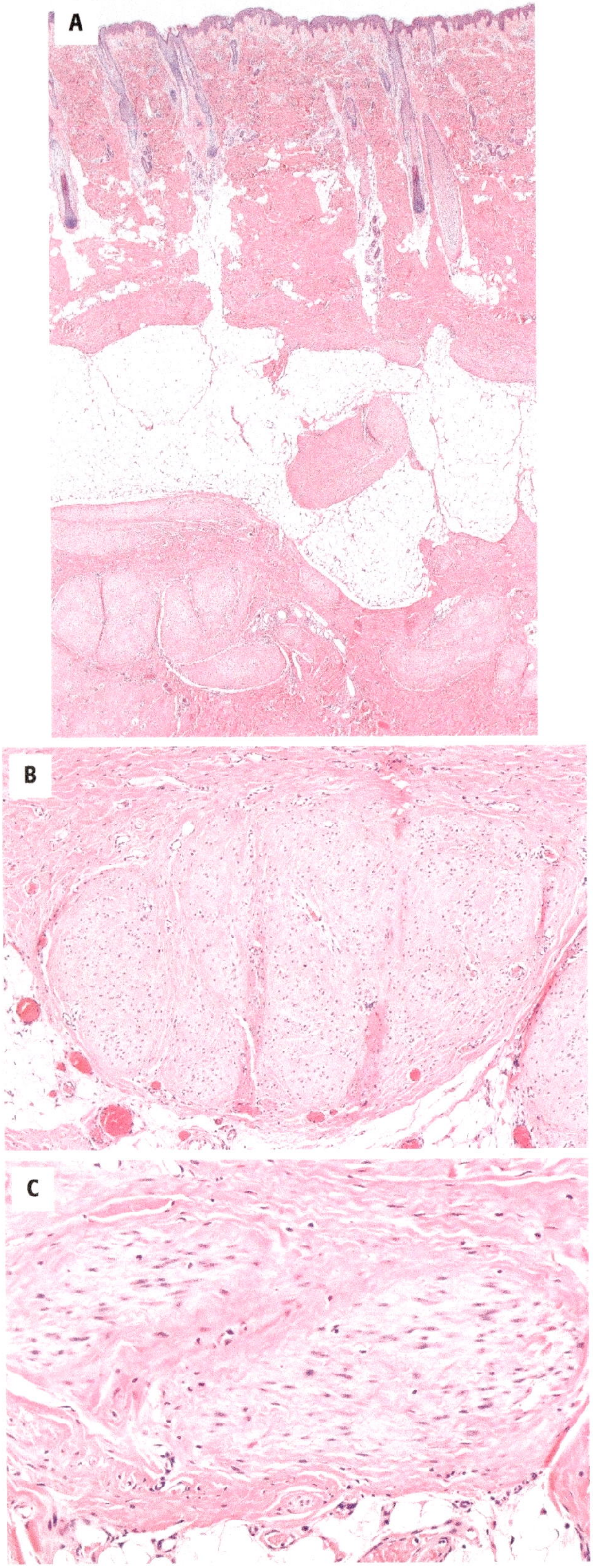

FIG. 14.21

Plexiform myofibroblastoma. **A,** Distinctly plexiform, infiltrative growth through the subcutaneous fibroadipose tissue and reticular dermis. **B,** Fascicles and nodules of cytologically bland eosinophilic fibroblastic/myofibroblastic cells with oval or elongated nuclei resembling fibromatosis. **C,** Myxoid stroma containing bland fibroblastic cells. *(Photographs courtesy of Drs. David Papke and Christopher Fletcher, Brigham and Women's Hospital.)*

Histopathologic Features

NTF is a paucicellular, poorly circumscribed lesion composed of thick, haphazardly arranged collagen bundles entrapping adipose tissue, with a characteristic cracking artifact and preservation of subcutaneous elastic fibers (Fig. 14.22A and B). A classic but inconsistent feature is the presence of entrapped nerves and traumatic neuroma-like changes at the periphery of the lesion. The sparce fibroblasts are short with small oval nuclei and inconspicuous nucleoli. The fibroblasts are positive for CD34 and negative for nuclear expression of β-catenin.

Differential Features

Gardner fibroma is a histologically nearly identical lesion that occurs in patients with familiar adenomatous polyposis/FAP due to germline *APC* gene mutations that result in aberrant activation of β-catenin pathway.

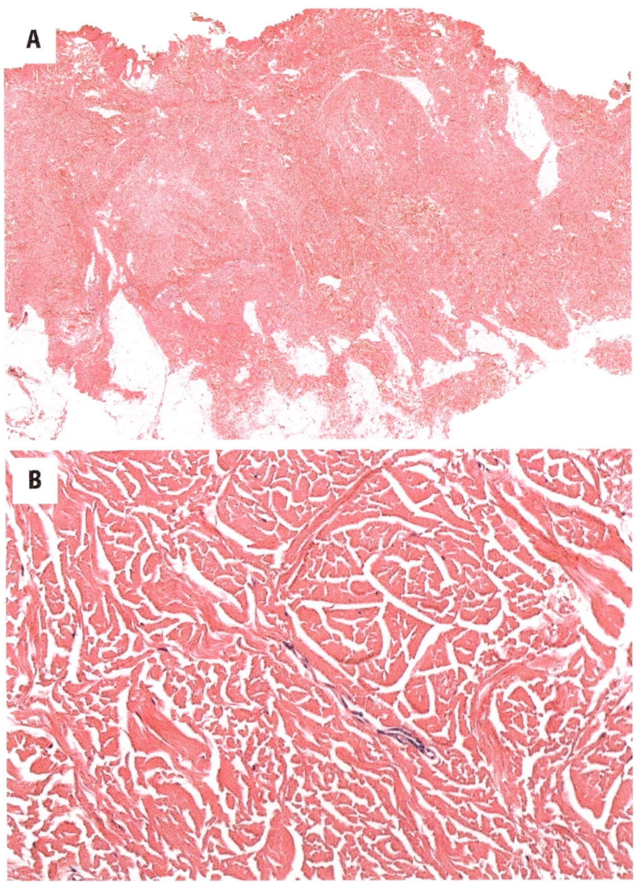

FIG. 14.22

Nuchal-type fibroma. **A,** A paucicellular, poorly circumscribed lesion containing haphazardly arranged thick collagen bundles with a cracking artifact, entrapping adipose tissue. **B,** The lesion is composed of short, widely spaced fibroblasts with small oval nuclei and inconspicuous nucleoli.

Gardner fibromas affect younger patients and have a wider anatomical distribution outside of the upper neck area; these lesions will be positive for β-catenin by IHC. Elastofibroma is a morphologically overlapping lesion that along with coarse bundles of collagen shows distinctive abnormal, fragmented elastic fibers and typically affects the scapular lesion.

Prognosis and Treatment

Nuchal fibroma is benign, with a small risk of local recurrence following an incomplete excision.

ELASTOFIBROMA

Clinical Findings

Elastofibroma is a benign soft tissue pseudotumor with a strong female predilection that typically occurs in the subscapular region of older adults and may be bilateral. Elastofibroma has a strong association with a history of repetitive trauma such as in the setting of intense manual labor.

Histopathologic Features

Elastofibromas are unencapsulated, poorly circumscribed paucicellular lesions composed of bland fibroblasts, thick collagen, and degenerated elastic fibers that have a characteristic serrated and beaded appearance, which can be highlighted with an elastic stain (Fig. 14.23A–C). The stroma is collagenous but may show areas of edema or myxoid change.

Differential Diagnosis

Elastofibroma is often mistaken for normal fibroconnective tissue with edema and scarring and the possibility of a mass-forming lesion is dismissed; therefore, awareness of the characteristic appearance of the elastic fibers in routine histologic sections is important. Nuchal fibroma appears similar at scanning magnification but lacks the degraded elastic fibers. Desmoplastic fibroblastoma, or collagenous fibroma, is a more deeply seated (deep subcutis, fascia, or skeletal muscle) paucicellular collagenous tumor that may appear similar to elastofibroma at low power. However, this tumor has a predilection for male patients, usually affects extremities, and is composed of distinctly different, slightly hyperchromatic

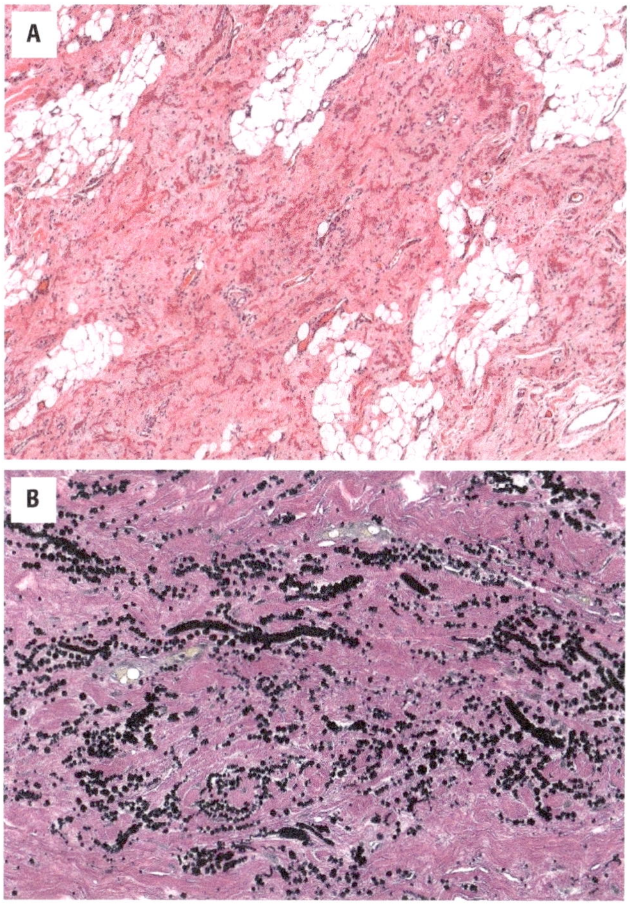

FIG. 14.23
Elastofibroma. **A,** An unencapsulated, poorly circumscribed paucicellular collagenous lesion containing very distinctive serrated degenerated elastic fibers that can be highlighted by elastic stain (**B**).

bipolar or stellate myofibroblasts with small nucleoli (Fig. 14.24). Desmoplastic fibroblastoma lacks distinctive altered elastic fibers. Desmoplastic fibroblastoma is variably positive for SMA and shows recurrent *FOSL1* and *FOS* rearrangements that can be detected using FOSL1 IHC.

Treatment and Prognosis

Elastofibromas are benign and typically do not recur even after an incomplete excision.

SCLEROTIC FIBROMA (STORIFORM COLLAGENOMA)

Clinical Findings

This benign fibrous lesion usually presents in adults as a solitary flesh-colored papule or nodule, most

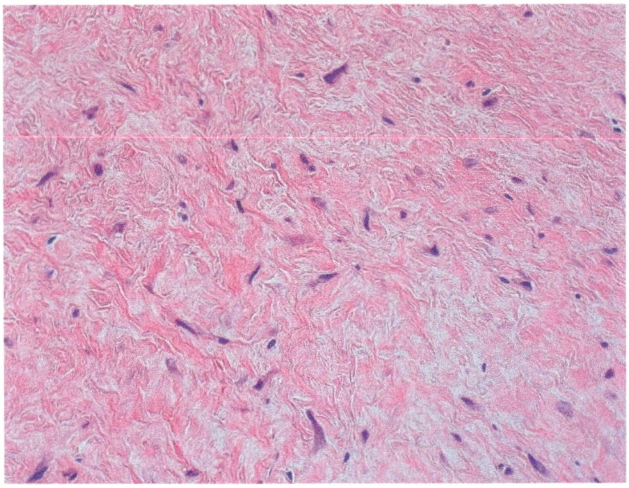

FIG. 14.24
Desmoplastic fibroblastoma composed of slightly hyperchromatic bipolar or stellate myofibroblasts with small nucleoli growing singly in a sclerotic background.

commonly on the arms or head and neck region. Multiple lesions may occur in the setting of phosphatase and tensin homolog (PTEN) hamartoma tumor syndrome including Cowden's syndrome.

Histopathologic Features

Sclerotic fibroma is a paucicellular, sharply circumscribed dermal nodule often with an epidermoid collarette. It is composed of bland spindled to stellate cells growing in a storiform fashion in a dense collagen matrix producing a distinctive wood grain–like or a plywood-like pattern with prominent intervening clefts (Fig. 14.25A and B). Occasional multinucleated cells are present. The spindle cells are diffusely positive for CD34 and variably express SMA, while S100 and EMA are negative.

SCLEROTIC FIBROMA—DISEASE FACT SHEET

Clinical Findings
- Solitary flesh-colored papule on the arms or head and neck
- Multiple lesions in the setting of PTEN hamartoma/Cowden's syndrome

Histopathologic Features
- Circumscribed dermal nodule with an epidermoid collarette
- Storiform spindled to stellate cells in a dense collagen matrix
- Plywood-like pattern with prominent intervening clefts

IHC/Molecular
- Diffuse CD34, variable SMA

Differential Diagnosis
- Soft tissue perineurioma
- Dermatofibroma

IHC, Immunohistochemistry; *PTEN*, phosphatase and tensin homolog; *SMA*, smooth muscle actin.

Differential Diagnosis

The differential diagnosis of sclerotic fibroma includes sclerotic and soft tissue perineurioma, which can also be CD34 positive but is distinguished by expression of markers of perineural differentiation such as EMA, claudin-1, and GLUT1. DF can be distinguished based on the more typical polymorphous appearance due to the mixture of fibrohistiocytic cells, Touton-type giant cells, foamy histiocytes and hemosiderin deposits, and a distinctly different, stellate tumor periphery showing fingerlike entrapment of the dermal collagen. This contrasts with the sharply outlined periphery of the sclerotic fibroma.

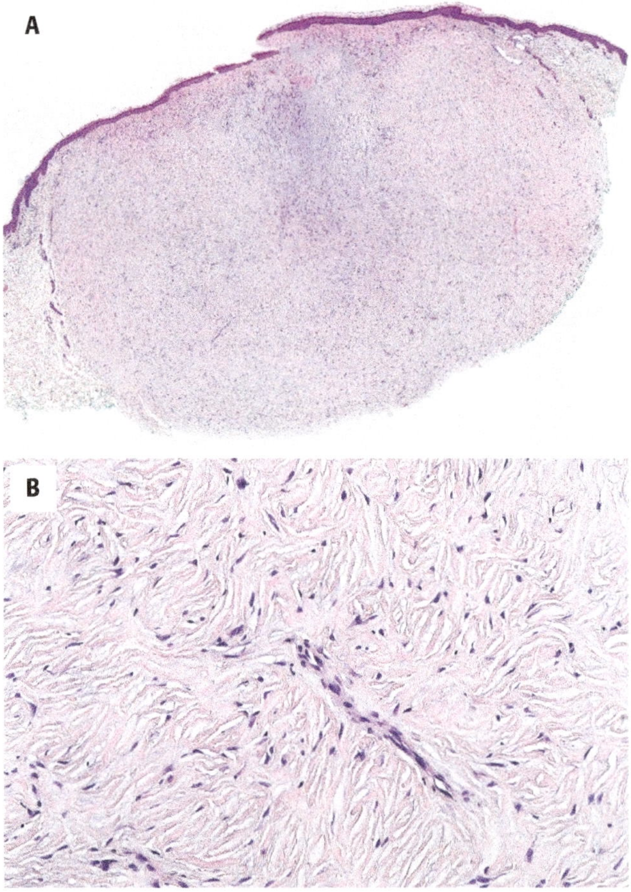

FIG. 14.25
Sclerotic fibroma. **A,** A paucicellular, sharply circumscribed dermal nodule with an epidermoid collarette. **B,** Bland spindled to stellate fibroblasts forming whorls in a densely collagen matrix with prominent intervening clefts imparting a distinctive plywood-like appearance.

Prognosis and Treatment

Sclerotic fibroma is a benign lesion cured by simple excision.

FIBROUS HAMARTOMA OF INFANCY

Clinical Findings

FHI presents as a subcutaneous mass on the trunk or limbs but any site including head and neck, scrotum, and breast has been reported. Mean age at presentation is approximately 15 months; a significant proportion of cases occurs at birth. Boys are affected more frequently than girls.

Histopathologic Features

FHI displays a pathognomonic triphasic morphology consisting of (1) infiltrative fascicles of cytologically bland fibroblastic cells, (2) aggregates of small round to fusiform or stellate primitive mesenchymal cells in a myxoid stroma, and (3) varying amounts of adipose tissue (Fig. 14.26A and B). Recently reported histologic variations include giant cell fibroblastoma-like areas and very rare tumors with sarcomatoid features. By IHC, the spindled fibroblasts are positive for SMA and may show focal CD34 expression, more so in sclerotic areas, while the primitive spindle cell component is negative for these markers. Molecular genetic findings are inconsistent, with some cases showing complex karyotypes and copy number gains, especially in those rare cases with sarcomatoid phenotype; there are no recurrent balanced translocations or diagnostic point mutations.

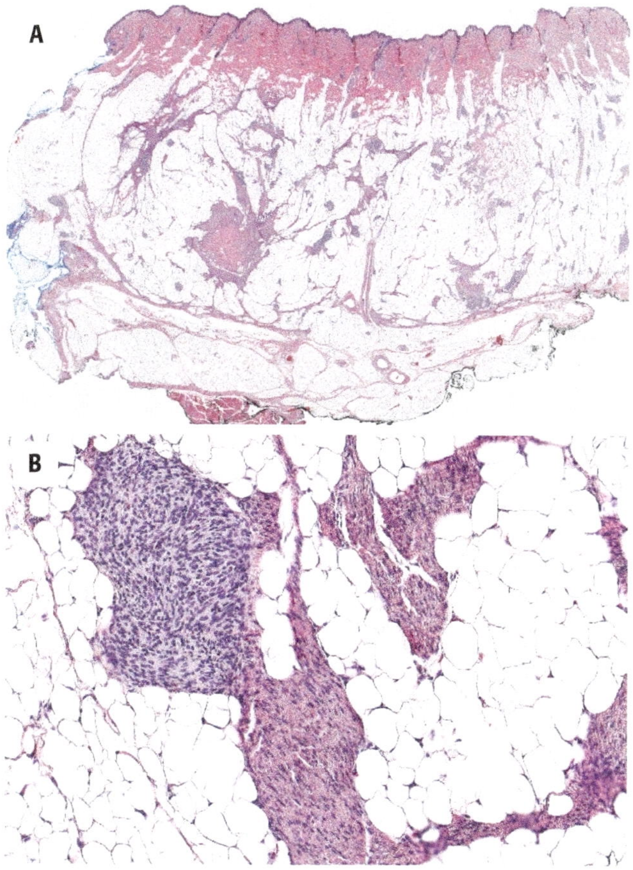

FIG. 14.26

Fibrous hamartoma of infancy. **A,** A dermal and subcutaneous circumscribed but unencapsulated mass. **B,** A pathognomonic triphasic morphology consisting of infiltrative fascicles of cytologically bland fibroblastic cells, basophilic nodules of primitive mesenchymal cells in a myxoid stroma, and mature adipose tissue.

FIBROUS HAMARTOMA OF INFANCY—DISEASE FACT SHEETS

Clinical Findings
- Subcutaneous mass on the trunk, limbs, head and neck
- Infants and children in the first few years of life

Histopathologic Features
- Triphasic morphology
  - Infiltrative fascicles of cytologically bland fibroblastic cells
  - Aggregates of small round or spindled stellate primitive mesenchymal cells in a myxoid stroma
  - Varying amounts of adipose tissue
  - Sarcomatoid features: very rare

IHC/Molecular
- SMA (myofibroblastic pattern); focal CD34 expression
- Primitive spindle cell component is negative for most markers
- No single pathognomonic genetic alteration

Differential Diagnosis
- Fibroblastic connective tissue nevus
- Dermatomyofibroma
- Myofibroma/myofibromatosis
- Lipofibromatosis
- Lipofibromatosis-like neural tumor

SMA, Smooth muscle actin.

Differential Diagnosis

The presence of immature mesenchymal aggregates is distinctive and separates FHI from its closest childhood mimics including FCTN, dermatomyofibroma, desmoid fibromatosis, lipofibromatosis, lipofibromatosis-like neural tumor (LF-NT), and myofibroma/myofibromatosis. Lipofibromatosis presents as an overgrowth syndrome clinically and has only a fibroblastic and an adipocytic component, with characteristic vacuolated "blister" cells at the interface between the two. Desmoid fibromatosis is a solid infiltrative mass of fibroblasts, with a broad, pushing border into the displaced subcutaneous adipose tissue rather than intermingling of various components, and has beta-catenin gene alterations. Myofibroma and myofibromatosis show biphasic architecture with lighter and darker staining myofibroblastic cells, strong expression of SMA, and, in a subset of cases, *RELA* fusions. FCTN and dermatomyofibroma are plaque-like, predominantly dermal lesions (rather than subcutaneous masses), with limited involvement of the subcutis. LF-NT shows a coexpression of CD34 and S100 and has *NTRK1* and related *TRK* family gene fusions.

MYOFIBROBLASTIC TUMORS WITH *USP6* GENE REARRANGEMENT

NODULAR FASCIITIS

Clinical Findings

Nodular fasciitis is a self-limiting neoplasm that presents as a rapidly growing subcutaneous nodule with a predilection for the upper extremities, trunk and head and neck, but it may occur at any anatomic site. All age groups are affected. Antecedent history of trauma is present in the minority of cases.

Histopathologic Features

Most cases are centered in the subcutis, but dermal involvement is common, and rare cases occur primarily in the dermis. Nodular fasciitis is a circumscribed or only focally infiltrative mass composed of spindled myofibroblasts with elongated, tapered nuclei with indistinct eosinophilic cytoplasmic processes growing loosely in a tissue culture–like growth pattern or in vague fascicles. The spindle cells are admixed with scattered lymphocytes and extravasated red blood cells. Most cases show varying cellularity and myxoid stroma, which sometimes shows cystic breakdown, or show keloidal collagen. Numerous plump, reactive-appearing vessels are present (Fig 14.27A and B). Osteoclast-type giant cells, focal aneurysmal bone cyst–like changes, and occasionally, new bone formation can also occur in keeping with the recent observations that nodular fasciitis, aneurysmal bone cyst, and myositis ossificans are related diseases unified by *USP6* gene rearrangements. Involution may result in a paucicellular lesion with hyalinized stroma. Necrosis is rare but should not stop from making the diagnosis in an otherwise classic case. Nuclear pleomorphism is not observed. Mitotic activity is brisk, but atypical mitotic figures are absent. With very rare exceptions that yet need to be further understood, overtly malignant cytologic features with nuclear pleomorphism, coarse chromatin, or large nucleoli are not a feature of nodular fasciitis. By IHC, SMA is expressed in a myofibroblastic pattern while desmin, CD34, S100, SOX10, and cytokeratins are negative. Molecular genetic studies show *USP6* gene fusions, most often with *MYH9* and less commonly, variant partners.

MYOFIBROBLASTIC TUMORS WITH *USP6* REARRANGEMENTS—DISEASE FACT SHEET

Nodular Fasciitis

- Rapidly growing subcutaneous nodule on limbs, trunk, head and neck
- Circumscribed mass with focal infiltration
- Loose myofibroblastic fascicles in a myxoid stroma
- Bland tapered nuclei and eosinophilic cytoplasm, normal mitotic figures
- Keloidal collagen, extravasated red blood cells, osteoclasts
- IHC: SMA in a "tram-track" myofibroblastic pattern
- Differential diagnosis
  - Cellular dermatofibroma/fibrous histiocytoma
  - Fibromatosis
  - Inflammatory myofibroblastic tumor

Fibroma of Tendon Sheath

- Slow-growing nodular mass attached to tendons of hands and feet
- Low or modest cellularity
- Loosely arranged bland myofibroblastic cells in a fibromyxoid stroma
- Crescent-shaped vessels at the periphery
- Bland tapered nuclei and eosinophilic cytoplasm, normal mitotic figures
- IHC: SMA in a "tram-track" myofibroblastic pattern
- *USP6* gene fusions in cellular fibroma of tendon sheath
- Differential diagnosis: superficial fibromatosis

Myositis Ossificans

- Painful enlarging nodule in skeletal muscle or fascia
- Mineralization on imaging
- Fasciitis-like proliferation of mitotically active myofibroblasts
- New bone formation with osteoblastic rimming and gradual maturation
- toward well-formed lamellar bone at the periphery
- Osteoclasts, aneurysmal bone cystlike changes, hyaline cartilage
- IHC: SMA in a "tram-track" myofibroblastic pattern
- Differential diagnosis: osteosarcoma

Fibroosseous Tumor of the Digits

- Small, painful nodule on the proximal phalanx of the fingers and toes
- Mineralization on imaging
- Fasciitis-like myofibroblastic proliferation with haphazard woven bone
- Osteoclasts, aneurysmal bone cystlike changes, hyaline cartilage
- IHC: SMA in a "tram-track" myofibroblastic pattern
- Differential diagnosis
  - Reactive periosteal new bone formation
  - Bizarre parosteal osteochondromatous proliferation
  - Subungual exostosis
  - Osteosarcoma

IHC, Immunohistochemistry; *SMA*, smooth muscle actin.

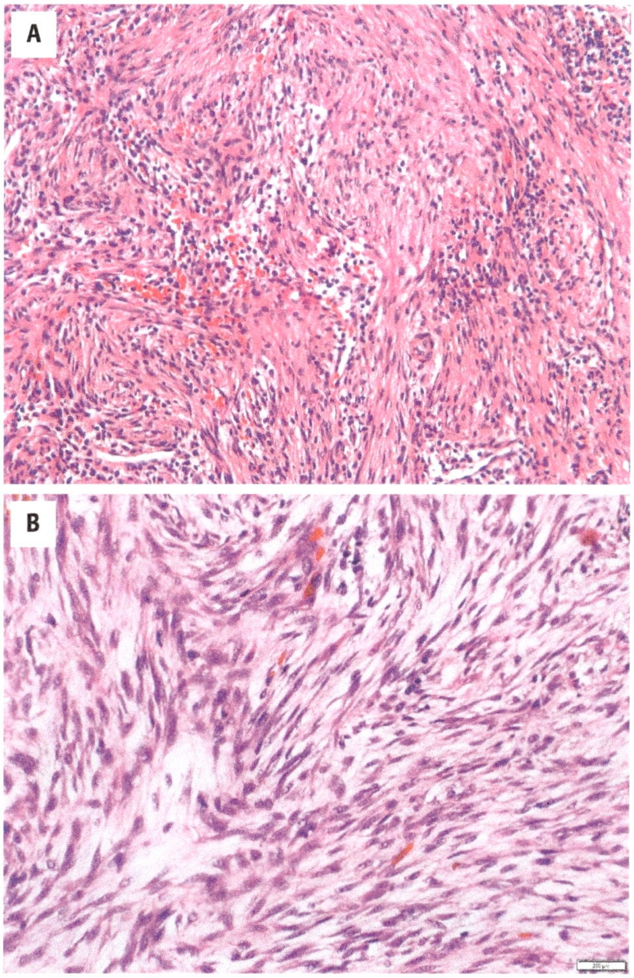

FIG. 14.27

Nodular fasciitis. **A,** Spindled myofibroblasts growing loosely in a tissue culture–like pattern or in vague fascicles in a variably myxoid stroma containing scattered lymphocytes and extravasated red blood cells. **B,** The constituent cells are myofibroblasts with uniform tapered nuclei, fine chromatin, and small nucleoli. Numerous plump, reactive-appearing vessels are present.

FISH testing for *USP6* gene rearrangements is a widely commercially available test.

Differential Diagnosis

Benign cellular FH can look very similar to nodular fasciitis, as both lesions show a focally infiltrative, somewhat stellate edge and myofibroblastic differentiation. Cellular FH shows at least focal peripheral collagen trapping, which is not a feature seen in association with nodular fasciitis, and typically lacks myxoid stroma. Desmoid fibromatosis, also a myofibroblastic proliferation, can show nodular fasciitis-like areas with or without keloidal collagen but can be distinguished by the predominance of long, sweeping fascicles, and a markedly infiltrative edge. Widespread myxoid stroma and microcystic changes are uncharacteristic. In difficult cases, FISH studies *USP6* gene fusion or molecular studies to identify confirmatory features of fibromatosis (exon 3 mutations in *CTNNB1* or alterations of the APC gene) can be performed. IMT can resemble nodular fasciitis but typically is more uniformly cellular tumor lacking significant myxoid stroma or cystic change and has a uniformly brisk lymphoplasmacytic inflammatory infiltrate and, in most cases, a very sharply defined edge. IMT is driven by *ALK* gene fusions with corresponding overexpression of ALK by IHC. Finally, owing to its loosely fascicular architecture and misleading immunophenotype, nodular fasciitis can look very similar to low-grade myofibroblastic sarcoma, spindle cell/sclerosing rhabdomyosarcoma, leiomyosarcoma, and other spindle cell sarcomas as well as sarcomatoid/spindle cell SCC. These lesions are uncommon, requiring a high index of suspicion. With very rare exceptions, cytology is key to distinguish nodular fasciitis from any superficial sarcoma as nuclear pleomorphism, coarse chromatin, prominent nucleoli, or atypical mitotic figures are a feature of nodular fasciitis. Identification of *USP* gene alteration by FISH or reverse transcription polymerase chain reaction (RT-PCR) or robust expression of any lineage-specific markers such as cytokeratins, schwannian (S100, SOX10), melanocytic, or myogenic markers (desmin, h-caldesmon, myogenin, MyoD1) in context of this differential diagnosis will argue against nodular fasciitis.

Prognosis and Treatment

While excision is traditionally performed, nodular fasciitis is an entirely benign, self-limited process that resolves spontaneously and is not expected to recur. Exceptionally rare cases of malignant nodular fasciitis defined by the presence of *USP6* gene rearrangement have been reported to date, and these cases require further study.

FIBROMA OF TENDON SHEATH

Clinical Findings

Fibroma of tendon sheath presents as a slow-growing nodular mass, usually on the hands and feet, firmly attached to the underlying tendon.

Histopathologic Features

Fibroma of tendon sheath is a circumscribed but unencapsulated mass that can be thought of as a paucicellular and more collagenized version of nodular fasciitis. The lesion consists of loosely arranged, cytologically banal myofibroblastic cells with elongated, tapered nuclei and indistinct eosinophilic cytoplasm. These cells are set in a variably myxoid or collagenized background containing characteristic slitlike crescent-shaped reactive vessels, mostly at the periphery of the lesion (Fig. 14.28A and B). More cellular and fascicular examples are indistinguishable from classic nodular fasciitis short of the location. As with all lesions in the *USP6* gene-rearranged tumor family, cellular fibromas of tendon sheath may show osteoclast-type giant cells, aneurysmal bone cyst–like changes and new bone formation. Rarely, degenerative-type nuclear atypia can occur. By IHC, the lesional cells show expression of SMA in a myofibroblastic pattern while desmin, CD34, cytokeratins, S100 and SOX10 are negative. Cellular fibromas of tendon sheath contain *USP6* gene rearrangements and can be regarded essentially as tenosynovial nodular fasciitis.

Differential Diagnosis

Superficial fibromatosis can be distinguished based on the more uniformly cellular, monotonous, and deeply infiltrative fascicles of fibroblastic cells separated by wavy collagen fibers; myxoid stroma is not characteristic. Tenosynovial giant cell tumor (discussed below) has a similar clinical presentation but a completely different histologic composition including epithelioid or plasmacytoid mononuclear cells, osteoclast-type giant cells, lymphocytes, foamy histiocytes, and hemosiderin deposits.

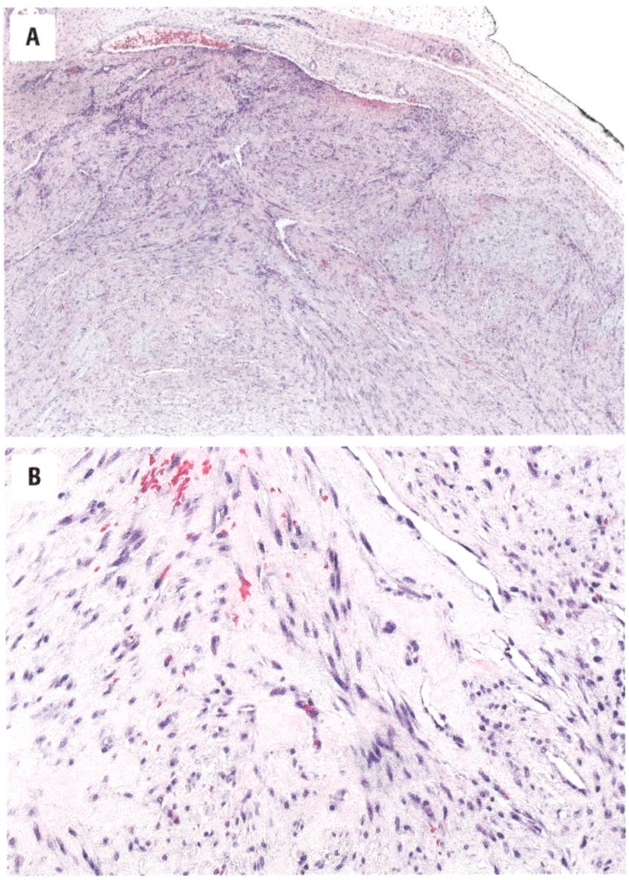

FIG. 14.28
Fibroma of tendon sheath. **A,** A circumscribed but unencapsulated mass with slitlike crescent-shaped reactive vessels. **B,** Fasciitis-like myofibroblastic proliferation with elongated, tapered nuclei and indistinct eosinophilic cytoplasm set in a myxocollagenous stroma.

Prognosis and Treatment

Fibroma is a benign tumor with a tendency for local recurrence (approximately 10% of cases) as they are usually marginally excised.

MYOSITIS OSSIFICANS AND FIBROOSSEOUS TUMOR OF THE DIGITS

Myositis ossificans and fibroosseous tumor of the digits are two other benign, self-limiting neoplasms in the *USP6*-rearranged tumor family that in contrast to classic nodular fasciitis, also feature a prominent component of reactive woven bone.

Clinical Findings

Myositis ossificans presents as a painful enlarging nodule in skeletal muscle, subcutis, or at a level of fascia where it is known as "fasciitis ossificans". Fibroosseous tumor of the digits, originally described under the name "florid reactive periostitis of the tubular bones of the hands and feet" presents as a small, painful nodule on the proximal phalanx of the fingers and toes; there may be an association with repetitive trauma/labor. Radiologic studies, if performed, will show mineralization.

Histopathologic Features

Myositis ossificans and fibroosseous tumor of the digits have the same microscopic appearance characterized by a central fasciitis-like proliferation of mitotically active myofibroblastic cells with tapered nuclei, open chromatin, and wispy eosinophilic cytoplasm transitioning to a zonal pattern of new bone formation with prominent osteoblastic rimming and gradual maturation toward a well-formed lamellar bone at the periphery (Fig. 14.29A–C). In myositis ossificans, the zonation process with time will produce a radiologically distinct zone of peripheral mineralization with central lucency; in fibroosseous tumor of the digits, the woven bone is more haphazardly distributed

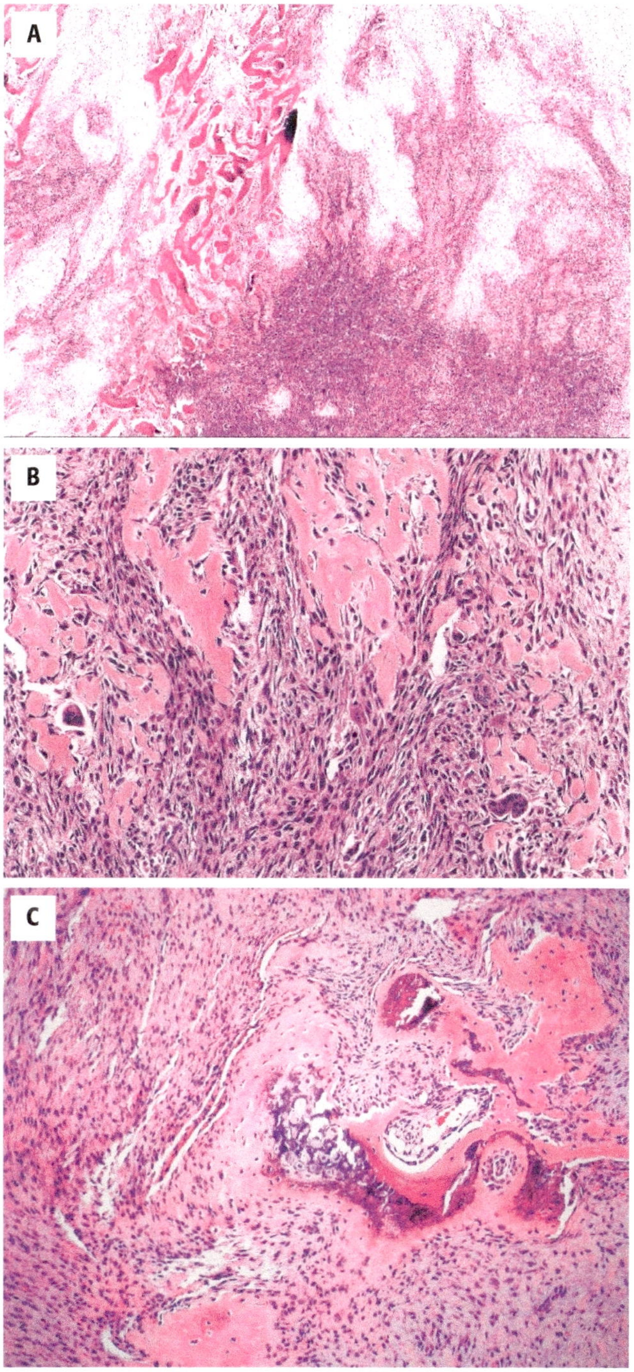

FIG. 14.29

A and **B**, Myositis ossificans showing a fasciitis-like proliferation of myofibroblastic cells with tapered nuclei, open chromatin, and wispy eosinophilic cytoplasm transitioning to a zonal pattern of reactive new bone formation with gradual maturation toward lamellar bone at the periphery. **C**, Fibroosseous tumor of the digits showing haphazardly distributed myofibroblastic and reactive bone components.

throughout the lesion. Osteoclast-type giant cells and aneurysmal bone cystlike changes containing large pools of blood may be present; when the latter feature dominates the histologic features, such cases prompted designation as a "soft tissue aneurysmal bone cyst." Hyaline cartilage undergoing enchondral ossification may be present; such areas closely resemble healing fracture. Long-standing lesions may progress toward a fully mature lamellar bone with little recognizable precursor spindle cell component. Spindle cells express SMA ("tram-track" pattern) and are negative for desmin, S100, CD34, and pan-cytokeratin. FISH or NGS testing will show *USP6* gene rearrangements like those seen in classic nodular fasciitis and aneurysmal bone cyst of the bone.

Differential Diagnosis

Reactive periosteal new bone formation in the setting of long-standing pressure ulcer or trauma lacks the cellular, fasciitis-like component and aneurysmal bone cyst-like changes. Extraskeletal or metastatic osteosarcoma can be distinguished based on the haphazardly distributed neoplastic osteoid that rarely exhibits significant maturation or a zonal distribution, and the overt cytologic atypia and pleomorphism of the constituent spindle cells. The differential diagnosis of fibroosseous tumor of the digits includes two other lesions frequently affecting phalanges: subungual exostosis and a bizarre parosteal osteochondromatous proliferation (BPOP or Nora lesion). Subungual exostosis is a benign osteochondroma-like soft tissue tumor that arises from the periosteum of the subungual region of the distal phalanx. Subungual exostosis is usually less cellular, has a characteristic radiologic appearance, and often includes a prominent cartilaginous cap while the cellular, fasciitis-like areas seen in fibroosseous tumor of the digit are uncharacteristic. The signature characteristic of BPOP is the presence of haphazardly arranged irregular islands of hyaline cartilage with clusters of enlarged, atypical and often binucleated chondrocytes. The cartilage undergoes enchondral ossification and produces a characteristic basophilic stroma. The spindle cell component of BPOP can resemble fibroosseous tumor of the digits; however, the cartilage in the latter lesion is generally infrequent, and atypical cartilage is not a feature.

Prognosis and Treatment

Both lesions are benign, with a very low risk of local recurrence following simple excision.

PROLIFERATIVE FASCIITIS AND PROLIFERATIVE MYOSITIS

Clinical Findings

Proliferative fasciitis is very similar in its clinical manifestation to nodular fasciitis but tends to affect slightly older patients. It tends to occur as a subcutaneous mass at sites of trauma on the extremities, especially the forearm, and is usually less than 5 cm in size. A similar lesion at the level of skeletal muscle is termed proliferative myositis.

Histopathologic Features

Proliferative fasciitis has a less circumscribed, more infiltrative pattern of growth and can mimic sarcoma at scanning magnification. The lesion consists of cytologically banal fasciitis-like fibroblastic cells growing in a loose, tissue culture–like pattern in a myxoid or collagenous background. The hallmark of proliferative fasciitis is the presence of large, plasmacytoid myofibroblasts with eccentric nuclei, prominent nucleoli, and abundant eosinophilic cytoplasm that resemble ganglion cells. The hallmark of proliferative fasciitis is ganglion-like myofibroblasts characterized by their large vesicular nuclei, prominent nucleoli, and abundant cytoplasm (Fig. 14.30A and B). These cells are typically absent in nodular fasciitis. Pediatric cases of proliferative fasciitis may be almost exclusively composed of these ganglion-like cells and show greater cytologic atypia and even focal necrosis, mimicking a malignant neoplasm. By IHC, the spindled and ganglion-like cells are positive for SMA reflecting their myofibroblastic differentiation; CD34, cytokeratin, desmin, and S100 protein are typically negative. Molecular studies showed *FOS* gene rearrangements that can be detected by FISH, NGS or with the use of c-FOS antibody; in contrast to nodular fasciitis, *USP6* gene rearrangements are not identified.

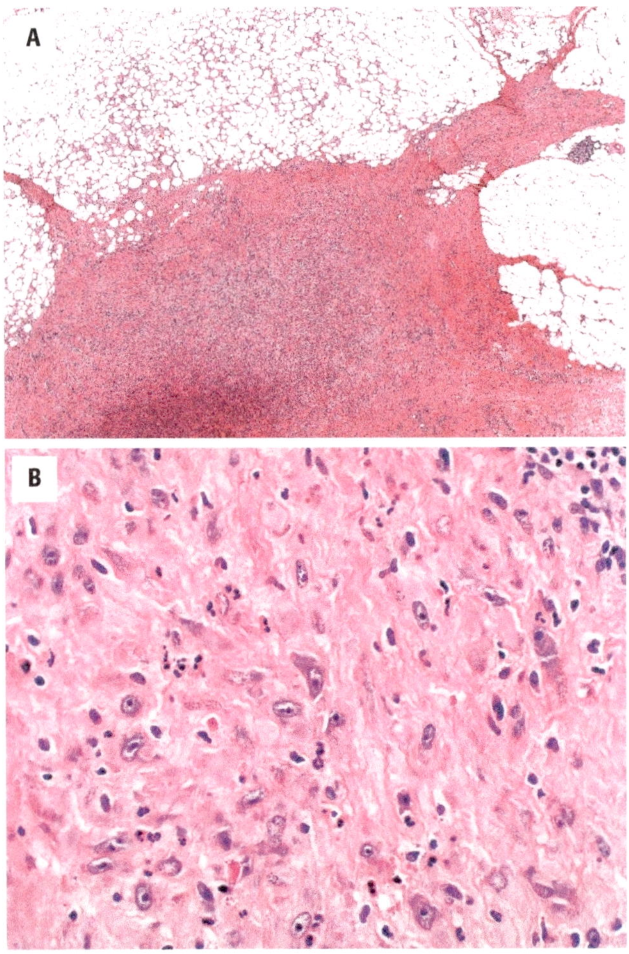

FIG. 14.30

Proliferative fasciitis. **A,** A somewhat infiltrative mass-like process in the subcutaneous adipose tissue. **B,** Ganglion-like large, plasmacytoid myofibroblasts with eccentric nuclei and prominent nucleoli growing loosely in a fibromyxoid stroma.

Differential Diagnosis

Because of the infiltrative edge and large ganglion-like myofibroblasts, the differential diagnosis usually includes sarcomas with epithelioid or epithelioid and pleomorphic morphology, especially pleomorphic or epithelioid rhabdomyosarcoma, epithelioid sarcoma, myxofibrosarcoma as well as true epithelial and melanocytic neoplasms. Coarse chromatin, nuclear pleomorphism, and atypical mitotic figures in context of this differential diagnosis argue against proliferative fasciitis. Application of lineage-specific markers can resolve the above differential diagnosis. The differential diagnosis with inflammatory myofibroblastic sarcoma (MIFS) is more problematic as both tumors can show similar ganglion-like cells. MIFS is very ill-defined tumor with a deeply infiltrative edge that extends far beyond the gross boundaries of the lesion. In difficult cases, identification of *BRAF* or *VGLL3* gene alterations present in MIFS or *FOS* gene rearrangements in proliferative fasciitis may help.

Prognosis and Treatment

Proliferative fasciitis is self-limiting process that recurs very rarely and requires no therapy.

PERICYTIC (PERIVASCULAR) TUMORS

This family of tumors includes myofibroma(tosis), myopericytoma, glomus tumor, and angioleiomyoma, which form a morphologic continuum characterized by a distinctive perivascular growth of myoid cells and point mutations in *PDGFRB* or *NOTCH* (*NOTCH1*, *NOTCH2*, and *NOTCH3*) family gene fusions to *CARMN* (microRNA-143 and microRNA-145). While each lesion has distinctive features, many cases have combined morphology. An emerging group within this category is *GLI1*-altered neoplasms, including pericytoma with t(7;12) and *ACTB::GLI1* fusion and nested glomoid tumor with *GLI1* fusions and amplifications. *GLI1*-altered neoplasms occur in superficial, deep, and visceral locations and are beyond the scope of this chapter.

MYOFIBROMA AND CELLULAR MYOFIBROMA WITH *RELA* FUSIONS

Clinical Findings

Myofibroma(tosis) belongs to a family of pericytic/perivascular tumors and forms a morphologic spectrum with myopericytomas and glomus tumors. Myofibromas usually appear in the first 2 years of life but can arise in adults, often with a male predominance. Tumors arise as solitary nodules in the skin and subcutis, most frequently in the head and neck followed by trunk and limbs. Myofibromatosis presents as multifocal infiltrative masses, almost exclusively in infants and very young children, and may also involve skeletal muscle, bone, or visceral organs. Tumors involving the skin often have a violaceous appearance that may be clinically mistaken for a vascular neoplasm.

MYOFIBROMA—DISEASE FACT SHEET

Clinical Findings

- ▸▸ Solitary myofibroma
  - Solitary nodule in the head and neck, trunk, limbs
  - Children and adults
- ▸▸ Myofibromatosis
  - Multifocal infiltrative masses in infants and children
  - Skin, subcutis, skeletal muscle, bone and viscera

Histopathologic Features

- ▸▸ Myofibroma
  - Well-circumscribed nodule
  - Biphasic architecture: small, spindled cells surrounding HPC-like vessels alternating with nodules of myoid cells with elongated nuclei and eosinophilic cytoplasm
- ▸▸ Cellular myofibroma
  - Increased cellularity, fascicular growth pattern, mitotic activity
  - Ischemic necrosis
- ▸▸ Myofibromatosis
  - Infiltrative cellular fascicles making biphasic architecture less apparent
  - Increased mitotic activity and areas of ischemic-type necrosis

IHC/Molecular

- ▸▸ Positive SMA, h-caldesmon; negative desmin; cellular myofibroma is positive for desmin
- ▸▸ Myofibroma and myofibromatosis: somatic point mutations in *PDGFRB* and *NOTCH3*
- ▸▸ Cellular myofibroma: *SRF::RELA* fusions

Differential Diagnosis

- ▸▸ Nodular fasciitis
- ▸▸ Desmoid fibromatosis
- ▸▸ Low-grade spindle cell sarcoma

IHC, Immunohistochemistry; *SMA*, smooth muscle actin.

Histopathologic Features

Myofibromas are well-circumscribed and nodular/lobular with a distinctive biphasic growth pattern. The lesion contains immature appearing, plump spindled cells surrounding branching, hemangiopericytoma-like vessels; these areas alternate with fascicles and bundles of larger, myoid-like cells with elongated nuclei and eosinophilic cytoplasm, set in a variably myxoid or hyalinized stroma (Fig. 14.31A). Variable mitoses are present. Cellular myofibromas and infantile myofibromatosis are more infiltrative tumors, with increased cellularity and fascicular growth pattern that makes the biphasic architecture less apparent. Cellular myofibromas more often show atypical features including increased mitotic activity and areas of ischemic-type necrosis but lack pleomorphism, atypical mitotic figures, and tumor coagulative necrosis (Fig. 14.31B and C). Tumor cells are positive for SMA, MSA, and h-caldesmon and typically negative for desmin, except for the newly characterized cellular variant, which can show diffuse desmin expression. CD34, myogenin, S100, and cytokeratins are negative. Molecular studies identified somatic point mutations *PDGFRB* and *NOTCH3* in myofibromas and germline alterations in these genes in familial forms of myofibromatosis. Cellular myofibromas show recurrent gene fusions, with *SRF::RELA* fusions being the most common, and combined with the more prominently fascicular morphology, likely represent a distinct entity from the rest of the tumors in this family.

Differential Diagnosis

The differential diagnosis varies depending on which component is most prominent. Tumors with a prominent fascicular myoid component need to be distinguished from nodular fasciitis, cellular DF, leiomyoma, desmoid-type fibromatosis, low-grade myofibroblastic sarcoma, and leiomyosarcoma. While all these lesions will express SMA, none shows biphasic architecture and hemangiopericytoma-like vessels, which help to identify a myofibroma. When the hemangiopericytoma-like areas dominate, the differential diagnosis includes myopericytoma, solitary fibrous tumor (SFT), glomus tumor and, in particular, cellular examples, SS. Myopericytoma may represent a morphologic continuum with a myofibroma but is often intravascular, lacks the biphasic appearance, and shows a rather whorled arrangement of the lesional myoid cells around staghorn vessels. SFT can be distinguished based on the characteristic expression of CD34 and STAT6. SS typically shows a greater degree of cellularity, monotonous fascicular arrangement, more overt nuclear atypia, and brisk mitotic activity—features not encountered in a myofibroma. FISH or NGS testing to identify the pathognomonic

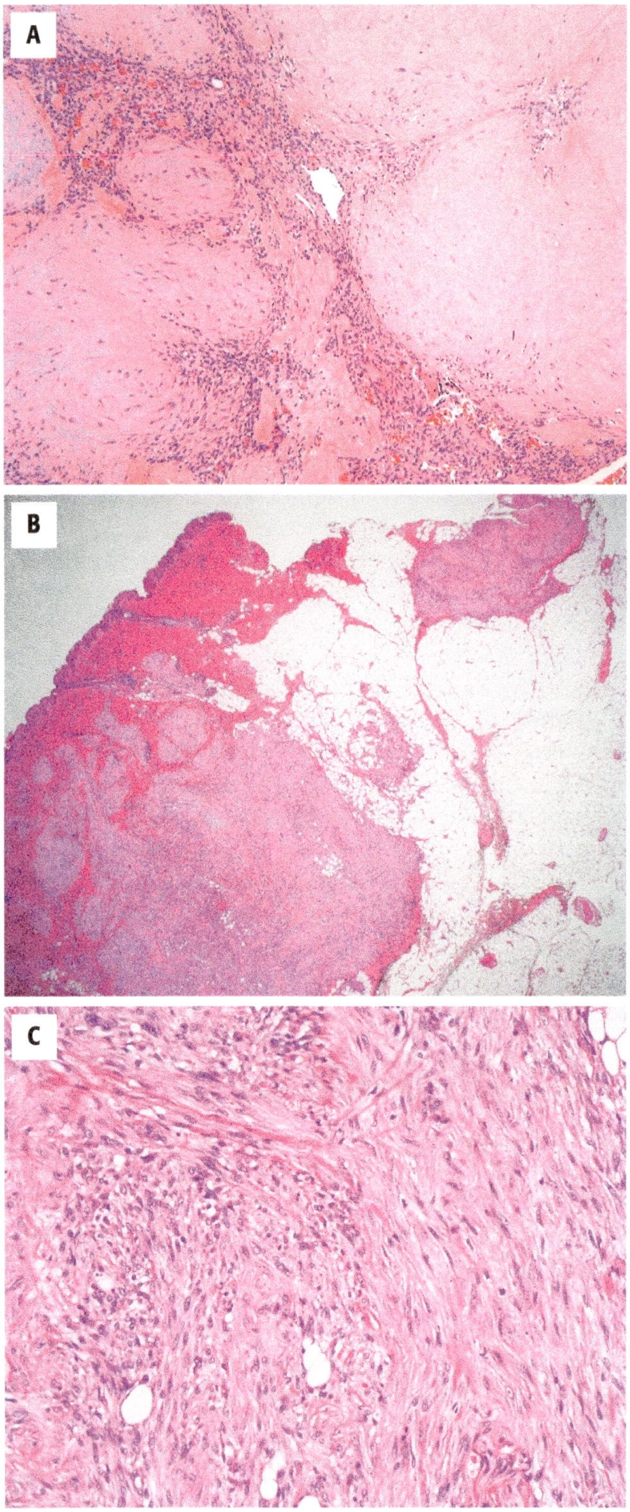

FIG. 14.31

A, Solitary myofibroma. A circumscribed biphasic mass with an immature small spindle cell component containing HPC-like vessels alternating with nodules and fascicles of larger, myoid-like cells with elongated nuclei and eosinophilic cytoplasm. **B,** Infantile myofibromatosis showing an infiltrative multinodular growth. **C,** Increased cellularity, fascicle formation, and mitotic activity with frequent loss of biphasic architecture are characteristic of both infantile myofibromatosis and cellular myofibromas.

SS18::SSX1, *SS18::SSX2*, or *SS18::SSX4* gene fusions or IHC for SS18-SSX fusion-specific antibody (E9X9V) and an SSX-specific antibody (E5A2C, directed at the C terminus of SSX) is diagnostic of SS. Cellular myofibromas may be confused with low-grade leiomyosarcoma, which shows elongated nuclei with hyperchromasia and pleomorphism and which expresses desmin, or low-grade myofibroblastic sarcoma, which displays cytologic atypia. Identification of *PDGFRB* mutation (seen in myofibroma and myofibromatosis) and *SRF::RELA* fusion in cellular myofibroma would help in discriminating it from these mimics.

Prognosis and Treatment

Solitary myofibromas often spontaneously resolve and do not recur after conservative excision. Infantile myofibromatosis can be life threatening. Cellular myofibromas can have atypical features that do not appear to adversely affect outcome. Given the gain of function *PDGFRB* alterations seen in severe multicentric myofibromatosis, tyrosine kinase inhibitors (imatinib) may be therapeutically beneficial.

MYOPERICYTOMA

Clinical Findings

Myopericytoma manifests as a slowly growing and often painful dermal or subcutaneous nodule on the extremities of the adults. It shows differentiation toward perivascular myoid cells and forms a morphologic spectrum with myofibroma.

Histopathologic Features

Myopericytoma is a well-circumscribed, multinodular and often entirely intravascular tumor composed of plump myoid cells with oval, bland nuclei and eosinophilic cytoplasm arranged in a prominently concentric fashion around blood vessels (Fig. 14.32A and B). Another common pattern is a so-called cavernous pattern with whorled or streaming growth around ectatic or hemangiopericytomatous vessels (Fig. 14.32C). Similar to myofibroma, a multifocal intravascular or perivascular growth may occur (myopericytomatosis), and very rare cases may show fascicular growth pattern, marked mitotic activity, cytologic atypia, and pleomorphism justifying classification as malignant myopericytoma. Such cases maintain the perivascular growth pattern and may show focal areas of a more conventional myopericytoma. The spindle cells are positive for SMA and h-caldesmon and negative for CD34, desmin, S100, SOX10, cytokeratin,

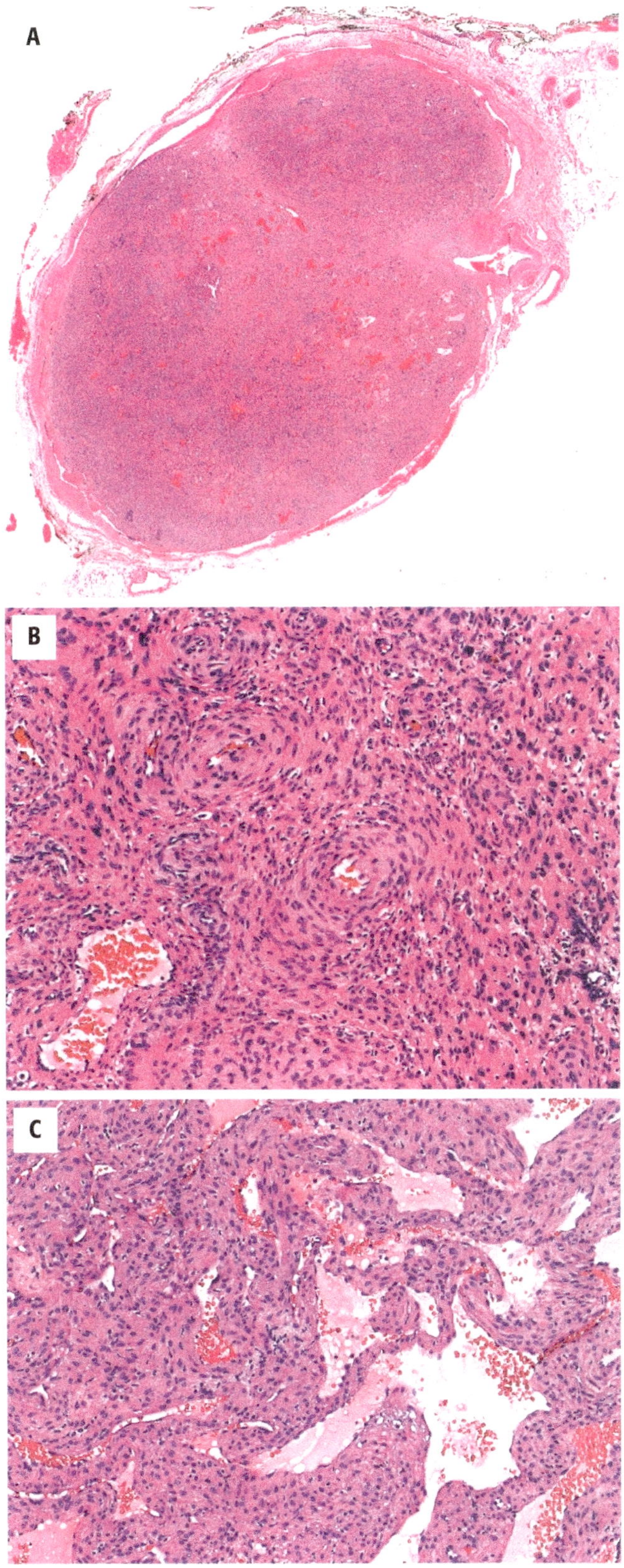

FIG. 14.32

Myopericytoma. **A** and **B,** A well-circumscribed intravascular tumor composed of plump myoid cells with oval, bland nuclei and eosinophilic cytoplasm arranged in a prominently concentric fashion around blood vessels. **C,** A "cavernous pattern" with prominent ectatic or hemangiopericytomatous vessels.

and STAT6. Like other entities in the pericytic tumor family, *PDGFRB* and *NOTCH3* alterations may occur in solitary myopericytomas and myopericytomatosis.

Differential Diagnosis

Myofibroma may be distinguished based on a biphasic appearance (nodules of eosinophilic myoid cells in a myxohyaline stroma juxtaposed on hemangiopericytoma-like areas). Glomus tumor will show very similar vasculature, but the myoid cells are cuboidal in shape with round, completely uniform nuclei and sharply outlined cytoplasmic borders, in contrast to the spindle cells with indistinct borders in myopericytoma. Angioleiomyoma and myopericytoma may be particularly difficult to distinguish; an easy way to think about it is that angioleiomyoma has a fully developed smooth muscle phenotype, with densely eosinophilic cytoplasm, sharp cytoplasmic borders, and desmin expression, which is not typically seen in tumors with a more pericytic phenotype, such as myofibroma and myopericytoma. SFT can be distinguished based on the characteristic expression of CD34 and STAT6. Atypical and malignant myopericytoma may be confused with SS; the latter can be distinguished based on cytokeratin immunoreactivity, FISH or NGS testing for the pathognomonic *SS18::SSX1*, *SS18::SSX2*, or *SS18::SSX4* gene fusions or IHC for SS18-SSX fusion-specific antibody (E9X9V) and an SSX C-terminus–specific antibody E5A2C.

Prognosis and Treatment

Because of the intravascular growth and multifocality, myopericytoma is more prone to local recurrence than other tumors in this family, with the conservative excision remaining the treatment mainstay.

ANGIOLEIOMYOMA

Clinical Findings

Angioleiomyoma presents as a subcutaneous, classically painful nodule around ankles and feet and, less often, head and neck region of middle-aged adults. They are typically small.

Histopathologic Features

Angioleiomyoma is a well-circumscribed nodule composed of bundles of well-differentiated smooth muscle arranged concentrically or radially around variably sized blood vessels which may be slitlike, venous (with well-developed thick smooth muscle wall), or ectatic and branching reminiscent of some examples of myopericytoma (Fig. 14.33A and B). The nuclear features are very bland, and mitotic figures are rare. Myxoid change, thrombosis, and dystrophic calcifications may occur. The tumor cells are positive for SMA, calponin, and h-caldesmon and will typically show desmin expression, in keeping with the more fully developed smooth muscle phenotype in contrast to myofibromas, myopericytomas, and glomus tumors. Like other entities in the pericytic tumor family, *PDGFRB* and *NOTCH* alterations may occur.

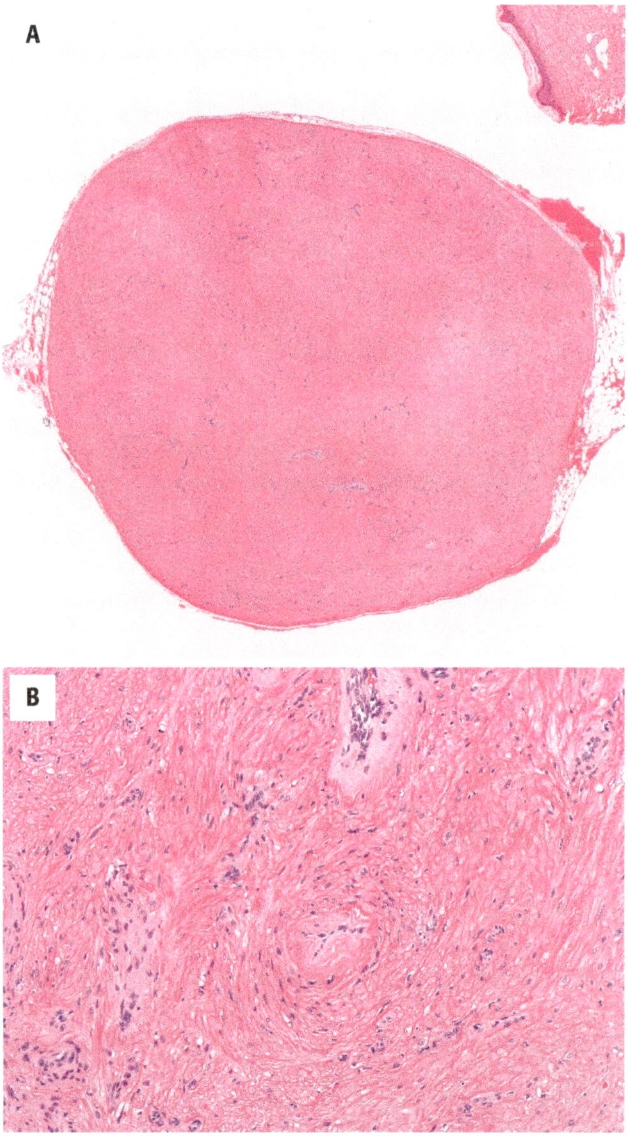

FIG. 14.33

Angioleiomyoma. **A,** A well-circumscribed subcutaneous eosinophilic nodule. **B,** Bundles of well-differentiated, bland smooth muscle arranged concentrically or radially around prominent blood vessels.

Differential Diagnosis

Pilar and nipple leiomyomas are typically dermis-based, symmetric but not circumscribed and consist of discontinuous intersecting bundles of banal smooth muscle each resembling pilar smooth muscle. The vascular pattern is not prominent. Most tumors that are labeled generically as "leiomyoma" the skin represent either a pilar leiomyoma or an angioleiomyoma. The distinction from myopericytoma may be impractical since these tumors represent a histologic spectrum. Cutaneous perivascular epithelioid cell tumor (PEComa) can be distinguished based on the perivascular or solid growth of predominantly epithelioid cells with clear cytoplasm, round nucleus, and small nucleolus, and a coexpression of melanocytic markers such as HMB45, MART, Melan-A, and less commonly, S100. Leiomyosarcomas of either pilar or subcutaneous vascular origin can be distinguished based on the presence of readily appreciable nuclear hyperchromasia, mitotic activity, and infiltrative growth pattern.

Prognosis and Treatment

Angioleiomyomas are benign and cured by simple local excision. Recurrences are rare.

GLOMUS TUMOR AND GLOMUVENOUS MALFORMATION

Clinical Findings

Glomus tumors classically present as small painful nailbed-based nodules in adult patients, although they can present as relatively large (up to 3 to 5 cm or more) painless subcutaneous masses at other sites including proximal extremities, trunk, or even visceral locations, of which the most famous is the GE junction. Glomuvenous malformation (formerly known as glomangioma) presents as multifocal, blanching irregular vascular stain, nodule, or plaque, involving limbs and trunk. This condition is due to a loss-of-function mutation in *GLMN* (glomulin) gene, with an autosomal dominant pattern of inheritance.

Histopathologic Features

Glomus tumors are circumscribed lesions composed of strikingly uniform, eosinophilic cuboidal cells with very uniform bland nuclei, surrounding branching or

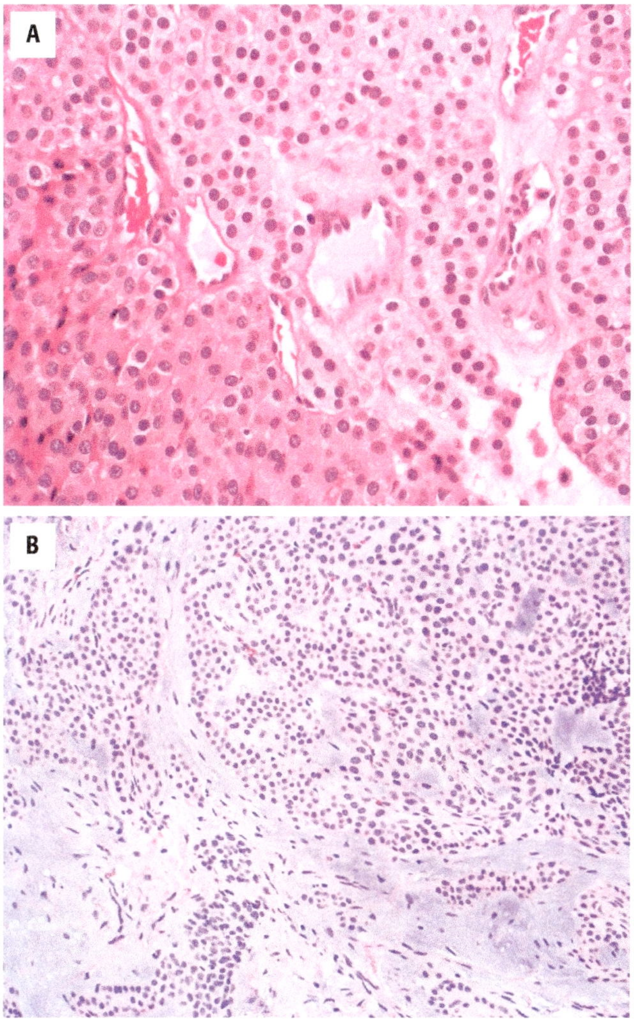

FIG. 14.34

Glomus tumor. **A,** Uniform, eosinophilic cuboidal cells with round nuclei, surrounding branching or slitlike vessels. **B,** Myxoid stroma is relatively common and can mimic adnexal neoplasms.

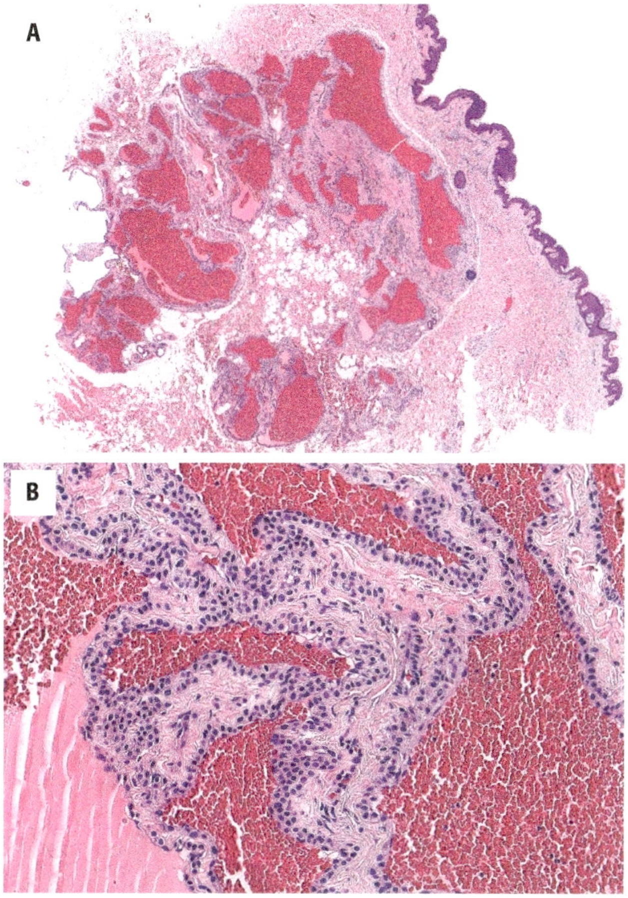

FIG. 14.35

A and **B,** Glomuvenous malformation consisting of large, dilated veins lined by a thin layer of glomus cells.

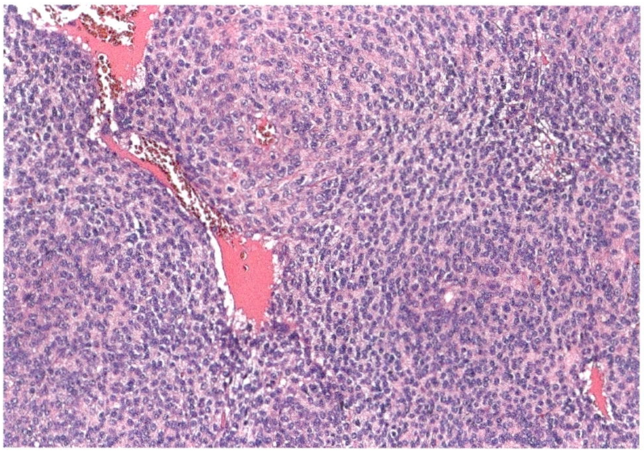

FIG. 14.36

Malignant glomus tumor with increased cellularity and sheets of atypical round cells with brisk mitotic activity. The overall monotonous architecture with perivascular growth pattern is still recognizable.

slitlike vessels. These cells differentiate toward a specialized perivascular myoid cell of the glomus body, responsible for thermoregulation. Myxoid stroma is relatively common (Fig. 14.34A and B). Cytologic atypia and mitotic activity are virtually nonexistent except of occasional degenerative-type atypia (so-called symplastic glomus tumor). Glomuvenous malformations are less circumscribed and show large, dilated veins lined by a thin layer of glomus cells, imparting the appearance of a venous malformation at scanning magnification (Fig. 14.35A and B). Rare glomus tumors with a substantial smooth muscle component are termed glomangiomyomas. Malignant glomus tumors are very rare, typically occur in the setting of a large deep soft tissue mass or a known long-standing benign precursor and can be recognized based on two patterns: an architecturally conventional glomus tumor but with increased cellularity and sheets of atypical round cells with brisk mitotic activity, atypical mitotic figures and/or necrosis or a conventional glomus tumor transitioning into a frank pleomorphic or spindle cell sarcoma (Fig. 14.36). Established criteria for malignancy include marked nuclear atypia, mitotic count >5/50 high-power fields

(HPF), atypical mitotic figures, and large size and deep location. Glomus cells can be highlighted by SMA, calponin, and collagen type IV, which shows a distinctive net-like pattern of basement membrane accentuation. Cytokeratins, S100, desmin, CD34, CD31, and ERG are negative. Malignant glomus tumors still maintain some SMA and collagen type IV expression, although it may be focal. Sporadic glomus tumors have *CARMN::NOTCH* fusions and *PDGFRB* gene alterations, while *GLMN* mutations characterize glomuvenous malformations. A subset of malignant glomus tumors may show BRAFV600E mutations, *ATRX* loss, or *CDKN2A* deletions.

Differential Diagnosis

The diagnosis of conventional glomus tumor is usually straightforward. Cases with prevalent myxoid stroma can be confused with benign adnexal tumors such as spiradenoma, hidradenoma, or mixed tumor (chondroid syringoma). A simple cytokeratin stain resolves the problem. Glomuvenous malformations may be mistaken for a hemangioma or a venous malformation because of their prominent dilated vascular component, including bona fide large veins, and more subtle investment of glomus cells. Recognition of the distinctive clinical picture is helpful. Malignant glomus tumor needs to be taken through a spindle or pleomorphic cell sarcoma algorithm with exclusion of rhabdomyosarcoma (positive for desmin, myogenin, MyoD1), leiomyosarcoma (coexpression of desmin and SMA), and undifferentiated round cell sarcomas (Ewing sarcoma and variant round cell sarcomas, poorly differentiated SS, malignant SFT) by application of C99, cytokeratins, EMA, STAT6, and appropriate genetic studies, which, depending on the platform, may also identify a *NOTCH3* mutation.

FIBROBLASTIC AND MYOFIBROBLASTIC TUMORS WITH *RB1* DELETION

Tumors in this section share histopathologic features, which include dermal/subcutaneous location, the presence of spindled or pleomorphic (myo)fibroblasts admixed with thick collagen bundles, frequent presence of mast cells, robust CD34 immunoreactivity, and a variable adipocytic component. Genetically, they show a high frequency of somatic Retinoblastoma 1 (*RB1*) deletions on 13q14.2, indicating that RB1 loss is involved in pathogenesis. This alteration can be detected as a loss of nuclear expression with RB1 antibody. Fibroblastic tumors are covered here while lipomatous tumors (spindle cell and pleomorphic lipoma, atypical spindle cell/pleomorphic lipomatous tumor, and pleomorphic liposarcoma) are discussed further in the chapter. Superficial angiofibroma, another neoplasm in this tumor spectrum occurs in vulvovaginal region in female patients or anogenital or scrotal lesion in men.

PLEOMORPHIC FIBROMA

Clinical Findings

A solitary, slow-growing dome-shaped papule affecting extremities followed by the trunk and head and neck in adult patients. Clinically, they can resemble a skin tag, a nevus, or a neurofibroma.

MYOFIBROBLASTIC TUMORS WITH *RB1* DELETION—DISEASE FACT SHEET

Pleomorphic Fibroma

- ►► Clinical findings
  - Solitary dome-shaped papule on limbs, trunk, head and neck of adults
- ►► Histopathologic features
  - Scattered spindled, stellate, and pleomorphic fibroblasts and multinucleated giant cells
  - Densely collagenous stroma without adnexal structures
- ►► IHC/molecular
  - CD34, SMA positive, loss of nuclear expression of RB1
  - *RB1* deletions on 13q14.2
- ►► Differential diagnosis
  - Atypical fibroxanthoma
  - Atypical fibrous histiocytoma

Myofibroblastoma

- ►► Clinical findings
  - Subcutaneous mass in the breast, groin, axilla, trunk in adults
- ►► Histopathologic features
  - Short spindle cells arranged in somewhat parallel fascicles
  - Thick, keloid-like, or ropey collagen fibers
  - Interspersed mast cells
  - Variable adipocytic component
- ►► IHC/molecular
  - CD34, variable desmin, SMA, ER/PR, loss of nuclear expression of RB1
  - *RB1* deletions on 13q14.2
- ►► Differential diagnosis
  - Solitary fibrous tumor
  - Schwannoma
  - DFSP

Superficial Acral Fibromyxoma

- ►► Clinical findings
  - Periungual nodule on fingers and toes, or on palms, heels in adult patients
- ►► Histopathologic features
  - Polypoid dermal nodule with infiltration into the subcutis
  - Ill-defined margin, bone involvement possible
  - Spindle or stellate bland fibroblasts growing loosely in vague fascicles in alternating collagenous and myxoid stroma
  - Conspicuous small, regular vessels

- IHC/molecular
  - CD34 positive, SMA and EMA variably positive, loss of nuclear RB1 expression
  - *RB1* deletions on 13q14.2
- Differential diagnosis
  - Acquired digital fibrokeratoma (acral fibrokeratoma)
  - Myxoid nerve sheath tumors
  - Low-grade fibromyxoid sarcoma (LGFMS)
  - *EWSR1-SMAD3* rearranged fibroblastic tumor

DFSP, Dermatofibrosarcoma protuberans; *EMA*, epithelial membrane antigen; *ER*, estrogen receptor; *IHC*, immunohistochemistry; *PR*, progesterone receptor; *SMA*, smooth muscle actin.

Histopathologic Features

Well-circumscribed, polypoid, dermal lesions composed of widely scattered spindled, stellate, and pleomorphic multinucleated giant cells resembling those seen in pleomorphic lipoma (Fig. 14.37A and B). Mitotic figures are rare, and atypical mitotic figures are almost never seen. The stroma is usually densely collagenous, but myxoid change may be seen and rarely is a prominent feature. Adnexal structures are absent. In addition to CD34 expression and loss of RB1 expression, the cells may express SMA. Desmin, cytokeratins, S100, and SOX10 are negative.

Differential Diagnosis

Atypical fibroxanthoma (AFX) is more cellular, has a greater degree of nuclear atypia and conspicuous mitotic activity, and is usually seen on sun-damaged skin of elderly patients. Atypical FH is also more cellular, shows more typical benign FH with peripheral collagen trapping, and is usually CD34-negative. *RB1* loss is not typical for either lesion.

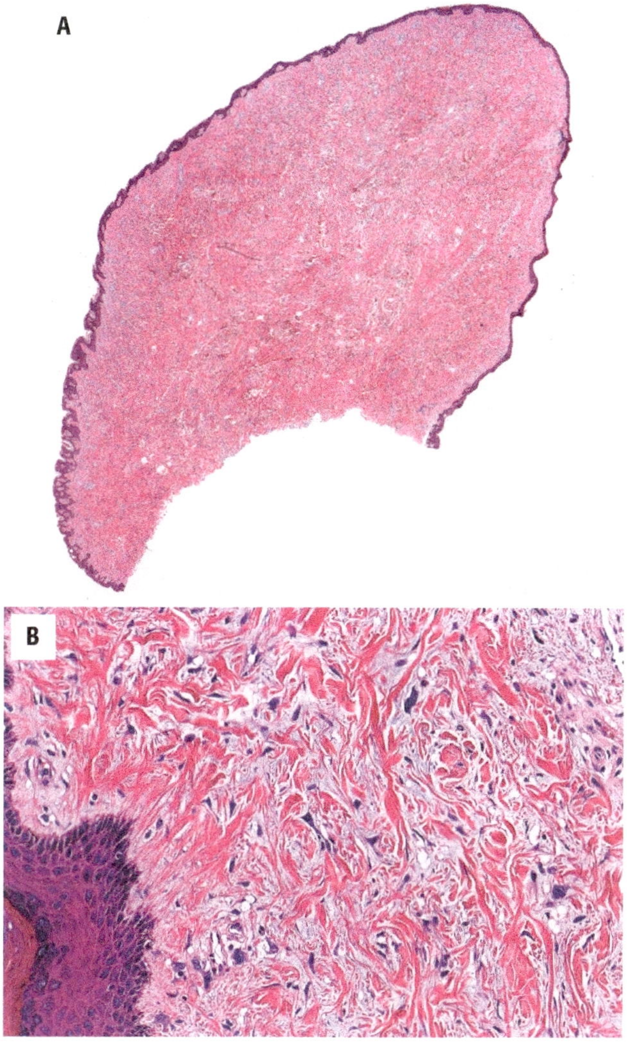

FIG. 14.37

Pleomorphic fibroma. **A,** A well-circumscribed polypoid dermal lesion without adnexal structures. **B,** Stellate fibroblasts and pleomorphic multinucleated giant cells scattered in a densely collagenous stroma.

MYOFIBROBLASTOMA

Clinical Findings

Myofibroblastoma is a benign tumor seen predominantly in middle-aged to elderly patients with a roughly equal incidence in males and females. Myofibroblastoma presents as a painless, slowly growing mobile subcutaneous mass in the breast, the inguinal region and groin, axilla, trunk, and, rarely, the extremities or retroperitoneum.

Histopathologic Features

Myofibroblastomas consist of short spindle cells arranged in somewhat parallel fascicles and interspersed with brightly eosinophilic collagen that can be thick, keloid-like, or thin and "ropey," reminiscent of their close relative, spindle cell lipoma. The spindle cells show ovoid nuclei and pale eosinophilic cytoplasm with indistinct cytoplasmic borders. The vasculature may be inconspicuous or branching resembling SFT (Fig. 14.38A and B). Interspersed mast cells are often present, and chondroid, osseous, or smooth muscle metaplasia may occur. There is no appreciable nuclear atypia above and beyond occasional degenerative changes. Mitotic figures are rare or absent, and there is no necrosis. The adipocytic component is highly variable and can be entirely absent or quite extensive, and such lesions are essentially indistinguishable from spindle cell lipoma. The epithelioid variant of myofibroblastoma is composed of cords, nests, or trabeculae of polygonal or plasmacytoid fibroblastic cells (Fig. 14.38C). Deciduoid, myxoid, leiomyomatous, and palisaded

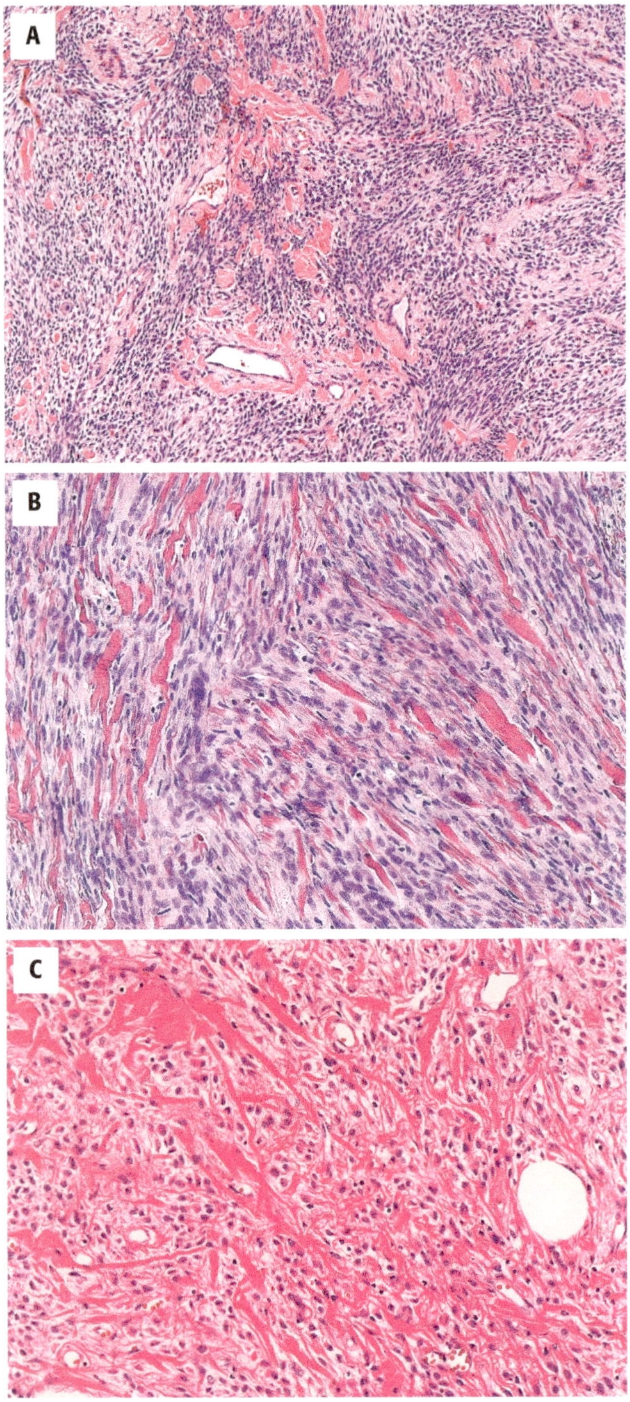

FIG. 14.38
Myofibroblastoma. **A,** Fascicles of short spindle cells interspersed with brightly eosinophilic ropey collagen. **B,** Bland spindle cells with ovoid nuclei and pale eosinophilic cytoplasm with indistinct cytoplasmic borders. **C,** Epithelioid myofibroblastoma composed of cords and trabeculae of polygonal fibroblastic cells.

variants have been described. In addition to CD34 expression and loss of RB1 that characterizes the entire group, myofibroblastoma is often positive estrogen, progesterone, and androgen receptors and, consistent with its myofibroblastic lineage, desmin, SMA, and calponin. S100 expression is rare and SOX10, STAT6, and cytokeratins are negative.

Differential Diagnosis

The differential diagnosis includes other CD34-positive bland fibroblastic tumors. SFT is a particularly close mimic but can be distinguished by positive STAT6 expression. Palisaded myofibroblastoma can mimic schwannomas but can be readily distinguished based on the presence of abundant collagen (collagen is uncommon in schwannomas) and lack of SOX10 expression; likewise, myofibroblastoma with myxoid change can resemble neurofibroma, in which case documentation of schwannian differentiation in a subset of cells by S100 or SOX10 immunostains and entrapped axons by neurofilament is helpful. Distinction from spindle cell lipoma has very little clinical relevance since myofibroblastomas and spindle cell lipomas belong to the same tumor family (based on their shared 13q14 region deletions). A more significant problem is that adipocyte-rich myofibroblastoma may appear rather infiltrative and mimic DFSP. DFSP is also diffusely positive for CD34 but is reliably negative for estrogen and progesterone receptor and does not show RB1 loss by IHC. In problematic cases, testing for the *COL1A1::PDGFRB* fusion (DFSP) may be performed, but this is rarely necessary. Epithelioid myofibroblastoma can mimic an infiltrative carcinoma such as metastatic lobular carcinoma of the breast or gastric signet ring cell carcinoma but can be readily distinguished using cytokeratin immunostaining.

SUPERFICIAL ACRAL FIBROMYXOMA (DIGITAL FIBROMYXOMA)

Clinical Findings

SAF most commonly arises in periungual regions of fingers and toes in adult patients. Rare cases were reported on the palm, heel, and nonacral sites. Clinically, this is a solitary, slow-growing nodule that may be painful.

Histopathologic Features

SAF is centered in the dermis and may abut the epidermis, resulting in a polypoid, exophytic appearance or may infiltrate the subcutaneous adipose tissue. The margins are usually ill defined and rarely, the underlying bone may be involved. Morphologically, it is composed of spindle or stellate cells growing loosely or in a vague fascicular pattern. The stroma characteristically shows alternating myxoid and collagenous areas (Fig. 14.39A–C). The vasculature is conspicuous, showing small, regular vessels. Cytologically, the cells show bland nuclear

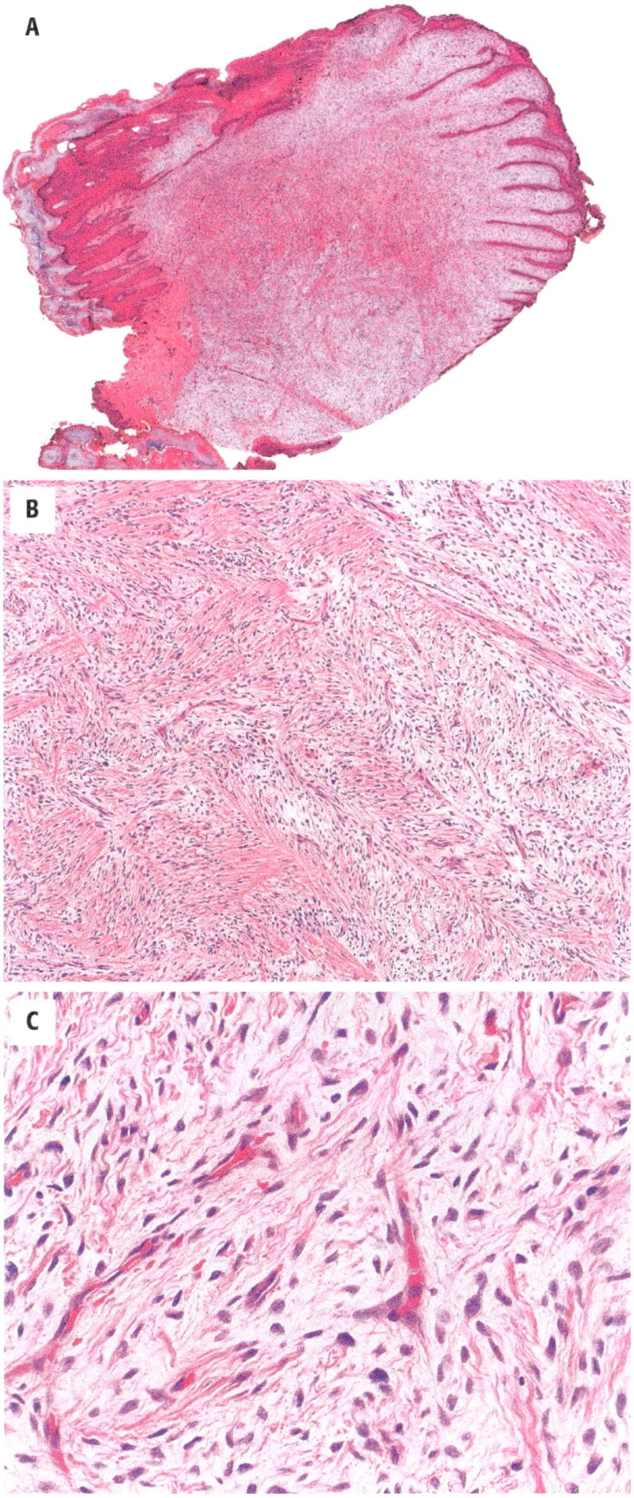

FIG. 14.39

Superficial acral fibromyxoma. **A,** A polypoid lesion centered in the dermis and an infiltrative border with the subcutaneous adipose tissue. **B,** Spindle or stellate cells with bland nuclear features growing loosely or in a vague fascicular pattern interspersed with ropey collagen bundles. The stroma characteristically shows alternating myxoid and collagenous areas. **C,** Conspicuous vessels are present in myxoid zones. Nuclear atypia of the "degenerative" type may occur.

features with small oval nuclei, inconspicuous nucleoli, and amphophilic cytoplasm. Mast cells are present. Nuclear atypia of the "degenerative" type and occasional multinucleated cells as well as cartilaginous and osseous metaplasia were reported. Mitotic figures are usually inconspicuous, and necrosis or vascular invasion is not seen. As is the case with the rest of the tumors in this category, SAF is positive for CD34 and shows loss of RB1 expression. A smaller proportion of cases may express EMA and SMA. S100, desmin, cytokeratins, and MUC4 are negative.

Differential Diagnosis

While several other superficial fibroblastic lesions with myxoid stroma enter the differential diagnosis of SAF, they are very rare at acral sites. Superficial angiomyxoma is more uniformly myxoid and shows conspicuous perivascular inflammatory infiltrates, including neutrophils. Myxoid nerve sheath tumors can be distinguished based on the presence of schwannian cells with hyperchromatic and wavy (neural) nuclei and immunoreactivity for S100 and SOX10. Acquired digital fibrokeratoma (acral fibrokeratoma) has a similar clinical presentation but is a smaller, less cellular, and more heavily collagenized lesion showing vertically oriented sparce spindle cells and collagen bundles. The presence of myxoid stroma and infiltration of subcutis are not typical for acquired digital fibrokeratoma. Low-grade fibromyxoid sarcoma (LGFMS) may occur in superficial locations, although fingers and toes are usually spared but is typically positive for MUC4. Myxoid DFSP may enter the differential diagnosis of SAF based on the presence of diffuse CD34 immunoreactivity; however, the clinical presentation (DFSP rarely arises in acral locations) and identification of more typical storiform areas help distinguish DFSP from SAF. *EWSR1-SMAD3* rearranged fibroblastic tumor (ESFT), another distinctive fibroblastic tumor with predilection for hands and feet (see below) has alternating cellular and hyalinized zones, lacks thick or ropey collagen bundles that characterize all tumors in the *RB1*-deleted family, and is positive for ERG while CD34 is negative. All of the above mimics lack RB1 gene deletion.

Prognosis and Treatment

Except for the pleomorphic liposarcoma, all fibroblastic and fatty tumors in the *RB1*-deleted tumor family are benign and typically cured by simple excision. SAF has a greater propensity for local recurrence in about one-quarter of cases, particularly in incompletely excised lesions.

CUTANEOUS MYXOMA AND SUPERFICIAL ANGIOMYXOMA

Clinical Findings

Outside of the well-established intramuscular myxoma with *GNAS* mutation, the descriptive term "myxoma" is used for benign superficial lesions that occur over a wide age range with a slight male predominance, as small dermal nodules most commonly on the trunk, lower extremities, and head and neck region. When the vascular component is conspicuous and accompanied by scattered neutrophils, such lesions are referred to as superficial angiomyxomas. Cutaneous myxomas and superficial angiomyxomas may occur either sporadically or in association with Carney complex, in which case these lesions are often multiple and present as multiple lesions on the ears, nipple, or eyelids in early adulthood. Carney's complex is an autosomal dominant condition associated with abnormalities in chromosomes 2p16 and 17q, involving mutations in the *PRKAR1A* gene. In addition to cutaneous myxomas, patients with Carney's complex also frequently develop cardiac myxomas, myxoid fibroadenomas, spotty pigmentation, endocrine overactivity, psammomatous melanotic schwannomas, and large-cell calcifying Sertoli cell tumors. Cutaneous myxoma may be the first manifestation of Carney's complex.

Histopathologic Features

Sporadic myxomas and myxomas associated with Carney's complex are essentially identical. They are characterized by a paucicellular proliferation of bland, oval to spindled cells embedded within an abundant myxoid matrix. Superficial angiomyxoma is notably more vascular, with scattered curvilinear blood vessels and a sprinkle of perivascular mixed inflammatory cells, of which the most unique are neutrophils (Fig. 14.40A and B). Another interesting feature is the presence of epithelial elements that can range from epidermoid cysts to strands of compressed basaloid epithelium (Fig. 14.40C). The cystic epithelial elements often show induction of follicular epithelium. Myxomas and angiomyxomas are variably positive for SMA and consistently negative for CD34, desmin, cytokeratins, S100, and SOX10.

Differential Diagnosis

The benign entities on the differential diagnosis include focal dermal mucinosis, digital mucous cyst, and dermal nerve sheath myxoma. Focal dermal mucinosis is a bland,

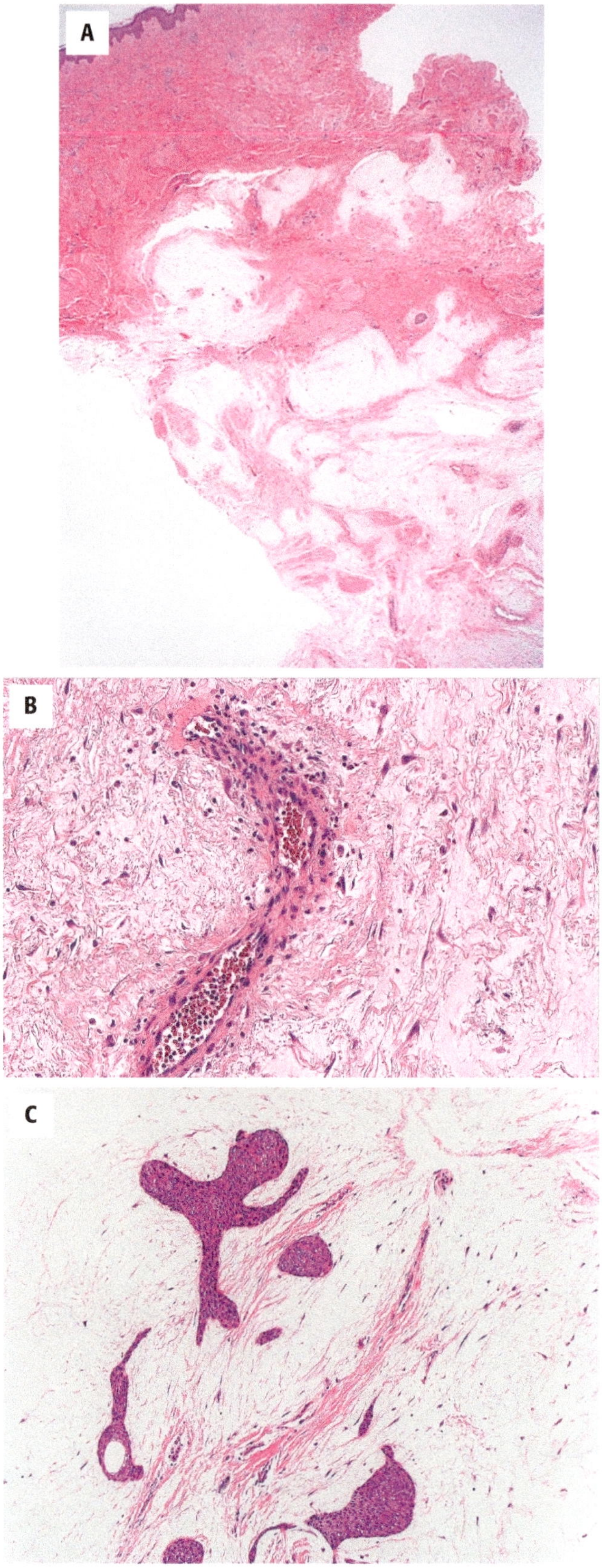

FIG. 14.40

Superficial angiomyxoma. **A,** A diffusely myxoid, paucicellular dermal and subcutaneous lesion growing in a multinodular, infiltrative pattern. **B,** Bland spindle cells surrounding prominent curvilinear blood vessels with a sprinkle of perivascular neutrophils. **C,** Entrapped epithelial elements.

hypocellular myxoid nodule that is cytologically similar to myxomas but lacks supporting tumor vasculature. Digital mucous cysts have similar morphology as focal dermal mucinosis but typically occur at the nail base of fingers and toes. Digital mucous cysts are traumatic lesions that connect to the underlying joint capsule and pathogenetically related to ganglion cysts. Myxoid neurofibromas tend to be more cellular than myxomas; show wavy, slightly hyperchromatic neural-type nuclei; and are immunoreactive for S100 protein and SOX10. Dermal nerve sheath myxoma (also known as myxoid neurothekeoma, discussed in the following) shows a characteristic multinodular growth pattern with multipolar Schwann cells containing long cytoplasmic processes and is also diffusely positive for schwannian markers. The only malignant lesion that has a real possibility of being mistaken for myxoma or superficial angiomyxoma is a low-grade myxofibrosarcoma given its characteristically subcutaneous location, relatively paucicellular stroma, curvilinear vasculature, and sparse chronic inflammation, although neutrophils are unusual. An important pitfall is that the infiltrative, multinodular growth pattern is very similar in both superficial angiomyxoma and myxofibrosarcoma but the latter has a greater degree of nuclear atypia, even in low-grade examples.

Prognosis and Treatment

Myxomas and angiomyxomas are benign lesions but may persist or recur locally. Recognizing the possible syndromic association with Carney complex represents an important clinical point since cardiac imaging may be needed to identify an occult cardiac myxoma.

SELECT GENE FUSION-DRIVEN FIBROBLASTIC NEOPLASMS WITH PREDILECTION FOR SKIN AND SUBCUTIS

LIPOFIBROMATOSIS

Clinical Findings

Lipofibromatosis is a rare tumor that occurs in the pediatric population, usually in the first year of life, with male predominance. Approximately 20% of cases are congenital. Tumors typically involve the hands and feet and clinically raise suspicion for an overgrowth syndrome. Prior to 2000, it was called infantile fibromatosis of nondesmoid type.

Histopathologic Features

Lipofibromatosis comprises mature adipose tissue with bland fibroblasts embedded in collagenous stroma forming septa that intercalate among the adipocytes. The atrophic adipocytes at the interface of adipose tissue and fibroblasts appear as small univacuolated cells (so-called blister cells); lobular architecture is preserved, and atypia and conspicuous mitoses are absent (Fig. 14.41A and B). The spindled cells may express CD34, CD99, and SMA. There is variable staining for S100, EMA, and muscle-specific actin. Desmin and cytokeratins are negative. Molecular profiling identified gene fusions that encode receptor tyrosine kinases (RTK) such as *BRAF*, *EGFR*, *PDGFRB*, *RET*, and *ROS1* or ligands to the epidermal growth factor receptor (*FN1-EGF*, *FN1-TGFA*), with downstream activation of the PI3K-AKT-mTOR pathway. These results place lipofibromatosis in the growing family of pediatric fibroblastic spindle cell tumors with RTK alterations.

LIPOFIBROMATOSIS-DISEASE FACT SHEET

Clinical Findings

- Infiltrative tumor on hands and feet in infants and young children

Histopathologic Features

- Mature adipose tissue with intercalating fascicles of bland fibroblasts
- Preservation of overall lobular architecture
- Small univacuolated cells (so-called blister cells)

IHC/Molecular

- Variable CD34, CD99, SMA, S100, EMA
- Receptor tyrosine kinase (*BRAF*, *EGFR*, *PDGFRB*, *RET*, and *ROS1*) or *FN1* fusions

Differential Diagnosis

- Fibrous hamartoma of infancy
- Lipofibromatosis-like neural tumor
- Desmoid fibromatosis
- Hemosiderotic fibrolipomatous tumor (HFLT)

EMA, Epithelial membrane antigen; *IHC*, immunohistochemistry; *SMA*, smooth muscle actin.

Differential Diagnosis

The main alternative diagnostic considerations include FHI, superficial and desmoid fibromatosis, and LF-NT and related low-grade tyrosine-kinase (TRK) gene fusion-driven mesenchymal neoplasms. FHI is distinguished based on the presence of immature mesenchymal aggregates with myxoid stroma along with the fibrous and fatty components and usually does not involve the distal extremities. Desmoid fibromatosis represents a solid proliferation of fibroblasts in long fascicles with dense collagen deposits and relatively little intermingled fat, mostly at the periphery of the pushing border of the mass and shows β-catenin gene alterations

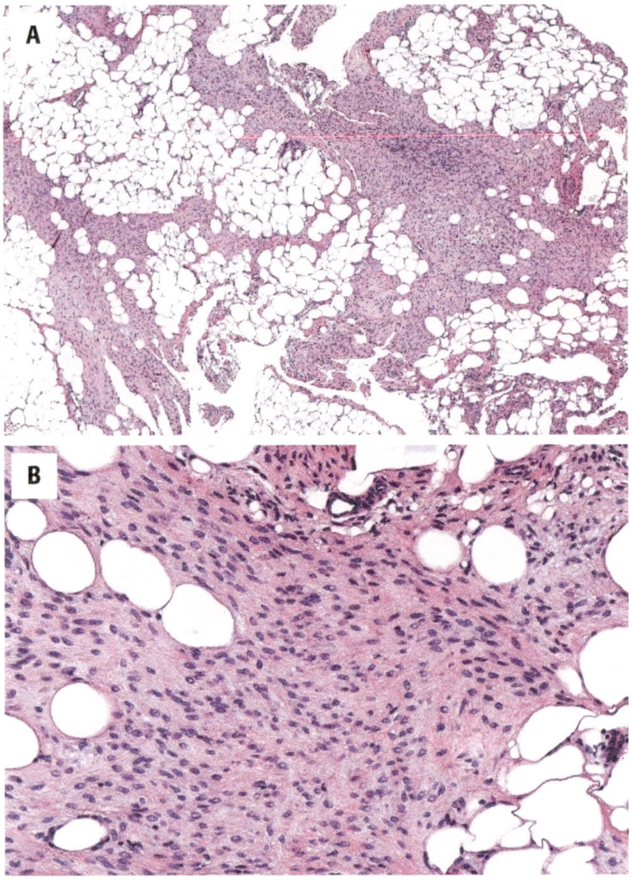

FIG. 14.41
Lipofibromatosis. **A,** Adipose tissue diffusely infiltrated by fibroblastic fascicles which, however, maintain the lobular architecture. **B,** The fibroblasts show bland nuclear features and low mitotic activity. Characteristic atrophic univacuolated adipocytes ("blister cells") are present at the interface with the fascicles.

with resultant nuclear overexpression by IHC. Superficial fibromatosis, which affects distal extremities, typically presents in older patients with contracting bands. FHI shows a component of primitive mesenchymal cells with a myxoid stroma and usually does not involve the distal extremities. Hemosiderotic fibrolipomatous tumor (HFLT) that also affects limbs and is composed of cytologically banal spindle cells with intracytoplasmic hemosiderin deposits, which percolate between the adipocytes, can closely resemble lipofibromatosis. However, HFLT presents in adults, contains giant cells and hemosiderin deposits, not typical of lipofibromatosis, lacks "blister" cells, and has an entirely different genetic composition with alterations of *TGFBR3* and *MGEA5* genes.

Prognosis and Treatment

The long-standing preferred treatment modality for lipofibromatosis was surgical approach; however, local recurrences are common due to the difficulty in obtaining clear margins, and in extensive limb involvement, surgery may be impractical. The treatment approach is changing with identification of potentially targetable RTK fusions in this disorder. Despite high rate of local recurrence, metastases do not occur.

LIPOFIBROMATOSIS-LIKE NEURAL TUMOR

Clinical Findings

LF-like neural tumor is an extremely rare, recently described tumor whose biology is still being defined. It tends to occur in infants, children, and young adults, primarily on the arms and legs, typically in the dermis and subcutis. It can appear pigmented clinically. The clinical presentation and the histologic findings overlap significantly with the classic lipofibromatosis.

Histopathologic Features

These tumors are poorly circumscribed and demonstrate a moderately cellular, somewhat haphazard and highly infiltrative arrangement of spindled cells arranged in loose fascicles in the dermis and subcutis. Cells are mildly atypical, with ill-defined pale cytoplasm and small monomorphic nuclei with inconspicuous nucleoli. Scattered lymphocytes are commonly seen, with occasional lymphoid aggregates or follicles. Staghorn vessels and perivascular hyalinization can also be seen. Pleomorphism is absent to minimal and mitotic rate is typically low; necrosis is usually absent (Fig. 14.42A and B). These tumors most commonly harbor *NTRK1* gene fusions. Tumors most often, but not always, show a coexpression of CD34 and S100 in the absence of SOX10 staining, as well as pan-TRK by IHC. There is morphologic and molecular overlap with the expanding pediatric and adult soft tissue tumors that show fascicular, low-grade malignant peripheral nerve sheath tumor (MPNST)–like and infantile fibrosarcoma (IFS)–like morphology and a spectrum of kinase fusions including *NTRK1,2,3, RET, ROS1, MET, ALK*, and *BRAF*.

Differential Diagnosis

The main differential diagnosis includes DFSP, neurofibroma, superficial ALK-rearranged SAMS, lipofibromatosis, and FHI. A practical approach in this setting is to recognize that LF-NT and related kinase fusion-driven tumors often (albeit somewhat inconsistently) display a partial neural immunophenotype, with coexpression of S100 and CD34 without SOX10 expression and may be positive for TRK by IHC. In contrast, DFSP, a gene fusion-driven but purely fibroblastic tumor likely derived from a

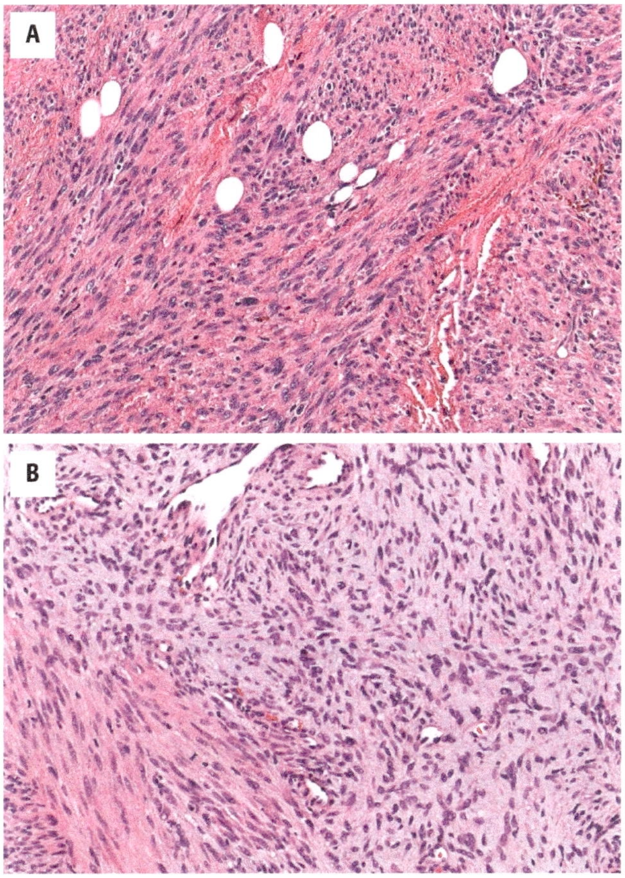

FIG. 14.42
Lipofibromatosis-like neural tumor. **A,** Moderately cellular fascicles of spindled fibroblastic cells with ill-defined pale cytoplasm and small monomorphic nuclei. **B,** Some examples show myxoid stroma and prominent vasculature. Pleomorphism is absent, and mitotic rate is low.

dermal-based fibroblastic precursor, is robustly positive for CD34 only. Neurofibromas show a true schwannian component with expression of all three markers (CD34, S100, and SOX10). SAMS is also positive for CD34 and S100, but it lacks TRK immunoreactivity. Instead, SAMS shows biphasic morphology and expresses ALK by IHC, in keeping with the driver *ALK* gene rearrangements. Lipofibromatosis has long fascicle of proliferative fibroblasts in the septa of adipose tissue and may variably coexpress CD34 and S100; this tumor lacks any degree of nuclear atypia, branching or hyalinized vessels and is negative for TRK by IHC as it lacks *NTRK1* gene fusion. However, as discussed above, there is increasing molecular evidence to place classic lipofibromatosis, LF-NT, and other similar RTK-altered pediatric fascicular tumors into the same family. FHI is relatively more organoid and has triphasic morphology including the presence of primitive, rounded, or stellate cells with myxoid stroma and mature adipose tissue. In FHI, CD34 and SMA may variably highlight fibroblastic component, S100 is positive only in adipocytic cells and TRK is negative. HFLT is also an infiltrative neoplasm composed of CD34-positive fascicles of cytologically banal spindle cells permeating subcutaneous tissue. In contrast to LF-NT, HFLT is an adult tumor and contains prominent cytoplasmic and stromal hemosiderin deposits, may contain fibrinous thrombi and osteoclast-type giant cells, is negative for S100, and harbors *TGFBR3* and *MGEA5* gene alterations.

Prognosis and Treatment

LF-NT is a low-grade tumor, with potential for local recurrence and reportedly, very rare metastases, and is managed with complete excision if feasible. TRK-targeted therapy, such as larotrectinib, has been shown to be useful in treating LF-NT and other *TRK* fusion-positive tumors. As this is an evolving entity, collective experience is limited.

EWSR1::SMAD3 REARRANGED FIBROBLASTIC TUMOR

Clinical Findings

ESFT is a distinctive benign dermal/subcutaneous fibroblastic tumor that usually arises in the hands and feet. There is a female predilection and wide age range.

Histopathologic Features

At low magnification, these tumors are nodular to somewhat infiltrative and show zonation pattern with areas of bland spindled cells arranged in intersecting fascicles of intermediate length, and hypocellular areas with stromal hyalinization. The cells have cigar-shaped to tapered and wavy nuclei without nucleoli (Fig. 14.43A–C). The fibroblastic cells have a peculiar immunophenotype with expression of ERG, while CD34, SMA, S100, and SOX10 are negative. ESFT is defined by fusion of *EWSR1* (exon 7) with *SMAD3* (exon 5).

Differential Diagnosis

The differential diagnosis of ESFT is broad, primarily comprising rare tumors from the fibroblastic/myofibroblastic category such as lipofibromatosis (diffuse architecture with intermingled adipose tissue and negative ERG), calcifying aponeurotic fibroma (CAF, more haphazardly arranged fascicles, distinctly infiltrative edge and grungy purple calcifications), and LF-NT (negative ERG, coexpression for S100 and CD34 without SOX10, and *NTRK1*, *ROS1*, and *ALK* rearrangements), myofibroma/myofibromatosis (plumper cells with biphasic

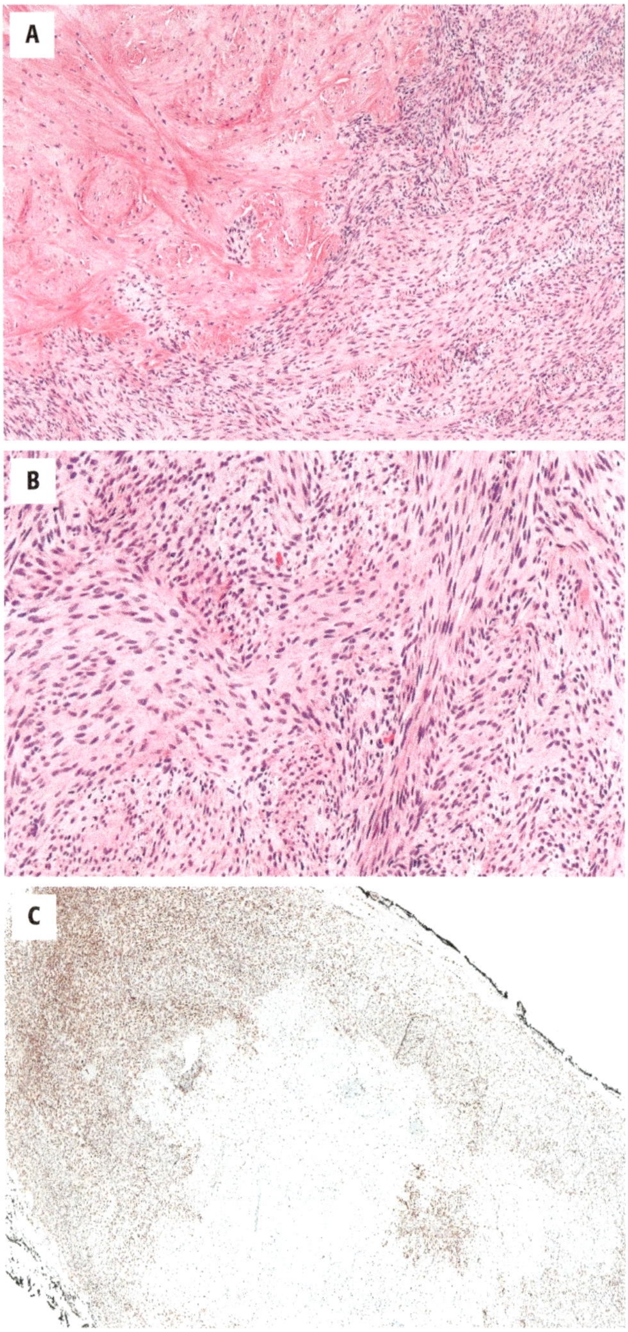

FIG. 14.43

EWSR1::SMAD3 rearranged fibroblastic tumor. **A,** Nodular and somewhat infiltrative lesion with biphasic appearance with areas of bland spindled cells arranged in intersecting fascicles of intermediate length, and hypocellular areas with stromal hyalinization. **B,** The cells have cigar-shaped to tapered and wavy nuclei without nucleoli. **C,** Nuclear expression of ERG is characteristic.

architecture containing small, primitive appearing spindle cells surrounding branching HPC-like capillaries, positive for SMA and desmin, negative for ERG), infantile digital fibroma/fibromatosis (lacks hyaline areas, shows distinctive eosinophilic inclusions, and is negative for ERG), palmar/plantar fibromatosis (presentation as volar surface mass/contraction, lacks zonation pattern, individual cells are separated by strikingly parallel, thin refractile collagen fibers, positive for SMA and negative for ERG), and monophasic SS (focal cytokeratin and EMA positivity, calcifications, negative for ERG).

Prognosis and Treatment

These tumors are treated with excision but are prone to recur locally. Metastasis has not been reported, although collective experience is limited.

OSSIFYING FIBROMYXOID TUMOR

Clinical Findings

Ossifying fibromyxoid tumor (OFMT) is a distinctive, translocation-associated mesenchymal neoplasm which occurs mostly in male, middle-aged adults (age range 10–88 years) as a solitary, well-circumscribed painless mass involving the superficial tissues of the limbs, trunk, and head and neck. Rarely, it involves unusual sites like the skeletal muscle, body cavities, thyroid gland, and breast. The median size is 3 to 4 cm.

OSSIFYING FIBROMYXOID TUMOR—DISEASE FACT SHEET

Clinical Findings

- Subcutaneous mass in adult patients, with wide anatomic distribution

Histopathologic Features

- Circumscribed mass with a fibrous pseudocapsule
- Peripheral shell of mature lamellar bone
- Epithelioid or spindled cells arranged in cords, nests, sheets, and trabeculae
- Myxoid, collagenous, hyalinized, or chondroid stroma
- Uniform oval nuclei with fine chromatin and delicate pinpoint nucleoli
- Malignant OFMT: high nuclear grade or high cellularity and a mitotic count of >2/50 HPF
- Atypical OFMT: a mitotic count of >2/50 HPF alone or high cellularity or moderate nuclear atypia with a mitotic count of ≤2/50 HPF

IHC/Molecular

- S100 (70%–90%), desmin (10%–40%), MUC4 (25%)
- Variable SMA, p63, GFAP, CD10; TFE3 in *TFE3*-rearranged cases
- Focal EMA and cytokeratins in malignant cases
- *PHF1* (most common); variant fusions involving *BCOR*, *BCORL1*, *KDMA2*, and *TFE3* genes

Differential Diagnosis

- Myoepithelial tumors
- Epithelioid schwannoma
- Low-grade fibromyxoid sarcoma
- Osteosarcoma (in cases of malignant OFMT)

EMA, Epithelial membrane antigen; *GFAP*, glial fibrillary acidic protein; *IHC*, immunohistochemistry; *OFMT*, ossifying fibromyxoid tumor; *SMA*, smooth muscle actin.

Histopathologic Features

OFMT is circumscribed and has a fibrous pseudocapsule. Focal infiltrative growth and microscopic satellite nodules may be present. The classic feature of OFMT is a peripheral shell of mature lamellar bone present in up to 85% of cases. The tumor is variably cellular and is composed of epithelioid or spindled cells arranged in corded, nested, trabecular, or sheetlike patterns, with variable proportions of myxoid, fibrous, hyalinized or chondroid stroma (Fig. 14.44A and B). In addition to the classic shell of lamellar bone at the periphery, deposits of woven bone without embedded tumor cells are often present. Microcystic changes, fascicle formation, and rhabdoid-like morphology may rarely occur. Irrespective of the growth pattern, all OFMTs show strikingly similar, uniform oval nuclei with fine chromatin and delicate pinpoint nucleoli (Fig. 14.44C). These nuclear features are one of the most helpful clues for identifying OFMT. In most cases, there is virtually no mitotic activity. Scattered nuclear atypia of degenerative type may be present.

Rare malignant OFMTs may arise de novo or from a more typical benign OFMT precursor. An outcome-based risk stratification system dividing OFMTs into typical, atypical, and malignant forms has been proposed based on diffuse nuclear atypia, high cellularity, and mitotic rate >2/50 HPF. Malignant OFMT is defined as having high nuclear grade (Fig. 14.44D) or a

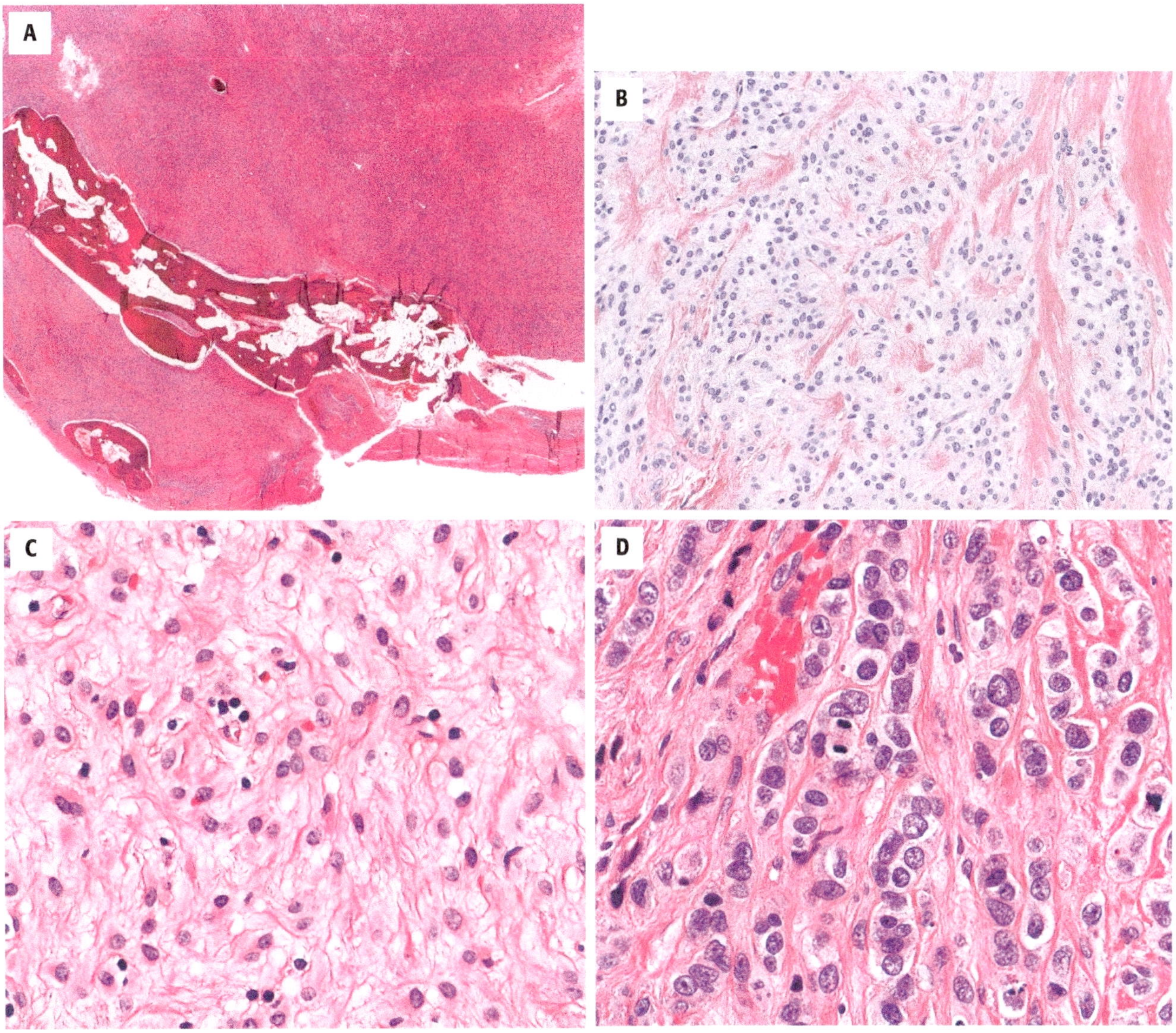

FIG. 14.44

Ossifying fibromyxoid tumor (OFMT). **A,** A circumscribed neoplasm with a fibrous pseudocapsule and a peripheral shell of mature lamellar bone. **B,** Nested growth pattern in a myxocollagenous background. **C,** Corded growth pattern with uniform oval nuclei with fine chromatin and delicate pinpoint nucleoli that are characteristic of all OFMT variants. **D,** Malignant OFMT with increased cellularity, diffuse nuclear atypia, and mitotic activity.

combination of high cellularity and a mitotic count of >2/50 HPF. Cases meeting one atypical feature such as a mitotic count of >2/50 HPF alone or high cellularity or moderate nuclear atypia with a mitotic count of ≤2/50 HPF are considered atypical OFMTs. By IHC, OFMT has a complex immunophenotype with expression of S100 (70% to 90% of cases), desmin (10% to 40% of cases), MUC4 (25% of cases) and inconsistent immunoreactivity for SMA, p63, glial fibrillary acidic protein (GFAP), CD10, estrogen receptor (ER), and progesterone receptor (PR). EMA and cytokeratins may show focal expression, although only in a minority of cases and more often in malignant OFMT. OFMTs are negative for melanocytic markers, SOX10, CD34, and CD31. Mosaic loss of INI1 expression can be observed in a subset of cases due to hemizygous deletions of SMARCB1. Up to 85% of OFMTs (including typical, atypical, and malignant cases) have recurrent gene rearrangements, most commonly involving *PHF1* on 6p21 with a variety of partners. Less common variant fusions involve *BCOR*, *BCORL1*, *KDMA2*, and *TFE3* genes. Most of the above genes participate in epigenetic regulation and histone modification. Accumulating evidence suggests that OFMTs with variant non-*PHF1* fusions and those with *PHF1-TFE3* fusion behave more aggressively. FISH to detect *PHF1* rearrangements is a useful ancillary diagnostic technique as is *TFE3* FISH or TFE3 protein IHC that will detect *PHF1-TFE3* rearranged tumors. *PHF1* and variant fusions can be detected by commercially available next-generation sarcoma fusion panels.

Differential Diagnosis

Myoepithelial tumors (myoepithelioma and myoepithelial carcinoma) are the closest mimic as these tumors also consist of epithelioid or spindled cells arranged in various combinations of reticular, trabecular, and nested patterns, within a fibromyxoid stroma. Cartilaginous and osseous differentiation may occur in myoepithelial tumors but it rarely takes the form of a peripheral rim of mature lamellar bone as seen in OFMT. Markers of myoepithelial differentiation such as p63, SMA, and particularly S100 protein are of limited value, because they are also expressed in OFMT. However, strong diffuse expression of keratins, EMA, and SOX10 would favor a myoepithelial tumor since these markers are expressed in only a handful of OFMTs and usually only focally. *PHF1* gene rearrangement has not been observed in myoepithelial tumors, which, in contrast, may demonstrate rearrangements of *EWSR1* (~80% of cases), *FUS*, and *PLAG1*. Since the array of gene fusions in both neoplasms is quite broad, a commercially available sarcoma fusion assay will likely surpass individual FISH probes for an accurate diagnostic classification.

Epithelioid schwannomas resemble OFMT, because they are also composed of epithelioid cells arranged in a nested or trabecular pattern, have hyalinized or myxoid stroma, and often lack Antoni A areas. Both tumors can be positive for S100 and can show inactivation of SMARCB1/INI1, which is seen in 42% of epithelioid schwannomas. The nuclei in epithelioid schwannomas are more irregular and reniform in appearance, and metaplastic ossification or desmin expression is entirely uncharacteristic. The presence of a conventional schwannoma component with hyalinized vasculature, a true capsule with EMA or GLUT1-positive perineurial cells, and very strong, diffuse immunoreactivity for SOX10 favors epithelioid schwannoma.

LGFMS, which also often presents as a well-circumscribed firm tumor in the subcutis, can be distinguished based on a prominent whorled/storiform arrangement of constitutive tumor cells and characteristic arcades of vessels in myxoid zones. By IHC, LGFMS is often positive for EMA and negative for S100. MUC4, a sensitive and specific marker of LGFMS can be positive in 20% to 30% of OFMT, although the staining is usually focal and weak. Diagnostically challenging cases of LGFMS can be distinguished from OFMT by testing for *FUS*, *EWSR1*, and *YAP1* rearrangements (present in LGFMS) and/or PFH1 rearrangements by FISH or NGS. Epithelioid MPNSTs typically lack a peripheral shell of lamellar bone and desmin immunoreactivity and show strong and diffuse S100 and SOX10 expression. Homozygous SMARCB1/INI loss is characteristic of epithelioid MPNSTs, while INI1 is usually retained or lost in a mosaic pattern in OFMT. Finally, OFMT cases with a more diffuse, lacelike, or random pattern of woven bone deposition and atypical or malignant histology can be mistaken for extraosseous or metastatic osteosarcoma. Marked atypia and nuclear pleomorphism favor osteosarcoma as these features are not typical of OFMT, even in malignant cases. The presence of desmin, S100, or substantial cytokeratin expression in this context would also argue against osteosarcoma.

Treatment and Prognosis

Typical OFMTs recur or metastasize very rarely (0%–4% and 0%–6%, respectively, based on various series), while malignant OFMTs show local recurrence in 22% and metastasis in 12.5% of cases. Because adverse events were reported even in cases with the typical low-grade morphology, all OFMTs at present are regarded as neoplasms of uncertain malignant behavior. The treatment for typical OFMTs is a complete surgical resection. Malignant OFMTs are best managed by a multidisciplinary sarcoma team. The data on chemotherapy use in OFMT are very sparse.

ANGIOFIBROMA OF SOFT TISSUE

Clinical Findings

Soft tissue angiofibroma occurs over a broad age range and shows a female predominance. Tumors present as painless superficial or sometimes deep-seated masses most often involving upper and lower extremities; median size is 5 cm.

Histopathologic Features

Soft tissue angiofibroma is a circumscribed tumor with focal infiltration into the surrounding soft tissue. It consists of bland, nondescript fibroblastic cells with ovoid nuclei, uniform chromatin, and pale eosinophilic cytoplasm, set within a loose myxoid to collagenous connective tissue matrix. Thick collagenous bands are uncharacteristic. The signature finding in this lesion is a rich network of evenly spaced, curvilinear to branched small caliber vessels. Additional vascular patterns may also be present, including medium- to large-sized staghorn vessels, perivascular collagen deposition, and fibrinoid necrosis (Fig. 14.45A and B). Nuclear atypia is typically absent short of degenerative type or ischemic changes, and mitotic figures are inconspicuous. As is often the case with translocation-driven neoplasms, soft tissue angiofibroma has a complex immunophenotype with frequent expression of ER and CD163, EMA (50%) and, in about 10% to 20% of cases, SMA, desmin, and CD34 (often focally). Cytokeratins, S100 and SOX10, are consistently negative. Focal and weak STAT6 expression has been reported in 7% of cases. Molecularly, soft tissue angiofibroma harbors *NCOA2-AHRR* fusion in more than half of the cases; less common variant fusions with *GTF21* and *ETV4*, and GAB1-ABL1 fusion were also described. NCOA2 IHC is a very sensitive albeit nonspecific marker of soft tissue angiofibroma.

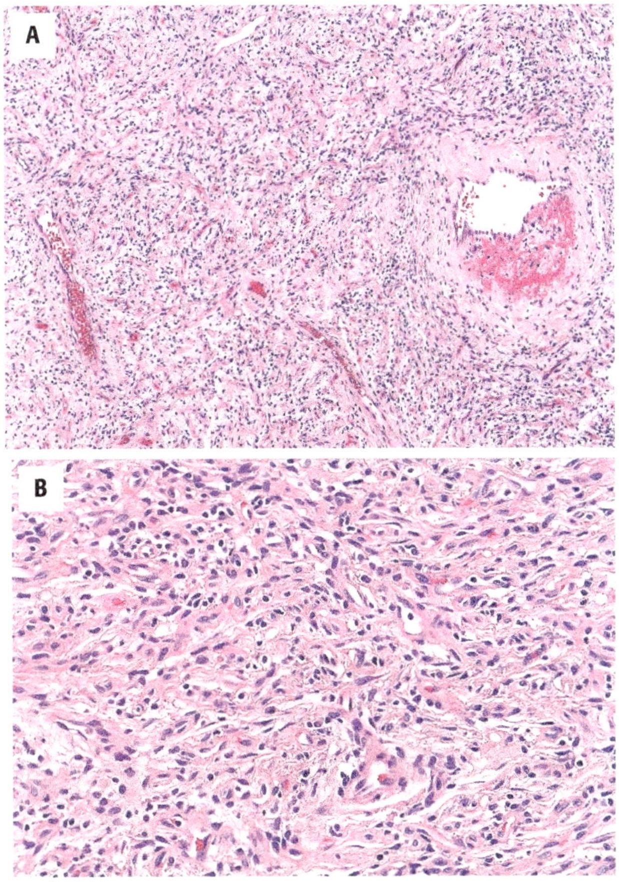

FIG. 14.45

Soft tissue angiofibroma. **A,** A fibroblastic tumor with striking vasculature including evenly spaced small caliber vessels, staghorn vessels, and large vessels with fibrinoid necrosis. **B,** Bland, nondescript fibroblastic cells with ovoid nuclei and pale eosinophilic cytoplasm growing loosely in a fibromyxoid stroma.

Differential Diagnosis

A staghorn vascular pattern in soft tissue angiofibroma can closely mimic an SFT. SFTs are usually more cellular and collagenous than soft tissue angiofibroma and show strong, diffuse STAT6 expression in contrast to only focal and weak staining in less than 10% of soft tissue angiofibroma cases. Myofibroblastoma has an overlapping immunoprofile (SMA, desmin, and ER) and may occasionally show a prominent vascular pattern, though not typically to the extent seen in soft tissue angiofibroma. Rb IHC (lost in myofibroblastoma) or molecular testing (for rearrangements in *NCOA2* for soft tissue angiofibroma) can be performed to aid in diagnosis. Prominent thick collagen bundles that are seen in both myofibroblastoma and SFT, and the extent of CD34 immunoreactivity seen with these tumors, are not characteristic of soft tissue angiofibroma. On the malignant side, soft tissue angiofibroma can mimic LGFMS and myxoid liposarcoma. LGFMS is positive for MUC4 by IHC, which is highly sensitive and specific in this setting, and will show *FUS*, *EWSR1*, or *YAP1* gene rearrangements in contrast to *NCOA2* gene rearrangement in soft tissue angiofibroma. The vasculature of myxoid liposarcoma is somewhat different with very delicate, arborizing capillaries without pericytes or secondary patterns that nearly always present in angiofibroma of soft tissue. The constituent cells are more epithelioid or comma-shaped and may show lipoblastic differentiation. Molecular testing shows *DDIT3* gene rearrangements.

Prognosis and Treatment

Soft tissue angiofibromas are benign, with a small risk of local recurrence. Treatment is surgical excision.

SUPERFICIAL CD34-POSITIVE FIBROBLASTIC TUMOR/*PRDM10*-REARRANGED SOFT TISSUE TUMOR

Clinical Findings

Superficial CD34-positive fibroblastic tumor/*PRDM10*-rearranged soft tissue tumor is a distinctive soft tissue tumor that typically presents as a painless cutaneous or subcutaneous mass on the trunk or proximal extremities of young to middle-aged adults.

Histopathologic Features

Microscopically, this is a densely cellular, unencapsulated, circumscribed to infiltrative neoplasm comprising fascicles and sheets of pleomorphic tumor cells. The cells are large, plump, and spindled to epithelioid with large, atypical nuclei and abundant, densely eosinophilic, "glassy" cytoplasm with distinct cytoplasmic borders. Alternatively, the cells may have foamy, granular, or vacuolated lipoblast-like cytoplasm. The striking feature is the degree of nuclear atypia, with enlarged, hyperchromatic bizarre nuclei and prominent, inclusion-like nucleoli. The spindle cells are admixed with numerous chronic inflammatory cells, and lymphoid aggregates may be present at the periphery of this tumor (Fig. 14.46A and B). Despite the cytologic atypia that resembles sarcoma, the mitotic count is typically very low (<1/10 HPF) as is Ki-67 proliferative index. Focal necrosis may be present. A subset of cases shows prominent dilated and hyalinized vessels resembling those seen in pleomorphic hyalinizing angiectatic tumor (PHAT). As the name implies, this tumor is characterized by a distinctive immunophenotype, namely strong,

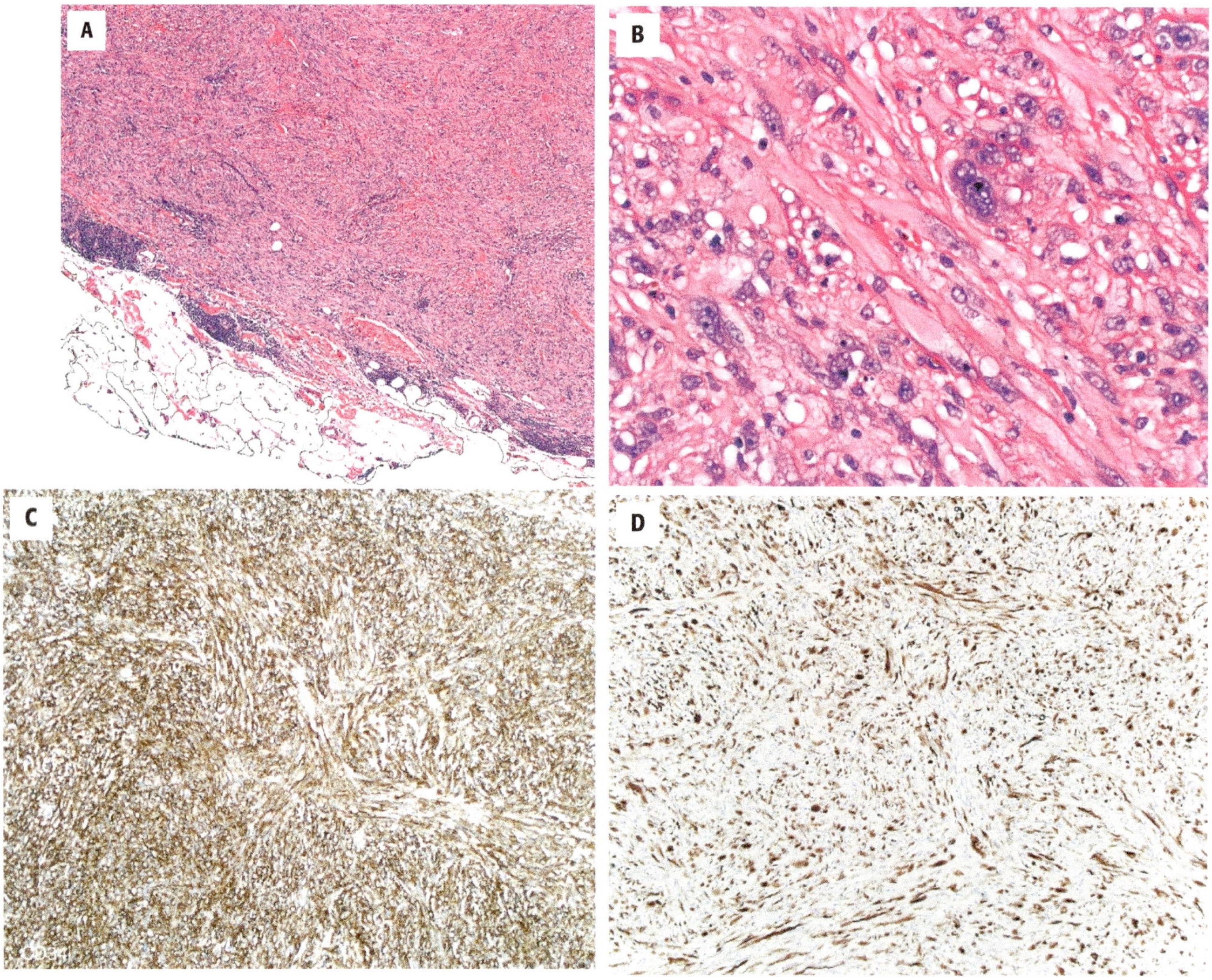

FIG. 14.46

Superficial CD34-positive fibroblastic tumor. **A,** Cellular unencapsulated neoplasm with a cuff of lymphoid aggregates centered in the subcutis. **B,** The tumor is composed of pleomorphic cells with large, atypical nuclei, prominent nucleoli, and eosinophilic "glassy" cytoplasm. A prominent inflammatory component is present. The tumor cells diffusely express CD34 (**C**) and are positive for cytokeratins (**D**).

diffuse expression of CD34 and CADM3 (cell adhesion molecule 3 or Syn-CAM3); in addition, there is focal expression of cytokeratins, desmin, and WT-1 (Fig. 14.46C and D). Vascular markers (CD31, ERG), S100, and markers of smooth muscle differentiation (SMA, h-caldesmon) are negative. Most SCD34FT harbor alterations in *PRDM10* gene, which encodes for a zinc-finger transcriptional regulator. *PRDM10* gene alterations have been initially described separately in a morphologically and immunophenotypically similar superficial neoplasm termed "*PRDM10*-rearranged soft tissue tumor". In addition to the well-circumscribed sheets and fascicles of spindled and pleomorphic cells with low mitotic activity and brightly eosinophilic or granular cytoplasm, ectatic blood vessels with fibrinous material, and lipoblast-like cells seen in SCD34FT, PRDM10-STT can show myxoid change and metaplastic bone. However, there is increasing evidence arguing that both SCD34FT and *PRDM10*-rearranged soft tissue tumor represent a single entity.

Differential Diagnosis

The most important differential diagnosis includes cutaneous tumors with pleomorphic and epithelioid pattern, most notably AFX, dermal pleomorphic sarcoma (undifferentiated pleomorphic sarcoma/UPS of the skin) and myxofibrosarcoma, and some cases of this tumor were likely mislabeled as such in the past. A simple but very effective rule is that in all of the above, the nuclear atypia is accompanied by mitotic activity, whereas the mitotic count is very low or absent in SCD34FT. Myxoinflammatory fibroblastic sarcoma (MIFS), characterized by similar pleomorphic cells with enlarged nuclei, inclusion-like nucleoli, a prominent inflammatory component, and a very low mitotic activity, typically presents in the distal extremities and has a more prominent inflammatory infiltrate, a more pronounced myxoid stroma and a more significant pattern of tissue infiltration that often extends far beyond the gross boundaries of the tumor. Focal CD34 and CADM3 expression can rarely be seen in all the above mimics; however, robust CD34 expression and coexpression of cytokeratins is uncharacteristic. Epithelioid sarcoma has a similar immunophenotype (frequent coexpression of CD34 and cytokeratin); however, the morphologic appearance of the superficial CD34-positive fibroblastic tumor is much more pleomorphic than that of an epithelioid sarcoma, and INI1 expression is retained. SCD34FS and PHAT (discussed below) may share dilated hyalinized vessels and expression of CD34 and CADM3. However, PHAT lacks the distinctive "glassy" cytoplasm and often shows areas of HFLT at the periphery, which consist of bland spindled cells infiltrating adipose tissue, with variable stromal myxoid change, small, injured blood vessels containing fibrinous thrombi, and conspicuous hemosiderin deposits. The plump, eosinophilic spindle cells that express cytokeratins may resemble those seen in pseudomyogenic hemangioendothelioma (PHE, discussed in the following), particularly in a limited biopsy specimen. However, the latter tumor is often multifocal, has less nuclear pleomorphism, and demonstrates true vascular differentiation (ERG+) while being negative for CD34 by IHC.

Prognosis and Treatment

This tumor is presently considered to be of borderline malignant potential with very rare lymph node metastases, which appear to play no prognostic role, and a small risk for local recurrence. The mainstay of treatment is surgical excision.

PLEOMORPHIC HYALINIZING ANGIECTATIC TUMOR

Clinical Findings

PHAT is a somewhat underrecognized slow-growing subcutaneous or dermal neoplasm of middle-aged adults with the potential for local recurrence and, in rare cases, progression to a higher-grade sarcoma. PHAT has a predilection for the lower extremities but can also involve the upper extremities, trunk, or head and neck or exceptionally rare visceral sites such as male breast, with an average size of 5 to 6 cm. PHAT may be clinically mistaken for a hematoma or a vascular neoplasm.

Histopathologic Features

PHAT is a vaguely circumscribed, infiltrative mass composed of spindled or pleomorphic cells surrounding clusters of very characteristic thin-walled dilated vessels with subendothelial and intraluminal amorphous fibrin deposits or hyalinized vessel walls. The cells range from hyperchromatic and spindled to strikingly pleomorphic and may show frequent intranuclear inclusions. The mitotic activity in PHAT is characteristically very low (0 to 1/50 HPF). Hemosiderin deposits can be seen in macrophages or in the cytoplasm of the lesional cells. Scattered inflammatory cells are usually present (Fig. 14.47A and B). Many PHATs at the periphery show areas reminiscent of HFLT. These areas are composed of cytologically banal spindle cells with intracytoplasmic and stromal hemosiderin deposits, which infiltrate

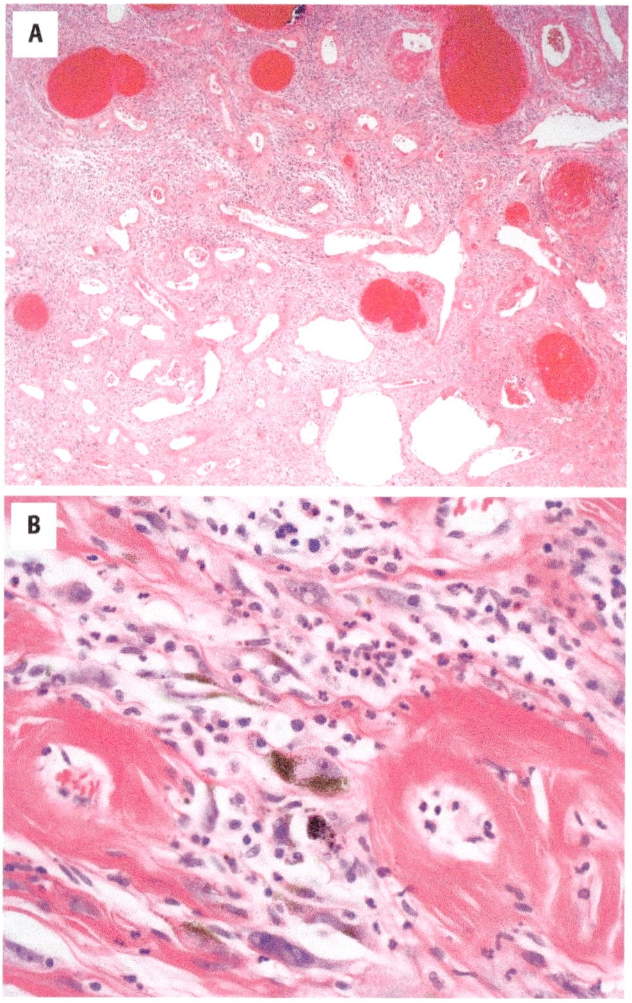

FIG. 14.47

Pleomorphic hyalinizing angiectatic tumor. **A,** An infiltrative mass composed of spindled or pleomorphic cells surrounding clusters of dilated hyalinized vessels with subendothelial and intraluminal fibrin deposits. **B,** The cells show conspicuous atypia and pleomorphism but lack mitotic activity. Intracytoplasmic and stromal hemosiderin deposits and scattered inflammatory cells are characteristic.

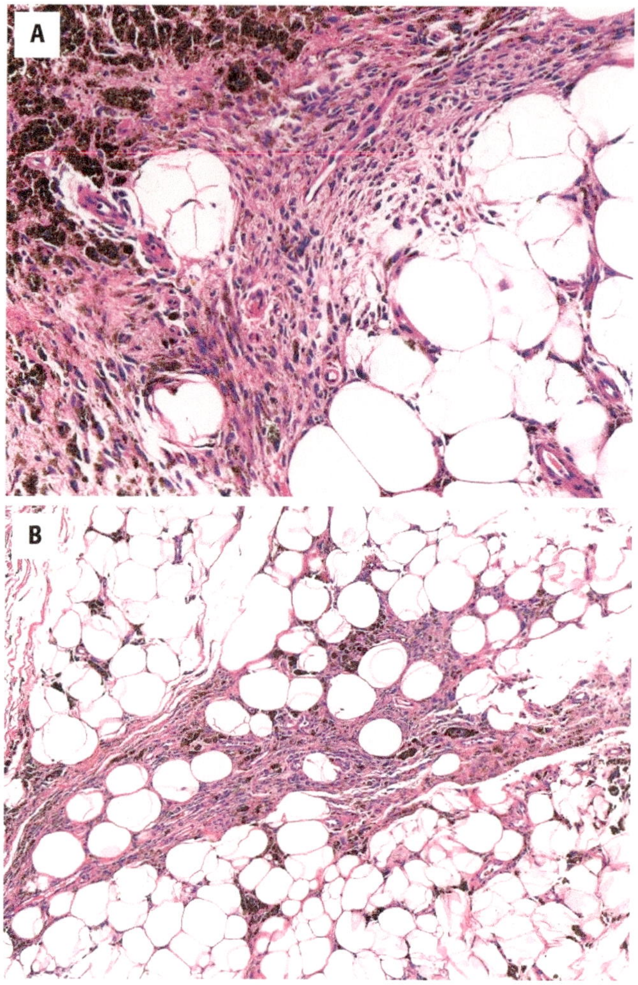

FIG. 14.48

Hemosiderotic fibrolipomatous tumor. **A** and **B,** Sheets and small fascicles of cytologically banal fibroblastic cells with intracytoplasmic and stromal hemosiderin deposits, which infiltrate between the adipocytes in a manner resembling lipofibromatosis or dermatofibrosarcoma protuberans.

between the adipocytes in a manner resembling lipofibromatosis or DFSP, and often containing small, damaged vessels with fibrin thrombi (Fig. 14.48A and B). This finding can be of diagnostic utility. Rarely, PHAT may progress to a sarcoma of higher histologic grade, especially in the setting of local recurrence. The sarcomatous components associated with PHAT often have myxoid stroma and a prominent inflammatory infiltrate resembling MIFS or myxofibrosarcoma, or a solid, undifferentiated spindle cell sarcoma-like morphology. Most PHATs are diffusely positive for CD34 and negative for S100 protein, SMA, desmin, and vascular markers CD31 and ERG. As discussed in the previous section, a subset of tumors may express CADM3. Molecular studies showed alterations in *OGA* (*MGEA5*) and *TGFBR3* genes, especially in tumors showing mixed features of PHAT and HFLT and, less consistently, in classic PHAT—a finding that provides further support for the relatedness of these two tumors. These alterations can be detected by FISH, but these unique probes are sparsely available and rarely needed for the diagnosis.

Differential Diagnosis

PHAT may be confused with a schwannoma with degenerative ("ancient") change, which often contains clusters of hyalinized vessels, inflammatory aggregates, and pleomorphic Schwann cells. In contrast to PHAT, schwannomas are well-circumscribed and encapsulated lesions without a HFLT-like component at the periphery. S100 and SOX10 proteins are diffusely expressed in schwannomas and are consistently negative in PHAT. Owing to the striking degree of nuclear atypia and pleomorphism often seen in PHAT, it can be misdiagnosed as undifferentiated pleomorphic sarcoma; however, PHAT lacks mitotic activity which invariably accompanies nuclear atypia in standard pleomorphic soft tissue sarcomas. Identification of a bona fide spindle cell sarcoma with myxoid stroma and an increase in mitotic activity in association with a recognizable classic PHAT indicates sarcomatous progression. MIFS typically presents in the distal extremities and may show similar pleomorphic cells with enlarged nuclei, inclusion-like nucleoli, a prominent inflammatory component, and a very low mitotic activity. MIFS has a more pronounced myxoid stroma and an overtly infiltrative growth pattern that does not appear circumscribed at scanning magnification. In contrast to PHAT, MIFS lacks distinctive vessels with fibrinoid necrosis. MIFS is often characterized by *VGGL3* and *BRAF* gene alterations, but the presence of alterations in *OGA* (*MGEA5*) and *TGFBR3* genes in pure MIFS devoid of PHAT or HFLT-like morphology has been controversial. The differential diagnosis with superficial CD34 positive fibroblastic tumor is discussed in the preceding section.

Treatment and Prognosis

Because of its infiltrative nature, PHAT is associated with a significant (30%–50%) risk of local recurrence and is therefore considered to represent a tumor of intermediate malignant potential. Limited studies indicate that PHAT may undergo transformation to a higher-grade sarcoma and acquire metastatic potential. The optimal treatment approach is complete surgical excision with tumor-free margins, although it might be difficult to achieve.

HEMOSIDEROTIC FIBROLIPOMATOUS TUMOR

Clinical Findings

Initially thought to represent a reactive process related to trauma, HFLT is a true neoplasm that manifests as a slowly growing subcutaneous mass or plaque, with a tendency to affect the dorsal surface of the ankle, foot, or hand in female patients.

Histopathologic Features

HFLTs are infiltrative neoplasms composed of ill-defined fascicles of bland fibroblastic cells that percolate through adipose tissue in a streaming, nodular, or diffuse pattern reminiscent of DFSP or lipofibromatosis. However, in contrast to these histologically similar processes HFLT contains prominent hemosiderin deposits that can be found in the stroma, in macrophages, and in the cytoplasm of the spindle cells. Small, injured capillary vessels that contain fibrinous thrombi are another distinctive feature. Myxoid stroma, inflammatory cells, and osteoclast-type giant cells may be present. HFLT-like areas can be found at the periphery or admixed with otherwise typical examples of PHAT (Fig. 14.48A and B).

Like PHAT, rare HFLT cases may progress to a sarcoma of higher histologic grade, especially in the setting of local recurrence. The sarcomatous components associated with both PHAT and HFLT often have myxoid stroma and a prominent inflammatory infiltrate that superficially resemble MIFS but tend to show more frequent solid component and a higher nuclear grade. HFLT is positive for CD34 and negative for S100, SMA, and desmin. Similar to PHAT, HFLT harbors a recurrent t(1;10) (p22;q24) rearrangement involving the *TGFBR3* and *OGA* (*MGEA5*) genes and may show *VGGL3* gene amplification. TGFBR3 and MGEA5 gene rearrangements have also been found in tumors showing mixed features of HFLT and PHAT and, less consistently, in classic PHAT, findings that further support the view that PHAT and HFLT may be related. FISH for TGFBR3 and MGEA5 rearrangements can be used in diagnostically challenging cases.

Differential Diagnosis

HFLT must be separated from three similarly infiltrative, bland fibroblastic CD34-positive lesions: DFSP, lipofibromatosis, and LF-NT. DFSP has a more uniform appearance than HFLT and lacks hemosiderin deposits and injured capillary vessels. Fatty infiltration in DFSP occurs at the edge of the tumor, whereas in HFLT, the adipocytic component is intimately admixed with the lesional cells and may dominate the histologic picture. FISH for *PDGFB* rearrangement of DFSP can be employed in difficult cases. In the pediatric population, lipofibromatosis and LF-NT can be distinguished based on the more monotonous appearance of the constituent spindle cells and, in case of classic lipofibromatosis, collections of small univacuolated cells at the interface between the adipocytic and spindle cell components. Osteoclast-type giant cells, fibrinous thrombi, and hemosiderin deposits are not typical of lipofibromatosis and are very rare in LF-NT. All three tumors are positive for CD34; however, LF-NT shows coexpression of S100 protein and TRK; by molecular testing, a spectrum of kinase fusions, most often involving *NTRK1,2,3*, *RET*, *ROS1*, *MET*, *ALK*, and *BRAF* can be seen. Similar alterations as well as alterations involving *EGFR* or its ligands are also being increasingly recognized in classic lipofibromatosis, but none of these are characteristic of HFLT. Mistaking HFLT for a reactive spindle cell proliferation in the setting of hematoma or prior injury remains the most significant diagnostic pitfall.

Prognosis and Treatment

The rate of local recurrence is relatively high (30%–50%) due to difficulty of complete local excision. Like PHAT, metastases have not been reported in HFLT. However, the tumor may acquire potential for metastasis with progression to a higher-grade sarcoma.

BENIGN FIBROHISTIOCYTIC OR HISTIOCYTOID TUMORS

DERMATOFIBROMA (BENIGN FIBROUS HISTIOCYTOMA) AND VARIANTS

DF or benign FH is a common benign mesenchymal tumor of the skin, which may show a spectrum of differentiation toward fibroblasts, myofibroblasts, or histiocytes.

Clinical Findings

DF manifests as a small, slowly growing, painless, tan to red-brown papule or nodule most often found on the extremities of adults, but the tumor can occur at any age and site. The tumors are usually small (around 1 cm in diameter) but variant FHs can attain a very large size.

Histopathologic Features

Classic DF is a somewhat circumscribed dermal spindle cell tumor, with a rim of uninvolved dermis that separates most tumors from the overlying epidermis, which frequently shows hyperplasia and basilar hyperpigmentation (Fig. 14.49A). The dermal-epidermal junction overlying a DF may show a trichoblastic proliferation that can be mistaken for a BCC on a superficial shave biopsy (Fig. 14.49B). Most classic DFs are restricted to the dermis, but extension into the superficial subcutaneous fat is not uncommon, especially in variant tumors. At the periphery of the lesion, the tumor cells interdigitate around preexisting collagen fibers of the reticular dermis in a characteristic pattern of "collagen trapping" present in most variants of this tumor (Fig. 14.49C). Cytologically, a DF is composed of a heterogeneous population of oval to fusiform fibroblastic and fibrohistiocytic cells that, despite banal nuclear features, produce an impression of a polymorphous tumor. The cells are arranged in a random or vaguely storiform pattern. Foamy histiocytes, multinucleated giant cells, dendritic cells, and hemosiderin-laden macrophages are frequently admixed with the spindle cells (Fig. 14.49D and E). Mitotic figures can be seen. Based on the appearance of the cells, lipidized (ankle-type), clear cell, granular cell, palisading, myxoid, and keloidal DFs were described, of no clinical consequence. However, several variants of FH differ significantly from the classic DF and are clinically meaningful tumors with greater risk of local recurrence and rare but well documented metastases.

DERMATOFIBROMA—HISTOPATHOLOGIC FEATURES

Classic Dermatofibroma

- Dermal spindle cell tumor with a storiform pattern
- Heterogenous composition: plump fibroblasts, histiocytes, dendritic cells
- Secondary elements: hemosiderin, lymphocytes, Touton giant cells, foamy histiocytes
- Spindle cells wrap around dermal collagen at the periphery
- Overlying epidermal changes:
  - Epidermal hyperplasia
  - Basaloid follicular induction
  - Basal cell hyperpigmentation
- IHC: Positive: CD68/CD163, factor XIIIa (dendritic cells); negative: CD34

Clinically Significant Variants with Greater Risk of Local Recurrence

Cellular Dermatofibroma

- Stellate lesion in deep dermis with frequent subcutaneous involvement
- Limited infiltration along fibrous septa
- Monotonous fascicles of plump spindle cells with eosinophilic cytoplasm
- Brisk normal mitotic activity; rare necrosis
- IHC: variable SMA, desmin; CD34 is negative except the periphery

Angiomatoid Dermatofibroma

- Basophilic cellular tumor at scanning magnification
- Blood-filled dilated spaces lined by attenuated tumor cells
- Polymorphous cellular composition like classic dermatofibroma
- IHC: same as classic dermatofibroma

Atypical Dermatofibroma

- Atypical hyperchromatic and pleomorphic cells with increased mitotic figures
- Multinucleated tumor cells with atypical nuclei ("monster" cells)
- IHC: same as classic dermatofibroma

Deep Dermatofibroma

- Deep dermis or subcutis
- Circumscribed periphery with frequent lymphoid aggregates
- Whorls or short fascicles of relatively monotonous fibroblastic cells
- Staghorn/HPC-like vessels
- IHC: variable SMA, desmin, CD34

Differential Diagnosis

- Classic DF: DFSP, dermatomyofibroma, scar, sclerosing nevus
- Cellular DF: DFSP, leiomyosarcoma, nodular fasciitis
- Atypical DF: pleomorphic fibroma, AFX
- Deep DF: solitary fibrous tumor, inflammatory myofibroblastic tumor

AFX, Atypical fibroxanthoma; *DF*, dermatofibroma; *DFSP*, dermatofibrosarcoma protuberans; *IHC*, immunohistochemistry; *SMA*, smooth muscle actin.

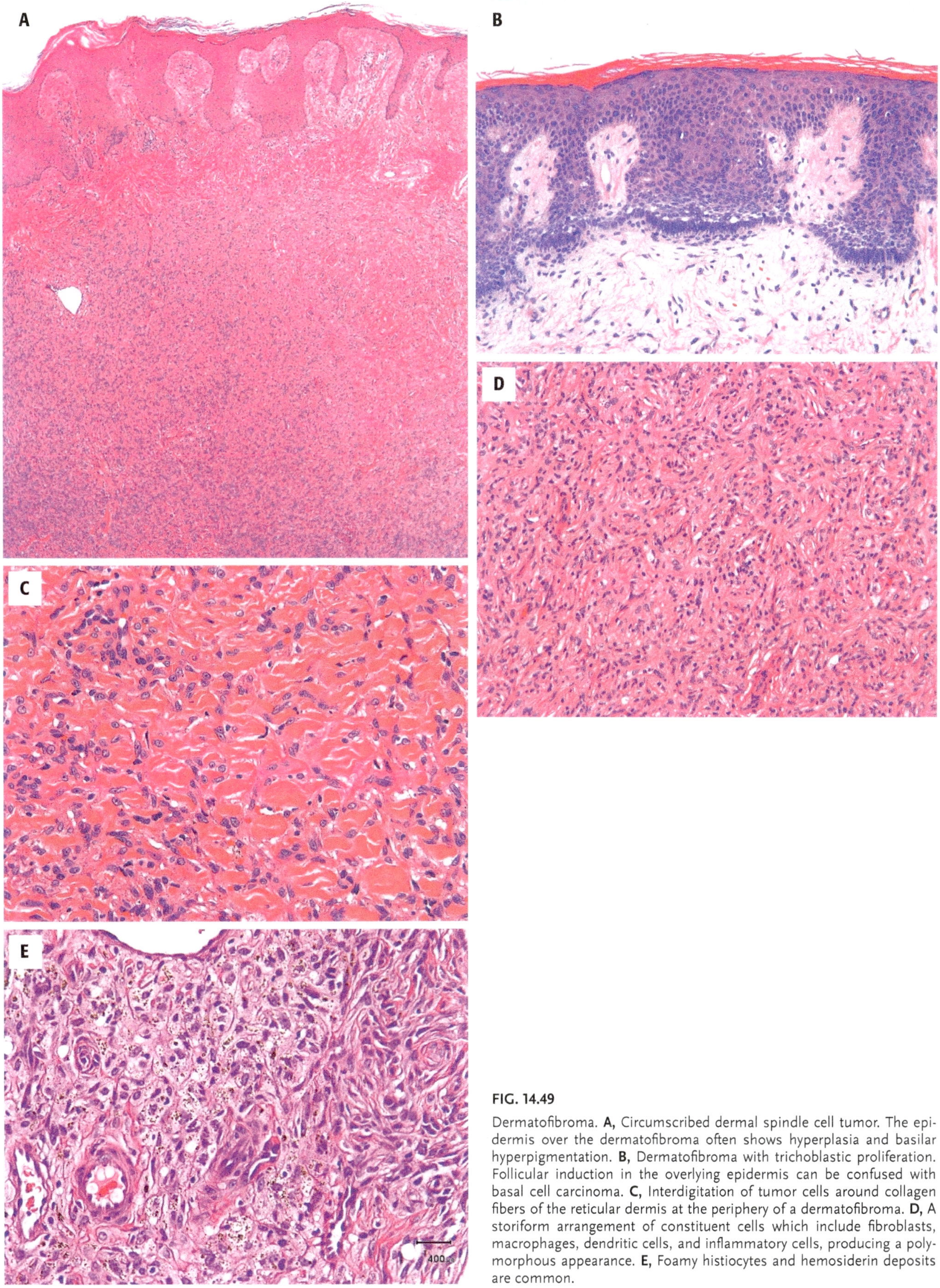

FIG. 14.49

Dermatofibroma. **A,** Circumscribed dermal spindle cell tumor. The epidermis over the dermatofibroma often shows hyperplasia and basilar hyperpigmentation. **B,** Dermatofibroma with trichoblastic proliferation. Follicular induction in the overlying epidermis can be confused with basal cell carcinoma. **C,** Interdigitation of tumor cells around collagen fibers of the reticular dermis at the periphery of a dermatofibroma. **D,** A storiform arrangement of constituent cells which include fibroblasts, macrophages, dendritic cells, and inflammatory cells, producing a polymorphous appearance. **E,** Foamy histiocytes and hemosiderin deposits are common.

As the name implies, cellular DF, also known as cellular FH, is more densely cellular and fascicular compared with classic DF It is typically a deeper-seated, stellate-shaped tumor that frequently involves the subcutis growing along fibrous septa. Cytologically, the tumor is more monomorphous resembling fibrosarcomatous DFSP, with a fascicular arrangement of spindled myofibroblastic cells with oval nuclei and pale eosinophilic cytoplasm, conspicuous mitotic activity (5 to 10/10 HPF) and at times, focal necrosis (Fig. 14.50A and B). However, in contrast to DFSP, cellular benign FH displays the typical collagen trapping at the periphery and lacks the diffuse infiltrative "honeycomb" subcutaneous growth pattern of the former. Of note, various secondary elements that are typically present in conventional benign DF (inflammatory cells, foamy histiocytes, giant cells, and hemosiderin deposits) are uncommon in cellular DF. However, cellular DF may coexist with other DF variants including the atypical and aneurysmal variant, making the diagnosis more straightforward. Cellular FH may occasionally show focal CD34 immunoreactivity, particularly at the periphery of the tumor where the tumor cells intercalate between dermal fibroblasts, as well as focal immunostaining for SMA and desmin, not seen in conventional DFs. Factor XIIIa, frequently used by dermatopathologists to detect a second population of dendritic cells within the lesion, is often negative in cellular FH.

Aneurysmal DF is characterized by large blood-filled spaces lined by compressed tumor cells in conjunction with otherwise typical histologic features of a DF (Fig. 14.51A and B). Hemosiderin-laden macrophages are often found in this variant. Atypical FH, also referred to as DF with monster cells, shows features of typical DF but contains a subpopulation of cells with large, hyperchromatic and pleomorphic nuclei and multinucleated cells (Fig. 14.52). Mitotic activity may be high, and atypical forms may be present. Deep FH is characterized by a purely subcutaneous and well-circumscribed tumor composed of bundles of palely eosinophilic fibrohistiocytic cells and often containing branching hemangiopericytomatous vessels and lymphoid aggregates at the periphery. Molecular findings identified recurrent fusions of protein kinase C genes *PRKC-B* and *PRKC-D* genes, with *LAMTOR1* being a common partner, in conventional, cellular, and aneurysmal FH further supporting the assertion that these tumors represent a histologic spectrum of the same entity.

A

B

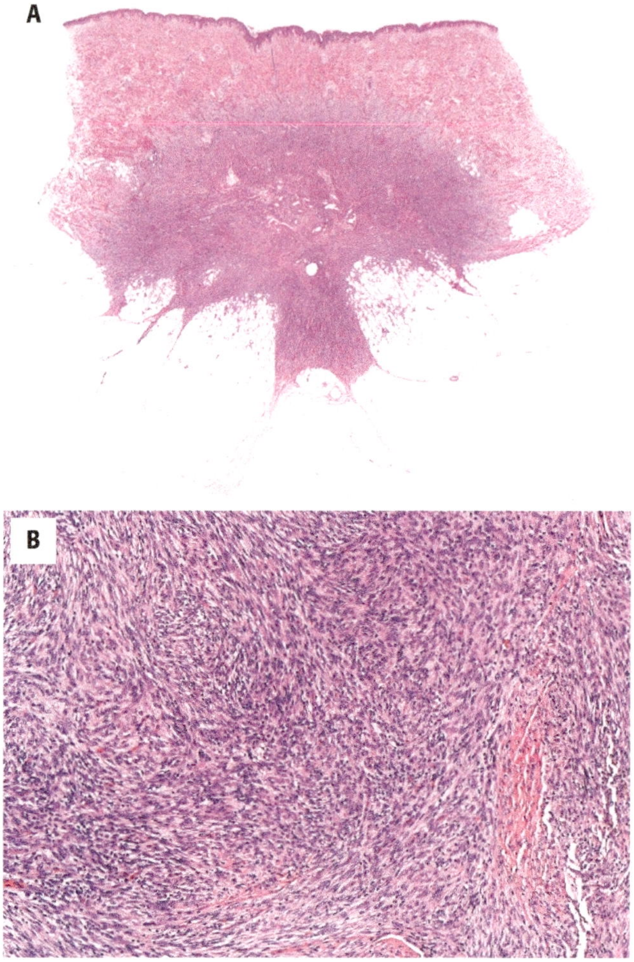

FIG. 14.50

Cellular dermatofibroma/cellular fibrous histiocytoma. **A,** A stellate-shaped tumor at the interface between dermis and subcutis with focal infiltration along the interlobular septa. **B,** Monomorphic fascicles of spindled myofibroblastic cells with oval nuclei, pale eosinophilic cytoplasm, and noticeable mitotic figures.

Differential Diagnosis

The principal differential diagnosis is DFSP, which can be separated by the more monotonous appearance of the lesional cells and a more diffuse pattern of infiltration incorporating individual adipocytes; the overlying epidermis is often atrophic. CD34 immunostaining is typically strongly positive in DFSP and negative in DF, although it might be positive at the lesional periphery where the lesional cells intermingle with dermal collagen. Lipidized versions of DF need to be distinguished from xanthoma and xanthogranuloma. Those lesions contain many more foamy histiocytes and lack a fibroblastic component and a peripheral collagen trapping. Atypical FH needs to be distinguished from AFX and pleomorphic dermal sarcoma. The latter two lesions typically occur on the sun-damaged skin of the head and neck region in older adults and lack the conventional DF component or peripheral collagen trapping seen in variants of DF, including atypical.

Cellular DF can appear quite alarming and maybe misdiagnosed as malignancy. In particular, cellular DF can closely resemble atypical dermal smooth muscle tumors and leiomyosarcomas, further confounded by frequent desmin and SMA expression. However, like its

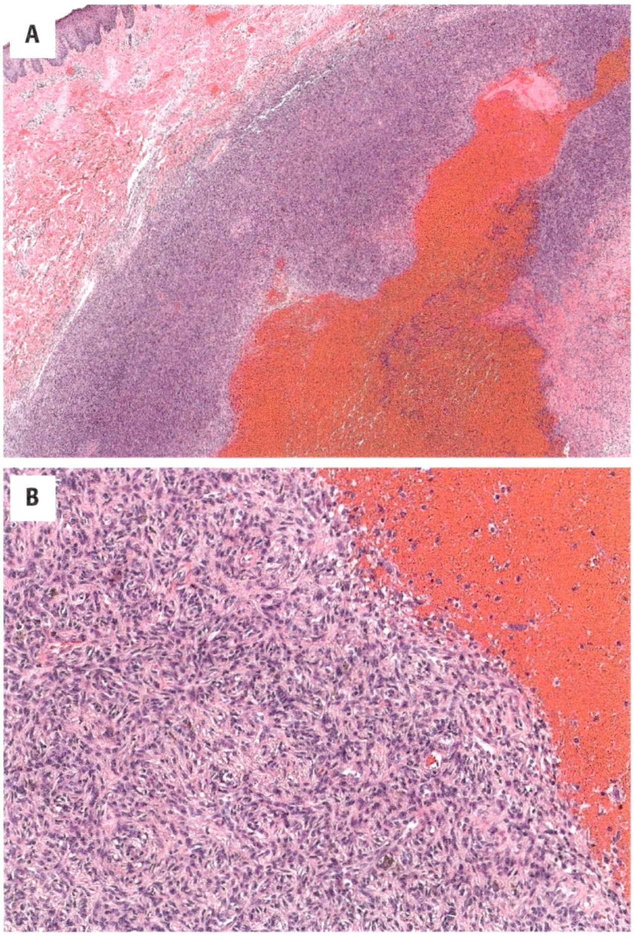

FIG. 14.51

A and **B**, Aneurysmal fibrous histiocytoma characterized by large blood-filled spaces lined by compressed tumor cells in conjunction with otherwise typical polymorphous appearance of the conventional dermatofibroma. Hemosiderin-laden macrophages are common.

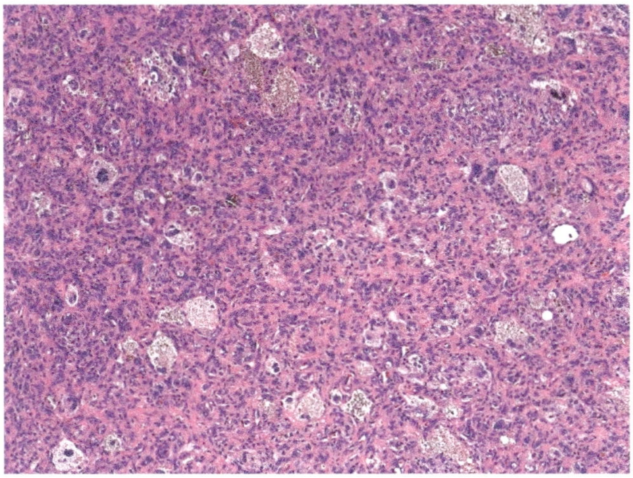

FIG. 14.52

Atypical fibrous histiocytoma showing large, hyperchromatic, and pleomorphic cells and multinucleated cells in a lesion with features otherwise typical of dermatofibroma. Mitotic activity may be conspicuous in this variant.

conventional counterpart, cellular DF consistently shows collagen trapping and in more superficial cases, also epidermal hyperplasia, features that are not seen in its smooth muscle mimics. Same principles apply when distinguishing cellular FH from conventional and fibrosarcomatous DFSP; cellular FH may be positive for CD34, usually at the periphery of the lesion, but in contrast to DFSP, it often co-expresses SMA and desmin. Difficult cases may be confirmed by FISH or molecular analysis targeting *COL1A1::PDGFRB* fusions.

Spindle cell metaplastic carcinoma can be distinguished based on the presence of cytokeratin expression and the presence of key pathognomonic histological features mentioned above (i.e., collagen trapping, epidermal hyperplasia). On the benign end of the spectrum, more cellular examples of nodular fasciitis might be especially difficult to separate from cellular DF as both lesions will show fascicular myofibroblastic architecture and a mildly infiltrative edge. FISH testing for *USP6* gene rearrangement can be employed in situations in which expectant management is considered, as cellular DF will tend to progress with time if not excised, whereas nodular fasciitis will likely regress.

Prognosis and Treatment

Conventional DF and variants are cured by simple excision. Cellular FH is associated with approximately 25% risk of nondestructive local recurrence and very rare metastases, typically in the setting of multiple recurrences. Atypical and aneurysmal FH may also recur; however, the risk is higher in tumors that also have cellular FH component. Therefore, these variants are ideally treated by complete local excision.

EPITHELIOID FIBROUS HISTIOCYTOMA AND NONNEURAL GRANULAR CELL TUMOR

Epithelioid FH and nonneural granular cell tumor (NNGCT, formerly known as primitive polypoid granular cell tumor) were once thought to represent variants of the conventional DF and granular cell tumor, respectively. Now they are considered to be distinct and possibly related entities defined by *ALK* gene rearrangements.

Clinical Findings

Epithelioid FH presents as a skin-colored or erythematous polypoid lesion on the extremities of young adults. NNCGT has an overlapping clinical presentation but may also involve other sites such as head and neck region.

EPITHELIOID FIBROUS HISTIOCYTOMA—DISEASE FACT SHEET

Clinical Findings
- ▸▸ Polypoid lesion on the extremities of young adults.

Histopathologic Features
- ▸▸ Polypoid lesion with an epidermal collarette
- ▸▸ Sheets of uniform epithelioid or stellate cells in a collagenous background
- ▸▸ Eccentric grooved or convoluted nucleus with open chromatin and a small nucleolus
- ▸▸ Ample eosinophilic cytoplasm

IHC/Molecular
- ▸▸ Positive for factor XIIIa in the tumor cells, not intervening dendritic cells
- ▸▸ Variable EMA, negative cytokeratins, S100, SOX10, desmin
- ▸▸ Recurrent *ALK* gene fusions resulting in robust expression of ALK by IHC

Differential Diagnosis
- ▸▸ Syncytial myoepithelioma
- ▸▸ Epithelioid schwannoma
- ▸▸ Nevi and melanoma
- ▸▸ Superficial ALK-rearranged spindle cell neoplasm (SAMS)

ALK, Anaplastic lymphoma kinase; *EMA*, epithelial membrane antigen; *IHC*, immunohistochemistry; *SMA*, smooth muscle actin.

Histopathologic Features

Epithelioid FH is a polypoid lesion with an epidermal collarette. It is composed of uniform epithelioid to polygonal to stellate cells growing in sheets in a collagenous background such that the boundaries of individual cells are well appreciated. The cells contain eccentric, enlarged, and somewhat convoluted nucleus with open chromatin and a small nucleolus, and ample eosinophilic cytoplasm (Fig. 14.53A and B). There is no significant cytologic atypia, and mitotic figures are sparce. The tumor cells diffusely express factor XIIIa in contrast to the conventional DF where factor XIIIa picks up a second population of dermal dendritic cells that invest the lesion. EMA may be positive but cytokeratins, S100, SOX10, desmin, and SMA are usually negative. NNGCT is a similarly polypoid lesion that may have a collarette, but it has a somewhat different appearance with sheets of spindled cells with eosinophilic and granular cytoplasm, oval, mildly atypical nuclei, and some mitotic activity (Fig. 14.53C and D). The prominent spindling is the main histologic difference from epithelioid FH. Angulated or branching vessels with peripheral accentuation may be present in both tumors. NNGCT may express NKI-C3 and is negative for cytokeratins, S100, SOX10, desmin, and SMA. Both tumors demonstrate the presence of recurrent *ALK* gene fusions in >90% of cases, with partners including *SQSTM1*, *VCL*, and *DCTN1* resulting in robust expression of ALK by IHC (Fig. 14.53E and F).

Differential Diagnosis

The differential diagnosis of an epithelioid FH is with other epithelioid cutaneous tumors, including Spitz nevi and malignant melanoma, syncytial myoepithelioma, and epithelioid schwannoma. Syncytial myoepitheliomas, like epithelioid FH, present as red-brown (at times polypoid) papules clinically and appear as well-circumscribed epithelioid dermal tumors histologically. Both tumors are negative for cytokeratins; however, syncytial myoepitheliomas robustly express EMA, frequently coexpress S100 and are negative for ALK. *EWSR1::PBX3* fusions occur in nearly all tumors, and *EWSR1* FISH testing can be helpful diagnostically. Epithelioid schwannomas can be distinguished based on the deeper location and overt tumor circumscription, robust expression of schwannian markers, and loss of SMARCB1/INI-1 expression, while ALK IHC in these tumors is negative. Spitz nevi (of which some can harbor *ALK* gene rearrangements) and melanoma are best distinguished based on the identification of junctional melanocytic component and expression of melanocytic markers (S100, SOX10, Melan-A) that are not present in epithelioid FH. NNGCT must be separated from the conventional granular cell tumor; the latter is a true schwannian neoplasm with expression of SOX10, S100, and inhibin driven by mutations in vacuolar proton transporter genes *ATP6AP1* and *ATP6AP2*. Conventional granular cell tumor shows less atypia than NNGCT and is negative for ALK. Cellular neurothekeoma may show similar spindled cells with granular cytoplasm and NKI-C3 expression; however, cellular neurothekeoma shows a distinctly nested growth pattern rather than forming solid sheets of spindle cells and lacks *ALK* gene alterations. Finally, superficial ALK-rearranged SAMS may enter the discussion based on the presentation as an extremity-based dermal tumor and ALK immunoreactivity. However, these lesions typically show biphasic appearance with cords, whorls, or loose fascicles of spindled to epithelioid neoplastic cells set in a prominent myxohyaline stroma. In contrast to epithelioid FH and NNGCT, SAMS co-expresses CD34 and S100.

Prognosis and Treatment

Epithelioid FH and nearly all NNGCT reported to date behave in a benign fashion, with rare recurrences. Locoregional recurrence and lymph node metastasis was reported in rare cases of NNGCT; however, the data on the behavior of this tumor considering molecular classification are still emerging.

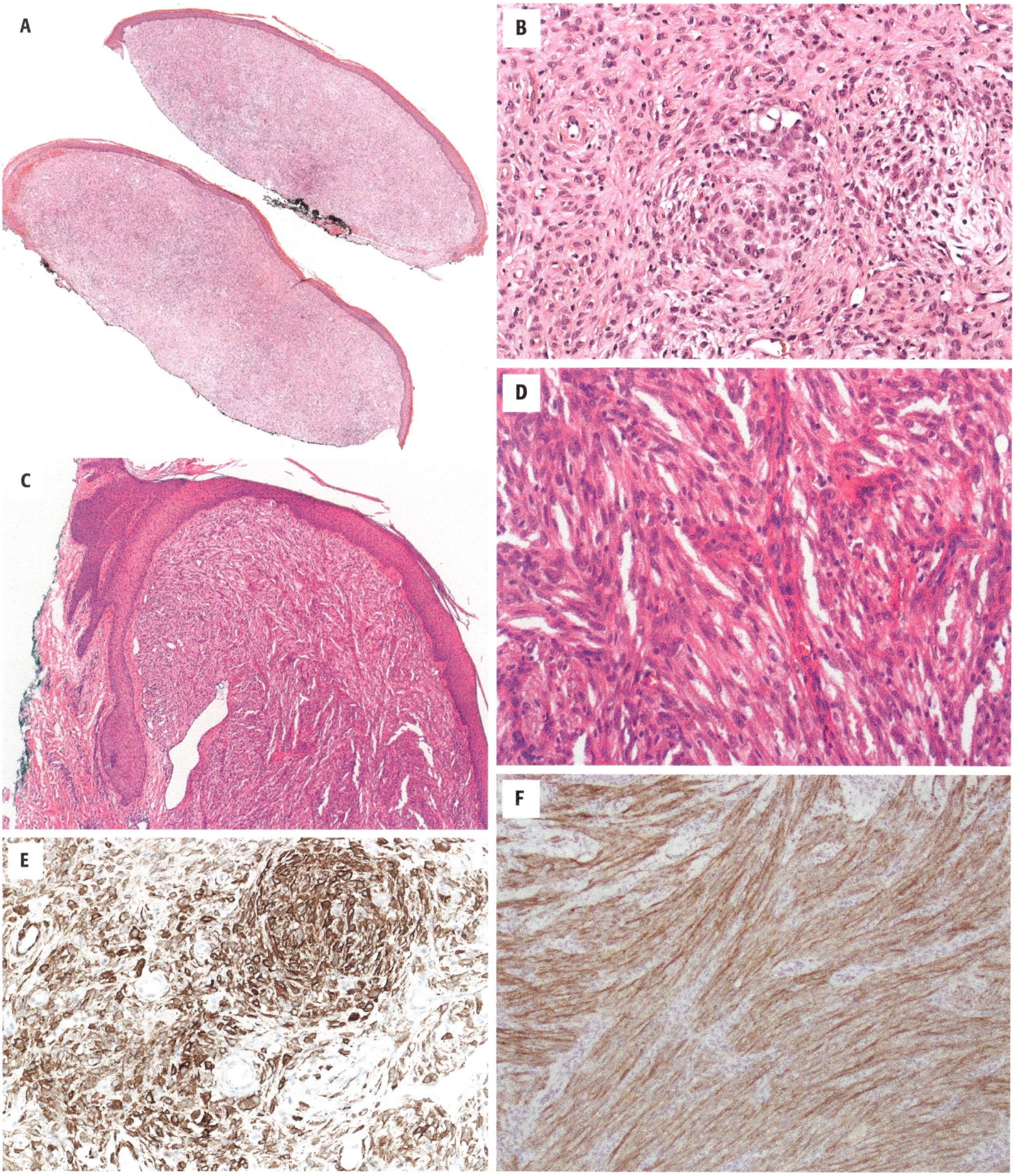

FIG. 14.53

Epithelioid fibrous histiocytoma. **A,** A circumscribed, exophytic lesion with an epidermal collarette. **B,** Uniform epithelioid, polygonal, or stellate cells with convoluted nuclei, growing in sheets in a collagenous background. **C,** Nonneural granular cell tumor (NNGCT) presenting as a polypoid lesion with a collarette. **D,** Sheets of spindled cells with eosinophilic granular cytoplasm, mildly atypical oval nuclei, and mitotic activity (**C** and **D**). Both epithelioid FH (**E**) and NNGCT (**F**) show robust expression of ALK.

CELLULAR NEUROTHEKEOMA

Clinical Findings

Cellular neurothekeoma is a distinctive fibrohistiocytic tumor that presents as a slowly enlarging cutaneous mass on the face or extremities of children and young adults, with a female predilection.

Histopathologic Features

Cellular neurothekeoma is composed of spindle or epithelioid cells arranged in a distinct lobular or nested pattern in the dermis. Extension into the superficial subcutis is possible. Cytologically, the tumor cells demonstrate oval, bland nuclei with uniform chromatin and abundant eosinophilic cytoplasm with indistinct cytoplasmic borders. The stroma is fibrous or myxoid, and occasional cases may show hemorrhage, hemosiderin deposits, or osteoclast-type giant cells within the nodules (Fig. 14.54A and B). Atypical features may include significant nuclear pleomorphism, mitotic activity, a focally infiltrative growth pattern, and rarely, perineural and lymphovascular invasion. None of these features appear to negatively impact the behavior. The tumor cells are positive for NKI-C3, CD10, and microphthalmia transcription factor (MITF) (variably). They are also frequently positive for PGP9.5, but this marker lacks sufficient discriminatory power to be useful. Some tumors also express CD68, CD163, and SMA. TFE3 expression has also been documented although this requires further understanding. SOX10, S100, CD34, desmin, and pancytokeratin are negative.

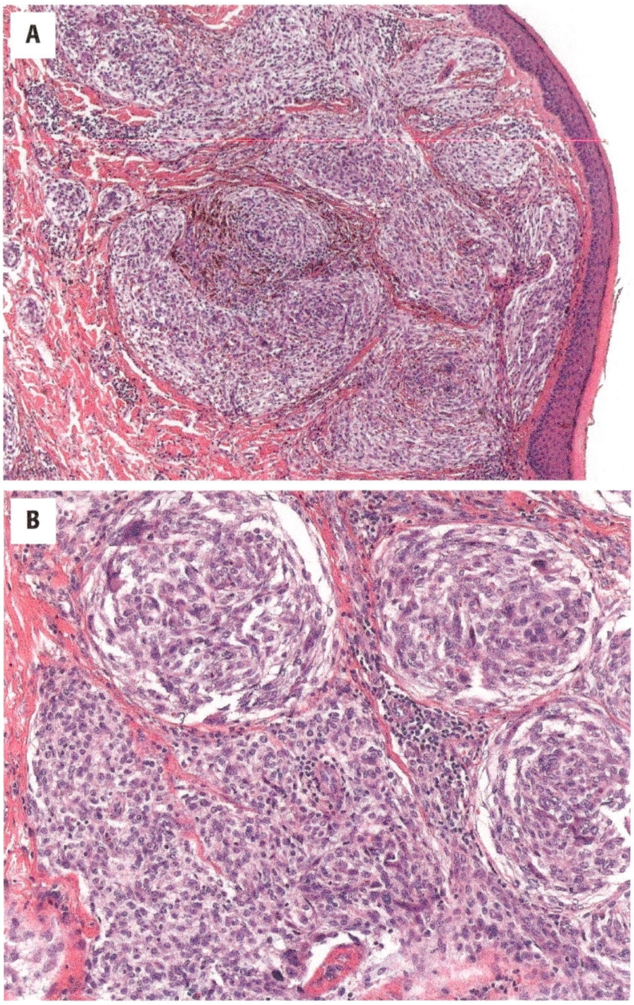

FIG. 14.54

Cellular neurothekeoma. **A,** Spindle or epithelioid cells in a nested pattern in the dermis. **B,** Cytologically, the tumor cells show oval, bland nuclei with uniform chromatin and abundant eosinophilic cytoplasm with indistinct cytoplasmic borders. Stromal hemosiderin deposits and osteoclast-type giant cells are present.

Differential Diagnosis

Melanocytic tumors can be distinguished based on expression of SOX10, S100, and MART/HMB45. Benign FHs lack distinct lobular growth pattern, show typical tumor interface with collagen trapping, and lack robust NKI-C3 expression even if CD10, PGP9.5, CD68, and CD163 expression can be seen in both tumors. Dermal nerve sheath myxoma (formerly known as myxoid neurothekeoma, discussed below) is similar in name only as it is a multinodular benign nerve sheath tumor with diffusely myxoid stroma and distinctive schwannian cells with multipolar processes that express S100 and SOX10. The individual tumor nodules of cellular neurothekeoma can look very similar to PFHT, but the latter prefers different anatomic regions (extremities) and typically extends into the deep soft tissue or skeletal muscle. PFHT is characteristically a biphasic neoplasm possibly driven by a neoplastic cell with CSF1 overexpression, composed of nodules of histiocytic cells and multinucleated giant cells separated by infiltrative fibromatosis-like fascicles; the latter component is not observed in cellular neurothekeoma. In contrast, myxoid stromal changes, which are commonly found in association with cellular neurothekeoma, are rarely seen with PFHT. Mitotic figures and some pleomorphism may be seen in association with a benign cellular neurothekeoma.

Prognosis and Treatment

Cellular neurothekeomas are benign. Conservative complete excision of atypical variants is generally recommended because of limited knowledge about the long-term recurrence potential of such lesions. Current evidence suggests that only a handful of tumors recur.

TENOSYNOVIAL GIANT CELL TUMOR

Clinical Findings

Tenosynovial giant cell tumors arise from synovium or related structures such as tendons, ligaments, and bursae and can be divided into two forms that have the same histologic appearance but different growth pattern. The localized, extraarticular type of tenosynovial giant cell tumor is also referred to as giant cell tumor of the tendon sheath. This tumor generally occurs in young to middle-aged adults, more frequently in women, and most commonly affects interphalangeal region of the fingers where it presents as a slow-growing mass fixed to the tendon sheath. Diffuse-type tenosynovial giant cell tumor, also termed pigmented villonodular synovitis, is a soft tissue equivalent of the intraarticular process with locally invasive, multinodular growth in periarticular soft tissues in the vicinity of large joints, often around the knee region, although small tubular bones of hands and feet can also be affected. Both forms of tenosynovial giant cell tumor are considered to represent a true neoplasm and are characterized by a recurrent translocation t(1;2)(p13;q37) resulting in *CSF1-COL6A3* fusion.

Histopathologic Features

Tenosynovial giant cell tumors are usually lobular, partially encapsulated, exophytic masses attached to the tendon sheath. There are five components present in variable proportions: round to oval mononuclear cells with oval eccentric nuclei, inconspicuous nucleoli and amphophilic cytoplasm, osteoclast-type giant cells, chronic inflammatory cells, lymphocytes, and hemosiderin deposits (Fig. 14.55A and B). The latter may form a ring within the cytoplasm of mononuclear cells. Cellular density and the amount of osteoclast-type giant cells is variable. Mitotic figures are common and can be brisk but significant atypia, sheetlike growth, and atypical mitotic figures are not seen and should prompt a consideration for rare malignant tenosynovial giant cell tumor, or an altogether different diagnosis. By IHC, clusterin and desmin can be expressed in the mononuclear cells, while the histiocytic and monocytic derivatives are highlighted by CD68, CD163, CD45, and MITF, which can be misleading.

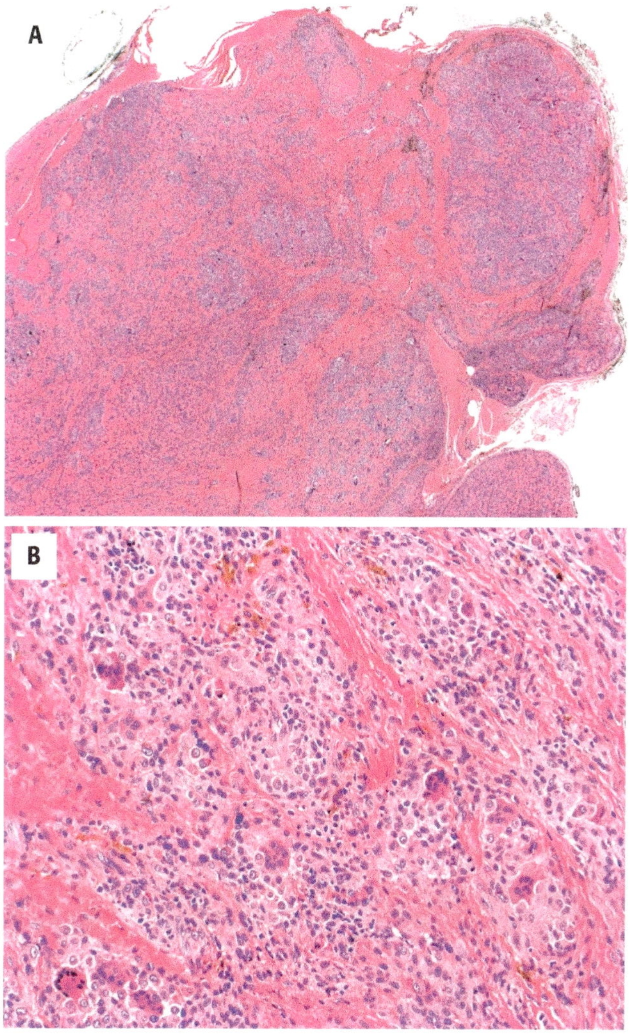

FIG. 14.55

Tenosynovial giant cell tumor. **A,** A multinodular mass attached to a tendon. **B,** Five components are present in variable proportions: oval to plasmacytoid mononuclear cells with eccentric nuclei, osteoclast-type giant cells, chronic inflammatory cells, lymphocytes, and hemosiderin deposits.

Differential Diagnosis

The giant cell tumor of soft tissue (GCT-ST) (also known as giant cell tumor of low malignant potential; see the following) does not typically involve the periarticular locations, has a distinctly multinodular growth pattern with thick intervening fibrous septa, a more prominent spindle cell component with nuclear features resembling those seen in osteoclast-type giant cells, and often a shell of metaplastic bone. Osseous metaplasia is distinctly uncommon in tenosynovial giant cell tumor. Tendinous xanthomas could be considered in the differential diagnosis in tumors in which xanthoma cells are particularly prominent, but xanthoma cells would be the only component in this tumor type. While also frequently polymorphous, DFs can be readily distinguished based on the spindled appearance of the lesional cells, characteristic superficial dermal appearance with fingerlike tissue interface, and overlying epidermal hyperplasia. DFs rarely share the clinical presentation of tenosynovial giant cell tumor.

Prognosis and Treatment

Tenosynovial giant cell tumor is a benign but prone to local recurrence, particularly for the diffuse-type tumors as complete excision is very difficult to achieve. Surgical excision remains the treatment of choice for both localized and diffuse type, although medical options targeting the CSF1 receptor are being explored.

ANGIOMATOID FIBROUS HISTIOCYTOMA

Clinical Findings

Angiomatoid FH (AFH) occurs in children and young adults as a solitary mass in the subcutis or deep dermis, most commonly in the extremities. Clinically, the lesion may resemble a hematoma, hemangioma, or a benign cyst and may grow rapidly due to intralesional hemorrhage. They may be associated with a variety of systemic manifestations, including fevers, weight loss, anemia, polyclonal gammopathy, and rarely a Castleman's disease–like lymphadenopathy. These systemic symptoms are attributed to cytokine production by the tumor because the systemic findings resolve shortly after the curative excision.

Histopathologic Features

At scanning magnification, AFH is a circumscribed subcutaneous tumor surrounded by a dense fibrous capsule and a chronic lymphocytic infiltrate which may include lymphoid follicle and germinal center formation and therefore be mistaken for a lymph node. The blood-filled cystic spaces lined by flattened tumor cells for which this tumor is named are present in most but not all cases (Fig. 14.56A and B). Cases without the large cystic spaces show at least some evidence of focal hemorrhage or hemosiderin deposits. The tumor cells may be either spindled, growing in a variety of patterns, including sheets, meningioma-like whorls, and short fascicles, or histiocytoid in appearance. Although the tumor cells are typically cytologically bland, with uniform oval nuclei and vesicular chromatin, occasional cases may show striking pleomorphism, which does not appear to have clinical significance (Fig. 14.56C). The mitotic rate is variable and can be striking in atypical AFH. Some cases have prominent myxoid stroma with reticular or corded arrangement of the cells (Fig. 14.56D). AFH have a unique immunophenotype, with variable coexpression of desmin, EMA, CD99, and CD68 and sometimes SMA. S100, SOX10, CD34, CD31, and ERG are consistently negative. ALK may on occasion be expressed, but there is no ALK rearrangement.. At the genetic level, AFHs are characterized by *EWSR1::CREB1* (over 90%), followed by *EWSR1::ATF1* (10%) and *FUS::ATF1* (<1%) gene fusions. These are amenable to diagnostic testing by *EWSR1* or *FUS* FISH.

ANGIOMATOID FIBROUS HISTIOCYTOMA—DISEASE FACT SHEET

Clinical Findings

- Dermal or subcutaneous mass in children and young adults
- Systemic symptoms (fevers, weight loss, anemia) due to cytokine production

Histopathologic Features

- Dense fibrous capsule
- Lymphoid aggregates with germinal centers at the periphery
- Blood-filled cystic spaces that can mimic a hematoma
- Sheets and whorls of spindled, epithelioid or histiocytoid cells
- Mild atypia and normal mitotic figures

IHC/Molecular

- Variable expression of desmin, EMA, CD99, CD68, SMA, and ALK
- *EWSR1::CREB1*, *EWSR1::ATF1* and *FUS::ATF1* fusions

Differential Diagnosis

- Aneurysmal dermatofibroma
- Pleomorphic and spindle cell sarcoma
- Malignancy metastatic to a lymph node

ALK, Anaplastic lymphoma kinase; *EMA*, epithelial membrane antigen; *IHC*, immunohistochemistry; *SMA*, smooth muscle actin.

Differential Diagnosis

Aneurysmal benign FH also occurs in the extremities of young adults and can present as a hemorrhagic nodule; however, it lacks a fibrous capsule and elsewhere shows typical features of DF including peripheral collagen trapping, epidermal hyperplasia and a more polymorphous cell population with siderophages and foamy macrophages. CD99, desmin, and EMA expression is uncharacteristic. The dense capsule and the surrounding lymphoid infiltrate seen in AFH may impart the appearance of a metastatic neoplasm in a lymph node. However, the pseudocapsule surrounding the lesional cells of AFH does not have subcapsular sinuses or afferent lymphatics that would indicate a true nodal architecture. AFH can easily be distinguished immunohistochemically from vascular neoplasms by lack of staining for vascular markers CD31, CD34, or ERG. Cytologically atypical cases may be diagnosed as a high-grade pleomorphic sarcoma as was the case when this lesion was originally described; however, the peripheral circumscription with lymphoid aggregates is a great clue to the correct diagnosis as sarcomas with pleomorphic phenotype rarely involve lymph nodes with exception for rhabdomyosarcoma, which can be distinguished based on the concurrent expression of markers of skeletal muscle differentiation including myogenin and MyoD1. Myxoid tumors with

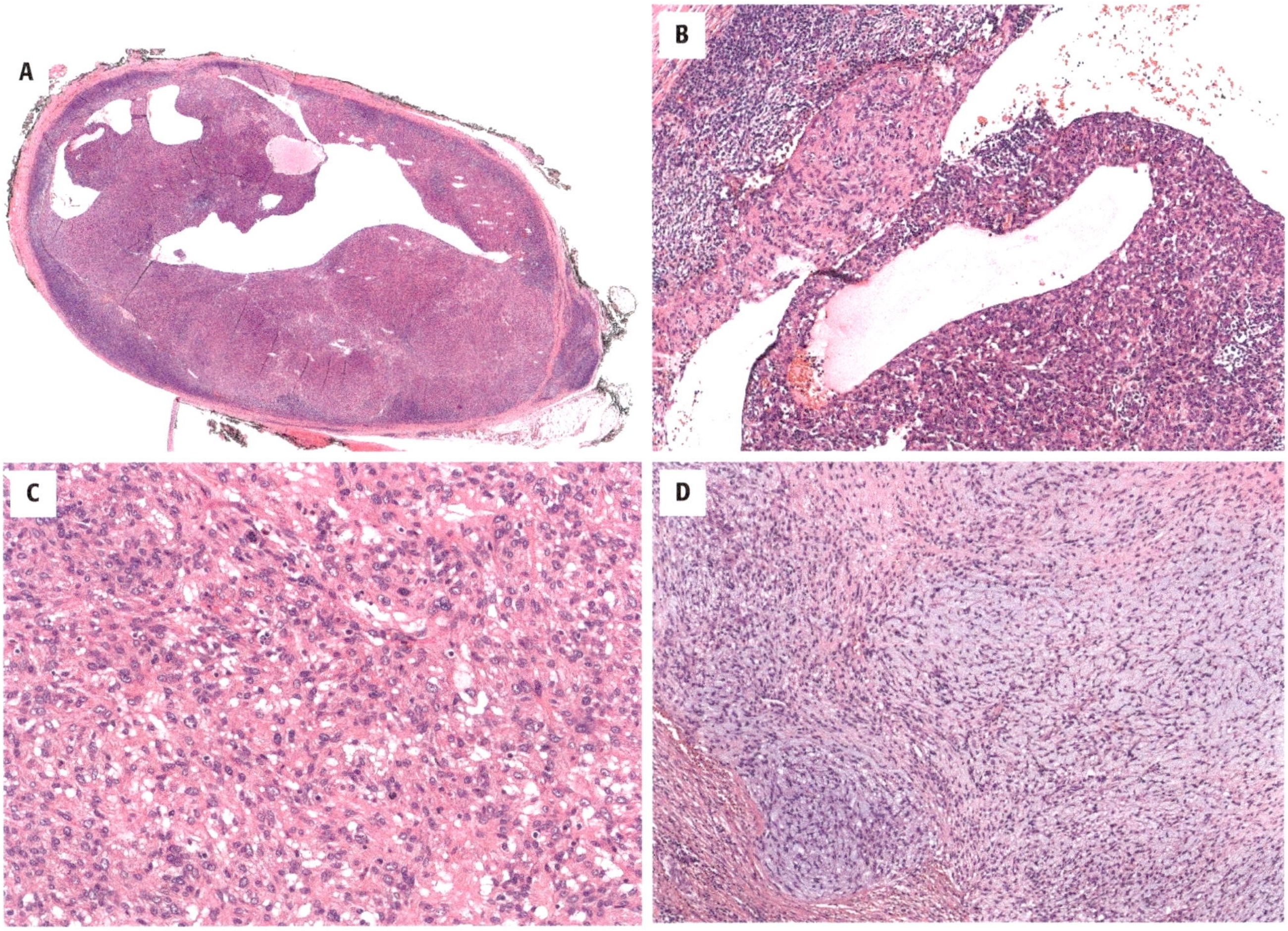

FIG. 14.56

Angiomatoid fibrous histiocytoma. **A,** A circumscribed tumor with a dense fibrous capsule and a chronic lymphocytic infiltrate. **B,** Blood-filled cystic spaces lined by flattened tumor cells. **C,** Histiocytoid spindle tumor cells growing in sheets, whorls, and short fascicles. There is mild atypia. **D,** Some cases have prominent myxoid stroma with reticular or corded arrangement of the cells.

reticular or corded growth pattern may be especially tricky as they resemble myoepithelial tumors, LGFMS, extraskeletal myxoid chondrosarcoma, OFMT, and other gene fusion-driven neoplasms with the so-called myoepithelial appearance and a highly variable malignant potential. In this context, none of the immunohistochemical stains will provide the needed diagnostic resolution, and we recommend that myxoid AFH is confirmed by FISH or molecular analysis.

Prognosis and Treatment

Once thought to be a sarcoma based on the initial description of this tumor leading to a designation as "angiomatoid malignant fibrous histiocytoma," AFH has an indolent clinical course with 10% to 15% risk of local recurrence and only a very low risk of metastasis, mostly to regional lymph nodes. Owing to this now recognized more indolent or low-grade behavior, AFH is now placed in a tumor of uncertain behavior category. Surgical excision remains the mainstay of therapy.

SYNCYTIAL MYOEPITHELIOMA

Clinical Findings

Cutaneous syncytial myoepithelioma is a distinctive subtype with a predilection for intraepidermal growth. These tumors usually present on the skin of the upper and lower extremities or head and neck as small (median, 0.8 mm) painless polypoid nodules. Truncal skin and exceptionally rare osseous and deep soft tissue locations have been reported.

Histopathologic Features

Syncytial myoepitheliomas are relatively well-circumscribed, unencapsulated nodules centered in the dermis and abutting the overlying epidermis and may show subcutaneous extension. They are composed of solid sheets of spindled, epithelioid, or histiocytoid cells with bland oval nuclei and eosinophilic cytoplasm without distinct cell borders, imparting a distinctive syncytial

SYNCYTIAL MYOEPITHELIOMA—DISEASE FACT SHEET

Clinical Findings

- Intraepidermal nodule on the skin of the upper and lower extremities

Histopathologic Features

- Circumscribed, unencapsulated nodule abutting epidermis
- Spindled, epithelioid, or histiocytoid cells with syncytial appearance
- Oval, bland nuclei, inconspicuous mitotic figures
- Chondroosseous or adipocytic metaplasia

IHC/Molecular

- EMA positive but cytokeratin usually negative
- Variable myoepithelial markers S100, SOX10, p63, GFAP, and calponin
- Recurrent *EWSR1::PBX3* gene fusions

Differential Diagnosis

- Nevi and nevoid melanoma
- Epithelioid fibrous histiocytoma
- Cellular neurothekeoma

EMA, Epithelial membrane antigen; *GFAP*, glial fibrillary acidic protein; *IHC*, immunohistochemistry.

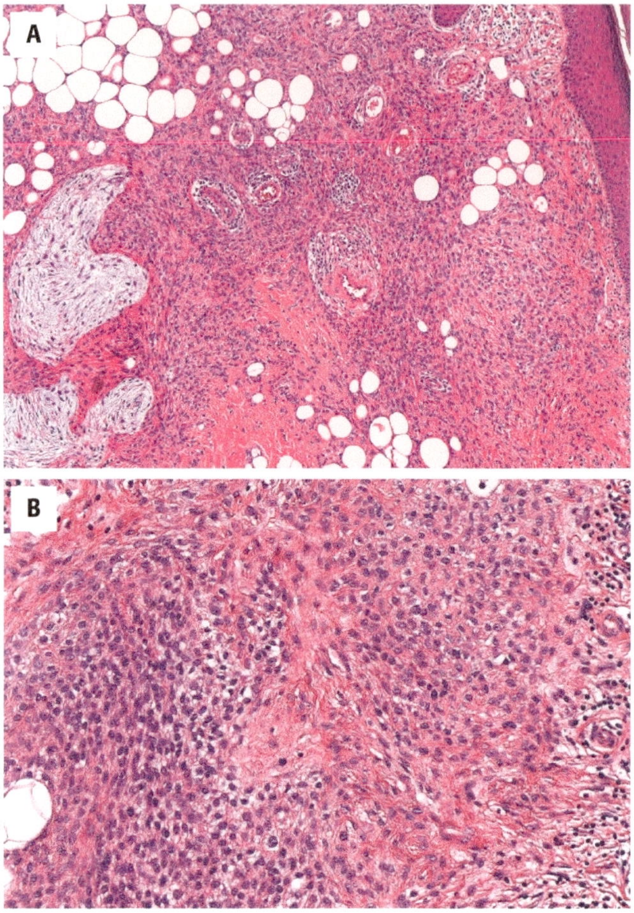

FIG. 14.57

Syncytial myoepithelioma. **A,** Dermal-based nodule abutting epidermis and extending into subcutis. Small myxoid islands and prominent adipocytic metaplasia is present. **B,** Sheets of cytologically bland, spindled, epithelioid to histiocytoid cells without distinct cell borders, imparting a syncytial appearance.

appearance. There is no tubuloductal differentiation as seen in cutaneous mixed tumors, but entrapped epithelial structures may occur (Fig. 14.57A). Multinucleated cells can occur. Mitotic figures are uncommon, and there is no necrosis or vascular invasion. Myxohyaline stroma typical of cutaneous mixed tumor is not a feature of syncytial myoepithelioma, but the latter may show small myxoid islands and chondroosseous or adipocytic metaplasia (Fig. 14.57B). Recognition of adipocytic metaplasia and epithelial entrapment in these tumors is important, as these features can be misinterpreted as infiltrative growth, giving the impression of a more aggressive neoplasm. Prominent lymphoid aggregates may be seen, usually at the tumor periphery. The immunoprofile of syncytial myoepitheliomas differs from cutaneous mixed tumor and myoepithelial tumors. Syncytial myoepitheliomas frequently express EMA and S100 protein and can be variably positive for other myoepithelial markers like SOX10, p63, GFAP, and calponin. However, cytokeratin expression is uncommon (approximately 10%) and is rarely diffuse. The INI1 expression pattern is uncertain. Recurrent *EWSR1::PBX3* gene fusions have been identified in syncytial myoepitheliomas.

Differential Diagnosis

Melanocytic neoplasms, such as nevoid melanomas, can be distinguished based on the expression of melanosome-based melanocytic markers such as HMB45 and Melan-A and, in difficult cases, FISH for EWSR1 gene rearrangement or *EWSR1::PBX3* gene fusion detected by NGS. Epithelioid FH usually presents as a well-circumscribed dermal nodule with an epidermal collarette, is composed of cytologically bland epithelioid or plasmacytoid cells with frequent binucleation, and can be positive for EMA. However, epithelioid FH lacks a distinctive syncytial growth pattern; rather, the cells are dispersed in a prominent collagenous stroma containing variable vessels with the boundary of each cell clearly visible. Adipocytic metaplasia is not characteristic of epithelioid FH. IHC is helpful as most EFHs show strong diffuse staining with factor XIIIa and ALK and are consistently negative for S100 protein and other myoepithelial markers. Cellular neurothekeoma has histiocytoid cells that are arranged in a distinctive nodular or plexiform growth pattern separated by fibrous bands rather than forming syncytia. Cellular neurothekeoma lacks S100 protein, EMA, and other myoepithelial marker expression and does not have an *EWSR1* gene rearrangement. Juvenile xanthogranulomas might arguably resemble syncytial myoepithelioma if they lack Touton-type giant cells; however, even in the absence of the latter juvenile xanthogranulomas are more polymorphous in appearance and contain foamy histiocytes and inflammatory cells such as eosinophils. They are negative for S100 protein, EMA, and myoepithelial markers and some may show *BRAF*V600E mutations detectable by IHC.

Prognosis and Treatment

Syncytial myoepitheliomas are benign, with a very low risk of local recurrence following simple excision.

LOCALLY AGGRESSIVE AND MALIGNANT FIBROBLASTIC/ MYOFIBROBLASTIC TUMORS

DERMATOFIBROSARCOMA PROTUBERANS AND GIANT CELL FIBROBLASTOMA

Clinical Findings

DFSP is a relatively common dermal or subcutaneous neoplasm of intermediate malignancy that has a predilection for the trunk and proximal extremities in young to middle-aged adults, though some cases can occur in very young children. DFSP presents as a nodular, red to tan to purple cutaneous mass, often in a background of a plaque or a scar, with slow but persistent growth; rapid growth may be associated with transformation to fibrosarcomatous DFSP. Giant cell fibroblastoma, for a while believed to represent a separate entity, is a version of DFSP with predilection for very young children and a distinctive morphology; however, both tumors share hybrid features and have the same molecular alterations indicating their relatedness.

Histopathologic Features

Microscopically, DFSP is characterized by an epicenter in the dermis and subcutaneous tissue with markedly infiltrative growth in the form of both infiltrative tumor septa as well as entrapment of individual adipocytes, forming the characteristic "honeycombed" appearance. The tumor cells are monotonous, bland-appearing fibroblastic spindle cells arranged in a storiform to the whorled pattern (Fig. 14.58A). Myoid nodules, composed of pink bundles or whorls of spindled cells, are an occasionally encountered, and nuclear palisading reminiscent of that seen in a schwannoma can be seen. Myxoid stroma rich in small vessels is not uncommon and is a predominant in some cases (Fig. 14.58B). Atrophic variant presents as a superficial plaque-like growth and may be mistaken for compressed normal tissue or nonneoplastic atrophic changes. DFSP colonized by melanin-containing dendritic cells can appear pigmented (Bednar tumor, Fig 14.58C). Giant cell fibroblastoma is a relatively paucicellular variant that consists of ovoid fibroblastic cells and scattered multinucleated tumor cells with a characteristic pericellular stromal clefting. Myxoid changes and areas of conventional DFSP can occur (Fig. 14.58D and E). Mitotic activity is inconspicuous and cytological atypia is minimal at best. By contrast, fibrosarcomatous DFSP shows a densely fascicular to herringbone monotonous growth pattern with moderate nuclear atypia and an elevated mitotic index. Fibrosarcomatous DFSP can paradoxically show a pushing tumor border with the exclusion of adipocytes within the interior of the tumor and corresponding loss of the "honeycombed" appearance seen in conventional DFSP (Fig. 14.59A and B). The background conventional DFSP is often compressed and may be underappreciated during surgical procedures or gross assessment of margins. By IHC, DFSP is diffusely and strongly positive for CD34 and is negative for SMA (except the myoid nodules), desmin, S100, SOX10, STAT6, and cytokeratins. There is usually no second factor XIIIa–positive cellular

DERMATOFIBROSARCOMA PROTUBERANS—DISEASE FACT SHEET

Clinical Findings

- Children and young adults
- Slow-growing cutaneous mass, plaque or scar on trunk and extremities

Histopathologic Features

- Diffusely infiltrative tumor with entrapment of individual adipocytes
- Monotonous, bland fibroblasts in a storiform pattern
- Myxoid stroma with prominent branching vessels
- Giant cell fibroblastoma:
  - Hypocellular tumor with ovoid fibroblastic cells and multinucleated tumor cells with pericellular clefting
- Fibrosarcomatous DFSP
  - Monotonous fascicles of spindle cells in a "herringbone" pattern
  - Moderate nuclear atypia and increased mitotic figures

IHC/Molecular

- Diffuse CD34 expression; negative for factor XIIIa, SMA, desmin, S100, SOX10, STAT6
- *COL1A1::PDGFRB* gene fusion or variant *COL6A3::PDGFD* fusion

Differential diagnosis

- Dermatofibroma
- Diffuse neurofibroma
- Fibroblastic connective tissue nevus
- Perineurioma
- Monotonous fascicular sarcomas (MPNST, synovial sarcoma, sarcomas with receptor tyrosine kinase gene fusions, fibrosarcoma)

DFSP, Dermatofibrosarcoma protuberans; *IHC*, immunohistochemistry; *SMA*, smooth muscle actin.

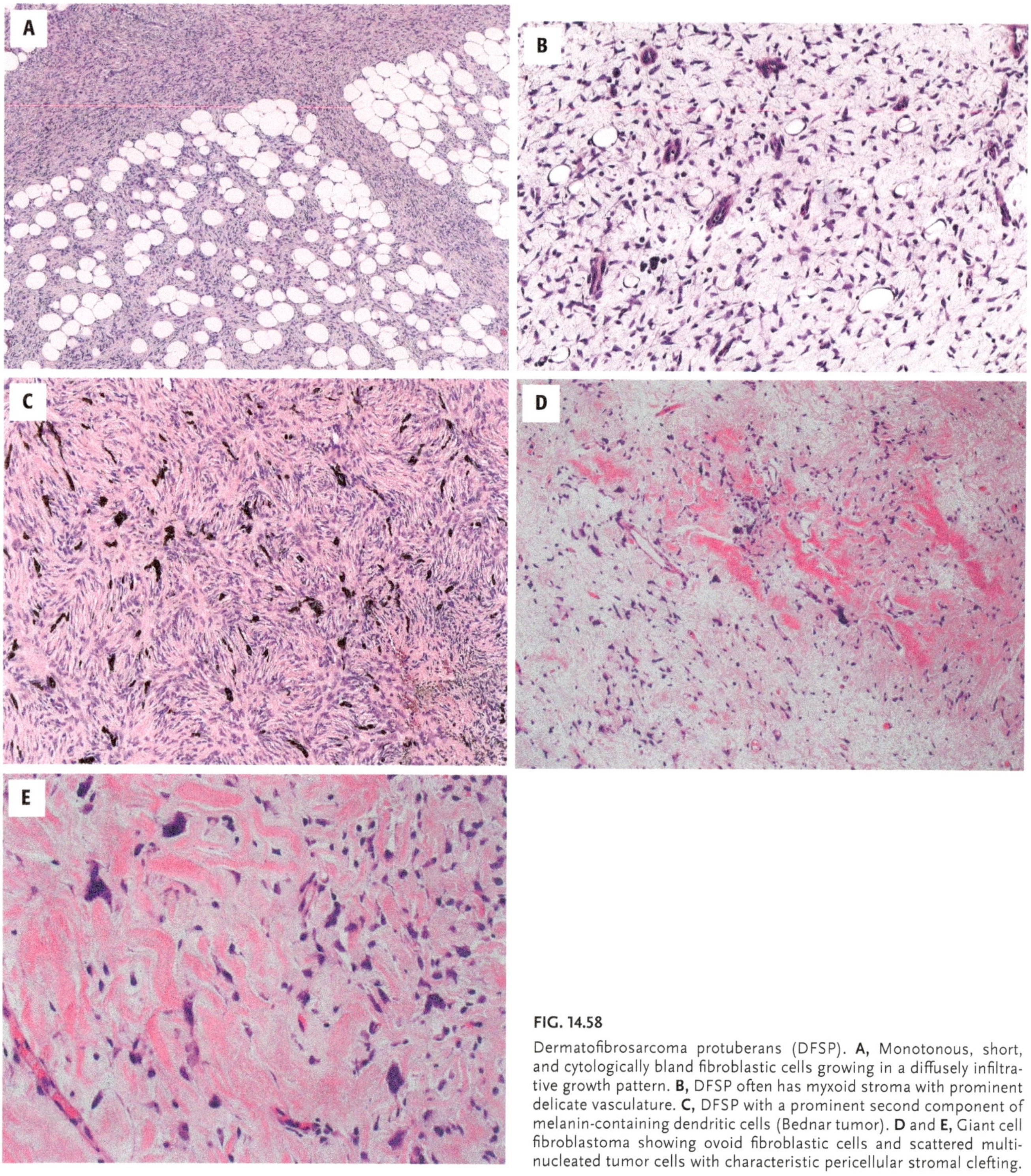

FIG. 14.58

Dermatofibrosarcoma protuberans (DFSP). **A,** Monotonous, short, and cytologically bland fibroblastic cells growing in a diffusely infiltrative growth pattern. **B,** DFSP often has myxoid stroma with prominent delicate vasculature. **C,** DFSP with a prominent second component of melanin-containing dendritic cells (Bednar tumor). **D** and **E,** Giant cell fibroblastoma showing ovoid fibroblastic cells and scattered multinucleated tumor cells with characteristic pericellular stromal clefting.

population, although this finding is not very reliable. CD34 expression can be patchy or absent in fibrosarcomatous DFSP. Molecular studies show the canonical *COL1A1::PDGFRB* gene fusion, which is retained in the fibrosarcomatous component. A novel variant *COL6A3::PDGFD* fusion has been described in cases with predilection for female breast, which still results in downstream expression of *PDGFRB*.

Differential Diagnosis

DFSP VERSUS CONVENTIONAL AND CELLULAR FIBROUS HISTIOCYTOMA

The distinction from the conventional DF based on a combination of classic features (a symmetric lesion with

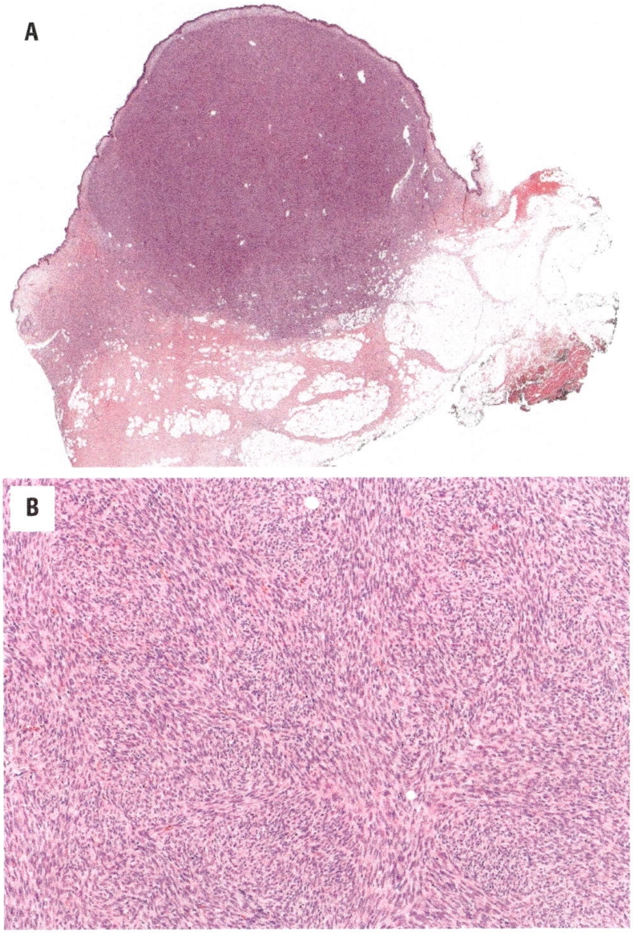

FIG. 14.59
Fibrosarcomatous dermatofibrosarcoma protuberans (DFSP). **A,** A cellular, relatively circumscribed tumor with compressed conventional DFSP at the periphery. **B,** Cellular fascicles arranged in a herringbone pattern with moderate nuclear atypia and increased mitotic activity.

epidermal hyperplasia, polymorphous cell composition, and limited peripheral tissue infiltration with collagen trapping) in combination with negative CD34 stain. The distinction from cellular FH is more problematic as the latter often has the monotonous, vaguely fascicular, and somewhat more infiltrative appearance with frequent subcutaneous extension, and variable CD34 immunoreactivity. One of the most helpful clues in this differential diagnosis is that cellular DF is also positive for desmin and SMA, markers that are consistently negative in all variants of DFSP.

DFSP VERSUS PERIPHERAL NERVE SHEATH TUMORS

With the impressive extent of subcutaneous involvement, diffuse neurofibroma may appear strikingly similar to DFSP; however, the cells lack the whorled growth pattern. While neurofibromas consist predominantly of CD34-positive fibroblasts, careful examination helps identify slightly hyperchromatic Schwann cells with coarse, wavy nuclei. In contrast, the whorled pattern predominates in soft tissue perineurioma and hybrid schwannomas/perineuriomas, and such cases are often diffusely CD34 positive. Soft tissue perineurioma and hybrid tumors are sharply circumscribed neoplasms with limited infiltration and often a pseudocapsule—a phenomenon not seen in DFSP. The cellular components may be discerned by morphology or by IHC for S100 and SOX10 (Schwann cells) and EMA, GLUT1, and claudin-1 (perineurial cells).

DFSP VERSUS FIBROBLASTIC CONNECTIVE TISSUE NEVUS

Plaque-like and atrophic variants of DFSP may resemble FCTN (discussed above). Both lesions demonstrate fascicles and bundles of bland spindle cells percolating the dermis and extending into the subcutis. However, DFSP can be distinguished based on the whorled growth pattern, absence of epidermal hyperplasia, and strong, diffuse CD34 immunoreactivity. Identification of giant cell fibroblastoma-like areas or other patterns of DFSP is very helpful, as is more diffuse subcutaneous infiltration in the latter as opposed to occasional adipocytes incorporated into the dermal portion of the lesion seen in FCTN.

DFSP VERSUS CD34-POSITVE MYOFIBROBLASTIC TUMORS, MYXOID LIPOSARCOMA AND LOW-GRADE MYXOFIBROSARCOMA

Spindle cell lipoma and its cousin, myofibroblastoma, can be distinguished based on a circumscribed growth pattern, thick or ropey refractile collagen fibers, variable expression of SMA and desmin, and loss of RB1 by IHC. SFT also shows variable degree of SMA expression and shows nuclear expression of STAT6. Myxoid DFSP looks strikingly similar to myxoid liposarcoma as the cells look similar and entrapped adipocytes can be mistaken for lipoblasts. However, careful examination of myxoid liposarcoma will show true multivacuolated lipoblasts, pools of myxoid material and a more uniform, delicate plexiform vasculature. Myxoid liposarcoma is negative for CD34 and harbors *DDIT3* gene rearrangements. Low-grade myxofibrosarcoma can be distinguished based on an uneven distribution of cellularity, more coarse vessels and importantly, cytologic pleomorphism that can be appreciated at low power even in the low-grade tumors. Myxofibrosarcoma is typically negative for CD34 and lacks *PDGFRB* gene rearrangements.

FIBROSARCOMATOUS DFSP VERSUS OTHER SARCOMAS WITH FIBROSARCOMATOUS PATTERN

Perhaps the most difficult differential diagnosis for a pure fibrosarcomatous DFSP at any site is an adult fibrosarcoma, from which fibrosarcomatous DFSP derives its name. Both tumors can look histologically identical, being composed of long and monotonous cellular fascicles, and both are variably positive for CD34. There is increasing evidence that most adult fibrosarcomas are also driven by various RTK gene fusions, most often involving *NTRK*, *RET*, or *ALK*, as opposed to the *PDGFRB* gene fusions seen in fibrosarcomatous DFSP. In an excisional specimen, the presence of an often compressed, conventional DFSP component at the periphery will give away the diagnosis; however, in small biopsy material, molecular testing for these rearrangements may be the only means for separating these pathogenetically related entities. As fusion-specific targeted therapies are available for both adult fibrosarcomas and fibrosarcomatous DFSP, this distinction has therapeutic implications in advanced or unresectable disease. Other mimics such as malignant SFT, spindle cell MPNST, SS, and atypical dermal smooth muscle tumor/leiomyosarcoma can be distinguished by application of appropriate lineage-specific immunostains. These are covered in detail elsewhere in this text. It is helpful to remember that fibrosarcomatous DFSP is negative for STAT6, S100, SOX10, and cytokeratins and virtually never expresses muscle markers to a significant extent. In all the diagnostic dilemmas described above, molecular or FISH testing for the pathognomonic *PDGFRB* gene fusion can be used to confirm the diagnosis of DFSP.

Prognosis and Treatment

All variants of conventional DFSP have a high rate of local recurrence (20%–50%) and therefore require wide local excision for optimal control. Metastases in conventional DFSP are exceedingly rare. By contrast, fibrosarcomatous DFSP can develop systemic metastases in 10% to 15% of cases. FNCLCC grading scheme is not applied to fibrosarcomatous DFSP because the degree of cytologic atypia or mitotic activity in this context are not predictive of metastasis. Targeted therapies are also available for patients with DFSP, making a distinction from its mimickers clinically relevant.

PLEXIFORM FIBROHISTIOCYTIC TUMOR

Clinical Findings

PFHT is rare, deep dermal or subcutaneous mass of the extremities predominantly in children and adolescents, with female predilection. It presents as slow-growing plaques or ill-defined fixed nodules, up to 3 cm in greatest dimension.

Histopathologic Features

PFHT displays as a poorly circumscribed, plexiform growth pattern (Fig. 14.60A). It has a biphasic appearance, being composed of multiple small nodules of histiocytoid cells in association with bandlike fascicles of bland fibroblastic cells that mingle with the histiocytoid nodules. The nodules contain round to oval mononuclear histiocytoid cells and osteoclast-like giant cells (Fig. 14.60B). There can be significant variation in the relative proportion of the spindle cell and histiocytic components in any given tumor. In the original description of the tumor, approximately 40% of cases showed the classic bimorphic appearance; another 40% showed a predominance of the histiocytic component, and 20% showed primarily a fibroblastic growth pattern. Mitotic activity in PFHT is typically low. The histiocytic cells show strong CD68, CD163, CD11c expression, while the spindle cells show membranous SMA expression in keeping with a myofibroblastic phenotype. Recent molecular

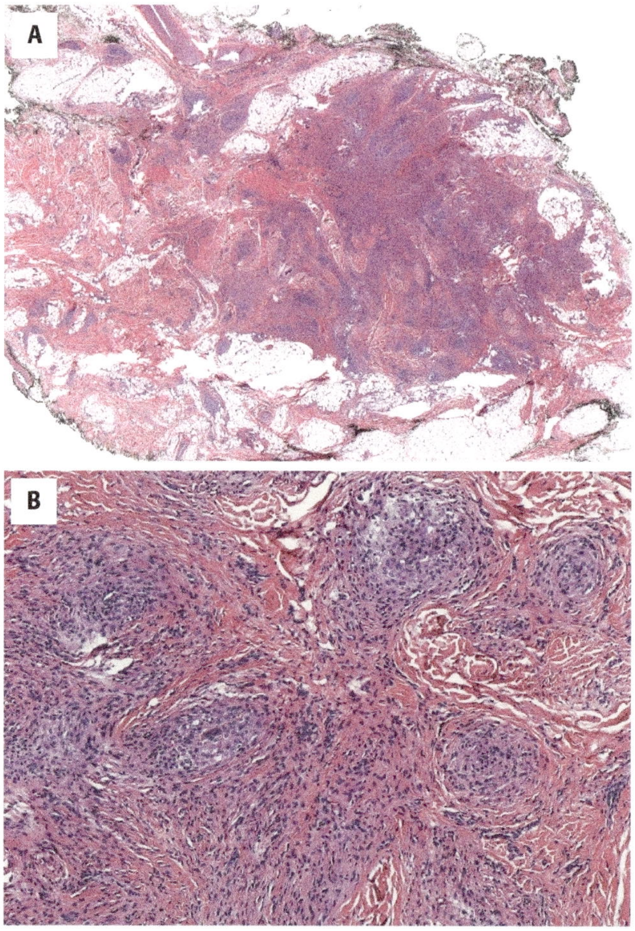

FIG. 14.60

Plexiform fibrohistiocytic tumor (PFHT). **A,** A poorly circumscribed, infiltrative subcutaneous tumor with a plexiform growth pattern. **B,** Biphasic appearance of PFHT with multiple small nodules of histiocytoid cells connected by fascicles of bland fibroblastic cells. The nodules contain round to oval mononuclear histiocytoid cells and osteoclast-like giant cells.

studies indicate that the neoplastic mononuclear histiocytoid cell may over express CSF1 but in contrast to the tenosynovial giant cell tumor, lack underlying *CSF1* gene rearrangements implying a different mechanism.

Differential Diagnosis

The differential diagnosis includes soft tissue tumors with plexiform growth pattern. The individual nodules of rounded cells and osteoclasts seen in PFHT can be indistinguishable from the tumor nodules of GCT-ST but the latter are typically much larger and more coarse, separated by thick fibrous bands rather than by an infiltrative fascicular component seen in PFHT. Like the giant cell tumor of bone, osteoclast-type giant cells dominate the picture in GCT-ST and obscure the nondescript mononuclear component. Metaplastic bone or aneurysmal bone cyst–like changes are supportive of GCT-ST. A predominantly fibroblastic growth pattern in a PFHT must be distinguished from lipofibromatosis and plexiform myofibroblastoma, with which it shares the clinical presentation as a superficial mass in young adults and a distinctly plexiform growth pattern with infiltration of deep subcutis at scanning magnification. However, the nodules of PFHT containing pale histiocytoid cells admixed with osteoclast-type giant cells are usually at least focally present in most cases and are not characteristic of the other entities. Cellular neurothekeoma is a superficial cutaneous tumor that, similar to PFHT, has a distinctly nodular growth pattern but typically not plexiform as the nodules are surrounded by collagenized stroma rather than proliferative fibroblastic fascicles. In contrast to PFHT, most cellular neurothekeomas are superficial tumors confined to the dermis and composed of larger, more epithelioid cells with eosinophilic cytoplasm in contrast to small histiocytic cells and myofibroblasts of the former. Myxoid stromal changes, which are commonly found in association with cellular neurothekeoma, are rarely seen with PFHT. Occasionally, it can be difficult to distinguish predominantly histiocytic PFHT from cellular neurothekeoma and predominantly fibroblastic PFHT from plexiform myofibroblastoma, particularly in partial biopsies, and it is likely that some of the pure histiocytoid and pure fibroblastic examples of PFHT described in the past indeed represent these other entities. By IHC, both cellular neurothekeoma and PFHT tumors express CD10 and NKI-C3 while MITF, present in cellular neurothekeomas, is typically negative in PFHT.

Prognosis and Treatment

PFHTs typically behave in an indolent fashion and may recur locally, but the risk of metastatic disease is exceptionally low and thus perhaps does not justify an overzealous wide excision of this very low-grade tumor. There is no role for chemotherapy or radiation therapy.

GIANT CELL TUMOR OF SOFT TISSUE

Clinical Findings

GCT-ST is a distinctive superficial mesenchymal neoplasm morphologically identical, but pathogenetically unrelated to giant cell tumor of bone. GCT-ST presents as a painless slowly growing subcutaneous or deep-seated nodule in adult patients, most often in the distal limbs followed by the trunk and head and neck region. Mean size is 3 cm.

Histopathologic Features

At scanning magnification, GCT-ST presents as multiple circumscribed nodules separated by thick fibrous bands (Fig. 14.61A). These nodules are composed of numerous osteoclast-type giant cells and an inconspicuous mononuclear component with round, plasmacytoid, or spindled cells with amphophilic cytoplasm, vesicular nuclei, and small nucleoli (Fig. 14.61B). The mononuclear cells are the neoplastic component in this tumor, which induce osteoclast recruitment by a RANKL-dependent mechanism. The stroma is highly vascular. Peripheral or septal metaplastic bone formation, aneurysmal bone cystlike changes, extravasated red blood cells, stromal fibrosis, and hemosiderin deposits are very common. Vascular invasion can be present but as is the case with giant cell tumors of bone, vascular invasion is not predictive of aggressive behavior. Mitotic activity in GCT-ST is often quite brisk, but as a general rule, atypical mitotic figures, significant nuclear atypia, and pleomorphism are uncharacteristic and, when present, should raise suspicion for an osteosarcoma or sarcomatoid carcinoma with an osteosarcomatous component. GCT-ST can be variably and usually focally immunoreactive for S100, SMA, SATB2, and p63, while osteoclast-type giant cells pick up CD68 and CD163. Cytokeratins and melanocytic markers are consistently negative. In contrast to giant cell tumors of bone, GCT-ST does not have H3F3A G34W mutation.

Differential Diagnosis

The differential diagnosis with PFHT is described in the previous section. Giant cell tumor of bone is very similar morphologically to GCT-ST but can be distinguished by

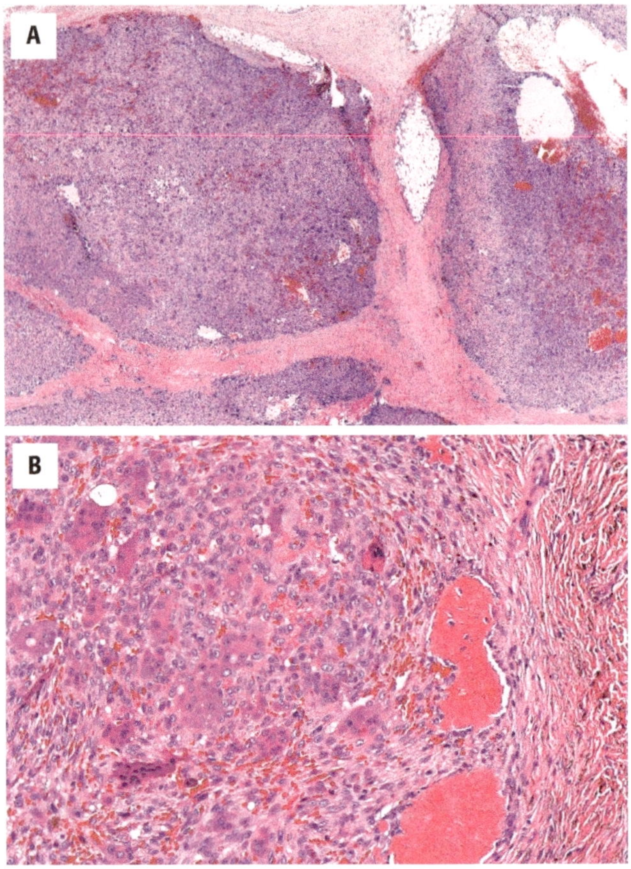

FIG. 14.61

Giant cell tumor of soft tissue. **A,** Circumscribed coalescing nodules separated by thick fibrous bands. **B,** Numerous osteoclast-type giant cells admixed with bland mononuclear cells with amphophilic cytoplasm, vesicular nuclei, and small nucleoli. The stroma is highly vascular.

H3F3A G34W IHC. The key differential diagnosis is with telangiectatic osteosarcoma, primary or metastatic. Like GCT-ST, extraskeletal osteosarcoma often develops aneurysmal bone cystlike changes and contains numerous osteoclast-type giant cells. However, the presence of lacelike immature osteoid deposits intimately associated with the tumor cells (in contrast to the well-developed rim of mature metaplastic bone in GCT-ST) favors osteosarcoma. But the key histologic clue to osteosarcoma is overt cytologic atypia, pleomorphism, and atypical mitotic figures that are not present in GCT-ST. Same principle applies to undifferentiated pleomorphic sarcoma with osteoclast-type giant cells. Sarcomatoid SCC with heterologous differentiation can be distinguished by the appropriate morphologic or immunophenotypic evidence of epithelial differentiation or identification of in situ carcinoma.

Prognosis and Treatment

GCT-ST is considered a tumor of uncertain malignancy, with a risk of local recurrence of approximately 10% to 15% and exceptionally rare metastases that do not justify regarding GCT-ST as a malignant neoplasm. No single histologic feature is predictive of behavior as tumors with overtly malignant nuclear features are classified as other tumor types. The treatment of choice is complete local excision.

MALIGNANT FIBROBLASTIC AND MYOFIBROBLASTIC TUMORS

ATYPICAL FIBROXANTHOMA AND DERMAL PLEOMORPHIC SARCOMA (UNDIFFERENTIATED PLEOMORPHIC SARCOMA OF THE SKIN)

Clinical Findings

AFX is a cutaneous tumor that presents as a papule or nodule on sun-damaged skin of elderly patients, typically in the head and neck region, particularly scalp. The overlying

ATYPICAL FIBROXANTHOMA—DISEASE FACT SHEET

Clinical Findings
- Rapidly growing papule or nodule on sun-damaged skin of elderly patients
- Commonly face, scalp particularly scalp

Histopathologic Features
- Circumscribed tumor with a pushing margin limited to the dermis
- Pleomorphic stellate, spindled, epithelioid, multinucleated cells
- Overt nuclear atypia, pleomorphism, atypical mitotic figures
- Epidermal collarette, ulceration, peritumoral chronic inflammation
- Background solar damage

IHC/Molecular
- SMA in a myofibroblastic pattern; nonspecific CD10, CD68
- UV signature, p53 and *TERT* promoter mutations

Differential Diagnosis
- Dermal pleomorphic sarcoma which looks like AFX but invades subcutis or shows vascular and perineural invasion
- Spindle cell squamous cell carcinoma
- Malignant melanoma
- Atypical dermatofibroma
- Other cutaneous pleomorphic sarcomas
  - Leiomyosarcoma
  - Pleomorphic rhabdomyosarcoma
  - Osteosarcoma
  - Pleomorphic liposarcoma

AFX, Atypical fibroxanthoma; *IHC*, immunohistochemistry; *SMA*, smooth muscle actin; *UV*, ultraviolet.

epidermis may be ulcerated, and the clinical appearance can be confused with common cutaneous malignancies such as BCC or SCC. Dermal pleomorphic sarcoma (undifferentiated pleomorphic sarcoma of the skin) represents a clinical and histologic continuum and is distinguished based on the depth of invasion or other parameters indicating aggressive growth.

Histopathologic Features

AFX is a dermal tumor composed of pleomorphic stellate to spindled and epithelioid cells with atypical hyperchromatic nuclei and amphophilic cytoplasm (Fig. 14.62A and B). The tumor cells can have a random arrangement or a fascicular to storiform growth pattern. A clear-cell variant exists (Fig. 14.62C). Background skin shows significant solar damage. Mitotic figures, including atypical forms, are usually present. The cytology of AFX is indistinguishable from undifferentiated sarcoma. The key distinction is based on the architecture: AFX is a relatively circumscribed tumor with a pushing margin confined to the dermis. Chronic inflammatory infiltrate and an epidermoid collarette may be present at the periphery of the tumor. AFX is usually confined to the dermis. A tumor with features of AFX, but subcutaneous involvement should be designated as pleomorphic dermal sarcoma (Fig. 14.63A and B). The tumor cells of AFX are positive for CD10 and p53. Some tumors show immunoreactivity for SMA. Cytokeratins, EMA, p40, desmin, S100, SOX10, and CD34 are negative. Molecular studies identify a variety of recurrent mutations associated with ultraviolet (UV) signature (C->T mutations in dipyrimidines) and p53—a mutational spectrum shared between AFX and dermal pleomorphic sarcoma.

Differential Diagnosis

- Dermal pleomorphic sarcoma is distinguished from AFX based on the architecture: invasion of the subcutis, vascular, or perineural invasion; necrosis; presence of satellite nodules; involvement of the periosteum are all features that should prompt classification as dermal pleomorphic sarcoma.
- Melanoma (positive for S100, SOX10, melanocytic markers, in situ component)
- Sarcomatoid SCC (positive for 34BE12, MNF116, CK 5/6, p63, in situ component)
- Extraskeletal osteosarcoma: identification of malignant osseous or cartilaginous matrix
- Pleomorphic leiomyosarcoma and rhabdomyosarcoma, which will show characteristic expression of desmin, smooth muscle–specific markers (SMA, h-caldesmon,

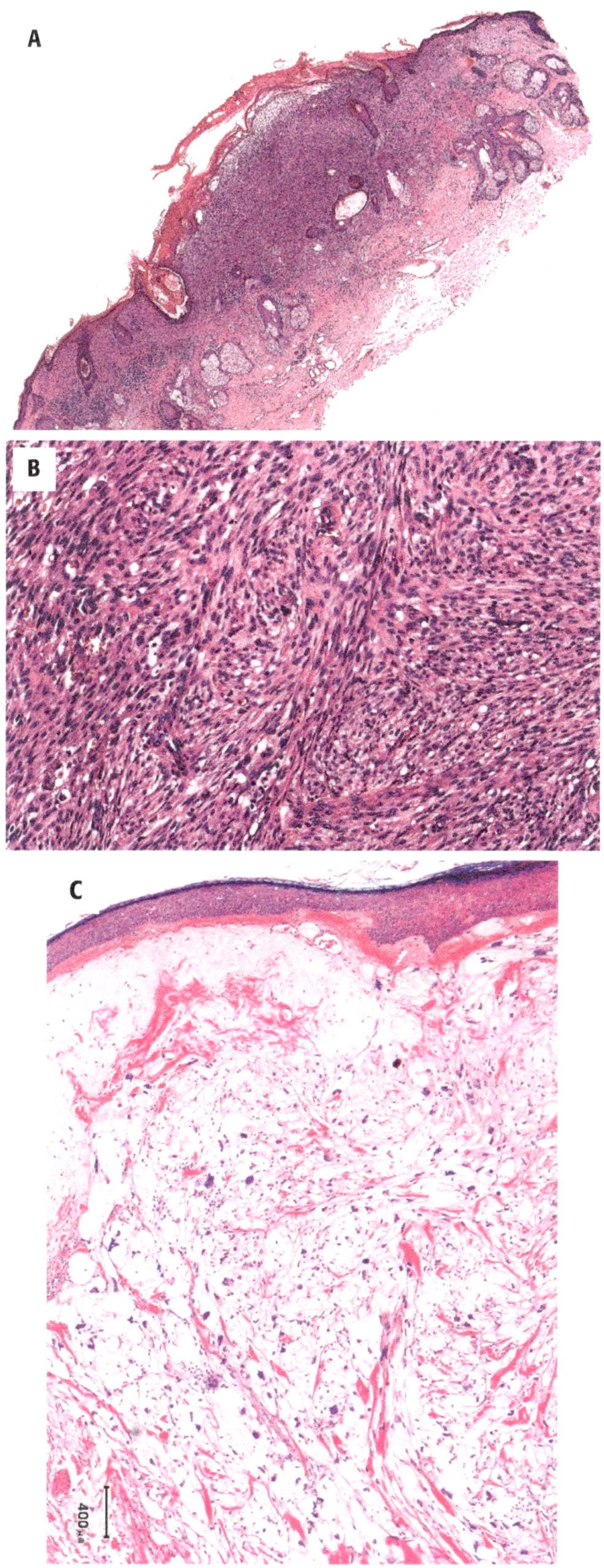

FIG. 14.62

Atypical fibroxanthoma (AFX). **A,** The tumor is confined to the dermis and occurs in the background of solar damage. **B,** Pleomorphic spindle cells with atypical hyperchromatic nuclei, amphiphilic cytoplasm and frequent mitotic figures arranged in fascicles. **C,** Clear-cell variant of AFX.

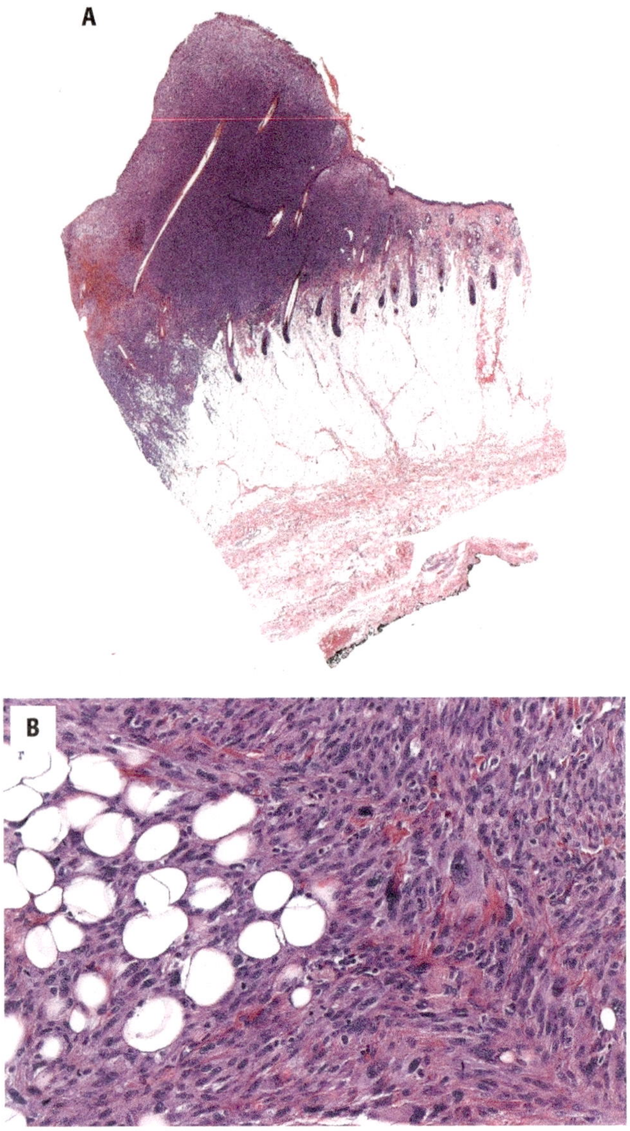

FIG. 14.63
Dermal pleomorphic sarcoma. **A,** The tumor is based on the dermis but shows infiltration of the subcutaneous tissue. **B,** Spindled to pleomorphic, mitotically active tumor cells forming fascicles and sheets. The cytology alone cannot separate dermal pleomorphic sarcoma from atypical fibroxanthoma.

and smooth muscle myosin heavy chain), or skeletal muscle markers (myogenin, MyoD1)
- Pleomorphic liposarcoma: identification of characteristic pleomorphic lipoblasts admixed with the spindle cell or pleomorphic component.

Differential Diagnosis

AFX and dermal pleomorphic sarcoma are a diagnosis of exclusion. The differential diagnosis includes malignant melanoma, sarcomatoid SCC, and a variety of dermal pleomorphic sarcomas. Although AFX is often ulcerated, the overlying epidermis is otherwise intact, and identifying an in situ carcinoma or an intraepithelial melanocytic proliferation would help to exclude carcinoma and malignant melanoma. Melanoma can be identified by positive staining for S100 protein or other markers of melanocytic differentiation. If cytokeratin immunoreactivity is noted, especially in the setting of associated actinic keratosis, a tumor, which otherwise could pass as an AFX, is best classified as poorly differentiated (spindled cell or sarcomatoid) SCC. Although broadly reactive antibodies such as to pan-cytokeratins AE1/AE3 identify most cases of spindled cell SCC, antibodies directed against high-molecular-weight cytokeratin such as 34βE12, CK5/6, or MNF116 are a better first-line choice because many spindled cell SCCs express only high-molecular-weight cytokeratins. Pleomorphic leiomyosarcoma and rhabdomyosarcoma can be distinguished based on the expression of desmin combined with smooth muscle–specific markers (SMA, h-caldesmon, and smooth muscle myosin heavy chain) or skeletal muscle markers (myogenin, MyoD1). Pleomorphic liposarcoma may be distinguished based on the presence of characteristic pleomorphic lipoblasts with overtly atypical nuclei. Extraskeletal osteosarcoma can be distinguished based on the presence of malignant lacelike osseous or cartilaginous matrix. Myxofibrosarcoma (see below) demonstrates distinctive multinodular growth pattern and myxoid stroma with distinctive curvilinear vessels. Another important differential diagnostic consideration, especially in context of a head and neck sarcoma, is radiation-associated sarcoma, which can take any of the above forms.

Once the competing epithelial, melanocytic, and mesenchymal mimics have been ruled out, the distinction between AFX and superficial pleomorphic undifferentiated sarcoma (also known as dermal pleomorphic sarcoma) is strictly based on anatomic level of invasion. The term AFX should be restricted to tumors limited to the dermis and with a pushing margin, which often requires examination of a completely excised specimen. We apply the term dermal pleomorphic sarcoma to cytologically similar tumors that extend into the subcutis or primarily present in deep soft tissue with extension superficially into the dermis because these tumors have a high risk for local recurrence and some risk for metastasis. The presence of tumor necrosis, infiltration of the subcutis, perivascular or perineural invasion, satellite nodules, or fascial/periosteal involvement is not compatible with the diagnosis of AFX, and such lesions should be classified as pleomorphic sarcoma.

Prognosis and Treatment

The similarities in the genetic signature indicate that AFX and dermal pleomorphic sarcoma represent a histologic continuum induced by UV damage. However, when strictly defined based on the parameters outlined above, completely resected AFX behave in a benign fashion essentially without any significant risk of local recurrence or metastasis. In our experience, most tumors labeled as AFX that develop local recurrence or systemic metastases were meeting criteria for dermal pleomorphic sarcoma at the time of original biopsy/excision.

Complete excision with negative margins is requisite treatment. Dermal pleomorphic sarcoma will require a wide excision and, depending on the depth of invasion, also possibly additional local control measures such as adjuvant radiation; therefore, these tumors are best managed by a multidisciplinary sarcoma team.

MYXOFIBROSARCOMA

Clinical Findings

Myxofibrosarcoma is one of the most common sarcomas in older adults, with a peak in the sixth to eighth decades of life. Most of these tumors arise in the subcutaneous tissue of the extremities; trunk and head and neck locations are very uncommon. Myxofibrosarcoma most commonly presents as a slowly enlarging painless multinodular mass with substantial infiltration along the underlying fascial planes.

Histopathologic Features

Myxofibrosarcomas grow in a multinodular pattern and have a very infiltrative border.

Cytologically, myxofibrosarcomas are composed of variably pleomorphic and hyperchromatic spindled or stellate cells distributed in a prominent myxoid matrix. The cells often cluster around distinctive curvilinear vessels (Fig. 14.64A and B) and may show mucin-containing cytoplasmic vacuoles mimicking lipoblasts (Fig. 14.64C). Areas of solid growth reminiscent of pleomorphic undifferentiated sarcoma and scattered inflammatory cells and

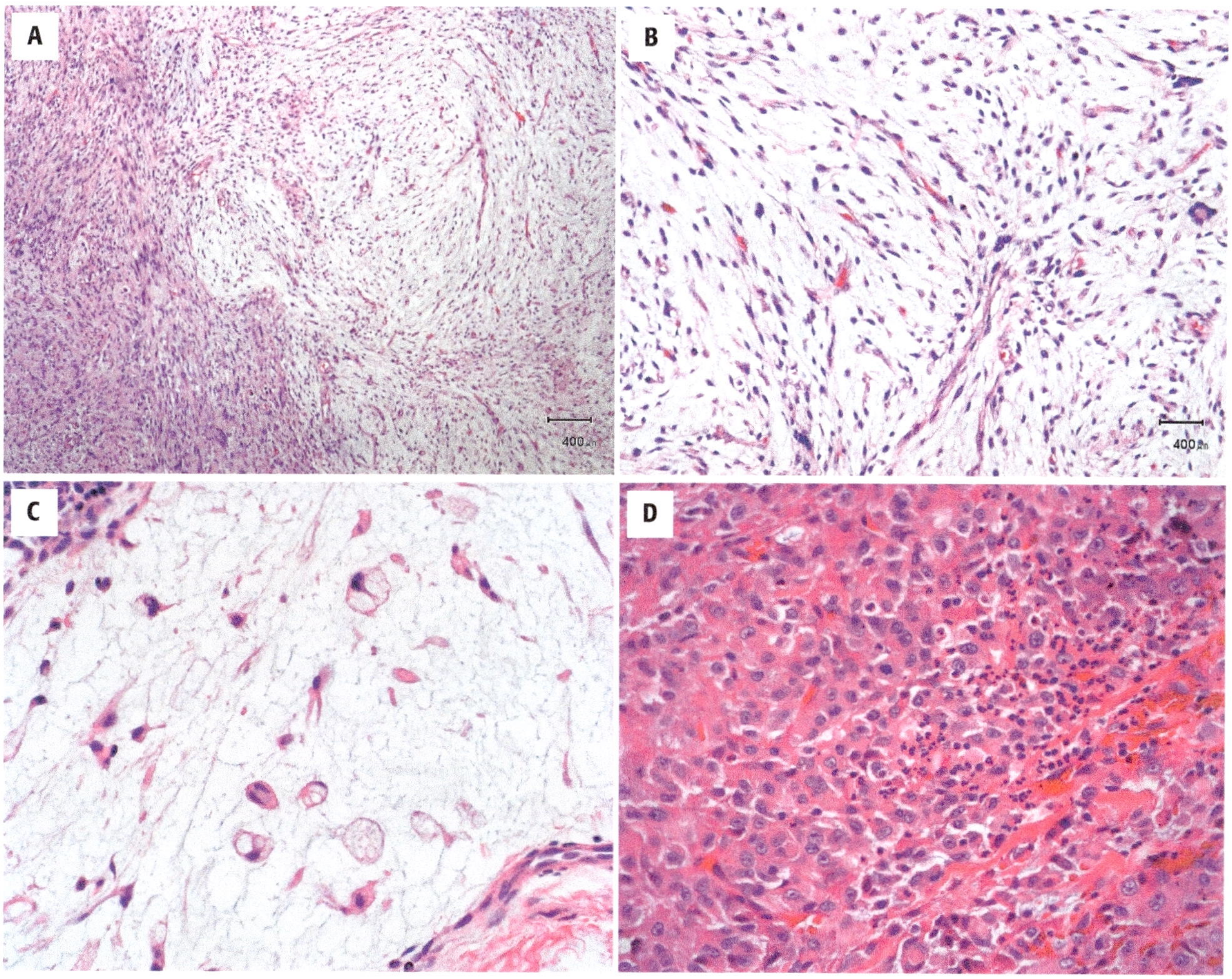

FIG. 14.64

Myxofibrosarcoma. **A,** Nodular spindle cell proliferation of variable cellular density in a myxoid stroma. **B,** Pleomorphic tumor cells are scattered around prominent curvilinear vessels. **C,** Mucin-containing tumor cells in myxofibrosarcoma resembling lipoblasts (so-called pseudolipoblasts). **D,** Epithelioid variant of myxofibrosarcoma reminiscent of carcinoma or malignant melanoma.

lymphoid aggregates are often present. An epithelioid variant has also been described, with the tumor cells resembling carcinoma or malignant melanoma (Fig. 14.64D). MFS can present at a range of histological grades, from low-grade to high-grade tumors that can be graded based on FNCLCC grading scheme. IHC in myxofibrosarcoma is nonspecific and of limited value.

Focal SMA immunoreactivity may be present consistent with myofibroblastic differentiation. Molecular genetic studies show complex karyotype with inconsistent structural and numerical alterations; there are no disease-defining molecular characteristics for this tumor type.

Differential Diagnosis

The differential diagnosis of low-grade myxofibrosarcoma includes other cutaneous tumors with myxoid stroma such as cutaneous myxoma and angiomyxoma, myxoid nerve sheath tumors (myxoid neurofibroma and dermal nerve sheath myxoma), and LGFMS. Low-grade myxofibrosarcoma can be mistaken for myxoma or superficial angiomyxoma as both tumors occur in the subcutis, have paucicellular, diffusely myxoid stroma and curvilinear vasculature with sparse chronic inflammation and display an infiltrative, multinodular growth pattern. As a rule, even in low-grade myxofibrosarcoma, the degree of nuclear atypia usually exceeds that of myxoma or superficial angiomyxoma. Myxoid neurofibroma and dermal nerve sheath myxoma can be easily separated based on Schwann cell marker expression such as S100 and SOX10. LGFMS is usually well circumscribed with alternating fibrous and myxoid areas. Cytologically, LGFMS is a far less pleomorphic tumor, even compared with the low-grade examples of myxofibrosarcoma. Immunohistochemical staining for MUC4 and genetic studies for *FUS* and *EWSR1* gene rearrangement can help in difficult cases (see later discussion). MIFS, a distinctive and exceptionally highly infiltrative low-grade sarcoma with predilection for the subcutaneous tissue of acral sites can look very similar to the classic myxofibrosarcoma as it is also composed of myxoid infiltrative nodules of pleomorphic spindle to epithelioid cells with large, viral inclusion-like nucleoli and a prominent inflammatory infiltrate that can obscure the underlying nature of the tumor (Fig. 14.65). Diffuse atypia, mitotic activity of more than 1 to 2/10 HPF, and a solid growth pattern would favor myxofibrosarcoma over MIFS. Molecular testing may aid in challenging cases as MIFS often harbor *BRAF* fusions, *VGLL3* amplifications, and in cases that show hybrid features with HFLT (see above), also *TGFBR3* and *OGA* (*MGEA5*) gene fusions. *BRAF* and *VGGL3* alterations are amenable to testing by FISH and can also help distinguishing MIFS from benign inflammatory conditions or granulomatous inflammation. MIFS is a highly infiltrative neoplasms, but it lacks metastatic potential.

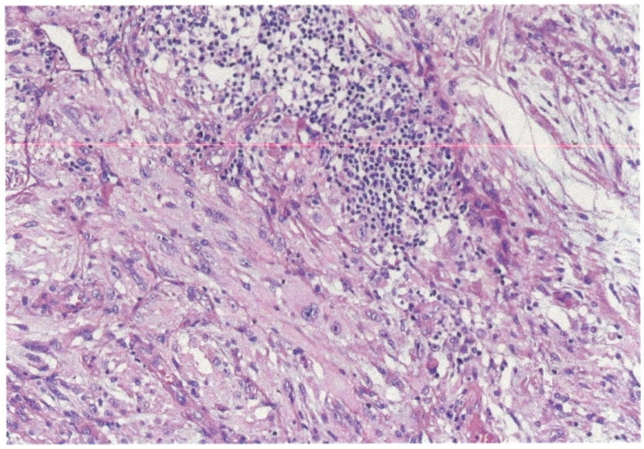

FIG. 14.65
Myxoinflammatory fibroblastic sarcoma composed of myxoid infiltrative nodules of pleomorphic spindle to epithelioid cells with large, viral inclusion-like nucleoli and a prominent inflammatory infiltrate. Despite nuclear pleomorphism, mitotic activity is inconspicuous.

However, in the setting of a confirmed prior diagnosis of MIFS, the presence of more conventional myxofibrosarcoma-like or solid areas indicates sarcomatous progression and therefore some potential for systemic metastasis proportionate to the grade of the tumor.

The differential diagnosis of a high-grade myxofibrosarcoma includes other pleomorphic sarcomas. The presence of multinodular growth pattern with myxoid nodules containing typical vessels, and a "null" immunophenotype help to establish the diagnosis of high-grade myxofibrosarcoma in this setting.

Prognosis and Treatment

Myxofibrosarcomas of all grades have a high rate of local recurrence (50% to 60%). Low-grade myxofibrosarcomas practically never metastasize, but higher-grade tumors acquire a significant metastatic potential (approximately 30%). Recurrences may be associated with higher nuclear grade. Regardless of tumor grade, excision with wide margins is essential to minimize the risk of local recurrence. Because of the degree of infiltration through the subcutaneous fibrous septa, careful preoperative mapping of the tumor edges by radiology is typically performed. The infiltrative growth pattern of myxofibrosarcoma often makes margin interpretation very problematic, especially in low-grade tumors as they can be extremely difficult to distinguish from reactive fibroblasts.

LOW-GRADE FIBROMYXOID SARCOMA

Clinical Findings

LGFMS, also known as Evans tumor, is a distinctive gene fusion-driven fibroblastic neoplasm that occurs predominantly in young adults or children as a deep, subfascial or intramuscular mass, although up to 20% of cases occur superficially, usually on the lower limbs. The size varies from 2 to 3 cm to >10 cm.

Histopathologic Features

LGFMS is characterized by alternating densely collagenous and myxoid areas containing short, cytologically bland fibroblasts arranged in a fascicular to whorled pattern. The cytologic features are deceptively banal; mitotic figures are usually inconspicuous, and there is no necrosis. This collagenous pattern with whorled or vaguely fascicular appearance predominates in most tumors. Two additional histologic features of LGFMS can greatly aid in its recognition. The first is the presence of curvilinear vessels which are most pronounced in the areas with myxoid stroma (Fig. 14.66A–C). The second is the occasional presence of collagenous rosettes composed of a core of densely hyalinized stroma surrounded by a rim of palisading spindle to epithelioid tumor cells (Fig. 14.66D). This variant morphology is often referred to as hyalinizing spindle cell tumor with giant rosettes. LGFMS expresses MUC4, which is highly sensitive and specific in this setting, being present in nearly 100% of LGFMS. There may be a variable expression of EMA, SMA, or S100 in these tumors. Cytokeratins and CD34 are negative. Genetically, LGFMS harbors *FUS::CREB3L2* fusions and less commonly, *FUS::CREB3L1*, *EWSR1::CREB3L1* and *EWSR1:: CREB3L2* fusions. *YAP1* and *KMT2A* variant fusions were also described, and these tumors are negative for MUC4 expression. Many of these rearrangements as well as MUC4 immunoreactivity are also shared by sclerosing epithelioid fibrosarcoma (SEF), a deep-seated, aggressive sarcoma with a corded pattern of epithelioid tumor cells. Testing for *FUS*, *EWSR1*, and *YAP1* gene rearrangements (the latter is present as part of many commercially available next-generation sarcoma fusion panels) may be necessary to capture the diagnostic alteration.

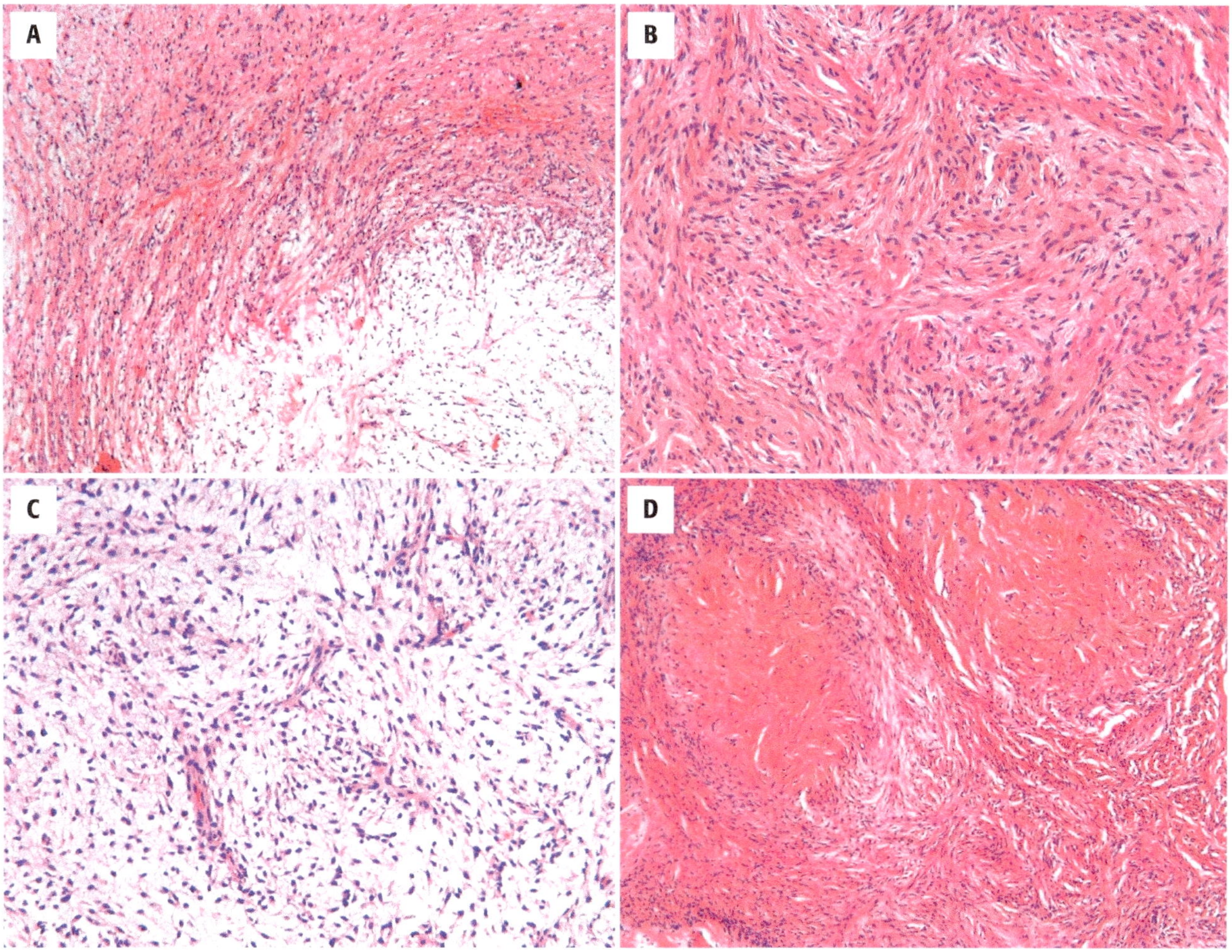

FIG. 14.66

Low-grade fibromyxoid sarcoma. **A,** Abrupt transition from the fibrous to myxoid zones. **B,** Storiform or fascicular growth pattern in fibrous zones. **C,** Myxoid zones frequently have arcades of curvilinear vessels and more stellate tumor cells. **D,** Giant collagen rosettes with eosinophilic collagen surrounded by round to oval tumor cells.

Differential Diagnosis

Because LGFMS is notoriously bland-looking, other clinically significant fibroblastic tumors can closely mimic LGFMS including myofibroblastoma, desmoid fibromatosis, DFSP, SFT, soft tissue perineurioma, and hybrid peripheral nerve sheath tumors. All the above mimics are expected to be negative for MUC4. CD34 can also serve as a quick screening tool as it is diffusely positive in myofibroblastoma, SFT, perineurioma, and DFSP but generally negative in LGFMS. Positive staining for STAT6 by IHC is virtually diagnostic for SFT in this setting; conversely, MUC4 is negative in SFT. Perineuriomas, hybrid nerve sheath tumors, and LGFMS can be positive for EMA; however, perineuriomas typically express other markers of perineurial differentiation (GLUT1, claudin-1), while the Schwann cell component in hybrid tumors can be picked up by S100 and SOX10 immunostains. In difficult cases, confirmatory testing for rearrangements involving FUS, EWSR1, or YAP1 is required in establishing the diagnosis of LGFMS.

Prognosis and Treatment

LGFMS is a full-fledged sarcoma with a relatively indolent short-term behavior but a substantial (50% or more) risk of late lung metastases and death. This is especially true for cases diagnosed prior to the widespread recognition of this entity as a true sarcoma that may have not received complete excision. LGFMS should be treated by an oncologic resection, and a life-long follow-up is required to monitor for late metastases.

LIPOMATOUS TUMORS

BENIGN TUMORS

LIPOMA

Clinical Findings

One of the most common soft tissue tumors, lipomas manifest in middle-aged and older adults as slow-growing painless subcutaneous masses on the upper back, extremities, and head and neck region.

Histopathologic Features

Lipomas are composed of mature benign adipocytes with hardly any variation in size and shape separated by very thin interlobular fibrous septa. Most lipomas are covered by a thin fibrous capsule that often separates from the tumor during tissue processing and is usually not seen in histologic sections. Areas of fat necrosis are common. Secondary changes may occur including fibrous component (fibrolipoma), myxoid change (myxolipoma), and chondroosseous metaplasia (chondroosseous lipoma).

Differential Diagnosis

In the setting of fat necrosis and atrophy, a decrease in amount of intracytoplasmic fat can cause nuclear enlargement mimicking lipoblasts and raising concern for an ALT/WDL. However, atrophic adipocytes lack the multiple fat vacuoles indenting the nucleus seen in true lipoblasts and still have a relatively open chromatin, sometimes with an intranuclear vacuole rather than an overtly hyperchromatic atypical fibroblasts with coarse chromatin seen in ALT. A simple and very helpful rule that ALT/WDLs are exceptionally rare in the superficial locations.

Prognosis and Treatment

Lipomas (ordinary or special subtypes of lipomas) do not need surgical removal other than for cosmetic, symptomatic, or diagnostic purposes (e.g., excisional biopsy to exclude an atypical lipomatous tumor or other neoplasm).

NEVUS LIPOMATOSUS SUPERFICIALIS

Clinical Findings

Nevus lipomatosus superficialis presents as solitary or multiple polypoid to plaque-like lesions, most often involving the buttocks, upper thighs, or lower back in children and young adults. Solitary lesions can be clinically indistinguishable from a fibroepithelial polyp (skin tag).

Histopathologic Features

Nevus lipomatosus is a hamartomatous lesion characterized by the presence of mature adipose tissue in the reticular and papillary dermis accompanied by verrucous or papillomatous hyperplasia of the overlying epidermis a decrease or absence of dermal adnexal structures. The adipocytes are often accentuated around small dermal blood vessels. Subcutis is usually not involved.

Differential Diagnosis

Skin-colored polypoid skin lesions including fibroepithelial polyp (acrochordon or skin tag), angiokeratoma, neurofibroma, smooth muscle hamartoma, and others may enter the clinical differential diagnosis of a solitary nevus lipomatosus. Most of these have distinctly different morphology covered elsewhere in this book; however, a fibroepithelial polyp with fatty metaplasia and a dermal fibrolipoma can indeed look very similar histologically and require clinical correlation for the correct diagnosis of nevus lipomatosus.

Prognosis and Treatment

This is a benign tumor that does not require treatment except for cosmetic reasons.

ANGIOLIPOMA

Clinical Findings

One or more often, multiple painful subcutaneous nodules in young adults, most commonly in the extremities followed by the trunk. The pain can be quite intense, especially in individuals with multiple lesions. Rare cases of autosomal dominant familiar angiolipomatosis have been reported.

Histopathologic Features

Angiolipomas are small (smaller than 2 cm) encapsulated tumors composed of mature fat in association with a proliferation of benign, thin-walled capillaries that are surrounded by pericytes and may contain fibrin thrombi (Fig. 14.67). The proportion of the different components can be quite variable in individual tumors, and cellular angiolipomas (defined as predominantly vascular component) can be difficult to distinguish from a capillary hemangioma. Angiolipomas often contain recurrent activating p.E545A PIK3CA mutations, implying a pathogenetic role of PI3K/AKT pathway. Low-level single-nucleotide mutations in *PRKD2* gene, a part of proteinase C complex pathway, have also been reported but are of uncertain significance.

Differential Diagnosis

The differential diagnosis depends on the proportion of the two components. Tumors with few vessels can be confused with conventional lipoma. Tumors predominantly composed of the vascular component can be confused with hemangiomas or Kaposi sarcoma. However, unlike angiolipoma, these lesions are not encapsulated and usually do not have the microthrombi that are so characteristic of angiolipoma.

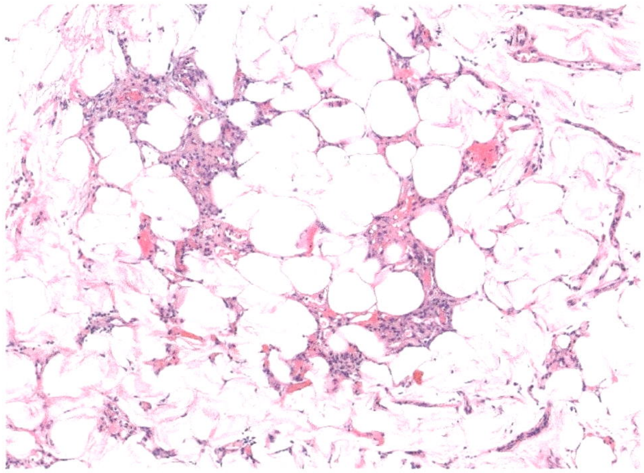

FIG. 14.67
Angiolipoma composed of mature fat in association with a proliferation of benign, thin-walled capillaries that are surrounded by pericytes and contain fibrin thrombi.

Prognosis and Treatment

Surgery is curative and eliminates symptoms; targeted therapies used in vascular malformations such as *PIK3CA* inhibitors may be considered in individuals with numerous lesions not amenable to surgery.

CHONDROID LIPOMA

Clinical Findings

Chondroid lipomas present as slow-growing, subcutaneous, or deep-seated masses involving proximal limbs or limb girdles, most often in adult women.

Histopathologic Features

Chondroid lipomas are well-circumscribed tumors with a lobular architecture. The tumor cells are eosinophilic or vacuolated, imparting a lipoblast-like appearance, and are embedded in a myxohyaline matrix (Fig. 14.68). A less common variant consists of more spindled in appearance cells with granular cytoplasm but similar nuclei and frequent vacuolization. Nuclear features are bland, and there is no significant mitotic activity. A subset of chondroid lipomas have a well-developed

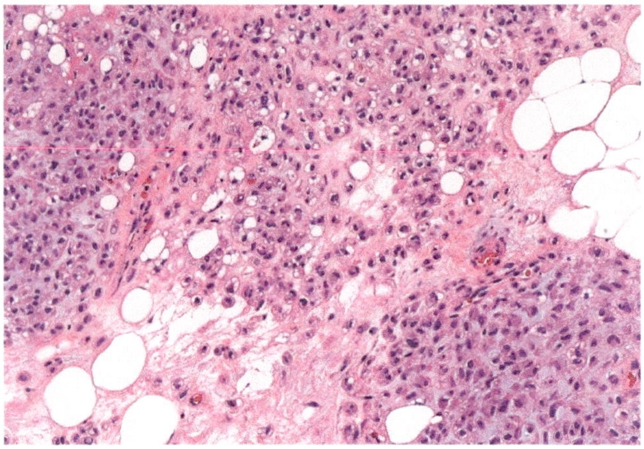

FIG. 14.68
Chondroid lipoma characterized by eosinophilic and vacuolated tumor cells embedded in a myxohyaline matrix.

vasculature with thick-walled vessels admixed with ectatic thin-walled vessels. The lesional adipocytes are variably positive for S100 and characteristically express cyclin D1. Molecular alterations in chondroid lipoma are a result of t(11;16)(q13;p13) translocation with *C11orf95::MRTFB* fusion and downstream activation of transcription factor SRF.

Differential Diagnosis

The combination of vacuolated cells and myxohyaline matrix raises consideration of cartilaginous tumors, including soft tissue chondroma, myoepithelioma, and myxoid liposarcoma. Soft tissue chondroma is largely restricted to the hands and feet and demonstrates hyaline cartilage differentiation and distinctive purple grungy calcifications; lipoblasts are uncharacteristic. Myoepithelial tumors can be distinguished based on the presence of true ductal differentiation (as is the case with chondroid syringoma) or demonstration of the myoepithelial immunophenotype with coexpression of cytokeratins or EMA and myoepithelial markers such as S100, SOX10, SMA, p63, or GFAP. Myxoid liposarcoma rarely arises in the subcutis and is characterized by more prominent myxoid component and branching capillary vasculature. The constituent cells of myxoid liposarcoma are round or comma shaped and small, with little cytoplasm and absence of vacuolization other than scattered true lipoblasts. Identification of the *DDIT3* gene characteristic of myxoid liposarcoma is helpful.

Treatment and Prognosis

Chondroid lipoma is benign with very rare recurrences. Surgical excision is curative

LIPOBLASTOMA AND LIPOBLASTOMATOSIS

Clinical Findings

Lipoblastoma is a tumor of infants and young children (first 3 years of life) that occurs as a solitary lesion (lipoblastoma) or, exceptionally rarely, as a diffuse form (lipoblastomatosis). Adult cases have been described but are exceptionally rare. The solitary form presents as a trunk or extremity-based mass clinically indistinguishable from conventional lipoma. Some cases arise in the deep soft tissues. Lipoblastomatosis is an infiltrative process that extensively involves the subcutis and often, the underlying skeletal muscle.

Histopathologic Features

The morphologic essence of lipoblastoma is that it recapitulates the appearance of fetal fat. The tumor is distinctly lobulated and is composed of primitive, cytologically bland spindle cells and lipoblasts within a myxoid matrix containing plexiform vasculature—an appearance that mimics conventional myxoid liposarcoma. Recurrent lesions are composed of mature fat or demonstrate a more prominent fibrous component reminiscent of lipofibromatosis (Fig. 14.69A and B). Molecular studies show that most lipoblastomas have *PLAG1* (8q11-13) gene fusions with a variety of partners and, rarely, polysomy 8 or *HMGA2* alterations. These may be confirmed by PLAG1 IHC. Conventional immunostains play no role in the diagnosis.

Differential Diagnosis

The most important differential diagnosis is with myxoid liposarcoma which can be morphologically indistinguishable in some cases. Myxoid liposarcoma usually has greater cellularity and a greater degree of nuclear atypia (although condensation of cellularity at the periphery of the lobules is typical of both) and is characterized by a *DDIT3* gene rearrangement, not present in lipoblastomas. However, the key to the differential diagnosis is the age of the patient: myxoid liposarcomas are exceedingly rare in early childhood when most of the lipoblastomas occur. FHI can be distinguished by its typical triphasic appearance including immature mesenchymal component in myxoid stroma, fascicles of bland myofibroblastic cells, and mature adipose tissue. Lipofibromatosis consists of mature fat percolated by small fascicles of bland fibroblastic cells, but it typically lacks myxoid stroma, a lobular growth

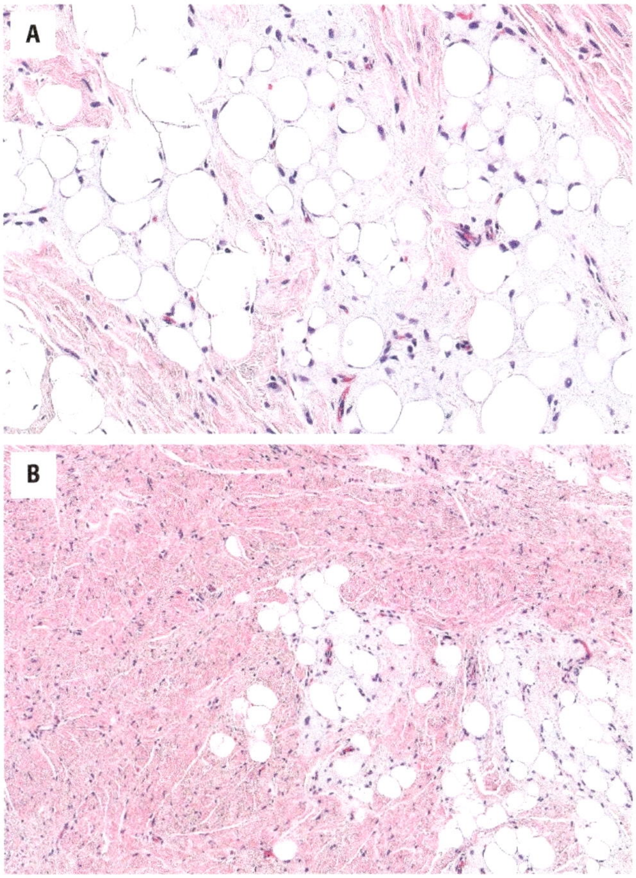

FIG. 14.69

Lipoblastoma. **A,** The tumor is distinctly lobulated and consists of cytologically bland primitive spindle cells and lipoblasts embedded in a myxoid matrix containing delicate plexiform vasculature. **B,** Recurrent lesions are composed of mature fat or may show a prominent fibrous component reminiscent of lipofibromatosis.

pattern, and prominent capillary vasculature of lipoblastoma. Both FHI and lipofibromatosis lack *PLAG1* gene rearrangements. Finally, lipoblastoma-like features of myxoid changes with increased vascularity can occasionally be seen in nonneoplastic adipose tissue in association with lipodystrophy or lipoatrophy.

Prognosis and Treatment

Lipoblastoma is a benign entity and is cured by simple excision. Lipoblastomatosis frequently recurs and requires a wide excision to achieve negative margins owing to its infiltrative growth pattern.

HIBERNOMA

Clinical Findings

Hibernomas are superficial, slow-growing subcutaneous fatty tumors with brown fat differentiation. These tumors occur in the extremities and trunk of young adult patients and rarely affect deep skeletal muscle or bone. Hibernomas are hardly ever seen in retroperitoneal, mediastinal, axillary, or deep pelvic locations. Hibernomas have two distinctive features that may cause clinical alarm: increased fibrous stroma with high vascularity leading to radiologic misinterpretation as ALT, and FDG high metabolic activity resulting in a PET-avid lesion that may be concerning for malignancy.

Histopathologic Features

Hibernomas are quite distinctive being composed of variably eosinophilic brown fat cells with centrally located bland round nuclei, numerous uniform cytoplasmic vacuoles that do not indent the nucleus to the same extent that lipoblasts do, and sharply outlined cell borders. These tumors are rich in vessels and can contain small capillaries or large vessels in accentuated fibrous septa (Fig. 14.70). Conventional white fat component is invariably present and may dominate the histologic picture requiring diligent sampling to detect the brown fat cells. Some cases show myxoid stroma and cellular spindling resembling myxolipoma or spindle cell lipoma. Brown fat differentiation may be detected by CD10 or adipophilin immunostains or, if available, an antibody to the uncoupling protein-1 (UCP1) involved in thermogenesis. Hibernomas are characterized by translocations and interstitial deletions of 11q13 with concomitant deletions of the tumor suppressor genes *MEN1* and *AIP*; it appears that the loss of AIP function upregulates UCP1 inducing brown fat differentiation in preexisting white fat cells.

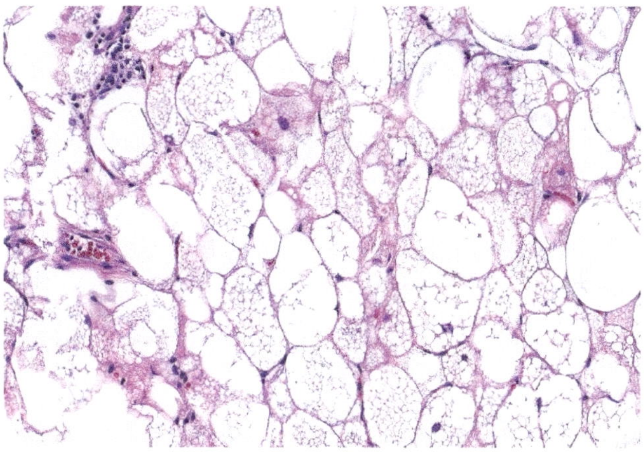

FIG. 14.70

Hibernoma composed of variably eosinophilic brown fat cells with centrally located bland round nuclei, numerous cytoplasmic vacuoles, and sharply outlined cell borders.

Differential Diagnosis

Atypical lipomatous tumor may show focal hibernomatous differentiation but are distinguished by the presence of atypical hyperchromatic stromal fibroblasts, true lipoblasts and *MDM2* gene amplification. In context of a superficial tumor, the presence of convincing brown fat component favors hibernoma over lipoma.

Prognosis and Treatment

Hibernomas are benign and cured by surgical excision.

BENIGN LIPOMATOUS TUMORS WITH RB1 DELETION

Once considered to represent separate entities, RB1-deleted tumor family includes a spectrum of benign fibroblastic and lipomatous tumors that share common histologic features, including dermal or subcutaneous location, the presence of spindled or pleomorphic (myo)fibroblasts admixed with thick collagen bundles, frequent mast cells, robust CD34 immunoreactivity, and a variable adipocytic component. Genetically, they show a high frequency of somatic Retinoblastoma 1 (*RB1*) deletions on 13q14.2, indicating that RB1 loss is involved in pathogenesis. This alteration can be detected as a loss of nuclear expression with RB1 antibody. The lipomatous tumors (spindle cell and pleomorphic lipoma, atypical spindle cell/pleomorphic lipomatous tumor and pleomorphic liposarcoma) are discussed below, while fibroblastic tumors (pleomorphic fibroma, SAF, myofibroblastoma) are discussed earlier in this chapter. Superficial angiofibroma, another neoplasm in this family, occurs in the vulvovaginal region in female patients or anogenital or scrotal lesion in men.

SPINDLE CELL AND PLEOMORPHIC LIPOMA

Clinical Findings

Spindle cell lipoma and pleomorphic lipoma classically present as a solitary subcutaneous nodule in the head and neck region of middle-aged and elderly adults, with a marked predilection for male patients. However, they can arise in virtually any anatomic location including proximal and distal limbs, and oral cavity, and can involve both dermis and subcutis. Such atypical presentations are especially common in women.

Histopathologic Features

Spindle cell lipomas are composed of three components: mature adipocytes, short bundles of spindle cells with short oval nuclei and pale eosinophilic wispy cytoplasm, and thick wiry collagen fibers (Fig. 14.71A). The stroma can be collagenous or myxoid. These components are variably distributed from tumor to tumor, and some have almost no fat (so-called fat-poor variant that can be mistaken for another SAMS). Cases with abundant myxoid stroma are relatively hypocellular but rich in small delicate vessels and can resemble myxoid DFSP or myxoid liposarcoma. More unusual appearances include a so-called pseudoangiomatous variant, with stromal breakdown mimicking ectatic vessels (Fig. 14.71B), and plexiform variant. Pleomorphic lipomas are identical tumors in every aspect except for the presence of pleomorphic fibroblasts with hyperchromatic nuclei that can be single or form multinucleated floret-like giant cells (Fig. 14.72). Mast cells are conspicuous in most cases, and both tumors can have lipoblasts. IHC is sometimes

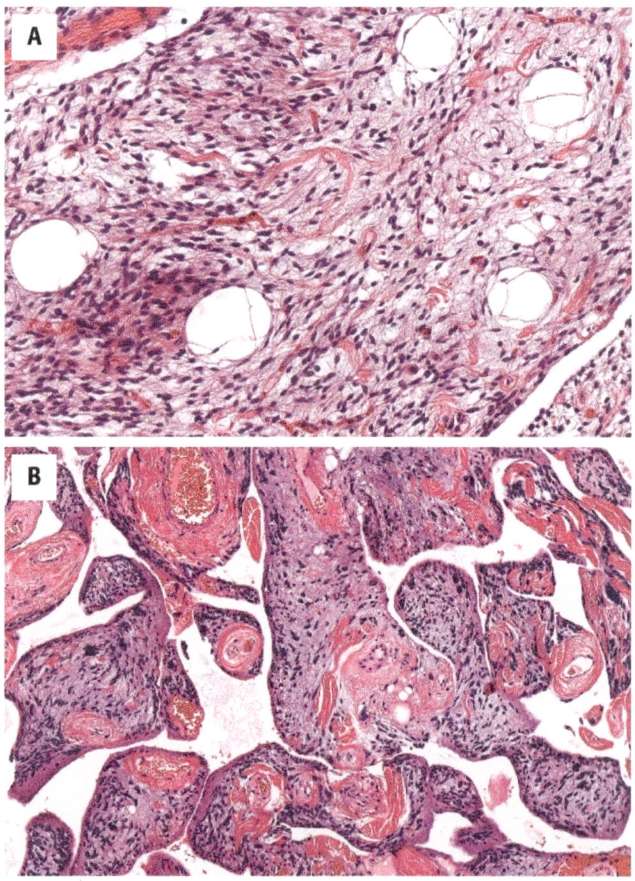

FIG. 14.71

Spindle cell lipoma. **A,** The tumor shows an admixture of mature adipocytes, bundles of spindle cells with short oval nuclei and eosinophilic wispy cytoplasm, and thick wiry collagen fibers. **B,** A pseudoangiomatous variant shows prominent myxoid stroma with stromal breakdown mimicking ectatic vessels. Mast cells frequently occur.

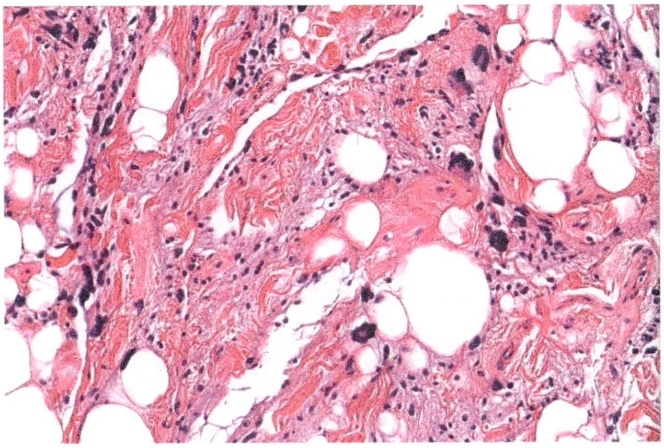

FIG. 14.72
Pleomorphic lipoma showing prominent pleomorphic fibroblasts with hyperchromatic nuclei and multinucleated floret-like giant cells in a background of what otherwise is a typical spindle cell lipoma. Mast cells are conspicuous.

useful in the diagnosis of spindle cell or pleomorphic lipoma, especially in relatively "fat-free" examples because constituent spindle cells are diffusely positive for CD34 and show loss of nuclear RB1 expression in keeping with the *RB1* gene deletions. S100 protein, SMA, and desmin are generally negative.

Differential Diagnosis

Benign nerve sheath tumors (neurofibroma, hybrid schwannoma/perineurioma) can mimic spindle cell lipoma as these lesions, especially neurofibroma, are rich in fibroblasts, often have myxoid stroma, thick collagen bundles, and mast cells, and are CD34 positive. The distinction can be easily made based on the coexpression of Schwann cell markers S100 and SOX10 in the spindle cell component and retained RB1 IHC. Myxoid spindle cell lipoma may simulate DFSP in a small biopsy, but it lacks the characteristic storiform growth pattern and deeply infiltrative edge of the latter. RB1 expression is retained in DFSP. Rare examples with myxoid stroma and prominent capillary vasculature may be mistaken for a superficial presentation of a myxoid liposarcoma. Myxoid liposarcoma is usually negative for CD34 and consistently shows *DDIT3* gene rearrangement that can be identified by FISH or NGS. SFT, which is very rare above the fascia, can be distinguished based on the presence of areas of alternating cellularity, prominent hemangiopericytomatous vasculature, and diffuse STAT6 expression.

Pleomorphic lipoma needs to be distinguished from ALT/WLD, which looks very similar morphologically but has a characteristically different presentation as a large mass deep in the musculature or in retroperitoneum, pelvis, or mediastinum. Areas resembling typical spindle cell lipoma are identified in most cases of pleomorphic lipoma. In an unusual clinical scenario (such as head and neck ALT/WDL, which may present more superficially due to lack of fascial planes between subcutaneous tissue and muscle) genetic testing for *MDM2* or *CDK4* gene amplification can be performed. The distinction of spindle cell and pleomorphic lipoma from each other and the remaining fibroblastic tumors in the *RB1*-deleted family (such as myofibroblastoma, pleomorphic fibroma, and cellular angiofibroma) has little clinical relevance as these tumors are essentially different faces of the same benign process, with variable amounts of adipocytes and preferred location being the main difference. However, these tumors need to be distinguished from atypical spindle cell/pleomorphic lipomatous tumor (discussed below) because of the impact on management.

Prognosis and Treatment

Spindle cell and pleomorphic lipomas are benign, with minimal risk of local recurrence following simple excision.

ATYPICAL SPINDLE CELL AND PLEOMORPHIC LIPOMATOUS TUMOR

Clinical Findings

ASCPLT is a recently delineated benign lipomatous tumor also characterized by *RB1* gene deletions that resembles spindle cell and pleomorphic lipoma but has several important histologic differences affecting the rate of local recurrence. ASCLTs occur as a relatively large (average size 5 cm) subcutaneous or, less often, deep-seated mass on the extremities, trunk or head and neck region. Visceral sites are rarely involved.

Histopathologic Features

ASCPLT fundamentally contains the same components as spindle cell and pleomorphic lipoma: variable amounts of adipocytes, CD34-positive fibroblastic spindle or pleomorphic cells, thick collagen bundles, fibromyxoid stroma, lipoblasts, and mast cells. The key histologic features that place these tumors into a separate category include infiltrative margin, increased cellularity with vaguely fascicular growth pattern, marked variation in size of individual adipocytes, more conspicuous nuclear atypia and hyperchromasia in spindle cells and bizarre atypical pleomorphic lipoblasts—in other words, any features that upon review would prompt a

ATYPICAL SPINDLE CELL AND PLEOMORPHIC LIPOMATOUS TUMOR—DISEASE FACT SHEET

Clinical Findings

- Subcutaneous or deep-seated mass on the extremities, trunk or head and neck

Histopathologic Features

- Same components as spindle cell and pleomorphic lipoma
  - Fibroblastic spindle or pleomorphic cells
  - Thick or ropey collagen bundles
  - Fibromyxoid stroma, lipoblasts, mast cells
- Infiltrative margin, increased cellularity with vaguely fascicular growth pattern
- Marked variation in size of individual adipocytes
- Conspicuous nuclear atypia and hyperchromasia in spindle cells
- Bizarre, atypical pleomorphic lipoblasts

IHC/Molecular

- CD34 positive, variable desmin and SMA, loss of nuclear RB1 (>70%)
- Somatic retinoblastoma 1 (*RB1*) deletions on 13q14.2
- Negative for *MDM2* and *CDK4* gene amplification.

Differential Diagnosis

- Spindle cell and pleomorphic lipoma
- Atypical lipomatous tumor/well-differentiated liposarcoma
- Pleomorphic liposarcoma

IHC, Immunohistochemistry; *SMA*, smooth muscle actin.

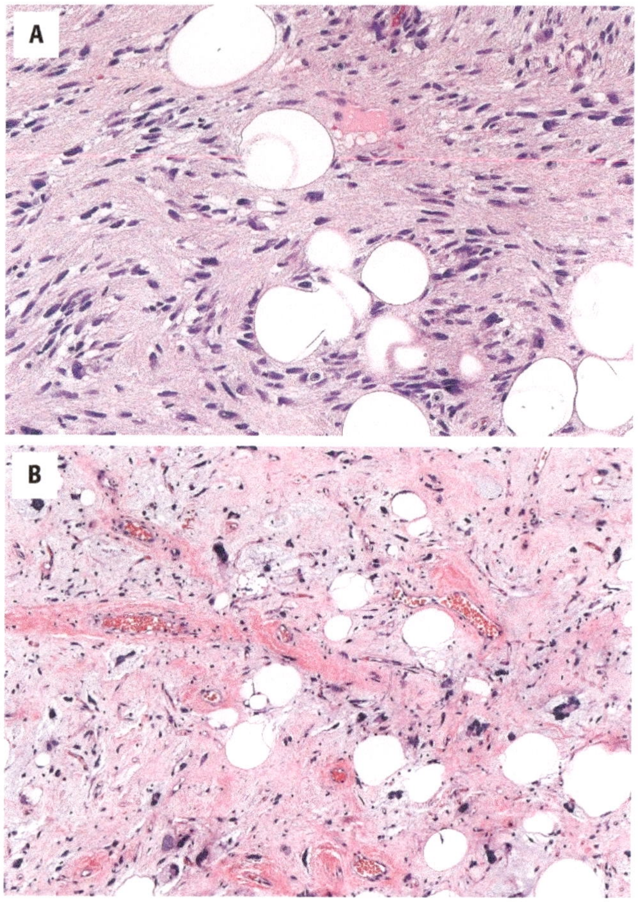

FIG. 14.73

Atypical spindle cell/pleomorphic lipomatous tumor. **A,** Cellular fascicles of mildly atypical spindle cells, adipocytes, and wispy collagen bundles growing in a fibrous stroma. **B,** Conspicuous nuclear atypia and hyperchromasia, variation in size of individual adipocytes and lipoblasts that prompt a consideration of an atypical lipomatous tumor/well-differentiated liposarcoma but are negative for *MDM2* gene amplification.

consideration of an ALT/WDL or a pleomorphic liposarcoma (Fig. 14.73A and B). Cases located on the hands and feet tend to have abundant myxoid stroma. Mitotic activity in order of 1 to 3/10 HPF can be encountered (mitotic figures are virtually nonexistent in classic spindle cell and pleomorphic lipoma). At the same time, solid growth, diffuse atypia and pleomorphism, brisk mitotic activity, or necrosis are not observed and, if present, should prompt the diagnosis of pleomorphic liposarcoma. ASCPLTs are positive for CD34, variably positive for desmin, and show loss of RB1 in over 70% of cases. S100 variably highlights adipocytic component. These tumors do not have *MDM2* and *CDK4* gene amplification.

Differential Diagnosis

Spindle cell and pleomorphic lipomas are distinguished based on size, circumscribed growth pattern, and lack of atypical features outlined above. ALT/WDL can look remarkably similar to a point that we often perform FISH testing for *MDM2* gene amplification before the diagnosis of ASCPLT is made. However, the clinical presentation is quite different: ALT/WDLs are almost always deep-seated tumors (skeletal muscle, retroperitoneum, pelvis, mediastinum) in contrast to ASCPLT which is often subcutaneous. Areas of frank sarcomatous growth indicative of dedifferentiation in ALT/WDL are not compatible with the diagnosis of ASCPLT. The difference between ASCPLT and pleomorphic liposarcoma is discussed below.

Prognosis and Treatment

ASPLT is regarded as a benign entity with a low recurrence rate (10%–15%) in incompletely excised lesions but without potential for dedifferentiation or metastasis.

EMERGING BENIGN LIPOMATOUS AND FIBROLIPOMATOUS TUMORS

The reader is referred to specialized text for the discussion of novel and emerging fibrolipomatous tumors including *lipoblastoma-like tumor* and *fibrosarcoma-like lipomatous neoplasm*, representing the same tumor spectrum with predilection for vulvovaginal region and mosaic or complete RB1 loss, and *PLAG1-rearranged fibroblastic tumor* that occurs almost exclusively in young children, and may represent a predominantly fibrous variant of lipoblastoma.

LOCALLY AGGRESSIVE AND MALIGNANT LIPOMATOUS TUMORS

Liposarcomas occur predominantly in the deep soft tissue but may involve the subcutis; a detailed discussion is beyond the scope of this text. Primary dermal liposarcomas are exceptionally rare.

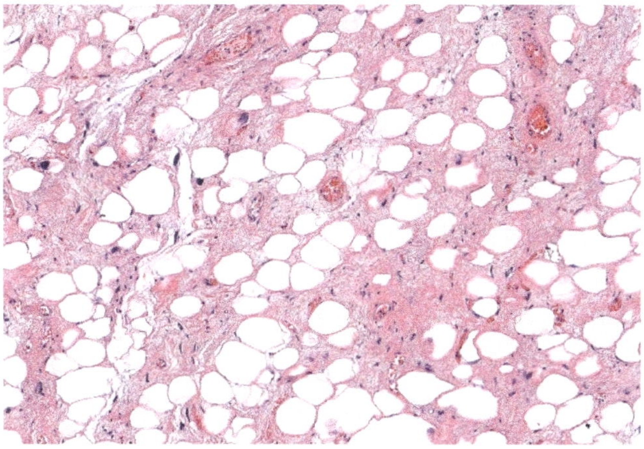

FIG. 14.74

Atypical lipomatous tumor with expansion of fibrous septa containing neoplastic atypical hyperchromatic stromal fibroblasts, variation in size of individual adipocytes, and rare lipoblasts.

ATYPICAL LIPOMATOUS TUMOR

Clinical Findings

ALT/WDL represent a locally aggressive, nonmetastasizing lipomatous tumor with potential for dedifferentiation. Most cases of ALT/WDL occur in the deep soft tissue, but some arise in the subcutis, such as in the head and neck region where there is an incomplete presence of fascia. Extremity-based tumors are labeled *atypical lipomatous tumor* rather than *well-differentiated liposarcoma* (a term used for mediastinal, retroperitoneal, deep pelvic, and scrotal tumors) because of the usual indolent behavior of the former. However, this distinction is based largely on completeness of excision, and fundamentally, atypical lipomatous tumors are the same neoplasm as their retroperitoneal or mediastinal counterparts. Rare, atypical lipomatous tumors of the subcutis have a similar presentation as conventional lipomas.

Histopathologic Features

ALT is a mature lipomatous neoplasm with adipocytes of varying sizes and shapes, characteristic neoplastic atypical hyperchromatic stromal fibroblasts, and rare lipoblasts. The atypical hyperchromatic spindled fibroblasts are often found in expanded fibrous septa within the tumor (Fig. 14.74). Lipoblasts may be entirely absent and are not a prerequisite for the diagnosis. Dedifferentiated liposarcoma is a progression of ALT/WDL to a nonlipomatous sarcoma with a variety of spindled, myxoid, or pleomorphic patterns and varying histologic grade, which is associated with metastatic potential. This phenomenon is exceptionally rare in superficial ALTs. Conventional IHC is not helpful and may be deceiving as the tumor cells are often positive for CD34 and can variably express SMA and desmin. However, immunostaining for MDM2 and CDK4 may be employed in this context. ALT/WDLs are driven by a classic structural alteration in the form of a supernumerary ring and giant marker chromosome derived from 12q14-q15 region and leading to amplification of *MDM2*, *CDK4*, *CPM*, and other genes. FISH testing for *MDM2* gene amplification (or its equivalent using microarray and NGS platforms) is highly accurate in distinguishing ALT from its lipomatous mimics.

Differential Diagnosis

Conventional lipoma with fat necrosis and atrophy can mimic ALT/WDL. However, atrophic adipocytes lack the multiple fat vacuoles indenting the nucleus seen in true lipoblasts and still have a relatively open chromatin, sometimes with an intranuclear vacuole rather than an overtly hyperchromatic atypical fibroblasts with coarse chromatin seen in ALT. A simple and very helpful rule that ALT/WDLs are exceptionally rare in the superficial locations. The differential diagnosis with pleomorphic lipoma and ASCPLT is discussed in the above section.

Prognosis and Treatment

Atypical lipomatous tumors tend to be indolent. Wide excision is generally curative, but local recurrence can occur. Dedifferentiated liposarcoma represents a transition from ALT/WDL to a sarcoma lacking adipocytic differentiation. The latter may have pleomorphic, spindle cell, or myxoid appearance and varying histologic grade (most often, high grade). Unlike well-differentiated liposarcoma, dedifferentiated liposarcoma has the capacity for metastasis. Dedifferentiation, however, is exceptionally rare in superficial tumors.

PLEOMORPHIC LIPOSARCOMA

Clinical Findings

While generally uncommon, pleomorphic liposarcoma is the most common subtype of liposarcoma to be encountered as a primary cutaneous or subcutaneous liposarcoma, typically affecting limbs, trunk, or head and neck of older patients, with a median size of 2 cm. A subset of pleomorphic liposarcomas with myxoid stroma often occurs in younger patients with Li-Fraumeni's syndrome.

Histopathologic Features

Pleomorphic liposarcoma is a high-grade undifferentiated pleomorphic sarcoma containing pleomorphic lipoblasts, which are definitionally required to make the diagnosis but can be very focal justifying thorough sampling (Fig. 14.75). A predominantly epithelioid proliferation of cells with eosinophilic cytoplasm that superficially resemble adrenal cortical tumors may be seen in approximately 25% of tumors. Myxoid stroma is common and abundant in some cases resembling high-grade myxoid liposarcoma or myxofibrosarcoma. By IHC, the lesional cells are positive for CD34 and variably positive for SMA (myofibroblastic pattern) while pleomorphic lipoblasts may express S100. Pleomorphic liposarcomas are characterized by complex numerical and structural chromosomal abnormalities including deletion of 13q14.2-q14.3 region, which can result in loss of RB1 expression by IHC in up to 60% of cases. *T53* gene alterations are also common. Pleomorphic liposarcomas do not show amplification of *MDM2* or *CDK4* genes that typify well-differentiated and dedifferentiated liposarcoma.

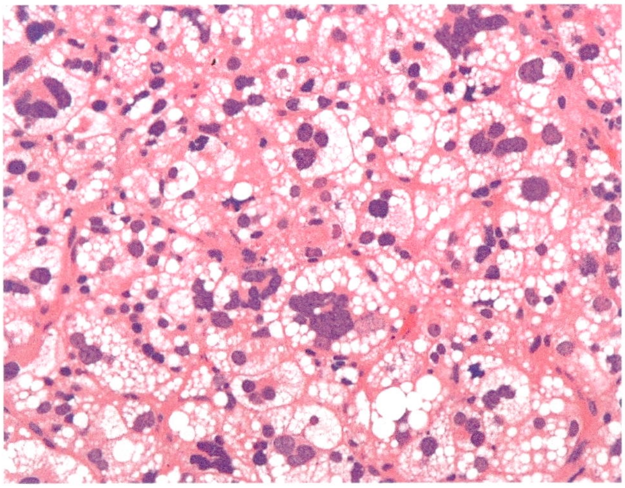

FIG. 14.75

Pleomorphic liposarcoma composed of overtly atypical pleomorphic lipoblasts in the background of undifferentiated pleomorphic or spindle cell sarcoma.

Differential Diagnosis

Recognition of pleomorphic lipoblasts is required for diagnosis and can separate pleomorphic liposarcomas from other dermal pleomorphic tumors including dermal pleomorphic sarcoma (undifferentiated spindle cell sarcoma of the skin), AFX, and high-grade myxofibrosarcoma. Dedifferentiated liposarcoma may contain pleomorphic lipoblasts along with the spindle cell or pleomorphic sarcoma component; however, these tumors are nearly uniformly deep-seated except special sites that lack a well-developed fascia like head and neck and show consistent *MDM2* gene amplification while RB1 expression is retained. The differential diagnosis with other fatty tumors in RB1 deletion tumor family (pleomorphic lipoma and atypical spindle cell pleomorphic lipomatous tumor) can be challenging because of the overlapping morphology. The presence of solid growth pattern with sheets or fascicles of spindled or pleomorphic cells with diffuse atypia, mitotic activity, atypical mitotic figures or necrosis—in other words, features that justify a general classification as sarcoma—will favor pleomorphic liposarcoma above any other mimics.

Prognosis and Treatment

Although pleomorphic liposarcoma of deep soft tissue is an aggressive tumor with a 5-year survival rate of 20% to 60%, superficial examples involving the dermis or subcutis appear to behave in an indolent fashion with a low risk of metastasis when completely excised.

MYXOID LIPOSARCOMA

Clinical Findings

Myxoid liposarcoma typically presents as a deep-seated mass in middle-age or older adult patients. Subcutaneous tumors comprise less than 20% of all cases, and primary dermal tumors are very rare. However, myxoid liposarcoma tends to metastasize to unusual, adipose tissue-rich sites such as skin, and the possibility of metastatic disease should always be excluded.

Histopathologic Features

Superficial myxoid liposarcoma forms circumscribed, lobulated nodules composed of short spindle or comma-shaped cells with mild atypia, lipoblasts, and variably maturing adipocytes in abundant myxoid stroma containing delicate, plexiform vasculature. The myxoid stromal material can sometimes form small pools or cystic spaces. Uni- and multivacuolar lipoblasts are often present but not required for diagnosis (Fig. 14.76A and B). The mitotic activity is very low, and usually there is no necrosis. This appearance recapitulates immature fetal fat. In contrast, high-grade myxoid liposarcoma (formerly, round cell liposarcoma) consists of hypercellular sheets of primitive round tumor cells with enlarged, hyperchromatic nuclei, increased mitotic activity, and necrosis, which obscure the characteristic plexiform vasculature (Fig. 14.77). In these instances, the presence of at least focal myxoid areas is the key to the diagnosis. It is generally accepted that a high-grade component greater than 5% of the tumor is needed to render the diagnosis of high-grade myxoid liposarcoma.

Myxoid liposarcoma is characterized by a t(12;16) *FUS::DDIT3* or a t(12;22) *EWSR1:: DDIT3* gene fusions that show no prognostic significance; these fusions can be picked up diagnostically by FISH, RT-PCR, or a commercial gene fusion NGS panel. Secondary alterations such as copy number gain, *T53, TERT, CDKN2A*, and other alterations may occur, more often in high-grade myxoid liposarcomas. IHC plays no diagnostic role although antibodies labeling DDIT3 fusion oncoprotein are being explored.

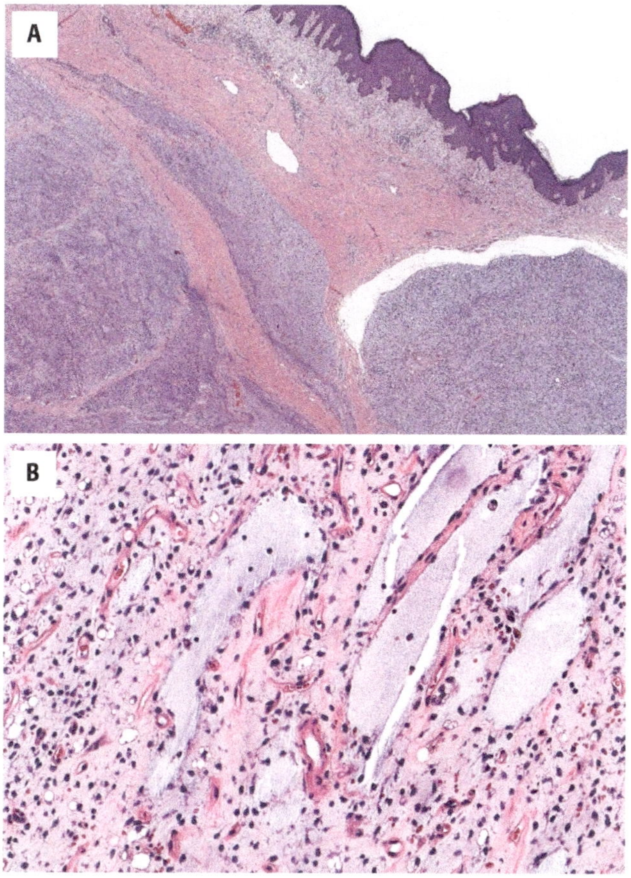

FIG. 14.76

Superficial myxoid liposarcoma. **A,** Circumscribed, lobulated subcutaneous tumor with diffusely myxoid stroma. **B,** Short spindle or comma-shaped cells admixed with lipoblasts in abundant myxoid stroma containing delicate, plexiform vasculature. Small pools or cystic spaces resembling pulmonary edema are often present.

Differential Diagnosis

Superficial myxoid liposarcoma can be confused with the myxoid variant of DFSP (discussed above), myxoid spindle cell lipoma, low-grade myxofibrosarcoma, and lipoblastoma. Myxoid DFSP, defined by the presence of myxoid stromal change in >50% of the tumor, can look strikingly similar to myxoid liposarcoma as this is also a relatively hypocellular tumor composed of short, mitotically quiescent spindle or stellate cells distributed loosely in a prominently myxoid stroma containing delicate vasculature. The most helpful feature is the presence of a conventional storiform component with a diffusely infiltrative edge, which is present in most myxoid DFSP cases, even if focal. Lipoblasts are uncharacteristic of myxoid DFSP but must be distinguished from entrapped mature adipocytes. The involvement of the dermis, a prominent feature in DFSP, is very rare in superficial myxoid liposarcoma. CD34 expression is helpful as most myxoid liposarcomas are

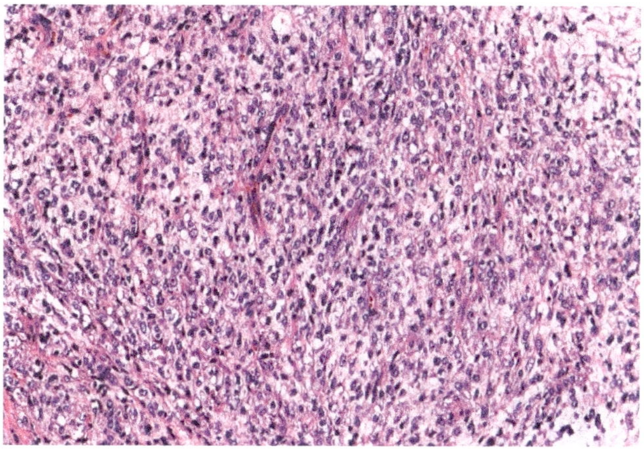

FIG. 14.77

High-grade myxoid liposarcoma (formerly, round cell liposarcoma) consists of hypercellular sheets of primitive round tumor cells obscuring plexiform vasculature, with enlarged, hyperchromatic nuclei, increased mitotic activity, and necrosis.

negative for this marker. The pitfall in this context lies in mistaking CD34-positive dermal fibroblasts for tumor cells. Identification of diagnostic *DDIT3* or *EWSR1* and/or the *COL01A-PDGFB* (specific for DFSP) gene rearrangements helps resolve challenging cases. Low-grade myxofibrosarcoma (discussed above) typically presents as a subcutaneous, lobulated mass in older patients. Myxofibrosarcoma shows infiltrative, multinodular growth pattern, larger and coarser vasculature with perivascular condensation of tumor cells, and nuclear pleomorphism appreciable even in low-grade tumors. Tumor cells containing intracytoplasmic mucin (so-called pseudolipoblasts) may occur but true lipoblastic differentiation does not occur. The high-grade component of myxofibrosarcoma has the appearance of pleomorphic sarcoma, in contrast to the primitive round cell appearance of high-grade myxoid liposarcoma. A pleomorphic sarcoma component is exceptionally rare in myxoid liposarcoma, likely a result of true dedifferentiation. *DDIT3* gene rearrangement is not seen in myxofibrosarcoma. Myxoid spindle cell lipomas are often fat-poor and feature prominent branching capillary vasculature very closely resembling myxoid liposarcoma. The presence of eosinophilic ropey collagen fibers, clusters of spindle cells, positive CD34, and loss of RB1 expression by IHC and the absence of *DDIT3* gene alterations are diagnostic of spindle cell lipoma. The differential diagnosis with lipoblastoma is discussed above.

Prognosis and Treatment

Myxoid liposarcoma is prone to local recurrence (10%–20%) and a relatively high rate of synchronous and metachronous systemic metastases (up to 60% in high-grade tumors) to fat-rich sites such as bone marrow, skin and subcutis, and retroperitoneum. These tumors are very sensitive to radiation therapy, which is often used neoadjuvantly prior to curative surgical excision, and chemotherapy including anthracycline and trabectedin regimens.

MYOGENIC TUMORS

BENIGN NEOPLASMS

PILAR LEIOMYOMA

Clinical Findings

Cutaneous leiomyomas arising from the arrector pili muscle and related leiomyomas of the smooth muscle of the nipple-areola complex present as slightly protuberant, well-circumscribed, pinkish-tan nodules in adults, usually less than 2 cm in size. They may be tender or change size with hormonal fluctuations (in the case of nipple leiomyoma). Overlying skin changes or nipple discharge are uncharacteristic. Nipple leiomyomas have a slight female predilection and are usually single although in male patients they may be bilateral.

BENIGN CUTANEOUS SMOOTH MUSCLE TUMORS—DIFFERENTIAL DIAGNOSIS

Pilar Leiomyoma

- Well-circumscribed, tan nodule on the limbs, trunk or nipple of adults
- Multiple lesions in autosomal dominant hereditary leiomyomatosis and renal cell carcinoma syndrome (HLRCC, Reed's syndrome)
  - Germline mutations of the fumarate hydratase (*FH*) gene
  - Multiple cutaneous and uterine leiomyomas
  - Renal cell carcinoma
  - Urothelial and prostate cancer, Leydig cell tumor
- Short, disorganized bundles of benign smooth muscle in the dermis
- Infiltrative growth between dermal collagen fibers
- Nucleoli, perinuclear eosinophilic inclusions, or degenerative-type nuclei in *FH*-deficient tumors
- Positive for desmin, SMA, caldesmon, smooth muscle myosin heavy chain
- Loss of cytoplasmic FH expression in *FH*-deficient tumors
- Differential diagnosis
  - Cutaneous leiomyosarcoma (atypia, mitotic figures, subcutaneous involvement)
  - Cutaneous PEComa
  - Smooth muscle hamartoma
  - Dermatomyofibroma

Angioleiomyoma

- Benign neoplasm in the pericytic tumor family
- Tender subcutaneous nodule around ankles and feet in middle-aged adults
- Bundles of benign smooth muscle bundles radiating around prominent vessels
- Thrombosis, myxoid change, and dystrophic calcifications
- Circumscribed edge
- Positive for SMA, calponin, h-caldesmon and desmin
- *PDGFRB* and *NOTCH* alterations
- Differential diagnosis
  - Pilar leiomyoma
  - Leiomyosarcoma

Smooth Muscle Hamartoma

- Congenital plaque in the lumbosacral region of infants or small children
- Crop of small papules that may contain coarse hair
- Linear arrangement of smooth muscle bundles in the dermis without forming a mass
- Epidermal hyperplasia
- Differential diagnosis
  - Becker's nevus
  - Dermatomyofibroma
  - Pilar leiomyoma

PEComa, Perivascular epithelioid cell tumor; *SMA*, smooth muscle actin

Cutaneous leiomyomas are often multiple occurring in crops. The clinical importance of recognizing multiple leiomyomas is that they may be the first manifestation of the hereditary leiomyomatosis and renal cell carcinoma syndrome (HLRCC, also known as Reed's syndrome), an autosomal dominant disorder due to germline mutations of the fumarate hydratase (*FH*) gene. This disorder manifests as multiple cutaneous and uterine leiomyomas, renal cell carcinoma, and a variety of other tumors including urothelial and prostate cancer, Leydig cell tumor, and others.

Histopathologic Features

Cutaneous and nipple leiomyomas are composed of short, disorganized bundles of benign smooth muscle that fill the reticular dermis and resemble pilar smooth muscle. While symmetric and circumscribed at low magnification, pilar leiomyomas have a somewhat infiltrative edge, percolating between dermal collagen fibers. In larger tumors, this feature is usually focally present at the tumor periphery. The tumor cells have elongated, blunt-ended nuclei, uniformly distributed chromatin and brightly eosinophilic cytoplasm with crisp cytoplasmic membranes, and the occasional presence of perinuclear cytoplasmic vacuoles (Fig. 14.78A and B). The vasculature is inconspicuous. There is no cytologic atypia or pleomorphism, and mitotic figures are very rare. Smooth muscle tumors associated with HLRCC may have a somewhat more prominent nucleoli or degenerative-type (symplastic) nuclear changes in the form of multinucleated cells with smudged chromatin, but these findings are not as reliable as the knowledge of clinical history and multiple lesions. The tumor cells express desmin, SMA, h-caldesmon, and smooth muscle myosin heavy chain and may occasionally express focal cytokeratin. Nipple leiomyomas may somewhat inconsistently express ER and PR receptors, which are not usually seen in pilar leiomyoma. S100, SOX10, p63, and melanocytic markers are negative. Loss of FH expression by IHC can be used as a quick screen to identify patients possibly affected by HLRCC and has a sensitivity of approximately 80%.

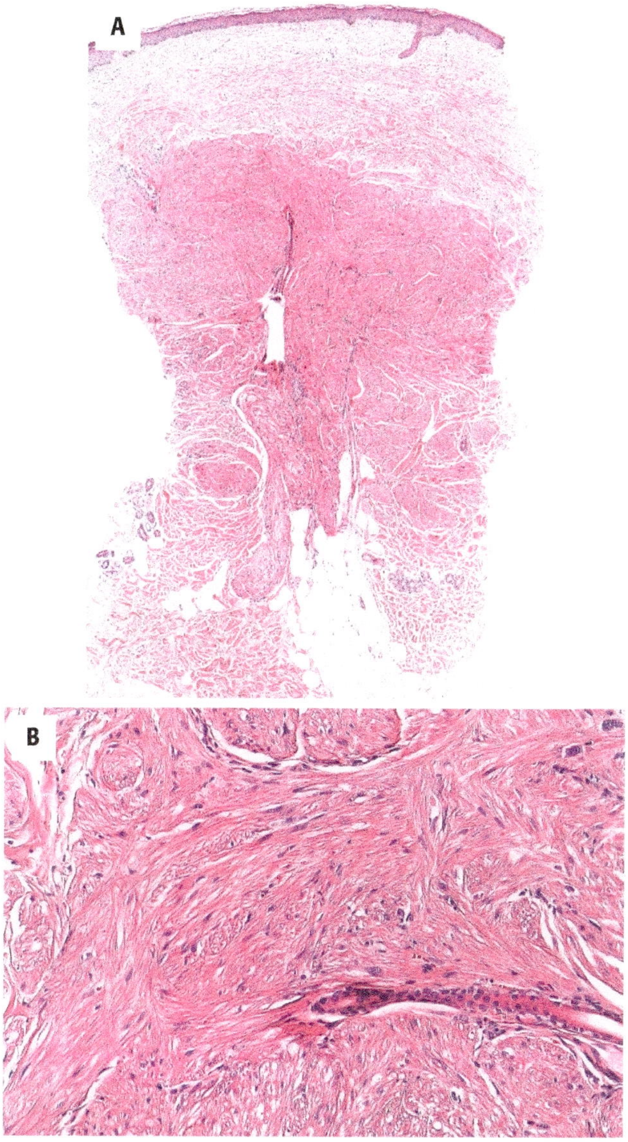

FIG. 14.78

Pilar leiomyoma. **A,** Dermal-based tumor with a stellate, somewhat infiltrative configuration. **B,** Short, disorganized bundles of benign smooth muscle resembling pilar smooth muscle.

Differential Diagnosis

Smooth muscle hamartoma (see below) is a congenital lesion with randomly arranged and widely separated discrete bundles of smooth muscle in the dermis and overlying epidermal hyperplasia. Angioleiomyoma, a benign neoplasm in the pericytic tumor family, is a distinctly circumscribed and somewhat deeper-seated, well-circumscribed nodule composed of bundles of well-differentiated smooth muscle arranged concentrically or radially around variably sized blood vessels. This contrasts with the discontinuous and somewhat infiltrative bundles of smooth muscle without angiocentricity seen in pilar leiomyoma. Dermatomyofibroma represents a myofibroblastic proliferation with bundles of bland spindle cells in a distinctly parallel arrangement to the epidermis. It lacks strong and diffuse staining for desmin, caldesmon, and smooth muscle myosin, in keeping with its myofibroblastic phenotype. Nerve sheath tumors including superficial schwannoma, solitary circumscribed neuroma, and conventional granular cell tumor can be easily distinguished by Schwann cell markers. Cutaneous PEComas show more epithelioid cells with round nuclei, small distinct nucleoli and pale eosinophilic or clear cytoplasm, and a coexpression of melanocytic markers such as HMB45. The differential diagnosis with atypical intradermal smooth muscle neoplasm/cutaneous leiomyosarcoma is discussed below.

Prognosis and Treatment

Pilar and nipple leiomyomas are benign and cured by simple excision.

SMOOTH MUSCLE HAMARTOMA

Clinical Findings

This is a congenital lesion that presents as an indurated plaque accompanied by a crop of small papules that may contain coarse hair, in the lumbosacral region of infants or small children.

Histopathologic Features

Smooth muscle hamartoma consists of randomly arranged bundles of smooth muscle in the dermis and is often accompanied by epidermal hyperplasia (Fig. 14.79). In contrast to pilar leiomyoma, the fascicles of smooth muscle are more widely separated by dermal collagen rather than forming a mass.

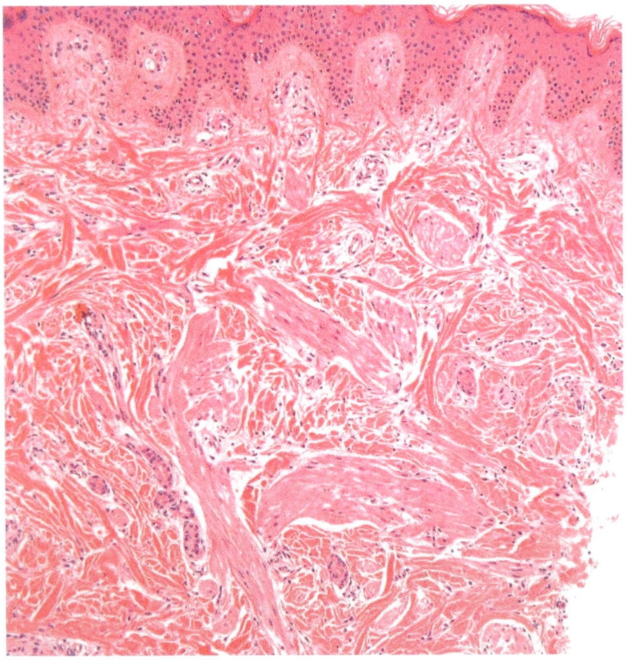

FIG. 14.79
Smooth muscle hamartoma consists of randomly arranged fascicles of smooth muscle percolating the dermis without forming a mass. The lesion is often accompanied by epidermal hyperplasia.

Differential Diagnosis

Becker's nevus can also show an increased number of smooth muscle bundles; however, it presents later in life (around puberty) and has a very prominent hypertrichosis that is readily recognized in clinic. The degree of epidermal changes associated with Becker's nevus (elongation of rete pegs with associated hyperpigmentation) is not as prominent in smooth muscle hamartoma.

Prognosis and Treatment

Smooth muscle hamartoma is benign and cured by excision for cosmetic reasons or definitive diagnosis.

RHABDOMYOMATOUS MESENCHYMAL HAMARTOMA

Clinical Findings

Rhabdomyomatous mesenchymal hamartoma is a rare congenital lesion that most often occurs on the central head (chin) of infants and young children, although it might not come to clinical attention until early adulthood when it is removed for diagnosis or cosmetic reasons.

Histopathologic Features

The lesion consists of a nodule of elongated bundles of mature striated muscle admixed with connective and adipose tissue and skin appendages in the reticular dermis (Fig. 14.80).

Differential Diagnosis

The biggest challenge, in our opinion, is to recognize the presence of this lesion in the first place, as it can blend with the adjacent normal tissue of the head and neck region with its typical intermingling of subcutaneous tissue and skeletal muscle. Nodular arrangement of skeletal muscle in reticular dermis or a juxtaposition of skeletal muscle fiber against a hair shaft will argue in favor of the lesion. Rhabdomyomas

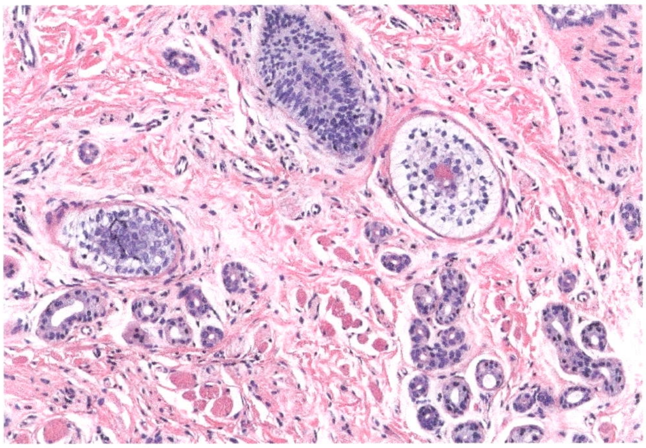

FIG. 14.80
Rhabdomyomatous mesenchymal hamartoma presents as elongated bundles of mature striated muscle admixed with connective and adipose tissue and skin appendages in the reticular dermis.

virtually always have a component of immature spindled or epithelioid rhabdomyoblasts with bland nuclear features.

Prognosis and Treatment

Rhabdomyomatous mesenchymal hamartoma is benign and cured by local excision.

MALIGNANT NEOPLASMS

DERMAL LEIOMYOSARCOMA

Clinical Findings

Cutaneous leiomyosarcomas present in older adults, with predilection for male patients, as solitary, somewhat lobulated protuberant tan-red nodules, usually less than 2 cm in size (range 0.3–5 cm), which, just like pilar leiomyomas, can be painful. Subcutaneous leiomyosarcomas originating from vascular smooth muscle present as palpable masses.

Histopathologic Features

Leiomyosarcomas are composed of cellular intersecting fascicles of smooth muscle cells with blunt-ended hyperchromatic nuclei and brightly eosinophilic cytoplasm with well-defined cell borders and occasional perinuclear vacuoles. Leiomyosarcomas have increased cellularity and nuclear atypia and hyperchromasia often appreciable at scanning magnification, accompanied by varying degree of mitotic activity, necrosis, and vascular invasion (Fig. 14.81A and B). Frank pleomorphism, dystrophic calcifications, and stromal hyalinization can be observed. For prognostic purposes, a distinction must be made between a cutaneous leiomyosarcoma originating from pilar smooth muscle and a subcutaneous leiomyosarcoma of vascular origin. Cutaneous leiomyosarcoma has a similar configuration as pilar leiomyoma, showing a poorly circumscribed lesion centered on the dermis, with a somewhat infiltrative growth of intersecting smooth muscle bundles and variable involvement of the subcutis. Cutaneous leiomyosarcomas of lower nuclear grade that are completely confined to the dermis or show only very minimal involvement of the subcutis and no vascular invasion tend to behave substantially better than their deep-seated counterparts. For these lesions, a designation as "atypical intradermal smooth muscle neoplasm" has been proposed, provided that the

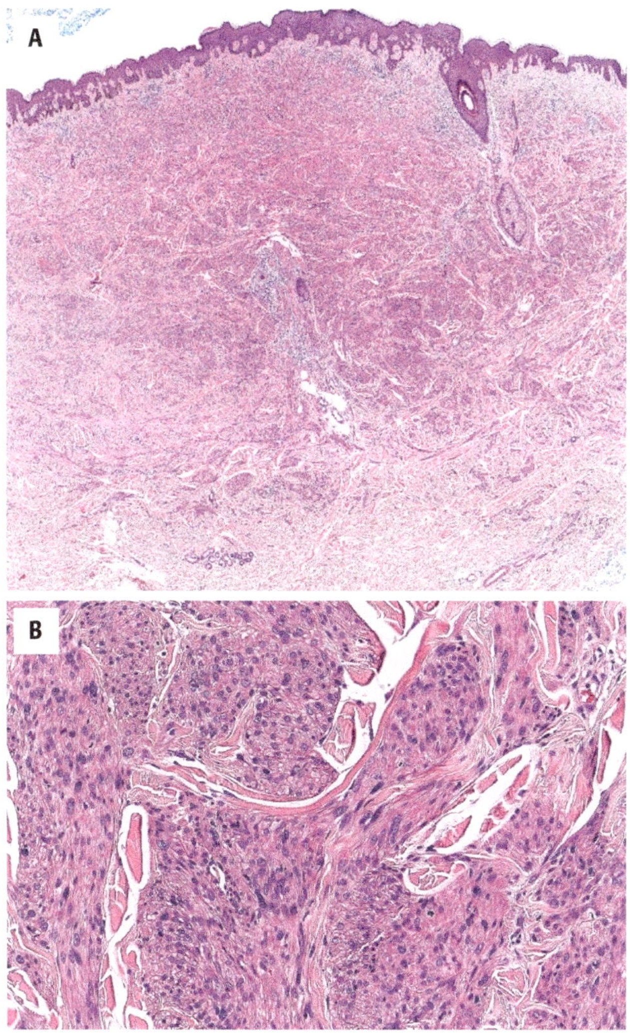

FIG. 14.81
Cutaneous leiomyosarcoma. **A,** Cellular intersecting fascicles of smooth muscle cells with somewhat infiltrative edge resembling pilar leiomyoma. **B,** The tumor shows increased cellularity, nuclear atypia, and mitotic activity.

interface with the subcutis can be adequately examined. Subcutaneous leiomyosarcomas arising from vascular smooth muscle are primarily centered on the subcutis and form a more sharply outlined solid mass rather than discontinuous bundles. Aggressive growth with pushing margin, a significant infiltration of the subcutis and vascular invasion is characteristic. Leiomyosarcomas of vascular smooth muscle are comparable in every way to their somatic soft tissue counterparts and should be graded according to the FNCLCC grading system. By IHC, leiomyosarcomas are variably positive for SMA, desmin, h-caldesmon, and smooth muscle myosin heavy chain, and the extent and intensity of immunostaining generally correlates with the degree of differentiation. Inconsistent expression of estrogen and PR can be present. Approximately 40% to 50% of leiomyosarcomas can be positive for cytokeratins.

Differential Diagnosis

Pilar leiomyoma is architecturally a very similar lesion which is confined to the dermis and can be distinguished by banal nuclear features and lack of mitotic activity or necrosis. AFX and dermal pleomorphic sarcoma are (myo)fibroblastic tumors which do not have smooth muscle phenotype either by morphology or by immunostaining. These tumors may show focal SMA expression in a typical myofibroblastic "tram-track" pattern, but they lack robust cytoplasmic SMA, caldesmon, or smooth muscle myosin expression and are usually negative, or only focally positive for desmin. Spindle cells SCCs and spindle cell melanomas rarely display a true smooth muscle differentiation and can be distinguished by identification of a precursor in situ component or appropriate epithelial and melanocytic markers. Cellular FH can be distinguished by the presence of peripheral collagen trapping, low-grade nuclear atypia, more basophilic cytoplasm of the lesional cells with indistinct borders, and a myofibroblastic pattern of myogenic marker expression.

Prognosis and Treatment

Subcutaneous leiomyosarcomas are aggressive and behave similarly to their somatic soft tissue counterparts, with tumor size, grade, and completeness of surgical resection determining the outcomes. The prognosis of cutaneous leiomyosarcomas tends to be much more favorable due to the smaller size, superficial location, and resectability of these tumors. Atypical smooth muscle tumors strictly confined to the dermis or with only very limited subcutaneous involvement have approximately 30% to 40% chance of local recurrence but very rare metastases. Based on these observations, the term "atypical intradermal smooth muscle neoplasm" was proposed for these lesions, emphasizing the need for complete surgical excision to minimize the risk of local recurrence while avoiding potential overtreatment. Whatever the preferred terminology, it appears that the best treatment strategy for dermal-based cutaneous leiomyosarcomas is complete surgical excision with negative margins, whereas subcutaneous leiomyosarcomas should be treated by a multimodality approach.

RHABDOMYOSARCOMA

Cutaneous rhabdomyosarcomas are very rare, and the reader is referred to the corresponding soft tissue and pediatric pathology literature for a comprehensive review of this topic and a contemporary molecular classification. Of the established morphologic subtypes of rhabdomyosarcoma (embryonal, alveolar, spindle cell/sclerotic, epithelioid, pleomorphic), pleomorphic rhabdomyosarcoma merits a brief mention here as it may manifest in the extremities or head and neck region of elderly patients and mimic other pleomorphic sarcomas that arise in the skin.

Histopathologic Features

Pleomorphic rhabdomyosarcoma is a high-grade pleomorphic sarcoma with a component of sheets of large spindled, epithelioid, or pleomorphic rhabdomyoblasts with round or pleomorphic nuclei and ample eosinophilic cytoplasm that may contain recognizable striations (Fig. 14.82). The tumor cells are diffusely positive for

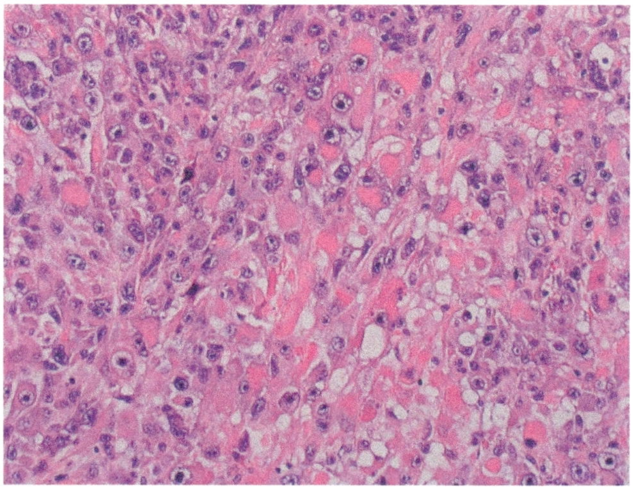

FIG. 14.82

Pleomorphic rhabdomyosarcoma showing sheets of large spindled, epithelioid, and pleomorphic rhabdomyoblasts with ample eosinophilic cytoplasm in the background of undifferentiated spindle cell or pleomorphic sarcoma.

desmin and show variable nuclear expression of myogenin and MyoD1. SMA and cytokeratins may be focally positive, while melanocytic markers are negative. Pleomorphic rhabdomyosarcoma is associated with a complex array of copy number alterations and point mutations, often involving *TP53*, and may occur in patients with Li-Fraumeni's syndrome. No single genetic alteration is pathognomonic for this rhabdomyosarcoma subtype.

Differential Diagnosis

Pleomorphic rhabdomyosarcoma should always be included when encountering a dermal pleomorphic sarcoma candidate with brightly eosinophilic cytoplasm and ruled out by application of a screening desmin immunostain with reflex for myogenic transcription factors myogenin and MyoD1 if desmin is diffusely positive. Spindle cell/sarcomatoid SCC and melanoma are other principal diagnostic considerations, and both can show a heterologous rhabdomyoblastic component. The distinction should be accomplished by a careful examination for the precursor lesion or in situ disease, and identification of epithelial or melanocytic phenotype and, in case of malignant melanoma, BRAFV600E expression.

Prognosis and Treatment

Even in superficial locations, pleomorphic rhabdomyosarcoma is an aggressive sarcoma and should be treated by complete excision with additional recommendations by the multidisciplinary sarcoma team.

NERVE SHEATH TUMORS AND TUMOR-LIKE REACTIONS

BENIGN LESIONS

TRAUMATIC NEUROMA

Traumatic neuromas manifest as a small, firm mass in the area of previous trauma and are often painful. They occur in areas of previous trauma. Histologically, the lesions are composed of a disorganized collection of hyperplastic axons and Schwann cells embedded in a scar (Fig. 14.83). Adjacent connective tissue may show nonspecific reactive vascular and fibroblastic proliferation and myxoid changes. Traumatic neuromas may be confused with mucosal neuromas of MEN type IIB syndrome, which lack an associated scar and history of trauma. Morton neuroma (localized interdigital neuritis), sometimes confused with traumatic neuroma, is a painful degenerative process affecting plantar nerve in the third metatarsal interspace due to compression by connective tissue resulting from chronic mechanical injury. This process is characterized by perineurial and endoneurial fibrosis and depletion of axons in association with thrombosis and hyaline arteriolosclerosis and reactive vascular and fibroblastic changes in the adjacent connective tissue. There are no prominent hyperplastic changes like those seen in traumatic neuroma, and oftentimes, the nerve itself is not present in the surgical debulking specimens. Both lesions are benign with surgical treatment performed only for pain relief or to alleviate compression.

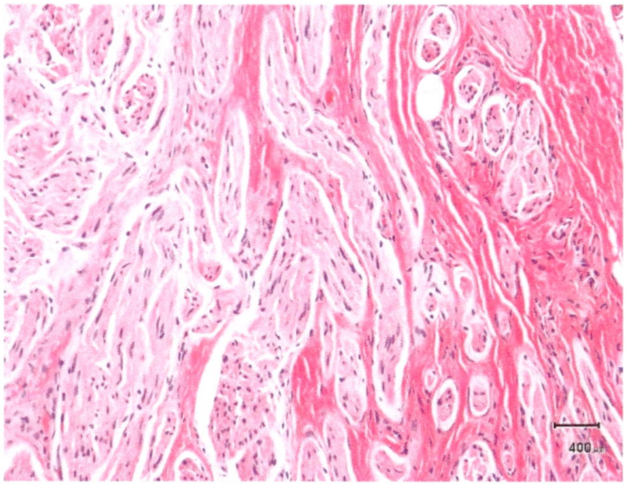

FIG. 14.83
Traumatic neuroma showing a disorganized collection of hyperplastic axons and Schwann cells embedded in a scar tissue.

RUDIMENTARY POLYDACTYLY

Rudimentary polydactyly presents as a small nodule usually at the base of the fifth finger and is often bilateral. It is histologically characterized by a disorganized proliferation of small nerves and Meissner corpuscles in fibrous connective tissue (Fig. 14.84). It should be distinguished from traumatic neuroma, which is associated with a scar and lacks Meissner corpuscles.

SOLITARY CIRCUMSCRIBED NEUROMA (PALISADED ENCAPSULATED NEUROMA)

Clinical Findings

Solitary circumscribed neuroma presents as a solitary flesh-colored dermal nodule in middle-aged adults, almost always in the face in close proximity to mucocutaneous junctions such as oral mucosa or eyelids.

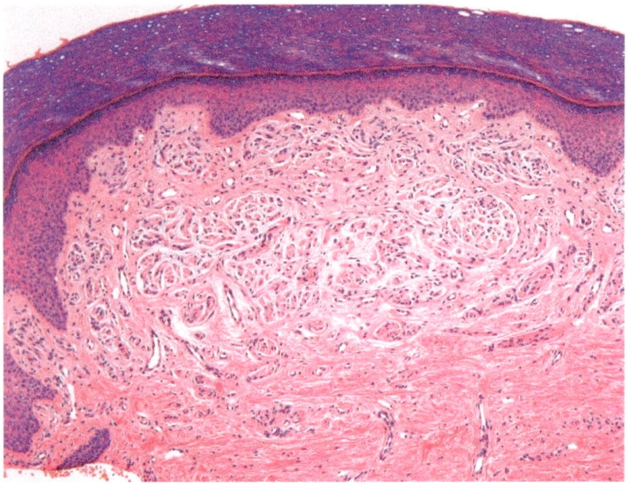

FIG. 14.84

Rudimentary polydactyly characterized by a disorganized proliferation of small nerves and Meissner corpuscles in fibrous connective tissue.

SOLITARY CIRCUMSCRIBED NEUROMA—DISEASE FACT SHEETS

Clinical Findings

- Solitary flesh-colored dermal nodule in the face of adult patients
- Close to mucocutaneous junctions (oral mucosa, eyelids)

Histopathologic Features

- Circumscribed dermal tumor with a partial fibroblastic capsule
- Fascicles of benign Schwann cells with wavy nuclei and occasional palisading
- Conspicuous intratumoral clefts

IHC: Positive for S100 and SOX10; neurofilament highlights small intralesional axons

Differential Diagnosis

- Schwannoma

IHC, Immunohistochemistry.

Histopathologic Features

Solitary circumscribed neuroma is a circumscribed tumor often partially surrounded by a thin fibroblastic capsule. The tumor is composed of fascicles of Schwann cells with wavy, slightly hyperchromatic nuclei and amphophilic cytoplasm with indistinct cytoplasmic borders (Fig. 14.85A and B). Occasional nuclear palisading is present. Intratumoral clefts are conspicuous. The spindle cells diffusely express schwannian markers S100 and SOX10, while neurofilament highlights small axons within the lesion.

Differential Diagnosis

Schwannoma is the main and somewhat frustrating differential diagnosis as both lesions are composed of

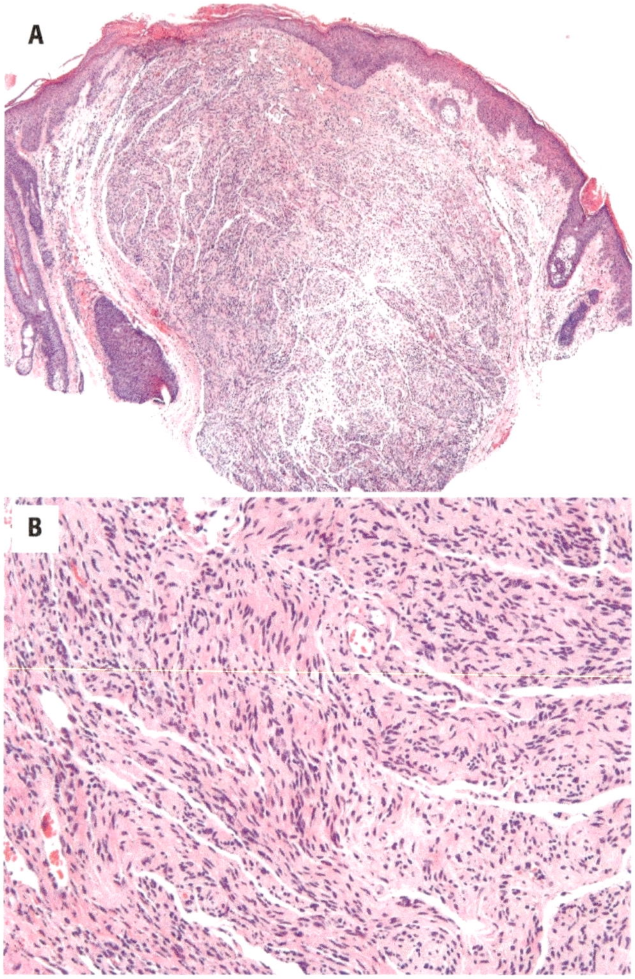

FIG. 14.85

Solitary circumscribed neuroma. **A,** A circumscribed tumor with bundles of tumor cells separated by intratumoral clefts. **B,** Fascicles of Schwann cells with wavy hyperchromatic nuclei and amphophilic cytoplasm with indistinct cytoplasmic borders.

cytologically identical benign Schwann cells without other components. Schwannomas have a well-developed capsule and lack the prominent intratumoral clefts typical of solitary circumscribed neuroma. In contrast to the more monotonous look of solitary circumscribed neuroma, schwannoma shows more variability in the cellular density with alternating Anthoni A and Anthony B areas and prominent hyalinized vessels. These features are not typical for solitary circumscribed neuroma. Neurofilament would typically highlight axons present only at the periphery of the tumor.

SCHWANNOMA

Clinical Findings

Schwannomas manifest as a solitary lesion in the dermis or subcutis in middle-age to older adults and most

SCHWANNOMA—DISEASE FACT SHEET

Clinical Findings

- ▸▸ Solitary lesion in the dermis or subcutis
- ▸▸ Sporadic or associated with the following syndromes:
  - Autosomal dominant neurofibromatosis type II (vestibular schwannomas)
  - Schwannomatosis: multiple schwannomas, germline *SMARCB1* mutations

Histopathologic Features

- ▸▸ Classic schwannoma
  - Circumscribed tumor with a fibrous capsule containing perineurial cells
  - Hypercellular (Antoni A) and hypocellular (Antoni B) areas
  - Cystic changes and inflammatory cells in Antoni B areas
  - Schwann cells with wavy nuclei and fibrillary amphophilic cytoplasm
  - Thick-walled hyalinized vessels
  - Secondary elements: hemorrhage, stromal hyalinization, hemosiderin deposits, and "degenerative" nuclear atypia
- ▸▸ Classic schwannoma variants
  - Cellular: Antoni A areas with a fascicular growth pattern
  - Plexiform: plexiform growth of Antoni A areas
  - Microcystic reticular: corded growth pattern in a diffusely myxoid stroma
  - Neuroblastoma-like: solid or rosette-like arrangement of round Schwann cells
- ▸▸ Epithelioid schwannoma
  - Epithelioid cells with eccentric raisinoid nuclei in a lobular configuration
  - Myxohyaline stroma with hyalinized vessels

IHC/Molecular

- Diffuse, strong S100 and SOX10
- Perineurial cells in the tumor capsule are positive for EMA, GLUT1, or claudin-1
- Inactivating mutations of *NF2*
- *SMARCB1* and *LZTR1* alterations in familial and sporadic schwannomatosis
- ▸▸ Mosaic INI-1 loss in neurofibromatosis type 2–associated multiple schwannomas due to loss of one copy of *SMARCB1* gene on 22q11
  - *SMARCB1* alterations with loss of INI-1 expression in sporadic epithelioid schwannoma

Differential Diagnosis

- ▸▸ Classic schwannoma
  - Neurofibroma
  - Solitary circumscribed neuroma
  - Hybrid schwannoma/perineurioma
  - Malignant peripheral nerve sheath tumor in cases of cellular schwannoma
- ▸▸ Epithelioid schwannoma
  - Myoepithelial tumor
  - Ossifying fibromyxoid tumor
  - Epithelioid fibrous histiocytoma

EMA, Epithelial membrane antigen; *GLUT1*, glucose transporter 1; *IHC*, immunohistochemistry.

often originate from the peripheral nerves in the skin, head and neck region, or extremities, although they can occur in many visceral sites and body cavities. Pain or paresthesia may be present owing to compression of the underlying nerve by the tumor, but most schwannomas are asymptomatic and often discovered incidentally. Most schwannomas are solitary and sporadic; multiple tumors are associated with autosomal dominant neurofibromatosis type II (vestibular schwannomas) and schwannomatosis, which is characterized by multiple schwannomas but without vestibular involvement, and germline mutations in *SMARCB1* gene.

Histopathologic Features

Schwannomas are circumscribed tumors surrounded by a fibrous capsule containing compressed perineurial cells. Schwannomas are characterized by varying cellularity with hypercellular (Antoni A) areas alternating with relatively hypocellular (Antoni B) areas (Fig. 14.86A and B). The hypocellular areas may show cystic change and contain chronic inflammatory cells. Cytologically, the tumor is composed of typical Schwann cells with slightly hyperchromatic spindled, wavy nuclei, and fibrillary amphophilic cytoplasm with indistinct borders. Thick-walled hyalinized vessels are often present within the tumor. Hemorrhage, stromal hyalinization, hemosiderin deposits, and "degenerative" nuclear atypia are very common. Cellular shwannoma consists mostly of Antoni A areas and has a fascicular growth pattern with a mild increase in atypia, mitotic figures, and even necrosis, raising the possibility of a sarcoma. Rarely, the tumor can be composed of discrete, mostly hypercellular thinly encapsulated Antony A nodules arranged in a distinctly plexiform growth pattern (plexiform schwannoma) (Fig. 14.87). Plexiform schwannoma can occur in patients with neurofibromatosis type II or schwannomatosis but not neurofibromatosis type 1 (NF-1). Microcystic reticular schwannoma has a diffusely myxoid stroma with corded growth pattern of schwannian cells and frequent microcyst formation (Fig. 14.88). This lesion lacks the biphasic appearance and hyalinized vasculature of the conventional schwannoma. Other uncommon histologic variations include neuroblastoma-like features with solid or rosette-like arrangement of mostly small round Schwann cells that resemble small blue cell tumors but lack atypia or proliferative activity (Fig. 14.89). The cells are strongly, diffusely positive for S100 and SOX10, while CD34 is either completely negative or present at the tumor periphery in the subcapsular zones. The presence of perineurial cells (highlighted by EMA, GLUT1, or claudin-1) and entrapped axons (highlighted by neurofilament stain) is also limited to the tumor capsule and the subcapsular zones. Both sporadic and syndromic conventional schwannomas may have inactivating mutations of *NF2*. Familial and sporadic forms of

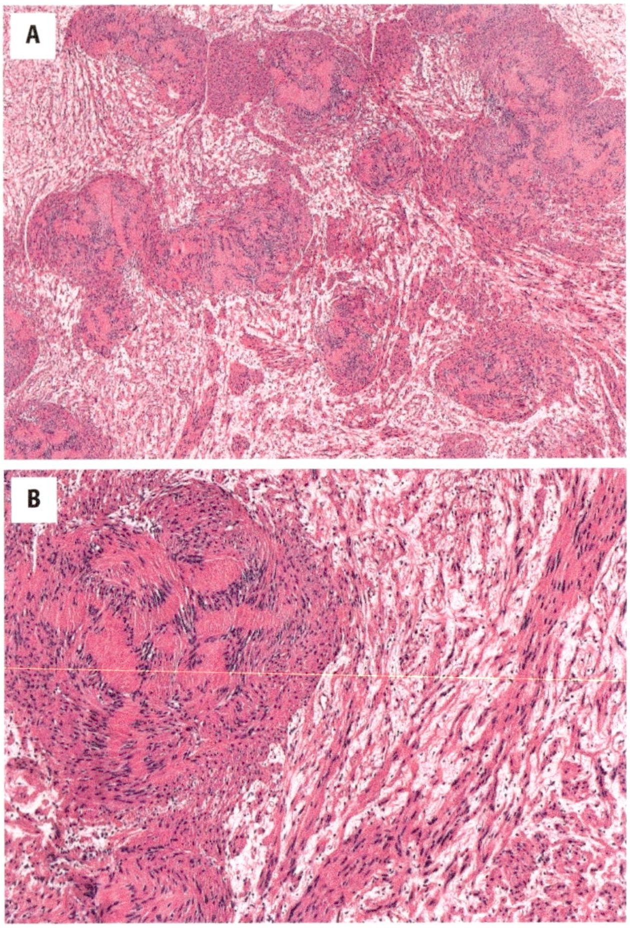

FIG. 14.86

Schwannoma. **A,** Hypercellular (Antoni A) areas alternating with hypocellular (Antoni B) areas, which contain myxoid stroma and inflammatory cells. **B,** Both components consist of Schwann cells with slightly hyperchromatic wavy nuclei and fibrillary amphophilic cytoplasm with indistinct borders. The tumor cells are arranged in a palisaded fashion (Verocay bodies).

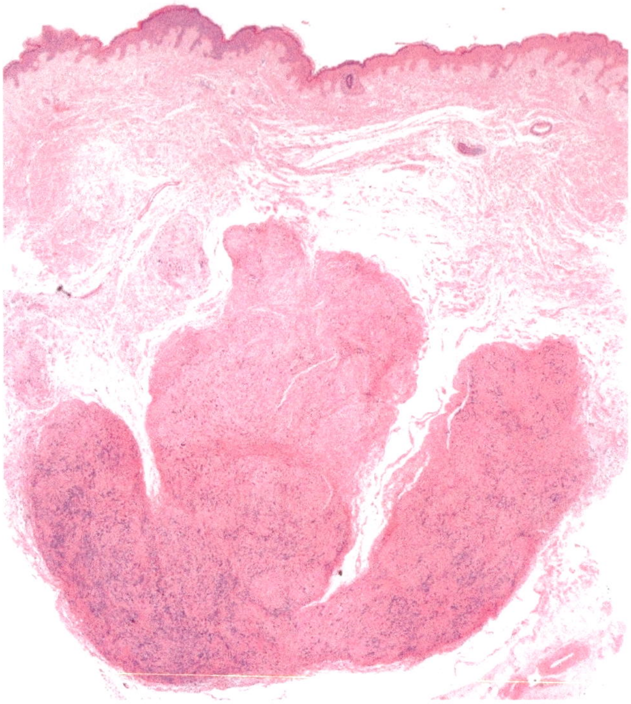

FIG. 14.87

Plexiform schwannoma composed of discrete, thinly encapsulated Antony A nodules arranges in a distinctly plexiform growth pattern.

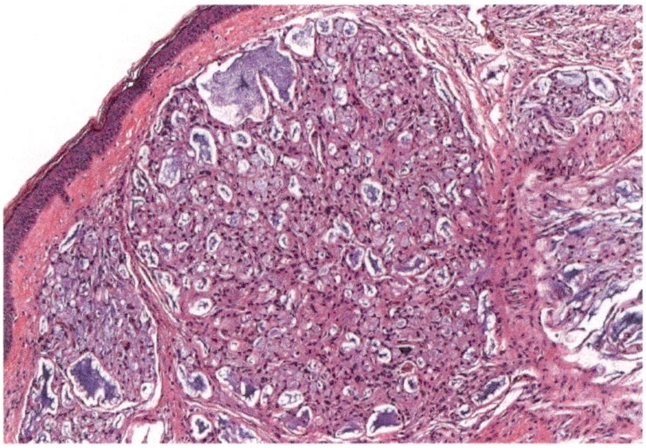

FIG. 14.88

Microcystic reticular schwannoma with corded growth pattern and frequent microcyst formation in a prominent myxoid stroma.

schwannomatosis contain *SMARCB1* and *LZTR1* alterations. Mosaic loss of INI-1 expression can also occur in neurofibromatosis type 2–associated multiple schwannomas due to the concurrent loss of one copy of *SMARCB1* gene, which is located upstream to *NF2* on chromosome 22q11.

Epithelioid schwannoma is a distinct variant composed of epithelioid Schwann cells with eccentric, somewhat raisinoid appearing nuclei, arranged in a lobular configuration in a myxohyaline background (Fig. 14.90A and B). These tumors are usually encapsulated and may show hyalinized vessels, but often lack Antoni A and Antoni B areas. Up to 42% of sporadic epithelioid schwannomas show *SMARCB1* alterations with loss of INI-1 expression by IHC.

Differential Diagnosis

Neurofibroma is usually unencapsulated and, in contrast to schwannoma, which is made only of Schwann cells, shows a mixture of components including mostly CD34-positive fibroblasts, Schwann cells, thick wavy collagen fibers, myxoid zones with inflammatory cells, and mast cells. Perineurial cells and axons are inconspicuous on hematoxylin and eosin (H&E)–stained sections but can be seen scattered throughout the tumor with the use of perineurial markers and neurofilament. The same rules apply to the distinction of plexiform schwannoma and plexiform neurofibroma. Solitary circumscribed neuroma lacks capsule, Antoni A and Antoni B components and hyalinized vasculature but instead may show characteristic cracking between the bundles of Schwann cells.

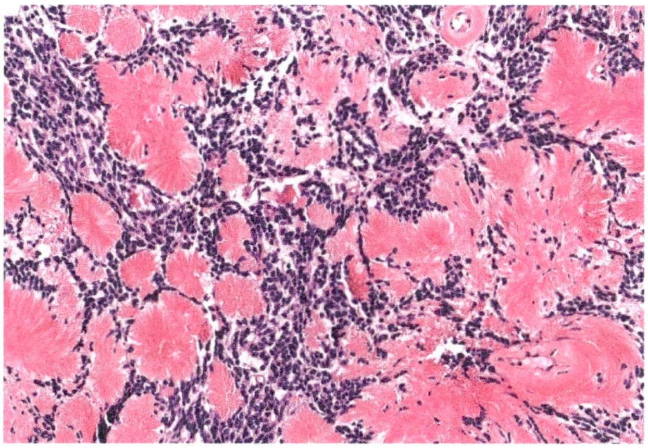

FIG. 14.89

Neuroblastoma-like variant of schwannoma with solid or rosette-like arrangement of mostly small round Schwann cells that resemble small blue cell tumors but lack atypia or proliferative activity.

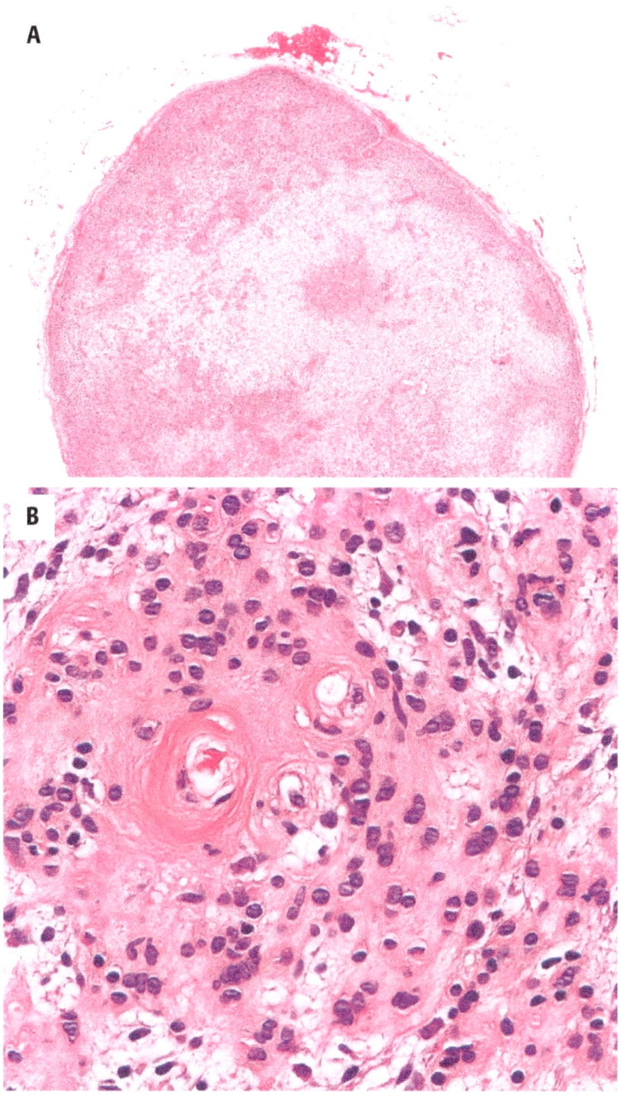

FIG. 14.90

Epithelioid schwannoma. **A,** Circumscribed neoplasm with a capsule and areas of alternating cellularity resembling conventional schwannoma. **B,** Epithelioid Schwann cells with eccentric raisinoid nuclei, arranged in a lobular configuration in a myxohyaline stroma containing prominent vessels.

Cellular schwannoma may raise suspicion for a conventional MPNST; the latter can be distinguished by lack of substantial S100 and SOX10 expression and loss of H3K27me3 immunostaining. Hybrid schwannoma/perineurioma will have a biphasic appearance with alternating whorls of perineurial cells and Schwann cells; this lesion is typically rich in collagen (in contrast to the standard schwannoma that contains very thin pericellular collagen that is not conspicuous in routine histologic sections) and shows expression of Schwann cell and perineurial markers (GLUT1, EMA, claudin-1) in each of the two cell populations. Hybrid schwannomas perineuriomas often show *VGLL3* and sometimes variant gene fusions. Epithelioid schwannomas need to be distinguished from cutaneous myoepithelial tumors, which can be separated based on the presence of a myoepithelial phenotype (coexpression of cytokeratin, EMA, and myoepithelial markers p63, GFAP, and SMA along with SOX10 and S100). Epithelioid schwannomas can resemble OFMT, because the latter is also composed of epithelioid cells arranged in a nested or trabecular pattern in a myxohyaline stroma. Both tumors can be positive for S100 and can show inactivation of *SMARCB1*/INI1. The nuclei in epithelioid schwannomas are more irregular and reniform in appearance, and metaplastic ossification or desmin expression is entirely uncharacteristic. OFMT is a gene fusion-driven neoplasm, with *PHF1* (6p21) gene being the most common. The presence of a conventional schwannoma component with hyalinized vasculature, a true capsule with EMA- or GLUT1-positive perineurial cells, and very strong, diffuse immunoreactivity for SOX10 favors epithelioid schwannoma. Epithelioid FH is a more superficial tumor that lacks expression of schwannian markers or loss of SMARCB1/INI-1 expression; instead epithelioid FH is positive ALK in keeping with the underlying *ALK* fusions. The distinction from epithelioid MPNST is based largely on the degree of nuclear atypia, mitotic activity and necrosis as both tumors are diffusely S100/SOX10 positive and can show loss of *SMARCB1*/INI-1.

Prognosis and Treatment

With exception to morbidity related to the syndromic manifestations such as vestibular schwannoma, these tumors are benign and cured by simple excision. Cutaneous and subcutaneous schwannomas virtually never recur.

NEUROFIBROMA

Clinical Findings

Neurofibroma presents as a solitary flesh-colored papule or nodule (*solitary or localized type*), plaque-like

DIAGNOSTIC CRITERIA FOR NEUROFIBROMATOSIS TYPE 1

Two or more of the following in a patient without a parent with neurofibromatosis type 1:

- Six or more café-au-lait macules >5 mm in prepubertal and over 15 mm in postpubertal patients
- Axillary or inguinal freckling
- Two or more neurofibromas of any type or one plexiform neurofibroma
- Optic pathway glioma
- Two or more iris Lisch nodules or two or more choroidal abnormalities detected by optical coherence tomography/near-infrared reflectance imaging
- Osseous lesions such as sphenoid dysplasia, anterolateral bowing of the tibia, pseudarthrosis
- A pathogenic germline heterozygous neurofibromin 1 (*NF1*) variant

One or more of the above in a patient with a parent with neurofibromatosis type 1

From Legius, E., Messiaen, L., Wolkenstein, P., Pancza, P., Avery, R. A., Berman, Y., et al. (2021). Revised diagnostic criteria for neurofibromatosis type 1 and Legius syndrome: an international consensus recommendation. *Genetics in Medicine*, 23(8), 1506–1513.

thickening (*diffuse type*) of the skin, or multinodular mass (*plexiform type*). Plexiform neurofibroma is nearly always associated with neurofibromatosis. Localized and diffuse neurofibromas are usually sporadic but may also occur in neurofibromatosis. Cutaneous neurofibromas occur in young or middle-aged adults and have a wide anatomic distribution.

Histopathologic Features

Localized neurofibromas are typically small superficial unencapsulated tumors composed of all components of the peripheral nerve including spindle Schwann cells wavy slightly hyperchromatic nuclei, fibroblasts, entrapped axons, and perineurial cells embedded in a wiry collagenous matrix (Fig. 14.91A and B). A perifollicular distribution is common in the head and neck region. Myxoid ground substance also makes up part of the stroma separating the collagen bundles. Occasionally, atypical cells in the absence of significant mitotic activity are seen, especially in NF1-associated tumors. This feature by itself is not indicative of malignant transformation. Mast cells are frequently seen scattered within the tumor. No true fibrous capsule is present. Pseudomeisserian differentiation, Schwann cell-rich nodules, and areas of increased cellularity without fascicle formation can be seen. Plexiform neurofibromas represent a segmental bulbous expansion of the endoneurium by a neurofibromatous process; tangential cuts of this process produce an impression of plexiform growth (Fig. 14.92A and B). Plexiform neurofibromas are initially confined by the perineurium but quickly extend into the adjacent soft tissue in a diffuse pattern. Diffuse neurofibromas have a strikingly infiltrative growth pattern with extensive involvement of the subcutis which resembles DFSP at scanning magnification (Fig. 14.93). Conventional neurofibromas show either no atypia or sporadic nuclear atypia that can be appreciated at scanning magnification. The histologic criteria for malignancy in neurofibroma have been best established for patients with NF1, where such changes often occur in a stepwise progression, but these criteria can be applied to sporadic tumors as well and include the following:

1. Neurofibroma with atypia: scattered hyperchromatic "ancient" nuclei without mitotic activity
2. Cellular neurofibroma: increase in cellularity without fascicle formation or mitotic activity
3. Atypical neurofibromatous neoplasm of uncertain biological potential (ANNUBP): Schwann cell neoplasm with two or more of the following: cytologic

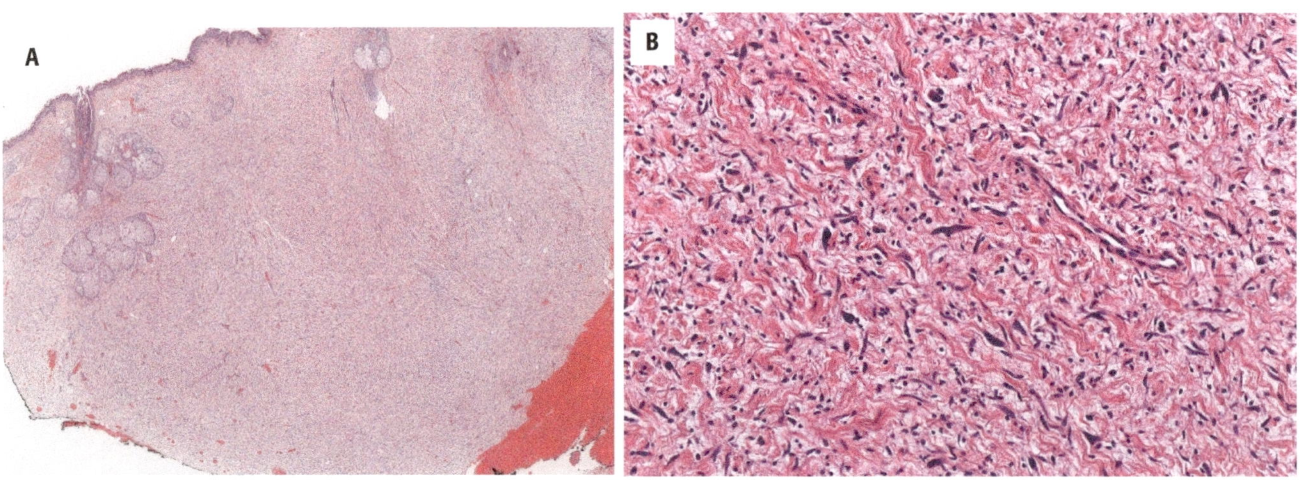

FIG. 14.91

Cutaneous neurofibroma. **A,** A circumscribed but unencapsulated superficial dermal tumor with a mildly infiltrative edge. **B,** Neurofibroma is composed of all components of the peripheral nerve including spindle Schwann cells, fibroblasts, entrapped axons and perineurial cells embedded in a wiry collagenous matrix or myxoid stroma. Sporadic hyperchromatic Schwann cells with degenerative-type atypia can occur.

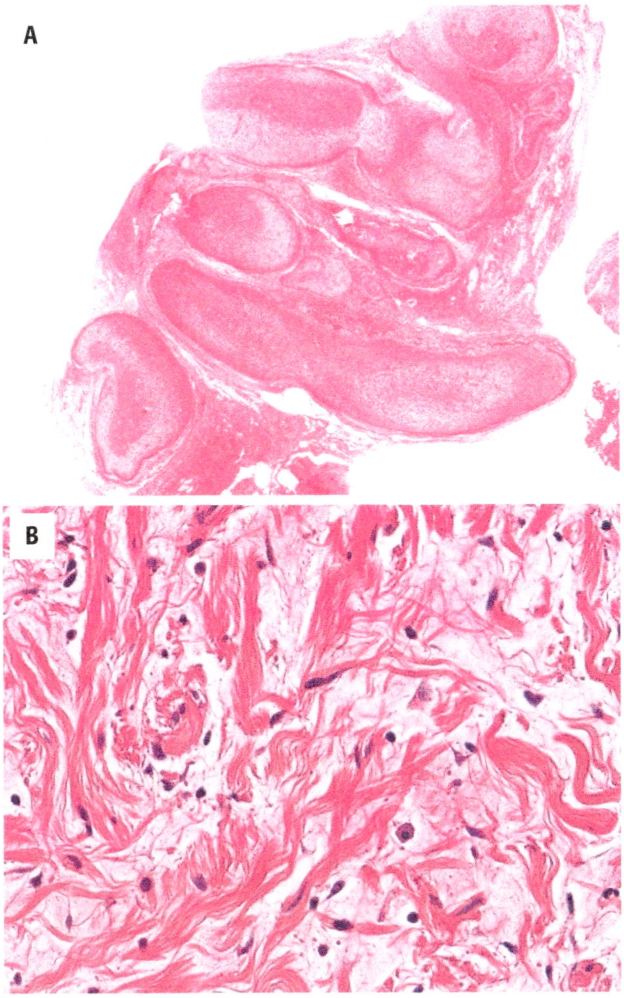

FIG. 14.92

Plexiform neurofibroma. **A,** A segmental bulbous expansion of the endoneurium by a neurofibromatous process with tangential cuts producing the appearance of plexiform growth. **B,** Myxoid stroma with prominent ropey collagen bundles is common.

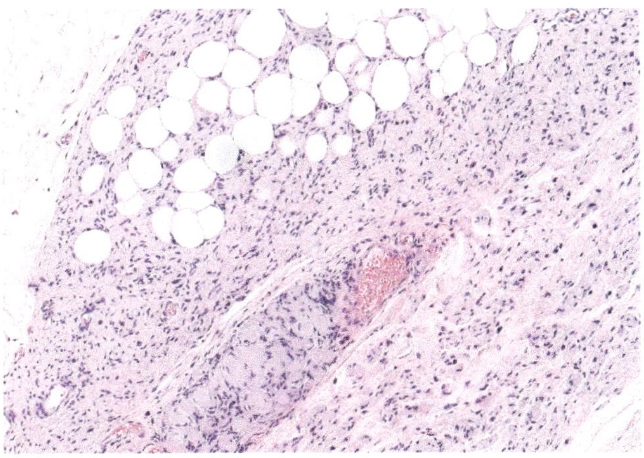

FIG. 14.93

Diffuse neurofibroma with a strikingly infiltrative growth pattern and extensive involvement of the subcutis mimicking dermatofibrosarcoma protuberans.

atypia, loss of neurofibromatous architecture (fascicle formation), hypercellularity, and <3 mitotic figures/10 HPF

4. Low-grade MPNST: ANNUBP and 3 to 9 mitotic figures/10 HPF and no necrosis
5. High-grade MPNST: ANNUBP with 10 or more mitotic figures/10 HPF or 3 to 9 mitotic figures/10 HPF AND necrosis

In keeping with the various components of neurofibroma, S100 and SOX10 are positive in Schwann cells, CD34 is positive in fibroblasts and neurofilament and perineurial markers EMA, GLUT1, or claudin-1 variably highlight entrapped axons and scattered perineurial cells, respectively. Neurofibroma-derived neoplastic Schwann cells harbor both germline and somatic inactivating mutations in the *NF1* gene on 17q11.

Differential Diagnosis

Neurotized nevus can be distinguished by the presence of focal epithelioid melanocytes, nests, or pigment in the superficial dermis; the myxoid or collagenous stromal changes are uncharacteristic. DF differs from neurofibroma by greater cellularity, a more fibrotic stroma, storiform growth pattern, plump histiocytoid cells, and a lack of staining for S100 or SOX10. In contrast to neurofibroma, schwannomas are encapsulated tumors with areas of alternating cellularity and characteristic large hyalinized vessels. Schwannomas are composed principally only of Schwann cells; thus, CD34-positive fibroblasts and lesional axons and perineurial cells are uncharacteristic except the subcapsular area. Solitary circumscribed neuroma is also composed only of Schwann cell population and can show characteristic cracking between cell bundles; myxoid change and collagenous stroma containing fibroblasts are uncharacteristic. Diffuse neurofibroma with diffuse subcutaneous infiltration can look very similar to DFSP and will show positive staining for CD34; however, recognition of Schwann cell component either by morphology or by application of S100 and SOX10 immunostains. Plexiform neurofibromas may need to be distinguished from plexiform schwannomas. Patchy (versus diffuse) S100 immunoreactivity, scattered axons, and a known clinical association with NF1 in plexiform neurofibromas help to separate them from plexiform schwannoma. Hybrid schwannoma/perineurioma will have a biphasic appearance with alternating whorls of perineurial cells and Schwann cells; this lesion is typically rich in collagen (in contrast to the standard schwannoma that contains very thin pericellular collagen that is not conspicuous in routine histologic sections) and show expression of Schwann cell and perineurial markers (GLUT1, EMA, claudin-1) in each of the two cell populations. Hybrid schwannomas perineuriomas often show *VGLL3* and sometimes variant gene fusions.

Prognosis and Treatment

Neurofibromas are benign, and localized and intraneural tumors are typically cured by local excision. Malignant transformation is rare in sporadic cases except for patients with NF1. The histologic criteria for MPNST from a precursor neurofibroma are outlined above.

PERINEURIOMA

Perineuriomas are tumors with differentiation toward the perineural cells of the nerve sheath. They can occur as intraneural, extraneural, and mucosal tumors affecting colonic mucosa. Only the extraneural soft tissue perineurioma is discussed here.

Clinical Findings

Perineuriomas are sporadic soft tissue tumors most commonly presenting in the subcutaneous tissue of the extremities and trunk in adult patients of all genders. Pure dermal and deep soft tissue presentations may occur but are uncommon. Sclerosing perineuriomas have a particular predilection for acral sites. There is no syndromic association.

Histopathologic Features

Soft tissue perineuriomas present as small- to medium-sized (4 cm) circumscribed but unencapsulated firm masses. They are composed of uniform, thin perineurial-like cells with slender, elongated nuclei and faintly eosinophilic cytoplasm with long bipolar processes, which sometimes can only be appreciated with the use of perineurial markers. These cells are arranged in whorls or fascicles in a collagenous stroma (Fig. 14.94A and B). There is characteristically no atypia aside from scattered cells with degenerative ancient change, or mitotic activity. Reticular growth pattern with myxoid stroma may occur. Sclerosing perineurioma is composed of cords of small epithelioid to spindle cells in a corded pattern in a densely collagenous stroma (Fig. 14.95). By IHC, the tumor cells are diffusely positive for perineurial markers EMA, claudin-1, and GLUT1, and positive for CD34 in half of the cases. Schwann cell markers S100 and SOX10 are negative in pure perineurioma. Molecular studies show recurrent deletions of *NF2* on 22q12 deletions and *NF1* on 17q11 deletions.

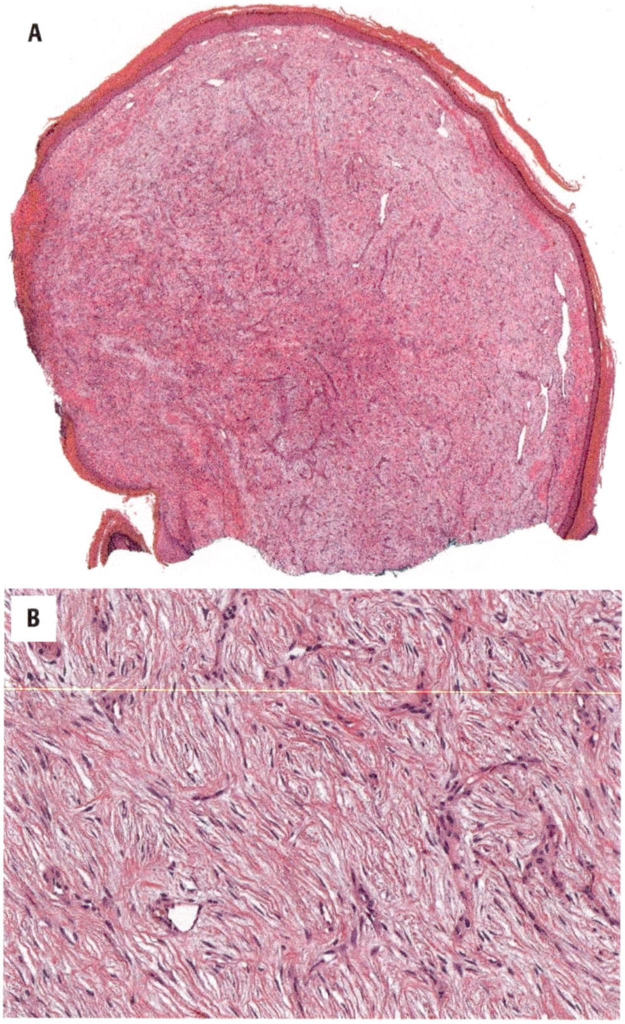

FIG. 14.94

Soft tissue perineurioma. **A,** Uniform, thin, perineurial-like cells arranged in whorls or fascicles in a collagenous stroma. **B,** Perineurial cells show slender, elongated nuclei and faintly eosinophilic cytoplasm with long bipolar processes.

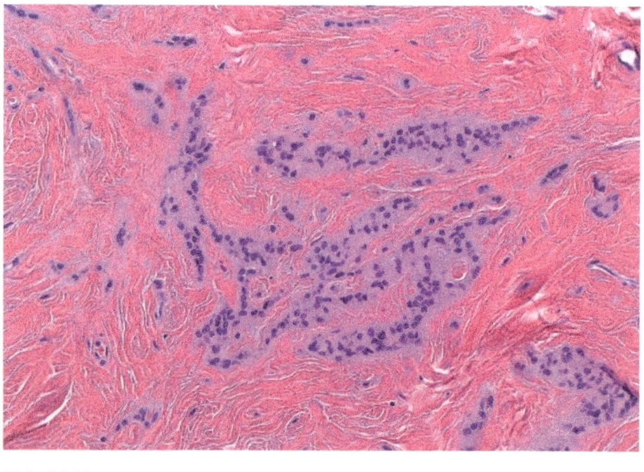

FIG. 14.95

Sclerosing perineurioma is composed of cords of small epithelioid cells in a densely collagenous stroma.

Differential Diagnosis

Localized neurofibromas, schwannomas, and hybrid schwannomas/perineuriomas can be distinguished by a morphologic or immunohistochemical identification of Schwann cell component, which is not present in a pure perineurioma. It should be noted though that all the above tumors will have scattered perineurial cells. DFSP can be distinguished based on the infiltrative rather than circumscribed growth pattern and lack of perineurial marker expression. LGFMS can express EMA; however, in contrast to perineurioma, LGFMS has a more prominent vasculature, especially in the myxoid zones, and may show hyalinized rosettes. The constituent cells are MUC-4–positive fibroblasts with a gene fusion, most frequently *FUS::CREB3L2*.

Prognosis and Treatment

Soft tissue and sclerosing perineuriomas are benign tumors with a very low risk of local recurrence. Exceptionally rare MPNSTs with perineurial differentiation have been described, and those demonstrate overtly malignant features permitting accurate managerial classification. Treatment is simple excision.

HYBRID SCHWANNOMA/PERINEURIOMA

Clinical Findings

The clinical presentation is typically that of a painless subcutaneous mass similar to the conventional benign nerve sheath tumors including schwannomas, soft tissue perineuriomas, and localized neurofibromas.

Histopathologic Features

Hybrid schwannoma/perineurioma is typically a circumscribed, unencapsulated tumor centered on the subcutis, although rare cases may show partially infiltrative growth pattern resembling diffuse neurofibroma or DFSP. The tumor has both features of schwannoma and perineurioma, although whether these tumors truly are of peripheral nerve sheath derivation is under debate. Constituent cells are arranged in a storiform, whorled, or vaguely fascicular growth pattern with an intervening and sometimes distinctly parallel arrangement of typical Schwann cells with wavy hyperchromatic nuclei and perineurial cells with very slender, pale nuclei, and wispy cytoplasm with long bipolar processes (Fig. 14.96A and B). These components are variably admixed within each tumor. Because of the perineurial component, hybrid tumors have a distinctly collagenous background. The nuclear atypia is limited to scattered ancient-type changes, and mitotic activity is low. By IHC, S100 and SOX10 highlight Schwann cells, whereas perineurial markers EMA, claudin-1, and GLUT1 highlight perineurial cells. CD34 is often positive. Molecular studies show that hybrid schwannomas/perineuriomas harbor recurrent gene fusions, most often involving *VGLL3* gene with a variety of partners.

HYBRID SCHWANNOMA/PERINEURIOMA—DISEASE FACT SHEET

Clinical Findings
- Painless subcutaneous mass

Histopathologic Features
- Unencapsulated subcutaneous tumor
- Storiform or fascicular growth pattern in a collagenous background
- An intervening arrangement of Schwann cells with wavy hyperchromatic nuclei and perineurial cells with slender nuclei and wispy cytoplasm with long bipolar processes

IHC/Molecular
- Schwann cells markers S100 and SOX10, frequent CD34
- Perineurial cells highlighted by EMA, claudin-1, and GLUT1
- Recurrent gene fusions involving *VGLL3* gene with a variety of partners

Differential Diagnosis
- Schwannoma
- Perineurioma
- Dermatofibrosarcoma protuberans
- Low-grade fibromyxoid sarcoma

EMA, Epithelial membrane antigen; *GLUT1*, glucose transporter 1; *IHC*, immunohistochemistry.

Differential Diagnosis

The differential diagnosis is essentially the same as for the soft tissue perineurioma described above.

Prognosis and Treatment

Hybrid schwannomas/perineuriomas are benign tumors with a small risk of local recurrence following an incomplete excision.

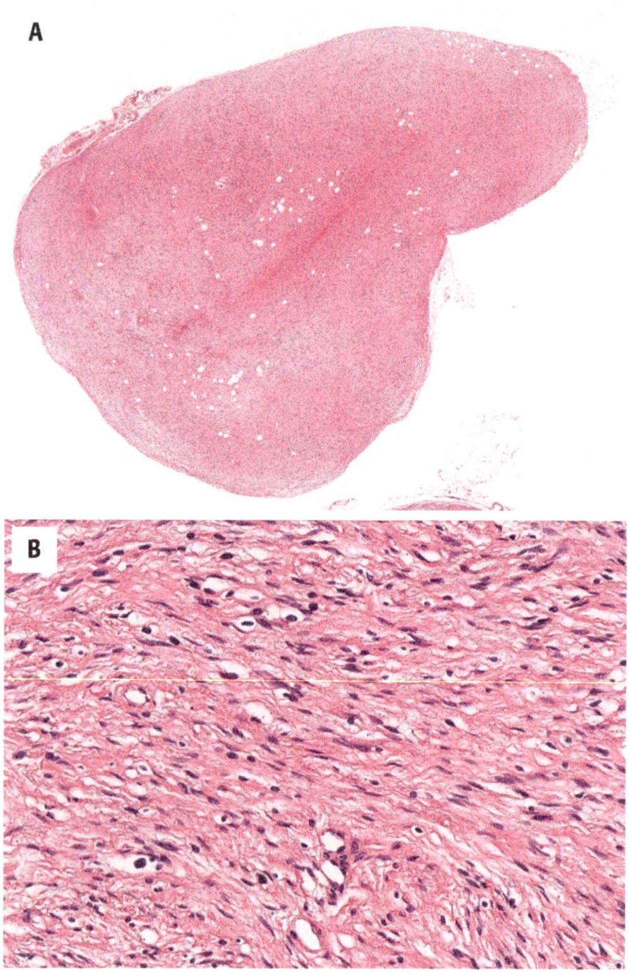

FIG. 14.96

Hybrid schwannoma/perineurioma. **A,** A circumscribed, unencapsulated tumor centered on the subcutis with a monotonous appearance and a collagenous background. **B,** Cells are arranged in a storiform or vaguely fascicular growth pattern with an intervening arrangement of typical Schwann cells with wavy hyperchromatic nuclei and perineurial cells with slender, pale nuclei and wispy cytoplasm with long bipolar processes.

GRANULAR CELL TUMOR

Clinical Findings

Granular cell tumors usually present in middle-aged adults as solitary painless nodules but can be multiple in about 10% of cases. Skin and mucosal involvement is quite common, with tongue being the most frequent site. The vast majority are sporadic, although associations with Noonan's syndrome and NF-1 have been reported.

Histopathologic Features

Granular cell tumors are poorly circumscribed and unencapsulated lesions with a somewhat infiltrative appearance. It is composed of highly characteristic large cells with round to oval nuclei and abundant distinctly granular eosinophilic cytoplasm arranged in sheets, ribbons, and nests that can be separated by fibrous bands. The cells form syncytia with indistinct cytoplasmic borders (Fig. 14.97). The overlying epidermis or squamous epithelium often shows prominent pseudoepitheliomatous hyperplasia, which sometimes may be mistaken for an SCC. Most benign granular cell tumors are small (smaller than 2 cm). Significant cytologic atypia and mitotic figures are usually absent. Malignant examples of granular cell tumor defined by necrosis, spindling, pleomorphism, prominent nucleoli, and mitotic activity >2/10 HPF exist but are exceptionally rare. Granular cell tumors show neuroectodermal differentiation and are immunoreactive for S100, SOX10, CD68, CD163, NKI-C3, and inhibin. Molecular studies show unique among soft tissue tumors loss-of-function mutations in V-ATPase–related genes *ATP6AP1* and *ATP6AP2* genes, which serve as endosomal regulatory proteins.

Differential Diagnosis

Rhabdomyomas can be differentiated by the presence of cross-striations and the expression of desmin and negative S100 and SOX10 immunostains. Hibernoma can be distinguished by the presence of admixed mature and vacuolated adipocytes and by its clinical presentation as a relatively large subcutaneous or deep soft tissue mass. Nonschwannian tumors may have extensive granular cell change, including DF, DFSP, smooth muscle tumors, AFX, and dermal pleomorphic sarcoma, but these can be distinguished chiefly based on the absence of schwannian phenotype by IHC. Cellular neurothekeoma may also be positive for CD68 and NKI-C3; however, these

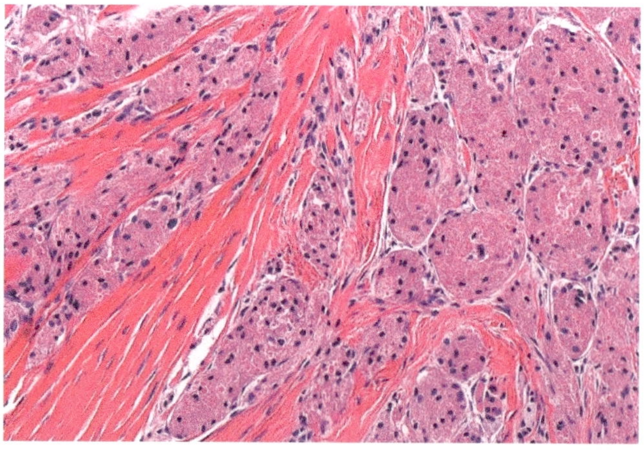

FIG. 14.97

Granular cell tumor is a somewhat infiltrative lesion composed of sheets of large cells with round to oval nuclei and abundant granular eosinophilic cytoplasm. The cells form syncytia with indistinct cytoplasmic borders.

tumors are negative for S100 and SOX10. A rare but important mimic of granular cell tumor, especially in the tongue or orbit in young children, is alveolar soft part sarcoma (ASPS). ASPS is composed of well-formed nests of plump epithelioid to cuboidal tumor cells separated by delicate vascular septa rather than forming syncytia with ill-defined borders as seen in granular cell tumors. The tumor cells are usually positive for TFE3 by IHC in keeping with the pathognomonic *ASPL1::TFE3* fusion and are negative for S100, SOX10, and inhibin. NNGCT, once thought to belong to the conventional granular cell tumor family, is now thought to represent a variant of epithelioid FH. NNGCT (discussed earlier in this text) are more slender and fascicular then the conventional granular cell tumors, lack S100, SOX10, and inhibin expression and instead show *ALK* gene rearrangements and ALK immunoreactivity. Finally, the overlying epithelial hyperplasia can sometimes be mistaken for SCC, especially in superficial biopsies.

Prognosis and Treatment

The great majority of granular cell tumors are benign but can show a small risk of local recurrence following an incomplete excision. Malignant granular cell tumors behave very aggressively with a high rate of systemic metastases.

DERMAL NERVE SHEATH MYXOMA

The term neurothekeoma has been applied to two tumor types: (1) a bona fide nerve sheath tumor, now termed dermal nerve sheath myxoma and (2) a tumor of uncertain differentiation, the cellular neurothekeoma (discussed above).

Clinical Findings

Dermal nerve sheath myxoma typically occurs in the dermis and subcutis of the extremities of middle-aged adults with a slight female predilection.

Histopathologic Features

Dermal nerve sheath myxoma shows a very distinctive multinodular growth pattern subdivided by fibrous septa. Cytologically, the lesions are composed of bland, spindled, stellate, or vacuolated cells with long cytoplasmic processes and abundant, diffuse myxoid stroma (Fig. 14.98A and B). There is no atypia, and mitotic activity is generally absent.

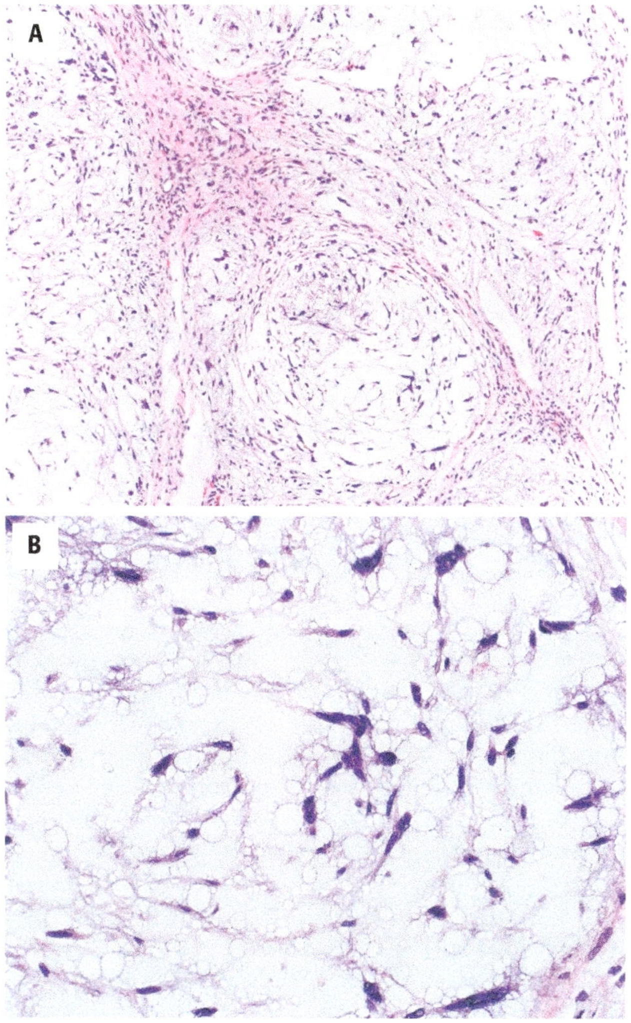

FIG. 14.98
Dermal nerve sheath myxoma. **A,** A distinctive multinodular growth pattern subdivided by fibrous septa. **B,** Cytologically banal, spindled, stellate, or vacuolated Schwann cells with long cytoplasmic processes and abundant, diffuse myxoid stroma.

The lesional cells are strongly, diffusely positive for S100 and SOX10, in keeping with Schwann cell differentiation. Perineurial markers may highlight entrapped perineurial cells in the fibrous capsule.

Differential Diagnosis

Cutaneous myxoma and superficial angiomyxoma lack the distinctive, sharply circumscribed nodules and vacuolated cells of dermal nerve sheath myxoma and lack expression of Schwann cell markers. Dermal nerve sheath myxoma can be distinguished from a low-grade myxofibrosarcoma by its bland cytology, lack of curvilinear vessels, and S100/SOX10 immunoreactivity. Plexiform neurofibromas with myxoid stroma contain wiry collagen bundles and are only patchy positive for S100 protein in keeping with the proportion of Schwann cells within the lesion. Identifying a precursor nerve in the middle of a nodule is a very helpful diagnostic feature of plexiform neurofibroma.

Prognosis and Treatment

Nerve sheath myxomas are benign. Conservative excision is generally performed; however, due to the multinodular growth pattern complete excision is difficult and recurrences are quite common.

ECTOPIC (EXTRACRANIAL) MENINGIOMA

Ectopic meningiomas are meningothelial tumors usually found in the head and neck area. Ectopic meningiomas overlap with meningothelial hamartomas, which represent developmental, nonneoplastic arachnoid rests and are usually found on the scalp along the lines of skeletal closure. Histologically, ectopic meningiomas are very similar to their intracranial counterparts characterized by nodules or whorls of meningothelial cells, sometimes with psammoma bodies (Fig. 14.99). Meningiomas are immunoreactive for EMA. By definition, ectopic meningiomas have no connection with an underlying intracranial tumor.

NASAL GLIAL HETEROTOPIA

Glial heterotopia, also called ectopic glial tissue or glial choristoma, most commonly occurs on the bridge of the nose of newborns and infants. Rarely they may connect to the brain through the cribriform plate and be associated with rhinorrhea. Glial heterotopia is composed of mature glial tissue with astrocytes in an eosinophilic fibrillary background (Fig. 14.100). These lesions are positive for GFAP and neurofilament. Glial heterotopia is considered to represent a congenital cranial malformation and not a neoplasm. These lesions usually do not connect to the cerebrum and are cured by simple excision. If there is evidence of such a connection, these lesions need to be approached with caution to avoid potential complications such as infection.

MALIGNANT NEOPLASMS

MALIGNANT PERIPHERAL NERVE SHEATH TUMOR

Clinical Findings

MPNST is a highly aggressive sarcoma that may occur sporadically or in association with NF-1 or prior radiation therapy. Primary tumors arising in the dermis or subcutis are rare and present as mass lesions in adults that may be associated with pain. In contrast, epithelioid MPNSTs (E-MPNSTs) predominantly occur in the subcutaneous tissue on the extremities of adult patients.

Histopathologic Features

Classic MPNST belongs to the so-called monotonous fascicular tumor category, being composed of sweeping fascicles of hyperchromatic spindled cells that often have wavy nuclear contours and basophilic cytoplasm. Varying cellularity with hypercellular zones alternating with less cellular, myxoid areas, as well as perivascular

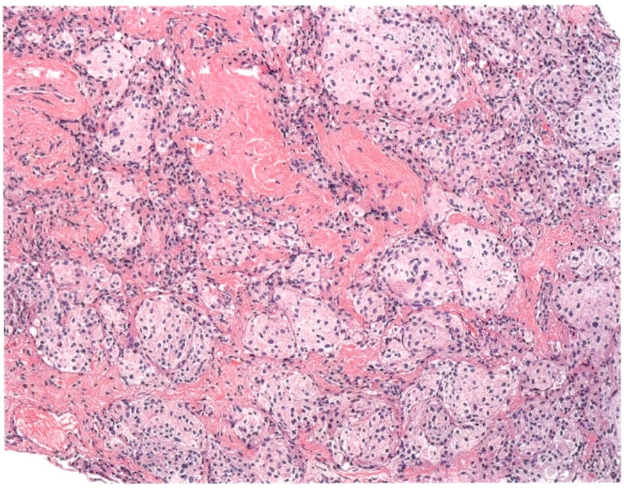

FIG. 14.99

Ectopic showing nodules or whorls of benign meningothelial cells in the dermis and subcutis, sometimes with psammoma bodies. *(Photograph courtesy of Dr. Andrew L. Folpe.)*

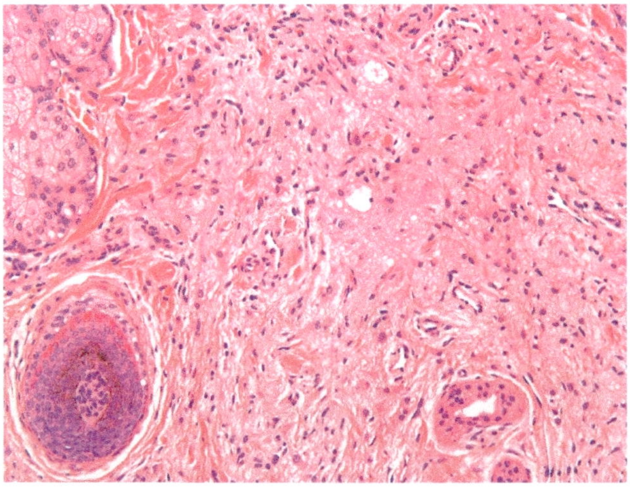

FIG. 14.100

Glial heterotopia is composed of mature glial tissue with benign astrocytes in an eosinophilic fibrillary background.

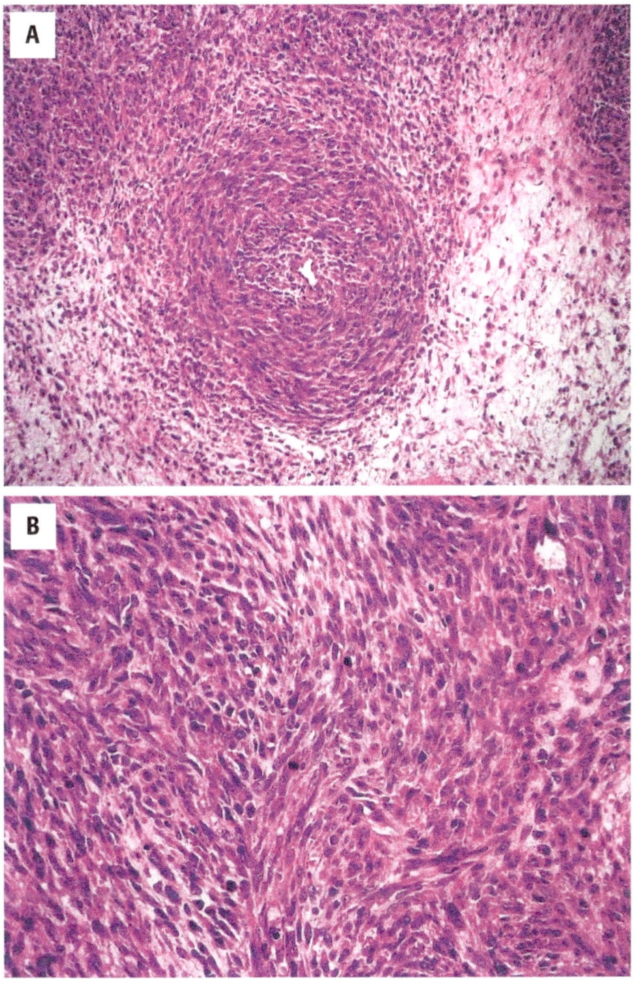

FIG. 14.101

Classic malignant peripheral nerve sheath tumor. **A,** Hypercellular zones alternating with less cellular, myxoid areas; perivascular condensation is common. **B,** Cellular fascicles of overtly atypical, hyperchromatic spindled cells with wavy nuclear contours and basophilic cytoplasm, arranged in a herringbone or sweeping pattern. Mitotic activity is high, and there is often necrosis.

condensation are common (Fig. 14.101A and B). Heterologous differentiation is also common taking the form of gland formation or a heterologous component including rhabdomyoblastic (Triton tumor), osteosarcomatous, chondrosarcomatous, or angiosarcomatous differentiation. Precursor neurofibroma or, with some luck, an intimate association with the originating nerve may be identified—both features can serve as definitive histologic criteria for MPNST. Classic MPNSTs have overt nuclear atypia, brisk mitotic activity, and frequent necrosis making classification as malignancy relatively straightforward. However, low-grade MPNSTs arising from a precursor neurofibroma in the setting of NF-1 can be more challenging to call out as they start as a relatively low-grade tumor, with greater degree of cytoplasmic eosinophilia and low mitotic count. The earliest morphologic clue indicating histologic progression is fascicle formation which contrasts with the loose arrangement of Schwann cells and fibroblasts in the precursor neurofibroma. The diagnosis and grading of MPNSTs in the setting of NF-1 is based on the criteria for malignancy listed in the above section on neurofibroma. By IHC, classic MPNSTs are variably positive for S100, SOX10, and CD34 but usually not to the extent seen in the benign nerve sheath tumors or in spindle cell malignant melanoma, its closest mimic. Most classic MPNSTs show relatively focal or altogether absent staining with S100 and SOX10. Focal cytokeratin expression is not uncommon and can be misleading. Heterologous elements can be highlighted by antibodies directed against the varying elements (e.g., desmin in rhabdomyoblasts).

Advances in molecular genetics showed that most classic MPNSTs (sporadic, NF-1, and radiation treatment-associated) are driven by alterations in the EED or SUZ12 components of the chromatin remodeling polycomb repressive complex 2 (PRC2), with downstream loss of trimethylation of the H3K27 histone leading to upregulation of cellular growth and proliferation. Loss of H3K27 trimethylation (H3K27me3) can be detected by IHC and is of some albeit limited diagnostic utility. Other frequent alterations in MPNST include *NF1* (sporadic or inherited via NF-1 syndrome) and *CDKN2A/B* pathways.

Epithelioid variant of MPNST (E-MPNST) is a pathogenetically distinct malignant nerve sheath tumor composed of atypical epithelioid cells growing in sheets or nests in a myxocollagenous stroma, with round, vesicular nuclei, prominent nucleoli, and abundant eosinophilic or amphophilic cytoplasm (Fig. 14.102). E-MPNST may be regarded as a malignant counterpart to epithelioid schwannoma, with overt nuclear atypia, brisk mitotic activity, atypical mitotic figures, and necrosis. In contrast to the conventional MPNSTs, E-MPNSTs are diffusely, strongly positive for S100 and SOX10. Like epithelioid schwannomas, E-MPNSTs show *SMARCB1*

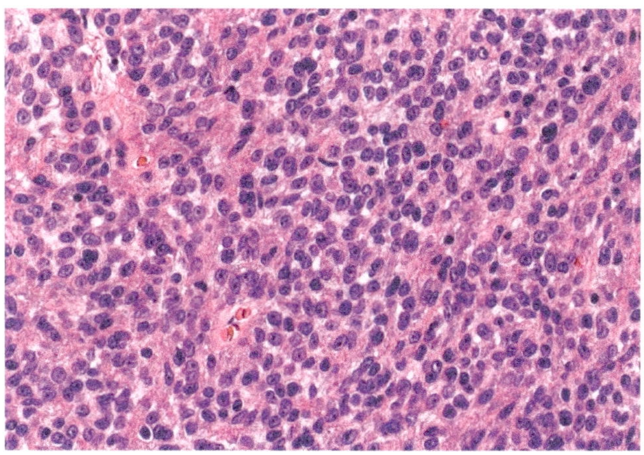

FIG. 14.102

Epithelioid malignant peripheral nerve sheath tumor consists of atypical epithelioid cells with abundant eosinophilic cytoplasm growing in sheets or nests in a myxocollagenous stroma. There is overt nuclear atypia with round, vesicular nuclei, prominent nucleoli, and mitotic activity.

(22q11.23) gene inactivation which results in loss of INI-1 expression by IHC. *SUZ12* and *EED* mutations with the resultant loss of H3K27me3 is not characteristic of E-MPNST.

Differential Diagnosis

In the skin and the subcutis, the most important differential diagnosis of both classic and E-MPNST is with a nodular conventional and spindle cell (often neurotropic) melanoma. This distinction is further complicated by the phenotypic plasticity of melanoma to a point that an MPNST-like variant of melanoma essentially recapitulates the features of classic MPNST including alterations in *NF1* and CDKN2A/B genes. Melanoma tends to be a dermal-based tumor arising in sun-damaged skin of the head and neck in elderly patients. MPNST tends to be a deep soft tissue–based tumor nodule associated with nerve trunks. Identification of a precursor nerve or a neurofibroma or a junctional component or melanoma in situ is the most reliable histologic feature to separate the two. Other features favoring melanoma include (1) tumor center located in the dermis, (2) the presence of lymphoid aggregates, (3) strong and diffuse staining for S100 and SOX10 proteins as classic MPNSTs express these markers only weakly and focally, and (4) presence of molecular aberrations (UV signature mutations, driver mutations) typical of melanoma. Of note, up to a third of malignant melanomas may show loss of H3K27me3. The distinction from the epithelioid MPNSTs could be even more problematic as these tumors tend to show diffuse expression of SOX10 and S100. Epithelioid MPNSTs more often show myxoid stroma, lack *BRAF* alterations, and instead show loss of SMARCN1/INI-1 expression.

Classic MPNST should be distinguished from other monotonous fascicular sarcomas, in particular monophasic spindle cell SS, fibrosarcomatous DFSP, and fibrosarcoma-like neoplasms with RTK fusions. Conventional high-grade MPNST demonstrates a greater degree of cytologic atypia, necrosis, and mitotic activity than seen in the above mimics and is also more likely to have myxoid stroma and perivascular condensation of the tumor cells. However, individual examples of these tumors can be indistinguishable from one another on morphologic grounds unless a precursor neurofibroma is identified. SS is best eliminated based on the pathognomonic *SS18::SSX1*, *SS18::SSX2*, or *SS18::SSX4* gene fusions or IHC for SS18-SSX fusion-specific antibodies. It should be noted that S100 protein is expressed in approximately one-third of SSs. Fibrosarcomatous DFSP often contains a conventional storiform DFSP component, is diffusely positive for CD34, and shows retained H3K27me3 expression; challenging cases may be resolved by testing for *PDGFRB* gene alterations. MPNST and various RTK-driven fibrosarcomas (such as those with *NTRK1/2/3*, *RET*, *BRAF*, *ROS*, *ALK* fusions) often coexpress S100 and CD34; however, SOX10 is uniformly negative in these tumors but is frequently expressed in MPNST. H3K27me3 staining by IHC, which is often lost in sporadic cases of MPNST, would be expected to be retained in these tumors; rearrangements in the above-mentioned kinase-encoding genes would strongly favor kinase fusion-based fibrosarcoma.

The distinction of incipient low-grade MPNST from neurofibroma and other benign nerve sheath tumors can be accomplished based on the criteria outlined in the previous section of this chapter. Of note, in contrast to the conventional high-grade MPNST, loss of H3K27me3 occurs in less than half of low-grade MPNSTs.

Prognosis and Treatment

Classic high-grade MPNST is an aggressive malignancy with a substantial risk of progression and systemic metastasis, especially when arising in NF-1 patients. Deep location, high-grade, and high tumor stage are adverse prognostic parameters, as is loss of H3K27me3, although all MPNSTs, including those in superficial locations, should be treated by a multidisciplinary team. Prognosis of epithelioid MPNSTs is better with a relatively low risk of local recurrence and systemic metastasis, irrespective of the tumor size, and many such tumors can be cured by complete local excision.

SOFT TISSUE NEOPLASMS WITH MELANOCYTIC DIFFERENTIATION

PERIVASCULAR EPITHELIOID CELL TUMOR

Clinical Findings

Cutaneous PEComas account for roughly 9% of all PEComas. They usually appear on the extremities or trunk as firm, tan, or pink-colored small (<2 cm) cutaneous nodules or plaques and are clinically reminiscent of FH. The age span is broad with a peak in middle-aged adults.

Histopathologic Features

Cutaneous PEComas are composed of nests, sheets, or cords of epithelioid, polygonal, or less often, spindled cells with abundant clear or granular eosinophilic cytoplasm surrounded by delicate capillary vessels. The cells have round, vesicular nuclei with small but very

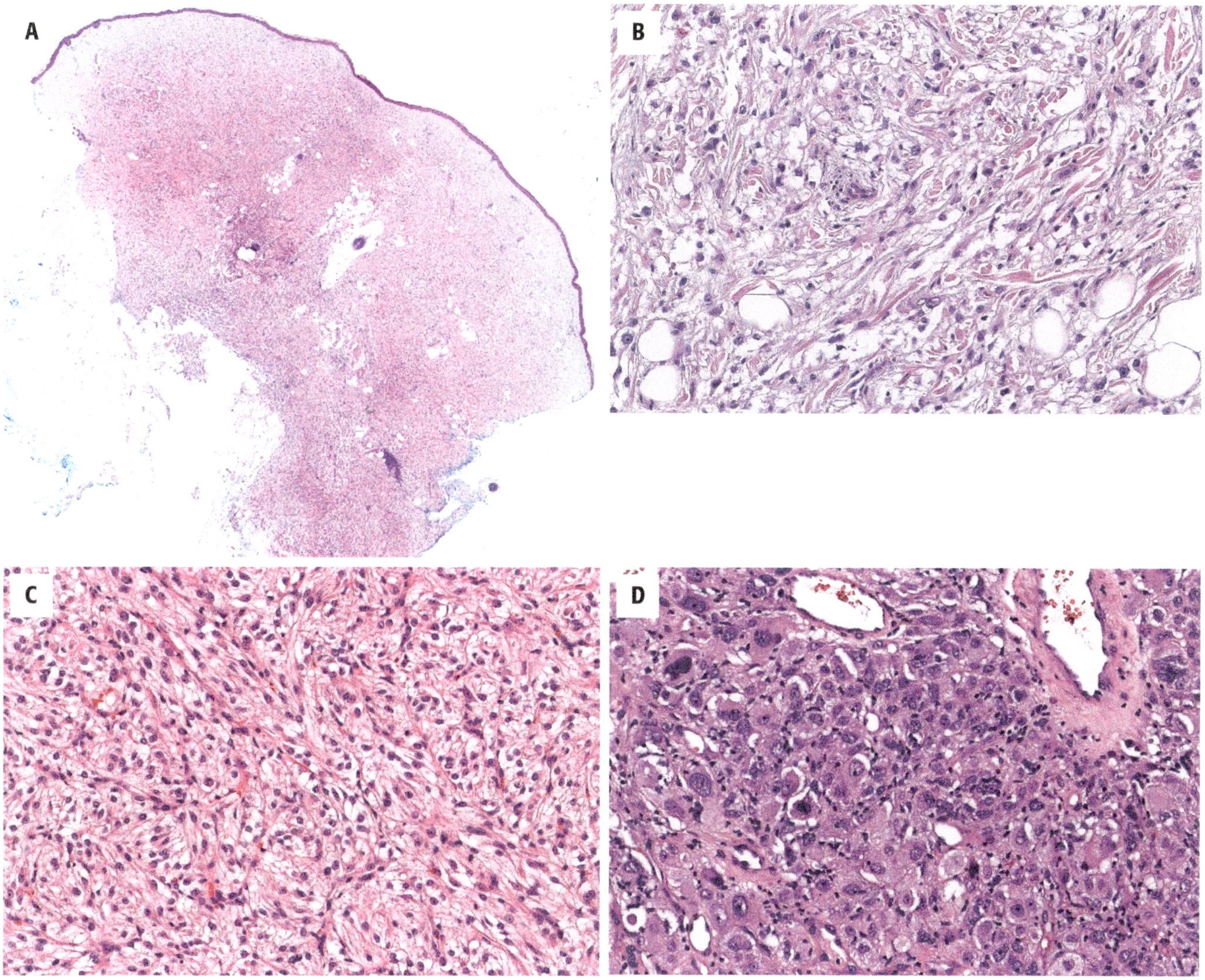

FIG. 14.103

Cutaneous perivascular epithelioid cell tumor (PEComa). **A,** A symmetric dermal lesion with a somewhat infiltrative edge resembling fibrous histiocytoma. **B** and **C**, Nests and sheets of epithelioid and spindled cells with abundant clear or granular eosinophilic cytoplasm, round nuclei, and small nucleoli separated by delicate fibrous septa. **D,** Cutaneous malignant PEComa showing high nuclear grade and mitotic activity.

distinct nucleoli (Fig. 14.103A–C). Perivascular growth pattern, with the tumor cells abutting the overlying endothelium, is characteristic, although this feature is easier to appreciate in cases with a more fibrous background. Cutaneous PEComas typically have a somewhat infiltrative edge and often show dermal collagen trapping at the periphery, reminiscent of benign FH. A mild degree of cellular pleomorphism is typical of PEComas at all sites, and multinucleated wreath-like giant cells with peripherally located nuclei can be seen. The mitotic count is typically very low (<1/10 HPF).

Cutaneous malignant PEComas are rare and recapitulate features seen in their deep soft tissue and visceral counterparts (Fig. 14.103D). The proposed histological criteria for malignancy in deep soft tissue PEComas include size >5 cm, an infiltrative growth pattern, high nuclear grade, mitotic activity >1/50 HPF, necrosis, and vascular invasion. PEComas lacking any of these features are classified as benign, those with 2 or more features as malignant, and those with only nuclear pleomorphism/giant cells (so-called symplastic PEComas) or size >5 cm as having uncertain malignant potential. It remains unclear whether this classification scheme is equally applicable to cutaneous PEComas due to the scarcity of published cases.

By definition, PEComas demonstrate variable coexpression of melanocytic markers (HMB45, MITF, NKI/C3 (CD63), Melan-A/MART1, PNL2, and S100) and markers of smooth muscle differentiation (desmin, SMA, caldesmon, and calponin) and also express cathepsin K. HMB45, MITF, and cathepsin K are the most sensitive melanocytic markers in cutaneous PEComa, with HMB45 showing the typical scattered strong immunoreactivity (Fig. 14.104). PEComas with *TFE3* alterations show diffuse HMB45 and TFE3 expression, but MITF and Melan-A expression can be focal or negative. S100 protein expression is seen focally in a

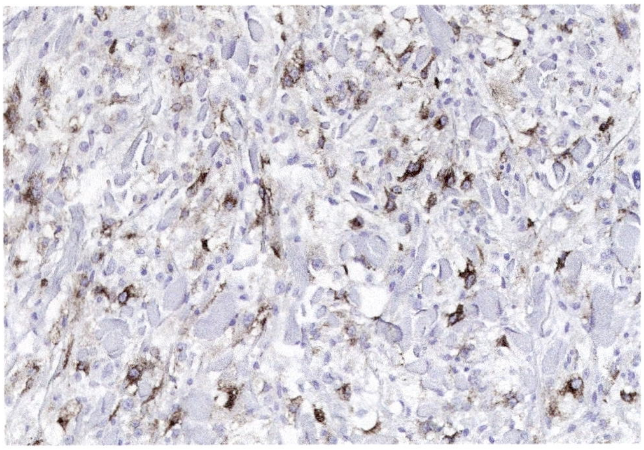

FIG. 14.104

Typical scattered strong pattern of HMB45 immunoreactivity in cutaneous perivascular epithelioid cell tumor.

minority of cases and SOX10 is universally negative. PEComas with epithelioid morphology, including the TFE3-rearranged cases, tend to show a more diffuse expression of HMB45, whereas expression of muscle markers can be very focal or negative. PEComas with a spindled component are more likely to show muscle marker expression. The most helpful smooth muscle markers in cutaneous PEComas are desmin and SMA, while calponin and caldesmon are seen with low frequency (10% to 15%). Cytokeratins and EMA are negative in PEComas.

Most sporadic and TSC-associated visceral and soft tissue PEComas are associated with *TSC1* (9q34) or *TSC2* (16p13.3) alterations, the most common being loss of heterozygosity in the *TSC2* locus. This results in a downstream upregulation of the mTOR pathway. A smaller subset of PEComas harbors oncogenic fusions of the *TFE3* (Xp11.2) gene, a member of MiT family, with a variety of partners, with TFE3 or indirect MITF upregulation driving the melanocytic phenotype. *TFE3*-rearranged and *TSC1/2* mutations in PEComas appear to be mutually exclusive.

Primary cutaneous PEComas very rarely contain *TSC1/2* alterations and do not have *TFE3* fusions, and their mechanisms continue to be explored. Of note in this context is the recent characterization of a cutaneous clear-cell melanocytic neoplasm with *MITF* fusions to *ACTB* or *ACTG1* members of *ACTIN* family (*ACTIN::MITF* fusions) resulting in direct MITF activation. Like cutaneous PEComas, these tumors also present as the extremity-based cutaneous nodules and have indolent behavior. These tumors also share significant morphologic overlap with cutaneous PEComas as they consist of nests of neoplastic cells with ample clear cytoplasm, distinct cell borders, and round nuclei with distinct nucleoli, entrapping dermal collagen bundles (Fig. 14.105A–C). At the same time, clear-cell cutaneous melanocytic neoplasms with *ACTIN::MITF* fusion lack *TFE3* or *TSC1/2* alterations and show strong, diffuse expression of S100 in half of the

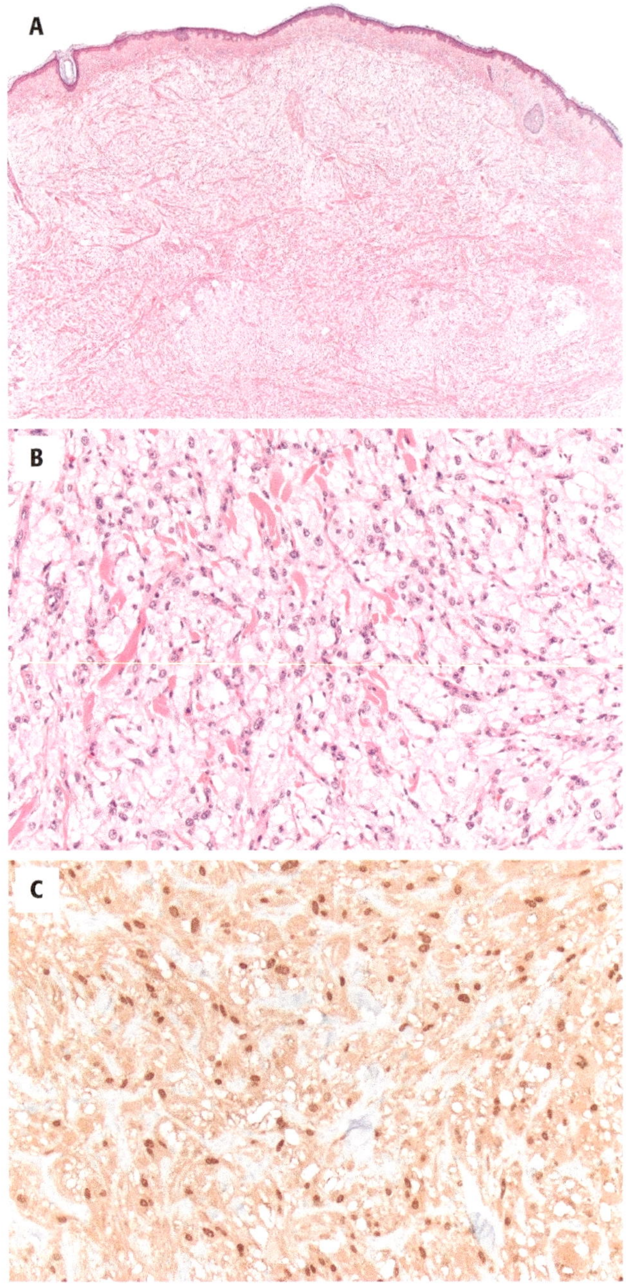

FIG. 14.105

Cutaneous clear-cell melanocytic neoplasm with *ACTIN::MITF* fusion. **A,** Extremity-based polypoid cutaneous nodule. **B,** Nests of neoplastic cells with ample clear cytoplasm, distinct cell borders, and round nuclei with small nucleoli, entrapping dermal collagen bundles. **C,** Strong nuclear immunolabeling with microphthalmia transcription factor antibody.

cases, and essentially no smooth muscle marker expression, indicating that they are likely distinct from cutaneous PEComas.

Differential Diagnosis

The differential diagnosis of cutaneous PEComa and the clear-cell cutaneous melanocytic neoplasms with

ACTIN::MITF fusion is essentially the same and includes tumors with clear or granular cytoplasm. Unlike PEComas, granular cell tumors demonstrate a more syncytial arrangement of constituent cells, the absence of a prominent vasculature, and a lack of nucleoli. The tumor cells are uniformly strongly positive for S100 protein and SOX10, express inhibin, and are negative for HMB45, Melan-A, desmin, and SMA. Myoepitheliomas with clear-cell morphology have a somewhat overlapping immunophenotype because the markers of myoepithelial differentiation S100, SMA, and calponin can also be expressed in cutaneous PEComas. However, myoepithelial tumors can be readily distinguished from PEComas by coexpression of cytokeratins and EMA and lack of HMB45 or MITF immunoreactivity. DF/benign FH can look strikingly similar, especially at scanning magnification, because of the intermingling arrangement of the tumor cells with dermal collagen but can be readily distinguished by lack of expression of melanocytic markers. Malignant melanoma with clear or balloon cell features is an epidermis-based tumor with a radial growth phase, intraepidermal pagetoid spread, robust expression of SOX10 and S100, and frequent presence of BRAFV600E immunoreactivity. Metastatic carcinomas with clear-cell features, primarily, clear-cell renal cell carcinoma of the kidney, should be readily distinguished by application of cytokeratins, immunostains, and negative melanocytic work up.

Treatment and Prognosis

Most cutaneous PEComas as well as cutaneous clear-cell melanocytic neoplasms with *ACTIN::MITF* fusion reported to date behave in a benign fashion, even if rare cases met the histologic criteria for malignancy. Reports of lymph node or systemic metastases are exceptionally rare, and large studies detailing the behavior of histologically malignant cutaneous PEComa are currently lacking. Complete excision is the treatment of choice for benign PEComas. Malignant visceral and soft tissue PEComas are best treated by a multidisciplinary sarcoma team, with a combination of surgery, radiation, and chemotherapy, including possible use of mTOR pathway inhibitors, although applicability of these modalities to rare malignant cutaneous PEComas remains underreported.

CLEAR-CELL SARCOMA OF SOFT TISSUE

Clinical Findings

Clear-cell sarcoma most often occurs in the second to fourth decade of life with a predilection for the ankle and foot, as a slowly growing, deep soft tissue mass with an attachment to tendons, aponeuroses, or fasciae. Occasionally, it may arise in the dermis. Cutaneous CCS also tends to occur in the distal extremities and has rarely been reported on the trunk, proximal limbs, or head and neck region. Average size is <2 cm.

Histopathologic Features

CCS is composed of nests and fascicles of uniform spindle to fusiform cells separated by fibrous septa. The overlying dermis is usually uninvolved but in cutaneous CCS, which is centered on the dermis, the epidermis may be ulcerated. Nests of tumor cells at the dermal-epidermal junction and an intraepidermal pagetoid spread may occur. Despite the name, the cytoplasm is palely eosinophilic and finely granular, resembling that of a cellular blue nevus or spindle cell melanoma. True optically clear cytoplasm is very rare. The cells are overtly atypical with large vesicular nuclei and prominent nucleoli but without significant pleomorphism, very similar to those seen in spindle cell malignant melanoma (Fig. 14.106A and B). The mitotic rate is highly variable, and the stroma is usually sclerotic. Multinucleated wreath-like tumor giant cells when present are a very helpful diagnostic feature (Fig. 14.107). Melanin pigment is seen in a minority of cases. Rare morphologic variations have been described such as rhabdoid features, bizarre pleomorphism, alveolar architecture due to cellular dyshesion, and a seminoma-like pattern. Clear-cell sarcomas diffusely express S100 protein and, in most cases, coexpress the melanocytic markers Melan-A, HMB45, SOX10, MITF, and NKI/C3. Synaptophysin, CD57, EMA, CD34, and CD117 (c-KIT) expressions have been observed in a minority of cases but cytokeratins, desmin, and SMA are usually negative. The key genetic event in clear-cell sarcoma is a *EWSR1* gene fusion with members of the CREB family transcription factors, most commonly *EWSR1::ATF1* fusion, and *EWSR1::CREB1* or *EWSR1::CREM* fusions in the minority of cases. The downstream effect of these fusions in clear-cell sarcoma is constitutive cAMP-independent transcription of MITF that drives the melanocytic phenotype. The fusion can be detected by FISH, RT-PCR, or NGS. Additional alterations such as *TP53* mutations may occur.

Differential Diagnosis

It is essential to distinguish CCS from other neoplasms with melanocytic phenotype. Cutaneous or metastatic spindle cell melanoma can be virtually identical to CCS. The monotonous appearance of the tumor nests (in contrast to the more heterogeneous appearance with more pleomorphism in spindle cell melanomas) and

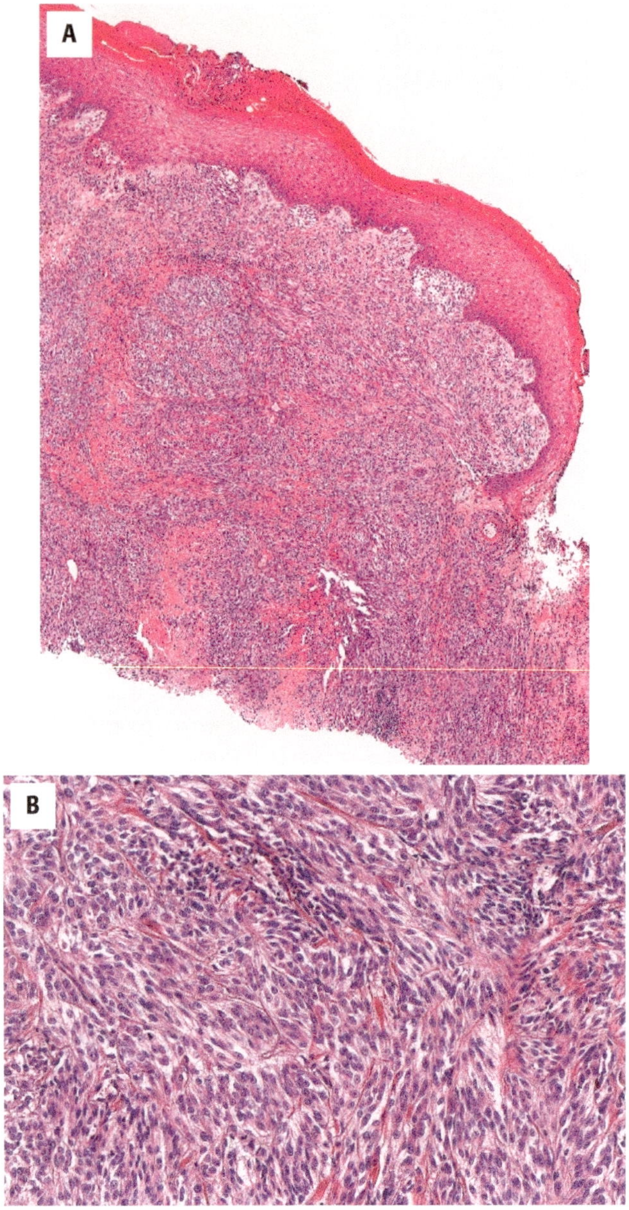

FIG. 14.106

Clear-cell sarcoma. **A,** Ulcerated dermal and subcutaneous nodule abutting the epidermis. **B,** Nests and fascicles of uniform spindle to fusiform cells separated by fibrous septa, with palely eosinophilic cytoplasm and monotonous yet atypical nuclei with prominent nucleoli.

wreath-like giant cells favor CCS. A junctional or lentiginous component is more typical of melanoma but tumor nests at the dermal-epidermal junction, intraepidermal involvement, and pagetoid spread have all been observed in a primary cutaneous CCS. Melanomas are negative for *EWSR1* gene rearrangements, while *BRAF*, *KIT*, or *NRAS* mutations that typify most cutaneous melanomas do not occur in clear-cell sarcoma.

An emerging novel cutaneous melanocytic tumor with *CRTC1::TRIM11* fusion (CMTCT) is an entity that can closely resemble CCS, cellular blue nevus, and metastatic spindle cell melanoma. A comprehensive discussion of this lesion is beyond the scope of this

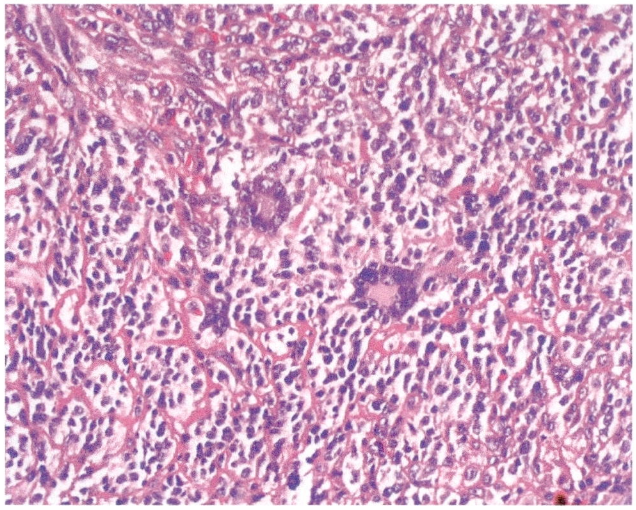

FIG. 14.107

Clear-cell sarcoma. Multinucleated wreath-like tumor giant cells are uncommon but very helpful diagnostic clue.

chapter, but it also often presents an extremity-based dermal nodule and consists of nests or short fascicles of monomorphic, epithelioid to spindle cells with amphophilic cytoplasm and prominent nucleoli (Fig 14.108). CMTCT is also positive for SOX10 and S100, with variable expression of HMB45 and Melan-A. While the presence of multinucleated wreath-like giant cells and a more overt nuclear atypia and mitotic activity argue in favor of CCS, the completely objective distinction between these two very phenotypically similar neoplasms might not be achieved without molecular analysis for the *EWSR* or *CRTC1::TRIM11* fusions. Awareness of this emerging entity is important due to its relatively indolent behavior compared with both melanoma and clear-cell sarcoma.

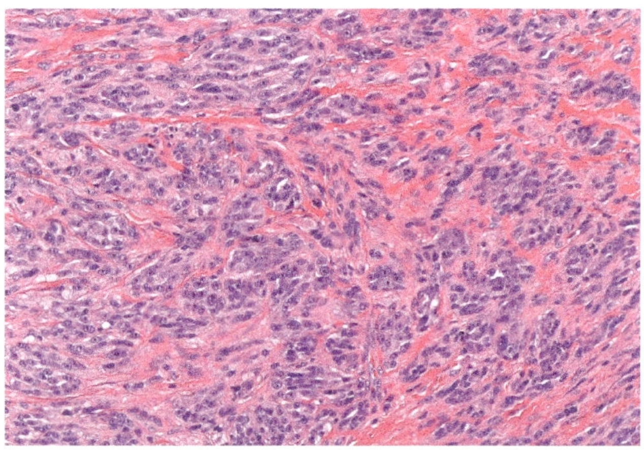

FIG. 14.108

Cutaneous melanocytic tumor with *CRTC1::TRIM11* fusion is an extremity-based dermal nodule that consists of nests or short fascicles of monomorphic, epithelioid to spindled melanocytic cells with amphophilic cytoplasm, and prominent nucleoli. The appearance overlaps with clear-cell sarcoma and cutaneous melanoma. *(Photographs courtesy of Drs. David Papke and John Hanna.)*

Amelanotic cellular blue nevus can resemble clear-cell sarcoma because of the increased cellularity, nested arrangement of uniform spindle cells surrounded by fibrous septa, scattered multinucleated giant cells, and multinodular involvement of dermis and subcutis. Identification of a second population of slender dendritic melanocytes, like those seen in common blue nevi, helps to distinguish cellular blue nevus from CCS. Most cellular blue nevi also lack the cytologic atypia and mitotic activity of CCS. In addition, blue nevi, including malignant blue nevi, lack *EWSR1* rearrangements.

Cutaneous PEComa and cutaneous clear-cell melanocytic neoplasms with *ACTIN::MITF* fusion (discussed above) can be distinguished based on the presence of the delicate capillary vasculature seen in association with the nests of tumor cells, more clear or granular cytoplasm, and the characteristic interdigitating growth pattern through the dermal collagen which resembles collagen trapping of DF. Cutaneous PEComas coexpress markers of melanocytic and smooth muscle differentiation (SMA, desmin, and caldesmon), the latter of which is consistently negative in CCS and lacks *EWSR1* gene rearrangements. Cutaneous clear-cell melanocytic neoplasms with *ACTIN::MITF* fusion can be positive for S100 but lack *EWSR1* gene rearrangements.

Prognosis and Treatment

CCS has a protracted clinical course but ultimately behaves aggressively, with approximately 40% risk of local recurrence a high rate of lymph node and systemic metastases, most often to the lungs and bones. The 5-year overall survival is 40% to 60%. Adverse prognostic features include large size, necrosis, local recurrence, and, in some reports, lymph node metastasis. The behavior of cutaneous CCS appears to be similar, although the number of reported cases with available follow-up is small.

MISCELLANEOUS SARCOMAS OF UNCERTAIN DIFFERENTIATION

SYNOVIAL SARCOMA

Clinical Findings

SS usually presents as an extremity-based asymptomatic or tender soft tissue mass in adolescents or young adults (median age 39 years), but SS spans a broad age range and may occur at virtually any anatomic site. The tumors range in size from minute to over 10 cm in greatest dimension.

Histopathologic Features

The signature histologic characteristic of SS is partial epithelial differentiation.

SSs are broadly divided into three main subtypes: monophasic (pure spindle cell), biphasic (spindle cell and epithelial component), and poorly differentiated (small round cell morphology). The monophasic SS consists of monotonous fascicles of basophilic spindle cells with uniform elongated vesicular nuclei with evenly distributed chromatin, scant cytoplasm, and indistinct cell borders arranged in a so-called herringbone pattern (Fig. 14.109A). The stroma contains delicate wiry collagen fibers or little intervening collagen, but can be markedly fibrous, hyalinized, or myxoid. Cystic changes, areas of hemorrhage, prominent branching staghorn-like vessels and mast cells are common. Biphasic SS shows an admixture of a monotonous spindle cells and epithelial cells forming glandular and papillary structures lined by cuboidal or columnar cells with similar nuclear features (Fig. 14.109B). Calcifications are common (approximately 30%, Fig. 14.109C). Pure monophasic epithelial tumors are very rare (<1%). Squamous metaplasia, ossification, rhabdoid features, granular cell change, and primary intraneural location may occur. Poorly differentiated SS consists of sheets of small cells with rounded atypical nuclei, variable nucleoli, scant cytoplasm, frequent mitotic figures, and areas of necrosis resembling an undifferentiated round cell sarcoma (Fig. 14.110). Both monophasic and biphasic SSs express variable combinations of epithelial markers including cytokeratins and EMA. CD34 is reliably negative. CD99 is seen in approximately 70% of SS. A third of cases may express S100. Genetically, SS is defined by a reciprocal t(X;18)(p11.2;q11.2), with pathognomonic *SS18::SSX1*, *SS18::SSX2*, or, rarely, *SS18::SSX4* or cryptic gene fusions, with downstream effects on SWI/SNF chromatin remodeling complexes. These alterations can be detected by FISH, RT-PCR, or NGS. There is no prognostic correlation with monophasic versus biphasic histology or the type of fusion transcript. Novel fusion-specific antibodies, an SS18-SSX fusion-specific antibody (E9X9V), and an SSX-specific antibody (E5A2C, directed at the C terminus of SSX) have demonstrated excellent sensitivity and specificity for SS.

Differential Diagnosis

The main differential diagnostic considerations are monotonous malignant spindle cell tumors arising from the overlying skin (i.e., spindle cell melanoma or fibrosarcomatous DFSP), conventional MPNST, and SFT.

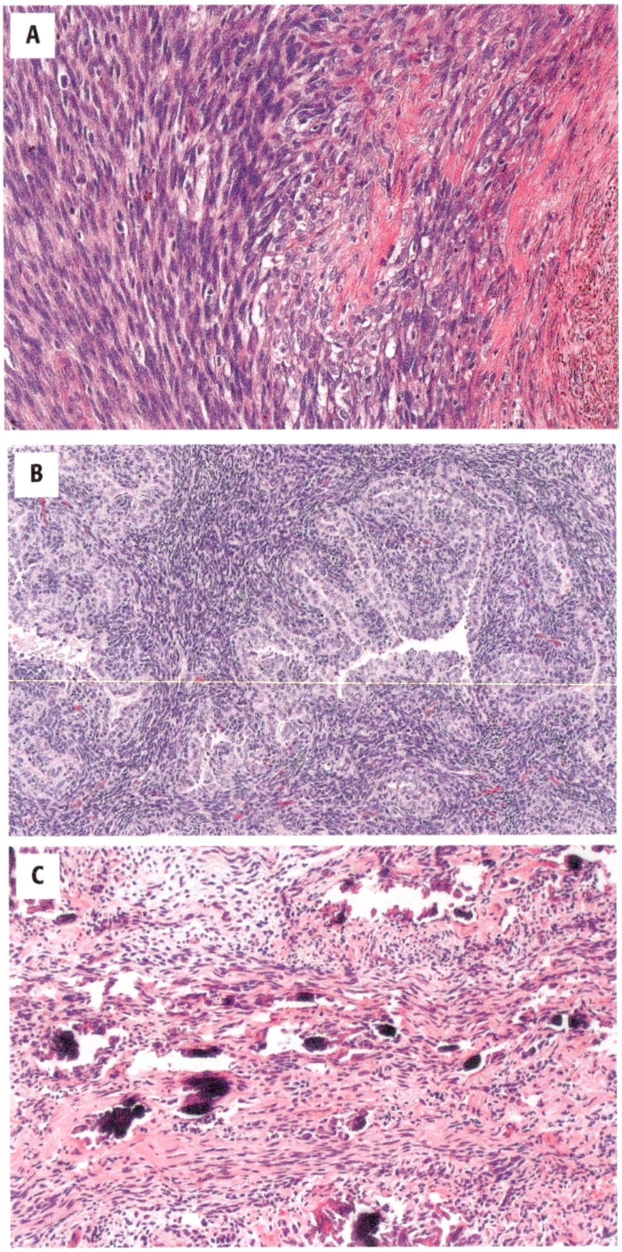

FIG. 14.109

A, Monophasic spindle cell synovial sarcoma composed of fascicles of basophilic spindle cells arranged in a herringbone pattern. The cells have elongated vesicular nuclei, evenly distributed chromatin, and scant cytoplasm. Delicate intercellular collagen fibers are present. **B,** Biphasic synovial sarcoma showing monotonous spindle cells and cuboidal or columnar epithelioid cells forming complex glandular and papillary structures. **C,** Lesional calcifications are common.

Spindle cell melanoma affects an older patient population and morphologically may display a focally nested growth pattern and a junctional component. S100 is of limited value in this context, although strong, diffuse expression would favor spindle cell melanoma. SOX10 is a very helpful marker because it is positive in most melanomas and is usually negative in SS. The most helpful histologic clue to separate fibrosarcomatous DFSP from SS is identification of a conventional DFSP component. CD34 can serve as a quick screening tool as

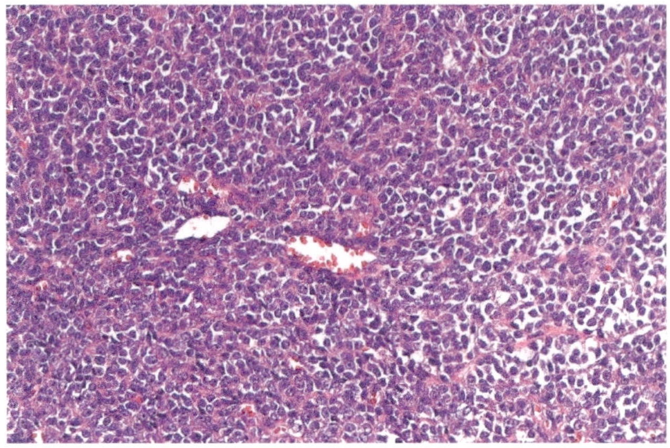

FIG. 14.110

Poorly differentiated synovial sarcoma with sheets of undifferentiated small round cells with frequent mitotic figures.

it is consistently negative in SS. SS with prominent collagenous stroma and staghorn vessels can be mistaken for SFT, but the latter can be readily distinguished by STAT6 expression. MPNSTs and SS may be virtually identical histologically, and both tumors can express S100. Unlike SS, MPNSTs are more often positive for SOX10 and the majority of cases show loss of H3K27me3 by IHC. FISH, RT-PCR, or IHC using the above-mentioned fusion-specific SS19-SSX and SSX-CT antibodies for SS gene fusions are extremely helpful, as these tests are negative in the histologic mimics of SS.

Prognosis and Treatment

SSs behave aggressively despite a protracted clinical course, with late local recurrences and systemic metastases, most commonly to the lungs, lymph nodes, and bones. An overall 5-year survival is approximately 60%. Large tumor size (>5 cm), visceral location, and poorly differentiated tumor morphology are associated with aggressive course, while the most favorable outcomes are seen in small fibrous and extensively calcified SSs of hands and feet, as they are amenable to complete excision. Surgical excision is the treatment of choice for localized disease, while a multimodal approach, including radiation therapy, conventional chemotherapy, tyrosine kinase inhibitors (imatinib, pazopanib), or immunotherapy targeting NY-ESO-1 and other biomarkers, can be used for locally advanced and metastatic disease.

EPITHELIOID SARCOMA

Clinical Findings

There are two types of ES: the conventional, or distal-type, and the proximal-type, which has a predilection for proximal or axial locations, rhabdoid morphology and aggressive behavior. Both types are characterized by mutations in the *SMARCB1/hSNF5/INI1* gene on chromosome 22q11.

Distal-type ES presents over a wide age range, with a peak incidence in the second to third decades, and manifests as a firm, slowly growing subcutaneous nodule, plaque, or nonhealing ulcer in the distal extremities, especially the fingers, hands, and forearms. Distal-type ES tends to grow along nerve trunks, fascial planes, and tendons, accounting for the very high rate of local recurrence (80%–90%). Proximal-type ES typically occurs as a deep-seated mass in a relatively older population, usually in the fourth decade and above. Common sites include the proximal limbs and limb girdles, as well as the pelvis, perineum, head and neck, and mediastinum.

EPITHELIOID SARCOMA—DISEASE FACT SHEET

Clinical findings

- Distal type: nodules or ulcers on distal extremities of young adults
- Proximal type: pelvic region or proximal extremities in older adults

Histopathologic Features

- Distal type
  - Eosinophilic epithelioid cells surrounding a zone of central geographic necrosis or fibrosis
  - Mild atypia and mitotic activity
  - Perineural and vascular invasion
- Proximal type
  - Large epithelioid cells with round eccentric nuclei and prominent nucleoli
  - Eosinophilic cytoplasm with a perinuclear rhabdoid inclusion
  - Overt nuclear atypia, mitotic activity and necrosis

IHC/Molecular

- Positive for cytokeratins, EMA with negative cytokeratin 5/6, and CD34 (60%)
- *SMARCB1/INI-1* inactivation with loss of nuclear INI-1 expression by IHC

Differential diagnosis

- Distal type
  - Granulomatous inflammation
  - Pseudomyogenic hemangioendothelioma
  - Cutaneous adnexal carcinoma or squamous cell carcinoma
- Proximal type
  - Malignant melanoma
  - Epithelioid angiosarcoma
  - Epithelioid malignant peripheral nerve sheath tumor
  - Myoepithelial carcinoma

EMA, Epithelial membrane antigen; *IHC*, immunohistochemistry.

Histopathologic Features

Distal-type ES is an infiltrative dermal or subcutaneous nodular process with ill-defined margins. There is often a zone of central geographic necrosis or fibrosis with a palisaded arrangement of the tumor cells resembling granuloma annulare or an infectious granuloma (Fig. 14.111A). Cytologically, distal-type ES is composed of relatively uniform epithelioid or spindled cells arranged in nests or cords. The cells have round to oval nuclei, vesicular chromatin, inconspicuous nucleoli, and abundant eosinophilic cytoplasm resembling histiocytes (Fig. 14.111B). Nuclear atypia ranges from mild to severe but is deceptively bland in most cases, and mitotic activity is usually low (<5/10 HPF). Perineural and vascular invasion, when present, are helpful in establishing the diagnosis. Cellular spindling and variable amounts of chronic inflammation and fibrosis are often present. Hemorrhage, necrosis, angiomatoid change, calcifications, and osseous or cartilaginous metaplasia may rarely occur.

Proximal-type ES is a large, subcutaneous, or deep-seated mass composed of sheets of large, overtly atypical and mitotically active epithelioid cells with round nuclei, prominent nucleoli, and dense abundant eosinophilic cytoplasm which may show a perinuclear

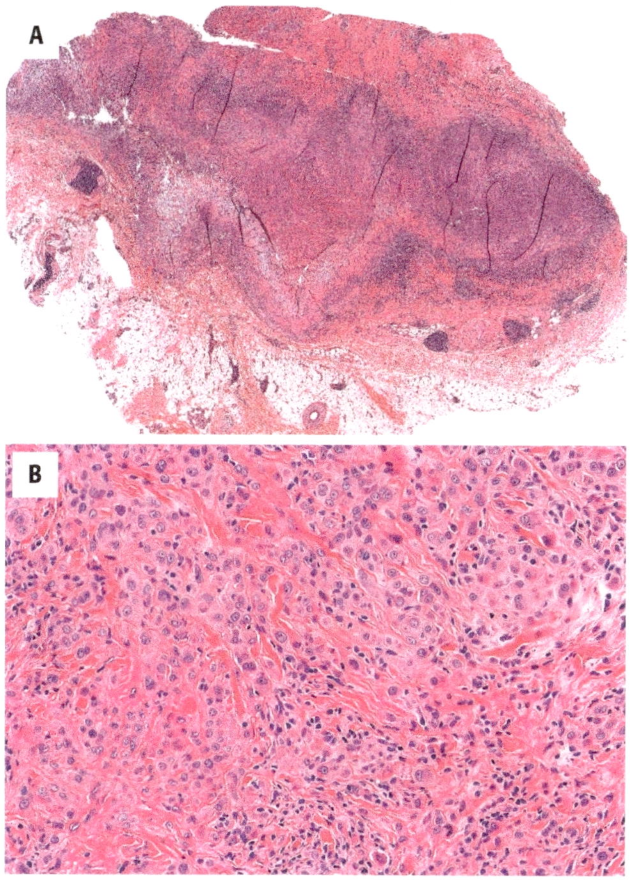

FIG. 14.111

Distal-type epithelioid sarcoma. **A,** Dermal or subcutaneous nodule with a zone of central geographic necrosis or fibrosis. **B,** Sheets of mildly atypical uniform epithelioid cells with round to oval nuclei, small nucleoli, and abundant eosinophilic cytoplasm resembling histiocytes. Mitotic figures are scant.

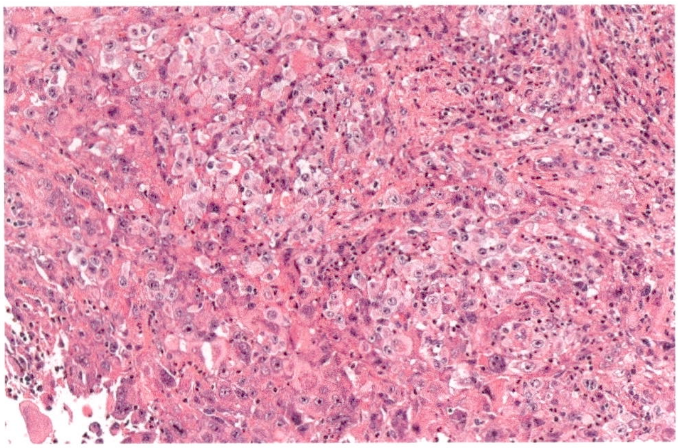

FIG. 14.112

Proximal-type epithelioid sarcoma. Sheets of large, overtly atypical and mitotically active epithelioid cells with round nuclei, prominent nucleoli, and dense eosinophilic cytoplasm.

accentuation in the form of a hyaline eosinophilic rhabdoid inclusion (Fig. 14.112). Ultrastructurally, these inclusions are composed of whorls of cytokeratin intermediate filaments. Most distal and proximal-type ES express cytokeratins and EMA, but immunoreactivity for cytokeratin 5/6 is usually absent. Approximately 60% of all cases are positive for CD34. SMA, S100, and clone-dependent ERG expression may be seen. Factor XIIIa may occasionally be positive in spindled ES, which may lead to diagnostic confusion with FHs. Both types of ES are characterized by inactivation of *SMARCB1/hSNF5/INI-1 gene* on chromosome 22q11, which encodes a subunit of the SWI/SNF chromatin remodeling complex. This results in loss of nuclear expression of SMARCB1 (INI1) in greater than 90% of all cases. Other subunits of SWI/SNF complex are rarely affected.

Differential Diagnosis

Granulomatous inflammatory processes (e.g., granuloma annulare, rheumatoid nodule, and necrobiosis lipoidica), infectious granulomas, and benign fibrohistiocytic tumors are the most significant mimics. Nuclear atypia, which is usually at least focally present in distal-type ES, is the most helpful histologic clue. IHC readily resolves challenging cases as the histiocytes in the non-neoplastic granulomatous proliferations and FHs express CD68 and CD163, lack cytokeratin and EMA immunoreactivity, and retain nuclear INI1 expression. A high index of suspicion for distal-type ES should be maintained in any distal extremity lesion from a young patient, especially if the clinical history suggests a long-standing, recurrent, or otherwise unusual process.

Cutaneous adnexal carcinoma or SCC, which have substantial immunohistochemical overlap with distal-type ES, usually lack a zone of geographic necrosis with peripheral palisading. By IHC, adnexal and SCCs are negative for CD34 and retain nuclear expression of INI1. SCCs typically express CK5/6, unlike distal-type ES.

Pseudomyogenic hemangioendothelioma (HE, also known as epithelioid sarcoma-like hemangioendothelioma) is an epithelioid vascular neoplasm of intermediate malignancy that also may arise in the distal extremities of young adults and present as multifocal disease. Pseudomyogenic HE is composed of sheets or fascicles of plump, cytokeratin-positive epithelioid or spindled cells with abundant eosinophilic cytoplasm, mild nuclear atypia, and low mitotic activity, all of which may be seen in distal-type ES. It differs from ES by its prominent fascicular myoid component and lack of a nodular growth pattern and geographic necrosis with peripheral palisading. Both tumors express cytokeratins, but unlike ES, pseudomyogenic HE is also positive for vascular markers ERG and CD31 (50% to 80%), is negative for CD34 and EMA, has retained INI1 expression, and shows nuclear expression of FOSB, a product of pathognomonic SERPINE1/FOSB rearrangement.

Proximal-type ES is readily recognizable as a malignancy, but it can closely mimic other malignant cutaneous tumors with epithelioid morphology. Amelanotic melanoma can be distinguished by melanocytic markers, lack of cytokeratin and CD34 expression, and retained INI1 expression. Epithelioid angiosarcoma often has a solid growth pattern like proximal-type ES and may express cytokeratins and CD34. However, epithelioid angiosarcoma consistently expresses additional vascular markers (ERG and CD31) and retains nuclear INI1 expression. Epithelioid MPNST frequently shows loss of INI1 expression, but this tumor often has prominent myxoid stroma, features not usually seen in proximal-type ES, and are positive for SOX10 and S100 and negative for cytokeratins. Myoepithelial carcinoma is a more morphologically heterogenous tumor that typically co-expresses cytokeratins and markers of myoepithelial differentiation such as p63, SMA, GFAP, and/or S100 and is negative for CD34. Approximately 80% of cases show rearrangement of *EWSR1*. A potential pitfall is that myoepithelial carcinoma shows loss of INI1 expression in approximately 50% of cases.

Prognosis and Treatment

Distal ES shows a protracted clinical course, with late metastases in up to 50% of patients, most commonly involving the lymph nodes and lung and less often, bones and skin (especially the scalp). The 5-year overall survival is 65% to 78% and up to 92% in children. Proximal-type ES behaves aggressively with rapid progression and early systemic metastases in up to 75% of patients. The treatment of choice for both distal and proximal-type ES is radical excision; adjuvant radiotherapy and chemotherapy have been used with some success. Although sometimes performed, the benefit of lymph node dissection or sentinel lymph node biopsy in epithelioid sarcoma remains uncertain.

SELECT UNDIFFERENTIATED ROUND CELL SARCOMAS

Advances in molecular profiling led to the expansion and refined classification of undifferentiated round cell sarcomas—a change that is gradually translating into differences in medical management. In addition to the classic Ewing sarcoma, pathogenetically distinct small round cell tumors of the soft tissue and bone involving other gene fusions have been well characterized and include *CIC*-rearranged sarcoma, sarcoma with *BCOR* genetic alterations, and undifferentiated round cell sarcomas with *EWSR1*-non-ETS gene fusions (such as *EWSR1::NFATC2* and *EWSR1::PATZ1*). Ewing sarcoma and *CIC*-rearranged sarcoma manifest in the skin with a reasonable frequency and are briefly discussed in this section. For an in-depth review of these and other undifferentiated round cell sarcomas, the reader is referred to the dedicated soft tissue pathology sources.

CUTANEOUS EWING SARCOMA

Cutaneous Ewing sarcoma, like its bone and deep soft tissue and visceral counterparts, has a broad age distribution with a peak in young adults (second to fourth decade) and a wide anatomical distribution. Awareness is important as these tumors are readily mistaken for more common cutaneous neoplasms. Histologically, classical Ewing sarcoma is characterized by sheets of uniform, oval to round tumor cells with a high nuclear-to-cytoplasmic ratio and even, finely stippled chromatin. Nuclear pleomorphism, hyperchromasia, and prominent nucleoli are uncharacteristic (Fig. 14.113A and B). Neural differentiation in the form of Homer-Wright rosettes may occur. The tumor cells show a crisp, membranous staining pattern for CD99, but the latter should not be used as a sole diagnostic marker due to its very poor specificity. NKX2-2 has greater specificity than CD99 for Ewing sarcoma. An important pitfall is that Ewing sarcoma, including cutaneous examples, can express common markers used in cutaneous pathology including cytokeratins, neuroendocrine markers, S100, p40, SOX10 as well as FLi1 and ERG that correspond to the fusions involving the respective genes but lack specificity. Classic Ewing sarcoma is characterized by gene fusions between members of the ETS family of genes and members of the FET (*FUS*, *EWSR1*, *TAF15*) family of genes. The most common of these is the *EWSR1-FLI1* fusion, followed by the *EWSR1-ERG* fusion.

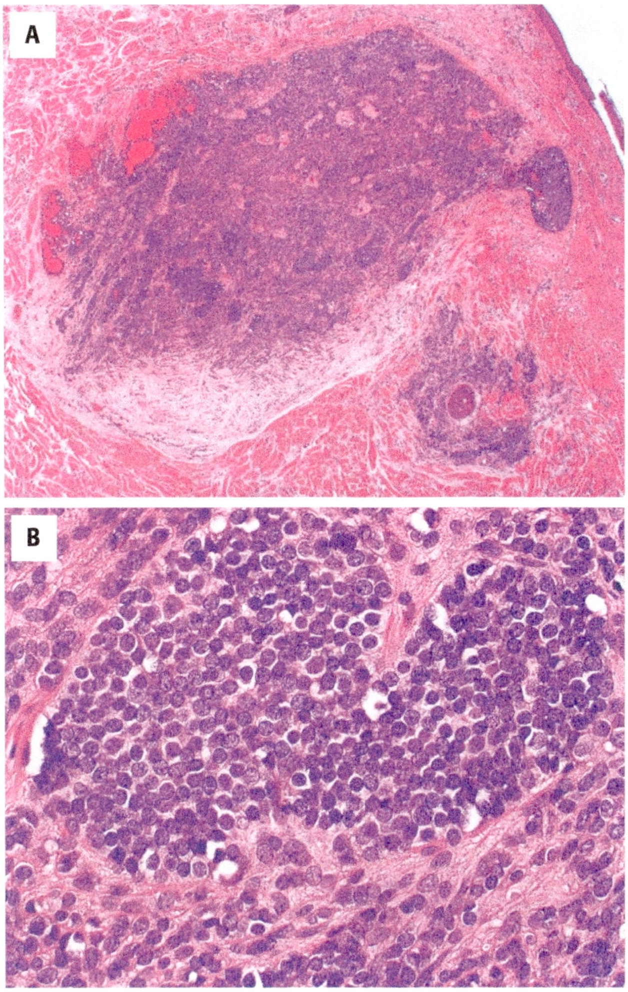

FIG. 14.113
Cutaneous Ewing sarcoma. **A,** A basophilic nodule centered on the dermis. **B,** Sheets of uniform, oval to round tumor cells with even, finely stippled chromatin.

Molecular ancillary testing for the identification of one of these fusions by FISH, RT-PCR, or an NGS fusion panel is required for a definitive diagnosis.

CIC-REARRANGED SARCOMA

Formerly regarded as a variant of Ewing sarcoma, undifferentiated round cell sarcomas with *CIC* gene rearrangements represent a distinct clinicopathologic entity with a significantly more aggressive clinical course than Ewing sarcoma. These tumors arise predominantly in the deep soft tissue and viscera; superficial cases involving dermis and subcutis comprise less than 10% of all cases. Histopathologically, these tumors are composed of undifferentiated round cells with pale eosinophilic or clear cytoplasm growing in solid sheets or nodules separated by fibrous bands. Large areas of geographic necrosis are typical, and myxoid stroma is common. In contrast to the relatively tame, monotonous appearance

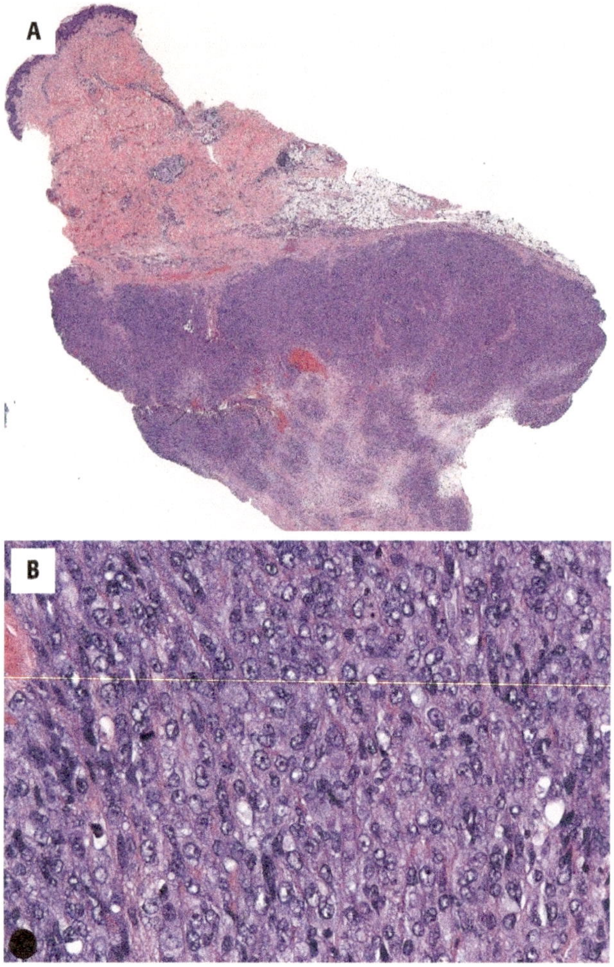

FIG. 14.114

CIC-rearranged sarcoma. **A,** A subcutaneous tumor composed of solid sheets of basophilic cells. **B,** Overtly atypical tumor cells with pale eosinophilic or clear cytoplasm, vesicular chromatin, some degree of pleomorphism, prominent nucleoli, and brisk mitotic activity.

of the classic Ewing sarcoma, the cells in *CIC*-rearranged sarcoma have overtly atypical nuclei with vesicular chromatin, some degree of pleomorphism, prominent nucleoli, and brisk mitotic activity (Fig. 14.114A and B). *CIC*-rearranged sarcomas express CD99 in a focal, heterogenous, and often cytoplasmic pattern and are positive for WT1 while NKX2.2 is negative. The downstream effect of *CIC::DUX4* fusion is transcriptional upregulation of *ETV1/4/5* genes; accordingly, ETV4 antibody shows superior specificity to other immunostains for the diagnosis of *CIC*-rearranged sarcoma with the caveat that it may be negative with non-*DUX4* partners. DUX4 antibody is also positive in cases with *CIC::DUX4* fusion. In general, a combination of nuclear WT1 and ETV4 expression, especially in conjunction with a heterogenous pattern of CD99 expression, provides excellent discriminatory value in suggesting the diagnosis of *CIC*-rearranged sarcoma ahead of confirmatory molecular or FISH testing. *CIC::DUX4* gene fusion is present in 95% of *CIC*-rearranged tumors as a result of either t(4;19) or t(10;19) translocations; rare partners include *FOXO4*, *LEUTX*, *NUTM1*, and *NUTM2A*. The sensitivity of FISH testing for *CIC* gene rearrangements is approximately 75% to 80%.

Differential Diagnosis

CIC-rearranged sarcoma should be considered any time the diagnosis of cutaneous Ewing sarcoma is suspected and can be favored over Ewing sarcoma based on the following features: (1) overt nuclear atypia with geographic necrosis and brisk mitotic activity; (2) patchy, weak or heterogenous pattern of CD99 expression; (3) expression of WT-1, ETV4 and DUX4, and negative NKX2.2 (when these antibodies are available); and (4) a confirmation of *CIC* gene fusions by either NGS or FISH as opposed to the ETS-FET fusions (*EWSR1::FLI1* or *EWSR1::ERG*) seen in Ewing sarcoma. Both sarcomas need to be distinguished from a broad range of morphologically similar cutaneous tumors, including Merkel cell carcinoma, lymphoblastic lymphoma, poorly differentiated SS, malignant melanoma, alveolar rhabdomyosarcoma, and malignant glomus tumor. The helpful features of some of these tumors are presented in Table 14.2 although it is important to emphasize that these features as well as expression of cytokeratins, S100, SOX10, EMA, and CD99 can be seen in many cutaneous malignancies, including undifferentiated sarcomas, ultimately requiring molecular or FISH testing for diagnostic confirmation.

Prognosis and Treatment

When treated by a multidisciplinary team, superficial Ewing sarcoma tends to show highly favorable outcomes, with 2% to 3% rate of systemic metastasis and overall survival >90%. In contrast, superficial *CIC*-rearranged sarcomas behave just as aggressively as their deep-seated counterparts, with local recurrence and systemic metastases in over 60% of patients and less than 40% overall survival rate, which is significantly less than both superficial and deep-seated Ewing sarcoma. Both tumors should be treated by a multimodality therapy including a wide local excision.

CUTANEOUS VASCULAR TUMORS

BENIGN VASCULAR NEOPLASMS: HEMANGIOMAS

Benign vascular lesions in the skin can be divided into hemangiomas and vascular malformations. Hemangiomas are typically acquired clonal vascular neoplasms.

TABLE 14.2

Differential Diagnosis of Select Cutaneous Round Cell Sarcomas

	Ewing Sarcoma	CIC-Rearranged Sarcoma	Poorly Differentiated Synovial Sarcoma	Alveolar Rhabdomyosarcoma	Precursor Lymphoblastic Leukemia	Merkel Cell Carcinoma	Malignant Glomus Tumor
Peak age	2nd–4th decade	3rd–4th decade	3rd–4th decade	1st–2nd decade	Broad and subtype-specific; most common in children	7th–8th decade	2nd–4th decade
Anatomic distribution	Metadiaphysis of bones, soft tissues of extremities, trunk	Soft tissues of the trunk, pelvis, extremities	Periarticular soft tissue of extremities but can be any anatomic site	Soft tissues of extremities, head and neck, pelvis/perineum	No site-specific predilection; concurrent involvement of bone, lymph nodes	Head and neck, extremities, concurrent lymph node metastases	Proximal limbs, visceral sites; distal cutaneous involvement is rare
Cell shape	Round	Round, plasmacytoid, rhabdoid	Spindled to round or ovoid	Round; a second population of large rhabdomyoblasts with eosinophilic cytoplasm	Round	Round	Round, spindled or pleomorphic
Distinctive architectural features	Monotonous sheets; Homer-Wright rosettes	Nodules separated by fibrous bands; myxoid or hyaline stroma, geographic necrosis	Delicate pericellular collagen; HPC-like vasculature, calcifications with the spindle cell precursor component	Sheets or nests separated by delicate septa with characteristic central dyshesion	Monotonous sheets with significant tissue infiltration	Monotonous sheets with significant tissue infiltration	Circumscribed mass; a precursor low-grade glomus tumor can be identified; HPC-like vasculature
Nuclear features	Monotonous with uniform chromatin	Vesicular with prominent nucleolus	Monotonous with variable nucleoli	Vesicular chromatin, prominent nucleoli	Finely dispersed chromatin	Finely dispersed uniform chromatin	Variably coarse or open with prominent nucleoli
Mitotic activity	Low	Brisk	Variable	Brisk	Variable	Variable	Brisk
IHC	Diffuse, membranous CD99, NKX2.2, fusion-dependent ERG and FLI1, variable and focal cytokeratin	ETV4, WT1, patchy and heterogenous CD99 expression; variable and focal cytokeratin	Cytokeratin, EMA, *SS18* fusion-specific antibodies, frequent CD99 (pitfall), S100 (30%)	Diffuse desmin, myogenin, MyoD1 expression; variable CD99 (pitfall); variable and focal cytokeratin	Diffuse, membranous CD99 (pitfall), TdT, CD34, precursor B and T-cell lymphoblastic markers	Diffuse cytokeratin staining; dot-like pattern of CK20 expression, Merkel cell polyoma virus (80%), variable CD99 and TdT (pitfall)	Patchy SMA, collagen type IV
Molecular findings	ETS-FET family fusions, most common *EWSR1::FLI1* or *EWSR1::ERG*	*CIC* fusion with *DUX4* (most common) or *FOXO4*, *LEUTX*, *NUTM1* and *NUTM2A*	*SS18::SSX1*, *SS18::SSX2* or *SS18::SSX4* fusions	*PAX3::FOXO1* or *PAX7::FOXO1* fusions	Broad spectrum of subtype-specific fusions	Merkel cell polyoma virus or UV damage signature with *TP53* and *Rb1* mutations	*CARMN::NOTCH* fusions, *PDGFRB* gene alterations, BRAFV600E mutations (subset), ATRX loss or CDKN2A deletions (subset)

Malformations are thought to be caused by mosaic mutations that occur during embryologic development of the vasculature and are present at birth, although clinical manifestations of a malformation may occur years later. The discussion of vascular anomalies is beyond the scope of this chapter.

Clinical Findings

Hemangiomas typically present as a single or multiple red, tan, or purple stains, macules, or nodules in the skin of children or adults. In contrast to the malformations that may require a multidisciplinary approach for diagnosis and clinical care, most hemangiomas are diagnosed clinically and/or histopathologically and cured by simple excision.

Histopathologic Features

Features shared by most hemangiomas include overall circumscription, well-formed and well-spaced vascular channels line by a single layer of bland endothelial cells and diffuse investment by pericytes (which can be highlighted by SMA immunostain). Exception to this are lesions with lymphatic phenotype, which often show a more diffuse or ill-defined growth pattern and often lack pericytes; the lymphatic phenotype can be appreciated using lymphatic markers PROX-1 and D2-40. The terminology used below reflects the 2018 International Society for the Study of Vascular Anomalies (ISSVA) classification.

HEMANGIOMAS WITH GNAQ/GNA11 MUTATIONS

CHERRY ANGIOMA OR *CAMPBELL DE MORGAN* SPOT

Clinical Findings

Cherry angiomas present as asymptomatic slightly raised erythematous papules on the extremities, trunk, or head and neck of adult patients and can be numerous.

Histopathologic Features

Cherry angiomas are vaguely polypoid and consist of thin-walled, dilated capillaries in the papillary dermis lined by bland endothelial cells without multilayering or mitotic activity. Intravascular organizing thrombi and stromal hyalinization may be present but in contrast to pyogenic granuloma, stromal inflammation is uncharacteristic. Cherry angiomas lack lymphatic marker expression, and have a thin, attenuated pericyte layer. Capillary and venulocapillary malformations may appear very similar in superficial biopsies but are distinguished based on their clinical presentation. Cherry angiomas were thought to represent telangiectasia in the past, but now are established as benign vascular neoplasms with recurrent *GNA14/GNAQ/GNA11* mutations.

BENIGN HEMANGIOMAS WITH *GNAQ/GNA11/GNAQ14* MUTATIONS—DISEASE FACT SHEET

Cherry Angioma

- Bright red asymptomatic papules on the limbs, trunk or head and neck of adults
- Thin dilated capillaries in the papillary dermis lined by bland endothelial cells
- Attenuated pericytes, stromal hyalinization

Congenital Nonprogressive Hemangioma

- Fully formed at birth
- Rapid involution (RICH), partial involution (PICH) or persistent growth without involution (NICH)
- Dermis, subcutis, and viscera but spare deep skeletal muscle
- Capillary lobules separated by fibrous stroma and stellate interlobular vessels
- Large feeding and draining vessels
- Mitotically quiescent small, slightly hyperchromatic "hobnailed" endothelial cells
- Secondary features: fibromyxoid stroma, hemosiderin, extramedullary hematopoiesis
- Negative for GLUT1 and lymphatic markers D2-40 and PROX-1

Anastomosing Hemangioma

- Deep axial and visceral sites, uncommon in superficial locations
- Complex, anastomosing capillary-sized vessels percolating through the adipose tissue
- Mitotically quiescent small, slightly hyperchromatic "hobnailed" endothelial cells
- Eosinophilic hyaline globules, thrombosis, extramedullary hematopoiesis
- Negative for GLUT1 and lymphatic markers D2-40 and PROX-1

GLUT1, Glucose transporter 1.

CONGENITAL NONPROGRESSIVE HEMANGIOMA

Clinical Findings

Congenital nonprogressive hemangiomas are fully formed at birth. Subsequently, they may either rapidly involute, usually within the first 6 months of life (rapidly involuting congenital hemangioma [RICH]), persist without any involution (noninvoluting congenital hemangioma [NICH]) or partially involute (PICH). These lesions occur in the dermis, subcutis, and viscera but spare deep skeletal muscle. There is no gender predilection. By imaging, these are also high-flow lesions without arteriovenous shunting.

Histopathologic Features

Congenital nonprogressive hemangiomas are composed of capillary lobules containing stellate interlobular vessels and separated by fibrous stroma. The lobules coalesce around a fibrous core containing prominent large interlobular feeding and draining vessels that can resemble a vascular malformation (Fig. 14.115A). At high power, the capillaries have a distinctive appearance with open lumina lined by small, rounded, slightly hyperchromatic "hobnailed" nuclei without significant atypia or mitotic activity (Fig. 14.115B). The stroma is fibrous or myxoid and, in contrast to the infantile hemangioma, the adnexal structures are typically destroyed. Calcifications, thrombi, hemosiderin deposits, and extramedullary hematopoiesis are common. Regressed lesions leave a scar. Congenital nonprogressive hemangiomas lack lymphatic phenotype and are negative for GLUT1 expression. They contain recurrent *GNAQ* and *GNA11* mutations.

Differential Diagnosis

The differential diagnosis is primarily with three other lesions that occur in the pediatric population: pyogenic granuloma, infantile hemangioma, and a superficial manifestation of an AVM. Pyogenic granuloma looks very similar as it is also composed of well-defined lobules of small capillaries in a fibrous stroma. Clinical presentation is very helpful in this distinction as pyogenic granuloma is an acquired and often eruptive vascular proliferation. Stellate intralobular and large interlobular draining vessels are not characteristic of pyogenic granuloma. Infantile hemangioma lacks the intralobular stellate vessels of congenital nonprogressive hemangioma and shows preservation of adnexal structures and no stromal scarring. The capillaries of infantile hemangioma are quite different showing plump, oval, mitotically active endothelial cells during the proliferative phase and flattened endothelium with thick, hyalinized basement membranes containing apoptotic dust during the involutional phase. The clinical history and immunophenotype (GLUT1+) of infantile hemangioma are very helpful features for making this distinction. AVM will contain large feeding and draining vessels, and both lesions will show a high-flow pattern by Doppler imaging. However, arteriovenous shunting is not characteristic of congenital nonprogressive hemangioma. Stromal fibrosis, myxoid change, and reactive vascular proliferation are common in AVMs, but these vessels do not form well-defined capillary lobules and lack the distinctive dark hobnailed endothelial cells seen in congenital nonprogressive hemangioma. A multidisciplinary approach is the key to establishing the correct diagnosis.

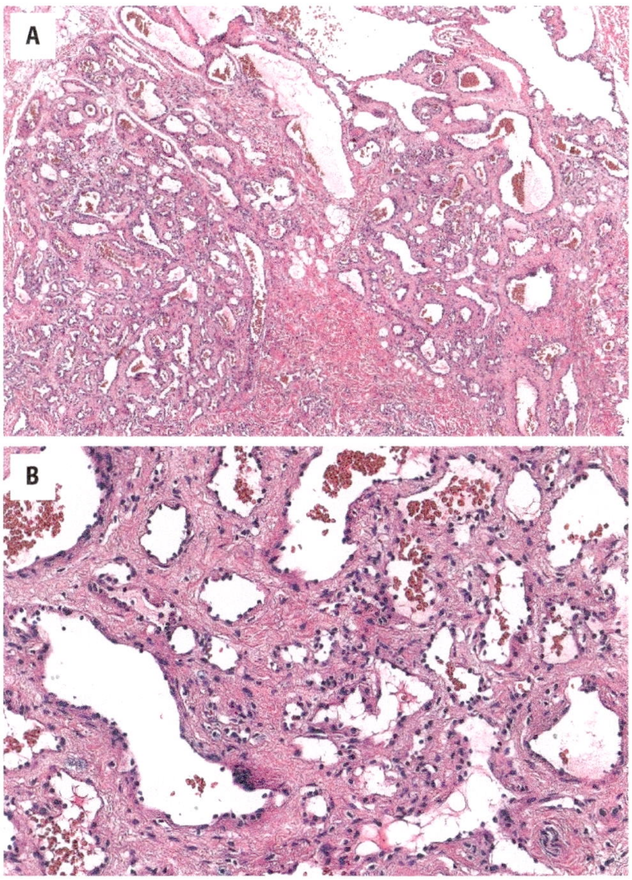

FIG. 14.115
Congenital nonprogressive hemangioma. **A,** Capillary lobules coalescing around a fibrous core containing interlobular feeding and draining vessels. **B,** The capillaries show open lumina lined by small, rounded, slightly hobnail nuclei without atypia or mitotic activity.

ANASTOMOSING HEMANGIOMA

Clinical Findings

First described in the genitourinary system in 2009, anastomosing hemangioma (AH) usually occurs in adults and has a wide anatomic distribution involving visceral locations, such as the liver, gastrointestinal (GI) tract, female genital tract, and deep soft tissue, particularly in the perinephric and paraspinal area. Superficial/subcutaneous presentations are rare, but awareness is important as the anastomosing growth pattern of this tumor can mimic angiosarcoma.

Histopathologic Features

AH are composed of relatively complex, anastomosing sinusoidal capillary-sized vascular channels forming vague lobules that may coalesce around or protrude into the lumen of large vessels. The vascular channels are lined by small, slightly hyperchromatic and mitotically quiescent endothelial cells, which are a signature

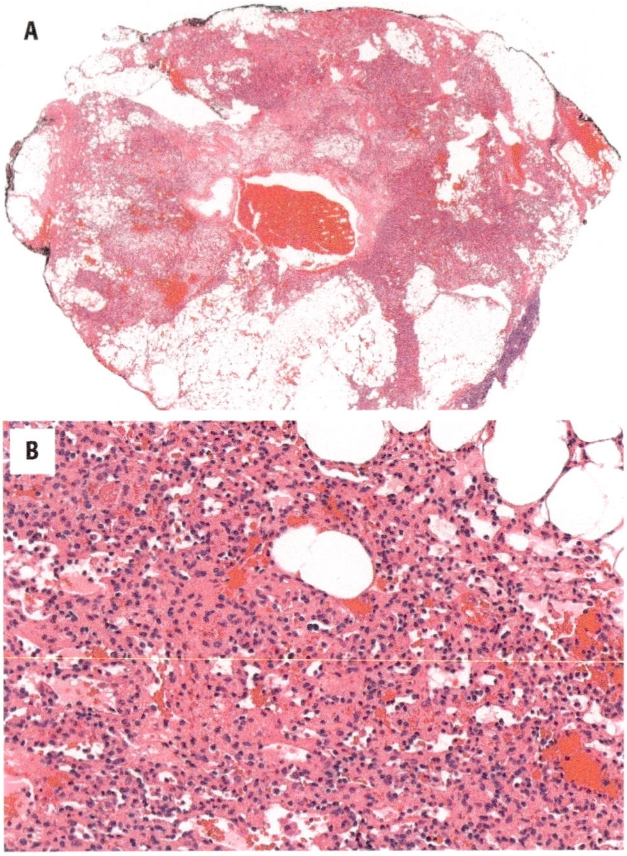

FIG. 14.116
Anastomosing hemangioma. **A,** Vascular lesion with a complex architecture and a somewhat infiltrative, anastomosing growth pattern through the subcutaneous tissue. **B,** The vascular channels are lined by small, slightly hyperchromatic and mitotically quiescent endothelial cells.

feature of *GNAQ/GNA11/GNA14*-mutated benign vascular neoplasms and are essentially identical to the endothelial cells seen in congenital nonprogressive hemangioma and cherry angioma (Fig. 14.116A and B). Eosinophilic hyaline globules, fibrin thrombi, and islands of extramedullary hematopoiesis may occur. AH lacks lymphatic marker expression.

Differential Diagnosis

AH can show an impressively infiltrative growth or protrude into the lumen of large vessels. These features can be alarming and raise suspicion for an angiosarcoma but the latter typically has a greater degree of nuclear atypia, frequent endothelial multilayering and mitotic activity, and lacks pericytic investment. The distinction from congenital nonprogressive hemangioma is based on the clinical presentation as a congenital lesion present at birth; the distinction from infantile hemangioma can be accomplished using GLUT1 immunostain.

INFANTILE HEMANGIOMA

Clinical Findings

Infantile hemangioma, formerly known as *juvenile hemangioma* or *cellular hemangioma of infancy*, is the most common pediatric soft tissue tumor, seen in approximately 5% to 10% of children, with a female predilection. Infantile hemangioma most often presents as a cutaneous or subcutaneous tumor in the head and neck, trunk, or extremities or may affect genital or visceral sites such as liver, GI tract, or upper aerodigestive tract. Based on the 2018 ISSVA classification, infantile hemangiomas are divided into focal, multifocal, segmental, and indeterminate subtypes. Segmental infantile hemangioma may be associated with PHACES or LUMBAR syndromes. Deep skeletal muscle is typically spared. All infantile hemangiomas share the same clinical course. They present shortly after birth as an erythematous to bluish macule, undergo rapid growth during the first year of life stabilizing around 5 to 7 months (proliferative phase), and then involute slowly over the course of several years (involution phase). Most cutaneous infantile hemangiomas are readily recognized clinically and regress spontaneously without treatment. Rarely, life-threatening complications, superimposed infection, or cosmetic and functional deformities may occur. Few patients present with consumptive hypothyroidism due to the expression of type 3 iodothyronine deiodinase. By imaging, infantile hemangiomas are high-flow lesions that lack the shunting that typifies AVMs. Infantile hemangiomas are infrequently biopsied except in clinically ambiguous cases or for cosmetic reasons.

Histopathologic Features

Infantile hemangioma generally fits the generic label of "lobular capillary hemangioma," and some cases are probably labeled as such. However, the lesions have very distinctive appearance that depends upon the phase in which the lesion is biopsied. In the proliferative phase, infantile hemangioma consists of lobules of densely packed, plump, mitotically active capillaries surrounded by pericytes and separated by delicate fibrous septa (Fig. 14.117A). The growth is nondestructive and spares normal tissue elements like adipose tissue, adnexal structures, and nerves. Reactive stromal changes in the form of fibrosis, myxoid change, or granulation tissue that characterize pyogenic granuloma, congenital nonprogressive hemangioma, and vascular malformations do not occur in infantile hemangioma. The capillaries are surrounded by a thin basement membrane and form small rounded lumina which can be obscured by rapidly proliferating endothelial cells (Fig. 14.117B). In the involutional phase, the endothelial cells and pericytes

INFANTILE HEMANGIOMA—DISEASE FACT SHEET

Clinical Findings

- ▸▸ Common (5% to 10% of children), cutaneous or subcutaneous tumor
- ▸▸ Segmental infantile hemangioma may be associated with Posterior fossa abnormalities, Hemangioma, Arterial lesions, Cardiac abnormalities and Eye or Endocrine abormalities (PHACES) or Lower-body hemangioma, Urogenital abnormalities, Myelopathy, Bone deformities, Anorectal malformations, and Renal anomalies (LUMBAR) syndrome
- ▸▸ Present shortly after birth with proliferative phase during the first year of life followed by involution over several years

Histopathologic Features

- ▸▸ Proliferative phase
  - Plump, mitotically active capillaries with small obscured lumina
  - Prominent pericytes and thin basement membrane
  - Nondestructive growth sparing adnexal structures and nerves
- ▸▸ Involutional phase
  - Attenuated endothelial cells with open lumina
  - Thick and hyalinized basement membrane, increased mast cells
  - Apoptotic dust within the basement membrane
  - Completely hyalinized residual capillaries in end-stage lesions

IHC/Molecular

- ▸▸ Expression of placental markers GLUT1, CD15, Lewis-Y antigen, CCR6, FcYRII, and merosin
- ▸▸ This phenotype is unique to infantile hemangioma

Differential Diagnosis

- ▸▸ Pyogenic granuloma
- ▸▸ Congenital nonprogressive hemangioma (NICH, RICH)
- ▸▸ Kaposiform hemangioendothelioma
- ▸▸ Small vessel vascular malformations

GLUT1, Glucose transporter 1; *IHC*, immunohistochemistry; *NICH*, noninvoluting congenital hemangioma; *LUMBAR*, Lower-body hemangioma, Urogenital abnormalities, Myelopathy, Bone deformities, Anorectal malformations, and Renal anomalies; *PHACE*, Posterior fossa abnormalities, Hemangioma, Arterial lesions, Cardiac abnormalities and Eye or Endocrine abnormalities; *RICH*, rapidly involuting congenital hemangioma.

become more attenuated, resulting in open capillary lumina, while the basement membranes become thick and hyalinized. A characteristic feature is the presence of apoptotic dust within the basement membrane and an increased number of mast cells (Fig. 14.117C). Features of both the proliferative and involutional phases often coexist within the same lesion. In end-stage lesions, residual capillaries become completely hyalinized (so-called ghost vessels) while the large feeding and draining vessels persist (Fig. 14.117D) mimicking a vascular malformation. Infantile hemangiomas have a unique immunophenotype shared only by the placental vasculature including expression of GLUT1, an erythrocyte glucose transporter protein, CD15, and unique placental markers such as Lewis-Y antigen, CCR6, FcYRII, and merosin. Since GLUT1 is not expressed in reactive vascular proliferations, other benign hemangiomas, and most vascular malformations, it is a very useful immunohistochemical marker for the diagnosis of infantile hemangioma and is expressed in all stages of this lesion.

Differential Diagnosis

Pyogenic granuloma typically occurs at an older age and can be distinguished from infantile hemangioma based on its thick fibrous stroma with reactive changes separating tumor lobules, and the lack of GLUT1 immunoreactivity. Highly cellular proliferative phase examples can be mistaken for a more aggressive neoplasm such as kaposiform hemangioendothelioma-tufted angioma (KHE/TA) or angiosarcoma. Pediatric angiosarcomas are very rare and can be distinguished based on complex architecture, infiltrative growth pattern, greater nuclear atypia, and the lack of a pericytic layer. An important diagnostic pitfall is the frequent expression of GLUT1 in angiosarcomas. Separation of end-stage examples of infantile hemangioma from vascular malformations is best accomplished by correlation with the clinical and radiologic findings and IHC for GLUT1. The distinction from the congenital nonprogressive hemangioma (NICH and RICH) is described above.

Prognosis and Treatment

Accurate histologic diagnosis is very important as clinically significant infantile hemangiomas uniquely respond to topical and systemic β-blockers.

PYOGENIC GRANULOMA (LOBULAR CAPILLARY HEMAGIOMA)

Clinical Findings

The term "pyogenic granuloma" is a misnomer as these lesions have neither an infectious etiology nor granulomatous inflammation, which is why the lesions are typically reported by pathologists as locular capillary hemangioma. However, the latter term, while morphologically correct, is not specific, since various pediatric and adult hemangiomas have lobular capillary architecture. For this reason, the term pyogenic granuloma is advantageous and may be preferable, especially in children where the distinction between different types of hemangiomas has important treatment implications. Pyogenic granuloma is an acquired, typically solitary polypoid erythematous nodule that occurs at any age, most commonly in the head and neck (including the oral and nasal mucosa) and the extremities. They are

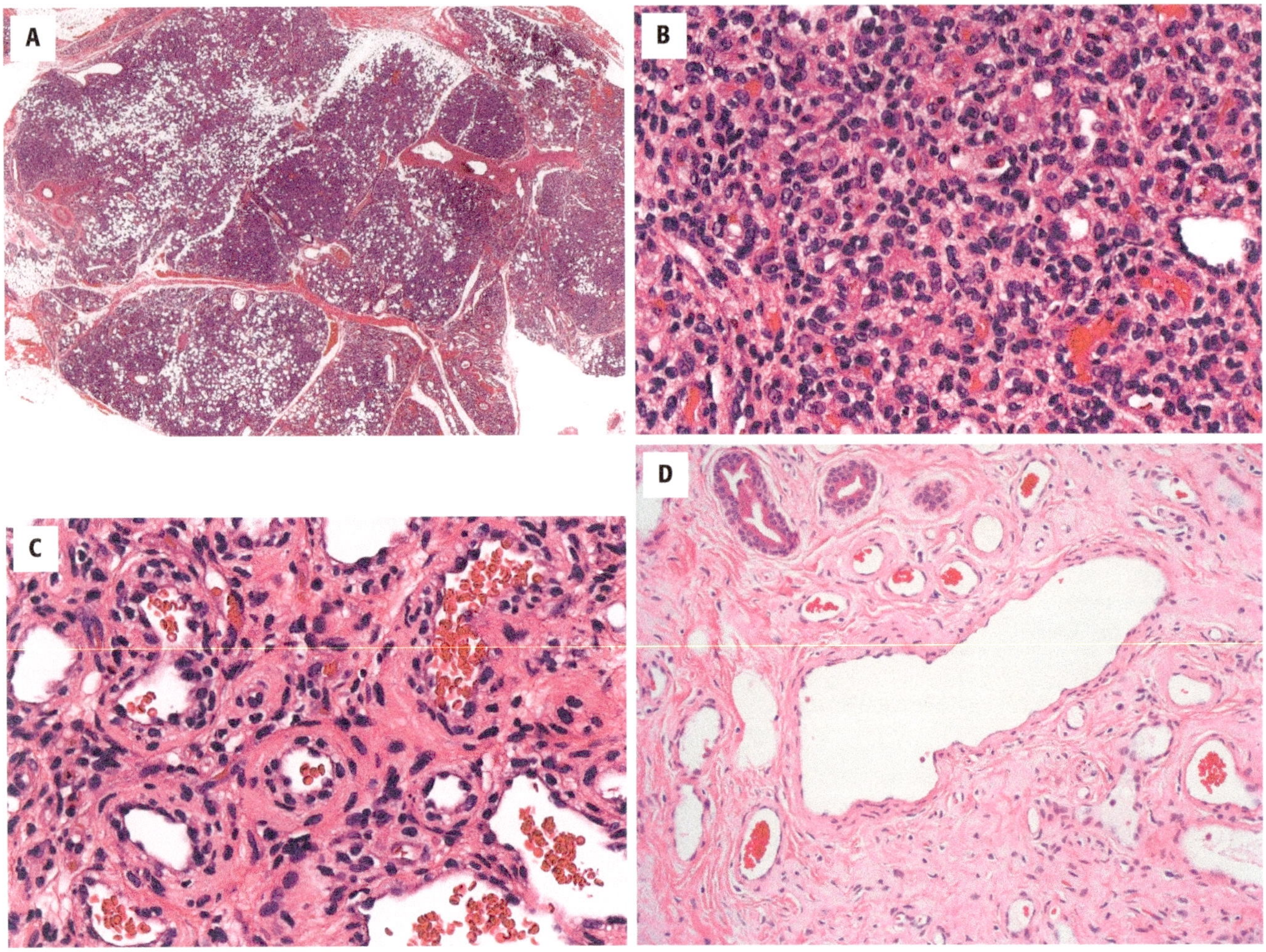

FIG. 14.117
Infantile hemangioma (IH). **A,** IH has a lobular configuration and shows a nondestructive growth pattern sparing normal tissue elements. **B,** Proliferative phase IH showing densely packed, plump, mitotically active capillaries surrounded by pericytes and separated by delicate fibrous septa. **C,** Involution phase IH with attenuation of the endothelial cells and pericytes, which results in open capillary lumina and thick hyalinized basement membrane. Apoptotic dust and mast cells are common. **D,** In end-stage lesions, residual capillaries become completely hyalinized while the large feeding and draining vessels persist.

typically solitary, with only rare multiple/eruptive forms described.

Histopathologic Features

Microscopically, pyogenic granulomas are composed of distinct lobules of closely packed mitotically active capillaries, often surrounding larger feeder vessels (Fig. 14.118A and B). Superficial lesions often have an epidermal collarette and if ulcerated, will show an associated brisk inflammatory reaction and granulation tissue. The stroma is fibrous or fibromyxoid, with a variable amount of inflammatory cells. Intravascular pyogenic granulomas consist of closely packed capillaries arising within a wall of a vein; these lesions tend to lack significant inflammation. Mutations in *BRAF*, *RAS*, and *GNA14* occur in pyogenic granuloma.

Differential Diagnosis

The diagnosis of pyogenic granuloma in adults is rarely problematic. Cherry hemangiomas (see above) can have an epidermal collarette but lack the closely packed vessels and inflammation often seen in pyogenic granuloma. Exuberant pyogenic granulomas in sun-damaged skin can be confused with angiosarcoma, in part because of the brisk mitotic rate, cellularity, and mild cytologic atypia but recognition of the lobular architecture and the lack of infiltrative growth help to exclude angiosarcoma. The presence of a pericytic layer that can be highlighted by a SMA stain is also helpful for making this distinction. On occasion pyogenic granulomas may be confused with BA and Kaposi sarcoma. The clinical context (compromised immune system) and the presence of cytoplasmic amphophilic granular material containing the

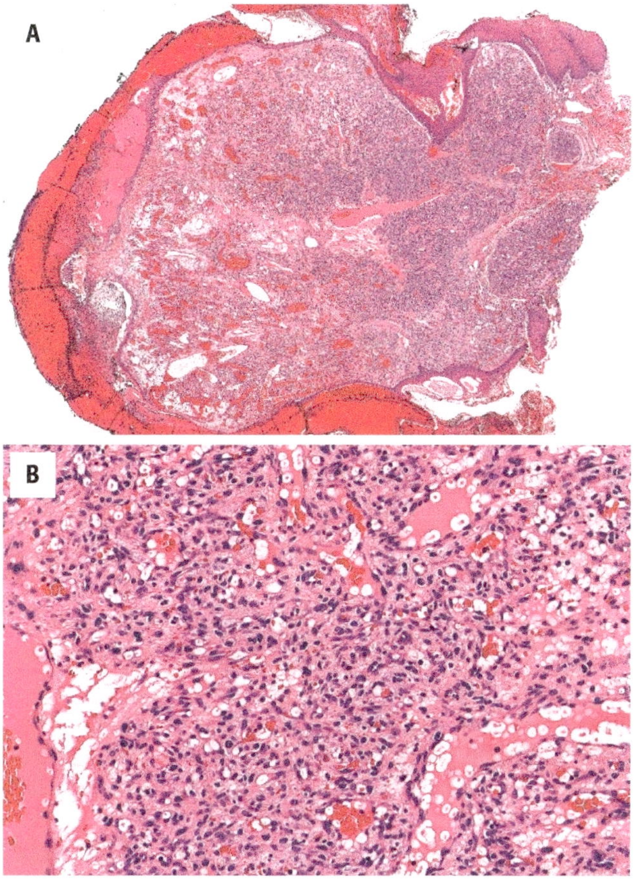

FIG. 14.118

Pyogenic granuloma. **A,** Lobules of closely packed mitotically active capillaries, often surrounding larger feeder vessels. Superficial lesions often have an epidermal collarette. **B,** Brisk inflammatory reaction, granulation tissue changes, and myxoid stroma may occur.

microorganism allows for its distinction of BA from pyogenic granuloma, while the diagnosis of an angioma-like variant of Kaposi sarcoma can be supported by immunoreactivity for HHV8.

SINUSOIDAL HEMANGIOMA

Clinical Findings

Sinusoidal hemangioma presents as a solitary subcutaneous or deep dermal nodule or plaque on the trunk, breasts, or extremities.

Histopathologic Features

Microscopically it manifests as circumscribed collection of markedly attenuated interanastomosing channels imparting a sieve-like appearance at low power and often showing pseudopapillary projections like those

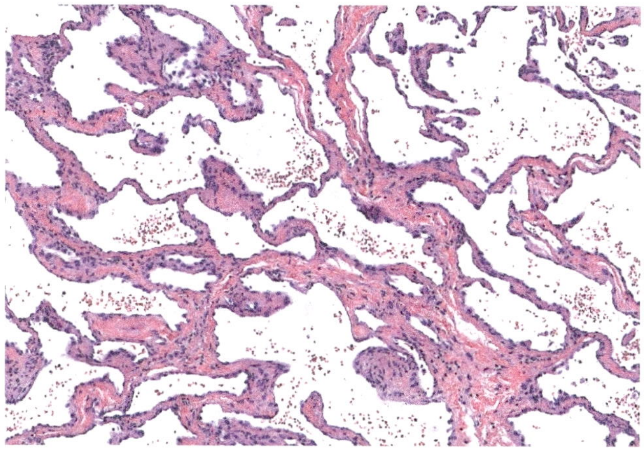

FIG. 14.119

Sinusoidal hemangioma shows attenuated interanastomosing channels imparting a sieve-like appearance at low power and often showing pseudopapillary projections.

seen in papillary endothelial hyperplasia (Fig. 14.119). Recent evidence suggests that sinusoidal hemangioma and papillary endothelial hyperplasia may share aberrant angiogenesis (sprouting and intussusceptive angiogenesis), which leads to vessel segmentation and papillary formation. Thrombosis and calcifications may occur.

Differential Diagnosis

Venous malformations, in the past often referred to as venous hemangiomas, also present a well-circumscribed collection of multiple, ectatic thin-walled vessels, lined by bland mitotically inactive endothelial cells. Thrombosis, dystrophic calcifications, and papillary endothelial hyperplasia may also occur. However, at high magnification these vessels most often contain a variable amount of irregular, disorganized smooth muscle and lack internal elastic lamina, consistent with veins (Fig. 14.120). Asymmetric fibromyxoid intimal thickening may be present. Correlation with the imaging impression is very useful in this context. Telangiectatic vascular channels filled with blood and lined by mitotically quiescent cells can be seen in a variety of hemangiomas, vascular malformations, organizing thrombi as well as in some aggressive vascular tumors such as kaposiform, retiform, and composite hemangioendothelioma (CHE) and even in Kaposi sarcoma and in angiosarcomas. Therefore, a scrutiny for an underlying vascular pattern is critical before a lesion with conspicuous dilated thinned vascular channels can be labeled as a sinusoidal hemangioma or a venous malformation. Many of the above lesions with a prominent thin dilated vascular component were historically labeled "cavernous hemangioma." We believe that cavernous hemangioma is more of a histologic pattern rather than a distinct clinicopathological entity and recommend avoiding using this term diagnostically.

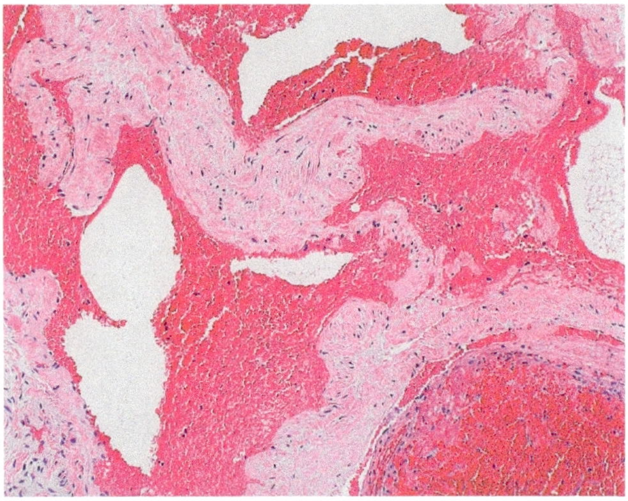

FIG. 14.120
Venous malformation showing ectatic thin-walled veins, lined by bland mitotically inactive endothelial cells and containing variable amount of irregular, disorganized smooth muscle.

Prognosis and Treatment

Sinusoidal hemangiomas are benign. Venous malformations, although benign, may cause significant morbidity depending on the size and anatomic distribution and should be treated by an interdisciplinary vascular anomaly group.

ANGIOKERATOMA AND OTHER HYPERKERATOTIC VASCULAR LESIONS

Clinical Features

Angiokeratoma is a benign acquired cutaneous vascular lesion with a somewhat different clinical presentation depending on age and anatomic site. These anatomic variations include:

- *Angiokeratoma of Fordyce*: solitary or multiple red to violaceous papules most commonly on the scrotum, penis, inner thighs, and vulva of older adults.
- *Angiokeratoma of Mibelli:* a wartlike lesion over bony prominences on the hands and feet of children and young adults, possibly related to trauma.
- *Solitary angiokeratoma* (most common): a solitary papule on the lower limbs of young male patients.
- *Angiokeratoma circumscriptum* is a type of congenital capillary malformation presenting as coalescing erythematous papules or plaques on the extremities of children, most commonly, thigh and buttock.
- *Angiokeratoma corporis diffusum*: multiple papules in a "bathing suit" distribution, typically, though not always, associated with Fabry disease, an X-linked deficiency of α-galactosidase A.

Histopathologic Features

Angiokeratomas consist of ectatic, thin-walled capillary vessels lined by flat, nonproliferative endothelium. The vessels are limited to the superficial dermis and typically herniate into the overlying dermal papilla producing an appearance of a vessel trapped within the epidermis. The overlying epidermis shows acanthosis and hyperkeratosis (Fig. 14.121). Angiokeratomas are negative for lymphatic markers D2-40 and PROX-1.

Differential Diagnosis

The fundamental differential diagnosis is with two other hyperkeratotic vascular lesions: verrucous venous malformation (VVM, formerly known as verrucous hemangioma) and cutaneous lymphatic malformation (formerly "lymphangioma circumscriptum"). Both lesions can look nearly identical to angiokeratoma in superficial biopsies as they also contain ectatic, thin-walled vessels filling the papillary dermis and "herniating" into an acanthotic and hyperkeratotic epidermis. The key histologic difference is the depth of involvement. Angiokeratomas are restricted to the upper dermis. In VVM, in addition to the angiokeratoma-like superficial dermal component, there is a florid proliferation of small venules in a lobular configuration involving the subcutis, while reticular dermis is often spared (Fig. 14.122A–C). VVMs are associated with somatic *MAP3K3* mutations. In lymphatic malformations, the vessels also extend deeper into papillary dermis and

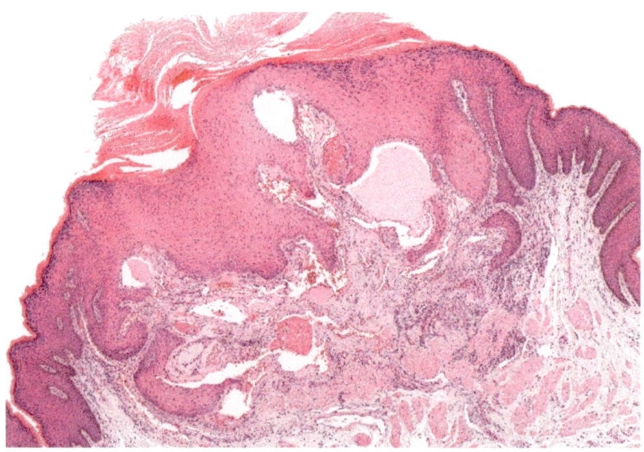

FIG. 14.121
Angiokeratoma consists of thin-walled dilated capillary vessels lined by flat endothelium. The vessels are limited to the superficial dermis and herniate into the overlying dermal papilla producing an appearance of a vessel trapped within the epidermis. The overlying epidermis shows acanthosis and hyperkeratosis.

often involve the reticular dermis and subcutis. The easiest way to separate cutaneous lymphatic malformations (see below) from the other two mimics is staining for lymphatic markers PROX1 and podoplanin (D2-40), as both angiokeratomas and VVMs are negative for these markers.

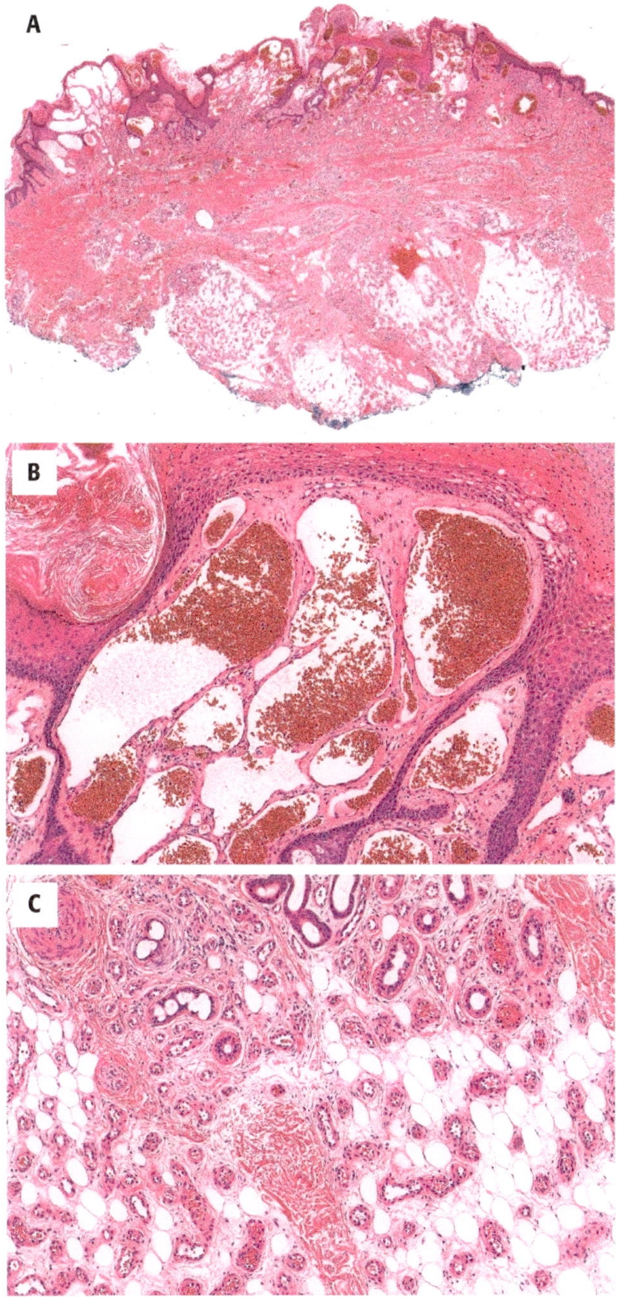

FIG. 14.122

Verrucous venous malformation. **A,** A hyperkeratotic vascular lesion involving dermis and subcutis. **B,** Angiokeratoma-like superficial dermal component. **C,** Florid proliferation of small venules in a lobular configuration involving the subcutis, while reticular dermis is often spared.

CUTANEOUS LYMPHATIC MALFORMATION

Clinical Findings

"Lymphangioma circumscriptum" and "cutaneous lymphangioma" are former terms for a localized cutaneous lymphatic malformation. The use of these terms is discouraged. Cutaneous lymphatic malformations can be sporadic or syndromic and manifest at birth or in infancy as crops of hyperkeratotic tan to yellow to red papules or vesicles. The lesions tend to localize in one area and usually involve the limb girdles, buttocks, or oral cavity, but any site can be affected. Cutaneous lymphatic malformations can be limited to the dermis, involve subcutaneous tissue, or represent a superficial component of a deeper-seated generalized lymphatic malformation or a complex vascular malformation, especially the venous subtype. Consultation with a multidisciplinary vascular malformation team is very valuable in this context.

Histopathologic Features

All lymphatic malformations can be divided based on the size of the dilated vascular channels into microcytic(<1 cm), macrocytic (≥1 cm), or combined subtypes, although these terms are most often used radiologically. Cutaneous and subcutaneous lymphatic malformations are usually microcystic. Microscopically, lymphatic malformations display features characteristic of a lymphatic phenotype, namely, irregularly angled vessels without significant smooth muscle or pericytic investment containing pale proteinaceous material, occasional lymphocytes, valve structures, and perivascular lymphoid aggregates (Fig. 14.123A and B). Lymphatic channels frequently contain red blood cells or organizing thrombi related to trauma, hemorrhage or from communication with the venous channels and thus can mimic venous malformations. The overlying epidermis is often acanthotic and hyperkeratotic, and the superficial lymphatic channels herniate into the dermal papillae like those seen in angiokeratoma and VVM discussed above. The endothelial cells express markers of lymphatic differentiation: podoplanin (D2-40), PROX1, and LYVE-1. Lymphatic malformations are most often associated with mosaic *PIK3CA* mutations.

Differential Diagnosis

Venous malformation, which can be distinguished based on the thicker caliber vessels with more prominent smooth muscle walls, and lack of expression of markers

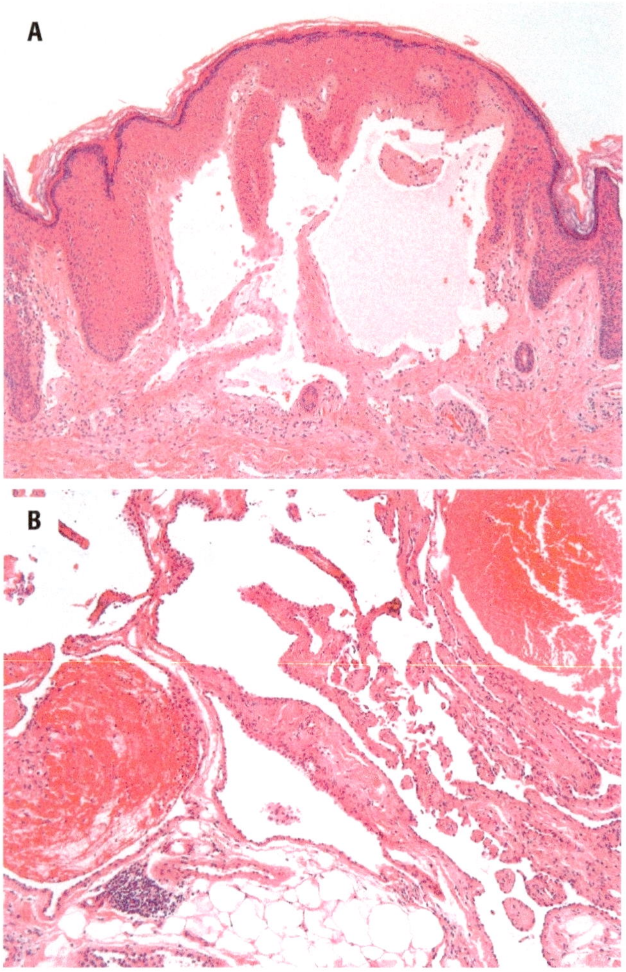

FIG. 14.123

A, Cutaneous lymphatic malformation showing dermal-based, thin irregular vessels without pericytes. The lymphatic channels herniate into the dermal papillae like those seen in angiokeratoma and verrucous venous malformation discussed above. **B,** Subcutaneous lymphatic malformation showing dilated lymphatics containing pale proteinaceous material, occasional lymphocytes, valve structures, and perivascular lymphoid aggregates.

of lymphatic differentiation. The distinction from angiokeratoma and VVM is described above.

HOBNAIL HEMANGIOMA

Clinical Features

Also known as targetoid hemosiderotic hemangioma, this lesion most often presents on the extremities of young to middle-aged adults. The classic, although not very common, clinical presentation is a central erythematous macule or papule surrounded by a pale ring and an ecchymotic halo, which fades with time. There is some debate whether this lesion represents a hemangioma or a type of lymphatic malformation, but it is grouped with hemangiomas in the latest 2018 ISSVA classification.

Histopathologic Features

Hobnail hemangiomas are wedge-shaped tumors centered on the upper dermis and composed of dilated vessels lined by bland and mitotically inactive hobnail endothelial cells. Focal intravascular papillae are common. Pericytes are absent. In the reticular dermis, the vessels become more compressed and slitlike and may show a somewhat dissecting growth pattern. Scattered lymphocytes, extravasated red blood cells, and hemosiderin deposits are common (Fig. 14.124A and B). The vessels show lymphatic phenotype with expression of PROX-1 and D2-40.

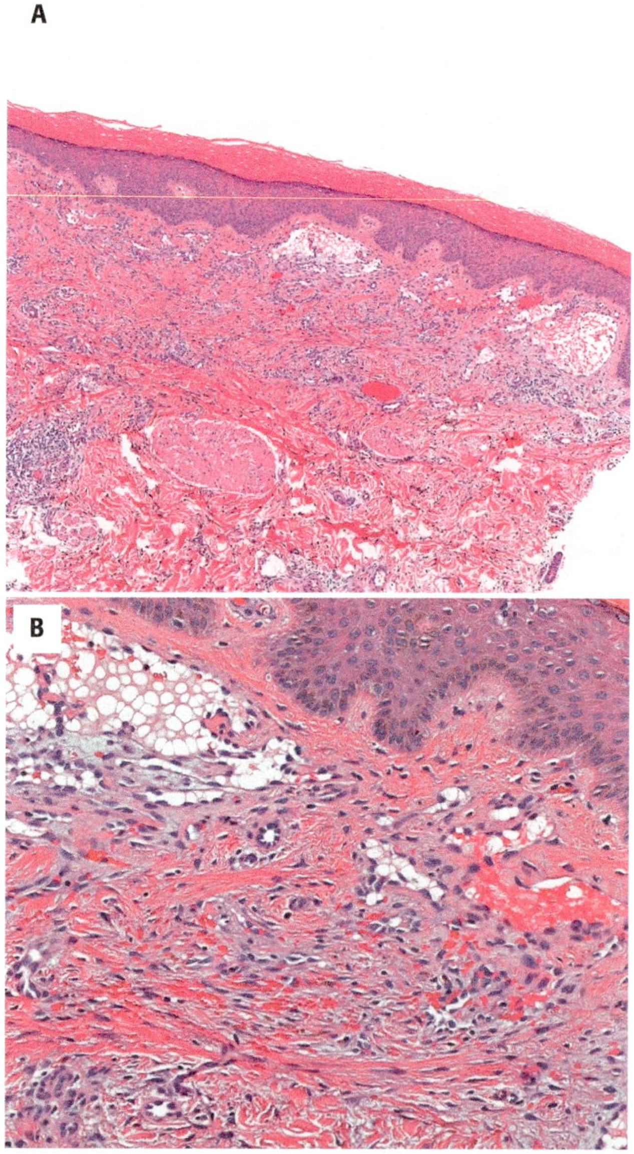

FIG. 14.124

Hobnail hemangioma. **A,** A wedge-shaped tumor centered on the upper dermis and composed of dilated vessels lined by bland and mitotically inactive hobnail endothelial cells. **B,** The vessels are more compressed and slitlike and may show a somewhat alarming dissecting growth pattern in the deeper dermis. Scattered lymphocytes, extravasated red blood cells, and hemosiderin deposits are common.

Differential Diagnosis

Hemangioendotheliomas with hobnail endothelial cells (retiform and CHE and papillary intralymphatic angioendothelioma [PILA]/Dabska tumor) can look similar. These tumors are discussed in detail below, but they are all characterized by a very complex vascular growth pattern and some degree of cytologic atypia beyond what is seen in hobnail hemangioma. A variant of postradiation AVL can closely resemble hobnail hemangioma both clinically and pathologically, but this entity occurs in previously irradiated skin, usually in the setting of treatment for breast cancer. Angiosarcoma has greater architectural complexity, multilayering of endothelial cells, nuclear atypia, and mitotic activity. Of note, all the above lesions, including angiosarcoma, may show lymphatic phenotype with expression of lymphatic markers D2-40 and PROX-1.

SPINDLE CELL HEMANGIOMA

Clinical Features

Spindle cell hemangioma has a rather classic presentation as red to violaceous, often multiple nodules on the distal limbs of children and adult patients. Spindle cell hemangiomas can arise sporadically or in association with nonhereditary Maffucci's syndrome, which includes also venous malformations, multiple enchondromas, and an increased risk of chondrosarcoma.

Histopathologic Features

Spindle cell hemangioma is an irregular, architecturally complex lesion, with overall circumscription at scanning magnification. Spindle cell hemangiomas consist of two principal components. One component shows prominent cavernous vascular spaces lined by bland endothelium, often with thrombosis and phlebolith formation. The second component is a proliferation of compressed spindled and mitotically active endothelial cells arranged in a somewhat fascicular fashion reminiscent of Kaposi sarcoma, numerous pericytes, and vacuolated epithelioid endothelial cells sometimes referred to as "blister" cells (Fig. 14.125A–C). Most spindle cell hemangiomas are at least partially intravascular, and a preexisting vessel wall is often present at the periphery. IHC is helpful in appreciating the vascular components and the presence of SMA-positive pericytes. Spindle cell hemangiomas often express markers of lymphatic differentiation such as podoplanin/D2-40 and PROX-1. Both sporadic and Maffucci's syndrome–associated cases have mutations in the isocitrate dehydrogenase (*IDH1* and *IDH2*) genes; this mutation is highly specific for this hemangioma subtype.

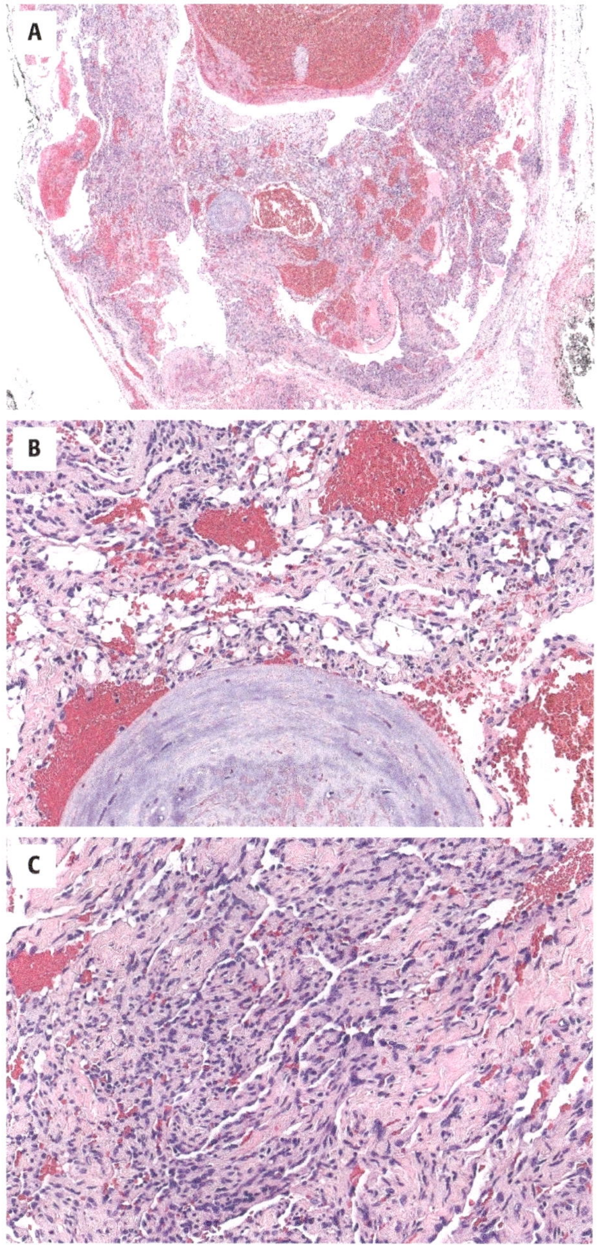

FIG. 14.125

Spindle cell hemangioma. **A,** A circumscribed intravascular architecturally complex lesion. **B,** Cavernous vascular spaces lined by bland endothelium, with thrombosis and phleboliths. **C,** Spindled, mitotically active endothelial cells arranged in a somewhat fascicular fashion reminiscent of Kaposi sarcoma and surrounded by numerous pericytes. Vacuolated epithelioid endothelial cells sometimes referred to as "blister" cells are present.

Differential Diagnosis

The key differential diagnosis is with Kaposi sarcoma because of the similar appearing, relatively low-grade spindle cell endothelial component. Kaposi sarcoma does not have the varying combinations of histologic features seen in spindle cell hemangioma and with rare exceptions, lacks dilated cavernous spaces and phleboliths. Kaposi sarcoma can be objectively diagnosed based on the positive HHV8 immunostain. Complex lymphatic and venolymphatic malformations may show significant overlap with spindle cell hemangioma; however, clinical and imaging findings and mutation profile of these lesions allow distinction.

EPITHELIOID HEMANGIOMA

Clinical Features

Epithelioid hemangiomas of the skin typically affect young to middle-aged women. Most occur in the head and neck region, but the anatomic distribution is wide. They may be solitary or multiple.

Histopathologic Features

The classic cutaneous manifestation has a lobular architecture with closely packed capillaries associated with a larger feeder vessel. Often admixed with the vascular proliferation is an inflammatory infiltrate of lymphocytes, eosinophils, and histiocytes, a manifestation that is also known as angiolymphoid hyperplasia with eosinophilia (EH-ALHE) (Fig. 14.126A and B). Peripheral eosinophilia can occur in approximately 20% of these cases.

The capillary vessels are lined by plump polygonal (often referred to as "tombstone-like") endothelial cells with abundant eosinophilic cytoplasm that can fill the vessels' lumina. The nuclei are slightly enlarged with fine chromatin and often have a distinct, but not prominent nucleolus. Mitotic figures are not uncommon. Cases of epithelioid hemangioma involving deep soft tissue, bone, or the penis typically have a less prominent inflammatory component and tend to have a more solid growth pattern with only a few well-formed capillaries in the center. A solid, sheetlike growth of epithelioid endothelial cells with minimal inflammatory component is also seen in the solid variant of cutaneous EH, originally described under the separate rubric of "cutaneous epithelioid angiomatous nodule" (Fig. 14.126C). A population of small, well-formed vascular channels in a slightly myxoid stroma may be present at the periphery of these solid lesions. Occasionally, epithelioid hemangioma can present as an intravascular tumor analogous to intravascular pyogenic granuloma.

The endothelial cells of EH express ERG, CD31, or CD34. Like other epithelioid vascular tumors, they may

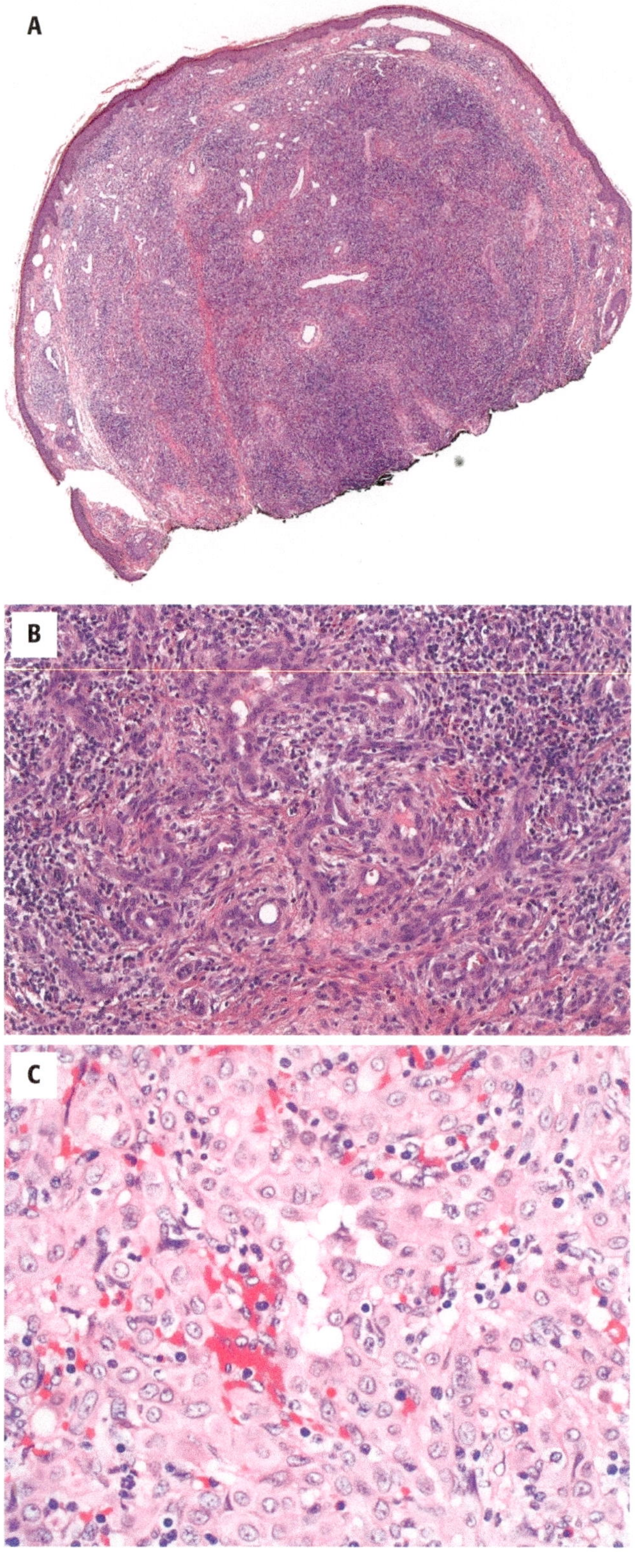

FIG. 14.126

Epithelioid hemangioma of angiolymphoid hyperplasia with eosinophilia. **A,** Closely packed capillaries in a lobular architecture admixed with a florid inflammatory infiltrate of lymphocytes, eosinophils and histiocytes. **B,** The vessels are lined by plump polygonal endothelial cells with abundant eosinophilic cytoplasm. **C,** A solid variant of cutaneous EH (also known as cutaneous epithelioid angiomatous nodule) shows sheetlike growth of epithelioid endothelial cells with minimal inflammatory component and rare vascular channels.

express cytokeratins. Rearrangements of the *FOS* and *FOSB* gene with a variety of partners have been identified in approximately 30% of cases. A subset of cutaneous EH of the head and neck harbor *GATA6::FOXO1* fusions. These alterations have not been identified in EH of ALHE type. FOS or FOSB IHC can be positive, albeit somewhat inconsistently, in up to 70% of EH, including EH of ALHE, but is rarely required for the diagnosis.

Differential Diagnosis

Classic epithelioid hemangioendothelioma (EHE) with *WWTR1::CAMTA1* fusion displays and infiltrative growth pattern with epithelioid endothelial cells arranged in cords and nests within a myxohyaline stroma. Eosinophils and vasoformative architecture are usually absent. However, EHE with *YAP1::TFE3* fusion may resemble epithelioid hemangioma due to its more vasoformative appearance and abundant eosinophilic cytoplasm. These tumors have greater cytologic atypia than classic epithelioid hemangioma, and express TFE3 by IHC, which can be utilized in diagnostically challenging cases. IHC can also help in the distinction of epithelioid hemangioma from classic EHE, since the latter expresses CAMTA1 protein, a product of *WWRT1::CAMTA1* fusion. Epithelioid angiosarcomas are architecturally more complex, infiltrative tumors and show greater cytologic atypia than EH. Pseudomyogenic (epithelioid sarcoma-like) hemangioendothelioma grows in solid sheets, does not form vascular channels, and has a distinctive myoid spindle cell component, with coexpression of cytokeratins and vascular markers CD31 and ERG but negative CD34. A *SERPINE1::FOSB* fusion is present in PHE/epithelioid sarcoma-like hemangioendothelioma that has not been found in EH, which shows *FOS* or *FOSB* fusions with other partners. EH-ALHE is often confused with Kimura disease. The latter appears to be a separate, distinctly entity. Kimura disease is prevalent in Asian male patients and is characterized by lymphadenopathy, often around the ears, in association with peripheral eosinophilia, but in the absence of a distinct soft tissue mass. The affected lymph nodes may contain numerous eosinophils and an associated vascular proliferation, but the telltale vessels of epithelioid hemangioma containing plump polygonal cells with abundant eosinophilic cytoplasm, filling vascular lumina, are not characteristic of Kimura disease, which typically has more flattened, reactive angioproliferative-type capillaries. Other inflammatory and neoplastic processes associated with florid cutaneous lymphoid hyperplasia, such as IgG4-related sclerosing diseases, or primary cutaneous follicular center-cell lymphoma, also lack the distinctive epithelioid endothelial cells seen in EH.

Prognosis and Treatment

Epithelioid hemangioma is benign, although local recurrence occurs in up to 40% of cases. There is no risk of metastasis.

OTHER ANGIOMA SUBTYPES

ACQUIRED PROGRESSIVE LYMPHATIC ANOMALY

Acquired progressive lymphatic anomaly or lymphangioma (APL) is a rare lymphatic anomaly that presents as a slowly progressing red to brown macule or plaque on the extremities both children and adults and can be quite large. It consists of a proliferation of irregular, bland lymphatic channels involving the dermis and subcutis and growing in a dissecting pattern parallel to the dermal collagen bundles (Fig. 14.127). The lesional cells show lymphatic phenotype with expression of PROX-1 and D2-40. Due to the dissecting growth pattern and lack of well-developed pericytes, APL can closely resemble a well-differentiated cutaneous angiosarcoma and patch stage Kaposi sarcoma. APL generally lacks the atypia, endothelial multilayering and mitotic activity seen in angiosarcoma and can be separated from Kaposi sarcoma by application of HHV8 latent nuclear antigen-1 immunostain. APL is benign and may be completely excised if small but larger, progressive lesions often require nonsurgical options such as laser therapy or vascular targeting systemic agents such as sirolimus.

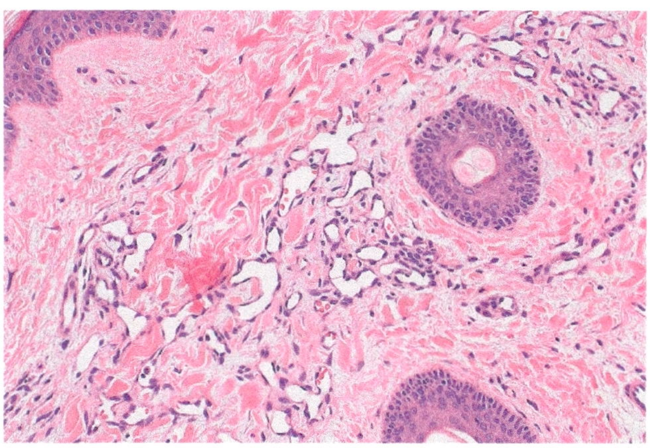

FIG. 14.127
Acquired progressive lymphatic anomaly/lymphangioma showing irregular, bland lymphatic channels growing in a dissecting pattern parallel to the dermal collagen bundles.

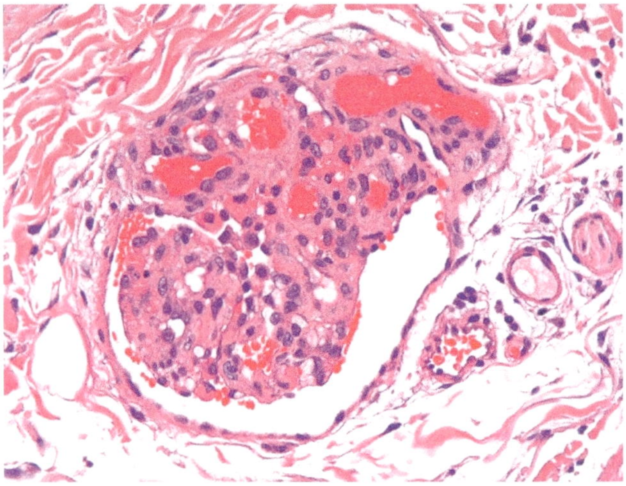

FIG. 14.128

Glomeruloid hemangioma showing an intravascular proliferation of densely packed capillaries, resembling a renal glomerulus. The capillaries contain eosinophilic, PAS-positive hyaline globules composed of polyclonal immunoglobulin.

GLOMERULOID HEMANGIOMA

Glomeruloid hemangioma is a classic cutaneous marker of POEMS (polyneuropathy, organomegaly, endocrinopathy, M-protein, and skin changes) syndrome. Patients present with multiple erythematous papules involving the trunk and extremities.

Glomeruloid hemangioma has a very distinctive appearance consisting of discrete dilated vessels within the dermis containing an intravascular proliferation of densely packed capillaries, resembling a renal glomerulus (Fig. 14.128). The capillaries contain eosinophilic, periodic acid-Schiff (PAS)–positive hyaline globules composed of polyclonal immunoglobulin. TA (see below) may superficially resemble glomeruloid hemangioma but the latter lacks intravascular growth and hyaline globules, and in contrast to the glomeruloid hemangioma, is positive for the lymphatic markers.

MICROVENULAR HEMANGIOMA

Microvenular hemangiomas occur as solitary or, rarely, multiple and eruptive red to violaceous papules on the trunk and extremities of young adults. Hormonal fluctuations such as pregnancy or oral contraceptive use may play a role. Histologically, microvenular hemangiomas have a relatively symmetric, wedge-shaped appearance and consist of thin-walled, irregular, compressed venules and capillaries that infiltrate between the collagen bundles of the reticular dermis imparting architectural complexity and thus raising suspicion for malignancy (Fig. 14.129A and B). The vessels may infiltrate into arrector pili muscle. However, the vessels are

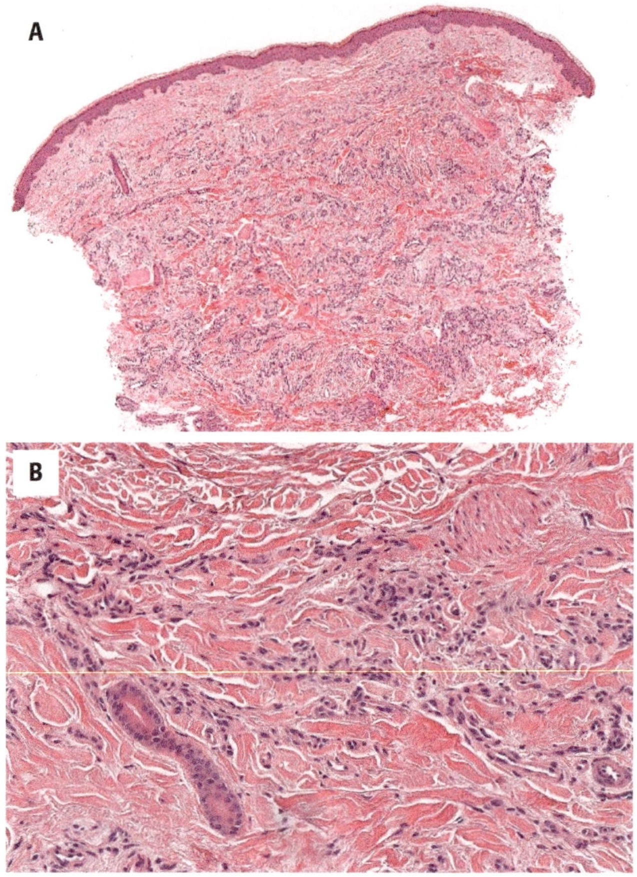

FIG. 14.129

Microvenular hemangioma. **A,** Symmetric, wedge-shaped vascular lesion composed of thin-walled, irregular, and compressed venules and capillaries. **B,** In the reticular dermis, the lesion infiltrates between the collagen bundles raising suspicion for malignancy. There is a prominent pericytic layer and no significant atypia.

invested by a readily visible pericyte layer and show no significant atypia or mitotic activity. There is no lymphatic marker expression. Patch stage of Kaposi sarcoma is a clinically significant mimic but can be distinguished based on the presence of spindle cell component, a lymphoplasmacytic infiltrate and expression of HHV8 latent nuclear antigen 1 (LANA-1). The deeper dermal component of hobnail hemangioma can look very similar to microvenular hemangioma but the former also has dilated vascular lumina lined by protruding endothelial cells and a lymphatic phenotype with expression of D2-40 and PROX-1.

ARTERIOVENOUS HEMANGIOMA

The so-called arteriovenous hemangioma, sometimes referred to as acral arteriovenous tumor or cirsoid aneurysm, is an acquired, small papule on the face or distal extremities, most often in middle-aged adults. These lesions are well-circumscribed, limited to the dermis and are composed of thick- and thin-walled veins and

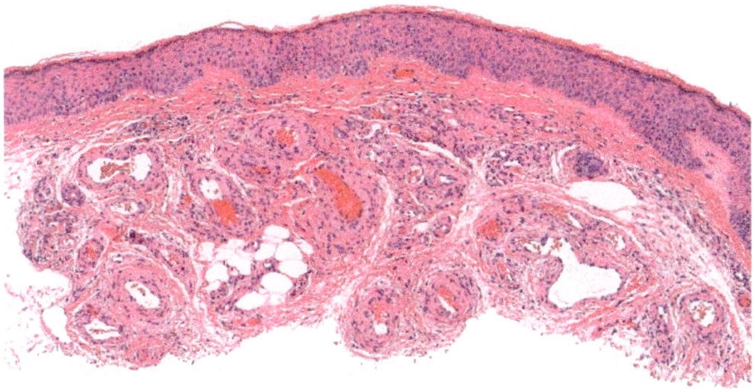

FIG. 14.130

Arteriovenous hemangioma (acral arteriovenous tumor or cirsoid aneurysm) showing thick-walled veins and indeterminate-type vessels that resemble but probably do not represent arteries. The lesion is well-circumscribed and limited to the dermis.

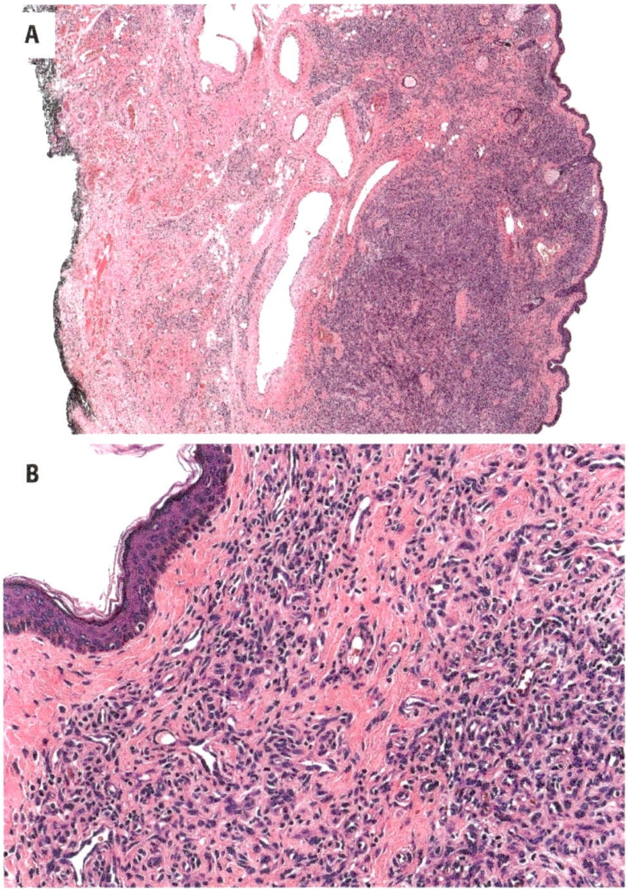

FIG. 14.131

Arteriovenous malformation. **A,** Thick-walled, larger caliber arteries and veins in a floridly proliferative background of smaller vascular channels including capillaries, arterioles, and venules. **B,** In response to the tissue ischemia, the stroma shows reactive fibromyxoid change and a reactive capillary-type proliferation resembling acroangiodermatitis (Stewart-Bluefarb syndrome).

indeterminate-type vessels that resemble but probably do not represent arteries as they lack internal elastic layer (Fig. 14.130). The etiology of these lesions is uncertain, but they do not appear to represent true AVMs as they lack evidence of arteriovenous shunting and associated tissue ischemia and are clinically indolent, although bleeding can occur. Simple excision is curative.

The term "cirsoid aneurysm" can be confusing as this term is also applied to denote large, clinically significant and cosmetically disfiguring AVMs of the scalp. In contrast to the arteriovenous hemangiomas that are limited to the dermis, AVMs at all sites usually involve the dermis and subcutis and, possibly, underlying structures. They show a combination of thick-walled, larger caliber arteries and veins in a floridly proliferative background of smaller vascular channels that can include capillaries, arterioles, and venules. In response to the high-flow environment with arteriovenous shunting, tissue ischemia, and arterial embolization prior to resection, the stroma shows reactive fibromyxoid change and often has a superimposed reactive capillary-type proliferation resembling acroangiodermatitis (Stewart-Bluefarb syndrome) (Fig. 14.131A and B). Organizing thrombi, a sign of a slow-flow vascular anomaly, are uncharacteristic of AVMs. The landscape of genetic alterations in AVMs is broad; sporadic cases most commonly show *MAP2K1* alterations.

LOCALLY AGGRESSIVE AND MALIGNANT VASCULAR TUMORS

KAPOSIFORM HEMANGIOENDOTHELIOMA AND TUFTED ANGIOMA

Clinical Features

KHE is an aggressive vascular tumor of intermediate malignancy that usually occurs in the first 2 years of life and may be congenital. KHE usually affects dermis and subcutis, but the deep soft tissues, spleen, retroperitoneum, and bone may also be involved. Superficial tumors present as large, red to violaceous, ill-defined masses. KHE often manifests as severe consumptive coagulopathy with profound and sustained thrombocytopenia, hypofibrinogenemia, and elevated D-dimer (Kasabach-Merritt syndrome) secondary to the development of platelet microthrombi within the tumor vessels. TA represents a smaller, more superficial example of KHE. TA usually presents in infants and small children as a solitary erythematous to violaceous dermal plaque or nodule, while a significant consumptive coagulopathy is seen in approximately 10% of patients. TA in adult patients is very rare.

Histopathologic Features

KHE is a cellular, ill-defined neoplasm composed of coalescing nodules of plump spindled endothelial cells

KAPOSIFORM HEMANGIOENDOTHELIOMA/TUFTED ANGIOMA—DISEASE FACT SHEET

Clinical Findings

- Ill-defined violaceous masses in dermis and subcutis, deep soft tissues in children
- Severe consumptive coagulopathy (Kasabach-Merritt syndrome)
- Tufted angioma presents in infants and small children as a solitary violaceous dermal plaque or nodule with consumptive coagulopathy in 10% of cases

Histopathologic Features

- Coalescing nodules of plump spindled and slitlike endothelial cells
- Crescent-shaped dilated lymphatic at the periphery of the nodules and within the stroma
- Mild atypia and mitotic activity
- Tufted angioma: round nodules of capillaries with a crescent-shaped vessel widely
- dispersed through the dermis in a "cannonball" fashion
- Platelet microthrombi in both forms

IHC/Molecular

- Positive for podoplanin/D2-40, LYVE-1, and Prox1
- Activating somatic mutations in *GNA14* in both forms

Differential Diagnosis

- Kaposi sarcoma
- Proliferative phase of infantile hemangioma
- Congenital nonprogressive hemangiomas (RICH and NICH)

IHC, immunohistochemistry; *NICH*, noninvoluting congenital hemangioma; *RICH*, rapidly involuting congenital hemangioma.

with a distinctive crescent-shaped dilated lymphatic at the periphery of the nodules. Similar vessels are also present within the stroma.

The periphery of the nodule shows fascicles of spindled endothelial cells and slitlike capillary vessels resembling Kaposi sarcoma, whereas the central portions contain more epithelioid endothelial cells surrounded by pericytes and often containing platelet microthrombi (Fig. 14.132 A and B). The endothelial cells show mild atypia and mitotic figures. Extravasated red blood cells and hemosiderin deposits are common. TA, in essence, is a KHE without the solid spindle cell component. It consists of identical, closely packed round nodules of basophilic capillaries that bulge into a crescent-shaped dilated vessel at the periphery of the lobule and may contain platelet microthrombi. However, because the solid spindle cell component that would incorporate these nodules into a large, mass-forming lesion of KHE is not present, the capillary nodules in TA are widely dispersed in the dermis in a so-called cannonball pattern that gave this lesion its distinctive name (Fig. 14.133A and B). TA/KHE have a unique and diagnostically useful pattern of lymphatic marker expression such that the spindled endothelial cells and the crescent-shaped vessels at the periphery of the nodules are positive for

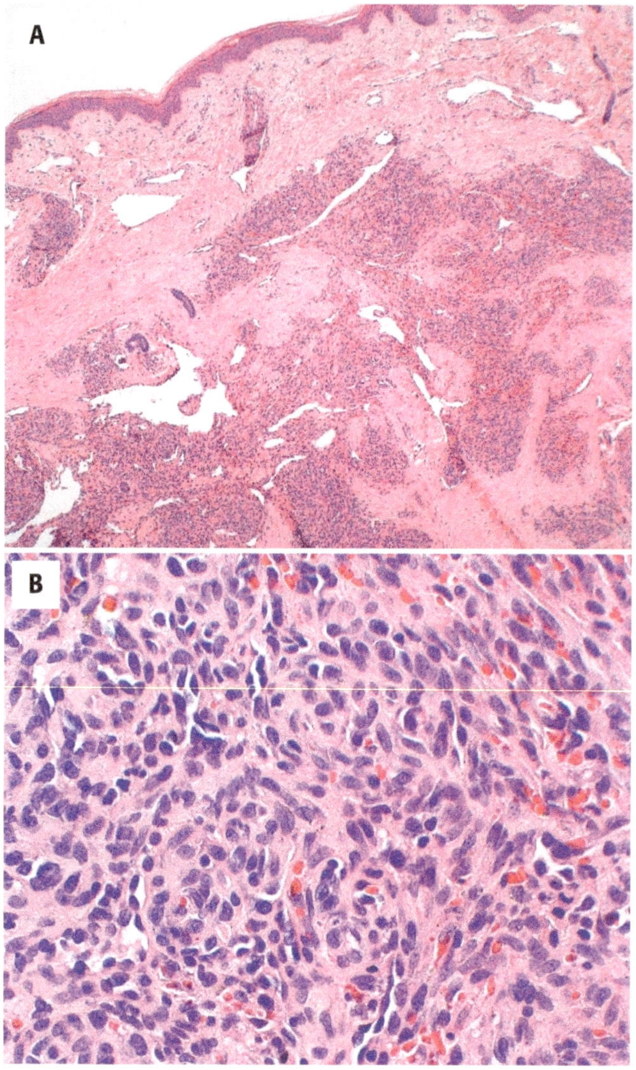

FIG. 14.132

Kaposiform hemangioendothelioma. **A,** Coalescing nodules of plump spindled endothelial cells with a distinctive crescent-shaped dilated lymphatic channels at the periphery of the nodules. **B,** Spindled and epithelioid endothelial cells and slitlike capillary vessels resembling Kaposi sarcoma and often containing platelet microthrombi. Mild atypia and mitotic figures are often present.

podoplanin/D2-40, LYVE-1, and Prox1 whereas the epithelioid capillaries in the center of the nodules do not express lymphatic markers. GLUT1 is negative. Molecular analysis shows activating somatic mutations in *GNA14* in both KHE and TA.

Differential Diagnosis

Kaposi sarcoma is extraordinarily rare in infants and young children and does not have the lobular architecture with peripheral crescent-shaped lymphatic channels, or the epithelioid component containing platelet microthrombi that are seen in KHE. Plasma cell infiltrates and HHV-8 expression do not occur in KHE.

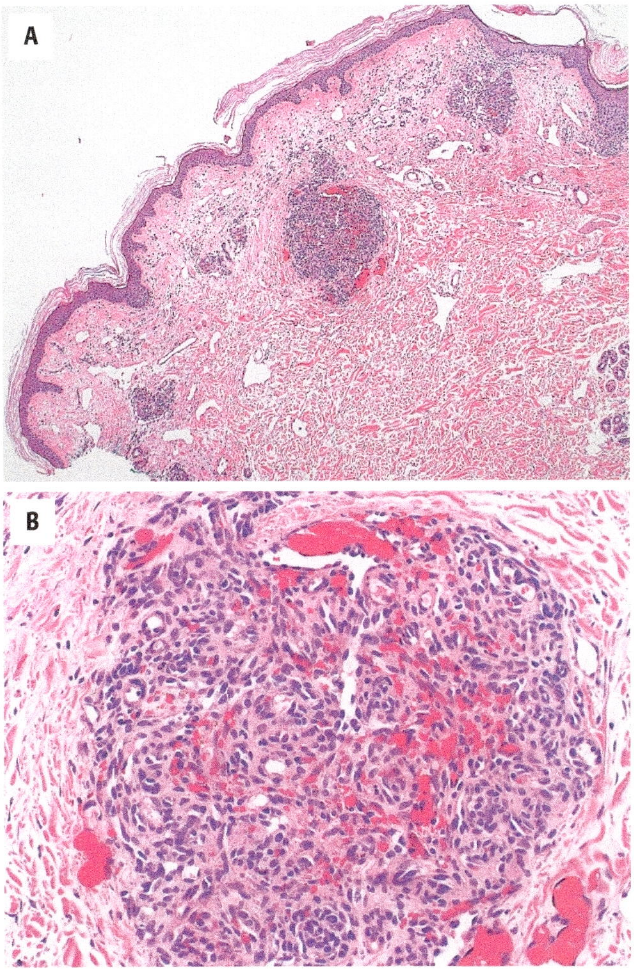

FIG. 14.133

Tufted angioma. **A,** The capillary nodules are widely dispersed in the dermis in a so-called cannonball pattern. **B,** The individual nodules consist of mostly epithelioid endothelial cells and slitlike capillary vessels containing platelet microthrombi.

The proliferative phase of infantile hemangioma shows a non-destructive growth pattern, lacks a spindle and epithelioid cell component and the distinctive perilobular crescentic vessels. Difficult cases can be resolved by utilizing a combination of GLUT1 (positive in infantile hemangioma, negative in kaposiform hemangioendothelioma/tufted hemangioma) and D2-40 or PROX-1 (positive in KHE/TA, negative in infantile hemangioma) immunostains. In young children, congenital nonprogressive hemangiomas (RICH and NICH) and pyogenic granuloma can closely resemble TA as both have discrete lobules of lesional capillaries and fibrous stroma containing large irregular stromal vessels. However, these lesions lack a solid spindle cell component, mitotic activity, and lymphatic phenotype of TA/KHE. The location of the feeding vessel is usually in the center of the lobules in congenital nonprogressive hemangioma and in many pyogenic granulomas, whereas TA/KHE have a crescent-shaped vessel at the lobule periphery.

Prognosis and Treatment

TA/KHEs are prone to local recurrence and may spread to lymph nodes. The lesions can stabilize over the years but typically do not involute. Distant metastases and malignant transformation do not occur. Mortality is almost invariably due to complications from the underlying coagulopathy, which may result in life-threatening hemorrhage. Multimodality treatment is usually employed and includes surgery for small superficial lesions and a variety of nonsurgical options, including conventional chemotherapy, intralesional or systemic steroids or interferon alpha therapy, radiation, and more recently, mTOR pathway inhibitor sirolimus. Platelet transfusions in TA/KHE paradoxically increase platelet trapping and worsen any thrombocytopenia.

PSEUDOMYOGENIC (EPITHELIOID SARCOMA-LIKE) HEMANGIOENDOTHELIOMA

Clinical Features

PHE most often involves extremities of adult male patients and is often multifocal at presentation, characteristically involving multiple tissue planes, including underlying bone. The lesions present as skin-colored nodules or ulcers resembling the distal epithelioid sarcoma.

PSEUDOMYOGENIC HEMANGIOENDOTHELIOMA—DISEASE FACT SHEET

Clinical Findings

- Multifocal skin-colored nodules or ulcers on extremities of adult patients
- Often involves multiple tissue planes

Histopathologic Features

- Sheets or fascicles of epithelioid or spindle cells with abundant eosinophilic cytoplasm
- Fibromyxoid stroma that may contain neutrophils
- No vasoformative architecture
- Mild nuclear atypia and very low mitotic activity

IHC/Molecular

- Coexpression of cytokeratin (AE1/3) and markers vascular differentiation Fli1 and ERG
- CD31 is seen in 50% to 80% of cases; CD34 is consistently absent
- Recurrent *SERPINE::FOSB*, *ACTB::FOSB* and rare variant *FOSB* fusions
- Nuclear FOSB expression

Differential Diagnosis

- Distal-type epithelioid sarcoma
- Spindle cell carcinoma of either cutaneous or adnexal origin

ERG, ETS family-related gene.

Histopathologic Features

PHE is composed of sheets or fascicles of plump, epithelioid or spindle cell with abundant eosinophilic cytoplasm, mild nuclear atypia, and very low mitotic activity (<1/10 HPF). The stroma is fibrous or myxoid (Fig. 14.134A and B). There is no vasoformative architecture. Neutrophils are often present and represent a helpful diagnostic clue. PHE has a unique immunophenotype, with a consistent expression of cytokeratin (AE1/3) and nuclear markers of vascular differentiation Fli1 and ERG, while CD31 is seen in 50% to 80% of cases and CD34 is consistently absent. Nuclear expression of SMARCB1/INI1 is retained. While some degree of SMA expression may occur in these tumors, desmin, high-molecular-weight cytokeratins, S100 and SOX10 are negative. Molecular studies show recurrent *SERPINE::FOSB* and *ACTB::FOSB* gene fusions, as well as rare variant *FOSB* fusions with *WWTR1*, *EGFL7*, and *CLTC*. The fusions can be which detected by nuclear staining with FOSB antibody, a useful diagnostic adjunct.

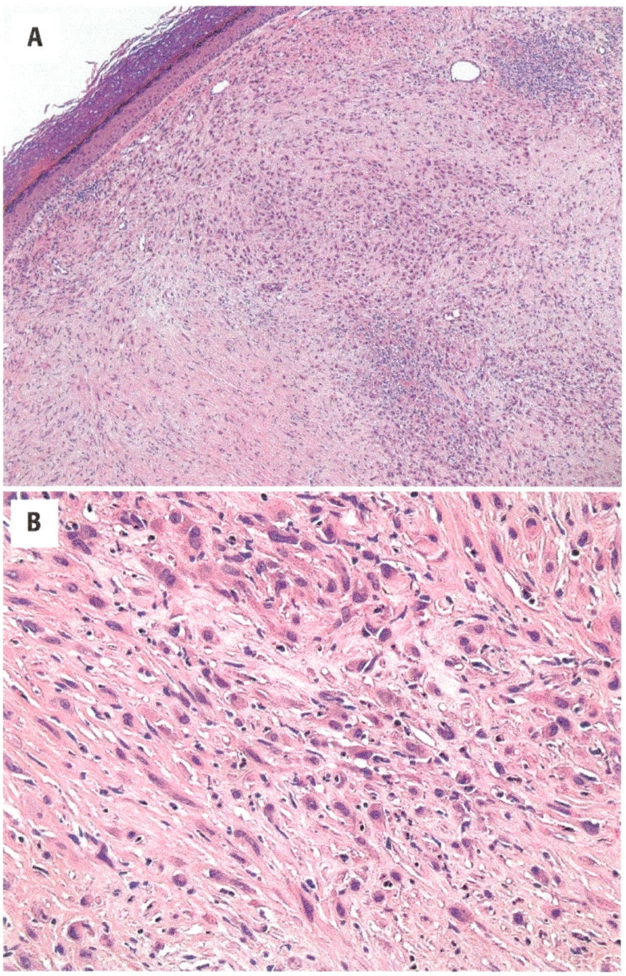

FIG. 14.134

Pseudomyogenic hemangioendothelioma. **A,** A nonvasoformative lesion composed of sheets or fascicles of plump, epithelioid, or spindle cells with abundant eosinophilic cytoplasm growing in a fibromyxoid stroma. **B,** The tumor cells have mild nuclear atypia, and very low mitotic activity.

Differential Diagnosis

The distinction from the distal-type epithelioid sarcoma can be quite difficult as both tumors show plump, cytokeratin-positive epithelioid or spindle cell with abundant eosinophilic cytoplasm, mild nuclear atypia, and low mitotic activity. On morphologic grounds, the prominent fascicular myoid component and lack of a nodular growth pattern with geographic necrosis and peripheral palisading would favor PHE. Epithelioid sarcoma is negative for vascular markers ERG and CD31 and, in contrast to PHE, is often positive for CD34 and shows loss of nuclear INI-1 expression.

Nuclear expression of FOSB, a product *of SERPINE1::FOSB* rearrangement, is not typical. Cutaneous fascicular tumors with muscle phenotype (low-grade leiomyosarcoma or spindle cell rhabdomyosarcoma), IMT or LF-NT, can be separated by application of pan-muscle markers such as desmin, smooth muscle–specific markers (smooth muscle myosin, caldesmon), skeletal muscle markers MyoD1 and myogenin, ALK, and combination of CD34 and S100 coexpression, respectively, or application of appropriate molecular analysis. A feature that we find very useful in this distinction is that PHE grows predominantly in sheets with only loose fascicular arrangement and does not form compact sweeping or intersecting fascicles that typify the above mimics. Finally, as is the case with other epithelioid vascular tumors, cytokeratin expression in PHE can be a significant diagnostic pitfall leading to misinterpretation as spindle cell carcinoma of either cutaneous or adnexal origin. This distinction can be accomplished by application of high-molecular-weight cytokeratins and p40, which are usually negative in the PHE, vascular markers, and, whenever necessary, FOSB immunostain.

Prognosis and Treatment

PHE has a rather high rate of local recurrence (approximately 60%) due to the multifocal growth pattern, but lymph node or systemic metastases to lungs, bone, or soft tissue are very rare. Surgery is the treatment of choice but may be very difficult or impossible in selected cases, due to multifocal presentation. Unresectable lesions can be targeted by mTOR pathway inhibitors such as sirolimus or everolimus.

RETIFORM HEMANGIOENDOTHELIOMA AND COMPOSITE HEMANGIOENDOTHELIOMA

Clinical Features

Retiform hemangioendothelioma (RHE) and CHE are rare vascular neoplasms of intermediate malignancy that occur in the skin and subcutaneous tissue of the distal extremities of children and young adults; less common locations include head and neck, trunk, and genital area. There may be an association with a precursor lymphatic malformation.

Histopathologic Features

RHE consists of architecturally complex, thin, stellate-shaped or branching vessels reminiscent of the rete testis lined by uniform, slightly hyperchromatic cuboidal or hobnail endothelial cells (Fig. 14.135A and B). An associated lymphocytic infiltrate is often present. The nuclear atypia is mild, and the mitotic activity is very low. Composite hemangioendothelioma represents an admixture of a component of RHE and an epithelioid component somewhat reminiscent of EHE. The latter pattern is composed of nests or sheets of plump epithelioid endothelial cells with eosinophilic cytoplasm often containing an intracytoplasmic vacuole (Fig. 14.136). Other components described in this lesion include solid spindled cell areas, vasoformative areas with low-grade nuclei reminiscent of well-differentiated angiosarcoma, and ectatic vascular channels lined by bland endothelial cells reminiscent of spindle cell hemangioma, sinusoidal hemangioma, or venous malformation. Retiform and composite hemangioendotheliomas are positive for vascular markers CD31 and ERG, variably express markers of lymphatic differentiation D2-40 and PROX-1 and can show expression of neuroendocrine marker synaptophysin. CHE with neuroendocrine marker expression (neuroendocrine CHE) may be associated with a more nested cytologic architecture and a more aggressive clinical course, although the data on this subset of CHE is still accumulating. Genetically, one-third of retiform and CHEs demonstrate *YAP1* gene rearrangements including *YAP1::MAML2* gene fusions. This can be demonstrated by loss of the YAP1 C-terminus expression by IHC.

Differential Diagnosis

EHE (discussed below) and angiosarcoma are the most important differential diagnostic considerations.

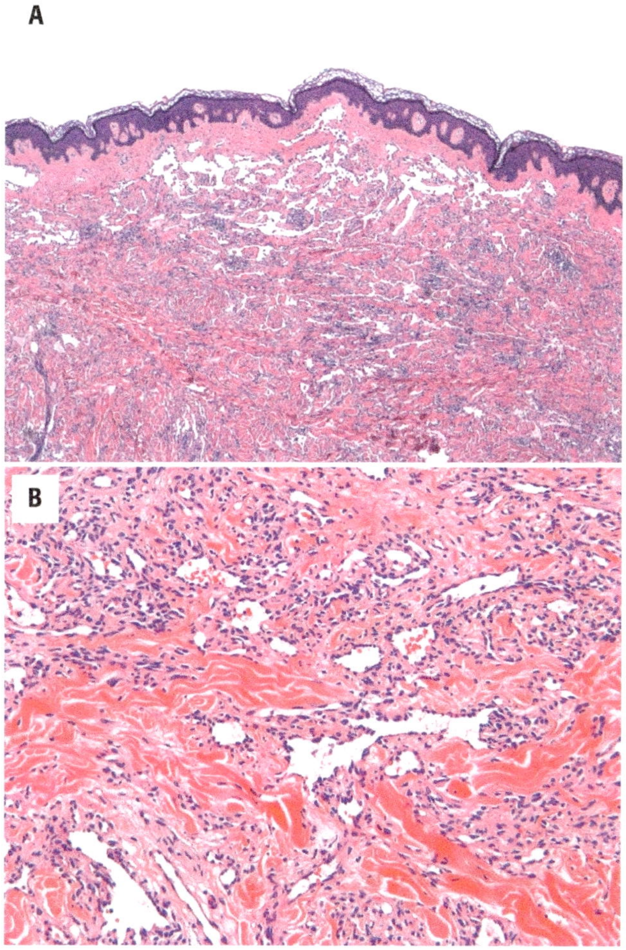

FIG. 14.135

Retiform hemangioendothelioma. **A,** Stellate-shaped or branching vessels reminiscent of the rete testis growing in a complex pattern in the dermis and subcutis. **B,** The vessels are lined by uniform, slightly hyperchromatic cuboidal or hobnail endothelial cells with mild nuclear atypia and inconspicuous mitotic figures.

EHE has similar epithelioid vacuolated endothelial cells, but they are usually arranged in a corded growth pattern or singly in a prominent myxohyaline matrix; this distinctive stroma is not seen in CHEs. There is also no evidence of a WWTR1-CAMTA1 fusion in CHEs, either by IHC, FISH, or RT-PCR. Distinction from angiosarcomas can be extraordinarily challenging. Angiosarcomas have overt cytologic atypia, endothelial multilayering, mitotic activity, and necrosis and lack the distinctive synaptophysin expression of RHE and PILA.

Prognosis and Treatment

Both retiform and CHEs behave in an indolent fashion but will slowly recur locally in a substantial proportion of cases, unless widely excised. While both retiform and CHE can show variable expression of neuroendocrine

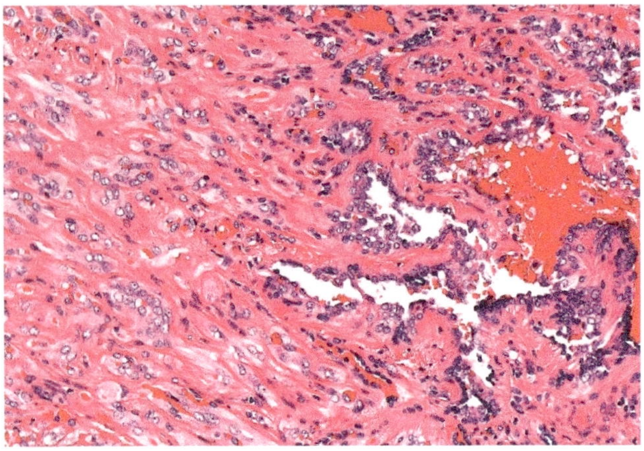

FIG. 14.136

Composite hemangioendothelioma has a component of retiform hemangioendothelioma and an epithelioid component consisting of nests or sheets of plump epithelioid endothelial cells with eosinophilic cytoplasm.

markers, neuroendocrine CHE tends to behave in a more aggressive fashion with distant metastasis to bone, lung, liver, or brain. However, the data on the prognosis of both neoplasms are still accumulating. Surgery is the treatment of choice.

PAPILLARY INTRALYMPHATIC ANGIOENDOTHELIOMA

Clinical Features

PILA, also known as Dabska tumor, is a rare superficial lymphatic vascular neoplasm of uncertain malignant potential, with characteristic intravascular growth. These lesions typically affect proximal or distal extremities, trunk, or head and neck region, and like other hobnailing hemangioendotheliomas, often occur in the background of a lymphatic malformation.

Histopathologic Features

PILA consists of thin, dilated lymphatic vessels with intraluminal papillary projections containing thin hyalinized cores lined by cuboidal-to-columnar, uniform, hobnailed endothelial cell without significant atypia or mitotic activity. Some of the papillae can appear to float within the vascular lumina due to tangential sectioning. Proteinaceous material and scattered intraluminal lymphocytes are often seen, in keeping with lymphatic differentiation. The surrounding stroma is fibrotic and contains lymphoid aggregates (Fig. 14.137). The endothelial cells show lymphatic phenotype with expression of podoplanin/D2-40 and PROX-1.

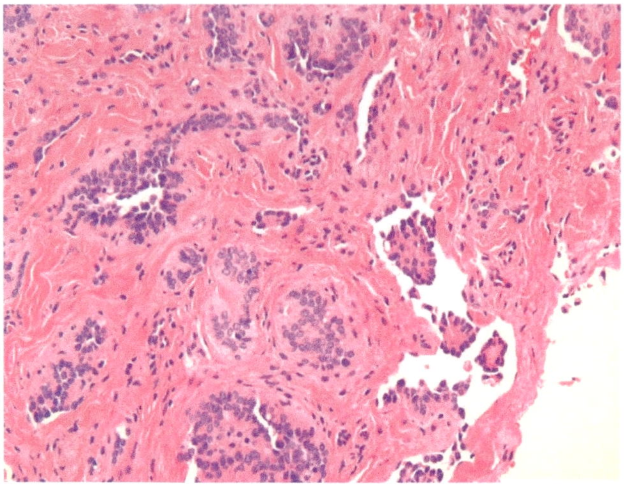

FIG. 14.137

Papillary intralymphatic angioendothelioma consists of thin, dilated lymphatic vessels with intraluminal hyalinized papillary structures lined by cuboidal-to-columnar, uniform, hobnailed endothelial cell without significant atypia or mitotic activity.

Differential Diagnosis

Cutaneous lymphatic malformation and hobnail hemangioma will show similar dilated vascular channels lined by hobnailing endothelial cells and containing proteinaceous material and scattered lymphocytes; however, PILA stands out based on the markedly increased intravascular architectural complexity with formation of papillary growth pattern, not characteristic of either of the above mimics. RHE (discussed below) may show papillary intravascular growth but typically shows a slit-like infiltrative growth pattern rather than mostly intravascular growth of PILA. Glomeruloid hemangioma can be distinguished based on the presence of intracytoplasmic hyaline globules that are composed of immunoglobulin, and lack of lymphatic marker expression. Angiosarcomas would typically show greater nuclear atypia, endothelial multilayering, and mitotic activity, and a greater degree of stromal infiltration relative to the predominantly intraluminal growth of PILA. Finally, PILA is an important morphologic mimic of multifocal lymphangioendotheliomatosis with thrombocytopenia (MLT), a rare and clinically significant generalized vascular anomaly that occurs predominantly in infants and manifests as multiple cutaneous, soft tissue, brain and visceral nodules, thrombocytopenia, and GI or intracerebral bleeding. Systemic therapy including targeted therapeutics such as sirolimus or everolimus is required. Biopsies of the MLT lesions show dilated lymphatics with a prominent intraluminal papillae lined by cytologically bland hobnail endothelial cells indeed appearing very similar to PILA. Knowledge of the clinical presentation is therefore crucial in making the diagnosis of PILA as the latter is usually a single lesion in otherwise healthy individual or an individual with a known precursor lymphatic malformation.

Prognosis and Treatment

PILA behaves in an indolent fashion and may recur locally, unless completely resected. Lymph node and systemic metastases are exceptionally rare, and an aggressive presentation, in the right clinical context, should raise suspicion for MLT.

EPITHELIOID HEMANGIOENDOTHELIOMA

Clinical Features

EHE typically occurs in adult patients, with a slight female predilection, and most commonly involves soft tissue and less often, bone, liver, and lung. In the skin, EHE has a nondescript presentation as a skin-colored nodule that lacks the erythematous to violaceous color of most cutaneous vascular tumors. EHEs are often multifocal and can show clinical evidence of metastatic disease at presentation.

Histopathologic Features

The pathologic features of EHE are dependent on the type of underlying gene fusion. The majority of EHEs are driven by *WWTR1::CAMTA1* fusion. These tumors display a cord-like or nested growth pattern of epithelioid endothelial cells embedded in a myxohyaline stroma. Well-formed vessels are not present; however, the endothelial cells frequently show individual intracytoplasmic vacuoles (so-called blister cells) that may contain red blood cells (Fig. 14.138A and B). Deep-seated tumors are often associated with a preexisting vessel and can be seen growing within and expanding the lumen, but intravascular growth is less common in cutaneous examples. The nuclear features are relatively bland and mitotic figures are low in approximately half of the cases; the other half is regarded as malignant or grade II sarcoma if based on at least two of the following criteria: moderate to marked nuclear pleomorphism, increased mitotic activity >2 mitotic figures/10 HPF and necrosis. EHEs with *YAP::TFE3* fusions are relatively uncommon and show a vasoformative architecture with plump, well-formed vascular channels lined by epithelioid cells with abundant eosinophilic to amphophilic cytoplasm similar to the cells seen in other *TFE3*-rearranged neoplasms. EHEs are immunoreactive for vascular markers CD31, CD34, and ERG and depending on the fusion subtype, may show either CAMTA1 or TFE3 expression. Importantly, approximately 25% of cases will also show immunoreactivity for cytokeratins, an important pitfall. As mentioned above, the genetic hallmark of EHE is a recurrent *WWTR1::CAMTA1* or, in a small subset, a *YAP1::TFE3* gene fusion. WWTR1 (TAZ) and YAP1 represent transcriptional co-activators downstream of the Hippo pathway and act as a promoter for the oncogenic activation of both CAMTA1 and TFE3 in endothelial cells.

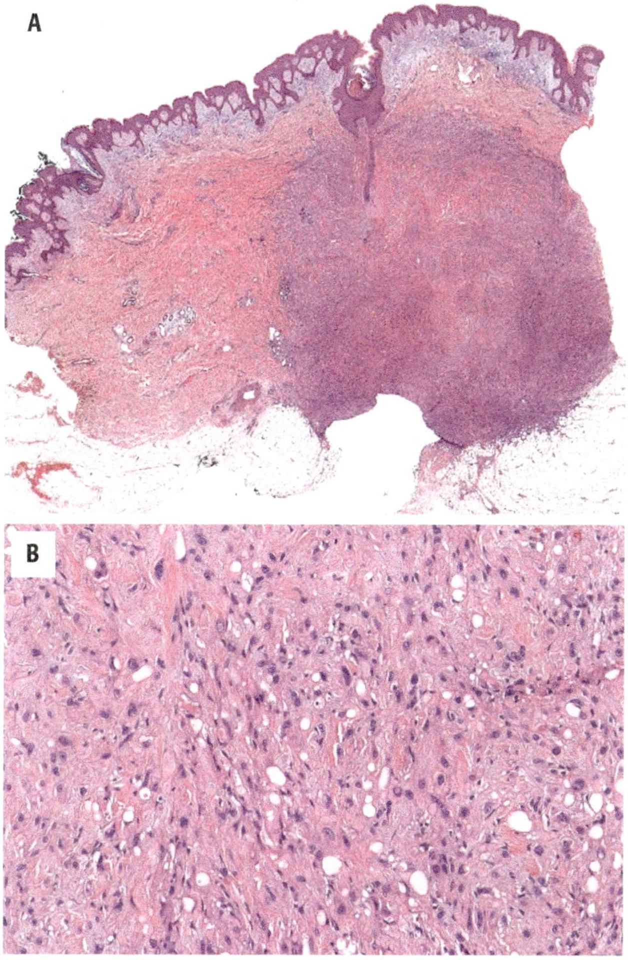

FIG. 14.138

Epithelioid hemangioendothelioma. **A,** An ill-defined cutaneous nodule. **B,** Epithelioid endothelial cells with cord-like or nested growth pattern in a myxohyaline stroma. Well-formed vessels are not present but the endothelial cells may show intracytoplasmic vacuoles containing degenerating red blood cells.

Differential Diagnosis

The differential diagnosis of EHE includes epithelioid sarcoma, pseudomyogenic (epithelioid sarcoma-like) hemangioendothelioma, and poorly differentiated adenocarcinoma. Epithelial sarcoma typically has a more solid, nodular proliferation of epithelioid cells often with foci of central necrosis reminiscent of necrotizing granulomas.

Epithelioid sarcoma demonstrates strong keratin and EMA immunoreactivity, and approximately 50% to 60% of cases are positive for CD34. While clone-specific ERG expression can be seen in some epithelioid sarcomas, the latter are negative for CD31, CAMTA1, and TFE3 and show loss of INI-1 (SMARCB1) expression. Pseudomyogenic (epithelioid sarcoma-like) hemangioendothelioma has a more solid, sheetlike growth pattern of epithelioid-to-spindled cells and is consistently negative for CD34, CAMTA1, and TFE3 antibodies. Poorly differentiated adenocarcinoma, especially metastatic lobular carcinoma of the breast or signet ring cell adenocarcinoma of the upper gastrointestinal tract, often shows cord-like arrangement of tumor cells and intracytoplasmic vacuoles but can be distinguished based on the application of cytokeratins and lack of vascular marker expression. Cutaneous mixed tumors and related myoepitheliomas can also have a cord-like-to-nested growth pattern and have a similar appearing stroma. Evidence of true ductal lumen formation, when present, can aid in the distinction, as EHE does not demonstrate ductal differentiation. While both tumors can be positive for cytokeratins, myoepithelial tumors are negative for vascular markers and show coexpression of myoepithelial markers such as SMA, SOX10, and p63/p40.

Prognosis and Treatment

EHEs of both types are regarded as low-grade sarcomas, with approximately 70% multifocal disease at presentation and metastases to regional lymph nodes or the lungs in 20% to 30% of cases. The overall mortality is about 10% to 20%. While curative resection is the mainstay of treatment for most unifocal localized cases (this may include lobectomy or liver transplant for visceral disease), multifocal disease can be treated with expectant management or multimodality chemotherapy regimens including conventional cytotoxic agents, targeted therapeutics, and immunotherapy. EHEs at all sites are best managed by the multidisciplinary sarcoma team.

KAPOSI SARCOMA

Clinical Features

Kaposi sarcoma has five clinical forms:

- *Classic* sporadic form that occurs in elderly men of Eastern European or Mediterranean descent and is generally associated with indolent clinical course.
- *Endemic* African form that occurs in non-HIV–infected children and adults in equatorial Africa and is associated with slightly more aggressive behavior.
- *Epidemic* AIDS-associated form: Kaposi sarcoma is one of the AIDS-defining diseases; generally worse prognosis unless immunosuppression is corrected.
- *Iatrogenic* form in the setting of non-AIDS–related immunosuppression, such as organ transplantation, immunosuppressive therapy, or other medical reasons; generally worse prognosis unless immunosuppression is corrected.
- Emerging *nonepidemic* form occurring in men who have sex with men but who are HIV-seronegative and have no apparent immunodeficiency; this form is largely cutaneous and is associated with a better prognosis.

All forms of Kaposi sarcoma present with violaceous patches, plaques, or nodules that may be limited to the skin or coincide with lymph node, mucosal or visceral involvement. Kaposi sarcoma is driven by HHV8, which is detected in all clinical forms.

KAPOSI SARCOMA—DISEASE FACT SHEET

Clinical Findings

- Violaceous patches, plaques, or nodules limited to the skin or with concurrent lymph node, mucosal or visceral involvement

ClinicalForms

- *Classic:* older men of Eastern European/Mediterranean descent; indolent course
- *Endemic:* non-HIV–infected children and adults in equatorial Africa; more aggressive course
- *Epidemic AIDS-associated:* aggressive course unless immunosuppression is corrected
- *Iatrogenic:* due to non-AIDS–related immunosuppression for other medical reasons: worse prognosis unless immunosuppression is corrected
- *Nonepidemic:* cutaneous disease in HIV-seronegative men who have sex with men, without apparent immunodeficiency; favorable prognosis

Histopathologic Features

- Slit like small irregular vessels dissecting between collagen bundles
- Promontory sign: entrapment of preexisting vessels and adnexal structures
- Solid sheets of spindle cells with slitlike vascular lumina and extravasated erythrocytes
- Lymphocytes and particularly plasma cells are characteristic
- Intracellular hyaline globules
- Monotonous nuclei with little atypia; pleomorphism is rare (anaplastic Kaposi sarcoma)

IHC/Molecular

- Positive for CD34, CD31, ERG, and often, lymphatic markers PROX-1 and D2-20
- HHV-8 latent nuclear antigen 1 (LANA-1)

Differential Diagnosis

- Spindle cell angiosarcoma
- Spindle cell hemangioma
- Kaposiform hemangioendothelioma/tufted angioma

AIDS, Acquired immunodeficiency syndrome; *ERG*, ETS family-related gene; *HIV*, human immunodeficiency virus; *IHC*, immunohistochemistry.

Histopathologic Features

Early forms show small irregular vessels dissecting between collagen bundles and sometimes incorporating preexisting vessels and adnexal structures (so-called promontory sign). As the tumor evolves from plaque to patch to nodule stage, the vessels become more irregular in shape and evolve into solid sheets of spindle cells with slitlike vascular lumina and extravasated erythrocytes (Fig. 14.139A and B). Lymphocytes and plasma cells are seen at the periphery. Hyaline globules representing degenerating erythrocytes are seen within solid areas of the tumor. Most cases consist of uniform spindle cells with monotonous nuclei and little atypia. A small subset of cases shows overt nuclear pleomorphism, increased mitotic activity, and necrosis (referred to as anaplastic Kaposi sarcoma), which appears to be due to gain of chromosomes 7, 11, 19, and 21 with downstream effect being upregulation of cyclin-dependent signaling pathways. By IHC, Kaposi sarcoma stain with standard vascular markers and often displays lymphatic phenotype; the frequency of CD34 expression is higher than in other vascular malignancies. The most useful immunostain in the diagnosis is directed against HHV-8 LANA-1, which is both a sensitive and specific marker of Kaposi sarcoma.

Differential Diagnosis

Spindle cell angiosarcoma typically has more nuclear atypia and mitotic activity, with the rare caveat of pleomorphic/anaplastic Kaposi sarcoma as outlined above. Spindle cell hemangioma, as discussed earlier, has a less infiltrative pattern of growth, best appreciated at scanning magnification, and demonstrates a more complex architecture including the characteristic ectatic vascular spaces, phleboliths, and vacuolated endothelial cells ("blister" cells). KHE/TA may be distinguished based on a characteristic clinical presentation as an infiltrative mass in infants and young children, often accompanied by thrombocytopenia, the characteristic lobular growth pattern of the lesional capillaries, absent plasma cells, and only partial lymphatic phenotype. Finally, lesions of Kaposi sarcoma may show an angiomatoid or a

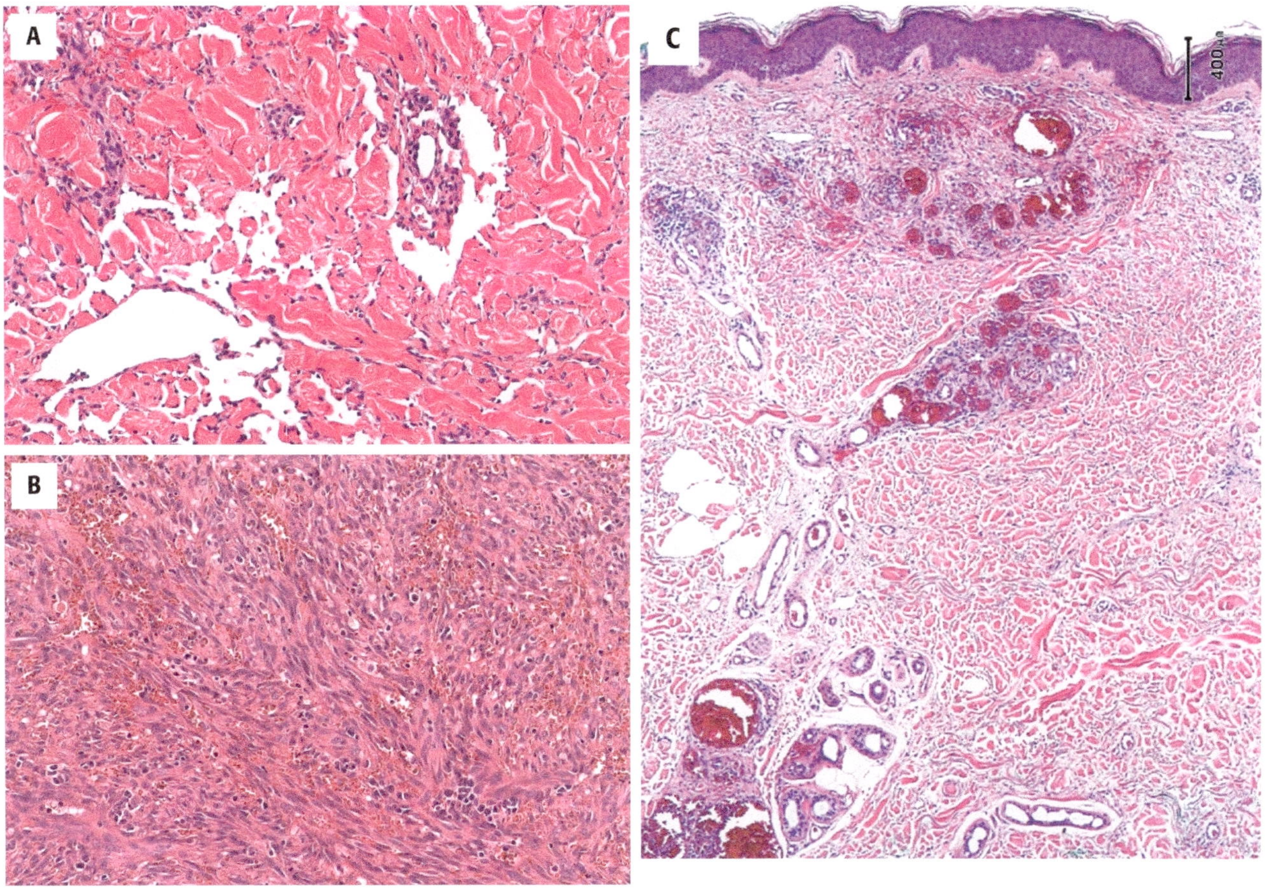

FIG. 14.139

Kaposi sarcoma. **A,** Small irregular vessels dissecting between the collagen bundles. **B,** Solid sheets of spindled endothelial cells with slitlike vascular lumina and extravasated erythrocytes. Plasma cells are quite characteristic. Hyaline globules representing degenerating erythrocytes are seen within solid areas of the tumor. **C,** Kaposi sarcoma with a deceptive angiomatous growth pattern.

lymphatic malformation-like pattern with thin, cystically dilated vessels (Fig. 14.139C). Such lesions can be confused with acquired progressive lymphangioma, lymphatic malformations, and ordinary hemangioma in limited biopsy samples and require a careful review of the clinical presentation. Kaposi sarcoma can be distinguished from all the above mimics by HHV8 immunostain.

Prognosis and Treatment

The clinical course is dependent on the subtype of the disease and how well the underlying immunosuppression can be corrected. Many patients have a relatively indolent course, with low mortality rate. Advanced disease in the setting of AIDS or anaplastic Kaposi sarcoma is associated with a significantly worse prognosis. Surgical therapy plays little role in the management of Kaposi sarcoma. Treatment options depend on the extent of disease and the clinical course and may include observation topical modalities such as cryotherapy for local control and radiation, chemotherapy, or both. Combined antiretroviral therapy is the mainstay of treatment in AIDS patients. There are no HHV8-specific therapies at present.

ANGIOSARCOMA

Clinical Features

Cutaneous angiosarcomas arise as either primary cutaneous tumors or secondary tumors related to radiation therapy or chronic lymphedema. Primary cutaneous angiosarcoma, with few exceptions, presents in the sun-damaged skin of the head and neck as a bruise-like areas or solitary or multiple violaceous nodules and/or plaques. Radiation and lymphedema-associated tumors have a broad distribution and arise in the skin of the radiation field, with an average latency of 5 years. The breast is the most common site. Lymphedema-associated angiosarcoma can be seen secondary to any cause of chronic lymphedema, such as morbid obesity or lymphedema secondary to filariasis.

ANGIOSARCOMA—DISEASE FACT SHEET

Clinical Findings

- Primary cutaneous tumor in the UV-exposed sites
- Secondary due to radiation therapy or chronic lymphedema
- Solitary or multiple bruise-like or violaceous nodules and/or plaques

Histopathologic Features

- Complex anastomosing vessels lined by atypical endothelial cells
- Dissecting growth pattern
- Intratumoral hemorrhage
- Solid, nonvasoformative growth in spindle and epithelioid angiosarcoma
- Mild to severe nuclear atypia, endothelial multilayering, mitotic activity
- Unique histologic patterns in cutaneous radiation-associated angiosarcoma
  - Radiation dermatitis–like pattern
  - Capillary lobule pattern

IHC/Molecular

- Vascular markers CD31, ERG, and CD34 (low sensitivity); frequent D2-40/PROX-1 expression
- MYC expression and *MYC* amplification by FISH in postradiation angiosarcoma
- Sporadic tumors show alterations in angiogenesis-related pathways (*PTPRB, PLCG1, KDR, FLT4*), *RAS, BRAF, TP53* mutations, and *CDKN2A* deletions
- *CIC* gene alterations
- *MYC* amplification in postradiation angiosarcoma

Differential Diagnosis

- Vasoformative tumors
  - Hemangiomas and vascular malformations
  - Reactive angioendotheliomatosis
  - Papillary endothelial hyperplasia
  - Postradiation atypical vascular lesion
- Nonvasoformative tumors
  - Spindle cell squamous cell carcinoma and adnexal carcinomas
  - Malignant melanoma
  - Atypical fibroxanthoma/dermal pleomorphic sarcoma
  - Proximal-type epithelioid sarcoma

ERG, ETS family-related gene; *IHC*, immunohistochemistry; *UV*, ultraviolet.

Histopathologic Features

Angiosarcoma is a poorly circumscribed, highly infiltrative tumor with a wide range of microscopic appearances, but they can all be boiled down to two principal patterns: a vasoformative pattern and a nonvasoformative pattern, which can be spindled, epithelioid, or both. The vasoformative pattern consists of complex vessels lined by atypical endothelial cells with enlarged hyperchromatic nuclei that dissect through the dermal collagen. Multilayering of endothelial cells lining lumina and papillae formation are commonly seen (Fig. 14.140A and B). The cytologic atypia associated with the complex vessels can be very mild or severe. The nonvasoformative patterns include solid sheetlike, spindle cell, and epithelioid areas, for which the helpful histologic clue is intratumoral hemorrhage. In these tumors, the vasoformative slitlike channels can usually be seen at the periphery of the tumor (Fig. 14.141). Epithelioid angiosarcoma consists of round cells with relatively abundant cytoplasm mimicking carcinoma or melanoma and may either form complex vascular channels or present as solid sheets (Fig. 14.142). Secondary

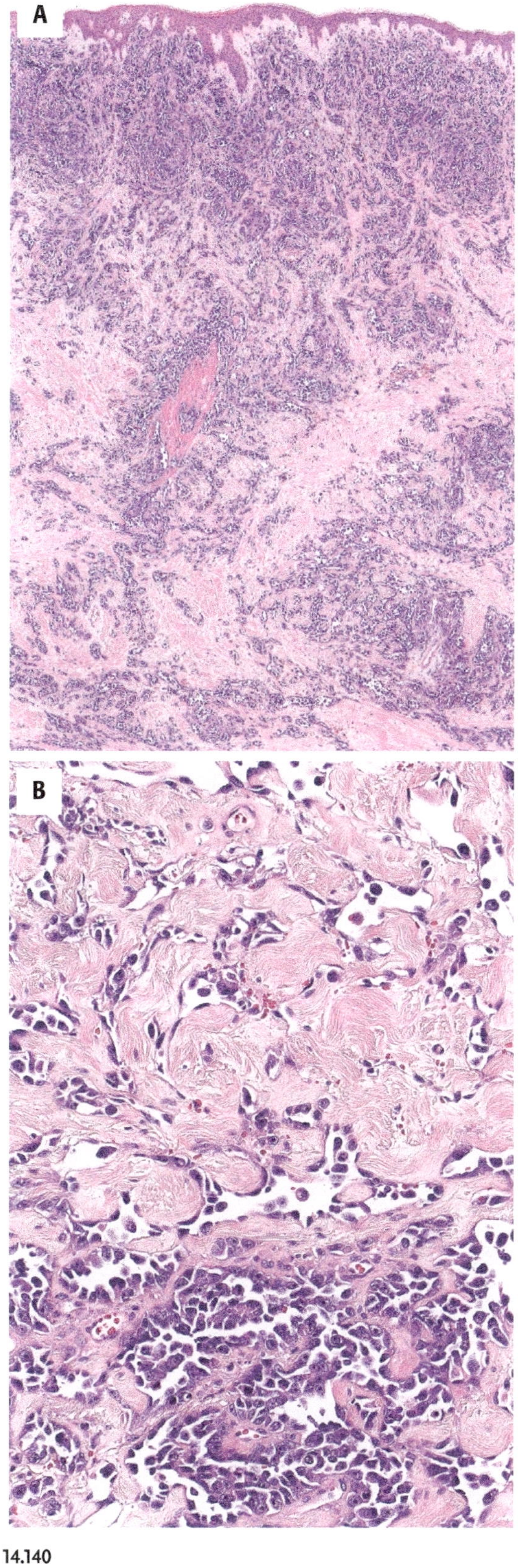

FIG. 14.140

Angiosarcoma. **A,** An infiltrative vascular neoplasm dissecting through the dermis and subcutis. **B,** The vessels are lined by atypical endothelial cells with endothelial multilayering, intravascular papillae, overt nuclear atypia, and mitotic activity.

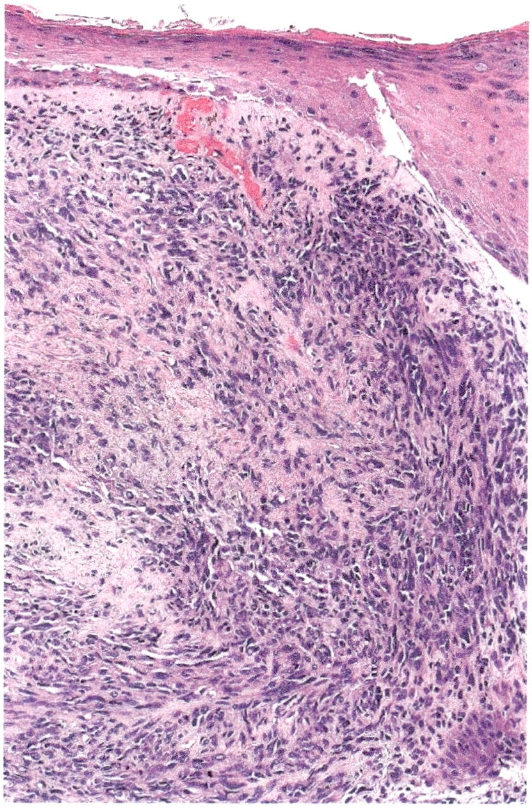

FIG. 14.141

Spindle cell angiosarcoma showing solid sheets of neoplastic cells with only subtle vasoformative architecture.

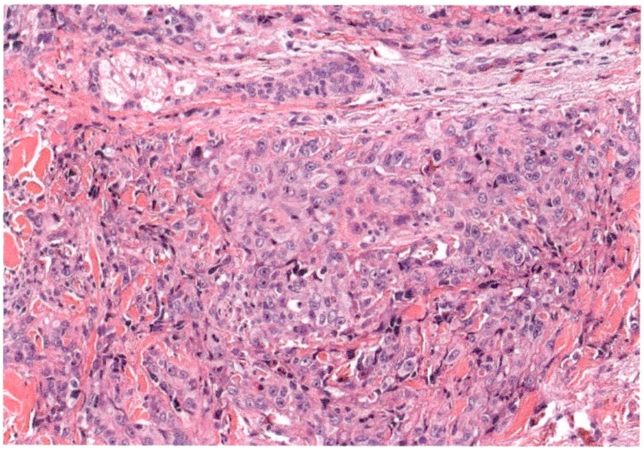

FIG. 14.142

Epithelioid angiosarcoma consists of round cells with relatively abundant cytoplasm mimicking carcinoma or melanoma.

angiosarcomas have the same range of histologic features as primary angiosarcoma. Two unusual histologic patterns have been described in cutaneous radiation-associated angiosarcoma of the breast: the so-called radiation dermatitis–like pattern and the capillary lobule pattern. The radiation dermatitis–like pattern is sparsely cellular with individual cells and noncomplex vessels recognized as malignant essentially only by cytologic atypia (Fig. 14.143A and B). The rare capillary lobule

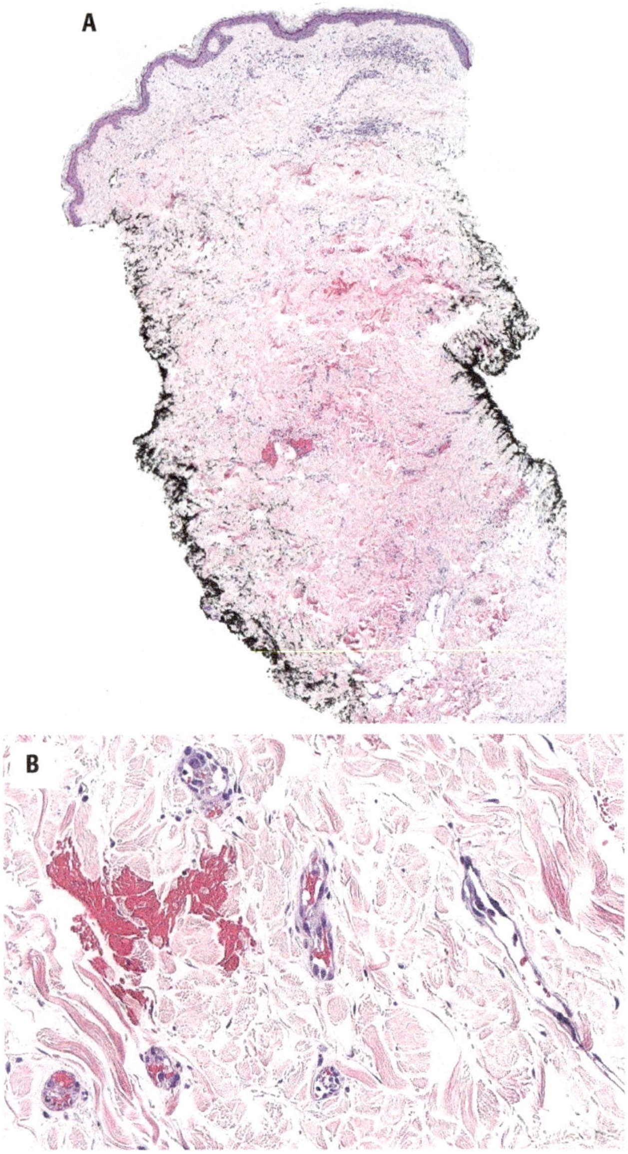

FIG. 14.143

Radiation dermatitis–like pattern of angiosarcoma. **A,** Very sparsely cellular lesion with mild chronic inflammatory infiltrate mimicking radiation dermatitis at scanning magnification. **B,** Noncomplex vessels recognized as malignant by marked cytologic atypia.

pattern shows distinct nodules of atypical vessels somewhat reminiscent of the cannonball pattern of TA.

Both sporadic and secondary angiosarcomas routinely express vascular markers CD31 and ERG. CD34 has lower sensitivity for angiosarcoma although it may be superior in the predominantly spindled examples. A notable pitfall is expression of CD31 by macrophages and sometimes T-lymphocytes. Expression of lymphoid markers podoplanin (D2-40) and PROX-1 is common. Epithelioid angiosarcomas can express cytokeratins, EMA, and CD30, sometimes quite impressively, presenting potential sources of diagnostic confusion. Unlike postradiation and lymphedema-associated angiosarcoma, primary cutaneous angiosarcoma is typically negative for MYC expression by IHC and *MYC* amplification by FISH.

Angiosarcomas are genomically complex tumors with heterogenous molecular alterations. Most sporadic tumors show alterations in angiogenesis-related pathways (*PTPRB, PLCG1, KDR, FLT4*) as well as *RAS, BRAF, TP53* mutations and *CDKN2A* deletions. *TP53* mutations are common in primary cutaneous angiosarcoma showing UV signature. A small subset of epithelioid angiosarcomas with aggressive behavior shows *CIC* gene alterations akin to those seen in *CIC*-rearranged round cell sarcomas. By contrast, more than 90% of radiation-associated angiosarcoma contain *MYC* amplification, which can be detected by FISH, chromogenic in situ hybridization, or by nuclear c-MYC expression by IHC.

Differential Diagnosis

For the clearly vasoformative tumors, the distinction from the benign vascular proliferations can be accomplished by the presence of complex vascular architecture, endothelial atypia, mitotic activity, and lack of pericytic investment. In sun-damaged skin, the index of suspicion for angiosarcoma should be high. Spindled and epithelioid nonvasoformative tumors need to be distinguished from sarcomatoid SCC and other poorly differentiated carcinomas, melanoma, AFX, and pleomorphic dermal sarcoma. Identification of the intratumoral hemorrhage and atypical vascular channels often present at the periphery of spindled or epithelioid angiosarcoma is very helpful. An important pitfall in this context is that angiosarcomas, particularly epithelioid angiosarcoma, can aberrantly express cytokeratins; however, expression of p40 and CK5/6 is uncharacteristic. The rest of the above differential diagnosis can be accomplished by application of vascular markers and melanocytic markers. The distinction between epithelioid angiosarcoma and proximal-type epithelioid sarcoma (both of which can be positive for cytokeratins and ERG) can be accomplished by concurrent expression of CD31 and retained nuclear INI-1 expression. The distinction from the postradiation AVL is discussed below.

Prognosis and Treatment

All angiosarcomas are aggressive neoplasms irrespective of the nuclear grade, with a high rate of local recurrence due to the notorious difficulty to achieve clear margins, and metastasis to lungs and lymph nodes. The overall survival rate in the range of 50% to 60%. Both primary and radiation-associated angiosarcomas are best treated by a multidisciplinary approach, with wide local excision remaining the mainstay of therapy.

RADIATION-INDUCED ATYPICAL VASCULAR LESION

Clinical Features

Postradiation AVLs occur in the radiation field on the skin of the breast in women treated with adjuvant radiation therapy for breast cancer. Like radiation-associated angiosarcoma, they may occur as early as one year to many years after treatment. AVLs manifest as small solitary or multiple (0.1–6 cm) skin-colored to erythematous papules, nodules, or crops of vesicles resembling cutaneous lymphatic malformations. This clinical picture is rather distinct from the appearance of cutaneous postradiation angiosarcoma in most cases, and this should be communicated to the dermatopathologist.

Histopathologic Features

AVLs are relatively well-circumscribed and symmetrical lesions with a wedge-shaped silhouette, usually confined to the papillary and superficial-to-mid reticular dermis. Subcutaneous extension is very rare. The superficial portion typically contains the more dilated lymphatic-type vascular spaces whereas in the deeper component, the vessels are compressed and may show a dissecting pattern between the collagen bundles. The vessels are lined by a single layer of endothelial cells. Some cases have papillary projections formed by the underlying stroma or slightly hyperchromatic hobnail endothelial cells resembling those seen in hobnail hemangioma (Fig. 14.144A and B). Complex dissecting growth pattern, endothelial multilayering, blood lakes, epithelioid morphology, and mitotic figures are entirely uncharacteristic and should prompt a consideration of angiosarcoma. By immunophenotype, AVLs are most often of lymphatic type, with expression of D2-40 and PROX-1. Unfortunately, precisely because of the lymphatic phenotype, AVLs often lack a well-defined pericytic layer—a generally reliable tool in separating benign vascular proliferations from angiosarcoma. Molecular studies showed infrequent *RAS* or *TERT* promoter alterations. Importantly, there is no *MYC* amplification and no MYC expression by IHC, with the caveat that intervening benign vascular channels or inflammatory cells may show sporadic focal staining.

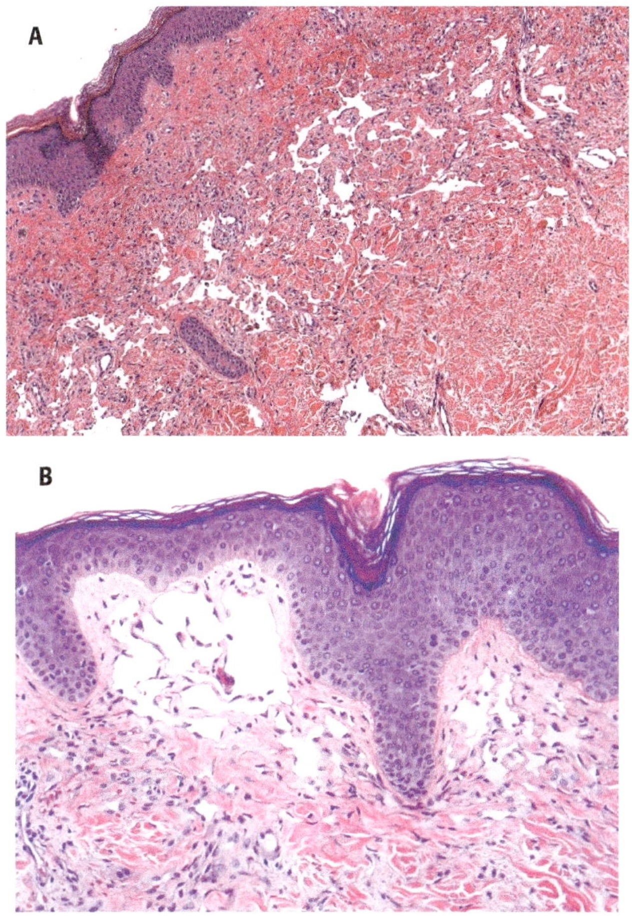

FIG. 14.144
Postradiation atypical vascular lesion. **A,** Symmetric lesions with a wedge-shaped silhouette confined to the papillary and superficial reticular dermis and composed of cytologically banal lymphatic channels. **B,** The deeper component may show compressed vessels with a somewhat dissecting pattern through the collagen bundles. Intravascular papillary projections or slightly hyperchromatic hobnail endothelial cells resembling those seen in hobnail hemangioma are present.

Differential Diagnosis

The principal differential diagnosis is with well-differentiated postradiation angiosarcoma. The relative circumscription of AVLs, bland cytology, and lack of multilayering typically allow distinction in most cases. However, the entire lesion needs to be visualized, particularly the base, before a diagnosis of AVL can be confidently made. Ancillary studies to detect *MYC* amplification or MYC expression are very useful with the caveat outlined above; difficult cases can be confirmed by *MYC* FISH.

Prognosis and Treatment

Clinically, AVLs are benign lesions and do not recur if completely excised. New AVLs can develop over time. Conservative excision is often recommended to ensure that the entire lesion is examined, and the area of concern should be monitored for the development of radiation-associated angiosarcoma.

TUMORS WITH CALCIFICATIONS, OSSEOUS, AND CARTILAGINOUS DIFFERENTIATION

Soft tissue tumors with FN-1 receptor tyrosine kinase fusions.

CALCIFYING APONEUROTIC FIBROMA

Clinical Features

CAF is a rare tumor of the distal extremities that occurs in association with aponeuroses, tendons, and fascia, typically in children and adolescents. It most commonly involves the palmer hands and fingers, followed by the plantar feet and toes, and less often the wrist or ankle. Rare examples have been reported proximal to this. The lesions present as a painless mass or swelling that grows slowly over time.

Histopathologic Features

Tumors are fairly circumscribed and arranged in heterologous lobules around irregular deposits of calcium. Lobules show zonal distribution of nodular, fibrocartilaginous calcified areas with palisaded epithelioid fibrohistiocytic cells, chondroid cells, and scattered osteoclast-like giant cells, surrounded by bland, infiltrative spindled cells in a fibrous stroma. The spindled cells are arranged in thin swirling fascicles and can have fibromatosis-like features. Staghorn-like vessels can be seen, and no significant cytologic atypia or mitoses are identified (Fig. 14.145A and B). They stain with SMA in a membranous myofibroblastic-like pattern, as well as CD99. S100 stains chondroid areas surrounding calcified areas. Tumors have been shown to harbor recurrent *FN1* gene fusions with RTK *EGF*.

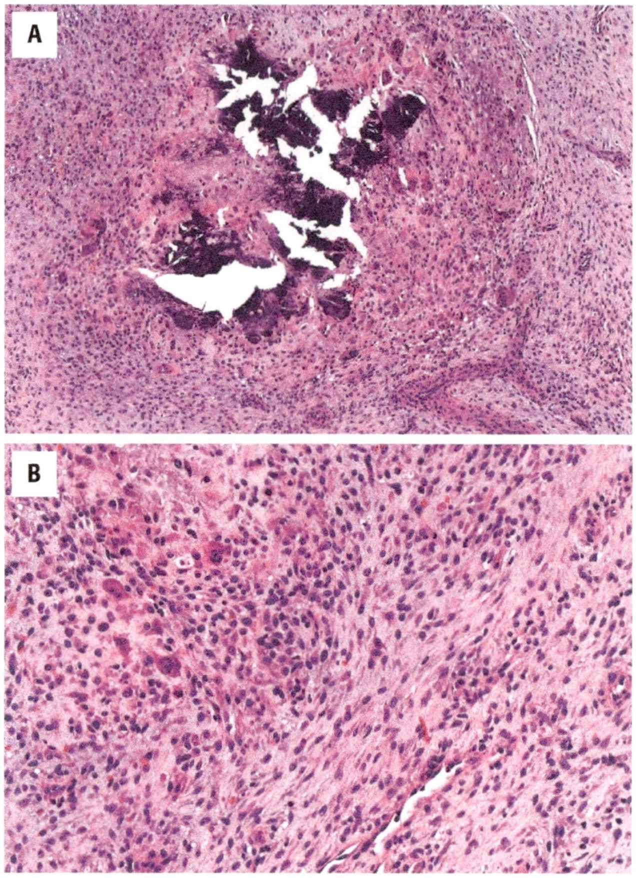

FIG. 14.145

Calcifying aponeurotic fibroma. **A,** Heterogenous cellular proliferation arranged around irregular deposits of calcium. **B,** Zonal distribution of nodular calcified areas containing palisaded epithelioid fibrohistiocytic cells, chondroid cells, and scattered osteoclast-like giant cells, surrounded by bland, infiltrative spindled cells in a fibrous stroma.

Differential Diagnosis

The main differential diagnoses are IBF, ganglion cyst, and schwannoma. IBF also occurs on the digits of children and shows bland spindled cells. However, calcium deposits are not identified, and characteristic intracytoplasmic inclusions are noted. Ganglion cysts are usually on the dorsal wrist. They are relatively more cystic and hypocellular. Schwannomas lack the heterologous cell types seen in CAF (spindled fibroblasts, epithelioid fibrohistiocytic cells, chondroid cells, and giant cells), although they also demonstrate variable cellularity and palisading. They stain diffusely for SOX10 and S100, which can be helpful to discriminate in small biopsies.

Prognosis and Treatment

CAF is benign, but can be locally aggressive, with a tendency to recur, due to its infiltrative nature. Complete excision is the treatment of choice.

SOFT TISSUE CHONDROMA

Clinical Features

Soft tissue chondromas occur in the hands and feet of adults typically.

Histopathologic Features

Tumors show a distinctive lobulated appearance at low power and comprise plump chondrocytic tumor cells with fine punctate or grungy calcification, focal fibrosis,

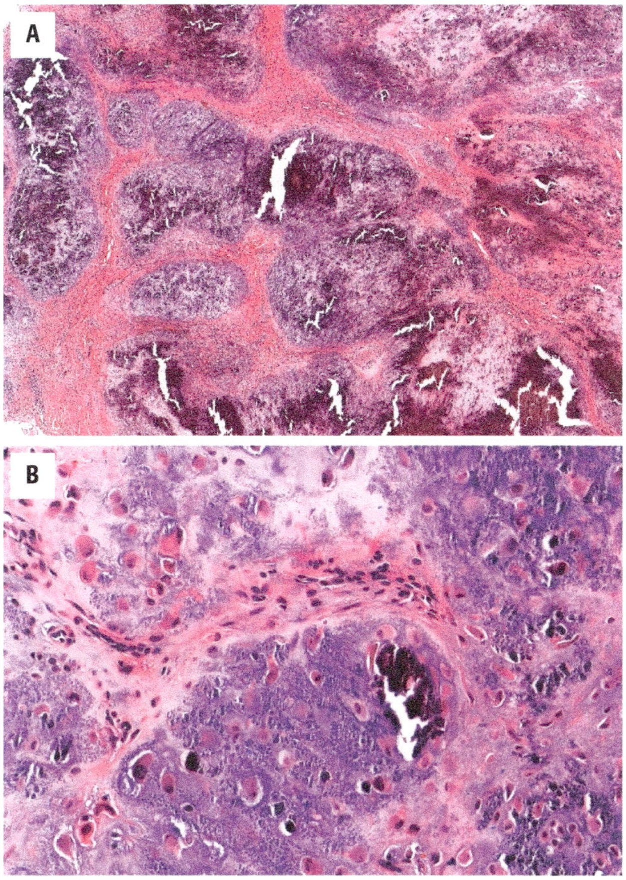

FIG. 14.146
Soft tissue chondroma. **A,** A circumscribed and lobulated appearance with grungy purple calcifications at low power. **B,** The lobules contain plump chondroid cells as well as focal fibrosis, and variable osteoclast-like giant cells and histiocyte-like cells. There is mild nuclear atypia; mitotic figures are rare.

and variable osteoclast-like giant cells, histiocyte-like cells, and vacuolated cells which can resemble lipoblasts. Nuclear hyperchromasia is common (Fig. 14.146A and B). *FN1* fusion to *FGFR1* or *FGFR2* has been described in soft tissue chondroma especially in cases showing dirty to lacy (chondroblastoma-like) calcification.

Differential Diagnosis

The differential diagnosis includes CAFs, synovial chondromatosis, and, rarely, myofibroma and chondrosarcoma. CAFs are relatively more infiltrative, with fascicles of plump spindled cells and coarsely clumped, hypocellular calcified regions. Synovial chondromatosis is a locally aggressive neoplasm composed of multiple nodules of hyaline cartilage, which may coalesce and present as an extraarticular soft tissue mass. However, synovial chondromatosis consists of pure hypocellular hyaline cartilage, which may undergo enchondral ossification or dystrophic calcifications, but it lacks the spindle cell component, histiocyte-like epithelioid cells, or the purple grungy calcifications seen in soft tissue chondroma. Synovial chondromatosis has a predilection for larger joints such as the knee and harbors *FN1::ACVR2A* fusion. Solitary myofibroma (descried above) may appear similar at scanning magnification, but these lesions do not contain grungy calcifications; rather, the similarity is due to the biphasic appearance of myofibroma with basophilic or palely eosinophilic nodules containing myoid spindle cells in a myxoid stroma that stand out against the background of nondescript primitive mesenchymal spindle cells and small HPC-like vessels. Chondrosarcomas rarely occur in the small tubular bones of hands and feet and can extend in the soft tissue; these tumors show an overt hyaline cartilage differentiation, high-grade nuclear features, and an infiltrative and destructive growth pattern. Grungy calcifications are uncharacteristic.

Prognosis and Treatment

Tumors are benign and treated with conservative excision.

FN1 alterations have been increasingly recognized in a variety of mesenchymal neoplasms with a predilection for hands and feet and an overlapping morphology, including chondroid differentiation, variable spindle, epithelioid or histiocytoid cells, osteoclast-type giant cells, and, most notably, distinctive blue or purple grungy or chicken wire calcifications. In addition to the CAF, soft tissue chondroma and synovial chondromatosis described above, this family of tumors includes phosphaturic mesenchymal tumor (PMT) characterized by *FN1::FGFR1* or *FN1::FGF1* fusions and overproduction of FGF23 leading to osteomalacia, chondroid tenosynovial giant cell tumor of the temporomandibular joint, calcium pyrophosphate dehydrate (CPPD) deposition disease (also known as pseudogout), and a recently delineated calcified chondroid mesenchymal neoplasm (CCMN). A detailed discussion of these rare entities is beyond the scope of this chapter.

OSTEOMA CUTIS

Clinical Features

Osteoma cutis presents as an asymptomatic solitary or multiple firm asymptomatic papules or plaques. Solitary osteoma cutis is by far the most common form and typically occurs as a reactive process in association with other conditions including trauma (foreign bodies, hematoma, puncture sites), inflammatory conditions such as diabetes mellitus, acne or morphea, or as a secondary ossification of cutaneous tumors such as pilomatrixoma, chondroid syringoma, soft tissue chondroma, or BCC. Multiple cutaneous osteomas are seen in Albright hereditary osteodystrophy.

Histopathologic Features

Osteoma cutis is a dermal nodule composed of mature bone, often with fatty marrow (Fig. 14.147). Osteoblastic rimming is rare except in Albright hereditary osteodystrophy.

The diagnosis of osteoma cutis does not pose diagnostic difficulty although recognition of the underlying lesion might be very important. Osteoma cutis does not typically have a significant woven bone component, cellularity, osteoclastic activity, cytologic atypia, or mitotic activity; accordingly, these findings should raise possibility of osteosarcoma (see below).

CUTANEOUS MANIFESTATIONS OF MALIGNANT MATRIX-FORMING NEOPLASMS

OSTEOSARCOMA

Osteosarcoma involving the skin is almost always seen in the setting of metastasis, heterologous osteosarcomatous differentiation in a (squamous cell) carcinoma, or an extension from the underlying bone (for example, on the scalp), although rare cases of primary cutaneous tumors have been reported. To qualify for the diagnosis, the tumor must contain overtly atypical spindle to epithelioid osteoblastic cells with pleomorphism and mitotic activity in association with lacelike immature malignant osteoid (Fig. 14.148A and B). A chondroblastic component of high histologic grade is often present (Fig. 14.148C). Understanding of the clinical presentation and recognition of an intraepithelial component and immunohistochemical stains for high-molecular-weight cytokeratins and p40 are helpful to distinguish osteosarcoma from sarcomatoid SCC because

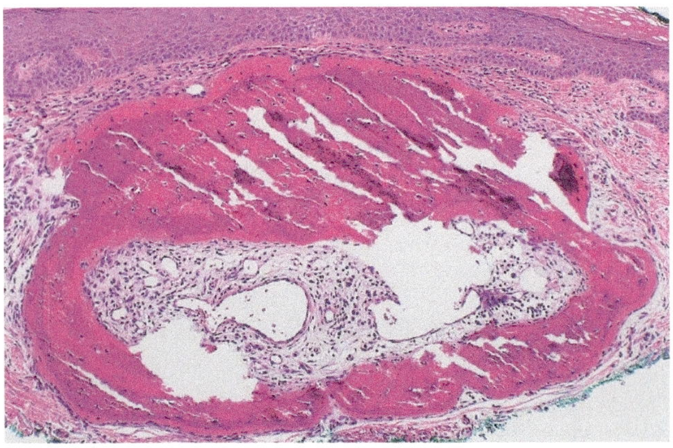

FIG. 14.147

Osteoma cutis presenting as a dermal nodule composed of mature woven to lamellar bone and fatty marrow.

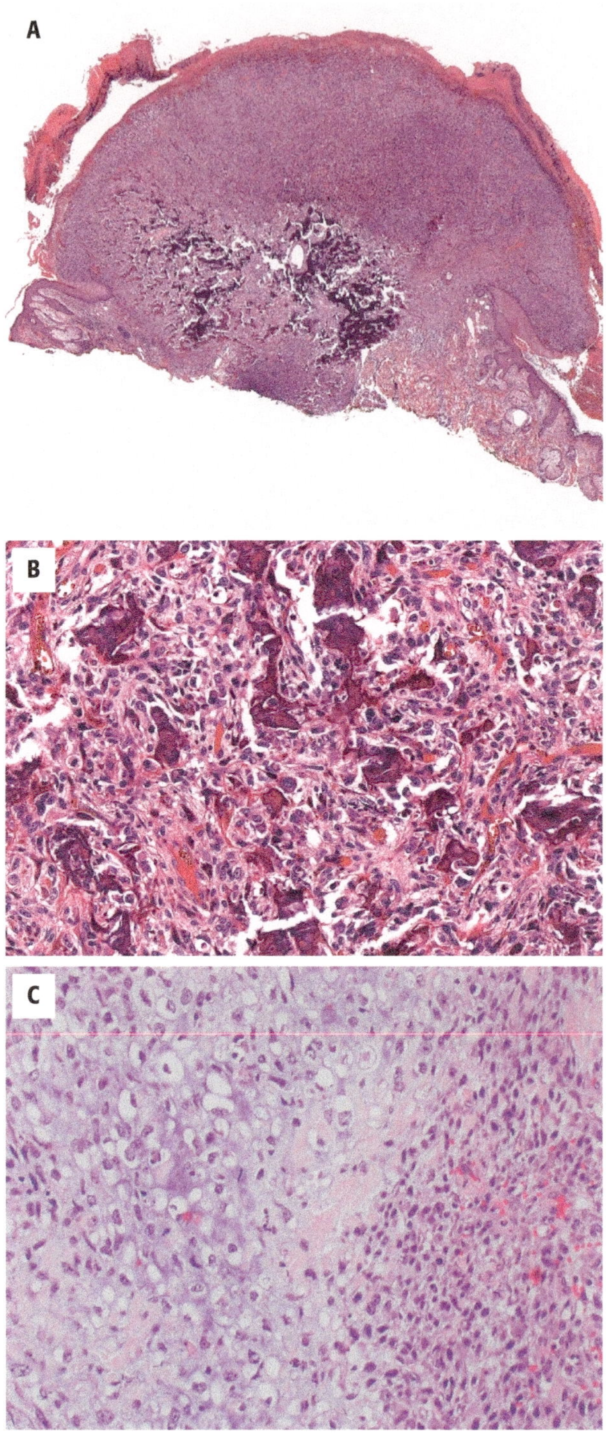

FIG. 14.148

Cutaneous osteosarcoma. **A,** A well-circumscribed densely cellular dermal nodule. **B,** Overtly atypical spindle to epithelioid osteoblastic cells with pleomorphism and mitotic activity in association with lacelike immature malignant osteoid. **C,** Chondroblastic osteosarcoma with a cartilaginous component of high histologic grade.

osteosarcoma is typically negative for these markers, although sporadic focal expression of low-molecular-weight cytokeratin may occur.

Prognosis and Treatment

Osteosarcoma, including primary osteosarcoma of the skin, is potentially aggressive with frequent metastasis to the lungs. Too few primary cutaneous osteosarcomas have been described to determine prognosis and the most effective treatment modalities; generally, an approach similar to that for extraskeletal osteosarcomas can be employed including a wide local excision with or without (neo)adjuvant chemotherapy.

CONVENTIONAL CHONDROSARCOMA

Cutaneous involvement of chondrosarcoma is almost exclusively seen in the setting of either metastasis or a direct extension from underlying deep soft tissue or bone mass. They typically manifest as subcutaneous nodules. Conventional chondrosarcoma consists of nodules of hyaline cartilage of varying histologic grade (Fig. 14.149). Dedifferentiated chondrosarcoma demonstrates a high-grade spindle cell or pleomorphic sarcoma component juxtaposed on the areas of conventional, typically low-grade chondrosarcoma. This contrasts with the chondroblastic osteosarcoma, where both components are typically high grade. The mutational profile of chondrosarcomas depends on the underlying etiology. Primary central chondrosarcomas most often contain alterations of *IDH1/2* genes, whereas those arising from a precursor osteochondroma or synovial chondromatosis may show *EXT1/2* or *FN-1* alterations. Molecular testing is rarely necessary for the diagnosis. Treatment for chondrosarcoma typically includes surgery/metastasectomy and this tumor is relatively resistant to chemotherapy and radiation therapy except in cases of dedifferentiated chondrosarcoma.

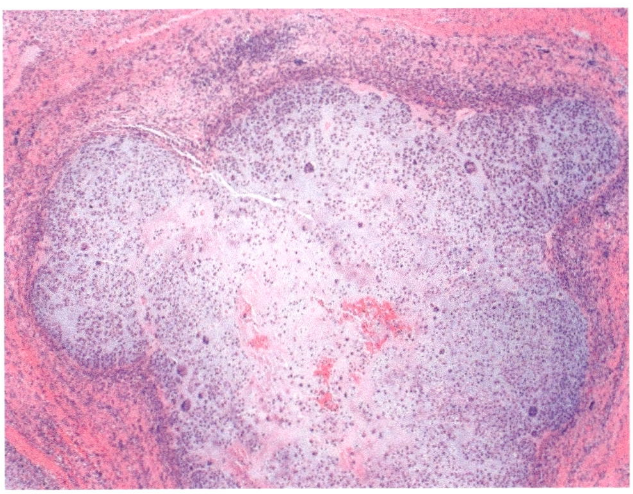

FIG. 14.149
Metastatic chondrosarcoma showing a well-circumscribed nodule of hyaline cartilage with increased cellularity and mild atypia.

CHORDOMA

Clinical Features

Chordomas occur in middle-age and older adults in the bones of axial skeleton, most commonly the sacrum followed by the sphenooccipital region. Chordomas present as a slowly growing mass causing chronic pain or symptoms related to compression of adjacent structures. Extraosseous/extraaxial chordomas are rare and often occur in the soft tissue in the vicinity of large joints or as intraarticular/intraosseous masses. Skin involvement typically represents a manifestation of metastatic disease or a locoregional recurrence.

Histopathologic Features

Chordomas consist of nests or cords of epithelioid cells with round or oval nucleus and abundant pale vacuolated cytoplasm (so-called physaliphorous cells) in a diffusely myxoid stroma (Fig. 14.150A and B). Conventional chordoma has low-grade nuclear atypia and scant mitotic activity. Poorly differentiated chordoma, often occurring in pediatric patients or young adults, is associated with rhabdoid morphology, high-grade nuclear features, and *SMARCB1/INI-1* deletions; similar features have also been observed in extraosseous chordomas. Dedifferentiated chordoma consists of a high-grade spindle cell or pleomorphic sarcoma juxtaposed on the low-grade conventional chordoma precursor. By IHC, chordomas coexpress low-molecular-weight cytokeratins, EMA, S100, and show characteristic expression of notochord marker brachyury. Dedifferentiated component may lose brachyury or cytokeratin expression. Poorly differentiated chordomas show a loss of INI-1.

Differential Diagnosis

Chordoma needs to be distinguished from chondrosarcoma, chondroid syringoma (mixed tumor of the

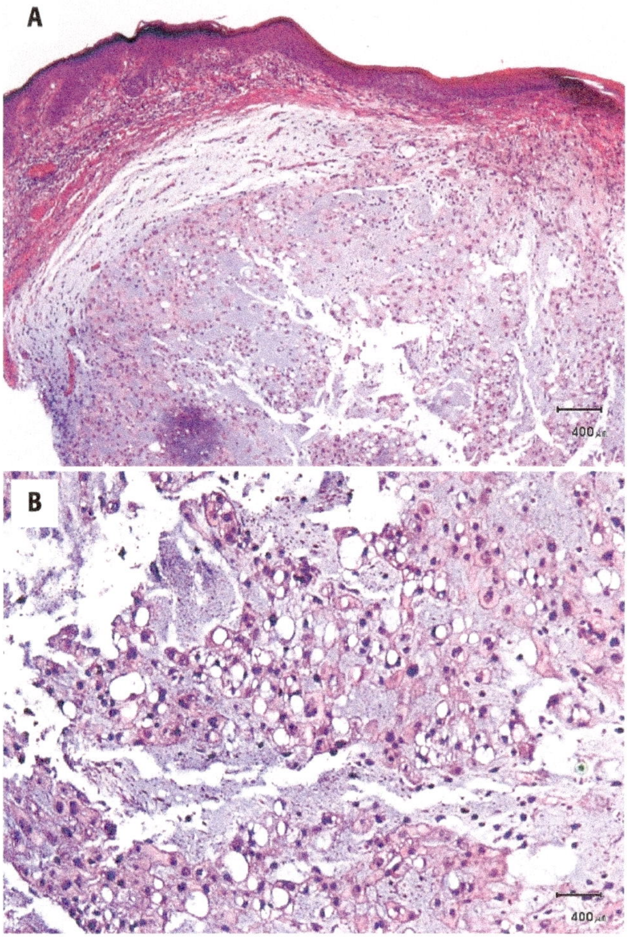

FIG. 14.150

Metastatic chordoma. **A,** A modestly cellular chondromyxoid nodule is present in the dermis. **B,** The nodule is composed of large epithelioid cells with vacuolated cytoplasm (physaliphorous cells) and relatively low-grade nuclei. Mitotic activity is inconspicuous.

skin), and metastatic mucinous carcinoma. In the absence of the classic physaliferous appearance or relevant history suggesting metastatic disease, immunostaining for brachyury is very helpful as it is positive in chordomas and absent in their mimics, even if other immunostains (cytokeratins, S100) can be expressed in all of these lesions.

Prognosis and Treatment

Surgery is the treatment of choice; however, the rates of local recurrence are very high. Resectability with a negative margin remains the most important prognostic factor for conventional chordoma. Poorly differentiated and dedifferentiated chordomas behave very aggressively. The role of radiation and chemotherapy in this disease is very limited.

SUGGESTED FURTHER READING

Agaram, N. P. (2022). Evolving classification of rhabdomyosarcoma. *Histopathology, 80*(1), 98–108.

Agaram, N. P., Zhang, L., Jungbluth, A. A., Dickson, B. C., & Antonescu, C. R. (2020). A molecular reappraisal of glomus tumors and related pericytic neoplasms with emphasis on NOTCH-gene fusions. *American Journal of Surgical Pathology, 44*(11), 1556–1562.

Agaram, N. P., Zhang, L., Sung, Y. S., Chen, C. L., Chung, C. T., Antonescu, C. R., & Fletcher, C. D. (2016). Recurrent *NTRK1* gene fusions define a novel subset of locally aggressive lipofibromatosis-like neural tumors. *American Journal of Surgical Pathology, 40*(10), 1407–1416.

Antonescu, C. R., Dickson, B. C., Sung, Y. S., Zhang, L., Suurmeijer, A. J. H., Stenzinger, A., Mechtersheimer, G., & Fletcher, C. D. M. (2020). Recurrent YAP1 and MAML2 gene rearrangements in retiform and composite hemangioendothelioma. *American Journal of Surgical Pathology, 44*(12), 1677–1684.

Antonescu, C. R., Sung, Y. S., Zhang, L., Agaram, N. P., & Fletcher, C. D. (2017). Recurrent SRF-RELA fusions define a novel subset of cellular myofibroma/myopericytoma: A potential diagnostic pitfall with sarcomas with myogenic differentiation. *American Journal of Surgical Pathology, 41*(5), 677–684.

Cellier, L., Perron, E., Pissaloux, D., Karanian, M., Haddad, V., Alberti, L., & de la Fouchardière, A. (2018). Cutaneous melanocytoma with CRTC1-TRIM11 fusion: Report of 5 cases resembling clear cell sarcoma. *American Journal of Surgical Pathology, 42*(3), 382–391.

Dachy, G., de Krijger, R. R., Fraitag, S., Théate, I., Brichard, B., Hoffman, S. B., Libbrecht, L., Arts, F. A., Brouillard, P., Vikkula, M., Limaye, N., & Demoulin, J. B. (2019). Association of PDGFRB mutations with pediatric myofibroma and myofibromatosis. *JAMA Dermatology, 155*(8), 946–950.

de la Fouchardiere, A., Pissaloux, D., Tirode, F., Karanian, M., Fletcher, C. D. M., & Hanna, J. (2021). Clear cell tumor with melanocytic differentiation and ACTIN-MITF translocation: Report of 7 cases of a novel entity. *American Journal of Surgical Pathology, 45*(7), 962–968.

Dermawan, J. K., Azzato, E. M., Goldblum, J. R., Rubin, B. P., Billings, S. D., & Ko, J. S. (2021). Superficial ALK-rearranged myxoid spindle cell neoplasm: A cutaneous soft tissue tumor with distinctive morphology and immunophenotypic profile. *Modern Pathology, 34*(9), 1710–1718.

Doyle, L. A., Mariño-Enriquez, A., Fletcher, C. D., & Hornick, J. L. (2015). ALK rearrangement and overexpression in epithelioid fibrous histiocytoma. *Modern Pathology, 28*(7), 904–912.

Fetsch, J. F., Miettinen, M., Laskin, W. B., Michal, M., & Enzinger, F. M. (2000). A clinicopathologic study of 45 pediatric soft tissue tumors with an admixture of adipose tissue and fibroblastic elements, and a proposal for classification as lipofibromatosis. *American Journal of Surgical Pathology, 24*(11), 1491–1500.

Huang, S. C., Zhang, L., Sung, Y. S., Chen, C. L., Krausz, T., Dickson, B. C., Kao, Y. C., Agaram, N. P., Fletcher, C. D., & Antonescu, C. R. (2015). Frequent FOS gene rearrangements in epithelioid hemangioma: A molecular study of 58 cases with morphologic reappraisal. *American Journal of Surgical Pathology, 39*(10), 1313–1321.

Iwamura, R., Komatsu, K., Kusano, M., Kubo, C., Inaba, Y., Shiba, E., Nawata, A., Tajiri, R., Matsuyama, A., Matoba, H., Koga, K., Takeda, M., Itami, H., & Hisaoka, M. (2023). PDGFRB and NOTCH3 Mutations are detectable in a wider range of pericytic tumors, including myopericytomas, angioleiomyomas, glomus tumors, and their combined tumors. *Modern Pathology, 36*(3), 100070.

Jo, V. Y., Antonescu, C. R., Dickson, B. C., Swanson, D., Zhang, L., Fletcher, C. D. M., & Demicco, E. G. (2019). Cutaneous syncytial myoepithelioma is characterized by recurrent EWSR1-PBX3 fusions. *American Journal of Surgical Pathology, 43*(10), 1349–1354.

Jo, V. Y., Antonescu, C. R., Zhang, L., Dal Cin, P., Hornick, J. L., & Fletcher, C. D. (2013). Cutaneous syncytial myoepithelioma: Clinicopathologic characterization in a series of 38 cases. *American Journal of Surgical Pathology, 37*(5), 710–718.

Kao, Y. C., Suurmeijer, A. J. H., Argani, P., Dickson, B. C., Zhang, L., Sung, Y. S., Agaram, N. P., Fletcher, C. D. M., & Antonescu, C. R. (2020). Soft tissue tumors characterized by a wide spectrum of kinase fusions share a lipofibromatosis-like neural tumor pattern. *Genes Chromosomes & Cancer, 59*(10), 575–583.

Ko, J. S., Marusic, Z., Azzato, E. M., Farkas, D. H., Van Arnam, J., Seiwerth, S., Fritchie, K., Patel, R. M., Rubin, B. P., & Billings, S. D.

(2020). Superficial sarcomas with CIC rearrangement are aggressive neoplasms: A series of eight cases. *Journal of Cutaneous Pathology*, *47*(6), 509–516.

Libbrecht, S., Van Dorpe, J., & Creytens, D. (2021). The rapidly expanding group of *RB1*-deleted soft tissue tumors: An updated review. *Diagnostics (Basel, Switzerland)*, *11*(3), 430.

Liu, Y. J., Wang, W., Yeh. J., Wu, Y., Mantilla, J. G., Fletcher, C. D. M., Ricciotti, R. W., & Chen, E. Y. (2021). Calcified chondroid mesenchymal neoplasms with FN1-receptor tyrosine kinase gene fusions including FGFR2, FGFR1, MERTK, NTRK1, and TEK: A molecular and clinicopathologic analysis. *Modern Pathology*, *34*(7), 1373–1383.

Llamas-Velasco, M., Itlinger-Monshi, B., Flucke, U., & Mentzel, T. (2022). Dermal lipofibromatosis-like neural tumor. *Journal of Cutaneous Pathology*, *49*(6), 525–531.

Nihous, H., Baud, J., Azmani, R., Michot, A., Perret, R., Mayeur, L., de Pinieux, G., Milin, S., Angot, E., Duquenne, S., Geneste, D., Lucchesi, C., Le Loarer, F., & Bouvier, C. (2022). Clinicopathologic and molecular study of hybrid nerve sheath tumors reveals their common association with fusions involving VGLL3. *American Journal of Surgical Pathology*, *46*(5), 591–602.

Papke, D. J., Jr, Al-Ibraheemi, A., & Fletcher, C. D. M. (2020). Plexiform myofibroblastoma: Clinicopathologic analysis of 36 cases of a distinctive benign tumor of soft tissue affecting mainly children and young adults. *American Journal of Surgical Pathology*, *44*(11), 1469–1478.

Perez-Atayde, A. R., Debelenko, L., Al-Ibraheemi, A., Eng, W., Ruiz-Gutierrez, M., O'Hare, M., Croteau, S. E., Trenor, C. C., 3rd, Boyer, D., Balkin, D. M., Barclay, S. F., Hsi Dickie, B., Liang, M. G., Chaudry, G., Alomari, A. I., Mulliken, J. B., Adams, D. M., Kurek, K. C., Fishman, S. J., & Kozakewich, H. P. W. (2022). Kaposiform lymphangiomatosis: Pathologic aspects in 43 patients. *American Journal of Surgical Pathology*, *46*(7), 963–976.

Thangaiah, J. J., Dashti, N. K., Agaimy, A., Fritchie, K., & Folpe, A. L. (2022). Plexiform fibrohistiocytic tumor: A clinicopathological and immunohistochemical study of 39 tumors, with evidence for a CSF1-producing "null cell" population. *Virchows Archiv: An International Journal of Pathology*, *481*(5), 739–750.

WHO Classification of Tumours International Agency for Research on Cancer. *Soft tissue and bone tumors* (5th ed.). Lyon: 2020.

15 Hematopoietic Neoplasms

Klaus J. Busam • Melissa P. Pulitzer

Hematopoietic neoplasms are dysregulated and/or neoplastic growths of the cells that make up the primary, secondary, and tertiary lymphoid organs of the immune system and cellular components of blood. Immune cells in the skin may exist as "innate" (skin-derived constituent) cells or adaptive (skin-homing/visiting) cells. Hence, hematopoietic neoplasms that are primary to the skin compartment are believed to develop in place from either skin resident or skin-homing precursor cells. Hematopoietic neoplasms that arise outside of the skin from any primary (bone marrow, thymus), secondary (lymph node, spleen), or tertiary (gut mucosa, tonsils, respiratory mucosa) lymphoid organs may also involve the skin. For historical purposes, certain histiocytic and dendritic cell neoplasia are described separately in a chapter on histiocytoses.

This chapter deals predominantly with primary cutaneous B- and T-cell lymphomas, that is, tumors of B and T cells that initially or primarily affect the skin, and reactive lymphoid infiltrates, which may simulate a lymphoma (so-called pseudolymphoma). Later sections of this chapter also address secondary cutaneous B- and T-cell lymphomas, that is, lymphomas that originate from an extracutaneous site and affect the skin, as well as hematopoietic infiltrates derived from nonlymphoid lineages that involve the skin.

Lymphomas and Lymphoproliferative Disorders Discussed in This Chapter

Primary Cutaneous T-Cell Lymphoma/Lymphoproliferative Disorders

- Mycosis fungoides and its variants
- Lymphomatoid papulosis
- Primary cutaneous anaplastic large cell lymphoma
- Subcutaneous panniculitis–like T-cell lymphoma
- CD8+ aggressive epidermotropic cytotoxic T-cell lymphoma
- CD4+ small or medium T-cell lymphoproliferative disorder
- Acral CD8+ T-cell lymphoproliferative disorder
- Primary cutaneous γδ T-cell lymphoma
- Primary cutaneous peripheral T-cell lymphoma, NOS

Secondary Cutaneous T-Cell Lymphoma

- Adult T-cell leukemia/lymphoma
- Extranodal natural killer T-cell lymphoma
- Hydroa vacciniforme-like lymphoma
- Angioimmunoblastic T-cell lymphoma
- Peripheral T-cell lymphoma, NOS

Primary Cutaneous B-Cell Lymphoma

- Marginal zone lymphoma
- Follicle center lymphoma
- Diffuse large B-cell lymphoma (DLBCL), leg type

Secondary Cutaneous B-Cell Neoplasms

- EBV-associated DLBCL
- Intravascular large B-cell lymphoma
- Lymphomatoid granulomatosis
- Other germinal center, high-grade, postgerminal center DLBCL
- Cutaneous (extraosseous) plasma cell neoplasm
- Mantle cell lymphoma
- Chronic lymphocytic leukemia

CUTANEOUS LYMPHOMAS AND BENIGN MIMICS

Cutaneous lymphomas may behave in an indolent fashion and remain limited to the skin in their disease manifestation. Indeed, in most recent edition of the World Health Organization (WHO) fascicle on *Haematolymphoid Tumours* and *Skin Tumours*, select indolent lymphomas were renamed "lymphoproliferative disorders" (LPDs) to reflect their usually indolent self-limited course. These LPDs can sometimes be pathologically indistinguishable from reactive infiltrates with clinically known inflammatory etiologies (so-called "pseudolymphomas"). However, there are also categorically aggressive types of cutaneous lymphomas that are likely to progress to involve extracutaneous sites and that are often lethal, separating them from the most common intermediate prognosis lymphomas that tend to recur and/or progress through therapy with a high disease-specific survival. The nomenclature used in this chapter mainly adheres to the 5th edition of the *World Health Organization Classification of Tumours – Haematolymphoid Tumours*, synchronized with the 4th edition of the *Skin Tumour* classification.

CUTANEOUS T-CELL LYMPHOMA

The majority (≈80%) of primary skin lymphomas are cutaneous T-cell lymphomas (CTCLs) which have an incidence of approximately 8 per million as per

United States Surveillance, Epidemiology, and End Results (SEER) registry data, including entities denoted as cutaneous LPDs. Different types of CTCLs/LPDs are recognized by distinct clinical and pathologic features. The most common type of CTCL is mycosis fungoides (MF). The CD30+ CTCL/LPDs including anaplastic large cell lymphoma (ALCL), lymphomatoid papulosis (LyP), and intermediate "borderline" cases, in addition to the primary cutaneous CD4+ small or medium T-cell lymphoproliferative, are more common compared to other non-MF CTCLs (5%–9% vs. less than 1%). The diagnosis of CTCL can be confounded by overlap in pathophysiology and presentation with benign inflammatory dermatosis and may be stalled by the presence of other immune deficiency–related neoplasms including solid tumors which commonly co-occur.

T-Cell Neoplasms Involving Skin

Usually Indolent Clinical Behavior
- Mycosis fungoides (MF): patch and plaque stage
  - Pagetoid reticulosis (localized disease)
  - Folliculotropic MF, early stage
  - Hypopigmented MF
- Primary cutaneous CD30+ T-cell lymphoproliferative disorders
  - CD30+ anaplastic large cell lymphoma
  - Lymphomatoid papulosis
- Subcutaneous panniculitis–like T-cell lymphoma
- Primary cutaneous CD4+ small or medium T-cell lymphoproliferative disorder
- Primary cutaneous acral CD8+ T-cell lymphoproliferative disorder

Aggressive Clinical Behavior
- Mycosis fungoides (MF), tumor stage, with and without large cell transformation
- Primary cutaneous CD8+ aggressive epidermotropic cytotoxic T-cell lymphoma
- Cutaneous γδ T-cell lymphoma

T-Cell Lymphomas with Both Extracutaneous and Skin Disease
- Sézary syndrome
- Adult T-cell leukemia/lymphoma
- Extranodal NK/T-cell lymphoma, nasal type
- T-lymphoblastic and T-prolymphocytic lymphoma
- Angioimmunoblastic T-cell lymphoma/peripheral T-cell lymphoma, NOS
- Hydroa vacciniforme-like lymphoma

PRIMARY CUTANEOUS T-CELL LYMPHOMA

MYCOSIS FUNGOIDES

Clinical Findings

MF accounts for approximately 70% of CTCL cases in the SEER data from 1973 to 2002. The annual age-adjusted incidence rate of MF has been reported to be approximately 6 per 1 million persons. MF is more commonly seen in men than women. It usually affects adults but may be seen in teens and rarely in children. The typical clinical presentation is that of persistent patches with a slight scale or a wrinkled surface. It is often accompanied by pruritus. The lesions may be pink to flesh-colored, hyperpigmented or hypopigmented, and have round to oval or annular morphology (Figs. 15.1–15.4). Spontaneous resolution and/or expansion of areas may result in bizarre and arcuate to polycyclic shapes (Fig. 15.5). Lesions may be atrophic (Fig. 15.6) and associated with variegated color and telangiectasia (poikiloderma vasculare atrophicans–like appearance) or they may be purpuric (Fig. 15.7). As the disease progresses, plaque

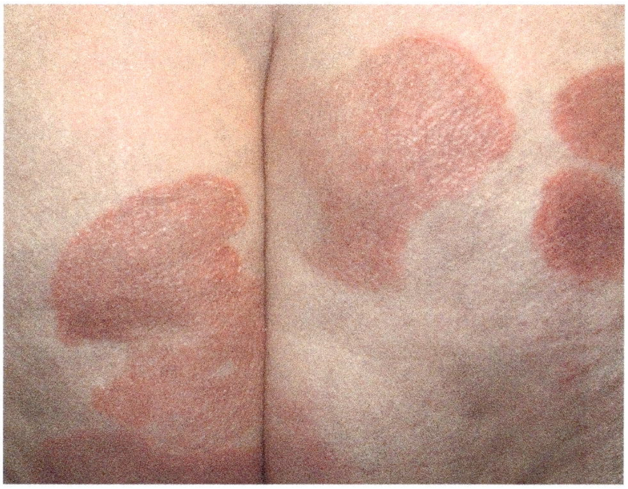

FIG. 15.1
Erythematous patch lesions of mycosis fungoides.

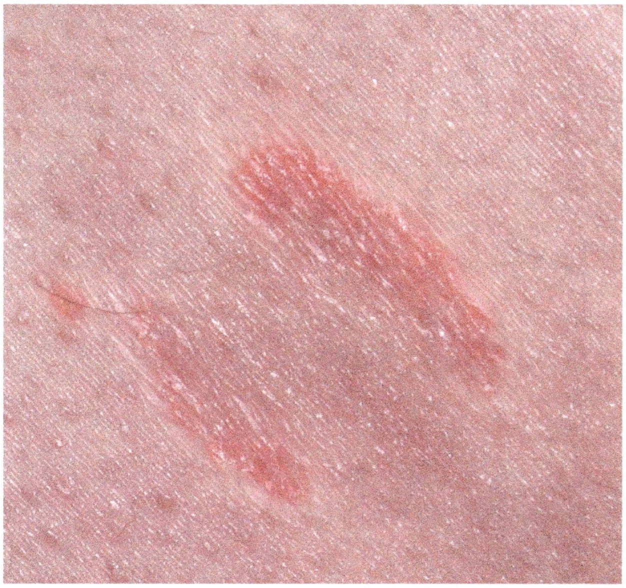

FIG. 15.2
Annular lesion of mycosis fungoides.

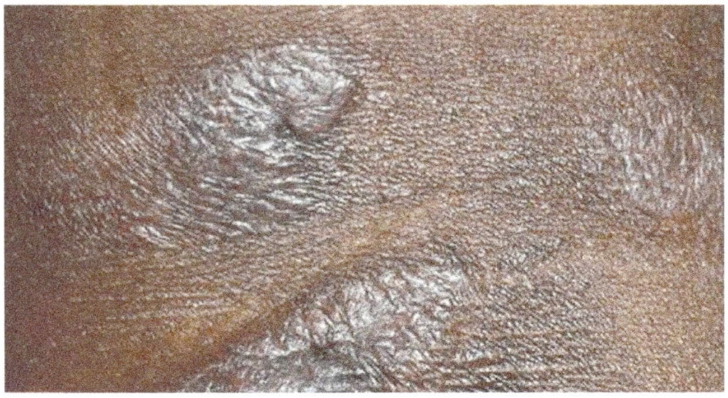

FIG. 15.3
Plaque lesion of mycosis fungoides.

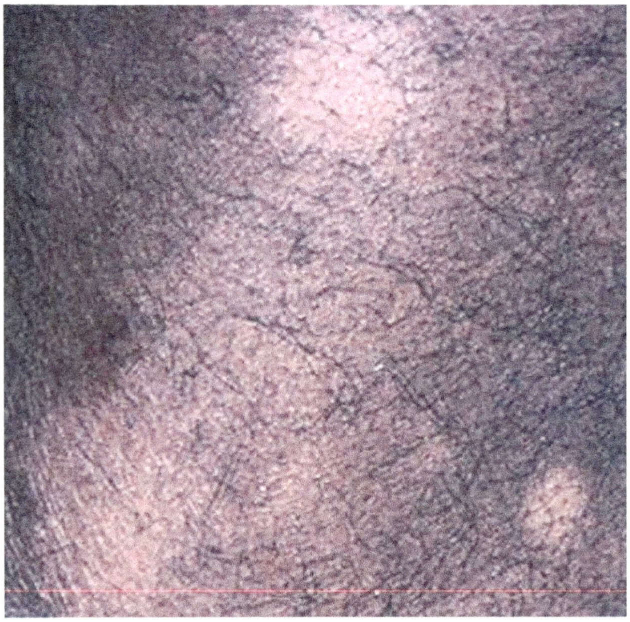

FIG. 15.4
Hypopigmented patches of mycosis fungoides.

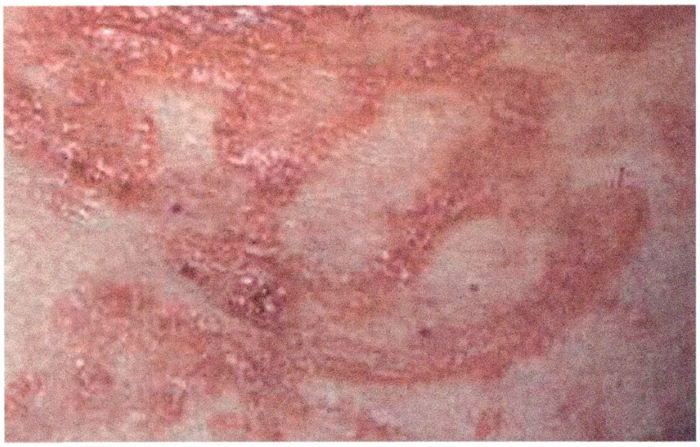

FIG. 15.5
Polycyclic lesion of mycosis fungoides.

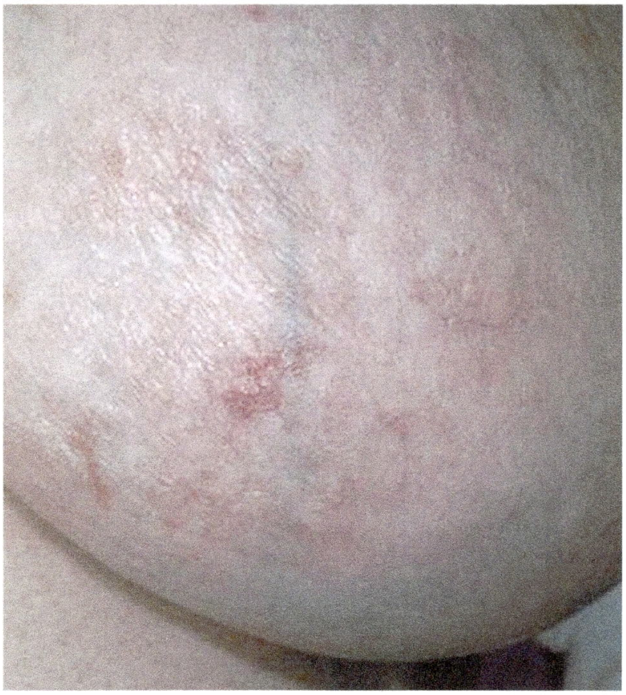

FIG. 15.6
Atrophic mycosis fungoides.

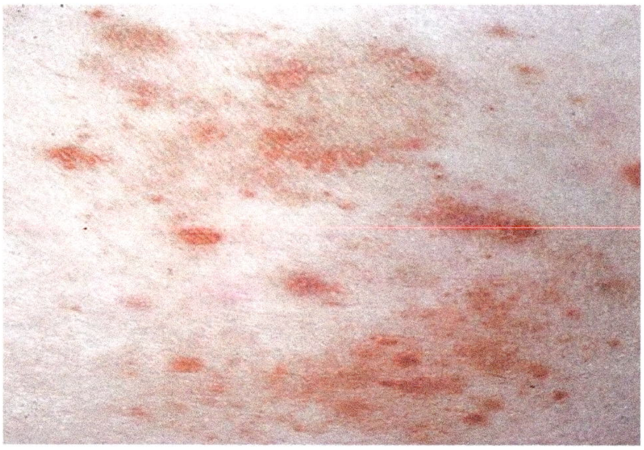

FIG. 15.7
Pigmented purpuric mycosis fungoides.

and tumor lesions may develop. MF may also manifest as erythroderma.

Patch and plaque lesions of MF tend to affect double-covered sites or follow a bathing trunk distribution (hip, buttock, groin, and breast). However, axillary or periaxillary and truncal lesions are also common. Some patients have persistent isolated patches only, but more commonly, the eruption progresses to a combination of generalized patches and plaques. A spectrum of different clinical phenotypes (patches, plaques, or tumors of variable size and shape) may be seen simultaneously. In advanced disease, lymph nodes, the peripheral blood, and less frequently visceral organs may be involved by lymphoma.

Several clinical variants of patch lesions of MF have been described. *Hypopigmented MF* (see Fig. 15.4) is typically seen in patients with darker skin tones but is also a common presentation in children and adolescents. It should be distinguished from pityriasis alba,

MYCOSIS FUNGOIDES—DISEASE FACT SHEET

Patient Group

- Typically adult patients in sixth decade of life
- Male-to-female ratio of 1.6 to 2 : 1

Site of Involvement

- May occur anywhere but preferentially affects bathing trunk (sun-protected) areas

Clinical Findings

- Erythematous wrinkled, atrophic, or scaly patches
- Indurated plaques and tumors, which may be ulcerated
- Papules based around hair follicles are the most common clinical variant (folliculotropic)
- Pruritus common
- Unresponsive to topical therapies attempted for inflammatory dermatoses
- Unusual variants: hypopigmented; palmoplantar; pigmented purpuric, poikilodermatous; bullous; guttate, verrucous, ichthyosiform, unilesional

Staging

- Stage I: skin involvement only
  - T1: less than 10% of body surface area involved; no tumor lesions
  - T2: greater than or equal to 10% of body surface area involved; no tumor lesions
  - T3: presence of tumor lesion(s) greater than or equal to 10 mm in diameter
- Stage II
  - IIa: T1 to T2 and clinically abnormal lymph nodes, histopathology Dutch grades 1 to 2
  - IIb: T3 and any node status
- Stage III: generalized erythroderma (T4: greater than or equal to 80% skin surface involved)
  - May or may not have nodal or low blood tumor burden
- Stage IV: any T with one of:
  - Abnormal lymph nodes with Dutch grades 3 to 4 histology (N3)
  - Pathologically confirmed nodal or visceral involvement (M1)
  - High blood tumor burden (Sézary count >1000/mL)

Prognosis

- Often protracted indolent course for stage I
- Poor prognosis for stage IV

Treatment

- Topical steroids, PUVA, radiation, nitrogen mustard for skin lesions
- Chemotherapy or biologic response modifiers for stage IIb to IV disease
- Allogeneic hematopoietic stem cell transplantation

PUVA, Psoralen and ultraviolet A.

vitiligo, and other causes of hypopigmentation. In *MF palmaris et plantaris* (*palmoplantar MF*), the lesions are hyperkeratotic; concentrated on acral sites, especially the palms and soles; and may simulate a keratoderma. The *pigmented purpura variant* of MF is characterized by cayenne pepper–colored or purpuric macules and patches (Fig. 15.7). Such lesions may be indistinguishable from benign pigmented purpuric dermatosis. MF should be considered if there are multiple purpuric lesions on the buttock or sites other than the lower extremities. Smaller papulosquamous lesions simulating small plaque parapsoriasis or pityriasis lichenoides represent less common variants of MF. Rarely, *bullous* lesions of MF can be seen in a background of patch and plaque lesions. Bullous MF may arise with or without a background of classic MF lesions or may be targetoid in appearance, simulating erythema multiforme. *Papuloerythroderma of Ofuji* is a variant of MF characterized by erythematous, flat-topped, coalescent papules, with erythroderma-like aspects over the chest, abdomen, and limbs, sparing the skin folds of the trunk and pressure areas (deck-chair sign).

Histopathologic Features

An infiltrate of morphologically atypical small- to intermediate-sized lymphocytes, which tend to be located along or within the epidermis (*epidermotropism*), is characteristic of MF. In a classic early patch or plaque lesion of MF, lymphocytes infiltrate the epidermis where they may or may not form small intraepidermal aggregates known as *Pautrier microabscesses*. A mixture of neoplastic and reactive lymphocytes extend below the epidermis in a bandlike (lichenoid) or superficial perivascular pattern (Fig. 15.8). The epidermis may show psoriasiform hyperplasia with hyperkeratosis and parakeratosis in a lenticular distribution (Fig. 15.9A). A common aspect of epidermotropism is the presence of solitary lymphocytes aligned along the dermal-epidermal junction

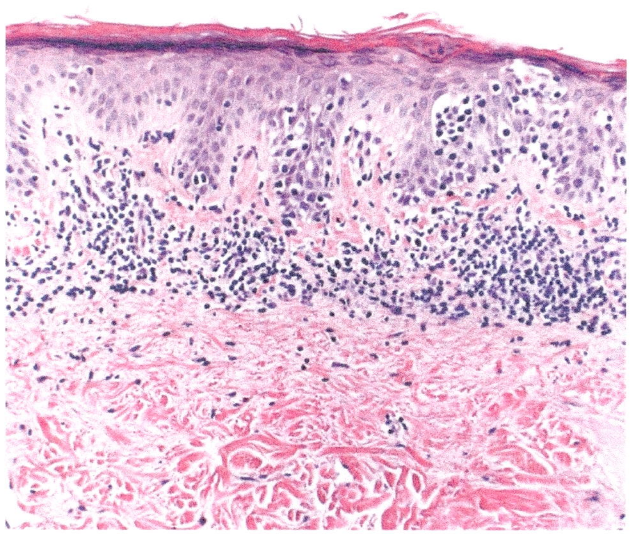

FIG. 15.8

Mycosis fungoides. Lichenoid pattern with atypical epidermotropic lymphocytes and Pautrier's microabscesses.

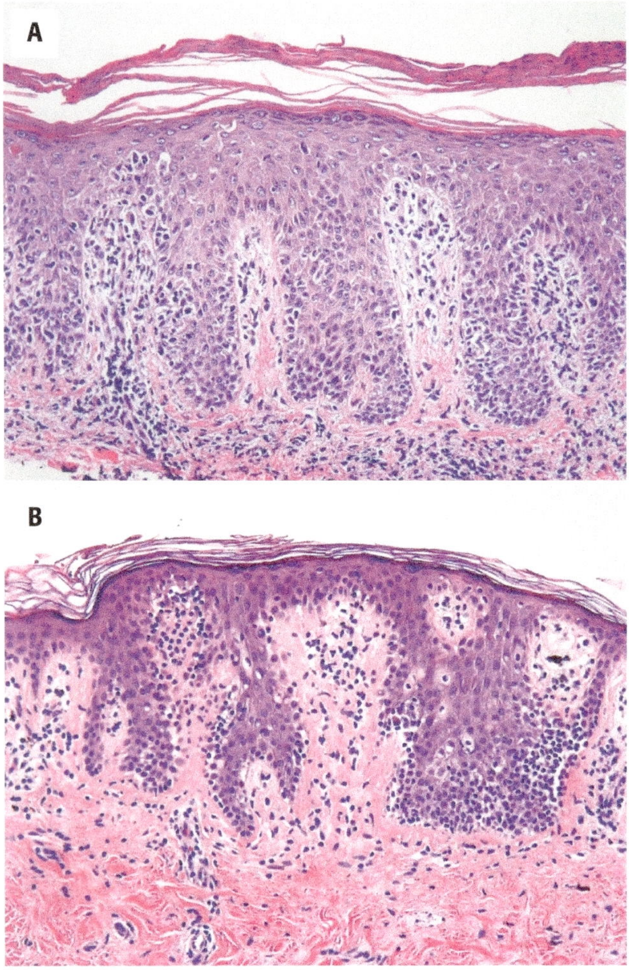

FIG. 15.9

Mycosis fungoides. **A,** Psoriasiform pattern with atypical epidermotropic lymphocytes. **B,** Hyperchromatic lymphocytes are peppered along elongated rete ridges.

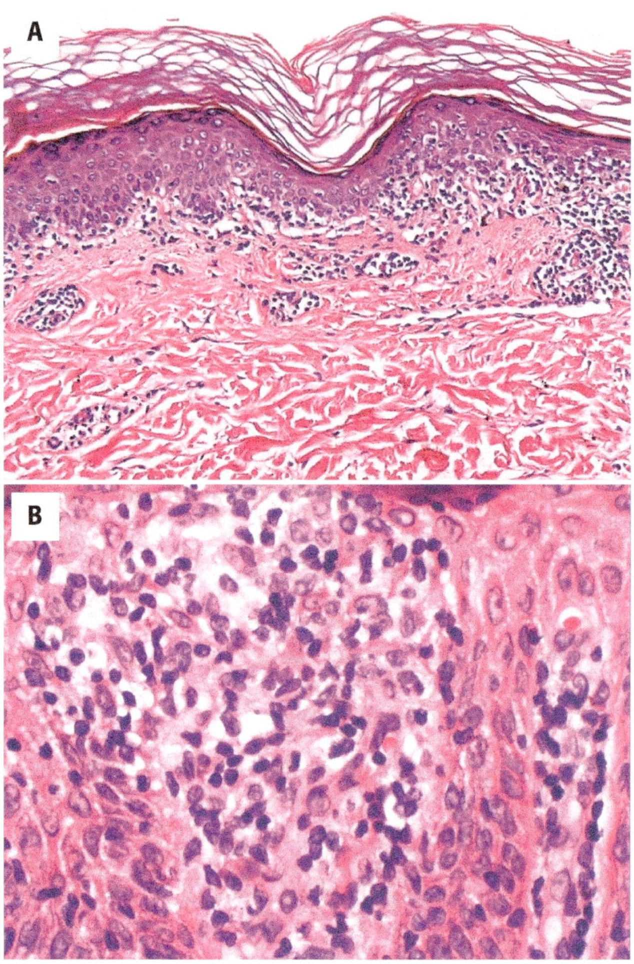

FIG. 15.10

Mycosis fungoides. **A,** Lymphocytes are lined up ("tag along") at the dermal-epidermal junction. **B,** The epidermotropic lymphocytes have hyperchromatic nuclei.

(Figs. 15.9B and 15.10A). Lymphocyte atypia is characterized by a hyperconvoluted, hyperchromatic nucleus. Slits and crevices within the nucleus give it a cerebriform appearance (Fig. 15.10B). Sometimes the lymphocytes are surrounded by perinuclear clearing or halo. While nuclear atypia may on occasion be striking, it is neither sensitive nor specific for the diagnosis. Clinical correlation and ancillary data are often needed for diagnosis.

The lymphocytes tend to collect in a relatively "passive" epidermis without significant spongiosis or Civatte body formation (although neither of these findings can exclude MF). There are varying degrees of epidermal atrophy and rete hyperplasia. In early MF, there is a mild, irregular proliferation of rete ridges. The stratum corneum tends to be subtly altered, by compaction, with mild parakeratosis. Often the biopsy of an early patch lesion of MF lacks a number of classic features and reveals subtle or equivocal histologic findings. The papillary dermis may be peppered by atypical lymphocytes admixed with nonatypical lymphocytes. A helpful clue to the diagnosis of early MF is the presence of lymphocytes aggregating in dermal papillae. In more well-developed lesions, there is a more intense band-like lymphocytic infiltrate, with fibroplasia of the papillary dermal collagen (Fig. 15.11). The papillary dermal fibrosis has been referred to as *wiry* or *fettuccine-like* collagen bundle alteration. However, early, treated, or recurrent disease may lack this feature. Lymphocytes may also be distributed around superficial dermal vessels. An admixture of eosinophils, histiocytes, and (at times) plasma cells may be seen.

As plaque and tumor lesions develop, the dermal infiltrate becomes denser, and Pautrier's microabscesses are lost (Fig. 15.12). In tumor lesions of MF, the infiltrate involves most of the reticular dermis (Fig. 15.13) or may even extend into the subcutis. Tumor lesions tend to have more cells with intermediate to large nuclei (Figs. 15.13 and 15.14). The number of large lymphocytes (greater than or equal to four times the size of a small lymphocyte) present can be prognostically relevant, although this finding associates with higher stage.

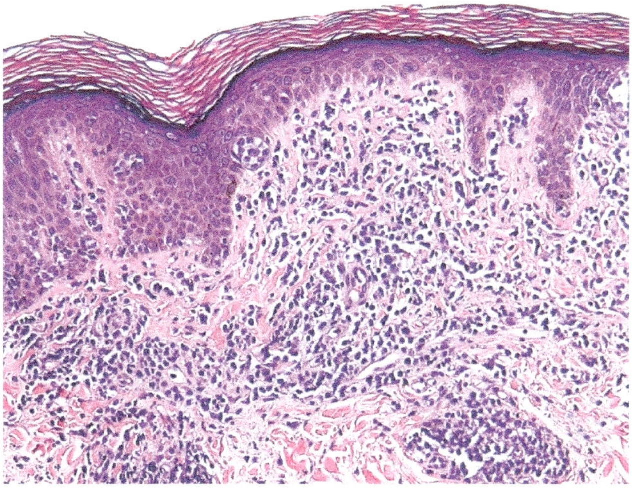

FIG. 15.11

Mycosis fungoides. Plaque lesion with hyperchromatic epidermotropic lymphocytes and papillary dermal fibrosis with "wiry" collagen bundles.

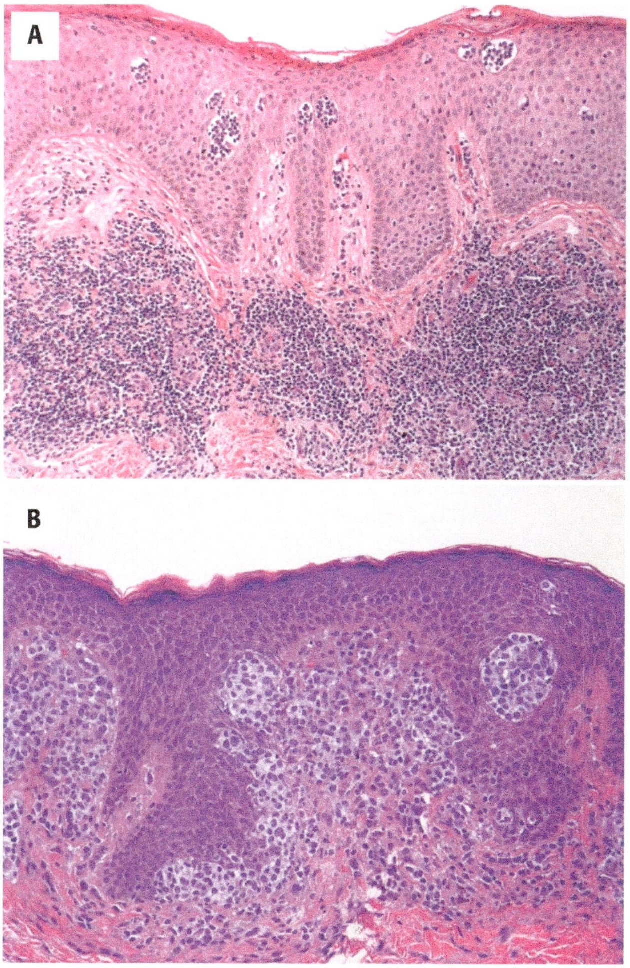

FIG. 15.12

Mycosis fungoides. **A,** Plaque lesion with several Pautrier's microabscesses of small- to intermediate-sized hyperchromatic lymphocytes. **B,** Plaque lesion with large lymphocytes.

MYCOSIS FUNGOIDES—PATHOLOGIC FEATURES

Histopathologic Features

- Variable epidermal changes: atrophy or psoriasiform hyperplasia, parakeratosis
- Bandlike lymphocytic infiltrate with epidermotropism
- Lymphocyte atypia (hyperchromatism, cerebriform nuclei, perinuclear halos)
- Wiry dermal collagen
- Unusual histologic variants: pigmented purpuric, interstitial, granulomatous, poikilodermatous

Ancillary Studies

- Immunophenotype
  - Usually CD4-predominant T-cell infiltrate
  - May show loss of CD7 or other T-cell antigens (CD2, CD5)
  - May show CD30-positive for cytotoxic (CD56, TIA) transformation

Molecular Studies

- Clonal T-cell receptor (TCR) gene rearrangement (may not be detectable in early lesions)*

Differential Diagnosis

- Drug reaction (e.g., phenytoin, immunomodulators)
- Chronic eczema
- Psoriasis
- Lichenoid keratosis
- Lichenoid pigmented purpuric dermatosis

*TCR sequencing can increase the specificity compared to fragment analysis by PCR, and assist with tracking small amounts of residual disease during therapy, the clinical significance of which is not yet understood.

The term *large cell transformation* is applied when the percentage of large cells exceeds 25% of the lesional lymphocyte population or when the large cells form discrete nodules. Large cell transformation is thought to be associated with worse outcomes, but that may be related to the fact that it tends to occur more often in tumor lesions. It can also be seen in patch or plaque lesions where its prognostic significance is uncertain (Fig. 15.12B). Large cells may be negative or positive for CD30 (Fig. 15.14). CD30 immunoreactivity, however, may also be seen in nontransformed lesions of MF.

Hypopigmented MF may have morphologic atypia similar to patch lesions of classic MF, but there is often a cytotoxic interface alteration with vacuolar alteration, and diminished melanin pigment in lesional epidermis compared with adjacent clinically uninvolved skin. The lesional lymphocytes are more often of the CD8+ T-cell subset. The lymphocytic infiltrate may be less intense, and the epidermis less acanthotic. Some variants of *palmoplantar MF* may show more prominent epidermotropism in addition to marked hyperkeratosis and epidermal hyperplasia. *Pigmented purpura MF* shows overlap features with lichenoid pigmented purpura, including erythrocyte extravasation, hemosiderin deposition, and often a subtle interface reaction (Fig. 15.15A). *MF with lichenoid features* does not have a clinical presentation

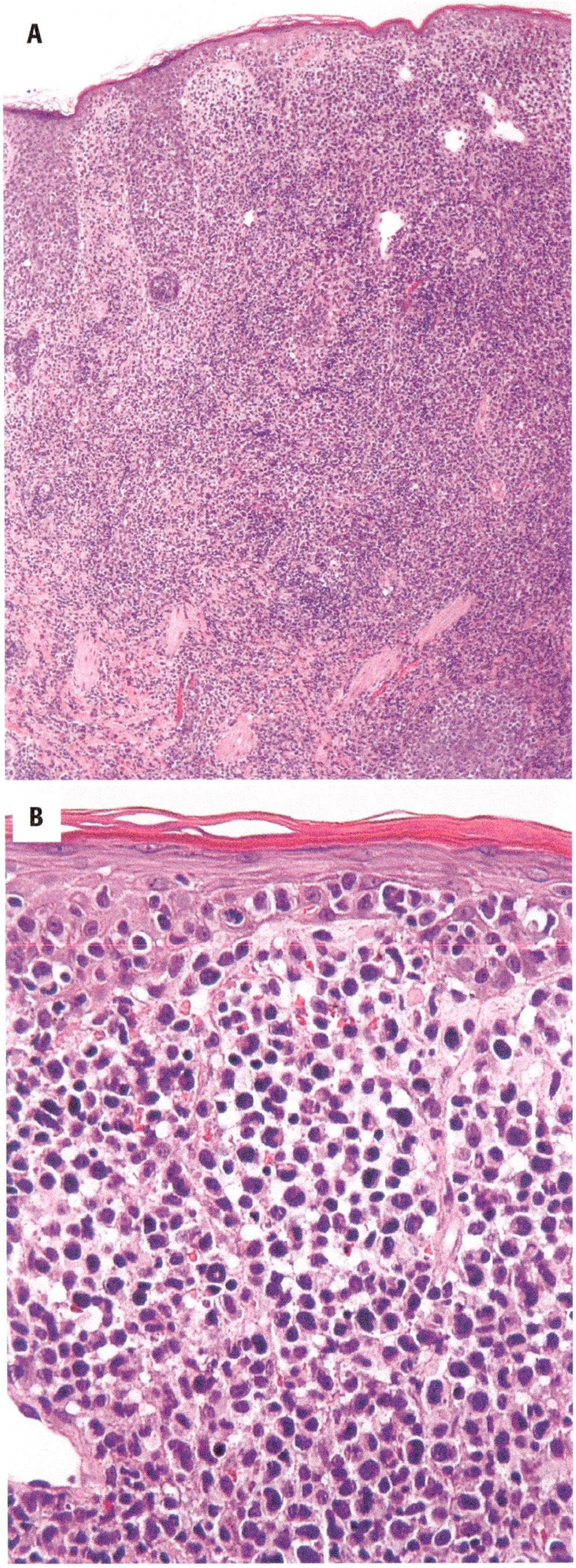

FIG. 15.13

Mycosis fungoides. **A,** Tumor lesion with dense nodular dermal lymphoid infiltrate. **B,** The tumor is predominantly composed of large lymphocytes, indicating large cell transformation.

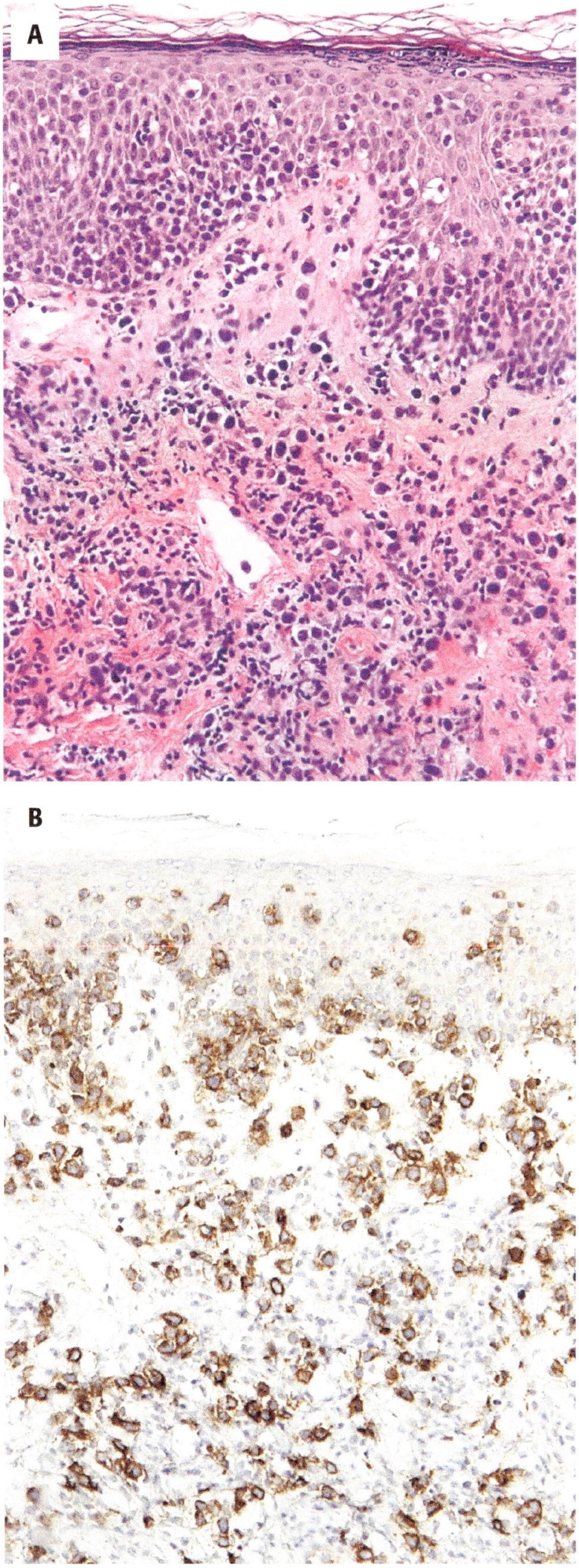

FIG. 15.14

Mycosis fungoides, tumor lesion, with CD30-positive large cell transformation. **A,** Large lymphocytes are present. **B,** The large cells are positive for CD30.

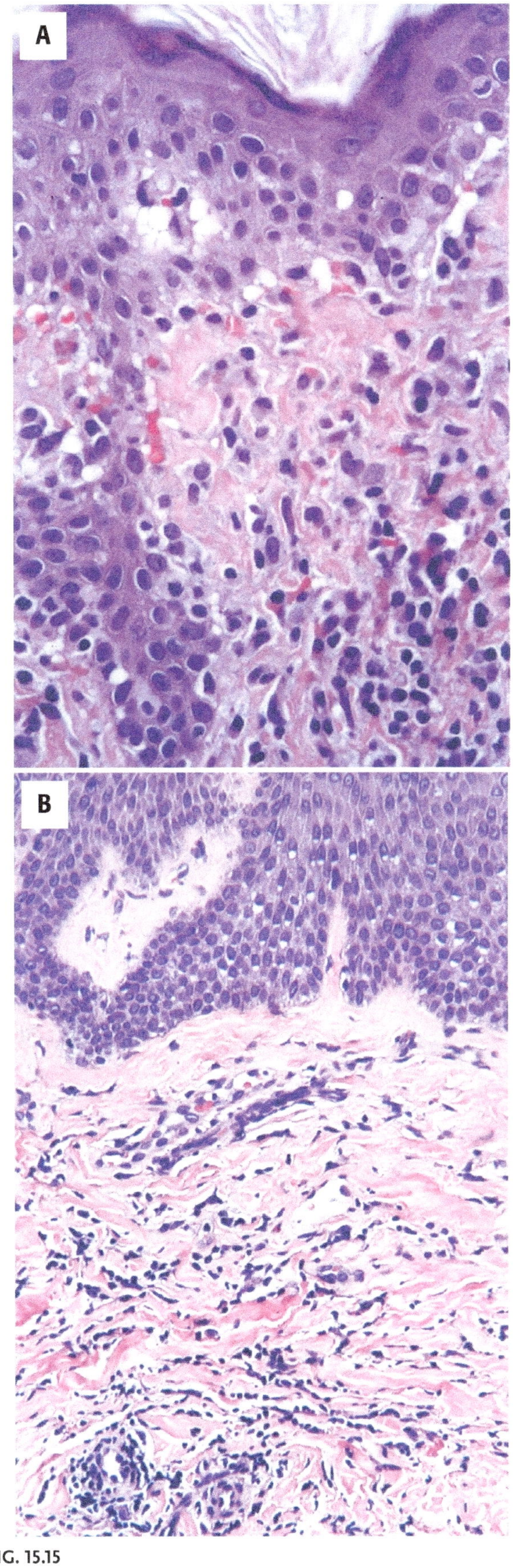

FIG. 15.15
Variants of mycosis fungoides. **A,** Purpuric patch lesion with extravasated red blood cells. **B,** Interstitial pattern of distribution of lymphocytes.

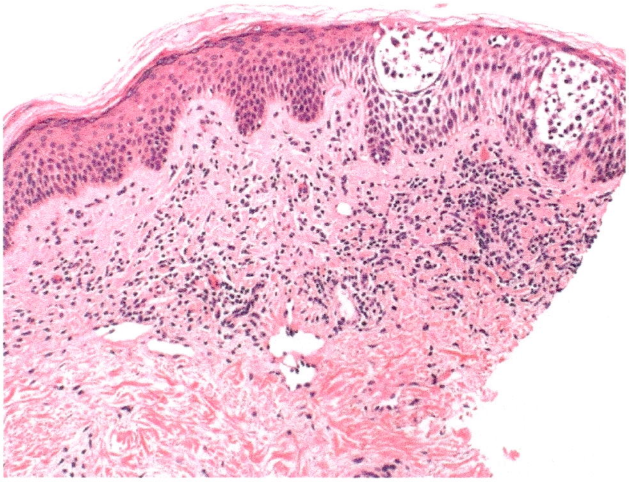

FIG. 15.16
Eczematous mycosis fungoides. There is bandlike infiltrate. The epidermis shows spongiosis.

that is distinct from classic MF but histologically shows features of a lichenoid tissue reaction, including vacuolar and liquefactive basal keratinocyte alteration with dyskeratosis and colloid body formation, overlapping with hypopigmented and CD8+ MF variants. *Interstitial MF* clinically looks similar to patch stage MF but lacks a significant scale or other epidermal changes. Histologically, there are few, if any, lymphocytes within or near the epidermis. Atypical lymphocytes permeate the reticular dermis in an interstitial pattern (Fig. 15.15B). *Bullous MF* may show either an intraepidermal blister resulting from confluence of Pautrier's microabscesses or a separation plane at the dermal-epidermal junction resulting from marked involvement by loosely cohesive neoplastic lymphocytes. The blister cavity contains atypical lymphocytes. There may be changes of MF at the edge of a blister. Spongiotic or eczematous variants of MF also exist (Fig. 15.16).

MF, especially tumor lesions thereof, may be accompanied by a prominent granulomatous inflammatory reaction (*granulomatous MF*) and lead to possible diagnostic confusion with drug eruptions, infection, sarcoidosis, or other nonneoplastic processes.

Ancillary Studies

A diagnosis of MF is usually made on routine histology alone in conjunction with the clinical presentation. In diagnostically difficult, controversial, or histopathologically subtle cases, establishing the immunophenotype might help support the diagnosis. Immunohistochemical studies are also helpful to distinguish MF from other T-cell lymphomas involving the skin.

IMMUNOHISTOCHEMISTRY

Immunohistochemical stains permit assessment of the helper: suppressor ratio (CD4 : CD8) and detection of antigen loss. Results need to be interpreted with caution because early disease or sparsely populated biopsies may not demonstrate classic immunophenotypic aberrations because of a population of suppressor host response.

Prototypical lesions of MF show an increase in the CD4 : CD8 ratio (Fig. 15.17). However, this ratio is more useful for flow cytometric interpretation of MF, as it is difficult to visually "gate" the purely neoplastic population using immunohistochemistry (IHC) on formalin-fixed paraffin-embedded (FFPE) tissues, which prove the presence or absence of lymphoma. In early patch lesions of MF, the CD4 : CD8 ratio may be similar to reactive infiltrates, in which the ratio tends to range from 1 : 1 to 3 : 1. A CD4 : CD8 ratio of greater than 10 : 1 in the appropriate clinical and histologic context may support a diagnosis of MF. Although the immunophenotype of classic MF is CD3(+), CD2(+), CD4(+), T-cell receptor (TCR) β(+), CD45 RO(+), TCRγδ(−), there are also cases that are CD8+/CD4−, CD8+/CD4+, CD4−/CD8−, TCRγδ(+), and/or TCR β(−).

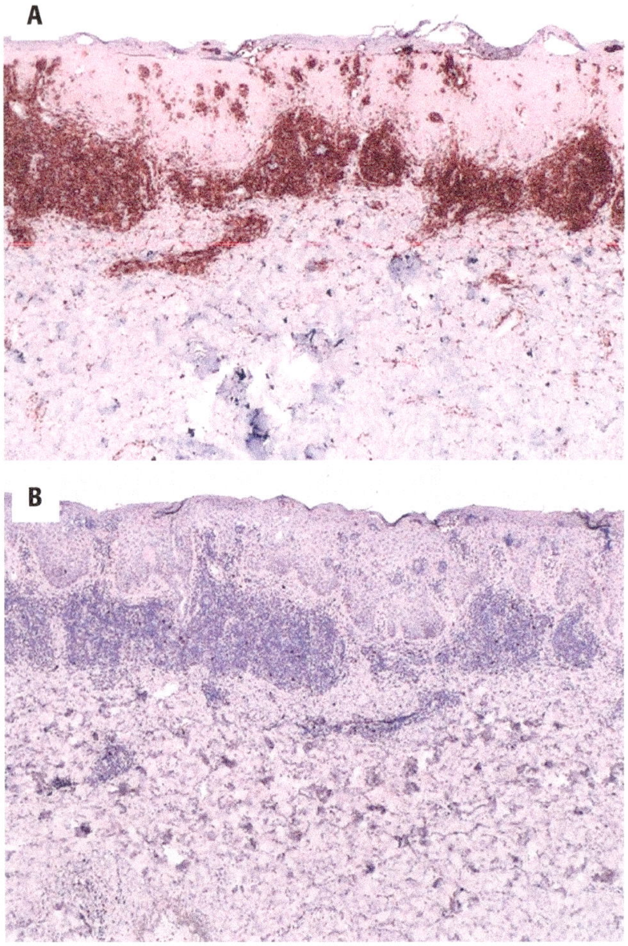

FIG. 15.17

Mycosis fungoides. **A,** There is a predominance of CD4-positive lymphocytes. **B,** Immunostain for CD8.

A reduction in staining for maturation T-cell markers such as CD7 or CD5 is commonly seen in MF; however, partial loss of CD7 can also occur in nonneoplastic inflammatory dermatoses. Even in bona fide MF, loss of CD7 staining may at times be seen only in late, histopathologically obvious lesions. The identification of unexpectedly strong and diffuse CD7 may, however, serve as a clue to consider a different CTCL or extracutaneous TCL within the differential diagnosis. Similarly, the identification of CD4−/CD8−, TCR β(−), or TCRγδ(+), immunophenotype should serve to reevaluate for a more aggressive TCL. As these histopathologic mimics may require significantly different therapeutic approaches, a limited panel of IHC is reasonable to perform in the case of new or changing clinical presentations.

The identification of a clonal T-cell population in suspect lesions of αβ-MF can often be confirmed by demonstrating restricted expression of the TCR constant region using antibodies to TRB-C1. This technique works best when the atypical cells are morphologically and/or spatially distinct. Close attention is warranted in mixed/inflamed infiltrates with scattered atypical cells and in posttreatment settings with low tumor burden. False positives may occur in reactive processes with nonneoplastic small clones.

MOLECULAR STUDIES

In many cases of MF, a monoclonal rearrangement of the TCR gene can be demonstrated by polymerase chain reaction (PCR) fragment analysis or next-generation sequencing (NGS), but results from clonality tests should be interpreted with caution, and integrated with longitudinal clinical and repeat molecular data. Although the detection of a T-cell clone may be used as additional evidence in support of MF if the clinical and histologic findings favor lymphoma, it does not represent unequivocal proof thereof because clonal T-cell populations may occur in nonneoplastic conditions, such as arthropod bites, eczema, or drug reactions. Likewise, the lack of detection of a T-cell clone in early or histologically subtle patch lesions of MF does not exclude the diagnosis because false-negative results occur in approximately 40% of early lesions of MF.

Differential Diagnosis

The differential diagnosis of MF depends on the clinical and histopathologic presentation. In early disease, all variants may show histopathologic overlap with inflammatory dermatoses including those related to antiviral immunity in the era of COVID-19, and with cutaneous reactions to the increasingly common immunomodulatory agents used for other health conditions. Indeed, current models of disease pathogenesis support the evolution of MF as dependent upon a context of antigenic exposure and related chronic inflammatory states.

MYCOSIS FUNGOIDES VERSUS ECZEMA

For patch lesions of MF, the most common problem is their distinction from chronic eczema, such as atopic, nummular, or allergic contact dermatitis. Spongiosis or the absence of epidermotropic atypical lymphocytes favors chronic eczema, but spongiosis may also occur in MF, and topical treatment with steroids may lead to temporary absence of epidermotropism. The pattern of papillary dermal fibrosis and cytology of lymphocytes are helpful features. The wiry collagen bundles often seen in MF are usually not found in eczema. Hyperchromatic cerebriform lymphocytes favor MF over eczema.

MYCOSIS FUNGOIDES VERSUS PSORIASIS

MF may also be difficult to distinguish from psoriasis. Attention to subtle histologic clues (e.g., neutrophils in stratum corneum, hypervascular dermal papillae) and clinical context (associated other features of psoriasis, family history) lead to the correct diagnosis in many cases. Of note, MF may rarely evolve in the context of a long-standing history of psoriasis, whether related to the patient's own immune microenvironment or to therapy/immunomodulator-related clonal selection. Such cases require in-depth review of sequential clinical, morphologic, and molecular data.

MYCOSIS FUNGOIDES VERSUS DRUG REACTION

Histopathologic features identical to MF can also be seen in association with a drug reaction, in particular after the use of phenytoin and/or other anticonvulsants, antihypertensives, selective serotonin reuptake inhibitors (SSRIs), and many immune-modifying agents. Clinical correlation (history of medication use) is essential to avoid a misdiagnosis. In the case of particular immunomodulatory medications such as mogamulizumab, TCR sequencing may assist in the pathologic distinction of a lymphogranulomatous drug reaction from recurrent CTCL.

MYCOSIS FUNGOIDES VERSUS TINEA

Dermatophyte infections can be associated with histopathologic features that simulate various patterns that can be found in patch lesions of MF. Therefore it is prudent practice to include a fungal stain in the workup of possible patch lesions of MF with only mild lymphoid atypia.

MYCOSIS FUNGOIDES VERSUS PIGMENTED PURPURA

The *pigmented purpura variant of MF* can be difficult to differentiate from persistent lichenoid pigmented purpura, and patients may undergo several biopsies until a diagnosis of MF can be established. Cerebriform atypia in the epidermis and dermis, in conjunction with a clinical presentation of generalized involvement or lesions above the lower extremities, favors MF. As with psoriasis, rare cases of MF can arise in a background of pigmented purpuric dermatosis, requiring in-depth review of longitudinal clinicopathologic data for diagnosis.

MYCOSIS FUNGOIDES VERSUS LICHENOID DERMATITIS

The *lichenoid variant of MF* shows overlap features with other lichenoid reactions such as lichen planus, lichen planus–like keratosis, lupus, lichenoid drug reaction, or pityriasis lichenoides chronica. Civatte bodies tend to be rare in lesions of MF but may be present. The presence of hyperchromatic cerebriform lymphocytes, lymphocytes with halos, or wiry papillary dermal collagen bundles favors lymphoma. Clinical correlation is essential. As with psoriasis and pigmented purpura, cases of pityriasis lichenoides may rarely evolve to MF via clonal selection in a background of chronic inflammation, requiring comprehensive longitudinal clinicopathologic correlation review for diagnosis.

MYCOSIS FUNGOIDES VERSUS VITILIGO

Hypopigmented MF may have overlap with early vitiligo and often occurs in individuals with dark skin, making it difficult to distinguish these entities even with clinicopathologic correlation. Furthermore, both entities may have a CD8 immunophenotype. Epidermotropism, hydropic degeneration of basal cells, partial loss of pigment, preservation of some melanocytes (noted with hematoxylin and eosin [H&E], SOX-10, or Melan-A), presence of lymphocytes within the papillary dermis, increased density of the dermal infiltrate, and wiry fibrosis of the papillary dermal collagen were shown to be detected with a significantly higher incidence in hypopigmented MF versus vitiligo. On the other hand, focal thickening of the basement membrane, complete loss of pigmentation, total absence of melanocytes, and absence or sparseness of lymphocytes in the dermal papillae were seen much more frequently in vitiligo.

LARGE CELL TRANSFORMATION ARISING IN MYCOSIS FUNGOIDES VERSUS PRIMARY ANAPLASTIC LARGE CELL LYMPHOMA

Some cases of MF with large cell transformation may show CD30 expression in the atypical cells. Clinical history (of MF, concurrent patch, or plaque lesions) and histopathologic context (adjacent features of classic MF) are needed for the distinction of lymphoma representing large cell transformation of MF from a primary cutaneous CD30-positive ALCL. This issue is important prognostically because patients with a primary cutaneous CD30-positive ALCL have longer survival times and distinct therapeutic algorithms versus those in whom the CD30-positive tumor represents MF with large cell transformation. The distinction can be particularly problematic since the two conditions may coexist as well.

Prognosis and Treatment

The majority of classic MF patients have an indolent clinical course over years to decades. The prognosis of the disease is defined by its stage. Patients with stage T1 disease (less than 10% of the body surface area involved by MF with no tumor lesions) have a survival time similar to that of an age-, sex-, and race-matched population. Poor prognostic factors include age older than 60 years, advanced stage (tumors, nodal, peripheral blood, or visceral involvement), and large cell transformation in the context of tumor lesions. When extracutaneous involvement or tumor evolution with or without large cell transformation occurs, the expected survival period is usually less than 2 years.

Several treatment options are available, depending on the stage or extent of skin involvement. Topical therapies include nitrogen mustard, carmustine (BCNU), high-potency topical steroids, and topical retinoids such as tazarotene and imiquimod. Ultraviolet (UV) light, especially UVA in conjunction with psoralen (PUVA) and narrow-band UVB, is often used. Current Food and Drug Administration–approved systemic medications are retinoids bexarotene, tazarotene, HDAC inhibitors vorinostat, and targeted therapy interleukin (IL)-2 inhibitor denileukin diftitox, brentuximab (targeting CD30), HDAC inhibitors romidepsin, and rituximab (JAK inhibition). Other frequently used systemic medications include interferon, other oral retinoids (e.g., isotretinoin), methotrexate, and pralatrexate. Immune response modifiers and targeted therapies such as lenalidomide, programmed cell death 1 (PD1)-inhibitors, and C-C chemokine receptor type 4 (CCR4) inhibitors are used for patients with advanced disease. Extracorporeal photopheresis may be used if there is significant peripheral blood involvement. Chlorambucil, liposomal doxorubicin, or gemcitabine may be used in advanced disease. Electron beam therapy is frequently used in generally refractory skin disease, either alone or in conjunction with other therapies. A combination of these biologic therapies is often used if there is generalized or advanced disease. Combination chemotherapy is typically reserved for advanced disease or patients who no longer respond to biologic modifiers. Some patients may undergo bone marrow and allogeneic stem cell transplantation for recalcitrant advanced-stage CTCL.

FOLLICOTROPIC MYCOSIS FUNGOIDES WITH OR WITHOUT FOLLICULAR MUCINOSIS

Folliculotropic mycosis fungoides (FMF) is a variant of MF in which the neoplastic T-cell infiltrate preferentially involves the hair follicles, at least in the early stages of the disease.

This may or may not be associated with mucinous degeneration of the follicular epithelium, which is termed *follicular mucinosis* (FM) and which is not specific to FMF.

Clinical Findings

FMF is much less common than classic MF. Isolated lesions of benign FMF may occur in children as well as in adults. FMF with or without mucinosis typically occurs in adults, with a male predominance. In contrast with classic MF, in which the "double-covered" sites are more frequently involved, in FMF, the lesions are concentrated in the head and neck region (Fig. 15.18). Very early lesions may show minimal changes that include follicular-distributed mild erythema or flesh-colored papules or patches of alopecia with follicular prominence. Other clinical presentations include various acneiform sequelae of follicular alteration, such as comedones, fine white follicular spines (Fig. 15.18), milia or small infundibular cysts, and foreign body reactions to

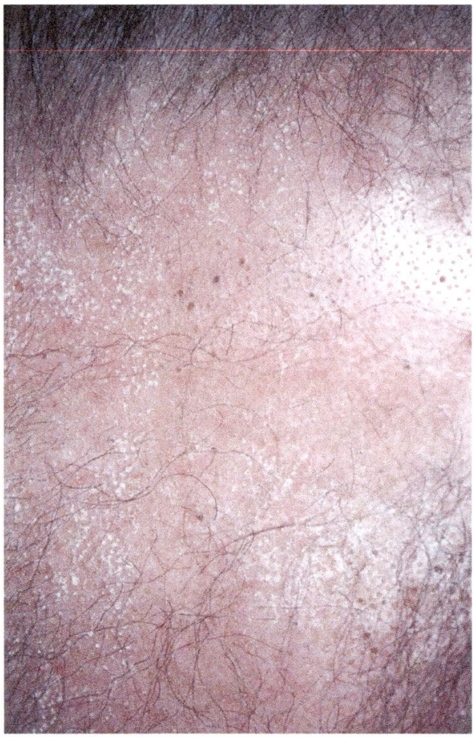

FIG. 15.18

Folliculotropic mycosis fungoides presenting as alopecia associated with follicular spines and comedones.

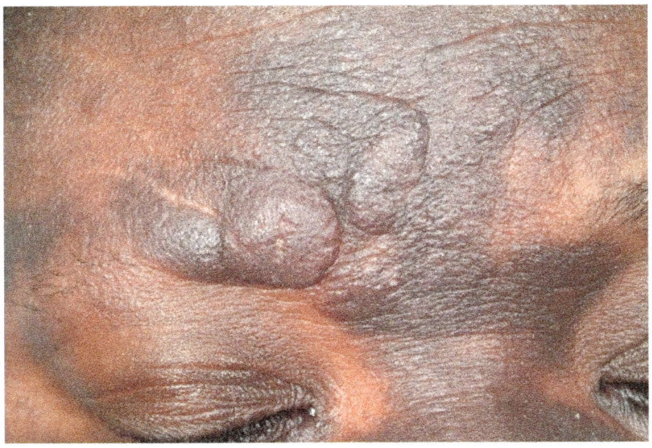

FIG. 15.19
Plaque lesions of folliculotropic mycosis fungoides.

follicular rupture. In advanced disease, mucinorrhea, tumid plaques, and nodules may be seen, and when associated with loss of eyebrow hair, a leonine facies may ensue (Fig. 15.19). Lesions of FMF typically arise as a pink solitary or oligolesional indurated or somewhat translucent-appearing erythematous plaque on the head and neck with alopecia. Features of FMF may coincide or collide with classic lesions of MF.

Histopathologic Features

Follicular mucinosis refers to the presence of mucinous edema within the follicular epithelium (Fig. 15.20). There may be a mild lymphocytic infiltrate without atypia. In well-developed lesions of FMF, hyperchromatic cerebriform lymphocytes are dispersed within the follicular epithelium and along the follicular dermal junction, with variable degrees of mucinosis or spongiosis. In pure cases of FMF, there is no or minimal epidermal involvement ("sparing of the interfollicular epidermis") (Fig. 15.21). However, commonly, the interfollicular dermis and epidermis may also be involved. There may be alteration of the follicle, resulting in comedonal changes, keratin plugging, or follicular rupture (Fig. 15.21).

In advanced lesions (as opposed to early lesions described earlier), there is a dense infiltrate of atypical lymphocytes involving the follicles as well as the epidermis and particularly, filling the dermis. Eosinophils are often abundant and may be associated with eosinophilic spongiosis. Follicular distortion and rupture result in a granulomatous component, potentially simulating a reactive infiltrate.

Ancillary Studies

The immunophenotype is similar to that of classic MF and a high CD4 : CD8 ratio is typical. Clonal TCR gene

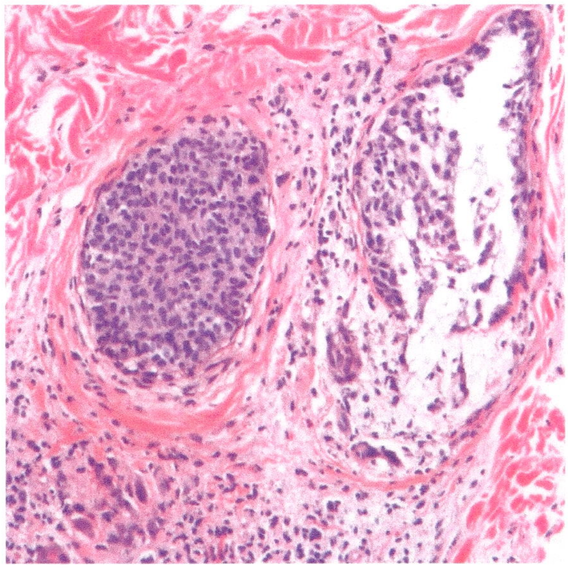

FIG. 15.20
Follicular mucinosis. Intrafollicular mucin is present as well as a sparse lymphocytic infiltrate.

rearrangement is often detected but may be negative in early disease. Ancillary studies cannot reliably distinguish benign FM from folliculotropic lymphoma.

Differential Diagnosis

FMF can be difficult to diagnose. In the absence of cerebriform nuclear atypia, it may be impossible to distinguish FMF from benign FM. Clinically, solitary or few lesions limited to the head and neck area in a younger patient population have been reported to occur more often in patients with limited benign FM.

Early lesions of FMF may also be confused with lymphocyte-rich follicular inflammatory processes, including lupus erythematosus (LE) and rosacea. Because spongiosis may be present in FMF, it may be confused with an eczematous dermatitis. Even in advanced disease, the presence of eosinophils and secondary changes such as spongiosis or granulomatous reactions to follicular rupture may simulate cutaneous lymphoid hyperplasia (CLH).

Prognosis and Treatment

The prognosis is thought to be worse for the follicular variant of MF than for classic MF in patch or plaque stage. Patients with FMF have been found to have a 5-year survival rate that is similar to patients with tumor-stage MF; however, this poor survival applies most aptly to patients with the histologically advanced categorization of FMF and does not apply to early/mild FMF with superficial follicular involvement and slight perivascular infiltrates.

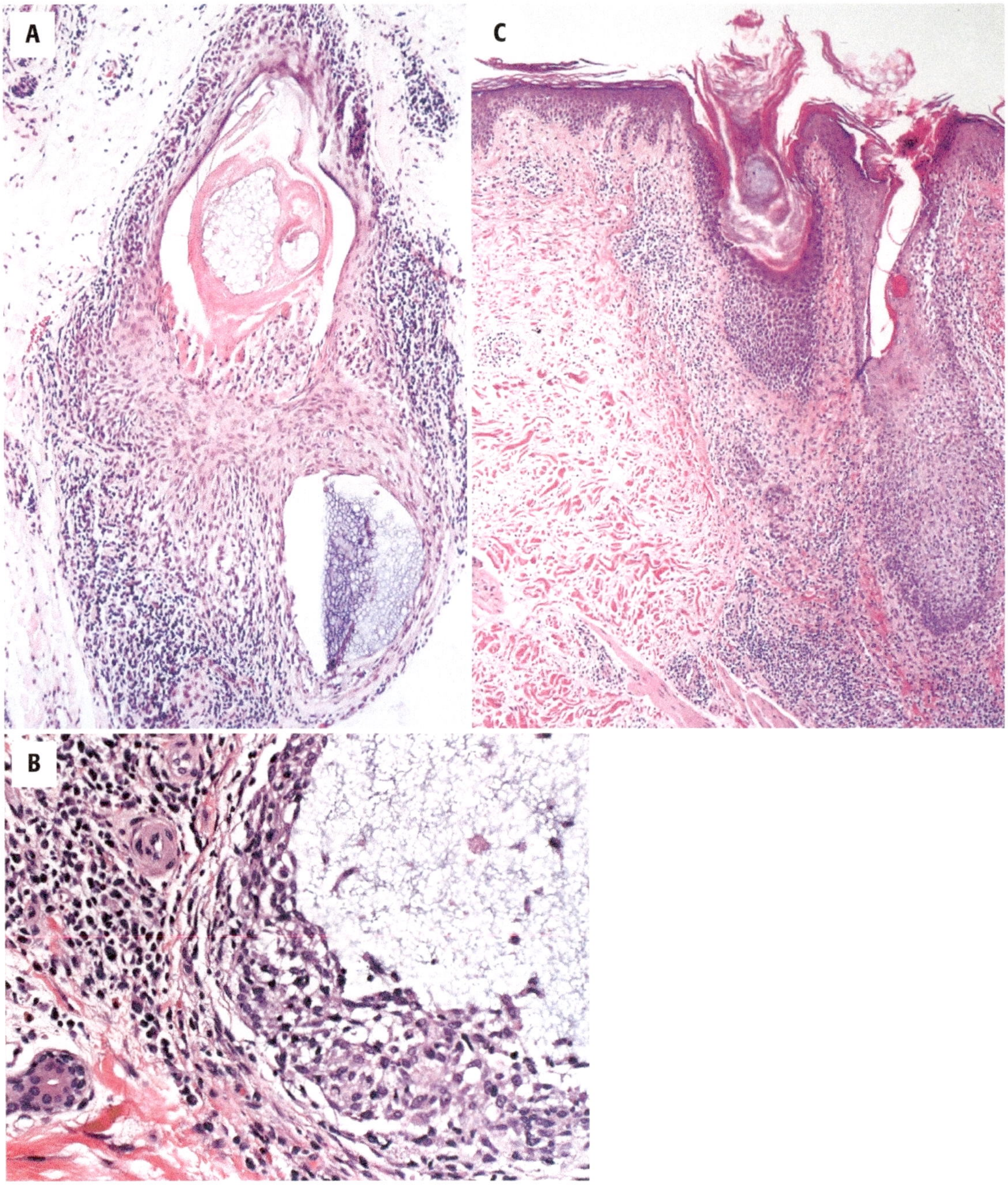

FIG. 15.21

Folliculotropic mycosis fungoides with follicular mucinosis. **A,** Intrafollicular mucin is associated with a folliculotropic atypical lymphocytic infiltrate. **B,** The lymphocytes are atypical and manifest around as well as within the follicular epithelium. **C,** Follicular ostia may be ectatic and the infiltrate may spill over to the adjacent epidermis.

Treatment is similar to that of classic MF, requiring multimodality therapy, often in conjunction with PUVA.

SYRINGOTROPIC MYCOSIS FUNGOIDES

This variant of MF is characterized by epitheliotropism of the eccrine apparatus. It can arise alone or in conjunction with classic or FMF.

Clinical Findings

Clinically, there are initially discrete red-brown macules with minimal scale, concentrated on the extremities, palms, and soles (Fig. 15.22). There may be anhidrosis. As the lesions advance, these eccrine-distributed lesions may merge into scaly patches and plaques (Fig. 15.23). Alopecia and follicular accentuation may be present. Often the lesions are solitary.

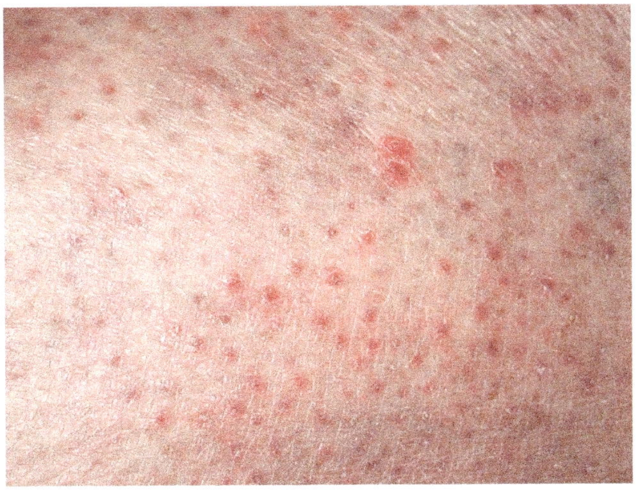

FIG. 15.22
Syringotropic mycosis fungoides manifesting as multiple small red papules.

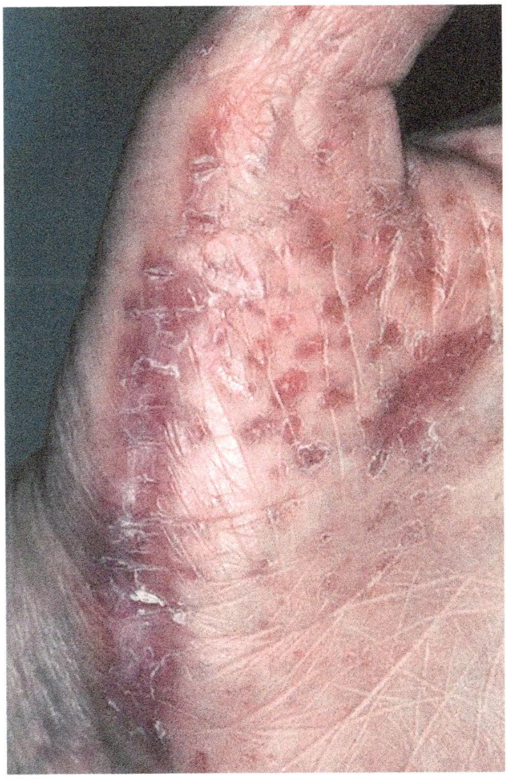

FIG. 15.23
Syringotropic mycosis fungoides manifesting as erythematous macules and plaques on the hand.

Histopathologic Features

There is a syringotropic atypical lymphocytic infiltrate (Fig. 15.24). This may arise alone or in conjunction with patch or plaque lesions of MF. The diagnostic features may not be apparent if an eccrine duct is not present in the sections, and one must be sure to specifically assess for this possibility by evaluating the deep eccrine

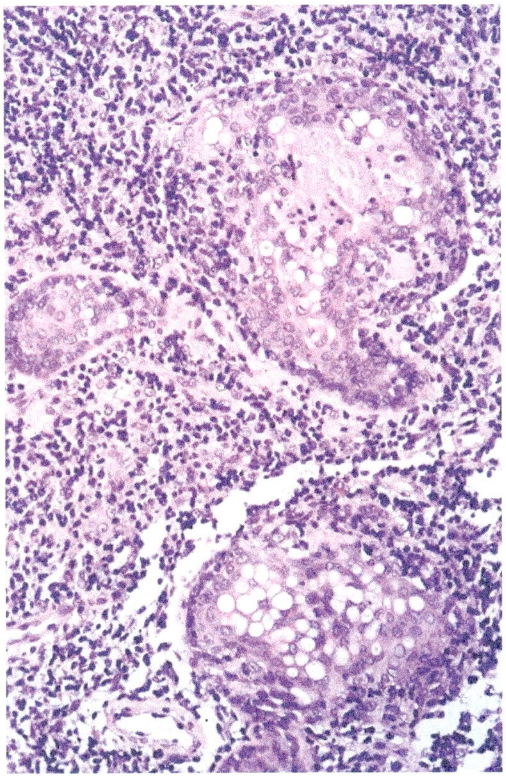

FIG. 15.24
Syringotropic mycosis fungoides with many atypical lymphocytes involving the sweat ducts.

coils. The eccrine ducts and glands are infiltrated and surrounded by atypical T lymphocytes. Eccrine gland hyperplasia may give rise to complex epithelial structures with a cribriform pattern of ductal hyperplasia or squamatization ("syringometaplasia").

Differential Diagnosis

The differential diagnosis of syringotropic MF includes a lymphoid drug eruption, lupus, or lichen striatus, all of which may involve the eccrine duct. If an eccrine gland is not present in the sections, the lymphocytic infiltrate may be too sparse to render a diagnosis of lymphoma, simulating "normal skin" or a nonspecific perivascular dermal hypersensitivity reaction. If there is a prominent dermal component and one does not recognize the syringotropism, the differential diagnosis includes a peripheral T-cell lymphoma or atypical CLH.

Prognosis and Treatment

Currently, there is no strong evidence that the presence of syringotropism has an impact on prognosis or treatment.

PAGETOID RETICULOSIS

Pagetoid reticulosis (PR) is a variant of MF that derives its name from the histologic feature of prominent intraepidermal (pagetoid) distribution of atypical lymphocytes.

Clinical Findings

Oligolesional or solitary PR (Woringer-Kolopp disease) is characterized by one or few, usually indolent, scaly to keratotic lesions, often occurring on the extremities. Historically, a disseminated variant of PR has been referred to as *Ketron-Goodman disease.* The latter is associated with a more aggressive clinical course and is now considered as a different subtype of CTCL, termed *primary cutaneous aggressive CD8 epidermotropic CTCL.*

Histopathologic Features

PR is characterized by a lymphocytic infiltrate that predominantly localizes to within the epidermis and the dermal-epidermal junction (Fig. 15.25A). Lymphocytes may be hyperchromatic cerebriform or show perinuclear halos. Typically, many atypical lymphocytes are distributed in a "buckshot" scattered pattern at all layers of the epidermis. However, not all unilesional forms of MF show prominent pagetoid epidermotropism. Some lesions display a bandlike pattern with involvement of both epidermis and superficial dermis (Fig. 15.25B) and only limited pagetoid invasion of the lower spinous cell layer.

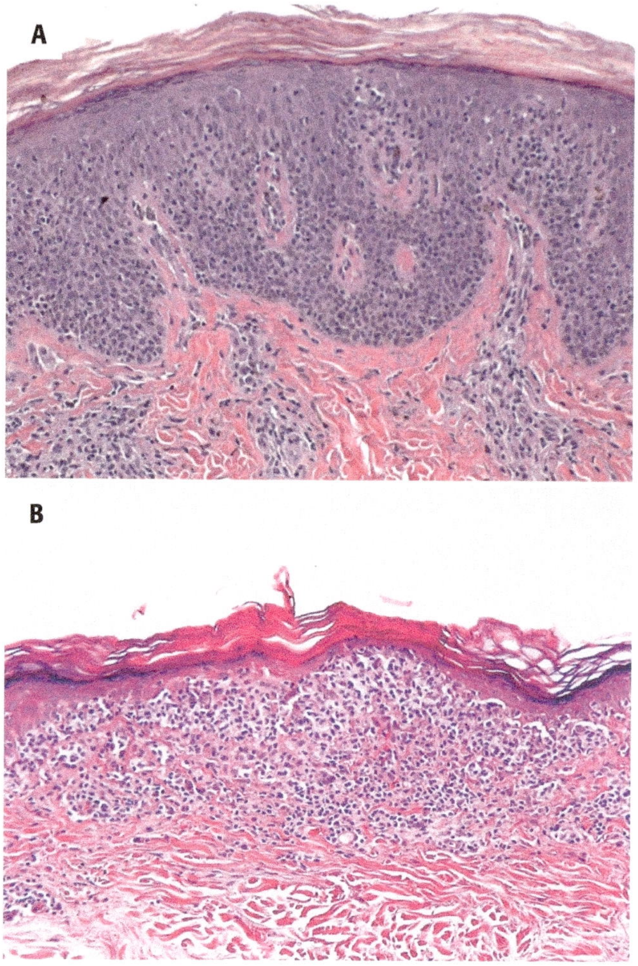

FIG. 15.25

Pagetoid reticulosis. **A,** Most of the atypical lymphocytes are clustered at the dermal-epidermal junction. **B,** Hyperchromatic lymphocytes show irregular nuclear contours.

Ancillary Studies

The infiltrate is immunopositive for CD3 and CD5. In contrast with classic MF, many of the cases show a predominance of CD8-positive cells within the epidermis. CD7 and CD2 expression may be lost.

Differential Diagnosis

Histopathologically, it is difficult to distinguish PR from the aggressive epidermotropic CD8 cytotoxic CTCL variants, although the latter may show a more pleomorphic infiltrate. PR is more likely than aggressive epidermotropic CD8+ cytotoxic CTCL to show expression of CCR4 and CD45RO, and to exhibit reduction of CD7. Fluorescence in situ hybridization (FISH) or molecular evidence of JAK2 fusion is not known in PR and may be useful to favor the aggressive lymphoma.

Lesions of clinically more classic MF, palmoplantar MF, hypopigmented MF, and rare CD8+ LyP may also show histopathologic, immunophenotypic, and molecular features of PR. Clinical correlation is essential to distinguish such cases from PR.

Prognosis and Treatment

Solitary or oligolesional variants typically have an indolent course. Simple surgical excision may suffice. Local radiation therapy or topical steroids may also be used.

GRANULOMATOUS SLACK SKIN

Granulomatous slack skin (GSS) is a recognized clinical-pathologic variant of MF, and it is distinct from "granulomatous" MF. The latter refers to a microscopic variant, in which there is a granulomatous or sarcoidal component to the infiltrate in a patient with otherwise classic MF or Sézary syndrome.

Clinical Findings

GSS is very rare. It generally affects patients at a younger age than classic MF and may manifest in the teens to young adulthood. The characteristic manifestation is that of lax skin or atrophic or pendulous plaques in the axillary and inguinal folds. Initially, lesions are indurated plaques, which slowly become wrinkled.

Histopathologic Features

There is a pandermal and subcutaneous infiltrate of atypical lymphocytes admixed with evenly distributed epithelioid and multinucleated giant cells, many of which contain numerous nuclei (Fig. 15.26). The multinucleated giant cells demonstrate prominent elastophagia and lymphophagocytosis (emperipolesis). Eosinophils and plasma cells are often present. Epidermotropism is usually minimal to absent.

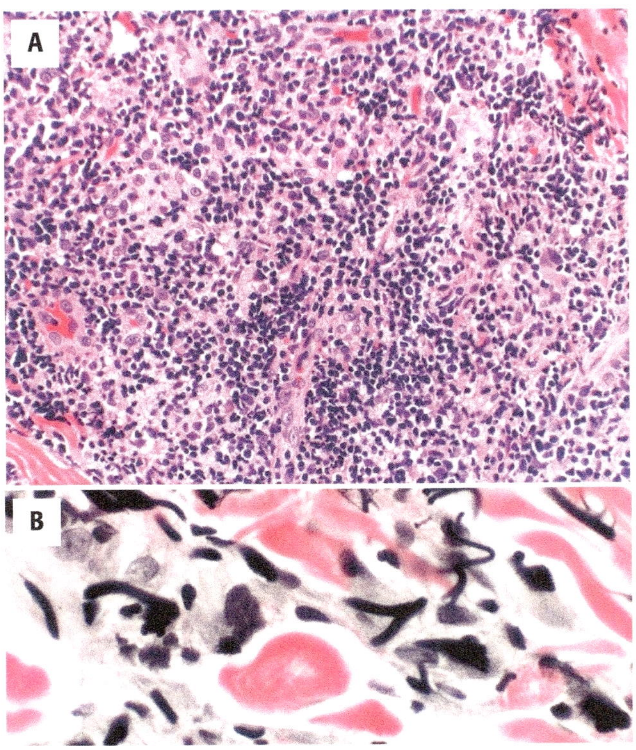

FIG. 15.26
Granulomatous slack skin. **A,** An atypical lymphocytic infiltrate is associated with a granulomatous reaction with emperiopolesis. **B,** Elastophagocytosis is seen (Verhoeff-van Gieson stain).

Ancillary Studies

Elastic tissue stains demonstrate loss of elastic fibers. IHC shows a CD4-predominant T-cell infiltrate. There may be loss of CD5 and CD7. These tumors typically show monoclonal rearrangements of the TCR.

Differential Diagnosis

Multinucleated giant cells with numerous nuclei, emperipolesis, elastophagia, and lymphocyte atypia are a distinct constellation of features that help differentiate GSS from other granulomatous and lymphoid infiltrates, such as granulomatous infiltrates in MF, infectious causes of granulomatous infiltrates, granulomatous hypersensitivity reactions, and CLH with anetoderma. The latter can be excluded by immunophenotyping, demonstrating a mixed T- and B-cell infiltrate. GSS does not tend to show an admixture of neutrophils, epithelioid histiocytes, and necrosis, which may be seen in infectious granulomata.

Prognosis and Treatment

Patients with GSS tend to have a protracted clinical course. Various topical and systemic agents listed earlier for MF may be tried, although the lesions may be difficult to completely eradicate. If the lesions are localized, radiation therapy or surgical excision may be helpful. The main concern is the development of a secondary extracutaneous lymphoma, which is reported to occur with this subgroup. Treatment is similar to that of MF.

SÉZARY SYNDROME

Sézary syndrome represents the leukemic form of CTCL characterized by erythroderma, lymphadenopathy, and neoplastic T cells (Sézary cells) in the skin, lymph nodes, and blood.

Clinical Findings

Patients have erythroderma (Fig. 15.27A), often associated with edema, induration, and scaling of the skin. Palmar or plantar keratoderma is often present. Lower eyelid ectropion, alopecia, and nail dystrophy may also be seen. In advanced disease, lymph node as well as systemic organ involvement including oropharynx, lungs, and central nervous system (CNS) may occur.

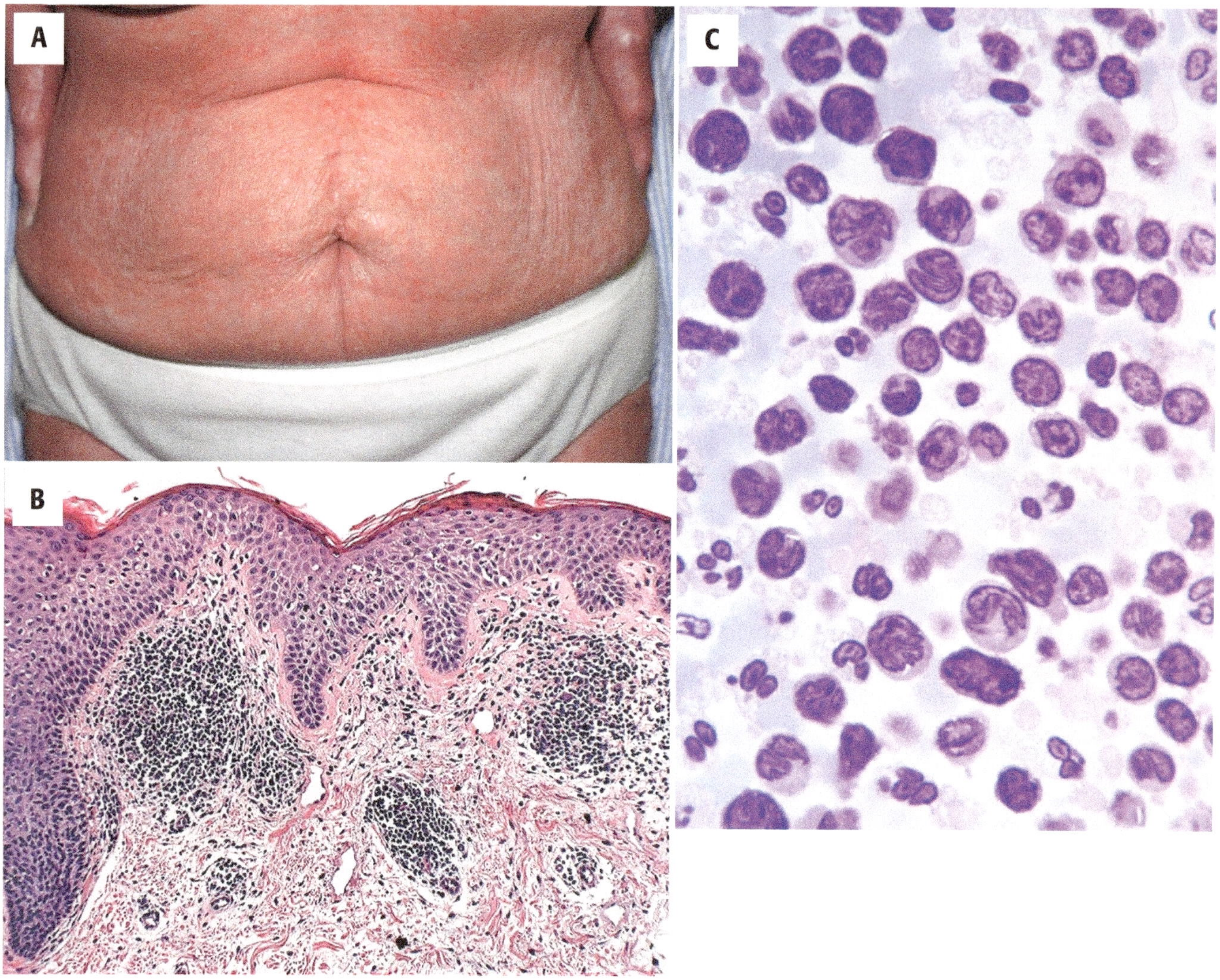

FIG. 15.27
Sézary syndrome. **A,** Erythroderma. **B,** Lymphocytic infiltrate with epidermotropism and mild spongiosis. **C,** Sézary cells in peripheral blood (buffy coat).

Histopathologic Features

The histopathology of Sézary syndrome is often more subtle than in classic MF. Often there is a perivascular lymphocytic infiltrate in the upper dermis, with mild acanthosis (Fig. 15.27B). The lymphocytes in Sézary syndrome display cytologic atypia, with a spectrum of larger cerebriform cells (Sézary cells) and smaller hyperchromatic lymphocytes with cerebriform nuclear contours (Lutzner cells). Eosinophils and plasma cells may accompany the lymphocytic infiltrate. Epidermotropism and cerebriform lymphoid atypia may be prominent but are often subtle. Frequently, the epidermis shows foci of mild spongiosis, making a distinction from erythrodermic eczema difficult without correlation with assessment for peripheral blood involvement and clinical context (history and laboratory data).

Ancillary Studies

The diagnosis of Sézary syndrome requires documentation of neoplastic T cells in the peripheral blood in the context of erythroderma. Since the histology in the skin may be more subtle, one clue to assess the peripheral blood is an elevated CD4 : CD8 ratio of lymphocytes in the skin. In general, IHC on these infiltrates shows a partial T-follicle helper phenotype with strong PD1 labeling. CCR4 is positive. TRBC1 IHC should show clonal restriction (predominantly positive or negative staining) in the atypical cells.

Evaluation of the peripheral blood is typically done by flow cytometry, but morphologic assessment by peripheral blood smear or buffy coat analysis may also support the diagnosis (Fig. 15.27C). The number of hyperconvoluted or Sézary cells required for a diagnosis of Sézary syndrome depends on the presence of other diagnostic features. Current criteria for the diagnosis of

Sézary syndrome include an absolute Sézary cell count of at least 1000 cells/mm^3; immunophenotypical abnormalities, including a CD4/CD8 ratio of 10 or higher (measured by flow cytometry), CD4+/CD7− cells ≥40%, CD4+/CD26− cells ≥30%; or the documentation of a T-cell clone in the blood.

Differential Diagnosis

The differential diagnosis includes erythroderma because of other causes, such as atopic dermatitis, psoriasis, pityriasis rubra pilaris, mastocytosis, and drug reactions. It is not always possible to distinguish between lymphoma and non–lymphoma-related erythroderma on histologic grounds alone if there is only mild lymphoid atypia. Examination of the peripheral blood and clinical correlation are critical for a final diagnosis. Adult T-cell leukemia/lymphoma (ATLL) (see the following) may show histology indistinguishable from Sézary syndrome. It is best distinguished by documenting human T-lymphotropic virus 1 (HTLV-1) lymphocyte infection and multilobated lymphocytes in the peripheral blood.

Prognosis and Treatment

Patients with erythrodermic CTCL or Sézary syndrome have a poorer prognosis than patients with early patch or plaque disease, with a 5-year survival rate of approximately 11%, but this is dependent on tumor-node-metastasis-blood (TNMB) stage. Treatment usually entails multimodality therapy using a combination of regimens outlined for skin-restricted CTCL, often in conjunction with extracorporeal photopheresis and systemic therapy (bexarotene, interferon, or chemotherapy).

PRIMARY CUTANEOUS CD30-POSITIVE LYMPHOPROLIFERATIVE DISORDERS

The CD30-positive LPD spectrum includes LyP, ALCL, and "borderline" lesions.

LYMPHOMATOID PAPULOSIS

Clinical Findings

LyP presents as a chronic, recurrent, self-healing eruption of papules that progress to papulonecrotic lesions before resolving (Fig. 15.28). People of all ages

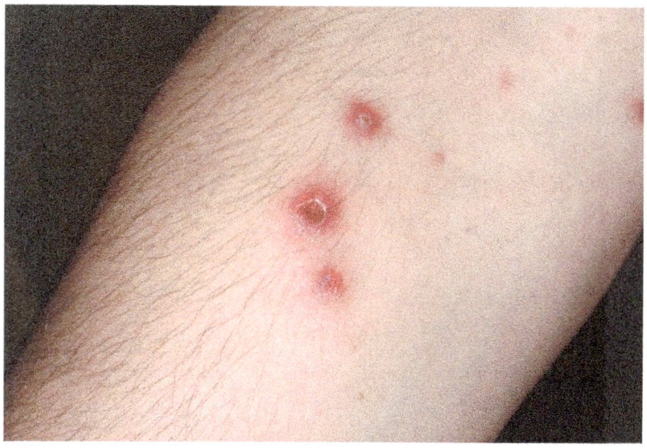

FIG. 15.28
Lymphomatoid papulosis. Erythematous and crusted papules.

can be affected, including children, but LyP has a peak incidence in the fifth decade of life. Typically, the lesions occur in crops and are found in different stages of evolution at clinical examination. Erythematous papules with scale crust may become ulcerated and necrotic. The eruption of LyP may recur over many years to decades. The most commonly affected sites include the trunk and proximal extremities; however, lesions may be seen on the face, palms, soles, and scalp. The lesions may be restricted to one region of the body or limb. Oral mucosal involvement is rare. Papules (less than 1 cm in size) are the most characteristic presentation. However, the presence of nodules measuring 1 to 2 cm is not uncommon. If nodules are present, this raises concerns for progression to or coexistence of ALCL or may lead to a designation of a borderline lesion if no definitive distinction between LyP and ALCL can be made. Lesions of LyP may heal with postinflammatory dyschromia or an atrophic scar. Resolution tends to occur within 3 to 6 weeks, but they may not completely regress for several months. Some studies have reported that 5% to 20% of patients have a concurrent or preceding diagnosis of Hodgkin's or non-Hodgkin's lymphoma (often MF or ALCL) or may develop such in the future. However, this may be an overestimate related to reported bias.

Histopathologic Features

There is a spectrum of histopathologic features associated with LyP, which in part depend on the evolutionary stage of the lesion. The most typical architectural pattern of the infiltrate is a wedge shape with the broad base of the wedge aligning with the epidermis (Fig. 15.29). Associated epidermal hyperplasia, ulceration, spongiosis, and focal epidermal necrosis are

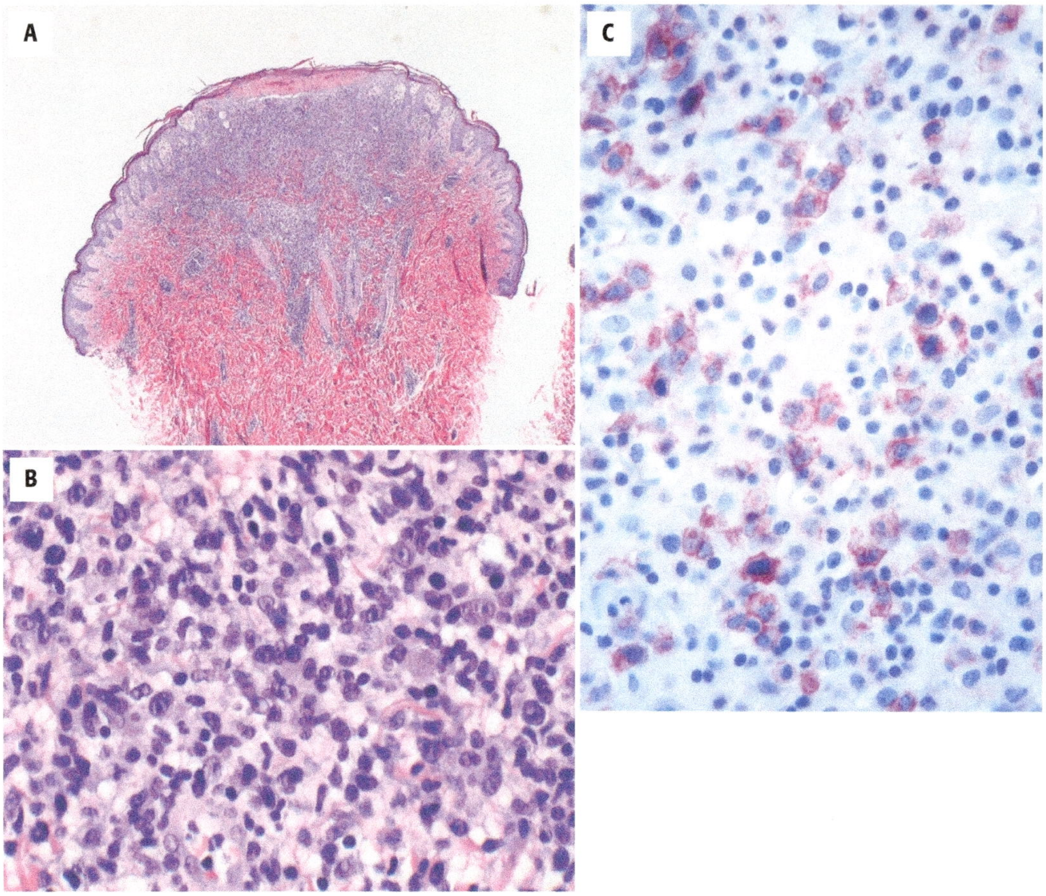

FIG. 15.29

Lymphomatoid papulosis. **A,** Papular lesion with wedge-shaped lymphocytic infiltrate. **B,** A mixed infiltrate of small and large lymphocytes is present. **C,** The subpopulation of large cells is positive for CD30.

LYMPHOMATOID PAPULOSIS—DISEASE FACT SHEET

Patient Group

- May occur at any age but most often in mid-adult life

Site of Involvement

- No site predilection; often on the trunk and extremities

Clinical Findings

- Small papules and papulonecrotic lesions that appear in crops
- May be asymptomatic or pruritic
- Lesions tend to resolve spontaneously between 2 and 6 weeks
- Waxing and waning of this process may last for decades

Prognosis

- Often chronic indolent disease
- No impact on life expectancy
- May be associated with lymphoma (mycosis fungoides, anaplastic large cell lymphoma, Hodgkin's disease) in 5% to 15% of affected individuals

Treatment

- Topical steroids, especially for pruritic lesions
- Phototherapy
- Therapy is not necessary in many cases
- Low-dose methotrexate

common. Hair follicles may be involved and may be dystrophic. The lymphocytic infiltrate usually involves both the epidermis and dermis. It is typically composed of a mixture of large cells, small- to intermediate-sized atypical lymphocytes, and a polymorphous background of neutrophils and eosinophils in variable proportions. Anaplastic binucleate cells with prominent nucleoli, similar to Reed-Sternberg cells of Hodgkin's disease, may be seen.

Subtypes of LyP with letters from A to F LyP have been reported, referring to variations in the architectural, cytomorphologic, and immunophenotype of the lymphoid infiltrate. The main value of these subtypes is for pathologists to be aware of the spectrum of histopathologic features that can be associated with LyP. In type A, the infiltrate is polymorphous, being composed of lymphocytes, neutrophils, and eosinophils admixed with large histiocyte-like CD30-positive lymphocytes. CD30 is generally positive in less than 50% of the infiltrate. Type B LyP is similar (or identical in appearance) to papular MF because the infiltrate is composed predominantly of smaller cerebriform lymphocytes (Lutzner cells) aligned along the dermo-epidermal junction, often demonstrating prominent epidermotropism.

In the past, these cells were said to be negative for CD30; however, with recent improvements in immunohistochemical techniques and reagents, some type B LyP cases may also be CD30 positive. Type C LyP is composed of a more exuberant population of large atypical CD30-positive cells in clusters and sheets, often histologically indistinguishable from ALCL on small biopsies (Fig. 15.30). Type D LyP is a lichenoid and epidermotropic form of LyP characterized by CD8-positive, αβ T cells expressing cytotoxic markers. The histopathologic findings are similar to what one sees in biopsies of primary cutaneous CD8-positive aggressive epidermotropic T-cell lymphoma (AETCL). LyP type E is ulcerated, usually self-healing lesions, which are characterized by an angioinvasive and angiodestructive infiltrate of small- to medium-sized CD8-positive and CD30-positive T cells. Type F LyP refers to a folliculotropic pattern of LyP. LyP comprising γδ T cells has been increasingly reported and should be considered in the correct clinical setting.

Ancillary Studies

Immunoreactivity for CD30, typically in a membranous pattern with occasional focal cytoplasmic and/or Golgi staining, is characteristic (Fig. 15.31). The small- to intermediate-sized lymphocytes are often predominantly composed of CD4-positive cells, but there is considerable variation in the CD4:CD8 ratio. Antigen deletion (CD7, CD2, CD3, CD5) may be seen. Type B LyP may be negative for CD30. Some lesions (particularly in type D LyP) may express CD56 or cytotoxic markers, such as T-cell intracytoplasmic antigen 1 (TIA-1) or granzyme B. PCR analysis may or may not demonstrate the presence of a T-cell clone. Chromosomal rearrangement of the DUSP22 locus on 6p25.3 can be identified with FISH in a subset of LyP cases, often predicted by a biphasic (small intraepidermal atypical cells and large dermal cells) morphology.

Differential Diagnosis

As described earlier, the differential diagnosis of individual lesions of LyP depends on the morphology of the biopsied lesion; for example, the need to distinguish *type B LyP versus MF (especially MF of the papular variant)*,

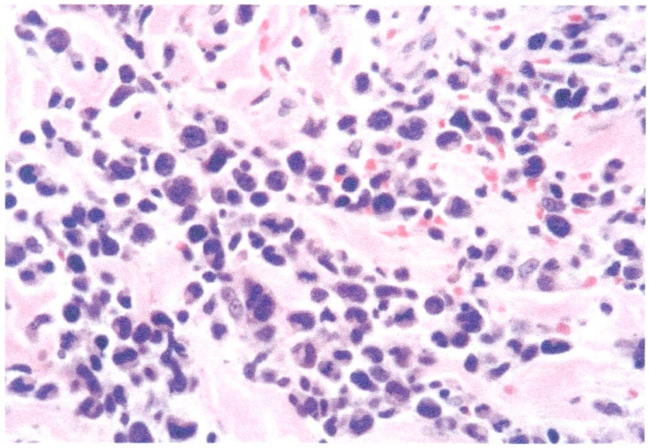

FIG. 15.30
Predominance of large lymphocytes of type C lymphomatoid papulosis.

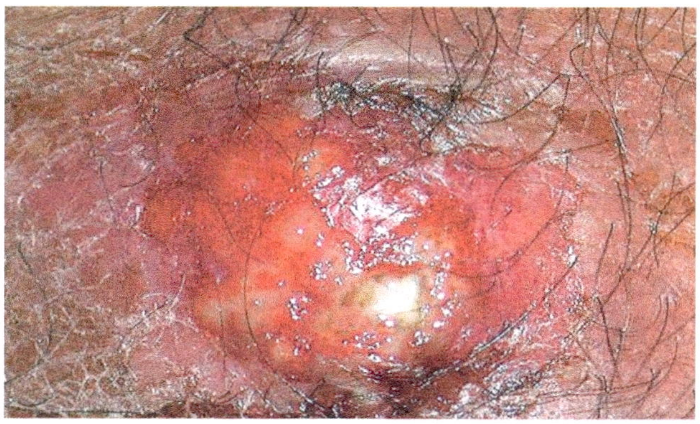

FIG. 15.31
Erythematous nodule of anaplastic large cell lymphoma.

Lymphomatoid Papulosis Types and Their Differential Diagnosis

LyP Type	Frequency	Histopathology	Immunophenotype	Differential Diagnosis
A	75%	Scattered large cells	CD30+, CD4+, CD8−	ALCL, tumor MF, drug reaction, arthropod bite
B	<5%	Epidermotropic small cells	CD30−, CD4+, CD8−	MF
C	<10%	Sheets of large cells	CD30+, CD4+, CD8−	ALCL, MF
D	<5%	Lichenoid/ epidermotropic	CD30+, CD4−, CD8+	CD8+ AETCL, PR, MF
E	<5%	Angioinvasive	CD30+, CD4−, CD8+	Extranodal NKTCL, PTCL, NOS
F	<1%	Folliculotropic	CD30+, CD4+, CD8−	Folliculotropic MF

AETCL, Aggressive epidermotropic T-cell lymphoma; *ALCL*, anaplastic large cell lymphoma; *LyP*, lymphomatoid papulosis; *MF*, mycosis fungoides; *NKTCL*, natural killer T-cell lymphoma; *NOS*, not otherwise specified; *PR*, pagetoid reticulosis; *PTCL*, peripheral T-cell lymphoma.

type C LyP versus ALCL, or type D LyP versus CD8-positive AETCL. Ultimately for such cases, correlation with the clinical presentation and course is imperative for the correct diagnosis. If multiple small papular lesions evolve *and spontaneously regress*, a diagnosis of LyP can be made confidently, irrespective of the proportion of CD30-positive large cells or cytotoxic CD8-positive epidermotropic cells. Diagnostic problems usually arise when only a few lesions are present that are intermediate in size (1–3 cm), which may persist longer but eventually involute weeks or months after biopsy. If such a lesion rich in CD30-positive large cells eventually clinically regresses and involutes, one should still consider LyP. Because ALCL may also self-involute, a provisional category of a "borderline lesion" of CD30-positive lymphoproliferative disease has been proposed for diagnostically difficult lesions.

A special problem is the presence of LyP-like lesions that have developed within a patch or plaque of MF. If large CD30-positive cells are present, the differential diagnosis is that of *secondary LyP in MF versus large cell transformation of MF*. Knowledge of the clinical context and evolution of the lesion(s) is necessary for the correct diagnosis. If a patient has a history of LyP or has multiple other lesions of LyP, a small CD30-positive cluster within a patch or plaque of MF should not be too quickly interpreted as large cell lymphoma and should be considered to be LyP unless the lesion persists and grows as would be expected for large cell transformation.

Clinically and histopathologically, LyP may show overlap with *pityriasis lichenoides et varioliformis acuta (PLEVA)*. PLEVA tends to have a higher number of lesions and a shorter overall course of the disease. Although classic PLEVA differs from LyP, some patients with PLEVA may have lesions with histology that is difficult to distinguish from LyP. Furthermore, PLEVA may exhibit CD30 positivity. A clear separation between LyP and PLEVA is not always possible. LyP and PLEVA may also coexist. Persistence of a clonal T-cell gene rearrangement, documented by PCR, or suggested by IHC for TRBC1 can help to favor LyP.

When considering LyP and reviewing immunostains for CD30, one should bear in mind that CD30-positive cells can be seen in many nonneoplastic lymphocyte-mediated disorders such as *hypersensitivity reactions from an arthropod bite or a drug*. The large CD30-positive cells tend to be fewer in these lesions than in LyP, but the clinical history is the key element to making the distinction in appearance to papular MF because the infiltrate is composed predominantly of smaller cerebriform lymphocytes, which are frequently negative for CD30 and demonstrate prominent epidermotropism. Type C LyP is composed of a more prominent population of atypical CD30-positive cells that may be in clusters and sheets, simulating ALCL (Fig. 15.30). Other less frequent features include lymphocytic vasculitis, marked epidermal hyperplasia, and prominent involvement of follicular epithelium. A syringotropic variant, a band-like presentation similar to MF, and associated keratoacanthoma have also been described.

Prognosis and Treatment

LyP is a chronic condition that may last decades. Patients with LyP will not die from this condition but may have morbidity related to an associated lymphoma. Treatment of LyP is not always necessary. LyP responds to PUVA, interferon, methotrexate, brentuximab vedotin, and systemic retinoids, but because none of these modalities or chemotherapy has been proved to alter the natural history, the condition recurs after discontinuing therapy. Associated cutaneous CD30-positive lymphoma, MF, and systemic Hodgkin's or non-Hodgkin's lymphoma are seen in 5% to 20% of cases. These neoplasms may occur concurrent with, before, or after a diagnosis of LyP.

PRIMARY CUTANEOUS ANAPLASTIC LARGE CELL LYMPHOMA

Clinical Findings

ALCL, previously referred to as Ki-1 lymphoma or CD30-positive lymphoma, is a neoplasm composed of CD30-positive lymphocytes. Primary cutaneous ALCL is restricted to the skin, but similar tumors may occur in the skin secondarily from systemic ALCL. Primary ALCL may affect any age but is rare in children. Lesions are usually solitary nodules (greater than 1–2 cm) (Fig. 15.31), tumors, or plaques that frequently ulcerate or become necrotic. The extremities are frequently involved as several grouped nodules or papules confined to a region or in multiple anatomic sites. Spontaneous regression may be seen in approximately 40%. Such tumors may arise in a patient with LyP or MF before or after diagnosis of LyP or MF. Tumors with the appearance of an ALCL arising in the context of MF are by convention regarded as large cell transformation, an interpretation that is often supported by shared clonal TCR gene rearrangements.

Histopathologic Features

The histology of ALCL can be similar to that described for LyP. However, the lesions tend to be larger and extend more deeply (Fig. 15.32). There are often dense cohesive sheets of CD30-positive cells present comprising the

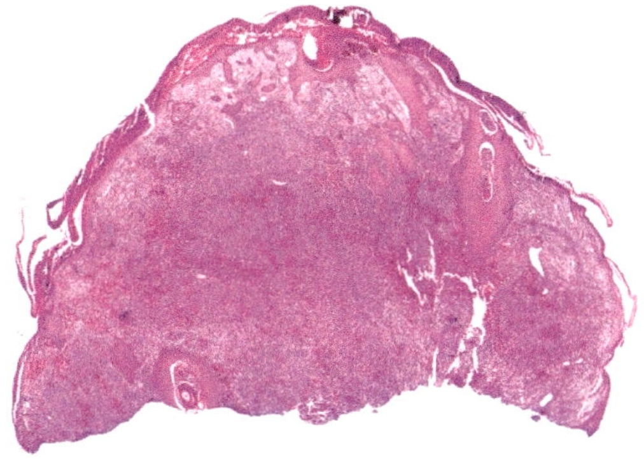

FIG. 15.32
Silhouette of an anaplastic large cell lymphoma. A dense infiltrate is associated with epidermal hyperplasia.

PRIMARY CUTANEOUS ANAPLASTIC LARGE T-CELL LYMPHOMA—DISEASE FACT SHEET

Patient Group
- ▸▸ Primary cutaneous anaplastic large cell lymphoma (ALCL) tends to affect middle-aged or older individuals
- ▸▸ May rarely be seen in children
- ▸▸ Men are more often affected than women
- ▸▸ Systemic ALCL tends to affect young adults as well as elderly people

Site of Involvement
- ▸▸ Head, extremities, and buttock

Clinical Findings
- ▸▸ Usually solitary rapidly growing nodule with ulceration
- ▸▸ Nodules are reddish brown and indurated

Prognosis
- ▸▸ Favorable prognosis with a 5-year survival rate of 90%
- ▸▸ May spontaneously regress

Treatment
- ▸▸ Radiation therapy
- ▸▸ Simple excision for localized solitary skin lesion
- ▸▸ Biologic therapy such as brentuximab vedotin for multifocal disease

majority of the lesional cell population (Fig. 15.33). Tumor nodules most often appear to be situated in the dermis; however, clusters of the cells may involve intratumoral vessels, or large portions of the tumor may be present intravascularly. Most often the atypical lymphocytes are medium to large in size, with classic intranuclear protrusions, horseshoe- or kidney bean-shaped nuclei, and multinucleation comprising the "hallmark cells" seen in all ALCL (Fig. 15.34). However, the infiltrates may alternatively be composed of small pleomorphic cells. Admixed eosinophils or neutrophils may be numerous. There may be less involvement of the epidermis than in LyP, but acanthosis and secondary epidermal changes with exocytosis or ulceration are also common with ALCL. The pseudoepitheliomatous epidermal hyperplasia overlying lesions of ALCL can occasionally be so exuberant as to simulate squamous cell carcinoma.

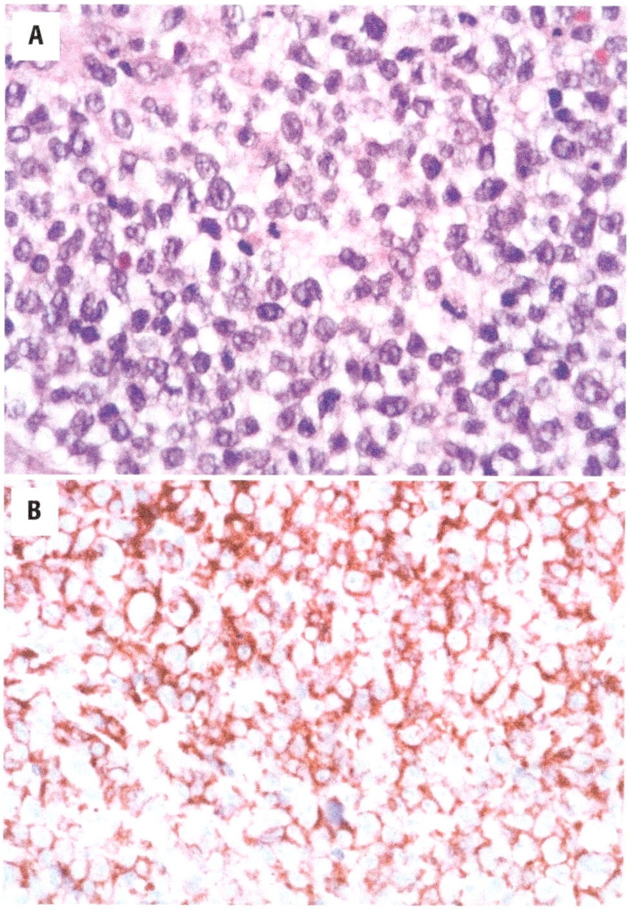

FIG. 15.33
CD30-positive large cell lymphoma. **A,** The infiltrate is composed of large cells. **B,** They are immunoreactive for CD30.

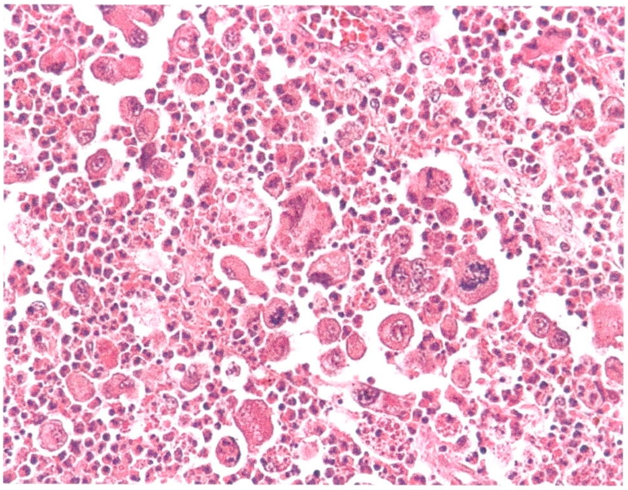

FIG. 15.34
The large anaplastic cells are intermingled with numerous neutrophils and eosinophils.

PRIMARY CUTANEOUS ANAPLASTIC LARGE T-CELL LYMPHOMA—PATHOLOGIC FEATURES

Histopathologic Features

- Dense nodular or diffuse infiltrate by large atypical mononuclear cells, rarely small
- Epidermotropism common
- Secondary surface changes common: ulceration, epidermal hyperplasia
- Variable associated mixed inflammatory cell infiltrate of lymphocytes, histiocytes, neutrophils, and eosinophils

Ancillary Studies

- Immunophenotype
  - Large cells are positive for CD30
  - Variable expression of T-cell markers
  - Negative for ALK

Molecular Studies

- Clonal TCR gene rearrangement presents in most cases (>90%)
- DUSP22 rearrangement in 20% to 25% c-ALCL, but does not rule out systemic ALCL

Differential Diagnosis

- Mycosis fungoides with CD30+ cells (with or without large cell transformation)
- Type C LyP
- Secondary involvement of the skin by systemic anaplastic large cell lymphoma
- Leukemia or mast cell neoplasia with immunoreactivity for CD30
- Nonlymphoid tumors: melanoma, poorly differentiated carcinoma

Ancillary Studies

Immunohistochemical staining reveals a CD2, CD3, CD4, and CD45RO+ lymphoid infiltrate with numerous (>75%) CD30-positive cells. Loss of pan T-cell antigens may be found, most commonly, CD3, warranting the use of more than one pan T-cell antigen in an evaluatory panel. T cells demonstrate an αβ phenotype (TCR-alpha and TCR-beta expression). The t(2;5) chromosomal translocation, identified by anaplastic large cell kinase positivity, which is seen in anaplastic lymphoma kinase (ALK)-positive systemic ALCL, is typically not present in primary cutaneous CD30-positive lymphoma. However, of the rare t(2;5) rearranged primary cutaneous ALCL cases that have been described, many are in pediatric patients. Strong nuclear labeling with ALK IHC is seen in these tumors. In contrast, ALK translocations with variant partners can sometimes be seen in primary cutaneous ALCL which correspond to a dim cytoplasmic labeling pattern on ALK IHC. P63 translocations are exceedingly rare in primary cutaneous ALCL. DUSP22-IRF4 locus translocations, which may be suggested by LEF1 protein expression, are common (20% to 25% of primary cutaneous ALCL). Primary cutaneous ALCL is also typically negative for CD 15/Leu-M1 and epithelial membrane antigen (EMA) (although occasional staining can be seen). Rare tumors may coexpress CD30 and CD56 or show γδ expression.

Differential Diagnosis

ALCL is best distinguished from LyP by clinical correlation, the latter representing small papular lesions that spontaneously involute. The lesions of bona fide CD30-positive ALCL tend to be nodular and persist.

After a diagnosis of CD30-positive lymphoma has been made, the issue arises whether it is primary or secondary skin involvement by nodal lymphoma. The latter, if ALK positive, are often also positive for EMA and cytotoxic markers and usually harbor a t(2 : 5) translocation. The identification of a DUSP-22IRF4 translocation slightly favors a primary cutaneous ALK-negative ALCL over an ALK-negative systemic ALCL. However, molecular or cytogenetic studies for DUSP22 and TP63 gene rearrangements are relevant for prognosis for patients with cutaneous and extracutaneous ALK-negative ALCLs. In that setting the presence of a DUSP22 gene rearrangement is generally prognostically favorable, while the presence of TP63 gene rearrangement is unfavorable.

ALK-negative systemic ALCL tends to be clinically more aggressive. Appropriate staging may help to resolve the distinction quickly (e.g., lymphadenopathy and B symptoms are common). Complete clinical staging of all CD30-positive ALCL in skin may not be necessary, but at least radiologic imaging is suggested for most cases. Bone marrow staging is not generally recommended for solitary skin lesions. Careful clinical examination is paramount for the identification of any clues of a systemic lymphoma.

A variety of lymphomas can have overlapping features with ALCL on routine H&E-stained sections, including tumor-stage MF with large cell transformation, peripheral T-cell lymphomas, natural killer (NK) cell lymphoma, leukemia, and diffuse large B-cell lymphoma. Furthermore, nonlymphoid neoplasms, such as amelanotic melanoma or poorly differentiated carcinoma, may be confused with ALCL on occasion. A panel of immunostains and attention to clinical context (e.g., history of MF) usually allow for a definitive diagnosis. As previously discussed, a CD30-positive large cell lymphoproliferative lesion in the context of MF is by convention accepted as transformation of MF and not a second lymphoma.

Prognosis and Treatment

The prognosis is favorable in primary cutaneous CD30-positive lymphomas irrespective of the cytology of the tumor cells. Therapy for patients with primary cutaneous CD30-positive lymphoma includes surgical excision, irradiation of the tumor, and treatments similar to advanced MF.

OTHER CUTANEOUS T-CELL LYMPHOMA

There are a number of CTCLs other than MF and ALCL. They represent less than 10% of all CTCLs. As a group, these tumors tend to be nonepitheliotropic. Most of them are more aggressive than MF or ALCL. The classification of these tumors is currently evolving as more cases are being described. In the WHO-European Organization for Research and Treatment of Cancer (EORTC) classification, this category includes subcutaneous panniculitis–like T-cell lymphoma (SPTCL); extranodal NK/T-cell lymphoma (ENKTCL), nasal type; and primary cutaneous peripheral T-cell lymphomas and CD4+ and CD8+ LPDs. The latter include primary cutaneous aggressive epidermotropic CD8-positive T-cell lymphoma, cutaneous $\gamma\delta$ T-cell lymphoma, CD8+ indolent acral, and primary cutaneous CD4-positive small-/medium-sized T-cell LPDs.

SUBCUTANEOUS PANNICULITIS–LIKE T-CELL LYMPHOMA

Clinical Findings

SPTCL is a cytotoxic $\alpha\beta$ T-cell lymphoma that preferentially involves the subcutaneous fat and exhibits a typically indolent clinical course. Occasional fatal outcomes have been reported and are most frequently due to the systemic impact of hemophagocytic lymphohistiocytosis (HLH). Autoimmune comorbidities are common (25%) and may play a role in the pathogenesis. A subset of SPTCL (at least 25%) arises in the background of a germline HAVCR2 mutation which causes misfolding of the surface immune checkpoint protein T-cell immunoglobulin mucin 3 (TIM3) putatively removing regulation of peripheral tolerance.

SPTCL has a predilection for females and may present in children or young adults as subcutaneous indurated nodules, tumors, and indurated or atrophic plaques, which may be solitary but more frequently are multiple. Ulceration is uncommon but may occur. The proximal lower and upper extremities are frequently involved, but lesions may also affect the trunk and rarely the head and neck region. Spontaneous regression has been reported. Constitutional symptoms, such as fever, weight loss, night sweats, and malaise, may be seen, especially if there is associated HLH.

Histopathologic Features

A nodular and diffuse sheetlike infiltrate of lymphocytes eradicates fat lobules (Fig. 15.35), often also extending into interlobular septae. Although the overlying dermis and epidermis are usually spared by dense tumoral infiltrates, frequently a scant mid to deep perivascular dermal lymphoid infiltrate is present. Rimming of adipocytes by tumor cells (protrusion of tumor cells into adipocyte cytoplasm) is a classic feature but is not specific and may be absent. There may be angiocentricity of tumor cells within and adjacent to fat lobules. The tumor cell population is most often pleomorphic and composed of small, medium, and large hyperchromatic atypical lymphocytes with frequent mitotic activity. However, in some biopsies or in early lesions, lymphoid atypia may be inconspicuous making diagnosis difficult. There may be many apoptotic tumor cells with prominent karyorrhexis. There is often an admixture of histiocytes. Multinucleated histiocytes may be seen engulfing lymphocytes (emperipolesis), and there may also be erythrocytophagia, leading to the presence of debris or cell-filled "bean-bag cells." Histiocytes form loose or well-defined granulomas. On occasion, the granulomatous component may predominate, making recognition of the lesion as a lymphoma more difficult. Fat necrosis with microcystic alteration of the adipocytes is characteristic. It is helpful when lymphoid follicles with germinal centers, mucin, and plasma cells are absent. However, because of overlap with autoimmune entities (whether due to evolution to clonal disease, or concomitant autoimmunity), sometimes these features can be present.

Ancillary Studies

Immunohistochemical staining of SPTCL typically demonstrates a T-cell α/β phenotype (CD2, CD3, βF1/TCR-beta positive) and a cytotoxic phenotype (CD8, TIA-1/GMP-17, granzyme B, and perforin positive). Loss of antigens such as CD5 and CD7 is common. TRBC1 IHC is monoclonally restricted in atypical cells. Unlike many other T-cell lymphomas primary to skin, CCR4 is negative. Markers for Epstein-Barr virus (EBV) are negative. CD56 is usually negative. When positive, it may portend a worse prognosis. PCR for $\alpha\beta$ TCR gene rearrangement usually reveals T-cell clonality. HAVCR2-mutant-related TIM3 alterations can be identified by a prominent dot-like immunohistochemical labeling pattern and confirmed by sequence analysis (although not clinically routinely performed).

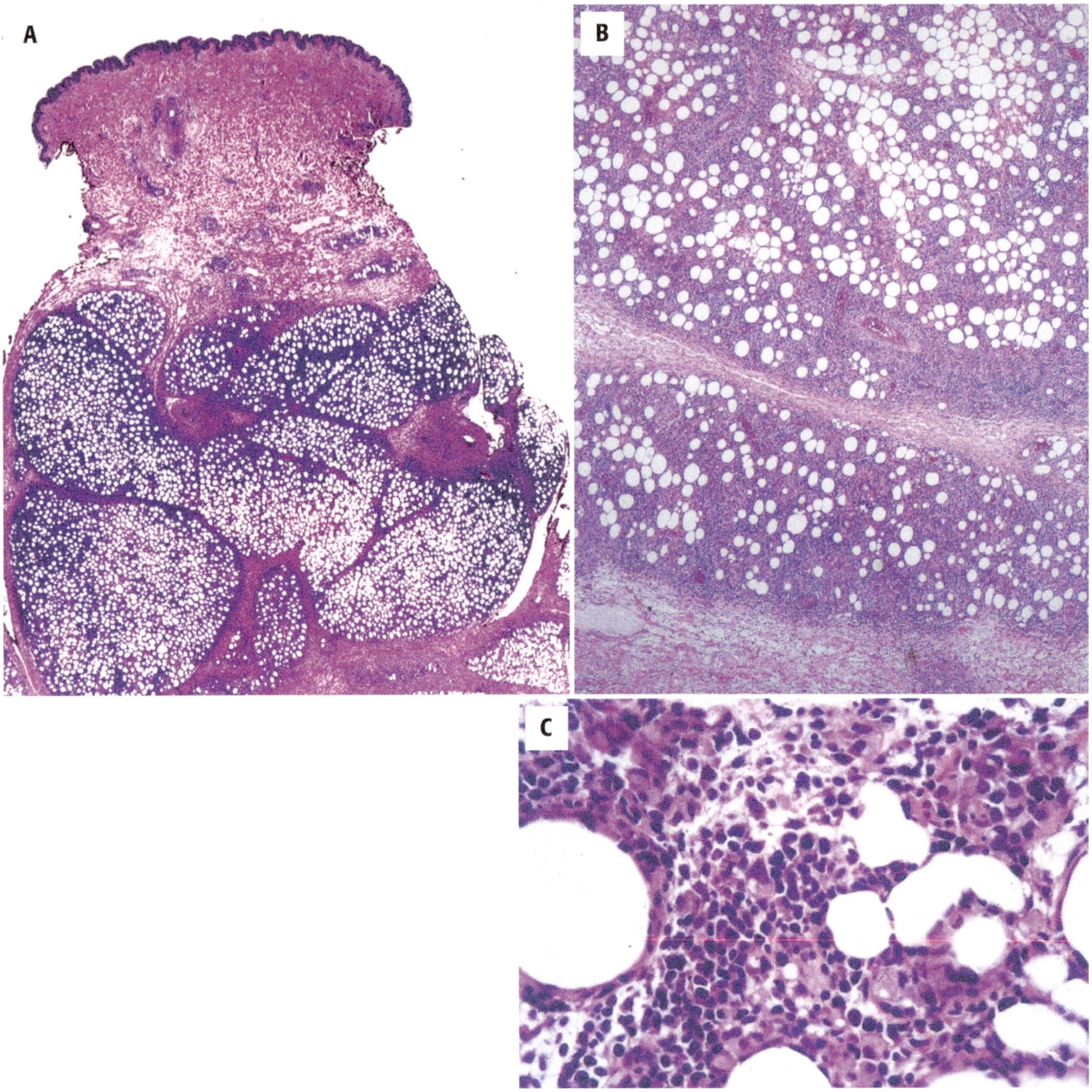

FIG. 15.35

Subcutaneous panniculitic T-cell lymphoma. **A,** Scanning magnification reveals an infiltrate in the subcutis. **B,** Dense sheets of lymphocytes are present. **C,** The lymphocytes are atypical.

Differential Diagnosis

The differential diagnosis includes the spectrum of lymphocyte-predominant lobular panniculitis.

Lupus panniculitis can be difficult to differentiate from SPTCL, especially in the early stages of SPTCL, when cytologic atypia of lymphocytes may not be prominent. Generally, a well-developed interface dermatitis, mucin deposition, a heavy B-cell population with germinal center formation and hyalinization of fat lobules, and plasma cells favor LE. However, mild vacuolar interface dermatitis and periadnexal dermal lymphocytes and few plasma cells can also rarely be seen in SPTCL, particularly in cases with autoimmune overlap, or precursor lesions. The fat alteration in SPTCL shows more necrosis and less hyalinization. LE lacks the striking karyorrhexis, atypia, and erythrocytophagy that typify SPTCL. Prominent atypia and extensive rimming of adipocytes by atypical lymphocytes is typical of lymphoma. However, overall there is significant overlap histologically and clinically such that, on an initial biopsy, a reliable distinction between LE and SPTCL may not be possible.

If there is a prominent histiocytic component, subcutaneous panniculitic T-cell lymphoma (SPCTL) might simulate *infectious panniculitis*, especially if there is prominent karyorrhexis and necrosis. The presence of neutrophils favors infection. Many cases of *cytophagic histiocytic* (or *macrophagic*) *panniculitis* likely represent

SUBCUTANEOUS PANNICULITIS–LIKE (αβ) T-CELL LYMPHOMA—DISEASE FACT SHEET

Patient Group

- Usually young adults, female predominant

Site of Involvement

- Extremities and trunk

Clinical Findings

- Subcutaneous nodules, usually in adults, but can occur in children
- May be associated with systemic symptoms

Prognosis

- 5-year survival rate of ≈80%
- Dissemination to mesentery, perinodal fat, and bone marrow is rare
- Hemophagocytic lymphohistiocytosis associated with a poor prognosis

Treatment

- Biologic therapy
- Radiotherapy
- Chemoablative therapy with stem cell transplant if HLH

SUBCUTANEOUS PANNICULITIS–LIKE (αβ) T-CELL LYMPHOMA—PATHOLOGIC FEATURES

Histopathologic Features

- Infiltration of fat lobules by atypical lymphocytes
- Rimming of fat by lymphocytes
- Emperipolesis, karyorrhexis, erythrocytophagia
- Associated granulomatous reaction common

Ancillary Studies

- Immunophenotype
- Usually positive for CD3, CD7, CD8, TIA-1, and βF-1
- CCR4, TCR γδ, and EBV negative
- Clusters of lymphocytes with elevated Ki-67

Molecular Studies

- Clonal TCR gene rearrangement detectable in most cases

Differential Diagnosis

- Other lymphomas with subcutaneous involvement, in particular γδ T-cell lymphoma or natural killer lymphoma
- Pseudolymphomas, in particular lupus panniculitis, or infection

SPTCL. However, the reaction pattern of macrophagic panniculitis can also represent a nonneoplastic process, for example, as a manifestation of a hemophagocytic syndrome after a viral infection.

Given the differences in prognosis, SPTCL also should be distinguished from other variants of lymphoma, which may involve the subcutis, such as NK-cell lymphoma (positive for CD56 or EBV) or γδ peripheral T-cell lymphoma. Secondary involvement of the subcutis by a nodal lymphoma (e.g., diffuse large B-cell lymphoma) can readily be distinguished by clinical context (adenopathy, history of lymphoma, and IHC).

Prognosis and Treatment

The 5-year survival rate of patients with CD8-positive α/β SPCTL is 80%. SPTCL has been shown to respond to irradiation, chemotherapy with doxorubicin, denileukin diftitox, cyclosporine, and retinoids. Systemic corticosteroids may provide benefit in nonaggressive cases. More aggressive therapy including hematopoietic stem cell transplant may be required in the context of HLH.

PRIMARY CUTANEOUS CD8-POSITIVE AGGRESSIVE EPIDERMOTROPIC CYTOTOXIC T-CELL LYMPHOMA

Primary cutaneous CD8-positive aggressive epidermotropic cytotoxic T-cell lymphoma is a rare but distinct subgroup recognized under the WHO-EORTC as a clinically high-grade lymphoma manifesting histologically as a prominently epidermotropic CD8-positive T-cell lymphoma with cytotoxic protein expression, high proliferation index, and necrosis of adjacent tissue.

Clinical Findings

These patients have rapidly evolving heterogeneous, often generalized skin lesions, including erythematous scaling and erosive patches, plaques, papules, nodules, and tumors. Surface changes include verrucous hyperkeratosis, hemorrhagic ulceration, and necrosis. There is frequent involvement of the oral cavity, with dissemination to unusual sites such as the testis, lungs, and CNS without lymph node involvement.

Histopathologic Features

There is an infiltrate of atypical hyperchromatic epidermotropic pleomorphic small, medium, or large lymphocytes that may show immunoblastic morphology. The epidermis may be hypertrophic or atrophic, with marked interface alteration, including dyskeratosis, single-cell necrosis, and junctional karyorrhexis as well as secondary changes such as spongiosis and ulceration. Involvement of the dermis and subcutis may be seen, with destruction of adnexa, angiocentricity, and angiodestruction.

Ancillary Studies

The immunophenotype is CD3+, CD8+/−, CD45RA+, βF1+, CD7+, CD2−, CD5−, EBV−, TCR γδ−, CCR4+/− with positive staining for cytotoxic granules (TIA1+, granzyme B, perforin). CD56 is usually negative, although rare positive cases have been reported.

Immunostains for pSTAT3 and pSTAT5 may be positive. FISH or anchored RNA-sequencing gene fusion analysis may reveal JAK2 fusions. Other less common fusions or gains in copy number implicating genes in JAK/STAT signaling pathways can be identified. A clonal TCR gene rearrangement is usually found.

Differential Diagnosis

A CD8-positive immunophenotype may be seen in various presentations of CTCL, including PR, hypopigmented (and rarely classic) MF, LyP type D, and SPTCL. Notably, each of these groups exhibits a more indolent behavior; therefore it is critical to appropriately distinguish them from aggressive epidermotropic CD8-positive cytotoxic T-cell lymphoma, which easily can be achieved with a clinical examination or correlation. Notably, the histology of the former entities tends to be more low grade than the latter. Other clues are helpful: MF is typically CD45RO positive and is more strongly positive for CCR4 than AETCL while AETCL shows more retention of CD7. SPTCL is not typically epitheliotropic and is negative for CCR4.

The clinical and histologic features may overlap with γδ CTCL. To distinguish the two, the demonstration of CD8 and βF1/TCR-αβ and CCR4-positivity favors the aggressive epidermotropic CD8-positive cytotoxic T-cell lymphoma. A CD4/CD8 null phenotype along with γ or δ positivity (with βF1/TCR-αβ-negativity) favors a γδ CTCL.

Finally, because cytotoxic granules may be present in NK cells, CD56 (and EBV nontranslated RNAs [EBER]/EBV) staining should be performed to exclude an NK-cell lymphoma.

Prognosis and Treatment

The prognosis is usually poor despite treatment with multimodality biologic modifier therapy or chemotherapy.

PRIMARY CUTANEOUS CD4-POSITIVE SMALL OR MEDIUM T-CELL LYMPHOPROLIFERATIVE DISORDER

Primary cutaneous CD4-positive small or medium T-cell LPD is a low-grade, typically solitary clonal lymphoid proliferation that exhibits a T-follicular helper (TFH) immunophenotype. Although the nosologic classification of this entity is yet unclear, the key clinical difficulty is in distinguishing these lesions prospectively from the early stages of more aggressive peripheral T-cell lymphomas. The distinction from a benign proliferation of lymphocytes (pseudolymphoma, e.g., CLH) is less important due to the shared indolent behavior and therapeutic approach for both entities.

Clinical Findings

Patients are typically adults in the sixth decade of life who present with solitary (Fig. 15.36A) or oligolesional erythematous to violaceous nodules, tumors, or plaques that arise de novo without evolution from or concurrent association with lesions of classic MF. Most tumors arise in the head and neck region, but tumors may also occur on the trunk or extremities.

Histopathologic Features

Tumors are most commonly composed of a dense nodular and diffuse infiltrate of pleomorphic small- to medium-sized atypical lymphocytes in the dermis (Fig. 15.36B), often with extension into the subcutis. Although folliculo- or adnexotropism is routine in these cases, epidermotropism is vanishingly rare. Current literature admits a second architectural variant arranged as a superficial dermal band with periadnexal extension. In either case, the lymphocytes may show an admixture of cerebriform, hyperchromatic, immunoblastic, and anaplastic features. Larger-sized lymphocytes should be limited to a very small subpopulation (<40% of the infiltrate), if seen at all. Mitoses may be seen but are not numerous.

Ancillary Studies

The lymphocytes stain positively for CD4 with infrequent loss of pan T-cell antigens. Ki-67 proliferation indices are typically less than 25%. TFH markers including PD-1 (most common), ICOS, CXCL13, and bcl-6 may be seen, often in a "rosetting" pattern, sometimes around solitary dispersed blastlike CD30+ cells. There is often a prominent component of CD20-positive B cells. A mixed inflammatory background may be present, including plasma cells, eosinophils, and histiocytes. EBER-ISH is negative. Molecular studies for clonal TCR gene

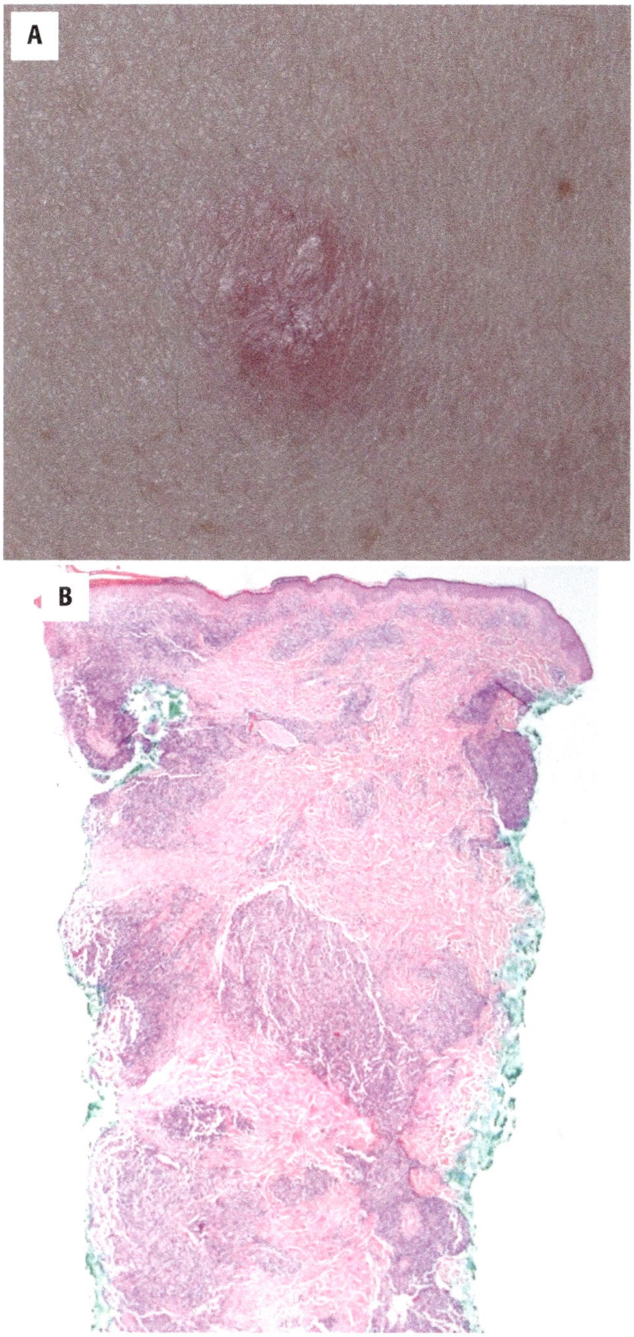

FIG. 15.36

Small/medium pleomorphic T-cell lymphoma. **A,** Erythematous nodule. **B,** Dense infiltrate of lymphocytes in dermis.

rearrangement are important for the diagnosis. Rarely a B-cell clone may also be identified.

Differential Diagnosis

Importantly, these tumors should be distinguished from more aggressive CD4-positive variants of peripheral T-cell lymphoma, such as tumor-stage MF, ATLL, and peripheral T-cell lymphoma, not otherwise specified (NOS, primary cutaneous or systemic). Clinical and serologic data are helpful to distinguish the first two. Multilesional or rapidly evolving tumors or nodules, the finding of more than 30% to 40% large cells, the absence of a reactive CD8-positive T-cell population, or a high proliferation index have been suggested as features favoring a *PTCL NOS.*

Indolent small- or medium-sized CD8-positive lymphoid proliferations with predilection for the ear, face, or acral sites bear some clinical similarity to CD4-positive small- or medium-sized T-cell LPD. These are distinguished by a more monomorphic cytology on H&E, sparing of the epidermis/adnexa by tumor nodules, and by the predominance of CD8-positive T cells.

Although individual lesions may be as indolent as a persistent bite or hypersensitivity reaction, their clinical persistence in the absence of inciting factors such as a medication or arthropod bite and the finding of clonality is used to classify the lesions as LPD. A conservative treatment approach with these lesions is usually best for the patient.

Prognosis and Treatment

Excision or radiotherapy may be used for solitary lesions.

PRIMARY CUTANEOUS ACRAL CD8-POSITIVE T-CELL LYMPHOPROLIFERATIVE DISORDER

This group of LPDs is comprised of dermal infiltrates of clonal medium-sized CD8+ T cells forming a slowly growing nonulcerated papule or nodule of middle-aged or elderly adults, typically involving acral sites.

Clinical Findings

Lesions most commonly present as solitary papulonodules at acral sites including the ear, nose, hands, and feet.

Histopathologic Features

Histopathologically, there is a dense diffuse dermal infiltrate, often sparing the epidermis and adnexae (resulting in a grenz zone). Cells are monomorphous, with moderate nuclear pleomorphism and only rare mitotic figures. Few to no intervening mixed inflammatory cells are seen.

Ancillary Studies

Tumors are comprised of TCR αβ-positive, CD3-positive, and CD8-positive T cells which often show a dot-like Golgi pattern with an antibody to CD68 and which may be CD99+. Some loss of pan-T-cell markers (CD2, CD5, CD7) is typical. Markers of a nonactivated cytotoxic T-cell are present (TIA1), but cells are negative for activation markers (granzyme B or perforin). TFH markers (e.g., PD1) are negative, although B-cell aggregates may be seen. CD30, EBER-ISH, and CD56 are negative. The Ki-67 labeling index is usually low.

Differential Diagnosis

These lesions should not be confused with CD8-positive AETCL. The latter has a more dramatic clinical presentation and aggressive course and is histopathologically characterized by epidermotropism, a high mitotic rate, activation markers granzyme B and perforin, JAK/STAT signaling pathway alterations, and not uncommonly by ulceration. CD8+ peripheral T-cell lymphoma (primary to the skin or systemic) is sometimes considered when the dermal infiltrates are comprised of larger cells with high mitotic rates, cytotoxic activation markers, and tissue damage more suggestive of an aggressive activated cytotoxic process (ulceration, hemorrhage, angiocentricity, necrosis). Clinical correlation is needed, with staging analysis in such cases.

Prognosis and Treatment

Local recurrences are rare. The lesions are often cured by simple excision or radiation.

PRIMARY CUTANEOUS γδ T-CELL LYMPHOMA

Primary cutaneous γδ T-cell lymphomas are rare monoclonal lymphoproliferations of γδ T cells within the skin and subcutis. While characteristically high grade, there are variable clinical manifestations within this group of lymphomas, purportedly correlating to skin compartment involved and specific γδ subset of origin (Vδ1 vs. Vδ2).

Clinical Findings

Patients may present at any age, but the median age of this disease is in the seventh decade of life, more often in men. The most common presentation is of thick plaques (Fig. 15.37A), some of which may simulate panniculitis, or MF-like patches and plaques. Dermal nodules or tumors can also be seen. Lesions tend to ulcerate (Fig. 15.37B). The legs, torso, and arms are common; however, any site may be involved. Constitutional symptoms are frequent, with associated autoimmune syndromes sometimes identified. Mucosal or extracutaneous involvement may occur. Nodal and bone marrow involvement is quite rare. Patients may have associated systemic symptoms (lactate dehydrogenase [LDH] is often high) and develop a lymphoma-associated hemophagocytic syndrome/lymphohistiocytosis (fever, pancytopenia, coagulopathy, hyperbilirubinemia, and organomegaly), which is frequently fatal. The coexistence of second lymphomas or carcinomas is occasionally noted.

Histopathologic Features

There is a broad spectrum of histologic patterns, ranging from a superficial pagetoid infiltrate to predominantly intradermal or subcutaneous nodular lesions. Most cases involve all parts of the skin. A common feature is a lichenoid or interface component with necrotic keratinocytes. The appearance of the lymphocytes is variable, tending to range from small to medium in size in most lesions but also at times ranging from medium to large in others. The nuclei tend to be elongated and twisted, with clumped chromatin; the cytoplasm appears faintly granular. Features of cytotoxicity, including hemorrhage, necrosis, and vasculitis (with angiocentricity and angioinvasion), are often seen. When the lesion presents as panniculitis, there may be an admixed granulomatous component, with notable cytophagocytosis. Perineural invasion and follicotropism can occasionally be seen.

Ancillary Studies

The tumor cells are immunopositive for CD3, CD2, one or more cytotoxic proteins (TIA-1, perforin, granzyme B, sometimes in an atypical Golgi pattern), and γ M1 and/or TCR-delta (Fig. 15.37C). TCR alpha and beta (βf1) are negative. CD56 is positive in approximately half of the cases. Tumors are most often negative for CD4, CD5, CD7, and CD8 (CD4/CD8 "double negative"). However, occasionally CD8 is expressed and may vary between lesions in the same patient. CD30 can be positive partly or completely, in a subset of cases. EBER-ISH/EBV is negative. There is clonal rearrangement of the TCR γ gene but not the TCR β gene.

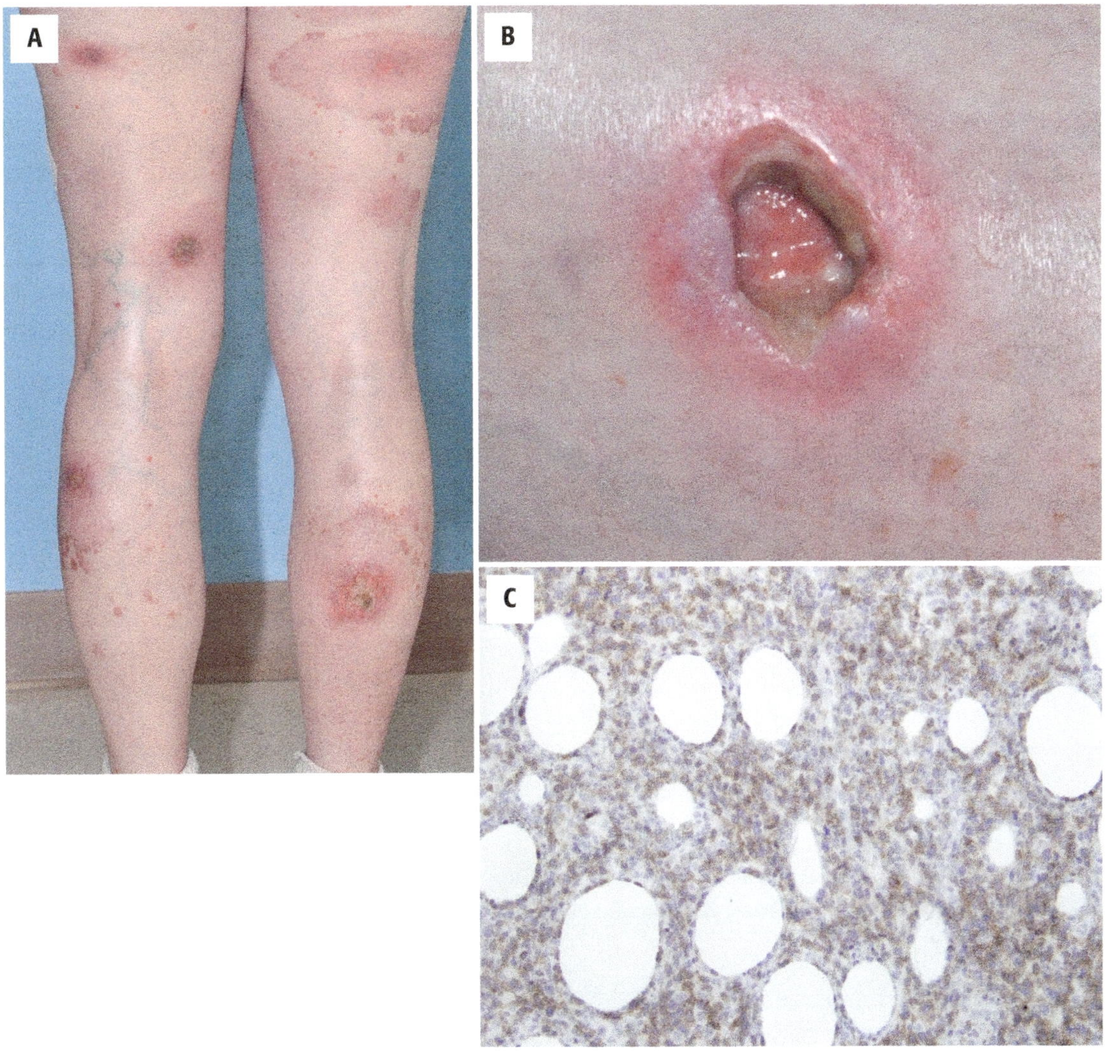

FIG. 15.37
γδ Lymphoma. **A,** Multiple plaques. **B,** Ulcerated nodule. **C,** Dense infiltrate of tumor cells in the subcutis with immunoreactivity for TCR γ.

Prognosis and Treatment

A diagnosis of γδ lymphoma usually implies a poor prognosis, with a median survival time of approximately 30 months and a 5-year overall survival rate of 20%. No therapies have shown significant results; multiagent chemotherapy and/or radiation do not typically result in sustained remission. Allogeneic stem cell transplantation may prolong remission.

PRIMARY CUTANEOUS PERIPHERAL T-CELL LYMPHOMA, NOS

This rare and rather haphazard group of lymphomas is comprised of primary CTCLs that do not meet the criteria/match the characteristics of the previously described well-characterized lymphomas or lymphoproliferative disorders.

Clinical Findings

Clinical manifestations range from disseminated nodules and papules on the trunk and limbs to oligolesional or unilesional tumors. While more common in the sixth decade of life, these poorly characterized CTCLs have been reported in all age groups. By definition, systemic involvement is not present at the time of diagnosis, although the lesions may disseminate systemically over time.

Histopathologic Features

Histopathologic features vary. Infiltrates are typically dense and composed of medium to large cells. If epidermal involvement is present, it is often focal and/or associated with deeper infiltrates. Cytotoxic tissue alteration is occasionally present.

Ancillary Studies

CD2 and CD3 are typically expressed, with most cases composed of CD4+ T cells. Variants including CD4−/CD8− and CD4+/CD8+ are seen. Cases can show a TFH phenotype with PD1, ICOS, CXCL13, bcl-6 and/or CD10, and/or expression of CD20. EBER-ISH/EBV markers are negative. CD30 is not prominent.

Differential Diagnosis

The differential diagnosis is broad. Clinicopathologic correlation is paramount.

Prognosis and Treatment

Prognosis is poor. Mean overall survival rates are between 2 and 6 years. Aside from occasional cases of unilesional disease treated by excision or radiation, therapies have not shown significant results.

SECONDARY T-CELL LYMPHOMA (EXTRACUTANEOUS T-CELL LYMPHOMA INVOLVING SKIN)

The spectrum of nodal or other extracutaneous lymphomas with secondary skin involvement is very broad and beyond the scope of this chapter. We only discuss herein four types: ATLL, hydro vacciniforme-like T-cell lymphoma, angioimmunoblastic T-cell lymphoma (AITL), and peripheral T-cell lymphoma, NOS.

ADULT T-CELL LEUKEMIA/LYMPHOMA

ATLL is an aggressive lymphoid neoplasm associated with HTLV-1, often characterized by systemic disease without cutaneous involvement. Cutaneous involvement without systemic disease at presentation is, however, the second most common presentation of ATLL, with fewer cases of cutaneous ATLL developing in the context of previously known systemic lymphoma. Fifty percent of all patients with ATLL develop skin lesions at some point during the course of disease.

Clinical Findings

ATLL is endemic in Japan, the Caribbean, South America, the Middle East, and parts of Central Africa, corresponding to areas in which there is a high prevalence of HTLV-1 infection. It is typically seen in adults after several years of viral infection. Only up to 5% of infected individuals develop ATLL. There are four main subtypes: acute, chronic, smoldering, and lymphoma. The *acute form* is most common and is diagnosed by exclusion of the other types. It is characterized by a leukemic presentation with fever, marked leukocytosis, lymphadenopathy, high LDH, hepatosplenomegaly and other organ involvement, and hypercalcemia with lytic bone lesions. Skin involvement may only be present in half of the cases and is manifested as tumors, papules (Fig. 15.38), or plaques, which arise rapidly without transition from a patch stage (although patches are occasionally seen). Erythroderma and purpuric lesions may also manifest. The *chronic form* has milder clinical symptoms, with a prolonged clinical course, but is characterized as either favorable or unfavorable depending upon LDH, blood urea nitrogen (BUN), and albumin levels. These patients have normal calcium levels and less generalized organ involvement, with the exception of hepatosplenomegaly and adenopathy. There is a chronic lymphocytosis of greater than 10%, but the cells are less atypical. The *smoldering form* may present with skin-predominant disease, with minimal or absent circulating cells (less than 5%), normal calcium levels and LDH, and minimal organomegaly and adenopathy. Patients with the *lymphoma form* of ATLL present with nodal disease without a leukemic phase or lymphocytosis. Acute, lymphoma, and unfavorable chronic types are considered to be aggressive variants of ATLL, while the smoldering and favorable chronic types are low grade. Regardless of initial presentation, all subtypes are susceptible to superimposed infection. One-half of indolent cases will evolve to aggressive disease within a 5-year period.

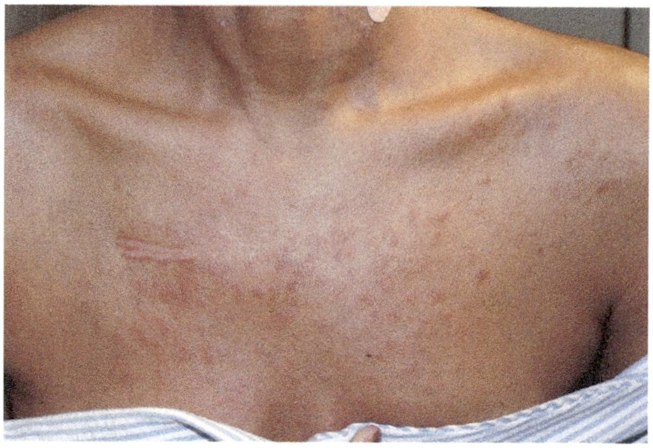

FIG. 15.38
Numerous erythematous papules in a patient with adult T-cell leukemia/lymphoma.

ADULT T-CELL LEUKEMIA/ LYMPHOMA—DISEASE FACT SHEET

Patient Group

- ▸▸ Affects 1% to 5% of individuals infected by human T-lymphotropic virus 1
- ▸▸ Endemic in certain regions (e.g., Caribbean islands, Southwest Japan)

Site of Involvement

- ▸▸ Skin, lymph nodes, lung, liver, spleen, bone, CNS, and other sites
- ▸▸ A variant with disease limited to the skin exists

Clinical Findings

- ▸▸ Acute leukemic form (≈two-thirds of cases): lymphadenopathy, lymphocytosis, lung and other organ involvement, lytic bone, and skin lesions
- ▸▸ Chronic: lymphadenopathy and skin involvement; no hypercalcemia
- ▸▸ Smoldering: abnormal lymphocytes of 3% or less with proviral integration; no lymphadenopathy; skin lesions may be present
- ▸▸ Lymphoma-type: lymphadenopathy in the absence of lymphocytosis; skin lesions in approximately one-third of patients
- ▸▸ Cutaneous lesions manifest as nodules, papules, plaques, macules, purpura, or erythroderma

Prognosis and Treatment

- ▸▸ Acute leukemic form: poor prognosis (average survival time, 6 months)
- ▸▸ Smoldering form and favorable chronic forms are less aggressive (average survival time, 2 years)
- ▸▸ Chemotherapy or interferon plus antiretroviral drugs

Regarding cutaneous presentation, nodulotumoral types of lesions are most common and correlate with the lymphoma (aggressive) clinical variant in terms of outcomes. Next most common skin lesions include plaques and papules, while erythroderma and purpura are the least common type of skin lesions.

Histopathologic Features

The histology of ATLL in the skin shows significant overlap with MF. As a general rule, these lesions appear histologically to be a higher-grade lymphoma than most cases of MF. Because biopsies often are taken from papular or nodular lesions, the infiltrates are often dense and diffuse. Epidermotropism is very common and may be exuberant (Fig. 15.39) even in tumor lesions, unlike MF. Angiocentrism, perineural localization, and folliculo- or adnexotropism are frequent. Cytologically, ATLL is commonly composed of a large cell population. Multilobation is characteristic but is often not as well appreciated as in the peripheral blood smears (Fig. 15.40). Multinucleated giant cells and follicular mucin are not uncommonly seen. The chronic form of ATLL may have a less prominent and less atypical infiltrate.

ADULT T-CELL LEUKEMIA/LYMPHOMA—PATHOLOGIC FEATURES

Histopathologic Features

- ▸▸ Epidermotropic infiltrate similar to mycosis fungoides
- ▸▸ Polylobated nuclei (flower cells) are characteristic
- ▸▸ The tumor cell infiltrate may extend deeply, involving the subcutis

Ancillary Studies

- ▸▸ The neoplastic T cells are immunopositive for CD3, CD4, and CD25
- ▸▸ Have clonal integration of human T-lymphotropic virus 1 proviral DNA

Differential Diagnosis

- ▸▸ Mycosis fungoides
- ▸▸ Lymphomatoid drug reaction

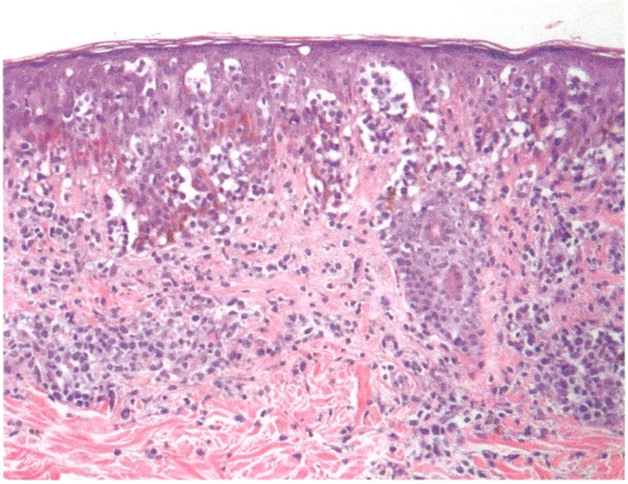

FIG. 15.39

Adult T-cell leukemia/lymphoma. An epidermotropic atypical lymphocytic infiltrate is present.

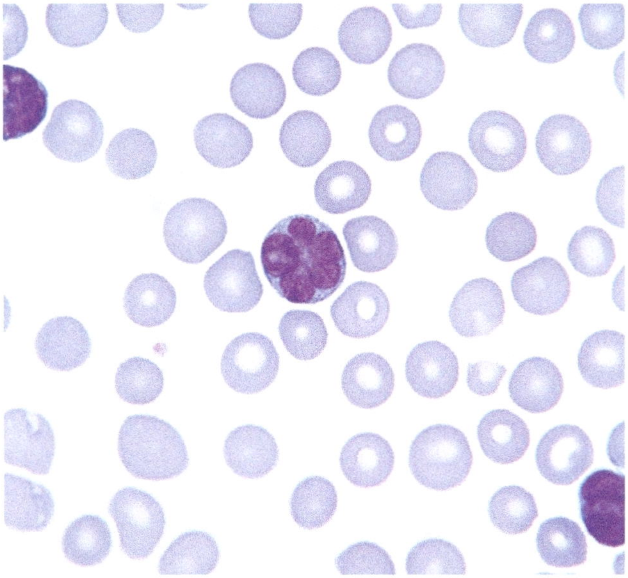

FIG. 15.40

Adult T-cell leukemia/lymphoma. Peripheral blood smear with atypical lymphocyte with hyperlobated nucleus.

Ancillary Studies

The neoplastic lymphocytes are positive for CD3, CD4, and CD25. CD7 and CD8 are usually negative. By IHC, CD4:CD8 ratios are often strikingly high, with estimated values greater than 20 : 1. CCR4 is typically positive, and CD30 has been found to be present in more than half of ATLL lesions, particularly in the Caribbean population. Fox-P3 is often present in these cases. PCR for clonal TCR gene rearrangement is usually positive. Molecular studies can confirm clonal integration of HTLV-1 provirus in the host genome, but this is not standard of care in the United States. HTLV-1 correlation typically comes from the finding of positive serologic tests.

Differential Diagnosis

The main differential diagnosis is that of MF. Clinically, the initial lesions of ATLL are papules or nodules rather than patches. Patients usually give a history of acute onset and rapid progression, although occasionally those with the "smoldering" variant of ATLL may undergo a more protracted initial course of disease. Documentation of HTLV-1 infection is necessary and usually is used clinically to make the distinction, although it is recognized that individuals from HTLV-1 endemically infected areas may also develop MF. Histologically, features of a high-grade lymphoma (large cells and marked epithelial, vascular, and neural destruction) along with multilobation or nucleation, high CD4:CD8 ratios, and strong CD25 or CD30 expression suggest the possibility of ATLL rather than MF, although MF can sometimes exhibit these features.

The acute presentation of generalized papules may suggest a lymphomatoid drug or eruption or viral exanthem. The cytologic and architectural atypia and immunophenotype should point toward a diagnosis of ATLL.

Prognosis and Treatment

The acute form is associated with a poor prognosis. Despite chemotherapy, the majority of patients die within less than 1 year. For the chronic type, the overall mean survival period is approximately 2 years. The smoldering form, when considered retrospectively, has a treatment and survival profile similar to that of MF, but these patients as well as the chronic type may transform to the acute phase. Overall, patients presenting with skin disease before systemic disease show a median survival time of less than 3 years; therefore aggressive therapies may be warranted earlier in the course of disease.

EXTRANODAL NATURAL KILLER T-CELL LYMPHOMA (NASAL OR DE NOVO PRIMARY NONNASAL TYPES)

This is an aggressive lymphoma characterized by an EBV-infected population of cells with an NK or T-cell immunophenotype that typically occurs in the nasal cavity or nasopharynx. Cases that present simultaneously or metachronously in the skin are classified as "nasal type," while primary skin presentation of ENKTCL without concurrent or eventual nasopharyngeal involvement is characterized as "nonnasal."

Clinical Findings

ENKTCL is rare. It affects adults with a male predominance. It is more common in East Asia and Central and South America. Most patients present with multiple skin lesions; dissemination of nasal type is similar to that of nonnasal subset; usually plaques or nodules on the trunk or extremities (Fig. 15.41). The tumors often ulcerate (Fig. 15.42). A clue to the diagnosis is persistent cellulitis or a nonhealing ulcer involving the face. Signs of nasal blockage or difficulty with ingestion or speech are common in the nasal type. Constitutional symptoms, including fever, weight loss, and malaise, are often seen and at times are accompanied by the hemophagocytic syndrome.

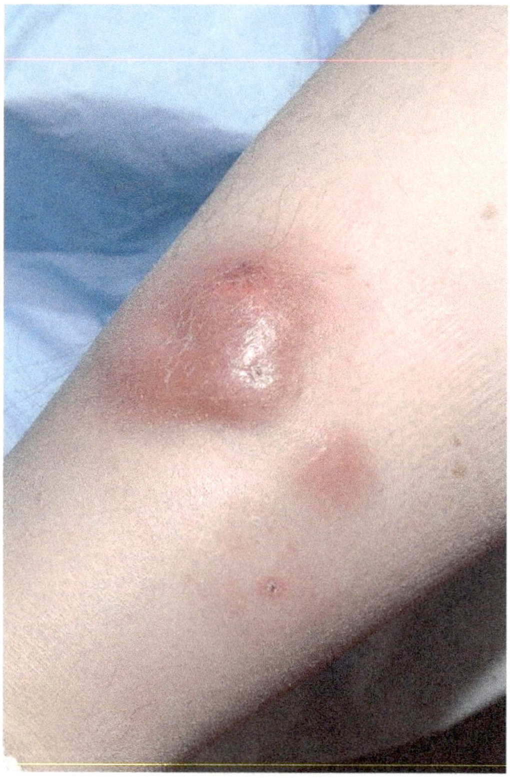

FIG. 15.41

Nodule of natural killer/T-cell lymphoma.

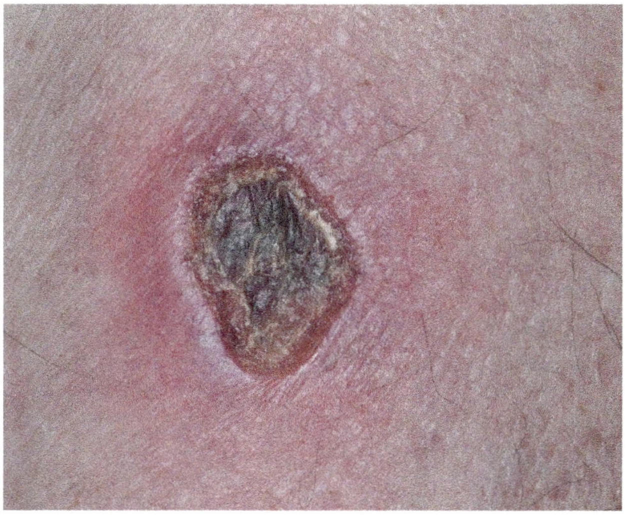

FIG. 15.42
Ulcerated lesion of natural killer/T-cell lymphoma.

Histopathologic Features

There is a nodular to diffuse dermal and frequently subcutaneous infiltrate of markedly atypical pleomorphic small, medium-sized, and large lymphocytes. There may be epidermotropism and adnexotropism. Angiocentricity is often seen (Fig. 15.43). There may be angiodestruction and zonal tumor necrosis. Commonly, one can find admixed inflammatory cells, including histiocytes, plasma cells, and eosinophils. In early lesions, the findings may be less florid, and the finding of clusters of markedly atypical perivascular and interstitial mononuclear cells can be a clue to the presence of cutaneous involvement.

Ancillary Studies

Neoplastic cells may be either T or NK cells in which in situ hybridization for EBER pathognomonically demonstrates the virus. Most cases of either type are positive for CD2, CD3ε (cytoplasmic CD3), and CD56 (Fig. 15.43). Cytotoxic marker expression (granzyme, perforin, and TIA-1) is common and CD30 may be expressed. In T-cell cases, additional markers include surface CD3 and TCR proteins (αβ, γδ, TRβC-1), and molecular studies demonstrate monoclonal TCR gene rearrangements. These tumors may be CD8+. Of note, current standard IHC on FFPE use antibodies for CD3 label both surface CD3 and cytoplasmic CD3ε and do not easily distinguish NK versus T-cell phenotype; flow cytometry, a broader panel of IHC or molecular studies for TCR, can make this distinction; however, the prognostic significance is uncertain. IHC for EBV latent membrane protein-1 (LMP) is less reliable than EBER-ISH. While a number of distinct molecular alterations have been identified in these lymphomas, mostly evidence of mutation or phosphorylation affecting JAK/STAT signaling in a particular case bears upon potential for therapeutic targeting at the current time.

Differential Diagnosis

The most challenging differential diagnosis of ENKTCL, nasal type, is that of a *blastic plasmacytoid dendritic cell neoplasm*. These tumors exhibit an architectural pattern of leukemic infiltrate (diffuse, interstitial, periadnexal, and perivascular) that may become quite dense and tumoral, often associated with hemorrhage in the dermis. Cells are fairly large and blastic in appearance. CD4 and CD56 are positive, and CD3 is negative. TCR genes do not exhibit clonal rearrangements. The finding of CD123 or TCL-1 positivity and absence of EBV favor this entity over an NK/T-cell lymphoma.

CD4-positive, CD56-positive tumor or plaque lesions of *MF* can be distinguished from NK/T-cell lymphomas by TCR protein positivity, EBV negativity, and clonal T-cell gene rearrangements, as well as clinical context. *CD30-positive ALCL* may also be CD56 positive and CD3 negative but exhibits clonal rearrangements of the TCR as well as EBV negativity. *SPTCL* can occasionally be CD56 positive but is EBV negative with clonal T-cell gene rearrangements. Indolent EBER-positive cases of SPTCL have been documented, particularly in the Asian population, and the significance of this finding is unclear. Miscellaneous other peripheral T-cell lymphoma subtypes such as *CD56-positive γδ TCL* or *hydroa vacciniforme lymphoproliferative disorder*, which may be either CD56 negative or positive, usually require a broad panel of immunomarkers and an appropriate clinical history to make a distinction.

Prognosis and Treatment

Patients with cutaneous NK/T-cell lymphoma often have a poor clinical outcome, with frequent progression of disease to nonnodal sites, despite aggressive chemotherapy. Overall there is a 50% 5-year mortality rate; the median survival time, however, is less than 1 year, especially if there is extracutaneous disease at presentation. Patients with skin-restricted disease at presentation may have a median survival time of 27 months.

HYDROA VACCINIFORME LYMPHOPROLIFERATIVE DISORDER

This neoplasm represents a rare cutaneous EBV-associated LPD primarily affecting T cells in children. It

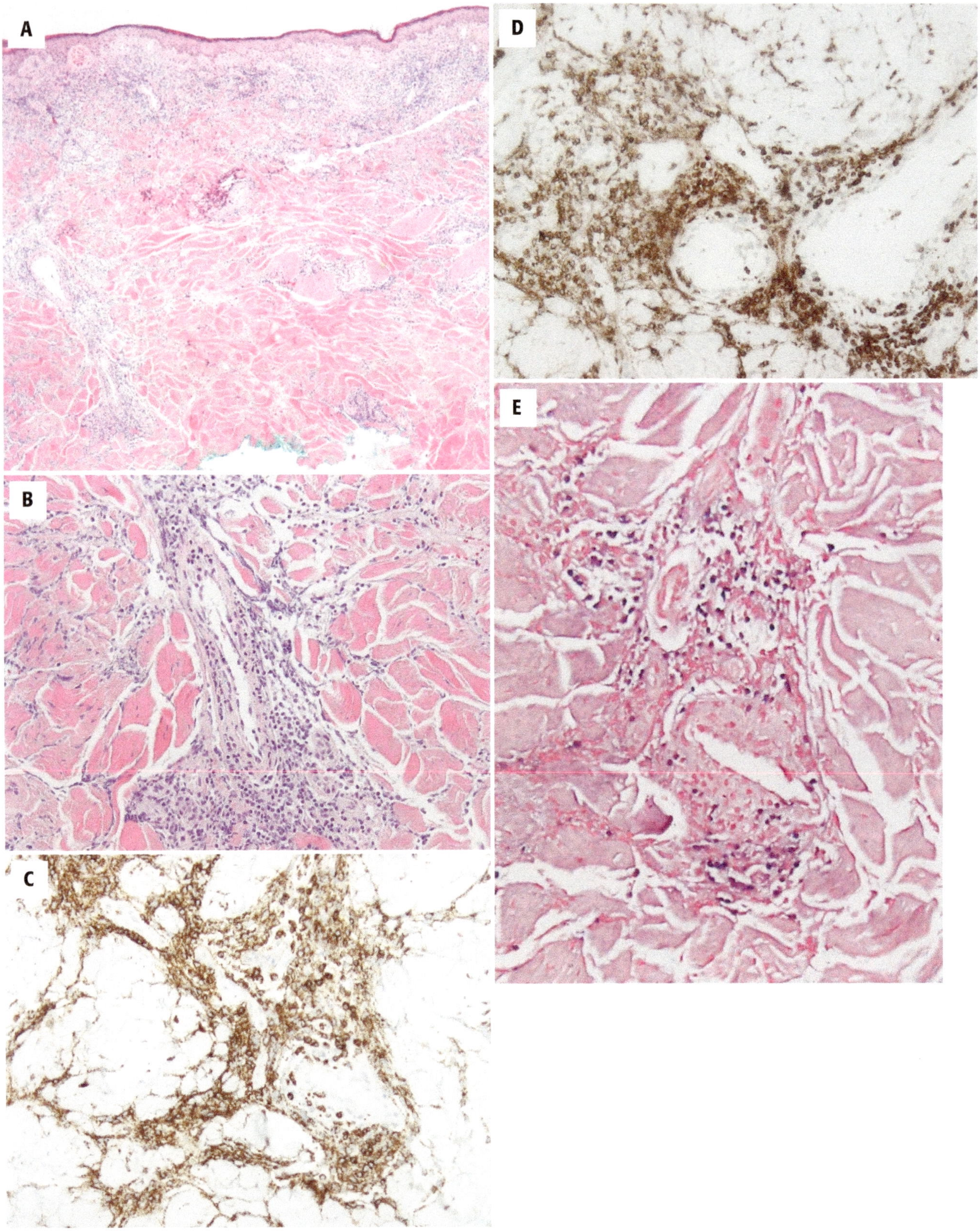

FIG. 15.43

Natural killer/T-cell lymphoma. **A,** Infiltrate of atypical lymphocytes in dermis. **B,** The lymphocytes are centered around and infiltrate vessel walls (angiocentric growth). **C,** They stain for CD3. **D,** They stain for CD56. **E,** They are positive for Epstein-Barr virus by in situ hybridization.

is considered a chronic relapsing form of chronic active EBV infection of T-cell or NK-cell type (CAEBV); the severity is related to the immunologic response of the individual. Most reported cases are from South America and Asia. In classic forms, lesions are seasonal (recur in spring and summer), when children typically present with a papulovesicular eruption of sun-exposed areas (face and extremities). In contrast, in systemic forms, the lesions are not entirely UV dependent/localized and may demonstrate liver, spleen, and lymph node involvement. These cases may arise in patients with severe hypersensitivity to mosquito bites. Individual lesions tend to ulcerate and heal as scars. Constitutional symptoms and abnormal liver function are common in the systemic form. The histology reveals an angiocentric dense lymphoid infiltrate, most commonly composed of T cells (CD8, CD4+/CD8+, or CD4+) with EBER positivity, cytotoxic marker expression, and monoclonal T-cell gene rearrangements. Less commonly, an NK-cell immunophenotype is seen. Classic cases may resolve, particularly in young patients. For those with systemic disease, the prognosis is poor.

NODAL T-FOLLICULAR HELPER T-CELL LYMPHOMA

AITL is by far the most common type of nodal T-follicular helper cell lymphoma, a rare peripheral T-cell lymphoma derived from CD4-positive T-follicular helper cells, featuring prominent high endothelial venules and follicular dendritic cells, and frequently involving the skin.

Clinical Findings

Patients with AITL typically present in middle-age to elderly with lymphadenopathy and generalized symptoms relating to infiltration of the spleen, liver, and bone marrow. Skin is one of the more common extranodal sites of involvement. Cutaneous manifestations are highly variable ranging from a morbilliform pruritic rash to purpuric eruption, papules, nodules, or plaques mostly without ulceration.

Histopathologic Features

There is a broad range of histopathologic manifestations that include robust perivascular or dense dermal lymphoid aggregates immediately prompting an immunohistochemical workup for lymphoma classification as well as subtle manifestations simulating drug reaction (a classic pitfall). Polymorphous backgrounds are present with plasma cells, histiocytes, immunoblasts, and eosinophils. Plasma cell infiltrates may be prominent. Granulomas may be present. Epidermotropism is not characteristic, but exocytosis may be seen.

Ancillary Studies

The neoplastic infiltrate can be sparse and is positive for pan T-cell markers (CD2, CD3, CD4, CD5, CD7+/−) of the αβ subset (TCR-beta/βf1 and TCR-alpha positive) and TRBC1 restricted. The cells are strongly positive for PD1 (in contrast to background dim positive reactive cells) and are commonly positive for ICOS. While CXCL13 and CD10 are more specific for the diagnosis of AITL, they are fairly uncommon in skin lesions. Bcl-6 may be positive. In situ hybridization for EBER may be positive in a subset of cases but is not required. CD20 highlights aggregates of B cells often associated with the TFH cells, many of which may be large. CD30+ large immunoblastic cells are often present and may be rimmed by CD4+/PD1+ tumor cells in rosettes. Plasma cells can be monoclonal or polyclonal upon analysis of kappa/lambda light chain expression. Monoclonal T-cell gene rearrangements can usually be identified. Immunoglobulin heavy-chain (IgH) gene rearrangements can be seen in some cases of clonal synchronous or metachronous evolution to B-cell lymphoma of varying types.

Differential Diagnosis

For dermatopathologists a main challenge is to recognize manifestations of AITL that clinically and/or histopathologically simulate a drug reaction. Slightly high density of medium- to large-sized cells in a perivascular distribution may serve as a clue to perform additional studies.

Cutaneous infiltration by AITL with robust peripheral blood involvement can be somewhat favored over Sézary syndrome when the clinical features are not obvious, if careful assessment of the patient's lymph node architectural patterns demonstrates the characteristic high endothelial venules (HEV) and follicular dendritic cell (FDC) findings. Identification of additional characteristic patterns of nodal TFH lymphoma may also require an excisional lymph node biopsy. Strong expression of multiple TFH markers, or of CXCL13 and CD10, suggests AITL versus Sézary syndrome. Molecular studies demonstrating RHOA p.G17V and IDH2 p.R172 mutations can be further used to support the diagnosis of AITL/nodal TFH cell lymphoma.

Prognosis and Treatment

The prognosis is variable, but usually unfavorable. Treatment choices include chemotherapy and stem cell transplantation.

PERIPHERAL T-CELL LYMPHOMA, NOT OTHERWISE SPECIFIED

Patients may present with a T-cell lymphoma involving the skin that cannot be identified neither as a primary CTCL nor as a specific systemic mature NK-cell or T-cell lymphoma such as NKTCL, ATLL, ALCL, or nodal TFH/AITL. Furthermore, unlike primary cutaneous peripheral T-cell lymphoma, NOS, these heterogeneous T-cell lymphomas have previously or contemporaneously identified nodal or systemic disease supporting extracutaneous origin. Most of these patients have an aggressive clinical course. We refer readers to hematopathology books and literature reviews for more details on these peripheral T-cell lymphomas.

CUTANEOUS T-CELL PSEUDOLYMPHOMA

There is a broad range of reactive T-cell infiltrates that may simulate the clinical or histologic appearance of a T-cell lymphoma. A few of them are listed here. Some are discussed in the differential diagnosis of various lymphomas. Lesions resulting in morphologic overlap with epidermotropic CTCL include lichenoid keratosis, chronic eczema, tinea, pigmented purpuric dermatitis, infestation, arthropod bites, CD8-positive human immunodeficiency virus (HIV)-associated atypical LPD, and drug reactions (in particular phenytoin-induced lymphocytic infiltrates), which may be indistinguishable from MF by light microscopy.

HIV-associated atypical CD8-positive LPD typically shows lining up of CD8-positive lymphocytes along the basal layer of the epidermis.

CD30-positive medium-sized or large cells may be present in a number of reactive T-cell infiltrates, such as arthropod bites or infestation-related infiltrates. Persistent bite reactions and florid hypersensitivity reactions, such as to scabies, may also simulate the pattern and immunophenotypic findings seen in peripheral T-cell lymphoma.

Subcutaneous lymphomas may show overlap with miscellaneous lymphocytic reactive panniculitis, in particular lupus profundus or spider bite reactions.

REACTIVE T-CELL INFILTRATES THAT MAY SIMULATE A T-CELL LYMPHOMA

- Drug reactions such as pseudo–mycosis fungoides induced by phenytoin
- Lichenoid keratosis
- Chronic eczematous dermatitis
- Arthropod bite reactions
- Infestation
- Atypical reactive T-cell infiltrates associated with viral infections

CUTANEOUS B-CELL LYMPHOMA

As with T-cell lymphomas, with B-cell lymphomas, the designation *primary cutaneous* refers to a lymphoma that manifests in the skin only, with no evidence of extracutaneous involvement at the time of diagnosis, as established by a workup, including body imaging, laboratory evaluation (including LDH), and bone marrow biopsy. Most primary cutaneous B-cell lymphomas (PCBCLs) remain confined to the skin for years. In a small subset of patients, however, the lymphoma eventually also involves lymph nodes, bone marrow, or other organs as the disease progresses. Several (indolent and aggressive) variants of PCBCL have been described. While also referring to other B-cell lymphoma types, this section of the chapter focuses on primary cutaneous marginal zone B-cell lymphoma (PCMZL), primary cutaneous follicle center lymphoma (PCFCL), and primary cutaneous diffuse large B-cell lymphoma, leg type (PCDLBCL).

INDOLENT VARIANTS OF PRIMARY CUTANEOUS B-CELL LYMPHOMA

The two common indolent variants of PCBCL include PCFCL and PCMZL. PCFCL constitutes slightly more than half of PCBCLs. PCMZL accounts for approximately one-third. Clinically, both types of lymphomas are managed similarly as low-grade PCBCL, which is why their prognosis and treatment are discussed together herein.

PRIMARY CUTANEOUS MARGINAL ZONE LYMPHOMA

Primary cutaneous marginal zone lymphoma, also known in a current classification as *primary cutaneous marginal zone lymphoproliferative disorder*, is a low-grade lymphoproliferation comprised of small centrocyte-like B cells of marginal zone phenotype, plasma cells, and reactive T cells. The spectrum of PCMZL includes lesions that have historically also been termed *primary cutaneous plasmacytoma, immunocytoma,* or *cutaneous lymphoid hyperplasia with monotypic plasma cells.* Some lesions of PCMZL arise in the dermis after the introduction of external antigen (e.g., tattoos or vaccinations), suggesting a role for antigenic stimulation. Infection, particularly that of *Borrelia burgdorferi,* appears to precede the development of some PCMZL, specifically in Europe.

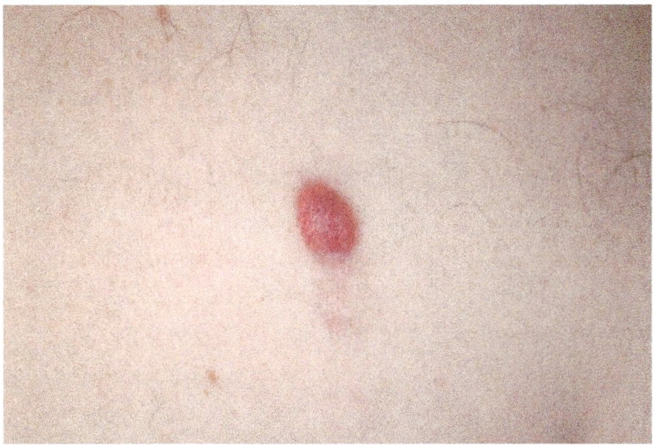

FIG. 15.44

Cutaneous marginal zone lymphoma presenting as an erythematous nodule.

Clinical Findings

Lesions of PCMZL present as erythematous to plum-colored papules, nodules, or plaques (Fig. 15.44) or a combination of lesions, frequently on the extremities (arms more often than legs) and trunk. Head and neck presentation may be found. Multifocal disease is common. Solitary lesions may simulate basal cell carcinoma or an insect bite reaction. Spontaneous remission may be noted and may be associated with anetoderma. Recurrences are common, especially if there is multifocal disease. Progression to disseminated disease is very rare.

MARGINAL ZONE B-CELL LYMPHOMA—DISEASE FACT SHEET

Patient Group

- Adults (median age, 53 years)
- May occur in children
- Male-to-female ratio of 2 : 1
- May be associated with *Borrelia* infection (Europe), tattoo, vaccine site

Site of Involvement

- Most common trunk and upper extremities; less often the head and neck
- Manifests frequently with multifocal lesions

Clinical Findings

- Red to violaceous papules, nodules, or plaques

Prognosis

- Cutaneous recurrences common
- Extracutaneous spread rare
- Excellent prognosis: 5-year survival rate greater than 95%

Treatment

- Localized disease: excision, local radiotherapy, or antibiotics
- Multifocal disease: antibiotics, steroids, local radiotherapy, rituximab, or chemotherapy
- Consider watch and wait

Histopathologic Features

There is typically a dense dermal infiltrate of lymphocytes, which spares the epidermis and is separated from it by a *grenz zone* of uninvolved tissue. The pattern of distribution may be nodular (Fig. 15.45), perivascular, or interstitial (Fig. 15.46). Well-formed or disorganized lymphoid follicles with germinal centers are almost always present which can complicate the interpretation of immunophenotype in small biopsy specimens. Identification of tingible body macrophages can help to identify the reactive nature of these germinal centers. The neoplastic and intermingled reactive infiltrates often extend down follicular adventitia, forming vertical columns. Perieccrine involvement may also be seen and can be prominent (Fig. 15.47). The infiltrate tends to be top heavy initially but with time may be broad and dense in its deep component, especially when it extends into the subcutis. Cytologically, the lymphocytes are small to intermediate in size with centrocytic features (Fig. 15.48). Centroblasts and immunoblasts are often admixed. Small clusters, dense aggregates, or single units of plasma cells are common at the periphery of the B-cell infiltrates as well as surrounding neighboring superficial vasculature. If plasma cells are numerous, Dutcher bodies, or periodic acid-Schiff–positive intranuclear or intracytoplasmic inclusions, are usually seen. Clusters of plasmacytoid dendritic cells (pDCs) are common at the periphery of tumor nodules. There may also be an admixture of eosinophils and histiocytes, including occasional granulomas or multinucleated giant cells.

MARGINAL ZONE B-CELL LYMPHOMA—PATHOLOGIC FEATURES

Histopathologic Features

- Nodular or diffuse pattern with grenz zone
- Dense dermal infiltrate of small lymphocytes (centrocyte-like)
- Often admixed with many reactive small T cells
- Reactive germinal centers common
- Plasma cells often located at periphery of the infiltrate

Ancillary Studies

- Marginal zone cells
  - Positive for CD20, CD79a, bcl-2
  - Negative for CD5, CD10, bcl-6, cyclin D1, usually CXCR3 (if class switched)
- Plasma cells
  - Evidence of light chain restriction
  - Evidence of heavy chain class-switched IgG, IgA, or IgE in 90%
  - Non–class-switched variant express IgM but few plasma cells
  - Positive for CD138, CD79a, MUM1/IRF-4

Molecular Studies

- Immunoglobulin heavy chains clonally rearranged

Differential Diagnosis

- Primary cutaneous follicular center lymphoma
- Reactive lymphoid hyperplasia

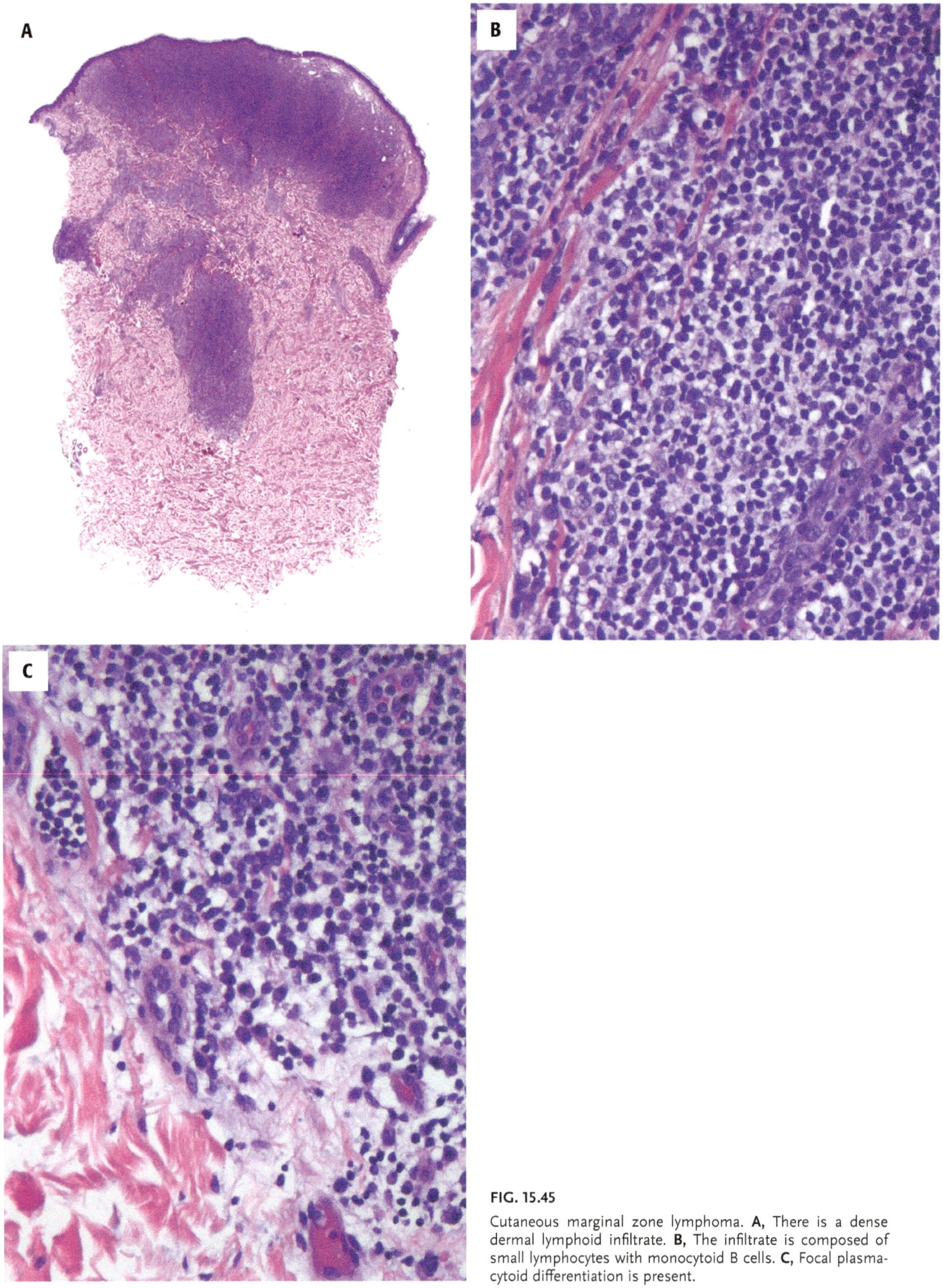

FIG. 15.45

Cutaneous marginal zone lymphoma. **A,** There is a dense dermal lymphoid infiltrate. **B,** The infiltrate is composed of small lymphocytes with monocytoid B cells. **C,** Focal plasmacytoid differentiation is present.

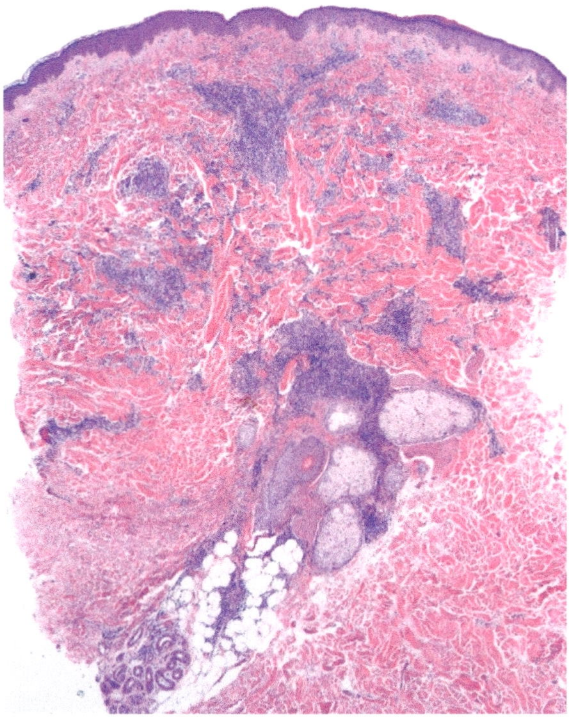

FIG. 15.46

Cutaneous marginal zone lymphoma. Some lesions show an interstitial or perivascular pattern.

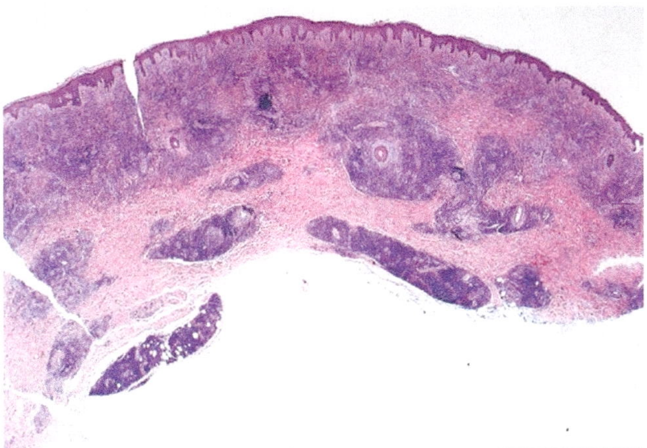

FIG. 15.47

Cutaneous marginal zone lymphoma with adnexotropism.

Ancillary Studies

Immunohistochemical stains for CD20, CD79a, or PAX-5 confirm an increased density of B cells and may reveal a multinodular or sheetlike arrangement of B cells (Fig. 15.49). There is almost always an admixture of reactive T cells. Although there are usually more B cells than T cells, in early lesions, T cells may outnumber B cells. CD79a is helpful in highlighting the plasma cells

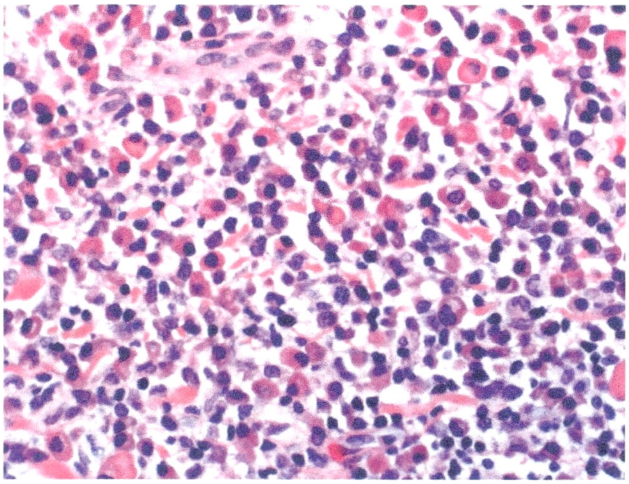

FIG. 15.48

Primary cutaneous marginal zone lymphoma. Many mature plasma cells are present.

(negative for CD20), particularly in cases that may have undergone prior anti-CD20 therapies. The neoplastic B cells of PCMZL coexpress bcl-2 or CD43. They are negative for CD5, CD10, cyclin D1, and bcl-6. However, the reactive germinal centers show positive staining, defined by complete or disrupted CD21+ follicular dendritic cell structures, and are positive for bcl-6 and CD10. Reactive T cells may also label for bcl-2. κ and λ often demonstrate light chain restriction manifested by a κ:λ ratio greater than 6 or λ:κ ratio of 2 or more. This can be assessed by IHC (Fig. 15.50) or in situ hybridization (Fig. 15.51). Most (90%) of cases demonstrate evidence of class switching in the plasma cells (IgG, IgA, IgE); these cases are CXCR3 negative. Non–class-switched cases tend to be more diffuse CXCR3 and IgM+ lesions, with fewer T cells and plasma cells. Occasional CD30+ large cells are noted in cases surrounded by PD1+ T-cell rosettes.

PCR analysis often reveals a clonal rearrangement of the IgH gene. However, a 25% to 30% false-negative rate may be seen. In addition, clonality is no proof of the presence of a lymphoma because it may be detected in CLH (*pseudolymphoma*). At times, when there is a dense T-cell infiltrate associated with the lymphoma, PCR studies may even suggest a positive T-cell clone and distract from the correct diagnosis of B-cell lymphoma.

Differential Diagnosis

PCMZL should be distinguished from PCFCL and CLH. The distinction from PCFCL is best made with a panel of immunomarkers and attention to cytologic features (cleaved cells of PCFCL), and peripheral plasma cell clusters in MZL. If there are follicles, IHC may distinguish between reactive germinal centers of PCMZL and the neoplastic follicles of PCFCL. CD21 highlights the

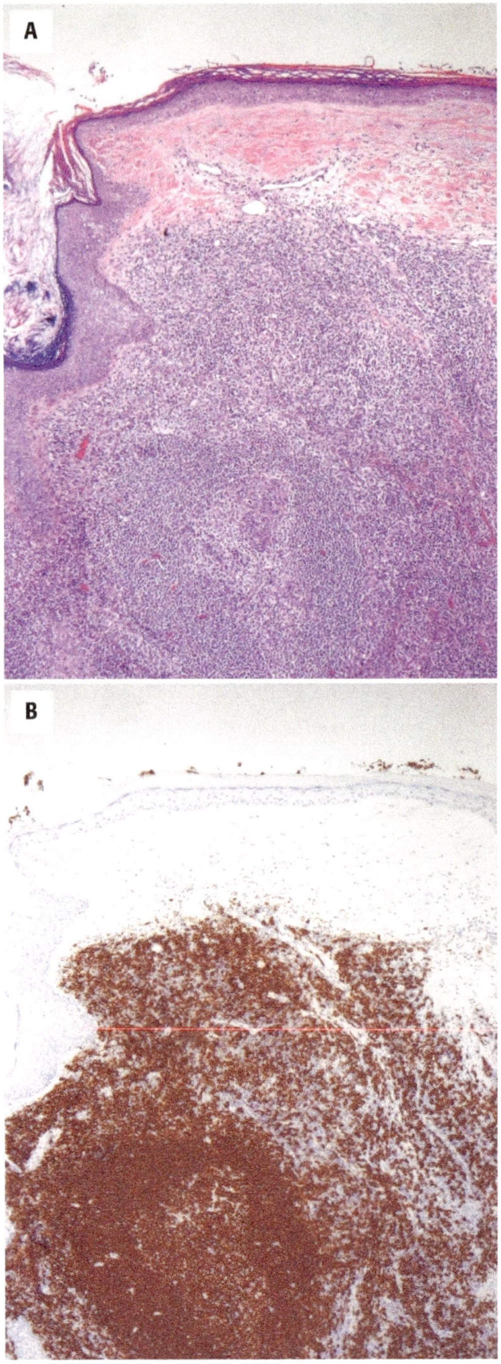

FIG. 15.49

Cutaneous marginal zone lymphoma. **A,** A dense infiltrate of lymphocytes with a grenz zone. **B,** Dense sheets of CD20-positive B cells are present, expanding and extending beyond a germinal center.

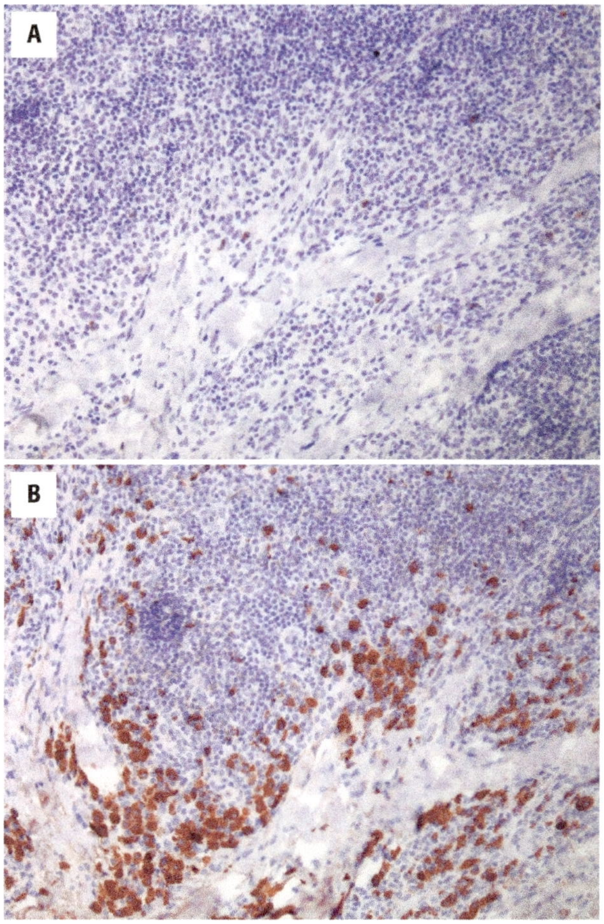

FIG. 15.50

Cutaneous marginal zone lymphoma. Evidence of light chain restriction. **A,** Immunostain for κ; only rare cells are positive. **B,** Immunostain for lambda—numerous cells are positive (vast excess of λ over κ).

follicular network. In PCMZL, it may identify inconspicuous follicles that have been "overrun" by the lymphoma cells. This, in conjunction with a prominent plasmacellular component at the periphery of the follicles, favors a diagnosis of marginal zone lymphoma. Bcl-6 is positive in the follicles in both, but the positive cells are not limited to the follicle in PCFCL.

Cutaneous B-cell pseudolymphoma shows an increased number of B cells but usually lacks dense nodular or sheetlike aggregates of CD20-positive cells. It is further discussed later.

Immunomarkers for the Classification of Common Cutaneous B-Cell Lymphomas

	CD20	Bcl-6	Bcl-2	CD10	MUM1
PCMZL	+	−	+	−	V
PCFCL	+	+	−	V	−
FCL, secondarily involving skin	+	+	+	+	−
PCLBCL, LT	+	V	+	−	+

+, Immunopositive; −, immunonegative; *FCL*, follicle center lymphoma; *MUM1*, multiple myeloma oncogene 1; *PCFCL*, primary cutaneous follicle center lymphoma; *PCLBCL, LT*, primary cutaneous diffuse large B-cell lymphoma, leg type; *PCMZL*, primary cutaneous marginal zone B-cell lymphoma; *V*, variably positive or negative.

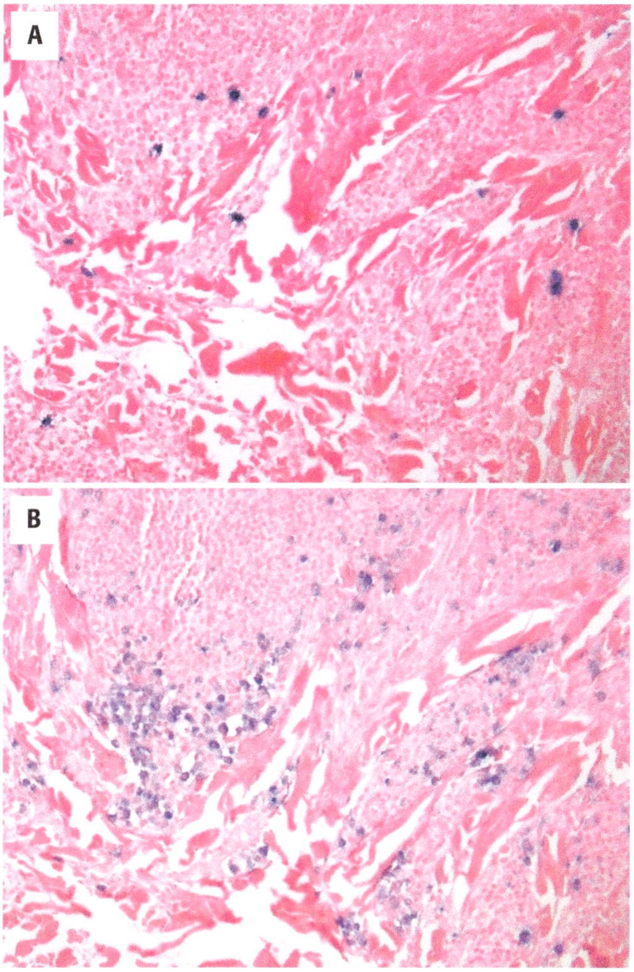

FIG. 15.51

Cutaneous marginal zone lymphoma. Evidence of light chain restriction. **A,** In situ hybridization for κ; only rare cells are positive. **B,** In situ hybridization for λ; numerous cells are positive (vast excess of λ over κ).

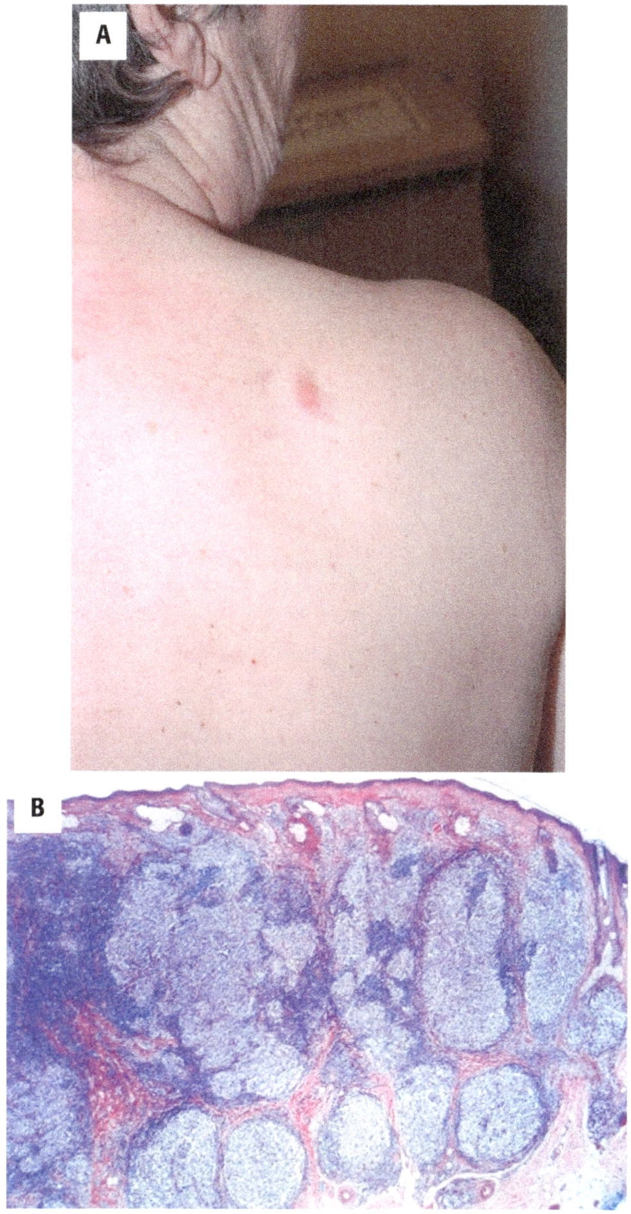

FIG. 15.52

Cutaneous follicle center lymphoma. **A,** Erythematous nodule. **B,** Dense multinodular lymphocytic infiltrate in the dermis and superficial subcutis.

PRIMARY CUTANEOUS FOLLICLE CENTER CELL LYMPHOMA

Clinical Findings

Individual lesions of PCFCL may present similar to PCMZL as a solitary erythematous to plum-colored nodule. However, in contrast with PCMZL, lesions of PCFCL predominantly affect the head and neck region or trunk (Fig. 15.52). Furthermore, lesions are usually solitary or regionally clustered; multiple lesions at different sites (common in PCMZL) are rare.

Histopathologic Features

Typically, there is a dense nodular to diffuse lymphocytic infiltrate in the dermis that may extend into the subcutis (Figs. 15.52 and 15.53). A grenz zone separating the epidermis from the dermal infiltrate is common. The infiltrate is usually composed of predominantly small- to intermediate-sized cleaved lymphocytes (centrocytes), although cases with more prominent centroblastic component can be found.

The B cells are usually admixed with a variably dense component of reactive T lymphocytes and a minor component of larger cleaved and noncleaved lymphocytes with more prominent nucleoli (centroblasts, immunoblasts).

Nodular follicular aggregates lack tangible body macrophages and a well-developed marginal and mantle zone typical of well-formed germinal centers. As in PCMZL, there may be a concentration of this process around the follicles and eccrine coils. In larger tumors or well-established lesions, there is a predominance of

CUTANEOUS FOLLICLE CENTER LYMPHOMA—DISEASE FACT SHEET

Patient Group
- Adults (median age, 58 years)
- Male-to-female ratio of 1:8

Site of Involvement
- Scalp, forehead, or trunk

Clinical Findings
- Solitary or clustered papules, nodules, or plaques
- Multifocal lesions in ≈15%

Prognosis
- Cutaneous recurrences in less than 25%
- Extracutaneous spread in less than 10%
- Excellent prognosis: 5-year survival: 95%

Treatment
- Localized disease: surgical removal or local radiotherapy
- Multifocal disease: radiotherapy or rituximab
- Consider watch and wait

CUTANEOUS FOLLICLE CENTER CELL LYMPHOMA—PATHOLOGIC FEATURES

Histopathologic Features
- Dense dermal infiltrate with grenz zone
- Follicular (5%), follicular and diffuse (30%), and diffuse (60%) pattern
- Intermediate to large lymphocytes (centrocytes)
- May be admixed with many reactive T cells

Ancillary Studies
- Immunophenotype
  - Positive for CD20, CD79a, bcl-6, CD10 (variable)
  - Negative or dim for bcl-2, MUM1/IRF-4

Molecular Studies
- Clonally rearranged immunoglobulin genes
- Usually negative for t(14;18)

Differential Diagnosis
- Primary cutaneous marginal zone lymphoma
- Follicular lymphoma secondarily involving the skin
- Pseudolymphoma

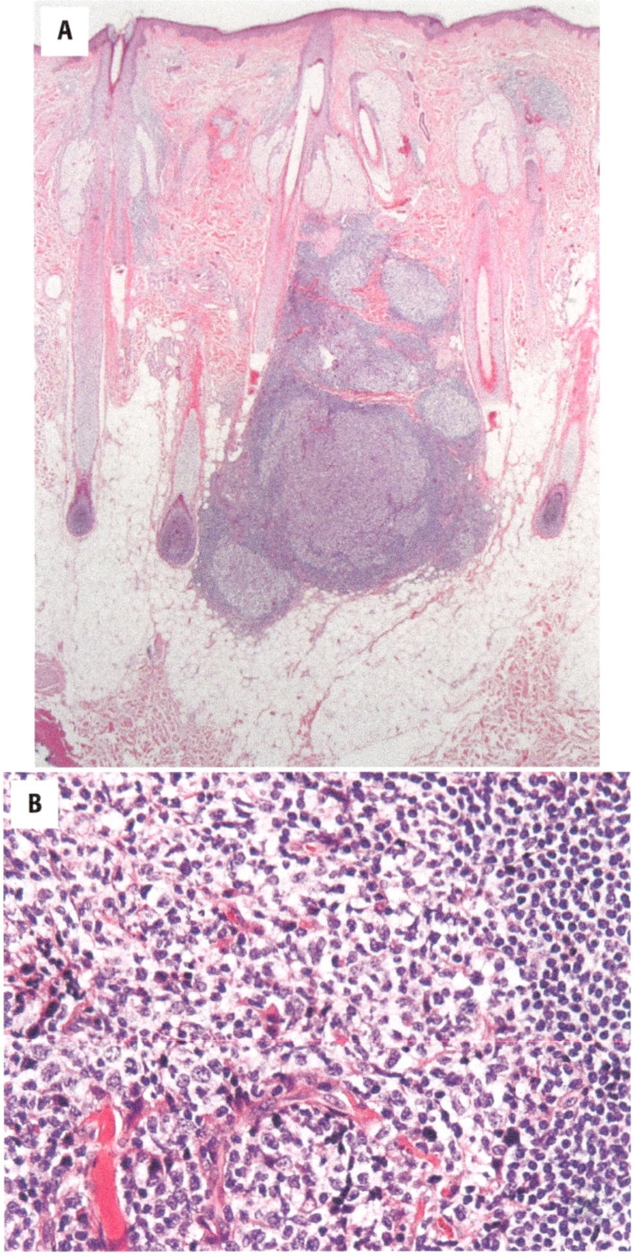

FIG. 15.53
Cutaneous follicular lymphoma. **A,** Nodular lymphoid infiltrate in the skin of the scalp. **B,** The infiltrate is composed of cleaved lymphocytes of various sizes.

large centrocytes, with an admixture of centroblasts and immunoblasts, and a minimally reactive T-cell component. If large lymphocytes appear numerous, one should consider entertaining suspicion for a diffuse large B-cell lymphoma.

Ancillary Studies

The lymphocytes are positive for CD20, CD79a, PAX-5, and bcl-6 along with other germinal center markers MEF2b, LMO2, or HGAL. CD5 and CD43 are often negative. CD21 may highlight an organized or disrupted follicular network in the more nodular variants. IHC for Ki-67 may show a diminished proliferation rate or a nonpolarized pattern, in contrast to reactive follicles in these networks; however, this is not as reliable in PCFCL as with systemic FCL. As with PCMZL, there is typically a predominance of B cells, but early or recurrent disease may also show a high density of T cells. Tumors with a follicular growth pattern typically express CD10. However, lesions with a diffuse architecture tend to be negative for CD10. Light chain restriction cannot as easily be demonstrated as with PCMZL and is often not detected. PCFCLs are usually negative for bcl-2, although they may show dim positivity (less than T-cell intensity), and if there is a T-cell–rich reactive infiltrate, bcl-2 positivity of T cells can be confusing. PCR studies tend to be positive for B-cell clonality in fully developed lesions but may be falsely negative in early lesions.

Differential Diagnosis

PCFCL may be confused with other B-cell lymphomas, in particular PCMZL. When the presence of a B-cell lymphoma is suspected because of dense aggregates of CD20-positive cells, the detection of plasmacytoid differentiation, evidence of light chain restriction, and coexpression of B cells for bcl-2 favor PCMZL, but staining for bcl-6 suggests PCFCL. The distinction between PCMZL and PCFCL is usually straightforward but can be difficult at times if in a given biopsy sample there is only minimal plasmacytoid differentiation and the interpretation of coexpression for bcl-2 is difficult because of numerous associated T cells (which normally express bcl-2).

The most important decisions, however, are whether or not a lymphoma is present, whether its features suggest a low- or high-grade neoplasm, and whether it is primary cutaneous or a nodal-based lymphoma secondarily involving the skin. Currently, after a diagnosis of a primary cutaneous low-grade B-cell lymphoma is made, further distinction between PCMZL and PCFCL is of limited relevance for treatment and prognosis.

On the other hand, it is important prognostically to distinguish a PCFCL from secondary involvement of the skin by follicular or other types of B-cell lymphomas, such as mantle cell lymphoma (positive for CD5 and cyclin D1 or SOX-11, which is negative in both PCMZL and PCFCL). Demonstration of bright bcl-2 and bcl-6 positivity of the neoplastic B cells favors secondary FCL. Clinical correlation and staging are recommended in these cases.

If there is a diffuse infiltrate of large round cells, a diagnosis of diffuse large B-cell lymphoma, "leg type" (DLBCLL), should be considered. DLBCLL typically has a blastic morphology with large cells with round cell morphology and prominent nucleoli and are also typically positive for MUM-1/IRF-4, IgM and bcl-2, both of which are usually negative in primary cutaneous follicle center cell lymphoma.

Differentiating low-grade PCBCL (PCMZL or PCFCL) from CLH (or pseudolymphoma) can be quite difficult. The latter can be seen in situations of chronic antigenic stimulation that may be localized (e.g., tattoo reaction, chronic arthropod bite reaction) or systemic (e.g., medication). A specific etiology is often not apparent. Molecular studies are of limited value because clonality may not be detectable in early lesions of lymphoma, and clonality may be detected in some cases of CLH. Reactive CLH is discussed more in the following at the end of the section on cutaneous B-cell lymphomas (CBLs).

Prognosis and Treatment

Both PCFCL and PCMZL have an excellent prognosis, with a 5-year survival rate that reportedly ranges from approximately 95% and 98% to 100%, respectively. The presence of a single versus multiple cutaneous lesions is important. The disease-free survival rate of patients with a PCBCL of either marginal zone or follicular center cell type with a single lesion is significantly higher than those with regional or disseminated lesions (5-year disease-free survival rate, 62% vs. 44%; 5-year overall survival rate, 97% vs. 85%, respectively). Clinical recurrences and additional lesions are common. Nearly half of patients with PCFCL or PCMZL experience relapse after the first treatment. Nearly one-fourth have two or more relapses during follow-up. The disease relapse is nearly always confined to the skin. In the few who develop extracutaneous involvement, there is usually also concomitant cutaneous relapse.

Although the higher incidence of relapses occurs in the first 4 years after diagnosis, a constant 2% to 6% risk of relapse has been observed even beyond 10 years, and the disease-free survival rate shows a plateau only after 15 years from the date of response. The risk of relapse after the achievement of complete clinical response is independent from the treatment used to obtain the response and is significantly lower in patients with a single cutaneous lesion than in those with either regional or disseminated cutaneous involvement.

Treatment includes surgical excision, radiation, intralesional or topical steroids, rituximab (anti-CD20), or chemotherapy. Disseminated cases require chemotherapy often in conjunction with radiation or treatment with anti-CD20 monoclonal antibody. Some cases of PCMZL are associated with infection with *B. burgdorferi* infection and thus may respond to antibiotics.

AGGRESSIVE VARIANTS OF CUTANEOUS B-CELL LYMPHOMA

DIFFUSE LARGE B-CELL LYMPHOMA, LEG TYPE

DLBCLL is an aggressive subtype of CBL that can be distinguished from other types of primary CBLs by a combination of clinical, histologic, and immunohistochemical features. This lymphoma often manifests as multiple lesions on the legs of elderly women and was initially referred to as DLBCL "of the leg" in the EORTC classification, at which point the characteristic

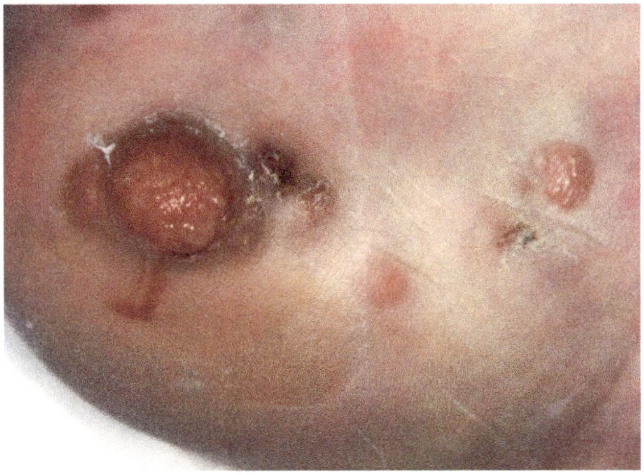

FIG. 15.54
Large B-cell lymphoma, leg type. An ulcerated nodule is present.

sheets of large lymphocytes with round cell morphology were thought to be specific for that site. It is now known that lymphomas with the same pathologic and aggressive clinical features may also arise at other sites.

Clinical Findings

The lesions typically manifest most commonly in elderly women on the legs as multiple or solitary erythematous to plum-colored nodules, plaques, or tumors (Fig. 15.54). However, similar lesions may also be found at sites other than the leg.

PRIMARY CUTANEOUS LARGE B-CELL LYMPHOMA, LEG TYPE—DISEASE FACT SHEET

Patient Group
- Usually elderly individuals (median age, 78 years)
- Male-to-female ratio of 0:5

Site of Involvement
- Lower leg(s)
- Sites other than the leg in 10% to 15%

Clinical Findings
- Red or violaceous nodules

Prognosis
- Cutaneous recurrences common
- Extracutaneous spread common
- Unfavorable prognosis: 5-year survival rate of 50% or less
- Presence of multiple lesions at presentation is an adverse risk factor

Treatment
- Chemotherapy
- Local radiotherapy
- Rituximab

Histopathologic Features

There is a nodular or diffuse infiltrate of large round to oval lymphocytes (centroblasts and immunoblasts) (Fig. 15.55). They typically lack nuclear cleaves. The tumor cells exhibit an activated germinal center immunophenotype. They are immunopositive for B-cell markers, such as CD20 and CD79a; however, in contrast with primary cutaneous large follicular center cell lymphomas, the cells are positive for bcl-2. Positive staining for MUM-1/IRF-4, MYC, and Fox-P1 is also characteristic. Cytoplasmic IgM, IgD, and HGAL staining may be seen with monotypic light chain expression. Some lesions stain for bcl-6, but CD10 is usually negative. The MIB-1 labeling index is high. T cells are few.

Differential Diagnosis

DLBCLL should be distinguished from diffuse presentations of *primary cutaneous follicular center cell type*. A morphologic clue for diffuse non–leg-type follicular lymphoma is the presence of cleaved nuclei. Definitive distinction is done by IHC. Molecular identification of MYD88 mutation can also favor DLBCL-LT.

EBV+ diffuse large B-cell lymphoma, a fairly indolent EBV-related lymphoma thought to be related to age-related immunosenescence, can also mimic leg-type lymphoma. The distinction is made by the identification of EBER or EBV-LMP1 positivity, implicating EBV. CD20 may be variable in these patients, and CD30 is typically positive, sometimes CD15.

Primary cutaneous large cell lymphomas also should be distinguished from EBV-positive mucocutaneous ulcer or other immune-associated B-cell lymphoproliferations, primary cutaneous large cell lymphomas (ALCL, peripheral T-cell lymphomas), secondary involvement of the skin by extracutaneous large cell lymphomas, leukemia cutis, and nonhematopoietic malignancies (e.g., malignant melanoma, poorly differentiated carcinoma).

Prognosis and Treatment

DLBCLL has a poor prognosis, with a 5-year rate survival of around 50%. Compared with FCL and MZL, DLBCLL has been shown to have statistically significant lower complete response rates, higher incidence of multiple cutaneous relapses and extracutaneous spreading, shorter time to progression, and shorter overall survival rates.

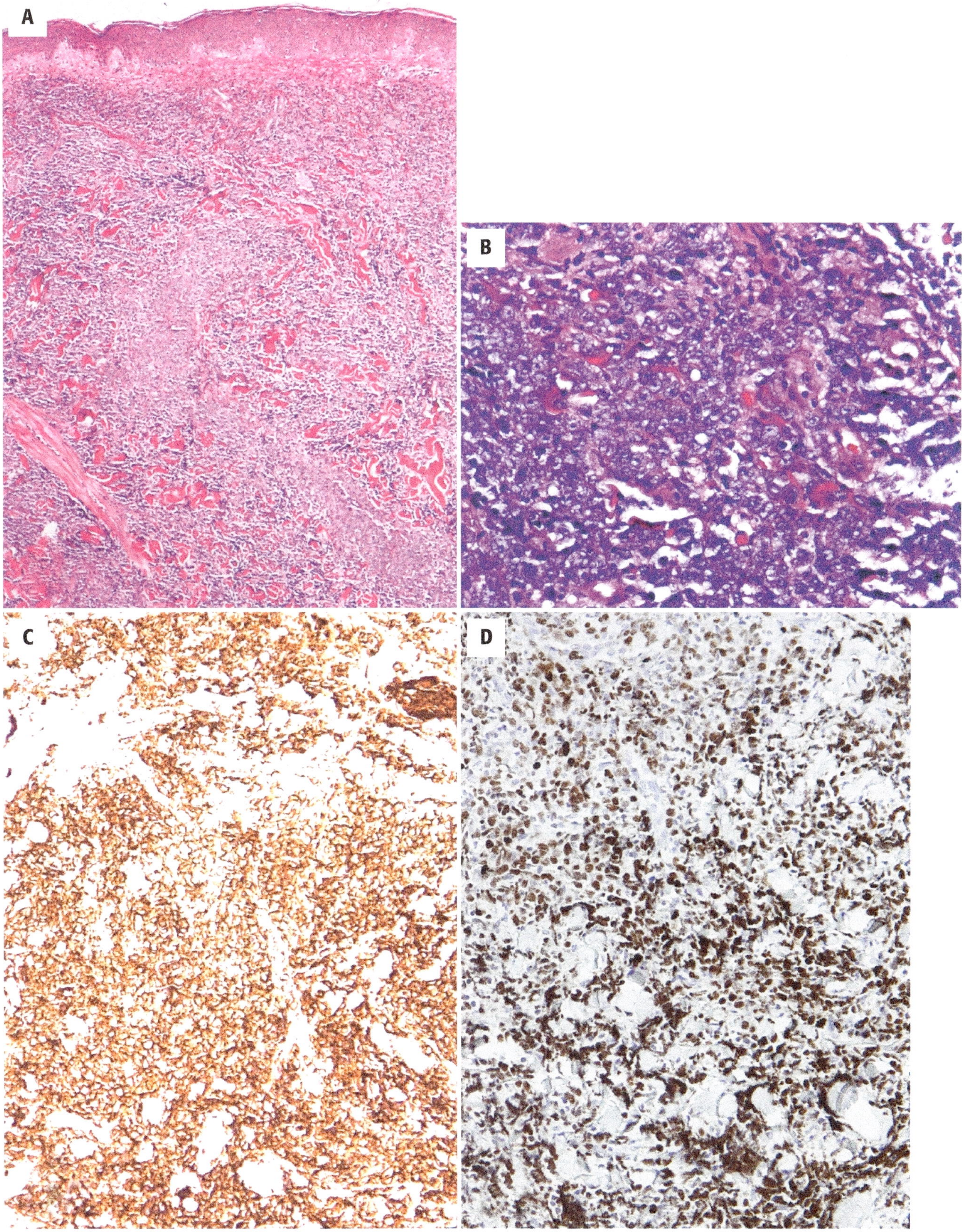

FIG. 15.55

Large B-cell lymphoma, leg type. **A,** Sheets of large lymphocytes are present in the dermis. **B,** The large lymphocytes have oval nuclei without cleaves. **C,** The tumor cells are positive for CD20. **D,** The nuclei of the tumor cells label for MUM1.

PRIMARY CUTANEOUS LARGE B-CELL LYMPHOMA, LEG TYPE—PATHOLOGIC FEATURES

Histopathologic Features

- Diffuse infiltrate of large nonepidermotropic lymphocytes with round cell morphology
- Few reactive T cells

Ancillary Studies

- Immunophenotype
  - Positive for CD20, CD79a
  - Usually positive for bcl-2, MUM-1/IRF4, Fox-P1, bcl-6
  - Usually negative for CD10

Molecular Studies

- Immunoglobulin heavy gene rearrangement
- IgH, MYC, or bcl-6 translocation
- MYD88 hotspot mutations
- Deletion of 9p21.3 (CDKN2A and CDKN2B gene loci) is associated with a more unfavorable prognosis

Differential Diagnosis

- Large cell lymphoma of non-leg type

MISCELLANEOUS OTHER B-CELL LYMPHOMAS AFFECTING THE SKIN

Other B-cell lymphomas or plasma cell neoplasms may predominantly or (usually) secondarily (as part of multiorgan disease) affect the skin. A few of them are briefly mentioned here.

EBV-POSITIVE DIFFUSE LARGE B-CELL LYMPHOMA

This EBV-associated lymphoma typically occurs in elderly patients, particularly when it involves the skin, but all ages can be affected. It is an aggressive lymphoma with a median survival time of approximately 2 years. The histopathologic picture is most commonly that of a polymorphous more often than monomorphous diffuse large B-cell lymphoma, often with angiocentricity and geographic necrosis, and with labeling for EBV (EBER in situ hybridization and EBV-LMP1) (Fig. 15.56). CD79a, MUM1, and CD30 are usually

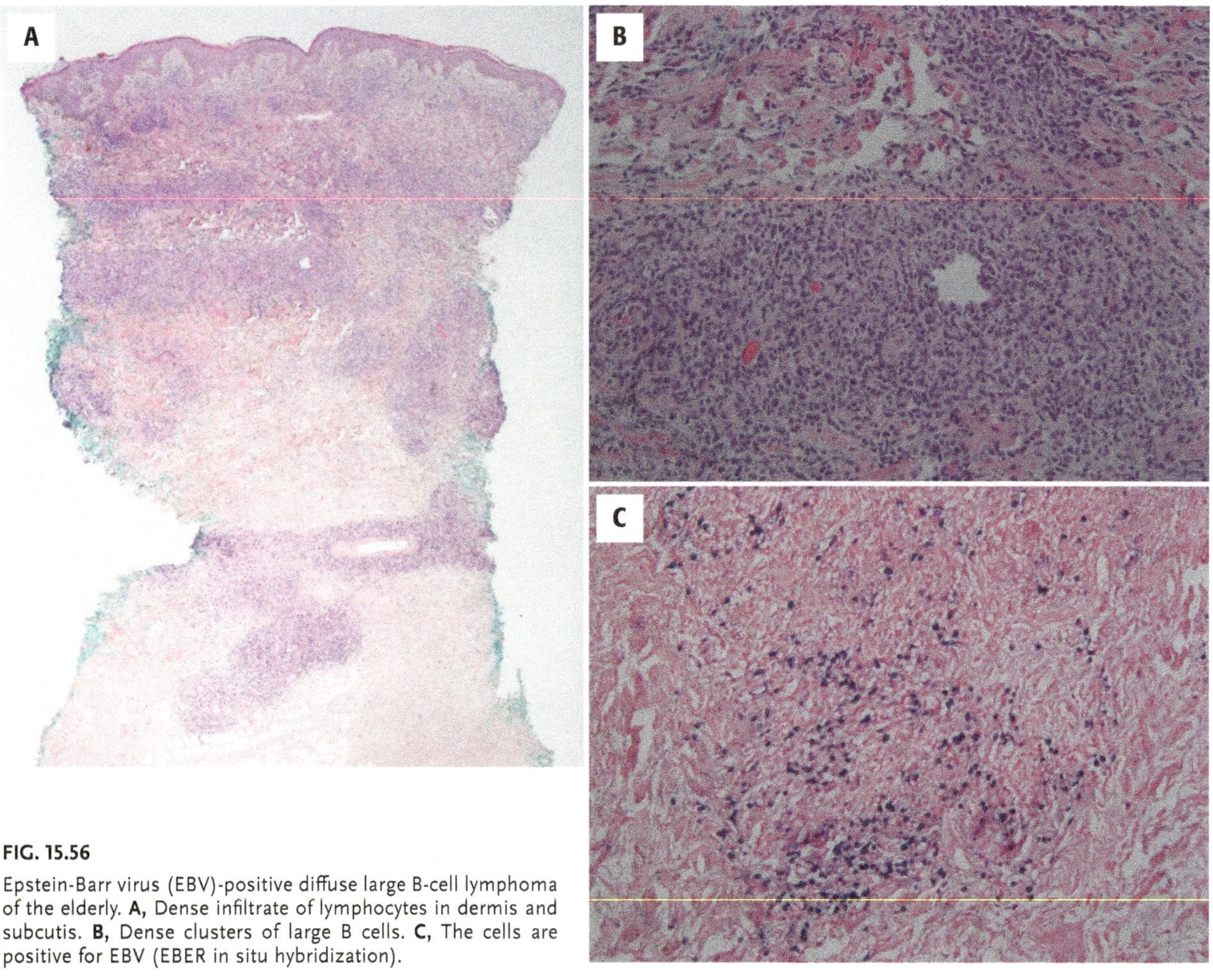

FIG. 15.56

Epstein-Barr virus (EBV)-positive diffuse large B-cell lymphoma of the elderly. **A,** Dense infiltrate of lymphocytes in dermis and subcutis. **B,** Dense clusters of large B cells. **C,** The cells are positive for EBV (EBER in situ hybridization).

positive in the tumor cells. Some lesions may show loss of CD20, which may lead to diagnostic confusion.

INTRAVASCULAR LARGE B-CELL LYMPHOMA

This subtype is characterized by the accumulation of atypical large B-cell lymphocytes in the vascular lumina. Skin can be exclusively involved (cutaneous variant, with better outcomes) or show involvement as part of the classic subtype in which systemic symptoms co-occur.

Patients present with indurated violaceous plaques, which may simulate panniculitis or a peau d'orange type of appearance, often on the lower extremities and trunk. Patches and telangiectatic lesions have also been described, and there are rare reports of this tumor populating the vessels of cutaneous angiomas. Frequent CNS dissemination and lung involvement are seen. Random skin biopsy can sometimes reveal disease even in the absence of clinical lesions.

Histopathologically, the dermal vessels are dilated and expanded by large intraluminal atypical lymphoid cells (Fig. 15.57). There may be vasoocclusion with secondary angiomatosis. In some cases, these atypical cells may extend into the extravascular dermis. The subcutis may also be involved. The cells are positive for B-cell markers. MYD88 or CD79B hotspot mutations are commonly identified.

The 5-year survival rate is less than 50%, although it may be better if the disease remains limited to the skin presentations (3-year overall survival rate, 56% versus 22%). Chemotherapy with rituximab is the treatment of choice.

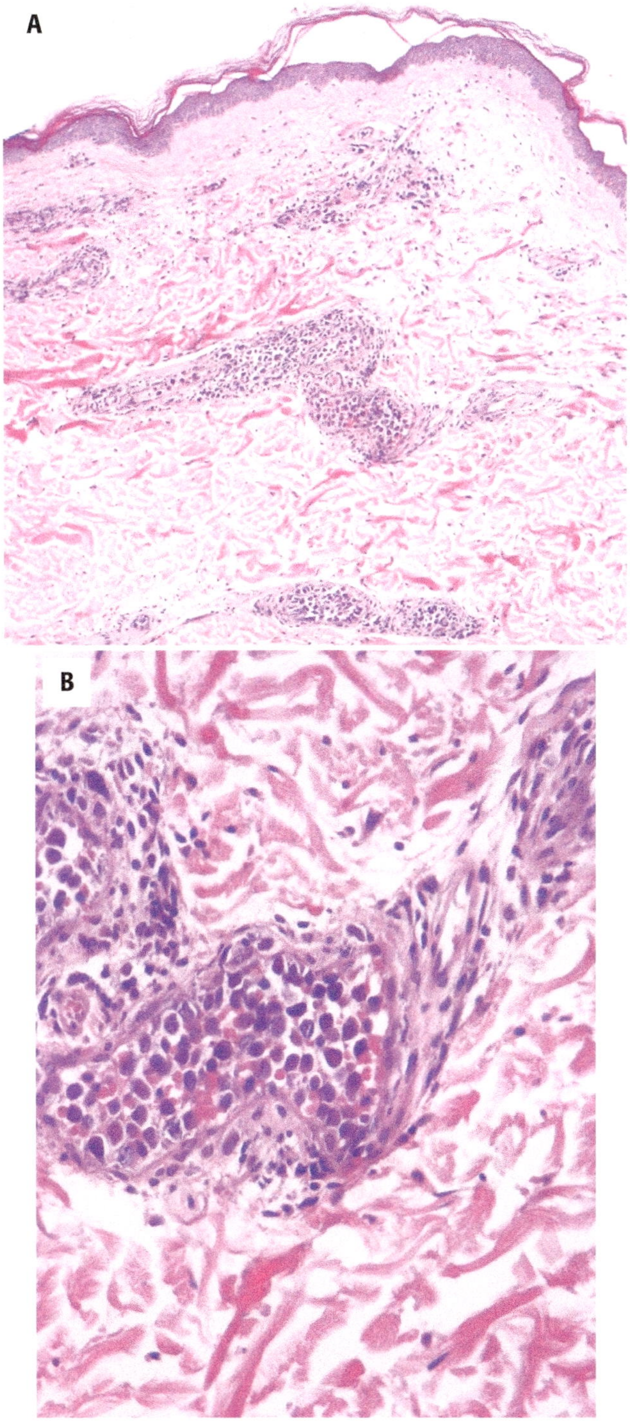

FIG. 15.57
Intravascular lymphoma. Typical large lymphocytes are present within dermal blood vessels (**A** and **B**).

CUTANEOUS (EXTRAMEDULLARY) PLASMACYTOMA

Plasmacytoma refers to a neoplasm of plasma cells. Extramedullary plasmacytoid neoplasms primarily or only manifesting in the skin are currently classified as plasma cell neoplasms within the *WHO Haematolymphoid Tumor 5th Edition Classification* and within the International Consensus Classification, or as primary cutaneous marginal zone lymphoma in the *WHO Skin Tumors 5th Edition Scheme*. Multiple myeloma and Waldenström's macroglobulinemia should be excluded by serum protein and immunoglobulin electrophoresis, radiographic skeletal survey, and bone marrow biopsy.

Although primary cutaneous disease is usually indolent, secondary involvement of the skin by multiple myeloma usually reflects advanced disease and is associated with a poor prognosis. Anaplastic variants of plasmacytoma may be difficult to recognize because their plasmacytoid differentiation is not readily apparent on routine H&E-stained sections. However, they typically occur in the setting of a patient with a known history of multiple myeloma. Knowledge of the clinical setting and confirmation of the plasmacytoid differentiation of the cells by immunostains (CD79a, CD38, and CD138 EMA) lead to the correct diagnosis. IgG or IgA are most often positive.

LYMPHOMATOID GRANULOMATOSIS

Lymphomatoid granulomatosis refers to an angiocentric and destructive EBV-associated B-cell LPD. The lymphoma usually spares the lymph nodes and spleen and tends to affect the upper respiratory tract. The skin is the second most common extrapulmonary site after CNS, but other sites such as kidney or liver may also be infiltrated. Cutaneous involvement rarely occurs without pulmonary disease. Skin disease usually manifests as multiple dermal or subcutaneous papules or nodules with or without ulceration. Lymphomatoid granulomatosis is characterized by angiocentricity and angiodestruction. Features of lymphocytic necrotizing vasculitis are commonly found. Skin biopsies of lesions of lymphomatoid granulomatosis often show only rare large EBV-positive B cells. They are usually outnumbered by T cells. There may also be a granulomatous reaction.

The disease usually affects adults, men more often than women. Most patients with higher-grade disease have an aggressive clinical course, although lower-grade disease can be indolent. Death is usually because of complications from lung disease. Some patients may experience spontaneous regression of tumors or have a waxing and waning course.

MANTLE CELL LYMPHOMA

This type of B-cell lymphoma tends to affect middle-aged to elderly patients. Most of them present with adenopathy, but gastrointestinal disease is also common. Cutaneous involvement is rare but may represent an initial manifestation of the disease as multiple papules or nodules on the trunk or extremities.

The lymphocytes of mantle cell lymphoma are intermediate in size. Similar to most B-cell lymphomas infiltrating the skin, the neoplastic cells tend to spare the epidermis, allowing for a grenz zone. In contrast with other B-cell lymphomas discussed so far, mantle cell lymphoma almost always overexpresses cyclin D1, which can be confirmed immunohistochemically. SOX-11 and CD5 are also usually positive. Of note LEF1 can be positive in blastoid or pleomorphic morphologies, a pitfall in the differential diagnosis with chronic lymphocytic leukemia (CLL) in the skin. Most of the tumors carry a t(11;14) translocation involving CCND1 and IgH genes, which can be detected by FISH.

CUTANEOUS B-CELL "PSEUDOLYMPHOMA"

B-cell pseudolymphoma is a controversial term which refers to the spectrum of reactive B-cell predominant lymphoid infiltrates in the skin, which may histopathologically simulate a B-cell lymphoma. These lesions are currently called "reactive B-cell–rich lymphoid proliferations" in the 5th edition *Skin* book from the WHO. Polyclonal B-cell–rich lymphocytic infiltrates may clinically or histologically simulate the appearance of a B-cell lymphoma.

Clinical Findings

The clinical spectrum parallels the appearance of lymphoma. Typically, a single or few persistent erythematous papules or nodules are present, which may or may not be associated with pruritus. However, disseminated lesions may also occur, albeit only very rarely. The lesions may represent a persistent insect bite, drug reaction, or reaction related to infection (e.g., *Borrelia* spp.). However, many times a precise etiology is difficult to establish. Typically, the patient is otherwise healthy. With time and discontinuation of the allergic stimulus, the lesions go away but may recur and on rare occasions progress to a low-grade B-cell lymphoma.

Histopathologic Features

Similar to lymphoma, there is a dense infiltrate of lymphocytes. It is often (Fig. 15.58), but not always, "top heavy," that is, the infiltrate tends to be wider in the horizontal dimension in the superficial dermis than in the deep dermis or subcutis. A *grenz zone* is often present but may be absent because of an associated reactive T-cell infiltrate, which is diagnostically helpful. Reactive germinal centers may be seen. The infiltrate is typically polymorphous with a mixed population of small- to intermediate-sized lymphocytes, histiocytes, plasma cells, and polymorphonuclear cells. The proportion of each of these components can be highly variable. Eosinophils, for example, may be numerous or absent.

Commonly, there are reactive stromal changes (fibrosis or edema). Endothelial cells may appear reactive (swollen), and there may be evidence of minor vascular damage (e.g., hemorrhage, fibrin).

REACTIVE B-CELL–RICH LYMPHOPROLIFERATIONS (B-CELL "PSEUDOLYMPHOMA")

- Hypersensitivity reactions (e.g., medication, arthropod, or spider bites; tattoos; vaccinations)
- Infection (e.g., *Borrelia* spp., syphilis)
- Connective tissue disease (e.g., inflammatory morphea, tumid lupus)
- Plasmacytosis

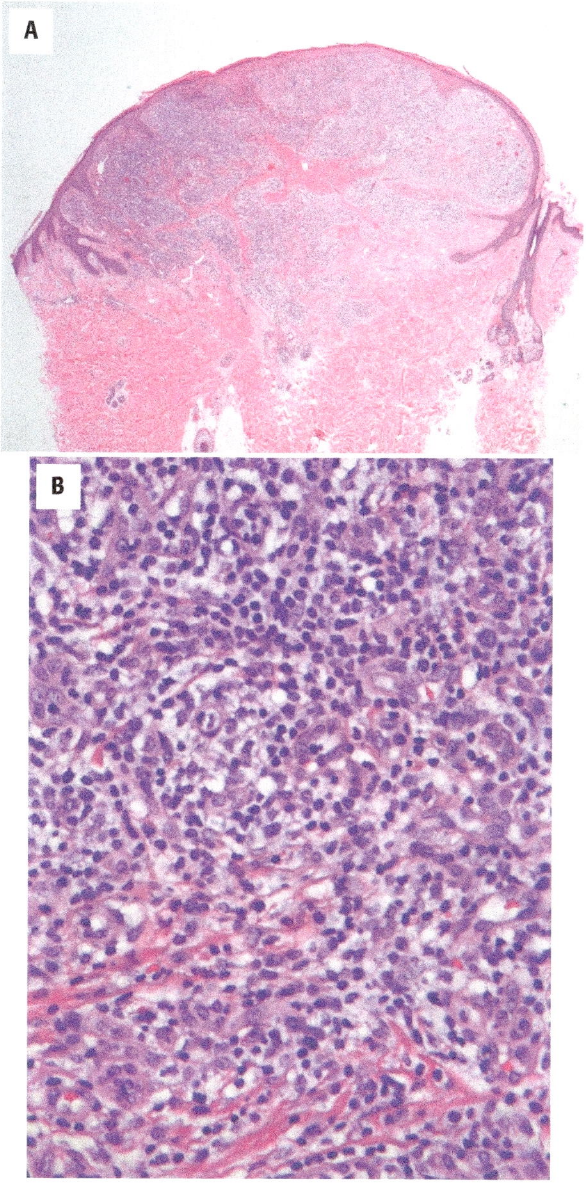

FIG. 15.58

Pseudolymphoma. **A,** There is a superficial dermal "top-heavy" inflammatory cell infiltrate. **B,** It is composed of mixed infiltrate of small lymphocytes, histiocytes.

Ancillary Studies

IHC for a panel of B- and T-cell markers and evidence of light chain restriction is necessary for the distinction of a B-cell pseudolymphoma from lymphoma. Molecular studies (PCR test for IgH gene rearrangements or in situ hybridization for λ or κ) may also be helpful.

Differential Diagnosis

Immunohistochemical analysis of a pseudo–B-cell lymphoma usually reveals a mixed population of T and B cells. If only isolated scattered CD20-positive B cells are present in a dense dermal infiltrate, it is easy to exclude a B-cell lymphoma. Lack of aberrant antigen expression (e.g., CD20-positive cells also express bcl-2) is also reassuring for a diagnosis of pseudolymphoma. The distinction of B-cell lymphoma from pseudolymphoma is more difficult when there are multiple small clusters of CD20-positive B cells or large dense sheetlike aggregates thereof.

Molecular studies may then be necessary. They usually fail to reveal evidence of clonality in the majority of pseudolymphomas. However, exceptions exist. False-positive test results occur also with reactive B-cell infiltrates. Occasionally, PCR studies for the workup of B-cell lymphoma versus pseudolymphoma may even suggest the presence of a T-cell population, which may lead to diagnostic confusion. Such "clonal" T-cell populations can be present in bona fide pseudolymphomas (e.g., drug-induced eruption with subsequent disappearance of the lesion after cessation of the medication).

When the clinical and histologic findings are not unequivocal, it may be prudent to report an infiltrate descriptively as "atypical" and defer the final diagnosis until later in time when additional clinical or histologic evidence permits a more definitive assessment.

CUTANEOUS PLASMACYTOSIS

This disease manifests clinically as persistent brown patches on the trunk or upper extremities (Fig. 15.59). Histopathologically, there may be a perivascular or nodular lymphoplasmacellular infiltrate (Fig. 15.59) with many mature polyclonal plasma cells. Affected patients may have associated systemic findings (fever, adenopathy, hypergammaglobulinemia). Some patients develop systemic plasmacytosis characterized by multiorgan involvement by polyclonal plasma cell–rich infiltrates. The disease is typically associated with elevated IL-6 levels. Therapy targeting IL-y may be beneficial in some cases.

INFILTRATION OF THE SKIN BY HEMATOPOIETIC STEM CELL AND PLASMACYTOID DENDRITIC CELL NEOPLASMS

Leukemia represents a large group of neoplasms of bone marrow–derived blood cells, usually white blood cells (leukocytes). Principally this group can be divided into acute and chronic forms and further subclassified according to the types of blood cells affected. Acute forms of leukemias are characterized by the rapid increase of immature blood cells. They may occur in children (acute leukemias represent the most common cause of cancer-related death in children in the United States) or adults.

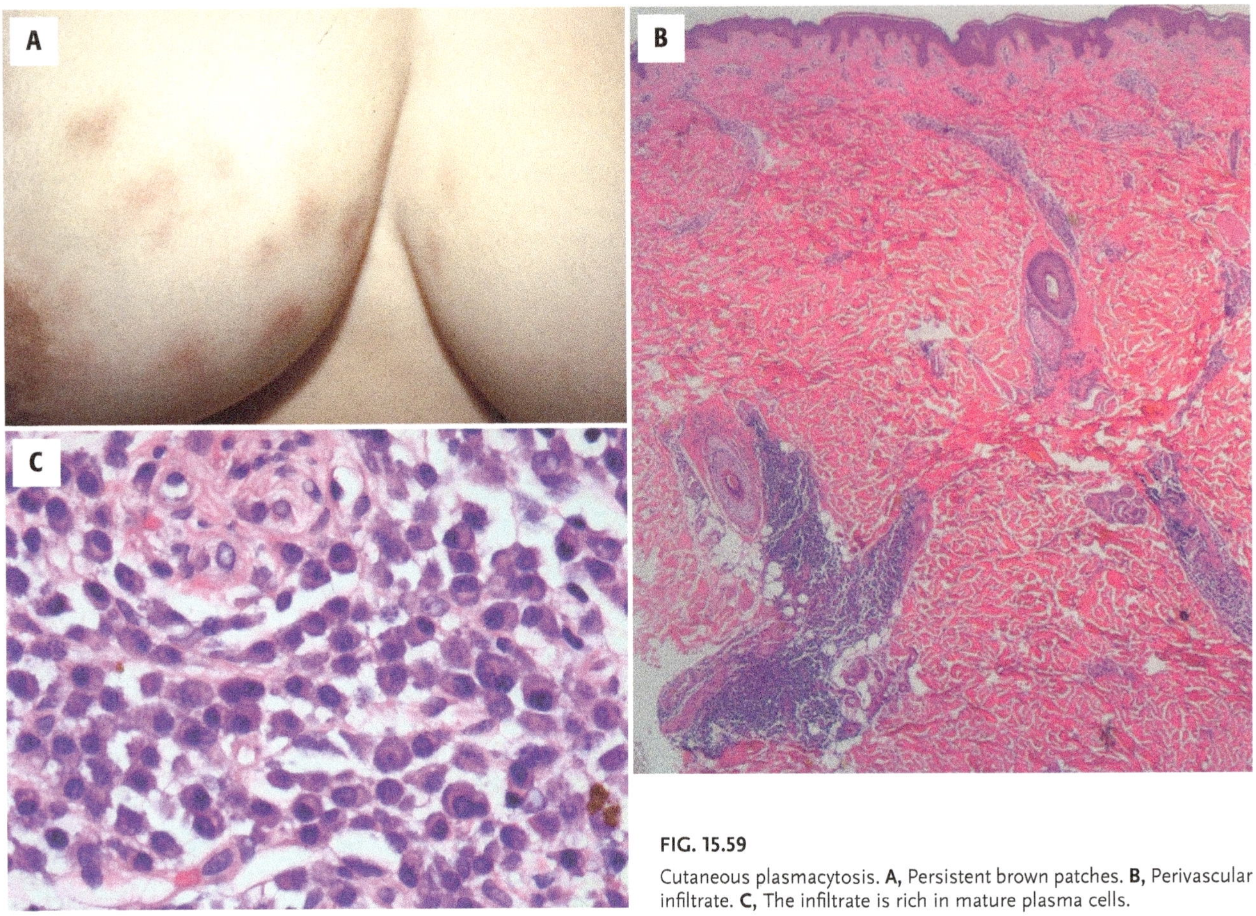

FIG. 15.59
Cutaneous plasmacytosis. **A,** Persistent brown patches. **B,** Perivascular infiltrate. **C,** The infiltrate is rich in mature plasma cells.

Chronic leukemia represents an excessive production and circulation of relatively mature albeit abnormal blood cells. It typically develops over months, years, or even decades and preferentially affects older individuals. Of note, seemingly chronic myeloproliferative and myelodysplastic neoplasms can involve the skin with or without progression to acute/blast phases.

While a detailed discussion of leukemia is beyond the scope of this chapter, with regard to cell type, a main distinction is between *lymphocytic/lymphoblastic* (lymphocyte precursor/differentiation) and *myeloid* (precursor for polymorphonuclear cells, red blood cells, and platelets) proliferations and neoplasms most simply referred to as leukemias. There are many subcategories within each group. The following discussion focuses on the cutaneous manifestation of the most common leukemias, particularly those that are seen involving skin.

The most common type of leukemia in children is acute lymphoblastic leukemia (ALL). The two most common forms of leukemias in adults are CLL and acute myelogenous leukemia (AML).

SUBTYPES OF LEUKEMIA CUTIS (REPRESENTATIVE AND GENERAL)

Myeloid Neoplasms and Proliferations:
- Acute myeloid leukemia (myeloid or myelomonocytic) (AML)
- Chronic myeloid leukemia
- Chronic myelomonocytic leukemia
- Myelodysplastic neoplasms ("MDS" per current classification acronyms)

Lymphoid Neoplasms and Proliferations:
- B-cell leukemia/lymphomas
  - Precursor B-cell neoplasms (B-lymphoblastic leukemias)
  - Mature B-cell neoplasms (chronic lymphocytic leukemia [CLL], monoclonal B-cell lymphocytosis [MBL])
  - Hairy cell leukemia
- T-cell leukemia/lymphomas
  - Precursor T-cell neoplasms (lymphoblastic leukemia)
  - Mature T-cell neoplasms (adult T-cell leukemia/lymphoma [ATLL], T-cell prolymphocytic leukemia, aggressive NK-cell leukemia, T and NK large granular lymphocytic leukemia)

CHRONIC LYMPHOCYTIC LEUKEMIA

Among the adult population of the United States, CLL is the most common form of leukemia. It is also the most prevalent because of its relatively longer survival rate. In the age group of 50- to 75-year-old adults, the incidence of CLL is between 15 and 20 individuals per 100,000 population, with the age of diagnosis at the lower end in non-White populations.

Clinical Findings

Men are nearly twice as likely as women to develop CLL. Lymphadenopathy is the most common finding, although splenomegaly can occur. Patients with CLL often show a predisposition to repeated infection and fatigue. They may have associated constitutional symptoms (e.g., fever, weight loss) or autoimmune hemolytic anemia.

Skin involvement by CLL may be clinically occult (incidental detection in a surgical specimen or biopsy for an unrelated lesion, such as squamous cell carcinoma) or manifest in a broad spectrum of clinical appearances, including pale pink macules, papules, nodules, tumors, plaques, erythroderma, or bullous lesions. Infiltration of herpes simplex virus infections or zoster scars and Mohs surgery sites may be seen.

Some authors have suggested that the latter presentation may represent a physiologic response (recruitment of blood cells, which includes leukemic cells) to the antigenic stimulus rather than an indication of leukemia exacerbation (primary expansion of neoplastic cells into the skin).

CHRONIC LYMPHOCYTIC LEUKEMIA—DISEASE FACT SHEET

Patient Group

- Usually older individuals
- Men more often affected than women

Site of Involvement

- Most patients present with adenopathy
- Bone marrow and peripheral blood (anemia/cytopenias and lymphocytosis)
- Skin involvement is rare (2%) but may be the initial manifestation

Clinical Findings

- Multiple erythematous macules, papules, plaques, or nodules
- May also be papulovesicular or manifest as paronychia
- May be clinically occult but seen incidentally in a skin biopsy occasionally in association with nonmelanoma skin cancer

Prognosis

- Prognosis depends on stage (Rai and Binet staging systems assess involvement of anemia or thrombocytopenia and lymph node regions involved)
- Most patients have an indolent course
- Transformation to large cell lymphoma may occur (Richter transformation), with intermediate forms of histologic progression (e.g., prolymphocytic progression occupying an intermediate prognostic space)
- TP53 alterations, Ig gene rearrangement and IGHV gene SHM status, and chromosomal alterations del(11q), del(13q), del(17p), and trisomy 12 show prognostic significance

Treatment

- Patients with low-risk stable disease only require periodic follow-up
- Chemotherapy or monoclonal antibodies (or both) for selected patient groups

Histopathologic Features

There is a variably dense dermal infiltration of small, monomorphous, round lymphocytes (Figs. 15.60 and 15.61). The pattern of distribution may be patchy, perivascular, periadnexal, or pandermal nodular or diffuse, with extension into the subcutis. Reactive T cells may be admixed with neoplastic B cells.

Ancillary Studies

The neoplastic cells are positive for CD79a (weak), CD20, PAX5, and LEF1. They are variably positive for CD23. Aberrant staining for CD5 and CD43 may be seen. MUM1 can be seen in proliferation centers. PCR is positive for a clonal B-cell population.

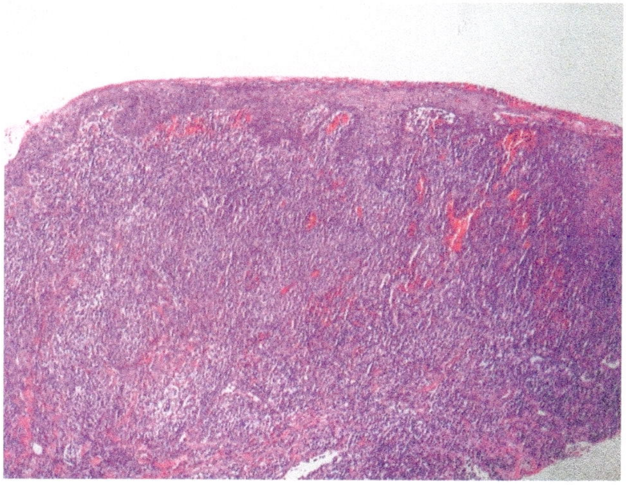

FIG. 15.60

Chronic lymphocytic leukemia. There is a dense infiltrate of small lymphocytes in the dermis.

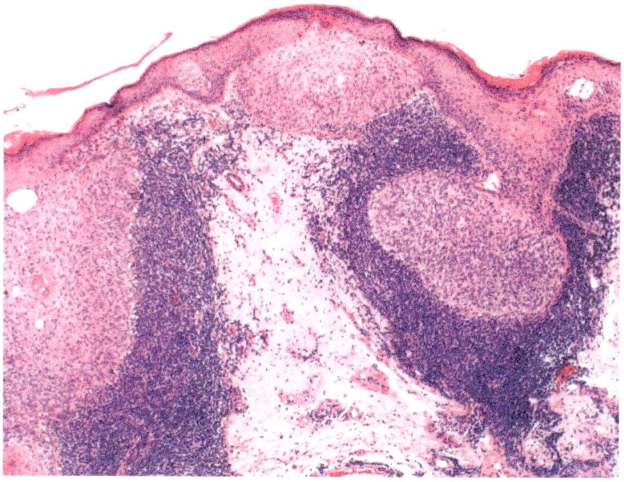

FIG. 15.61

Chronic lymphocytic leukemia incidentally detected in a biopsy for squamous cell carcinoma.

CHRONIC LYMPHOCYTIC LEUKEMIA—PATHOLOGIC FEATURES

Histopathologic Features

- Small round lymphocytes with condensed chromatin
- The pattern of distribution is variable (diffuse, patchy, perivascular, nodular)
- There may be many admixed T cells and/or eosinophils
- There may be an association with granulomatous reaction

Ancillary Studies

- The neoplastic lymphocytes are
  - Immunopositive for CD5, CD43, CD23, CD20, LEF1
  - Immunonegative for CD10, cyclin D1
- The neoplastic lymphocytes show immunoglobulin gene rearrangement

Differential Diagnosis

- Hypersensitivity reaction
- Other lymphomas

Differential Diagnosis

The lymphocytes are small and well differentiated. At times, infiltrate is incidentally present in association with another process, such as a carcinoma. Often, a reactive process is suspected at first, but CLL is readily distinguished from reactive infiltrates by the presence of dense sheets of small round well-differentiated lymphocytes that are immunoreactive for CD20.

On the other hand, not all dense lymphocytic infiltrates that occur in patients with CLL represent leukemia. Hypersensitivity reactions do occur in patients with CLL and may at times be florid (exaggerated hypersensitivity reaction), simulating a lymphoma on H&E-stained sections (Fig. 15.62). Reactive infiltrates usually show a predominance of T cells, with few or no B cells.

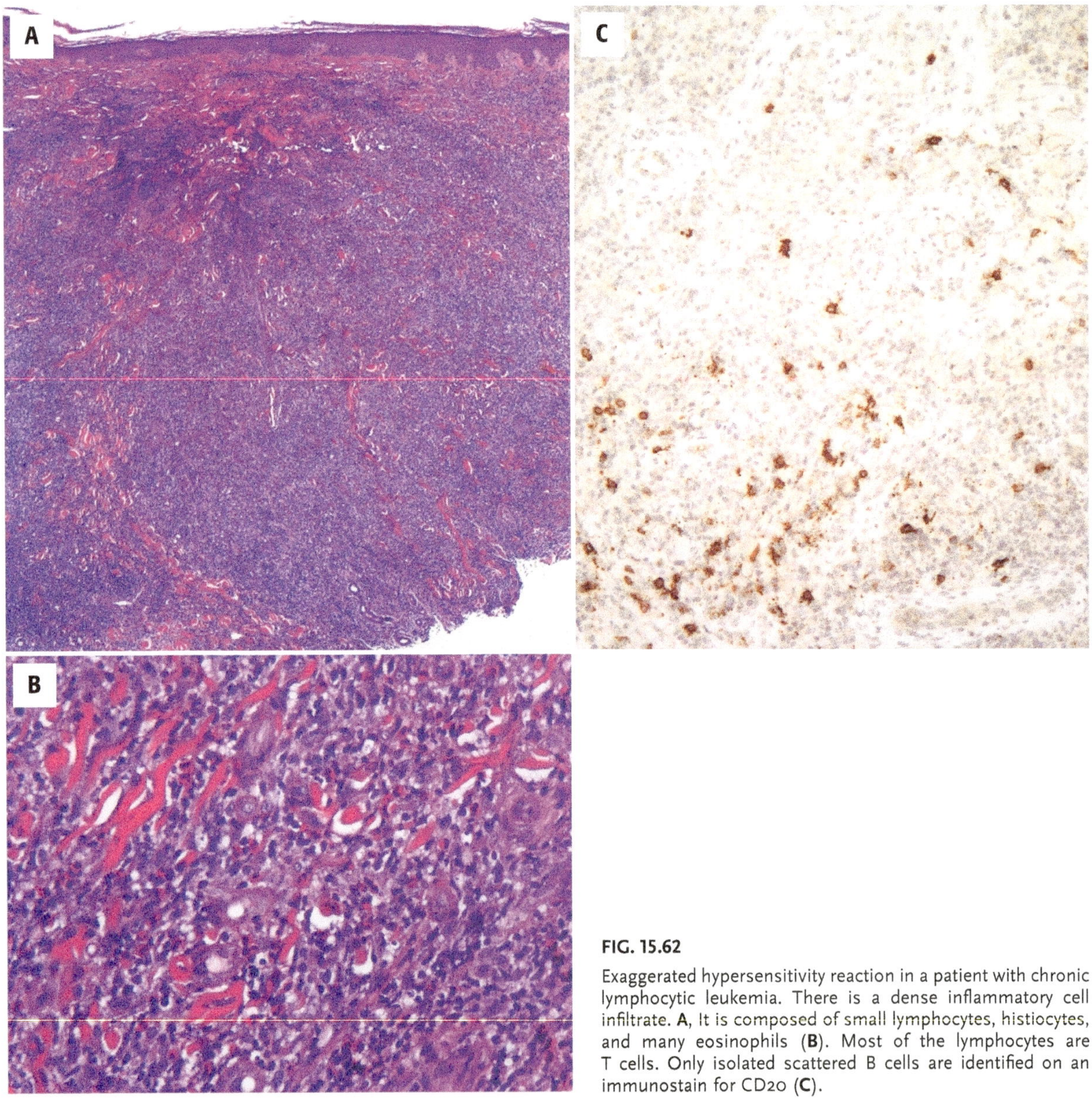

FIG. 15.62

Exaggerated hypersensitivity reaction in a patient with chronic lymphocytic leukemia. There is a dense inflammatory cell infiltrate. **A**, It is composed of small lymphocytes, histiocytes, and many eosinophils (**B**). Most of the lymphocytes are T cells. Only isolated scattered B cells are identified on an immunostain for CD20 (**C**).

Prognosis and Treatment

Various staging systems have been developed for patients with CLL, taking into account laboratory data (e.g., lymphocytosis, hemoglobin, and platelets) and physical findings (e.g., extent of lymphadenopathy or organomegaly). Most patients with CLL fall into a low-risk group with chronic indolent disease and should not be treated with chemotherapy unless they are symptomatic or there is evidence of disease progression. In addition to conventional chemotherapy, monoclonal antibodies (e.g., alemtuzumab or rituximab) have been found to be effective.

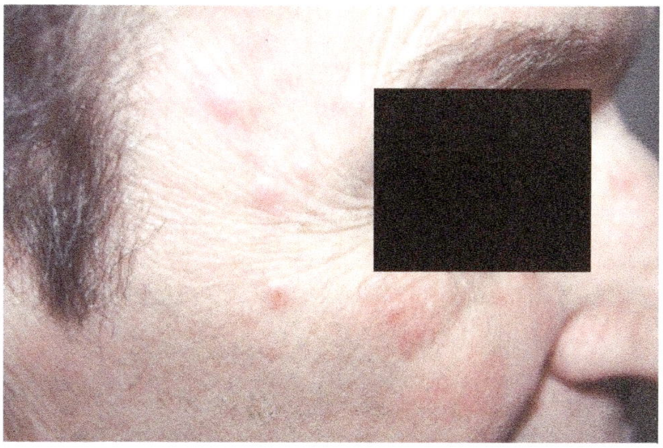

FIG. 15.63
Myeloid leukemia cutis. Multiple erythematous papules are seen.

MYELOID LEUKEMIA

Patients with myeloid leukemia may have a number of cutaneous eruptions related to leukemia that, however, do not represent direct infiltration of neoplastic myeloid cells of the skin. Such reactions include (Sweet's-like) neutrophilic dermatosis and florid (exaggerated) hypersensitivity reactions. Direct infiltration of the skin by leukemic cells is often referred to as "specific" cutaneous lesions. Specific cutaneous leukemic infiltrates have been reported in 10% to 50% of patients with AML of the French-American-British (FAB) classification subtypes M4 and M5 (acute myelomonocytic and acute myeloblastic/monocytic leukemia) and up to 10% of patients with AML-FAB subtypes M0, M1, M2, and M3 (e.g., AML with minimal differentiation, without maturation and with maturation)—although these data may shift when considering AMLs with specific genetic abnormalities. Cutaneous lesions in patients with chronic myeloid leukemia (CML) are rare, occurring in fewer than 2% of individuals affected by CML.

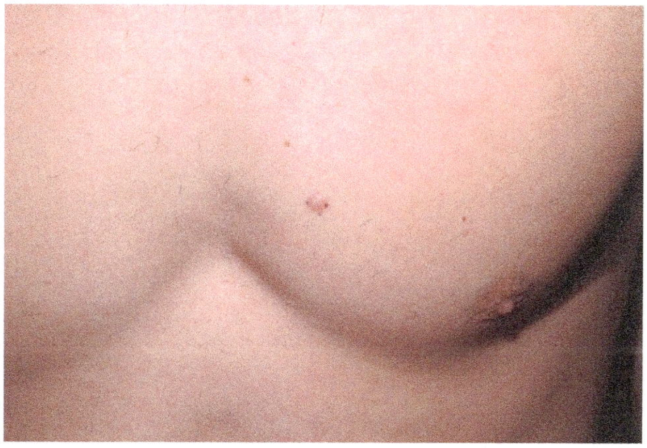

FIG. 15.64
Myeloid leukemia cutis. A solitary nodule is present.

Clinical Findings

In patients with AML, specific cutaneous lesions may present before, simultaneously with, or after a diagnosis of leukemia has been made. In aleukemic leukemia cutis, the skin lesions occur without hematologic evidence of leukemia.

Clinically, there are often multiple erythematous to violaceous or hemorrhagic papules, nodules, and plaques, but solitary lesions are also seen (Figs. 15.63 and 15.64). Ulceration, crusting, and bulla may occur. There may be a generalized macular and papular eruption, but lesions may be quite subtle. The lesions often occur on the trunk and extremities, but the head and neck region or any site may be involved. The interval between diagnosis of systemic leukemia and leukemia cutis ranges from approximately 0 to 13 months, and this may be the first sign of hematologic malignancy. Concurrent extramedullary involvement of noncutaneous sites may be seen. Gingival hyperplasia because of infiltration of leukemic cells is a feature seen in AML and acute myelomonocytic leukemia (AMML). In addition, there can be unusual sites of involvement, such as the orbit and pharynx. Solitary tumorlike infiltrates of myeloid leukemic cells have been historically referred to as *granulocytic sarcoma* or *chloroma*.

CML usually affects older individuals. Leukemic infiltration of the skin is rare. The clinical spectrum of individual lesions is variable. Typically, specific skin lesions develop after a diagnosis of CML has already been established, usually within a period of 36 to 72 months after the diagnosis.

Histopathologic Features

A spectrum of histologic features can be seen in myeloid leukemia cutis, ranging from dense infiltrates of poorly differentiated blasts to paucicellular infiltrates of variably

ACUTE MYELOID LEUKEMIA CUTIS—DISEASE FACT SHEET

Patient Group

- ►► Children and adults
- ►► Risk factors include smoking, exposure to toxic materials or drugs (chemotherapy), Down syndrome, and Fanconi anemia

Site of Involvement

- ►► Scalp, face, trunk and extremities, mucous membranes (gums, conjunctiva)

Clinical Findings

- ►► Systemic symptoms (fever, malaise, fatigue, weight loss)
- ►► Variable: erythematous macule(s), papule(s), nodule(s), or plaque(s); purpuric or vasculitic or urticarial presentation
- ►► Often diagnosed in the setting of known acute myelogenous leukemia or a history of myelodysplasia
- ►► May occur in patients with no evidence of extracutaneous disease (aleukemic leukemia cutis)
- ►► Skin involvement most often seen with acute myelomonocytic leukemia (AMML; French-American-British [FAB] M4) and monoblastic/monocytic leukemia (acute monocytic leukemia [AMOL]; FAB M5)

Prognosis

- ►► Depends on subtype and chromosomal aberrations

Unfavorable Prognostic Factors

- ►► Age older than 60 years
- ►► Certain chromosomal abnormalities
- ►► Prior treatment with radiation or chemotherapy

Treatment

- ►► Chemotherapy
- ►► Hematopoietic stem cell transplantation

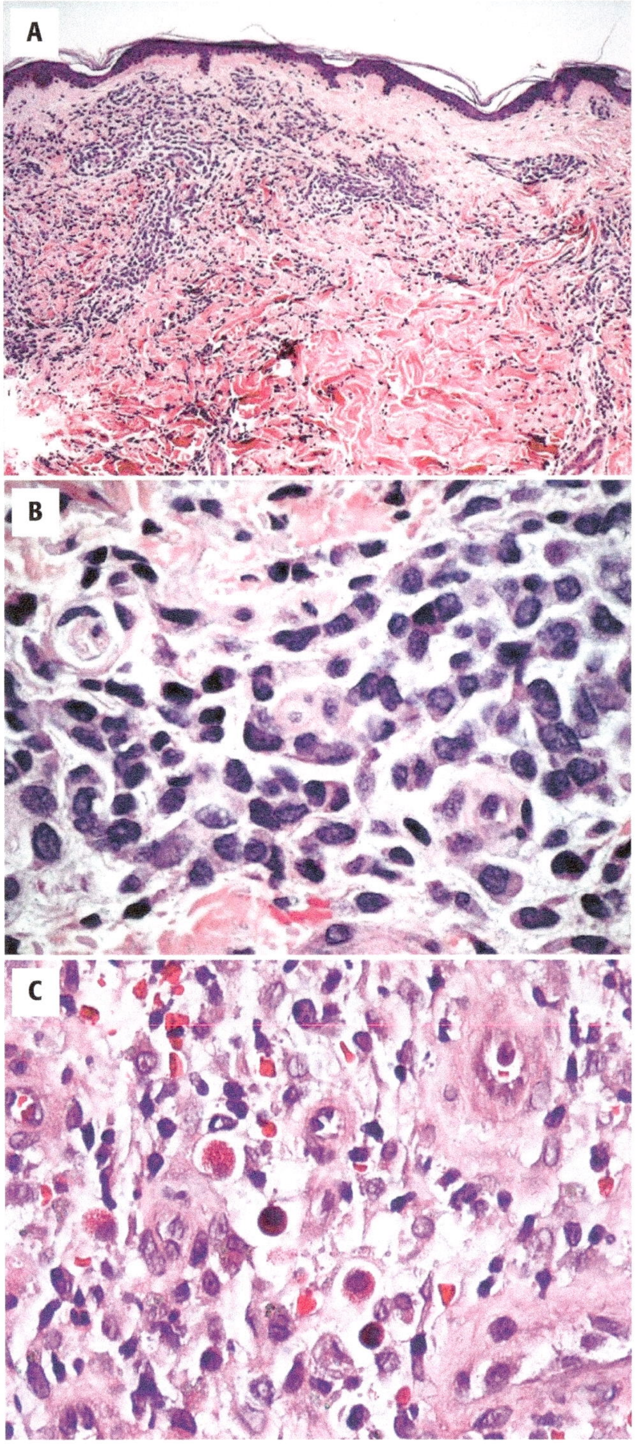

FIG. 15.65

Myeloid leukemia cutis. There is a mononuclear cell infiltrate in a perivascular and interstitial pattern. **A,** The infiltrate is composed of immature myeloid cells (**B**). The presence of mononuclear immature eosinophils is a helpful diagnostic clue (**C**).

mature and immature myeloid cells, which may be admixed with reactive inflammatory cells, such as T cells and histiocytes. In AML, one often finds a diffuse dermal infiltrate of immature mononuclear cells that permeate a passive reticular dermis, sparing the epidermis (Fig. 15.65). The infiltrate may be perivascular, periadnexal, and interstitial. Commonly, there is evidence of minor vascular damage. Frank necrotizing small vessel vasculitis may also be seen. Extension into the subcutaneous tissue may occur, but the upper papillary dermis is usually spared.

A characteristic feature is that of trickling of neoplastic cells between the collagen bundles in a horizontal single-cell arrangement. There may be concentric "cuffing" of the neoplastic cells around the vessels and adnexa, especially with M4 and M5. AML may histologically present as cellular tumors or be subtle in the form of a leukemic vasculitis or folliculitis with admixed lymphocytes and histiocytes.

The nuclear features vary depending on the subtype of leukemia or level of maturation arrest. In M1 and M2, often there are larger mononuclear cells, or atypical myeloblasts and myelocytes, characterized by eccentrically placed basophilic nuclei with distinct nucleoli and scant cytoplasm. In M4 and M5, there tend to be medium-sized round to oval mononuclear cells or atypical monocytoid cells, with eosinophilic cytoplasm and indented, bilobular, or reniform basophilic nuclei. In some cases, there

ACUTE MYELOID LEUKEMIA CUTIS—PATHOLOGIC FEATURES

Histopathologic Features

- Infiltrate of immature myeloid cells in dermis
- Perivascular, interstitial and/or nodular infiltrate
- Mononuclear eosinophils are a helpful diagnostic clue

Ancillary Studies

- Variably positive for CD43, muramidase, myeloperoxidase, CD68, CD33
- Often positive for ERG; blasts may be positive for CD117, CD34
- Negative for CD3, CD20, CD56, CD4, TCF4

Differential Diagnosis

- Reactive infiltrate with left shift among myeloid cells (e.g., infection, drug reaction, histiocytoid variant of neutrophilic dermatosis)
- Plasmacytoid dendritic cell neoplasm (positive for CD123 and TCF4)
- CD30+ anaplastic large cell lymphoma

is a predominance of small or large neoplastic cells. The presence of immature mononuclear eosinophils is a helpful diagnostic clue, especially in the setting of admixed reactive cells. CML is more pleomorphic, with a variable mixture of mature and immature granulocytic cell lines, including myelocytes, metamyelocytes, and segmented neutrophils. Mononuclear cells may also be seen. The infiltrates in both AML and CML demonstrate apoptosis and frequent and occasionally atypical mitoses.

Ancillary Studies

Results from bone marrow biopsies and aspirates and peripheral blood analysis, including flow cytometry and cytogenetic analysis, are most critical for the classification of myeloid leukemias. Ancillary studies routinely applied directly to skin tissue biopsies include special chemical stains (e.g., Giemsa), IHC, and FISH. Targeted anchored multiplex RNA seq and NGS assays can confirm and sometimes diagnose leukemias with specific genetic abnormalities in skin tissues when access to extracutaneous tissues is challenging.

The purpose of the former studies (IHC and enzyme histochemistry) is to highlight the line of differentiation, which is diagnostically needed (e.g., for the distinction of myeloid leukemia from lymphoblastic leukemia or lymphoma). Special stains cannot distinguish many cases of reactive infiltrates from neoplastic ones (e.g., bona fide myeloid leukemia versus left shift secondary to infection). In typical cases with a history or concurrent bone marrow biopsy documenting the type of leukemia, ancillary studies are usually not necessary. However, special stains are helpful when there is insufficient clinical information or the histology is suboptimal (e.g., crush artifacts rendering evaluation of cytologic features more difficult).

Stains that highlight myeloid differentiation include naphthol AS-D chloroacetate-esterase (NASD), muramidase, CD33, and myeloperoxidase (MPO). A Giemsa stain highlights granules. Many lesions, but not all of them, are positive for these myeloid markers. The neoplastic cells of AML are also usually immunoreactive for CD43 and LCA (CD45RA). They tend to be negative for lymphoid markers, such as CD3, CD20, and CD30. However, staining for some lymphoid markers, such as CD4 or CD56, may be seen in AML. Acute myeloblastic leukemia may be immunoreactive for CD34, CD117 (Fig. 15.66), but results with these markers are quite variable and not uncommonly negative, especially in monocytoid leukemias. Anti-CD68 (KP1; PGM1), CD163, and Mac 387 help document monocytoid differentiation. Occasionally, transdifferentiation of myeloid leukemias, whether primary or due to therapy, may eventuate in the identification of a leukemia of a different lineage (e.g., B-cell or histiocytic), which may share underlying molecular features.

IHC also helps distinguish myeloid from hairy cell leukemia. The neoplastic cells of hairy cell leukemia are immunopositive for TRAP, CD20, CD79a, CD25, CD11c, and CD103 but negative for CD23, CD5, and CD10.

IHC for ERG can help for the distinction of leukemia from reactive infiltrates because reactive inflammatory cells usually lack expression of this marker, but many leukemia cells are strongly positive. A stain for TCF4 helps distinguish myeloid leukemia from a pDC neoplasm.

Differential Diagnosis

The differential diagnosis depends on the leukemia subtype. There are no microscopic or immunohistochemical features to definitively distinguish the FAB subtypes or differentiate AML from CML. All subtypes may show cytomorphic features identical to lymphoma, especially in cases of weak or negative MPO or lysozome, and positive LCA, UCHL-1, and CD43. In this situation, one may also perform immunostains for T- and B-cell markers, fragment analysis or TCR/IgH sequencing, FISH, or targeted genomic assays as appropriate for the specific case.

For example, an immunophenotype with positive staining for MPO, lysozyme, CD45, and CD43 and lack of staining for CD20 and CD3 is characteristic of myeloid leukemia cutis. When there is blastic morphology, pDC neoplasm needs to be considered as well as on occasion a possible nonhematopoietic neoplasm, such as poorly differentiated carcinoma and melanoma. They can usually be readily identified with immunostains. Rarely, leukemic infiltrates may show granulomatous features, leading to possible confusion with benign granulomatous infiltrates. Other leukemias may show divergent histiocytic differentiation.

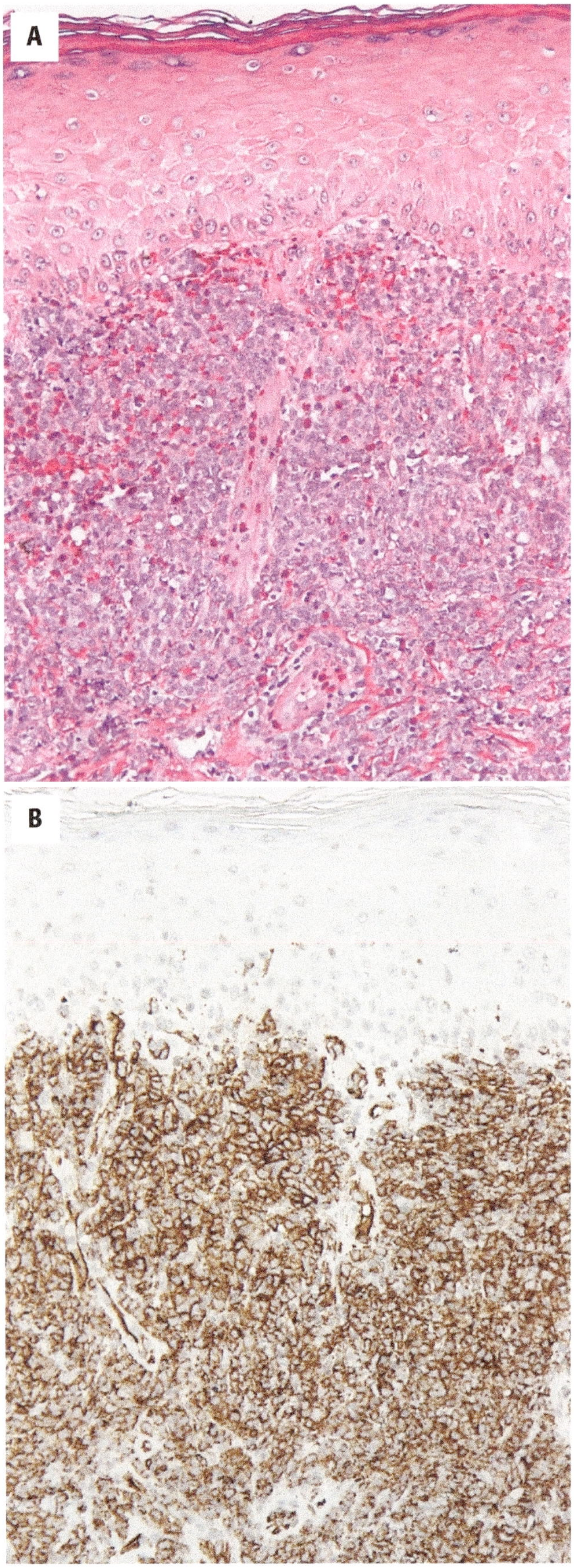

FIG. 15.66
Myeloid leukemia cutis. **A,** Dense dermal infiltrate of blasts. **B,** The neoplastic cells are immunoreactive for CD34.

If a drug rash occurs in a patient with a high number of circulating leukemic cells or if the number of blasts is very small or diluted by an associated reactive infiltrate, such as from a folliculitis, AML may be difficult to distinguish from a "left shift" related to infection or a drug reaction. Furthermore, new drugs such as isocitrate dehydrogenase (IDH) inhibitors may induce differentiation of AML cells to a more neutrophilic morphology. A related diagnostic problem is the histiocytoid variant of Sweet's syndrome. Clinical correlation and careful assessment of cell maturity are essential. Leukemia often occurs after a long history of myeloid dysplasia or anemia. In some cases, leukemia cutis may be the first manifestation of leukemia (aleukemic leukemia). Bone marrow biopsies and peripheral blood samples may only confirm months later that unequivocal leukemia is present. Positive labeling for ERG can help support the diagnosis of leukemia because strong ERG expression is not a feature of a reactive left shift.

CML can be difficult to distinguish from neutrophilic infiltrates, such as infection or noninfectious neutrophilic dermatoses. Clinical context is critical. Leukemic infiltrates related to CML are usually slowly progressing, but infectious lesions or lesions of neutrophilic dermatosis (Sweet's syndrome) tend to be of more rapid onset and respond to antibiotics or steroids, respectively.

Prognosis and Treatment

The prognosis depends on the subtype of leukemia, patient age, and stage. For AML, medical care includes various regimens of chemotherapy and bone marrow transplantation. For patients with chronic-phase CML, imatinib is the treatment of choice.

PLASMACYTOID DENDRITIC CELL NEOPLASM

The neoplastic cells are devoid of common T-cell, B-cell, NK-cell, and myeloid lineage markers. They are derived from pDCs. Blastic plasmacytoid dendritic cell neoplasm (BPDCN) shows disease characteristics similar to leukemias and can develop in patients with a history of (or concurrent) myelodysplastic syndrome or CML, and may be divergently expressed with chronic myelomonocytic leukemia (CMML), sharing mutational profiles, which is why the disease is discussed in this chapter along with leukemia.

Clinical Findings

Patients present with solitary or multiple bruise-like or brown nodules and plaques (Fig. 15.67). Oral

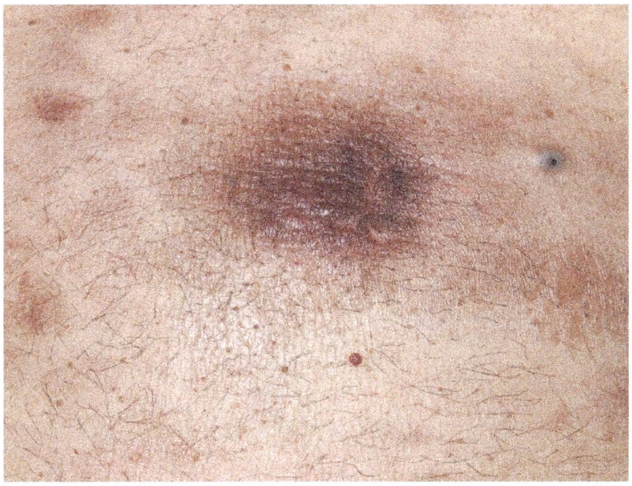

FIG. 15.67
Plasmacytoid dendritic cell neoplasm. Multiple *(brownish)* papules and plaques are present.

mucosal lesions, which may be ulcerous, are common. Constitutional symptoms, hepatosplenomegaly, and hemophagocytic syndrome may be seen. Approximately half of patients present with marrow or nodal disease, and those presenting initially with skin-limited disease frequently disseminate to lymph nodes, marrow, blood, and visceral organs.

Histopathologic Features

There is a dermal or subcutaneous infiltrate of intermediate-sized cells with blastic morphology characterized by finely dispersed chromatin and nonprominent nucleoli (Fig. 15.68). Mitotic figures are easily identified. Angiodestruction and necrosis as often seen with NK lymphomas are usually absent.

PLASMACYTOID DENDRITIC CELL NEOPLASM—DISEASE FACT SHEET

Patient Group
- Middle-aged or elderly adults

Site of Involvement
- Skin, lymph nodes, bone marrow, and central nervous system (CNS)

Clinical Findings
- Solitary or multiple skin nodules

Site of Involvement
- Skin, lymph nodes, bone marrow, and CNS

Prognosis and Treatment
- Poor; usually rapid progression
- Most patients die or relapse within a few years
- Chemotherapy

Ancillary Studies

The lymphocytes are immunopositive for CD123, CD4, CD56, and TCF4. They may also be positive staining for CD7, CD68, and terminal deoxynucleotidyl transferase (TdT). CD3 and CD8 are usually negative. Cytotoxic proteins are not seen, and EBV is negative. The TCR gene is germline.

Differential Diagnosis

Because of the blastic morphology and expression of CD56 in leukemia, pDC neoplasm needs to be differentiated from myelomonocytic leukemia cutis. TCF4 is often helpful for this distinction. pDC neoplasm may also need to be distinguished from NK and NK–T-cell lymphomas. An additional consideration is the mature pDC proliferations that occur in the context of myeloid neoplasms, frequently seen in skin, which should be negative or only show dim CD56.

Prognosis and Treatment

The prognosis is generally poor for most patients, with a median survival period of 14 months. Remission with hyper-CVAD (fractionated cyclophosphamide, vincristine, doxorubicin, and dexamethasone) alternating with high-dose methotrexate-cytarabine has been reported, but patients frequently relapse.

PLASMACYTOID DENDRITIC CELL NEOPLASM—PATHOLOGIC FEATURES

Histopathologic Features
- Diffuse dermal infiltrate with grenz zone
- Dense monotonous infiltrate of medium-sized mononuclear cells with clumped chromatin (blastlike appearance)
- Frequent mitotic figures

Ancillary Studies
- Immunophenotype
  - Positive for CD4, CD56, CD123, TCF4
  - Variably positive for CD2, CD7, TdT, CD34
  - Negative for CD3, muramidase, myeloperoxidase

Molecular Studies
- Germline TCR
- Negative for EBV

Differential Diagnosis
- Myeloid leukemia
- Other lymphomas, in particular, NK-cell lymphomas and peripheral TCL
- Mature plasmacytoid dendritic cell proliferations associated with myeloid neoplasms

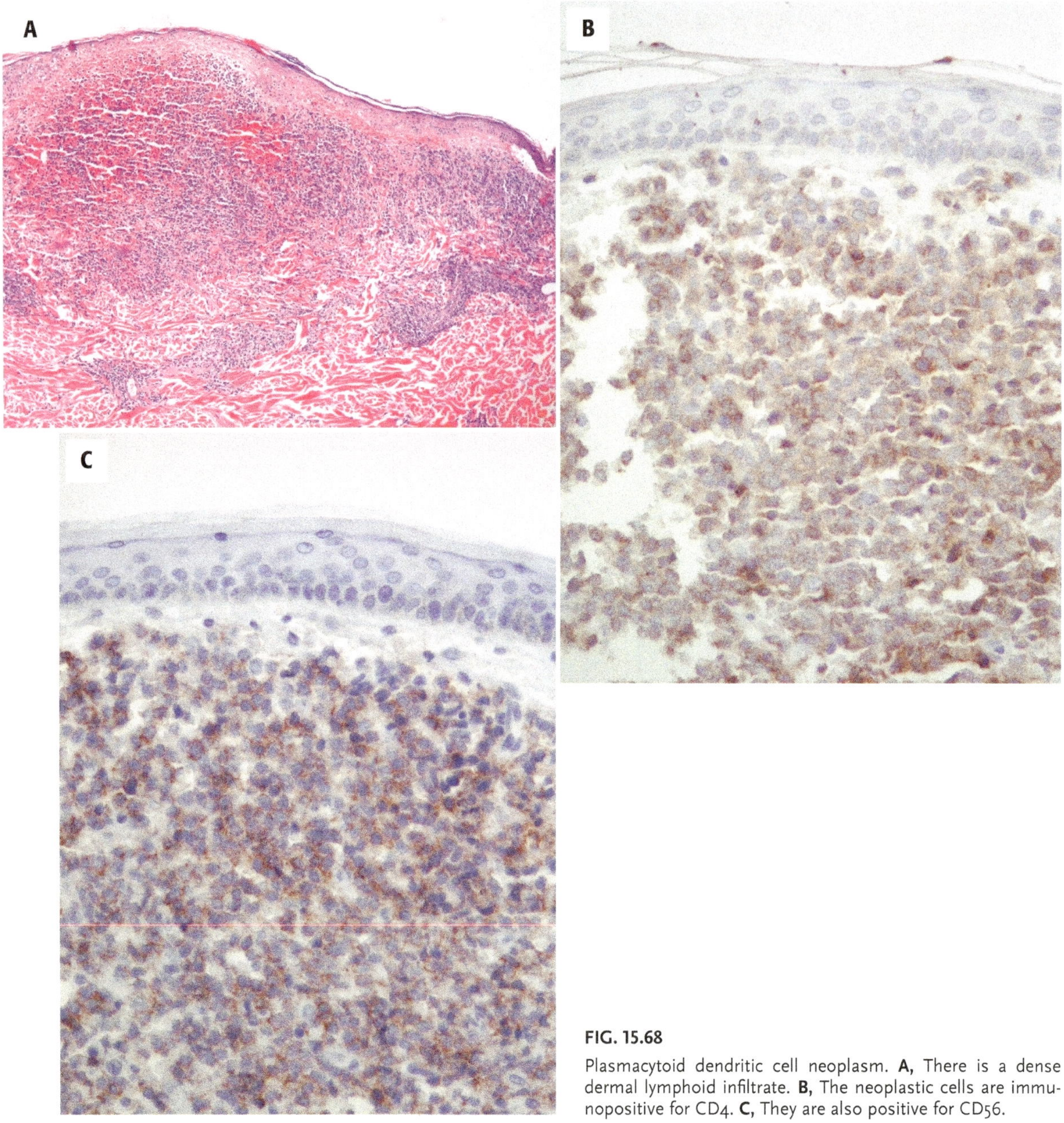

FIG. 15.68
Plasmacytoid dendritic cell neoplasm. **A,** There is a dense dermal lymphoid infiltrate. **B,** The neoplastic cells are immunopositive for CD4. **C,** They are also positive for CD56.

MAST CELL INFILTRATES

MASTOCYTOSIS

Mastocytosis refers to a spectrum of conditions in which mast cells accumulate in varying amounts in the skin, bone marrow, and visceral organs. The majority of patients have cutaneous mastocytosis (CM) with disease limited to the skin and an indolent clinical course. A minority of patients have systemic mastocytosis, which may also be indolent but can be clinically aggressive. Systemic mast cell disease may also be associated with non–mast cell hematologic neoplasms or present as mast cell leukemia. The following section focuses on cutaneous mast cell disease. Readers are referred to textbooks of hematopathology to learn more about systemic mast cell disease.

CUTANEOUS MASTOCYTOSIS

Clinical Findings

CM may manifest as maculopapular cutaneous mastocytosis (MPCM), diffuse CM, or solitary mastocytoma (SM) of the skin (Fig. 15.69). CM, especially urticaria pigmentosa (UP), may be familial, with an autosomal dominant inheritance pattern. Rare families carry germline c-kit mutations. CM may present at birth. A peak incidence is during infancy. Another peak occurs in young adulthood.

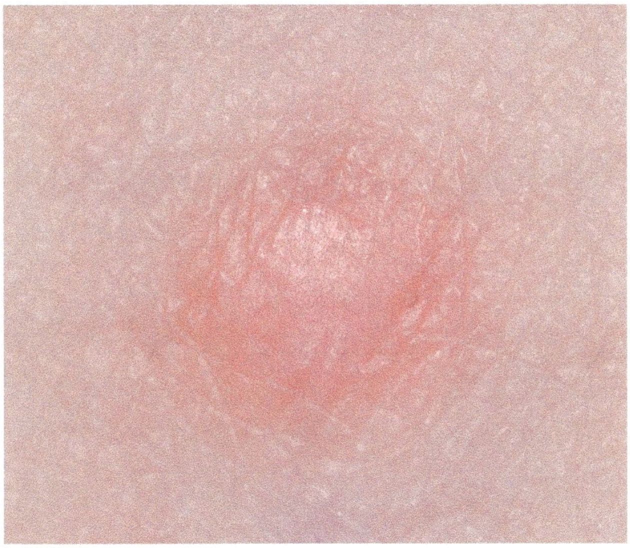

FIG. 15.69
Solitary mastocytoma.

Lesions that develop during childhood tend to regress, but adult-onset lesions tend to persist.

A clinical feature common to all forms of CM is a positive Darier's sign. It means that stroking of a lesion of CM leads to localized swelling (because of mast cell degranulation). Many lesions are also associated with pruritus or hyperpigmentation. Urtication of lesions may lead to blister formation.

MPCM may manifest as UP or *telangiectasia macularis eruptiva perstans* (TMEP). UP refers to the clinical presentation of diffuse brown or red-brown to tan nonscaly macules and papules disseminated on the trunk and extremities. TMEP presents as an erythematous patch that may be in a capelike distribution on the upper back or as erythematous-tan macules with telangiectases.

In diffuse mastocytosis, patients present with brownish indurated erythroderma. In infancy, when these patients present, bullae formation is common, and this presentation may be referred to as bullous mastocytosis. The lesions themselves may be itchy or asymptomatic. If there is a significant amount of mast cell infiltration of the skin, especially if there is associated SM, there may be symptoms related to mast cell degranulation and histamine release, such as flushing, diarrhea, and palpitations.

SM typically occurs in children as a lightly pigmented nodule. Individual lesions may also present as multiple papules or large plaques.

CUTANEOUS MASTOCYTOSIS—DISEASE FACT SHEET

Spectrum of Cutaneous Mastocytosis
- Urticaria pigmentosa
- Maculopapular cutaneous mastocytosis
- Diffuse cutaneous mastocytosis
- Mastocytoma

Patient Group
- 75% of patients are children
- The remainder of affected patients are usually middle-aged adults

Site of Involvement
- Majority of patients have disease confined to the skin
- Extracutaneous sites include bone marrow, lymph nodes, spleen, lung, and gastrointestinal tract

Signs and Symptoms
- Pruritus is common
- Darier's sign is typical

Prognosis
- Good prognosis if disease is confined to the skin
- Solitary lesions in children usually regress
- Tumors in adults are more persistent
- Less favorable clinical course for some aggressive variants of systemic mastocytosis or mastocytosis associated with hematologic malignancy

Treatment
- No treatment of small solitary lesion needed
- Solitary lesions in adults may be excised
- Chemotherapy for aggressive variants

Histopathologic Features

The histologic features are variable, but the common feature is an increased density of mast cells in the dermis. These cells are mononuclear, with a central or somewhat eccentrically placed nucleus, and generous, subtly granular cytoplasm. Sometimes, the cells have a "fried egg" appearance. Spindled or dendritic morphology may also be seen.

In early lesions of UP or mastocytoma, mast cells tend to show a perivascular distribution and preference for the papillary dermis. They may eventually form dense dermal nodular or diffuse aggregates (Fig. 15.70). Scattered eosinophils are commonly associated with CM. The epidermis often shows basal cell hyperpigmentation. In TMEP, there is a very sparse perivascular mast cell infiltrate in the upper dermis associated with telangiectases (Fig. 15.71). These MCs are often spindled and thus may be nearly inconspicuous on routine sections.

Ancillary Studies

Mast cells are recognizable on routine H&E staining but may require special stains for confirmation because similar morphology can be seen in other mononuclear cells, such as nevomelanocytes, and other hematologic infiltrates, such as lymphocytes, monocytes, and histiocytes.

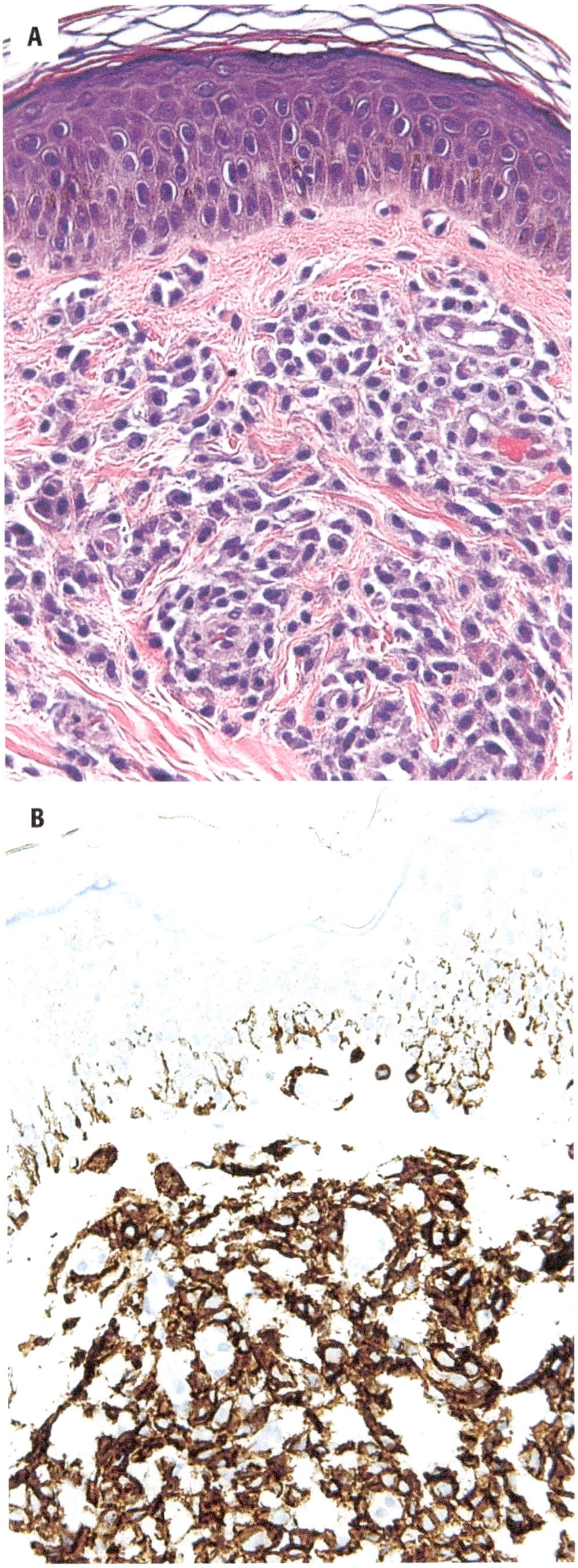

FIG. 15.70

Urticaria pigmentosa. **A,** Dense infiltrate of mast cells in the superficial dermis. **B,** They are immunoreactive for tryptase.

CUTANEOUS MASTOCYTOSIS—PATHOLOGIC FEATURES

Histopathologic Features

- Mastocytoma/urticaria pigmentosa: tumorous aggregates of mast cells in dermis
- Telangiectasia macularis eruptiva perstans (TMEP): increase density in perivascular and interstitial mast cells

Ancillary Studies

- Special stains: mast cells show metachromasia with toluidine blue and Giemsa
- Immunohistochemistry: mast cells are immunoreactive for CD117 and tryptase

Differential Diagnosis

- Mastocytoma: melanocytic nevus, leukemia, lymphoma
- Dermatitis with nonspecific increase in mast cells (e.g., hypersensitivity reaction)

Mast cells stain metachromatically with Giemsa. Toluidine blue also stains mast cells. The Leder stain, or naphthol AS-D, stains mast cells a brilliant red color. IHC is now often used with c-kit (CD117). This is especially helpful in evaluating for TMEP, in which the infiltrate is quite sparse and the mast cells may be fusiform and difficult to identify. Tryptase is especially helpful in assessing bone marrow infiltrates.

Because adult patients with CM are more likely to have SM, additional workup for possible systemic disease or associated hematologic malignancies may be indicated. Such additional tests include serum tryptase and bone marrow biopsies.

Differential Diagnosis

A mastocytoma may be confused with lymphoma, leukemia cutis, or a melanocytic nevus. In biopsies of TMEP, the mast cell infiltrate may be very sparse, and the changes may look similar to those of normal skin. In these cases, staining for c-kit may be helpful in detecting an increased number of mast cells. Lesions of UP or TMEP may also be mistaken for hypersensitivity reactions (and vice versa) because the latter can be accompanied by an increased density of mast cells. There may be variable numbers of eosinophils. However, hypersensitivity reactions are not as monomorphous as mast cell proliferative lesions. The infiltrate tends to be more polymorphous with eosinophils, lymphocytes, and histiocytes. There is overlap with the upper limit of normal number of mast cells in the skin and lower limit of numbers seen in TMEP and in systemic mastocytosis. The numbers of normal mast cells in the skin also vary with the anatomic site, so borderline cases should be correlated with systemic evaluation for mast cell overproduction.

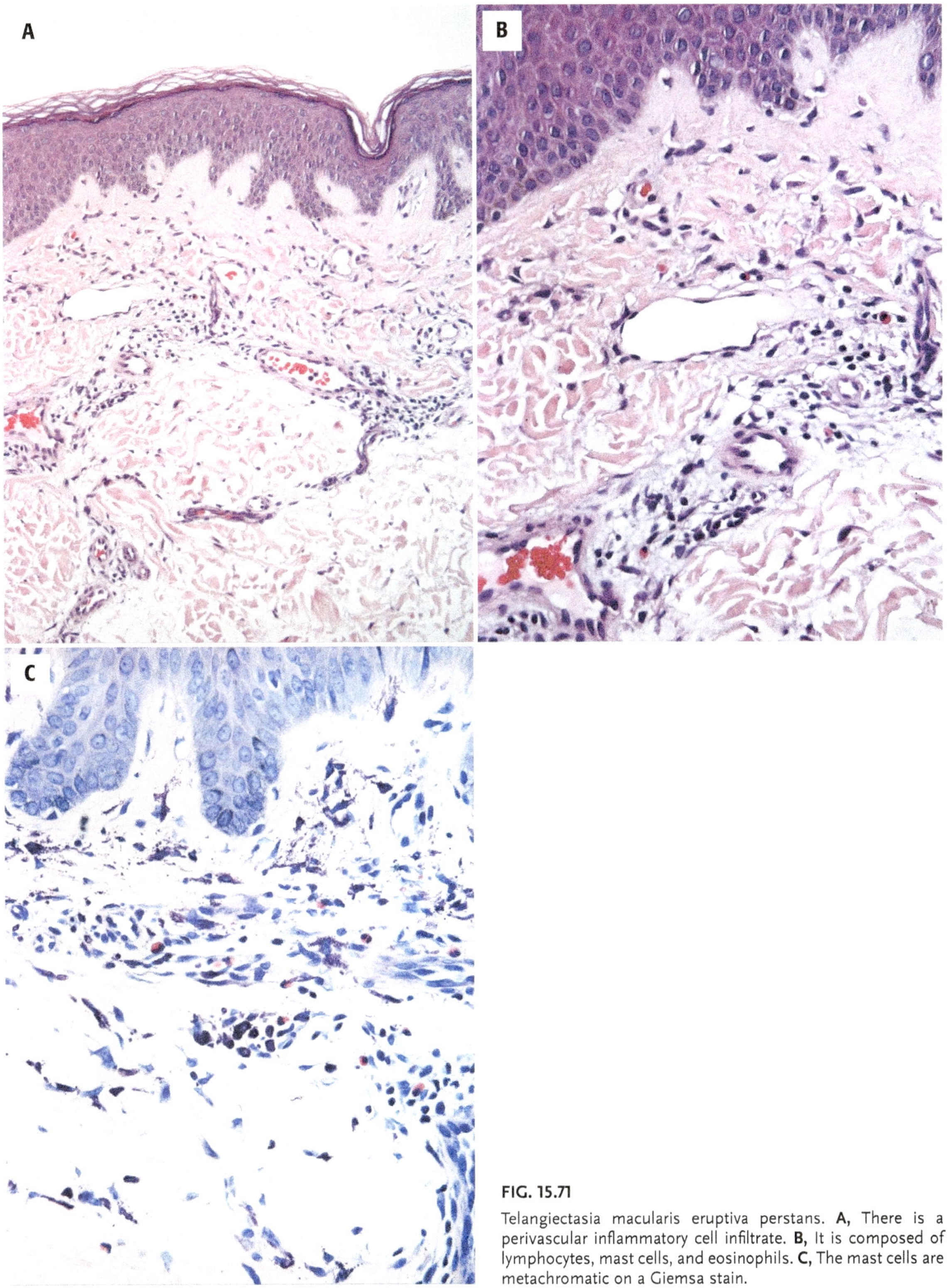

FIG. 15.71
Telangiectasia macularis eruptiva perstans. **A,** There is a perivascular inflammatory cell infiltrate. **B,** It is composed of lymphocytes, mast cells, and eosinophils. **C,** The mast cells are metachromatic on a Giemsa stain.

Prognosis and Treatment

CM is most often diagnosed in children, in whom systemic disease is rarely seen, and the lesions usually self-resolve by adolescence. Lesions of mastocytosis may resolve with anetoderma. In adults, mast cell disease tends to persist and is more likely to progress to SM. Overall survival is rarely affected, except for the few patients with aggressive SM or SM associated with hematologic malignancies.

Treatment of CM is directed toward symptoms (e.g., pruritus). PUVA may provide benefit. Solitary persistent nodules and plaques may be excised.

ACKNOWLEDGMENT

This current chapter represents an updated version of the prior edition's chapter. The author and editors wish to thank Drs. Junkins-Hopkins and Myskowski for their prior contributions.

SUGGESTED FURTHER READING

Alaggio, R., Amador, C., Anagnostopoulos, I., Attygalle, A. D., Araujo, I. B. O., Berti, E., Bhagat, G., Borges, A. M., Boyer, D., Calaminici, M., Chadburn, A., Chan, J. K. C., Cheuk, W., Chng, W. J., Choi, J. K., Chuang, S. S., Coupland, S. E., Czader, M., Dave, S. S., de Jong, D., ... Xiao, W. (2022). The 5th edition of the World Health Organization classification of haematolymphoid tumours: Lymphoid neoplasms. *Leukemia*, *36*(7), 1720–1748. doi:10.1038/s41375-022-01620-2. Erratum in: Leukemia, 37(9), 1944–1951, 2023.

Dummer, R., Vermeer, M. H., Scarisbrick, J. J., Kim, Y. H., Stonesifer, C., Tensen, C. P., Geskin, L. J., Quaglino, P., & Ramelyte, E. (2021). Cutaneous T cell lymphoma. *Nature Reviews. Disease Primers*, *7*(1), 61. doi:10.1038/s41572-021-00296-9.

Goyal, A., LeBlanc, R. E., & Carter, J. B. (2019). Cutaneous B-cell lymphoma. *Hematology/Oncology Clinics of North America*, *33*(1), 149–161. doi:10.1016/j.hoc.2018.08.006.

Hague, C., Farquharson, N., Menasce, L., Parry, E., & Cowan, R. (2022). Cutaneous T-cell lymphoma: Diagnosing subtypes and the challenges. *British Journal of Hospital Medicine (London, England: 2005)*, *83*(4), 1–7. doi:10.12968/hmed.2021.0149.

Jawed, S. I., Myskowski, P. L., Horwitz, S., Moskowitz, A., & Querfeld, C. (2014). Primary cutaneous T-cell lymphoma (mycosis fungoides and Sézary syndrome): Part I. Diagnosis: Clinical and histopathologic features and new molecular and biologic markers. *Journal of the American Academy of Dermatology*, *70*, 205.e1–205.e16, 2014.

Jawed, S. I., Myskowski, P. L., Horwitz, S., Moskowitz, A., & Querfeld, C. (2014). Primary cutaneous T-cell lymphoma (mycosis fungoides and Sézary syndrome): Part II. Prognosis, management, and future directions. *Journal of the American Academy of Dermatology*, *70*, 223.e1–223.e17, 2014.

Kim, Y. H., Willemze, R., Pimpinelli, N., Whittaker, S., Olsen, E. A., Ranki, A., Dummer, R., Hoppe, R. T., & ISCL and the EORTC. (2007). TNM classification system for primary cutaneous lymphomas other than mycosis fungoides and Sézary syndrome: A proposal of the International Society for Cutaneous Lymphomas (ISCL) and the Cutaneous Lymphoma Task Force of the European Organization of Research and Treatment of Cancer (EORTC). *Blood*, *110*, 479–484, 2007.

Kinney, M. C., & Jones, D. (2007). Cutaneous T-cell and NK-cell lymphomas. The WHO-EORTC classification and the increasing recognition of specialized tumor types. *American Journal of Clinical Pathology*, *127*, 670–686.

Martinez-Cabriales, S. A., Walsh, S., Sade, S., & Shear, N. H. (2020). Lymphomatoid papulosis: An update and review. *Journal of the European Academy of Dermatology and Venereology*, *34*(1), 59–73. doi:10.1111/jdv.15931.

Mitteldorf, C., & Kempf, W. (2020). Cutaneous pseudolymphoma-a review on the spectrum and a proposal for a new classification. *Journal of Cutaneous Pathology*, *47*(1), 76–97. doi:10.1111/cup.13532.

Parsi, M., Go, M. S., & Ahmed, A. (2023). Leukemia Cutis. [Updated 2023 Jul 17]. In *StatPearls* [Internet]. Treasure Island, FL: StatPearls Publishing. https://www.ncbi.nlm.nih.gov/books/NBK541136/

Senff, N. J., Noordijk, E. M., Kim, Y. H., Bagot, M., Berti, E., Cerroni, L., Dummer, R., Duvic, M., Hoppe, R. T., Pimpinelli, N., Rosen, S. T., Vermeer, M. H., Whittaker, S., Willemze, R., European Organization for Research and Treatment of Cancer, & International Society for Cutaneous Lymphoma. (2008). European Organization for Research and Treatment of Cancer and International Society for Cutaneous Lymphoma consensus recommendations for the management of cutaneous B-cell lymphomas. *Blood*, *112*, 1600–1609, 2008.

Suárez, A. L., Pulitzer, M., Horwitz, S., Moskowitz, A., Querfeld, C., & Myskowski, P. L. (2013). Primary cutaneous B-cell lymphomas: Part I. Clinical features, diagnosis, and classification. *Journal of the American Academy of Dermatology*, *69*, 329.e1–329.e13, 2013.

Sukswai, N., Lyapichev, K., Khoury, J. D., & Medeiros, L. J. (2020). Diffuse large B-cell lymphoma variants: An update. *Pathology*, *52*(1), 53–67. doi:10.1016/j.pathol.2019.08.013.

Valent, P., Akin, C., Hartmann, K., Alvarez-Twose, I., Brockow, K., Hermine, O., Niedoszytko, M., Schwaab, J., Lyons, J. J., Carter, M. C., Elberink, H. O., Butterfield, J. H., George, T. I., Greiner, G., Ustun, C., Bonadonna, P., Sotlar, K., Nilsson, G., Jawhar, M., Siebenhaar, F., ... Metcalfe, D. D. (2021). Updated diagnostic criteria and classification of mast cell disorders: A consensus proposal. *Hemasphere*, *5*(11), e646. doi:10.1097/HS9.0000000000000646.

Willemze, R., Cerroni, L., Kempf, W., Berti, E., Facchetti, F., Swerdlow, S. H., & Jaffe, E. S. (2019). The 2018 update of the WHO-EORTC classification for primary cutaneous lymphomas. *Blood*, *133*(16), 1703–1714. doi:10.1182/blood-2018-11-881268. Erratum in: Blood, 134(13):1112, 2019.

Histiocytoses 16

Melissa P. Pulitzer • Bijal Amin • Klaus J. Busam

DEFINITION OF TERMS

The term *histiocyte* (literally translated from Greek as "tissue cell") was used by Aschoff and Kiyono to designate mononuclear phagocytes. The mononuclear phagocyte system includes dendritic cells (DCs), monocytes, and macrophages. The term histiocyte is nowadays generally used as a morphologic term referring to tissue-resident macrophages.

Macrophages are involved in the clearance of pathogens and cellular debris. They are usually oval-shaped. The cytoplasm may vary from foamy to eosinophilic to ground glass. There may be multinucleated giant cells of the Touton type (ring of nuclei with peripheral lipid accumulation and an eosinophilic center) or foreign body type (multiple haphazardly arranged nuclei).

DCs play a role in antigen presentation and the activation of T cells. Microscopically they have a star-like appearance with several thin cytoplasmic projections. DCs are subclassified into plasmacytoid and myeloid DCs.

Histiocytoses comprise a spectrum of neoplastic proliferations of DCs or macrophages. Historically, histiocytic infiltrates affecting the skin have been divided as Langerhans cell (LHC) (DC) versus non-LHC (macrophage) histiocytosis (LCH). The largest group of non-LCH is the xanthogranuloma family, which includes benign cephalic histiocytosis, juvenile xanthogranuloma (JXG), xanthoma disseminatum (XD), generalized eruptive histiocytosis (GEH), and progressive nodular histiocytosis. Other non-LCH include multicentric reticulohistiocytosis (MRH), reticulohistiocytoma, and cutaneous Rosai-Dorfman disease (RDD).

The contemporary classification of histiocytoses takes into account not only the phenotype of the tumor cells and clinical context but also molecular findings.

HISTIOCYTOSES—CLASSIFICATION

- L Group
  - LCH
  - ICH
  - ECD
  - Mixed LCH/ECD
- C Group
  - Cutaneous non-LCH
  - XG family (AXG, JXG, GEH, other)
  - Non-XG family (cutaneous RDD, NXG, other)
  - Cutaneous non-LCH with systemic involvement
- R Group[a]
  - Familial RDD
  - Sporadic RDD
- H Group[a]
  - Primary HLH
  - Secondary HLH
  - HLH of unknown origin
- M Group[a]
  - Primary malignant histiocytosis
  - Secondary malignant histiocytosis

[a]HLH, malignant histiocytoses, and extracutaneous RDD are not further discussed in this chapter.

AXG, Adult xanthogranuloma; *ECD*, Erdheim-Chester disease; *GEH*, generalized eruptive histiocytosis; *HLH*, hemophagocytic lymphohistiocytosis; *ICD*, indeterminate cell histiocytosis; *JXG*, Juvenile xanthogranuloma; *LCH*, Langerhans cell histiocytosis; *NXG*, necrobiotic xanthogranuloma; *RDD*, Rosai-Dorfman disease; *XG*, Xanthogranuloma.

Adapted and modified from Emile, J. F., Abla, O., Fraitag, S., Horne, A., Haroche, J., Donadieu, J., Requena-Caballero, L., Jordan, M. B., Abdel-Wahab, O., Allen, C. E., Charlotte, F., Diamond, E. L., Egeler, R. M., Fischer, A., Herrera, J. G., Henter, J. I., Janku, F., Merad, M., Picarsic, J., Rodriguez-Galindo, C., ... Histiocyte Society (2016). Revised classification of histiocytoses and neoplasms of the macrophage-dendritic cell lineages. *Blood*, 127, 2672–2681.

L GROUP HISTIOCYTOSES

LANGERHANS CELL HISTIOCYTOSIS

Langerhans cells (LHCs) are antigen-presenting cells. Langerhans cell histiocytosis (LCH) refers to a clonal neoplastic disease of LHC. LHC hyperplasia is a non-neoplastic reactive proliferation of LHC, which may be seen in infectious or allergic reactions or scabies and can be confused with LCH. The incidence of LCH is approximately 5 to 10 cases per 1 million children and 1 to 2 cases per 1 million adults.

Clinical Findings

Characteristic clinical manifestations include lytic bone lesions, skin rash, ear drainage, soft tissue and lymph node swelling, and gum hypertrophy. Severe systemic disease may lead to cytopenias, hepatosplenomegaly, and decreased liver function, with associated higher risk for

CLINICAL SPECTRUM OF LANGERHANS CELL HISTIOCYTOSIS

Letterer-Siwe Disease
- Typically young children
- Disseminated disease
- Cutaneous lesions common; may clinically simulate seborrheic dermatitis

Hand-Schüller-Christian Disease
- Triad of lytic skull lesion, hypopituitarism, and diabetes insipidus
- Cutaneous lesions in approximately one-third of patients

Eosinophilic Granuloma
- Isolated granulomas, often in lung
- Rare cutaneous involvement

Miscellaneous Nonclassic Variants
- Isolated or clustered cutaneous papules at any age

mortality. The clinical manifestations of LCH have historically been described as four separate disease entities. However, it is now recognized that each of these entities represents a clinical variant within a spectrum of findings found in this one disease process. It has been proposed to replace the historical nomenclature with an attribution of extent of disease, such as low-risk single or multisystem disease versus high-risk multisystem disease.

LETTERER-SIWE DISEASE

Letterer-Siwe disease represents a disseminated form of Langerhans cell disease (LCD) that usually affects children in the first year of life, but it can be seen in any age, including adults. There are pinkish-yellow to red-brown coalescent scaly papules, plaques, and patches over seborrheic areas, including the scalp, groin, nasolabial folds, perioral area, and upper trunk. Less commonly, there are pustules, petechiae, erosions, or ulcerated nodules. The skin lesions are accompanied by systemic symptoms of fever, lymphadenopathy, weight loss, pancytopenia, and hepatosplenomegaly.

HAND-SCHÜLLER-CHRISTIAN DISEASE

Hand-Schüller-Christian disease is more common in older children. The characteristic triad of features includes osteolytic skull lesions, hypopituitarism with diabetes insipidus, and exophthalmos. Skin lesions are seen in approximately one-third of cases; there are papules and nodules, possibly eroded or ulcerated, in the intertriginous areas.

EOSINOPHILIC GRANULOMA

This form of LCD is more common in older children and adults and is characterized by bone lesions; skin involvement is rare.

CONGENITAL SELF-HEALING RETICULOHISTIOCYTOSIS (HASHIMOTO-PRITZKER)

This rare form is seen at birth or in neonates. Solitary or multiple papules, vesicles, or nodules, possibly ulcerated, are located on the head, trunk, palms, and soles. There is usually spontaneous resolution over weeks to months, possibly leaving behind areas of hyperpigmentation or hypopigmentation. However, congenital selfhealing reticulohistiocytosis (CSHR) may progress toward a Letterer-Siwe clinical picture.

Many clinical presentations do not neatly fit into any of the "classic" variants of LCD, such as limited localized maculopapular cutaneous disease (Fig. 16.1).

Histopathologic Features

The common histologic feature is the accumulation of cells with abundant amphophilic or eosinophilic cytoplasm and large, vesicular folded, lobulated, or reniform nuclei without prominent nucleoli in the papillary dermis and epidermis (Fig. 16.2) and, in nodular forms, in the reticular dermis. There are often accompanying nonhistiocytic inflammatory cells, including lymphocytes, eosinophils, and neutrophils. Occasionally, a more granulomatous pattern with occasional xanthomatous cells and multinucleated giant cells may be seen.

Ancillary Studies

Immunohistochemistry is important for the correct diagnosis of LCH. LHCs are immunoreactive for CD1a, S100, and Langerin (CD207) (Fig. 16.3). They are also positive for CD43 and CD4. They are negative for CD68.

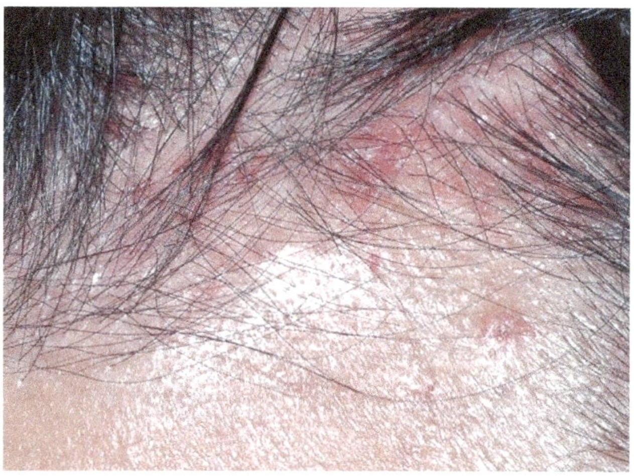

FIG. 16.1
Cutaneous Langerhans cell disease manifesting as erythematous macules and papules.

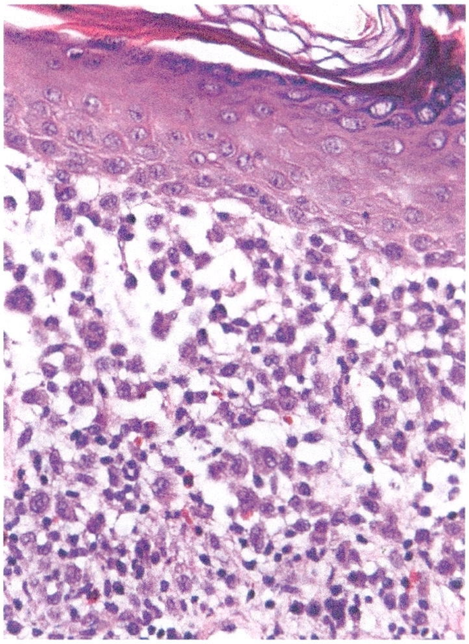

FIG. 16.2
Cutaneous Langerhans cell disease. Dense infiltrate of mononuclear cells with reniform nuclei in dermis and epidermis.

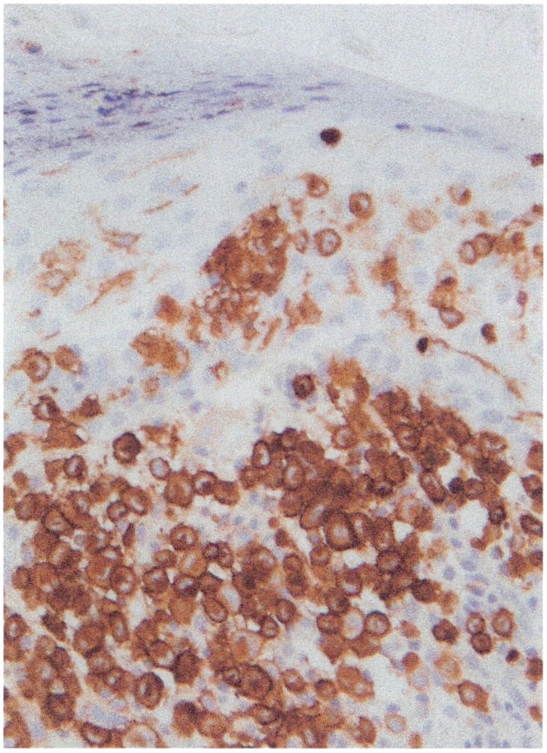

FIG. 16.3
The mononuclear Langerhans cells in the dermis and epidermis are immunopositive for CD1a.

Electron microscopy demonstrates characteristic racquet-shaped or rocket-shaped Birbeck granules (Fig. 16.4). Lesions of CSHR can also show myelinoid laminated inclusions, known as vermiform bodies. Electron microscopy is no longer needed for the contemporary diagnosis of LCH.

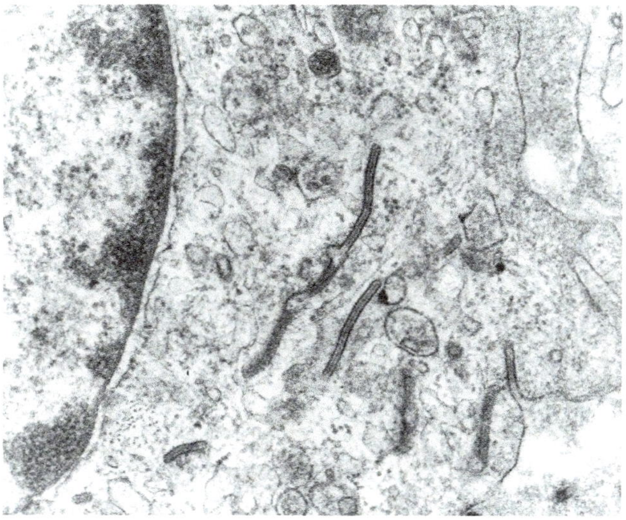

FIG. 16.4
Ultrastructure of Langerhans cells—Birbeck granules (racquet-shaped organelles) are present.

Immunohistochemistry using the monoclonal antibody VE1 can help document the presence or absence of the mutant BRAFV600E protein. This may facilitate selection of patients with symptomatic systemic disease for treatment with vemurafenib. Immunoreactivity may be weak (generally weaker than in metastatic melanoma cells carrying the same mutation).

Analysis by molecular methods, in particular next-generation sequence analysis, is currently the gold standard to determine the presence and type of an associated driver mutation. Activating mutations in the MAPK-ERG pathway genes are found in most cases of LCH. *BRAFV600E* mutations are detected in approximately 50% to 60%. Mutations in *MAP2K1* or rare other mutations in the MAPK pathway have also been reported. Mutations affecting other signaling pathways, such as *PIK3CA* or *PICK1*, have also been reported.

Differential Diagnosis

LHCs may be confused with non-Langerhans histiocytes or on occasion with a mast cell, immature or leukemic myeloid infiltrate, or even a melanocytic proliferation. Close attention to nuclear detail (reniform nucleus) is helpful. Immunostains allow for a ready distinction. While LHCs and LCH have distinct morphologic and immunophenotypic characteristics, some patients may have mixed or overlap histiocytosis, with some lesions displaying features of LCH and others displaying features of non-LHCs, such as in Erdheim-Chester disease (ECD) or in patients with RDD.

Langerhans Cell Histiocytosis Versus Xanthogranuloma

Reniform Nuclear Shape	Foamy Cytoplasm	Touton-type Giant Cells	Immunoprofile
LCH			
Common	Usually absent	Usually absent	+ S100P +CD1a +CD207 (Langerin)
XG			
Uncommon	Usually present	Usually present	−S100P −CD1a −CD207 +CD68

Reactive LHC hyperplasia may result from an allergic reaction, such as eczema, or a hypersensitivity reaction such as with scabies. The degree of LCH hyperplasia which may on occasion be florid, may be mistaken as LCH and lead to overtreatment. Whereas in LCH, there are typically dense clusters of LHCs, in reactive hyperplasia, LHCs tend to be more dispersed as solitary units, although there may be many of them in the dermis and epidermis admixed with lymphocytes and eosinophils. Molecular studies may be helpful in difficult cases. The detection of a driver mutation supports the diagnosis of LCH.

LCH also needs to be distinguished from Langerhans cell sarcoma. The latter is characterized by tumorous aggregates of cells with the immunophenotype of Langerhans cells displaying marked cytologic atypia.

Prognosis and Treatment

The disease course is variable and does not correlate with histopathology. Adverse prognostic features include age younger than 1 year (except in CSHR), organ dysfunction, and male gender. Complete remission occurs in 30%; the majority of patients have a chronic course. Systemic involvement may lead to severe morbidity and even death. Treatment strategies are related to the extent of disease. Patients with localized disease can be treated with simple excision, topical nitrogen mustard, oral thalidomide, or ultraviolet light therapy. A variety of chemotherapy agents, such as cladribine and cytarabine, steroids, and possibly bone marrow transplant, are used in cases of systemic disease. There is an emerging role for targeted therapy with BRAF and MEK inhibitors.

INDETERMINATE CELL HISTIOCYTOSIS

The term *indeterminate* is used for mononuclear cells, which share some, but not all, of the classic characteristics of LHCs. Similar to LHCs, they are immunoreactive for antibodies to CD1a and S100P but lack detectable Birbeck granules. It is postulated that the counterpart cell of this disorder is an immature LHC, that is, a DC before maturation in the lymph node.

Clinical Findings

This rare disorder occurs in both children and adults of each gender. It generally presents as a solitary, soft, erythematous, ulcerated nodule or as crops of firm, red-brown papules that develop over several months or years. Extracutaneous involvement has been documented.

Histopathologic Features

The dermis contains a well-circumscribed or diffuse infiltrate of histiocytes admixed with lymphocytic aggregates. The histiocytes have eosinophilic or granular cytoplasm.

Ancillary Studies

The histiocytes are immunoreactive for CD68, S100 protein, and factor XIIIa and weakly or focally positive for CD1a. They are negative for Langerin. No Birbeck granules are detectable by electron microscopy.

Differential Diagnosis

Other histiocytoses.

Prognosis and Treatment

Solitary lesions can be treated with simple excision. Multiple lesions are usually stable or only slowly progressive, and treatment is usually not necessary.

ERDHEIM-CHESTER DISEASE

Clinical Findings

ECD is a rare systemic histiocytosis with a mean age at diagnosis between 56 and 60 years of age. Morbidity is related to histiocytic infiltration of multiple organs. Sites that are commonly involved include bone, the CNS, cardiovascular system, lungs, retroperitoneum, and skin. More than 95% of patients have skeletal involvement. Bone pain is the most common first symptom of disease manifestation. Bilateral symmetric cortical osteosclerosis of the diaphyseal and metaphyseal regions of the long bones with increased uptake by scintigraphy is considered strongly suggestive of ECD. Xanthelasmas of the eyelid or periorbital region are the most common skin manifestation.

Histopathologic Features

The histopathologic spectrum of cutaneous lesions of ECD is variable. Most of them have the phenotype of a xanthelasma or xanthogranuloma. Some have the appearance of a fibrous histiocytoma. Some lesions manifest with the phenotype of a Langerhans cell histiocytoma.

Ancillary Studies

Depending on the phenotype, the cells may be immunoreactive for CD68 or display antigen expression of an LHC. Some patients have tumors with mixed LHC and non-LHC phenotypes.

Differential Diagnosis

Clinical context is essential for the correct diagnosis.

Prognosis and Treatment

The prognosis depends on the extent of and site of infiltration. CNS involvement is most problematic. Molecular analysis for a targetable driver mutation is important to assess treatment options. Many patients respond well to MEK kinase inhibitors.

C GROUP OF HISTIOCYTES

This group of histiocytoses is divided into xanthogranulomas and nonxanthogranulomatous families. The latter includes cutaneous RDD.

XANTHOGRANULOMA FAMILY

This family of histiocytic tumors includes JXG and adult xanthogranuloma (AXG) as well as miscellaneous other related neoplasms (benign cephalic histiocytosis, XD, generalized eruptive histiocytoma).

JUVENILE XANTHOGRANULOMA

Clinical Findings

JXG is the most common non-LHC histiocytosis. It is a normolipemic condition that presents congenitally in 15% to 30% of cases and within the first year of life in approximately 75% of cases. Identical lesions may also be seen in adults (AXG). Skin lesions are more often solitary but can be multiple, and they consist of well-demarcated, rubbery, reddish brown to yellow asymptomatic papules measuring 2 to 5 mm. They are located mostly on the upper body but have been documented in skin of all sites. Less commonly, there are shiny, translucent, red to yellow nodules, sometimes with telangiectasias, measuring 5 to 20 mm. Giant forms measuring greater than 20 mm in diameter have been reported. There is a male predominance, especially in cases with multiple skin lesions. Mucous membrane and extracutaneous involvement can occur, with or without accompanying skin lesions. The eye is the most common extracutaneous site; ocular lesions occur in 1% to 10%, are usually unilateral, and may precede skin lesions. Systemic involvement may occur, affecting the oropharynx, orbit, nasal and paranasal sinus areas, CNS, liver, spleen, lungs, bone marrow, testis, breast, or kidney. JXG may be associated with neurofibromatosis type I or with juvenile chronic myelogenous leukemia (JCML). Children with JXG and NF1 have a 20- to 30-fold higher risk of JCML.

Histopathologic Features

Early lesions demonstrate an unencapsulated, dense, monomorphic population of small- to intermediate-sized eosinophilic mononuclear cells in the papillary and reticular dermis (Fig. 16.5). Sometimes the nodular aggregate extends into, or occurs isolated within, the subcutaneous fat. Touton cells may not be evident in

JUVENILE XANTHOGRANULOMA—DISEASE FACT SHEET

- Most common form of non–Langerhans cell histiocytosis

Patient Group

- The majority of patients are infants or children
- May also present in adults (adult xanthogranuloma)

Site of Involvement

- Usually skin of upper part of body
- Eye
- Other (e.g., visceral, bone) sites may be involved

Clinical Findings

- Papular form (most common presentation)
  - Multiple small red, brown, or yellow papules
  - May be associated with neurofibromatosis and/or juvenile chronic myeloid leukemia.
- Nodular form (less common)
  - One or a few lesions (1- to 2-cm nodules)

Prognosis and Treatment

- Most lesions are selflimited and tend to disappear spontaneously
- Conservative excision for persistent lesions or for cosmetic reasons
- Rare cases with central nervous system involvement may be fatal

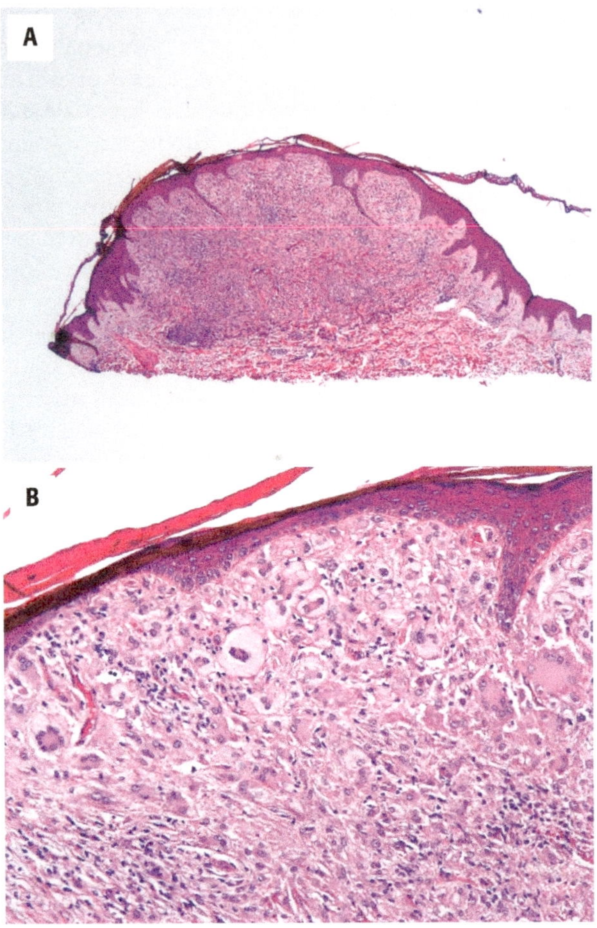

FIG. 16.5

Juvenile xanthogranuloma. **A,** Dermal infiltrate of mononuclear cells with eosinophilic or foamy cytoplasm. **B,** Touton-type giant cells are present.

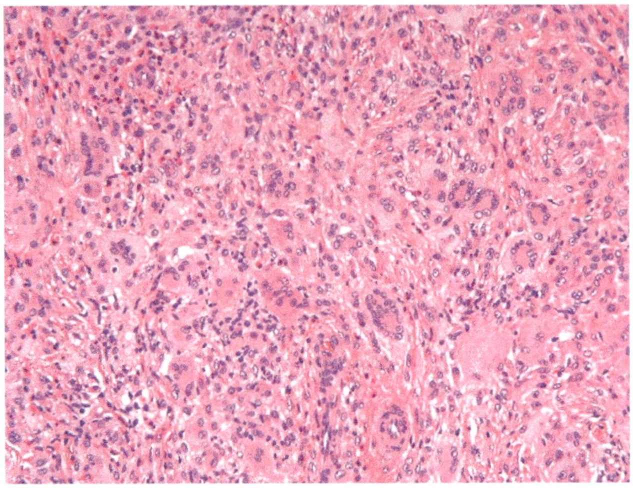

FIG. 16.6

Juvenile xanthogranuloma. Spindle and epithelioid cells with pink cytoplasm. Many eosinophils are present.

these early lesions. The nuclei are small, round, ovoid, or indented with inconspicuous nucleoli. In time, the cytoplasm becomes foamy, and multinucleation becomes more prominent. Both foreign body and Touton giant cells can be seen in variable numbers with or without an accompanying inflammatory infiltrate, usually lymphocytes and eosinophils (Fig. 16.6). Histiocytes may also become fusiform (Fig. 16.6). Mitotic figures can be seen. They are usually rare in older lesions but may readily be found in the superficial areas of early, nonlipidized lesions.

Ancillary Studies

The tumor cells of JXG demonstrate strong, granular, cytoplasmic staining for CD68 (Fig. 16.7). They are

JUVENILE XANTHOGRANULOMA—PATHOLOGIC FEATURES

Histopathologic Features

- Nodular dermal infiltrate of mononuclear cells
- Early lesions tend to show minimal lipidization (eosinophilic cytoplasm)
- Mature lesions contain histiocytes with foamy cytoplasm
- Touton-type giant cells are often seen
- Associated eosinophils are common

Ancillary Studies

- Immunopositive for CD68
- Immunonegative for CD1a
- Usually immunonegative for S100P

Differential Diagnosis

- Other histiocytoses (clinical correlation essential)
- Melanocytic tumors

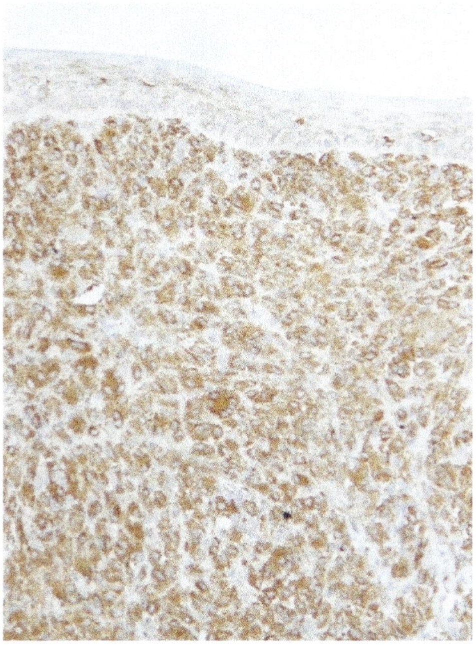

FIG. 16.7
Juvenile xanthogranuloma. The histiocytes are immunopositive for CD68.

frequently positive for HAM56 and CD4. There is often a subpopulation of cells positive for factor XIIIa. JXG is negative for CD1a. It usually is immunonegative for S100 protein, but staining for this marker may be seen occasionally.

Differential Diagnosis

JXG can be confused with melanocytic nevi or melanoma as well as other histiocytic proliferations. Confusion with melanocytic tumors is most likely with lesions lacking foamy or Touton-type giant cells. The presence of eosinophils may still provide a clue to a histiocytic rather than melanocytic tumor, although eosinophils may be less prominent in older lesions. Immunostains usually allow for a ready distinction. JXG is negative for the melanocyte differentiation antigens Melan-A/Mart-1 and tyrosinase. Differentiating JXG from a xanthomatized dermatofibroma may occasionally be difficult because Touton-type giant cells and even eosinophils may be seen in either entity. In these cases, the presence of peripheral "ropy" collagen fibers entrapped by stellate and triangular DCs may favor the latter diagnosis. CD4 positivity favors a diagnosis of JXG.

Prognosis and Treatment

Cutaneous lesions in children typically regress over a period of 3 to 6 years. Lesions in adults more often persist. Solitary lesions may be treated with simple excision or laser therapy. Recurrence of an excised lesion is frequent. Systemic disease is more difficult to treat, especially CNS involvement. Disseminated JXG is treated with various combinations of surgery, radiation, and chemotherapy protocols similar to those used for LHC histiocytosis. High-grade sarcomatous transformation and fatalities have been reported. Monitoring for JCML and ophthalmic evaluation in children younger than 2 years of age with multiple lesions is advised.

BENIGN CEPHALIC HISTIOCYTOSIS

Many consider benign cephalic histiocytosis to be an early form of JXG. The disease typically affects young children, usually between 2 and 34 months of age, and presents as multiple 2- to 3-mm reddish brown to yellow macules and papules on the head and upper body without systemic involvement. Usually there are few lesions, but uncommonly there can be hundreds. Rarely, it is associated with diabetes insipidus. Histologically the lesions are indistinguishable from JXG. The disease is generally selflimited and requires no treatment.

GENERALIZED ERUPTIVE HISTIOCYTOSIS

GEH is a rare disorder of normolipemic adults and children that presents as crops of numerous, diffuse, symmetric red-blue papules on the trunk and proximal extremities, sparing the flexural areas that eventually spontaneously involute. Mucous membrane involvement is less common than in XD. The histology is similar to JXG. The lesions are usually selflimited and do not require treatment.

XANTHOMA DISSEMINATUM

Clinical Findings

XD is a rare disorder that may affect children and adults. Numerous, symmetric reddish yellow or brown papules and nodules are found involving skin folds and on flexor areas of the head and upper body. They are initially discrete but over time coalesce into verrucous plaques. Lesions may resolve or persist. Mucosal and extracutaneous lesions are not uncommon, such as lesions of bone or the CNS. Involvement of the latter may lead to diabetes insipidus. Lipid levels are usually normal in these patients. There may be an associated monoclonal gammopathy.

Histopathologic Features

Typically, there is a nodular proliferation of histiocytes with round to oval nuclei and eosinophilic cytoplasm (Fig. 16.8). The histiocytes may have scalloped borders. With time, more foamy histiocytes and Touton-type giant cells appear.

Ancillary Studies

The histiocytes of XD are negative for CD1a but positive for CD68.

Differential Diagnosis

Clinical correlation is essential. Histologically, lesions of XD may be indistinguishable from lesions of xanthoma or xanthogranuloma. They can be distinguished from LCD morphologically and by immunohistochemistry.

Prognosis and Treatment

The prognosis depends on the extent and anatomic site of extracutaneous disease. Isolated skin lesions may be treated by locally destructive therapy.

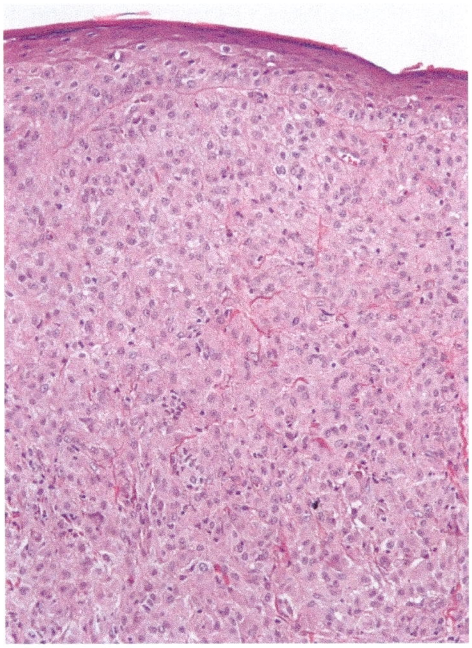

FIG. 16.8

Xanthoma disseminatum. Infiltrate of mononuclear cells with eosinophilic cytoplasm (indistinguishable from lesions of juvenile xanthogranuloma).

RETICULOHISTIOCYTOSIS (SOLITARY GIANT CELL RETICULOHISTIOCYTOMA AND MULTICENTRIC RETICULOHISTIOCYTOSIS)

Clinical Findings

Reticulohistiocytoma usually presents as an isolated red to yellow papule in the absence of other associated disease. Multiple lesions may also occur in the absence of systemic symptoms. MRH is a rare disease characterized by the presence of multiple cutaneous and mucous membrane lesions associated with arthropathy. Middle-aged white women are typically affected. The disease may on occasion represent a paraneoplastic process.

Histopathologic Features

There is a dense nodular aggregate of large multinucleated histiocytes with abundant eosinophilic, finely granular ground-glass cytoplasm (Fig. 16.9) containing diastase-resistant periodic acid-Schiff–positive material. The cytoplasm may be vacuolated or foamy. The nuclei are vesicular with distinct nuclear membranes and one to two prominent nucleoli. Other inflammatory cells, such as lymphocytes and eosinophils, may be present. Phagocytosis of collagen may be seen.

Ancillary Studies

The histiocytes are positive for CD68 and negative for CD1a and factor XIIIa. S100 is generally negative; however, S100-positive cases have been reported.

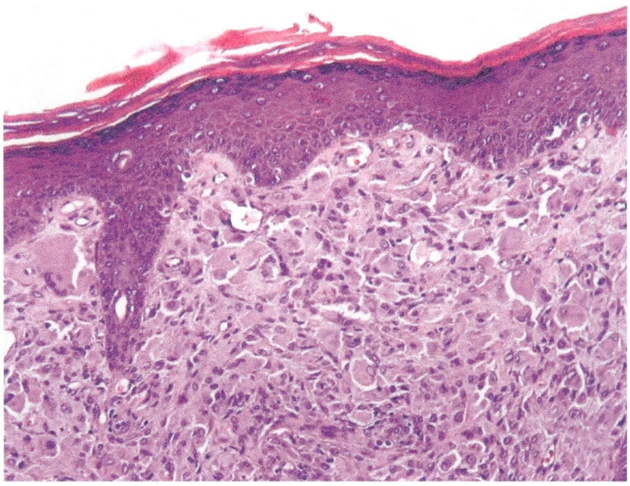

FIG. 16.9

Reticulohistiocytoma. Large histiocytes with abundant eosinophilic ground-glass cytoplasm.

Differential Diagnosis

A solitary lesion of reticulohistiocytoma may be confused with another histiocytic proliferation or a Spitz's nevus. Immunohistochemistry for melanocyte differentiation antigens should allow for a clear distinction from a melanocytic proliferation.

Prognosis and Treatment

Solitary lesions do not require therapy. For multicentric disease, treatment is primarily directed toward associated symptoms (arthropathy) and, if present, associated underlying malignancy. The cutaneous findings typically wax and wane. Spontaneous remission may occur.

CUTANEOUS ROSAI-DORFMAN DISEASE

It has been proposed to separate cutaneous RDD from classic RDD because of notable clinical and epidemiologic differences as well as molecular findings.

Clinical Findings

Classic RDD presents with lymphadenopathy, fever, and malaise. Patients are usually children and young adults; the mean age is approximately 20 years. It occurs more commonly in African patients with a slight male predominance. Anemia, leukocytosis, hypergammaglobulinemia, and an elevated erythrocyte sedimentation rate are frequently found. Extranodal disease occurs in approximately 40% of patients and can involve any organ. The skin is the most common extranodal site of the disease. "Primary" cutaneous RDD usually presents in adults (third and fourth decades of life). Women are twice as likely to be affected as men. It affects a higher proportion of Asians and fair-skinned individuals. They usually lack extracutaneous disease. Individual skin lesions may manifest as yellow to erythematous or brown papules, nodules, or plaques (Fig. 16.10), varying in size from less than 1 cm to 30 cm in diameter, and can be present on skin in any area.

Histopathologic Features

Cutaneous RDD usually manifests as a dense nodular lymphogranulomatous inflammatory process (Fig. 16.11). The histiocytes have abundant pale eosinophilic, or occasionally foamy, cytoplasm; indistinct cell borders; and large, vesicular nuclei with delicate nuclear membranes and a single prominent nucleolus. Multinucleation, atypia, and mitotic figures are not often seen. Emperipolesis, the presence of one or more intact leukocytes within histiocytes, is often cited as a hallmark feature of this disease but is not specific (can also be seen in lymphoma) and may not be prominent. Plasma cells are frequently present and clustered around postcapillary venules.

CUTANEOUS ROSAI-DORFMAN DISEASE—DISEASE FACT SHEET

Patient Group
- Adults with a mean age of 44 years
- Women to men = 2 : 1

Site of Involvement
- Skin of head and neck and extremities

Clinical Findings
- Skin lesions present as papules, nodules, or plaques

Prognosis and Treatment
- Usually selflimited with benign clinical course
- May regress spontaneously
- Persistent lesions can be removed surgically if symptomatic or for cosmetic reasons

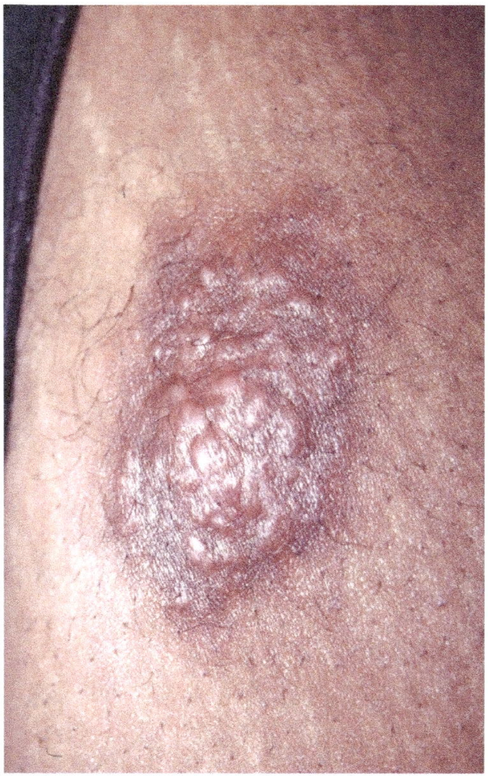

FIG. 16.10
Rosai-Dorfman disease. Brown plaque.

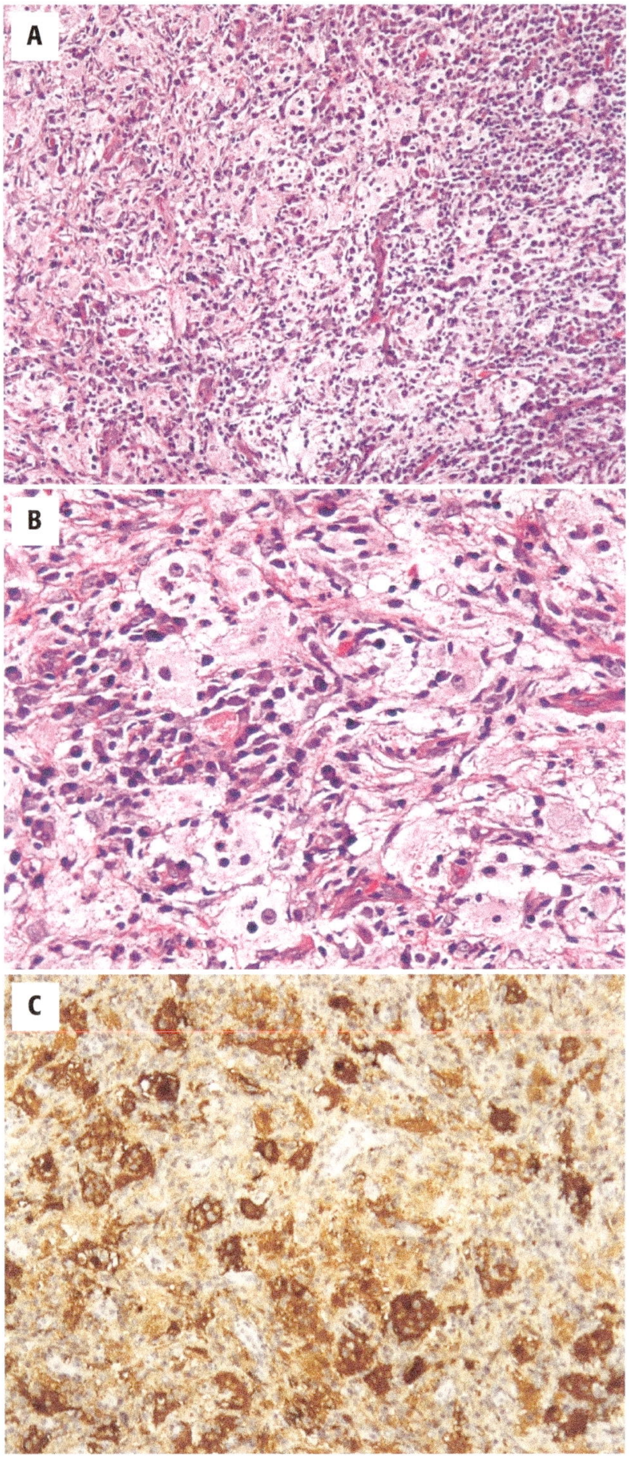

FIG. 16.11
Rosai-Dorfman disease. **A,** Xanthogranulomatous and lymphoplasma cellular infiltrate with large foamy histiocytes. **B,** Inflammatory cells are seen within the abundant cytoplasm of the histiocytes. **C,** The large histiocytes are positive for S100 protein.

Ancillary Studies

At least a subpopulation of the histiocytic infiltrate is positive for S100 protein. A subset of lesions of classic RDD has been found to be associated with various kinase mutations. Cutaneous RDD usually lacks detectable mutations.

Differential Diagnosis

The lesions need to be distinguished from an identifiable infection by cultures and special stains. At times, especially if the biopsy sample lacks a significant number of S100P-positive histiocytes, a definitive diagnosis may not be possible, and a diagnostic evaluation may need to be performed to exclude miscellaneous granulomatous processes, including a granulomatous lymphoma.

Prognosis and Treatment

Purely cutaneous RDD is generally selflimited and does not progress to classic RDD. Varying treatment modalities, including surgery, steroids, and radiation, have been tried, with variable success. In general, smaller lesions are more responsive to therapy.

HYPERLIPIDEMIA-ASSOCIATED XANTHOMA

Clinical Findings

Tuberous xanthomas are seen as yellow-red coalescent, soft papules, and firm nodules, most commonly on extensor surfaces, such as elbows, knees, knuckles, buttocks, and palms, manifesting with hypercholesterolemia, dyslipoproteinemia, and hypertriglyceridemia. Tendinous xanthomas manifest as deep-seated, freely mobile, firm nodules covered by normal-appearing skin. They typically affect the extensor

ROSAI-DORFMAN DISEASE—PATHOLOGIC FEATURES

Histopathologic Features

- Xanthogranulomatous infiltrate
- Associated plasma cells, lymphocytes, neutrophils
- Emperipolesis (leukocytes within cytoplasm of macrophages)

Ancillary Studies

- Immunopositive for CD68 and S100P (at least in a significant subpopulation of histiocytes)
- Polyclonal lymphocytic infiltrate
- Negative on special stains for microorganisms

Differential Diagnosis

- Infection
- Lymphoma

tendons of the hand and feet and the Achilles tendon, ligaments, and fascia, usually in the setting of hypercholesterolemia. Xanthelasma occurs on the eyelids idiopathically or in patients with hypercholesterolemia or dyslipoproteinemia; the incidence of elevated cholesterol is higher in young patients. Eruptive xanthomas manifest as many small papules that appear suddenly in crops over multiple areas of the body in patients with lipoprotein lipase deficiency, dyslipoproteinemia, hypertriglyceridemia, and diabetes mellitus.

Histopathologic Features

Tuberous xanthomas, tendinous xanthomas, and xanthelasma have similar findings, including nodules and small clusters of foamy macrophages between collagen bundles without or with only very few accompanying inflammatory cells (Fig. 16.12). Eruptive xanthomas tend to have fewer foamy cells and more of an accompanying inflammatory infiltrate, including lymphocytes, neutrophils, and macrophages. They are characterized by the presence of intracellular and extracellular lipid. Some may have a palisaded granulomatous appearance.

Prognosis and Treatment

These are benign lesions. Their diagnosis should prompt an evaluation for underlying hyperlipidemia or diabetes. Tuberous xanthomas sometimes resolve with treatment of underlying hyperlipidemias.

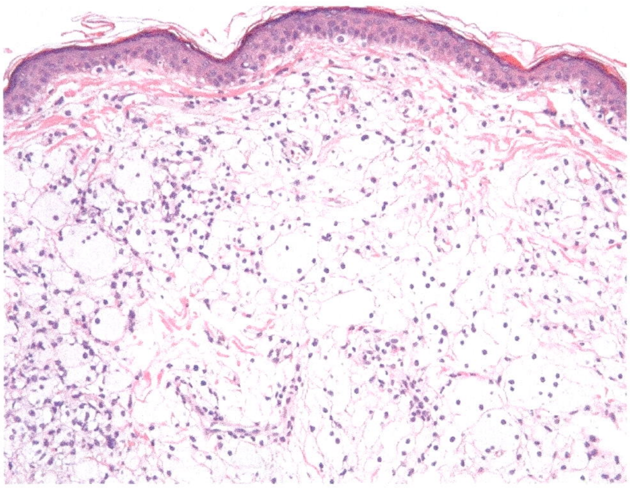

FIG. 16.12

Xanthoma. Nodular compact aggregate of foamy mononuclear cells. A few lymphocytes are also seen.

XANTHOMA NOT ASSOCIATED WITH HYPERLIPIDEMIA

Xanthomatous infiltrates may lead to papular skin lesions in normolipemic, otherwise healthy individuals. The spectrum of lesions includes solitary papular xanthoma or xanthelasma and verruciform xanthoma.

Papular xanthomas present as isolated sporadic yellowish papules. Xanthomatous papules or plaques affecting the eyelid are generally referred to as xanthelasma. In individuals with no lipid abnormalities, they may be sporadic or familial and commonly affect people of Asian or Mediterranean origin. They are histopathologically similar to xanthomas at other sites but often of lower cell density. Xanthomas and xanthelasmas usually contain mostly foamy mononuclear cells and few Touton giant cells. There may be associated lymphocytes. Verruciform xanthoma primarily affects the oral mucosa (Fig. 16.13). The histopathology of verruciform xanthoma is characterized by verruciform hyperplasia of the squamous mucosa with parakeratosis and a xanthomatous infiltrate filling the papillary stroma (Fig. 16.14).

Clinical correlation is needed to distinguish an isolated xanthoma from one related to hyperlipidemia. Verruciform xanthoma has a distinctive constellation of clinical and histologic findings (location in oral mucosa, associated with verrucous epithelial hyperplasia). The lesions may spontaneously regress or persist. Small lesions are often completely removed by the biopsy procedure.

DIFFUSE NORMOLIPEMIC PLANE XANTHOMA

Synonyms include generalized plane xanthoma and normolipemic plane xanthoma.

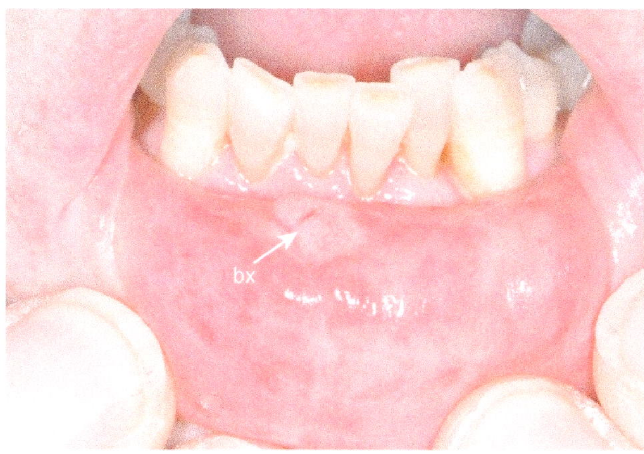

FIG. 16.13

Verruciform xanthoma. Verrucous plaque on oral mucosa.

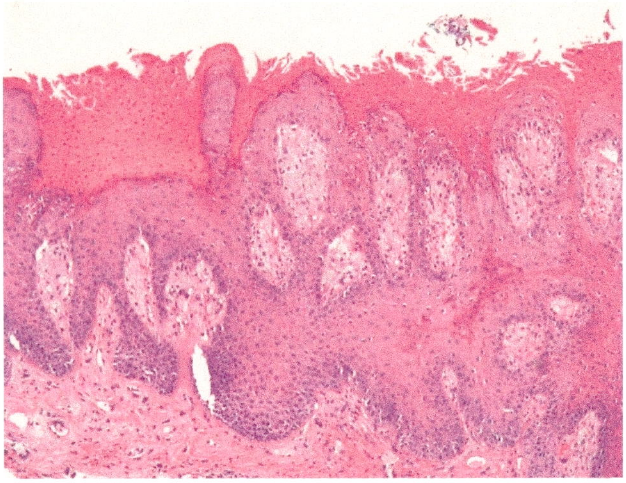

FIG. 16.14
Verruciform xanthoma. Verruciform epithelial hyperplasia with parakeratosis and xanthomatous infiltrate in papillary stroma.

These lesions are thought to be mediated by perivascular immunoglobulin deposition, as may be seen with certain systemic diseases.

Clinical Findings

Yellow to orange macules, papules, plaques, and nodules are present in the periorbital area, neck, trunk, and extremities of normolipemic patients (Fig. 16.15). Xanthelasma is usually also present. There is frequently, but not always, an association with systemic disease, most often a plasma cell neoplasm, monoclonal paraproteinemia, leukemia, or lymphoma. An association with cryoglobulinemia, erythrodermas, and many other conditions has also been described.

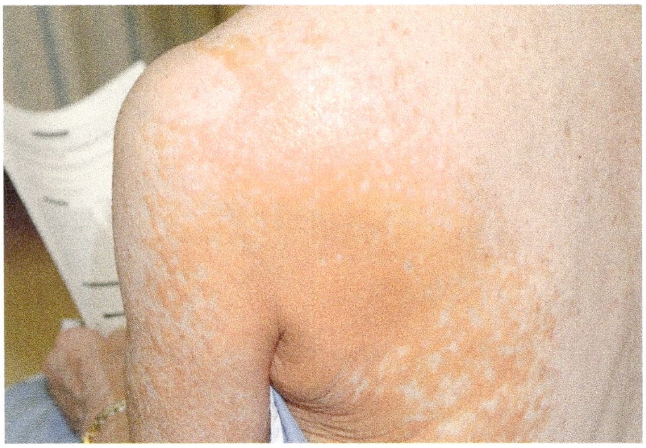

FIG. 16.15
Diffuse plane xanthomas. Multiple orange papules are present; some coalesce.

Skin lesions may precede these conditions by several years.

Histopathologic Features

There is perivascular deposition of foamy macrophages and Touton giant cells within the dermis and possibly extending into the subcutaneous tissue. Small foci of necrobiosis (degeneration or alteration of collagen) can be present.

Ancillary Studies

The foamy cells are positive for CD68 and factor XIIIa and negative for S100, CD1a, and MAC387.

Differential Diagnosis

Clinical correlation is needed to distinguish plane from other xanthomas. Plane xanthomas with focal necrosis may be difficult or impossible to distinguish from necrobiotic xanthogranuloma (NXG).

Prognosis and Treatment

The prognosis depends primarily on the nature of an associated lymphoproliferative process.

NECROBIOTIC XANTHOGRANULOMA

Clinical Findings

NXG typically affects elderly adults. There are usually multiple reddish-yellow papules, nodules, or plaques. They may be located in the periorbital area, extremities, or trunk. NXG has a strong association with paraproteinemia, usually IgG monoclonal gammopathy, and cryoglobulinemia.

Histopathologic Features

There are areas of necrobiosis (altered, dissolved-appearing collagen, with cellular debris) surrounded by granulomas (Fig. 16.16). Cholesterol clefts and Touton giant cells are often identified. Bizarre foreign body giant cells or giant cell asteroid bodies may be seen.

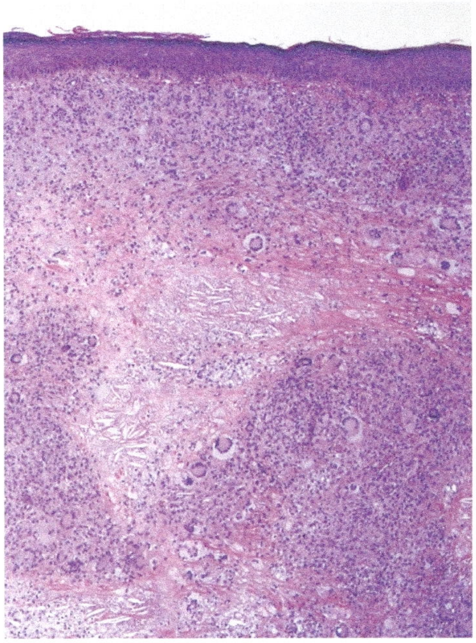

FIG. 16.16
Necrobiotic xanthogranuloma. An infiltrate of mononuclear histiocytes and Touton-type giant cells surrounds areas of necrobiosis with cholesterol clefts.

Ancillary Studies

The histiocytes are positive for CD68 and negative for S100 and CD1a. The histiocytes of ECD may harbor the BRAFV600E mutation.

Differential Diagnosis

NXG shows overlap with diffuse normolipemic plane xanthoma clinically and histologically. It needs to be distinguished from a granulomatous infectious process, granuloma annulare, and necrobiosis lipoidica.

Prognosis and Treatment

The lesions are chronic and can progress. Steroids and cytotoxic therapies have been tried with variable and limited success.

MALIGNANT HISTIOCYTIC NEOPLASMS

There are several rare malignant and usually aggressive neoplasms that include Langerhans cell sarcoma, histiocytic sarcoma, and hemophagocytic lymphohistiocytosis (HLH). In Langerhans cell sarcoma, Langerhans cells have pleomorphic nuclei and mitoses. HLH predominantly affects children. Many of them develop skin findings, typically characterized by a maculopapular rash. Due to the rarity of these disorders and limited scope of this textbook, the reader is referred to more specialized literature for more details.

SUGGESTED FURTHER READING

Abla, O., Jacobsen, E., Picarsic, J., Krenova, Z., Jaffe, R., Emile, J. F., Durham, B. H., Braier, J., Charlotte, F., Donadieu, J., Cohen-Aubart, F., Rodriguez-Galindo, C., Allen, C., Whitlock, J. A., Weitzman, S., McClain, K. L., Haroche, J., & Diamond, E. L. (2018). Consensus recommendations for the diagnosis and clinical management of Rosai-Dorfman-Destombes disease. *Blood*, *131*, 2877–2890.

Caputo, R., Marzano, A. V., Passoni, E., & Berti, E. (2007). Unusual variants of non-Langerhans cell histiocytoses. *Journal of the American Academy of Dermatology*, *57*(6), 1031–1035.

Emile, J. F., Abla, O., Fraitag, S., Horne, A., Haroche, J., Donadieu, J., Requena-Caballero, L., Jordan, M. B., Abdel-Wahab, O., Allen, C. E., Charlotte, F., Diamond, E. L., Egeler, R. M., Fischer, A., Herrera, J. G., Henter, J. I., Janku, F., Merad, M., Picarsic, J., Rodriguez-Galindo, C., ... Histiocyte Society. (2016). Histiocyte Society. Revised classification of histiocytoses and neoplasms of the macrophage-dendritic cell lineages. *Blood*, *127*, 2672–2681.

Khoury, J. D., Solary, E., Abla, O., Akkari, Y., Alaggio, R., Apperley, J. F., Bejar, R., Berti, E., Busque, L., Chan, J. K. C., Chen, W., Chen, X., Chng, W. J., Choi, J. K., Colmenero, I., Coupland, S. E., Cross, N. C. P., De Jong, D., Elghetany, M. T., Takahashi, E., ... Hochhaus, A. (2022). The 5th edition of the World Health Organization Classification of haematolymphoid tumours: Myeloid and histiocytic/dendritic neoplasms. *Leukemia*, *36*(7), 1703–1719.

Magro, C. M., Kazi, N., & Sisinger, A. E. (2018). Primary cutaneous histiocytic sarcoma: A report of five cases with primary cutaneous involvement and review of the literature. *Annals of Diagnostic Pathology*, *32*, 56–62.

Ozkaya, N., Rosenblum, M. K., Durham, B. H., Pichardo, J. D., Abdel-Wahab, O., Hameed, M. R., Busam, K. J., Travis, W. D., Diamond, E. L., & Dogan, A. (2018). The histopathology of Erdheim-Chester disease: a comprehensive review of a molecularly characterized cohort. *Modern Pathology*, *31*, 581–597.

Ronen, S., Keiser, E., Collins, K. M., Aung, P. P., Nagarajan, P., Tetzlaff, M. T., Curry, J. L., Ivan, D., Prieto, V. G., Hymes, S., Medeiros, L. J., & Torres-Cabala, C. A. (2021). Langerhans cell sarcoma involving skin and showing epidermotropism: A comprehensive review. *Journal of Cutaneous Pathology*, *48*, 547–557.

Zelger, B. W. H., & Burgdorf, W. H. (2001). The cutaneous "histiocytoses". *Advances in Dermatology*, *17*, 77–114.

Granuloma Annulare Versus Necrobiosis Lipoidica Diabeticorum Versus Necrobiotic Xanthogranuloma

	Mucin	Intervening Normal Dermis	Foamy Cells	Cholesterol Clefts
Granuloma annulare	Common	Typical	Absent	Absent
Necrobiosis lipoidica diabeticorum	Absent	Minimal	Absent	Absent
Necrobiotic xanthogranuloma	Absent	Minimal	Present	Present

17 Cutaneous Neuroendocrine (Merkel Cell) Carcinoma

Klaus J. Busam

Merkel cell carcinoma (MCC) is the eponymous term for primary neuroendocrine carcinoma of the skin, subcutis, or both.

MERKEL CELL CARCINOMA

Clinical Findings

MCC is uncommon. Depending on the geographic area its annual incidence ranges from 0.1 to 1.6 cases per 100,000 individuals. Its incidence is on the rise, having nearly doubled in the United States between 2000 and 2013. MCC typically occurs on chronically sun-damaged skin of elderly White individuals but can also occur in younger patients on sun-protected sites and in individuals with dark skin. The mean age at presentation is 61 years. Most tumors present on the extremities or the head and neck region. The buttocks are also not infrequently involved. Truncal tumors are rare. Approximately 10% of patients present with metastatic disease with no known primary tumor. There is an increased incidence of MCC in immunosuppressed patients (14-fold increased risk among patients with human immunodeficiency virus [HIV]; 10-fold increased risk after solid organ transplantation).

The clinical features of MCC are indistinctive in its early stage. MCC may present as a pink erythematous or violaceous papule, nodule (Fig. 17.1), or plaque or as deep-seated nodule or cystlike mass (Fig. 17.2). MCC is rarely recognized as such. Clinically, biopsies are usually submitted to rule out basal cell carcinoma (BCC), adnexal tumor, squamous cell carcinoma (SCC), cyst, or lipoma.

MERKEL CELL CARCINOMA—DISEASE FACT SHEET

Patient Group

- Mean age at presentation is 61 years
- Immunosuppressed patients
  - 14-fold increased risk in HIV-positive patients
  - 10-fold increased risk after organ transplantation

Site of Involvement

- Head and neck region
- Extremities

Clinical Findings

- Papule, pink, purple, or violaceous nodule, or "cystlike" dermal or subcutaneous mass

Etiology

- Merkel cell polyomavirus
- Chronic UV damage

Prognosis

- Depends on stage
- High recurrence risk for large tumors with lymphatic invasion

Treatment

- Surgical excision
- Radiation for nodal or locally recurrent disease
- Chemotherapy or immunotherapy for distant metastatic disease

Histologic Features

MCC typically presents under the microscope as a "blue" nodule in the dermis or subcutis (or both). It may be fairly circumscribed but more often shows an infiltrative growth pattern at its periphery (Figs. 17.3 and 17.4). The blue appearance relates to the composition of the tumor nodules of cells with minimal cytoplasm. A spectrum from small to intermediate and large cells has been described based on the nuclear size, the intermediate cell type being most common (Figs. 17.5–17.7). The cytology of the tumor cells is characterized by nuclei with a finely granular (salt and pepper) chromatin pattern. Dense hyperchromatic cells may be present, but the nuclei are often pale ("see-through" nuclei). Nuclear molding is often seen. On occasion, one may note rosettes. An Azzopardi phenomenon (crushed nuclei) may be found. Mitotic figures and apoptotic bodies tend to be numerous. Lymphatic tumor emboli are commonly identified at the periphery of many tumors. There may or may not be an associated lymphocytic inflammatory cell infiltrate of variable density. Some tumors show a combined phenotype of neuroendocrine carcinoma associated with a nonneuroendocrine tumor, most often SCC.

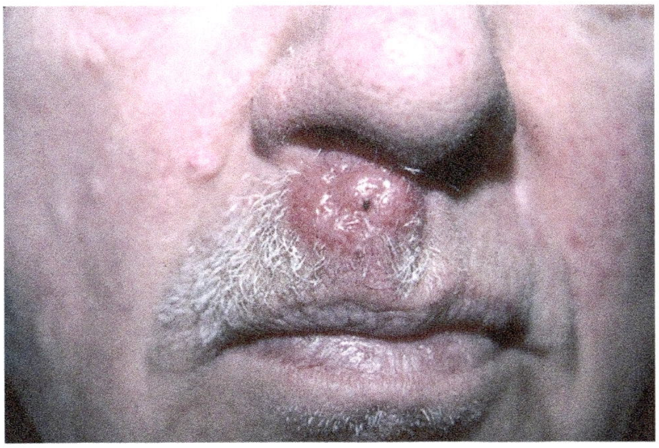

FIG. 17.1
Nodule of Merkel cell carcinoma above the upper lip.

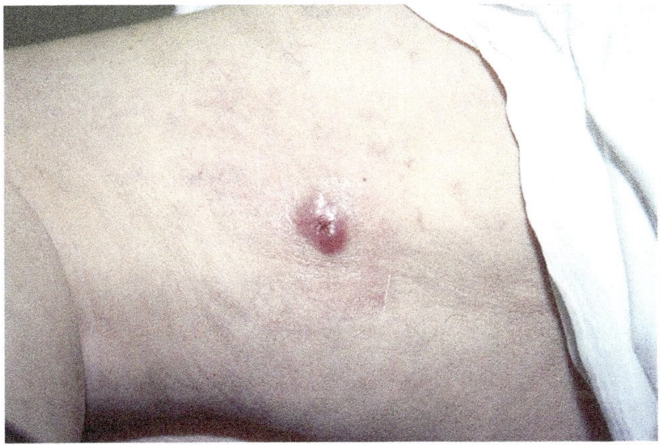

FIG. 17.2
Nodule of Merkel cell carcinoma clinically thought to be a cyst.

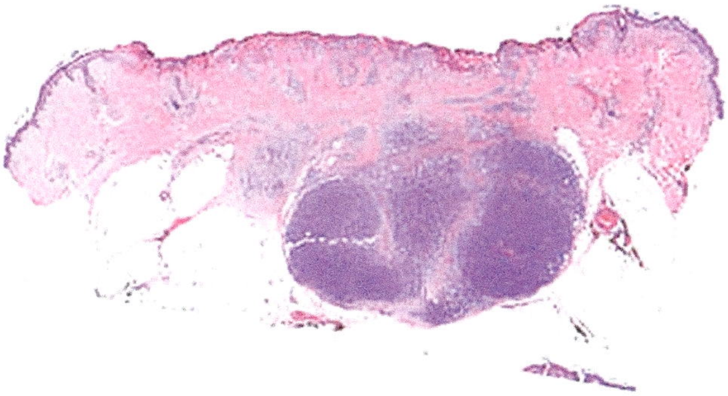

FIG. 17.3
Nodular growth pattern of Merkel cell carcinoma.

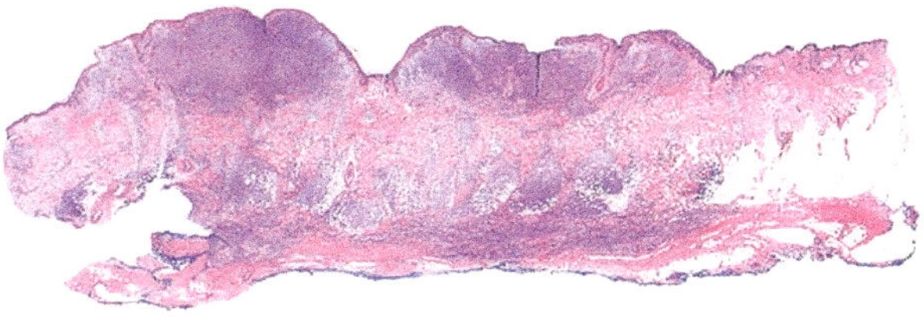

FIG. 17.4
Merkel cell carcinoma with a diffuse infiltrative growth pattern.

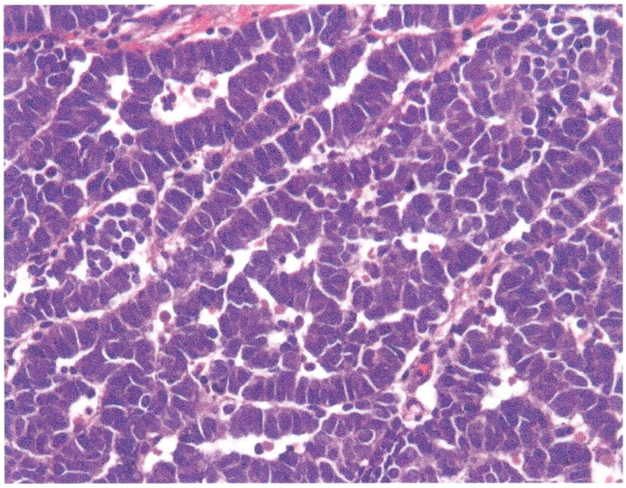

FIG. 17.5
Merkel cell carcinoma with large cell features.

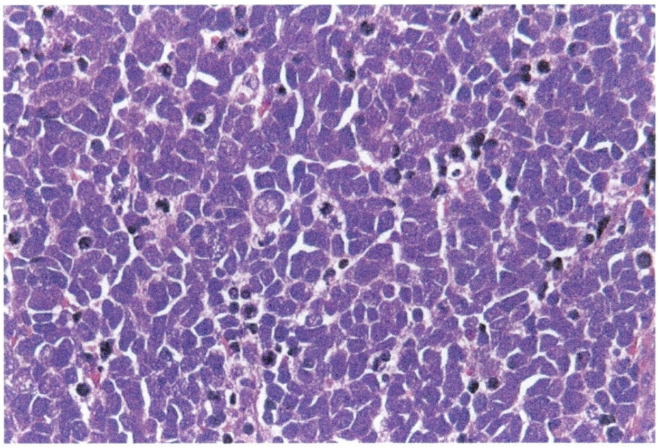

FIG. 17.6
Merkel cell carcinoma with intermediate cell features.

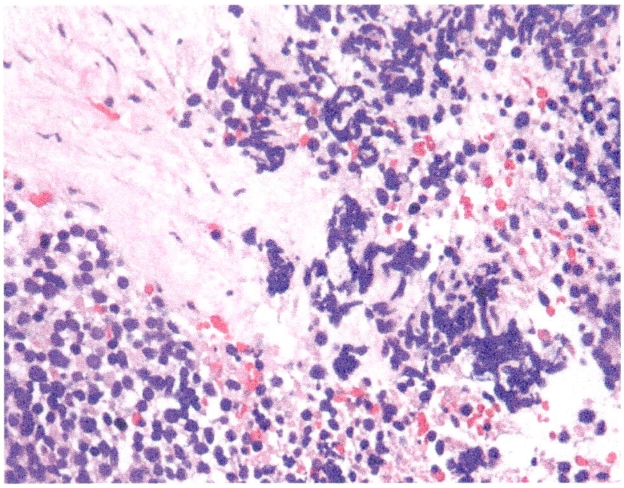

FIG. 17.7
Merkel cell carcinoma with small cell features.

MERKEL CELL CARCINOMA—PATHOLOGIC FEATURES

Histologic Features

- Most tumors present as dermal or subcutaneous "blue" nodule
- Fewer than 10% are combined—most often with SCC
- Growth patterns
  - Nodular circumscribed
  - Nodular infiltrative (most common)
  - Diffusely infiltrative
- Cytology
  - Nuclei with fine salt and pepper chromatin pattern
  - Nuclear size variable: small, intermediate (most common), and large
  - Cytoplasm: scant
  - Mitotic and apoptotic figures common

Ancillary Studies

- Immunohistochemistry
  - Positive for cytokeratins, in particular CK20, often with a dot-like perinuclear pattern
  - Positive for neuroendocrine markers (INSM1, chromogranin, synaptophysin)
  - Positive for neurofilament (dotlike pattern)
  - Positive with CM2B4 or AB2 (MCPyV large T-antigen)
  - Negative for TTF-1

Molecular Studies

- Positive for MCPyV
- Low mutation burden in virus-associated tumors
- Mutations common in tumors not associated with MCPyV, especially combined squamous and neuroendocrine carcinomas

Differential Diagnosis

- Primary versus metastatic MCC (clinical correlation)
- Metastatic extracutaneous small cell carcinoma (often positive for TTF-1)
- Basal cell carcinoma (palisading nuclei, fewer mitoses)
- Cutaneous Ewing sarcoma (positive for EWSR1-rearrangement)

EWS, Ewing sarcoma; *MCC*, Merkel cell carcinoma; *MCPyV*, Merkel cell polyomavirus; *SCC*, squamous cell carcinoma; *TTF*, thyroid transcription factor.

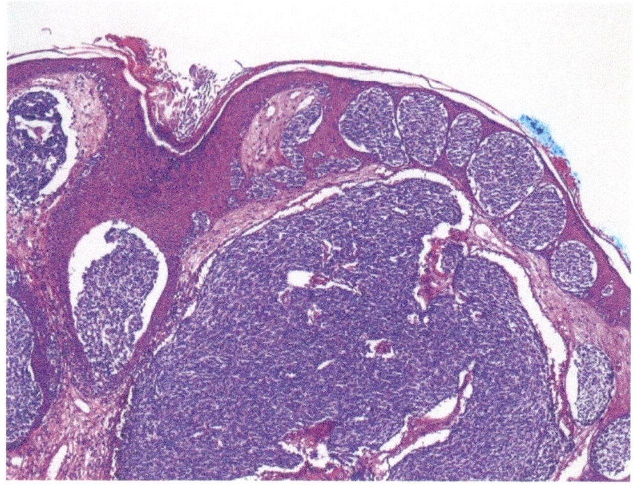

FIG. 17.8
Epidermotropic Merkel cell carcinoma.

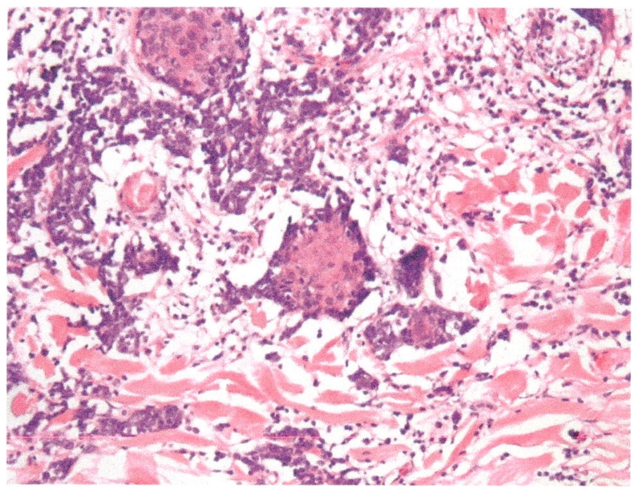

FIG. 17.9
Combined Merkel cell carcinoma and squamous cell carcinoma.

A trabecular "organoid" growth pattern may be present (see Fig. 17.5), but most often the tumor cells are dispersed as sheets lacking a distinct architectural arrangement. Cellular dyscohesion may be marked and give rise to a diffusely infiltrative lymphoma-like appearance.

Although most MCCs are entirely dermal or subcutaneous, some of them have an intraepidermal component (epidermotropic MCC) (Fig. 17.8). It is exceedingly rare to see MCC confined to the epidermis or hair follicles (MCC in situ). Some tumors surround adnexal structures. Classic MCC develops de novo and presents with a pure neuroendocrine phenotype. A subset of cutaneous neuroendocrine carcinomas, however, is found in association with other tumors, most often SCC, rarely BCC, atypical fibroxanthoma, or other adnexal tumors. Although collision lesions may occur, the intimate admixture of squamous and neuroendocrine features within the same tumor mass and the presence of transition areas indicate that at least a subset of cutaneous neuroendocrine carcinomas represent biphenotypic (combined) carcinomas (Fig. 17.9). In some cases the formation of neuroendocrine carcinoma is preceded by SCC at the same anatomic site and transition areas are still found after MCC is detected. The Merkel cell polyomavirus is not associated with combined squamous and neuroendocrine carcinomas. One may regard combined squamous and neuroendocrine carcinomas as dedifferentiated SCC, but they are usually grouped together with MCC and discussed as a combined MCC.

Ancillary Studies

IMMUNOHISTOCHEMISTRY

The tumor cells express epithelial markers (cytokeratins, such as Cam5.2, AE1 : AE3, CK20, 34BE12, Berep4,

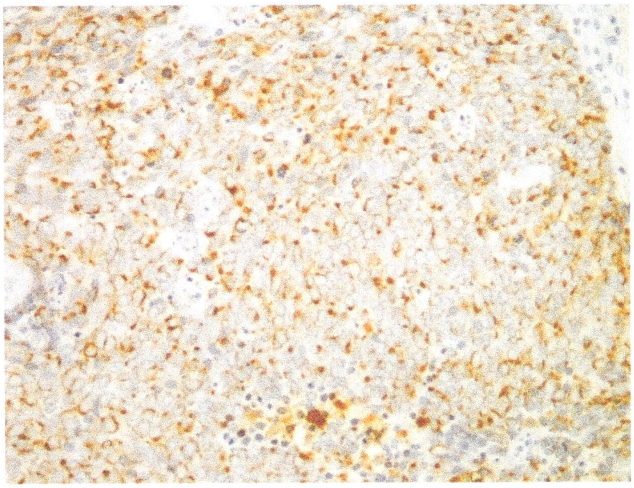

FIG. 17.10
Merkel cell carcinoma with paranuclear dotlike staining for CK20.

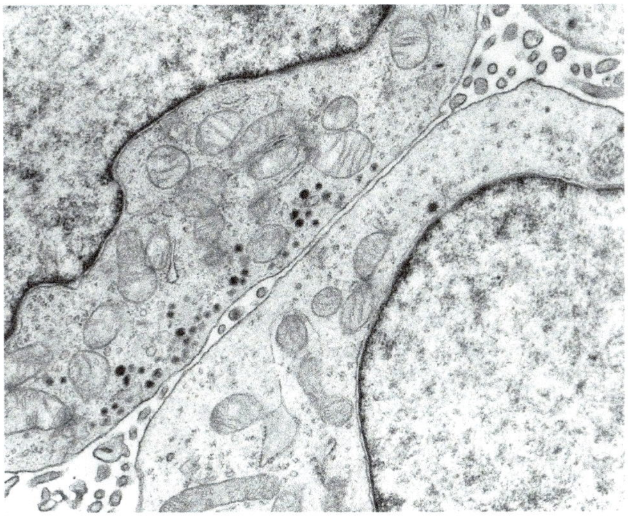

FIG. 17.11
Ultrastructure of Merkel cell carcinoma. Electron-dense neurosecretory granules are characteristic.

and EMA and occasionally CK7) and neuroendocrine markers (INSM1, chromogranin, synaptophysin, CD56). CK20 is particularly useful for diagnosis. The majority of MCCs (75% to 90% of cases) are at least focally positive for CK20, typically (i.e., not always) in a perinuclear dotlike pattern (Fig. 17.10). Neurofilament is another very useful diagnostic marker in the vast majority of MCCs. MCCs may also be positive for p63, CD99, Pax-8, or CD117, but these markers lack specificity for the differential diagnosis. In contrast with the majority of pulmonary and a subset of extrapulmonary (noncutaneous) neuroendocrine carcinomas, MCCs are usually negative for thyroid transcription factor-1 (TTF-1). Monoclonal antibodies (CM2B4 or AB2) can document the presence of Merkel cell polyomavirus in the majority of classic (pure) MCCs. Virus-negative tumors are usually positive for p53 and associated with loss of Rb.

When immunohistochemistry is used for the distinction of lymphoma from MCC, one needs to bear in mind that MCC may coexpress lymphoid markers, such as terminal deoxynucleotidyl transferase (TdT) of Pax-5.

ELECTRON MICROSCOPY

MCC is characterized by the presence of membrane-bound, 80- to 120-nm, dense core granules located in the cytoplasm at the periphery of the cells (Fig. 17.11). Round groups of intermediate filaments may be observed adjacent to the nucleus. Although electron microscopy (EM) has been useful historically, it is now no longer necessary for diagnosis.

MOLECULAR STUDIES

The presence of Merkel cell virus can be demonstrated by polymerase chain reaction (PCR) studies in the majority of pure MCCs. Virus-positive tumors have a low mutation burden. Virus-negative tumors tend to carry mutations, typically reflecting ultraviolet (UV) damage, in particular p53.

Differential Diagnosis

MCC may be confused with other primary cutaneous tumors, such as carcinomas with basaloid or small cell features (BCC, small cell or basaloid variant of sweat gland carcinoma, pilomatrix carcinoma), small cell variant of melanoma, cutaneous Ewing sarcoma, and lymphoma. The distinction may on occasion be difficult on a small biopsy sample, but attention to the presence or absence of the characteristic nuclear features associated with MCC and the use of immunohistochemical markers should lead to the correct diagnosis (Table 17.1).

TABLE 17.1
Immunostains Useful for the Distinction of Merkel Cell Carcinoma From Histologic Simulants

Marker	MCC	BCC	Lymphoma	Melanoma
CK20	+	–	–	–
CM2B4	+	–	–	–
Berep4	±	+	–	–
LYM	–	–	+	–
MDA	–	–	–	+

BCC, Basal cell carcinoma; *CK*, cytokeratin; *CM2B4*, antibody clone to Merkel cell polyomavirus large T-antigen; *LYM*, lymphoid makers: *LCA*, CD20 or CD3 (caution: Pax-5 or TdT may be expressed by Merkel cell carcinoma [MCC]); *MCC*, Merkel cell carcinoma; *MDA*, melanocyte differentiation antigens (S100P, SOX-10, tyrosinase, gp100, Mart-1/Melan-A).

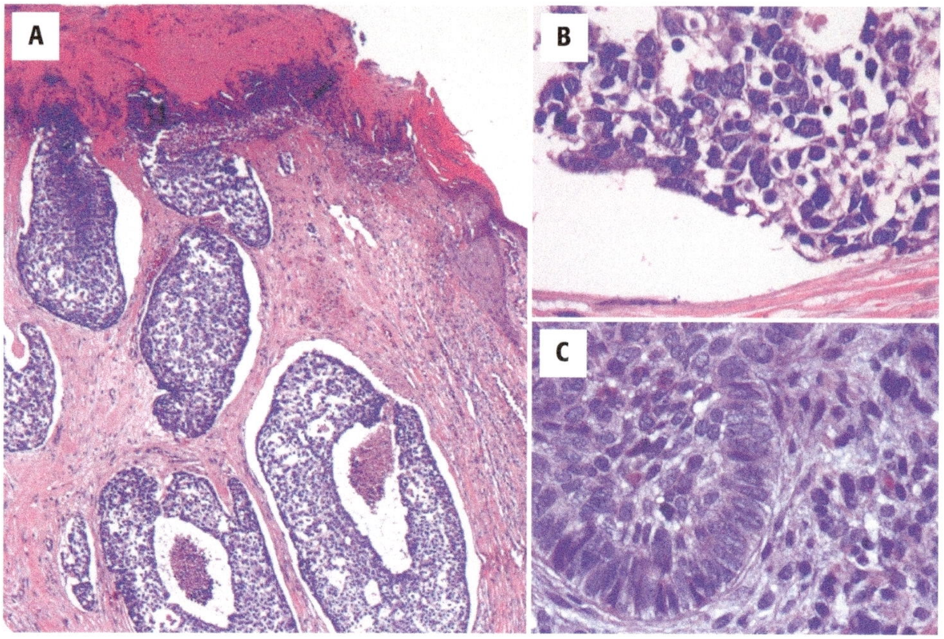

FIG. 17.12

Merkel cell carcinoma (MCC) simulating a basal cell carcinoma (BCC). **A,** MCC in the dermis with nodular growth. **B,** Clefts separate the tumor cells from the stroma, but the tumor cell nuclei lack polarity and overlap. **C,** BCC with peripheral palisading of its nuclei.

Confusion with BCC, for example, may occur when MCC displays a nodular growth pattern in the superficial dermis with clefts between nodules and stroma similar to BCC (Fig. 17.12). A diagnostic error, however, can be avoided when attention is paid to the cytologic features of the tumor cells. MCC lacks peripheral palisading. The tumor cell nuclei overlap and may show molding, and mitotic figures are more frequent.

The distinction of cutaneous Ewing sarcoma from MCC can be difficult because both tumors may express cytokeratins, neuroendocrine markers, and CD99. Molecular studies (fluorescence in situ hybridization for Ewing translocation or PCR studies for EWS-Fli-1 fusion product) help establish a diagnosis of suspected Ewing sarcoma.

MCC may on rare occasions also not be recognized because of a dense inflammatory cell infiltrate (Fig. 17.13), which may lead the diagnostic workup in the wrong direction (lymphoma or pseudolymphoma).

MCC may also be confused with neuroendocrine neoplasms metastatic to the skin, especially metastatic small cell carcinoma. If there is no known history of an extracutaneous neuroendocrine carcinoma and the tumor presents in the superficial dermis of sun-damaged skin with the characteristic light microscopic finding of intermediate-sized pale (see-through) nuclei with fine salt and pepper chromatin pattern, the diagnosis of MCC is almost certain because other neuroendocrine carcinomas with the exception of those of salivary gland origin rarely show the pale nuclear features typical of MCC. However, if a tumor shows cytologic features similar to small cell carcinomas of the lung, a definitive diagnosis requires immunohistochemical studies and clinical correlation. Typically, pulmonary small cell carcinomas are positive for TTF-1 and negative for neurofilament, but MCCs are usually positive for CK20 and neurofilaments but negative for TTF-1.

However, exceptions exist. Some pulmonary and extrapulmonary noncutaneous small cell carcinomas may also be positive for CK20, and some MCCs may be positive for both CK7 and CK20. Furthermore, not all lung tumors stain for TTF-1, and TTF-1 expression is not restricted to lung tumors but can also be seen in extrapulmonary neuroendocrine carcinomas, including a rare case of MCC with focal labeling. It also needs to be emphasized that not all MCCs are CK20 positive. Approximately 10% of them fail to stain for CK20. One can accept a CK20-negative tumor as MCC if the histology and marker studies (positive staining for other keratins, neurofilament, or neuroendocrine markers) support a neuroendocrine carcinoma and the clinical setting is consistent with a primary cutaneous origin. In CK20-negative cases, AE1/AE3 or other pan keratin markers often also label with a perinuclear dotlike pattern. Generally, a diagnosis of the most likely origin of a neuroendocrine carcinoma should not be based on immunohistochemical results alone. Correlation with histologic and clinical findings is paramount. Confusion of MCC with other metastatic well-differentiated neuroendocrine neoplasms of gastrointestinal, pancreatic, or pulmonary origin can usually be avoided by paying attention to the cytology (more atypia and mitotic figures in MCC compared with well-differentiated neuroendocrine neoplasms). The distinction from

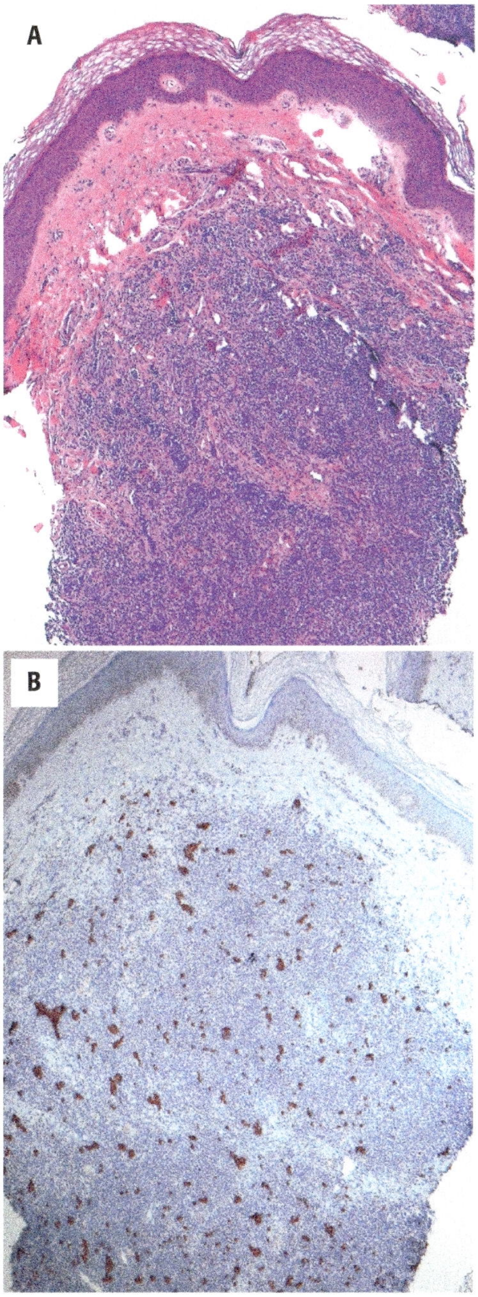

FIG. 17.13
Merkel cell carcinoma with dense lymphocytic infiltrate. **A,** Dense lymphoid infiltrate in the dermis. **B,** The tumor cells are highlighted by immunostain for CK20.

metastatic basaloid SCCs of the head and neck region usually requires immunohistochemical stains (paranuclear dotlike labeling for CK20 in the case of MCC but not metastatic basaloid SCC; both may be strongly positive for p16).

On occasion, primary MCC should be distinguished from metastatic MCC to the skin. Clinical history is essential here. A few histologic features can help, such as the presence of an associated SCC or a dense lymphocytic infiltrate, both of which favor a primary tumor. If a patient has more than one cutaneous MCC, even if they occur anatomically apart and separated chronologically by many years, the second lesion is most likely metastatic. Comparative genomic hybridization may be helpful to establish a relationship between two tumors, if there remain clinical doubts about two independent primary tumors versus metastatic disease.

Prognosis and Treatment

MCC is generally referred to as an "aggressive" tumor. However, it is not uniformly lethal. Overall survival rates in the literature range from 30% to 75%. In a study from Memorial Sloan-Kettering Cancer Center, the 5-year disease-specific survival rate was 64%. The most important prognostic parameter is stage. Multiple differemt staging systems have been proposed. All of them distinguish stages of primary skin tumor from regional nodal disease and distant metastases. According to the current American Joint Committee on Cancer (AJCC) staging system, size and depth of invasion determine the T-stage. T1 refers to tumors no more than 2 cm in greatest clinically measured diameter. Tumors larger than 2 cm, but no greater than 5 cm, are designated as T2. If the size is greater than 5 cm, the stage is T3, unless the tumor invades muscle, fascia, cartilage, or bone, in which case the tumor is upstaged to T4. Depending on the size of the primary tumor (≤2 cm or >2 cm), localized primary tumor limited to the skin or soft tissue is classified as stage I or II, respectively. Stage III defines regional metastatic disease to lymph node, skin, or soft tissue. Stage IV disease is defined as distant metastatic disease (i.e., tumor spread beyond the regional lymph nodes).

Approximately 20% to 30% of patients with MCC have lymph node involvement at the time of initial diagnosis (Fig. 17.14). An additional 30% to 50% of

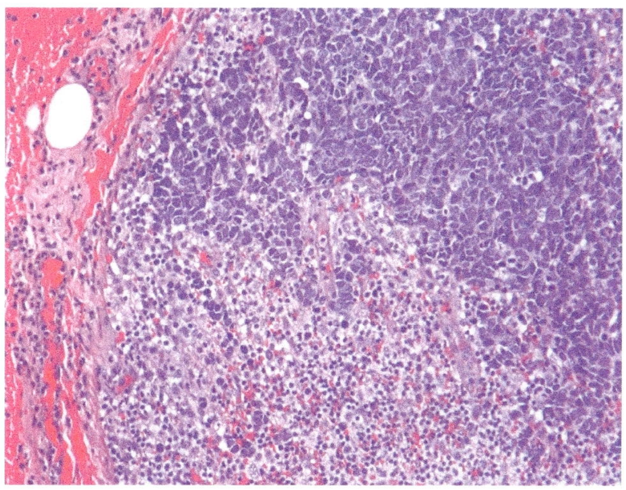

FIG. 17.14
Metastatic Merkel cell carcinoma in a sentinel lymph node.

patients have recurrence with nodal disease at some point. In an attempt to improve the accuracy of staging, sentinel lymph node (SLN) mapping and biopsy are offered at many cancer centers to patients with MCC. If no obvious tumor is found on the initial levels of a bisected SLN, additional levels and immunostains for CK20 or Cam5.2 can help identify small metastatic deposits. However, controversy exists about the prognostic value of micrometastatic disease.

With regard to pathology reports of primary MCC, the following features are prognostically relevant and therefore recommended to be included in the report: tumor size, depth of invasion (e.g., involvement of skeletal muscle and bone), and the presence or absence of lymphatic invasion. The viral status is also important: patients with tumors associated with the Merkel cell polyomavirus (best documented by immunohistochemistry using CM2B4 or AB2) have a better prognosis than those with virus-negative tumors.

Surgical excision is the mainstay of treatment for patients with MCC. However, the tumor is radiosensitive, which is why there is a role for radiation therapy for unresectable tumors and to control regional nodal disease or regionally recurrent tumor. Whether there should be a more general role for radiation therapy is controversial. Chemotherapy is an option for patients with stage IV disease, but its effects are usually short-lived. Immunotherapy on the other hand has found to be effective in many patients.

ACKNOWLEDGMENT

The current chapter is an updated version of a prior chapter, which contained contributions from Dr. Bijal Amin.

SUGGESTED FURTHER READING

Allen, P. J., Bowne, W. B., Jaques, D. P., Brennan, M. F., Busam, K., & Coit, D. G. (2005). Merkel cell carcinoma: Prognosis and treatment of patients from a single institution. *Journal of Clinical Oncology*, *23*, 2300–2309.

Allen, P. J., Zhang, Z. F., & Coit, D. G. (1999). Surgical management of Merkel cell carcinoma. *Annals of Surgery*, *229*, 97–105.

Bichakjian, C. K., Lowe, L., Lao, C. D., Sandler, H. M., Bradford, C. R., Johnson, T. M., & Wong, S. L. (2007). Merkel cell carcinoma: critical review with guidelines for multidisciplinary management. *Cancer*, *110*, 1–12.

Busam, K. J., Judge, M. J., Bichakjian, C. K., Coit, D., Kutzner, H., Requena, L., Scolyer, R. A., Stefanato, C. M., Wood, B. A., & Walsh, N. M. (2022). Dataset for the reporting of Merkel cell carcinoma: recommendations from the International Collaboration on Cancer Reporting (ICCR). *American Journal of Surgical Pathology*, *46*, 1583–1591.

Dinh, V., Feun, L., Elgart, G., & Savaraj, N. (2007). Merkel cell carcinomas. *Hematology/Oncology Clinics of North America*, *21*, 527–544.

Feng, H., Shuda, M., Chang, Y., & Moore, P. S. (2008). Clonal integration of a polyomavirus in human Merkel cell carcinoma. *Science*, *319*, 1096–1100.

Fields, R. C., Busam, K. J., Chou, J. F., Panageas, K. S., Pulitzer, M. P., Allen, P. J., Kraus, D. H., Brady, M. S., & Coit, D. G. (2011). Five hundred patients with Merkel cell carcinoma evaluated at a single institution. *Annals of Surgery*, *254*, 465–475.

Plaza, J. A., & Suster, S. (2006). The Toker tumor: Spectrum of morphologic features in primary neuroendocrine carcinomas of the skin (Merkel cell carcinoma). *Annals of Diagnostic Pathology*, *10*, 376–385.

Pulitzer, M. P., Amin, B. D., & Busam, K. J. (2009). Merkel cell carcinoma: Review. *Advances in Anatomic Pathology*, *16*, 135–144.

Walsh, N. M. (2001). Primary neuroendocrine (Merkel cell) carcinoma of the skin: Morphologic diversity and implications thereof. *Human Pathology*, *32*, 680–689.

Metastatic Tumors Involving the Skin

18

Nigel G. Maher • Richard A. Scolyer

Introduction

The involvement of the skin by metastatic malignancy is relatively uncommon but is important to recognize as it may have significant implications for both management and prognosis. A cutaneous metastasis may represent the first manifestation of an unrecognized internal malignancy or the first evidence of recurrence of a previously treated primary tumor. Determining the site of the primary tumor, if unknown, is often very difficult and sometimes impossible. However, certain primary sites may be suspected from the histopathologic features and the immunohistochemical and/or molecular profile of the cutaneous metastatic deposit.

Secondary tumors may involve the skin by direct spread from adjacent noncutaneous structures; by lymphatic or hematogenous spread; or, rarely, as a consequence of implantation following a surgical or other diagnostic procedure. While tumors involving the skin as a consequence of direct spread from adjacent noncutaneous structures are not true metastases, they may be misdiagnosed by the unwary as unusual primary cutaneous tumors unless the possibility of a noncutaneous origin of the tumor is considered. The presence of skin metastases usually occurs in the clinical setting of a known primary tumor, often with accompanying widespread visceral metastatic disease. In such cases, a pathologist, provided with a thorough and accurate clinical history, will usually have little difficulty in correctly recognizing non-primary tumors. In other situations, there is a real risk that a metastatic tumor may be incorrectly diagnosed; for example, when there is inadequate clinical information on the pathology request form; or when a metastasis is solitary, isolated, and presents a long time after the primary tumor was initially diagnosed; or when a cutaneous metastasis represents the first indication of an underlying visceral cancer or other tumor. Conversely, uncommon variants of primary cutaneous malignancies, including basal cell carcinoma, squamous cell carcinoma, and melanoma, may occasionally be mistaken for metastases. Misdiagnosis of a metastasis as a primary tumor or vice versa may result in inaccurate prognostic assessment, inappropriate management, and a potentially poorer clinical outcome. A high index of suspicion and careful clinicopathologic correlation are the key factors in preventing misdiagnosis.

Prevalence

Cutaneous metastases are relatively uncommon. The reported prevalence varies between studies, possibly both due to regional variation in cancer subtype prevalence and due to advances in cancer management over time. A recent retrospective study of 11,418 patients with solid malignancies by Teyateeti and others found only 33 (0.3%) had cutaneous metastases, mostly adenocarcinoma (70%). An older retrospective study of 4022 patients with metastatic visceral malignancy found that 10% had cutaneous involvement. Cutaneous metastases usually occur late in the course of disease, and in approximately 7% of cases this interval is greater than 5 years. As cancer patients live longer with advances in treatment, the incidence of cutaneous metastases is increasing. Melanoma and breast carcinoma are the most common tumor types to present with delayed metastases, including cutaneous metastases. While delayed breast cancer metastases usually occur in the setting of previous metastatic disease (particularly previous involvement of the regional lymph nodes draining the primary tumor), cutaneous metastases from melanoma are sometimes the first manifestation of metastatic disease in patients with a previously treated primary cutaneous melanoma. Occasionally a cutaneous metastasis occurs as the first clinical indication of an underlying internal malignancy, with the reported incidence ranging from 0.8% to 30% of all cutaneous metastases in different series. Clearly the latter situation represents the greatest challenge to accurate pathologic diagnosis.

Pathophysiology

Metastases develop following a complex series of interactions between the tumor and the host environment. Metastasis can occur only after the development in the primary tumor of a clone of tumor cells that possess the right combination of genetic and/or epigenetic aberrations to complete all the necessary steps for dissemination of malignant tumor cells followed by colonization (establishment and growth of tumor cells) at a new site. These steps include adhesion to and invasion through the basement membrane around the primary tumor, passage through the extracellular matrix, invasion of vessels, interaction of tumor cells with host lymphoid cells, extravasation, angiogenesis, and growth of the metastatic deposit (Table 18.1). Each step in this process is influenced by multiple factors, and at any one step in the sequence, the metastasizing cells may not survive. In recent years, some insight has been gained into the molecular mechanisms underlying the development of metastases and new metastasis-related genes have been identified. For example, several recent studies have shown the utility of biomarker assessment using a variety of techniques, including gene sequencing, gene expression, and microRNA expression studies, to determine genetic aberrations of metastases. However, many of these biomarkers require validation in large prospective studies before it would be appropriate to utilize them in routine clinical practice. Furthermore, targeted next-generation sequencing panels that can evaluate sequence alterations and copy number alterations in selected sets of cancer-associated genes are already being used in some institutions to profile tumors with the goal of identifying actionable therapeutic targets. In the near future, it may be possible to assess a primary tumor using such panels for validated genetic alterations that promote or suppress the development of metastases and which therefore have prognostic and therapeutic implications. Such panels may also provide important information in determining the primary site of origin of metastases when it is unknown or uncertain.

TABLE 18.1

Sequential Pathophysiologic Steps Involved in the Development of Cutaneous Metastases

Sequential Step	Pathophysiologic Event
1	Adhesion to and invasion through basement membrane
2	Detachment from primary tumor
3	Passage through extracellular matrix
4	Invasion of vessels
5	Interaction with host lymphocytes
6	Extravasation of tumor cells
7	Angiogenesis
8	Growth of metastatic deposit

Adapted from Cotran, R. S., Kumar, V., Collins, T. (Eds.) (1999). *Robbins pathologic basis of disease* (6th ed.). Philadelphia: WB Saunders.

CUTANEOUS METASTASIS—DISEASE FACT SHEET

Definition

- Cutaneous tumor deposits discontinuous with or distant to the primary tumor

Mechanisms of Development

- Lymphatic spread
- Hematogenous spread
- Direct spread from adjacent noncutaneous structures[a]
- Implantation following a surgical or diagnostic procedure[a]

Prevalence

- Occur in 0.3%–10% of patients with visceral cancer
- 0.8%–10% of cases are the first clinical indication ofhe reported incidence ranging from 0.8
- May occur at any age but is more common in the elderly

Types of Tumors

- Parallels the incidence of various tumors in each particular age, sex, and ethnic group
- In Western societies, the most common tumors in adults include:
  - In females: breast cancer, melanoma, colorectal cancer
  - In males: lung cancer, melanoma, colorectal cancer, prostate cancer

Anatomic Location

- Usually close to the primary site but may occur anywhere
- Often involve multiple locations

Clinical Features

- Usually multiple discrete, painless nodules of sudden onset
- Several nodules may be localized to one area
- Less commonly may present as a plaque, multiple papules, an area of alopecia, cellulitis, or mimicking a benign dermatologic condition

Presentations Associated With a High Risk of Misdiagnosis

- First manifestation of internal malignancy
- First evidence of recurrence of previously treated primary tumor
- History of previous malignancy not known

Biopsy Specimens

- Preferable biopsy size and type will vary depending on the type of tumor, the level of clinical suspicion, and range of necessary ancillary investigations
- Formal tissue biopsy is generally preferable but fine-needle biopsy is often adequate in certain circumstances (especially in melanoma)

Pathology

- Dermal localization of a carcinoma or melanoma raises suspicion that tumor could be a metastasis but is not definitive
- Metastasis usually shows histologic similarities to putative primary tumor (although sometimes it is more anaplastic)
- If unknown, certain primary sites may be suspected from morphologic features- see text for details
- Metastatic adenocarcinomas may be indistinguishable from primary cutaneous sweat gland carcinomas
- Metastatic melanoma is usually localized to the dermis/subcutis
- "Epidermotropic" metastatic melanoma (and so-called primary dermal melanoma) also occur and are only recognized by clinicopathologic correlation

Immunochemistry and Other Ancillary Investigations

- For a poorly differentiated malignant cutaneous tumor, initial workup to determine histogenesis (i.e., whether the tumor is a carcinoma, melanoma, sarcoma, or hemopoietic tumor) by panel of immunostains
- Ancillary investigations are of limited usefulness in determining whether an adenocarcinoma is of adnexal or metastatic origin. Exceptions include thyroid (thyroglobulin+, TTF-1+, PAX8+), lung (TTF-1+, NapsinA+, thyroglobulin−), prostate (PSA+, PAcP+, PMSA+, NKX3.1+)
- Immunochemistry that may help in determining the site of origin of neuroendocrine carcinomas: Merkel cell carcinoma is usually CK20+, CK7−, TTF-1−, subset MCPyV+; small cell lung carcinoma is usually CK7+, TTF-1+, CK20−
- Molecular tumor profiling using a variety of assays shows promise in assisting with the determination of the likely primary source of metastatic tumors

Prognosis

- Varies depending on the type of tumor and other clinical features
- Grave prognostic sign when associated with widespread dissemination

[a]Not a "true" metastasis but may appear clinically similar.
CK, Cytokeratin; *PAcP*, prostate acid phosphatase; *PMSA*, prostate membrane–specific antigen; *PSA*, prostate-specific antigen; *TTF*, thyroid transcription factor.

Sites of Origin

Cutaneous metastases are more common in older individuals, paralleling the increasing incidence of malignancy with increasing age. Furthermore, the type of malignancy metastasizing to the skin in patients of different ages and sexes is generally in keeping with the incidence of various tumors in each particular age and sex group. For example, in Western countries, the most common cutaneous metastases are breast cancer, melanoma, colorectal cancer, and lung cancer in females, and lung cancer, melanoma, colorectal cancer, and prostate cancer in males. Neuroblastoma and rhabdomyosarcoma are the most common cutaneous metastases in children, reflecting the incidence of these tumors in this age group. In children, approximately 50% of cutaneous malignant tumors are metastases rather than primary skin tumors, and cutaneous metastases represent the first clinical manifestation of disease in up to 84% of cases. Cutaneous metastases that are the first clinical manifestation of internal malignancy are most commonly carcinomas of the lung, kidney, and ovary because the primary tumors in these organs often remain clinically silent until late in their development.

ANATOMIC LOCALIZATION

Cutaneous metastases are most commonly observed in sites in the vicinity of the primary tumor but may occur anywhere. For example, breast cancers tend to metastasize to skin overlying the anterior chest wall or upper limbs, gastrointestinal cancers often involve skin of the anterior abdominal wall, and pelvic tumors have a predilection to involve the perineum or inguinal region.

Metastases to the umbilicus have been termed Sister Mary Joseph nodules in recognition of the nurse who is credited with recognizing the clinical significance of tumor nodules at this site. The underlying primary tumor is most commonly a gastric adenocarcinoma but occasionally carcinomas from other primary sites such as the large bowel, pancreas, breast, and female genital tract may also metastasize to the umbilicus. Scalp metastases account for up to 5% of all cutaneous metastases, and the most common sources are tumors from the breast, lung, kidney, and melanomas. Although a tumor deposit may involve the skin directly overlying the primary tumor after a diagnostic biopsy, presumably as a result of implantation of tumor cells, metastatic tumor deposits may also involve the skin at the sites of procedures distant to the primary tumor. It is speculated that this may occur as a consequence of the release of cytokines, growth factors, and other chemokines resulting in a "fertile soil" for the growth of metastases. An example of this phenomenon is melanoma metastasis occurring in a skin graft donor site. Metastases from primary tumors of the internal viscera to skin of the extremities are uncommon.

Clinical Features

Cutaneous metastases commonly present as multiple, discrete, painless nodules of sudden onset. Most lesions are less than 2 cm in diameter at presentation. Sometimes several nodules are localized to one area, but often the metastatic deposits involve more than one anatomic location. The presence of multiple, sometimes clustered, skin nodules should raise clinical suspicion of metastatic cutaneous deposits. Solitary metastases occur in approximately 10% of cases and are usually indistinguishable clinically from other skin lesions, particularly primary tumors. Occasionally a cutaneous metastasis may present as a plaque or an area of alopecia (Fig. 18.1) or resemble a dermatologic condition such as erythema annulare, lupus erythematosus, herpes zoster, or a condyloma. An inflammatory pattern resembling cellulitis or erysipelas ("carcinoma erysipelatoides") is occasionally observed in breast cancers involving the skin overlying the primary tumor, but this pattern may also occur at other sites and in association with metastases from many other tumor types. Other unusual cutaneous presentations of breast cancer include multiple telangiectatic papules, "peau d'orange" (representing dermal edema of the breast caused by obstruction of cutaneous lymphatics by tumor), and "carcinoma en cuirasse" (a large, intensely sclerotic plaque of confluent tumor).

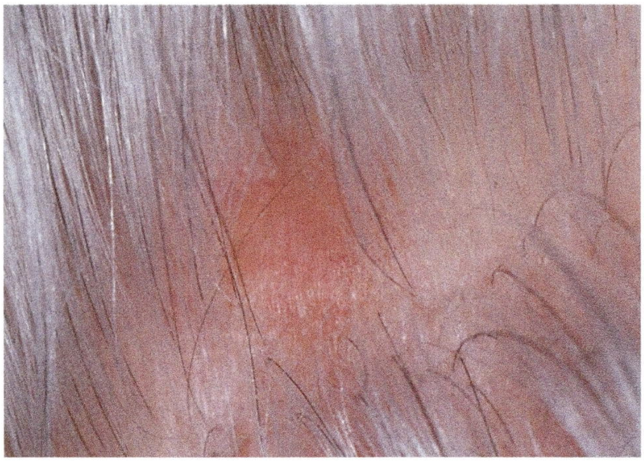

FIG. 18.1

Metastatic breast carcinoma involving skin of the scalp: clinical photograph. A pale plaque associated with a small area of alopecia is present. (Courtesy of Professor Scott W. Menzies, Sydney Melanoma Diagnostic Centre.)

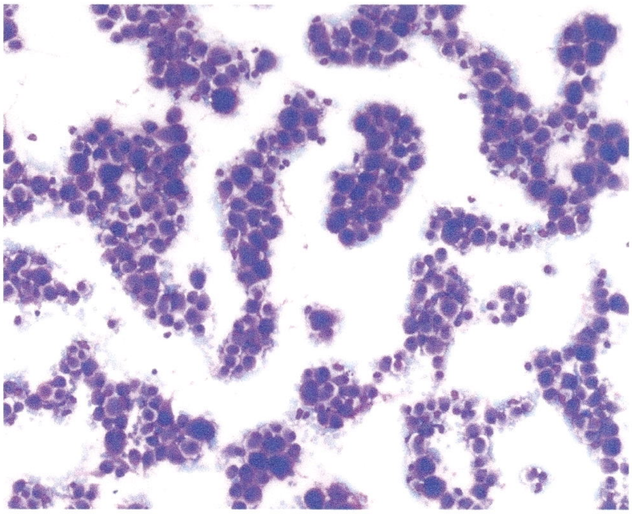

FIG. 18.2

Metastatic melanoma: fine-needle biopsy cytology. Low-power micrograph showing large numbers of dissociating pleomorphic epithelioid cells in a lightly blood-stained background (Diff-Quick stained smear).

Biopsy Specimens

An appropriate, well-processed biopsy is mandatory for accurate pathologic diagnosis. A formal tissue biopsy, rather than fine-needle biopsy material, is usually preferable for pathologic diagnosis of cutaneous metastases. In certain situations, however, the latter will suffice. The biopsy should provide a sample of the lesion that is large enough to allow diagnosis without the need for further biopsies. The size and type of an adequate biopsy will vary depending on the type of tumor, the level of clinical suspicion, and the range of necessary ancillary investigations. Punch, incisional, excisional, and occasionally shave biopsies may be adequate depending on the circumstances. The biopsy should be free of crush or fixation artifacts, and the tissue sections should be well prepared to avoid misdiagnosis; for example, crushed lymphoid cells may be misdiagnosed as cutaneous neuroendocrine carcinoma or metastatic small cell lung carcinoma. Misdiagnosis in this situation may have a profound adverse impact on the patient's treatment and subsequent outcome. In the setting of a known primary tumor and clinical suspicion of a metastasis, a fine-needle biopsy specimen, with the collection of additional material for appropriate ancillary investigations such as immunochemistry and genetic testing, may be sufficient for definitive diagnosis. For instance, in melanoma, which commonly metastasizes to skin/subcutis, abundant material is usually obtainable by fine-needle biopsy and the cytologic appearances are characteristic (Figs. 18.2 and 18.3). For epithelial malignancies, however, it is usually more difficult to distinguish between a primary tumor and a metastasis on a cytology specimen than on a tissue biopsy. Nonetheless, if the clinical suspicion is high and the patient is unfit or unwilling to undergo a formal tissue biopsy, fine-needle biopsy may offer a reasonable alternative. Fine-needle biopsy can also provide fresh tumor samples for molecular profiling using various genetic assays, which can assist in establishing the origin of metastases in morphologically challenging cases and for detecting biomarkers that predict response to various systemic therapies including monoclonal antibodies targeting oncogenic proteins or immune checkpoint inhibitors.

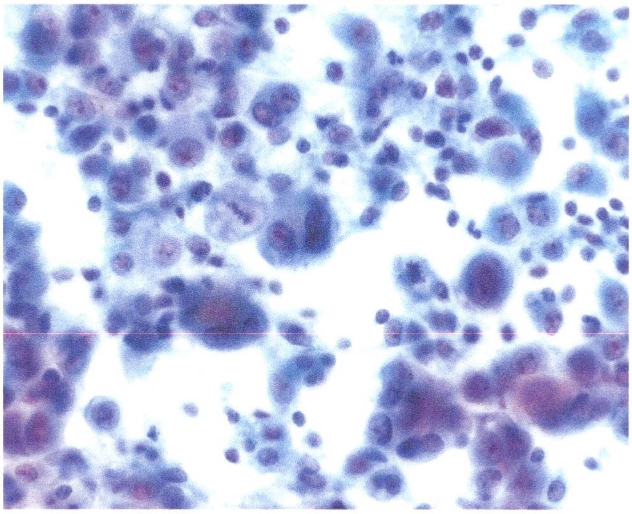

FIG. 18.3

Metastatic melanoma: fine-needle biopsy cytology. High-power micrograph showing large pleomorphic epithelioid cells with prominent nucleoli. Two mitotic figures are present. There is an occasional multinucleated tumor giant cell. No melanin pigment is apparent (Papanicolaou stained smear).

Pathology

GENERAL COMMENTS

To reduce the risk of a metastasis being misdiagnosed, an adequate clinical history is necessary when interpreting the pathology. Nevertheless, even in the absence of a history of a previous tumor, it is important that the pathologist be alert to histologic or other features suggesting that the tumor is in fact a secondary deposit and not an unusual primary tumor, as metastases may be the first clinical manifestation of an internal malignancy or the first metastasis of a previously treated primary tumor. As metastases usually show histopathologic similarities to the primary tumor (although they are sometimes more anaplastic), it is essential for pathologists, even specialized dermatopathologists, to have an adequate experience and knowledge of the morphologic appearances of tumors that arise at noncutaneous sites to avoid misdiagnosis. When no history of prior malignancy is supplied on the pathology request form, it may be necessary in some cases to ask the clinician specifically if the tumor could represent a metastasis. Histologic comparison of the metastasis with the putative primary tumor may be of value if the original slides are available. As detailed above, the age and sex of the patient and the location, distribution, and clinical appearance of the cutaneous tumor deposit may also be helpful in identifying a tumor as a metastasis and in suggesting a likely primary site if this is unknown.

Metastases are usually centered in the dermis and subcutis (Figs. 18.4 and 18.5), in contrast to primary carcinomas and melanomas, which, in most cases, involve the epidermis at least focally. The epidermis is usually uninvolved and separated from the underlying tumor by an uninvolved strip of superficial dermis, the so-called grenz zone. Although the dermal localization of a tumor may be helpful in distinguishing a metastasis from a primary tumor of epidermal origin, it is not definitive. Because primary cutaneous adnexal tumors are usually localized to the dermis and devoid of an epidermal component, dermal localization alone cannot be used to distinguish primary adnexal tumors from cutaneous metastases. It is particularly difficult and often impossible to distinguish an adenocarcinoma of sweat gland type from a metastasis on the basis of morphology or immunochemical profile. Furthermore, some primary melanomas may lack an epidermal component (so-called primary dermal melanomas) and may be diagnosed as melanoma metastases. Occasionally, specific melanoma subtypes (e.g., blue nevus–like melanoma) may arise in the dermis without an epidermal component. Regression, previous biopsy (such as a shave biopsy), or superficial treatment (such as cryotherapy) may all result in absence of the epidermal or junctional component of a primary cutaneous melanoma in a subsequent biopsy. Selective sampling of a large skin tumor may not reveal the epidermal origin of a primary tumor in the sections examined and may therefore result in misdiagnosis of a squamous cell carcinoma as an adnexal carcinoma or metastasis. In contrast, occasional metastases, such as so-called epidermotropic melanoma metastases, may involve the epidermis and dermis and display histopathologic features indistinguishable from a primary melanoma, and in this case, clinicopathologic correlation is necessary for accurate diagnosis. In the presence of prominent lymphovascular involvement by tumor (as is typically observed in inflammatory carcinoma of the breast), the possibility that the tumor could be a metastasis should always be considered (Fig. 18.6).

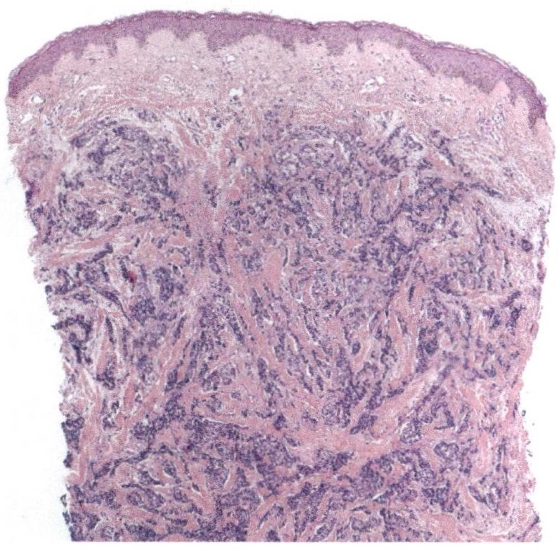

FIG. 18.4

Metastatic breast carcinoma of ductal type. Low-power micrograph of punch biopsy of skin showing cohesive clusters of pleomorphic epithelioid cells within the dermis.

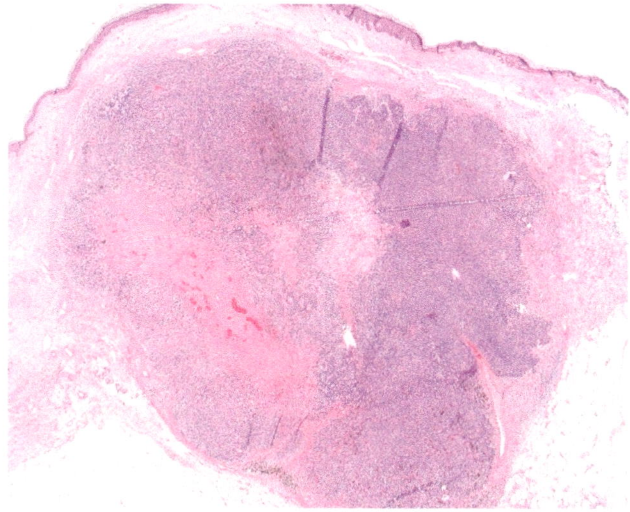

FIG. 18.5

Metastatic melanoma. Low-power micrograph showing a centrally necrotic tumor involving the dermis and subcutis. The uninvolved epidermis is separated from the underlying tumor by a so-called grenz zone of uninvolved dermis.

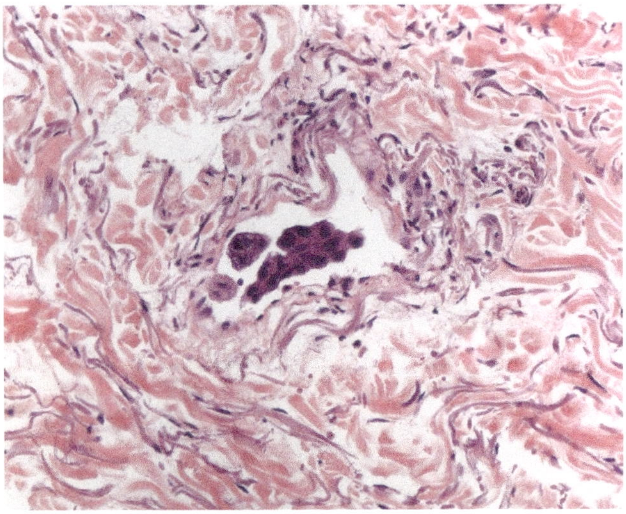

FIG. 18.6

Metastatic breast carcinoma of ductal type. High-power micrograph showing tumor within a dermal lymphatic channel.

TABLE 18.2

Potential Causes of the Pathologic Misdiagnosis of Cutaneous Metastases and Methods of Avoiding Them

Pitfall/Contributing Factor to Misdiagnosis	Solution
Inadequate/insufficient clinical information	1. Encourage provision of relevant clinical details on pathology request form 2. Ask the clinician specifically if tumor could represent a metastasis
Small, crushed, or inadequate biopsy or suboptimal sections	Ensure biopsy is of adequate size and type and sections are well prepared and stained
Misdiagnosis of metastasis as a rare type of primary skin adnexal tumor	Always consider the possibility of a metastasis before diagnosing a skin adnexal tumor
Misdiagnosis of a primary tumor as a metastasis	Clinicopathologic correlation (on some occasions the pathologic features of primary and secondary tumors (e.g., melanomas) may be indistinguishable)

Potential pitfalls and factors that may contribute to the misdiagnosis of cutaneous metastases and ways to avoid them are listed in Table 18.2.

ANCILLARY INVESTIGATIONS (INCLUDING IMMUNOCHEMISTRY AND TUMOR PROFILING)

The widespread availability of immunochemistry for identification of numerous antigens in formalin-fixed, paraffin-embedded tissue and the ease of correlation of immunohistochemical stains with conventional histopathology have resulted in immunochemistry largely replacing special histochemical stains and electron microscopy as aids to histopathologic diagnosis. In recent years, molecular methods such as in situ hybridization, gene mutation analysis, and gene microarray analysis have become more frequently utilized for pathologic diagnosis, prognostic assessment, and assisting in therapeutic decision-making. The usefulness of immunochemistry in improving the accuracy of pathologic diagnosis cannot be understated; however, it is a technique not without limitations and must always be interpreted in conjunction with assessment of morphology of the tumor and correlation with the clinical findings. Few, if any, of the currently available antibodies are totally specific for any one tumor or tissue type, and both the sensitivity and specificity of any immunostain may vary from laboratory to laboratory and between antibody clones. Malignant tumors may not express certain antigens that are characteristic of their normal cellular counterparts, and others may express antigens not normally present in their corresponding benign tissues. For example, occasionally metastatic melanomas may not stain for Melan A/ MART-1 and even S100 protein, while others may occasionally coexpress the muscle marker desmin. For such reasons, a panel of markers is necessary in most cases when a number of differential diagnostic possibilities are being considered. The initial approach to a poorly differentiated malignant tumor may involve the use of appropriate markers to determine the type of differentiation/histogenesis of the tumor (i.e., to confirm whether the tumor is a carcinoma, melanoma, sarcoma, germ cell or hemopoietic malignancy) (Table 18.3) with subsequent application of further immunostains to allow subclassification.

Immunochemistry may be useful not only in determining the type or differentiation of a tumor but also in determining its site of origin in some situations (Tables 18.4 and 18.5). Examples include distinguishing Merkel cell carcinoma of the skin from metastatic small cell neuroendocrine carcinoma of pulmonary origin; identifying adenocarcinomas of colorectal, gynecologic, thyroid, lung, and prostate origin; confirming the nature of some rare metastases such as metastatic germ cell tumors; and sometimes in suggesting that an adenocarcinoma may be a metastasis from the gastrointestinal tract or female genital tract. In some cases, immunochemistry may be able to establish whether a cutaneous tumor is primary or secondary; however, in some instances, even with an extensive panel of immunostains and taking into account other histologic features, it will not be possible to determine with complete certainty whether a poorly differentiated adenocarcinoma or squamous cell carcinoma is an unusual primary tumor or a metastasis. Even if a metastasis is suspected, only a list of the more likely sites of the primary lesion can be proffered. Combining the results of a panel of immunostains may improve their sensitivity and specificity but a definite answer may still not be possible. It is also essential that pathologists are aware of the range of tumors that may express any particular antigen in order to

TABLE 18.3

Immunostains Useful in Determining the Histogenesis/Line of Differentiation of a Poorly/Undifferentiated Malignant Cutaneous Tumor[b]

	TYPE OF TUMOR			
Antibody	Carcinoma	Melanoma	Sarcoma	Hemopoietic Tumor
Pan keratins	+/−	−	−/+	−
p40	+/−	−	−	−
EMA	+/−	−	−/+	−/+
S100	−/+	+/−	−/+	−
SOX10	−[c]	+/−	−/+	−
HMB45	−	+/−	−/+[a]	−
Melan A	−	+/−	−	−
BRAF V600E	−/+	+/−	−	−
NRAS Q61R	−	−/+	−	−
Vimentin	−/+	+	+	−/+
CD45	−	−	−	+
CD3	−	−	−	+/−
CD20	−	−	−	+/−
CD30	−	−	−	−/+

[a]Positive in clear-cell sarcoma.
[b]For identification of germ cell tumours, OCT 3/4, Glypican 3, CD30, AFP, beta-hCG and CD117 can be performed.
[c]Certain primary adnexal and metastatic carcinomas are SOX10 positive
+, Usually positive; +/−, often positive, sometimes negative; −/+, often negative, occasionally positive; −, usually negative; *EMA*, epithelial membrane antigen.

TABLE 18.4

Immunostains That May Be Helpful in Determining the Likely Primary Site of Origin of a Cutaneous Adenocarcinoma

	SITE OF ORIGIN OF PRIMARY ADENOCARCINOMA								
Antibody	Skin	Breast	Lung	Colorectal	Thyroid	Prostate	Gynecologic	Stomach	Pancreas
CK8/18	+	+	+	+	+	+	+	+	+
CK7	+	+	+	−/+	+	−/+	+	+/−	+/−
CK20	−	−	−	+/−	−	−/+	−/+	−/+	+/−
CEA	+/−	+/−	+/−	+/−	+/−	+/−	+/−	+/−	+/−
ER/PR	+/−	+/−	−	−	−	−	−	−	−
GATA3	+/−[a]	+	−	−	−	−	−	−	−
S100	−/+	−/+	−	−	−	−	−/+	−	−
GCDFP−15	+/−	+/−	−	−	−	−/+	−	−	−
TTF-1	−	−	+	−	+	−	−	−	−
NapsinA	−	−	+	−	−	−	+/−	−	−
PSA	−	−	−	−	−	+	−	−	−
NKX3.1	−	−/+[b]	−	−	−	+	−	−	−
PAcP	−	−	−	−	−	+	−	−	−
PMSA	−	−	−	−	−	+	−	−	−
Ca125	−	−/+	−/+	−	−/+	−	+/−	−/+	+/−
PAX8	−	−	−	−	+	−	+/−	−	−
CDX2	−	−	−	+/−	−	−	−/+	+/−	+/−
SATB2	−	−	−	+	−	−	−	−	−

[a]Particularly apocrine carcinoma.
[b]Positive in ~25% of lobular subtype.
+, Usually positive; +/−, often positive, sometimes negative; −/+, often negative, occasionally positive; −, usually negative; *ER*, estrogen receptor; *CEA*, carcinoembryonic antigen; *GCDFP*, gross cystic disease fluid protein; *PAcP*, prostate acid phosphatase; *PMSA*, prostate membrane–specific antigen; *PR*, progesterone receptor; *PSA*, prostate-specific antigen; *TTF-1*, thyroid transcription factor-1.

TABLE 18.5

Immunostains That May Be Helpful in Determining the Likely Primary Site of Origin of a Cutaneous Neuroendocrine Carcinoma

	SITE OF ORIGIN OF PRIMARY NEUROENDOCRINE CARCINOMA (HIGH GRADE)		
Antibody	Skin (Merkel)	Lung	Other
CK8/18	+	+	+
CK7	−	+	+
CK20	+/−	−	−
TTF-1	−	+	−/+
Chromogranin	+/	+/−	+/−
Synaptophysin	+/−	+/−	+/−
CD56	+	+	+
MCV T antigen	+/−	−	−

+, Usually positive; +/−, often positive, sometimes negative; −/+, often negative, occasionally positive; −, usually negative; *MCV*, Merkel cell polyomavirus; *TTF-1*, thyroid transcription factor-1.

avoid misinterpretation. Referring to up-to-date literature or frequently updated websites may also be helpful. Although the histopathology may not provide a definite answer on the site of origin of a metastatic tumor, certain histologic features may prompt further clinical investigation and ultimately provide critical information on which the patient's management depends.

Molecular profiling of metastases using various genetic assays (including gene expression profiling, reverse transcription polymerase chain reaction (RT-PCR), and targeted next-generation sequencing) may assist in establishing the primary tumor site of origin of metastases. The accuracy of these assays varies between studies and depends on the type of assay and the markers or combinations of markers that were used to classify the tumors according to their primary sites of origin. As these assays are validated, and with the increasing availability of genetic assays in many laboratories, molecular profiling will become more important in the algorithm for assessment of tumors from patients with cutaneous metastases.

SPECIFIC METASTASES

Metastatic tumors involving skin include carcinomas, melanomas, sarcomas, germ cell malignancies or cutaneous involvement by hemopoietic malignancies. Metastatic carcinomas are the most common and are also most problematic in determining their site of origin. They can be broadly categorized into adenocarcinoma, squamous, neuroendocrine, and miscellaneous carcinoma subtypes based on their microscopic appearance. Knowledge of the features characteristic of carcinomas from specific sites may be useful or even critical in directing further histologic and clinical investigations. This knowledge will be most useful when clinical information is incomplete or not available.

ADENOCARCINOMA

Metastatic adenocarcinomas involving the skin may appear very similar or even be indistinguishable on morphologic features from sweat gland carcinomas that are primary to the skin. As the latter are rare, the possibility that a tumor could represent a metastasis should always be considered before rendering a diagnosis of a skin adnexal carcinoma. The most common primary sites for metastatic adenocarcinomas involving the skin are breast, lung, and large bowel. Less common primary sites include stomach, prostate, pancreas, ovary, endometrium, and thyroid.

Cutaneous metastases from the breast have a variety of appearances that are often similar to the primary tumor, and hence comparison of histology may be helpful. The most common appearance is that of scattered, isolated, well-formed glands and solid nests of tumor cells (Fig. 18.7); however, similar appearances are also seen frequently in metastatic adenocarcinomas from the lung (Fig. 18.8), stomach, or pancreas. Sometimes the metastatic tumor, like the breast primary, is associated with abundant dense sclerotic collagenous stroma (Fig. 18.9). A linear pattern of tumor cells in single files dissecting between the dermal collagen bundles is characteristic of lobular carcinoma from the breast (Figs. 18.10–18.13) but a similar pattern may sometimes be seen in other tumors including gastric and prostatic adenocarcinomas and occasionally in large cell lymphomas or neuroendocrine carcinomas. So-called inflammatory carcinoma, which most commonly occurs in

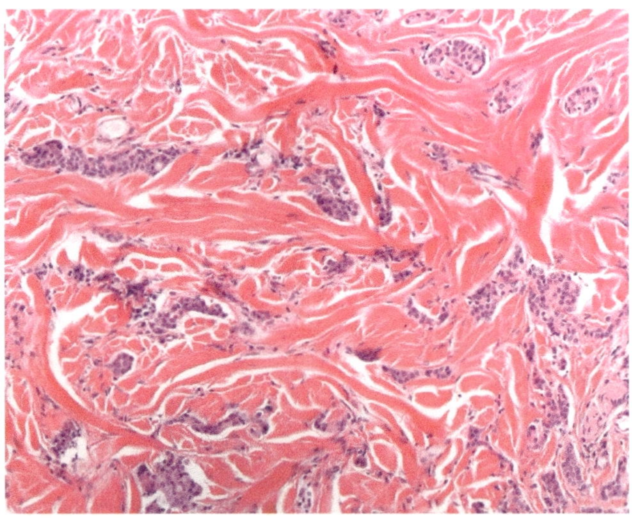

FIG. 18.7
Metastatic breast carcinoma of ductal type. Medium-power micrograph showing nests of tumor with focal gland formation.

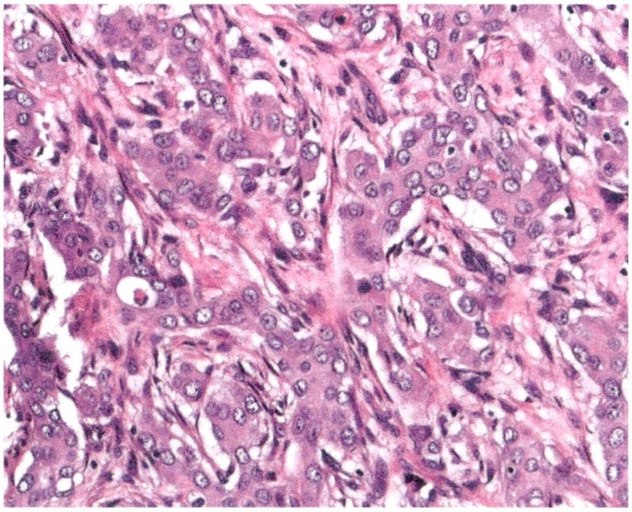

FIG. 18.8

Metastatic adenocarcinoma from the lung. High-power micrograph showing clusters of large pleomorphic epithelioid cells with focal gland formation.

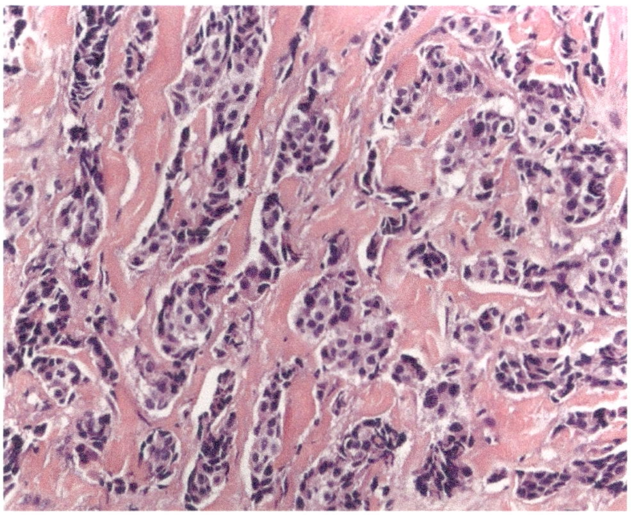

FIG. 18.9

Metastatic breast carcinoma of ductal type. Medium-power micrograph showing islands of tumor associated with surrounding dense sclerotic dermal collagenous stroma.

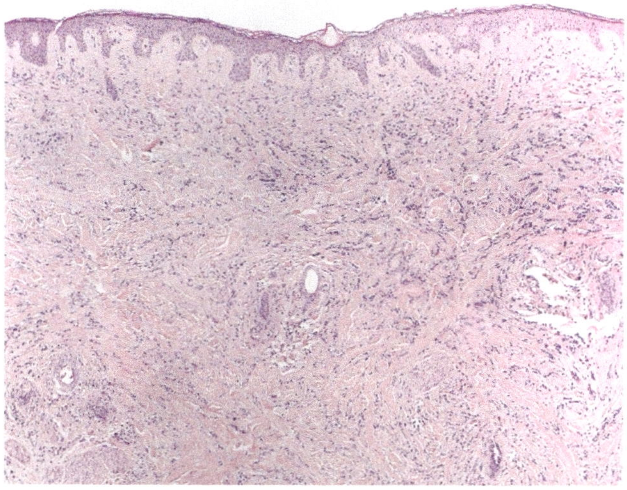

FIG. 18.10

Metastatic breast carcinoma of lobular type. Low-power micrograph showing single files and small clusters of cells. It is not possible to be certain from the morphologic appearance that this tumor is a carcinoma. Appropriate immunostains to exclude other possibilities (such as a large cell lymphoma, melanoma, or epithelioid sarcoma) are necessary (see Table 18.3).

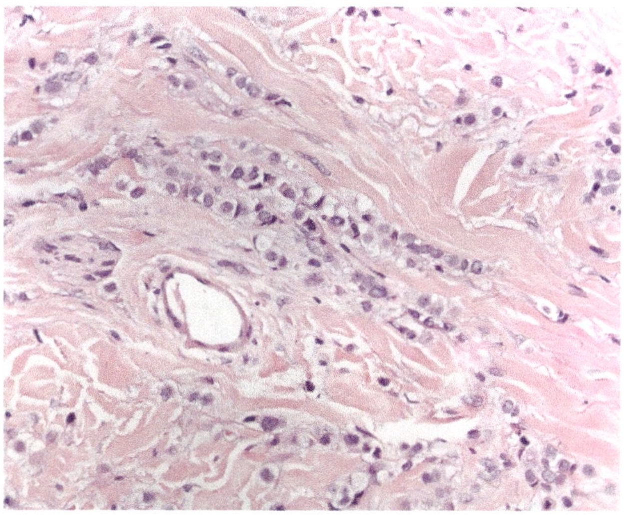

FIG. 18.11

Metastatic breast carcinoma of lobular type. Medium-power micrograph showing single files of large epithelioid cells dissecting between the dermal collagen bundles.

breast carcinoma involving the skin of the breast and/or chest wall, is characterized by the presence of numerous intralymphatic tumor deposits and dermal edema.

A well-differentiated glandular architecture with elongated cells, prominent peripheral palisading, and luminal necrosis is characteristic of adenocarcinoma of colorectal origin. Papillary differentiation within an adenocarcinoma may occur in primary sweat gland adenocarcinomas, as well as in metastases from the thyroid, lung, female genital tract, pancreas, breast, and large bowel. The presence of eosinophilic colloid-like material within the glandular spaces (Figs. 18.14–18.17) or nuclear clearing, grooves, and pseudoinclusions raises the possibility of a thyroid tumor and should prompt the use of appropriate confirmatory immunohistochemistry (see below). A signet ring cell appearance is characteristic of gastric adenocarcinoma, but less commonly may be observed in adenocarcinomas from any primary site including the skin. Mucinous adenocarcinoma (colloid carcinoma) is characterized by the presence of islands of cohesive tumor cells floating within abundant extracellular mucin. It may be present in adenocarcinomas of sweat gland origin or in metastases from any site, especially the breast, pancreas, stomach, large bowel, and prostate. Similarly, adenoid cystic carcinoma may represent a primary skin tumor or a

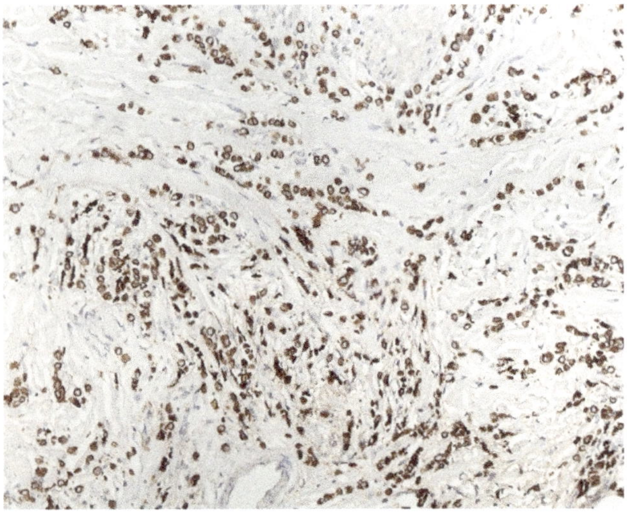

FIG. 18.12

Metastatic breast carcinoma of lobular type. Medium-power micrograph showing positive staining of tumor cells with the broad-spectrum anticytokeratin antibody AE1/AE3.

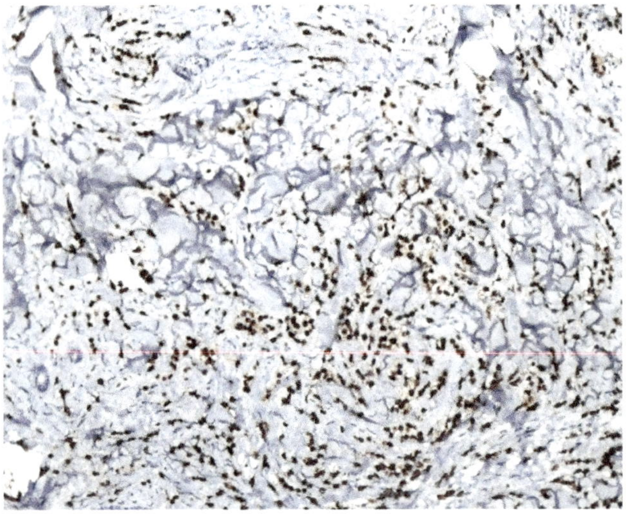

FIG. 18.13

Metastatic breast carcinoma of lobular type. Medium-power micrograph showing positive staining of tumor cells for estrogen receptor.

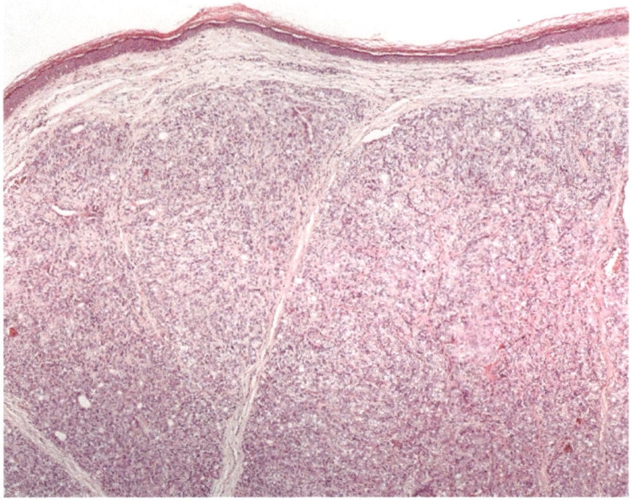

FIG. 18.14

Metastatic thyroid carcinoma of follicular type. Low-power micrograph showing clusters of epithelioid cells with focal follicle formation.

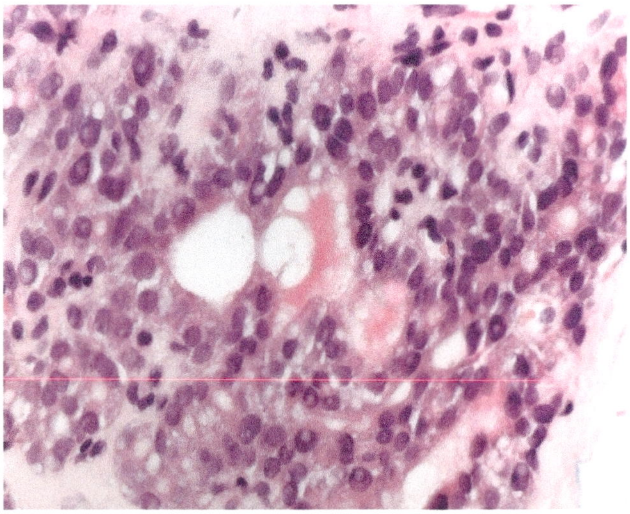

FIG. 18.15

Metastatic thyroid carcinoma of follicular type. High-power micrograph showing clusters of epithelioid cells with focal follicle formation and associated colloid.

metastasis from a salivary gland, respiratory tract, or other site. Rarely metastatic adenocarcinoma may show epidermotropism with involvement of the epidermis and, thus, may mimic superficial spreading melanoma, Paget disease, or pagetoid Bowen disease.

Metastatic clear-cell carcinoma is typically of renal origin and shows nests of clear cells within a richly vascular capillary network (Fig. 18.18). Nonetheless, metastatic carcinoma from almost any site, most commonly the lung, ovary, endometrium, pancreas, and cervix, may be composed predominantly of clear cells. Metastatic clear-cell carcinoma must be distinguished from primary skin tumors including clear-cell squamous cell carcinoma and various adnexal carcinomas such as sebaceous carcinoma, trichilemmal carcinoma, and clear-cell sweat gland tumors. Characteristic histologic features of these primary tumors mean that distinction is usually possible on morphologic grounds, but immunohistochemistry may also be useful.

Immunohistochemistry has only limited usefulness in determining whether an adenocarcinoma is of adnexal or metastatic origin, although there are a few exceptions (Table 18.4). A thyroid origin is supported by positive staining for thyroglobulin, thyroid transcription factor-1 (TTF-1), and PAX8. Prostate carcinoma is usually positive for prostate-specific antigen (PSA), prostate membrane–specific antigen (PMSA), prostatic acid phosphatase, and NKX3.1 and often negative for the cytokeratins (CK) CK7 and CK20. Lung adenocarcinomas (and some pulmonary large cell carcinomas) are

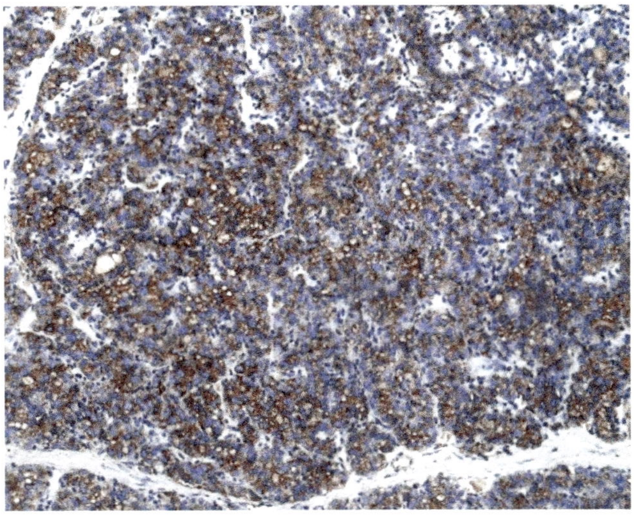

FIG. 18.16

Metastatic thyroid carcinoma of follicular type. Medium-power micrograph showing positive staining of tumor cells for thyroglobulin.

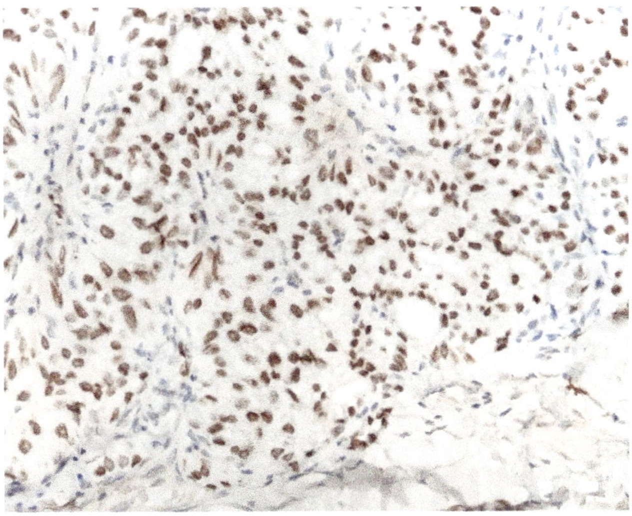

FIG. 18.17

Metastatic thyroid carcinoma of follicular type. High-power micrograph showing positive nuclear staining of tumor cells with the antibody TTF-1.

usually positive for TTF-1 and NapsinA. Distinguishing between a primary cutaneous malignant sweat gland tumor and metastatic breast carcinoma is challenging, as estrogen and progesterone receptors, mammaglobin, S100 protein, gross cystic disease fluid protein-15 (GCDFP-15), GATA3, and carcinoembryonic antigen (CEA) are often expressed in both these tumors, reflecting the close relationship between sweat glands and the glandular tissue of the breast. Differential staining for CK7 and CK20 has only limited value in the differential diagnosis of an adenocarcinoma in the skin. CK7 is usually positive in sweat gland tumors as well as in carcinomas from many other sites (including breast, lung, and the female genital tract), although it may be negative, particularly in more poorly differentiated tumors. CK20 may be more helpful as its expression in skin adnexal

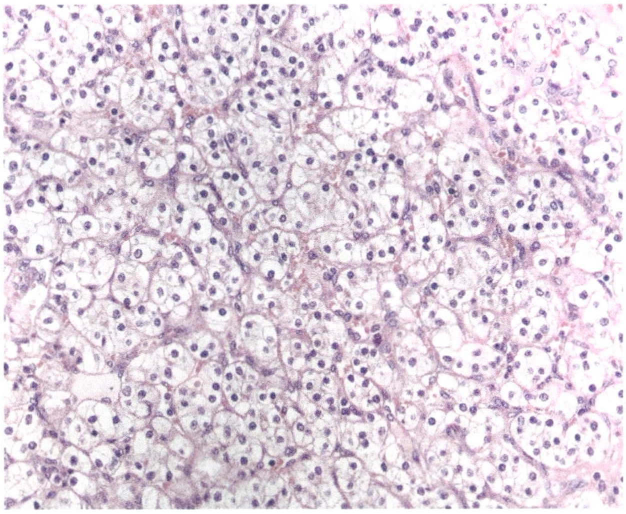

FIG. 18.18

Metastatic renal cell carcinoma of clear-cell type. Medium-power micrograph showing nests of large cells with clear cytoplasm. The nests are surrounded by thin-walled capillary-type blood vessels.

tumors is exceptionally rare, and CK20 is expressed in only a limited range of tumors; it is characteristic of colorectal adenocarcinomas (along with SATB2 and CDX-2) and is not uncommon in adenocarcinomas of the stomach and pancreas and urothelial tumors. CK5/6 and p63 have been reported to be more frequently positive in cutaneous adnexal carcinomas compared with metastatic adenocarcinomas involving the skin, although their low specificity will limit their usefulness in individual cases. Renal cell carcinomas are often positive for CD10, PAX2, PAX8, and epithelial membrane antigen (EMA), although the latter is also commonly expressed by other cutaneous clear-cell carcinomas, particularly sebaceous carcinoma and squamous cell carcinoma. Morphologic features are more useful in recognizing metastatic renal cell carcinoma, particularly that of the classic clear-cell type. Malignant mesothelioma may invade the skin of the chest wall or occasionally metastasize to the skin and hence may enter the differential diagnosis of a cutaneous adenocarcinoma. Epithelioid mesotheliomas are typically positive for calretinin, CK5/6, Wilms tumor protein (WT-1; nuclear staining), and D2-40 (podoplanin) and negative for CEA, BerEP4, MOC-31, BG-8, and cluster of differentiation (CD) 15.

SQUAMOUS CELL CARCINOMA

Metastatic squamous cell carcinoma may originate from a wide variety of sites including the lung, cervix, esophagus, oropharynx, and larynx as well as skin, and there are no specific morphologic features that are of assistance in determining the site of origin of the tumor. The presence of keratinization and well-formed intercellular bridges characterize well and moderately differentiated squamous cell carcinomas. It should be noted that focal keratinization may be present in a variety of other primary and secondary nonsquamous skin tumors, and this is a potential source of misdiagnosis. The tumors in which this is most likely to occur include basal cell carcinomas and skin adnexal tumors. As primary squamous cell carcinoma of the skin is much more common than cutaneous metastases of squamous cell carcinoma, lack of an identifiable epidermal origin should not be taken as definitive evidence that the tumor is a metastasis unless this is supported by an appropriate clinical history and multiple tissue blocks and/or sections have been examined. A primary squamous cell carcinoma of the skin may not show involvement of the epidermis if sampling is limited or if the epidermal component is present only focally. Cases of metastatic squamous cell carcinoma showing epidermotropism have been reported, making distinction from primary cutaneous squamous cell carcinoma extremely difficult. Careful clinicopathologic correlation is necessary to avoid misdiagnosis. Poorly differentiated squamous cell carcinomas may show only very focal evidence of squamous differentiation, identification of which may require extensive sampling. Like their primary cutaneous counterpart, metastatic spindle cell and anaplastic squamous carcinomas may be difficult to distinguish from melanoma or sarcoma on morphology, and immunohistochemistry may be necessary. It is important to recognize that spindle cell squamous cell carcinomas are usually negative with the antibody CAM5.2 (which recognizes the low-molecular-weight cytokeratins CK8 and CK18) and are often also negative with the broad-spectrum keratin marker AE1/AE3. However, stains for complex, high-molecular-weight CKs such as CK5/6 and MNF116 are positive and are usually required to avoid misdiagnosis.

While it is usually not difficult to recognize squamous cell carcinoma, occasionally it can be very difficult or impossible to determine with certainty whether the tumor represents a skin primary or a metastasis even with available clinical details. Immunohistochemistry and tumor morphology do not assist in determining whether a squamous carcinoma is a primary cutaneous tumor or a metastasis or, in the case of the latter, in determining its likely site of origin. On occasion, molecular studies may help by documenting the presence of ultraviolet (UV) mutation signature, thereby excluding an extracutaneous origin. In situ hybridization studies for the human papillomavirus (HPV) may also provide support for the likely metastatic status of a tumor, if it carries the same HPV type as a prior cervical or oral mucosal squamous cell carcinoma.

NEUROENDOCRINE CARCINOMAS

Neuroendocrine carcinomas may arise from any organ, although the lung and skin (Merkel cell carcinoma) are the two most common sites. Neuroendocrine differentiation is recognized morphologically by the presence of small- to intermediate-sized cells with high nuclear-to-cytoplasmic ratios, coarse granular nuclear chromatin, and inconspicuous nucleoli. Most cutaneous neuroendocrine carcinomas are high-grade tumors associated with frequent mitoses and apoptotic cells (Fig. 18.19). Small cell neuroendocrine carcinomas can be difficult to distinguish morphologically from other so-called small blue cell tumors such as lymphomas, Ewing sarcoma, rhabdomyosarcoma, and some cases of melanoma. Appropriate immunohistochemistry is usually necessary to confirm the epithelial nature of the tumor and to exclude the other possibilities (Table 18.6). Neuroendocrine carcinomas are usually positive with CAM5.2 and broad-spectrum cytokeratin antibodies such as AE1/AE3. Neuroendocrine differentiation can be confirmed by positive staining for neuroendocrine markers such as INSM1, chromogranin, synaptophysin, and CD56. The latter is less specific but more sensitive in high-grade neuroendocrine carcinomas. Immunohistochemistry can be useful in distinguishing metastatic small cell carcinoma of pulmonary origin from Merkel cell carcinoma, as the former is usually positive for CK7 and TTF-1 and negative for CK20, while the latter is typically positive for CK20 (Fig. 18.20) and negative for CK7 and TTF-1 (Table 18.5). A subset of Merkel cell carcinomas may also show positivity with immunohistochemistry for Merkel cell polyomavirus using the antibodies CM2B4 or AB2. A subset of primary salivary gland small cell carcinomas show a similar immunoprofile to Merkel cell carcinoma (i.e., CK20 positive, TTF-1 negative).

Medullary carcinoma of the thyroid gland is another neuroendocrine carcinoma that may rarely involve the skin. It usually expresses calcitonin (which can also be measured in the serum), enabling distinction from other neuroendocrine tumors.

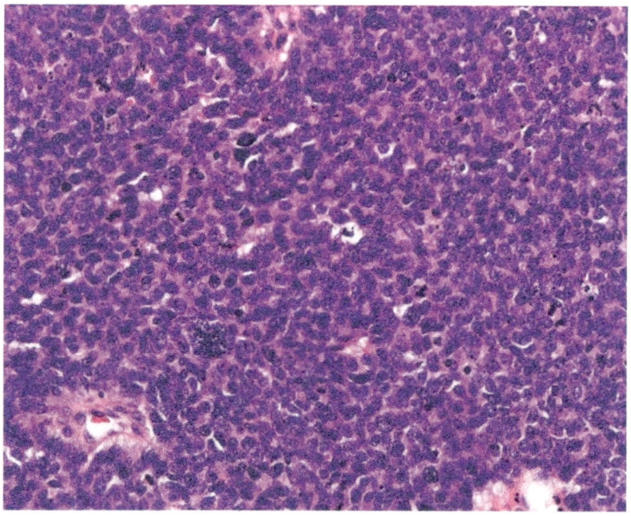

FIG. 18.19

Metastatic Merkel cell carcinoma. High-power micrograph showing tumor composed of sheets of cells with high nuclear-to-cytoplasmic ratio, granular chromatin, and mostly inconspicuous nucleoli. Frequent mitoses and apoptotic cells are present.

TABLE 18.6

Immunostains Useful in Determining the Histogenesis/Line of Differentiation of a Malignant "Small Round Blue Cell" Tumor Involving the Skin

	TYPE OF TUMOR					
Antibody	Small Cell NE Carcinoma	Melanoma	Lymphoma	Ewing Sarcoma	Rhabdomyosarcoma	Neuroblastoma
Keratins	+	−	−	−/+	−	−
Chromogranin	+/−	−	−	−	−	−
Synaptophysin	+/−	−	−	−	−	+/−
CD56	+	−/+	−/+	−/+	−/+	+
Neurofilament protein	+	−	−	−	−	+
Neuron-specific enolase	−	−/+	−	−	−	+
S100 protein	−	+	−	−/+	−	−/+
HMB45	−	+/−	−	−	−	−
Melan A	−	+/−	−	−	−	−
CD3	−	−	+/−	−	−	−
CD20	−	−	+/−	−	−	−
CD30	−	−	−/+	−	−	−
TdT	−	−	−/+	−	−	−
CD99	−	−	−/+	+ (membranous pattern)	−	−
FLI1	−	−/+	−/+[a]	+	−	−
Desmin	−	−	−	−	+/−	−
MyoD1	−	−	−	−	+	−
Myogenin	−	−	−	−	+/−	−

[a]Positive in 85% of lymphoblastic lymphomas, variable in others.
+, Usually positive; +/−, often positive, sometimes negative; −/+, often negative, occasionally positive; −, usually negative; *NE*, neuroendocrine; *TdT*, terminal deoxynucleotidyl transferase.

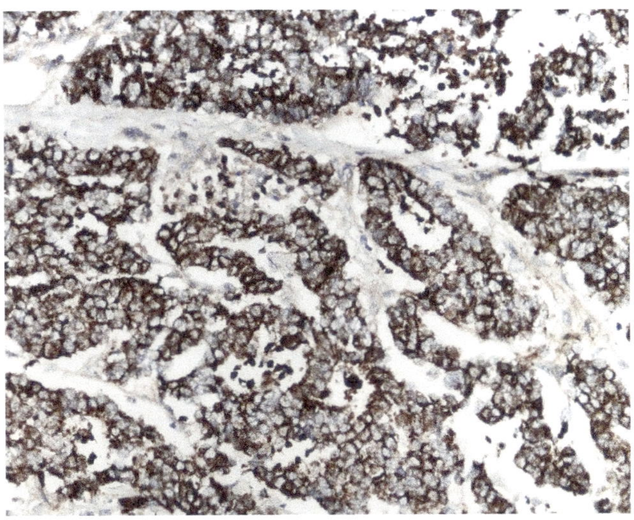

FIG. 18.20
Metastatic Merkel cell carcinoma. High-power micrograph showing positive staining of the tumor cells for CK20.

Low-grade neuroendocrine tumors (carcinoid tumors) are composed of uniform cells with abundant granular cytoplasm, with a nested or trabecular growth pattern and characteristically low mitotic activity. When such tumors involve the skin, they are almost always metastases, as primary low-grade neuroendocrine tumors of the skin are exceptionally rare. The most common primary sites are lung, appendix, small and large bowel, and stomach. While the neuroendocrine differentiation of the tumor can be confirmed by the use of appropriate immunohistochemistry, it may not be possible to determine the primary site of the tumor from either its morphology or its immunoprofile. However, in contrast to high-grade neuroendocrine carcinomas in which TTF-1 staining is not specific for a lung origin, in the context of well-differentiated neuroendocrine tumors (including carcinoid tumors), positive staining for TTF-1 suggests the possibility of a primary in lung, while positive staining for CDX-2 suggests the possibility of a gastrointestinal or pancreatic primary.

MELANOMA

Skin and subcutaneous tissues are common sites of metastasis for melanoma and the skin is often the first site of metastasis. The reported prevalence of melanoma metastases to the skin varies with the geographic variation in the incidence of melanoma and also depends on whether so-called local and in-transit metastases are included. In Australia, the country with the highest incidence of melanoma in the world, melanoma is the most frequent metastatic tumor in the skin. Local and in-transit metastases are distinguished by their proximity to the primary cutaneous melanoma site and usually occur in the skin between the primary site and the draining regional lymph nodes (Fig. 18.21). They probably represent outgrowths of intralymphatic tumor emboli into dermis or subcutis. Occasionally metastases may occur distal to the primary tumor site, possibly as a result of retrograde lymphatic or perivascular (angiotropic) spread. In the appropriate clinical context, the diagnosis of cutaneous deposits of metastatic melanoma is usually straightforward. In most cases, they differ from primary melanoma by the absence of an epidermal component, the presence of an uninvolved "grenz" zone of superficial dermis (Fig. 18.5), more frequent mitotic activity, and the frequent presence of an associated lymphoid infiltrate (Fig. 18.22). Occasionally, molecular analysis, and the identification of a common driver mutation between a primary melanoma and the suspected metastasis, may assist in the diagnosis. Epidermotropic metastatic melanoma, however, may be indistinguishable from primary melanoma and only by careful clinicopathologic correlation will the correct diagnosis be reached (Fig. 18.23). Furthermore, some primary melanomas may lack an epidermal component and may be diagnosed as melanoma metastases unless the possibility of a so-called primary dermal melanoma is considered and thorough correlation of the pathologic and clinical features is performed. If no melanin pigment is present, immunostains including for S100 protein, Melan A, HMB45, tyrosinase, SOX10, and/or MITF1 may be necessary to confirm that a cutaneous metastasis is melanoma.

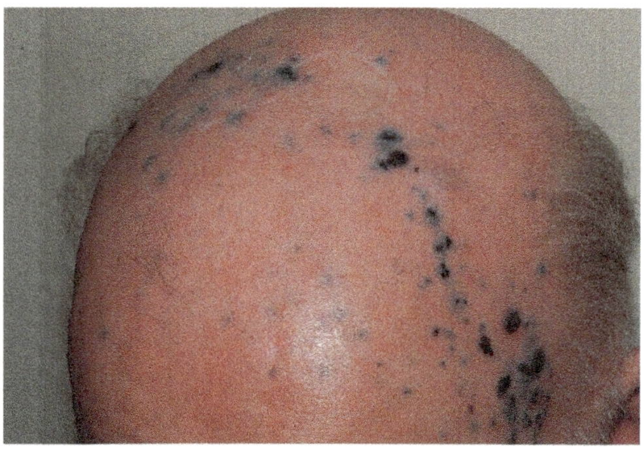

FIG. 18.21

Metastatic melanoma. Clinical photograph showing numerous cutaneous and subcutaneous deposits of tumor on the scalp. A skin graft at the primary cutaneous melanoma site is present on the top of the scalp. (Courtesy of Dr. Kerwin Shannon, Melanoma Institute Australia.)

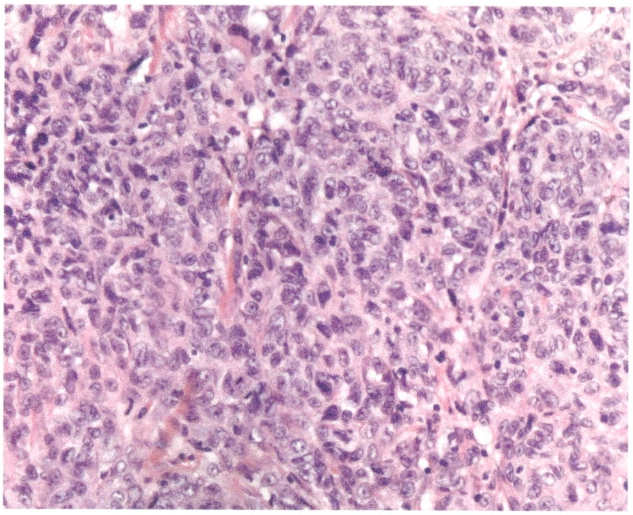

FIG. 18.22

Metastatic melanoma. High-power micrograph showing clusters of pleomorphic epithelioid cells within the dermis. In the absence of intracytoplasmic melanin pigment, an appropriate panel of immunostains would be necessary to confirm that the tumor is a melanoma and not a poorly differentiated carcinoma, lymphoma, or sarcoma (see Table 18.3).

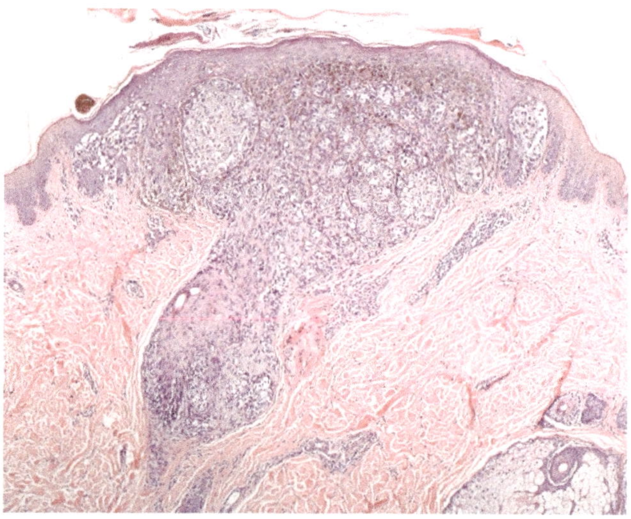

FIG. 18.23

Epidermotropic metastatic melanoma mimicking primary melanoma. Medium-power micrograph showing an epidermal and dermal components to the tumor. The diagnosis cannot be made without clinicopathologic correlation.

MISCELLANEOUS TUMORS

Hemopoietic tumors in the skin may originate there or may represent cutaneous involvement by leukemia, systemic lymphoma, or lymphoma originating in other sites. Clinicopathologic correlation is the only means of distinguishing between these possibilities and, as the prognosis is vastly different for morphologically similar tumors (e.g., primary cutaneous diffuse large B-cell lymphoma versus cutaneous involvement by nodal diffuse large B-cell lymphoma), and therefore the distinction is mandatory. Hemopoietic tumors are classified on the basis of their morphologic, immunophenotypic, molecular, and cytogenetic features, the details of which are beyond the scope of this chapter.

A wide variety of other tumors including mesotheliomas, germ cell tumors, various sarcomas, thymomas, odontogenic tumors, tumors of the central nervous system, adrenal tumors, paragangliomas, and cardiac myxomas have all been reported to metastasize to the skin on rare occasions. Careful morphologic examination, appropriate use of ancillary investigations, and, most importantly, thorough clinicopathologic correlation should allow accurate diagnosis.

SUGGESTED FURTHER READING

Gan, E. Y., Chio, M. T., & Tan, W. P. (2015). A retrospective review of cutaneous metastases at the National Skin Centre Singapore. *Australas J Dermatol*, *56*(1), 1–6.

Greco, F. A., Lennington, W. J., Spigel, D. R., & Hainsworth, J. D. (2013). Molecular profiling diagnosis in unknown primary cancer: accuracy and ability to complement standard pathology. *Journal of the National Cancer Institute*, *105*(11), 782–790.

Hainsworth, J. D., Rubin, M. S., Spigel, D. R., Boccia, R. V., Raby, S., Quinn, R., & Greco, F. A. (2013). Molecular gene expression profiling to predict the tissue of origin and direct site-specific therapy in patients with carcinoma of unknown primary site: A prospective trial of the Sarah Cannon research institute. *Journal of Clinical Oncology*, *31*(2), 217–223.

Lookingbill, D. P., Spangler, N., & Helm, K. F. (1993). Cutaneous metastases in patients with metastatic carcinoma: A retrospective study of 4020 patients. *Journal of the American Academy of Dermatology*, *29*(2 Pt 1), 228–236, 1993.

Lookingbill, D. P., Spangler, N., & Sexton, F. M. (1990). Skin involvement as the presenting sign of internal carcinoma. A retrospective study of 7316 cancer patients. *Journal of the American Academy of Dermatology*, *22*(1), 19–26.

Qureshi, H. S., Ormsby, A. H., Lee, M. W., Zarbo, R. J., & Ma, C. K. (2004). The diagnostic utility of p63, CK5/6, CK 7, and CK 20 in distinguishing primary cutaneous adnexal neoplasms from metastatic carcinomas. *Journal of Cutaneous Pathology*, *31*(2), 145–152.

Saeed, S., Keehn, C. A., & Morgan, M. B. (2004). Cutaneous metastasis: A clinical, pathological, and immunohistochemical appraisal. *Journal of Cutaneous Pathology*, *31*(6), 419–430.

Swetter, S. M., Ecker, P. M., Johnson, D. L., & Harvell, J. D. (2004). Primary dermal melanoma: A distinct subtype of melanoma. *Archives of Dermatology*, *140*(1), 99–103.

Teyateeti, P., & Ungtrakul, T. (2021). Retrospective review of cutaneous metastasis among 11,418 patients with solid malignancy: A tertiary cancer center experience. *Medicine (Baltimore)*, *100*(29), e26737.

Varadhachary, G. R., Talantov, D., Raber, M. N., Meng, C., Hess, K. R., Jatkoe, T., Lenzi, R., Spigel, D. R., Wang, Y., Greco, F. A., Abbruzzese, J. L., & Hainsworth, J. D. (2008). Molecular profiling of carcinoma of unknown primary and correlation with clinical evaluation. *Journal of Clinical Oncology*, *26*(27), 4442–4448.

Wagle, N., Berger, M. F., Davis, M. J., Blumenstiel, B., Defelice, M., Pochanard, P., Ducar, M., Van Hummelen, P., Macconaill, L. E., Hahn, W. C., Meyerson, M., Gabriel, S. B., & Garraway, L. A. (2012). High-throughput detection of actionable genomic alterations in clinical tumor samples by targeted, massively parallel sequencing. *Cancer Discovery*, *2*(1), 82–93.

Section 3

Pathology of Special Sites

Neoplastic and Nonneoplastic Disorders of the Nail Apparatus

19

Beth S. Ruben

Dermatopathology of the nail unit remains a somewhat esoteric and elusive subject for several reasons. Most dermatopathologists have little experience with material from this site, and little has been written comprehensively about this subject. Part of the difficulty stems from the fact that many dermatologic conditions affecting the nail unit are diagnosed on clinical grounds alone, in part owing to the reluctance of practitioners to perform biopsies at this site, especially if diagnostic lesions are present elsewhere on the skin, and of patients to submit to such a procedure. Clinicians and pathologists alike may also have limited knowledge of the normal anatomy of this site and of diseases that affect it. This has a tendency to result in suboptimal specimens and interpretation of them. Disorders at other cutaneous sites may have similar histologic appearance when expressing themselves in the nail unit, but there are some differences, as a result of the peculiarities of the nail anatomy, that may create diagnostic difficulty. This chapter reviews the gross and microscopic anatomy of the nail unit; describes methods of biopsy appropriate to this area and the types of specimens that result; and illustrates select more commonly encountered or distinctive inflammatory, infectious, and neoplastic disorders that affect it.

ANATOMY OF THE NAIL UNIT

GROSS ANATOMY

The nail unit includes the nail matrix and nail bed and their product, the nail plate. Important sheaths, including the cuticle, also produced by nail unit epithelium protect the nail from the environment (Fig. 19.1). Epithelial folds and grooves provide protection and framing. There are also fibrocollagenous supportive tissues and a distinctive onychodermis. Clinically, the lunula corresponds to the distal matrix. The proximal nail matrix lies well behind the proximal nail fold. The proximal nail fold may cover the matrix to varying degrees. The lunula can generally be observed best on the thumbs and hallux. The matrix produces the bulk of the nail plate. The cuticle (or false cuticle as it is also known) emanates from the proximal nail fold and adheres to the nail plate. The true cuticle, produced by the undersurface of the proximal nail fold (eponychium), is rarely visible but forms an important sheath to protect the nail unit. From the lunula to the onychodermal dermal band lies the nail bed. It makes a small contribution to the undersurface of the nail plate. The onychodermal band is the last point of attachment of the nail plate to the nail bed. The free edge of the nail covers the hyponychium, the most distal portion of the nail unit.

BASIC NAIL PHYSIOLOGY—DISEASE FACT SHEET

- Nail matrix: responsible for most of nail plate production
- Nail bed: assures nail plate adhesion
- Proximal nail fold: protects nail production
- Nail growth rate:
  - Fingernails: 3 mm/month
  - Toenails: 1 mm/month

Histologic Features

The nail matrix epithelium consists of gently rounded ridges, called mamelons, that are oriented longitudinally and angle toward the tip of the digit, becoming progressively flattened in transition to the nail bed epithelium (Fig. 19.2). The keratinocytes of the lower matrix are basaloid, and they flatten and become more eosinophilic as they keratinize abruptly along the keratogenous zone to form the nail plate. The nail plate, composed of hard and soft keratins, is formed via onychokeratinization, which has many similarities to trichilemmal keratinization. Keratinization is abrupt and occurs without a granular zone. There may be several normally inapparent layers in the nail plate.

The proximal matrix produces the superficial aspects of the plate (roughly one-third); the dorsal matrix produces a very thin surface layer of the plate, giving it its luster; and the distal matrix the remaining lower two-thirds, with a small contribution from the nail bed. These features explain how nail pitting occurs via insults to the proximal matrix and how proximal matrix damage produces more obvious nail plate deformity. The nail unit also shares some of the same

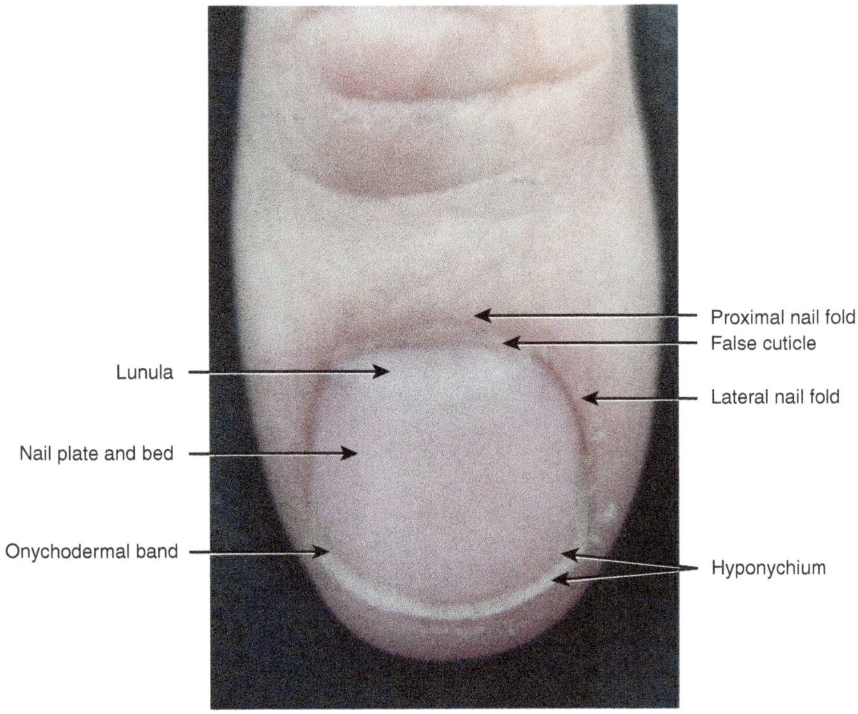

FIG. 19.1

Normal nail unit.

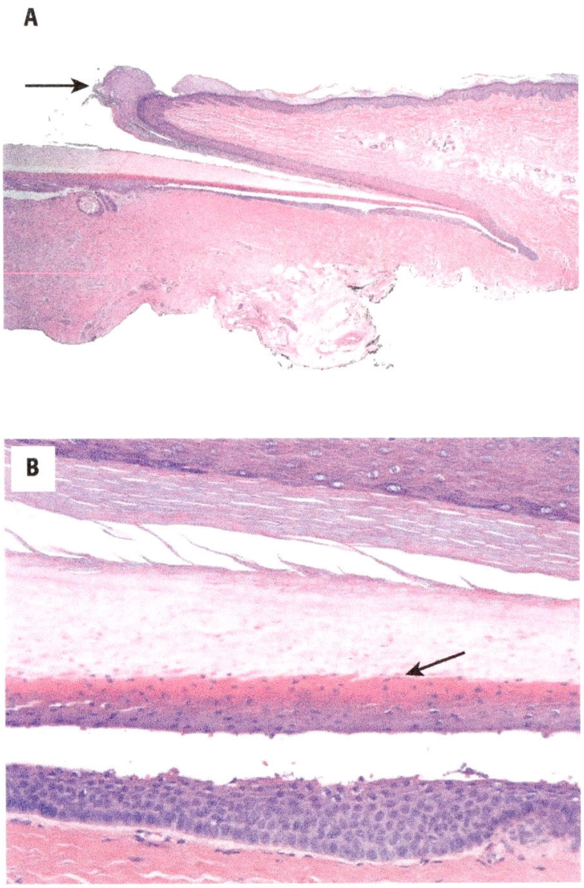

FIG. 19.2

Microscopic features of the proximal nail unit. **A,** Nail fold *(arrow)* and nail matrix (with incidental subungual epidermoid inclusion). **B,** Ventral surface of proximal nail fold (eponychium) with granular cell layer on top and matrix epithelium at the bottom. In between is the keratogenous zone *(arrow)* nail plate.

keratin subunits seen in hair. Unlike in keratinization of hair, there are no trichohyalinegranules, nor are there keratohyaline granules. In fact, keratohyaline granules or a granular zone of the nail matrix or bed are pathologic findings in the nail unit. These features can be seen nonspecifically in a variety of conditions, including psoriasis, lichen planus, trachyonychia, and onychomycosis, and can also be seen in the setting of trauma or neoplasms, which create pressure on the nail matrix or otherwise disrupt nail unit architecture. Nail matrix hypergranulosis as a response to various insults may be more analogous to parakeratosis at cutaneous sites.

The nail bed that occurs beyond the keratogenous zone of the matrix (Fig. 19.3) contains a thinner and more eosinophilic epithelium, whose parallel ridges (not rete) are oriented longitudinally and interdigitate in "tongue and groove" fashion with the underlying dermis. There is also interdigitation with the underside of the nail plate, producing longitudinal striations. This pattern of ridges can only be appreciated when examining transverse "cuts" through the nail bed (from side to side) and is thus often not evident in longitudinal biopsies. These architectural features lead to the appearance of splinter hemorrhages over the nail bed. Trauma to the distal vessels leads to hemorrhage, which accumulates in the grooves. Although the derivation of the nail plate has been a subject of debate among nail aficionados, many recent studies indicate that the nail matrix gives rise to the bulk of the nail plate, with only a scant contribution from the nail bed, mainly to its underside. The nail bed may make more of a contribution in the setting of certain diseases.

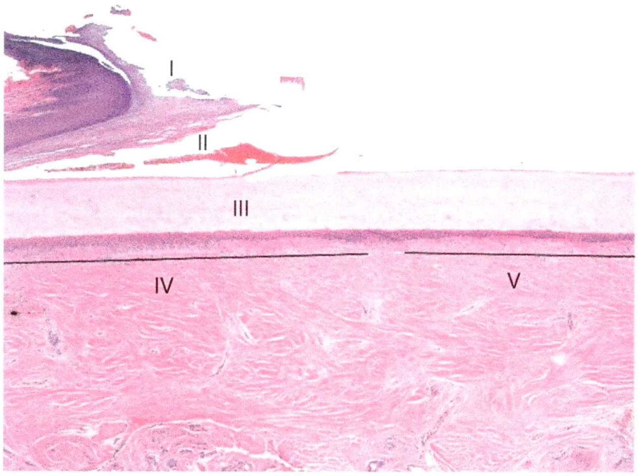

FIG. 19.3

Histologic features of the distal nail matrix, nail bed, and hyponychium. *I*, False cuticle; *II*, true cuticle; *III*, nail plate; *IV*, distal nail matrix; *V*, nail bed.

The framing of the nail unit consists of the proximal and lateral nail folds and grooves, which transition to the acral skin surrounding the nail unit. These provide structural support to the nail plate and protect it from trauma. The folds also give rise to the sheaths, which further protect the nail plate. The sheaths include the cuticles, hyponychium, and onychodermal band. The true cuticle arises from the ventral surface of the proximal nail fold (eponychium) and is formed of semihard keratin by onycholemmal keratinization. It blends with the surface of the nail plate. The solehorn, a barely visible zone that forms at the undersurface of the distal nail plate, is similar. The false cuticle (the one we generally think of as the cuticle) is visible as an extension of the apex of the proximal nail fold. It keratinizes, as does normal acral skin and the hyponychium. Chronic diseases, especially those that lead to cessation of nail growth or trauma to the proximal nail fold, lead to a loss of the cuticle and rounding up of the proximal nail fold, allowing for further damage to the nail unit, as in paronychia. The hyponychium is the distal counterpart to the eponychium, also forming a seal around the nail unit and a transition to the surrounding skin. It also keratinizes via a granular layer. The hyponychial attachment to the nail plate can be seen under the plate as the onychodermal band.

There is no distinct papillary or reticular dermis in the nail unit, nor is there subcutaneous fat except at its periphery on acral skin. There are also no adnexa in the nail unit except for sweat glands in the dorsal aspect of the proximal nail fold. There are specialized nerve endings in these areas, including Meissnerian and Pacinian corpuscles, as well as specialized vascular shunts, the glomus apparati. The dermis is often myxoid. Recent studies have suggested a specialized "onychodermis" of the nail unit.

BIOPSY TECHNIQUES AND NAIL BIOPSY PROCESSING

Sampling the nail unit presents special problems. A punch or shave biopsy on other cutaneous sites is relatively straightforward, but in the nail unit, there are unique considerations from a technical and functional standpoint. Some techniques are better than others as far as obtaining tissue suitable for diagnosis while preserving cosmesis and function for the patient. Damage to the nail matrix, especially the proximal matrix, can result in permanent nail dystrophy. The procured tissue must be handled with utmost care. Communication of the submitting clinician with laboratory staff and pathologists is essential for ensuring proper handling of the specimen.

Most commonly used biopsy techniques, such as punch, shave, or excision, can be used for nail unit sampling, but the barrier of the nail plate can present challenges to obtaining a biopsy suitable for interpretation. En bloc longitudinal excisional biopsy is the gold standard and usually mitigates some of the problems with disruption of the nail epithelium that can occur using other methods. This procedure generally includes the entire length of the nail unit, including proximal nail fold, nail matrix, nail bed, hyponychium, and nail plate. As in the case of excisional biopsies of melanocytic neoplasms elsewhere, such a procedure is optimal for allowing complete assessment of symmetry and circumscription of melanocytic lesions and to avoid compression artifact. They can also be very useful in evaluating nail dystrophy when it may not be clear clinically which component of the nail unit is responsible for it.

Nail matrix biopsies are often performed for evaluation of melanocytic lesions, which usually arise in the distal matrix, and for some inflammatory disorders. They can be obtained via a punch biopsy through the proximal nail fold and nail plate to the matrix, but this represents a somewhat blind technique because the area of pigmentation responsible for the pigmented band is not directly visualized. A preferable technique involves incising and retracting the nail fold to expose the proximal nail plate, transversely incising and gently removing the proximal plate, and then directly sampling the matrix by a punch or shave technique. Another technique involves avulsing the entire nail plate first to expose the underlying matrix and bed, at which point a punch or shave biopsy can be done. This has a tendency to cause more disruption to the underlying epithelium. And leaving the distal nail plate in place can be a benefit to function during the healing process. Regardless of the method, careful attention must be given to avoid crushing the delicate specimen containing the nail epithelium. The nail plate should also be submitted because a substantial amount of superficial epithelium may accompany it and hold diagnostic clues. Punch biopsies of the nail bed are often sufficient for diagnosis of inflammatory and some neoplastic conditions and may avoid resultant nail dystrophy.

Orientation of the specimen with respect to which area of the nail unit was sampled should also be provided to the laboratory, along with any specific instructions, to make sure the specimen is properly handled. Small biopsies benefit from being placed on a piece of cardboard or paper and then in formalin to preserve orientation of the nail matrix epithelium and prevent curling of thin specimens. Ideally, the pathologist should be closely involved in grossing these specimens or providing guidance to the laboratory team. When sectioning of the specimen is involved, a longitudinal plane is preferred to maintain orientation of all components of the nail unit. Although some softening techniques can help in preparing and processing the specimen if it contains nail plate, including calcium or sodium hydroxide preparation and cedarwood oil processing, it is unknown how these techniques might affect ancillary studies, such as immunoperoxidase staining of epithelium. There is certainly no place for decalcification per se unless bone is present. However, a simple technique can be done at the time of cutting paraffin-embedded sections and does not have notable secondary effects. Soaking the paraffin block briefly on a water bath can hydrate the nail plate, making the cutting smoother, and help prevent nail tissue from popping out of the paraffin block. Albumin can be used to help the sections remain on the slide during staining.

NAIL PLATE SAMPLES FOR DIAGNOSIS

Most pathologists have experience with this type of specimen, although they may not have received much training in how to interpret it. Common uses include diagnosis of onychomycosis, *Pseudomonas* infection, nail bed psoriasis (which can avoid deeper sampling and nail disruption), and nail plate hemorrhage versus melanin. Distal clippings or avulsed nail plate may be submitted.

Examination of nail clippings with periodic acid-Schiff with diastase digestion (PAS-D) or Gomori methenamine silver stain for diagnosis of onychomycosis (e.g., dermatophyte or tinea unguium, *Candida*, mold) is the most sensitive method for diagnosis (≈70%), more sensitive even than fungal culture, and much faster. It does not allow for identification of the precise organism(s), of course, although there may be some clues to the presence of nondermatophytes. If more specificity is desired, culture should also be performed. Treatment decisions often depend on whether dermatophytic fungi or yeast and mold are present and how extensive the infection is. It is important to sample the nail plate and subungual material when submitting such a specimen because subungual material usually harbors the microorganisms more consistently except in superficial infections (clinically, white superficial onychomycosis). If little subungual material is submitted, this can create a false-negative result. However, any part of the nail plate or all of it may be involved (Fig. 19.4). It is also important to examine each portion of nail submitted because sometimes hyphae are few in number, especially if there has been partial treatment. Longer septate hyphae and occasionally spores will be evident in dermatophytic infections. Ballooned forms can also be seen when degenerating fungi are present. Pigmented onychomycosis is an ever-increasing diagnosis as well, especially in warmer or tropical climates. This infection often creates "fungal melanonychia" because the fungal walls actually contain melanin. Thus it is a frequent mimicker of melanocytic neoplasms. This underscores the importance of submitting nail plate in cases of melanonychia. Molds such as *Scopulariopsis*, *Scytalidium*, and *Trichophyton rubrum nigricans* are often implicated in pigmented onychiomycosis, but many other molds such as *Aspergillus* and *Fusarium* may involve the nail. They may be encountered as large irregular branching, truncated, and sometimes perforating hyphae and spores. Candidal yeasts are often present under or within the nail plate (see Fig. 19.4). It had been a matter of debate as to whether they are true pathogens or more often colonizers of an abnormal nail unit, but more recently they are accepted as pathogenic organisms. Such infections may be more common in the setting of immunodeficiency. They are, as expected, usually manifest as smaller spores and pseudohyphae, with budding (Fig. 19.5). Incidental *Pityrosporon* from surrounding skin can be present as well. Bacteria are often present nonspecifically, especially if distal nail plate is submitted, but may be observed in paronychia. Exogenous material may also be observed, including nail polish.

Dermatophytoma is a recalcitrant form of onychomycosis that often presents in an atypical fashion as a mass lesion within or under the nail (or both) and is often loculated. Its structure may reflect the multiple layers of the nail plate. This arrangement is a type of biofilm or populations of microorganisms that adhere to surfaces in an environment organized to make the most use of nutrients and promote their own growth. They can secrete an extracellular matrix, which can create antimicrobial resistance. Fungi in this setting are often thick walled and contain spores and arthroconidia, and they may reproduce at a lower rate, also making them harder to treat. There can be a pure fungal biofilm or with mold and bacteria (see Fig. 19.5). This variant may require destructive modalities such as nail avulsion or debridement, and thus it is important for pathologists to mention this finding.

In pseudomonal infection the nail plate is often greenish clinically and has a characteristic lemon yellow to bright green hue in the lower nail plate histologically, caused by fluorescein produced by the bacterium

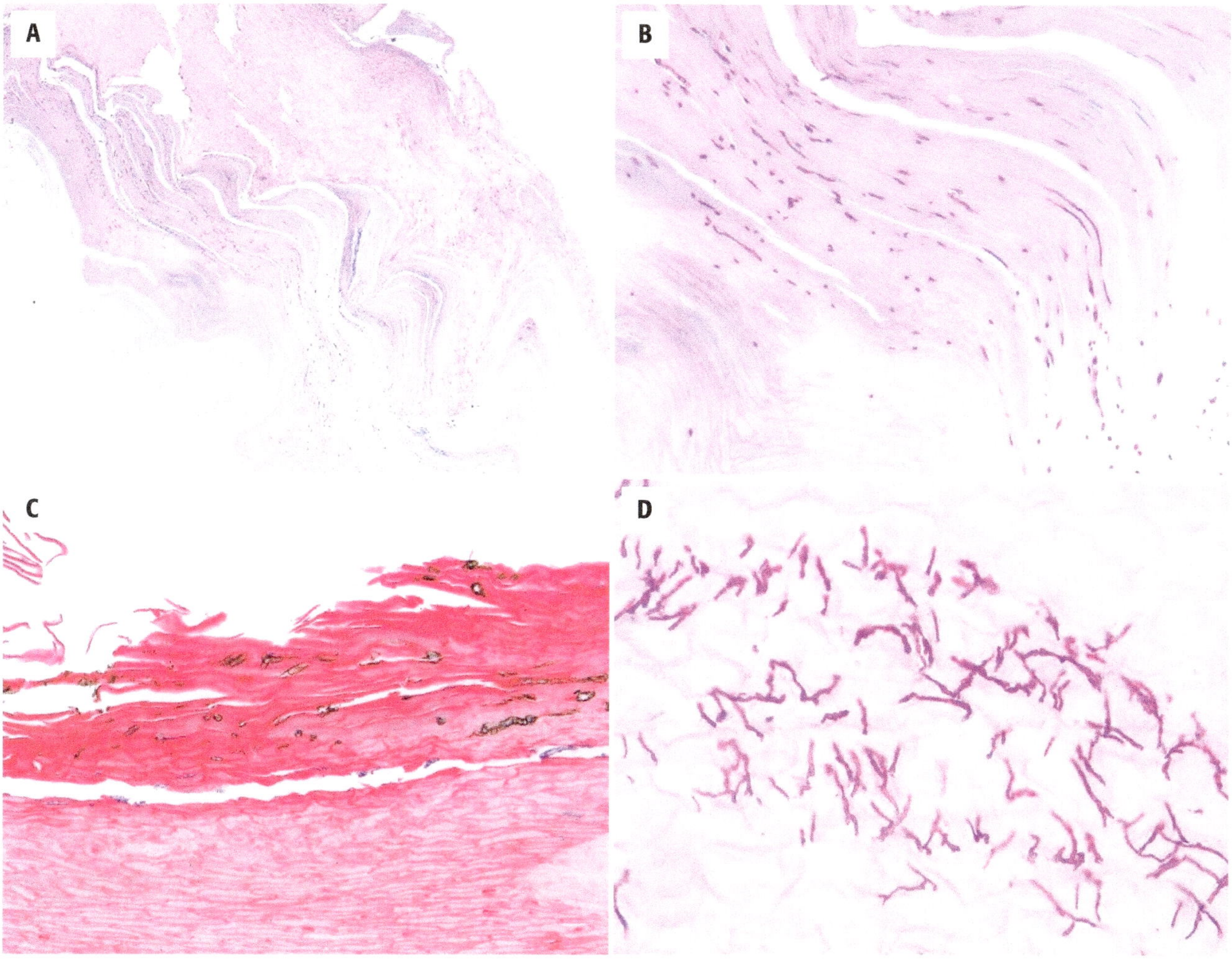

FIG. 19.4

Onychomycosis. **A** and **B,** Tinea unguium, with dermatophytic hyphae throughout the nail plate and within subungual debris (periodic acid-Schiff with diastase digestion [PAS-D] stains). **C,** Pigmented superficial onychomycosis with pigmented fungi embedded in the surface of the nail plate. **D,** Onychomycosis caused by mold, with irregular branching thick hyphae that perforate the nail plate at irregular angles (PAS-D stain).

(see Fig. 19.5). It also produces pyocyanin, which produces a blue color, together giving blue-green discoloration of the nail clinically. Do not expect to demonstrate the gram-negative organisms in the nail plate, however.

The findings in psoriasis of the nail can arise from involvement of the nail matrix or nail bed (discussed in more detail later). Especially in the case of a thickened nail plate, usually the result of nail bed disease, the avulsed or partially sampled plate alone can be used to make the diagnosis, an easier procedure with less morbidity for the patient. The thickened plate contains serum and more specifically neutrophils, often laminated between layers of the nail plate, with marked subungual parakeratosis with serum and neutrophils and occasional hemorrhage (Fig. 19.6). A PAS-D stain should be part of the evaluation to exclude onychomycosis, which can produce identical changes.

Distinction of subungual hemorrhage from melanin in the nail plate can often be made on clinical grounds and via dermatoscopy. A history of trauma and, better still, an irregular focus of pigment (not just a band) that may not arise from the matrix, with a ragged distal edge and importantly that grows out with the nail, are features supportive of subungual hemorrhage in the absence of other nail deformity. If a nail matrix biopsy does not seem justified, sampling the affected nail plate can be a first step. Often the presence of blood in the nail plate is readily apparent, in large or small loculations, under or within the nail plate (Fig. 19.7). Be aware that conventional iron stains, such as Perls' or Prussian blue stain, do not work in nail plate specimens. As blood is loculated in an avascular space, it is not degraded to hemosiderin, the form of iron "recognized" by these stains. Instead, a modified benzidine technique for hemoglobin can be used if needed to help localize small loculations if a careful review does not disclose them. Unmodified benzidine is a carcinogen and requires special procedures for its use, and so the modified technique is preferred. If no hemorrhage is identified, the nail can be stained with Fontana stain to

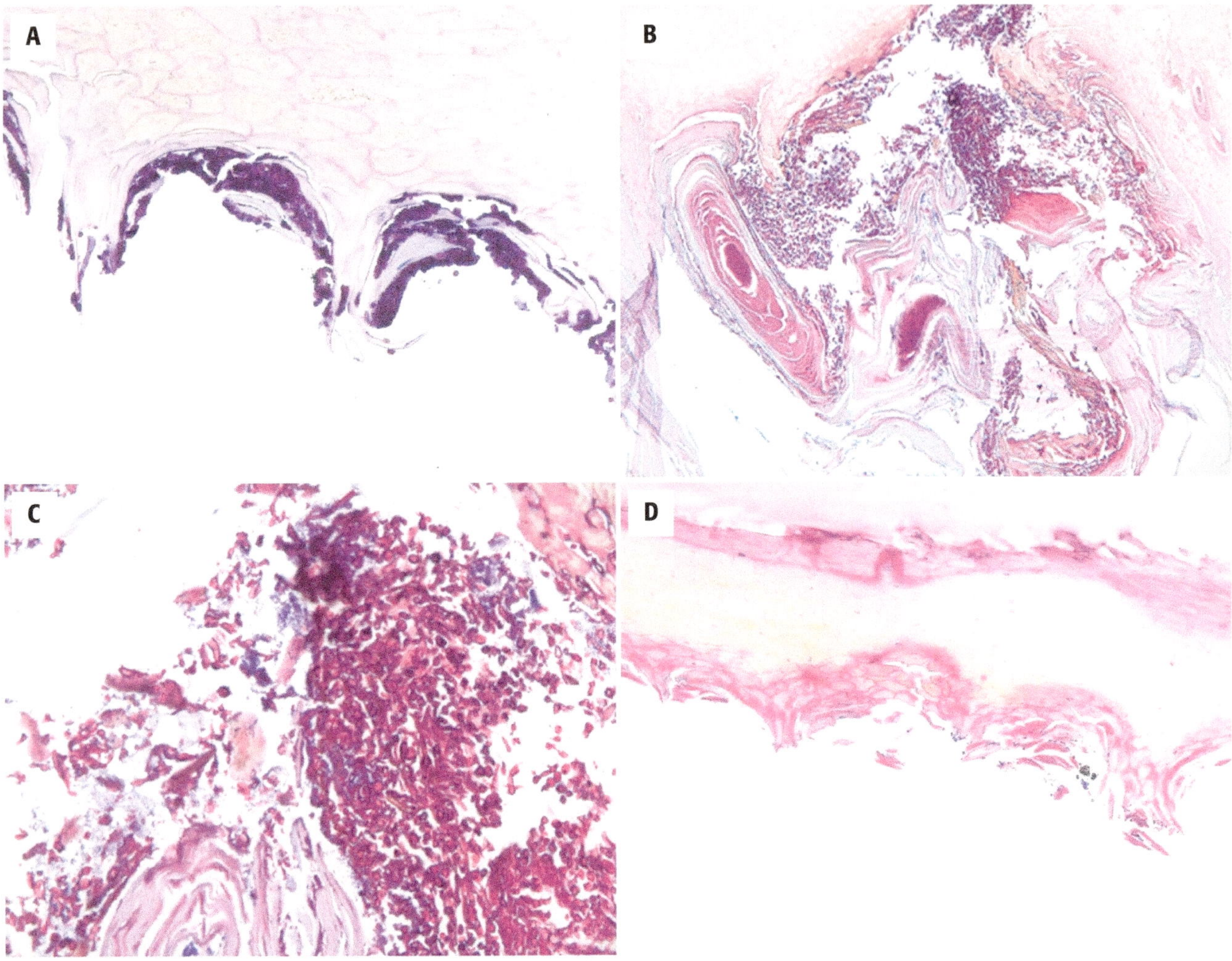

FIG. 19.5

A, Candidal onychomycosis, featuring small spores and pseudohyphae on the undersurface of the nail plate (periodic acid-Schiff with diastase digestion [PAS-D] stain). **B** and **C,** Dermatophytoma, a loculated mass of fungi or mold and bacteria, representing a recalcitrant form of onychomycosis (PAS-D stain). **D,** Pseudomonas infection, with the typical lemon-yellow hue of the nail plate caused by diffusible fluorescein pigment produced by the bacterium.

look for melanin. This stain must be titrated for use in nail plate to avoid dark brown staining that cannot be interpreted. Melanin granules can also be difficult to discern in many cases but when obvious are generally present in an orderly staggered array in nail plate in benign causes of melanonychia (see Fig. 19.7). Irregular globules can be concerning, but benign causes of melanonychia such as melanocytic nevi in children can sometimes produce them. A common pitfall in examining Fontana stains of nail plate is the presence of tiny air bubbles under the coverslip, which can be misinterpreted as melanin granules but are more refractile. As a final note, hemorrhage can be associated with melanoma or other nail neoplasms, and melanin can be found in the nail plate after trauma. Thus nail plate sampling is only a screening procedure, and any suspicious pigmentation is best biopsied in traditional and more ample fashion at its source.

INFECTIOUS DISEASE OF THE NAIL UNIT

As described earlier, the nail unit can be involved in various infectious diseases, including fungal infections such as onychomycosis and dermatophytoma, candidiasis, and bacterial infections such as *Pseudomonas* and as a sequela of paronychia. Crusted scabies can also involve the nail and sometimes be a reservoir for reinfection in treated patients.

INFLAMMATORY AND KERATOTIC DISEASES OF THE NAIL UNIT

Many dermatologic conditions may also involve the nail unit, but if lesions exist elsewhere, they are generally biopsied for diagnosis preferentially. The diseases discussed here may be the sole manifestations of their

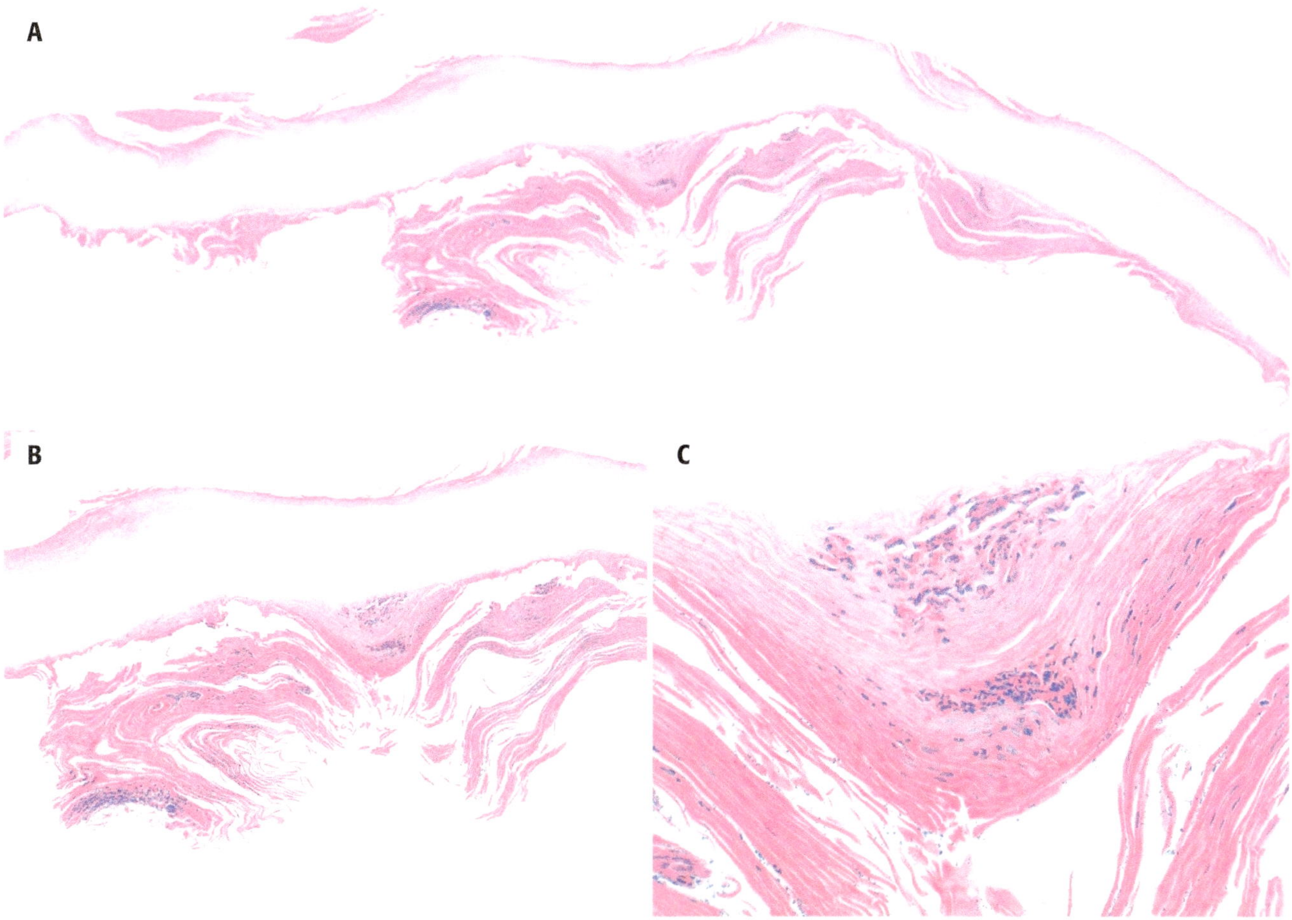

FIG. 19.6

Psoriasis. **A** to **C,** Nail clippings in nail bed psoriasis contain subungual hyper- and parakeratosis layered with serum and neutrophils and sometimes also contain hemorrhage. The same pattern can be observed in onychomycosis.

conditions or so commonly involved that a biopsy is more often undertaken.

PSORIASIS

Psoriasis can affect the nail matrix or nail bed, as well as periungual skin. Diagnostic findings are usually more evident in fingernails; toenail involvement is often identical clinically to onychomycosis. Clinically, when the proximal matrix is affected, there are superficial nail plate changes, such as pitting, crumbling, and roughening, that are rarely an impetus for biopsy. These findings result from zones of parakeratosis of varying extent on the surface of the nail plate. Involvement of the mid to distal nail matrix produces leukonychia (whitening), resulting from parakeratosis of the deeper aspects of the nail plate. "Oil spots" or "salmon patches" result from involvement of the nail bed, which can demonstrate spongiosis (not seen in typical cutaneous psoriasis), resultant accumulation of serum, parakeratotic subungual debris, and neutrophils, producing pink or orange to brown discoloration. Disease affecting the distal nail bed and hyponychium usually manifests as onycholysis (separation of nail plate from the bed) or subungual debris or thickening. Onycholysis and oil spots are commonly found adjacent to one another. Nail disease is often accompanied by psoriatic arthropathy.

Biopsies to prove psoriasis are generally taken from the nail bed because this zone is more commonly affected in severe disease in which treatment is contemplated, and a biopsy from this zone tends to produce less nail dystrophy. A longitudinal biopsy is often done, however, when it is unclear which compartment is responsible for the nail dystrophy. The affected epithelium demonstrates many similar features to psoriasis elsewhere (Fig. 19.8). The nail bed epithelium is acanthotic, with elongated and sometimes thin ridges and parakeratosis with serum and neutrophils. The epithelium may also be thin between ridges, and there are dilated capillaries within the superficial dermis, which also produce characteristic splinter hemorrhages, the nail unit equivalent of Auspitz sign. Unusual features include spongiosis, more often seen in acral psoriasis in general but usually still accompanied by neutrophils. Pustules may develop in so-called acrodermatitis of

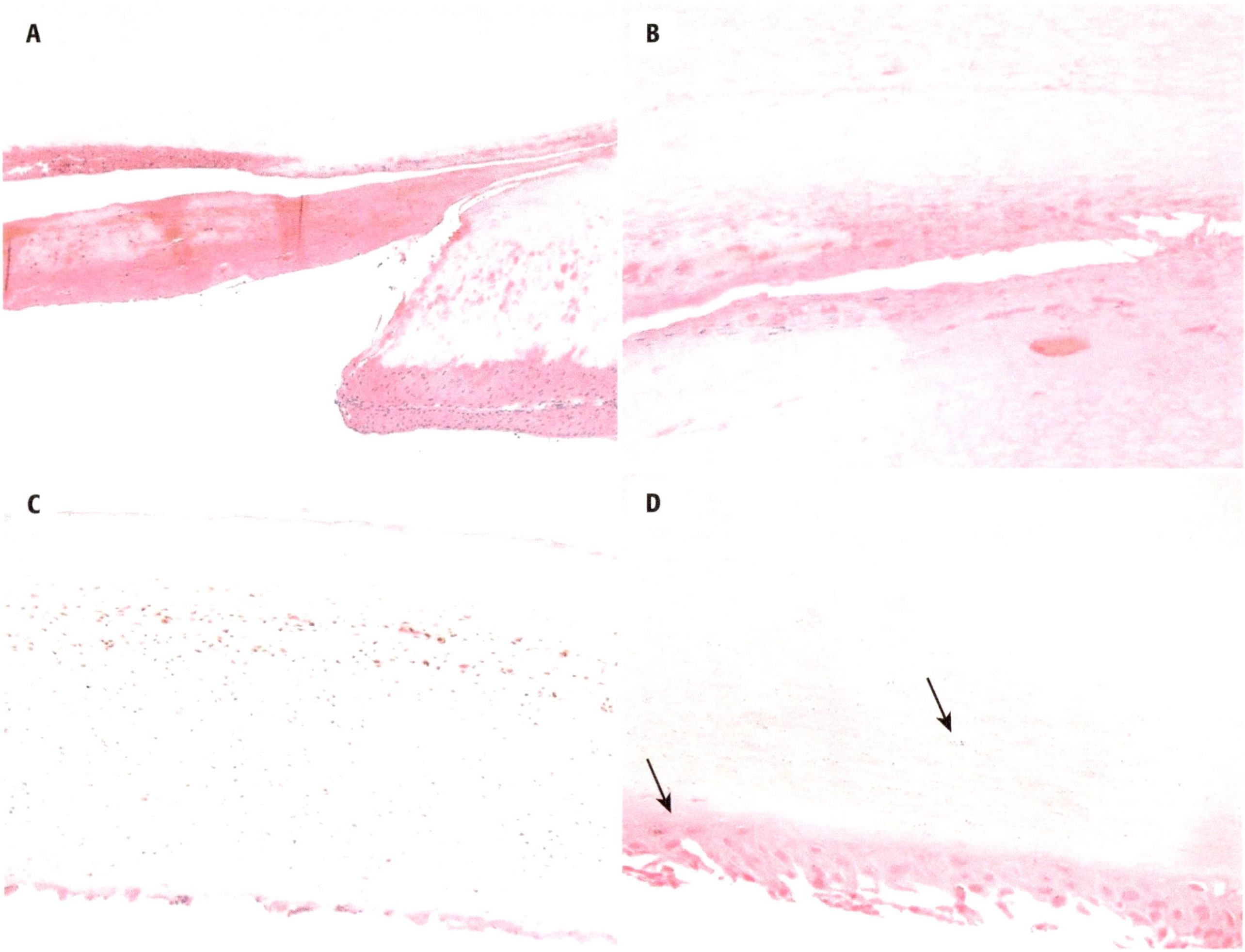

FIG. 19.7

A and **B**, Subungual hemorrhage, with a large collection and some smaller loculations of erythrocytes. **C**, Melanin within the nail plate, with granules of melanin in a somewhat periodic array. **D**, Melanin within the nail plate, with subtle pigmentation of the nail plate and attached nail bed epithelium, highlighted in a Fontana stain *(arrows)*.

Hallopeau (see Fig. 19.8). Also, chronic or onycholytic lesions may lose characteristic features, resembling lichen simplex chronicus (LSC), with hypergranulosis (never a normal finding on the nail bed), but still retain the elongate ridges expected in psoriasis. The clinical and histologic differential diagnosis includes mainly dermatophytosis and candidiasis, which should be excluded by PAS-D stain. Nail plate biopsies, as discussed earlier, can be helpful in this setting. Lichen planus and eczematous nail disease may also enter into the differential diagnosis.

LICHEN PLANUS

Lichen planus of the nails can present a variety of clinical features and may affect any or all parts of the nail unit. The most common findings are nail thinning and fissuring, longitudinal ridging and splitting, and trachyonychia. In late stages, dorsal nail pterygium may occur. As the epithelium is no longer able to produce nail plate, adherence of the proximal nail fold to nail matrix and bed essentially produces an irreversible syncytium, pterygium, resulting in permanent nail loss. The clinical and histologic findings in graft versus host disease of the nail unit are nearly identical.

Histologic findings in lichen planus of the nail are similar to those seen in cutaneous disease. Any portion or all of the nail unit can be affected, with a lichenoid lymphocytic infiltrate of varying intensity, necrotic keratinocytes along the junctional zone, hypergranulosis, and irregular hyperplasia of nail unit epithelium (Fig. 19.9). There may be striking hyperkeratosis and the nail plate may be disrupted in so-called onychorrhexis. In later lesions the epithelium may be thinned, with foci of hypergranulosis, and the infiltrate may be more limited. In such cases, it can be difficult to render the diagnosis. When severe damage has been done, the end-stage changes of pterygium are manifest by loss of normal architecture as above and scarring or loss of the matrix as it fuses with the nail bed and resultant loss of the nail plate (anonychia).

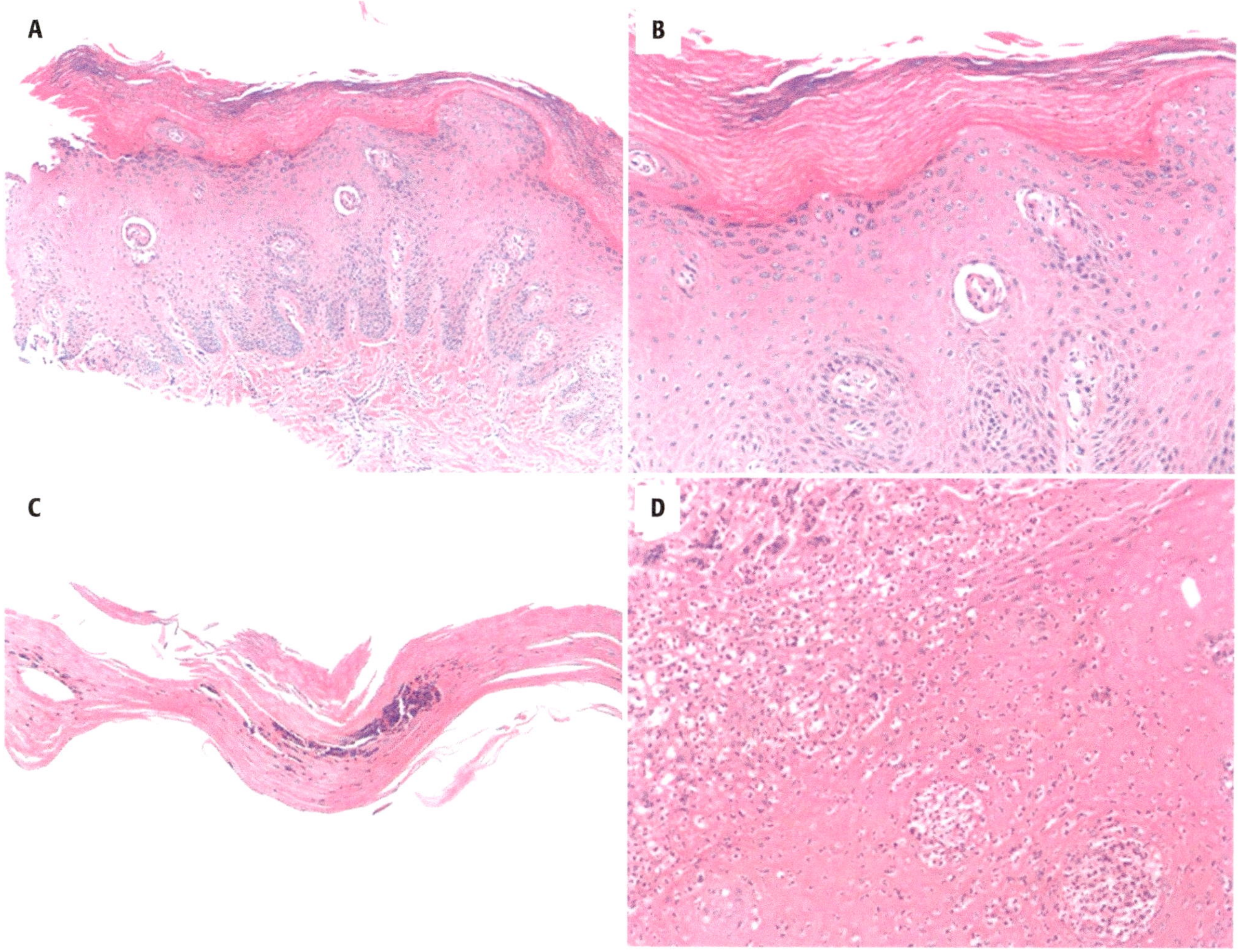

FIG. 19.8

Nail bed psoriasis. **A,** Epithelial hyperplasia, hyper- and parakeratosis with scattered neutrophils, and dilated superficial dermal vessels. **B,** Hypergranulosis and dilated vessel in papillary dermis. **C,** Detached cornified material with neutrophils and parakeratosis. **D,** Pustular psoriasis of nail bed from a patient who had onycholysis, with many neutrophils within the epithelium, forming spongiform pustules.

TRACHYONYCHIA

This term refers to thinning and roughening of the nail plate, with striation and distal splitting. It commonly involves many or all nails. A synonymous term is 20-nail dystrophy. This term has fallen out of favor, however, because this condition may involve fewer nails and is likely not a disorder in and of itself but may be the result of several diseases, including lichen planus, psoriasis, and spongiotic (eczematous) disorders. It can also be associated with alopecia areata. Biopsy is often useful in this setting to elucidate the underlying process.

LUPUS ERYTHEMATOSUS

Changes affecting the proximal nail folds, such as periungual telangiectasia, are well known as stigmata of connective tissue disease such as dermatomyositis and lupus erythematosus. Systemic lupus can also involve the nail in 25% of cases, presenting as distal onycholysis and nail bed hyperkeratosis. However, discoid lesions involving the nail unit are rare and consist of hyperkeratotic plaques. The histologic changes are lichenoid and similar to those seen elsewhere. As disease is never limited to only the nail unit, it is rarely biopsied.

LICHEN SIMPLEX CHRONICUS

As in cutaneous disease, LSC can be seen as a secondary event in diseases of the nail, such as psoriasis, or a result of overly aggressive nail hygiene or cosmesis (manicure, drummeling, artificial nails). It can also be a primary diagnosis as a consequence of onychotillomania (similar to prurigo nodularis in the skin). In the nail epithelium, as elsewhere, it produces epithelial hyperplasia, a granular zone or hypergranulosis, and hyperkeratosis. The nail plate may be dystrophic or lost. It is important to note that in many conditions in which the nail bed is

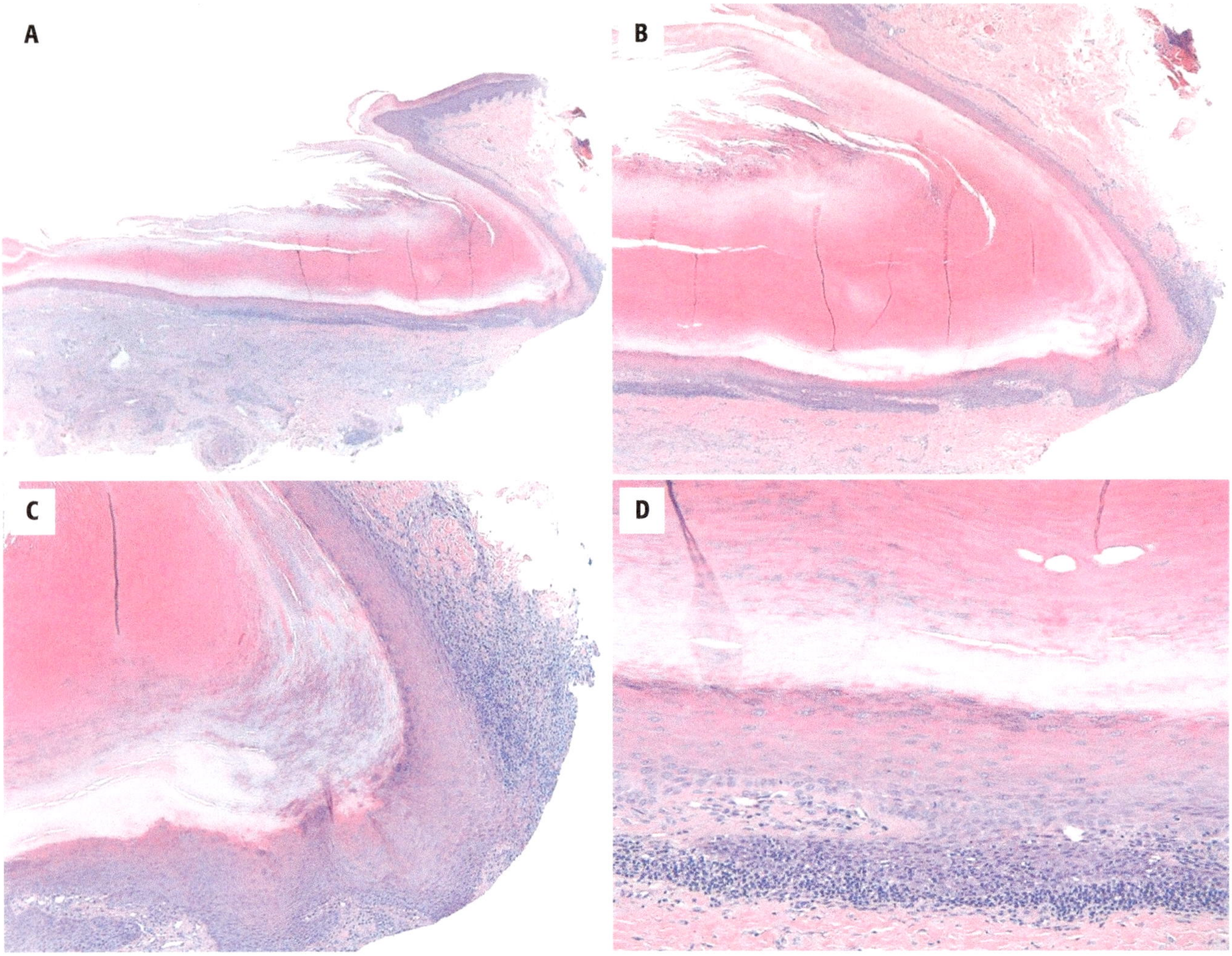

FIG. 19.9

Lichen planus. **A** to **D,** A longitudinal excision demonstrating a lichenoid lymphocytic infiltrate obscuring the junctional zone of nail unit epithelium; any portion or all of it can be involved. The epithelium, including the matrix, becomes thin, and the nail plate also becomes thin, with abnormal hypergranulosis and hyperkeratosis of the nail epithelium. As nail production ceases in more advanced cases, the proximal nail fold may adhere to the nail bed (pterygium).

exposed, for example, in onycholysis, the histologic appearance may be similar to LSC as the nail epithelium reverts to that of acral skin.

PITYRIASIS RUBRA PILARIS

The nails are almost never involved in isolation in this papulosquamous disorder, in contrast to psoriasis, and thus biopsies of affected nails are not done routinely. The diagnosis can be confirmed on skin biopsy instead. The clinical findings in pityriasis rubra pilaris of the nail are similar to those of psoriasis but without irregular pitting or oil spots. Studies have shown that the histologic changes consist of patchy parakeratosis mainly over the nail bed and affecting the nail plate, slightly thickened nail bed epithelium, foci of vacuolar change and spongiosis, and a sparse lymphocytic infiltrate. Hyperkeratosis and parakeratosis are present at the hyponychium. Samples of the distal nail plate can sometimes demonstrate the characteristic parakeratosis and hyperkeratosis. The lack of interspersed neutrophils can be helpful in excluding psoriasis or dermatophytosis.

PACHYONYCHIA CONGENITA

This form of autosomal dominant ectodermal dysplasia presents in the nail unit as massive subungual hyperkeratosis, leading to a curved and thickened nail plate. There are five variants, classified according to specific keratin defects. These may demonstrate associated conditions such as palmoplantar keratoderma, oral leukokeratosis, cysts, mild keratoderma, and other ectodermal defects. Occasional late presentations with isolated nail involvement have been reported. The pathology involves a hyperplastic nail bed, which displays papillated hyperplasia with hypergranulosis

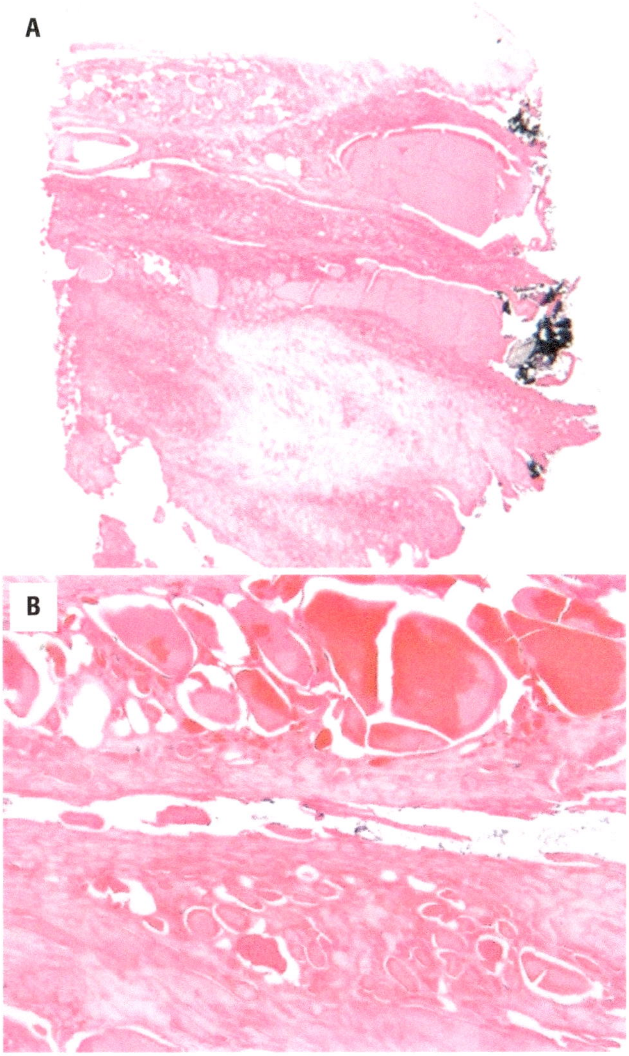

FIG. 19.10

Pachyonychia congenita. **A,** Nail clippings with massive subungual hyperkeratosis with serum. **B,** Hemorrhage.

and marked hyperkeratosis. The nail matrix is spared. Nail clippings can suggest the diagnosis in some cases, with massive subungual hyperkeratosis evident (Fig. 19.10).

MISCELLANEOUS CONDITIONS

Other mainly inflammatory conditions that can affect the nail unit include eczematous disease, pemphigus vulgaris, pemphigoid, erythema multiforme/toxic epidermal necrolysis, Darier's disease, Hailey-Hailey disease, keratosis punctata, keratoderma, yellow nail syndrome, Langerhans cell histiocytosis, lichen striatus, Sézary syndrome, punctate keratoderma, sarcoidosis, and amyloidosis, among others. Drugs, especially some chemotherapy agents, may also cause significant nail alterations.

NEOPLASMS AFFECTING THE NAIL UNIT

MELANOCYTIC NEOPLASMS OF THE NAIL UNIT

Probably the most common reason to perform biopsy of the nail matrix is in the evaluation of longitudinal melanonychia, or pigmented bands of the nail. When narrow and solitary, these are usually benign and the result of melanocytic activation, lentigines, or melanocytic nevi. Especially in the situation of an irregular, broad, or inhomogeneous band, the chief concern is exclusion of subungual melanoma. Nonmelanocytic conditions can also cause melanonychia, such as pigmented squamous cell carcinoma in situ (SCCIS) and some benign epithelial proliferations. Fungal melanonychia, as described earlier, can also cause confusion with a melanocytic neoplasm.

Clinical Findings

In addition to a basic understanding of the unique histology of the nail unit, one must also obtain as much clinical information as possible before attempting to evaluate any pigmented lesion of the nail unit. It is essential for this information to be provided on any requisition form, but if not, the pathologist should make every effort to obtain it. Most pigmented lesions biopsied display longitudinal melanonychia (a pigmented band) and arise from the distal matrix. Key clinical features useful in evaluating a pigmented band have been discussed in many publications and include if the band is solitary or if multiple bands are present, the width of the band, the homogeneity of the band, lateral demarcation of the band (border), Hutchinson's sign (periungual pigmentation), duration and any change over time, which digit and which hand (dominant?) affected, the age of the patient, any extenuating clinical history (drugs, pregnancy, baseline pigmentation, personal or family history of melanoma), and the findings on dermatoscopy. If only one piece of information is given, the width may be the most helpful, just as the size of a pigmented lesion at any other cutaneous site is particularly informative. However, it is important to recognize that even benign lesions may be broad.

Demographic data such as the age of the patient and the digit affected are also very important. For example, melanoma often arises in older individuals, and the thumb and hallux are more commonly affected, as is the dominant hand. It is exceptionally rare in children and most such lesions are in situ. It is helpful to know from where the pigment originates and its overall configuration. For example, if it does not involve the matrical zone or is irregular at its free edge, subungual hemorrhage may be its etiology instead of a melanocytic proliferation. The findings on dermatoscopy may also be quite helpful in that particular distinction, although there are limitations of this technique at this site for evaluation of melanocytic neoplasms. Direct intraoperative nail matrix dermoscopy is a technique that may prove more helpful in this context. A preoperative clinical photograph can be quite helpful. However, if only a small punch is taken from the proximal portion of the band, with the plate left intact, a postoperative photograph may still contain valuable clues with respect to the remaining band.

Most examples of melanocytic activation, lentigo, and nevus measure 3 to 5 mm or less in width, or less than 40% of the diameter of the involved nail plate; melanoma tends to display a wider or irregular band. A notable exception is a melanocytic proliferation in a young person, which may be broad but still benign, sometimes displaying complete melanonychia. In melanocytic activation, a narrow tan to gray band or bands are present. Melanocytic activation can be associated with trauma, endocrinopathy, pregnancy, medication, racial pigmentation, Laugier-Hunziker and Peutz-Jeghers syndromes, and a variety of conditions (both inflammatory and neoplastic) that disrupt the nail unit. Most lentigines and nevi display a narrow band with a tan to brown hue. A benign band is generally also relatively homogeneous with respect to color and color intensity, displays regular lines within it, and has sharp edges. Nevi in children may also display pigment globules, and zig-zag lines, as well as distal brush pigmentation of the hyponychium. Most pigmented lesions producing melanin arise in the distal nail matrix. In general, there should be no periungual pigmentation (Hutchinson's sign), with nevi in children a notable exception. Be aware, however, of the causes of pseudo-Hutchinson sign, which are discussed in more detail later. One common example consists of pigmentation transmitted from a heavily melanized matrical lesion through the proximal nail fold without actual extension of the melanocytic proliferation onto that area. This is generally confined only to the breadth of the pigmented band, however, and should not diffuse beyond it.

Although relatively uncommon, nail apparatus melanoma (NAM) has a poor prognosis, in part because of later diagnosis. Compared with melanoma at other sites, it has a disproportionately higher mortality rate. The 5-year survival rate ranges widely from 16% to 87%, depending on the series, with two larger series in the 51% to 55% range. It has been purported to affect patients of color with higher frequency than does conventional melanoma, but this concept has been called into question more recently, and larger epidemiologic studies may be needed to address this. It may be that this type of melanoma is proportionally more common in patients of color relative to conventional melanoma on sun-exposed sites. The relationship to sun exposure for this subtype has not been elucidated, but because the nail plate provides a modest barrier to ultraviolet penetration, this seems less likely. It is generally considered a subtype of acral melanoma. Most NAM arises in the thumb and great toe (hallux), and digits on the dominant hand are also more often affected. It can present in atypical clinical fashion, with nail dystrophy, and with or without abnormal pigmentation, especially if arising from the nail bed. This, of course, leads to late diagnoses and poor outcomes as a rule. In one larger study, the mean Breslow thickness at diagnosis was 4.8 mm. It may arise in the nail matrix or less often the nail bed. When nail matrix melanoma presents as melanonychia (as it does in roughly 75% of cases), it often produces a band wider than 3 mm, which has widened over time. A disturbing clinical finding is a band wider at the base than the distal edge of the nail, a sign of relatively rapid enlargement (the triangle sign). However, in children, this may occur in nevi. The band is often irregular and not crisp at its lateral margins and may be "streaky" or heterogeneous in color.

With time and involvement of the nail bed or periungual tissue, its irregularity becomes more obvious. Involvement of the proximal nail fold and sometimes the hyponychium (Hutchinson's sign, periungual pigmentation) is a fairly diagnostic clue, especially if the pigmentation is also irregular or diffuse. Hutchinson sign correlates histologically to melanoma in situ in many cases. Causes of pseudo-Hutchinson sign should be kept in mind, including melanocytic nevi and lentigines, SCCIS, drug-induced pigmentation, trauma, radiation, racial pigmentation, malnutrition, and hemorrhage, among others. Nail plate thinning or fissuring is another concerning feature when seen concurrently with abnormal pigmentation. If the tumor is allowed to progress, a nodule may develop, often with ulceration and nail plate destruction. In addition, amelanotic melanoma often originates in the nail bed, where melanocytes may not produce much melanin pigment. Such lesions are often mistaken for granulation tissue or pyogenic granuloma, squamous cell carcinoma (SCC), or an ingrown nail and thus may elude diagnosis for a prolonged period. An exceptional presentation of amelanotic melanoma in situ is as monodactylic nail dystrophy mimicking lichen planus. Desmoplastic melanoma of the nail unit has also been described. NAM in children is exceedingly rare. Even using accepted clinical criteria such as the ABCDEF (Asymmetry, Border irregularity, Color, Diameter, Evolution, Family history) rule and dermatoscopic information, the interobserver variation in clinical diagnosis is marked even among experts, and thus histologic examination remains the gold standard.

Histologic Findings

In addition to knowing the normal anatomy, one must also develop an understanding for the normal density of melanocytes and their distribution at this site, which differs from other cutaneous sites. In normal nail unit epithelium, the quantity of melanocytes is lower than in the skin, about 200/mm^2 compared with around 1150/mm^2, respectively. They also tend to be inconspicuous in normal matrix. Melanocytes may be found in a suprabasal position in the matrix, especially in the proximal matrix, where they are often located within the lower two to four cell layers. In the distal matrix, they are generally located in the first and second layers. Normally, many of them do not actively synthesize melanin, especially those in the proximal matrix. In the distal matrix, however, approximately 50% synthesize melanin. Melanocytes that normally reside in nail bed epithelium are even fewer (absent to 50/mm^2) and do not synthesize melanin. This serves as an explanation as to why melanoma arising from the nail bed tends to be amelanotic and thus a diagnostic difficulty.

From a practical point of view, it is important to have a grasp on the normal density of melanocytes along the basal layer to be able to assess if there is a significant increase, suggesting a melanocytic proliferation. The melanocyte density is generally measured over a 1-mm interval at the epidermal-dermal junction of the nail matrix or nail bed. In normal nails the density ranges from 4 to 9 melanocytes (mean, 7.7) per 1-mm segment of nail matrix epithelium. Normal matrical melanocytes are generally small and inconspicuous in routine sections, and some may display dendritic processes. They are best highlighted via immunoperoxidase stains, including SOX10, MITF (microphthalmia transcription factor-1), HMB45, and Melan A. Melan A and HMB45, as melanosome markers, often exaggerate the density of melanocytes, especially in a heavily melanized or dendritic nail melanocytic neoplasm. MITF and SOX10, as nuclear stains, give a more accurate assessment of density and location within the matrix. One interesting pitfall that the author has noted is that MITF also often labels the nuclei of keratinocytes in the upper keratogenous zone of the matrix. SOX10 may also fail on occasion and thus Melan A may be the most reliable. Using a red chromogen in heavily melanized proliferations in particular can be helpful in identifying melanocytes in a background of pigmented keratinocytes. It is important to note that S100 immunostain should not be used especially as a single stain because nail unit melanocytes tend not to express this antigen reliably.

MELANOCYTIC ACTIVATION (HYPERMELANOSIS)

Melanocytic activation is probably the most common cause of benign melanonychia in adults as confirmed in some studies. This consists mainly of hyperpigmentation of the nail matrix epithelium without an obvious increase in melanocytes. Melanocytic density can be highlighted in immunoperoxidase stains, such as SOX10, MITF, or Melan A, and use of a red chromogen or Giemsa counterstain is helpful in delineating the immunostain result in the midst of heavy melanization of keratinocytes. More subtle background pigmentation can be demonstrated in a Fontana stain because a longitudinal band may result even when the matrical pigmentation is rather limited histologically, although the band tends to be tan or gray. The melanocytes in this setting are often dendritic, and there may be scattered melanophages (Fig. 19.11).

MELANONYCHIA—DIFFERENTIAL DIAGNOSIS

Melanocytic

- Melanocyte activation (hypermelanosis)
- Nail unit lentigo
- Nail unit melanocytic nevus
- Nail unit melanoma

Nonmelanocytic

- Infection (e.g., fungal)
- Pigmented squamous cell carcinoma or benign pigmented epithelial proliferations
- Environmental factors (often leading to melanocytic activation)

LENTIGO (MELANOCYTIC HYPERPLASIA)

The simplest melanocytic proliferation of the matrix, as elsewhere on the skin, is the lentigo, also known as benign melanocytic hyperplasia. This has sometimes also been referred to by the confusing term *melanotic macule*. Some authors have also used this designation to refer to lesions compatible with melanocytic activation or hypermelanosis or to a group of lesions including both hypermelanosis and lentigo. Because this term, when applied to lesions at other cutaneous sites, indicates a lesion containing hyperpigmentation of the basal layer but no increase in melanocytes, it is best avoided in this setting.

Lentigo of the nail unit consists of a slight to moderate increase in the number of single matrical melanocytes (10–31 cells per mm in one study) without any demonstration of confluence. Dendritic melanocytes may be present. Cytologic atypia is absent or minimal (Fig. 19.12). Suprabasilar scatter of melanocytes should be only rarely observed and limited in extent. As in melanocytic activation, scattered melanophages may be present. Heavy melanization of the nail epithelium may limit assessment of melanocyte density in some cases in routine sections, and thus melanocytic markers may be needed, as discussed. It is important to recognize the difficulty in distinguishing this pattern from the earliest changes of melanoma in situ in some cases (discussed later), highlighting the necessity for correlation with the clinical findings.

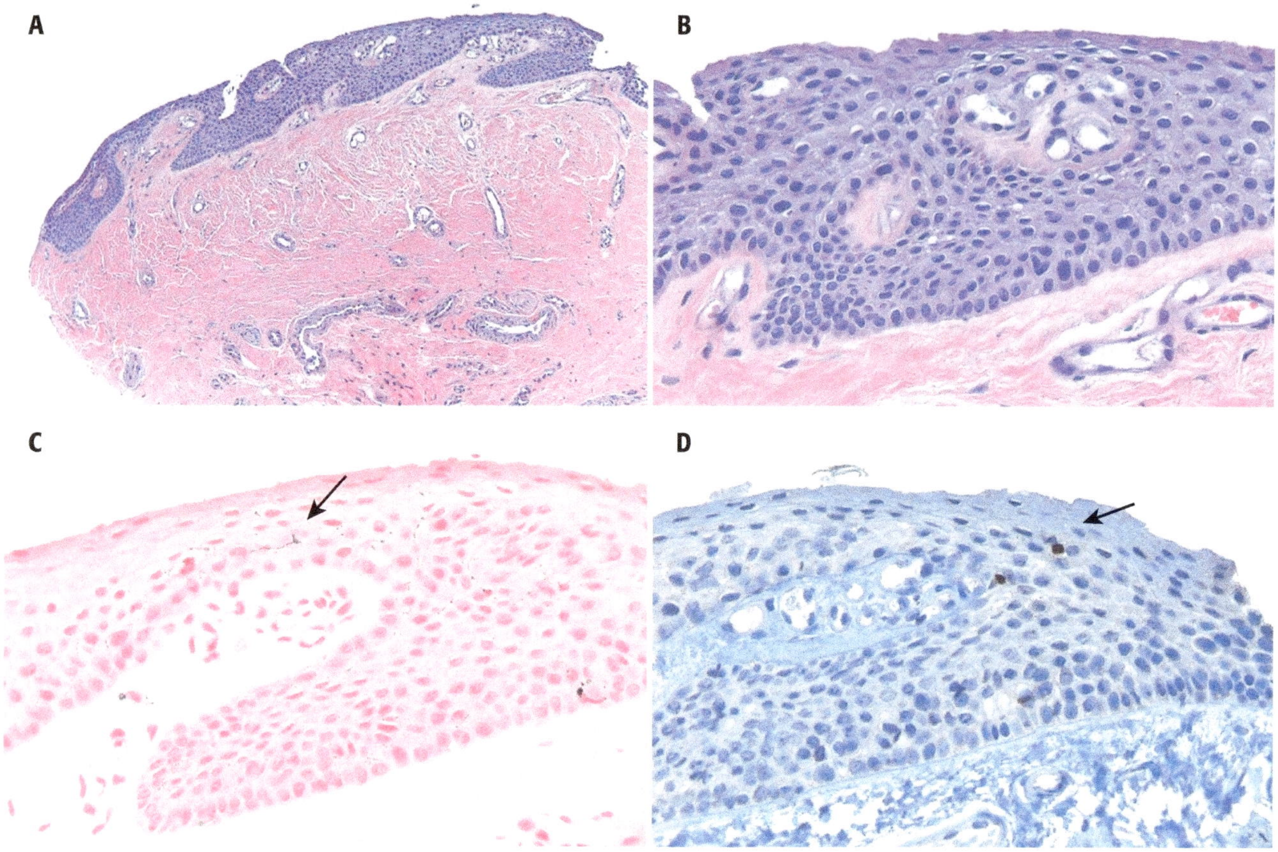

FIG. 19.11

Melanocytic activation. **A** and **B,** Normal matrix epithelium with normal melanocyte cell density and subtle melanin pigment deposition. **C,** Fontana stain highlights melanin pigment, including pigmented dendritic processes of melanocytes *(arrow)*. **D,** SOX10 immunoperoxidase stain illustrates rare basilar melanocytes in normal density *(arrow)*.

MELANOCYTIC NEVI

Nail matrix nevi are probably the most common cause of melanonychia in children. Nail matrix nevi are usually junctional and rarely compound. Most are of the "ordinary" type, although nevi with pigmented epithelioid melanocytes are fairly common, and blue nevi and Spitz nevi have been rarely reported. The nail unit is a "special site," and nevi in this area can display unusual features, many of which are similar to those observed in acral nevi. There may be a lentiginous pattern of melanocytes in early lesions. The nests are sometimes irregular and occasionally crowded, especially if the sections examined are longitudinal, and melanocytes may be present above the basal layer to a limited extent, particularly in children (Fig. 19.13). Melanocytes should not be present in general in the superficial aspects of the nail matrix epithelium. This is a worrisome feature seen more commonly in melanoma, but again, this may occur exceptionally in nevi. Melanocytes in the nail plate are also a function of suprabasilar scatter and may raise concern, especially in adults. Nail unit nevi may occasionally involve the periungual acral skin, and this is particularly true of congenital nevi or nevi in children. Compound nevi often contain dermal nests that are arrayed horizontally, perhaps a compressive effect of the hard overlying nail and relatively firm dermal tissue under the nail epithelium.

NAIL UNIT MELANOMA—DISEASE FACT SHEET

Incidence

- ►► Uncommon; ≈1% of melanomas

Affected Individuals

- ►► Typically age 50 to 70 years
- ►► Independent of skin color and sun exposure

Clinical Manifestations

- ►► Melanonychia
- ►► Hutchinson sign
- ►► Ulceration or bleeding
- ►► Nail dystrophy
- ►► ≈25% are amelanotic

Treatment and Prognosis

- ►► Prognosis depends on tumor thickness

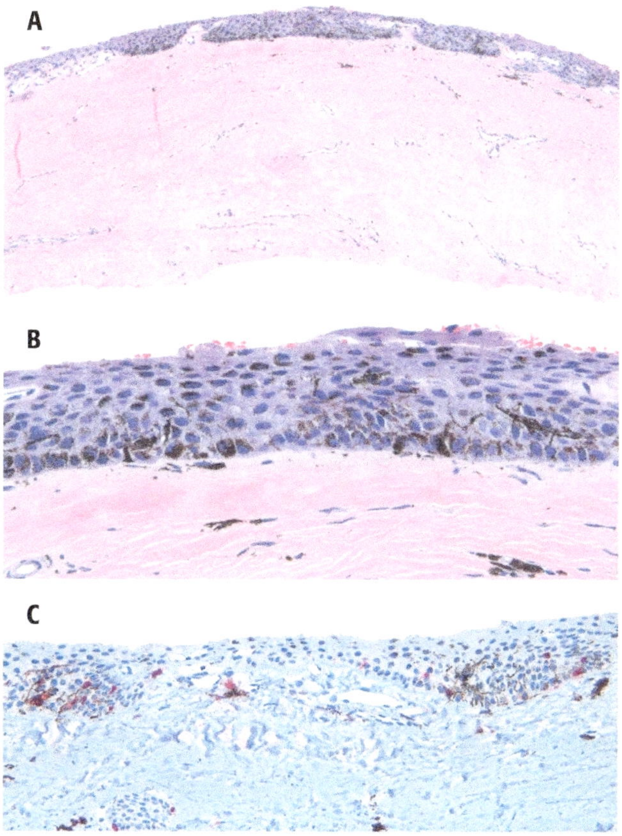

FIG. 19.12

Lentigo. **A,** A narrow zone of heavy melanization of nail matrix epithelium with dendritic and hyperpigmented melanocytes. **B,** Melanocytes at an increased density over normal matrix accompanied by melanophages. **C,** Melan A immunoperoxidase stain highlights the density and distribution of markedly dendritic melanocytes.

- ▸▸ Staging similar to other melanomas (no Clark's levels except V, periosteal)
- ▸▸ Conservative total nail unit excision for melanoma in situ and thin melanoma
- ▸▸ Distal phalanx amputation may be necessary for more extensive tumor

NAIL UNIT MELANOMA—PATHOLOGIC FEATURES

Microscopic Findings

- ▸▸ Asymmetric silhouette
- ▸▸ Usually predominance of solitary units in early lesions, higher density than in lentigo
- ▸▸ Pagetoid spread common, including melanocytes in nail plate
- ▸▸ Cytologic atypia, especially nuclear hyperchromasia
- ▸▸ Involvement of nail folds and/or nail bed or hyponychium (Hutchinson sign)
- ▸▸ Ulceration/nail plate destruction in later lesions
- ▸▸ Associated lichenoid inflammatory reaction

Differential Diagnosis

- ▸▸ Nail unit lentigo
- ▸▸ Nail unit nevus
- ▸▸ For amelanotic and/or spindled tumors: miscellaneous soft tissue neoplasms

NAIL UNIT/APPARATUS MELANOMA (SUBUNGUAL OR UNGUAL MELANOMA)

Criteria for the diagnosis of nail unit melanoma are still in evolution to a degree, as are prognostic factors. Larger studies are needed to address the latter. There is histologic discordance even among experts. Various criteria can be used to establish a diagnosis of melanoma, including poor circumscription, asymmetry, and involvement of eponychial and nail fold epithelium; the density of single intraepidermal melanocytes in sparse proliferations; and an irregular distribution of melanocytes, including confluence of nests, degree of suprabasal scatter, cytologic atypia, multinucleate melanocytes, a lymphocytic infiltrate, and anisodendrocytosis (variation of dendrite size, also seen in acral melanoma). Use of immunoperoxidase stains may be crucial to elucidating these features in some cases. The ability to evaluate salient features also hinges significantly on the quality of the tissue submitted. In a seminal study, the mean number of melanocytes in melanoma in situ was 58.9 per 1-mm interval along the epidermal-dermal junction (range, 39–136) compared with 15.3 (up to 31) for lentigo or benign melanocytic hyperplasia. However, as evidenced in these data, the upper limit of density in lentigines is not far off from the lower end observed in melanoma in situ in some cases, and thus melanocyte density alone cannot be used to make a diagnosis of melanoma in situ and is a diagnostic pitfall in some cases. Confluence of single melanocytes may be observed, and there is usually a predominance of single cells over nests in early lesions. If suprabasal scatter is marked and involves the superficial aspects of the matrical zone, this is worrisome (Figs. 19.14–19.16). It is thus crucial to examine any portions of nail plate for the superficial portions of the matrical keratogenous zone and nail bed epithelium, portions of which often remain attached to the nail plate when it is avulsed, because these may contain important diagnostic clues, including melanin and even melanocytes. Involvement of periungual or eponychial epithelium, as in Hutchinson sign, is an indicator of poor circumscription. Interestingly, cytologic atypia may not be marked in such areas. Sometimes only pigmentation is observed in Hutchinson sign in melanoma (diagnostic in other areas of the nail unit). Bear in mind that melanocytic nevi may involve the nail folds on occasion, as noted earlier. A lichenoid reaction can be seen more often in melanoma in situ than in lentigines. When intense, and in areas of regression, this can be mistaken for lichen planus in partial biopsies. PRAME (PReferentially expressed Antigen in MElanoma) immunostain has recently been shown to be effective for the diagnosis of nail unit melanoma and may be helpful in low cellularity lesions, but as elsewhere, false-positive results may occur.

Invasive nail unit melanoma displays many of the same features as observed elsewhere in the skin.

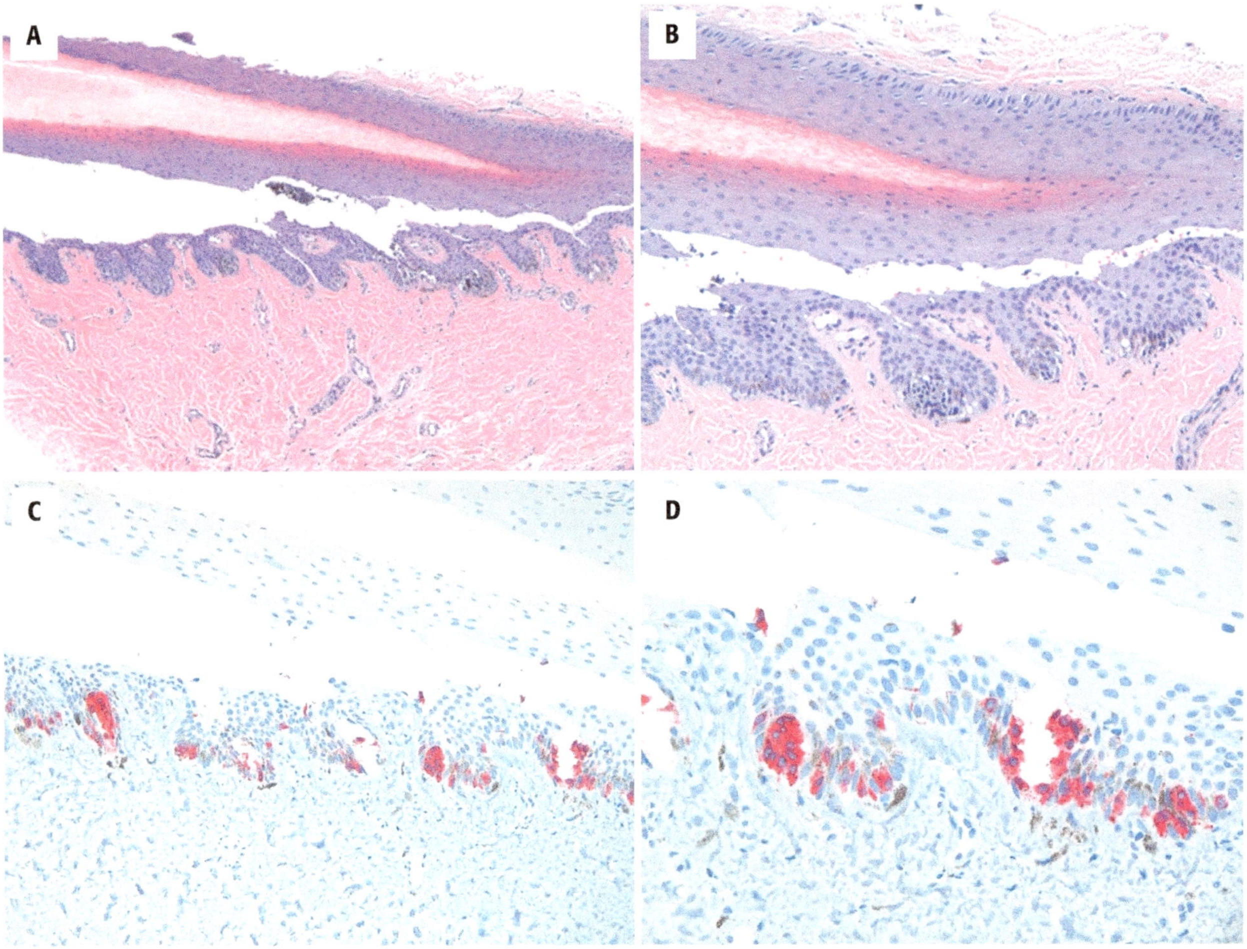

FIG. 19.13

Nevus. **A,** A well-circumscribed, mainly nested proliferation of melanocytes concentrated in the distal matrix. The cleft subjacent to the nail plate is a common cleavage plane in these specimens. **B,** Nests of bland melanocytes confined to the lower distal nail matrix, with basilar pigmentation. **C** and **D,** Discrete nests of melanocytes highlighted in a Melan A immunoperoxidase stain.

In addition to the findings noted in melanoma in situ at this site, the dermal component lacks adequate maturation, may display an irregular distribution of nests and syncytia, and may display an increased mitotic rate (see Figs. 19.15 and 19.16). Neurotropism and lymphovascular invasion may occur. Unusual variants also found in nail unit melanoma include nevoid melanoma, as well as myxoid, chondroid, neuroid, and desmoplastic types. Nail bed invasive melanoma is usually amelanotic, as noted earlier. In more advanced tumors, ulceration and loss of the nail are frequently noted.

Diagnostic reporting of nail unit melanoma by the dermatopathologist can be somewhat challenging. Breslow thickness is reported in the same manner, with a measurement from the most superficial epithelial layer visible to the thickest portion of the dermal component. Normally, there is no granular zone in the nail unit, although one frequently develops in disease states, including melanoma. The correlation of thickness and prognosis may not be the same as for melanoma elsewhere. Although no longer used in the current American Joint Committee on Cancer (AJCC) criteria for melanoma, Clark's anatomic levels cannot be established in the same manner because there is no distinct papillary dermis or subcutis in the nail unit proper. Level V has been reported as involvement of the phalangeal periosteum or bone. Apart from general AJCC staging criteria, no other significant prognostic factors have been established firmly, especially with respect to the primary tumor characteristics, and larger epidemiologic studies may better address those issues. Nonetheless, the author's practice is to record the prognostic features commonly reported in cutaneous melanoma as far as they apply to this site.

When a diagnosis of melanoma has been rendered, the surgical treatment may entail significant functional considerations. Although in the past, such a diagnosis might result in a Ray amputation, more conservative surgery is now emerging, including distal digital amputation, and for melanoma in situ and thin melanoma, total nail unit excision and grafting, possibly with some superficial bone removal, without amputation.

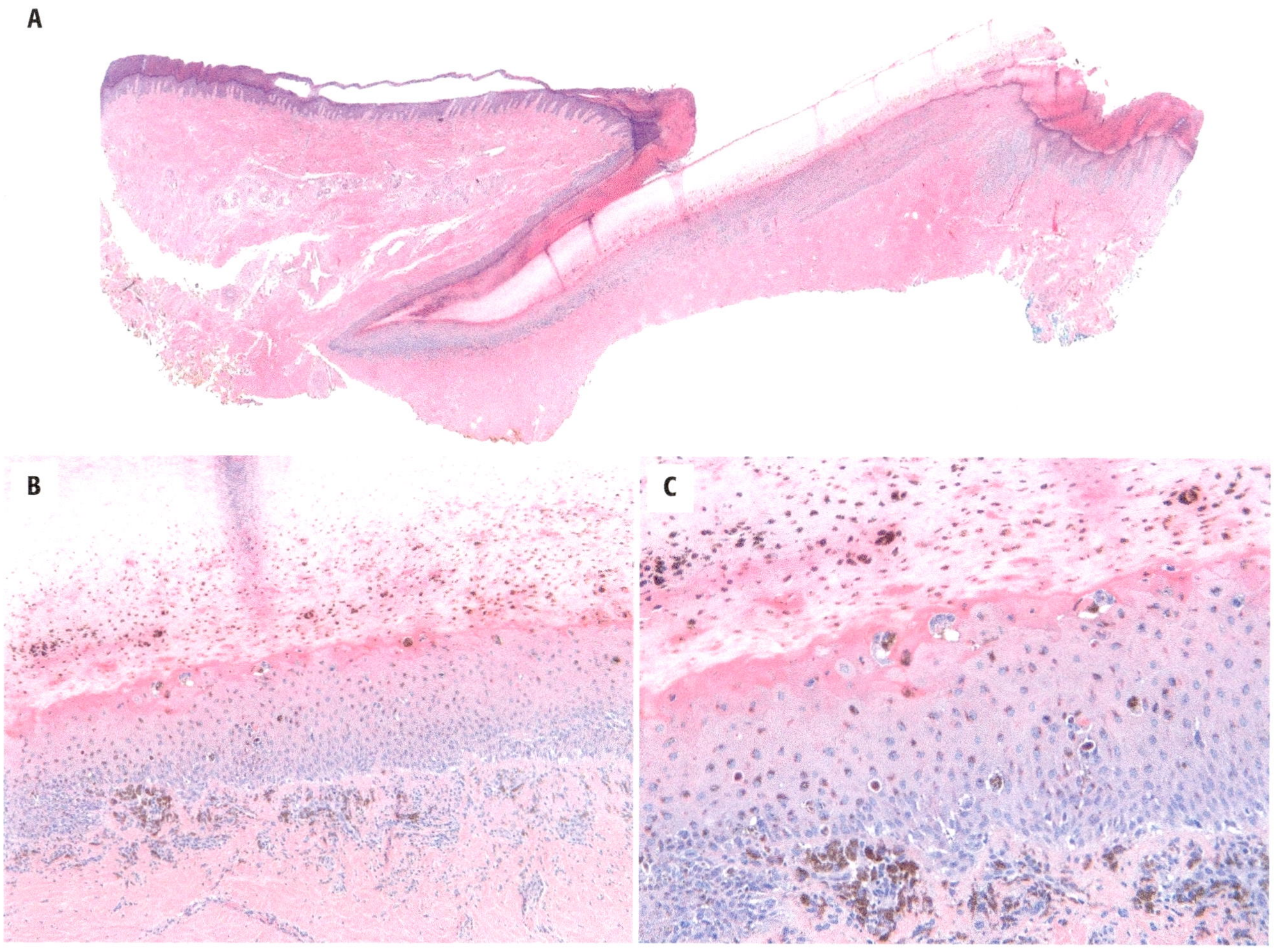

FIG. 19.14

Subungual melanoma in situ. **A,** En bloc longitudinal reexcision demonstrating diffuse involvement of nail matrix, nail bed, proximal nail fold, and hyponychium (the latter two correlating with Hutchinson's sign), with a lymphocytic infiltrate and areas of regression. **B,** Irregular distribution of atypical melanocytes singly and in clusters, with irregular pigment granules and globules within nail plate. **C,** Scatter of atypical melanocytes within the matrical epithelium.

Although some controversy exists as to which procedure is best, conservative surgery is being adopted increasingly to preserve functionality without affecting overall outcomes. With respect to assessing margins in a total nail unit excision, the pathologist should be alert to a common source of incomplete excision and that occurs at the proximal matrical zone, which also accounts for some of the debate as to which procedure is best for eradicating the tumor. This zone of the matrical epithelium is angled deeper within the dermis and lies very close to the distal phalanx (on average within 0.8 mm) and the extensor tendon of the distal digit and may be transected if attention is not paid to the surgical approach (Figs. 19.14 and 19.15). If this occurs, it can be a source of recurrences and formation of nail spicules, which can be problematic for the patient. The author's preference and the standard for grossing these whole nail unit specimens is longitudinal sectioning with orientation. The most lateral sections may need to be leveled if questions of margin adequacy result in such areas.

EPITHELIAL NEOPLASMS AND HYPERPLASIA

VERRUCA VULGARIS

This hyperplasia caused by human papillomavirus (HPV) usually arises from periungual acral skin at the proximal and lateral nail folds or the hyponychium, resembling verruca at other cutaneous sites, but may extend to the nail bed, producing nail dystrophy and hemorrhage. It rarely involves the nail matrix. Clinically, verruca vulgaris (VV) may mimic SCC. The histology is that of typical VV or myrmecia. There is papillated epidermal hyperplasia, with hypergranulosis and hyperkeratosis, as well as hemorrhage. Viropathic changes such as perinuclear vacuoles; coarse keratohyaline granules; and in the case of myrmecia, eosinophilic cytoplasmic inclusions may be present. Involutional warts may become endophytic and lose typical viropathic changes. It is important to remember that the nail unit epithelium may

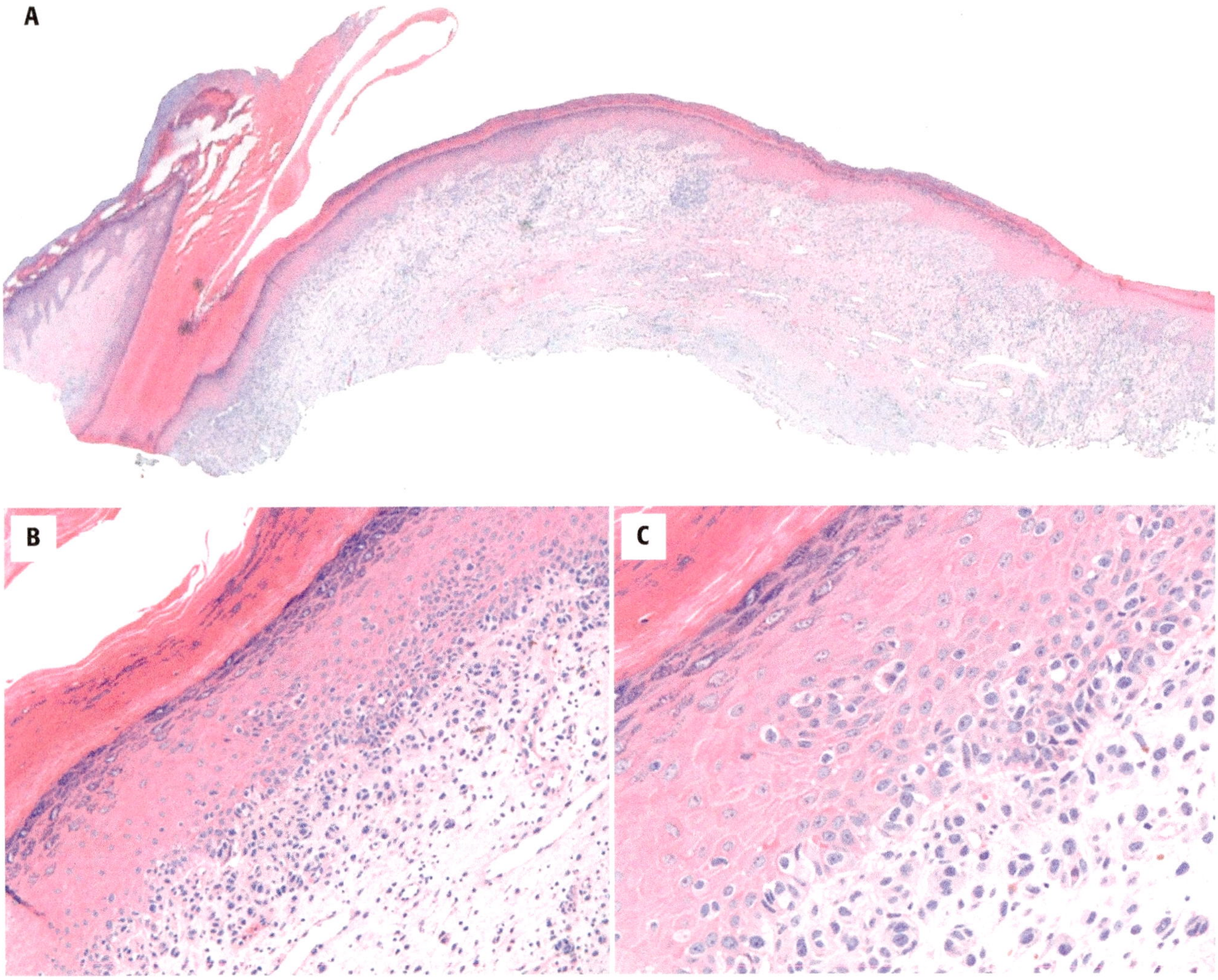

FIG. 19.15

Invasive melanoma. **A,** Involvement of the nail matrix and nail bed with loss of normal epithelial architecture and loss of the nail plate in that area. **B** and **C,** Atypical melanocytes arrayed irregularly within the nail bed epithelium and within the dermis without maturation with descent.

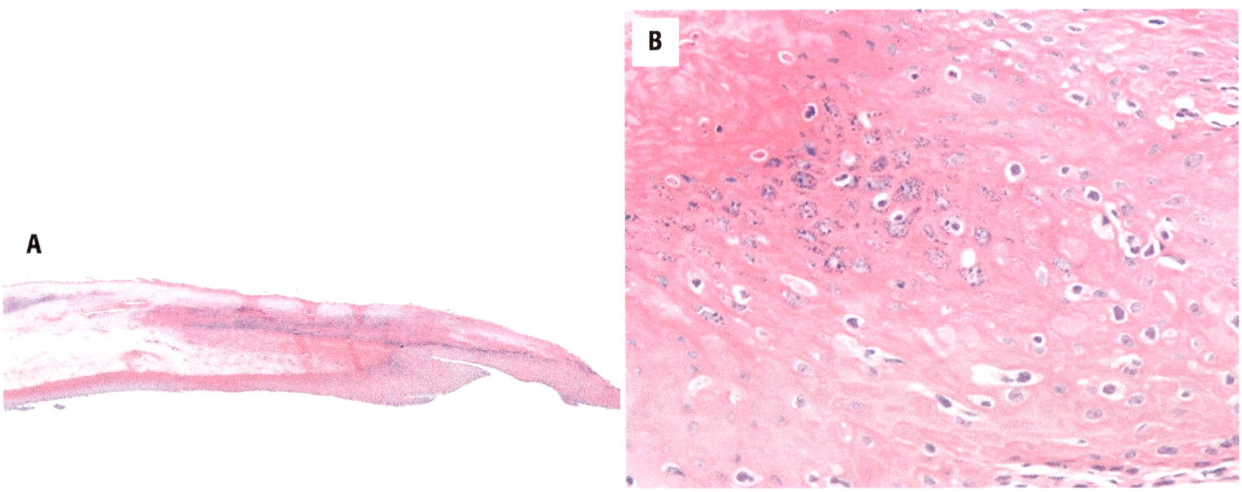

FIG. 19.16

Melanoma, nail plate. **A,** Avulsed nail plate. **B,** Melanocytes are displayed erratically throughout the epithelium.

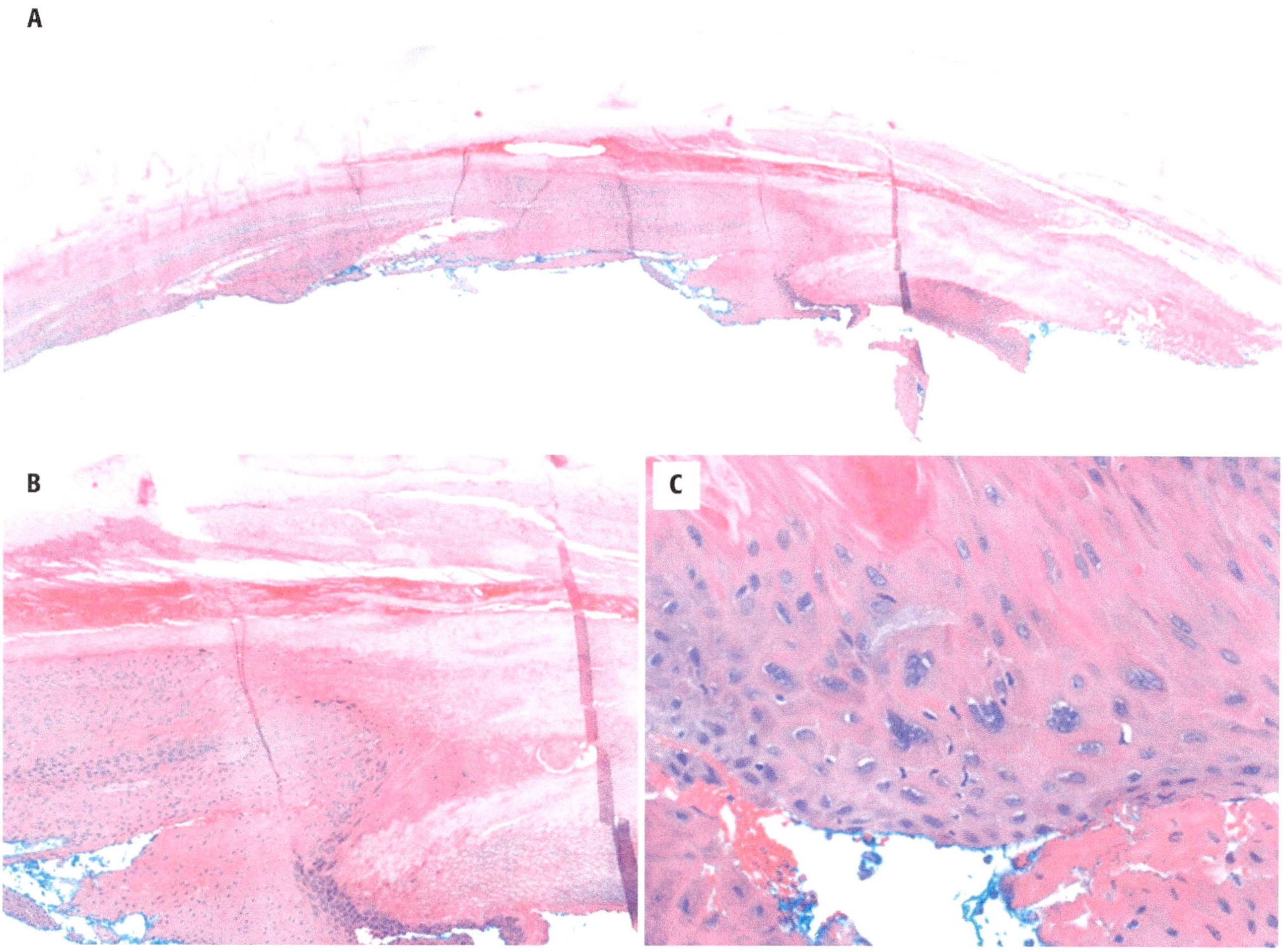

FIG. 19.17

Onychopapilloma. **A,** A longitudinal excision of a band of erythronychia showing a papillated and hyperplastic nail bed with subungual hemorrhage and hyperkeratosis, especially distally. **B,** Papillated hyperplasia of the distal nail bed and hyponychium with prominent parakeratosis and subungual hemorrhage and without koilocytic changes. **C,** Benign multinucleate keratinocytes in the hyperplastic distal nail bed epithelium with reactive changes.

become papillated nonspecifically in other conditions that disrupt it, both inflammatory and neoplastic, and thus a rigorous application of the clinical and histologic criteria is indicated. In addition, onychopapilloma, discussed next, is a common mimic.

ONYCHOPAPILLOMA

This is a fairly common benign entity, commonly causing erythronychia, or a pink to reddish longitudinal band, arising from the distal matrix and nail bed. It often displays distal subungual hyperkeratosis forming a spicule distally and is commonly associated with hemorrhage. Pigmented variants arise from melanocytic activation. Histologically, its features may vary, and it may be appreciable depending on the type of sample submitted. A longitudinal excision is best. If the nail plate has been avulsed and discarded, often containing superficial nail bed epithelium, it may be difficult to appreciate any abnormality in the subjacent nail bed. There are varying degrees of papillated epidermal hyperplasia and subungual hyper- and parakeratosis with hemorrhage, usually distally. So-called matrical metaplasia of nail bed has also been described, in which the proximal nail bed may resemble nail matrix, with retained nuclei similar to the keratogenous zone. Multinucleate keratinocytes may be observed in the nail bed distally, but cytologic atypia is not (Fig. 19.17). Unlike VV, which often originates in the nail folds and secondarily involves the nail bed, this entity does not involve the nail folds.

SQUAMOUS CELL CARCINOMA

Clinical Findings

SCC of the nail unit is the most common malignancy of the nail unit, yet it is still uncommon. Unusual clinical

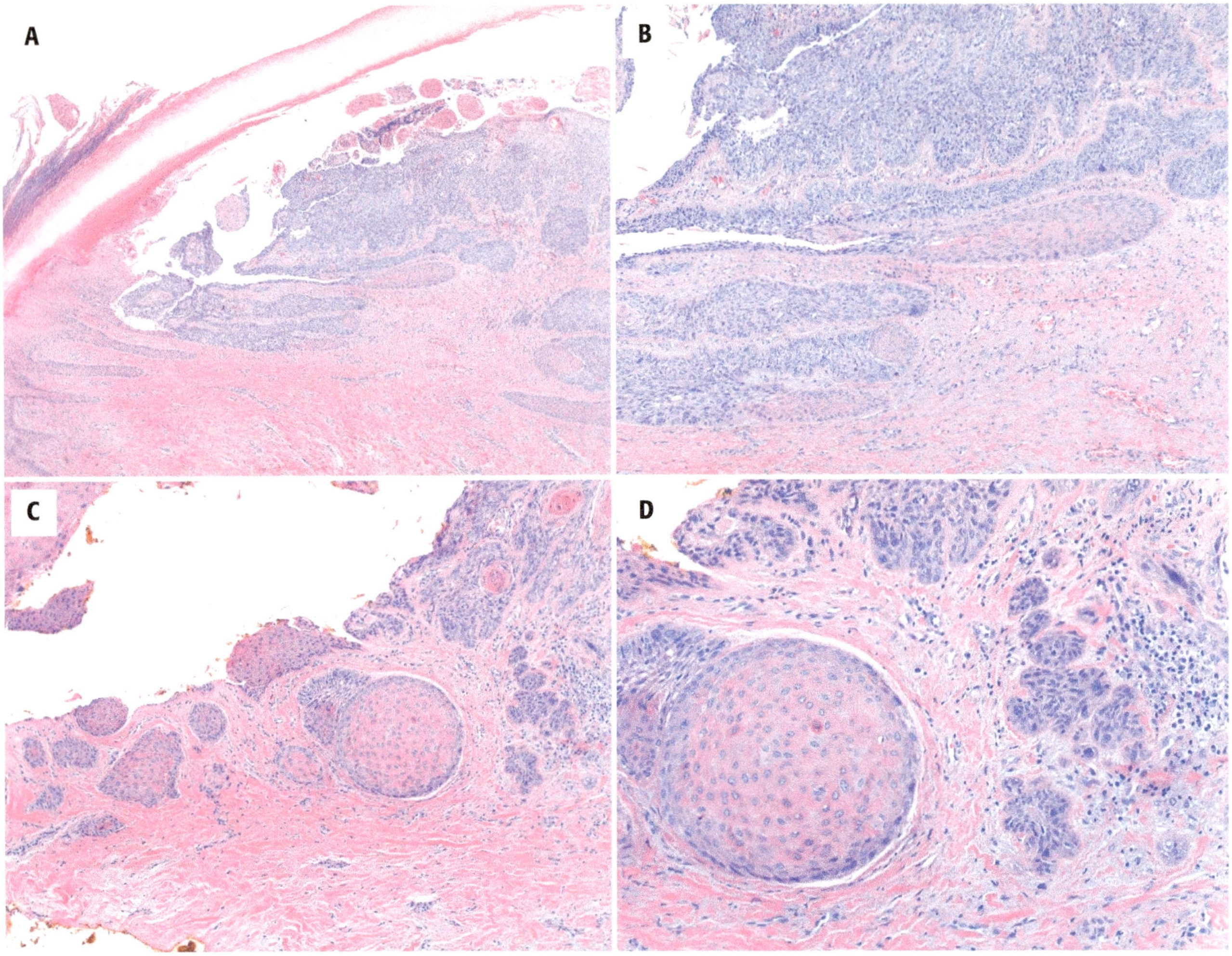

FIG. 19.18

Squamous cell carcinoma (SCC). **A,** In situ and invasive SCC involving the nail bed. **B,** Tumor replaces the nail bed epithelium and has basaloid features. **C** and **D,** Invasive carcinoma juxtaposed with bland aggregates of subungual epidermoid inclusions of nail bed epithelium.

presentations are the rule rather than the exception, leading to delayed diagnoses, and include nail dystrophy, onycholysis, ulceration, paronychia, oozing, subungual hyperkeratosis, nail loss, and rarely longitudinal melanonychia. Lesions often have a warty appearance and may be regarded as verruca clinically, also leading to delays in diagnosis. A monodactylic presentation of nail dystrophy is a helpful clinical clue, suggesting a neoplastic process over an inflammatory one. Men are more commonly affected than women, and the fingers are more often involved. HPVs of oncogenic subtypes have been implicated in many cases, just as in digital SCC in general. This association is also more common in the setting of human immunodeficiency virus infection. Other predisposing factors include chronic radiodermatitis, although the incidence of this condition is now more limited. Treatment using Mohs micrographic surgery is most commonly recommended as a tissue-sparing procedure. Amputation is rarely needed unless there is bone involvement, which is uncommon. Radiologic evaluation is suggested in long-standing lesions to exclude bony involvement.

Histologic Findings

The histologic features are similar to those of cutaneous SCC, and SCCIS is more common than invasive disease (Fig. 19.18). Viropathic changes may be encountered in HPV-driven disease. SCCIS involving the matrix can be a challenge because the matrix epithelium is basaloid and somewhat immature in appearance at baseline. One should look for characteristic features, including an increase in mitotic figures above the basal layer, dyskeratosis, and acanthosis, as well as parakeratosis with enlarged nuclei. Proliferation markers such as Ki-67 immunostain at this normally proliferative site may have limited utility in this setting, although they may be helpful in subtle nail bed SCCIS. More systematic studies of these entities with regard to the utility of staining subtle cases with p53 and p16 are needed.

KERATOACANTHOMA

By contrast, keratoacanthoma (KA) of the nail unit is relatively rare. The clinical presentation in the nail is similar to that of conventional SCC. However, KAs often display rapid growth, are painful, and cause underlying osteolysis or pressure erosion. Unlike KA at other sites, they do not display a tendency to involute, and thus excision is required.

Histologically, subungual KA also consists of a crateriform to lobular, papillated to endophytic proliferation of atypical pallid or eosinophilic keratinocytes (Fig. 19.19). In addition, KAs distinctively display many individually dyskeratotic keratinocytes, sometimes in clusters, which can calcify. The calcified corneocytes can occur within the epithelium or in the cornified portions of the tumor. This feature can be highlighted on von Kossa stain.

PAINFUL SUBUNGUAL TUMORS OF INCONTINENTIA PIGMENTI

Such tumors represent a late phase of incontinentia pigmenti. They are exceedingly painful and often involve multiple digits. Surgery and in some cases amputation were considered the mainstay of treatment for these debilitating tumors, especially if osteolysis is present, but retinoids have been adopted more recently as a nonsurgical approach with some success. Histologically, these neoplasms are practically indistinguishable from subungual KA (Fig. 19.20). Sometimes many eosinophils are evident in the infiltrate associated with the tumor, offering a small clue to the diagnosis, but these are often present in conventional KA.

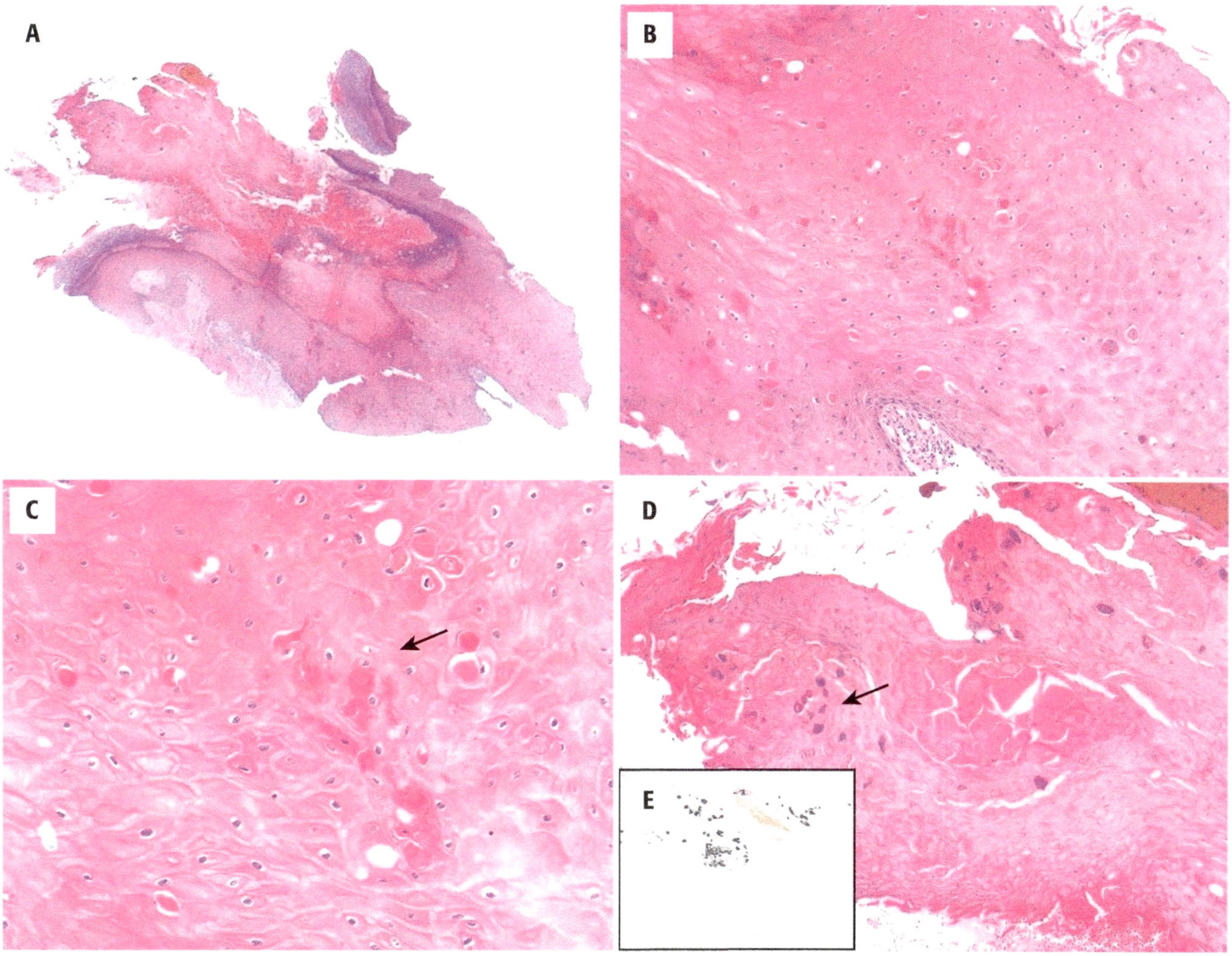

FIG. 19.19

Subungual keratoacanthoma. **A,** Crateriform squamous proliferation with central keratin plug and lobular growth. **B,** The tumor cells have abundant pale eosinophilic cytoplasm. **C,** Numerous often individually necrotic keratinocytes are present *(arrow)*. **D,** Calcified keratinocytes and corneocytes are common *(arrow)*. **E,** Calcium is highlighted by von Kossa stain.

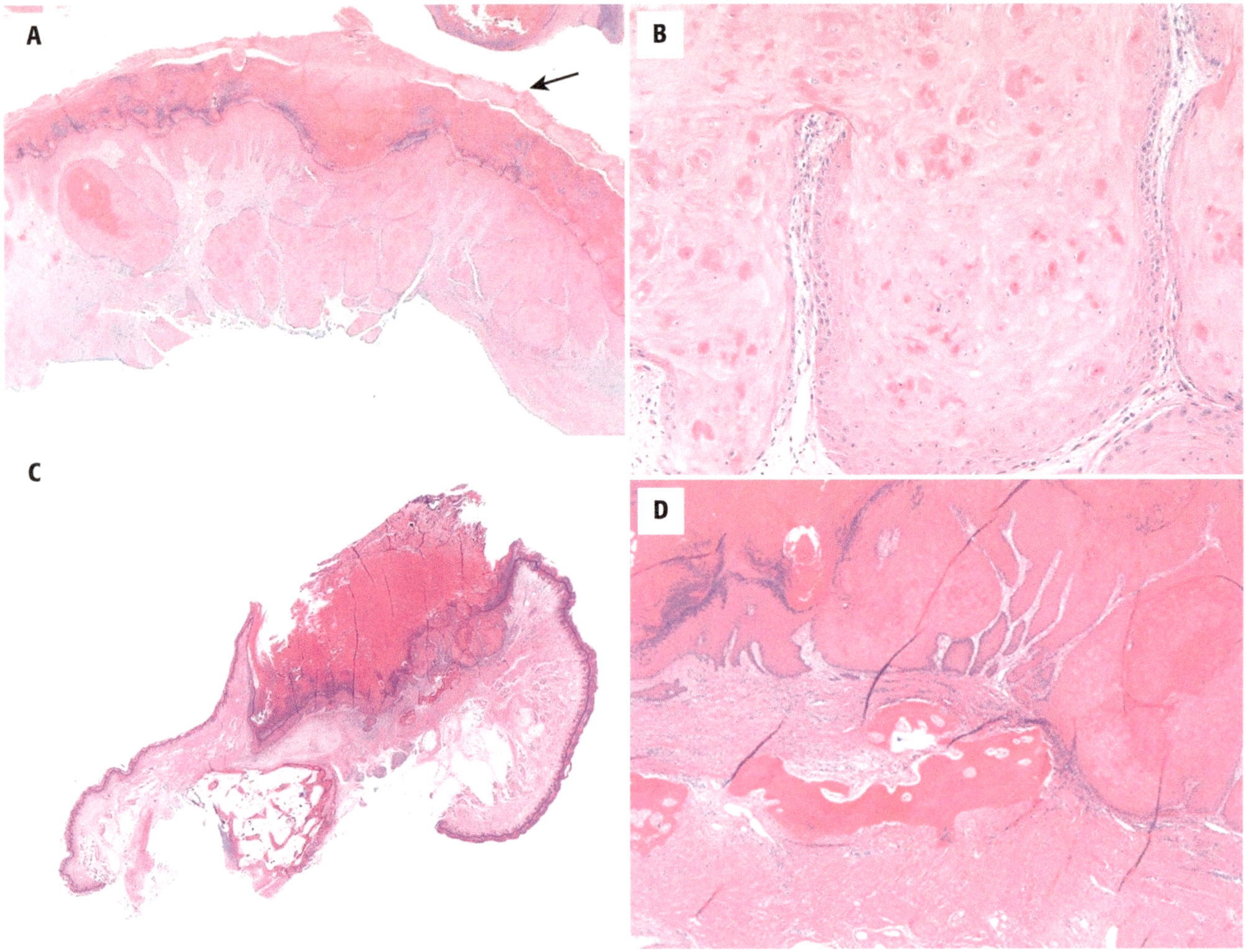

FIG. 19.20

Painful subungual tumors of incontinentia pigmenti. This lesion is indistinguishable from a keratoacanthoma. **A,** Tonguelike downward projections of keratinocytes. **B,** Keratinocytes with bland nuclei, abundant pale eosinophilic cytoplasm, and individually necrotic keratinocytes. **C,** Another cub-shaped squamous proliferation with extensive hyperkeratosis from the same patient. **D,** Downward lobular bulbous epithelial growth of well-differentiated keratinocytes with bland nuclear features extending to bone. There are associated inflammation and bone erosion (corresponding to osteolysis).

ONYCHOLEMMAL CARCINOMA

This exceptionally rare tumor of nail bed epithelium has also been referred to as malignant proliferating onycholemmal cyst. It is a slow-growing tumor that has a tendency, similar to subungual KA, to invade underlying bone. However, it has not been associated with metastasis. Unlike conventional SCC, it demonstrates a lobular growth pattern, cystic features, with foci of abrupt (onycholemmal) keratinization (Fig. 19.21). Some authors aver that this neoplasm should be classified more as an adnexal neoplasm, drawing analogies to trichilemmal and microcystic adnexal carcinoma, rather than simply conventional SCC. These authors also suggest that although it may not be possible to know, some reported examples of subungual KA might more appropriately be classified as onycholemmal carcinoma.

SUBUNGUAL EPIDERMOID INCLUSIONS

Although not neoplastic per se, subungual epidermoid inclusions can be seen in a variety of settings and are important to recognize because otherwise they can be mistaken for carcinoma histologically. They have also been referred to as onycholemmal cysts. They can be an incidental finding in other inflammatory or neoplastic conditions or can be associated with nail dystrophy, especially a shortened and dystrophic nail plate, in which they can mimic either primary inflammatory or neoplastic nail disease. There may be associated hyperkeratosis of the nail bed. A history of trauma is common, and there may be underlying bony abnormalities as well, such as exostoses.

Histologically, these are small rounded or elongate aggregates of keratinocytes that can be found under the

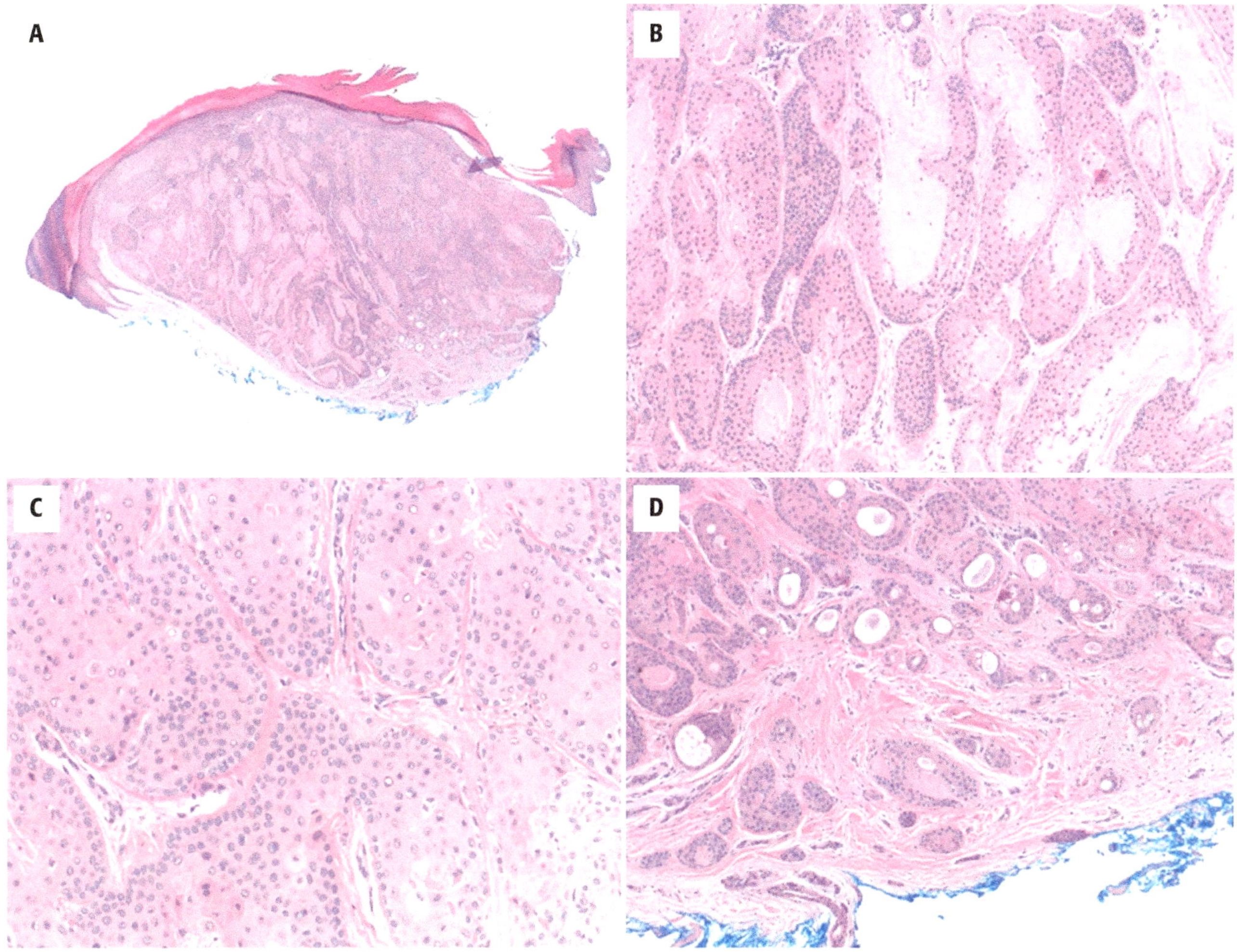

FIG. 19.21

Onycholemmal carcinoma. **A,** Nodule with infiltrative base. **B,** Lobular growth of keratinocytes. **C,** Keratinocytes with eosinophilic cytoplasm. **D,** Micronodular infiltrative growth at the base.

nail epithelium of the nail bed (see Figs. 19.18 and 19.22). They consist of eosinophilic keratinocytes and may form small cysts that may mimic ductal epithelium, forming an inner zone of keratinization. Whether these inclusions display genuine adnexal differentiation is a matter for further study. Calcification may also occur. They tend to be fairly superficial. A classification scheme for these has been proposed, although it is rarely used on a practical basis. A single large solitary cystic inclusion, often painful and associated with parrot-beak and clubbing deformity of the nail, and osteolysis, is referred to as an epidermoid implantation cyst. Multiple inclusions can be deemed type 1 or 2 depending on their extent, with type 1 being associated with limited clinical findings and superficial histology and type 2 with more notable clinical changes and more extensive aggregates histologically. It is important to recognize the less cystic variants because they can be mistaken for SCC or onycholemmal carcinoma in some instances. They tend to be quite bland cytologically and relatively superficial.

BASAL CELL CARCINOMA

Despite its frequency elsewhere, BCC is an exceedingly rare tumor of the nail unit, with only a handful of reported cases. As is the case for other nail tumors, they often have a misleading clinical appearance resembling a dermatitis, paronychia, fungal infection, or nonspecific ulcer with adjacent nail dystrophy. The histology is the same as elsewhere on the skin.

DISTINCTIVE TUMORS OF THE NAIL UNIT

ONYCHOMATRICOMA

Clinical Findings

Onychomatricoma (OM) is an uncommon and benign fibroepithelial proliferation of the nail unit. It typically presents as a nodule near the proximal nail fold, with

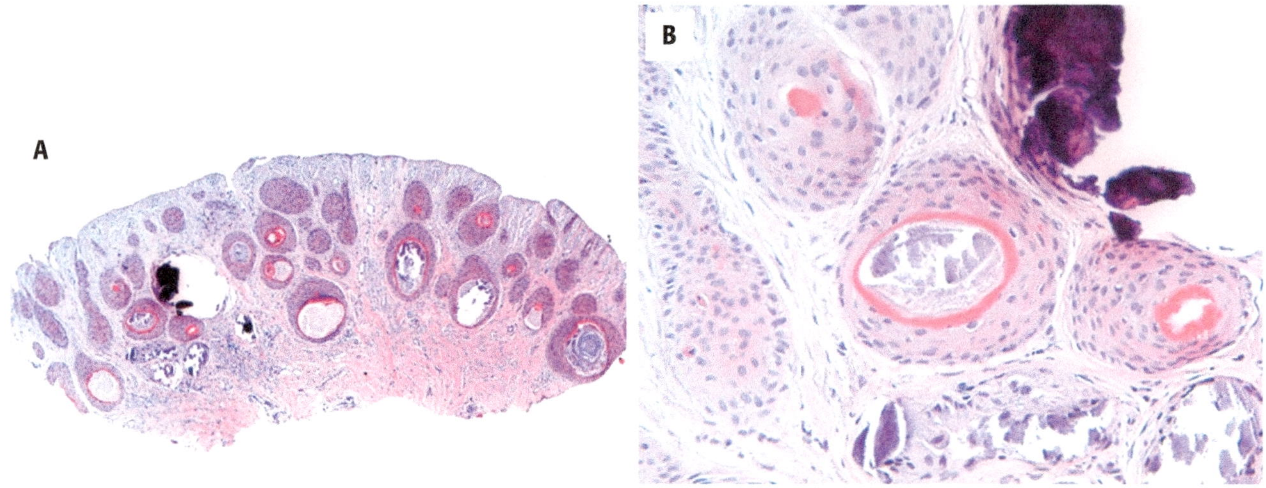

FIG. 19.22

Subungual epidermoid inclusions. **A,** Small superficial solid or solid microcystic aggregates of bland nail bed epithelium-like structures. **B,** Calcification may be present.

ONYCHOMATRICOMA—CLINICAL FINDINGS

Incidence
- Uncommon

Affected Individuals
- Typically age, 40 to 60 years but may occur at any age
- Male-to-female ratio: female predominance reported

Clinical Manifestations
- Nodule near proximal nail fold
- Yellow thickening of the nail plate
- Transverse overcurvature of the nail plate
- Splinter hemorrhages
- Holes in the proximal and free edge of the nail plate

Treatment and Prognosis
- Surgical removal
- Benign, may locally recur

ONYCHOMATRICOMA—PATHOLOGIC FEATURES

Microscopic Findings
- Fibroepithelial lesion
- Multiple fingerlike projections of matrical-type epithelium
- Fibrocellular stroma (may be cellular, myxoid, and contain pleomorphic mesenchymal cells)
- Thick nail plate with cavities containing serum

Differential Diagnosis
- Superficial acral fibromyxoma
- Cellular digital fibroma or fibrokeratoma
- Pleomorphic fibroma
- Angiofibroma

associated yellow thickening of the nail plate (also known as xanthopachyonychia), transverse overcurvature of the nail plate, and proximal splinter hemorrhages. It may involve a portion of the nail unit or all of it. The finding of holes in the free edge of the nail plate is another helpful clue. It most often affects the fingernails of middle-aged persons, more commonly women. The clinical differential diagnosis often includes VV, angiofibroma (periungual fibroma), and other tumors affecting the nail matrix. Pigmented OM can also be a cause of longitudinal melanonychia.

Histologic Findings

The complexities described in some writings on this entity are beyond the scope of this chapter, but in essence, it is a distinctive and thus fairly easy neoplasm to recognize if sampled amply or completely. If removed intact, it can be observed to contain both stromal and epithelial components of the matrix and possibly proximal nail bed. However, often the nail plate is avulsed, including much nail unit epithelium, in which case primary fibrous tumors such as angiofibroma, acquired digital fibrokeratoma (ADF), and superficial acral fibromyxoma are often considered instead.

The key histologic features include proximally, multiple fibroepithelial projections of the matrical zone, producing a thick keratogenous zone with V-shaped invaginations (appearing as normal matrix) (Fig. 19.23). There are also downward and inward projections of matrical epithelium forming deep channels interdigitating with epithelium ("glove-finger" appearance), and a fibrocellular stroma of variable cellularity, on occasion somewhat myxoid. Pleomorphic mesenchymal cells can occasionally be observed, but there is no evidence as to a sarcomatous counterpart per se (Fig. 19.24). These may reflect the same phenomenon as similar cells in the benign pleomorphic fibroma, for example. The nail bed may be slightly papillated.

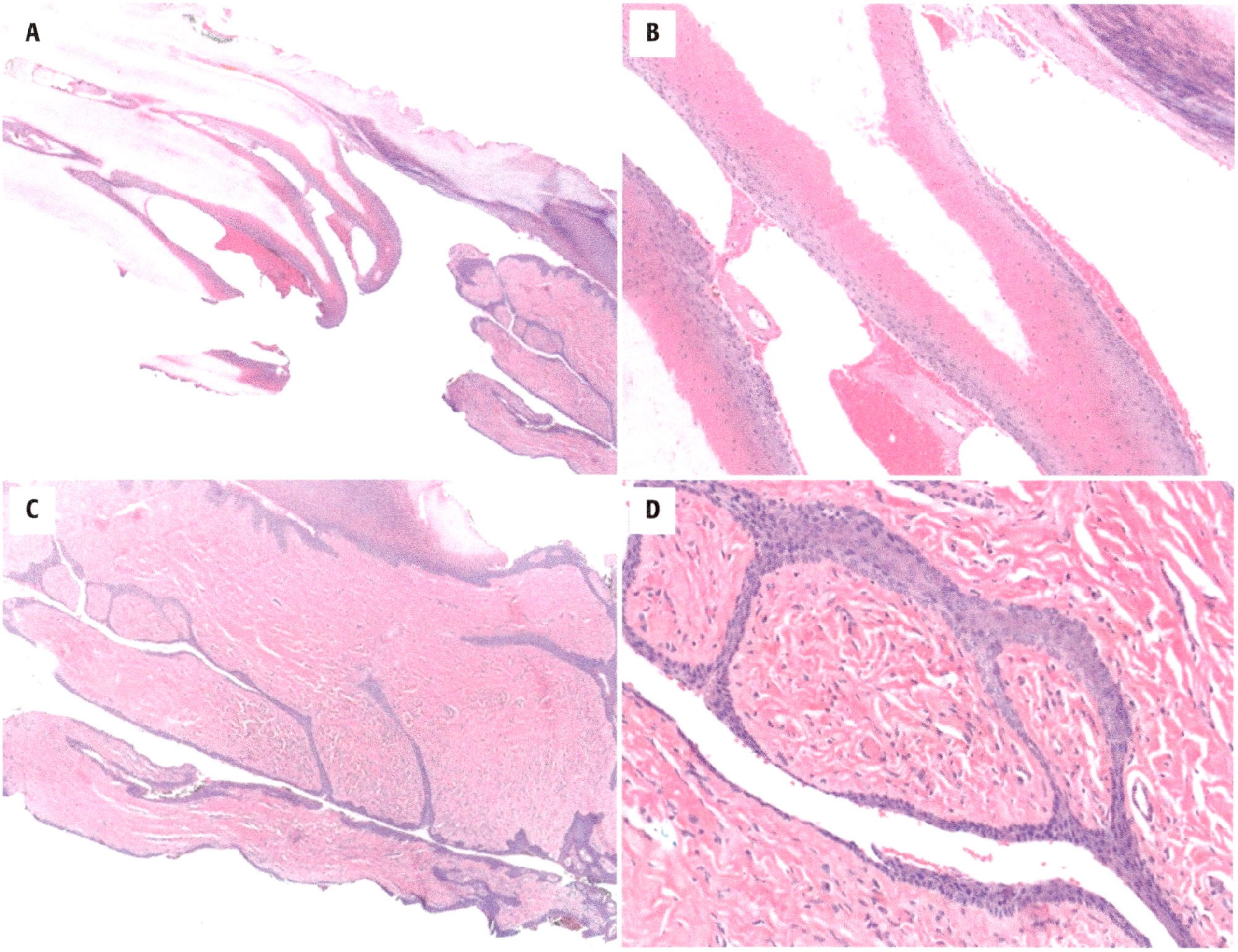

FIG. 19.23

Onychomatricoma. **A,** Distally, there is a thickened nail plate with serum and hemorrhage; proximally, there is an interdigitating fibroepithelial portion. **B,** There is reduplicated nail matrix epithelium, with the superficial aspects of the keratogenous zone apposed to the proximal nail plate. **C,** The proximal fibroepithelial portion consists of a fibrous stroma of varying cellularity. **D,** Cytologically bland matrical-type epithelium.

The nail plate beyond the lunula is thick, with cavities containing loculated serum, and often sometimes hemorrhage. It may contain some of the superficial papillations of the tumor, which in the author's experience are often edematous. Nail clippings, preferably oriented transversely, may be distinctive (see Fig. 19.24) and can be used to make the diagnosis if a surgical procedure is not desired. A keratin stain can highlight the epithelium sometimes included. The stromal cells in OM are CD34 positive, which is true of many other fibrous and neural proliferations on acral skin, but they are negative for CD99, S100 protein, and epithelial membrane antigen (EMA), making the distinction from superficial acral fibromyxoma and some neural neoplasms possible. CD13, a marker of onychofibroblasts, also stains stromal cells. When the tumor is viewed optimally en bloc, there is not much else that realistically enters the differential diagnosis.

ONYCHOCYTIC MATRICOMA

This is a more recently reported matrical proliferation that presents clinically with thickening and variable pigmentation of the nail plate (pachymelanonychia or xanthopachyonychia). It has been reported under the heading of subungual seborrheic keratosis as well. Onychoacanthoma or subungual longitudinal acanthoma has been proposed as an overarching term. Histologically, the authors of a 2012 paper describe three variants: acanthotic, papillomatous, and keratogenous. The most easily recognizable features are acanthosis of the nail matrix, with prekeratogenous and keratogenous cells in concentric array, forming squamous eddies (nail eddies) and small whorls of incipient nail plate (Fig. 19.25). There are variable pigmentation and melanocytic density, but it is low overall. The nail bed may be papillated and mimic verruca. The nail plate is thickened and may contain whorled

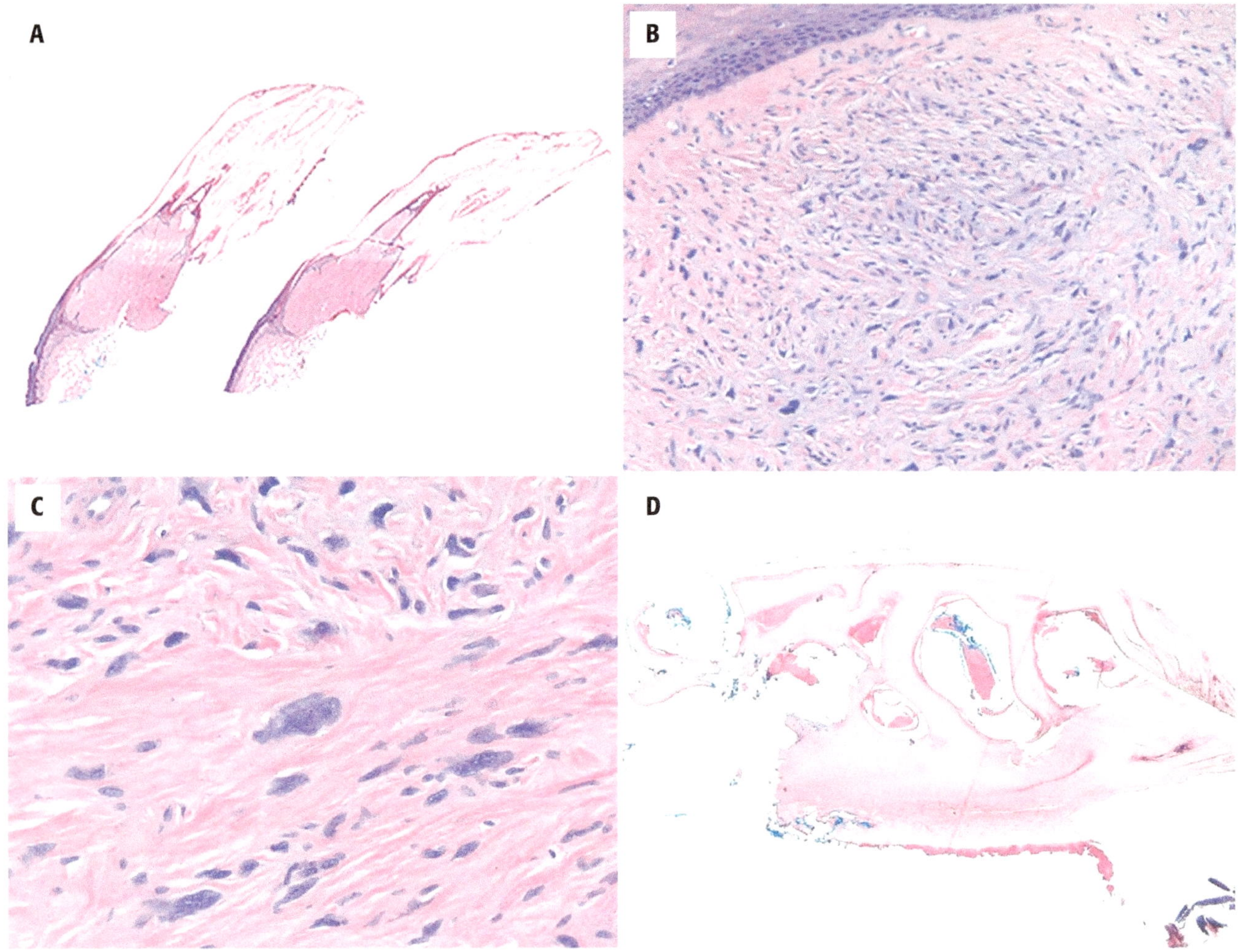

FIG. 19.24

Onychomatricoma. **A,** Tumor with prominent stromal growth. **B,** Hypercellular stroma with spindle and epithelioid cells. **C,** Occasional stromal cells show large pleomorphic nuclei or multinucleation. **D,** Distal nail clippings can be used to make the diagnosis. Especially if oriented transversely as in this case, the large loculations containing serum and often hemorrhage are fairly distinctive.

keratin. The clinical differential diagnosis includes OM, onychopapilloma, verruca, and SCCIS. The histologic differential diagnosis is mainly SCCIS and verruca. A malignant variant, onychocytic carcinoma has rarely been reported but whether this is a unique entity or a more basaloid variant of SCC is controversial.

FIBROUS AND SOFT TISSUE NEOPLASMS MORE COMMON IN THE NAIL UNIT

DIGITAL FIBROMAS

These include ADF and acral angiofibroma (periungual fibroma, also known as Koenen's tumor in the setting of tuberous sclerosis). There is considerable overlap among these entities. They all present as skin-toned papules, often with overlying hyperkeratosis, often in periungual areas, sometimes resting on the nail plate. This often produces a gutter in the nail plate. They are frequently mistaken for VV. Single or multiple lesions may be present, the latter in particular in the setting of tuberous sclerosis.

Histologically, they display varying degrees of fibrosis and telangiectasia, with ADF displaying in general more fibrosis, with haphazardly arrayed thick collagen bundles, and angiofibroma displaying a more prominent fibroblastic and sometimes vascular component. Stellate fibroblasts may be present. The stromal cells may label with CD34.

SUPERFICIAL ACRAL FIBROMYXOMA

Clinical Findings

This generally benign soft tissue neoplasm is an uncommon tumor of the nail unit. It is a slow-growing, painless

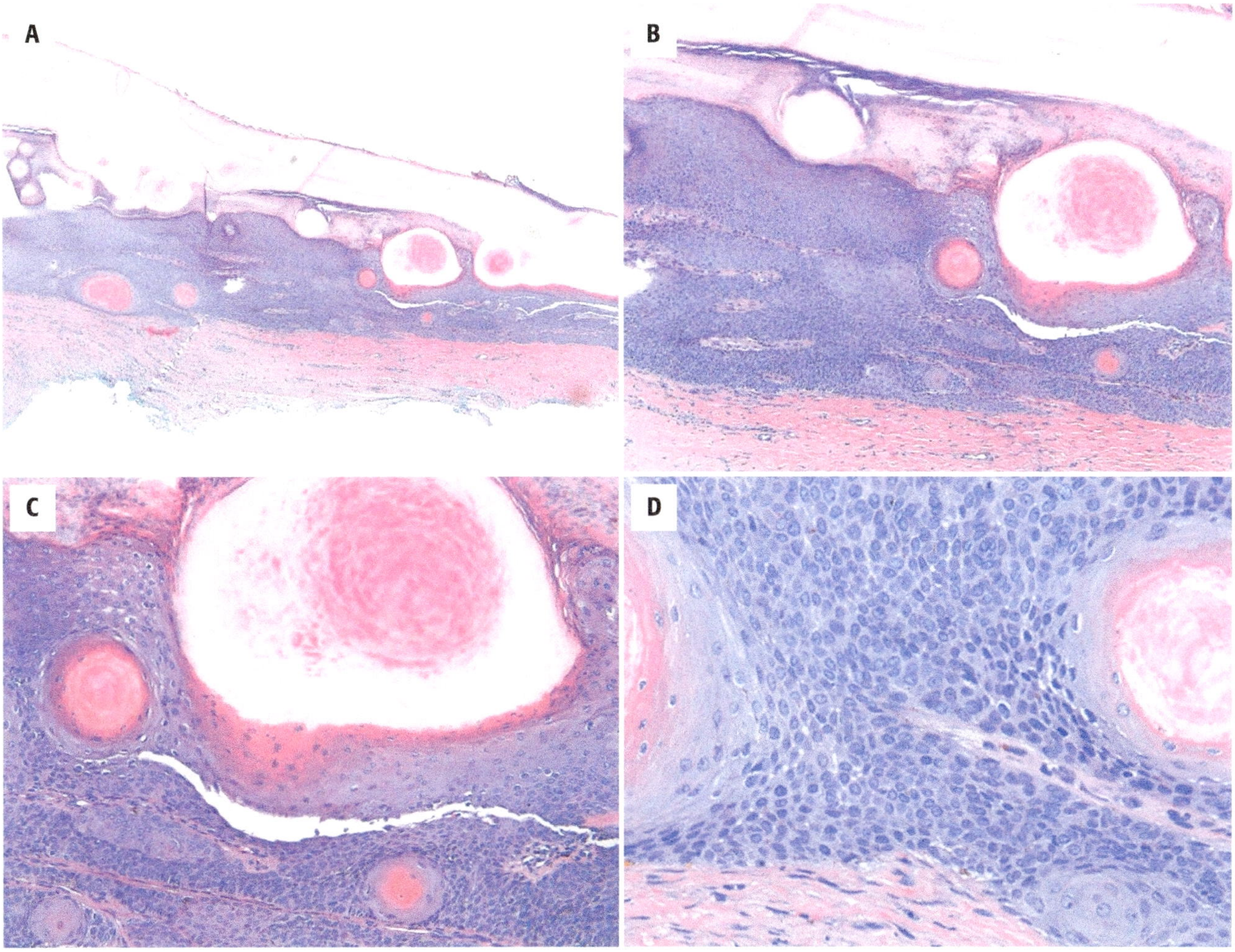

FIG. 19.25

Onychocytic matricoma. **A,** The tumor consists of an acanthotic matrical epithelium, forming small whorls of incipient nail plate. **B** and **C,** The tumor forms so-called prekeratogenous and keratogenous areas, recapitulating normal nail plate formation by the matrix. **D,** Pigmentation is often present, although melanocytes are not significantly increased in number. The basaloid epithelium may also be confused with carcinoma in situ.

nodule that has a predilection for the hands and feet, and involvement of the nail unit occurs in 50% of the cases. It may mimic an acral angiofibroma, and in one case report, occupied the entire nail unit.

Histologic Findings

They present as nonencapsulated dermal or subcutaneous proliferations of stellate or spindled fibroblastic cells, with occasional multinucleate forms, and only slight atypia if present. These are arrayed in nodular, loose storiform or fascicular patterns and contain a stroma that is myxoid, myxocollagenous, or collagenous, with accentuated vasculature and mast cells. Constituent cells stain with CD34 immunostain best and with EMA and CD99 more variably. One had weak positivity with S100. It is important to be familiar with this benign neoplasm because the differential diagnosis includes many benign and some malignant myxoid neoplasms, including myxoid neurofibroma, sclerosing perineurioma, superficial angiomyxoma, myxoid dermatofibrosarcoma protuberans, low-grade myxofibrosarcoma, and myxoinflammatory fibroblastic sarcoma. As noted earlier, it has sometimes been confused with OM when only the stroma of the latter is sampled.

GIANT CELL TUMOR OF THE TENDON SHEATH (PIGMENTED NODULAR TENOSYNOVITIS)

This is the second most common nonepithelial benign tumor of the hand. It may involve the distal digit but rarely involves the periungual areas. Only rare cases involving the nail unit have been described. Typically, it contains sheets of histiocytes, often foamy, and often with multinucleate osteoclast-like giant cells, hemorrhage, hemosiderin, siderophages, and sometimes a sclerotic stroma.

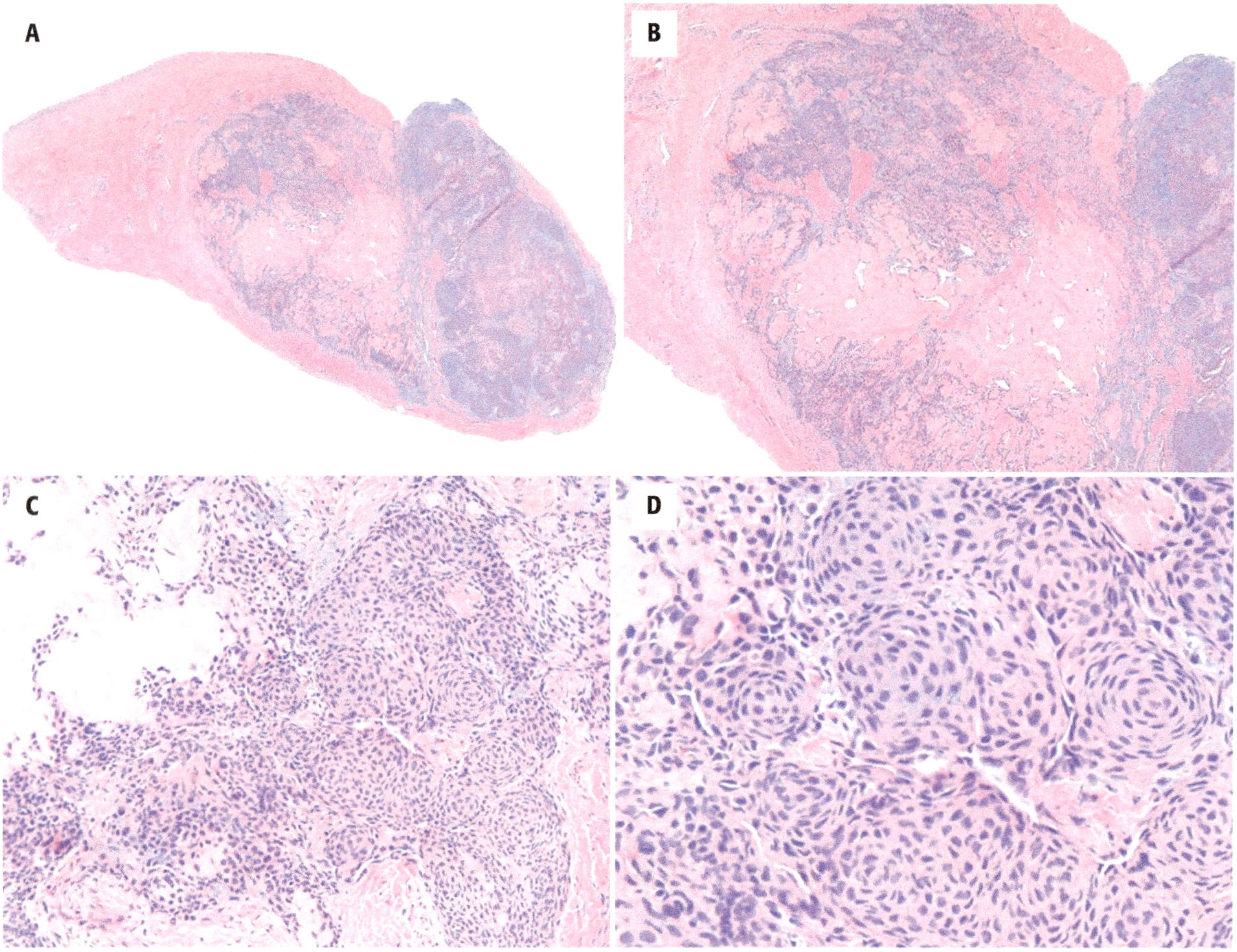

FIG. 19.26

Glomus tumor. **A,** Well-circumscribed subungual tumor. **B,** Areas of hypervascularity with ectatic vessels. **C,** The monomorphous modified smooth muscle cells are often associated with a fibrotic or sclerotic to myxoid stroma. **D,** The small, rounded uniform cells may be arrayed in a whorled pattern.

VASCULAR NEOPLASMS

PYOGENIC GRANULOMA (LOBULAR CAPILLARY HEMANGIOMA)

These common benign acral lesions can occur in a periungual or subungual location. They may arise because of trauma, an ingrown toenail, or underlying exostosis, and multiple lesions can occur as a side effect of retinoid treatment (i.e., isotretinoin, Soriatane, acitretin) and cast immobilization. The histologic features of a lobular capillary proliferation, with interlobular septa, are the same as elsewhere on the skin.

GLOMUS TUMOR

This is a benign proliferation of the modified smooth muscle cells seen in the glomus apparatus, a vascular shunt located on acral surfaces, but is frequently seen at other sites as well. Subungual tumors often present as tender nodules in the nail bed, which can cause nail dystrophy and sometimes erythronychia.

Histologically, it consists of a well-circumscribed nodule composed of small monomorphous glomus cells, sometimes aligned along larger vascular spaces. The stroma can be myxoid to fibrotic (Fig. 19.26). A symplastic variant with occasional larger atypical cells can also be seen in this setting.

MISCELLANEOUS NEOPLASMS REPORTED IN THE NAIL UNIT

A wide variety of other neoplasms have been reported at this location, of course, but in the interest of brevity, they cannot be discussed further; these include acantholytic acanthoma, lipoma, neurothekeoma, perineurioma, myxoid neurofibroma, osteochondroma, enchondroma, exostoses, papillary digital adenocarcinoma, and angiolymphoid hyperplasia.

SUGGESTED FURTHER READING

Amin, B., Nehal, K. S., Jungbluth, A. A., Zaidi, B., Brady, M. S., Coit, D. C., Zhou, Q., & Busam, K. J. (2008). Histologic distinction between subungual lentigo and melanoma. *American Journal of Surgical Pathology*, *32*(6), 835–843.

Baran, R., Moulonguet, I., Goettmann-Bonvallot, S., Encaoua, R., & Robert, C. (2018). Longitudinal subungual acanthoma: One denomination for various clinical presentations. *Journal of the European Academy of Dermatology and Venereology*, *32*(9), 1608–1613.

De Berker, D. (2013). Nail anatomy. *Clinics in Dermatology*, *31*(5), 509–515.

De Berker, D., Ruben, B. S., & Robert B. (2018). Chapter 1: Science of the nail apparatus. In: B. S. Ruben (ed.), *Baran and Dawber's diseases of the nails and their management* (5th ed.). Wiley Blackwell.

Delvaux, C., Richert, B., Lecerf, P., & André, J. (2018). Onychopapillomas: A 68-case series to determine best surgical procedure and histologic sectioning. *Journal of the European Academy of Dermatology and Venereology*, *32*(11), 2025–2030. doi:10.1111/jdv.15037.

Haneke, E. (2012). Ungual melanoma - controversies in diagnosis and treatment. *Dermatologic Therapy*, *25*(6), 510–524.

Lee, J. H., Lim, Y., Park, J. H., Lee, J. H., Jang, K. T., Kwon, E. J., & Lee, D. Y. (2018). Clinicopathologic features of 28 cases of nail matrix nevi (NMNs) in Asians: comparison between children and adults. *Journal of the American Academy of Dermatology*, *78*(3), 479–489. doi:10.1016/j.jaad.2017.08.052.

Perrin, C., Baran, R., Pisani, A., Ortonne, J. P., & Michiels, J. F. (2002). The onychomatricoma: Additional histologic criteria and immunohistochemical study. *American Journal of Dermatopathology*, *24*(3), 199–203.

Perrin, C., Cannata, G. E., Bossard, C., Grill, J. M., Ambrossetti, D., & Michiels, J. F. (2012). Onychocytic matricoma presenting as pachymelanonychia longitudinal. A new entity (report of five cases). *American Journal of Dermatopathology*, *34*(1), 54–59.

Richert, B., Theunis, A., Norrenberg, S., & André, J. (2013). Tangential excision of pigmented nail matrix lesions responsible for longitudinal melanonychia: Evaluation of the technique on a series of 30 patients. *Journal of the American Academy of Dermatology*, *69*(1), 96–104.

Ruben, B. S. (2014). Melanocytic lesions of the nail apparatus. In: R. Barnhill (ed.), *Pathology of melanocytic nevi and malignant melanoma* (3rd ed.). Springer.

Ruben, B. S. (2015). Pigmented lesions of the nail unit. *Seminars in Cutaneous Medicine and Surgery*, *34*(2), 101–108.

Ruben, B. S. (2018). Histology techniques for nails. In: *Scher and Daniel's nails diagnosis, surgery, therapy* (4th ed., pp. 29–38). Springer.

Thai, K. E., Young, R., & Sinclair, R. D. (2001). Nail apparatus melanoma. *Australasian Journal of Dermatology*, *42*(2), 71–81, quiz 82–83.

Werner, B., Fonseca, G. P., & Seidel, G. (2015). Microscopic nail clipping findings in patients with psoriasis. *American Journal of Dermatopathology*, *37*(6), 429–439.

Wlodek, C., Lecerf, P., Andre, J., Ruben, B. S., & de Berker, D. (2017). An international survey about nail histology processing techniques. *Journal of Cutaneous Pathology*, *44*(9), 749–756. doi:10.1111/cup.12976.

Yesudian, P. D., & de Berker, D. A. R. (2021). Inflammatory nail conditions. Part 1: Nail changes in psoriasis. *Clinical and Experimental Dermatology*, *46*(1), 9–15.

Yesudian, P. D., de Berker, D. A. R. (2021). Inflammatory nail conditions. Part 2: Nail changes in lichen planus and alopecia areata. *Clinical and Experimental Dermatology*, *46*(1), 16–20.

20 Neoplastic and Nonneoplastic Disorders of the Conjunctiva and Eyelid

Jasmine H. Francis • Klaus J. Busam • Brian P. Marr

NONNEOPLASTIC DISORDERS

INFLAMMATORY LESIONS

CONJUNCTIVITIS (INFECTIOUS AND NONINFECTIOUS)

Conjunctivitis is an inflammation of the conjunctiva that can manifest in both an acute and chronic form (persisting for 4 weeks or more). The etiology of the inflammation can include allergic, infectious (bacterial, viral, protozoal, parasitic), autoimmune, or autoreactive.

Clinical Findings

Conjunctivitis typically involves erythematous changes to conjunctiva, which may be accompanied by chemosis, discharge, or membranes. Depending on the etiology, the conjunctiva can present with a papillary (micropapillae with central vessels) or follicular reaction (slightly elevated, discrete, hypopigmented lesions with overlying or peripherally displaced vessels). Conjunctival inflammation can lead to a disturbance of the tear film and concomitant keratopathy (keratoconjunctivitis). In severe cases, conjunctival cicatrization and fibrosis can result in architectural changes to the fornix and eyelid.

Histologic Features

A conjunctival biopsy is often not needed but can be useful in characterizing conjunctivitis and distinguishing it from neoplastic disorders. As with any inflammatory process, the density, composition, and proportion of the inflammatory cells (lymphocytes, neutrophils, eosinophils, histiocytes, plasma cells) vary depending on the time course (early versus late), activity (acute versus chronic), and nature of the process (allergic versus infectious versus other). A suppurative neutrophil-rich infiltrate is typical of an acute bacterial infection, but lymphocytes and plasma cells are commonly seen in chronic conjunctivitis (Fig. 20.1). Chronic irritated lesions often display squamous metaplasia of the surface mucosa (Fig. 20.2). On occasion, a conjunctivolith may be seen in the mucosa (Fig. 20.3). A high number of eosinophils suggest an allergic hypersensitivity reaction. Except for the identification of an infectious organism, foreign body, or ruptured cyst, the cause of conjunctivitis can usually not be deduced from the histologic findings and depends on clinical correlation.

Ancillary Studies

Special stains and/or cultures for microorganisms (Gram, periodic acid-Schiff with diastase digestion [PAS-D], acid fast bacilli [AFB], Fite, Steiner) may assist in the identification of infectious organisms. Direct immunofluorescence studies are indicated for the workup of an autoimmune process, such as cicatricial pemphigoid. Immunohistochemical and molecular studies can help in the differential diagnosis of pseudolymphoma from lymphoma. Serologic studies may be needed to determine whether the conjunctivitis is part of a systemic process (e.g., connective tissue disease, Wegener's granulomatosis).

Differential Diagnosis

The differential diagnosis is broad. The process may be localized (primary conjunctivitis) or a manifestation of systemic process. A key issue is whether a conjunctivitis may be infectious in etiology or not because this directs further treatment. Special stains and cultures are helpful in this regard. If an infectious etiology can be excluded, inflammation may reflect an allergic reaction, autoimmune disease, or chronic irritation. A plasma cell–rich conjunctivitis may lead to concerns about a low-grade B-cell lymphoma (immunocytoma or marginal zone B-cell lymphoma). Immunohistochemical studies for light chain restriction and molecular tests for B-cell clonality can help establish a definitive diagnosis.

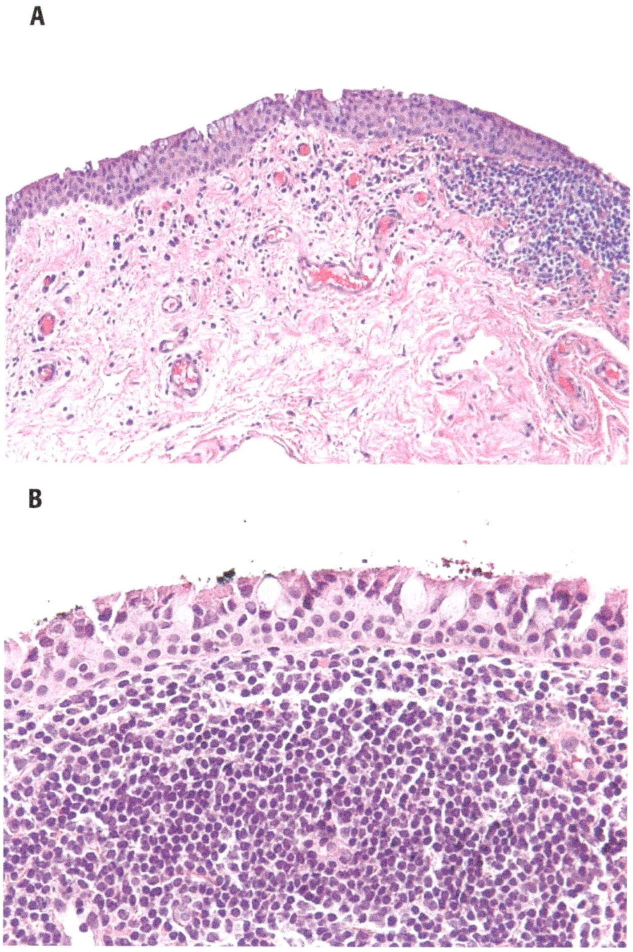

FIG. 20.1

Chronic conjunctivitis. **A,** Conjunctival mucosa with focal bandlike lymphoplasmacellular infiltrate. **B,** Dense infiltrate of lymphocytes and plasma cells.

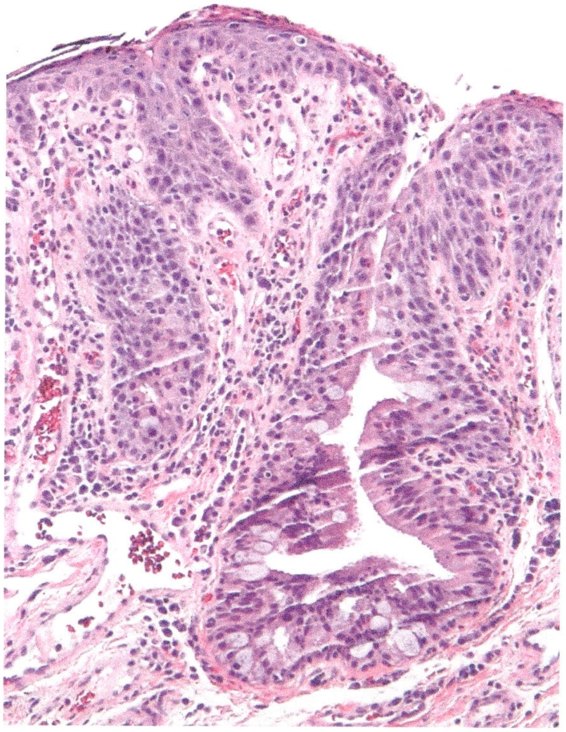

FIG. 20.2

Chronic conjunctivitis with squamous metaplasia.

Prognosis and Treatment

The etiology of the conjunctivitis dictates its appropriate treatment. Viral conjunctivitis can run its course and be managed with supportive measures such as lubricants, but other infectious causes benefit from both topical and oral antibiotics. Allergic conjunctivitis is treated by avoidance of the antigen, topical and systemic antihistamines, and mast cell stabilizers. Autoimmune or autoreactive causes benefit from steroids, immunomodulatory agents, and in some instances dapsone.

FOREIGN BODY GRANULOMA OR CHALAZION

Conjunctival foreign bodies can elicit focal inflammation. Similarly, a chalazion is a discrete granulomatous inflammatory lesion resulting from retained sebaceous material secreted from meibomian glands along the eyelid edge. It is also referred to as "lipogranuloma."

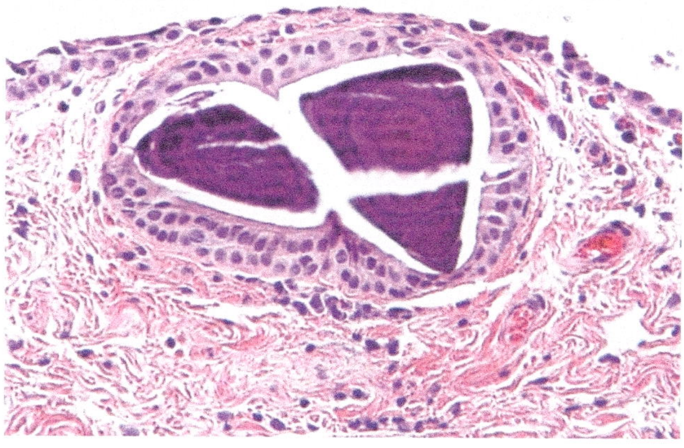

FIG. 20.3

Conjunctivolith.

Clinical Findings

Foreign body granulomas present as an elevated erythematous nodule that can incite circumscribing inflammatory

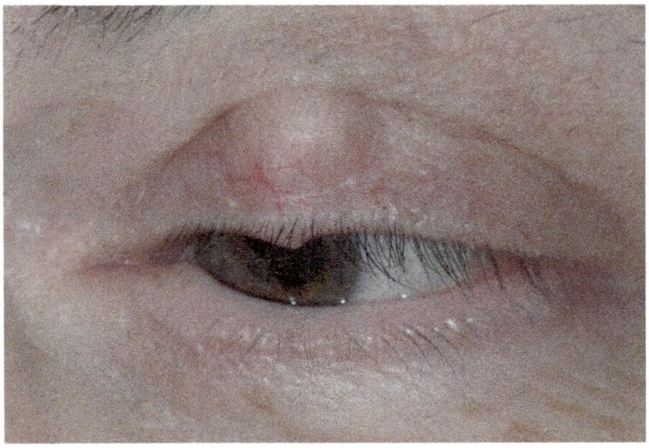

FIG. 20.4
Chalazion of the upper eyelid.

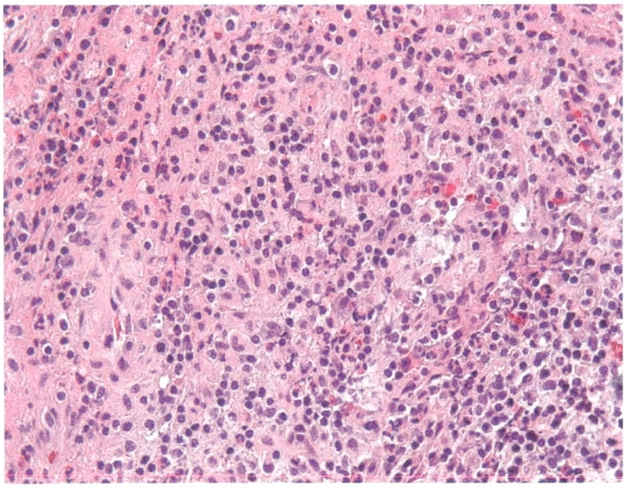

FIG. 20.5
Mixed cell inflammatory reaction with a granulomatous component.

reaction. Similarly, a chalazion is a discrete nontender nodule with overlying erythema and typically located close to the eyelid margin. An inspissated meibomian gland may be visualized (Fig. 20.4).

Histologic Features

The pathology of a chalazion usually shows a nodular mixed inflammatory cell infiltrate, typically with a prominent lymphogranulomatous component reaction, but neutrophils and plasma cells may also be present (Fig. 20.5). In later stages, there may be associated fibrosis.

Differential Diagnosis

The main differential diagnosis is with an infection and foreign body reaction. Special stains (PAS-D, AFB, Fite) can help exclude an infectious etiology. Examination for polarizable material is also prudent.

Prognosis and Treatment

Topical antiinflammatory agents can be helpful in treating the symptoms of a foreign body granuloma or chalazion. Alternatively, the granulomatous nodule can be surgically excised. The foreign body can be removed or warm compresses used to help expel the retained sebaceous material trapped in a chalazion.

CONNECTIVE TISSUE DISEASE (WEGENER'S GRANULOMATOSIS)

The conjunctiva is an uncommon site of involvement for connective tissue disease, occurring in approximately 5% to 15% of Wegener's granulomatosis cases.

Clinical Findings

In Wegener's granulomatosis, the palpebral conjunctiva and tarsus of the upper eyelid are common sites of disease. In its inflammatory stage, the conjunctiva appears hyperemic with granulomatous or ulcerative changes. The lesion may become necrotic with an avascular appearance and surrounding conjunctival injection and may progress to a fibrovascular proliferation and fibrous scar tissue. A concomitant episcleritis or scleritis is possible. Peripheral ulcerative keratitis may also occur, with dilated perilimbal vessels, peripheral cornea thinning, and epithelial defect (Fig. 20.6). Cicatricial changes can lead to alterations in eyelid architecture, including ectropion and entropion.

Histologic Features

The histologic changes associated with Wegener's granulomatosis of the conjunctiva usually involve a lymphoid infiltrate admixed with plasma cells, histiocytes, and eosinophils (Fig. 20.7). There may or may not be evidence of vascular damage. A necrotizing vasculitis is rarely seen.

Prognosis and Treatment

Conjunctival disease can be treated with both systemic and topical steroids and immunomodulatory agents.

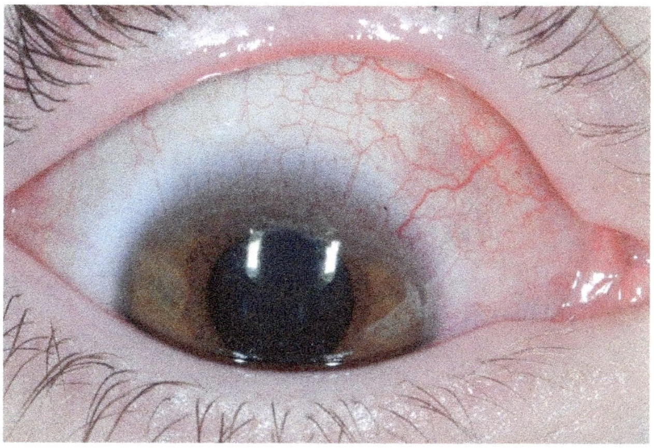

FIG. 20.6
Peripheral ulcerative keratitis of Wegener's granulomatosis.

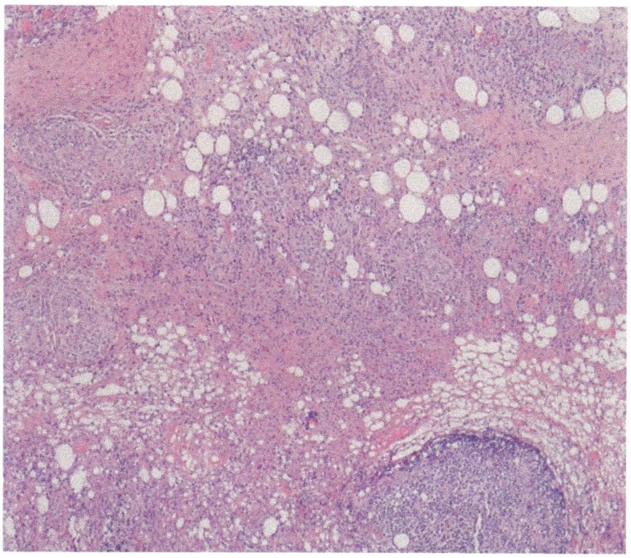

FIG. 20.7
Lymphogranulomatous reaction with focal mild vascular damage.

Epithelial defects of the cornea are covered with a topical antibiotic to prevent superinfection. An otolaryngologist should evaluate patients with conjunctival–tarsus involvement because there is an association with subglottic stenosis, which may lead to laryngeal obstruction and respiratory distress.

NONINFLAMMATORY LESIONS

DEGENERATIVE (SOLAR ELASTOSIS)

Prolonged exposure to ultraviolet (UV) light can result in solar damage to the conjunctiva, known as solar elastosis (and akin to actinic keratosis of the skin). Because of its predisposition from cumulative sun exposure, it is more common in individuals of advancing age.

Clinical Findings

Solar elastosis typically appears in the intrapalpebral space as a raised erythematous lesion, sometimes with yellow-white deposits (hyperkeratotic) or a pigmented appearance. Their elevated nature can disturb the tear film and result in keratoconjunctivitis.

Histologic Features

Solar elastosis is characterized by loss of pink material and fibers on routine sections and their replacement by homogeneous grayish material (Fig. 20.8).

Prognosis and Treatment

Symptoms of solar elastosis can be managed with lubricating or antiinflammatory preparations. Given the risk of malignant transformation, these lesions can also be surgically excised. Patients should be encouraged to protect their eyes from further UV light damage with the use of sunglasses.

PINGUECULAE AND PTERYGIUM

Both pingueculae and pterygium occur with advancing years and result from elastotic degeneration due to prolonged UV exposure (Fig. 20.9).

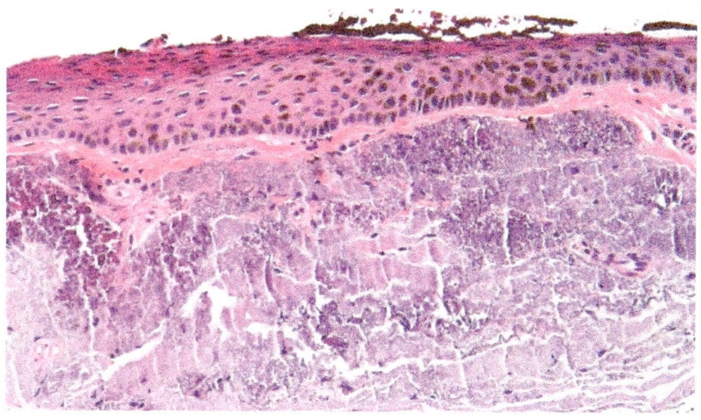

FIG. 20.8
Atrophic conjunctival mucosa with marked stromal solar elastosis.

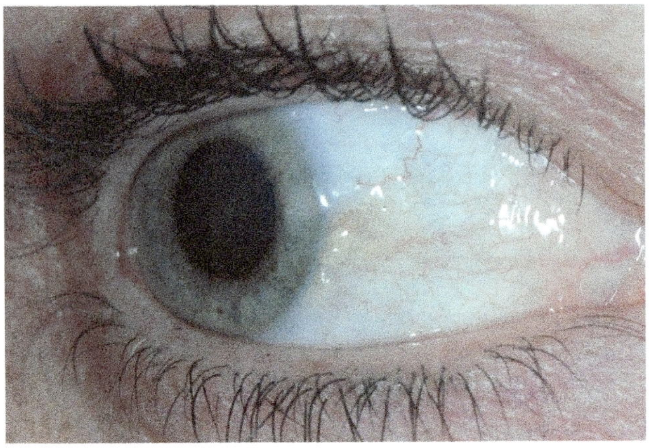

FIG. 20.9
Pinguecula.

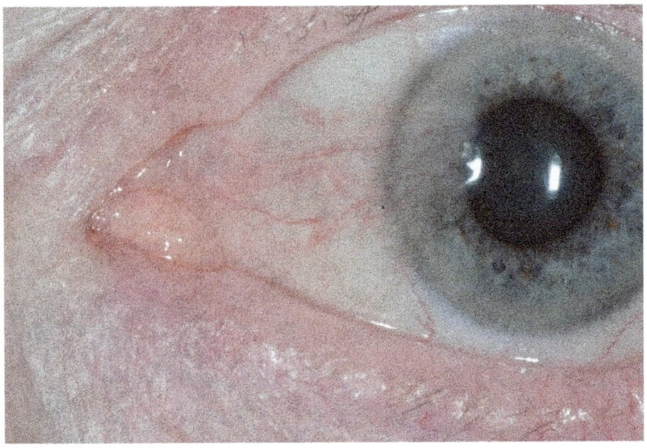

FIG. 20.10
Pterygium.

Clinical Findings

Both pingueculae and pterygium occur in the intrapalpebral space adjacent to the limbus. They typically develop over many years. They are not neoplasms but degenerative tissue alterations related to chronic sun damage. Pingueculae appear as small yellow-gray-white nodules with either an atrophic or thickened overlying epithelium. Pterygium crosses over the limbus and impinges onto the cornea in a winglike, triangular expansion (Fig. 20.10). It has a thickened, fibrovascular appearance.

Histologic Features

These lesions are usually not biopsied for diagnosis, but tissue may be removed surgically for symptomatic relief. The histologic findings usually reveal solar elastotic degeneration associated with nonspecific fibrosis and chronic inflammation.

Prognosis and Treatment

Treatment of pingueculae is unnecessary because they are typically asymptomatic and show either no or little growth. As it encroaches onto the cornea, a pterygium can interrupt the tear film or induce astigmatism. In this instance, it can be surgically excised and a conjunctival autograft sutured in place to reduce the likelihood of recurrence. On rare occasions, pingueculae and pterygium can incite an inflammatory reaction, which is best treated with a course of topical antiinflammatory drops.

AMYLOID

Conjunctival deposition of amyloid protein is a common process in healthy young and middle-aged adults without systemic amyloidosis. It is typically a primary localized entity but can less commonly result from prolonged, antecedent inflammation. It can also occur as an ophthalmic manifestation of systemic disease, such as multiple myeloma or lymphoma.

Clinical Findings

Amyloid deposition presents as a nodular or diffuse rubbery, waxy thickening of the conjunctiva (Fig. 20.11). It has a yellow-orange appearance and clings in a perivascular fashion. Whereas palpebral deposits usually signify a localized pathology, eyelid involvement is more commonly a systemic manifestation.

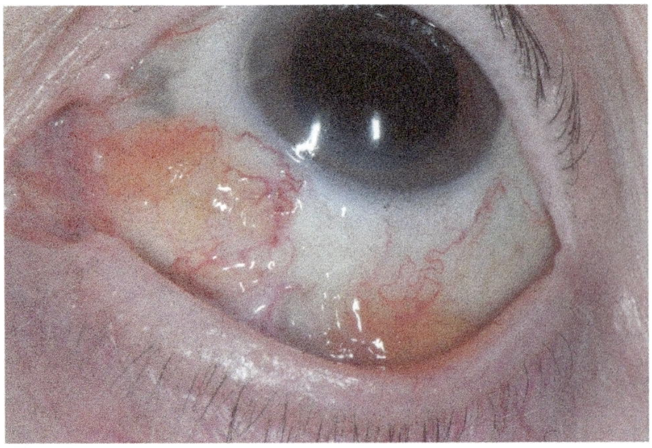

FIG. 20.11
Amyloid deposition of the conjunctiva.

Histologic Features

Amyloid material manifests on routine sections as hyaline amorphous pink material (Fig. 20.12).

Ancillary Studies

Special stains (toluidine blue, Congo red) can assist in documenting the presence of amyloid.

Prognosis and Treatment

Extensive, thickened deposition can disrupt the tear film and benefit from topical lubrication. Instances of larger, cosmetically undesirable lesions can be surgically excised.

CYSTS

Retention cysts of the conjunctiva are common and asymptomatic and previous surgery can be a predisposing feature.

Clinical Findings

Cysts appear as thin-walled, clear fluid-filled elevations more commonly on the palpebral conjunctiva (Fig. 20.13). They can form large solitary lesions or small cysts may form confluent clusters.

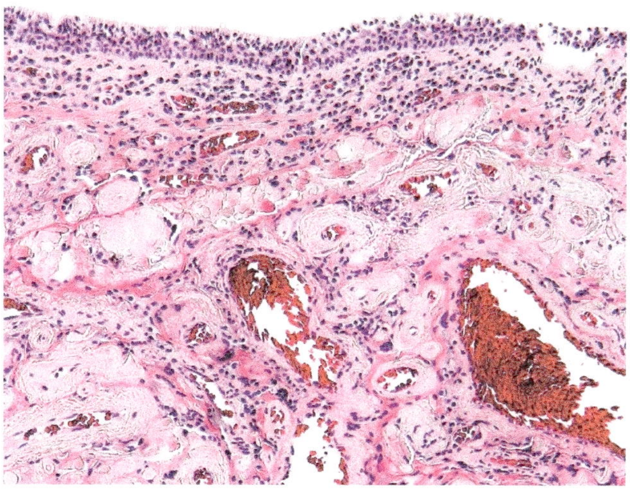

FIG. 20.12

Amyloid deposition of the conjunctiva. Hyaline material is present in the subepithelial stroma.

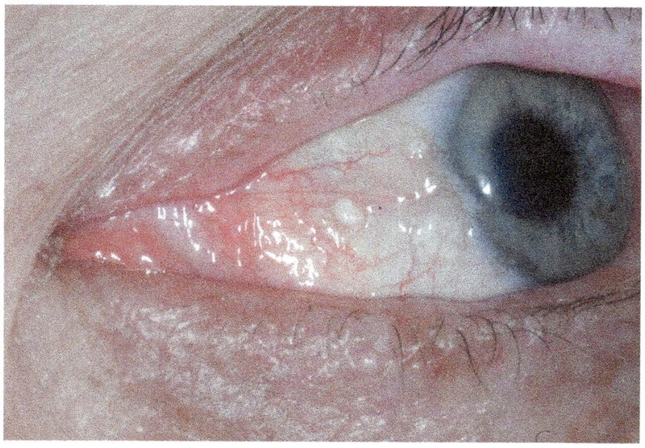

FIG. 20.13

Conjunctival cysts on the bulbar conjunctiva.

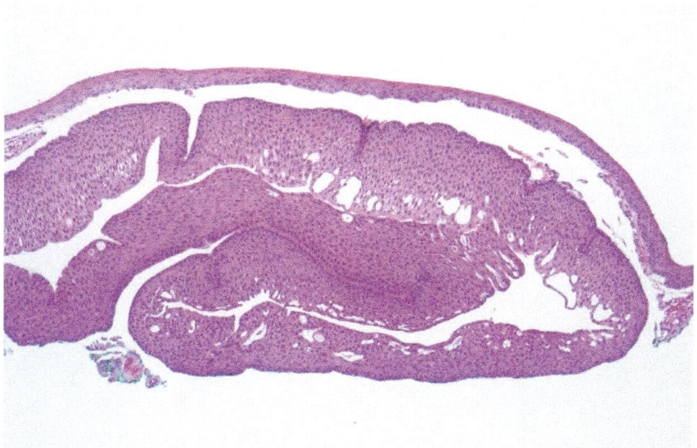

FIG. 20.14

Conjunctival cyst. Cystic invagination of conjunctival mucosa.

Histologic Features

Conjunctival cysts are lined by conjunctival-type mucosa, including columnar epithelium and goblet cells. Squamous metaplasia may be present. They usually appear as cystic invaginations of the surface mucosa in the superficial subepithelial stroma (Fig. 20.14).

Prognosis and Treatment

Because of their asymptomatic nature, cysts often require no treatment. However, they can be lanced by needle puncture to expel the fluid contents, but they may recur thereafter.

NEOPLASMS

SQUAMOUS LESIONS

SQUAMOUS PAPILLOMA

Clinical Findings

Squamous papillomas are benign epithelial proliferations usually related to human papillomavirus (HPV; conjunctival warts). They may be pedunculated or sessile. Pedunculated lesions tend to occur in children and young adults, most often located inferiorly in the fornix. Sessile lesions are more common in the bulbar conjunctiva of adults. They present as grayish-red soft lesions, may be multifocal, are associated with irritation and inflammation, and impair visual acuity.

Histologic Features

Lesions are characterized by papillomatous epithelial hyperplasia. Multiple branching fronds may emanate from a fibrovascular core (Fig. 20.15). Pedunculated lesions have a narrow stalk, sessile lesions, and a broad base. The epithelium is usually composed of nonkeratinizing squamous epithelium with variable number of admixed goblet cells. The fibrous cores are usually hypervascular with many ectatic vessels. Cytologic atypia is usually absent. HPV cytopathic changes (koilocytes, binucleated cells, raisinoid nuclei) may or may not be present.

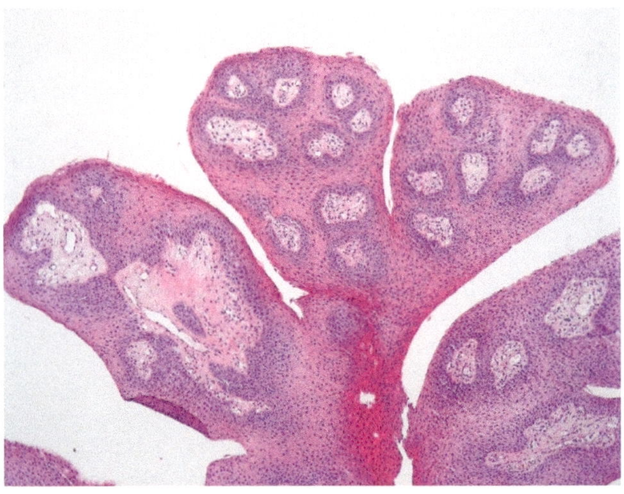

FIG. 20.15

Squamous papilloma. Papillomatous epithelial growth with fibrovascular cores.

Prognosis and Treatment

Symptomatic lesions are usually surgically removed. Similar to cutaneous warts, lesions may recur after local destruction or surgical removal.

OCULAR SURFACE SQUAMOUS NEOPLASIA

Ocular surface squamous neoplasia (OSSN) consists of corneal/conjunctival intraepithelial neoplasia (CCIN) and squamous cell carcinoma (SCC). Its incidence is between 0.2 and 20 cases per million and varies geographically, with some of the highest rates in Africa. The incidence in the United States is approximately $1/10^6$. Risk factors include older age, UV or toxin exposure, immunosuppression, HPV infection, male gender, and fair skin.

Clinical Findings

OSSN usually presents as a slowly progressive redness or irritation of the eye. Lesions are typically raised and hypervascular, occurring on the bulbar conjunctiva at the limbus and in the interpalpebral area. Isolated fornix and corneal lesions can occur but less frequently.

OCULAR SURFACE SQUAMOUS NEOPLASIA—DISEASE FACT SHEET

Incidence
- Depending on geographic area, 0.3 to $20/10^6$

Risk Factors
- Older age
- Male White individuals
- Chronic ultraviolet exposure
- History of smoking
- Human papillomavirus
- Immunosuppression
- Exposure to toxic compounds
- DNA repair defects

Clinical Appearance
- Sessile, fleshy, elevated lesion
- Leukoplakia
- Erythematous conjunctivitis like

Treatment
- Topical chemotherapy (mitomycin C, 5-fluorouracil)
- Surgery

Prognosis
- Local recurrence rate <5%
- Regional metastases <2%

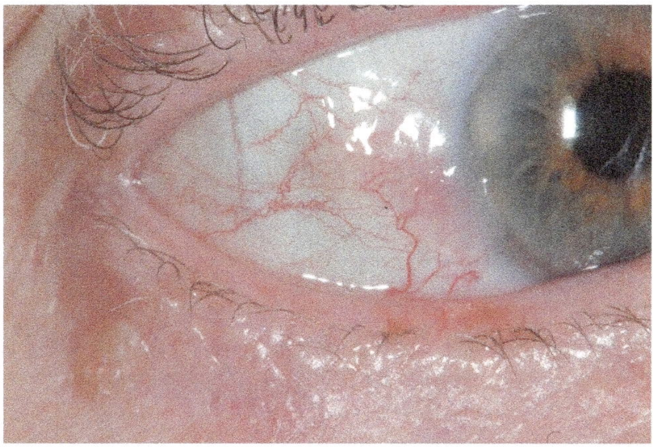

FIG. 20.16

Conjunctival intraepithelial neoplasia, clinical appearance.

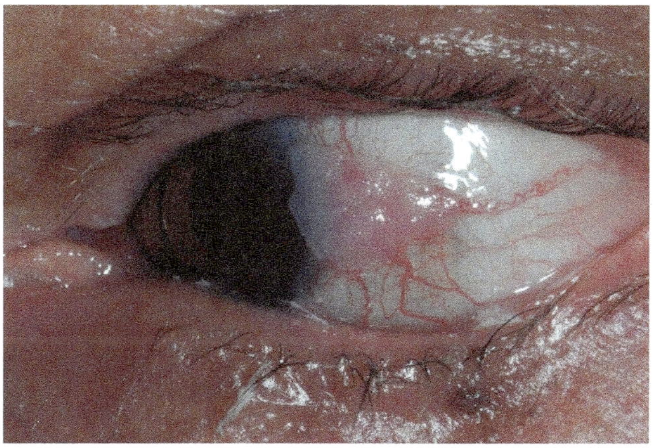

FIG. 20.17

Conjunctival intraepithelial neoplasia with overlying leukoplakia.

The surface of the lesion can appear fleshy or papillomatous or have overlying leukoplakia or a glazed appearance (Figs. 20.16 and 20.17). As they grow, they can extend onto adjacent cornea, conjunctiva, or skin or into the underlying sclera and orbit.

Histologic Features

CCIN is characterized by loss of polarity of keratinocytes and variable degrees of atypia (nuclear enlargement, hyperchromatism) involving the basilar (Fig. 20.18), suprabasilar epithelial compartment, or full thickness of the mucosa (Figs. 20.19 and 20.20). A grading system of CCIN from I to III exists depending on the extent of involvement of the epithelial cell layer by atypical tumor cells.

SCC of the cornea or conjunctiva is characterized by a downward growth of tumor below the level of the adjacent mucosa. It may have a solid lobular or an

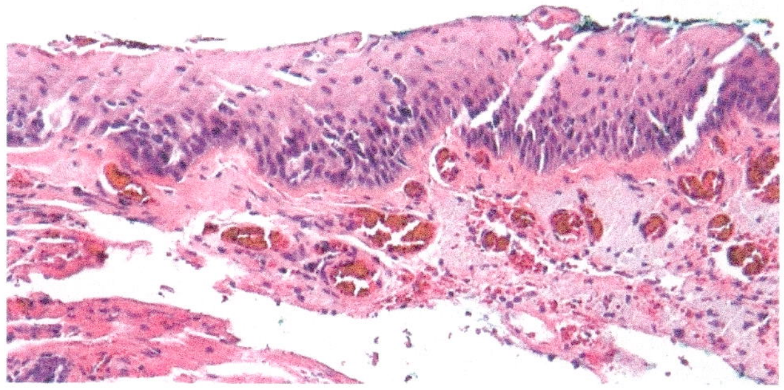

FIG. 20.18

Conjunctival intraepithelial neoplasm grade I to II. There is basilar and focal suprabasilar atypia.

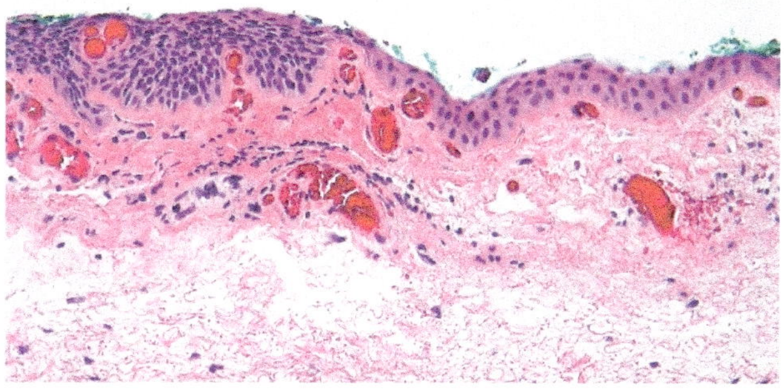

FIG. 20.19

Conjunctival intraepithelial neoplasia grade III (squamous cell carcinoma in situ [SCCIS]). There are patches of full-thickness epithelial atypia (basaloid SCCIS) alternating with benign squamous epithelium.

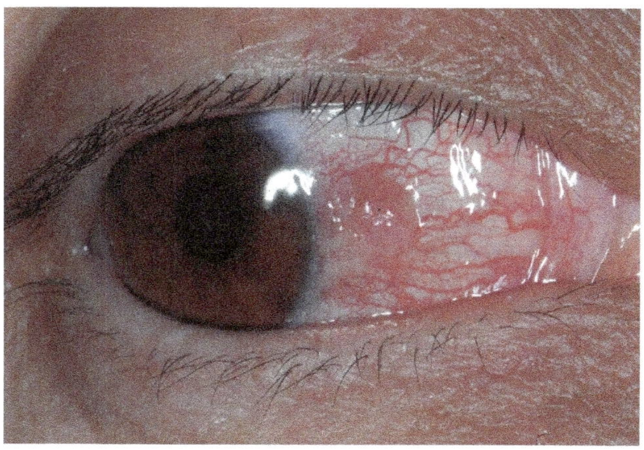

FIG. 20.20

Squamous cell carcinoma of the conjunctiva.

OCULAR SURFACE SQUAMOUS NEOPLASIA (OSSN)—PATHOLOGIC FEATURES

Features

- Noninvasive: conjunctival intraepithelial neoplasia (CIN)
- CIN I: epithelial atypia limited to lower third of mucosal thickness
- CIN II: epithelial atypia limited to lower two-thirds of mucosal thickness
- CIN III: full- or near full-thickness (more than two-thirds of the mucosal layer) atypia (high-grade dysplasia or squamous cell carcinoma in situ)

Invasive Carcinoma

- Bulky solid or infiltrative growth
- Degrees of differentiation (extent of keratinization): well, moderate, and poor
- Variants: conventional, clear cell, spindle cell, acantholytic, or basaloid

Immunohistochemistry

- Positive for AE1: AE3, p40
- Variably positive for epithelial membrane antigen, CK7, p16

Differential Diagnosis

- Sebaceous carcinoma
- Extramammary Paget's disease
- Melanoma
- Basal cell carcinoma with squamous metaplasia

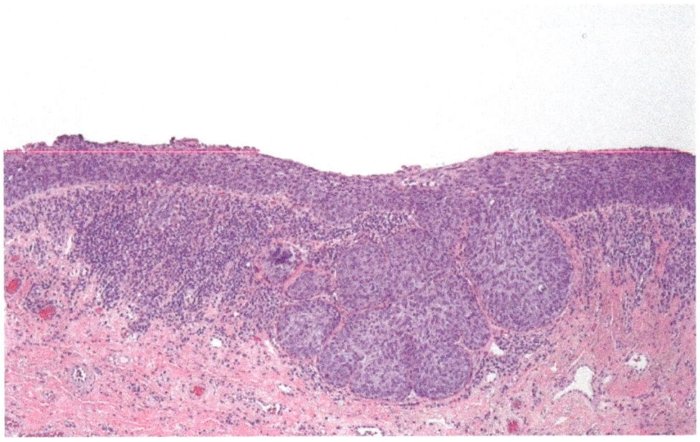

FIG. 20.21

Squamous cell carcinoma of the conjunctiva, basaloid type. There is in situ and invasive carcinoma with basaloid features. Invasive carcinoma grows downward below the level of the adjacent in situ carcinoma.

irregular jagged interface with the surrounding stroma. There may be an inflammatory or fibrosing reaction to the invasive tumor. Tumors may be keratinizing or not. Keratinizing tumors typically display a pink cytoplasm. Their tumor cells usually have elongated, angulated, or hyperchromatic nuclei. Abrupt maturation is common at the invasive front of the tumor. The spectrum of appearances of conjunctival SCC is similar to cutaneous SCC. HPV-associated SCCs of the conjunctiva often have a basaloid appearance (Fig. 20.21). Poorly differentiated tumors usually lack visible keratin and may require immunohistochemical studies for confirmation of the diagnosis.

Ancillary Studies

Ancillary studies used for the diagnosis of OSSN usually include immunohistochemical studies (e.g., for the diagnosis of poorly differentiated tumors or the distinction of SCC from sebaceous carcinoma) or to document association with HPV.

Differential Diagnosis

Intraepithelial neoplasia needs to be distinguished from squamous metaplasia with reactive atypia or reparative changes (pseudoepitheliomatous hyperplasia). It also needs to be distinguished from intraepithelial carcinoma of nonsquamous type, such as extramammary Paget's disease or intraepithelial sebaceous carcinoma (sebaceous carcinoma in situ).

The diagnosis of invasive well-differentiated SCC is usually straightforward. Poorly differentiated tumors are readily recognized as malignant but can be difficult to distinguish from a poorly differentiated sebaceous carcinoma. Immunostains, such as for adipophilin, can assist in the distinction of SCC from sebaceous carcinoma (Table 20.1).

Prognosis and Treatment

Treatment of OSSN involves surgery for well-circumscribed lesions and carries a low recurrence rate. Cryotherapy can

TABLE 20.1

Immunohistochemical Distinction of Sebaceous Carcinoma from Basal Cell Carcinoma and Squamous Cell Carcinoma

Antibody	Sebaceous CA	BCC	SCC	MCC
EMA	+	–	–	(+)
Berep4	+	+	–	(+)
Cam5.2	+	–	±	+
ADP	+	–	–	–
AR	+	±	±	–
CK20	–	–	–	+

ADP, Adipophilin; *AR*, androgen receptor; *BCC*, basal cell carcinoma; *EMA*, epithelial membrane antigen; *MCC*, Merkel cell carcinoma; *SCC*, squamous cell carcinoma.

be used in conjunction with surgery or by itself in addition to the use of topical chemotherapies and immunomodulators. Local radiation and brachytherapy have also been used for nonsurgical candidates. Corneal/CIN has a low rate of deeper invasion (3%–5%). With contemporary therapy, conjunctival SCC has a local recurrence rate of less than 5% and metastasizes to regional lymph nodes in fewer than 2% of patients. Metastatic disease is usually detected first in the adjacent preauricular, submandibular, or cervical lymph nodes. Risk for metastatic disease includes aggressive histologic features (poorly differentiated, basaloid, acantholytic, or spindle cell features; high mitotic index, size larger than 5 mm; lymphatic invasion; orbital or eyelid invasion).

MELANOCYTIC LESIONS

COMPLEXION-ASSOCIATED MELANOSIS

Complexion-related melanosis is a benign conjunctival pigmentation that occurs more frequently in patients with darkly pigmented skin. In one study, complexion-related melanosis was reported in 5% of the White population, 28% of the Hispanic population, 36% of the Asian population, and 93% of the Black population.

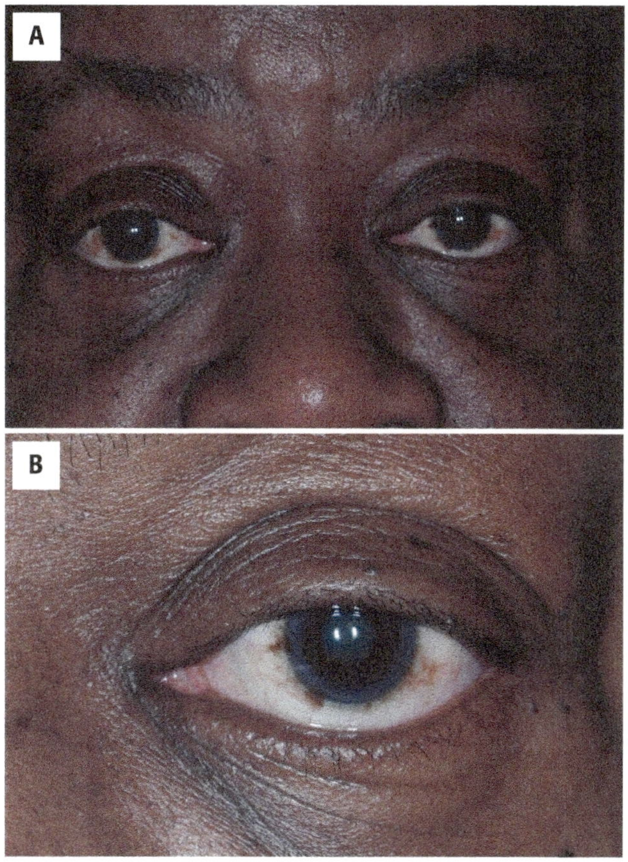

FIG. 20.22
A, Bilateral complexion-related melanosis. **B,** Higher magnification.

Clinical Findings

Complexion-associated melanosis consists of fine pigmentation, usually bilaterally; can be asymmetric; and is found most frequently in the limbal area (Fig. 20.22). It typically correlates with skin pigmentation being more frequent in dark-skinned individuals. The pigment does not have any intrinsic or feeder vessels nor does it extend on to the corneal epithelium or have significant thickness.

Histologic Features

Complexion-associated melanosis is rarely biopsied unless the clinical presentation is not straightforward and there is concern about a possible melanocytic neoplasm. The most important issue is confirmation that the melanocyte density is within normal limits and that there is therefore no evidence for a melanocytic neoplasm. The clinically visible pigment alteration is reflected by an increase in the deposition of melanin pigment in epithelial cells or stromal melanophages.

Prognosis and Treatment

Complexion-associated melanosis has no malignant potential and is observed without treatment. If rapid asymmetric irregular growth occurs, then a biopsy should be performed to distinguish it from primary acquired melanosis (PAM).

CONJUNCTIVAL MELANOCYTIC NEVUS

Conjunctival nevi are the most common pigmented tumors of the conjunctiva. They are typically asymptomatic and are usually noted at an early age because of cosmetic reasons or if they become inflamed.

Clinical Findings

Conjunctival nevi appear as elevated variably pigmented lesions on the conjunctiva. They are frequently found on the bulbar conjunctiva near the limbus but can occur on any part of the conjunctiva (Fig. 20.23). They have

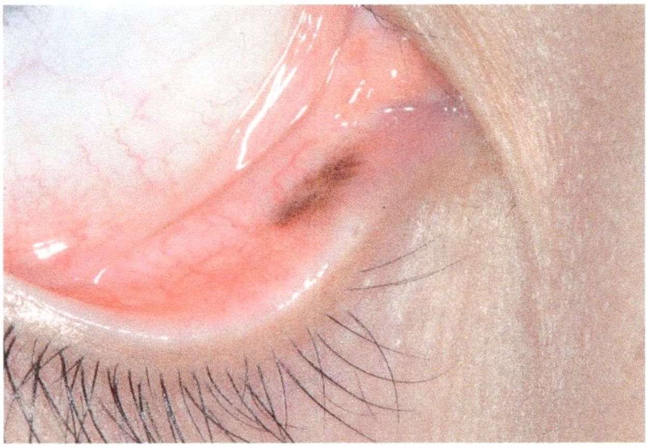

FIG. 20.23
Melanotic nevus of the palpebral conjunctiva.

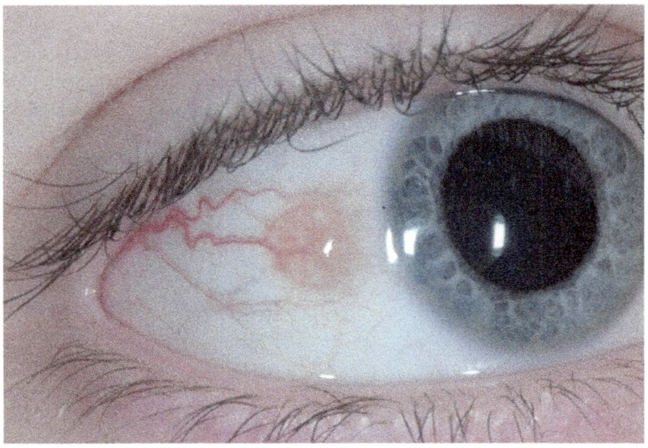

FIG. 20.24
Amelanotic nevus of the bulbar conjunctiva.

intrinsic vasculature, intrinsic cysts that can be pigmented or clear, and nondilated feeder vessels (Fig. 20.24). They do not extend over the limbus onto the cornea and are freely mobile with the conjunctiva. They can grow slowly during adolescence but are typically stationary during adulthood. Clinically, they can be classified as either congenital or acquired. A distinct variant is conjunctival melanocytosis (diffuse blue nevus), which is usually seen in the setting of nevus of Ota (nevus fuscoceruleus ophthalmomaxillaris) (Fig. 20.25).

Histologic Features

Conjunctival melanocytic nevi may be confined to the conjunctival mucosa ("junctional" nevus), involve both the mucosa and submucosa ("compound" nevus), or be present only in the stroma (subepithelial nevus). Most (nearly 80%) nevi of the conjunctiva are compound (Fig. 20.26), 10% to 15% are subepithelial, and 5% are junctional only. A typical feature of conjunctival nevi is the presence of epithelium with goblet cells forming invaginations into the stroma or small cysts (see Fig. 20.26). Such intralesional epithelial-lined cysts are found in approximately half of conjunctival nevi. The cytology of the melanocytes within a nevus may vary from large epithelioid to small epithelioid or fusiform. Fusiform melanocytes may display schwannian features. Melanocytic nevi of the conjunctiva may be pigmented or amelanotic. A lesion may be uniform in its cytology (e.g., predominantly small epithelioid), but there is often a mixture of cell types. Common (Fig. 20.27) and cellular variants of blue nevi may be seen. Some melanocytic nevi are inflamed and hypervascular and may be confused with an inflammatory process or angioma.

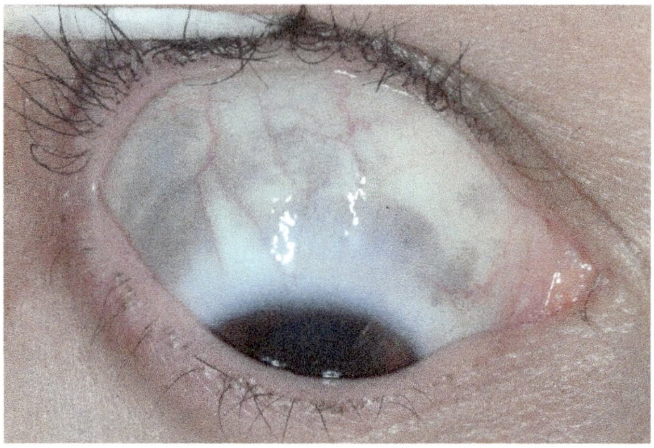

FIG. 20.25
Nevus of Ota involving the conjunctiva.

Analogous to cutaneous nevi, histologic variants of conjunctival nevi have been reported, including blue nevi (common and cellular blue nevi), Spitz's nevi, and balloon cell nevi, as well as combinations in phenotypes (combined nevi), such as ordinary and blue nevus, and ordinary nevi with a minor subpopulation of large pigmented epithelioid melanocytes (Fig. 20.28), spitzoid, or clear or balloon cells (Fig. 20.29). Melanocytic nevi of the conjunctiva usually display good evidence of maturation and lack mitotic figures.

Slightly more than half of the common types of conjunctival melanocytic nevi carry the *BRAFV600E* mutation. Others may harbor NRASQ61R mutations. Conjunctival melanocytic nevi usually lack cytogenetic aberrations.

Differential Diagnosis

The main distinction is from conjunctival melanoma. Features favoring a melanocytic nevus include sharp circumscription and lateral demarcation, evidence of

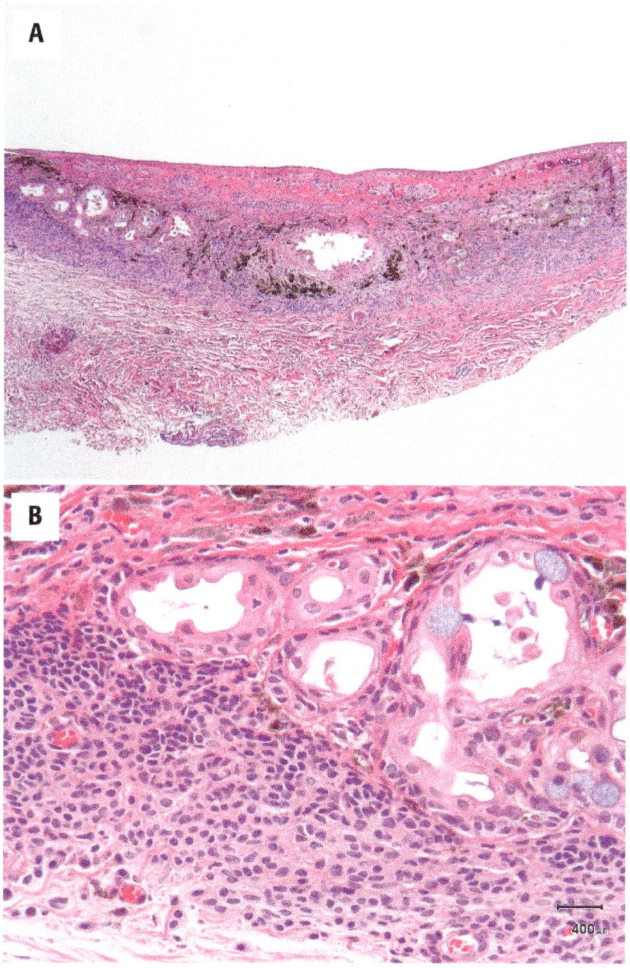

FIG. 20.26

Compound melanocytic nevus of the conjunctiva. **A,** The lesion is small with a symmetric silhouette. **B,** Cytologically bland melanocytes adjacent to epithelial cysts.

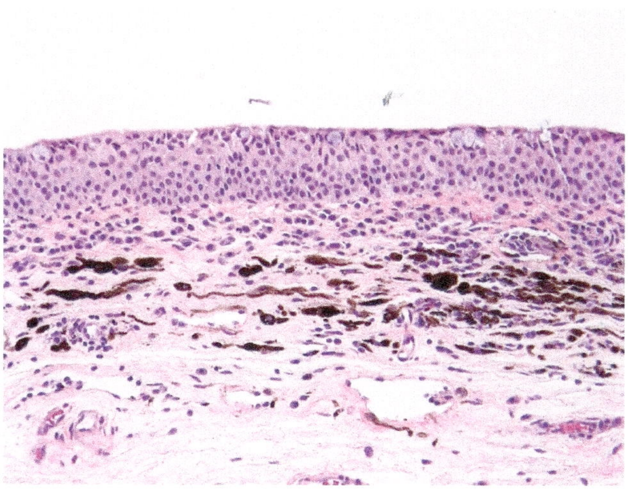

FIG. 20.27

Blue nevus of the conjunctiva. Slender bland pigmented fusiform and dendritic melanocytes and melanophages are seen in the subepithelial stroma.

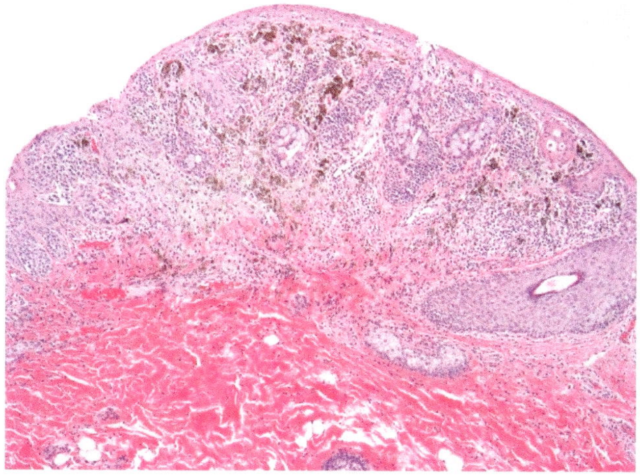

FIG. 20.28

Combined "inverted type A" nevus of the conjunctiva. There is a small population of large pigmented epithelioid melanocytes associated with an otherwise ordinary conjunctival nevus.

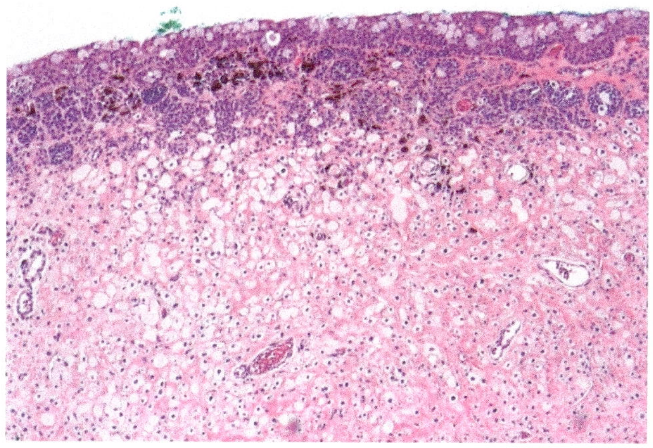

FIG. 20.29

Combined conjunctival nevus with a conventional small epithelioid and many clear cell melanocytes.

maturation, lack of mitotic figures, or pleomorphism. Caution is needed not to overemphasize one single diagnostic parameter. Disordered junctional growth with confluent nests can be seen in a melanocytic nevus and does not necessarily imply melanoma. Correlation with clinical findings (e.g., age of onset, anatomic location, clinical change) is important to arrive at the correct diagnosis. For diagnostically problematic cases, ancillary cytogenetic studies may be helpful. Cytogenetic methods tend to reveal copy number changes in melanoma but not in melanocytic nevi. Immunohistochemistry for PRAME (PReferentially expressed Antigen in MElanoma) can also be helpful. Nevi are usually negative, while melanomas are commonly positive.

Prognosis and Treatment

Malignant transformation is rare and occurs in less than 1% of conjunctival nevi. They are typically observed clinically or removed because of cosmetic reasons or mechanical irritation.

PRIMARY ACQUIRED MELANOSIS

Clinical Findings

PAM is acquired pigmentation of the conjunctiva that occurs more commonly in middle-aged White population. It accounts for 6% to 20% of pigmented conjunctival lesions. It can be found in up to 36% of White population and has the potential to evolve to melanoma.

PAM is asymptomatic and is usually noted on a routine eye examination or by the patient as a new slowly progressive pigmented lesion (Fig. 20.30). PAM can occur in any portion of the conjunctival surface as an area of irregular pigmentation, and its extent can be minimal (Fig. 20.31) or diffuse (Fig. 20.32). Pigmentation can also be seen traversing the limbus and extending onto the corneal epithelium. Histologic evaluation is needed to distinguish PAM without atypia from PAM with atypia.

HISTOLOGIC FEATURES OF PRIMARY ACQUIRED MELANOSIS WITHOUT ATYPIA

PAM without atypia is histopathologically characterized by increased melanin pigment deposition (hypermelanosis) in the conjunctival epithelium (with or without squamous metaplasia) (Fig. 20.33). Similar to a cutaneous lentigo or melanotic macule, there may be an associated lichenoid inflammatory reaction or scattered melanophages in the subepithelial stroma. The density of intramucosal melanocytes is within normal limits. The melanocytes are cytologically bland.

PRIMARY ACQUIRED MELANOSIS—DISEASE FACT SHEET

Affected Individuals

- Men > women
- Middle-aged to elderly adults
- Predominantly White population

Clinical Appearance

- Irregular brown macule or patch
- Treatment
- Topical mitomycin C

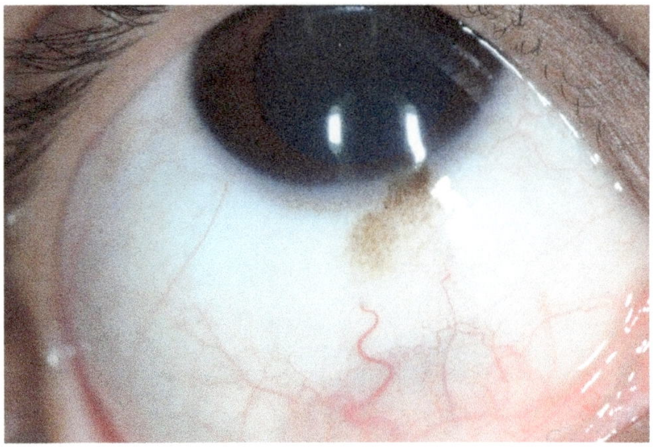

FIG. 20.30
Primary acquired melanosis (without atypia).

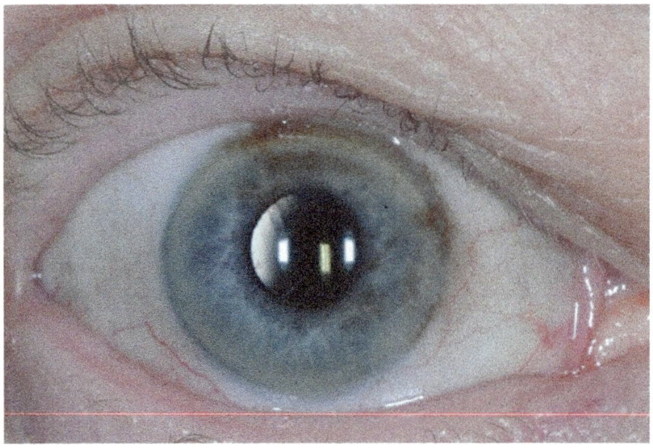

FIG. 20.31
Primary acquired melanosis (with atypia), localized.

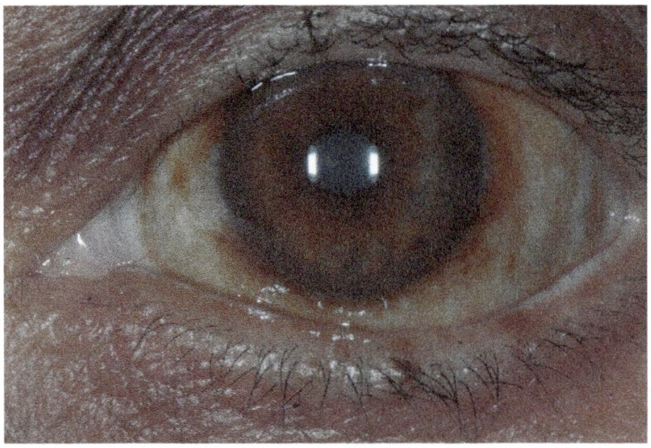

FIG. 20.32
Primary acquired melanosis (with atypia), diffuse.

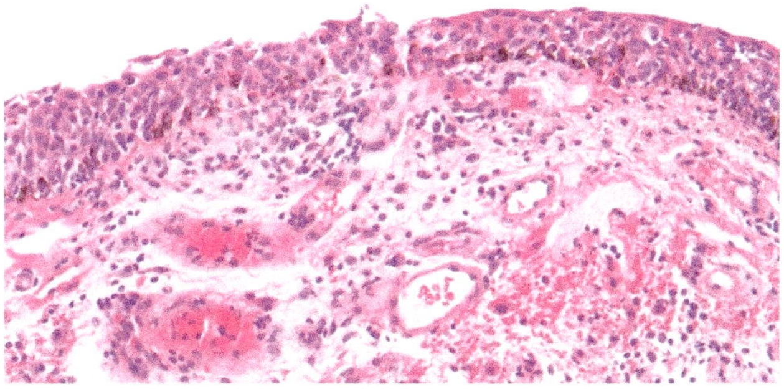

FIG. 20.33

Primary acquired melanosis with atypia. There is melanin pigment in (predominantly basilar) epithelial cells. The density and cytology of junctional melanocytes is within normal limits. Melanophages are seen in the subepithelial stroma.

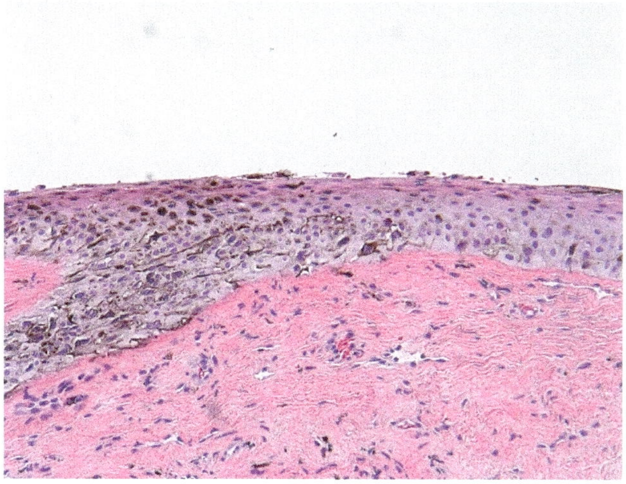

FIG. 20.34

Primary acquired melanosis with atypia. There is an increase in the density of solitary units of melanocytes within the mucosa associated with hyperpigmentation.

PRIMARY ACQUIRED MELANOSIS—PATHOLOGIC FEATURES

Primary Acquired Melanosis Without Atypia

- Hypermelanosis (melanin in melanocytes, epithelial cells, or macrophages)
- Melanocyte density within normal limits
- Melanocytes confined to epithelial stromal junction (no pagetoid spread)
- Little or no atypia of melanocytes

Primary Acquired Melanosis With Atypia (Conjunctival Melanocyte Intraepithelial Neoplasia)

- Hypermelanosis (melanin in melanocytes, epithelial cells, or macrophages)
- Increase in melanocyte density
- Melanocytes at epithelial stromal junction or above it (pagetoid spread)
- Atypia of melanocytes ranging from mild to moderate and severe

Histology of Primary Acquired Melanosis With Atypia or Conjunctival Melanocytic Intraepithelial Neoplasia

PAM with atypia has been entrenched in the ophthalmology literature, which is why we also use it herein. An alternate terminology in lieu of "PAM with atypia," which more accurately reflects the biology and pathology of the disease process, is "conjunctival intraepithelial melanocyte neoplasia" (C-MIN). The histopathologic hallmark of this process is an increase in the density of predominantly solitary units of melanocytes within the conjunctival mucosa, typically, but not always, associated with hypermelanosis (Figs. 20.34–20.36). As the lesion progresses, the tumor cell population becomes more cellular, usually accompanied by a higher degree of cytologic atypia (increased nuclear size, hyperchromatism). Melanocytes at the epithelial stromal junction become confluent and may form nests. Pagetoid spread

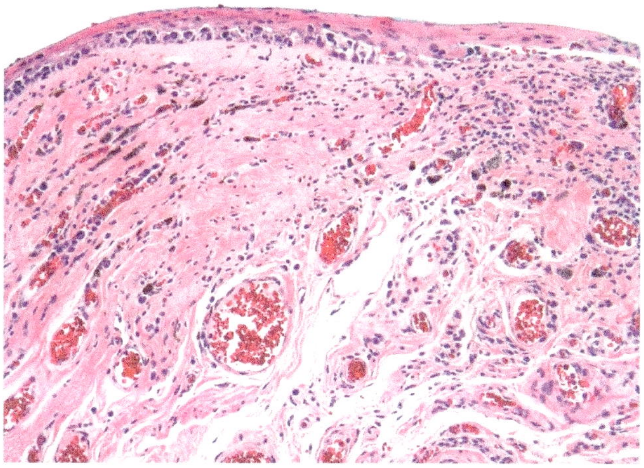

FIG. 20.35

Primary acquired melanosis with atypia (melanoma in situ). There is near confluency of atypical solitary units of melanocytes along the epithelial stromal junction of squamatized mucosa. Melanophages are present in the subepithelial stroma.

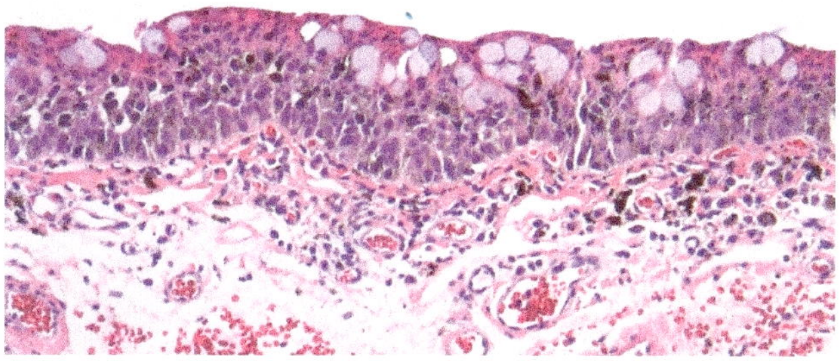

FIG. 20.36

Primary acquired melanosis with atypia (melanoma in situ). There is a high density of solitary units of atypical melanocytes in conjunctival mucosa.

may be noted within the mucosa. Grading systems have been proposed for both PAM with atypia (mild, moderate, and severe atypia; melanoma in situ) as well as C-MIN. The scoring system for C-MIN is based on the intraepithelial horizontal (melanocyte confluency or not) and vertical (pagetoid spread or not) growth pattern and degree of cytologic atypia. A score out of 10 is given. Accordingly, a C-MIN score of 0 implies "melanosis" only (i.e., in the absence of an increase in melanocyte density or cytologic atypia). A C-MIN score of 1 corresponds to "PAM with mild atypia," a C-MIN score of 2 or 3 to "PAM with moderate atypia," and a C-MIN score of 4 to "PAM with severe atypia." A C-MIN score of 5 or greater is equivalent to "conjunctival melanoma in situ." The argument has been made that in essence all variants of PAM with atypia (and implicitly most grades of C-MIN) may be regarded as conjunctival melanoma in situ (akin to lentigo maligna) and simply reflect more obvious versus more subtle or early evolving lesions thereof.

Prognosis and Treatment

The prognosis of PAM is variable and depends on the histopathologic degree of atypia as well as the extent of the pigmentation. PAM with no or mild atypia has no malignant potential, but 13% of patients with PAM with severe atypia will progress into melanoma. Seventy-five percent of conjunctival melanomas arise from a background of PAM. Treatment ranges from observation to excisional biopsy with cryotherapy or topical chemotherapy.

CONJUNCTIVAL MELANOMA

The incidence of conjunctival melanoma is 0.5 per million individuals in the United States. Conjunctival melanoma occurs more commonly in middle-aged White individuals. Conjunctival melanoma makes up 1.6% of noncutaneous melanoma. Its frequency has been increasing similar to cutaneous melanoma.

CONJUNCTIVAL MELANOMA—DISEASE FACT SHEET

Incidence
- 0.2 to $0.8/10^6$ White individuals per year

Median Age
- 60 years

Preferred Sites
- Perilimbal
- Bulbar
- Plica semilunaris

Associated Precursors
- 70% arise in association with primary acquired melanosis with atypia or conjunctival melanocytic intraepithelial neoplasia
- 25% arise from nevi
- 5% arise de novo

Clinical Appearance
- Irregular patch or nodule
- Variable pigmentation (red to brown)

Treatment
- Topical treatment for melanoma in situ
- Surgery for invasive melanoma
- Sentinel lymph node biopsy may be used for staging

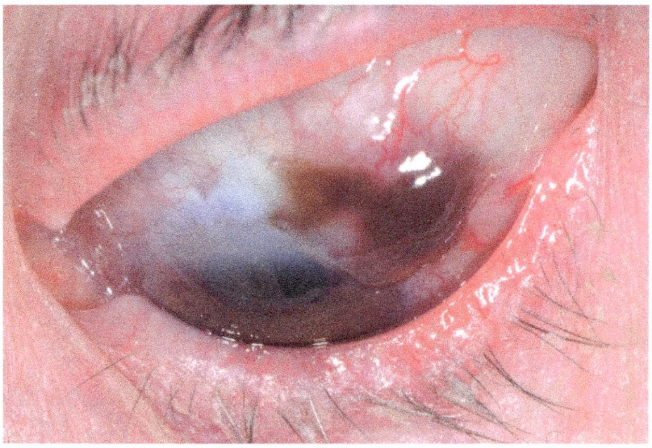

FIG. 20.37
Conjunctival malignant melanoma. Irregular brown plaque.

Clinical Findings

Conjunctival melanoma can occur in any portion of the conjunctival surface as an area of thickened irregular pigmentation and can be nodular or diffuse (Fig. 20.37). Conjunctival melanoma begins as an asymptomatic enlarging pigmented or amelanotic lesion with enlarged feeder vessels that can become progressively symptomatic. The lesion can grow onto the cornea or eyelid or extend into the orbit. Twenty percent of the lesions arise de novo, 5% arise from a conjunctival nevus, and 75% arise from preexisting PAM.

Histologic Features

Tumors usually display an asymmetric silhouette, with stromal infiltration by cytologically atypical melanocytes lacking maturation (Fig. 20.38). Pigmentation is variable (Figs. 20.39–20.41). Tumors may be composed of epithelioid melanocytes, fusiform cells, or mixture

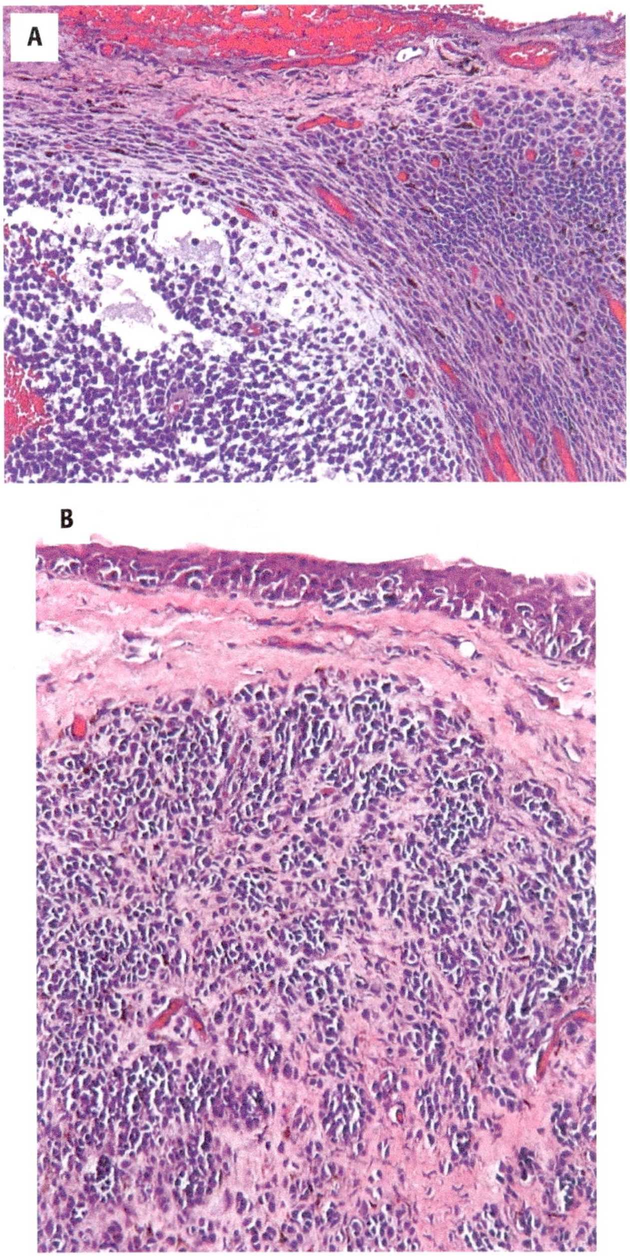

FIG. 20.38

Conjunctival melanoma. **A,** Invasive melanoma with nodule in the subepithelial stroma. **B,** Adjacent melanoma in situ and invasive melanoma with atypical tumor cells lacking maturation.

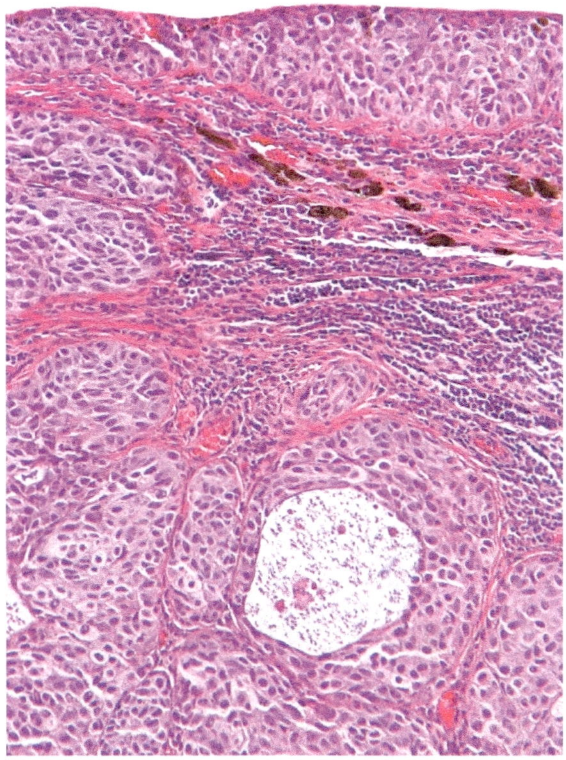

FIG. 20.39

Conjunctival melanoma in mucosa and submucosa. There are dense aggregates of atypical melanocytes. There is associated inflammation with melanophages.

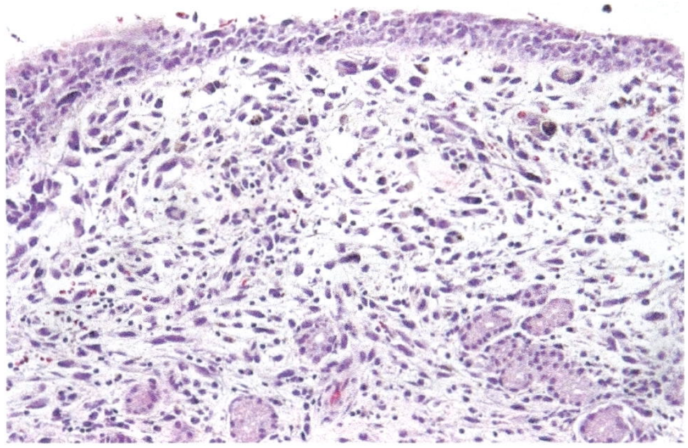

FIG. 20.40

Conjunctival melanoma with dispersed atypical single cells in edematous stroma.

thereof at variable proportions. Sheetlike growth in lieu of a nevoid nested growth pattern may be seen. Some tumors have a diffuse single-cell infiltrative pattern (Fig. 20.40). In tumors with prior topical surface treatments, an invasive tumor may arise in association with an intraductal melanoma population (Fig. 20.41). The mean and median tumor thickness at the time of diagnosis are both approximately 2 mm.

For adequate margin assessment and measurement of tumor thickness, it is important to maintain correct orientation and embedding of conjunctival biopsies. To this end, it is helpful for the surgeon to place the specimen on a paper mount and have the tissue handled by experienced individuals to minimize trauma and maintain proper orientation. Tangential sectioning may significantly compromise measurement of thickness and lead to false-positive margins. Melanoma in situ may grow along adnexal structures or ducts, which

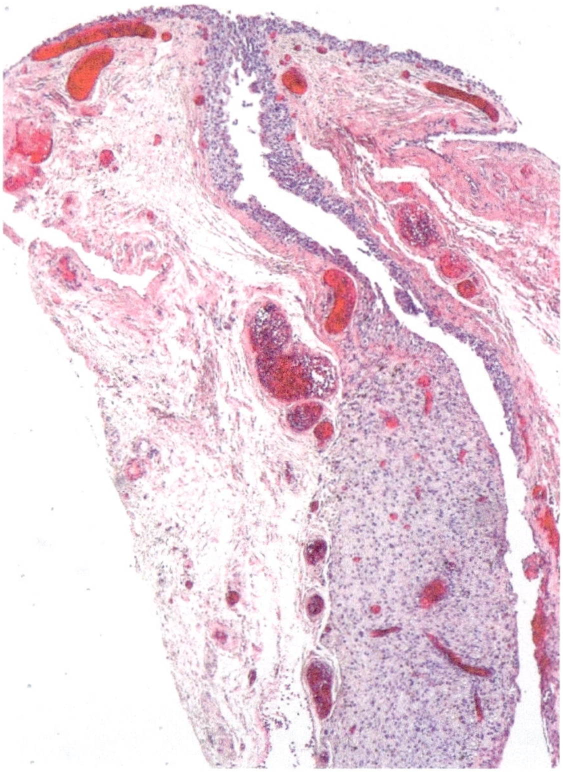

FIG. 20.41

Locally recurrent or persistent melanoma. Invasive tumor is associated with intraductal melanoma in situ.

CONJUNCTIVAL MELANOMA—PATHOLOGIC FEATURES

Features

- Asymmetry
- Ill-defined periphery
- Atypia and mitotic figures
- Limited or absent maturation

Ancillary Studies

- Immunohistochemistry similar to cutaneous melanoma
- Mutation profile similar to cutaneous melanoma
- Cytogenetic aberrations similar to cutaneous melanoma

Differential Diagnosis

- Conjunctival melanocytic nevus
- Metastatic melanoma
- Poorly differentiated carcinoma

is not to be confused with invasive melanoma. When lymphatic invasion is seen, it should be documented.

Some conjunctival melanomas carry the *BRAFV600E* mutation. Fewer tumors are associated with *NRASQ61R* mutations. Similar to cutaneous melanomas, a number of cytogenetic aberrations have been detected in conjunctival melanoma and the tumors tend to be diffusely positive for PRAME.

Ancillary Studies

Immunohistochemical markers for melanocyte differentiation antigens or epithelial or lymphoid markers may help distinguish an amelanotic melanoma from a poorly differentiated carcinoma or lymphoma. Diffuse PRAME expression favors melanoma over a nevus. Cytogenetic studies may also help to distinguish conjunctival nevi (they usually lack chromosomal copy number changes) from melanoma (they typically carry copy number changes). If a patient develops metastatic melanoma and there is limited or no readily accessible metastatic tumor tissue available for mutation analysis, the primary tumor can be studied by immunohistochemistry or molecular methods for the presence or absence of *BRAFV600E* mutation for treatment selection.

Prognosis and Treatment

The mortality rate from conjunctival melanoma ranges from 6% to 23% at 5 years depending on the extent of the lesion and disease stage. Metastatic conjunctival melanoma typically presents in the ipsilateral preauricular, submandibular, or cervical lymph nodes and then can be found in lung and brain most frequently. Certain clinical findings are associated with a poorer prognosis; they include lesions located in the fornix, caruncle, or tarsal conjunctiva and lesions with increased thickness (greater than 2 mm). Lesions are managed by surgical resection in conjunction with cryotherapy and or topical chemotherapy. Recurrence rates vary and can be as high as 26% at 5 years, especially if incisional biopsies were performed before definitive resection.

HEMATOLYMPHOID NEOPLASMS

XANTHOMA AND XANTHELASMA

This is a benign subcutaneous lipomatous eyelid lesion that is very common and has a slight female preponderance. In half of cases, there is evidence of systemic hyperlipidemia, particularly in younger men. Individuals with this entity may be at slightly higher risk of morbidity from cardiovascular disease.

Clinical Findings

Xanthelasma appears in middle-aged or older patients as bilateral, symmetric, single, or multiple yellow placoid lesions typically in the nasal portion of the upper eyelid (Fig. 20.42).

American Joint Committee on Cancer (AJCC) Classification of Conjunctival Melanoma

Primary Tumor (T)	
Tx	Primary tumor cannot be assessed
T0	No evidence of primary tumor
T(is)	Melanoma confined to the conjunctival epithelium
T1	Melanoma of the bulbar conjunctiva
T1a	<1 quadrant
pT1a	Tumor thickness <0.5 mm
T1b	>1 but <2 quadrants
pT1b	Tumor thickness >0.5–1.5 mm
T1c	>2 but <3 quadrants
pT1c	Tumor thickness >1.5 mm
T1d	>3 quadrants
T2	Melanoma of the palpebral, forniceal conjunctiva, or caruncle
T2a	<1 quadrant, not involving the caruncle
pT2a	Tumor thickness <0.5 mm
T2b	>1 quadrant, not involving the caruncle
pT2b	Tumor thickness >0.5–1.5 mm
T2c	<1 quadrant and involving the caruncle
pT2c	Tumor thickness >1.5 mm
T2d	>1 quadrant and involving the caruncle
T3	Melanoma with local invasion
T3a	Globe
T3b	Eyelid
T3c	Orbit
T3d	Paranasal sinus
T4	Melanoma with intracranial invasion
Regional Lymph Nodes (N)	
Nx	Regional lymph nodes cannot be assessed
N0a	No regional lymph node metastasis, status post (s/p) biopsy
N0b	No regional lymph node metastasis; no biopsy
N1	Regional lymph node metastasis
Distant Metastasis (M)	
M0	No distant metastasis
M1	Distant metastasis

Modified from Shields, C. L., Kaliki, S., Al-Dahmash, S. A., et al. (2012). American Joint Committee on Cancer (AJCC) clinical classification predicts conjunctival melanoma outcomes. *Ophthalmic Plastic and Reconstructive Surgery, 28*, 313–323.

Histologic Features

Lesions of xanthelasma are characterized by an infiltrate of pale foamy macrophages and variable number of lymphocytes (Fig. 20.43).

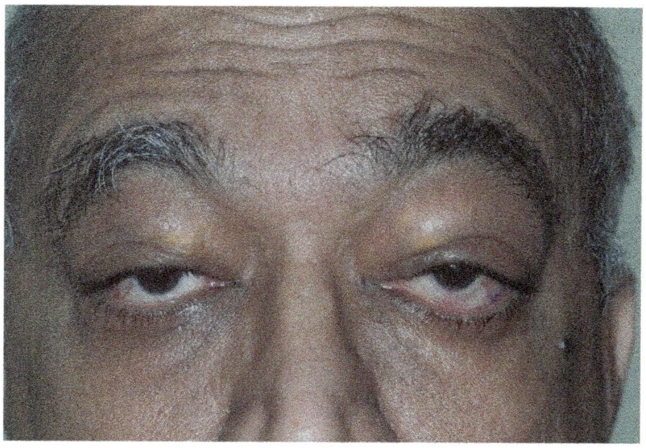

FIG. 20.42

Bilateral xanthelasma of the upper eyelids.

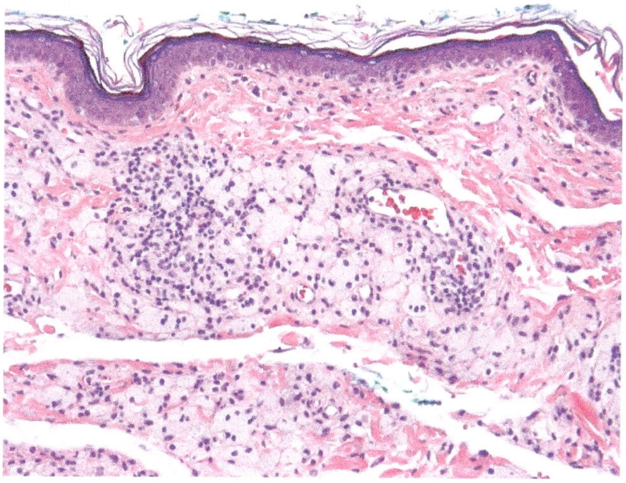

FIG. 20.43

Xanthelasma. There is an infiltrate of cytologically bland foamy histiocytes and a few lymphocytes.

Ancillary Studies

Immunohistochemical studies can verify the presence of macrophages (positive for CD68 and CD163). Immunohistochemistry and molecular studies for *BRAFV600E* can assist in treatment selection of patients in whom xanthelasma is a manifestation of Erdheim-Chester disease (ECD).

Prognosis and Treatment

Patients with this lesion warrant an assessment for hyperlipidemia and ECD. Because of their benign nature, eyelid lesions can be observed. Cosmetically undesirable lesions can be surgically excised, treated with topical acidic preparations, or ablated with erbium: yttrium aluminum garnet (YAG) or carbon dioxide laser. Regression can also be achieved with oral cholesterol-lowering agents. Patients with ECD and documented driver mutations may benefit from targeted therapy (e.g., BRAF or MEK inhibitors).

LYMPHOMA

Lymphoproliferative lesions of the conjunctiva span a broad spectrum from benign reactive hyperplasia to malignant lymphoma. Ocular adnexal lymphomas represent approximately 8% of extranodal lymphoma. The majority are localized to the conjunctiva and not associated with systemic disease, particularly in unilateral cases. In contrast, two-thirds of preseptal eyelid lesions have systemic involvement. Orbital lymphoma can extend anteriorly and have conjunctival involvement. The majority of ocular adnexal lymphoma is characterized by low-grade B cells and typically falls into the category of mucosa-associated lymphoma tumor (MALT).

Clinical Findings

Lymphoproliferative lesions of the conjunctiva appear as pink or salmon-colored lesions that are slightly elevated, with a soft or rubbery consistency and smooth or multinodular surface (Figs. 20.44 and 20.45). They typically present in the bulbar or forniceal conjunctiva and may be accompanied by lymphadenopathy.

Histologic Features

Lymphoma is typically recognized or at least suspected by a densely cellular infiltrate. If the tumor cells are large or pleomorphic, a malignant diagnosis is readily suspected and ancillary immunohistochemical studies ordered for further characterization of the neoplasm. If the lymphocytes are small and well differentiated, the diagnosis of lymphoma or pseudolymphoma may not be immediately obvious, and the final diagnosis may need to be deferred until results from marker or molecular studies have become available. The most common lymphoma of the conjunctiva is the low-grade B-cell lymphoma of marginal zone type.

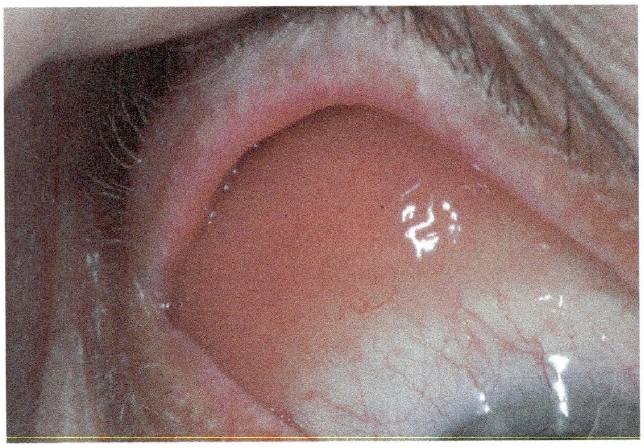

FIG. 20.44
Conjunctival lymphoma, salmon patch.

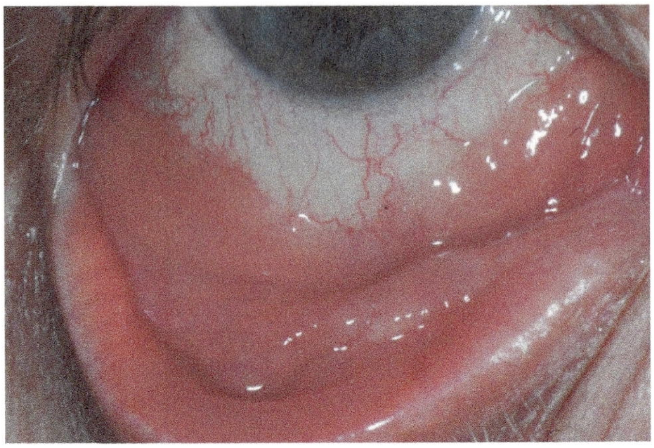

FIG. 20.45
Conjunctival lymphoma, forniceal involvement.

Prognosis and Treatment

Localized lesions can be surgically excised, treated with cryotherapy, and thereafter observed for progression or recurrence. Localized depots of steroids can be useful at debulking and minimizing conjunctival lesions. Larger lesions, particularly those of a malignant variant, can be treated with radiation or systemic chemotherapy. Instances that have systemic involvement can benefit from chemotherapy or rituximab (or both). Because of the increasing evidence that MALT lymphoma may result from chronic antigenic stimulation, there may be a role for antibiotics against *Helicobacter pylori* and *Campylobacter jejuni* and chlamydial infections. Approximately 15% of patients with unilateral disease have systemic involvement, in contrast to bilateral disease in which close to half of patients demonstrate systemic lymphoma.

LEUKEMIA

Leukemic infiltrates of the ocular structures are common, with the choroid being the most frequently affected site. Ocular adnexal infiltrates can occur, typically originate in the orbit, and extend anteriorly to the eyelids and conjunctiva. Granulocytic sarcomas or "chloromas" are myeloid leukemic infiltrations in children.

Clinical Findings

Leukemic infiltrates can present as a subconjunctival hemorrhage, or they can take on a similar appearance to lymphoma, although with a more pronounced red hue.

Histologic Features

Conjunctival involvement by leukemia is most often related to myeloid or myelomonocytic leukemia. There is typically an infiltrate of immature myeloid cells with blastlike or monocytoid features. Immunohistochemical studies can help exclude lymphoma. Myeloid or myelomonocytic leukemia is usually immunoreactive for CD43 and ETS family-related gene (ERG) and variably positive for CD34 (if blasts are present) or CD68 (monocytoid differentiation). The neoplastic cells are negative for CD3 and CD20.

Prognosis and Treatment

Leukemic infiltration of the conjunctiva is managed by treatment of the systemic disease, typically involving a suitable chemotherapeutic agent. Symptoms arising from disruption of the tear film benefit from topical lubricants. Low-dose radiation can be useful for cases refractory to systemic treatment.

GLANDULAR LESIONS

ONCOCYTOMA

The caruncle is located at the medial canthus adjacent to the plica semiluminarus and is partly composed of cutaneous constituents. An oncocytoma is a benign tumor of transformed glandular epithelial cells that can occur in the caruncle.

Clinical Findings

A caruncular oncocytoma presents in elderly individuals as a slow-growing, nontender mass with a bluish-red and cystic hue.

Histologic Features

An oncocytoma is characterized by a nodular or nodulocystic tumor lined by an epithelial and myoepithelial cell layer (Fig. 20.46). The tumor cells may grow in a solid, cribriform, or papillary pattern. The epithelial cells are characterized by abundant granular eosinophilic cytoplasm.

Prognosis and Treatment

Caruncular oncocytomas can be observed or surgically excised if unsightly in appearance.

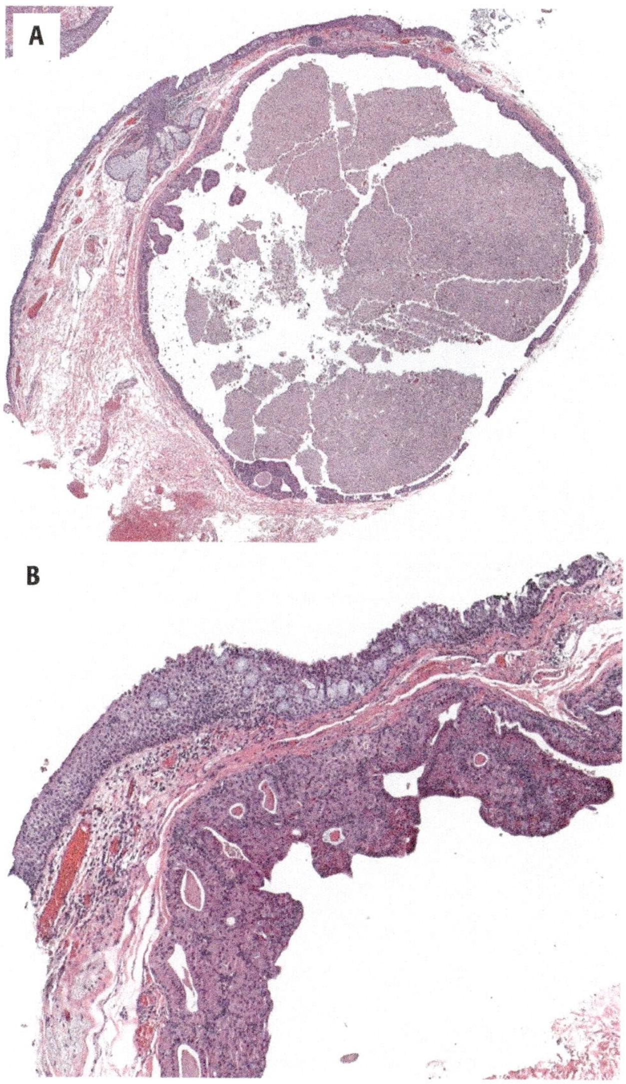

FIG. 20.46

Conjunctival oncocytoma. **A**, Nodulocystic epithelial tumor with papillary projections. **B**, The tumor cells have an eosinophilic granular (oncocytic) cytoplasm.

SEBACEOUS CARCINOMA

Periocular sebaceous carcinoma accounts for approximately 75% of all sebaceous carcinomas. In the periocular region, it originates from the glands of Zeis in the eyelid, the sebaceous glands of the caruncle, or the meibomian glands of the tarsus. Tumors can progress to involve the conjunctiva. Sebaceous carcinomas typically affect older individuals, although they have been found in younger patients with a history of head radiation and have an association with Muir-Torre syndrome. They are said to be slightly more common in women than in men.

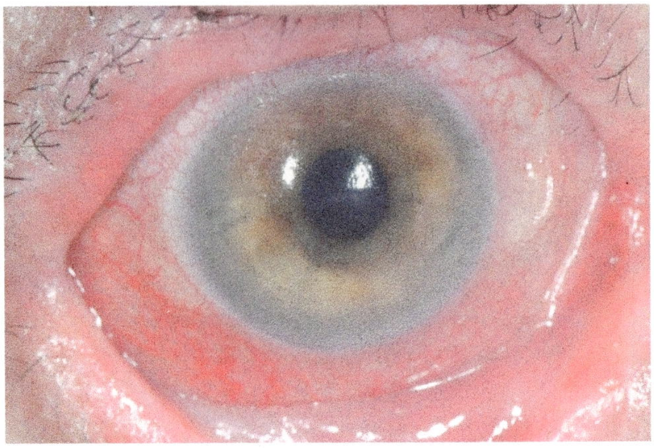

FIG. 20.47

Sebaceous carcinoma.

Clinical Findings

Sebaceous carcinoma has a tendency to mimic blepharoconjunctivitis or a chalazion, thus delaying its diagnosis (Fig. 20.47). It can present with a thickened erythematous eyelid and a localized, yellowish nodule. With time, it can progress to involve the entire eyelid, thus mimicking the appearance of unilateral blepharoconjunctivitis (Fig. 20.48). The cilia of the eyelid often become thickened (trichomegaly) or can be obliterated (madarosis). The upper eyelid is more frequently involved than the lower eyelid.

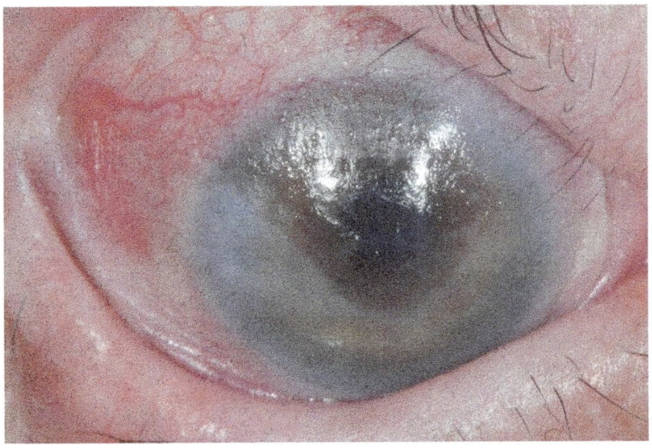

FIG. 20.48

Sebaceous carcinoma.

Histologic Features

Sebaceous carcinoma is characterized by malignant tumor cells with sebaceous differentiation. The tumor may display a predominantly nodular lobular growth pattern (Fig. 20.49) but may also display a diffusely infiltrative silhouette. The tumor cell aggregates are composed of atypical epithelial cells with variable extent of sebaceous differentiation (well, moderate, or poor). Well-differentiated tumors contain a predominant component of cells with clear to foamy vacuolated cytoplasm, albeit with atypical nuclei. Well-recognizable clear sebocytes tend to be a minor cell population in moderately differentiated tumors, where tumor cells with a higher nuclear-to-cytoplasmic ratio predominate. Nonetheless, evidence of sebaceous differentiation (foamy vacuolated cytoplasm with weblike appearance, scalloped hyperchromatic nuclei, or nuclei with vesicular chromatin) is not difficult to identify (Fig. 20.50). In poorly differentiated tumors, finding evidence of sebaceous differentiation is difficult. Immunostains are usually necessary and the sebaceous origin of the tumor is often deduced from association of the tumor with sebaceous glands and lack of associated other carcinoma that may secondarily involve sebaceous glands.

SEBACEOUS CARCINOMA—DISEASE FACT SHEET

Incidence
- 1.5% to 3% of eyelid malignancies in White individuals
- Up to one-third of eyelid malignancies in Asians

Patient Group
- Asians
- Middle-aged to elderly adults
- Women > men

Affected Site
- Most often Meibomian gland of upper eyelid

Clinical Appearance
- Nodule (may be mistaken for chalazion)
- Infiltrative with a conjunctivitis-like appearance

Treatment
- Surgical excision

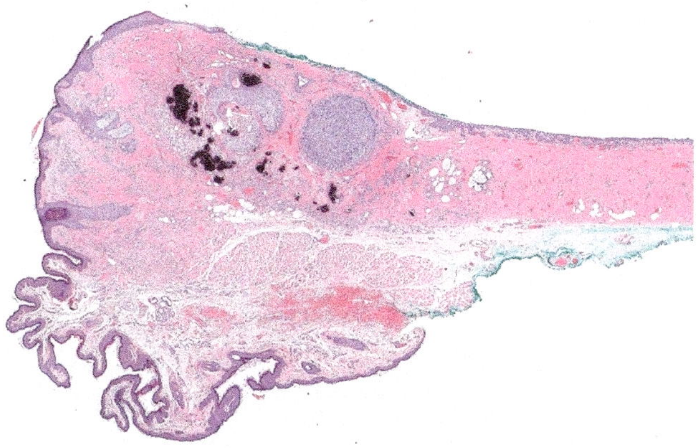

FIG. 20.49
Sebaceous carcinoma. Invasive tumor with sebaceous differentiation.

SEBACEOUS CARCINOMA—PATHOLOGIC FEATURES

Features

- Nodular or infiltrative silhouette
- Cytologic atypia and mitoses
- Cytologic evidence of sebaceous differentiation (lipidized cytoplasm with many microvacuoles; scalloped nuclei)
- May extend into and populate overlying conjunctiva

Immunophenotype

- Usually positive for epithelial membrane antigen, Berep4, CK7, Cam5.2
- Usually positive for adipophilin, androgen receptor, PRAME

Differential Diagnosis

- Squamous cell carcinoma
- Basal cell carcinoma
- Merkel cell carcinoma
- Metastatic carcinoma

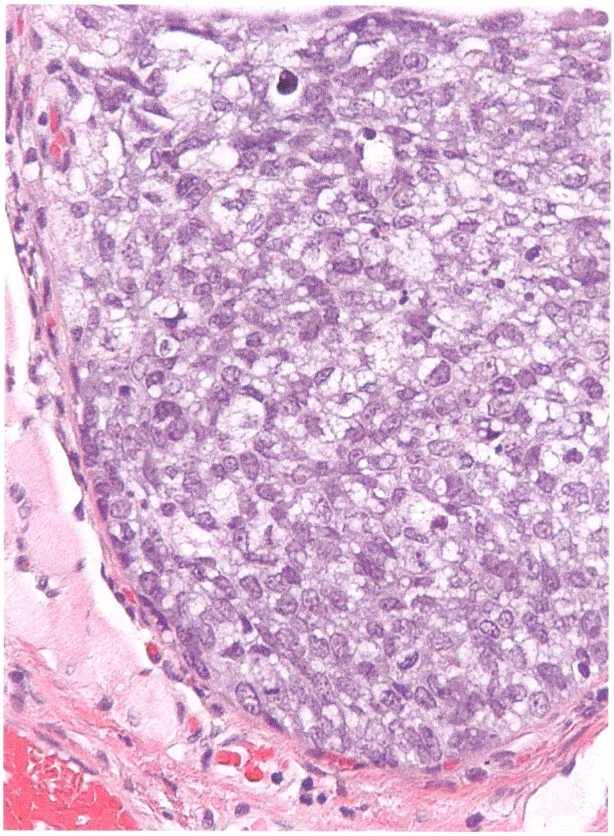

FIG. 20.50
Sebaceous carcinoma. Vacuolated lipidized cytoplasm and scalloped nuclei are characteristic features.

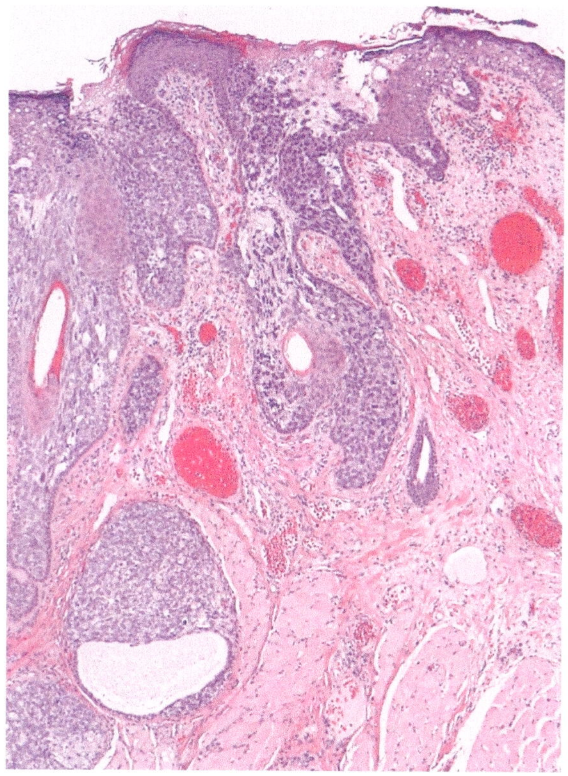

FIG. 20.51
Sebaceous carcinoma with extension into overlying mucosa.

Sebaceous carcinoma commonly extends into the overlying mucosa (Fig. 20.51) and may display prominent intramucosal pagetoid growth (Fig. 20.52). In the absence of well-documented underlying sebaceous carcinoma, the latter can be difficult to distinguish from primary pagetoid squamous cell carcinoma in situ (SCCIS).

Ancillary Studies

Immunohistochemical studies using cytokeratins and other epithelial markers (epithelial membrane antigen [EMA]) can help distinguish a poorly differentiated sebaceous carcinoma from a nonepithelial malignant tumor (lymphoma, melanoma). Immunohistochemical

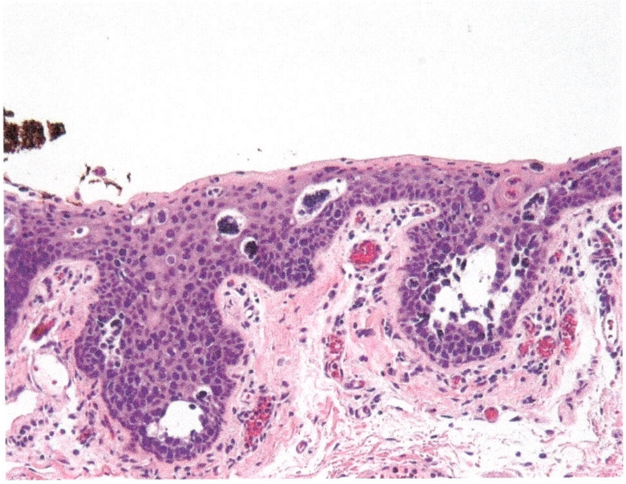

FIG. 20.52

Sebaceous carcinoma with intramucosal pagetoid growth.

studies can aid in the distinction of sebaceous carcinoma from basal cell carcinoma (BCC), SCC, or Merkel cell carcinoma (MCC). Whereas sebaceous carcinomas are typically positive for both EMA and Berep4, BCC is usually negative for EMA and SCC usually negative for Berep4 (Table 20.1). However, there are limitations: not all sebaceous carcinomas strongly express Berep4 or EMA throughout the tumor. Lipid stains can be helpful. However, they require frozen tissue. As a substitute for lipid stains, an antibody to a protein associated with lipid droplets may be used (adipophilin). It is a very sensitive marker but also not entirely specific for sebaceous differentiation. Additional useful markers (all with limitations) include androgen receptor (common in sebaceous carcinoma, not expected to be found in SCC) and carcinoembryonic antigen (CEA) (common in sebaceous carcinoma, usually absent in SCC).

Differential Diagnosis

The most common and difficult diagnostic issue related to sebaceous carcinoma is the distinction of intramucosal pagetoid sebaceous carcinoma from SCCIS, especially in the setting of a small superficial biopsy in the absence of known underlying sebaceous carcinoma. Careful attention to focal lipidized cytoplasm is helpful, but clear cell features and cytoplasmic vacuoles are not entirely specific for sebaceous carcinoma because such focal cytoplasmic features can also be found in SCC. Features of HPV effect (binucleation, koilocytes, raisinoid nuclei) favor SCC. Often immunohistochemical stains are needed. They may permit a distinction, but on occasion they may not, and a final diagnosis may need to be deferred until more of the clinical lesion has been reviewed under the microscope.

Prognosis and Treatment

Mapping biopsies can be useful in establishing the extent of disease and guide plans for appropriate treatment. Histologic prognostic features include tumor size, diffuse infiltrative pattern, extensive pagetoid intramucosal growth, and extension into adjacent anatomic structures. Nodular lesions can be resected with wide margins and frozen section control, but diffuse or invasive disease often requires orbital exenteration but may also benefit from radiation. Topical chemotherapeutic agents should be reserved for intraepithelial disease. Sebaceous carcinoma can be aggressive with high local recurrence rates and ability to metastasize to lymph nodes and systemically. Reported rates of metastases range from 15% to 25% of patients. Although the mortality rate is worse than for other conjunctival cancers, it has improved in recent years because of increased awareness.

ENDOCRINE MUCIN–PRODUCING SWEAT GLAND CARCINOMA

Endocrine mucin–producing sweat gland carcinoma is a rare neoplasm originating from sweat glands and having a predilection for periocular skin.

Clinical Findings

Endocrine mucin–producing sweat gland carcinoma typically affects elderly individuals, women more often than men. It usually occurs on the eyelid, especially the lower eyelid margin. Its clinical appearance is not specific. It may have a nodular flesh-colored appearance with a cystic clear or blue hue and intrinsic telangiectatic vessels. It can induce overlying madarosis. Lesions are usually not ulcerated. Clinically, they are typically submitted to rule out cyst, chalazion, or BCC.

ENDOCRINE MUCIN–PRODUCING SWEAT GLAND CARCINOMA—DISEASE FACT SHEET

Incidence

- Rare adnexal tumor
- Affected individuals
  - Middle-aged to elderly adults
  - Women > men

Clinical Appearance

- Red or flesh-colored nodule
- Slowly growing

Prognosis and Treatment

- Low-grade tumor with potential for local recurrence
- Complete surgical excision is usually curative

Histologic Features

The histologic features are distinct and characteristic. The tumor usually displays a nodular or nodulocystic silhouette with intranodular solid, cribriform, or papillary growth patterns by epithelioid cells (Fig. 20.53). The tumor cells tend to have round to oval nuclei with coarse granular chromatin and uniform nuclear membranes. The nucleo usually have a low grade appearance. A characteristic microscopic finding is the presence of intratumoral mucin, the amount of which is variable. Perineural invasion is usually absent.

Ancillary Studies

The tumor has a characteristic immunohistochemical profile. The tumor cells are strongly and diffusely positive for estrogen receptor (ER) and variably positive for Cam5.2, CK7, chromogranin, or synaptophysin (Fig. 20.54).

Differential Diagnosis

The most common diagnostic confusion is on a partial biopsy with BCC or a sweat gland adenoma. In contrast to BCC, endocrine mucin–producing sweat gland carcinoma usually lacks peripheral palisading. Another distinction is the distribution of mucin. There is more mucin and more copious amounts of mucin within tumor nodules, but in BCC, the mucin is usually more subtle and located in the stroma surrounding the tumor (except for the rare adenoidal variants of BCC). Immunohistochemical studies permit a definitive distinction from BCC. Although BCC is positive for Berep4, it usually negative for markers typically positive in endocrine mucin–producing sweat gland carcinoma, including ER, progesterone receptor (PR), Cam5.2, and CK7. Caution is necessary with regard to chromogranin and synaptophysin because both may be focally positive in BCC.

The distinction from apocrine adenomas can be problematic on a partial biopsy because endocrine mucin–producing sweat gland carcinoma may have

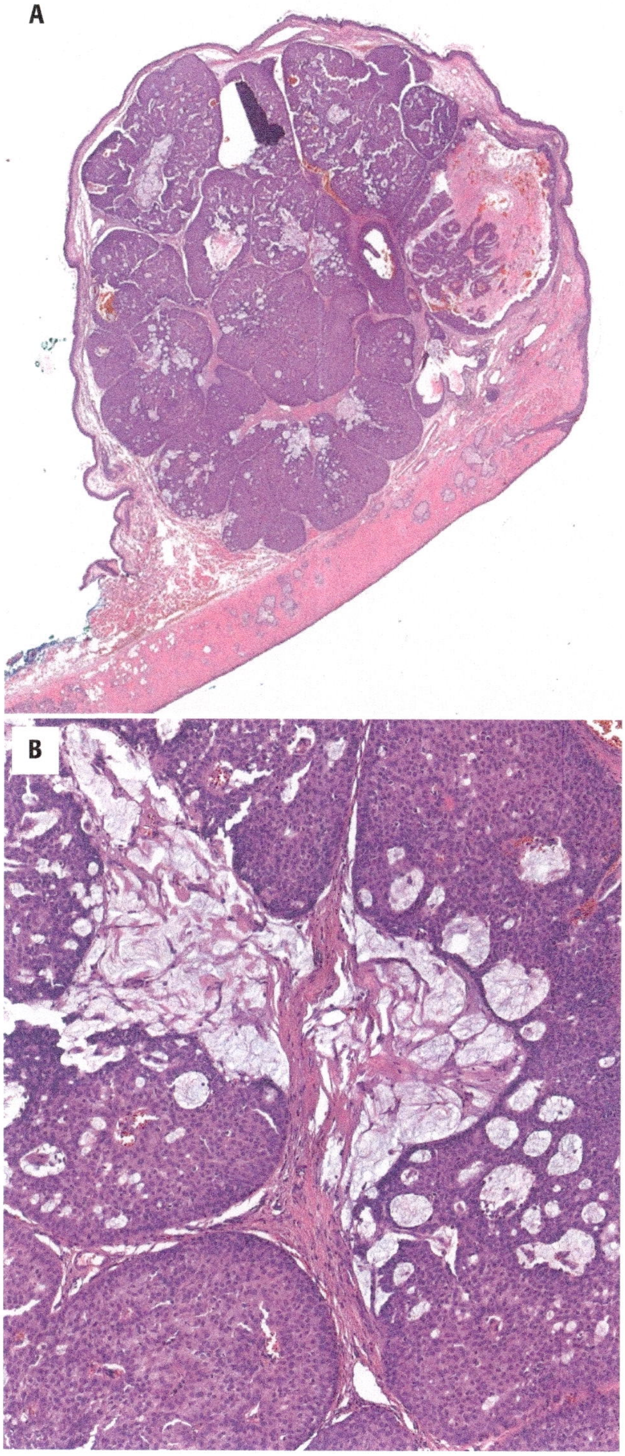

A

B

FIG. 20.53

Endocrine mucin–producing sweat gland tumor. **A,** Nodulocystic silhoutte with intratumoral papillary, cribriform, and solid growth patterns. **B,** The tumor is composed of epithelial cells with a high nuclear-to-cytoplasmic ratio. There is stromal mucin.

ENDOCRINE MUCIN–PRODUCING SWEAT GLAND CARCINOMA—PATHOLOGIC FEATURES

Features

- Nodulocystic silhouette
- Intratumoral cribriform, papillary of solid growth
- Well-differentiated adenoma-like appearance with low grade nuclei
- Intratumoral mucin

Immunohistochemistry

- Positive for CK7, estrogen receptor, and progesterone receptor
- Positive for INSM1 chromogranin, synaptophysin

Differential Diagnosis

- Basal cell carcinoma
- Papillary apocrine adenoma

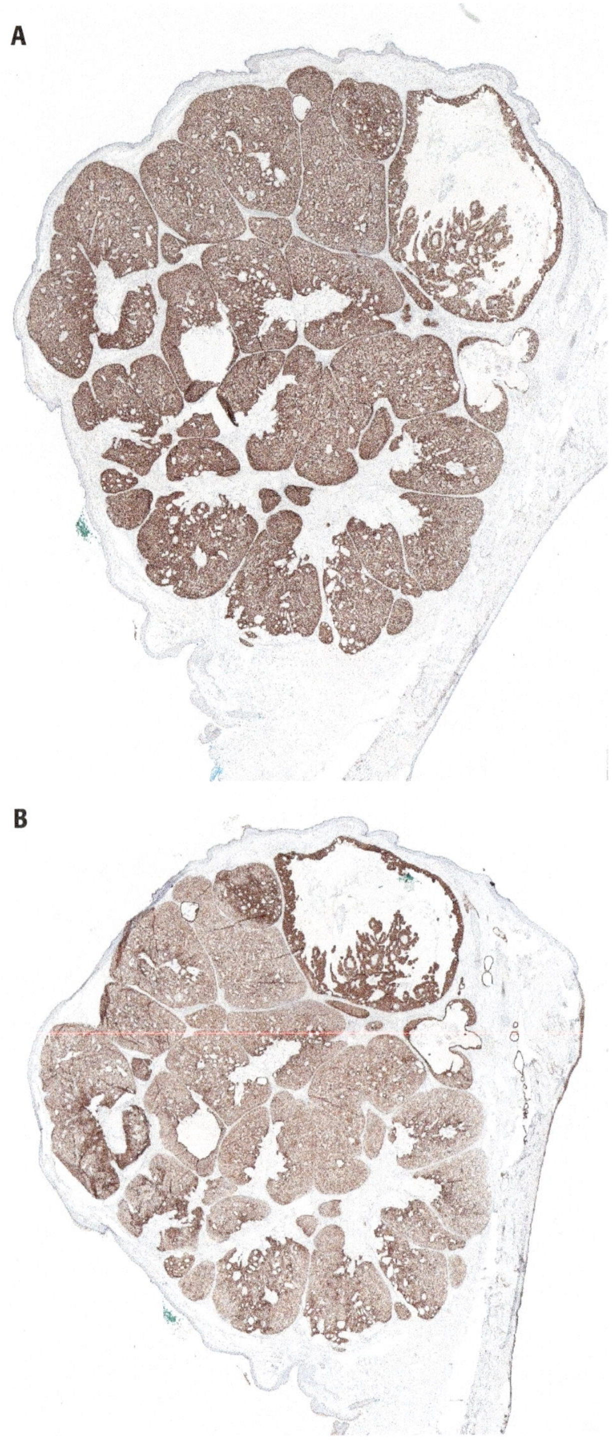

FIG. 20.54

Immunohistochemistry of endocrine mucin-producing sweat gland tumor. **A,** The tumor cells are strongly positive for estrogen receptor. **B,** The tumor cells are positive for CK7.

adenoma-like features (circumscribed growth, bland nuclei) and similar immunohistochemical characteristics (positive labeling for CK7, ER, and PR). Positive labeling for chromogranin or synaptophysin may help favor carcinoma because these markers are rarely expressed in adenomas. Review of the completely excised tumor usually permits a definitive distinction: adenomas are small, well-differentiated tumors composed of an epithelial and myoepithelial cell layer, usually without mitoses, atypia, or mucin and lacking an infiltrative interface with the surrounding stroma. Endocrine mucin-producing sweat gland carcinomas are more cellular tumors, usually with mitoses, mucin, and at least focal stromal infiltration.

On occasion, in a patient with a history of carcinoma elsewhere, such as mammary carcinoma, and a mitotically active tumor, one may also need to consider the possibility of metastatic carcinoma in the differential diagnosis.

Prognosis and Treatment

Endocrine mucin-producing sweat gland carcinomas can be locally excised with or without frozen sections. Alternatively, the Mohs procedure may be applied to ensure complete removal. The tumors are low grade. They may locally recur, especially with focally positive margins.

OTHER TUMORS

There are many other common benign tumors of the eyelid (e.g., hidrocystomas, nevi) and common or rare malignant tumors (e.g., BCC, MCC). The latter, when occurring in the skin of the eyelid, may extend into the conjunctiva or subconjunctival mucosa. Because these tumors primarily occur in the skin, they are described in other chapters of this book.

SUGGESTED FURTHER READING

Esmaeli, B., Nasser, Q. J., Cruz, H., Fellman, M., Warneke, C. L., & Ivan, D. (2012). American Joint Committee on Cancer T category for eyelid sebaceous carcinoma correlates with nodal metastasis and survival. *Ophthalmology*, *119*, 1078–1082.

Francis, J. H., Grossniklaus, H. E., Habib, L. A., Marr, B., Abramson, D. H., & Busam, K. J. (2018). BRAF, NRAS, and GNAQ mutations in conjunctival melanocytic nevi. *Investigative Ophthalmology & Visual Science*, *59*, 117–121.

Grossniklaus, H. E., Green, W. R., Luckenbach, M., & Chan, C. C. (1987). Conjunctival lesions in adults. A clinical and histopathologic review. *Cornea*, *6*, 78–116.

Hamam, R., Bhat, P., & Foster, C. S. (2009). Conjunctival/corneal intraepithelial neoplasia. *International Ophthalmology Clinics*, *49*, 63–70.

Kim, J. W., & Abramson, D. H. (2008). Topical treatment options for conjunctival neoplasms. *Clinical Ophthalmology (Auckland, N.Z.)*, *2*, 503–515.

Mulay, K., Aggarwal, E., & White, V. A. (2013). Periocular sebaceous gland carcinoma: A comprehensive review. *Saudi Journal of Ophthalmology*, *27*, 159–165.

Robinson, M. R., Lee, S. S., Sneller, M. C., Lerner, R., Langford, C. A., Talar-Williams, C., Cox, T. A., Chan, C. C., & Smith, J. A. (2003). Tarsal-conjunctival disease associated with Wegener's granulomatosis. *Ophthalmology*, *110*, 1770–1780.

Shields, C. L., & Shields, J. A. (2004). Tumors of the conjunctiva and cornea. *Survey of Ophthalmology*, *49*, 3–24.

Index

Page numbers followed by "f" indicate figures, "t" indicate tables, and "b" indicate boxes.

C

D

E

M

O